INFECTIONS OF THE CENTRAL NERVOUS SYSTEM

INFECTIONS OF THE CENTRAL NERVOUS SYSTEM

Editors

W. Michael Scheld, M.D.

*Professor of Internal Medicine
and Neurosurgery
Associate Chair for Residency Programs
Department of Internal Medicine
University of Virginia School of Medicine
Charlottesville, Virginia*

Richard J. Whitley, M.D.

*Professor of Pediatrics, Microbiology
and Medicine
Department of Pediatrics
University of Alabama
Birmingham, Alabama*

David T. Durack, M.B., D.Phil.

*Professor of Medicine, Microbiology
and Immunology
Department of Medicine
Duke University Medical Center
Durham, North Carolina*

Raven Press ❦ New York

Raven Press Ltd., 1185 Avenue of the Americas, New York, New York 10036

Made in the United States of America

Library of Congress Cataloging-in-Publication Data
Infections of the central nervous system/editors, W. Michael Scheld.
  Richard J. Whitley, David T. Durack.
      p. cm.
    Includes bibliographical references and index.
    ISBN 0-88167-766-3
    1. Central nervous system—Infections. 2. Virus Diseases.
  I. Scheld, W. Michael. II. Whitley, Richard J. III. Durack, David T.
    [DNLM: 1. Bacterial Infections. 2. Central Nervous System
  Diseases—microbiology. WL 300 I425]
  RC361.I49 1991
  616.8—dc20
  DNLM/DLC
  for Library of Congress   91-15028
                                                        CIP

*Notice: The editors and publisher of this work have made every effort to ensure that the
drug dosage schedules herein are accurate and in accord with the standards accepted
at the time of publication. Readers are advised, however, to check the product information sheet included in the package of each drug prior to administration to be certain
that changes have not been made in either the recommended dose or contraindications. Such verification is especially important with regard to new or infrequently used
drugs.*

To Suss and Sarah;
Salley, Kevin, Christopher, Jennifer, Katherine;
Carmen, Jeremy, Kim, Sunny, and Justin

Contents

Contributing Authors xi

Foreword xv
Robert G. Petersdorf

Preface xvii

1 Introduction: Approach to the Patient with Central Nervous System Infection 1
David T. Durack, Richard J. Whitley, and W. Michael Scheld

Part I: Viral Infections of the Central Nervous System and Related Disorders

2 Pathogenesis and Pathophysiology of Viral Infections of the Central Nervous System 7
Michael Schlitt, Robert B. Chronister, and Richard J. Whitley

3 Viral Meningitis and the Aseptic Meningitis Syndrome 19
Harley A. Rotbart

4 Encephalitis Caused by Herpesviruses, Including B Virus 41
Richard J. Whitley and Michael Schlitt

5 Arthropod-Borne Encephalitides 87
Richard J. Whitley

6 Meningitis and Encephalitis Caused by Mumps Virus 113
John W. Gnann, Jr.

7 Rabies 127
Richard J. Whitley and Mark Middlebrooks

8 Slow Viral Infections of the Human Nervous System 145
David M. Asher

9 Perinatal Viral Infections 167
Richard J. Whitley and Sergio Stagno

10 Neurological Manifestations of Infection with the Human Immunodeficiency Viruses 201
Bradley K. Evans, Diane K. Donley, and John N. Whitaker

11 Viral Vaccines that Protect the Central Nervous System 233
Mark F. Mangano and Stanley A. Plotkin

12 Guillain–Barré Syndrome 259
Gene Tenorio, Arie Ashkenasi, and John W. Benton

Part II: Mycoplasmal Infections of the Central Nervous System

13 Mycoplasmal Diseases of the Central Nervous System 283
Wallace A. Clyde, Jr.

Part III: Bacterial Infections of the Central Nervous System

14 Pathogenesis and Pathophysiology of Bacterial Infections of the Central
Nervous System 297
Allan R. Tunkel and W. Michael Scheld

15 Neonatal Bacterial Meningitis 313
Arnold L. Smith and Joel Haas

16 Acute Bacterial Meningitis in Children and Adults 335
Karen L. Roos, Allan R. Tunkel, and W. Michael Scheld

17 Rickettsiae and the Central Nervous System 411
Jerome H. Kim and David T. Durack

18 Tuberculosis of the Central Nervous System 425
Abigail Zuger and Franklin D. Lowy

19 Brain Abscess 457
Brian Wispelwey, Ralph G. Dacey, Jr., and W. Michael Scheld

20 Subdural Empyema 487
David C. Helfgott, Karen Weingarten, and Barry J. Hartman

21 Epidural Abscess 499
*Bruce G. Gellin, Karen Weingarten, Francis W. Gamache, Jr.,
and Barry J. Hartman*

22 Central Nervous System Complications of Infective Endocarditis 515
Patrick Francioli

23 Infections of Cerebrospinal Fluid Shunts 561
Bruce A. Kaufman and David G. McLone

Part IV. Central Nervous System Syndromes Mediated by Bacterial Toxins

24 Botulism 589
James M. Hughes

25 Tetanus 603
Thomas P. Bleck

26 *Bordetella pertussis* and the Central Nervous System 625
Erik L. Hewlett

Part V: Spirochetal Infections of the Central Nervous System

27 Central Nervous System Syphilis 639
Edward W. Hook III

28 Lyme Disease 657
Louis Reik, Jr.

Part VI: Fungal Infections of the Central Nervous System

29 Pathogenesis and Pathophysiology of Fungal Infections of the Central Nervous System 693
John R. Perfect and David T. Durack

30 Chronic Meningitis 703
Tarvez Tucker and Jerrold J. Ellner

31 Diagnosis and Treatment of Fungal Meningitis 729
John R. Perfect

32 Space-Occupying Fungal Lesions of the Central Nervous System 741
Kent Sepkowitz and Donald Armstrong

Part VII: Protozoal and Helminthic Infections of the Central Nervous System

33 Protozoal Infections of the Central Nervous System 767
J. Peter Cegielski and David T. Durack

34 Toxoplasmosis of the Central Nervous System 801
Carol S. Dukes, Benjamin J. Luft, and David T. Durack

35 Helminthic Infections of the Central Nervous System 825
Miriam L. Cameron and David T. Durack

Part VIII: Diagnostic Evaluation of Central Nervous System Infections

36 Cerebrospinal Fluid in Central Nervous System Infections 861
John E. Greenlee

37 Imaging of Intracranial Infections 887
Robert A. Zimmerman

Subject Index 909

Contributing Authors

Donald Armstrong, M.D.   *Infectious Disease Service, Memorial Sloan–Kettering Cancer Center, New York, New York 10021*

David M. Asher, M.D.   *Laboratory of CNS Studies, National Institute of Neurological Disorders and Stroke, Bethesda, Maryland 20892*

Arie Ashkenasi, M.D.   *Department of Pediatric Neurology, University of Alabama, Birmingham, Alabama 35294*

John W. Benton, M.D.   *Department of Pediatric Neurology, University of Alabama, Birmingham, Alabama 35294*

Thomas P. Bleck, M.D.   *Department of Neurology, University of Virginia School of Medicine, Charlottesville, Virginia 22908*

Miriam L. Cameron, M.D.   *Division of Infectious Diseases and International Health, Duke University Medical Center, Durham, North Carolina 27710*

J. Peter Cegielski, M.D.   *Division of Infectious Diseases and International Health, Duke University Medical Center, Durham, North Carolina 27710*

Robert B. Chronister, M.D.   *Department of Neuroanatomy, University of South Alabama, Mobile, Alabama 36688*

Wallace A. Clyde, Jr., M.D.   *Department of Pediatrics, University of North Carolina, Chapel Hill, North Carolina 27599*

Ralph G. Dacey, Jr., M.D.   *Department of Neurosurgery, Washington University School of Medicine, St. Louis, Missouri 63110*

Diane K. Donley, M.D.   *Department of Pediatrics, UAB School of Medicine, Birmingham, Alabama 35294, and Sparks Center for Developmental and Learning Disabilities, Birmingham, Alabama 35294*

Carol S. Dukes, M.D.   *Division of Infectious Diseases and International Health, Duke University Medical Center, Durham, North Carolina 27710*

David T. Durack, M.B., D.Phil.,   *Chief, Division of Infectious Diseases and International Health, Duke University Medical Center, Durham, North Carolina 27710*

Jerrold J. Ellner, M.D.   *Departments of Neurology and Medicine, University Hospitals of Cleveland, Case Western Reserve University, Cleveland, Ohio 44106*

Bradley K. Evans, M.D.   *Department of Neurology, UAB School of Medicine, Birmingham, Alabama 35294, and Department of Neurology, Birmingham Veterans Administration Hospital, Birmingham, Alabama 35294*

Patrick Francioli, M.D.   *Division of Hospital Preventive Medicine, Department of Internal Medicine, Division of Infectious Disease, Centre Hospitalier Universitaire Vaudois, Lausanne, Switzerland*

Francis W. Gamache, Jr., M.D.   *Department of Surgery, Cornell University Medical Center, New York, New York 10021*

Bruce G. Gellin, M.D.   *Department of Medicine, Division of Infectious Diseases, Cornell University Medical College, New York, New York 10021*

John W. Gnann, Jr., M.D.   *Departments of Medicine and Microbiology, Division of Infectious Diseases, University of Alabama at Birmingham, Birmingham, Alabama 35294*

John E. Greenlee, M.D.   *Neurology Service, Veterans Affairs Medical Center, Salt Lake City, Utah 84148, and Department of Neurology, University of Utah School of Medicine, Salt Lake City, Utah 84132*

Joel Haas, M.D.   *Division of Infectious Diseases and Department of Pathology, Children's Hospital and Medical Center, Seattle, Washington 98105*

Barry J. Hartman, M.D.   *Department of Medicine, Division of Infectious Diseases, Cornell University Medical College, New York, New York 10021*

David C. Helfgott, M.D.   *Department of Medicine, Division of Infectious Diseases, Cornell University Medical College, New York, New York 10021, and the Rockefeller University, New York, New York 10021*

Erik L. Hewlett, M.D.   *Division of Clinical Pharmacology, University of Virginia School of Medicine, Charlottesville, Virginia 22908*

Edward W. Hook III, M.D.   *Department of Medicine, Johns Hopkins University School of Medicine, Baltimore, Maryland 21205, and STD Clinical Services, Baltimore City Health Department, Baltimore, Maryland 21205*

James M. Hughes, M.D.   *Center of Infectious Diseases, Centers for Disease Control, Public Health Service, U.S. Department of Health and Human Services, Atlanta, Georgia 30333*

Bruce A. Kaufman, M.D.   *Department of Neurosurgery, St. Louis Children's Hospital, Washington University School of Medicine, St. Louis, Missouri 63110*

Jerome H. Kim, M.D.   *Division of Infectious Diseases and International Health, Duke University Medical Center, Durham, North Carolina 27710*

Franklin D. Lowy, M.D.   *Division of Infectious Diseases, Department of Medicine, Montefiore Medical Center and the Albert Einstein College of Medicine, Bronx, New York 10467*

Benjamin J. Luft, M.D.   *Division of Infectious Diseases, State University of New York—Stony Brook, Stony Brook, New York 11794*

Mark F. Mangano, M.D.   *Division of Infectious Diseases, The Children's Hospital of Philadelphia, Philadelphia, Pennsylvania 19104, and The Wistar Institute, Philadelphia, Pennsylvania 19104*

David G. McLone, M.D.   *Department of Neurosurgery, Children's Memorial Hospital, Northwestern University, Chicago, Illinois 60614*

Mark Middlebrooks, M.D.   *Departments of Pediatrics, Microbiology, and Medicine, University of Alabama, Birmingham, Alabama 35294*

John R. Perfect, M.D.   *Division of Infectious Diseases and International Health, Duke University Medical Center, Durham, North Carolina 27710*

Stanley A. Plotkin, M.D.   *Division of Infectious Diseases, The Children's Hospital of Philadelphia, Philadelphia, Pennsylvania 19104, and The Wistar Institute, Philadelphia, Pennsylvania 19104, and Departments of Pediatrics and Microbiology, The University of Pennsylvania, Philadelphia, Pennsylvania 19104*

Louis Reik, Jr., M.D.   *Department of Neurology, University of Connecticut Health Center, Farmington, Connecticut 06032*

Karen L. Roos, M.D. *Department of Neurology, Regenstrief Health Center, Indiana University Medical Center, Indianapolis, Indiana 46202*

Harley A. Rotbart, M.D. *Departments of Pediatrics (Infectious Diseases) and Microbiology/Immunology, University of Colorado School of Medicine and The Children's Hospital of Denver, Denver, Colorado 80262*

W. Michael Scheld, M.D. *Departments of Medicine and Neurosurgery, Associate Chair for Residency Programs, Division of Infectious Diseases, University of Virginia Health Sciences Center, Charlottesville, Virginia 22908*

Michael Schlitt, M.D. *Suite 310, 3915 Talbot Road South, Renton, Washington 98055. Former address: Department of Neurosurgery, University of South Alabama, Mobile, Alabama 36617*

Kent Sepkowitz, M.D. *Infectious Disease Service, Memorial Sloan–Kettering Cancer Center, New York, New York 10021*

Arnold L. Smith, M.D. *Division of Infectious Diseases and Department of Pathology, Children's Hospital and Medical Center, Seattle, Washington 98105*

Sergio Stagno, M.D. *Departments of Pediatrics, Microbiology, and Medicine, University of Alabama, Birmingham, Alabama 35294*

Gene Tenorio, M.D. *Department of Pediatric Neurology, University of Alabama, Birmingham, Alabama 35294*

Tarvez Tucker, M.D. *Departments of Neurology and Medicine, University Hospitals of Cleveland, Case Western Reserve University, Cleveland, Ohio 44106*

Allan R. Tunkel, M.D., Ph.D. *Department of Medicine, Division of Infectious Diseases, Medical College of Pennsylvania, Philadelphia, Pennsylvania 19129*

Karen Weingarten, M.D. *Department of Radiology, Division of Neuroradiology, Cornell University Medical College, New York, New York 10021*

John N. Whitaker, M.D. *Department of Neurology, UAB School of Medicine, Birmingham, Alabama 35294, and Department of Neurology, Birmingham Veterans Administration Hospital, Birmingham, Alabama 35294*

Richard J. Whitley, M.D. *Departments of Pediatrics, Microbiology, and Medicine, University of Alabama, Birmingham, Alabama 35294*

Brian Wispelwey, M.D. *Department of Medicine, Division of Infectious Diseases, University of Virginia Health Sciences Center, Charlottesville, Virginia 22908*

Robert A. Zimmerman, M.D. *Department of Radiology, Children's Hospital of Philadelphia, Philadelphia, Pennsylvania 19014*

Abigail Zuger, M.D. *Division of Infectious Diseases, Department of Medicine, Montefiore Medical Center and the Albert Einstein College of Medicine, Bronx, New York 10467*

Foreword

My long-standing personal interest in infections of the nervous system makes me excited about this book. Beginning in 1958 and twenty years thereafter I worked on experimental meningitis. I remember, in 1960, presenting some rather simple experiments to explain the fall in CSF sugar in experimental bacterial meningitis to the plenary session of the American Society for Clinical Investigation. Much has happened in the investigative world since those early days; the problem that I tried to rationalize in such simple terms over 30 years ago has turned out to be more complex, and still not altogether solved.

This book treats the subject matter extensively. What is known about central nervous system infections has increased exponentially and that volume of material is captured here. Although the editors apologize for restricting the number of references, I was impressed with the thoroughness of the authors' literature review and the up-to-date nature of the references they cite.

I am pleased that the material in this text includes a heavy emphasis on pathogenesis. In 1958, Dr. Donald Harter, a neurologist, and I reviewed what little was then known about the pathogenesis of bacterial meningitis. While considerable advances have occurred more recently, the core question of how and why microbes leave an infectious nidus in the periphery to nest in the central nervous system has not been answered; how they get there is also not clear. A better understanding of these issues would be beneficial for more effective prevention and treatment to take place.

An appealing feature of this book is the different background of the editors and authors. Infectious disease internists, pediatricians, neurologists and neurosurgeons, and imaging specialists are all involved. As a long-term editor of the infectious disease section of a textbook of general medicine, I was frequently involved in turf battles concerning where to place the discussion of some central nervous system infections, and sometimes, infections primarily affecting children were lost altogether. In this text, the editors have achieved an editorial balance that has not been achieved in other texts.

Perhaps the most influential change in the approach to central nervous system infections has been the development of new imaging technologies. In many countries, including ours, most patients with meningitis have CT or MRI scans as part of their diagnostic tests. The advent of new and more potent antimicrobials is also changing the treatment of bacterial meningitis. With viral central nervous system infections, the surface has barely been scratched. I agree with the editors that the mortality and morbidity outcomes of central nervous system infections remain unacceptably high. I am afraid that even with our more potent diagnostic and therapeutic arsenal, mortality and morbidity will not improve a great deal until we answer more definitively some of the enigmas posed by pathogenesis.

This book will surely become the "gold standard". I hope the editors will update the book frequently as further investigations answer some of the questions yet unanswered.

Robert G. Petersdorf

Preface

From the brain, and from the brain only, arise our pleasures, joys, laughter and jests, as well as our sorrows, pains, griefs and tears. . . . It is the same thing which makes us mad or delirious, inspires us with dread or fear, whether by night or by day, brings sleeplessness, inopportune mistakes, aimless anxieties, absent-mindedness, and acts that are contrary to habit. These things that we suffer all come from the brain, when it is not healthy, but becomes abnormally hot, cold, moist, or dry.

Hippocrates, *The Sacred Disease,* Section XVII

Every physician, almost, hath his favourite disease, to which he ascribes all the victories obtained over human nature. The gout, the rheumatism, the stone, the gravel, and the consumption have all their several patrons in the faculty; and none more than the nervous fever, or the fever on the spirits.

Henry Fielding, *Tom Jones,* Book II, Chapter 9

I hasten to give you a sketch of the spotted fever in this place. It made its first appearance about the beginning of January last; but the instances were few and distant from each other, until last week. Although it had proved fatal in most instances, seven only had died belonging to this town, previous to the 25th of February. Since that time the disorder has come upon us like a flood of mighty waters. We have buried eight persons within the last eight days. About twelve or fifteen new cases appeared on Thursday last; many of them very sudden and violent. This was the most melancholy and alarming day ever witnessed in this place. Seven or eight physicians were continually engaged in the neighborhood north of the meeting house, and I believe not one half hour passed in the forenoon without presenting a new case. Pale fear and extreme anxiety were visible in every countenance. . . ."

Reverend Festus Foster of Petersham, Massachusetts in a letter to the editor
of *The Worchester Spy,* 6 March 1810

These vignettes concerning central nervous system (CNS) infections come down to us over a span of 25 centuries. The Reverend Foster's graphic description of an outbreak of meningococcemia and meningococcal meningitis in the late winter of 1810 makes it easy to understand why these infections engendered fear among physicians and lay persons alike. Today, even with the comforts of vastly better knowledge and treatments, CNS infections continue to pose serious problems in health care. Some CNS infections are common, occurring either as sporadic cases or in epidemics. For example, major outbreaks of meningococcal disease have occurred in Africa and Asia during the past few years. Furthermore, despite the introduction of newer antimicrobial agents and diagnostic techniques, the mortality associated with some infections of the central nervous system remains high, particularly in tuberculous, pneumococcal, and gram-negative aerobic bacillary meningitis; rabies; tetanus; cryptococcal meningitis in patients with acquired immunodeficiency syndrome (AIDS); and Jakob–Creutzfeldt disease. The morbidity associated with CNS infections may be even more important than the death rate, especially in developing countries. Neurologic sequelae, elegantly described by Hippocrates above, may deprive survivors of hearing, intellect, or function, demeaning the quality of human life and burdening health resources and social services.

The distinctive nature and natural history of CNS infections set them somewhat apart from the mainstream of infectious diseases. The scope of today's knowledge of these infections can no longer be presented adequately within the confines of a subsection in a general textbook. Indeed, the understanding and management of CNS infections is evolving toward a subspecialty in its own right. For these reasons, a new major text seems justified—hence this book, devoted to a comprehensive coverage of human CNS infections.

The work is a comprehensive treatise for the advanced reader on all aspects of CNS infections. The book occupies a central niche between large general texts on pediatrics, medicine, neurology, neurosurgery, and infectious diseases on the one hand, and specialized single-subject treatises on the other. We have assembled an outstanding group of contributors, drawn from the ranks of internal medicine, pediatrics, neurology, neurosurgery, infectious diseases, epidemiology, virology, neuroradiology, and the basic neurosciences.

After a brief introduction that emphasizes the syndrome-oriented clinical approach to the patient with a CNS syndrome and fever, the book is divided into parts based on microorganisms. The major CNS pathogens (viruses, bacteria, fungi, and protozoa) receive the most attention, although rarer pathogens such as mycoplasmas, slow viruses, and helminths are also covered in depth. In keeping with our philosophy that advances in diagnosis, therapy, prognosis, and prevention require better understanding of the pathogenesis and pathophysiology of these disorders, an introductory chapter on these subjects is included in each of the major sections of the book. Within each section a syndromic approach has been maintained whenever possible, but in many instances we felt that specific diseases required separate coverage—for example, tetanus, neurosyphilis, and Lyme disease. In some sections we have separated processes that primarily present as meningitis or meningoencephalitis from those that usually present as focal CNS lesions. The book concludes with discussions on two major diagnostic modalities: (i) evaluation of the cerebrospinal fluid and (ii) neurodiagnostic imaging by computerized tomography and magnetic resonance imaging.

In choosing the contributors, we have sought individuals with clinical experience as well as with active basic and/or clinical investigative interests in their topic. We asked them to take a comprehensive approach, ranging from recent advances in molecular pathogenesis to the clinical manifestations, therapy, and prevention of CNS infections. We also established certain other ground rules. To gain a measure of unity among the chapters, each contributor was asked to write under common subheadings: history of the syndrome, epidemiology, etiology, pathogenesis and pathophysiology, pathology, clinical manifestations, approach to diagnosis, therapy, and prevention. We asked authors to provide an extensive but not exhaustive bibliography, emphasizing classical papers and recent (1985–1991) references while limiting each chapter total to 350 citations or less. We strongly encouraged the liberal use of tables, drawings, and photographs. Although a degree of overlap between chapters is inevitable (and sometimes even desirable) in a multiauthored volume, we have attempted to minimize redundancies as much as possible.

From its inception 3 years ago, we intended that this should be a "gold standard" reference text. We set out to bring together the best information from the best authors in the best format. Inevitably, the size and complexity of the field means that we will fall short in some areas. Recognizing this, we hope to develop and improve the book through future editions. Our ambition will remain the same: to present the best available comprehensive resource and reference text for all who deal with infections of the central nervous system.

W. Michael Scheld
Richard J. Whitley
David T. Durack

Acknowledgments

We thank everyone who has helped us in the preparation of this large book. Most importantly, we wish to thank all the authors for their outstanding contributions. Numerous other colleagues provided helpful discussion and criticism. We are particularly grateful to our secretaries: Eve Schwartz, Mona Bernhardt, Janet Routten, Mary Ann Howard, Nancy Boice and Sherlyn Burks. The editorial staff at Raven Press deserves our gratitude, especially Lisa Berger, Senior Medical Editor responsible for the project, Susan Lupack, Jeffrey Stier, Susan Berkowitz, and Jennifer DeSpain, who helped make the original idea for this text a reality. And finally, we thank our families for their tolerance and support during the interminable hours required to bring this undertaking to its end.

The Editors

Infections of the Central Nervous System,
edited by W. M. Scheld, R. J. Whitley, and
D. T. Durack, Raven Press, Ltd., New York © 1991.

CHAPTER 1

Introduction

Approach to the Patient with Central Nervous System Infection

David T. Durack, Richard J. Whitley, and W. Michael Scheld

Central nervous system (CNS) infections are notable for their diversity; they range from common to rare, from acute to chronic, and from trivial to fatal. Some are easily cured, whereas others lack any specific treatment. These infections share certain special characteristics.

Firstly, they occur within an anatomic closed space. Inside the rigid bony cage of the skull they are separated, immunologically, from the rest of the body. Thus, some important systemic immune responses may be excluded from the CNS while others are sequestered within it.

Secondly, the natural history of illnesses due to CNS infection often differs strikingly from that of those due to infection at other sites, even when caused by the same organisms. The obvious contrasts between a gram-negative bacterial infection of the urinary tract and meningitis caused by the same species illustrate this point. Likewise, polioviruses usually cause only mild systemic illness but, in some individuals, can cause devastating damage to motor neurons in the CNS.

Thirdly, many CNS infections cause high mortality or, if the patient survives, serious sequelae after resolution of the acute infection. For the many CNS infections which are treatable, prompt diagnosis and aggressive management are necessary to allow the best chance of recovery without sequelae.

D. T. Durack: Department of Infectious Diseases, Duke University Medical Center, Durham, North Carolina 27710.
R. J. Whitley: Departments of Pediatrics, Microbiology, and Medicine, University of Alabama, Birmingham, Alabama 35294.
W. M. Scheld: Division of Infectious Diseases, Department of Medicine, University of Virginia, Charlottesville, Virginia 22901.

An effective clinical approach to CNS infections must be tailored to these special characteristics. A logical and consistent method is possible, despite the diversity of presentations and problems encountered.

FOUR CARDINAL MANIFESTATIONS OF CNS INFECTION

The cardinal manifestations of CNS infection are four: fever, headache, alteration of mental status, and focal neurologic signs. Obviously, all of these features can sometimes be found in other, noninfectious CNS syndromes. Therefore, while their presence directs attention to the CNS, they are nonspecific. To narrow the differential diagnosis, other characteristics must be evaluated. The most helpful of these often is the time course of the illness.

NATURAL HISTORY OF CNS INFECTIONS

The time course of disease is especially important in the evaluation of diseases affecting the CNS. Their temporal profile is often distinctive, even unique. The remitting and relapsing course of multiple sclerosis provides a familiar example. The temporal profile of many CNS infections is equally distinctive. The date of onset, temporal relationship to predisposing factors, rate of progression, time to reach the peak of severity, time needed to respond to treatment, and rate of resolution are all highly informative. Thus, careful study of the natural history is of central importance in the clinical approach to CNS infections.

PHYSICAL EXAMINATION

Physical findings are of utmost importance in the evaluation of CNS infections. At the outset, a key question is: Does this patient have *any* definite abnormality on physical examination? Many patients who present with symptoms compatible with a CNS infection have no abnormal findings whatsoever on physical examination. In this situation, the patient may have functional disease, a psychiatric diagnosis, or a condition that does not involve the CNS. Alternatively, the patient may have an active CNS infection but no physical findings. This is an unusual situation, but when it occurs, diagnostic information will have to be sought in other directions. Once one or more definite physical abnormalities related to the CNS have been found, another key question arises: Does the patient have *focal* neurologic signs? Even a single focal finding shifts the differential diagnosis strongly towards important syndromes such as space-occupying lesions or herpes simplex encephalitis.

THE SYNDROME RECOGNITION APPROACH TO DIAGNOSIS

The spectrum of infectious agents that cause neural infections is remarkably broad. All the main human microbial pathogens can involve the CNS: viruses and viroids, mycoplasmas, bacteria, spirochetes, fungi, protozoa, and helminths. This range of potential pathogens is so large that often it is impractical to attempt an initial diagnosis by species of organism. Rather, it is necessary to begin by matching the clinical findings to one of the syndromes associated with CNS infections, then progress towards a specific etiologic diagnosis. Some of the characteristics of the main syndromes are displayed in Table 1.

The Acute Meningitis Syndrome

For many physicians, the acute meningitis syndrome is perhaps the most familiar among the CNS infections. Its dominant features are acute onset (over a few hours to a few days) of high fever, headache, photophobia, stiff neck, and altered mental state. The latter may range from simple irritability to confusion, obtundation, or coma. Vomiting may occur, especially in young children, but may be more characteristic of raised intracranial pressure than of meningitis itself. A history or complaint of headache is unlikely to be available if the patient is a young child. The etiology may be viral ("aseptic meningitis") or bacterial. The patient with an acute meningitis syndrome usually presents for medical evaluation within a few hours to days of onset; if correctly diagnosed and treated, this syndrome will improve within a few days.

The Subacute or Chronic Meningitis Syndrome

In contrast to acute meningitis, subacute and chronic meningitis syndromes run their course over weeks, months, or years. Although some of the clinical findings may be the same as for acute meningitis, the onset is usually gradual, often unrelated to any evident predisposing condition. Fever, while often present, tends to be lower and less hectic than in acute meningitis. The patient is more likely to present a picture of chronic general debility, as well as having symptoms referable to the CNS. Focal neurologic findings are more common than in acute meningitis but are less common than with space-occupying syndromes.

The Acute Encephalitis Syndrome

This syndrome shares many features with acute meningitis; indeed, the two conditions often coexist in the form of meningoencephalitis. The likelihood of mental change early in the disease prior to onset of obtundation or coma is greater than in acute meningitis. Seizures are much more likely to occur in encephalitis than in the meningitis syndromes. The patient is likely to have an associated systemic illness, with nausea and vomiting often being prominent. Clinical findings may reflect tropism of some viruses for specific locations in the CNS; for example, herpes simplex preferentially affects the temporal lobes.

The Chronic Encephalitis Syndrome

This shares many clinical features with acute encephalitis. However, the onset is gradual and the course is less hectic. The findings may be less dramatic or less severe than in acute disease, but they often progress gradually to severe disability or death. Relapses and recrudescences may occur over a long period. Chronic encephalitis evolves over weeks to months or years. The patient presents a picture of general debility rather than acute illness. Complications such as pressure sores, contractures, or dementia may develop during the course.

The Space-Occupying Lesion Syndrome

In these patients, the key findings result from a focal lesion and raised intracranial pressure. Onset may be acute, subacute, or chronic. Clinical manifestations such as headache, nausea, or vomiting often begin intermittently, but they progress in a crescendo to a crisis at about the time the patient is admitted to the hospital. This crisis may consist of (a) a focal or generalized seizure or (b) onset of obtundation progressing to coma.

TABLE 1. *Summary of features of the main CNS infection syndromes*

CNS infection syndrome	Onset	Duration	Intracranial pressure	General or focal seizures	Autonomic involvement	Extraneural findings	Mortality with modern treatment	Examples[a]
Acute meningitis	Sudden	Days	Raised	Yes	No	Yes	Low	Bacterial viral, or meningitis
Subacute meningitis	Gradual	Weeks to months	Raised	Yes	No	No	Moderate	Tuberculous, cryptococcal, or syphilitic meningitis
Chronic meningitis	Gradual	Months	Raised	Yes	No	No	High	Coccidioidomycosis, sporotrichosis, syphilis, enterovirus in immunodeficients
Acute encephalitis or encephalomyelitis	Sudden	Days	Raised	Yes	Yes	Yes	Variable	Measles, herpes simplex, rickettsial infections
Chronic encephalitis or encephalomyelitis	Gradual	Months to years	Raised	Yes	No	No	Variable	SSPE, HTLV-1 myelitis, HIV encephalitis, Lyme disease, syphilis
Space-occupying lesions	Intermittent symptoms	Weeks to years	Raised	Yes	No	No	Moderate	Brain abscess, cysticercosis, spinal or epidural abscess, subdural empyema
Toxin-mediated syndrome	Sudden	Days	Normal	No	Yes	No	Low to moderate	Tetanus, botulism
Postinfectious syndromes	Sudden or gradual	Days to weeks	Raised	Yes	Yes	No	Moderate	Postinfectious encephalomyelitis
Slow-virus syndromes	Insidious	Months to years	Normal	No	No	No	High	Jakob–Creutzfeldt disease, kuru, PML

[a] SSPE, subacute sclerosing panencephalitis; HTLV-1, human T-lymphotrophic virus 1; HIV, human immunodeficiency virus; PML, progressive multifocal leukoencephalopathy.

The focal neurologic signs obviously will depend upon the location of the lesion or lesions.

When a space-occupying lesion occurs in the spinal canal, a distinctive set of manifestations develops. Findings often develop in a typical sequential manner: first, localized back pain; second, nerve root pain with associated alteration in reflexes; third, motor weakness followed by sensory changes with bowel or bladder dysfunction; fourth, paralysis. Often, the fourth phase is accompanied by an improvement in pain even though the syndrome has progressed to its critical stage. Although this is a typical sequence, the rate of progression from one stage to the next is unpredictable. Because the frequency of permanent neurologic sequelae depends upon the stage and degree of damage inflicted before intervention, this syndrome presents an emergency which requires immediate diagnosis and therapy.

Toxin-Mediated Syndromes

Several distinctive syndromes can occur when microbial toxins that react specifically with neural tissue reach the CNS. The leading examples are tetanus and botulism. In the first, many of the findings result from overstimulation of neural cells, whereas in the second the main findings result from interruption of neural transmission. Of all the syndromes, toxin-mediated conditions are least likely to show the four cardinal manifestations of CNS manifestation: fever, headache, disturbance of consciousness, and focal neurologic signs. For example, botulism is characterized by absence of fever and normal consciousness in most patients, even when they are severely paralyzed.

Postinfectious Syndromes

Several important syndromes develop following microbial infections. The usual sequence begins with a common, often rather trivial, viral infection. Most patients recover uneventfully from such infections. Rarely, a serious postinfectious neurologic syndrome develops, presumably as an idiosyncratic reaction to the primary infection. Examples include Guillain–Barré syndrome, postinfectious encephalitis, postinfectious encephalomyelitis, and transverse myelitis. These reactions are presumably mediated in most cases by an immunologic response to the etiologic microbe or to antigens revealed as a result of the primary infection. The original etiologic agent often cannot be directly demonstrated in neural lesions. Although rare, these syndromes can be severe, even fatal. In a significant number of cases, the inciting infection may pass completely unnoticed, either because it was so mild or because some time passed before the development of the more serious neurologic complication.

Slow Virus Diseases

These unconventional infections cause unconventional syndromes. CNS slow virus infections develop insidiously, over months or longer. Patients show progressive signs of neuronal destruction, often affecting motor function severely. They do not become febrile and do not have raised intracranial pressure or seizures. Mortality is high.

This book will elaborate on these themes through a detailed description of individual infectious agents and the CNS diseases that they produce in humans.

PART I

Viral Infections of the CNS and Related Disorders

Infections of the Central Nervous System,
edited by W. M. Scheld, R. J. Whitley, and
D. T. Durack, Raven Press, Ltd., New York © 1991.

CHAPTER 2

Pathogenesis and Pathophysiology of Viral Infections of the Central Nervous System

Michael Schlitt, Robert B. Chronister, and Richard J. Whitley

Viral infections of the central nervous system (CNS) have attracted the attention of historians and physicians for millennia (1,2). With the exception of herpes simplex encephalitis (HSE) (3,4), the specific causes of neurologic syndromes of viral origin have been difficult (and often impossible) to identify. These CNS infections usually represent complications of a systemic viral illness. It must be emphasized that relative to the high incidence of viral infections of other organ systems, infection and disease of the CNS are unusual. Despite the relative infrequency of CNS viral infections, brain and spinal cord diseases are of great importance because of the nature of the organ system that is infected. Injured brain tissue recovers slowly (often incompletely) and regenerates minimally. Even in patients with completely reversible viral encephalopathies and encephalitides, a full return of function rarely occurs before 3 months have elapsed from the onset of illness.

Infections of the CNS may result in a variety of different clinical syndromes identified as meningitis, encephalitis, meningoencephalitis, or myelitis. Anatomic sites of involvement for each of these forms of infection are, respectively, the leptomeninges, brain parenchyma, a combination of both, or the spinal cord. Commonly, each of these terms is used to define a clinical syndrome(s) indicative of the extent of brain or peripheral nervous system involvement.

Over the last 20 years, with the introduction of anti-viral therapy, progress has been achieved in understanding manifestations, pathogenesis, diagnosis, and treatment of viral CNS diseases. However, much yet needs to be learned. Viruses invade the CNS by either a neural or a hematogenous route, depending on the specific virus and the clinical circumstances. The route of preference must relate to cell receptors, local and systemic immune responses, and inoculum size. The contributions of these factors, singularly and collectively, are unknown. Mechanisms of viral invasion into brain cells and, perhaps, establishment of latency within the CNS are poorly understood. Differences in the extent of viral replication leading to cytolysis in one instance versus nonproductive or chronic infection in another circumstance have only recently been related to specific viral genes and gene products. Understanding of the mechanisms involved in the maintenance and reactivation of latent herpesviruses is in its infancy. Nevertheless, an understanding of these issues will be essential if reactivation of virus is to be prevented. Experimental animal models of latent viruses in the CNS may be helpful in predicting long-term clinical outcome of humans who experience similar infections. For example, animals with experimental HSE which have survived several years will demonstrate temporal lobe sclerosis with persistent evidence of viral genetic sequences resident at the sclerotic site (M. Schlitt and R. B. Chronister, *unpublished observations*). The relationship between a latent infection and the development of sclerosis with the potential for seizure activity is unknown but needs to be addressed. Similarly, the means of transmission of virus within the CNS is debated, and it is probably different for different viral groups and/or viral disease states. Other than quantity of the virus, the basic mechanisms for CNS viral disease remain to be elucidated. Even in HSE where effective treatment is available, the severe morbidity or mortality rates remain at 50%.

M. Schlitt: 3915 Talbot Road, Renton, Washington 98055; formerly with the Department of Neurosurgery, University of South Alabama, Mobile, Alabama 36617.

R. B. Chronister: Department of Neuroanatomy, University of South Alabama, Mobile, Alabama 36688.

R. Whitley: Departments of Pediatrics, Microbiology, and Medicine, University of Alabama, Birmingham, Alabama 35294.

This chapter overviews the pathogenesis and pathophysiology of viral infections of the CNS. It will also consider basic mechanisms of replication in relation to neural tissue. The correlation of typical clinical syndromes associated with well-defined viral CNS disease with the underlying neurophysiological mechanisms will be considered as based on current neurobiological knowledge. Ultimately, diagnosis and treatment of infections of the CNS requires an understanding of the epidemiology, pathogenesis, and clinical manifestations of disease. This chapter provides such an overview, as an introduction to chapters on specific CNS viral infections.

OVERVIEW OF VIRAL INFECTIONS OF THE CNS

Most viral infections of the CNS either involve the meninges, as in aseptic meningitis, or cause a mild clinical syndrome of meningoencephalitis rather than the alarming forms of encephalitis. Encephalitis is an unusual complication of common viral infections (5–8). Thus, the ratio of persons with systemic viral illness to those in whom clinical CNS disease develops is inordinately high. In general, viral infections of the CNS can be considered in several distinct categories. These include a relatively benign inflammation of the meninges (aseptic meningitis), acute viral encephalitis, postinfectious encephalitis, slow viral infections of the CNS, and chronic degenerative diseases of the CNS of presumed viral origin. In addition, inflammation of the spinal cord and peripheral nerves such as myelitis or radiculomyelitis can cause other viral syndromes involving the nervous system.

Many viral pathogens cause CNS infections in humans (2). According to the Centers for Disease Control survey and other surveys, approximately 20,000 cases of encephalitis occur in the United States each year, most of them mild. There are probably an additional 40,000–60,000 cases of leptomeningitis associated with viral infections of the CNS (9,10). The two endemic causes of encephalitis in the United States are herpes simplex virus (HSV) and rabies virus. HSV accounts for approximately 10% of all cases of encephalitis in the United States (11,12). Rabies virus only causes encephalitis and is more common in developing countries.

Japanese B encephalitis is probably the most common epidemic viral infection of the CNS outside North America. In China alone, there are more than 10,000 cases annually despite childhood immunization (13,14). The development of effective vaccines to control diseases such as measles, mumps, rubella, and yellow fever has substantially decreased the incidence of acute encephalitis, meningitis, and the complication of postinfectious encephalomyelitis following these viral disorders. The control of poliomyelitis through vaccination has greatly decreased the incidence of poliovirus infection of the CNS (15). A few sporadic cases do occur as a consequence of vaccine-associated infection with poliovirus type 2 or type 3. Other members of the picornavirus family certainly have the potential to invade the brain, including coxsackievirus and echovirus (2,16–18). Usually these viruses cause a benign aseptic meningitis, but paralytic polio-like syndromes have been documented.

The arthropod-borne viruses [arboviruses, St. Louis encephalitis (SLE), eastern equine encephalitis, Venezuelan encephalitis, and La Cross virus infections] cause sporadic and epidemic CNS infections in the United States (19–23). Early identification and recognition of the specific cause of epidemics may lead to measures to prevent burgeoning mosquito populations which serve as vectors of infection (24). The recent outbreaks of SLE in Florida and Texas (1990) illustrate this point (25).

In the United States, postinfectious encephalomyelitis has commonly been associated with infections of the upper respiratory tract, particularly influenza. In Third World countries where vaccinations are not routine, measles is a major cause of postinfectious encephalomyelitis, accounting for as many as 100,000 cases worldwide (26).

The common and representative pathogens of the CNS, along with their associated clinical syndromes and route of progression to the brain, are summarized in Table 1. Most recognized virus groups can cause CNS diseases. Orthomyxoviruses (which include influenza) do not cause recognizable, acute neurologic syndromes; however, they do contribute to postinfectious encephalitis and can cause Reye's syndrome, a postinfectious metabolic disease. Similarly, adeno- and coronavirus infections are generally confined to the respiratory tract but also can result in a postinfectious syndrome. Before its

TABLE 1. *Pathogenesis of viral infections of the CNS; routes of viral access*

Pathway	Examples of viral pathogen
Hematogenous	Herpes simplex virus (newborn)
	Cytomegalovirus
	Epstein–Barr virus
	Polioviruses
	Coxsackieviruses
	Human immunodeficiency virus
	Mumps virus
	Echoviruses
	Lymphocytic choriomeningitis virus
	Arboviruses (usually)
	Paraviruses
Neuronal	Herpes simplex virus
	B Virus
	Varicella-zoster virus
	Rabies
Olfactory	Herpes simplex virus (?)

eradication, smallpox seldom produced intracranial infection. Essentially all of the other virus families [picorna-, toga-, retro-, rhabdo-, arena-, bunya-, rubi-, and reoviruses (among the RNA viruses) and parvo-, papova-, and herpesviruses (among the DNA viruses)] can and do cause CNS infections (with variable frequency).

Diseases caused by various virus groups can be classified into several different clinical syndromes. Toga-, arena-, paramyxo-, bunya-, retro-, and reoviruses (among the RNA viruses) and, rarely, adenoviruses (among the DNA viruses) can cause a panmeningoencephalitis without focal neurologic findings. For most of these syndromes, the mode of viral spread to the brain is thought to be hematogenous. Onset is rapid; these infections tend not to cause severe cortical disease and secondary brain destruction. Outcome has been shown to vary: Complete recovery usually occurs following western equine encephalitis, whereas high mortality is associated with eastern equine encephalitis. Rabies, varicella-zoster virus (VZV), and herpes simplex type 1 (HSV-1) in adults can cause characteristic focal infections of the brain. For rabies, the infection tends to be a non-necrotizing infection of the hippocampi, cerebellum, and mesencephalon; HSV-1, in contrast, causes a severe necrotizing mesial temporal, insular, and orbitofrontal destruction. VZV can cause a cerebellitis or involve cortical gray matter. For rabies, virus is transported to the brain by a neural route. Similarly, in most cases of HSE caused by HSV-1 beyond the newborn age, neural transmission occurs; however, the route (olfactory versus trigeminal) is controversial. Mumps, herpes simplex type 2 (HSV-2), arenaviruses, and the coxsackieviruses frequently cause aseptic meningitis or meningoencephalitis. With the exception of HSV-2, these other viruses are transported to the CNS by the bloodstream; HSV-2 infection of adults generally causes a meningitis during the primary infection, with transmission resulting from neural transport via sacral nerve roots. Recovery from these viral infections is nearly always complete, and cell destruction is usually minimal. HSV-2, cytomegalovirus (CMV), and the rubivirus, rubella, all can cause catastrophic brain infections in the fetus (rubella and CMV) or the neonate (HSV-2). For rubella and CMV, the route of transmission to the brain is hematogenous after transplacental infection, whereas either hematogenous or neuronal transport of virus can result from perinatal HSV-2 infections. Brain involvement is patchy, and tissue destruction is the rule.

In immunosuppressed patients, polyomaviruses occasionally cause a specific oligodendrogliopathy referred to as progressive multifocal leukoencephalopathy (PML). Diffuse patchy demyelination, occurring primarily in the subcortical white matter, is demonstrable pathologically. These viruses are acquired most often in childhood and remain latent throughout life. Reactivation leading to disease is associated with immunosuppression, especially impaired T-lymphocyte function. The virus has a particular affinity for the oligodendroglia which are converted from the usual physiologic function of myelin preservation to that of polyomavirus production. Viral replication is eventually lytic for the oligodendroglia cell. Cell culture is difficult; nevertheless, proof of a viral etiology for disease can be presumed by electron-microscopic examination of infected brain tissue (particularly the oligodendrocytes) and confirmed by molecular analyses.

Among the picornaviruses, poliovirus (and, occasionally, a few other enteroviruses) can cause a selective infection of motor neuron cells of the anterior horn of the spinal cord and the brainstem, resulting in clinical poliomyelitis. These viruses reach the spinal cord from the bloodstream after replication in the gastrointestinal tract, but they can be transported centrally by the splanchnic nerves as well. These infections tend to cause a cytolytic infection of the anterior horn cells of the spinal cord, leading to paralysis early and atrophy after the acute phase of replication. It should be remembered that although many individuals are infected with these viruses, few develop diseases.

Epstein–Barr virus, SV40, and BK (polyomaviruses) have been implicated causally in brain tumors. Viral latency is probably an important component in the cause of such syndromes; however, the mechanism by which these viruses are transported to the brain is unknown.

Measles virus and rubella can result in unique CNS syndromes. They can cause either an acute encephalomyelitis (which in the case of measles may be mediated by the immune system) or a progressive, slowly evolving disease. The disease associated with the measles virus is known as subacute sclerosing panencephalitis (SSPE), and that associated with the rubella virus is called progressive rubella panencephalitis (PRP). The route of access to the brain is hematogenous, but it should be noted that these diseases take months or years to develop and/or progress. For SSPE, there is a deficiency of M-protein (which is critical for the release of virus), and the viral infection is not rapidly cytolytic. PRP results in a more widespread brain destruction.

Of particular interest is the chronic, progressive, dementing encephalopathy occurring with human immunodeficiency virus (HIV) infection which leads to brain atrophy (27–33). Virus entry to the brain is mediated by mononuclear cells following hematogenous spread; white matter is most affected (34–37). The primary hematogenous cell infected is the monocyte–macrophage; this cell does not undergo lysis but, instead, mediates fusion with other monocytes and CD4-bearing cells to form multinucleated giant cells. As in lentiviral encephalitis, the infected macrophage may function as a "Trojan horse" within the CNS, mediating disease or being a site for persistent infection (38,39). It should be noted that HIV probably interacts with other viruses in the CNS, such as CMV. Myelin damage is thought to be due to a bystander effect from macrophage and giant cell dysfunction.

PATHOGENESIS OF VIRAL INFECTIONS OF THE CNS

Viruses generally gain access to the CNS by one of two routes, either hematogenous or neuronal (2,5–7,13,19,40). Clearly, hematogenous spread of virus to the CNS is the most common route and can result in an altered blood–brain barrier (19,41), best exemplified by arthropod-borne viral diseases (14,19,42,43). Fortunately, while humans are constantly exposed to environmental pathogens, innate host defenses successfully prevent disease in most circumstances.

Blood–Brain Barrier

Essential to the understanding of the dynamics of viral infections of the CNS and the drugs required for their treatment is an understanding of the blood–brain barrier. After first being described by Ehrlich (44), the observation that the intravenous administration of various dyes distributed evenly throughout the body (with the exception of the CNS) led to the postulate of a blood–brain barrier. As is best understood, the blood–brain barrier anatomically is defined according to cerebral capillary endothelial cell tight junctions (44–46). These tight junctions determine passive transfer of cellular and soluble components from the vascular tree across the blood–brain barrier. Transfer of soluble components is determined by lipid solubility, whereas the transport of cells or viruses is mediated by surface adhesion molecules or surface charge and cellular attachment proteins (47–50). Infections of the CNS can disrupt endothelial tight cell junctions, as evidenced by perivascular cuffing and by changes in cerebrospinal fluid (CSF) biochemical composition.

It was emphasized in a recent review (7) that in addition to the blood–brain barrier, a knowledge of CNS infection must also include an understanding of the interaction between blood, CSF, and brain parenchyma (48,51). The choroid plexus is the principal site for generation of CSF. Proteins, viruses, drugs, antibodies, and so on, can enter relatively easily into the interstitial spaces of the choroid plexus. However, these molecules may or may not pass through the lamina epithelialis of the choroid plexus (the site of the blood–CSF barrier) into the CSF (52,53). Transmission across the choroidal epithelial cells is dependent upon size and charge (54,55). Once a substance has entered the CSF, there is facile transfer across the ependyma into the brain parenchyma (56). As a consequence, the transfer of substances in a bidirectional fashion can occur with relative ease. These concepts are essential for understanding transmission of vi-

ruses across cellular borders into CSF and the brain parenchyma. Even more importantly, the access of drugs utilized to treat infections of the CNS into these privileged sites is modulated by these factors (7).

General Pathogenic Concepts

In general, neurologic infections only occur following viremia, direct viral inoculation (into muscle or nerve), or contact with free nerve endings in specialized tissues (e.g., in the olfactory system, in the enteric submucosa, or through trigeminal afferents to the lips and cornea). Low concentrations of virus introduced by peripheral inoculation are usually less effective or ineffective in causing productive viral infection of the brain—with the exceptions of rabies, diseases in certain immune-deficient hosts, or, perhaps, B virus. Lack of transmission from peripheral sites to the CNS is usually the consequence of local and systemic immune responses and the anatomy of the blood–brain barrier. However, once the virus does enter the nervous system, the incorporation of virus into parenchyma can be extremely rapid. In some experimental systems, as few as 1–10 viral particles are capable of producing fulminant viral encephalitis once they are in the CNS.

Hematogenous Spread

The most common route of viral access to the brain is hematogenous. Viral prototypes for hematogenous spread to the brain are the family of arboviruses and enteroviruses. The pathogenesis for hematogenous spread is displayed in Fig. 1. Utilizing enteroviral infections as one model, initial viral replication occurs in the gastrointestinal tract, usually in Peyer's patches. The initial round of replication is followed by a primary viremia with seeding of the reticuloendothelial system. Viral replication often occurs at the site of inoculation of the virus (e.g., the gastrointestinal tract for enteroviruses or subcu-

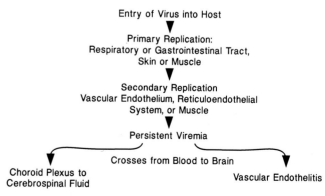

FIG. 1. Pathogenesis of viral infections of the CNS; hematogenous spread.

taneously and intramuscularly for togaviruses), with subsequent viremic spread to the reticuloendothelial system (especially liver, lymph nodes, and spleen). Once virus has reached the reticuloendothelial system, replication is terminated or can persist. Secondary viremia results in seeding of the CNS, as noted below. Subsequently, this secondary viremia can be cleared by the immune system rapidly. The rapidity of viral replication can overcome host defenses. Alternatively, viruses can become adherent to red cells (paramyxo- and togaviruses) or can multiply within white blood cells (mumps and measles viruses), thereby impeding attempts of the immune system to clear infection or, in some circumstances, to even recognize infection.

The actual pathophysiology of viral transport (active versus passive) from the bloodstream to brain tissue is less well understood. As noted above, brain capillaries are characterized by tight junctions between the endothelial cells. These endothelial cells are covered by astrocytic foot processes (with the exception of the Virchow–Robin space). This barrier is relatively impervious to all but highly lipid-soluble substances and nutrients (such as glucose) that are transported actively across endothelial membranes. Lipid-insoluble substances, including some viruses, usually have limited access to the brain. Nevertheless, viruses can diffuse through the cells, or some viruses can be actively taken up by infection of endothelial cells. Once across the blood–brain barrier, virus can be transported to neurons by either the brain interstitium or within the astrocyte. These alternatives are displayed in Fig. 1. Notably, it is presumed that passive viral transport across the blood–brain barrier is responsible for the clinical syndrome of aseptic meningitis. Alternatively, active transport across vascular endothelium can lead to cortical disease associated with encephalitis. Induction of Fc and C3 receptors on endothelial cells has been documented (41,57,58). Histopathologic examination of brain tissue under such circumstances indicates perivascular lymphocytic infiltrates. There may be gaps in the tight junctions enabling viruses to pass through, but this has not been shown conclusively. Similarly, it may be that hematogenous access depends upon contact between virus particles and circumferential organs— such as the area postrema, where the blood–brain barrier is deficient—in order for uptake to occur.

Neural or Myoneural Transmission

Viruses can enter the nervous system by peripheral intraneuronal routes, as exemplified by HSV and rabies (59–62). The prototype virus for neuronal transmission is rabies. An example is shown in Fig. 2. Rabies virus is inoculated into skin and/or muscle tissue of humans following a rabid animal bite, although cases of rabies due to inhalation of aerosolized virus have been reported.

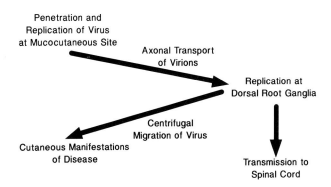

FIG. 2. Pathogenesis of viral infections of the CNS; neuronal transmission.

Furthermore, human-to-human transmission has occurred following corneal transplantation (63). Virus is excreted into the saliva of rabid animals from the salivary glands, where the virus buds from the acinar cells. Following a bite, the virus replicates locally in the myocytes and invades the myoneural junction and, hence, is transported centrally within the axons. A clinical finding which occurs in parallel with neuronal transmission of rabies is the development of paresthesia in the dermatome of the affected nerves. Upon reaching the spinal cord, virus is transported to areas of the brain (usually the hypothalamus and brainstem) which are connected to limbic structures where the virus replicates, though it does not cause cytolysis.

The olfactory system is unique among the cranial nerves and provides an alternative route for virus access to the CNS. Several features of the olfactory system are relevant. The first-order neurons undergo regeneration with an average lifespan per cell of 1 month. Furthermore, these first-order neurons are in contact with the ambient atmosphere via the olfactory mucosa. At this site the olfactory nerves ramify among the entodermally derived mucosa from the nostrils and immediately penetrate to the subarachnoid space. Aromatic substances dissolve in the fluid secreted by the Bowman glands; this fluid overlies the olfactory vesicles of the olfactory neurons. These substances thereby gain access to the olfactory neuron dendrites, and stimulation of these neurons produces the sensation of odor. Additionally, substances such as wheat-germ agglutinin are able to penetrate the subarachnoid space in this region (64). Notably, this area is deficient for the blood–brain barrier. Theoretically, virus gaining access to this watery fluid overlying the olfactory neurons could be transported by the bipolar neuron or enter the duct of the Bowman glands and be transported into the venous tubuloalveolar spaces as well as cells of the lamina propria. Events of viral replication are initiated in the olfactory neurons. Thus, virus (such as HSV-1) could gain access to the olfactory system by a direct neural route or by entrance through an area deficient in the blood–brain barrier, and from there it travels to the areas of innervation of the olfactory system.

REPLICATION OF VIRUS IN THE CNS

Association Between Clinical Disease and Selected Cells

The hallmark of all viral infections of the CNS is the acute onset of a febrile illness. The clinical manifestations of viral infections of the CNS reflect the extent of viral replication within brain tissue. These manifestations range from the relatively benign findings of aseptic meningitis (including headache, malaise, nuchal rigidity, and photophobia) to the more serious forms of encephalitis (including headache, fever, an altered level of consciousness, disorientation, behavioral and speech disturbances, and neurologic signs, sometimes focal but generally diffuse such as hemiparesis or seizures).

The clinical findings also reflect the progression of infection in the brain as the cells of the CNS become infected. The tropism of viruses for different CNS cell types can be used to illustrate this point (2,5–7). For example, polioviruses preferentially infect motor neurons, rabies virus selects neurons of the limbic system, and mumps virus can infect the ependymal cells of newborns. Infection of cortical neurons can lead to abnormal electrical activity and be associated with seizures or focal deficits. Demyelination may follow the destruction of oligodendroglia. The predisposition of HSV to infect the temporal lobes leads to clinical findings of aphasia, temporal lobe seizures, and focal neurologic defects. The basis for the replication of virus within these cell systems will be delineated according to general principles of viral replication.

Attachment and Entry

The details of viral absorption are an essential first step prior to replication and the development of CNS disease. Virus attachment and entry into the cell has been clarified considerably in recent years. Epstein–Barr virus (65), poliovirus (66), and HSV (67) have an attachment protein or binding domain on their surface which mediates interaction of the virus with a receptor domain on the host cell, as reviewed by Lentz (68). Interestingly, many of these host receptor domains are the same regions as those utilized by neurotransmitters or have a sequence homology recognized by the attachment or binding domain of the virus (69). In some cases, the actual binding is mediated by an intermediate molecule (70). Regardless of the binding sequence, viral attachment must be followed by viral absorption and, subsequently, replication (71).

Attachment proteins constitute the binding domain on the virus envelope and are usually highly conserved. In fact, certain neurotrophic viruses, such as poliovirus, appear to have the binding domain present in a depression on the virus surface (72). It has been hypothesized that binding domains (identified by unique amino acid sequences) in depressions such as these can be constant whereas the areas around the depression can be hypervariable (73). Other viruses such as foot-and-mouth disease virus have a binding loop of constant sequence projecting from its surface but within an antigenically dominant variable sequence (74). In these circumstances, antibodies cannot recognize the binding sequence. Obviously, the binding of the virus to the host cell is well determined for the virus; in fact, constant binding regions can exist in a virus known to have many strains. It has been suggested that some viruses facilitate the binding of other viruses (75).

As is apparent from the above discussion, the pathophysiologic role of specific receptors is essential to understanding virus–host interactions which lead to absorption and penetration. Of specific interest are those receptors that appear to be related to neurohumoral–neuromodulator–neurotransmitter receptors. Identified to date are the acetylcholine receptor for rabies virus (62) and the beta-adrenergic receptor for reovirus (76). Other receptors include proteins or sequences related to the immunoglobulin superfamily (77), such as the CD4 receptor for HIV (78). Importantly, CD4 receptors are also found on cells in the brain (79). Additional receptors include those for growth factors, such as (a) the epidermal growth factor receptor for vaccinia virus and (b) fibroblast growth factor receptor for HSV-1 (67). A preponderance of the latter receptor is localized to the nervous system (80). Thus, it appears that many viruses bind to receptors that are present in the CNS.

Once attached to the host cell by the respective attachment-protein–receptor domain, the virus envelope usually fuses with the host plasma membrane; then the virus enters the cell via receptor-mediated endocytosis (81,82). Nonenveloped viruses are endocytosed. In the latter case, the receptor–virus complex can become trapped within a clathrin-coated pit. At intervals of approximately 30 sec, a receptosome is formed from the bottom of the pit. The contents of such receptosomes are the entrapped viral proteins within the pit, which in this case would be the virus–receptor complex. After the virus-containing receptosome has gained entrance to the cell cytoplasm, the next step in the viral replication cycle is dependent upon whether the virus causes disruption of the receptosome membrane or, alternatively, fuses with the receptosome membrane (68). In the latter circumstance, the virus remains intact and discharges an unenveloped virus particle into the cytoplasm. Both events are thought to be substantially modulated by different values of cellular pH. It may well be that viruses have the ability to lower the cellular pH, thereby facilitating viral release into the cytosol.

Replication

After the virus successfully has gained access to the cytoplasm, the next steps in replication depend upon the nature of the viruses' nucleic acids (83). In the case of RNA viruses, replication of the nucleic acid occurs in the cytoplasm. There are several different mechanisms of viral replication which depend on whether or not the RNA is positive- or negative-stranded. Some viral systems require RNA polymerases exclusively, whereas for others RNA replication is due to cellular enzymes that are utilized by the viral genetic machinery. For negative-stranded RNA viruses, the first step is usually the production of a positive strand which serves as a template for copies of the genetic material and from which the virus proteins are coded. Obviously, this step is not required in positive-stranded RNA viruses. Through poorly understood mechanisms, beginning with the onset of translation of the viral genome, there is a marked decrease in the translation of host cell messenger RNAs. At least one positive-stranded RNA virus family—the retroviruses—contains a reverse transcriptase which is capable of using RNA as a template for DNA generation. The RNAs are coded from the DNA for transcription. This family of viruses has assumed great importance as the epidemic of acquired immunodeficiency syndrome (AIDS) has spread and with the recognition of CNS dementia syndromes.

DNA viruses tend (with some exceptions) to be transmitted through the cytoplasm to the cell nucleus. Within the nucleus, either virus or host (or both) are used to code proteins and, subsequently, genetic material. The first proteins or enzymes coded tend to be those which regulate the expression of the subsequent proteins. Enzymes important to replication of viral DNA tend to be coded next (in the case of HSV, thymidine kinase). Structural proteins which acquire glycosylated residues and which become the structural proteins for the viral capsid are usually assembled last. Encapsulation with completed glycoprotein processing is completed for herpesviruses within the Golgi. Viral assembly is completed by the acquisition of an envelope from either nuclear or cell membrane.

Cell-to-Cell Spread in the CNS

Despite interest in animal models dating back more than 50 years, a number of questions persist regarding the transmission of viruses through the CNS (84). In early studies using animal models, it was shown that HSV was transmitted from the site of inoculation to the neuroanatomic terminus of fibers innervating the site of inoculation (85). Based on these studies, the investigators suggested that neural, "axis cylinder" transmission existed and that this phenomena was the basis for "invasive proliferation." In 1974, investigators suggested that endoneural cells were responsible for the transport of the virus (86). However, in contrast to the peripheral nervous system, the exact mechanisms of HSV-1 transport to the CNS have been described only circumstantially. Recently, it has been shown to involve movement of the virus across defined neural pathways in what is most probably a transsynaptic transfer (87–91; R. B. Chronister and M. Schlitt, *unpublished observations*). It should be pointed out, however, that the majority of the evidence for transsynaptic transmission is circumstantial and not experimental in nature.

Important questions remain: Is the transport across synapses or across junctional complexes? Is there involvement of glial cells in the transport? Is there a vascular component to the transport, and, more significantly, is the transport tubulin-dependent? All these must be answered in greater detail before the contributions of axoplasmic transport to the travel of HSV in the CNS can be better understood. Several studies have sought to address these points and have shown that virus particles could be found within cell bodies and axons of a neural system, as well as within the glia—as had been reported earlier (86,92). Several investigators have suggested that cell-to-cell transmission is most important with glial cells advancing the infection toward the brain (93), whereas others have stressed that the role of axonal endoplasmic reticulum is important in this transport system (94). Recent technological improvements have allowed investigations of small amounts of virus in axons and at synapses (95). The timing of infection seems to be related to tubulin-dependent fast retrograde transport in axons (94). However, it may be that certain strains of virus travel anterogradely while others travel retrogradely (90). Interestingly, a virus that travels retrogradely can also be used to show specific anterograde connectivity but does so at transport rates considerably slower than at its retrograde rate (91). Whether this difference in rate is due to polarity of the tubulin or due to the use of specific transport motors, such as kinesin, is completely unknown.

As noted, recent studies suggest indeed that virus transport in the CNS is via axoplasmic transport (59) and not cell-to-cell. As noted above, HSV-1 transportation is probably tubulin-dependent, and viral transmission (for the most part) is in a retrograde direction. Furthermore, HSV-1 has a predilection for the synaptosome (96) which represents pre- and postsynaptic membranes and which may be analogous to the receptosome of the cell body. Therefore, once the virus gains access to the CNS, any free virus may be picked up by synaptic endings. Regardless of the route of uptake, there is little doubt that cell-to-cell transmission occurs only through specialized means (97).

However, the actual transsynaptic movement of HSV-1 has yet to be demonstrated. Recent experiments have demonstrated preferential uptake and transport of HSV-1 following olfactory bulb inoculation in the rabbit (98,99). Anatomic regions most likely to be infected by HSV-1 are the termini of the olfactory system—areas inferomedial to the rhinal sulcus. The resulting acute CNS infection is extensive, involving much of the olfactory cortices within reasonable proximity of the olfactory tuberculum. With time, there is immunocytochemical label in cells that are not contiguous with the labeled olfactory cortex; that is, certain regions are skipped while new cells are labeled. Furthermore, the cells that are labeled tend to be projection cells (i.e., larger, presumably cholinergic cells of the major islet of Calleja) but not the adjacent (smaller, GABAergic) interneurons. Examination of these animals has shown that HSV-1 can also involve the magnocellular regions of the basal forebrain (such as the nucleus basalis), scattered cells of the diagonal band of Broca, and large cells in the ventral pallidum. Interestingly, this work also demonstrated that the virus could not be detected (in positively infected animals) with immunohistochemistry prior to 3 days or after 14 days post-injection. The reasons for this time window are the following: (a) Early in the infection, there are very few virus particles in any given cell. (b) The antibodies used to label the virus are to the glycoprotein coat, and this component is one of the last proteins made by the virus. (c) With time, HSV becomes latent in surviving cells and can be demonstrated only by molecular methods such as in situ hybridization, polymerase chain reaction, or other molecular biologic assays.

During studies of cell-to-cell transmission of HSV, it was noted that glial cells were seldom labeled with the virus but still showed morphological changes indicating a reaction to the neuronal infection. Double-labeling studies indicate that glial cells become infected late in the disease when the neurons lyse. This observation raises a number of interesting questions. Why should the affinity of the virus for the neuronal compartments be greater than the affinity for the glial cell compartments? Perhaps there is a quantitative difference in receptosomes and clatharin-coated pits. Furthermore, why would the glial cell sequester virus and prevent its random spread? One of the functions suggested for the glial cells has been the isolation of synaptic transport to prevent nonspecific neuronal communication. Perhaps the limitation of viral spread has evolved in a similar way. Finally, one important difference between the neurons and the glial cells is the ability of the glial cell to replicate and the relative inability of the neurons to do so. Why should the cell population most able to recover be infected last? Are these cells more resistant, or does their interaction assist

in the establishment of latency and/or an immunologic response? These questions await further study.

PATHOPHYSIOLOGIC CORRELATES OF DISEASE MANIFESTATIONS

Seizures in HSE

Seizure disorders are frequent in HSE, occurring in approximately 40% of patients. Abnormal brain electrophysiology is far more common, occurring in most patients. Electroencephalographic patterns include focal slowing, spiking, and paroxysmal lateralizing epileptiform discharges. The cellular mechanisms for all seizure discharges are incompletely understood, and this applies in particular to HSE. Most current theories of epileptogenesis posit dysfunction of the smaller, inhibitory GABAergic neurons; yet recent studies show that HSV-1 preferentially infects larger, presumably excitatory, long projection neurons. While the seizures encountered in patients with HSE could be directly attributed to cellular destruction, other hypotheses warrant consideration.

An alternative hypothesis for epileptogenesis in this particular disease state is that the uptake of virus into the long projection neurons causes, along with other perturbations of the host cell machinery, a cessation or slowdown in those processes that retain acetylcholine within the nerve terminal. This excitatory neurotransmitter could leak from the cell processes and, ultimately, trigger a seizure focus. In addition to this disturbance, suboptimal uptake of acetylcholine by malfunctioning pre- and postsynaptic terminals could lead to a relative excess and, subsequently, abnormal electrical discharges. There could be a significant decrease in the synthesis of degradatory enzymes (such as acetylcholinesterase) as viral replication proceeds. Finally, chronic seizure foci are known to be hypometabolic during interictal periods, and perhaps the first result of viral infection—the inhibition of the cell's homeostatic mechanisms, all of which require energy to sustain—predisposes to disordered electrical discharges.

Neurologic Deficits (such as hemiplegia) in HSE

Focal neurologic deficits occur in approximately 95% of patients with biopsy-proven HSE. These deficits include dysphasia and hemiparesis. Dysphasia is not difficult to explain, since there is considerable variability in the locations of Wernicke's and Broca's areas in the temporal and frontal lobes, respectively, but hemiparesis is more difficult to explain. HSE in adults characteristically involves medial temporal and orbitofrontal cortex, and it has been incorrectly excluded when brain biopsy has been directed to other regions. Why, then, should motor neurons located at a distance from cells infected with HSV-1 cease to function properly and lead to hemiplegia?

Several potential reasons exist for this clinical picture. First, virus may exist in these cells at the time of the patient's presentation, but in too low a concentration and/or in a less infective form than would easily allow culture. Such a small viral load might be sufficient to cause neuronal malfunction, as outlined above. Second, cells in the amygdala, which is nearly always involved in HSE, are just two synapses removed from pyramidal cells in the motor cortex. Inappropriate function of these cells could easily lead to a persistence of the inhibitory tonus inciting the pyramidal system, the lysis of which is felt to be important in the initiation of voluntary movement. Third, a phenomenon similar to the spreading depression seen after manipulating brain tissue might be functional. Finally, primary cellular destruction may be the cause; however, neurologic signs often precede evidence of hemorrhagic necrosis.

Rabies Infection of the CNS

The classic manifestations of rabies have been well characterized and form the basis of one classic view of the CNS structures that control emotion (100). The areas of the brain involved are the hippocampus, hypothalamus, related limbic structures, and brainstem. In addition, limited inflammatory responses are typically seen in the basal ganglia. In rare cases, there is involvement of motor neurons (the so-called paralytic, or dumb, variant of the disease). Generally, all cases involving humans can be considered to be fatal (for exception see ref. 101), with the course of the disease progressing through various stages characterized by increasing neuronal involvement as a result of viral spread (102,103); ultimately the patient will die of respiratory arrest.

The mode of transport of the virus is undoubtedly via axoplasmic transport (104) but is temporally variable in humans, with a delay in symptom presentation ranging from 13 days to as much as 9 months. This variability may be accounted for by the type of neuronal transport involved. Anterograde transport is much slower than retrograde transport for at least some viruses (see above). Nonetheless, the argument for neuronal (and perhaps vascular) transport is compelling. For example, it is known that one of the early symptoms of the disease is pain and dysesthesia occurring in the branches of the nerves supplying the area of initial viral infection (105). This clearly suggests the sequestering of the virus in specific anatomic pathways or compartments. Unfortunately, once the virus enters the CNS proper, it replicates freely and then travels transneuronally, probably transsynaptically.

Given the symptoms and course of the disease, it is reasonable to speculate upon the specific route and transport of the virus spread. After initial replication, patients are characterized by increasing levels of excitement and autonomic dysfunction. The consensus view for the reasons behind this manifestation is increasing brainstem and hypothalamic involvement. Given the fact that structures in the brainstem and cell groups in the hypothalamus have widespread connectivity with extensive projections to the spinal cord, it is not surprising that these areas become involved in the disease. What is surprising, however, is that other areas with comparable projections do not exhibit such selective vulnerability. Once the hypothalamus is involved, the virus would undoubtedly travel via retrograde axoplasmic transport to the structures which provide the bulk of the input to this diencephalic structure. These structures include the hippocampus via the postcommissural fornix, the amygdala via the stria terminalis and amygdalofugal pathways, and the septal complex and basal forebrain via the medial forebrain bundle. From these structures, the whole of the limbic lobe would rapidly become involved as a result of the myriad of interconnections between these structures and the ones connected to the hypothalamus (106).

POSTINFECTIOUS ENCEPHALITIS

In the United States, postinfectious encephalomyelitis is most commonly associated with the occurrence of varicella and infections of the upper respiratory tract, particularly influenza (2). A late demyelination syndrome has been reported after HSV infections of the CNS (107). Worldwide, measles is the most important cause of postinfectious encephalitis (108,109). In what appears to be the consequence of perturbation of the immune response with postinfectious encephalomyelitis, patients have an invariably irreversible demyelinating syndrome. Why only certain patients develop a postinfectious encephalomyelitis syndrome remains to be explained. It is estimated that approximately 1.5 million children worldwide die yearly of measles and that 1 in 1000 cases results in postinfectious encephalomyelitis (26,109). Johnson and colleagues (13,109–116) determined that immunologic abnormalities accompanying acute infection are not simply due to immunosuppression, but are due to immunoregulatory failure as well. These observations may account, in part, for the autoimmune complications identified in some patients with postinfectious encephalomyelitis after measles.

Reye's syndrome can be considered a postinfectious complication leading to CNS complications, although the liver is the principal site of disease involvement. Illness is characterized by acute encephalopathy with fatty infiltration of the liver. It has been associated temporally with the occurrence of influenza B and VZV infections in the community. For example, a prospective Centers for Disease Control program identified clusters of influenza B infections which accounted for a total of 326 cases in the years 1962, 1967, 1969, and 1974 (117). Noticeably, for unexplained reasons the occurrence of disease was greater in rural populations than in urban ones (118). Recently, Reye's syndrome has unequivocally been associated with (a) the utilization of aspirin and (b) a subsequent metabolic biochemical defect of the liver leading to the acute encephalopathic changes. Thus, it cannot be considered a direct viral insult on the CNS.

CONCLUSION

Although much has been learned about the pathogenesis of viral infections of the CNS, a great deal of knowledge will probably be forthcoming. Progress in fundamental neuroscience will result in direct understanding of host–virus interaction in neuronal tissue. Such knowledge may allow improved prevention of severe and devastating viral CNS diseases.

ACKNOWLEDGMENTS

Original studies performed by the investigators were supported by grants from the National Institute of Allergy and Infectious Diseases (NO1-AI-62554), the Division of Research Resources (RR0023) of the National Institutes of Health, and the State of Alabama.

REFERENCES

1. Hughes SS. *The virus. A history of the concept.* New York: Science History Publications, 1977.
2. Johnson RT. *Viral infections of the nervous system.* New York: Raven Press, 1982.
3. Smith MG, Lennette EH, Reames HR. Isolation of the virus of herpes simplex and the demonstration of intranuclear inclusions in a case of acute encephalitis. *Am J Pathol* 1941;17:55–68.
4. Zarafonetis CJD, Smodel MC, Adams JW, Haymaker W. Fatal herpes simplex encephalitis in man. *Am J Pathol* 1944;20:429–455.
5. Johnson RT, Mims CA. Pathogenesis of viral infections of the nervous system. *N Engl J Med* 1968;278:23–30, 84–92.
6. Mims CA. *The pathogenesis of infectious disease.* London: Academic Press, 1976.
7. Griffin DE. Viral infections of the central nervous system. In: Galasso GJ, Whitley RJ, Merigan TC, eds. *Antiviral agents and viral diseases of man,* 3rd ed. New York: Raven Press, 1990;461–495.
8. Whitley RJ. Viral encephalitis. *N Engl J Med* 1990;323:242–250.
9. Beghi E, Nicolosi A, Kurland LT, Mulder DW, Hauser WA, Shuster I. Encephalitis and aseptic meningitis. Olmsted County, Minnesota, 1950–1981. I. Epidemiology. *Ann Neurol* 1984;16:283–294.
10. Centers for Disease Control. Summary of notifiable diseases United States, 1987. *MMWR* 1988;36:(54):1–59.
11. Olson LC, Buescher EK, Artenstein MS. Herpesvirus infections of the human central nervous system. *N Engl J Med* 1967;277:1271.
12. Goldsmith SM, Whitley RJ. Herpes simplex encephalitis. In: Lambert HP, ed. *Infections of the central nervous system.* Philadelphia: BC Decker, 1990; in press.
13. Johnson RT. The pathogenesis of acute viral encephalitis and postinfectious encephalitis. *J Infect Dis* 1987;155:359–364.
14. Rosen L. The natural history of Japanese encephalitis virus. *Annu Rev Microbiol* 1986;40:395–414.
15. Melnick JL. Poliomyelitis vaccines: an appraisal after 25 years. *Compr Ther* 1980;5:6–114.
16. Melnick JL. Enteroviruses: polioviruses, coxsackieviruses, echoviruses and newer enteroviruses. In: Fields BN, Knipe DM, Chanock RM, Hirsch MS, Melnick JL, Monath TP, Roizman B, eds. *Virology,* 2nd ed. New York: Raven Press, 1990;549–607.
17. Modlin JF. Poliovirus. In: Mandell GL, Douglas RG Jr, Bennett JE, eds. *Principles and practice of infectious diseases,* 3rd ed. New York: Churchill Livingstone, 1990;1365–1367.
18. Modlin JF. Coxsackievirus and echovirus. In: Mandell GL, Douglas RG Jr, Bennett JE, eds. *Principles and practice of infectious diseases,* 3nd ed. New York: Churchill Livingstone, 1990;1367–1383.
19. Johnson RT. Virus invasion of the central nervous system. A study of Sindbis virus infection in the mouse using fluorescent antibody. *Am J Pathol* 1965;46:929–943.
20. Luby JP. St. Louis encephalitis. *Epidemiol Rev* 1979;1:55–73.
21. Monath TP, Tsai TF. St. Louis encephalitis: lessons from the last decade. *Am J Trop Med Hyg* 1987;37:49S–59S.
22. Monath TP. Flaviviruses. In: Fields BN, Knipe DM, Chanock RM, Hirsch MS, Melnick JL, Monath TP, Roizman B, eds. *Virology,* 2nd ed. New York: Raven Press, 1990;763–814.
23. Peters CJ, Dalrymple JM. Alphaviruses. In: Fields BN, Knipe DM, Chanock RM, Hirsch MS, Melnick JL, Monath TP, Roizman B, eds. *Virology,* 2nd ed. New York: Raven Press, 1990;713–762.
24. Eldridge BF. Strategies for surveillance, prevention, and control of arbovirus diseases in western North America. *Am J Trop Med Hyg* 1987;37:77–86.
25. Hudson KL, et al. Update St. Louis encephalitis—Florida and Texas, 1990. *MMWR* 1990;39:756–779.
26. Assaad F. Measles: summary of worldwide impact. *Rev Infect Dis* 1983;5:452–459.
27. Ho DD, Rota TR, Schooley RT, et al. Isolation of HTLV-III from cerebrospinal fluid and neural tissues of patients with neurologic syndromes related to the acquired immunodeficiency syndrome. *N Engl J Med* 1985;313:1493–1497.
28. Hollander H, Levy JA. Neurologic abnormalities and recovery of human immunodeficiency virus from cerebrospinal fluid. *Ann Intern Med* 1987;106:692–695.
29. McArthur JC. Neurologic manifestations of AIDS. *Medicine* 1987;66:407–437.
30. Grant I, Atkinson JH, Hesselink JR, et al. Evidence for early central nervous system involvement in the acquired immunodeficiency syndrome (AIDS) and other human immunodeficiency virus (HIV) infections. *Ann Intern Med* 1987;107:828–836.
31. Jarvik JG, Hesselink JR, Kennedy C, et al. Acquired immunodeficiency syndrome magnetic resonance patterns of brain involvement with pathologic correlation. *Arch Neurol* 1988;45:731–738.
32. Navia BA, Cho E-S, Petito CK, Price RW. The AIDS dementia complex. II. Neuropathology. *Ann Neurol* 1986;19:525–534.
33. Navia BA, Jordan BD, Price RW. The AIDS dementia complex. I. Clinical features. *Ann Neurol* 1986;19:517–524.
34. Wiley CA, Schrier RD, Nelson JA, Lampert PW, Oldstone MBA. Cellular localization of human immunodeficiency virus infection within the brains of acquired immune deficiency syndrome patients. *Proc Natl Acad Sci USA* 1986;83:7089–7093.
35. Gabuzda DH, de la Monte SM, Ho DD, Hirsch MS, Rota TR, Sobel RA. Immunohistochemical identification of HTLV-III antigen in brains of patients with AIDS. *Ann Neurol* 1986;20:289–295.
36. Stoler MH, Eskin TA, Benn S, Angerer RC, Angerer LM. Human T-cell lymphotropic virus type III infection of the central nervous

system. A preliminary *in situ* analysis. *JAMA* 1986;256:2360–2364.

37. Koenig S, Gendelman HE, Orenstein JM, et al. Detection of AIDS virus in macrophages in brain tissue from AIDS patients with encephalopathy. *Science* 1986;233:1089–1093.

38. Pederson C, Nielsen CM, Vestergaard BF, Gerstoft J, Kroggaard K, Nielsen JO. Temporal relation of antigenaemia and loss of antibodies to core antigens to development of clinical disease in HIV infection. *Br Med J* 1987;295:567–569.

39. Ho DD, Rota TR, Hirsch MS. Infection of monocyte/macrophages by human T lymphotropic virus type III. *J Clin Invest* 1986;77:1712–1715.

40. Weiner LP, Fleming JO. Viral infections of the nervous system. *J Neurosurg* 1984;61:207–224.

41. Friedman HM, Macarak EJ, MacGregor RR, Wolfe J, Kefalides NA. Virus infection of endothelial cells. *J Infect Dis* 1981;143:266–273.

42. Albrecht P. Pathogenesis of neutropic arbovirus infections. *Curr Top Microbiol Immunol* 1968;43:44–91.

43. Johnson KP, Johnson RT. California encephalitis. II. Studies of experimental infection in the mouse. *J Neuropathol Exp Neurol* 1968;27:390–400.

44. Ehrlich P. Zur therapeutischen Bedeutung der substituirenden Schwefelsauregruppe. *Ther Monatsschr* 1887;1:88–90.

45. Reese TS, Karnovsky MJ. Fine structural localization of a blood–brain barrier to exogenous peroxidase. *J Cell Biol* 1967;34:207–217.

46. Brightman MW, Reese TS. Junctions between intimately apposed cell membranes in the vertebrate brain. *J Cell Biol* 1969;40:648–677.

47. Goldstein GW, Betz AL. Blood vessels and the blood–brain barrier. In: Asbury AK, McKhann GM, McDonald WI, eds. *Diseases of the nervous system.* Philadelphia: WB Saunders, 1986:172–184.

48. Pardridge WM, Oldendorf WH, Gancilla P, Frank HJL. Blood–brain barrier: interface between internal medicine and the brain. *Ann Intern Med* 1986;105:82–95.

49. Helmer ME. Adhesive protein receptors on hematopoietic cells. *Immunol Today* 1988;9:109–113.

50. Friedemann U. Permeability of the blood–brain barrier to neurotropic viruses. *Arch Pathol* 1943;35:912–931.

51. Brightman MW, Klatzo I, Olsson Y, Reese TS. The blood–brain barrier to proteins under normal and pathological conditions. *J Neurol Sci* 1970;10215–10239.

52. Maxwell DS, Pease DC. The electron microscopy of the choroid plexus. *J Biophys Biochem Cytol* 1956;2:467–481.

53. Van Deurs B, Koehler JK. Tight junctions in the choroid plexus epithelium: a freeze-fracture study including complementary replicas. *J Cell Biol* 1979;80:662–673.

54. Flegenhauer K. Protein size and cerebrospinal fluid composition. *Klin Wochenschr* 1974;52:1158–1164.

55. Griffin DE, Giffels J. Study of protein characteristics that influence entry into cerebrospinal fluid of normal mice and mice with encephalitis. *J Clin Invest* 1982;70:289–295.

56. Brightman MW. The intracerebral movement of proteins injected into blood and cerebrospinal fluid of mice. *Prog Brain Res* 1967;29:19–37.

57. Friedman HM, Cohen GH, Eisenberg RJ, Seidel CA, Cines DB. Glycoprotein C of herpes simplex virus 1 acts as a receptor for the C3b complement component on infected cells. *Nature* 1984;309:633–635.

58. Frank I, Friedman HM. A novel function of the herpes simplex virus type 1 Fc receptor: participation in bipolar bridging of antiviral immunoglobulin G. *J Virol* 1989;63:4479–4488.

59. Cook ML, Stevens JG. Pathogenesis of herpetic neuritis and ganglionitis in mice: evidence of intra-axonal transport of infection. *Infect Immun* 1973;7:272–278.

60. Baringer JR. Herpes simplex virus infection of nervous tissue in animals and man. *Prog Med Virol* 1975;20:1–26.

61. Kristensson K, Nennesmo I, Persson L, Lycke E. Neuron to neuron transmission of herpes simplex virus. Transport of virus from skin to brainstem nuclei. *J Neurol Sci* 1982;54:149–156.

62. Murphy FA. Rabies pathogenesis: a brief review. *Arch Virol* 1977;54:(4):279–297.

63. Houff SA, Burton RC, Wilson RW, Henson TE, London WT, Baer GM, Anderson LJ, Winkler WG, Madden DL, Sever JL. Human-to-human transmission of rabies virus by corneal transplant. *N Eng J Med* 1979;300:603.

64. Shipley MT, Adamek GD. Transport of molecules from nose to brain: transneuronal anterograde and retrograde labeling in the rat olfactory system by wheat germ agglutinin–horseradish peroxidase applied to the nasal epithelium. *Brain Res Bull* 1985;15:129–142.

65. Nemerow GR, Houghten RA, Moore MD, Cooper NR. Identification of an epitope in the major envelop protein of Epstein–Barr virus that mediates binding to the B lymphocyte FBV receptor (CR2). *Cell* 1989;56:369–377.

66. Murray MG, Bradley J, Yang X-F, Wimmer E, Moss EG, Racaniello VR. Poliovirus host range is determined by a short amino acid sequence in neutralization antigenic site 1. *Science* 1988;241:213–215.

67. Kaner RJ, Baird A, Mansukhani A, Basilico C, Summers BD, Florkiewicz RZ, Hajjar DP. Fibroblast growth factor receptor is a portal of cellular entry for herpes simplex virus type 1. *Science* 1990;248:1410–1413.

68. Lentz TL. The recognition event between virus and host cell receptor: a target for antiviral agents. *J Gen Vir* 1990;71:751–766.

69. Damian RT. Molecular mimicry revisited. *Parasitol Today* 1987;3:263–266.

70. Homsy J, Meyer M, Tateno M, Clarkson S, Levy JA. The Fc and not CD4 receptor mediates antibody enhancement of HIV infection in human cells. *Science* 1989;244:1357–1360.

71. Tardieu M, Epstein RL, Weiner HL. Interaction of viruses with cell surface receptors. *Int Rev Cytol* 1982;80:27–61.

72. Hogle JM, Chow M, Filman DJ. Three dimensional structure of poliovirus at 2.3 Å resolution. *Science* 1985;229:1358–1365.

73. Rossmann MG, Palmenberg AC. Conservation of the putative receptor attachment site in picornaviruses. *Virology* 1988;164:373–382.

74. Acharya R, Fry E, Stuart D, Fox G, Rowlands D, Brown F. The three-dimensional structure of foot-and-mouth disease virus at 2.9 Å resolution. *Nature* 1989;337:709–716.

75. Fuller SD, von Bonsdorff C-H, Simons S. Cell surface influenza hemagglutinin can mediate infection by other animal viruses. *EMBO J* 1985;4:2475–2485.

76. Co MS, Gaulton GN, Tominaga A, Homcy CJ, Fields BN, Greene MI. Structural similarities between the mammalian β-adrenergic and reovirus type 3 receptors. *Proc Natl Acad Sci USA* 1985;82:5315–5318.

77. White JM, Littman DR. Viral receptors of the immunoglobulin superfamily. *Cell* 1989;56:725–728.

78. Sattentau QJ, Weiss RA. The CD4 antigen: physiological ligand and HIV receptor. *Cell* 1988;52:631–633.

79. Funke I, Hahn A, Rieber EP, Weiss E, Riethmuller G. The cellular receptor (CD4) of the human immunodeficiency virus is expressed on neurons and glial cells in human brain. *J Exp Med* 1987;165:1230–1235.

80. Rifkin DB, Moscatelli D. Recent developments in the cell biology of basic fibroblast growth factor. *J Cell Biol* 1989;109:1–6.

81. Paulson JC. Interactions of animal viruses with cell surface receptors. In: Conn PM, ed. *The receptors,* vol 2. Orlando, FL: Academic Press, 1985;131–219.

82. Marsh M, Helenius A. Virus entry into animal cells. *Adv Virus Res* 1989;36:105–151.

83. Roizman B. Multiplication of viruses: an overview. In: Fields BN, Knipe DM, et al., eds. *Virology,* vol 1. New York: Raven Press, 1990;87–94.

84. Doerr R, Vochting K. Etudes sur le virus de la herpes febrile. *Rev Gen Ophthalmol* 1920;34:409–421.

85. Goodpasture EW, Teague O. Transmission of the virus of herpes febrilis along nerves in experimentally infected rabbits. *J Med Res* 1923;44:139–188.

86. Kristensson K, Ghetti B, Wisniewski HM. Study on the propagation of herpes simplex virus (type 2) into the brain after intraocular injection. *Brain Res* 1974;69:189–201.

87. Martin X, Dolivo M. Neuronal and transneuronal tracing in the trigeminal system using the herpes virus suis. *Brain Res* 1983;272:253–276.
88. Ugolini G, Kuypers HGJM, Simmons A. Retrograde transneuronal transfer of herpes simplex virus type 1 (HSV1) from motoneurones. *Brain Res* 1987;422:242–256.
89. Ugolini G, Kuypers HGJM, Strick PL. Transneuronal transfer of herpes virus from peripheral nerves to cortex and brainstem. *Science* 1989;243:89–91.
90. Rouiller EM, Capt M, Dolivo M, De Ribaupierre F. Neuronal organization of the stapedius reflex pathways in the rat: a retrograde HRP and viral transneuronal tracing study. *Brain Res* 1989;476:21–28.
91. Card JP, Rinaman L, Schwaber JS, Miselis RR, Whealy ME, Robbins AK, Enquist LW. Neurotropic properties of pseudorabies virus: uptake and transneuronal passage in the rat central nervous system. *Neuroscience* 1990;10(6):1974–1994.
92. Hurst EW. The newer knowledge of virus diseases of the nervous system: a review and interpretation. *Brain* 1936;59:1–34.
93. Anderson JR, Field HJ. The distribution of herpes simplex type 1 antigen in mouse central nervous system after different routes of inoculation. *J Neurol Sci* 1983;60:181–195.
94. Griffin JW, Watson DF. Axonal transport in neurological disease. *Ann Neurol* 1988;23:3–13.
95. Burrage TG, Tignor GH, Smith AL. Immunoelectron microscopic localization of rabies virus antigen in central nervous system and peripheral tissue using low-temperature embedding and protein A-gold. *J Virol Methods* 1983;7:337–350.
96. Vahlne A, Nystrom B, Sandberg M, Hamberger A, Lycke E. Attachment of herpes simplex virus to neurons and glial cells. *J Gen Virol* 1978;40:359–371.
97. Schaechter M, Schlessinger D. Strategies to study microbial pathogenesis. In: M Schaechter, G Medoff, D Schlessinger, eds. *Mechanisms of microbial disease.* Baltimore: Williams & Wilkins, 1989;164–176.
98. Schlitt M, Lakeman AD, Wilson ER, To A, Acoff RW, Harsh GR, Whitley RJ. A rabbit model of focal herpes simplex encephalitis. *J Infect Dis* 1986;153:732–735.
99. Schlitt M, Bucher AP, Stropp WG, Pindak F, Bastian FO, Jennings RA, Lakeman AD, Whitley RJ. Mortality in an experimental focal herpes encephalitis: relationship to seizures. *Brain Res* 1988;440:293–298.
100. Papez JW. A proposed mechanism of emotion. *Arch Neurol Psychiatry* 1937;38:725–743.
101. Hattwick MA, Weis TT, Stechschulte CJ. Recovery from rabies. A case report. *Ann Intern Med* 1972;76:931–942.
102. Maton PN, Pollard JD, Davis JN. Human rabies encephalomyelitis. *Br Med J* 1976;1:1038–1040.
103. Morrison AJ Jr, Wenzl RP. Rabies: a review and current approach for the physician. *South Med J* 1985;78:1211–1218.
104. Tsiang H. Evidence for an intraaxonal transport of fixed and street rabies virus. *J Neuropathol Exp Neurol* 1979;38:286–299.
105. Dyken PR. Viral infections of the nervous system. In: *Pediatric Neurologic Diseases.* 1989;475–515.
106. Chronister RB, White LE Jr. Fiberarchitecture of the hippocampal formation: anatomy, projections, and structural significance. In: Isaacson RL, Pribram KH, eds. *The hippocampus,* vol 1 New York: Plenum Press, 1975;9–37.
107. Koening H, Rabinowitz SG, Day E, Miller V. Post-infectious encephalomyelitis after successful treatment of herpes simplex encephalitis with adenine arabinoside: ultrastructural observations. *N Engl J Med* 1979;300:1089–1093.
108. Miller HG, Stanton JB, Gibbons JL. Para-infectious encephalomyelitis and related syndromes. *Q J Med* 1956;25:427–505.
109. Johnson RT, Griffin DE, Gendelman HE. Postinfectious encephalomyelitis. *Semin Neurol* 1985;5:180–190.
110. Graves M, Griffin DE, Johnson RT, Hirsch RL, Lindo de Soriano I, Roedenbeck S, Vaisberg A. Development of antibody to measles virus polypeptides during complicated and uncomplicated measles virus infections. *J Virol* 1984;49:409–412.
111. Hirsch RL, Griffin DE, Johnson RT, Cooper SJ, Linde de Soriano I, Roedenbeck S, Vaisberg A. Cellular immune responses during complicated and uncomplicated measles virus infections of man. *Clin Immunol Immunopathol* 1984;31:1–12.
112. Griffin DE, Moench TR, Johnson RT, Lindo de Soriano I, Vaisberg A. Peripheral blood mononuclear cells during natural measles virus infection: cell surface phenotypes and evidence for activation. *Clin Immunol Immunopathol* 1986;40:305–312.
113. Griffin DE, Hirsch RL, Johnson RT, Lindo de Soriano I, Roedenbeck S, Vaisberg A. Changes in serum C-reactive protein during complicated and uncomplicated measles virus infections. *Infect Immun* 1983;41:861–864.
114. Griffin DE, Cooper SJ, Hirsch RL, Johnson RT, Lindo de Soriano I, Roedenbeck S, Vaisberg A. Changes in plasma IgE levels during complicated and uncomplicated measles virus infections. *J Allerg Clin Immunol* 1985;76:206–213.
115. Johnson TR, Griffin DE, Hirsch RL, et al. Measles encephalomyelitis—clinical and immunologic studies. *N Engl J Med* 1984;310:127–141.
116. Gendelman HE, Pezeshkpour GH, Pressman NJ, et al. A quantitation of myelin-associated glycoprotein and myelin basic protein loss in different demyelinating diseases. *Ann Neurol* 1985;18:324–328.
117. Corey L, Rubin RJ, Hattwick MAW, et al. A nationwide outbreak of Reye's syndrome: its epidemiologic relationship to influenza B. *Am J Med* 1976;61:615–625.
118. DeVivo DC, Keating JP. Reye's syndrome. *Adv Pediatr* 1975;22:175–229.

Infections of the Central Nervous System,
edited by W. M. Scheld, R. J. Whitley, and
D. T. Durack, Raven Press, Ltd., New York © 1991.

CHAPTER 3

Viral Meningitis and the Aseptic Meningitis Syndrome

Harley A. Rotbart

The term "aseptic meningitis" refers to a clinical syndrome of meningeal inflammation in which common bacterial agents cannot be identified in the cerebrospinal fluid (CSF) (1,2). Implicit in the definition of aseptic meningitis is the benignity of the clinical course and the absence of signs of parenchymal brain involvement (encephalitis) or spinal cord inflammation (myelitis). Certain pathogens more commonly cause "pure" meningitis or "pure" encephalitis, whereas others are more likely to result in less discrete manifestations of central nervous system (CNS) infection and are described as meningoencephalitis or encephalomyelitis. This review will emphasize those organisms which most often cause the aseptic meningitis syndrome; pathogens responsible for encephalitic syndromes are discussed elsewhere in this volume. Suffice it to say, however, that overlap among the two groups of etiologic agents is significant and that both groups must be considered in the individual patient.

More than 7000 cases of aseptic meningitis are reported in the United States annually (2a); the actual incidence, including unreported cases, may be as much as 10-fold higher. The vast majority of cases are due to viral infections (Table 1); however, nonviral pathogens, including certain bacteria (which are not readily seen by stains and/or do not grow in standard culture systems), mycoplasmae, and fungi, may present in a manner identical to that of viruses. Autoimmune diseases, malignancies, and reactions to certain drugs occasionally are manifest as aseptic meningitis as well. The first viruses recognized to cause meningitis, mumps, lymphocytic choriomeningitis virus, and poliovirus are uncommon

causes in developed countries today. Initial series of aseptic meningitis included identification of a specific etiologic agent in only 25% of cases (3,4). With the discovery of the group B coxsackieviruses in 1948 (5), and with the advent of tissue culture in 1949 (6) permitting the convenient and efficient identification of the polioviruses and echoviruses, enteroviruses (EVs) quickly emerged as the leading recognizable cause of aseptic meningitis (Table 2). More recent series include identification of a specific viral pathogen in as many as 55–70% of cases when consistent diagnostic methodology is applied (7–9). Currently, in the vaccine era, non-polio EVs account for 80–85% of all cases of aseptic meningitis for which an etiologic agent is identified (10–15); conversely, aseptic meningitis is the most commonly identified syndrome associated with EV infections (16,17). The latter is due to the age distribution of EV meningitis, which affects very young children disproportionately (18), and to the difficulty in this age group of clinically distinguishing aseptic from bacterial meningitis. Hence, viral cultures, particularly of the CSF, are commonly obtained from children with meningitis, and EVs are frequently identified (18,19).

This chapter will review the aseptic meningitis syndrome, with an emphasis on the EVs. The overall epidemiology, pathogenesis, and clinical manifestations of aseptic meningitis mirror those of the EVs (Fig. 1) because of the striking numeric dominance of the latter among the etiologic agents. Less common pathogens and noninfectious causes of aseptic meningitis will be discussed more briefly, with particular attention to their distinguishing characteristics from the EVs. Many of those less common agents of aseptic meningitis (e.g., arboviruses, herpesviruses, and measles) are important etiologies of other CNS syndromes and will be discussed in great detail elsewhere in this volume.

H. A. Rotbart: Departments of Pediatrics (Infectious Diseases) and Microbiology/Immunology, University of Colorado School of Medicine and The Children's Hospital of Denver, Denver, Colorado 80262.

TABLE 1. *Etiologies of the aseptic meningitis syndrome and their current relative incidences*

Common
Viruses
    Enteroviruses
    Arboviruses[a]
    Herpes simplex virus type 2
Bacteria
    Borrelia burgdorferi (Lyme disease)[a]
    Partially treated bacterial meningitis (common pathogens)
    Parameningeal bacterial infection

Uncommon
Viruses
    Mumps
    Lymphocytic choriomeningitis virus
    Human immunodeficiency virus
Bacteria
    Mycobacterium tuberculosis
    Leptospira species[a]
Other
    Fungi[a] (including *Cryptococcus neoformans, Coccidioides immitis, Histoplasma capsulatum, Candida* species, *Blastomyces dermatitidis*)
    Mycoplasma pneumoniae

Rare
Viruses
    Herpes simplex virus type 1
    Varicella-zoster virus
    Cytomegalovirus
    Epstein–Barr virus
    Influenza A and B viruses
    Parainfluenza virus
    Measles
    Rotavirus
    Coronavirus
    Encephalomyocarditis virus
Other
    Brucella species
    Mycoplasma hominis
    Toxoplasma gondii
    Fungi (many)
    Autoimmune disorders
    Behcet's syndrome
    Drugs (including immunomodulators and antibiotics)
    Malignancy

[a] Incidence varies greatly with geographic region.

ENTEROVIRUSES

Virology and Pathogenesis

The EVs comprise nearly 70 distinct serotypes within the family Picornaviridiae ("pico" meaning small, "rna" for ribonucleic acid). The subgroups of EVs include the polioviruses, coxsackieviruses A and B, echoviruses, and the newer "numbered EVs" (Table 3). Like other picornaviruses, EVs are small (27–30 nm in diameter; 1.34 g/ml buoyant density), consisting of a simple viral capsid and a single strand of positive (message) sense RNA. The capsid contains four proteins, VP1–VP4, arranged in 60 repeating protomeric units of an icosahedron. Varia-

tions within capsid proteins VP1–VP3 are responsible for the antigenic diversity among the EVs; neutralization sites are most densely clustered on VP1 (20). VP4 is not present on the viral surface (21); rather, it is in close association with the RNA core, functioning as an anchor to the viral capsid. Destabilization of VP4 results in viral uncoating (see below). The atomic structures of two poliovirus serotypes, types 1 and 3, have recently been resolved by computerized crystallographic studies (22,23), and they reveal a deep cleft or canyon in the center of each protomeric unit into which the specific cellular receptor for the EVs fits when virus encounters a susceptible host cell.

The encapsidated RNA of the human EVs is approximately 7.4 kb in length and serves as a template for both viral protein translation and RNA replication, the latter being accomplished via a double-stranded replicative intermediate form of RNA (24). At the 5′ end of the genome is a virally coded, covalently linked polypeptide (VPg). The 3′ end of the viral RNA contains a poly-A tail of 60 or more bases in length. A single reading frame begins at approximately nucleotide 740 from the 5′ end and terminates at approximately nucleotide 7370, leaving 740 bases at the 5′ end and 70 bases at the 3′ end (just upstream from the poly-A tail) untranslated; these untranslated sequences are felt to be involved in viral regulatory activities such as replication and translation. A single polyprotein is translated from the open reading frame. Post-translational modification is accomplished by three virus-coded proteases, and it results in generation of the four capsid proteins, VPg, a polymerase, and the proteases themselves (reviewed in refs. 25,26).

Although genetic differences in the capsid-coding regions result in the wide variety of EV serotypes, great similarities exist among the genomes of many of the EVs in a number of other regions along the RNA, including (a) the untranslated sequences at the 5′ and 3′ ends and (b) the sequences coding for the polymerase, protease, and VPg proteins. Ten of the EV serotypes have been fully sequenced at the genomic level: poliovirus types 1, 2, and 3; coxsackieviruses A9, A21, B1, B3, and B4; and enteroviruses 70 and 72 (hepatitis A) (27–34). Other serotypes have been partially sequenced (35). Homology among serotypes which have not been fully sequenced has been documented by dot–blot hybridization experiments (36–39). Hepatitis A alone appears genetically dissimilar from the other EVs studied and may ultimately require reclassification. Hepatitis A is also one of the few serotypes which has not been associated with CNS infection.

The pathogenesis of EV infections has been studied at molecular, cellular, and organ system levels (20,25); although much has been learned, much more remains unexplained. EVs are acquired by fecal–oral contamination and, less commonly, by respiratory droplet. Most of what is known about the subsequent viral pathway

TABLE 2. *Viral causes of aseptic meningitis in selected large series[a]*

Investigators	Years	Number of cases	Entero-viruses P	Entero-viruses NPE	Arbo-viruses	Mumps	Herpes	LCM	Other	None	Consistent meth-odology[b]
Rassmussen (3)	1941–1946	374				15.3		11.2	No	73.5	Yes
Adair et al. (4)	1947–1952	480				13.3	5.3	9.7	No	74.8	Yes
Meyer et al. (7)	1953–1958	430	8.8	29.8	0.7	15.8	1.4	8.8	No	29	Yes
Lennette et al. (8)	1958	368	2	57		9	1		Yes[c]	31	Yes
Buescher et al. (9)	1958–1963	374	4.8	38.5	0.8	7.5	0.5	1.9	Yes[d]	43.5	Yes
Deibel and co-workers (11–15)	1972–1979	2382	0.5	24	1.4	1.2	2.7	0.5	Yes[e]	68.3	No

[a] P, polioviruses; NPE, non-polio enteroviruses; LCM, lymphocytic choriomeningitis virus.

[b] Consistent methodology: virologic and/or serologic studies performed by a single laboratory with most or all specimens subjected to all tests.

[c] 1% adenovirus.

[d] <1% each: measles, Epstein–Barr virus, influenza A.

[e] 1.4% influenza A, 1% adenovirus. <1% each: measles, cytomegalovirus, varicella-zoster virus, rubella, influenza B, parainfluenza, respiratory syncytial virus.

within the host was derived from experimental poliovirus infections in chimpanzees more than four decades ago (40,41). Although some replication occurs in the nasopharynx with spread to upper respiratory tract lymphatics, most of the viral inoculum is swallowed. The EVs distinguish themselves from the rhinoviruses, another large genus of picornaviruses, by being stable at acid pH, the characteristic responsible for the ability of the EVs to traverse the stomach en route to the site of primary infection in the lower gastrointestinal tract. There EVs presumably bind to specific receptors on enterocytes; it is unknown precisely which cells are suscepti-

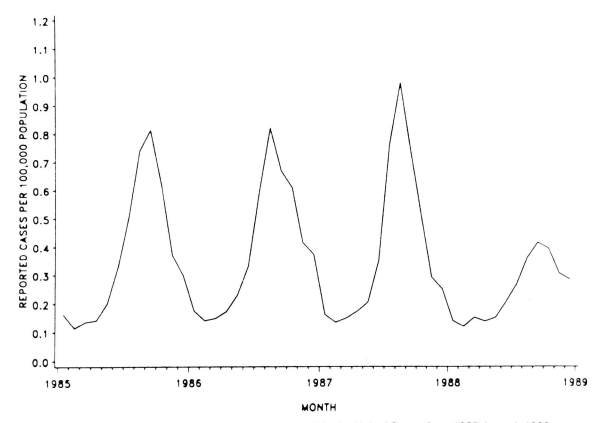

FIG. 1. The seasonal occurrence of aseptic meningitis in the United States from 1985 through 1988, as reported to the Centers for Disease Control (2a). The striking predominance of cases during the summer months reflects the predominance of enteroviruses as etiologic agents in aseptic meningitis.

TABLE 3. *The enteroviruses*

Subgroup	Serotypes
Poliovirus	1–3
Coxsackieviruses A	1–22, 24[a]
Coxsackieviruses B	1–6
Echoviruses	1–9, 11–27, 29–31[a]
Numbered enteroviruses	68–72

[a] Coxsackievirus A23 and echoviruses 10 and 28 have been reclassified.

ble and whether the so-called M cells responsible for reovirus uptake and penetration (42) are similarly involved during EV infection. The virus traverses the intestinal lining cells, perhaps with replication but without apparent cytopathicity, and reaches the Peyer's patches in the lamina propria where significant viral replication occurs. A minor viremia ensues, seeding numerous organ systems such as the CNS, liver, lungs, and heart. More significant replication at these sites results in a major viremia associated with the signs and symptoms of viral infection. If the CNS has not been seeded with the initial viremic episode, spread there may occur with the major viremia. Although fairly well established, viremia as the source of CNS infection has been long debated, with direct neural spread (43) suggested as an alternate hypothesis. The mechanism by which EVs leave the blood and enter the CNS is entirely unknown; "leakiness" in the vessels of the choroid plexus (meningitis) and/or of the parenchyma (encephalitis) is probably responsible, as opposed to active transport of viral particles across the blood–brain barrier. During clinical infections, EVs have been recovered from both the cellular and plasma fractions of the blood (44), and the more important of the blood compartments for establishing CNS infection are not known. *In vitro,* EVs are released into the media by infected cells and can survive cell-free for many days; hence cell association (e.g., monocytes or lymphocytes) may not be as important for CNS access as it is for other viruses (45).

The benign nature of EV meningitis has made human pathological data for this disease sparse. A report of a child who died of coxsackievirus B5 myocarditis with concomitant meningitis (46) describes inflammation of the choroid plexus of the lateral and fourth ventricles, fibrosis of the vascular walls with focal destruction of the ependymal lining, and fibrotic basal leptomeninges. Parenchymal findings were limited to moderate, symmetric dilation of the ventricles and an increase in number and size of subependymal astrocytes. The inflammatory reaction at the choroid plexus supports the concept of viremic spread to the CNS.

At the cellular level, the events of infection with polioviruses are well-studied; non-polio EVs probably have analogous cellular pathogenesis. The virus binds a specific cell receptor at a single viral capsid canyon site (47); this probably occurs first in the intestine. After subse-

quent progression of infection, this phenomenon will ultimately also occur at other target tissue sites. The human cellular receptor for enteroviruses maps to chromosome 19 and, for polioviruses at least, is a member of the "Ig superfamily" (48). Competition studies have shown that the polioviruses comprise one so-called receptor family and that the coxsackie B viruses comprise another. Coxsackie A21 does not displace, and is not displaced by, polioviruses or coxsackie B viruses, hence belonging to yet another family (49). Other EV serotypes have not been carefully studied. Following attachment of the virus, recruitment of additional cellular receptors occurs, and the virion is enveloped by cell membrane, bound now at multiple viral protomers (25). A steric shift in the capsid conformation occurs, resulting in extrusion of the VP4 viral protein and destabilization of the capsid structure (50,51). The now "uncoated" RNA is released freely into the cellular cytoplasm, where it rapidly binds to ribosomes and begins protein synthesis. A single polypeptide is produced, which is almost instantaneously autocleaved by viral proteases (25,26) to form all of the viral protein products, including those (such as the RNA-dependent RNA polymerase) required for viral RNA replication. Within 6 hours of infection, all host cell protein synthesis has been shut down by the EV, and the cell has become a factory for viral production (52). Infectious virions are released by cell lysis and spread to neighboring and distant cells via the surrounding growth media *in vitro* and via the blood *in vivo.*

Studies of molecular correlates of pathogenesis have been thus far limited to the polioviruses. The viral RNA of both neurovirulent and attenuated (vaccine) strains have been sequenced, and only a few differences exist between them. At least two single base changes are felt to be responsible for the attenuation of previously neurovirulent polioviruses (53). Following vaccination with attenuated strains, "back mutation" to virulence has been observed in the fecally shed virions recovered from normal children (54). Molecular neurovirulence determinants among the non-polio EVs have not yet been demonstrated; hence there is currently no genomic explanation for the increased frequency of aseptic meningitis observed with certain serotypes (see below). However, presence or absence of specific cellular receptors is unlikely to explain all of this heterogeneity, since variations in neurotropism exist even within receptor families. Coxsackievirus B6, for example, is a rare cause of CNS infection, in contrast to the other five coxsackie B viruses which are important causes of both meningitis and encephalitis (10).

Epidemiology

The EVs are worldwide in their distribution (55,56). While the polioviruses have been largely controlled in developed countries with introduction of vaccines, underdeveloped parts of the world continue to experience significant morbidity and mortality from those pathogens (57). In temperate climates, the EVs appear with a marked summer/fall seasonality; a high year-round incidence occurs in tropical and subtropical areas. It is felt that the fecal–oral spread of these agents is facilitated, particularly among children, during periods of warm weather and sparse clothing. In addition to transmission by direct person-to-person contact, EVs may be recovered from houseflies, wastewater, and sewage (20). Water sources clearly contribute to enterovirus 72 (hepatitis A) spread (58). Although shellfish concentrate other EVs as well, water- or seafood-related outbreaks of other serotypes have been difficult to identify. Each EV season in each part of the world is dominated by only a few of the serotypes (20,56). In the United States, the 15 most commonly occurring EVs account for more than 80% of all U.S. EV isolates (59). The annual determination of predominant serotypes is necessarily biased by the inability to readily grow numerous serotypes in tissue culture, particularly coxsackie A viruses. A role for these noncultivable agents in aseptic meningitis is implied by the 25–35% of CSF specimens each summer (from symptomatic patients) which fail to yield enterovirus (19). The predominant serotypes cycle with varying periodicity (10,59), a reflection of the availability of new susceptible host populations (especially children) within a community. Children are, indeed, the primary victims of EV aseptic meningitis (18). In a large Finnish cohort (60), an annual incidence of viral meningitis of 219/100,000 children less than 1 year of age was noted, as opposed to 19/100,000 in children between the ages of 1 and 4 years. The incidence dropped even further with increased age. The vast majority of identified viral pathogens were EVs. The youngest children are the most susceptible for the same reason they are most susceptible to many infections—the absence of previous exposure and immunity. Although EVs are also the most common cause of aseptic meningitis among adults, the incidence and severity of this disease (as well as the vigor with which a specific viral etiology is sought) are all lower in older age groups.

Among the many EV serotypes which cycle from year to year, certain serotypes are more commonly associated with aseptic meningitis than others. Among the most common U.S. EV isolates during the years 1970–1983 are also found the most common EV causes of meningitis, since isolates from patients with meningitis dominate the specimens submitted for typing each year (59). The predominant isolates during that 14-year period were (in decreasing order): echovirus 11; echovirus 9; coxsackievirus B5; echoviruses 30, 4, and 6; coxsackieviruses B2, B4, B3, and A9; echoviruses 3, 7, 5, and 24; and coxsackievirus B1 (59). The five serotypes most frequently isolated during each of the subsequent 5 years are shown in Table 4 (61–65). Polioviruses, once major causes of aseptic meningitis (only occasionally followed by para-

TABLE 4. *Most common enterovirus isolates 1984–1988[a]*

Year	1[b]	2	3	4	5	6
1984	E9[c]	E11	CB5	E30	CB2	CA9
1985	E11	E21	E6 = E7		CB2	CB4
1986	E11	E4	E7	E18	CB4 = CB5	
1987	E6	E18	E11	CA9	CB2	E9
1988	E11	E9	CB4	CB2	E6	CB5

[a] Data were taken from refs. 61–65.
[b] Most common isolate; "2" indicates second most common isolate, etc.
[c] E, echovirus; CB, coxsackievirus B; CA, coxsackievirus A.

lytic myelitis), are now rarely recovered from patients with aseptic meningitis (Table 2). Vaccine strains have been recovered from the CSF of occasional patients with CNS shunts in place who develop an aseptic meningitis syndrome shortly after immunization (66), and from as many as 10 persons annually in the United States who contract poliomyelitis following vaccination of themselves or of a close household contact (67). Coxsackievirus B5 and several of the echoviruses (serotypes 4, 6, 9, 11) are the most common non-polio causes of EV aseptic meningitis in the United States (10). Only a few EV serotypes have not been associated (virus recovered from the stool or throat) or confirmed (virus recovered from the CSF or blood) as the cause of aseptic meningitis (10,20,55,56). Those agents may well cause meningitis and not have been recognized because of difficulty in viral isolation methods for certain serotypes or because most EV isolates are never specifically serotyped. The observation that clinical stigmata do not significantly differ among the non-polio EVs causing aseptic meningitis (68), coupled with the limited quantities of typing serum pools (69), has made investigators increasingly content to identify individual cases or outbreaks as simply "an enterovirus" based on characteristic cytopathic effect in tissue culture (see below).

Host factors which predispose to EV meningitis, other than young age and immunodeficiency (see below), have been difficult to identify. Physical exercise, an established risk factor for paralytic poliomyelitis (70–72) and a hypothesized one for enteroviral myocarditis (73), may also predispose infected individuals to developing non-polio EV aseptic meningitis. Attack rates for aseptic meningitis among athletes have been higher than among other students during EV outbreaks (17,74). A male-to-female incidence ratio for EV infections of 1.3:1 to 1.5:1 has been reported (17). Individuals may develop more than one episode of EV meningitis (75,76); however, the same EV serotype has not been implicated twice in any one immunocompetent patient (77). Immunization with poliovirus vaccines does not protect against non-polio EV infections. Mixed infections involving EVs and other viruses (78) or bacteria (79) have been well described.

Clinical Manifestations

The clinical disease observed during EV meningitis varies with the host's age and immune status. Neonates are at risk for severe systemic illness of which meningitis or meningoencephalitis is commonly a part (80). Group B coxsackieviruses were associated with aseptic meningitis in 62% of infants less than 3 months of age in one study (81). Echoviruses identified in babies less than 2 weeks of age were associated with meningitis or meningoencephalitis in 27% of cases (82). In a recent prospective study of neonates (≤2 weeks of age) with proved EV infection, 75% had clinical and/or laboratory evidence of meningitis (M. J. Abzug, *personal communication*). The infected neonate appears to be at greatest risk for severe morbidity and mortality when signs and symptoms develop in the first days of life, suggesting a possible transplacental acquisition (81–83). Maternal illness has been reported in 59–68% of infected neonates (81–83); however, additional risk to the neonate associated with maternal illness has been difficult to establish. Even in the youngest patients, fever is ubiquitous, accompanied early by nonspecific signs such as vomiting, anorexia, rash, and/or upper respiratory findings (84). Neurologic involvement may or may not be associated with signs of meningeal inflammation, including nuchal rigidity and bulging anterior fontanelle. As the neonatal disease progresses, major systemic manifestations such as hepatic necrosis, myocarditis, and necrotizing enterocolitis may develop (80–83). Disseminated intravascular coagulation and other findings of "sepsis" result in a patient with illness indistinguishable from that due to overwhelming bacterial infection. The CNS disease may progress to a more encephalitic picture with seizures and focal neurologic findings suggestive of herpes simplex virus. The incidence of morbidity and mortality due to perinatal EV infections are not precisely known, but they may be as high as 74% and 10%, respectively (81). When death occurs, it is seldom (if ever) the result of CNS involvement, but rather the result of hepatic failure (echoviruses) or myocarditis (coxsackieviruses).

EV meningitis outside of the immediate (<2 weeks of age) neonatal period is rarely associated with severe disease or poor outcome. The natural history of typical EV meningitis is shown in Fig. 2 (68). Onset is usually sudden, and a fever of 38–40°C is the most consistent clinical finding, occurring in 76–100% of patients (18,85). The fever pattern may be biphasic, appearing first with nonspecific constitutional symptoms, followed by resolution and reappearance with the onset of meningeal signs. Nuchal rigidity is found in more than half of the patients, particularly in children older than 1–2 years of age (18,85). Headache is nearly always present in adults and children old enough to report it, and photophobia is also common. Nonspecific and constitutional signs and symptoms of viral infection, in decreasing order of occur-

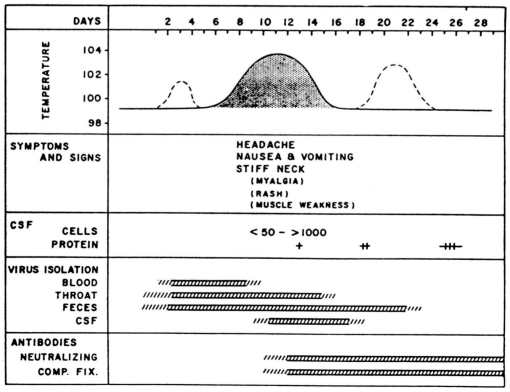

FIG. 2. The clinical course of enteroviral aseptic meningitis. (From ref. 68, with permission.)

rence, include vomiting, anorexia, rash, diarrhea, cough and upper respiratory findings (particularly pharyngitis), diarrhea, and myalgias (18,85). Aseptic meningitis with certain EV serotypes is associated with particular clinical stigmata; for example, hand–foot–mouth syndrome frequently occurs with EV 71 meningitis (86,87), and nonspecific rashes are especially common with echovirus 9 meningitis (88), although both incidental findings can occur with numerous other serotypes as well (10). Neurologic abnormalities are rare and, depending on the criteria used for identification of aseptic meningitis, may not occur at all. That is, because of the implicit benign clinical course associated with the diagnosis of aseptic meningitis, patients with abnormal neurologic findings are likely to be diagnosed with encephalitis or myelitis. Hence the literature on EV meningitis rarely includes more than 5% of patients with abnormal neurologic examinations. Febrile seizures are among those neurologic "abnormalities" which may complicate aseptic meningitis in children without implicating parenchymal brain involvement. The syndrome of inappropriate antidiuretic hormone was reported in 9 of 102 cases of EV meningitis in one study (89). A history of concomitant family illness is often obtained, including rashes and upper respiratory or gastrointestinal symptoms and, occasionally, meningitis (90). The duration of illness due to EV meningitis is usually less than 1 week, with many patients feeling better immediately after the lumbar puncture (91), presumably due to the reduction of intracranial pressure with fluid removal. Occasional adult patients may have symptoms which persist for several weeks (92), an observation not frequently made in children. The short-term prognosis of young children with EV meningitis early in life appears to be good; however, there is some controversy as to possible later sequelae. Learning disabilities and hearing loss have been reported in two long-term follow-up investigations (93,94). Limitations of those studies include their small sample size and the characteristics of the control populations. A more recent study found no long-term effects of EV meningitis in young infants (95).

The unique situation of a child or adult with absent or deficient humoral immunity illustrates an important "experiment of nature" with regard to EV infections of the CNS. Unlike other viruses which are largely contained by cellular immune mechanisms, the EVs are cleared from the host by antibody-mediated mechanisms. Agammaglobulinemic individuals infected with the EVs may develop chronic meningitis or meningoencephalitis lasting many years, often with fatal outcome (96). Although CSF culture-negative periods occur, evidence of persistent virus has been obtained using the polymerase chain reaction (97) (Fig. 3). Alteration of the viral genome over time in the same individual has also been documented (98). Approximately 50% of these infected patients also develop a rheumatologic syndrome,

most often dermatomyositis, which is also felt to be a direct result of EV infection of the affected tissues (96). Treatment with antibody preparations intravenously and intrathecally or intraventricularly has resulted in stabilization of some of these patients; however, viral persistence has been documented during therapy (96,97) (Fig. 3). With the availability of intravenous preparations of gammaglobulin and the early recognition of this syndrome, fewer patients appear to be progressing to chronic and debilitating infection. This phenomenon of antibody deficiency and serious EV infections may be relevant to patients other than those few with agammaglobulinemia. The severity of neonatal infection, for example, appears to be related to the presence or absence (in the baby) of maternal antibody to the infecting serotype (99). Older children and adults who develop severe EV diseases may have unproven susceptibility to infection due to specific antibody defects. EVs have been implicated in chronic diseases such as diabetes (100) and polymyositis/dermatomyositis (101,102); the presence of subtle antibody deficiencies to the EVs has not been studied in patients with those chronic illnesses, but an occasional patient has responded to therapy with gammaglobulin (103).

Laboratory Findings and Diagnosis

Of paramount importance in the diagnosis and management of meningitis is the establishment of etiology; specifically, bacterial (including partially treated meningitis and parameningeal infections) and other causes which have specific therapy available must be ruled out before viral meningitis can be assumed. Clues to the diagnosis of EV meningitis can be obtained from nonspecific CSF findings (Table 5) (104). Pleocytosis is almost always present, although EVs have been isolated from the CSF of patients (usually young infants) with clinical evidence of meningitis but no cells (83,105). CSF white blood cell counts may range as high as several thousand (106), but 100–1000 cells are the rule (85). The higher the white blood cell count in the CSF, the greater the chance of isolating the causative EV (107). Polymorphonuclear cells may predominate early in meningeal infection, usually giving way to a lymphocytic profile over the first 8–48 hours (107a). Hypoglycorrhachia and elevated CSF protein, if they occur, are usually mild (85), but extreme degrees of both have been reported (108). When controlled for age of the patient, low CSF glucose was much more common than high CSF protein in one study (109). Wide variations in all parameters, however, are the rule, even during an epidemic involving a single serotype (110,111). By definition, Gram's stain should be negative for bacteria; however, numerous cases of combined EV and bacterial cases have been reported (79), emphasizing the caution which must be taken in

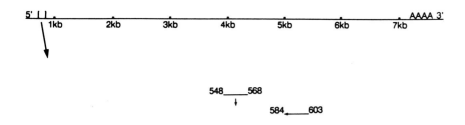

a

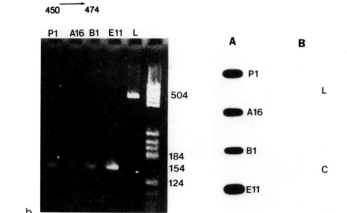

b

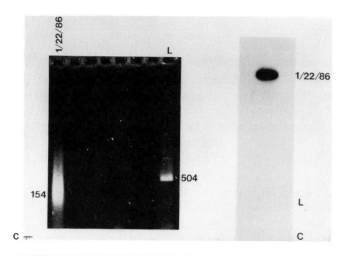

c

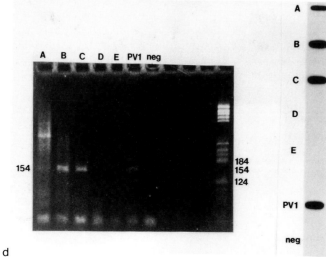

d

FIG. 3. The polymerase chain reaction (PCR) for detection of enteroviruses. (a) Schematic representation of the location on the 7.5-kb enteroviral genome of primers and probe used in the PCR reaction. Bracketed region at top is enlarged on the bottom half of the diagram. The horizontal arrows indicate the direction of priming, and the vertical arrow depicts the probe molecule which will detect the amplified segment without overlapping the sequences of the genome to which the primer molecules will bind. (b) Detection of four representative enterovirus serotypes by PCR. *Left-hand panel:* Agarose mini-gel showing a 154-base amplified segment for each of the four serotypes tested, along with a lambda-phage-control PCR which produces a 504-base amplified segment. The right-most lane is a size marker. *Right-hand panel:* Confirmatory slot–blot hybridization using the oligomeric probe, labeled with [32]P. P1, poliovirus type 1; A16, coxsackievirus A16; B1, coxsackievirus B1; E11, echovirus 11; L, lambda phage control; C, saline-negative control containing no DNA or RNA template but otherwise run exactly as the other specimens. (c) PCR assay of the CSF from a patient with agammaglobulinemia and chronic echovirus 11 meningoencephalitis. CSF became sterile (negative viral cultures) on January 21, 1986. The specimen shown, from January 22, 1986, was strongly positive by PCR for echovirus 11 RNA. *Left-hand panel:* Mini-gel analysis. *Right-hand panel:* Confirmatory slot–blot hybridization. The abbreviations are the same as in part b. (d) PCR analysis of five CSF specimens from patients with enteroviral aseptic meningitis (samples A, B, and C) or no CNS infection (samples D and E). Positive control is a virus stock of poliovirus type 1 (PV1) added to normal CSF. Negative (neg) control contains saline only (no DNA or RNA template). Controls were processed in a manner exactly the same as that of all other samples. Bands of 154 bases in length are seen following amplification of samples A, B, and C and of the PV1-positive control (*left-hand panel*). Slot–blot hybridization confirms those findings (*right-hand panel*).

TABLE 5. *Typical CSF patterns during meningitis[a]*

Pathogen	Number of WBCs	Pattern		
		Predominant cell	Glucose	Protein
Bacteria (common)	100's–1000's	Neutrophils	↓	↑
Viruses Leptospira Lyme disease Mycoplasma Mollaret's Kawasaki's Parameningeal[b] Partially treated[b]	10's–100's	Mononuclears	nl/sl↓	nl/sl↑
Mycobacteria Brucella Fungal Toxoplasma[c]	10's–100's	Mononuclears	↓	↑
Connective tissue disease Parameningeal[b] Partially treated[b]	10's–100's	Neutrophils	nl/sl↓	nl/sl↑

[a] WBCs, white blood cells; nl, normal; sl, slightly; ↓, decrease; ↑, increase.
[b] Either pattern may be seen.
[c] Glucose usually normal.

determining a viral etiology in a patient with meningitis. Utility in distinguishing viral (usually EV) meningitis from that due to bacteria has been claimed by various groups studying CSF immunoglobulin levels (112), serum-C-reactive protein (113,114), CSF lactic acid (115), and lactate dehydrogenase (116), as well as CSF interleukin 1β and CSF tumor necrosis factor (117,118). Of all these latter parameters, tumor necrosis factor may be the most specific for bacterial (versus aseptic) meningitis. In three reports studying CSF tumor necrosis factor detection in meningitis (117,118,118a), none of 50 cumulative patients with aseptic meningitis, as well as none of 19 patients without meningitis, had detectable levels of CSF tumor necrosis factor. This compared with 107 of 145 (74%) cumulative patients with detectable CSF tumor necrosis factor accompanying bacterial meningitis (117,118,118a). In contrast, while interleukin-1β concentrations were much higher in the CSF of patients with bacterial meningitis, detectable levels were still observed in the majority of patients with aseptic meningitis and in occasional patients without meningitis (118).

Specific virologic diagnosis of EV meningitis depends upon the recovery of virus from CSF in tissue culture (19,119). Although a non-polio EV isolated from throat or rectum of a patient with aseptic meningitis is suggestive, the mean shedding periods from those sites following infection are 1 week and several weeks, respectively (10). Hence, shedding from a past infection cannot be ruled out unless the virus is detected in nonpermissive sites, specifically the CSF or blood. Tissue culture has been the mainstay of EV diagnosis since Enders et al. (6) first reported success in growing poliovirus *in vitro;* however, the technique has limitations as a diagnostic modality. The sensitivity of tissue culture for EV serotypes is only 65–75% (19), largely a reflection of the inability to grow many coxsackievirus A serotypes (120). The latter require suckling mouse inoculations (paralysis of the animals indicates a positive culture), a technique too cumbersome to be employed by all but a few reference laboratories. The use of multiple cell lines improves the recovery of EVs (121,122), but it may not be cost-effective or efficient enough for most clinical settings. Furthermore, the titer of EVs in the CSF of patients with aseptic meningitis may be as low as 10^1–10^3 TCID$_{50}$ per milliliter of CSF (123), resulting in slower growth than observed with specimens of throat or rectal origin. Investigators report 3.7–8.2 days as the mean time for CSF EVs to grow in tissue culture (60,110); thus, by the time the results are available they are often moot in distinguishing viral from bacterial infection, since final bacterial culture results are usually available by 72 hr. Attempts at rapid diagnosis of EV infections using immunoassay techniques have been hampered by the lack of a common antigen among the many serotypes (124–126), although two recent studies report success in detecting numerous EV serotypes with polyclonal (127) or monoclonal antibodies (128). Complementary DNA nucleic acid probes derived from cloned sequences of polioviruses, coxsackie B viruses, and echovirus 9 have been prepared and demonstrated to detect multiple EV serotypes in dot–blot hybridization experiments (36–39). Although EVs were readily detected in CSF during reconstruction experiments (39), the clinical sensitivity was only 33% or less (129); occasional culture-negative specimens from patients with typical aseptic meningitis during EV outbreaks were positive by the hybridization assay (129). RNA probes for the EVs have been shown to be more sensitive (130), but still not of clinical utility in detecting CSF infections (131). The limiting variable in all of these hybridization-based assays is undoubtably the low titer of EVs in many CSF specimens from patients with aseptic meningitis (see above). Utilizing regions of known genomic conservation among the EV serotypes which have been fully sequenced, a pair of oligonucleotide primers were designed for polymerase chain reaction amplification of EV RNA (132,133). Eleven of 11 EV serotypes tested were successfully amplified by this method to produce cDNA sequences of predicted length, detectable within 2–4 hr (133) (Fig. 3). Preliminary clinical testing of 20 CSF specimens from patients with meningitis and controls indicates that this technique has the sensitivity and specificity required for a rapid diagnostic test for the EVs (134) (Fig. 3). Of 12 patients with the clinical diagnosis of aseptic meningitis, all were positive by polymerase chain reaction (PCR) for EV RNA; one patient with viral encephalitis was also EV-positive. Four children with bacterial meningitis and three with miscellaneous noninfectious illnesses were all negative for EV RNA by PCR (134). That study found PCR to be more sensitive, and equally specific, to concurrently run cell cultures for the diagnosis of EV meningitis, corroborating the increased sensitivity of PCR (versus culture) in detecting chronic EV meningoencephalitis, as noted above (98).

Other Neurologic Syndromes Associated with EV Infections

Several non-polio EVs have been associated with outbreaks of paralytic myelitis, including coxsackievirus A7 (135), EV 70 (136), and EV 71 (86,87). Sporadic cases of paralysis have been reported in association with isolation of an EV from the stool (10,135), a situation in which causality is difficult to establish because of the known prolonged fecal shedding period of the EVs.

Encephalitis due to the EVs is well known but is, nonetheless, a rare complication (4,7–9,11–15). Clinical manifestations are often indistinguishable from those of other viral encephalitides, including those due to herpes simplex and arboviruses. Cerebellar ataxia has occasionally been associated with EV infections, as have Guillain–Barré syndrome and transverse myelitis (10). All such associations suffer from the same difficulty in distinguishing pathogenicity of a throat or stool isolate from coincidental shedding.

Treatment and Prevention

Specific antiviral therapy for the EVs is not currently available for clinical use. Although a number of drugs have been developed with efficacy *in vitro* and in animal studies, these agents have not reached clinical trials, largely because of inadequate diagnostic methods for rapid identification and enrollment of infected patients. The "WIN" family of drugs, developed by the Sterling–Winthrop Research Institute, are agents which inhibit the uncoating of EVs (137–140). These drugs slip through a pore at the base of the receptor canyon (described above) and bind within a hydrophobic pocket beneath the canyon floor, preventing either (a) the steric change required by the EVs for uncoating or (b) viral binding to a cellular receptor (141,142). One of these drugs, disoxaril, protects mice from developing meningoencephalitis due to echoviruses (143); in addition, it cures mice of chronic EV meningitis in another experimental model (144). The drug, administered orally to infected mice, reduced the incidence of paralysis due to echovirus 9 (143), and it cleared persistent poliovirus type 2 CNS infection from cyclophosphamide-treated mice (144); both of these reactions occurred with minimal to no observed toxicity.

As noted above, clearance of EVs by the host is antibody-mediated; as might be expected, exogenously administered antibody has been useful in certain EV infections. Agammaglobulinemic patients with chronic EV meningitis or meningoencephalitis have shown stabilization and improvement during therapy with gammaglobulin, often administered by multiple routes (e.g., directly into the CNS) (96). Neonates with overwhelming EV sepsis, including meningitis, have received intravenous gammaglobulin, maternal plasma, and exchange transfusions in attempts to reverse their otherwise bleak course, with occasional success (81,82). A single randomized trial of intravenous gammaglobulin plus standard therapy versus standard therapy alone in neonates suspected of having EV infection in the first 2 weeks of life has been undertaken; however, too few patients have been enrolled to date for a definitive conclusion (M. J. Abzug, *personal communication*). Among those patients, 75% had clinical and/or laboratory evidence of meningitis.

Supportive care for the patient with EV meningitis is usually adequate to ensure complete recovery. Attention to fluid balance is necessary to avoid or ameliorate the syndrome of inappropriate antidiuretic hormone and/or brain edema. Electrolytes and, on occasion, urine and serum osmolality may require monitoring. Brain edema is a rare complication of EV meningitis, but it is readily managed with mannitol. Seizures may result from fever alone, or they may reflect direct viral or indirect inflammatory damage of brain parenchyma (in which case "encephalitis" is the more apt term). Phenytoin or phenobarbital are the preferred agents for managing this complication. A rapidly progressive, downhill course requiring more intensive support speaks strongly against an EV etiology, and other potentially treatable causes must be immediately considered (see below).

OTHER VIRAL PATHOGENS

Arboviruses

"Arbovirus" is a taxonomically defunct term which still has useful practical meaning, encompassing viral pathogens transmitted by arthropod vectors (145). Hundreds of such viruses have been identified worldwide, each with distinct seasonal and geographic characteristics determined by the biologic patterns of both the particular vector and the animal reservoirs. Although encephalitis is the most clinically significant and commonly recognized neurologic manifestation of infection (see Chapter 15), certain of the viruses also frequently cause aseptic meningitis as part of their disease spectrum; meningoencephalitis is common as well. The pathogenesis of these infections begins with subcutaneous inoculation by a mosquito or tick vector, followed by local tissue and lymph node replication, viremia, and, finally, invasion of deeper soft tissues, organs, and the CNS. As with many other neurotropic viruses, the exact route to the meninges and brain remains equivocal; however, animal models suggest viremic infection of olfactory nerves with subsequent neuronal spread (146). Hematogenous spread directly to the meninges and brain has not been ruled out as an important mechanism of infection (147,148). Seasonality and geographic distribution are determined by the life cycles and habitat of the vectors; hence most infections in this country occur during summer and fall—peak mosquito and tick seasons. Except during large epidemics, far fewer cases of summer/fall meningitis are due to arboviruses than to enteroviruses.

St. Louis encephalitis (SLE) virus, a flavivirus, is the most common vector-transmitted cause of aseptic meningitis. SLE virus, like other flaviviruses, is a positive (message)-sense, single-stranded RNA virus. Three structural proteins are recognized. They form the 40- to 50-nm spherical virion structure and express multiple antigenic epitopes (149). Originally recognized in the midwestern United States, SLE has now been identified as the cause of sporadic and epidemic meningitis and encephalitis throughout the Americas. Birds are the reservoir, and four different species of mosquitoes—each with a specific geographic distribution—are the principal vectors. Vector exposure may be more likely to occur indoors than outside, since poorly sealed residences appear to be a risk factor (150). Aseptic meningitis accounts for approximately 15% of all symptomatic cases of SLE; in children this figure may be as high as 35–60% (151), since younger patients tend to have milder forms of SLE-associated CNS disease. In contrast, patients over 60 years old rarely (5% or fewer cases) present with aseptic meningitis; 85% of symptomatic SLE virus infections in these individuals manifest as encephalitis (151). Fa-

talities also cluster in the older age groups (150,151). Other flaviviruses, such as those causing Japanese encephalitis, Murray Valley encephalitis, and West Nile fever, are far less commonly identified in cases of meningitis.

The California encephalitis group of viruses is composed of five viruses in the bunyavirus family. Three of these agents (La Crosse, Jamestown Canyon, and Snowshoe hare viruses) have been associated with aseptic meningitis. The bunyaviruses are 80- to 120-nm enveloped particles containing a negative-sense, single-stranded RNA genome. The RNA is present in three segments, each in its own nucleocapsid structure (152). La Crosse virus is endemic in forested regions (particularly around the Great Lakes) and primarily infects children (151). Approximately 50% of cases present with aseptic meningitis, intact sensorium, and no focal neurologic signs (153). Jamestown Canyon virus presents primarily as aseptic meningitis, with only rare cases of encephalitis (154).

The agent of Colorado tick fever (CTF) is an orbivirus, a member of the family Reoviridae. Of numerous orbiviruses in nature, the CTF agent is the only one which infects humans. Orbiviruses are double-stranded, segmented RNA viruses. The CTF agent differs from other orbiviruses not only in its host range, but also in the number of genomic RNA segments (12 versus 11 for other orbiviruses), its geographic distribution (mostly western and mountainous regions of the United States), and its tick vector (*Dermatocentor andersoni*) (155). The virion is nonenveloped, with an outer diameter of 80 nm and an inner core diameter of 50 nm. The virus is introduced by a tick bite, followed by a 3- to 6-day incubation period. Hematopoietic cells, principally erythrocytes, are the major targets wherein viral replication and dissemination occurs (155). A biphasic illness is characteristic; however, it is actually observed in only 50% of patients (156,157), consisting of initial sudden onset of high fever and headache with flu-like constitutional symptoms. Hepatosplenomegaly may occur, as well as gastrointestinal symptoms. Stiff neck and other meningeal signs occur in as many as 18% of confirmed CTF cases (158). Meningoencephalitis and encephalitis have also been reported (156,159), but they are less common than meningitis. The period of illness is usually brief (2–3 days). A peripheral leukopenia with relative lymphocytosis is common. A lymphocyte-predominant CSF pleocytosis and elevated protein are typically found in patients with neurologic manifestations. Certain patients will transiently improve (1–2 days), followed by a second phase of illness of equal or greater severity (lasting an additional 2–3 days). Severe sequelae and death have been reported (159), but they are rare. Typically, recovery is rapid and complete within 2 weeks. Many days to weeks following recovery and development of antibody, virus can be demonstrated to persist in circulating erythrocytes (160). Ongoing replication of virus in those cells has not been demonstrated. The overlapping seasonality of CTF with other arboviruses, as well as with enteroviruses, makes a high index of suspicion necessary for diagnosis. Laboratory diagnosis is best made by inoculation of blood (clot or unclotted cellular fraction) into suckling mice (160,161). Virus may also be detected in peripheral blood smears by indirect immunofluorescence (161). Paired acute and convalescent serology is useful for retrospective diagnosis; a number of techniques have been reported (162,163).

Specific therapy for arboviral meningitis does not currently exist. Supportive care, as for the enteroviruses, is usually effective.

Mumps

Virology and Pathogenesis

The mumps virus is a member of the family Paramyxoviridiae. No significant antigenic differences have been detected among isolates; hence only a single serotype is thought to exist (164). Mumps virions are enveloped, pleomorphic structures containing an inner ribonucleoprotein core structure composed of a single-stranded RNA of negative (anti-message) sense and at least two proteins, one of which is thought to be the RNA-dependent RNA polymerase (165). A third, larger protein may also be associated with the ribonucleoprotein core structure. Two surface glycoproteins are responsible for the neuraminidase, hemagglutination, and fusion properties of mumps virus which facilitate adsorption of the virion to host cells and penetration of the genetic material into the cells (165). Mumps RNA replication is via a positive-stranded intermediate which serves as both the template for negative-sense RNA replication and as messenger RNA for protein translation (165).

Mumps is acquired by the respiratory droplet route, with primary replication presumably occurring in the upper respiratory epithelium. Local viral invasion of the parotid gland via the duct epithelium accounts for the most prominent manifestation of infection, parotitis. Parotitis is not, however, required for, and may be incidental to, dissemination of the virus (166). Viremia can be documented (167) and is the likely means of spread to distant target organs; infection of circulating mononuclear cells may be important in this dissemination (168). The role of lymphatics and local nodes as intermediaries between the respiratory epithelium and blood is not clear. Viremia results in spread of mumps infection to the CNS, as well as to the kidneys, gonads, myocardium, pancreas, placenta, and breast milk. Meningitis is the most common neurologic manifestation of mumps in-

fection (169). Based on a hamster model of mumps meningoencephalitis, viral entry into the CNS is presumed to be via the egress of mumps-infected mononuclear cells across the choroid plexus endothelium (168). Secondary infection of choroidal epithelium results in release of virus into ventricular fluid, followed by spread to meningeal surfaces by the normal routes of CSF flow. Occasionally, spread of virus from infected ependymal cells to brain parenchyma occurs with resultant signs of encephalitis. Ependymal involvement at the aqueduct of Sylvius may result in obstructive hydrocephalus in rare cases of mumps meningitis (170). Meningitis and meningoencephalitis due to mumps are usually benign and self-limited diseases (169,171–173). The occasional fatalities demonstrate pathologic findings of demyelination near blood vessels (169) suggestive of an autoimmune process, as well as evidence of acute parenchymal involvement (174,175). Rare cochlear infection may result in deafness.

Epidemiology and Clinical Presentation

Like other respiratory viruses, mumps infections occur with increased incidence in the winter and spring months. In the pre-vaccine era, more than half of all children had antibodies to mumps (indicating past infection) prior to school entry. The highest incidence of infection occurs in school-age children (5–9 years old); however, a recent shift to older children and adolescents has been observed (176), attributable to an underimmunized population of children born between 1967 (when the vaccine was made available) and 1977 (when the vaccine was recommended for routine use) (176). The widespread use of the attenuated live-virus vaccine in the United States has resulted in a drop in incidence from 76.3 cases per 100,000 population in 1968, to 7.7 cases per 100,000 in 1978, to 2.1 cases per 100,000 in 1988 (67). Whereas mumps once was the leading identifiable cause of aseptic meningitis, the dramatic decline in total number of mumps infections, coupled with improved diagnostic tests for other viruses, has resulted in mumps meningitis being only rarely diagnosed in the United States today (Table 2). Symptomatic mumps is twice as frequent in males as in females, and neurologic involvement is three times more common in males; neither observation has been explained.

Aseptic meningitis is the most common neurologic complication of mumps. CSF pleocytosis occurs in more than 50% of patients with mumps parotitis (169), but most were not symptomatic of meningitis. Symptoms of meningitis are reported in 0–30% of all cases of mumps parotitis by 4–10 days of illness, but they may precede parotitis by as much as 7 days; half or more cases of mumps meningitis may not be associated with parotitis at all (172,177). The clinical manifestations of mumps aseptic meningitis are nonspecific and differ little from those of the EVs. However, because the average age of the patients with mumps is greater than that of patients with EV meningitis, certain signs and symptoms such as headache, nausea, vomiting, and meningismus are more elicitable and reported as more prominent with mumps meningitis. Fever is universal, usually lasting 3 days but occasionally persisting for a week (172). Bradycardia, drowsiness, lethargy, and anemia are all reported. Virtually by definition, the prognosis for rapid and full recovery from mumps meningitis is excellent (169, 171–173).

More significant neurologic involvement can occur. Encephalitis is described concomitantly with meningitis in as many as 35% of cases (172) or in as few as 4% (177). The differences appear to lie in both biologic variation and the criteria established for the designation of encephalitis. A full spectrum of parenchymal brain involvement has been seen with mumps infection, ranging from focal and generalized seizures to obtundation, delirium, and coma (169,171,173). In all but the most severe cases, full recovery is the rule. Occasional fatalities have been reported (174) and, as noted above, may sometimes represent autoimmune sequelae. Myelitis due to mumps has occasionally been reported (178), as has paralysis (179). Deafness appears to be a complication of mumps infection which is unrelated to meningitis or encephalitis.

Most, but not all, cases of symptomatic mumps meningitis have accompanying CSF pleocytosis, primarily mononuclear cells (169). Half of all patients have 500 or fewer cells per cubic millimeter, 75% of cases have fewer than 1000 cells per cubic millimeter, and the remainder of patients have fewer than 5000 cells per cubic millimeter. Exceptional cases with more than 5000 cells have been reported (169,173). Pleocytosis may persist for weeks. CSF protein has been reported as normal (<40 mg/100 ml) in more than half of all patients with mumps meningitis in some series (172,180,181), but it has been significantly elevated in the majority of cases in other studies (166). Glucose is normal in most patients, but it may be depressed (177,182). Opening pressure is usually normal.

The availability of reliable serologic testing for mumps virus infection accounted for the preeminence of mumps among cases of meningitis and meningoencephalitis for which an etiologic diagnosis could be made in the pre-tissue-culture era (3,4). Complement fixation (183) and hemagglutination inhibition were the mainstays and continue to be useful (184). Hemolysis-in-gel assays have been reported for mumps (185). Paired acute and convalescent serologic studies, specific IgM and IgG assays on a single specimen, and comparative CSF and serum antibody measurements all have roles in diagnosis of mumps meningitis. Mumps virus from CSF can be grown in tissue culture for at least a week following onset

of disease, but sensitivity of the technique is highly variable. Hemadsorption can be used to confirm cytopathic effect or to detect noncytopathic isolates in tissue culture.

Treatment and Prevention

There is no specific antiviral agent for mumps infections. Specific hyperimmune globulin reduced the incidence of orchitis in a single prospective controlled trial (186), but no benefit has been proven for neurologic syndromes. The currently used attenuated live-virus vaccine was made available in the United States in 1967 and recommended for routine use in this country in 1977. It is most commonly administered in combination with attenuated measles and rubella virus vaccines to children at 15 months of age. Immunity appears to be long-lasting without evidence of waning over time. Cost–benefit analysis has shown a benefit–cost ratio of nearly 40:1 using an approximation of actual mumps incidence without vaccination, including a reduction of more than 98% of cases of mumps meningoencephalitis (187). Rare cases of vaccine-associated mumps meningitis have been reported; there have been no sequelae (188–190).

Lymphocytic Choriomeningitis Virus

Lymphocytic choriomeningitis virus (LCMV), a member of the Arenavirus family, is an enveloped, single-stranded RNA virus of variable size and shape. At least three proteins are produced by the virus: One is associated with the nucleocapsid structure, and two are surface glycoproteins (191). Enzymatic activities have also been identified in viral preparations, including polymerase and transcriptase functions (191). LCMV was one of the earliest and seemingly most significant viruses to be associated with aseptic meningitis in humans (Table 2). Because of improved methods for detecting other meningitic viruses, and perhaps because of other undefined epidemiologic factors, LCMV is now rarely identified in humans; cases have not been reported in the literature for more than 10 years. LCMV is transmitted by rodents (hamsters, rats, mice); thus laboratory workers, pet owners, and individuals living under impoverished and nonhygienic circumstances have traditionally been at greatest risk (192,193). Ingestion of animal-urine-contaminated food or exposure of open wounds to dirt are presumed routes of transmission. Human-to-human transmission does not occur. Seroprevalence in the general community has never been adequately studied, but it is estimated at less than 0.1% (191). Since many cases of aseptic meningitis resolve without an etiologic agent being identified, an ongoing role for LCMV cannot be ruled out. The required high degree of suspicion is no longer present, and confirmatory laboratory tests are rarely performed.

The clinical manifestations of aseptic meningitis occur in only about 15% of patients with confirmed LCMV infections (192,193). The remainder of infected individuals are mildly ill with constitutional symptoms or are asymptomatic. Occasional severe neurologic disease (meningoencephalitis, encephalitis) has been reported (194), as have rare fatal cases (195). The course of meningitis and recovery is often prolonged, but permanent neurologic impairment is rare (7). CSF findings are indistinguishable from those of other viral causes of aseptic meningitis: mild pleocytosis (lymphocytes predominate), mildly elevated protein, and usually normal or slightly low glucose. Tissue culture, animal culture, immunoassay, and serologic techniques are all available (in research laboratory settings) for diagnosis.

LCMV has become an important agent for studying virus–host immune interactions. A recent review summarizes this large body of information (196).

Herpes Family Viruses

Neurologic complications are well known with herpes simplex types 1 and 2, varicella-zoster, and cytomegalovirus infections. Although aseptic meningitis has been reported with all of those pathogens (197–202), only that associated with herpes simplex viruses (HSVs) appears to be of numeric significance. The clinical course and outcome of aseptic meningitis (versus other neurologic disease) due to all of the herpes family viruses are uniformly good, and these patients are clinically indistinguishable from those with aseptic meningitis of other etiologies.

The most common syndrome of HSV-associated aseptic meningitis occurs concomitant with primary HSV-2 genital infection, or shortly thereafter (197–199). More than 33% of women and 11% of men in one study of primary HSV-2 infections developed an aseptic meningitis syndrome including CSF pleocytosis (199). Primary HSV-1 genital infection is less often associated with aseptic meningitis, and nonprimary genital infection with either HSV type rarely results in meningitis (199). Meningitis has also been reported with HSV-1 (203,204) in the absence of recent genital lesions; however, the recently appreciated high frequency of asymptomatic shedding of genital HSV may explain this apparent *de novo* HSV meningitis. Overall, HSV appears to account for approximately 1–3% of all cases of aseptic meningitis (205) (Table 2).

Meningitis is rarely diagnosed during acute chickenpox, although occasional cases have been suspected and, when CSF examination is performed, pleocytosis may be documented (205a). The benign course is typical of other aseptic meningitides. A better recognized, albeit also rare, syndrome is acute aseptic meningitis associated with herpes zoster (shingles) (205b–205d). CSF pleocytosis may occur in many patients with herpes zoster; however, they are usually asymptomatic of CNS disease. Clinically apparent herpes-zoster meningitis is generally benign, and it has been demonstrated in individuals with typical skin lesions as well as in some patients with no cutaneous manifestations; the latter syndrome is known as "zoster sine herpete." Virus has occasionally been isolated from the CSF of patients with herpes-zoster meningitis (205e), but the viral association has usually been by immunoassay and/or serologic techniques, particularly in the absence of typical skin lesions. Meningoencephalitis, postinfectious encephalopathy, and Reye's syndrome are all more common than aseptic meningitis as neurologic complications of varicella-zoster infections. Similarly, aseptic meningitis associated with Epstein–Barr virus and cytomegalovirus infections is rare but reported (201,205f), and other neurologic manifestations of both agents are far more common.

Mollaret's recurrent meningitis (see below) has been repeatedly studied for herpes family viruses. A single case associated with HSV-1 (206) and another associated with Epstein–Barr virus (207) have been reported.

Other Viruses

A variety of other viruses have been occasionally identified in a patient with the aseptic meningitis syndrome. Measles virus and adenovirus are well known to cause encephalitis and meningoencephalitis, particularly in immunocompromised patients. Occasional cases of aseptic meningitis due to adenoviruses in normal patients have been noted (11–15), and measles infection may be associated with pleocytosis in as many as 30% of uncomplicated cases in normal patients, usually without signs or symptoms of meningitis (208). Other respiratory viruses are rarely described in association with aseptic meningitis. A recent case of parainfluenza type 3 meningitis has been reported (209); a variety of neurologic syndromes have been described with influenza A and B infections, including aseptic meningitis (11–15,210). A single case of aseptic meningitis in association with rotavirus gastroenteritis has been noted (211). Encephalomyocarditis virus, a murine picornavirus, has been reported in a few patients with aseptic meningitis (212), but not within the past 25 years.

Two patterns of human immunodeficiency virus (HIV) meningitis have been described in infected patients without other HIV-associated CNS manifestations or evidence of secondary pathogens (213–215). The acute presentation pattern may occur as part of the primary infection (i.e., at seroconversion) or in an already infected patient. Headache, fever, and meningeal signs, usually resolving within 10 days, characterize this form. Other patients develop chronic headache and pleocytosis, without meningismus (213,216). These mild findings may persist for months. Progression of HIV meningitis to encephalopathy or to other CNS manifestations has not been shown, but the numbers of meningitis patients described in the literature remain small. Human T-lymphotrophic virus 1 (HTLV-1) meningitis has been described (217), but the case more closely fits the term "meningoencephalitis."

NONVIRAL PATHOGENS

The aseptic meningitis syndrome is defined by the absence of a readily identifiable bacterial etiology (1,2). Nevertheless, certain bacteria do present occultly with classic features of aseptic meningitis (Table 5). As one would predict based on the definition of aseptic meningitis, bacteria responsible for these occult presentations are not typically detected by Gram's stain of CSF; these include spirochetes, mycobacteria, and brucella. Partially treated bacterial meningitis (caused by common bacterial pathogens) and parameningeal (e.g., sinus) infection may also present in a manner similar to that of viral meningitis and must always be considered, since specific therapy is required.

Leptospirosis is an acute systemic vasculitic disease caused by a number of spirochetes in the *Leptospira* genus. Acquisition by humans is via contact with infected animal body fluids. Although more typically noted in the anicteric variety, meningitis is common in icteric leptospirosis (Weil's disease) as well (218,219). The CSF profile is indistinguishable from that due to common viruses, except that, overall, more patients develop elevated CSF protein than do patients with common viral meningitis. Leptospiral meningitis is benign and recovery is usually rapid regardless of therapeutic intervention, although prolonged symptoms have been occasionally observed (220).

Another important spirochetal cause of aseptic meningitis is *Borrelia burgdorferi*, the etiologic agent of Lyme disease. Transmitted by tick bite, this organism causes a three-stage disease, the second stage of which is characterized by disseminated infection and multisystemic involvement (221). Although headache and stiff neck may be part of stage 1 manifestations (along with the characteristic skin rash called "erythema chronicum migrans"), the CSF is usually normal at that time. At a median of 4 weeks following the recognition of disease, many patients develop an aseptic meningitis syndrome which may or may not be associated with concomitant or subsequent cranial and/or radiculoneuritis (222). Meningitis may be the first manifestation of Lyme disease, presumably because stage 1 infection goes unnoticed in those patients (222). Lymphocyte pleocytosis (median 166 white blood cells per cubic millimeter, 93% lymphocytes), modest protein elevation (median 79 mg/

dl), and normal glucose comprise the typical CSF profile (222). Prognosis for the meningitis component of Lyme disease appears good with appropriate antibiotic therapy; without therapy, a waxing and waning course over months to years may be observed. Development of more severe neurologic disease during stage 3 (late) illness is well known (221,223).

Aseptic meningitis is a relatively uncommon manifestation of secondary syphilis and of relapsing fever (borreliosis), two additional spirochetal illnesses found in humans. As with Lyme disease, more severe neurologic illness is of greater concern and of greater clinical significance in these illnesses.

The often subacute presentation of tuberculous meningitis may be the only clinically distinguishing feature of this disease. Seventy-five percent of patients with meningitis due to *Mycobacterium tuberculosis* have evidence of extrameningeal (usually pulmonary) disease; the remaining 25% present the most challenging diagnostic aspect of this disease and the most common explanation for delay in diagnosis and increased severity (224–226). In most cases, the pathogenesis of tuberculous meningitis involves the rupture of a subependymal tuberculoma into the subarachnoid space (227). The tuberculoma itself results from hematogenous dissemination of primary disease. The clinical spectrum ranges from benign (even self-resolving) cases (228) to progressive and fatal courses. In addition to almost universal meningismus, other neurologic findings may include altered levels of consciousness, Babinski's reflex, and cranial nerve palsies (229). CSF findings are stereotypic in late disease, with markedly elevated protein and decreased glucose. Earlier in the course, however, protein is often only modestly elevated and glucose may be normal. Confusing the diagnosis with enterovirus or mumps meningitis is not uncommon (229); dual infections with other pathogens have also been reported (230). Conversely, enterovirus infections can mimic tuberculous meningitis (108). Lymphocyte predominance with several hundred cells is typical for tuberculous meningitis, further complicating its distinction from viral infections.

CNS infections with brucella species are well described but are rare (230a). Meningoencephalitis is the usual presentation, and both acute and chronic forms have been reported. Antibiotic therapy is usually curative; however, some residual neurologic defects are the rule. Encephalitis, myelitis, and neuritis have also been described (230a).

Fungal meningitis is increasingly being recognized among immunocompromised hosts; however, fungi may infect the CNS of normal individuals as well and must be considered in any indolent, atypical aseptic meningitis syndrome (231). These pathogens often also cause meningoencephalitis, brain abscess, and/or granuloma formation in the CNS. Cryptococcus is the most commonly recognized cause of fungal meningitis (231). The presentation may mimic that of tuberculous meningitis or may present with concurrent signs of encephalitis or focal lesions. Histoplasma, blastomyces, and coccidioides infections of the CNS predominantly manifest as meningitis, most often in normal hosts (231). Candida meningitis can occur in normal and immunocompromised individuals. Although many fungal CNS infections occur in association with other organ system involvement, meningitis may present in isolation.

A variety of neurologic manifestations have been reported to be associated with *Mycoplasma pneumoniae* infections (232), among which aseptic meningitis is the most common. Clinically, this disease is impossible to distinguish from viral meningitis. Like typical viral infection, sequelae are not observed with mycoplasmal meningitis. Diagnosis is by serology, since the organism is difficult to culture from CSF (232). *Mycoplasma hominis* has been associated with cases of neonatal meningitis, usually in pre-term infants (233–235).

NONINFECTIOUS CAUSES OF THE ASEPTIC MENINGITIS SYNDROME

Patients with immune-mediated diseases and/or receiving immunomodulating drug therapy may develop an aseptic meningitis syndrome, often characterized by recurrent episodes. Meningitis has been described as the initial manifestation of systemic lupus erythematosus in several patients (236,237), but it has more often been regarded as part of the ongoing disease evolution. Two to four percent of lupus patients may develop aseptic meningitis during the course of their disease (236–239). In some of those patients, anti-inflammatory agents, particularly nonsteroidal anti-inflammatory drugs (NSAIDs), have been implicated (240–244). NSAIDs have also been reported in association with aseptic meningitis in patients with Sjögren's syndrome (245) or rheumatoid arthritis (246), as well as in some individuals with only serologic evidence of connective tissue disease (247). An occasional patient without clinical or serologic evidence of underlying disease has developed NSAID-associated meningitis (248). The effect of these therapeutics may be drug-specific rather than drug-mechanism-specific, since (a) not all NSAIDs have been reported to cause this syndrome and (b) certain patients developing aseptic meningitis after one NSAID tolerate other NSAIDs well (243). The pathogenesis of NSAID-associated aseptic meningitis appears to involve a cellular immune hypersensitivity reaction (249), a hypothesis supported by animal model experiments (250). The only distinguishing feature between connective tissue disease aseptic meningitis and viral meningitis is that the former tends to have a neutrophil-predominant CSF pleocytosis.

Other immune-modulating drugs have also been associated with aseptic meningitis in patients with underlying diseases other than that of connective tissue. Cytosine arabinoside (251), immune serum globulin (252), and the murine monoclonal antibody OKT3 used to reduce graft rejection (253,254) are examples. Antibiotics, particularly sulfa-containing compounds, have also been associated with aseptic meningitis, often (but not always) in patients with underlying connective tissue disease (255–257). Carbamazepine has caused aseptic meningitis in a similar setting (258).

Mollaret's meningitis is a rare disease characterized by recurrent, benign episodes of aseptic meningitis with symptom-free intervals between episodes (259,260). The disease is defined by the absence of an identifiable etiologic agent, although various pathogens have occasionally been identified in these individuals, including Epstein–Barr virus (207) and herpes simplex type 1 (206). This syndrome is to be distinguished from recurrent meningitis due to identifiable pathogens (75). Clinically, each episode is very similar to typical viral meningitis, with the exception of the laboratory finding (in certain patients) of cells resembling endothelial cells (in addition to a lymphocyte-predominant pleocytosis) in the CSF. Current investigators feel that these so-called Mollaret cells are likely to be monocytes (261); these cells are fragile, appear only transiently, and are of unknown importance.

Kawasaki disease, or mucocutaneous lymph node syndrome (262–264), is a disease of children which manifests as a systemic vasculitis; the etiology is unknown, but it is probably infectious. Characterized by prolonged fever, rash, mucous membrane changes, lymphadenopathy, and changes of the extremities (erythema, edema, and desquamation) (263,264), the major significance of this illness is the vasculitis of coronary arteries which develops in 15–25% of patients. Aseptic meningitis develops in 26–70% of patients with Kawasaki disease. It is benign and resolves with resolution of other systemic manifestations. This disease is endemic, with periodic epidemics, in Japan; children of Asian descent are at highest risk in the United States and elsewhere in the world.

REFERENCES

1. Wallgren A. Une nouvelle maladie infectieuse du système nerveux central? *Acta Paediatr Scand* 1925;4(Suppl):158–182.
2. Wallgren A. Die atiologie der enzephalomeningitis bei kindern, besonders des syndromes der akuten abakteriellen (aseptichen) meningitis. *Acta Paediatr Scand* 1951;40:541–565.
2a. Centers for Disease Control. Summary of notifiable diseases, United States, 1988. *MMWR* 1989;37:1–57.
3. Rassmussen AF Jr. The laboratory diagnosis of lymphocytic choriomeningitis and mumps. Presented at the Rocky Mountain Conference on Poliomyelitis, Denver, Colorado, December 16, 1946.
4. Adair CV, Gauld RL, Smadel JE. Aseptic meningitis, a disease of diverse etiology: clinical and etiologic studies on 854 cases. *Ann Intern Med* 1953;39:675–704.

5. Dalldorf G, Sickles GM. An unidentified, filtrable agent isolated from the feces of children with paralysis. *Science* 1948;108:61–62.
6. Enders JR, Weller TH, Robbins FC. Cultivation of the Lansing strain of poliomyelitis virus in cultures of various human embryonic tissues. *Science* 1949;109:85–87.
7. Meyer HM Jr, Johnson RT, Crawford IP, Dascomb HE, Rogers NG. Central nervous system syndromes of "viral" etiology. *Am J Med* 1960;29:334–347.
8. Lennette EH, Magoffin RL, Knouf EG. Viral central nervous system disease: an etiologic study conducted at the Los Angeles County General Hospital. *JAMA* 1962;179:687–695.
9. Buescher EL, Artenstein MS, Olson LC. Central nervous system infections of viral etiology: the changing pattern. *Res Publ Assoc Nerv Ment Dis* 1968;44:147–163.
10. Cherry JD. Enteroviruses: polioviruses (poliomyelitis), coxsackieviruses, echoviruses, and enteroviruses. In: Feigin RD, Cherry JD, eds. *Textbook of pediatric infectious diseases,* 2nd ed. Philadelphia: WB Saunders, 1987;1729–1841.
11. Deibel R, Barron A, Millian S, Smith V. Central nervous system infections in New York State: etiologic and epidemiologic observations, 1972. *NY State J Med* 1974;74:1929–1935.
12. Deibel R, Flanagan TD, Smith V. Central nervous system infections in New York State: etiologic and epidemiologic observations, 1974. *NY State J Med* 1975;75:2337–2342.
13. Deibel R, Flanagan TD, Smith V. Central nervous system infections: etiologic and epidemiologic observations in New York State, 1975. *NY State J Med* 1977;77:1398–1404.
14. Deibel R, Flanagan TD. Central nervous system infections: etiologic and epidemiologic observations in New York State, 1976–1977. *NY State J Med* 1979;79:689–695.
15. Flanagan TD, Deibel R. Central nervous system infections: etiologic and epidemiologic observations in New York State, 1978–1979. *NY State J Med* 1981;81:1346–1353.
16. McLean DM, Coleman MA, Larke RPB, McNaughton GA. Viral infections of Toronto children during 1965. I. Enteroviral disease. *Can Med Assoc J* 1966;94:839–843.
17. Moore M. Enteroviral disease in the United States, 1970–1979. *J Infect Dis* 1982;146:103–108.
18. Wilfert CM, Lehrman SN, Katz SL. Enteroviruses and meningitis. *Pediatr Infect Dis* 1983;2:333–341.
19. Wildin S, Chonmaitree T. The importance of the virology laboratory in the diagnosis and management of viral meningitis. *Am J Dis Child* 1987;141:454–457.
20. Melnick JL. Enteroviruses: polioviruses, coxsackieviruses, echoviruses, and newer enteroviruses. In: Fields BN, Knipe DM, eds. *Virology.* New York: Raven Press, 1990;549–605.
21. Wetz K, Habermehl K-O. Specific cross-linking of capsid proteins to virus RNA by ultraviolet irradiation of poliovirus. *J Gen Virol* 1982;59:397–401.
22. Hogle JM, Chow M, Filman DJ. Three-dimensional structure of poliovirus at 2.9 Å resolution. *Science* 1985;229:1358–1365.
23. Hogle JM, Filman DJ, Syed R, Chow M, Minor PD. Structural basis for serotypic differences and thermostability in poliovirus. In: Semler BL, Ehrenfeld E, eds. *Molecular aspects of picornavirus infection and detection.* Washington, DC: American Society of Microbiology Publications, 1989;125–137.
24. Baltimore D, Girard M. An intermediate in synthesis of poliovirus RNA. *Proc Natl Acad Sci USA* 1966;56:741–748.
25. Rueckert RR. Picornaviruses and their replication. In: Fields BN, Knipe DM, eds. *Virology.* New York: Raven Press, 1990;507–548.
26. Dewalt PG, Semler BL. Molecular biology and genetics of poliovirus protein processing. In: Semler BL, Ehrenfeld E, eds. *Molecular aspects of picornavirus infection and detection.* Washington, DC: American Society of Microbiology, 1989;73–93.
27. Toyoda H, Kohara M, Kataoka Y, Suganuma T, Omata T, Imura N, Nomoto A. Complete nucleotide sequences of all three poliovirus serotype genomes: implication for genetic relationship, gene function and antigenic determinants. *J Mol Biol* 1984;174:561–585.
28. Chang KH, Auvinen P, Hyypiä T, Stanway G. The nucleotide sequence of coxsackievirus A9; implications for receptor binding and enterovirus classification. *J Gen Virol* 1989;70:3269–3280.
29. Hughes PJ, North C, Minor PD, Stanway G. The complete nucleotide sequence of coxsackievirus A21. *J Gen Virol* 1989; 70:2943–2952.
30. Iizuka N, Kuge S, Nomoto A. Complete nucleotide sequence of the genome of coxsackievirus B1. *Virology* 1987;156:64–73.
31. Lindberg AM, Stalhandski POK, Pettersson U. Genome of coxsackievirus B3. *Virology* 1987;156:50–63.
32. Jenkins O, Booth JD, Minor PD, Almond JW. The complete nucleotide sequence of coxsackievirus B4 and its comparison to other members of the picornaviridae. *J Gen Virol* 1987;68:1835–1848.
33. Takeda N. Complete nucleotide and amino acid sequences of enterovirus 70. In: Ishii K, Uchida Y, Miyamara K, Yamazaki S, eds. *Acute hemorrhagic conjunctivitis etiology, epidemiology, and clinical manifestations.* Tokyo: University of Tokyo Press, 1989;419–424.
34. Cohen JI, Ticehurst JR, Purcell RH, Buckler-White A, Baroudy BM. Complete nucleotide sequence of wild-type hepatitis A virus: comparison with different strains of hepatitis A virus and other picornaviruses. *J Virol* 1987;61:50–59.
35. Werner G, Rosenwirth B, Bauer E, Seifert J-M, Werner F-J, Besemer J. Molecular cloning and sequence determination of the genomic regions encoding protease and genome-linked protein of three picornaviruses. *J Virol* 1986;57:1084–1093.
36. Hyypia T, Stalhandske P, Vainionpaa R, Pettersson U. Detection of enteroviruses by spot hybridization. *J Clin Microbiol* 1984;19:436–438.
37. Rotbart HA, Levin MJ, Villarreal LP. Use of subgenomic poliovirus DNA hybridization probes to detect the major subgroups of enteroviruses. *J Clin Microbiol* 1984;20:1105–1108.
38. Tracy S. A comparison of the genomic homologies among the coxsackievirus B group: use of fragments of the cloned coxsackievirus B3 genome as probes. *J Gen Virol* 1984;65:2167–2172.
39. Rotbart HA, Levin MJ, Villarreal LP, Tracy S, Semler BL, Wimmer E. Factors affecting the detection of enteroviruses in cerebrospinal fluid with coxsackievirus B3 and poliovirus type 1 cDNA probes. *J Clin Microbiol* 1985;22:220–224.
40. Bodian D. Emerging concept of poliomyelitis infection. *Science* 1955;122:105–108.
41. Bodian D. Poliomyelitis: pathogenesis and histopathology. In: Rivers TM, Horsfall FL Jr, eds. *Viral and rickettsial infections of man,* 3rd ed. Philadelphia: JB Lippincott 1954;479–518.
42. Wolf JL, Rubin DH, Finberg R, Kauffman RS, Sharpe AH, Trier JS, Fields BN. Intestinal M cells: a pathway for entry of reovirus into the host. *Science* 1981;212:471–472.
43. Wyatt HV. Provocation poliomyelitis and entry of poliovirus to the CNS. *Med Hypotheses* 1976;2:269–274.
44. Prather SL, Dagan R, Jenista JA, Menegus MA. The isolation of enteroviruses from blood: a comparison of four processing methods. *J Med Virol* 1984;14:221–227.
45. Peluso R, Haase A, Stowring L, Edwards M, Ventura P. A Trojan horse mechanism for the spread of visna virus in monocytes. *Virology* 1985;147:231–236.
46. Price RA, Garcia JH, Rightsel WA. Choriomeningitis and myocarditis in an adolescent with isolation of coxsackie B-5 virus. *Am J Clin Pathol* 1970;53:825–831.
47. Colonno RJ, Condra JH, Mizutani S, Callahan PL, Davies M-E, Murcko MA. Evidence for the direct involvement of the rhinovirus canyon in receptor binding. *Proc Natl Acad Sci USA* 1988;85:5449–5453.
48. Mendelsohn CL, Wimmer E, Racaniello VR. Cellular receptor for poliovirus: molecular cloning, nucleotide sequence and expression of a new member of the immunoglobulin superfamily. *Cell* 1989;56:855–865.
49. Lonberg-Holm K, Crowell RL, Philipson L. Unrelated animal viruses share receptors. *Nature* 1976;259:679–716.
50. DeSena J, Mandel B. Studies on the *in vitro* uncoating of poliovirus. II. Characterization of the membrane-modified particle. *Virology* 1977;78:554–566.
51. Guttman N, Baltimore D. A plasma membrane component able to bind and alter virions of poliovirus type 1: studies on cell-free alteration using a simplified assay. *Virology* 1977;82:25–36.
52. Ehrenfeld E. Picornavirus inhibition of host cell protein synthe-

sis. In: Fraenkel-Conrat H, Wagner RR, eds. *Comprehensive virology*. New York: Plenum Press, 1984;19:177–221.

53. Minor PD, Dunn G, John A, Phillips A, Westrop GD, Wareham K, Almond JW. Attenuation and reversion of the Sabin type 3 vaccine strain. In: Semler BL, Ehrenfeld E, eds. *Molecular aspects of picornavirus infection and detection*. Washington, DC: American Society of Microbiology, 1989;307–318.

54. Minor PD, John A, Ferguson M, Icenogle JP. Antigenic and molecular evolution of the vaccine strain of type 3 poliovirus during the period of excretion by a primary vaccinee. *J Gen Virol* 1986;67:693–706.

55. Wenner HA. The enteroviruses. *Am J Clin Pathol* 1972;57:751–761.

56. Grist NR, Bell EJ, Assaad F. Enteroviruses in human disease. *Prog Med Virol* 1978;24:114–157.

57. Assaad F, Ljungars-Esteves K. World overview of poliomyelitis: regional patterns and trends. *Rev Infect Dis* 1984;6:S302–S307.

58. Mason JO, McLean WR. Infectious hepatitis traced to the consumption of raw oysters; an epidemiologic study. *Am J Hyg* 1962;75:90–111.

59. Strikas RA, Anderson LJ, Parker RA. Temporal and geographic patterns of isolates of nonpolio enterovirus in the United States, 1970–1983. *J Infect Dis* 1986;153:346–351.

60. Rantakallio P, Leskinen M, von Wendt L. Incidence and prognosis of central nervous system infections in a birth cohort of 12,000 children. *Scand J Infect Dis* 1986;18:287–294.

61. Centers for Disease Control. Enterovirus surveillance—United States, 1984. *MMWR* 1985;33:388.

62. Centers for Disease Control. Enterovirus surveillance—United States, 1985. *MMWR* 1986;34:494–495.

63. Centers for Disease Control. Enterovirus surveillance—United States, 1986. *MMWR* 1987;35:503.

64. Centers for Disease Control. Enterovirus surveillance—United States, 1987. *MMWR* 1988;36:570–575.

65. Centers for Disease Control. Enterovirus surveillance—United States, 1988. *MMWR* 1989;37:516.

66. Gutierrez K, Abzug MJ. Vaccine-associated poliovirus meningitis in children with ventriculoperitoneal shunts. *J Pediatr* 1990;117:424–427.

67. Centers for Disease Control. Summary of notifiable diseases, United States, 1988. *MMWR* 1989;37:1–57.

68. Horstmann DM, Yamada N. Enterovirus infections of the central nervous system. *Res Publ Assoc Nerv Ment Dis* 1968;44:236–253.

69. Melnick JL, Wimberly IL. Lyophilized combination pools of enterovirus equine antisera: new LBM pools prepared from reserves of antisera stored frozen for two decades. *Bull WHO* 1985;63:543–550.

70. Russell WR. Poliomyelitis; pre-paralytic stage and effect of physical activity on severity of paralysis. *Br Med J* 1947;2:1023.

71. Russell WR. Paralytic poliomyelitis. The early symptoms and the effect of physical activity on symptoms and the course of disease. *Br Med J* 1949;1:465.

72. Horstmann DM. Acute poliomyelitis: relation of physical activity at the time of onset to the course of the disease. *JAMA* 1950;142:236–241.

73. Gatmaitan BG, Chason JL, Lerner AM. Augmentation of the virulence of murine coxsackievirus B-3 myocardiopathy by exercise. *J Exp Med* 1970;131:1121–1136.

74. Moore M, Baron RC, Filstein MR, et al. Aseptic meningitis and high school football players, 1978–1980. *JAMA* 1983;249:2039–2042.

75. Klemola E, Lapinleimu K. Multiple attacks of aseptic meningitis in the same individual. *Br Med J* 1964;1:1087–1090.

76. Nakao T, Miura R. Recurrent virus meningitis. *Pediatrics* 1971;47:773–776.

77. Chang T-W. Recurrent viral infection (reinfection). *N Engl J Med* 1971;284:765–773.

78. Balfour HH Jr, Seifert GL, Seifert MH Jr, et al. Meningoencephalitis and laboratory evidence of triple infection with California encephalitis virus, echovirus 11 and mumps. *Pediatrics* 1973;51:680–684.

79. Eglin RP, Swann RA, Isaacs D, Moxon ER. Simultaneous bacterial and viral meningitis. *Lancet* 1984;2:984.

80. Morens DM. Enteroviral disease in early infancy. *J Pediatr* 1978;92:374–377.

81. Kaplan MH, Klein SW, McPhee J, Harper RG. Group B coxsackievirus infections in infants younger than three months of age: a serious childhood illness. *Rev Infect Dis* 1983;5:1019–1032.

82. Modlin JF. Perinatal echovirus infection: insights from a literature review of 61 cases of serious infection and 16 outbreaks in nurseries. *Rev Infect Dis* 1986;8:918–926.

83. Lake AM, Lauer BA, Clark JC, Wesenberg RL, McIntosh K. Enterovirus infections in neonates. *J Pediatr* 1976;89:787–791.

84. Nogen AG, Lepow ML. Enteroviral meningitis in very young infants. *Pediatrics* 1967;40:617–627.

85. Singer JI, Maur PR, Riley JP, Smith PB. Management of central nervous system infections during an epidemic of enteroviral aseptic meningitis. *J Pediatr* 1980;96:559–563.

86. Ishimaru Y, Nakano S, Yamaoka K, et al. Outbreaks of hand, foot, and mouth disease by enterovirus 71. High incidence of complication disorders of central nervous system. *Arch Dis Child* 1980;55:583–588.

87. Gilbert GL, Dickson KE, Waters M-J, Kennett ML, Land SA, Sneddon M. Outbreak of enterovirus 71 infection in Victoria, Australia, with a high incidence of neurologic involvement. *Pediatr Infect Dis J* 1988;7:484–488.

88. Solomon P, Weinstein L, Chang TW, et al. Epidemiologic, clinical and laboratory features of an epidemic of type 9 echo virus meningitis. *J Pediatr* 1959;55:609–619.

89. Chemtob S, Reece ER, Mills EL. Syndrome of inappropriate secretion of antidiuretic hormone in enteroviral meningitis. *Am J Dis Child* 1985;139:292–294.

90. Faulkner RS, MacLeod AJ, Van Rooyen CE. Virus meningitis—seven cases in one family. *Can Med Assoc J* 1957;77:439–444.

91. Jaffe M, Srugo I, Tirosh E, Collin AA, Tal Y. The ameliorating effect of lumbar puncture in viral meningitis. *Am J Dis Child* 1989;143:682–685.

92. Lepow ML, Coyne N, Thompson LB, Carver DH, Robbins FC. A clinical epidemiologic and laboratory investigation of aseptic meningitis during the four-year period, 1955–1958. II. The clinical disease and its sequelae. *N Engl J Med* 1962;266:1188–1193.

93. Sells CJ, Carpenter RL, Ray CG. Sequelae of central-nervous-system enterovirus infections. *N Engl J Med* 1975;293:1–4.

94. Wilfert CM, Thompson RJ, Sunder TR, O'Quinn A, Zeller J, Blacharsh J. Longitudinal assessment of children with enteroviral meningitis during the first three months of life. *Pediatrics* 1981;67:811–815.

95. Bergman I, Painter MJ, Wald ER, Chiponis D, Holland AL, Taylor HG. Outcome in children with enteroviral meningitis during the first year of life. *J Pediatr* 1987;110:705–709.

96. McKinney RE Jr, Katz SL, Wilfert CM. Chronic enteroviral meningoencephalitis in agammaglobulinemic patients. *Rev Infect Dis* 1987;9:334–356.

97. Rotbart HA, Kinsella JP, Wasserman RL. Persistent enterovirus infection in culture-negative meningoencephalitis—demonstration by enzymatic RNA amplification. *J Infect Dis* 1990;161:787–791.

98. O'Neil KM, Pallansch MA, Winkelstein JA, Lock TM, Modlin JF. Chronic group A coxsackievirus infection in agammaglobulinemia: demonstration of genomic variation of serotypically identical isolates persistently excreted by the same patient. *J Infect Dis* 1988;157:183–186.

99. Modlin JF, Polk BF, Horton P, Etking P, Crane E, Spiliotes A. Perinatal echovirus infection; risk of transmission during a community outbreak. *N Engl J Med* 1981;305:368–371.

100. Barrett-Connor E. Is insulin-dependent diabetes mellitus caused by coxsackievirus B infection: a review of the epidemiologic evidence. *Rev Infect Dis* 1985;7:207–215.

101. Bowles NE, Sewry CA, Dubowitz V, Archard LC. Dermatomyositis, polymyositis, and coxsackie-B-virus infection. *Lancet* 1987;1:1004–1007.

102. Rosenberg NL, Rotbart HA, Abzug MJ, Ringel SP, Levin MJ. Evidence for a novel picornavirus in human dermatomyositis. *Ann Neurol* 1989;26:204–209.

103. Roifman CM, Schaffer FM, Wachsmuth SE, Murphy G, Gelfand EW. Reversal of chronic polymyositis following intravenous immune serum globulin therapy. *JAMA* 1987;258:513–515.

104. Karandanis D, Shulman JA. Recent survey of infectious meningitis in adults: review of laboratory findings in bacterial, tuberculous, and aseptic meningitis. *South Med J* 1976;69:449–457.

105. Yeager AS, Bruhn FW, Clark J. Cerebrospinal fluid; presence of virus unaccompanied by pleocytosis. *J Pediatr* 1974;85:578.

106. Miller SA, Wald ER, Bergman I, DeBiasio R. Enteroviral meningitis in January with marked cerebrospinal fluid pleocytosis. *Pediatr Infect Dis* 1986;5:706–707.

107. Dagan R, Jenista JA, Menegus MA. Association of clinical presentation, laboratory findings, and virus serotypes with the presence of meningitis in hospitalized infants with enterovirus infection. *J Pediatr* 1988;113:975–978.

107a. Feigin RD, Shackelford PG. Value of repeat lumbar puncture in the differential diagnosis of meningitis. *N Engl J Med* 1973;289:571–574.

108. Malcom BS, Eiden JJ, Hendley JO. ECHO virus type 9 meningitis simulating tuberculous meningitis. *Pediatrics* 1980;65:725–726.

109. Shohat M, Lerman-Sagie T, Levy Y, Nitzan M. Cerebrospinal fluid findings in infants with nonpolio enteroviral meningitis. *Isr J Med Sci* 1988;24:233–236.

110. Jarvis WR, Tucker G. Echovirus type 7 meningitis in young children. *Am J Dis Child* 1981;135:1009–1012.

111. Howden CW, Lang WR, Laws J. An epidemic of ECHO 9 virus meningitis in Auckland. *N Z Med J* 1966;65:763–784.

112. Kaldor J, Ferris AA. Immunoglobin levels in cerebro-spinal fluid in viral and bacterial meningitis. *Med J Aust* 1969;2:1206–1209.

113. Peltola HO. C-reactive protein for rapid monitoring of infections of the central nervous system. *Lancet* 1982;1:980–983.

114. Clarke D, Cost K. Use of serum C-reactive protein in differentiating septic from aseptic meningitis in children. *J Pediatr* 1983;102:718–720.

115. Controni G, Rodriguez WJ, Hicks JM, et al. Cerebrospinal fluid lactic acid levels in meningitis. *J Pediatr* 1977;91:379–384.

116. Neches W, Platt M. Cerebrospinal fluid LDH in 287 children, including 53 cases of meningitis of bacterial and nonbacterial etiology. *Pediatrics* 1968;41:1097–1103.

117. Leist TP, Frei K, Kam-Hansen S, Zinkernagel RM, Fontana A. Tumor necrosis factor-α in cerebrospinal fluid during bacterial, but not viral, meningitis: evaluation in murine model infections and in patients. *J Exp Med* 1988;167:1743–1748.

118. Ramilo O, Mustafa MM, Porter J, Sáez-Llorens X, Mertsola J, Olsen KD, Luby JP, Beutler B, McCracken GH Jr. Detection of interleukin 1β but not tumor necrosis factor-α in cerebrospinal fluid of children with aseptic meningitis. *Am J Dis Child* 1990;144:349–352.

118a. Arditi M, Manogue KR, Yogev R. CSF cachectin (TNF-α) activity in children with bacterial and aseptic meningitis. *Pediatr Res* 1989;25:117a.

119. Chonmaitree T, Baldwin CD, Lucia HL. Role of the virology laboratory in diagnosis and management of patients with central nervous system disease. *Clin Microbiol Rev* 1989;2:1–14.

120. Lipson SM, Walderman R, Costello P, Szabo K. Sensitivity of rhabdomyosarcoma and guinea pig embryo cell cultures to field isolates of difficult-to-cultivate group A coxsackieviruses. *J Clin Microbiol* 1988;26:1298–1303.

121. Dagan R, Menegus MA. A combination of four cell types for rapid detection of enteroviruses in clinical specimens. *J Med Virol* 1986;19:219–228.

122. Chonmaitree T, Ford C, Sanders C, Lucia HL. Comparison of cell cultures for rapid isolation of enteroviruses. *J Clin Microbiol* 1988;26:2576–2580.

123. Wilfert CM, Zeller J. Enterovirus diagnosis. In: de la Maza L, Peterson EM, eds. *Medical virology IV: proceedings of the 1984 international symposium on medical virology.* London: Lawrence Erlbaum Associates, 1985;85–107.

124. Herrmann JE, Hendry RM, Collins MF. Factors involved in enzyme-linked immunoassay of viruses and evaluation of the method for identification of enteroviruses. *J Clin Microbiol* 1979;10:210–217.

125. Yolken RH, Torsch VM. Enzyme-linked immunosorbent assay for detection and identification of coxsackie B antigen in tissue cultures and clinical specimens. *J Med Virol* 1980;6:45–52.

126. Yolken RH, Torsch VM. Enzyme-linked immunosorbent assay for detection and identification of coxsackieviruses A. *Infect Immun* 1981;31:742–750.

127. Romero J, Putnak JR, Wimmer E. The use of poliovirus proteins VP3 and 2C as group antigens for the detection of enteroviral infections by indirect immunofluorescence. *Pediatr Res* 1986; 20:319A.

128. Yousef GE, Brown IN, Mowbray JF. Derivation and biochemical characterization of an enterovirus group-specific monoclonal antibody. *Intervirology* 1987;28:163–170.

129. Rotbart HA. Human enterovirus infections—molecular approaches to diagnosis and pathogenesis. In: Semler B, Ehrenfeld E, eds. *Molecular aspects of picornavirus infection and detection.* Washington, DC: American Society of Microbiology, 1989;243–264.

130. Rotbart HA, Abzug MJ, Levin MJ. Development and application of RNA probes for the study of picornaviruses. *Mol Cell Probes* 1988;2:65–73.

131. Petitjean J, Quibriac M, Freymuth F, Fuchs F, Laconche N, Aymard M, Kopecka H. Specific detection of enteroviruses in clinical samples by molecular hybridization using poliovirus subgenomic riboprobes. *J Clin Microbiol* 1990;28:307–311.

132. Rotbart HA. Polymerase chain reaction of enteroviruses. In: Innis MA, Gelfand DH, Sninsky JJ, White TJ, eds. *PCR protocols: a guide to methods and applications.* Orlando, FL: Academic Press, 1990;372–377.

133. Rotbart HA. Enzymatic RNA amplification of the enteroviruses. *J Clin Micro* 1990;28:438–442.

134. Rotbart HA. Diagnosis of enteroviral meningitis with the polymerase chain reaction. *J Pediatr* 1990;117:85–89.

135. Grist NR, Bell EJ. Paralytic poliomyelitis and nonpolio enteroviruses: studies in Scotland. *Rev Infect Dis* 1984;6:S385–S386.

136. Wadia NH, Katrak SM, Misra VP, et al. Polio-like motor paralysis associated with acute hemorrhagic conjunctivitis in an outbreak in 1981 in Bombay, India: clinical and serologic studies. *J Infect Dis* 1983;147:660–668.

137. McSharry JJ, Caliguiri LA, Eggers HJ. Inhibition of uncoating of poliovirus by arildone, a new antiviral drug. *Virology* 1979; 97:307–315.

138. Zeichhardt H, Otto MJ, McKinlay MA, Willingmann P, Habermehl K-O. Inhibition of poliovirus uncoating by disoxaril (WIN 51711). *Virology* 1987;160:281–285.

139. Otto MJ, Fox MP, Fancher MJ, Kuhrt MF, Diana GD, McKinlay MA. *In vitro* activity of WIN 51711, a new broad-spectrum antipicornavirus drug. *Antimicrob Agents Chemother* 1985; 27:883–886.

140. Woods MG, Diana GD, Rogge MC, Otto MJ, Dutko FJ, McKinlay MA. *In vitro* and *in vivo* activities of WIN 54954, a new broad-spectrum antipicornavirus drug. *Antimicrob Agents Chemother* 1989;33:2069–2074.

141. Smith TJ, Kremer MJ, Luo M, et al. The site of attachment in human rhinovirus 14 for antiviral agents that inhibit uncoating. *Science* 1986;233:1286–1293.

142. Badger J, Minor I, Dremer MJ, Oliveira MA, Smith TJ, Griffith JP. Structural analysis of a series of antiviral agents complexed with human rhinovirus 14. *Proc Natl Acad Sci USA* 1988;85:3304–3308.

143. McKinlay MA, Frank JA Jr, Benziger DP, Steinberg BA. Use of WIN 51711 to prevent echovirus type 9-induced paralysis in suckling mice. *J Infect Dis* 1986;154:676–681.

144. Jubelt B, Wilson AK, Ropka SL, Guidinger PL, McKinlay MA. Clearance of a persistent human enterovirus infection of the mouse central nervous system by the antiviral agent disoxaril. *J Infect Dis* 1989;159:866–871.

145. Casals J. Arboviruses. *Am J Clin Pathol* 1972;57:762–770.

146. Monath TP, Cropp CB, Harrison AK. Mode of entry of a neurotropic arbovirus into the central nervous system: reinvestigation of an old controversy. *Lab Invest* 1983;48:399–410.

147. Johnson RT. *Viral infections of the nervous system* New York: Raven Press, 1982.

148. Albrecht P. Pathogenesis of neurotropic arbovirus infections. In: Arber W, Braun W, Cramer F, et al., eds. *Current topics in microbiology and immunology,* vol 43. National Institute for Neurological Diseases and Blindness, NIH. Berlin: Springer-Verlag, 1968;44–91.

149. Monath TP. Flaviviruses. In: Fields BN, Knipe DM, eds. *Virology*. New York: Raven Press, 1990;763–814.
150. Tsai TF, Canfield MA, Reed CM, et al. Epidemiological aspects of a St. Louis encephalitis outbreak in Harris County, Texas, 1986. *J Infect Dis* 1988;157:351–356.
151. Tsai TF, Monath TP. Viral diseases in North America transmitted by arthropods or from vertebrate reservoirs. In: Feigin RD, Cherry JD, eds. *Textbook of pediatric infectious diseases*, 2nd ed. Philadelphia: WB Saunders, 1987;1417–1456.
152. Schmaljohn CS, Patterson JL. Bunyaviridae and their replication, Part II: replication of Bunyaviridae. In: Fields BN, Knipe DM, eds. *Virology*. New York: Raven Press, 1990;1175–1194.
153. Balfour HH Jr, Siem RA, Bauer H, Quie PG. California arbovirus (LaCrosse) infections. I. Clinical and laboratory findings in 66 children with meningoencephalitis. *Pediatrics* 1973;52:680–691.
154. Srihongse S, Grayson MA, Deibel R. California serogroup viruses in New York State: the role of subtypes in human infections. *Am J Trop Med Hyg* 1984;33:1218–1227.
155. Emmons RW. Ecology of Colorado tick fever. *Annu Rev Microbiol* 1988;42:49–64.
156. Spruance SL, Bailey A. Colorado tick fever: a review of 115 laboratory confirmed cases. *Arch Intern Med* 1973;131:288–293.
157. Silver HK, Meiklejohn G, Kempe CH. Colorado tick fever. *Am J Dis Child* 1961;101:56–61.
158. Goodpasture HC, Poland JD, Francy DB, et al. Colorado tick fever: clinical, epidemiologic, and laboratory aspects of 228 cases in Colorado in 1973–1974. *Ann Intern Med* 1978;88:303–310.
159. Eklund CM, Kohls GM, Jellison WL, et al. The clinical and ecological aspects of Colorado tick fever. In: *Proceedings of the sixth international congress on tropical medicine and malaria*, vol 5. 1959;197–203.
160. Hughes L, Casper EA, Clifford C. Persistence of Colorado tick fever virus in red blood cells. *Am J Trop Med Hyg* 1974;23:530–532.
161. Emmons RW. Orbivirus (Colorado tick fever). In: Balows A, Hausler WJ, Lenette EH, eds. *Laboratory diagnosis of infectious diseases: principles and practice*. 1988;402–410.
162. Calisher CH, Poland JD, Calisher SB, Warmoth LA. Diagnosis of Colorado tick fever virus infection by enzyme immunoassays for immunoglobulin M and G antibodies. *J Clin Microbiol* 1985;22:84–88.
163. Emmons RW, Dondero DV, Devlin V, Lennette EH. Serologic diagnosis of Colorado tick fever. A comparison of complement-fixation, immunofluorescence, and plaque-reduction methods. *Am J Trop Med Hyg* 1969;18:796–802.
164. McCarthy M, Jubelt B, Fay DB, Johnson RT. Comparative studies of five strains of mumps virus *in vitro* and in neonatal hamsters. Evaluation of growth, cytopathogenicity and neurovirulence. *J Med Virol* 1980;5:1–5.
165. Wolinsky JS, Waxham MN. Mumps virus. In: Fields BN, Knipe DM, eds. *Virology*. New York: Raven Press, 1990;989–1011.
166. Kilham L. Mumps meningoencephalitis with and without parotitis. *Am J Dis Child* 1949;78:324–333.
167. Kilham L. Isolation of mumps virus from the blood of a patient. *Proc Soc Exp Biol Med* 1948;69:99–100.
168. Wolinsky JS, Klassen T, Baringer JR. Persistence of neuroadapted mumps virus in brains of newborn hamsters after intraperitoneal inoculation. *J Infect Dis* 1976;133:260–267.
169. Bang HO, Bang J. Involvement of the central nervous system in mumps. *Acta Med Scand* 1943;113:487–505.
170. Wolinsky JS. Mumps virus-induced hydrocephalus in hamsters: ultrastructure of the chronic infection. *Lab Invest* 1977;37:229–236.
171. Russell RR, Donald JC. The neurological complications of mumps. *Br Med J* 1958;78:27–30.
172. Azimi PH, Cramblett HG, Haynes RE. Mumps meningoencephalitis in children. *JAMA* 1969;207:509–512.
173. Levison H, Thordarson O. Mumps meningitis and meningoencephalitis. *Acta Med Scand* 1942;113:314–327.
174. Bistrian B, Phillips CA, Kaye IS. Fatal mumps meningoencephalitis: isolation of virus premortem and postmortem. *JAMA* 1972;222:478–479.
175. Poser CM. Disseminated vasculomyelinopathy. *Acta Neurol Scand* 1969;45(Suppl 37):1–44.
176. Centers for Disease Control. Mumps—United States, 1985–1988. *MMWR* 1989;38:101–105.
177. Johnstone JA, Ross CAC, Dunn M. Meningitis and encephalitis associated with mumps infection; a 10-year survey. *Arch Dis Child* 1972;47:647–651.
178. Scheid W. Mumps virus and the central nervous system. *World Neurol* 1961;2:117.
179. Lennett EH, Caplan GE, Magoffin RL. Mumps virus infection simulating paralytic poliomyelitis. A report of 11 cases. *Pediatrics* 1960;25:788–797.
180. Donald PR, Burger PJ, Becker WB. Mumps meningo-encephalitis. *S Afr Med J* 1987;71:283–285.
181. Strussberg S, Winter S, Friedman A, Benderly A, Kahana D, Freundlich E. Notes on mumps meningoencephalitis: some features of 199 cases in children. *Clin Pediatr* 1969;8:373–374.
182. Wilfert CM. Mumps meningoencephalitis with low cerebrospinal-fluid glucose, prolonged pleocytosis and elevation of protein. *N Engl J Med* 1969;280:855–859.
183. Enders JF, Cohen S. Detection of antibody by complement-fixation in sera of man and monkey convalescent from mumps. *Proc Soc Exp Biol Med* 1942;50:180.
184. Freeman R, Hambling MH. Serological studies on 40 cases of mumps virus infection. *J Clin Pathol* 1980;33:28–32.
185. Grillner L, Blomberg J. Hemolysis-in-gel and neutralization tests for determination of antibodies to mumps virus. *J Clin Microbiol* 1976;4:11–15.
186. Gellis SS, McGuiness AC, Peters M. A study of the prevention of mumps orchitis by gammaglobulin. *Am J Med Sci* 1945;210:661–664.
187. Koplan JP, Preblud SR. A benefit–cost analysis of mumps vaccine. *Am J Dis Child* 1982;136:362–364.
188. Thomas E. A case of mumps meningitis: a complication of vaccination? *Can Med Assoc J* 1988;138:135.
189. Cizman M, Mozetic M, Radescek-Rakar R, Pleterski-Rigler D, Susec-Michieli M. Aseptic meningitis after vaccination against measles and mumps. *Pediatr Infect Dis J* 1989;8:302–308.
190. McDonald JC, Moore DL, Quennec P. Clinical and epidemiologic features of mumps meningoencephalitis and possible vaccine-related disease. *Pediatr Infect Dis J* 1989;8:751–755.
191. McCormick JB. Arenaviruses. In: Fields BN, Knipe DM, eds. *Virology*. New York: Raven Press, 1990;1245–1267.
192. Deibel R, Woodall JP, Decher WJ, Schryver GD. Lymphocytic choriomeningitis virus in man. Serologic evidence of association with pet hamsters. *JAMA* 1975;232:501–504.
193. Vanzee BE, Doublas RG Jr, Betts RF, Bauman AW, Frazer DW, Hinman AR. Lymphocytic choriomeningitis in university hospital personnel. Clinical features. *Am J Med* 1975;58:803–809.
194. Hirsch MS, Moellering RC Jr, Pope HG, Poskanzer DC. Lymphocytic-choriomeningitis-virus infection traced to a pet hamster. *N Engl J Med* 1974;291:610–612.
195. Warkel RL, Rinaldi CF, Bancroft WH, et al. Fatal acute meningoencephalitis due to lymphocytic choriomeningitis virus. *Neurology* 1973;23:198–203.
196. Oldstone MBA, ed. Arenaviruses: biology and immunotherapy. In: *Current topics in microbiology and immunology*. Berlin: Springer-Verlag, 1987;134.
197. Olson LC, Buescher EL, Artenstein MS, Parkman PD. Herpesvirus infections of the human central nervous system. *N Engl J Med* 1967;277:1271–1277.
198. Craig CP, Nahmias AJ. Different patterns of neurologic involvement with herpes simplex virus types 1 and 2: isolation of herpes simplex virus type 2 from the buffy coat of two adults with meningitis. *J Infect Dis* 1973;127:365–372.
199. Corey L, Adams HG, Brown ZA, Holmes KK. Genital herpes simplex virus infections: clinical manifestations, course, and complications. *Ann Intern Med* 1983;98:958–972.
200. Echevarria JM, Martinez-Martin P, Téllez A, et al. Aseptic meningitis due to varicella-zoster virus: serum antibody levels and local synthesis of specific IgG, IgM, and IgA. *J Infect Dis* 1987;155:959–967.
201. Causey JQ. Spontaneous cytomegalovirus mononucleosis-like

syndrome and aseptic meningitis. *South Med J* 1976;69:1384–1387.

202. Duchowny M, Caplan L, Siber G. Cytomegalovirus infection of the adult nervous system. *Ann Neurol* 1979;5:458–461.

203. Cappel R, Klastersky J. Herpetic meningitis (type 1) in a case of acute leukemia. *Arch Neurol* 1973;28:415–416.

204. Hartford CG, Wellinghoff W, Weinstein RA. Isolation of herpes simplex from the cerebrospinal fluid in viral meningitis. *Neurology (Minneap)* 1975;25:198–200.

205. Skoldenberg B, Jeansson S, Wolontis S. Herpes simplex virus type 2 and acute aseptic meningitis: clinical feature of cases with isolation of herpes simplex virus from cerebrospinal fluids. *Scand J Infect Dis* 1975;7:227–232.

205a. Johnson R, Milbourn PE. Central nervous system manifestations of chickenpox. *Can Med Assoc J* 1970;102:831–834.

205b. Echeverria JM, Martinez-Martin P, Tellez A, et al. Aseptic meningitis due to varicella-zoster virus: serum antibody levels and local synthesis of specific IgG, IgM, and IgA. *J Infect Dis* 1987;155:959–967.

205c. Mayo DR, Booss J. Varicella zoster-associated neurologic disease without skin disease. *Arch Neurol* 1989;46:313–315.

205d. Karp SJ. Meningitis and disseminated cutaneous zoster complicating herpes zoster infection. *J Neurol Neurosurg Psychiatry* 1983;46:582–590.

205e. Gold E. Serologic and virus-isolation studies of patients with varicella or herpes-zoster infection. *N Engl J Med* 1966;274:181–185.

205f. Silverstein A, Steinberg G, Nathanson M. Nervous system involvement in infectious mononucleosis. *Arch Neurol* 1972;26:353–358.

206. Steel JG, Dix RD, Baringer JR. Isolation of herpes simplex virus type 1 in recurrent (Mollaret) meningitis. *Ann Neurol* 1982;11:17–21.

207. Graman PS. Mollaret's meningitis associated with acute Epstein–Barr virus mononucleosis. *Arch Neurol* 1987;44:1204–1205.

208. Hänninen P, Arstila P, Lang H, et al. Involvement of the central nervous system in acute, uncomplicated measles virus infection. *J Clin Microbiol* 1980;11:610–613.

209. Wong VK, Steinberg E, Warford A. Parainfluenza virus type 3 meningitis in an 11-month-old infant. *Pediatr Infect Dis J* 1988;7:300–301.

210. Paisley JW, Bruhn FW, Lauer BA, McIntosh K. Type A$_2$ influenza viral infections in children. *Am J Dis Child* 1978;132:34–36.

211. Wong CJ, Price Z, Bruckner DA. Aseptic meningitis in an infant with rotavirus gastroenteritis. *Pediatr Infect Dis* 1984;3:244–246.

212. Gajdusek DC. Review article—encephalomyocarditis virus infection in childhood. *Pediatrics* 1955;16:902–906.

213. Hollander H, Stringari S. Human immunodeficiency virus-associated meningitis: clinical course and correlations. *Am J Med* 1987;83:813–816.

214. Levy RM, Bredesen DE, Rosenblum ML. Neurological manifestations of the acquired immunodeficiency syndrome (AIDS): experience at UCSF and review of the literature. *J Neurosurg* 1985;62:475–495.

215. Ho DD, Sarngadharan MG, Resnick L, Dimarzo-Veronese F, Rota TR, Hirsch MS. Primary human T-lymphotropic virus type III infection. *Ann Intern Med* 1985;103:880–883.

216. Bredesen DE, Lipkin WI, Messing R, et al. Prolonged recurrent aseptic meningitis with prominent cranial nerve abnormalities: a new epidemic in gay men? *Neurology* 1983;33(Suppl 2):85.

217. Yokota T, Yamada M, Furukawa T, Tsukagoshi. HTLV-I-associated meningitis. *J Neurol* 1988;235:129–130.

218. Hubbert WT, Humphrey GL. Epidemiology of leptospirosis in California: a cause of aseptic meningitis. *Calif Med* 1968;108:113–117.

219. Lecour H, Miranda M, Magro C, et al. Human leptospirosis—a review of 50 cases. *Infection* 1989;17:10–14.

220. Edwards GA, Domm BM. Human leptospirosis. *Medicine* 1960;39:117–156.

221. Steere A. Lyme disease. *N Engl J Med* 1989;321:586–596.

222. Pachner AR, Steere AC. The triad of neurologic manifestations of Lyme disease: meningitis, cranial neuritis, and radiculoneuritis. *Neurology* 1985;35:47–53.

223. Halperin JJ, Luft BJ, Anand AK, et al. Lyme neuroborreliosis: central nervous system manifestations. *Neurology* 1989;39:753–759.

224. Auerbach O. Tuberculous meningitis. Correlation of therapeutic results with pathogenesis and pathologic changes; general considerations and pathogenesis. *Am Rev Tuberc* 1951;64:408.

225. Idriss ZH, Sinno AA, Kronfol NM. Tuberculous meningitis in childhood. Forty-three cases. *Am J Dis Child* 1976;130:364.

226. Smith AL. Tuberculous meningitis in childhood. *Med J Aust* 1975;1:57.

227. Rich AR, McCordock HA. Pathogenesis of tuberculous meningitis. *Bull Johns Hopkins Hosp* 1933;52:5.

228. Emond RTC, McKendrick GDW. Tuberculosis as a cause of transient aseptic meningitis. *Lancet* 1973;2:234–236.

229. Kennedy DH, Fallon RJ. Tuberculous meningitis. *JAMA* 1979;241:264–268.

230. Kalis NN, Donald PR, Burger PJ, Becker WB. Simultaneous occurrence of mumps meningoencephalitis and tuberculosis meningitis. *Pediatr Infect Dis J* 1989;8:476–477.

230a. Young EJ. Human brucellosis. *Rev Infect Dis* 1983;5:821–842.

231. Salaki JS, Louria DB, Chemel H. Fungal and yeast infections of the central nervous system: a clinical review. *Medicine* 1984;63:108–132.

232. Lind K, Zoffmann H, Larsen SO, Jessen O. *Mycoplasma pneumoniae* infection associated with affection of the central nervous system. *Acta Med Scand* 1979;205:325–332.

233. Roe O, Jorgen D, Matre R. Isolation of *Mycoplasma hominis* from cerebrospinal fluid. *Scand J Infect Dis* 1973;5:285–288.

234. Wheathall SR. *Mycoplasma* meningitis in infants with spina bifida. *Dev Med Child Neurol* 1975;17(Suppl 35):117–122.

235. Waites KB, Rudd P, Canupp K, et al. Colonization of cerebrospinal fluid in neonates by *Mycoplasma hominis* and *Ureaplasma urealyticum*. In: Program and Abstracts of the Sixth International Congress of the International Organization for Mycoplasmology, Birmingham, Alabama, August 26–31, 1986;11–95A.

236. Johnson RT, Richardson EP. The neurological manifestations of systemic lupus erythematosus. *Medicine* 1968;47:337–369.

237. Canoso JJ, Cohen AS. Aseptic meningitis in systemic lupus erythematosus: report of three cases. *Arthritis Rheum* 1975;18:369–373.

238. O'Connor JF, Mosher DM. Central nervous system involvement in systemic lupus erythematosus. *Arch Neurol* 1966;14:157–164.

239. Sands ML, Ryczak M, Brown RB. Recurrent aseptic meningitis followed by transverse myelitis as a presentation of systemic lupus erythematosus. *J Rheumatol* 1988;15:862–864.

240. Widener HL, Littman BH. Ibuprofen-induced meningitis in systemic lupus erythematosus. *JAMA* 1978;239:1062–1064.

241. Ballas ZK, Donta ST. Sulindac-induced aseptic meningitis. *Arch Intern Med* 1982;142:165–166.

242. Ruppert GB, Barth WF. Tolmetin-induced meningitis. *JAMA* 1981;245:67–68.

243. Greenberg GN. Recurrent sulindac-induced aseptic meningitis in a patient tolerant to other nonsteroidal anti-inflammatory drugs. *South Med J* 1988;81:1463–1464.

244. O'Brien WM. Adverse reactions to nonsteroidal anti-inflammatory drugs; diclofenac compared with other nonsteroidal anti-inflammatory drugs. *Am J Med* 1986;80(Suppl 4B):70–80.

245. Alexander EI, Provost TT, Stevens MB, Alexander GE. Neurologic complications of primary Sjögren's syndrome. *Medicine* 1982;61:247–257.

246. Bathon JM, Moreland LW, DiBartolomeo AG. Inflammatory central nervous system involvement in rheumatoid arthritis. *Semin Arthritis Rheum* 1989;18:258–266.

247. Ewert BH. Resident article: ibuprofen-associated meningitis in a woman with only serologic evidence of a rheumatologic disorder. *Am J Med Sci* 1989;297:326–327.

248. Lawson JM, Grady MJ. Ibuprofen-induced aseptic meningitis in a previously healthy patient. *West J Med* 1985;143:386–387.

249. Shoenfeld Y, Livni E, Shaklai M, Pinkas J. Sensitization to ibuprofen in systemic lupus erythematosus. *JAMA* 1980;244:547–548.

250. Berliner S, Weinberger A, Shoenfeld Y, et al. Ibuprofen may induce meningitis in (NZB × NZW)F1 mice. *Arthritis Rheum* 1985;28:104–107.

251. Thordarson H, Talstad I. Acute meningitis and cerebellar dysfunction complicating high-dose cytosine arabinoside therapy. *Acta Med Scand* 1986;220:493–495.

252. Kato E, Shindo S, Eto Y, et al. Administration of immune globulin associated with aseptic meningitis. *JAMA* 1988;259:3269–3270.

253. Martin MA, Massanari M, Nghiem DD, et al. Nosocomial aseptic meningitis associated with administration of OKT3. *JAMA* 1988;259:2002–2005.

254. Centers for Disease Control. Aseptic meningitis among kidney transplant recipients receiving a newly marketed murine monoclonal antibody preparation. *MMWR* 1986;35:551–552.

255. Carlson J, Wiholm B-E. Trimethoprim associated aseptic meningitis. *Scand J Infect Dis* 1987;19:687–691.

256. Farmer L, Echalin FA, Loughlin WC. Pachymeningitis apparently due to penicillin hypersensitivity. *Ann Intern Med* 1960;52:910–915.

257. Garagusi VF, Neefe LI, Mann O. Acute meningoencephalitis associated with isoniazid administration. *JAMA* 1976;235:1141–1142.

258. Hilton E, Stroh EM. Aseptic meningitis associated with administration of carbamazepine. *J Infect Dis* 1989;159:363–364.

259. Hermans PE, Goldstein NP, Wellman WE. Mollaret's meningitis and differential diagnosis of recurrent meningitis; report of case, with review of the literature. *Am J Med* 1972;52:128–140.

260. Mascia RA, Smith CW. Mollaret's meningitis: an unusual disease with a characteristic presentation. *Am J Med Sci* 1984;287:52–53.

261. Stoppe G, Stark E, Patzold U. Mollaret's meningitis: CSF-immunocytological examinations. *J Neurol* 1987;234:103–106.

262. Kawasaki T, Kosaki F, Okawa S, et al. A new infantile mucocutaneous lymph node syndrome (MLNS) prevailing in Japan. *Pediatrics* 1974;54:271.

263. Melish ME, Hicks RM, Larson EJ. Mucocutaneous lymph node syndrome in the United States. *Am J Dis Child* 1976;130:599–607.

264. Morens DM, Anderson LJ, Hurwitz ES. National surveillance of Kawasaki disease. *Pediatrics* 1980;65:21–25.

Infections of the Central Nervous System,
edited by W. M. Scheld, R. J. Whitley, and
D. T. Durack, Raven Press, Ltd., New York © 1991.

CHAPTER 4

Encephalitis Caused by Herpesviruses, Including B Virus

Richard J. Whitley and Michael Schlitt

Eight herpesviruses cause human disease; seven, including herpes simplex virus 1 (HSV-1), and herpes simplex virus 2 (HSV-2), cytomegalovirus (CMV), varicella-zoster virus, (VZV), Epstein–Barr virus (EBV), human herpesvirus 6 (HHV-6), and human herpesvirus 7 (HHV-7), are usual human pathogens. One simian herpesvirus, B virus (*Crypotetia crypta*), can also infect humans, resulting in devastating central nervous system (CNS) disease. These viruses share similar molecular and biologic characteristics, being double-stranded DNA viruses and having the unique ability to establish latency and be reactivated. These agents, among the most common encountered by humans, are frequent causes of CNS infections.

Since the first suggestions of herpes simplex encephalitis (HSE) by the Mathewson Commission in 1926 (1) and the subsequent description of the histopathologic changes seen in a case of herpes encephalitis (2), HSV has been recognized as the most common cause of sporadic fatal encephalitis in the United States (3). VZV, the causative agent in chickenpox and zoster (shingles), has been associated with a wide variety of neurologic complications, ranging from a benign cerebellar ataxia to fulminant and life-threatening encephalitis. Inadvertent infection with B virus in animal workers leads to severe CNS disease. Patients with acquired immunodeficiency virus [from human immunodeficiency virus (HIV)] infections may have unusual manifestations of CMV and EBV infections of the CNS. Infections of the CNS caused by HHV-6 and HHV-7 have not been documented at

this time. This chapter will summarize our knowledge of herpesvirus infections of the CNS; particular reference will be made to HSV, VZV, and B virus, since CNS infections with CMV and EBV are less well characterized.

GENERAL CHARACTERISTICS OF HERPESVIRUSES

All herpesviridae have a similar molecular structure. These viruses contain double-stranded DNA which is located at the central core. The DNA is surrounded by a capsid, consisting of 262 capsomers and providing icosapentahedral symmetry to the virus. The structure of a prototype herpesvirus, namely HSV, is shown in Fig. 1. Tightly adherent to the capsid is an amorphous tegument. Loosely surrounding the capsid is a lipid bilayer envelope. The overall size of herpes virions varies from 120 nm to approximately 300 nm, depending upon the virus. The envelope consists of polyamines, lipids, and glycoproteins. The glycoproteins confer distinctive properties to each virus, providing unique antigens to which the host is capable of responding.

Table 1 summarizes the herpesviruses known to infect humans, according to the three subfamilies (α, β, or γ) and genome characteristics. Herpesvirus DNA varies in molecular weight from approximately 80 to 150 million and consists of 120,000 to 230,000 base pairs. Base composition of herpesvirus DNA varies between 31% and 75% of guanine plus cytosine.

Herpesvirus DNA is divided into six groups arbitrarily classified A to F. For those herpesviruses which infect humans (group C, group D, and group E), unique genomic structures are demonstrable. In the group C genomes, as exemplified by EBV, the number of terminal reiterations divides the genome into several well-delineated domains. The group D genomes, such as

R. Whitley: Department of Pediatrics, Microbiology, and Medicine, University of Alabama, Birmingham, Alabama 35294.

M. Schlitt: 3915 Talbot Road South, Renton, Washington 98055; formerly with the Department of Neurosurgery, University of South Alabama 36617.

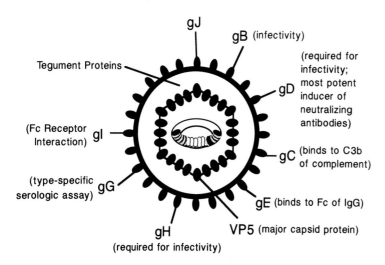

FIG. 1. Prototype herpesvirus with structure of HSV demonstrated. VP5, viral capsid protein 5; gB, glycoprotein B; gC, glycoprotein C; gD, glycoprotein D; gE, glycoprotein E; gG, glycoprotein G; gH, glycoprotein H; gI, glycoprotein I; gJ, glycoprotein J; IgG, immunoglobulin G.

VZV, have sequences from one terminus repeated in an inverted orientation internally. Thus, the DNA extracted from these virions consists of two equimolar populations. For group E viral genomes, such as HSV and CMV, the genomes are divided into internal unique sequences whereby both termini are repeated in an inverted orientation. Thus, the genomes can form four equimolar populations which differ only in the relative orientation of the two components.

Of all the herpesviruses, HSV-1 and HSV-2 are the most closely related, with approximately 50% genomic homology. Examples of differences in the molecular weight of these viruses are as follows: HSV-1 and HSV-2 have a molecular weight of approximately 100 million; EBV, 114 million; and CMV, 150 million. With the exception of HSV-1 and HSV-2, the structural and nonstructural proteins coded by the DNA of the human herpesviruses are not immunologically related. However, HSV-1 and HSV-2 share common types of proteins and, therefore, cross-antigenic reactions do occur.

The current classification of herpesviruses into subfamilies serves the purpose of identifying evolutionary relatedness as well as summarizing unique properties of each member. Three herpesviruses subfamilies exist: alpha, beta, and gamma herpesviruses. The members of

the alpha herpesvirus family are characterized by a very short reproductive cycle, prompt destruction of the host cell, and ability to establish latency, usually in sensory ganglia. This subfamily consists of HSV-1, HSV-2 and VZV. Beta herpesviruses have a host range restricted to tissues of human organs. In contrast to the reproductive life cycle of the alpha herpesviruses, that of the beta herpesviruses is long, with infection progressing slowly in cell culture systems. A characteristic of these viruses is their ability to form enlarged cells, as occurs with human CMV infection. These viruses can be maintained in a latent state in secretory glands, cells of the reticuloendothelial system (particularly lymphatic cells), and kidneys, among other tissues. Finally, the gamma herpesviruses (EBV) have the most limited host range. These viruses replicate in lymphoblastoid cells *in vitro* and can cause lytic infections in certain targeted cells. Latent virus often can be found in lymphoid tissue. Conceptually, HHV-6 should be classified as a gamma herpesvirus; however, it has a host range similar to that of a beta herpesvirus. Future studies will have to clarify its true classification and will also have to clarify the newly described HHV-7.

HERPES SIMPLEX VIRUS

History

Infections caused by HSV have been recognized since the time of ancient Greece. Greek physicians used the word "herpes" to mean creeping or crawling in reference to skin lesions. Likely, this word was used to describe a variety of skin conditions, ranging from cancer to shingles and probably even fever blisters. The Roman scholar Herodotus associated mouth ulcers and lip vesicles with fever (4) and called this event "herpes febrilis." Genital herpetic infections were described first by a physician to the French royalty, Astruc (5).

The transmissibility of these viruses was established

TABLE 1. *Selected viruses of the family Herpesviridae*

Common name	Subfamily	G + C (mole %)	Genome size (kilobase pairs)
Herpes simplex virus 1	α	67	152
Herpes simplex virus 2	α	69	152
Varicella-zoster virus	α	46	125
Epstein–Barr virus	γ	60	172
Cytomegalovirus	β	57	229
Human herpesvirus 6	NA	42	170
Human herpesvirus 7	—	—	—
B virus	α	75	107

a G + C, guanine plus cystosine.

unequivocally by passage of virus from human lip and genital lesions to either the cornea or the scarified skin of the rabbit (6). Goodpasture (7) further demonstrated that material derived from herpes labialis consistently produced encephalitis when inoculated onto the scarified cornea of rabbits.

Intranuclear inclusion bodies consistent with HSV infection were first demonstrated in the brain of a neonate with encephalitis by Smith et al. (2) in 1941. Virus was subsequently isolated from this brain tissue (2). The first adult case of HSE providing similar proof of viral disease (i.e., intranuclear inclusions in brain tissue and virus isolation) was described in 1944 by Zarafonetis et al. (8). The most striking pathologic finding in this patient's brain was apparent in the left temporal lobe, which demonstrated perivascular cuffs of lymphocytes and numerous small hemorrhages. This temporal lobe localization subsequently has been determined to be characteristic of adult HSE, and it differs from the patchy diffuse encephalitis of neonates with HSV brain infection.

In the mid-1960s, Nahmias and Dowdle (9) demonstrated two antigenic types of HSV; this distinction led to the clarification of the epidemiology of herpes infections. Viral typing allowed the demonstration that HSV-1 was primarily responsible for infections "above the belt" (including brain disease in adults), whereas HSV-2 was primarily responsible for infections "below the belt" and brain disease in neonates. Over the past 15 years our knowledge of HSV has expanded, particularly in the biochemistry of replication and resultant gene products as well as in the epidemiology, natural history, and pathogenesis of HSV infections.

Infectious Agent

Recent detailed reviews highlight the importance of these organisms as models of viral replication and as pathogens for human infection. A brief review of the specific characteristics of HSV is indicated (10–12). Our current understanding of the structure of HSV indicates that the genome has a molecular weight of approximately 100 million (13). The DNA encodes about 70 polypeptides, few of which are understood biologically (14). The DNAs of HSV-1 and HSV-2 are collinear with reasonable, but not identical, matching of base pairs. Of note, there is considerable overlap in the cross-reactivity between the HSV-1 and HSV-2 glycoproteins, although uniqueness can be demonstrated, as discussed below (10,15–18). Distinction between the two viral types can be demonstrated by restriction enzyme analyses of viral DNA patterns. This technique has been applied to epidemiologic investigations of human HSV infections.

Replication of HSV is characterized by the expression of three gene classes: immediate-early, early, and late, which are expressed temporally and in a rolling circle

sequence (19,20). A few relevant events will be noted. There are five immediate early genes, one of which is necessary for imitating viral replication. One other immediate-early gene, alpha-0, probably has a role in latency. The early gene products include those enzymes necessary for viral replication (such as HSV thymidine kinase), as well as the regulatory proteins. Current antivirals with a selective mechanism of action are activated at the level of early gene expression. Acyclovir is an example of such a drug, being transformed into an active monophosphate derivative by HSV thymidine kinase (21). Early gene expression coincides with an irreversible shut-off of host cellular macromolecular protein synthesis (20), which results in cell death. Structural proteins are usually of the late gene class (18,20). Assembly of the virus begins in the nucleus, and the envelope is acquired as the capsid buds through the inner lamella of the nuclear membrane, as shown in Fig. 2. Virus is transported

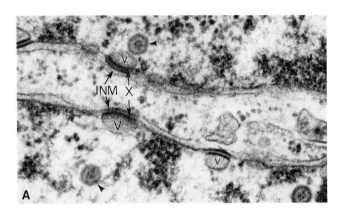

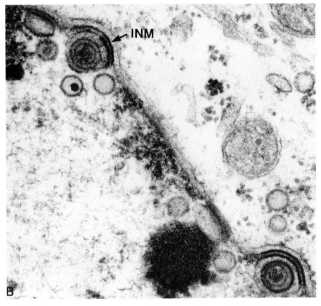

FIG. 2. Electron-microscopic maturation of HSV. **A:** Electron micrograph showing early vesiculation at the internuclear membrane (INM). **B:** Electron micrograph showing development of an encapsidated HSV at the INM. (Courtesy of S. Chatterjee, Ph.D.)

through the cytoskeleton to the plasma membrane, where lysis of the cell and release of progeny virions occurs. The replicative efficiency of HSV is poor, as indicated by the ratio of infectious to noninfectious virions.

The biologic properties of the eight glycoproteins gB, gC, gD, gE, gG, gH, gI, and gJ have been summarized and portrayed in Fig. 1 (10,18). Of relevance to CNS disease, glycoprotein D (gD) is related to viral infectivity and is the most potent inducer of neutralizing antibodies. Glycoprotein B (gB) is required for infectivity. Glycoprotein C (gC) binds to the C3b component of complement, whereas glycoprotein E (gE) binds to the Fc portion of immunoglobulin G (IgG). A deletion in gC enhances viral pathogenicity, particularly for the CNS (22). Glycoprotein G (gG) provides antigenic specificity to HSV and, therefore, results in an antibody response which allows for the distinction between HSV-1 (gG-1) and HSV-2 (gG-2). Glycoprotein I (gI) (23) is thought to be involved with gE at the Fc receptor. The role of glycoprotein J (gJ) is not well understood.

Pathology and Pathogenesis

General Pathologic Observations

The pathologic changes induced by replicating HSV are similar for both primary and recurrent infection but vary in the quantitative extent of cytopathology. The histopathologic characteristics of a skin lesion induced by HSV represent a combination of virus-mediated cellular death and associated inflammatory responses. Changes induced by viral infection include ballooning of infected cells and the appearance of chromatin within the nuclei

of cells; this is followed by degeneration of the cellular nuclei, generally within parabasal and intermediate cells of the epithelium. Cells lose intact plasma membranes and form multinucleated giant cells. If replication occurs within the skin (along with cell lysis), vesicular fluid containing large quantities of virus appears between the epidermis and dermal layer. In dermal substructures there is an intense inflammatory response, usually in the corium of the skin; this occurs more frequently with primary infection than with recurrent infection. With healing, the vesicular fluid becomes pustular with the recruitment of inflammatory cells, subsequently producing a scab. Scarring is uncommon, but it occasionally occurs in patients with frequently recurrent lesions.

Local lymphatics can show evidence of infection with intrusion of inflammatory cells because they drain infected secretions from the area of viral replication. The intensity of the inflammatory response is significantly less with recurrent disease. As host defenses are mounted, an influx of mononuclear cells can be detected in infected tissue.

Pathology of CNS Disease

The gross appearance of the brain in adults with HSE initially shows acute inflammation, congestion and/or hemorrhage, and softening, most prominently in the temporal lobes and usually disposed asymptomatically (24). Adjacent limbic areas show involvement as well. The meninges overlying the temporal lobes may appear clouded or congested. After approximately 2 weeks these changes proceed to frank necrosis and liquefaction as shown in Fig. 3.

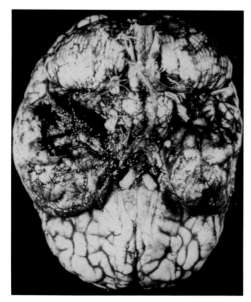
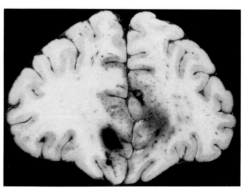

FIG. 3. Gross pathologic findings in HSE, illustrating hemorrhagic necrosis of the inferior medial portion of the temporal lobe.

Microscopically, involvement extends beyond areas that appear grossly abnormal. At the earliest stage the histological changes are not dramatic and may be non-specific. Congestion of capillaries and other small vessels in the cortex and subcortical white matter is evident; other changes are also evident, including petechiae. Vascular changes which have been reported in the area of infection include areas of hemorrhagic necrosis and perivascular cuffing (Fig. 4A and 4B). The perivascular cuffing becomes prominent in the second and third weeks of infection. Glial nodules are common after the second week (25). The microscopic appearance becomes dominated by evidence of necrosis and, eventually, inflammation; the latter is characterized by a diffuse perivascular subarachnoid mononuclear cell infiltrate, gliosis, and satellitosis–neuronophagia (24,26). In such cases, widespread areas of hemorrhagic necrosis, mirroring the area of infection, become most prominent. Oligodendrocytic involvement and gliosis (as well as astrocytosis) are common, but these changes develop very late in the disease course. Though found in only approximately 50% of patients, the presence of intranuclear inclusions supports the diagnosis of viral infection, and these inclusions are most often visible in the first week of infection. The intranuclear inclusions (Cowdry type A inclusions) are characterized by an eosinophilic homogeneous appearance often surrounded by a clear, unstained zone beyond which lies a rim of marginated chromatin, as shown in Fig. 5.

Pathogenesis: General Observations

The pathogenesis of human disease is dependent upon the intimate, personal contact of a susceptible individual (namely, one who is seronegative) with someone excreting HSV. Virus must come in contact with mucosal surfaces or abraded skin for infection to be initiated. With viral replication at the site of infection, the capsid is transported by neurons to the dorsal root ganglia, where, after another round of viral replication, latency is established. These events have been demonstrated in a variety of ani-

mal models, as reviewed elsewhere (27). Transport of the virion is by retrograde axonal flow (28). In some instances, replication can lead to severe CNS infection; however, more usually a host–virus interaction resulting in latency occurs. After latency is established, reactivation can occur with virus proliferation and shedding at mucocutaneous sites, appearing as skin vesicles or mucosal ulcers. Occasionally, primary infection can become systemic, affecting other organ systems besides the central and peripheral nervous systems. Such circumstances include: disseminated neonatal HSV infection with multiorgan involvement; multiorgan disease of pregnancy; and, infrequently, dissemination in patients undergoing immunosuppressive therapy. It is reasonable to presume that widespread organ involvement is the consequence of viremia in a host not capable of limiting replication to mucosal surfaces.

Infection with HSV-1, generally limited to the oropharynx, can be transmitted by respiratory droplets or through direct contact (by a susceptible individual) with infectious secretions (such as virus contained in orolabial vesicular fluid). Thus, initial replication of virus will occur in the oropharyngeal mucosa. Invariably, the trigeminal ganglia will become colonized and harbor latent virus; it is not clear why other cranial nerve systems (VII, IX, X, and XII) are not invaded successfully. On the other hand, acquisition of HSV-2 infection is usually the consequence of transmission via genital routes. Under these circumstances, virus replicates in the vaginal tract or on penile skin sites, with seeding of the sacral ganglia.

For individuals susceptible to HSV infections (namely, those without preexisting antibodies), first exposure to either HSV-1 or HSV-2 will result in that which is defined as a "primary" infection. The epidemiology and clinical characteristics of primary infection are distinctly different from those associated with recurrent infection. After the establishment of latency, a recurrence of HSV is known as "reactivated" or "recurrent" infection. This form of infection leads to recurrent vesicular lesions of the skin, such as HSV labialis or recurrent HSV genitalis. The status of our knowledge of latency and the subsequent events of reactivation are discussed

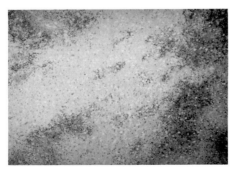
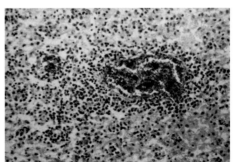

A B

FIG. 4. A: Hemorrhagic necrosis on microscopic examination. **B:** Perivascular cuffing on histopathologic examination of a patient with HSE.

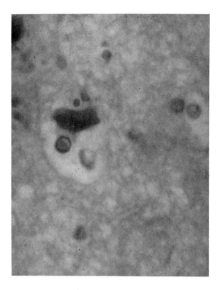 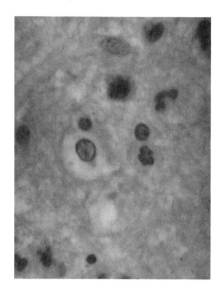

FIG. 5. Intranuclear inclusions.

below. Individuals with preexisting antibodies to one type of HSV can experience a first infection with the opposite virus type at a different site. Under such circumstances, the infection is known as an "initial" infection rather than as a primary one. An example of an initial infection would be an infection that occurs in those individuals who have preexisting HSV-1 antibodies (acquired after HSV gingivostomatitis) and who then acquire a genital HSV-2 infection. It should also be noted that reinfection with different strains of HSV can occur.

Pathogenesis of Latency

A most interesting property of all of the herpesviruses is their ability to become latent, persist in an apparent inactive state for varying durations of time, and be reactivated by a provocative stimulus, also as yet unequivocally specified (11,29–34). Thus, after infection, viral DNA (or a fragment thereof) persists in the host for the entire lifetime of the individual. As a biologic phenomenon, latency has been recognized since the beginning of this century (29,31–33,35–41). In 1905, Cushing (42) noted that patients treated for trigeminal neuralgia (by sectioning a branch of the trigeminal nerve) developed herpetic lesions along the innervated areas of the sectioned branch, as suggested previously by Goodpasture (43). Observations by Carlton and Kilbourne (44) and Pazin et al. (45,46), as well as by others (47), have demonstrated that microvascular surgery of the trigeminal nerve tract for tic douloureux resulted in recurrent herpetic lesions in over 90% of seropositive individuals. Axonal injury and attempts at excision of lesions have been associated with recurrences (48,49). Reactivation of la-

tent virus appears to be dependent upon an intact anterior nerve route and peripheral nerve pathways (50). No data exist to support that HSV is present in peripheral skin tissue in a latent state (32,51).

Recurrences appear despite the presence of both cell-mediated and humoral immunity. No virus can be isolated from patients during those times between recurrences, at or near the usual site of recurrent lesions. Recurrences are spontaneous, but there have been associations with physical or emotional stress, fever, exposure to ultraviolet light, tissue damage, and immune suppression (33,40,52,53). Herpes labialis develops three times more frequently in febrile patients than in nonfebrile controls (54,55). Viral DNA can be detected in neuronal tissue in the absence of cutaneous lesions (27,32,37, 56–60).

Recently, initial reports have suggested that maintenance of a latent state results from an antisense message that maps in the ICP0 region of the viral genome, known as the "latency-associated transcript" (LAT) (61). Subsequently, LAT has been identified in trigeminal ganglia collected from humans at the time of autopsy (62). Engineered viruses with genomic deletions in LAT have been used to infect mice and rabbits. Upon co-cultivation of the explanted ganglia from these animals, the mutant viruses could be reactivated (63,64). Thus, LAT is not a simple solution to the latency problem.

Latent virus has been retrieved from the trigeminal, sacral, and vagal ganglia of humans (29,35,36,56,60). Trigeminal ganglia have been found to harbor latent virus in approximately 50% of cases, which helps explain the observation of vesicles that recur on the vermillion border of the lip. Random screening of sacral ganglia indicated a positivity rate of about 10%. It is unknown whether HSV can become latent directly in human brain tissue as occurs in some animal models.

Pathogenesis of Encephalitis

The pathogenesis of HSE is only partly understood. It is apparent that both primary and recurrent HSV infections can cause disease of the CNS. From studies performed by the National Institute of Allergy and Infectious Diseases (NIAID) Collaborative Antiviral Study Group, it was learned that approximately one-third of the cases of HSE are the consequence of primary infection. For the most part, the patients with primary infection are less than 18 years of age. The remaining two-thirds of cases occur in the presence of preexisting antibodies, but only approximately 10% of patients have a history of recurrent herpes simplex labialis. Patients with preexisting antibodies are considered to have HSE as a consequence of reactivation of HSV (65). When the DNAs from the resulting peripheral and CNS isolates are compared by restriction endonuclease analyses, identity of the isolates is usually identical; however, this is not always the case. The virus isolated from the peripheral site is often different from that retrieved from the CNS (66). Thus, the issue of reactivation of virus directly within the CNS, the potential for enhanced neurotropism of certain viruses, and the selective reactivation and access of one virus by the trigeminal route or other routes to the CNS remain for further elucidation. However, as discussed below, it is unclear whether reaction can occur directly in the CNS, being localized initially to one temporal lobe.

The route of access of virus to the CNS in primary infection is a subject of debate, especially in humans. While studies performed over five decades ago defined pathways for HSV access to the brain in animals, including both the olfactory and trigeminal nerves among others (67), it is not clear which of these nerve tracts uniformly leads to HSV infection in the CNS of humans. The anatomic distribution of nerves from the olfactory tract into the limbic system, along with the recovery of virus from the temporal lobe (the site of apparent onset of HSE in the human brain), suggests that viral access to the CNS via this route is a tenable hypothesis. Reports in the literature have found electron-microscopic evidence that, in fact, this has been the case in some individuals with HSE (68–71). Animal model data support the contention that the olfactory tract provides one neurologic avenue for viral access to the CNS and causes localization of the infection in brain regions analogous to medial temporal structures in humans (72,73). Definitive proof for such progression in humans is lacking. No doubt the pathogenesis of human disease is far more complex than simple accession of virus by the olfactory tract; the immunologic status of the nasal passages and/or the "neurovirulence" of a given strain must play a role.

Reactivation of HSV, leading to focal HSE, is a similarly confusing problem from the standpoint of pathogenesis. While it is possible to demonstrate evidence of latent virus infection within infected brain tissue (74), the likelihood of reactivation at that site remains purely hypothetical. Reactivation of virus peripherally (namely, in the olfactory bulb or the trigeminal ganglion) with subsequent neuronal transmission to the CNS has been suggested (67,73,75,76). Nevertheless, a relevant observation is that with recurrent HSV labialis, whereby reactivation of virus from the trigeminal ganglia occurs, HSE is a very uncommon event. Furthermore, HSE does not occur more frequently in immunocompromised patients. These questions will provide important subjects for future investigations, particularly with the recent development of appropriate animal models and newer technology to study pathogenesis, such as the polymerase chain reaction.

Host immunity plays an important, but as yet undefined, role in the pathogenesis of HSE. It is possible that the CNS is particularly prone to HSV infection because intraneuronal spread may shelter virus from defense mechanisms. HSE is no more common in the immunosuppressed host than in the normal host; however, when it does occur, the presentation is atypical with a subacute but progressively deteriorating course (77). Mucocutaneous HSV infections, on the other hand, are much more common and severe in immunocompromised hosts (24).

Epidemiology

The epidemiology of HSV infections is multifaceted. Because the focus of this book is on CNS infections, only a brief review of HSV infections follows. The reader is referred to more complete reviews (78,79). HSVs are distributed worldwide and have been reported in both developed and underdeveloped countries, including remote Brazilian tribes (80). Animal vectors for human HSV infections have not been described; therefore, humans remain the sole reservoir for transmission of these viruses to other humans. Virus is transmitted from infected individuals to susceptible individuals during close personal contact. There is no seasonal variation in the incidence of infection. Because infection is rarely fatal and these viruses become latent, it is estimated that over one-third of the world's population has recurrent HSV infections and is, therefore, capable of transmitting HSV during episodes of productive infection. HSV diseases range from mild (even undiscernible) in the majority of patients, to sporadic, severe, and life-threatening disease in very few infants, children, and adults. Children, particularly those less than 5 years of age, are most often infected; however, primary infections can also occur in older individuals. With clinical illness, oropharyngeal disease, namely gingivostomatitis, usually is the manifestation. Primary infection in young adults has been associated with pharyngitis and, often, a mononucleosis-like syndrome (81). Like other herpesvirus infections, seroprevalence studies have demonstrated that acquisition of HSV-1 infection is related to socioeconomic factors. The association of HSV with primary gingivostomatitis—and its confirmation by Burnett and Williams (82), as further elucidated by Dodd et al. (83)—led to the definition of the natural history of infection, including the appearance of neutralizing antibodies (84), absence of virus shedding in children less than 6 months of age (85), and a higher rate of occurrence among individuals of lower socioeconomic status. Contemporary surveys document the viral shedding data, ranging from 2% to 5% (86–93).

Advances in antibody detection methodology have helped clarify the epidemiology of infection. Geographic location, socioeconomic status, and age all influence to a considerable extent the frequency of HSV infection. These associations were brought to light by several investigators (82,94–96), and these data have been summarized by Rawls and Campione-Piccardo (97). Utilizing antibody prevalence in developing countries, seroconversion occurs early in life, but with some minor differences between selected populations. In Brazilian Indians, HSV antibodies were present in over 95% of children by the age of 15 (98). Similarly, serologic studies performed in New Orleans demonstrated acquisition of antibodies in over 90% of children by the age of 15 (99). In developing countries such as Uruguay or in lower socioeconomic populations in the central United States, the appearance of antibodies occurred at similar but lower frequencies (99). These lower rates of acquisition of infection were particularly evident in the poor black communities of Atlanta and Houston (100–102). By 5 years of age, approximately one-third of patients had seroconverted; this frequency increased to 70–80% by early adolescence.

Predictably, middle-class individuals of industrialized societies acquired antibodies even later in life. Seroconversion occurred over the first 5 years of life in 20% of children; there was no significant increase until the second and third decades of life, at which time the prevalence of antibodies increased to 40% and 60%, respectively (103,104). Further support for the relationship of socioeconomic status to age of acquisition of primary infection is offered by a variety of other studies (81,105,106). One study of university students demonstrated that seroconversion of susceptible individuals occurred at an annual frequency of approximately 5–10% (81,107,108). In summary, these studies demonstrated a significantly lower prevalence of antibodies during childhood, adolescence, and even later in life in the relatively middle and upper socioeconomic classes. Primary infection occurred much earlier in life, generally very early, in children of underdeveloped countries as well as those of lower socioeconomic classes; however, in developed

countries and more affluent classes, primary infection was delayed until adolescence or, perhaps, even adulthood. Frequency of direct person-to-person contact, consistent with crowded living conditions associated with lower socioeconomic status, appeared to be the major mediator of infection.

Genital Herpes Simplex Infections

Because infections with HSV-2 are usually acquired through sexual contact, antibodies to this virus are rarely found before the age of onset of sexual activity. Although most genital HSV infections are caused by HSV-2, a recognizable but variable proportion is attributable to HSV-1 (109–112). The distinction in virus type is not insignificant, since genital HSV-1 infections are usually less severe clinically and recur less frequently (109,113). Sexual transmission is the primary route of the spread of HSV-2 (114–118). The major line of evidence supporting sexual transmission includes the demonstrated high probability of infection following sexual contact with patients having confirmed disease.

Sexually transmitted disease clinics provide the basis for prevalence data on genital HSV infections, particularly those in the United States, England, and Sweden (117,119–121). The number of new cases of genital HSV infections is estimated to be approximately 500,000 per year (121). This estimate is probably conservative at best. Since genital HSV infections are not reportable diseases in the United States, these numbers are estimates from a recent Institute of Medicine assessment of vaccine priorities (122). It has been suggested that the number of new cases of easily identifiable sexually transmitted diseases can serve to determine estimates of the number of cases of genital herpes. If the incidence of new cases is calculated from a ratio of five to 10 cases of gonorrhea to every one case of genital HSV, approximately 300,000 new cases would occur yearly in the United States (121,123,124). A report by Corey et al. (125) suggests a much higher rate of infection, namely a ratio of one case of genital herpes infection to 2.2 cases of gonorrhea. Such estimates would strikingly increase the frequency of primary disease. One difficulty in determining actual prevalence stems from the lack of an aforementioned national reporting system. Current estimates of individuals with genital herpetic infection in the United States alone range from as low as 10 million to as high as 30–40 million Americans (122,125). Predicated upon newer serologic methods for detection of prior HSV-2 infection, a more accurate estimate should set this range as 40–60 million cases of infected individuals in the United States (126).

Cytopathologic screening by Papanicolaou staining of clinical specimens adds another epidemiologic tool for the study of these problems (87,116,127). If these methods are employed along with virus isolation, the prevalence of genital HSV infections ranges from 0.09% to 0.24% in normal women (128–131). In contrast, rates of infection in individuals routinely attending sexually transmitted disease clinics vary between 0.002% and 3.3% (and sometimes as high as 7.0%) depending upon the population studied (130,132). It should be recognized that these studies were performed over a decade ago, when the prevalence of disease was probably lower than at present.

Women have been reported to have the highest rates of infection, particularly prostitutes and others with multiple sex partners. Among prostitutes, an interesting observation has been made relating the frequency of HSV shedding to age. The most sexually active prostitutes (age range 20–29 years) were most likely to excrete HSV (12%), whereas those in older age groups had a decreased frequency (6%) of viral excretion. Of note, one study found that the incidence of genital HSV infections in both indigent women and those of middle and upper socioeconomic classes appeared to be significantly lower than that found among women attending sexually transmitted disease clinics: 0.3% and 0.2%, respectively (133). As with HSV-1 infections of the mouth, HSV-2 can be excreted in the absence of symptoms at the time of primary, initial, or recurrent infection (134,135). The actual frequency of asymptomatic excretion of HSV-2 is unknown, but its occurrence creates a silent reservoir for transmission of infection.

In spite of prior difficulties encountered in determining type-specific antibodies, the appearance of HSV-2 antibodies reflects the time of exposure or, more simply, the acquisition of infection. The appearance of antibodies can be positively correlated with the onset of sexual activity (101,102,136), although crowded living conditions may indirectly contribute to antibody prevalence (130,137). If HSV-2 antibodies are sought in healthy women, there is a wide discrepancy in prevalence, ranging from 10% in the United States to 77% in Uganda (138). Up to 50–60% of lower socioeconomic populations in the United States and elsewhere develop antibodies to HSV-2 by adulthood (11). In contrast, 10–20% of individuals in higher socioeconomic groups are seropositive (105,139). Recently, seroepidemiologic studies performed by Nahmias and colleagues (140,141) have utilized type-specific antigen for HSV-1 and HSV-2 (glycoprotein G-1 and glycoprotein G-2, respectively) which identify antibodies to this virus in approximately 35% of middle-class women receiving care through an Atlanta Health Maintenance Organization. In a series of studies performed by the Nahmias group, the seroprevalence of HSV-2 increases from 6.9% at 15–29 years of age to 23.4% by the age of 60. If the populations are analyzed according to race, these percentages are 4.6%

and 19.7% for whites and 21.8% and 64.7% for blacks, respectively. Factors found to influence acquisition of HSV-2 include: sex (women more than men), race (blacks more than whites), marital status (divorced individuals more than single or married ones), place of residence (city greater than suburb). In addition, the number of sexual partners has also been reported to influence acquisition of infection (142–144).

The rate of primary infection has been determined for specific subpopulations within these epidemiologic studies. For a large southern university population, evidence of seroconversion to HSV-2 (namely, primary infection) occurred at a rate of approximately 1.0% per year (107). Parenthetically, seroconversion to HSV-1 occurred at a rate of 2.5% per year in this same college population. Other serologic studies have defined the incidence of HSV-2 infection. In one middle-class maternal population (20–30 years of age), primary infection occurred at a rate of 1.8% per year (139). Because the infection occurs primarily in adolescents and young adults, antibody prevalence rates increase most rapidly in those aged 20–29 years, followed by those sexually active but under 20 years of age.

Conversely, antibodies to HSV-2 are virtually nonexistent in nuns (97,101,132,142). As an interesting and provocative side-issue, a previous history of antibodies to either HSV-1 or HSV-2 may have an ameliorative effect on the expression of clinical disease (107,125,143,145–148). This suggestion is of importance because it relates to vaccine development.

Recurrent HSV-2 Infections

Recurrent genital infection is the largest reservoir for transmission of HSV-2. As with HSV-1 infection, recurrent HSV-2 infection can be either symptomatic or asymptomatic; however, recurrence is usually associated with a shorter duration of viral shedding and fewer lesions (109). The frequency of recurrences is somewhat higher in males than in females: 2.7 and 1.9 per 100 patient-days, respectively (109). Overall, several studies have implicated a frequency of recurrence as high as 60% (136,149). The type of genital infection, HSV-1 versus HSV-2, appears predictive of the frequency of recurrence (113,149,150). HSV-1 infection appears to recur less frequently than those caused by HSV-2. Ongoing epidemiologic investigations of genital HSV infections are addressing such issues as the age of acquisition, frequency of intercourse, number of sexual partners, and prior antibody status as well as the influence of socioeconomic conditions on disease manifestations.

A recent report has defined the frequency of recurrences in individuals with dual HSV-1 and HSV-2 infections (147,151). From this unique study it was learned that HSV-2 was more likely to recur than HSV-1, irrespective of the site of infection—namely, oropharynx versus genital tract.

HERPES SIMPLEX ENCEPHALITIS

Background

HSV infections of the CNS are among the most severe of all human viral infections of the brain. Currently, HSE is estimated to occur in approximately one in 250,000 to one in 500,000 individuals per year. At the University of Alabama at Birmingham, a medical center which accepts statewide referrals of patients with suspected HSE, the diagnosis of HSE was proven by brain biopsy at an average of 10 patients per year over a 10-year period. Alabama has a population of 3.3 million; thus, the projected incidence of clinically evident disease is approximately one (or more) in 300,000 individuals. A similar incidence was found in Sweden and England and is believed to be the approximate incidence in other industrialized countries as well (152,153). In the United States, HSE is thought to account for up to 10–20% of encephalitic viral infections of the CNS (154).

The economic cost of HSE is considerable. For 1983 the estimated medical costs of hospitalization alone for HSE in adults was over $25 million (155). The total medical cost of this disease is considerably higher because of the long-term care and support services required for many of the survivors.

HSE occurs throughout the year and in patients of all ages, with approximately one-third of cases occurring in patients younger than age 20 and approximately one-half in patients older than 50 (156). Caucasians account for 95% of patients with biopsy-proven disease. Both sexes are affected equally.

The severity of disease, as defined by the natural history of infection, is best determined by the outcome of patients who have received no therapy or who have been given an ineffective antiviral medication such as idoxuridine or cytosine arabinoside. In such situations, mortality is in excess of 70%; only approximately 2.5% of all patients with confirmed disease (9.1% of survivors) returned to normal function following recovery from their illness (157–161). Because brain biopsy with isolation of HSV from brain tissue was the method of diagnosis in these studies, it is likely that a far broader spectrum of HSV infections of the CNS actually exists. One British study has suggested milder forms of HSE which are associated with lower mortality and improved morbidity (162). Serologic evaluations were the basis for the diagnosis in this latter report, a problem which will be discussed below. Regardless, a spectrum of CNS disease caused by HSV must exist.

Although the clinical presentation, diagnosis, and outcome of patients with HSE have been considered for some time, the reported studies indicate extreme variability in the methods of diagnosis, mortality, morbidity, and the clinical course of disease. The studies performed in the United States by the NIAID Collaborative Antiviral Study Group have helped resolve some of these issues. The clarification of many of these issues has become possible because of a uniform diagnostic approach, namely, brain biopsy and subsequent isolation of HSV from brain tissue as the means of disease confirmation. Unequivocal diagnosis often has created both practical dilemmas (3,67,163) and intellectual controversies (156,164,165). This procedure has not been routinely employed in therapeutic, natural history, or diagnostic investigations performed outside the United States for the prospective evaluation of patients with focal encephalitis.

Diagnosis of Herpes Simplex Encephalitis

Several aspects relating to the diagnosis of HSE merit discussion: (a) the clinical presentation regarding the sensitivity and specificity of various clinical characteristics; (b) the need for brain biopsy to establish the diagnosis; (c) conditions which mimic HSE; and (d) the prospects of noninvasive means of diagnosis.

Because the NIAID Collaborative Antiviral Study Group required a positive brain biopsy for inclusion in its studies, a unique opportunity arose to evaluate clinical and neurodiagnostic characteristics of brain-biopsy-positive and brain-biopsy-negative patients (156). It is worth remembering that at the outset, all of these patients had clinical findings compatible with HSE. Of 202 patients who were evaluated for HSE, HSV was isolated from brain tissue of only 113 patients. Only four of the remaining patients had combinations of serologic and clinical findings suggestive of HSE.

Most patients with biopsy-proven HSE presented with a focal encephalopathic process, including (a) altered mentation and decreasing levels of consciousness with focal neurologic findings, (b) cerebrospinal-fluid (CSF) pleocytosis and proteinosis, (c) the absence of bacterial and fungal pathogens in the CSF, and (d) focal electroencephalographic, computed tomographic (CT), and/or technetium brain scan findings, as shown in Table 2. The use of magnetic resonance imaging (MRI) has not been adequately studied to date, although MRI will likely be a very useful diagnostic tool for other viral causes of CNS disease. The frequency of headache and CSF pleocytosis was higher in patients with proven HSE than in patients with other diseases of the CNS which mimicked HSE. A higher frequency of ataxia occurred in those individuals who had diseases which mimicked HSV infection of the CNS. Nearly uniformly, patients with HSE presented with fever and personality change.

TABLE 2. *Comparison of findings in "brain-positive" and "brain-negative" patients with herpes simplex encephalitis[a]*

	Number (%) of patients	
	Brain-positive	Brain-negative
Historical findings		
Alteration of		
consciousness	109/112 (97)	82/84 (96)
CSF pleocytosis	107/110 (97)	71/82 (87)
Fever	101/112 (90)	68/85 (78)
Headache	89/110 (81)	56/73 (77)
Personality change	62/87 (71)	44/65 (68)
Seizures	73/109 (67)	48/81 (59)
Vomiting	51/111 (46)	38/82 (46)
Hemiparesis	33/100 (33)	19/71 (26)
Memory loss	14/59 (24)	9/47 (19)
Clinical findings		
at presentation		
Fever	101/110 (92)	84/79 (81)
Personality change	69/81 (85)	43/58 (74)
Dysphasia	58/76 (76)	36/54 (67)
Autonomic dysfunction	53/88 (80)	40/71 (58)
Ataxia	22/55 (40)	18/45 (40)
Hemiparesis	41/107 (38)	24/81 (30)
Seizures	43/112 (38)	40/85 (47)
Focal	28	13
Generalized	10	14
Both	5	13
Cranial nerve defects	34/105 (32)	27/81 (33)
Visual field loss	8/58 (14)	4/33 (12)
Papilledema	16/111 (14)	9/84 (11)

[a] "Brain-positive" and "brain-negative" refer to positive or negative brain tissue culture findings. None of the differences were significant at the 5% level by χ^2 tests. CSF, cerebrospinal fluid.

Seizures, whether focal or generalized, occurred in only approximately two-thirds of all patients with proven disease. Thus, the clinical findings of HSE were nonspecific and did not allow for empirical diagnosis of disease predicated solely on clinical presentation. While clinical evidence of a localized temporal lobe lesion was often thought to be HSE, under the proper circumstances it has been learned that a variety of other diseases can be shown to mimic this condition.

Examination of the CSF is indicated in patients with altered mentation, provided that evidence of increased intracranial pressure does not prevent this procedure. In patients with HSE, CSF examination is nondiagnostic. It has been learned that patients with biopsy-proven disease have CSF findings similar to those from patients with other infections of the CNS. Invariably, the CSF white blood cell count is elevated, with a predominance of lymphocytes. The CSF protein is similarly elevated. The average white blood cell counts of CSF obtained from patients with HSE is 100 cells/μl. Similarly, the CSF protein averages approximately 100 mg/dl. Sequential evaluation of CSF specimens from patients with HSE indicates increasing cell counts and levels of pro-

tein. The presence of CSF red blood cells is not diagnostic for HSE.

Noninvasive neurodiagnostic studies have been utilized to support a presumptive diagnosis of HSE. These studies have included EEG, CT, and technetium brain scans. More recently, MRI scans have been utilized for diagnostic purposes, although the value of such scans remains to be established in carefully documented and controlled clinical situations. Studying focal changes of the electroencephalogram (EEG) appears to be the most sensitive of the noninvasive neurodiagnostic procedures (166–170). Characteristic findings on the electroencephalogram are spike-and-slow-wave activity and periodic lateralized epileptiform discharges (PLEDs), which arise from the temporal lobe. Early in the disease, the abnormal electrical activity usually involves one temporal lobe and then spreads to the contralateral temporal lobe as the disease evolves, usually over a period of 7–10 days. The sensitivity of the EEG has been defined as approximately 84%, but, unfortunately, a specificity of only 32.5% has been demonstrated in the NIAID Collaborative Antiviral Study Group trials.

CT scans initially show low-density areas with mass effect localized to the temporal lobe, which can progress to radiolucent and/or hemorrhagic lesions (171,172). Bitemporal disease is common in the absence of therapy, particularly late in the disease course. A characteristic CT scan with sequential distribution over time is shown in Fig. 6. When these neurodiagnostic tests are used in combination, the sensitivity can be enhanced; however, the specificity of these diagnostic procedures is inadequate. At the present time, none of these neurodiagnostic tests is uniformly satisfactory for diagnosing HSE; perhaps MRI will prove to be the best neurodiagnostic test.

Brain Biopsy

The most sensitive and specific means of diagnosis, at least at the present time, remains the isolation of HSV from tissue obtained at brain biopsy. While this diagnostic approach continues to be controversial, brain-biopsy complications, either acute or chronic in nature, are approximately 3%. Fears of potentiating acute illness (by incising the brain in a diseased area) or of causing chronic seizure disorders have not been substantiated by follow-up studies of NIAID Collaborative Antiviral Study Group patients.

Serologic Evaluation

Several strategies utilizing antibody production as a means of diagnosing HSE have been studied. Data from the NIAID Collaborative Antiviral Study Group were analyzed for comparison of serum and CSF antibody

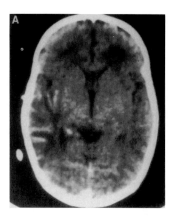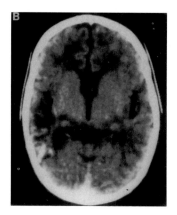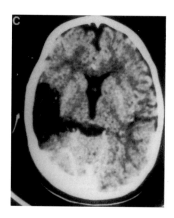

FIG. 6. Sequential CT examination of a patient with confirmed HSE.

production in patients with brain-biopsy-proven disease (86). Because the majority of patients were seropositive to HSV prior to their presentation with encephalitis, seroconversion, per se, was usually not helpful; fever alone can reactivate labial herpes. A fourfold rise in serum antibody was neither sensitive nor specific enough to be useful, although most of the brain-biopsy-negative patients who had a rise in serum antibody had a history of documented recurrent herpes labialis. A fourfold or greater rise in CSF antibody occurred significantly more often within a month after onset of infection in patients with biopsy-proven HSE: 85% versus 29% at 1 week. By 10 days after clinical presentation, however, only 50% of brain-biopsy-positive patients had a fourfold rise in CSF antibody. This test has been considered useful for diagnosis, but only retrospectively. The utilization of a serum-to-CSF-antibody ratio of ≤20 did not improve sensitivity during the first 10 days of disease.

Antigen Detection

Alternative noninvasive diagnostic procedures are in varying stages of development. A promising assay is the demonstration of antigens to glycoproteins gB, gD, and gE in CSF of patients with biopsy-proven disease (173). After the onset of clinical findings of HSE, the CSF has evidence of antigen to HSV as early as 5 days after disease onset in 65–75% of specimens tested. The assay is nearly 100% specific, and it increases in sensitivity as the disease progresses. It is conceivable that the availability of an antigen detection assay to be utilized on CSF will replace the uniform diagnosis of HSE by brain biopsy.

More recently, the application of polymerase chain reaction to CSF specimens from patients with suspect HSE appears to be useful (174).

Diseases Which Mimic HSE

In the most recent compilation of the NIAID Collaborative Antiviral Study Group data, 193 of 432 (45%) pa-tients undergoing brain biopsy had HSE (175). The remaining patients were evaluated for diseases which mimic HSE, as shown in Table 3. Thirty-eight had disease amenable to other forms of therapy, including brain abscess, tuberculosis, cryptococcal infection, and brain tumor. An additional 19 patients had diseases which were indirectly treatable, and another 38 patients had an alternative diagnosis established but for which there was no current therapy. Usually these patients had infections caused by viruses other than those in the herpesvirus family. The diagnosis of other treatable causes of encephalitis provides the most compelling support for brain biopsy of patients with a focal encephalopathic process. Thus, the future deployment of noninvasive diagnostic procedures must take into consideration those diseases which mimic HSV infection of the CNS and which require immediate medical intervention.

Other Neurologic Syndromes

HSV obviously involves areas of the nervous system other than the brain. Primary and recurrent genital herpes have been associated with neuritis localized to one extremity or even transverse myelitis. Neuritis evident in these patients can be associated with altered sensation of the lower extremities as well as dysesthesias, shooting pain, and motor impairment. Urinary and fecal incontinence have been reported in a few patients. Guillain–Barré syndrome and localized dermatomal rashes associated with acute neuritis have also been attributed to HSV infections.

Therapy

The first antiviral drug evaluated and the first one for which therapeutic usefulness was suggested in the literature was idoxuridine, a compound studied in the late 1960s and early 1970s (176–181). In 1972, the NIAID Collaborative Antiviral Study Group, in cooperation with the Boston Interhospital Viral Study Group, demon-

TABLE 3. *Diseases[a] which mimic herpes simplex encephalitis*

Treatable (N = 38)		Nontreatable (N = 57)	
Infection		Nonviral (N = 17)	
Abscess/subdural empyema		Vascular disease	11
Bacterial	5	Toxic encephalopathy	5
Listeria	1	Reye's syndrome	1
Fungal	2	Viral (N = 40)	
Mycoplasma	2	Togavirus infections	
Tuberculosis	6	St. Louis encephalitis	7
Cryptococcal	3	Western equine encephalitis	3
Rickettsial	2	California encephalitis	4
Toxoplasmosis	1	Eastern equine encephalitis	2
Mucormycosis	1	Other herpesviruses	
Meningococcal meningitis	1	Epstein–Barr virus	8
Tumor	5	Cytomegalovirus	1
Subdural hematoma	2	Others	
Systemic lupus erythematosus	1	Echovirus	3
Adrenal leukodystrophy	6	Influenza A	4
		Mumps	3
		Adenovirus	1
		Progressive multifocal leukoencephalopathy	1
		Lymphocytic choriomeningitis	2
		Subacute sclerosing panencephalitis	2

[a] Of 432 patients assessed.

strated that idoxuridine was both ineffective and toxic for patients with HSE (157). Toxicity was manifested as bone marrow suppression (neutropenia and thrombocytopenia) and secondary bacterial infection. These life-threatening complications developed in patients who received purportedly effective dosages of medication; thus, the therapeutic index (ratio of efficacy to toxicity) was unfavorable. As a consequence of this study, idoxuridine was no longer considered an acceptable therapeutic agent for the management of HSE. These early controlled studies of HSE demonstrated that uniform methods of data collection and uniform approaches to management of patients with HSE might establish earlier diagnoses and improve therapy.

Subsequent therapeutic trials defined vidarabine as a useful medication for the management of biopsy-proven HSE (160,161). In the first of a series of controlled studies of HSE, which utilized a double-blind, placebo-controlled study design, vidarabine therapy decreased mortality from 70% to 28% 1 month after disease onset —and from 70% to 44% 6 months later—for patients with biopsy-proven disease. This study of 28 patients was terminated for ethical reasons because of decreased mortality in the vidarabine recipients.

An open and uncontrolled study verified mortality and defined long-term morbidity. This follow-up study of nearly 100 patients with proven disease defined long-term mortality as 40%. Of importance, the variables of age and level of consciousness at the onset of therapy were proven to be major determinants of clinical outcome. Patients less than 30 years of age and with a more normal level of consciousness (lethargic as opposed to

comatose) were more likely to return to normal function after HSE than were older patients, especially those who were semicomatose or comatose, as illustrated in Fig. 7. From these data, it is apparent that older patients (greater than 30 years of age), whether comatose or semicomatose, had mortality rates which approached 70%—a figure very similar to that encountered in the placebo recipients of the previously cited studies. In patients less than 30 years of age, a more acceptable outcome was achieved, as evidenced by (a) a mortality rate of 25% and (b) a high percentage (40%) of individuals returning to normal function. Clearly, an important lesson learned from these trials was that if therapy is to be effective, it must be instituted prior to the onset of hemorrhagic necrosis of a dominant temporal lobe, or before widespread bilateral disease ensues, as reflected by deterioration of a patient's level of consciousness.

More recently, the NIAID Collaborative Antiviral Study Group has demonstrated that acyclovir is superior to vidarabine for the treatment of HSE (182). The design and mechanism of action of acyclovir have previously been discussed at length (183). The single criterion for inclusion in the study's database was the establishment of diagnosis by isolation of HSV from brain-biopsy tissue. Notably, this criterion is somewhat different from that of a similar study performed in Sweden which also compared these two medications. The NIAID study demonstrated that acyclovir decreased mortality to 19% 6 months after therapy. Importantly, 38% of patients, irrespective of age, returned to normal function. Scandinavian investigators, led by Dr. Birgit Skoldenberg, defined similar outcome, but in a smaller group of patients

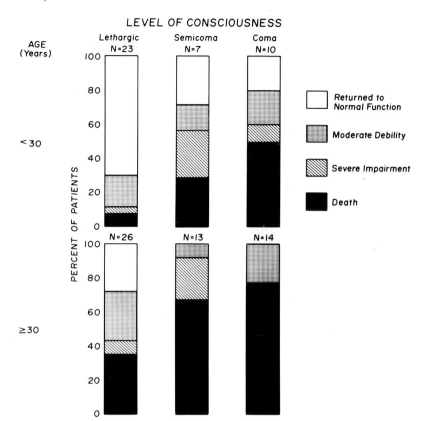

FIG. 7. Influence of level of consciousness and age on mortality and morbidity.

whose diagnoses were established by a variety of methods (153). Both studies taken together indicate that acyclovir is superior to vidarabine for the treatment of HSE.

As shown in Fig. 8, the data from the NIAID Collaborative Antiviral Study Group indicate a mortality of 55% at 6 and 18 months after the onset of treatment for patients who received vidarabine, as compared to 19% and 28% at 6 and 18 months after the onset of treatment for the acyclovir group. Late deaths in this study were not a consequence of either persistent or reactivated HSV infection of the CNS but occurred in patients who were severely impaired as a consequence of their disease.

The mortality rate following vidarabine therapy in this study was higher than that encountered in the original trials. A partial explanation for enhanced mortality in the vidarabine-treated group was that this group of patients consisted of older individuals who had a lower level of consciousness; both factors are known to be associated with higher mortality. When patient populations were compared according to specific age and level of consciousness, however, differences in therapeutic outcome were significant for long-term mortality (utilizing a two-tail test, $p = 0.04$).

Previous studies indicated that age and level of consciousness influenced long-term outcome. A more objective reflection of level of consciousness, the Glasgow coma score (GCS), rates patients according to motor, verbal, and sensory responses. As shown in Fig. 9, scores which approached normal predicted enhanced survival.

When GCS and age were assessed simultaneously, as illustrated in Fig. 10, a GCS of ≤6 led to a poor therapeutic outcome, irrespective of the agent which was administered or of the age of the patient (182).

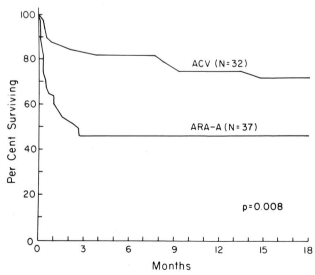

FIG. 8. Comparison of survival in patients with biopsy-proven HSE treated with vidarabine (ARA-A) or acyclovir (ACV); $p = 0.008$.

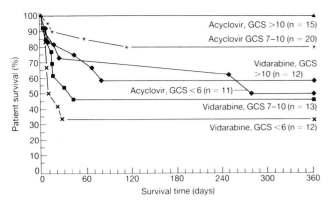

FIG. 9. Survival of biopsy-proven patients with HSE receiving acyclovir or vidarabine. GCS, Glasgow coma score.

Long-term morbidity following administration of an antiviral is of particular importance. Historically, the vidarabine studies indicated that approximately 15–20% of patients overall would develop normally following therapy of HSE on long-term follow-up. The current trial indicated that 13% of vidarabine recipients were left with no or minor sequelae, whereas those with moderate or severe sequelae and dead on follow-up were 22% and 65%, respectively. For acyclovir recipients, 38% of pa-

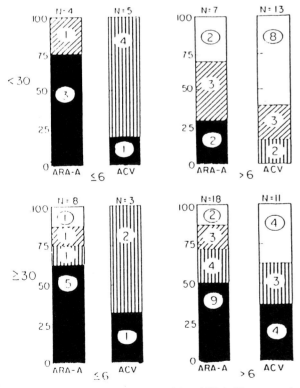

FIG. 10. Morbidity after vidarabine (ARA-A) or acyclovir (ACV) treatment of biopsy-proven HSE, according to age (<30 versus ≥30) and the Glasgow coma score (≤6 versus >6). The scale at the left side of each column indicates percentages (0–100). The number inside each oval denotes number of patients; □, normal and mild; ▨, moderate; ⫿, severe; ■, dead.

tients were normal or with minor impairment, 9% of patients had moderate sequelae, and 53% of patients were left with severe impairment or were dead. Currently, an open study of acyclovir is underway for biopsy-proven disease in order to verify long-term morbidity and mortality.

No patient entered into the NIAID trials suffered a relapse after completion of therapy. Nevertheless, when causes of fever other than HSE were excluded, such as bacterial pneumonia, urinary tract infection, etc., the median duration of an afebrile state was only 3.1 days at the completion of 10 days of treatment. Thus, a longer afebrile state might be considered desirable, thereby extending therapy to a minimum of 14 days. Relapse of HSE has been documented in a few patients following the administration of vidarabine (184,185); recently, relapse of HSE has also been reported after treatment with acyclovir (186). These reports are of concern. In only one case was reisolation of HSV achieved; however, few patients were rebiopsied. These reports of relapse support a longer duration of treatment. Demyelination syndromes have also been identified after successful treatment of HSE (187).

In defining the therapeutic index of a compound for the management of HSE, the denominator, or toxicity, becomes an important component of the equation. As shown in Table 4, the vidarabine recipients were more likely to develop laboratory abnormalities during the course of treatment than were the counterpart acyclovir recipients (50% versus 25%, $p = 0.04$).

The most significant laboratory abnormalities encountered among vidarabine recipients were as follows: a platelet count less than 100,000 (11%), an elevated serum glutamic-oxaloacetic transaminase greater than 250 IU (14%), and an elevated blood urea nitrogen (BUN) in excess of 30 mg/dl (11%). In contrast, 10% of acyclovir recipients experienced an elevated BUN, and 6% developed a creatinine in excess of 2 mg/dl. It should be emphasized that the administration of either drug was not associated with clinical evidence of toxicity and that these findings simply represented laboratory aberrations encountered during the course of management of these patients.

These findings indicate that the current therapy of choice for the management of HSE is acyclovir rather than vidarabine. Recently, a New Drug Application was approved by the Food and Drug Administration for utilization of this compound at a dosage of 10 mg/kg every 8 hr (30 mg/kg/day) for a period of only 10–14 days in the United States.

Future Directions

Acyclovir is the treatment of choice for biopsy-proven HSE, resulting in improved morbidity and mortality.

TABLE 4. *Abnormal laboratory values in 69 patients with biopsy-proven herpes simplex encephalitis*

Laboratory index[a]	Number of patients (%) treated with vidarabine	Number of patients (%) treated with acyclovir
Platelets (<100,000 cells/mm^3)	4 (11)	2 (6)
SGOT (>250 IU/dl)	5 (14)	1 (3)
BUN (>50 mg/dl)	4 (11)	3 (10)
White cells (<2500 cells/mm^3)	2 (6)	0 (0)
Total bilirubin (>3 mg/dl)	1 (3)	0 (0)
Creatinine (>3 mg/dl)	0 (0)	2 (6)
Combinations		
SGOT + bilirubin	1 (3)	0 (0)
White cells + platelets	0 (0)	0 (0)
BUN, platelets, +SGOT	1 (3)	0 (0)
Total	18 (49)	8 (25)

[a] SGOT, serum aspartate aminotransferase; BUN, blood urea nitrogen. To convert values for BUN to millimoles per liter, multiply by 0.357; to convert values for bilirubin and creatinine to micromoles per liter, multiply by 17.1 and 88.4, respectively.

Nevertheless, alternative therapeutic approaches must be developed. The development of sensitive and specific noninvasive diagnostic procedures may contribute to improved outcome by avoiding delays in the onset of therapy while awaiting a biopsy. However, the value of such procedures and their standardization remain to be established. A longer duration of therapy with current antiviral agents and at current or higher doses may be beneficial.

Another approach to the future therapy of HSE is the utilization of combination chemotherapy which has been deployed for the management of malignancy and certain other viral infections (188,189). Such approaches have been developed in order to decrease therapeutic failures, minimize potential for drug resistance, and potentially decrease dosages of medication to avoid toxic effects. The application of combination therapy to the treatment of viral infections has been studied *in vitro* as well as in animal model systems (190–196). Acyclovir and vidarabine have an additive effect for reduction of replication of both HSV-1 and HSV-2 in both systems; no antagonistic effect has been demonstrated (191).

Animal model data indicate that combination chemotherapy, utilizing acyclovir and vidarabine, have at least an additive and, perhaps, a synergistic effect for decreasing mortality, even when therapy is initiated *late* after infection. Similar animal model data have previously predicted the value of both acyclovir and vidarabine as single agents for treatment of HSE and support the potential utility of combination chemotherapy (195).

Combination chemotherapy may well have potential for decreasing the development of viral resistance. Resistant viral mutants can be generated easily in tissue culture systems and have appeared in immunodeficient humans (197–200).

New compounds with increased activity or increased lipophilicity, thereby allowing enhanced penetration of drug into the CNS, are being sought. Thus, future thera-

peutic efforts, at least initially, will use compounds presently in use, but they will be used either in combination (for longer duration) or in higher doses.

VARICELLA-ZOSTER VIRUS INFECTIONS

History

Varicella-zoster virus (VZV) causes two clinically distinct diseases. Varicella (chickenpox) is the primary disease which results from infection of a susceptible individual. Varicella—a ubiquitous, extremely contagious, and generally benign acute illness—is characterized by a generalized vesicular rash and occurs in epidemics. Recurrent infection results in the localized lesions of herpes zoster, or shingles, a common infection among the elderly. Shingles has been recognized since ancient times as a unique clinical entity because of the dermatomal vesicular rash; however, varicella was often confused with smallpox. Chickenpox and smallpox were differentiated by the clinical descriptions of Heberbed in 1867, as reviewed by Gordon and Meader (201). In 1975, Steiner (202) successfully demonstrated the transmissibility of VZV by inoculating vesicular fluid from an individual suffering from chickenpox into volunteers who subsequently developed the same disease. The infectious nature of VZV was further elucidated by von Bokay (203,204), who reported the occurrence of chickenpox in individuals who had close contact with others suffering from herpes zoster. In addition to close contact, the inoculation of vesicular fluid from patients suffering from herpes zoster into susceptible individuals resulted in chickenpox (205,206). Subsequent reports reinforced the infectivity of VZV (207), suggested that zoster was the consequence of reactivation of latent VZV (208), and noted intranuclear inclusions and multinucleated giant cells in biopsies of lesions from both clinical entities (209,210).

Weller and co-workers (211–215) first propagated VZV in tissue culture and demonstrated no biological or immunological differences between the viral agents isolated from patients with these two clinical entities. Restriction endonuclease cleavage patterns of VZV DNA have supported the epidemiological relatedness of VZV strains (216–219).

In 1974, chickenpox resulted in at least one million physician visits, and nearly half of these individuals required a second office appointment. Herpes zoster during the same year accounted for over 1.75 million physician visits, and nearly three-quarters of these patients required follow-up medical care.

Infectious Agent

VZV, being a member of the family Herpetoviridae, shares structural characteristics with other members of this family. The complete virion is approximately 150–200 nm in diameter; the capsid measures approximately 90–95 nm in diameter (220,221) and has a lipid-containing envelope with glycoprotein spikes (222). The molecular weight of VZV DNA is approximately 100×10^6 (222–224) and has a density of approximately 1.703–1.709 g/cm^3 after ultracentrification (224,225). Analysis of VZV DNA reveals a lower guanosine and cytosine composition as compared with that of other human herpesviruses (226,227). The genome contains 125,000 base pairs and is organized in a manner similar to that of other herpesviruses, having unique long (U_l; 105 kb) and unique short (U_s; 5.2 kb) regions of the genome (228). Five VZV glycoproteins have been identified: gp I, gp II, gp III, gp IV, and gp V. Viral infectivity can be neutralized by monoclonal antibodies directed against gp I, gp II, and gp III, as recently reviewed (229).

VZVs can be isolated in a variety of continuous and discontinuous cell culture systems of human and simian origin. A cellular cytopathic effect begins as a focal process with subsequent cell-to-cell spread, as shown in Fig. 11. Approximately 8–10 hr after infection, virus-specific immunofluorescence can be detected in cells adjacent to the initial focus of infection. Electron-microscopic studies show the appearance of immature viral particles within 12 hr of the onset of infection. Subsequently, as with HSV, the capsids form an envelope at the nuclear membrane and are released into the perinuclear space where large vacuoles are formed (220,230).

Pathology and Pathogenesis

General Observations

The histopathologic findings in human VZV infection, whether varicella or herpes zoster, are virtually identical. Skin disease is characterized by vesicles. Vesicles involve the corium and dermis. As viral replication progresses, the epithelial cells undergo degenerative changes characterized by ballooning, with the subsequent appearance of multinucleated giant cells and prominent eosinophilic intranuclear inclusions (203,231). These intranuclear inclusions have been called "Cowdry type A intranuclear inclusions" and are indicative of herpesvirus infections (232). Under unusual circumstances (disease in severely immunocompromised hosts), necrosis and hemorrhage may appear in the dermis. As the vesicle evolves, the collected fluid becomes cloudy with the appearance of leukocytes, degenerated cells, and fibrin. Ultimately, the vesicles either rupture or gradually become reabsorbed.

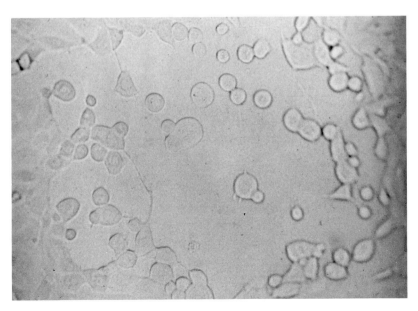

FIG. 11. Cytopathic effect of VZV infection.

Pathology of Encephalitis

Infection of the CNS can result in pathologic findings similar to those prominent in the skin, but with the addition of hemorrhagic necrosis, perivascular lymphocytic cuffing, and intranuclear inclusions.

Pathogenesis of VZV Infections: General Considerations

Primary VZV infections are the consequence of respiratory droplet spread. After presumed initial replication in the nasopharynx, a primary and secondary viremia is thought to ensue. With the secondary viremia, seeding of widespread organs, including skin, occurs. The potential mechanisms of pathogenesis for CNS disease are considered separately for each clinical manifestation, as noted below.

Reactivation of latent VZV infection results in a dermatomal rash of herpes zoster. The mechanism of reactivation is not understood. The cutaneous lesions and resultant pathology have been described above. The pathogenesis of herpes zoster involvement of the CNS will be considered below.

Epidemiology

Chickenpox

Several recent excellent reviews have summarized our knowledge of the epidemiology of VZV infections (233). Only a brief review will ensue. Humans are the only known reservoir for VZV. Chickenpox, being a primary infection, follows exposure of a susceptible or seronegative individual to VZV. Although it is assumed that the virus is spread by the respiratory route and replicates in the nasopharynx or upper respiratory tract, retrieval of virus from individuals incubating VZV has been uncommon. Varicella is endemic in the population at large; however, it becomes epidemic among susceptible individuals during seasonal periods, namely, late winter and early spring (207,234). Overall, chickenpox is a disease of childhood, with 90% of the cases occurring in children less than 10 years of age; this disease involves both sexes equally, and it occurs in individuals of all races (235). Intimate contact appears to be the key determinant for transmission; this is evident from infectivity data for household versus societal contacts, where the attack rates were 61–96% and 12%, respectively (234,236,237). The incubation period for chickenpox is generally regarded as 14–15 days (201,236), with a range of 10–20 days; this accounts for over 95% of cases (238). The secondary attack has been defined as 87% in siblings within the household after introduction of a primary case of varicella (238).

Herpes Zoster

As noted earlier, herpes zoster is the consequence of reactivation of latent VZV. It is characterized by excruciating pain in most adults and is localized within the dermatome of the vesicular eruption. The vesicular rash is unilateral in involvement in most patients, as shown in Fig. 12. The dermatomes most usually involved are from T3 through L4 (239,240). Involvement of cervical and facial dermatomes can have special complications. If the ophthalmic branch of the trigeminal nerve is involved, zoster ophthalmicus is a common complication which may result in blindness. Lesions of other branches of the trigeminal nerve (maxillary or mandibular branch) can result in intraoral involvement with lesions of the palate, tonsilar fossa, floor of the mouth, and the tongue. A Ramsay Hunt syndrome will occur if the geniculate ganglion is involved with vesicles on the pinna of the ear.

The specific stimulus responsible for the reactivation of herpes zoster is unknown, but zoster is associated with several temporal events. If herpes zoster occurs in the child, the course is generally benign and not associated with progressive pain or discomfort. In the adult, systemic manifestations, particularly acute neuritis and postherpetic neuralgia, can be debilitating. The onset of disease is heralded by pain within the dermatome that may precede, by approximately 24–48 hr or longer, the appearance of an erythematous rash which itself occurs before the onset of vesicular lesions. In the normal host, these lesions remain few in number and progress for a period of approximately 3–5 days before pustulating and scabbing. The total duration of disease is generally between 7 and 10 days; however, it may take as long as 3–4 weeks before the skin returns to normal. Patients at

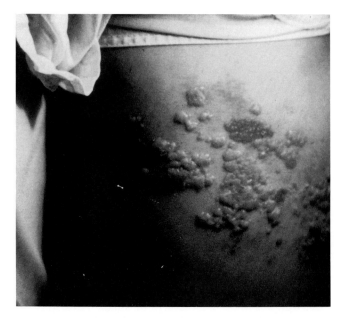

FIG. 12. Localized dermatomal rash of shingles.

greatest risk for developing herpes zoster are individuals suffering from Hodgkin's disease and non-Hodgkin's lymphoma as well as acquired immunodeficiency syndrome (AIDS). These patient populations are at increased risk for complications. The major complication with herpes zoster in the immunocompromised host is cutaneous dissemination and visceral involvement. A direct correlation exists between cutaneous dissemination and the appearance of visceral complications, including meningoencephalitis.

Over the past several years, herpes zoster has been documented in male homosexuals, intravenous drug abusers, and others with human immunodeficiency virus infections. While disease frequency is higher, visceral complications are uncommon.

Varicella-Zoster Virus Infections of the Central Nervous System

Varicella

The actual incidence of CNS complications with varicella is unknown. The observed incidence ranges from 0.1% to 0.75% in several series (241–244). Because many cases of varicella do not come to medical attention, any estimate of the frequency of neurologic complications is likely to be high. The CNS manifestations of chickenpox can be divided into four categories on the basis of the predominating neurologic abnormalities: (i) cerebellar ataxia, (ii) generalized meningoencephalitis, (iii) transverse myelitis, and (iv) aseptic meningitis (241,242,245,246). In addition, Reye's syndrome (encephalopathy with fatty infiltration of the liver) is a well-documented postinfectious CNS complication of varicella (247,248). However, this latter problem is now associated with concomitant salicylate therapy for fever. Guillain–Barré syndrome (polyradiculopathy and ascending paralysis) can occur, but this subject is considered in depth elsewhere (240,242). The following discussion is limited to the four neurologic complications of chickenpox previously listed and includes appropriate diagnostic and pathogenic concepts.

Cerebellar Ataxia

Cerebellar ataxia is the most common neurologic abnormality associated with varicella. Several earlier series support a frequency of cerebellar dysfunction in approximately one in 4,000 cases (241,245,246). Children can develop CNS abnormalities from several days before to 2 weeks after the onset of the rash, although neurologic symptoms often occur concomitantly with the rash. Symptoms consist of nausea, vomiting, and headache accompanied by nuchal rigidity and ataxia. Fever, if present, is usually moderate. Seizures are rare. In cases presenting before the development of the rash, the diagnosis may not be clinically apparent. Alternative diagnoses may include cerebellar tumors, obstructive hydrocephalus, and other infectious or parainfectious encephalitides (244).

The extent of the diagnostic evaluation in varicella-associated cerebellar dysfunction should be governed by the severity of the illness or the uncertainty of the diagnosis. In uncomplicated cases, the clinical presentation alone is sufficient to establish the diagnosis, and no further diagnostic evaluation is necessary. In more complicated situations, a CSF examination, an EEG, or a CT or MRI scan of the brain usually is warranted. The CSF is frequently normal, but a mild lymphocytic pleocytosis and elevated protein may occur in 20–30% of cases (245). Early in the course of the illness, polymorphonuclear (PMN) cells may be present (244,249). The CSF glucose is normal. The EEG demonstrates diffuse slow-wave activity in approximately 20% of cases and becomes normal as the symptoms resolve (245). The brain CT scan would be expected to be normal in cases of varicella-associated ataxia, although there are few such reports in the literature. Recent MRI studies have detected CNS abnormalities in apparent benign disease, although the number of patients evaluated is limited.

The cerebellar manifestations of chickenpox are usually self-limited, and most abnormalities resolve within several weeks. Mortality is low (0–5%) and correlates with the development of non-neurologic complications such as pneumonia (241,245). The majority of patients recover without apparent sequelae (241).

The pathogenesis of this syndrome remains an enigma, partly because of the lack of necropsy studies in a usually benign illness. Two basic mechanisms seem plausible: (i) direct viral involvement of the cerebellum and (ii) a parainfectious, immunologically mediated process analogous to that seen in association with other viral infections. Direct demonstration of the virus in brain or CSF by immunologic or electron-microscopic techniques has not been reported in varicella-associated cerebellar ataxia. Gershon et al. (250) demonstrated the presence of VZV antibodies in the CSF of three patients with unspecified CNS abnormalities in association with varicella. These antibodies were not detected in control patients who had varicella but no neurologic abnormality, perhaps reflecting intrathecal antibody production. Peters et al. (251) found evidence of VZV antigen in the CSF mononuclear cells of two patients with varicella-associated cerebellar ataxia. Both observations suggest CNS invasion and VZV replication. However, detailed studies are lacking, and the evidence for a viral invasion of the cerebellum is circumstantial. To our knowledge, there are no reports of isolation of VZV from the CSF of patients with cerebellar ataxia. There are no data in the literature to support or refute an immunologically mediated pathogenesis for varicella-associated ataxia.

Meningoencephalitis

A less common but frequently more severe CNS complication of chickenpox is meningoencephalitis or cerebritis. The actual incidence of encephalitis in chickenpox is low. Although earlier series suggested that up to 40% of patients with varicella-associated CNS dysfunction had encephalitis (245), it is likely that many of the cases were Reye's syndrome rather than infectious cerebritis (248,252). Excluding cases of Reye's syndrome, the clinical picture in varicella-associated encephalitis is similar to that seen in other encephalitides (247). Neurologic symptoms may occur from 11 days before to several weeks after the onset of the rash. Headache, fever, and vomiting are often accompanied by an altered sensorium. Seizures may occur in 29–52% of cases (240,245,253). Focal neurologic abnormalities can include cranial nerve dysfunction, aphasia, and hemiplegia (240).

In varicella-associated cerebritis, the CSF is frequently abnormal with a mild-to-moderate lymphocytic pleocytosis and elevated protein. Eighty percent of cases will have fewer than 100 cells per microliter (247). The protein is below 200 mg/dl. These findings are similar to those seen with cerebellar ataxia. However, in the one series that analyzed separately the CSF of patients with generalized cerebritis versus that of patients with cerebellar ataxia, the abnormalities were more pronounced in the patients with cerebritis.

The EEG is often diffusely abnormal in these cases. Focal abnormalities suggestive of epileptiform activity may occur even without clinical seizures (253). In patients who do have seizures, these EEG abnormalities tend to persist and are present in 43% of follow-up EEGs at 1 year (253).

In many of the previously published series, the mortality and morbidity data for varicella-associated encephalitis are clouded by the inclusion of cases of Reye's syndrome. The reported mortality varies from 0% to 35% (240–242,245,248). It is likely that the actual mortality in varicella cerebritis is low, with complete or nearly complete recovery in the majority of cases. Applebaum et al. (241) reported a 5% mortality in a series of 59 cases of varicella with CNS involvement. Two of the three deaths were associated with the development of pneumonia. Eighty percent of the survivors were discharged from the hospital without detectable sequelae. Of those patients with persistent abnormalities at discharge, several resolved with time.

Postmortem studies of the brain in fatal varicella cerebritis have been remarkable for the lack of distinctive histopathologic findings. Diffuse cerebral edema is generally present. Perivascular monocytic infiltration and demyelination have been seen in some cases, the latter suggesting a postinfectious demyelinating process (243). There are similarities in the histopathologic changes in experimental allergic encephalitis in animals produced by injection of lymphocytes sensitized to myelin basic proteins (252,254). Other cases have shown very little cellular reaction or demyelination (241). Intranuclear inclusions have been observed rarely in the brain following varicella. Nicholaides (255) reported a case of fatal infection with varicella pneumonia without clinical evidence of encephalitis in which intranuclear inclusions hemorrhagic necrosis and demyelination were seen in the brain tissue at postmortem examination. Takashima and Becker (256) reported two cases of fatal neonatal varicella in which viral involvement was demonstrated in brain tissue at postmortem examination. Although viral isolation from brain and CSF was not accomplished in these patients, the histopathologic findings suggest active viral replication.

Transverse Myelitis and Aseptic Meningitis

On rare occasions, varicella has been associated with an isolated weakness of the lower extremities, sphincter dysfunction, and abnormal deep tendon reflexes and extensor plantar reflexes. The CSF is characterized by a lymphocytic pleocytosis and elevated protein with a normal glucose. The completeness of recovery is variable (240,245). The pathogenesis of this neurologic complication is not known; however, immunologic mechanisms may be operant, as is suspected for other CNS manifestations of varicella.

The aseptic meningitis encountered with varicella is similar to many of the other viral meningitides (245). Fever and meningismus without evidence of cerebral dysfunction are suggestive of the diagnosis. CSF findings are typical of a viral meningitis with mild lymphocytic pleocytosis, slight elevation in the protein content, and normal glucose. Virus has not been cultured from the CSF. When not associated with encephalitis, the clinical course of this illness is benign with complete recovery expected.

Herpes Zoster

The neurologic complications of herpes zoster (shingles) are the subject of a number of reports. As in varicella, several distinct clinical syndromes have been described, including: (a) encephalitis (257–264), (b) ophthalmic zoster with contralateral hemiplegia (264–268), (c) myelitis (269–271), (d) multifocal leukoencephalopathy (272), (e) polyradiculitis (Guillain–Barré syndrome) (240,273), and (f) cranial and peripheral nerve palsies (238,271). The following discussion is limited to the first three syndromes and neuritis.

In general, the CNS complications of herpes zoster are associated with a higher morbidity and mortality than encountered with varicella. This may, in part, be a function of the patient's advanced age and the underlying diseases often associated with shingles. More is known about the pathogenesis of these syndromes than about that of the varicella-associated neurologic abnormalities because of the greater number of postmortem studies performed. Nevertheless, CNS complications in herpes zoster are uncommon, with immunocompromised patients being at greatest risk (274,275).

Encephalitis

Encephalitis is the most common CNS abnormality associated with herpes zoster. Risk factors for the development of this complication include advanced age, immunosuppression, and disseminated cutaneous zoster (275,276). In a series of patients reported by Jemsek et al. (258), 10 of 32 cases with disseminated herpes zoster were thought to have encephalitis. All but one of 12 cases with herpes-zoster-associated encephalitis (HZAE) were immunosuppressed. Mortality was 30% in this series. Other reviews (240) indicate a mortality ranging from 0% to 50%. Many deaths relate to the development of non-neurologic complications such as pneumonia. The incidence of long-term neurologic sequelae in survivors may be as high as 30% (241).

The clinical manifestations of HZAE are those of other infectious encephalitides. Altered mentation without other explanation in patients with either localized or disseminated herpes zoster is the most suggestive sign of CNS involvement. Fever may not be present. Other symptoms and signs of CNS disease include hallucinations, meningismus, ataxia, seizures, or motor paralysis. In most cases, evidence of CNS involvement begins within 1 or 2 weeks of onset of cutaneous disease, but this varies greatly (241,258,260,262,275). The occurrence of CNS symptoms may antedate the appearance of the rash by up to 21 days (241). In uncomplicated cases, recovery may take several weeks.

The diagnosis of HZAE is dependent on the presence of the characteristic rash or a recent history of zoster. Lumbar puncture frequently yields an abnormal CSF formula. A lymphocytic pleocytosis is common, as are elevated protein but a normal glucose. It should be noted that as many as 40% of cases of uncomplicated herpes zoster will also have an abnormal CSF, possibly reflecting a ganglionitis of the involved nerve root (241,277). Other diagnostic adjuncts in cases of HZAE include the EEG as well as the CT or MRI scan. Frequently, a diffuse slowing is evident on EEG without a specific abnormal focus (240,241,258,260). CT scans of the brain are usually normal in cases of generalized HZAE but are useful in excluding other possible etiologies of CNS symptoms (tumor, cerebrovascular accident, etc.).

In contrast to the varicella-associated neurologic syndromes, VZV has been cultured from the brain and CSF

in a number of cases of HZAE (249,277–282). Viral inclusions in glial cells, neurons, and arteries of the brain are well described in fatal cases (262,280,283,284). In addition, several investigators have demonstrated VZV antibodies and lymphocyte-associated VZV antigens in the CSF of patients with HZAE (242,278,285–287). Several autopsy studies have reported a granulomatous angiitis in cases of generalized herpes zoster encephalitis (283,288). Thus, the pathogenesis of varicella encephalitis and HZAE may differ.

Herpes Zoster Ophthalmicus and Contralateral Hemiplegia

A distinctive CNS manifestation that is sometimes seen in cases of ophthalmic zoster is contralateral hemiplegia. This syndrome has accounted for up to one-third of cases of CNS abnormalities in herpes zoster (275). Typically, zoster ophthalmicus precedes the appearance of hemiplegia by several weeks or more (268). In some cases, the onset of hemiplegia may be as late as 6 months after the rash has resolved (260,264). The pathogenesis of this disease is poorly understood but is thought to reflect viral involvement of the larger arteries of the CNS. In a postmortem examination of a patient treated with steroids, viral particles were demonstrated in sections of the larger arteries examined by electron microscopy (266). There were no light-microscopic findings suggestive of viral infection. The virus may gain access to the basilar structures of the brain via the trigeminal ganglia. Cerebral angiography in these cases often demonstrates unilateral arteritis or thrombosis of individual vessels (264,266,267,275). A CT scan may show evidence of cerebral infarction in some cases (266,267). The prognosis for recovery in this syndrome is variable. Reports of fatal cases appear in the literature, and mortality from this complication is probably underreported (266). The incidence of significant sequelae among survivors is not known.

Herpes-Zoster-Associated Myelitis

Myelitis associated with herpes zoster is an unusual complication of dermatomal disease. It occurs at approximately one-half the frequency of encephalitis (275). In a series of 1210 cases of herpes zoster evaluated at the Mayo Clinic over 9 years, only one case of herpes-zoster-associated myelitis was recorded (271). In some cases, the pathogenesis appears to involve a direct viral invasion of the spinal cord as demonstrated by the presence of viral inclusions and positive cultures for VZV (269,280). Other reports have implicated a vasculitic process with ischemic necrosis as a possible pathogenetic mechanism (262). An immunologic, parainfectious cause for spinal-cord destruction has been postulated by others (241). Onset may occur weeks to months after an acute episode of herpes zoster. The physical findings are those seen with any destructive lesion of the spinal cord (e.g., paralysis, altered sensation, loss of upper motor neuron regulation). Abnormalities in the CSF include a lymphocytic pleocytosis and elevated protein. The glucose is usually normal.

Several cases recorded in the literature have had progressive deterioration with ascending paralysis and extensive cord involvement present at postmortem exam (262,269). Patients who survive are frequently left with a residual neurologic deficit (270).

Neuritis

Cranial and peripheral nerve palsies are the most common neurologic manifestations of herpes zoster, occurring in the involved dermatome in 1–6% of cases (250,271). While not a CNS complication of VZV infection, the combination of acute neuritis and postherpetic neuralgia is an extremely debilitating neurologic complication of zoster both in the immunocompromised host and in the normal individual. Postherpetic neuralgia is uncommon in young individuals, but at least 50% of afflicted patients over the age of 60 will have persistent pain. The mean duration of pain is variable; it lasts for less than 6 months in most patients. About 5–10% of patients return to the physician with recurrent complaints persisting 6 months after the onset of infection (289). The incidence of this complication has prompted the evaluation of a variety of treatment regimens, including (a) long-term administration of narcotic analgesics, (b) attempts at altering the acute pain course with hopes of having an impact on the subsequent appearance of postherpetic neuralgia (steroids, amitriptyline, Prolixin, etc.), and (c) treatment of VZV with antiviral medications in order to shorten the extent of infection.

Diagnosis

Clinical

The diagnosis of chickenpox is clinical, predicated upon a proper history and characteristic lesions. Involvement of the CNS concomitant with the appearance of chickenpox leads the clinician to suspect viral infection of the brain; however, other potential etiologies should be excluded (such as Reye's syndrome or, rarely, concomitant bacterial infection).

Unilateral vesicular lesions in a dermatomal pattern lead the clinician to suspect a diagnosis of shingles. The diagnosis can be confirmed by isolation of virus from lesions. The optimal method for retrieval of virus is bedside inoculation of aspirated vesicular fluid into susceptible tissue culture cell lines. It has been reported that HSV

and coxsackievirus infections can masquerade as dermatomal vesicular lesions. In such situations, diagnostic viral cultures remain the best method for proving the etiology of the infection. The utilization of lesion scrapings and staining by Tzanck smear to demonstrate the presence of intranuclear inclusions and multinucleated giant cells is helpful in establishing a presumptive diagnosis of herpesvirus infection, as discussed earlier.

The diagnosis of VZV infection of the CNS in patients with chickenpox rests greatly on clinical association with overt cutaneous disease. Thus, the appearance of cerebellar ataxia in a patient with a classic chickenpox rash usually assures the diagnosis. Similarly, in the presence of a dermatomal vesicular rash and altered mentation, a diagnosis of HZAE is made.

Laboratory: Virus Isolation/Serologic Assessment

CNS infection with VZV is not usually substantiated by virus isolation from brain or neuronal tissue. Instead, the diagnosis is entertained by clinical findings. However, it may be that certain circumstances dictate the isolation of VZV from brain tissue, as would occur at necropsy. Experience with the isolation of VZV is derived, in large part, from its isolation from cutaneous lesions. These methods will be summarized.

Confirmation of the diagnosis of cutaneous VZV infection is possible only through isolation of virus in susceptible tissue culture lines or through the demonstration of seroconversion by antibody assessment. A rapid diagnostic impression can be obtained by scraping the base of the lesions in an attempt to demonstrate intranuclear inclusion bodies and multinucleated giant cells by Tzanck smear. These changes are not pathognomonic for VZV infection and require differentiation from other herpesvirus infections, specifically HSV. The ideal diagnostic confirmation is isolation of VZV from clinical specimens. It is important to emphasize that bedside collection and inoculation of specimens are imperative for recovery of virus in tissue culture. Vesicles should be aspirated with a tuberculin syringe containing viral transport media at the bedside and inoculated directly into susceptible cell lines. Cell lines suitable for isolation of VZV include either human embryonic skin–muscle tissue or foreskin fibroblasts. Although cytopathic effects can appear within 48–72 hr, it is more likely for them to appear approximately 7–10 days after inoculation of clinical specimens into the tissue. The description of the cytopathology has been noted previously. Unequivocal confirmation of the cytopathic effect can be achieved by neutralization with antibody in a complement-dependent neutralization assay or through fluorescent staining of the cell sheet.

In the past, serologic assessment of patients with VZV infections has focused on utilization of the complement-fixing (CF) antibody assay, although other approaches have included indirect immunofluorescence, fluorescent antibody to VZV membrane antigen (FAMA), complement-dependent neutralization, immune adherence hemagglutination (IAHA), enzyme-linked immunoabsorbance assay (ELISA), and radioimmunoassay. The CF assay has been replaced by more sensitive antibody detection procedures that utilize antigens prepared in alternative fashions (256,263,276,290). These assays have been reviewed for clinical utility elsewhere.

Treatment

Supportive Care

There is no specific therapy for either chickenpox or herpes zoster in the normal host. As a consequence, treatment is usually supportive. For patients with chickenpox, closely cropped finger nails to avoid scratching and associated secondary bacterial complications are important. Astringent soaks, antipyretics, and attention to secondary bacterial complications are all indicated. In contrast, the optimal approach for managing patients with herpes zoster is the appropriate administration of analgesics for control of pain. Cleansing of the lesions and frequent Burrow's solution soaks to the involved surface area are soothing and help to prevent secondary bacterial infection. With severe neuritis, it has been suggested that Elavil (amitriptyline hydrochloride) and Prolixin (fluphenazine hydrochloride), alone or in combination, are useful for amelioration of acute neuritis and may decrease the frequency of postherpetic neuralgia, but reports showing no efficacy also exist. In addition, administration of steroids has been reported to be useful in small controlled studies (291,292). Utilization of orally administered steroids may, however, delay healing in the primary dermatome (293). One recent large study concluded that pain was not beneficially influenced by the administration of corticosteroids (294). Severe unrelenting pain may necessitate nerve blocks.

Antiviral Therapy

Because of the recognized complications of both varicella and herpes zoster, several experimental antiviral treatments have been attempted in primarily immunocompromised patients but also in normal patients. It should be noted that treatment data have been derived from studies of patients with cutaneous disease and not specifically those with neurologic complications. These treatment data will be summarized.

The data from three antiviral trials of chickenpox are summarized in Table 5. The first successful antiviral chemotherapeutic agent for the management of chickenpox in the immunocompromised host was the drug vidarabine. In controlled investigations of 34 immunocompromised patients performed by the NIAID Collaborative Antiviral Study Group, a dosage of 10 mg/kg/day resulted in treated patients ceasing to form new lesions, and it enabled these patients to undergo defervescence more rapidly than their placebo counterparts (295). Importantly, the treated patients had a significantly lower incidence of life-threatening complications: 53% in placebo versus 5% in drug recipients ($p < 0.01$, Fischer exact test) (295). Thus, when therapy is instituted within 72 hr of the onset of chickenpox in the immunocompromised host, outcome is beneficially influenced (295).

A similar study model was employed for the evaluation of acyclovir (296). In this trial, therapy had no effect on cutaneous healing or fever; however, the administration of acyclovir did decrease the development of pneumonitis from 45% to 0%. No significant toxicity was reported. In spite of the lack of proof from large-scale controlled studies, the safety of acyclovir and its efficacy for other VZV infections have led to its preferential use in this disease. Acyclovir has been studied in adults with chickenpox who were considered to have normal immune systems. This clinical trial suggested that therapy was useful (297).

Interferons are a series of naturally occurring, low-molecular-weight glycoproteins that, among other func-

TABLE 5. *Therapy for chickenpox in immunocompromised patients*[a]

Demographics	Vidarabine (N = 19)	Leukocyte interferon (N = 23)	Acyclovir (N = 8)	Placebo (N = 48)
ALL or AML	12 (63%)	18 (78%)	6 (75%)	37 (77%)
Disease duration (days ± SEM)	1.7 ± 0.8	1.61 ± 0.50	2.2 ± 1.6	1.94 ± 1.08
Healing, time to lesion cessation (days ± SEM)	3.8 ± 1.1	3.8 ± 1.89	NR	5.45 ± 2.16
Visceral complications				
Postenrollment pneumonia	1 (5%)	3 (13%)	0	13 (27%)
Encephalitis	0	0	0	3 (6%)
Hepatitis	0	5 (22%)	0	9 (19%)
Overall	0	8 (35%)	0	25 (52%)
Mortality	0	2 (9%)	0	8 (17%)

[a] ALL, acute lymphoblastic leukemia; AML, acute myelocytic leukemia; NR, not reported.

tions, enhance host resistance to viral infection. High titers of interferon have been found in vesicle fluid from patients with varicella at the termination of illness, suggesting that interferon may play a role in the control of this disease (298). High dosages of interferon (leukocyte) have been shown to decrease the frequency of visceral complications and prevent progressive disease in children with varicella (299,300).

Specific therapeutic measures have been developed for treatment of herpes zoster in the immunocompromised host. Obviously, the high-risk patient with lymphoproliferative malignancy has the greatest need for parenteral antiviral therapy. At present, while three medications have been shown useful, only two therapies are of relevance. These therapeutic trials are summarized in Table 6. In two studies, vidarabine has been shown to accelerate the events of cutaneous healing, namely, cessation of new vesicle formation, time to total pustulation, and scabbing (293,301,302). Furthermore, therapy within 72 hr of onset prevents progression of lesion formation within the dermatome and allows gradual regression of the disease in the area involved. The most important advantage of administration of vidarabine to immunocompromised patients is the reduction of visceral complications from an overall frequency of 19% to 5% (293). Thus, early vidarabine therapy administered within 72 hr of lesion formation is effective in preventing complications and accelerating healing. Benefit can be achieved at a dosage of 10 mg/kg/day administered in standard intravenous solutions at a concentration of 0.5 mg/ml over 12 hr for 5 days.

A second therapeutic modality, but one which is not clinically useful at this time, is the administration of interferon. It has been employed successfully in a dose-escalating study of 90 patients with herpes zoster and an underlying malignancy (303). In this study, intramuscular administration of interferon at a dosage of $1-2 \times 10^6$ IU/kg resulted in (a) decreased vesicle formation in the primary dermatome and (b) a lowered frequency of cutaneous dissemination. The interferon-treated patients did not show a significant decrease in total healing time, but they did have significant amelioration of postherpetic neuralgia. Toxicity included fever, malaise, myalgia, and depressed leukocyte counts. The usefulness of leukocyte interferon for treatment of herpes zoster infections in the immunocompromised host may be expanded with the availability of recombinant-DNA-produced interferon.

A third treatment modality is the administration of intravenous acyclovir at dosages of 500 mg/m² every 8 hr for 7–10 days. Two studies, one placebo-controlled and the other a comparative trial with vidarabine, indicate that progressive disease is slowed in the immunocompromised host (304,305). In bone marrow transplant recipients, acyclovir therapy was superior to vidarabine treatment; in this study, all events of cutaneous healing and disease progression were statistically significantly improved with acyclovir therapy (305). Furthermore, a small comparative study of these two medications for disseminated zoster also suggested superiority of acyclovir therapy (306). Thus, intravenous acyclovir therapy has become the choice for patients at high risk for progressive disease and has replaced vidarabine in clinical practice.

As with CNS complications of chickenpox, no clinical trial has established the value of an antiviral agent for HZAE. Nevertheless, when confronted with a patient suffering from herpes zoster and clinical evidence of encephalitis, acyclovir is used empirically.

TABLE 6. *Therapeutic trials of antivirals for herpes zoster in immunocompromised hosts*[a]

	N	Days of new lesion formation	Dissemination/ progression of cutaneous disease	Visceral disease	Resolution of postherpetic neuralgia
Interferon (106)					
Drug	45	$p < 0.01$	$p < 0.025$	1/45	27/29
Placebo	45			6/45	21/29
				($p < 0.05$)	($p = 0.05$)
Vidarabine (164,166)					
Drug	47	$p = 0.004$	CNE	CNE	CNE
Placebo	40				
Drug	63	$p = 0.002$	5 (8%)	3 (5%)	35 (56%)
Placebo	58		14 (24%)	11 (19%)	10 (17%)
			$p = 0.014$	$p = 0.015$	$p = 0.047$
Acyclovir (16)					
Drug	52	NS	9/28	0/52	
Placebo	42		15/24	4/42	NS
			NS	($p = 0.04$)	
Acyclovir versus vidarabine (136)					
Drug	11	$p = 0.03$	$p = 0.016$	0	NS
Placebo	11			0	

[a] CNE, could not evaluate; NS, not significant.

Recently, several trials have reported the outcome of patients receiving oral (307–309)—400 to 800 mg five times daily—or intravenous acyclovir (310–312) for localized zoster in the normal host. Therapy accelerated, but variably so, the duration of lesion formation and time to healing but appears to have little effect on postherpetic neuralgia. Hopefully, ongoing trials will help clarify clinical utility.

Future Directions

The medical community is cognizant of the fact that chickenpox is benign in children but that it tends to cause more severe illness in adults. The same age parallel is appropriate for herpes zoster. The variable of immunosuppression increases the propensity of VZV infections to cause life-threatening illness. Individuals who develop herpes zoster while immunocompromised are at risk for the life-threatening complications of varicella pneumonitis, whereas the older individual, immunocompromised or not, may suffer from severe neuritis as well as postherpetic neuralgia.

Currently, antiviral treatment regimens are available only for the immunocompromised host. To date, successful and practical therapeutic approaches have involved the utilization of acyclovir and vidarabine for the management of disease. Evaluations of orally administered acyclovir for management of herpes zoster in the immunocompromised and normal host continue.

EPSTEIN–BARR VIRUS

History

The history of Epstein–Barr virus (EBV) infections parallels that of our clinical knowledge of infectious mononucleosis. In 1920, Sprunt and Evans (313) described an illness compatible with infectious mononucleosis. Subsequently, Downey and McKinlay (314) defined the hematologic parameters associated with infection. In 1932, Paul and Brunnell (397) found the heterophile antibodies in the sera of patients who served as controls for individuals with rheumatoid arthritis. Subsequently, Downey and McKinlay (314) defined the hematologic parameters associated with this infection. Virologic confirmation of EBV did not occur until the late 1950s and under somewhat different clinical circumstances. In 1958, Burkitt (315) identified a tumor of East African children which involved the jaw and which was classified as a lymphoma. In search of a virologic etiology, electron-microscopic studies of these lymphomas demonstrated the presence of viral particles resembling herpesviruses. However, it was not until 1966 that Drs. Gertrude and Werner Henle identified the antigens of EBV within infected cells (316,317). Subsequently, a

technician working with EBV in the Henle laboratory developed a mononucleosis-like illness, with confirmed serologic changes to EBV. These observations provided a documented serologic approach to this infection (318–320). Subsequent collaboration with Drs. Niederman and McCollum provided convincing proof of the association between EBV and mononucleosis.

During the 1970s, viral culture and molecular biologic techniques allowed for the identification of viral nucleic acids in tumors identified by Burkitt (315) as well as in nasopharyngeal carcinoma (321,322). In subsequent years, the spectrum of EBV infections in humans has expanded. We now recognize that EBV is a cause of (a) a B-cell lymphoproliferative disease (323–325) in immunosuppressed individuals and (b) oral leukoplakia in patients with AIDS (326–328). Proof of a relationship between EBV and the chronic fatigue syndrome is lacking (329). These viruses do not appear to infect the CNS at high frequency. Thus, only a brief summary of EBV will ensue.

Infectious Agent

EBV is a lymphotropic herpesvirus, being a member of the gamma Herpesviridae subfamily. EBVs are unique in their ability to replicate *in vitro* in B lymphocytes, resulting in continuous proliferation. These viruses, like other members of the herpesviruses family, establish latency and can be reactivated. The diameter of the virion is 122 nm, and that of the capsid is 80 nm. The guanosine and cytosine content is somewhat different from that of other herpesviruses, being 59% (330). The genome consists of approximately 175,000 base pairs and has been totally sequenced (331,332). Transcription of EBV DNA results in excess of 60 RNA species which conform to immediate-early, early, and late genes. The most abundant protein appearing in infected cells is viral capsid antigen (VCA) (333).

Pathology and Pathogenesis

EBV has the unique property of being able to infect and immortalize lymphocytes of immunoglobulin-producing lineage (B lymphocytes) (334). Infected cells possess specific receptors (CR2 for C3D) (335).

It is likely that EBV gains access to humans via the oropharynx, where it can be identified; this virus replicates in the salivary gland and exfoliated oral secretions, as well as in other localized cells of the area (321,325,336–344). It is estimated that approximately one in every 500 lymphocytes contains EBV during acute mononucleosis (339).

Two patterns of replication can be identified in humans: (i) lytic infection resulting in cell death and (ii) immortalization of infected cells with the establishment of a latent state. Detailed reviews have summarized the replication and pathogenesis of EBV infections (330,345,346). These replicative cycles will not be detailed; however, it is worth noting that at least eight genes have been identified as playing critical roles in the replication of latent virus. These include a series of EBV nuclear antigens (identified as 1–5), a leader protein, and a latent membrane protein (LMP), among others. The precise biological properties of each of these genes is not well-appreciated; however, functions of three have begun to be identified. These include: Epstein–Barr virus nuclear antigen (EBNA) 1, apparently responsible for replicating the episomal genome; EBNA-2, required for transformation; and LMP, which confers transformation characteristics on B cells. These latter events may be particularly relevant, since they relate to the association of EBV with transformed cells both in humans and animals (330,345,347–350).

Epidemiology

EBV is an ubiquitous agent with world-wide distribution. Socioeconomic status is a major determinant of acquisition of infection by EBV, especially early in life. Individuals of lower socioeconomic status and those living in crowded conditions are more prone to acquire infection early in life. Specifically, in countries with a high population density, over 90% of children will have acquired EBV before entry into school (351,352). In contrast, individuals of higher socioeconomic status do not acquire infection until adolescence or upon entry into college (345,353–365).

EBV is most notably associated with the infectious mononucleosis syndrome. The estimate of the incidence of mononucleosis in the United States is approximately 25–99 cases per 100,000 per year (366–370). A lower incidence has been reported in other countries (371). However, this may be a function of reporting differences. Infectious mononucleosis is characterized by fever, pharyngitis, cervical adenopathy, and splenomegaly. Routinely, patients report malaise. The clinical findings with infectious mononucleosis have been described in general textbooks of infectious diseases (346,372).

The incubation period for EBV infection appears to be between 4 and 7 weeks. Virus can be detected in the saliva in the majority of patients. Clearly, a viremic phase is associated with other manifestations of disease, including splenomegaly. Splenomegaly develops in 50% of patients, and a smaller percentage of patients will have hepatic enlargement; however, virtually all patients will have events of transient elevation of liver enzymes. The most characteristic laboratory abnormality is evidence of atypical lymphocytosis on the peripheral blood smear. This may appear late in the course of disease but, nevertheless, provides a basis for diagnosis.

Other prominent clinical syndromes attributed to EBV include associated malignancies, particularly Burkitt's lymphoma and nasopharyngeal carcinoma (373–378). EBVs in the immunocompromised host can cause a lymphoproliferative disease. Furthermore, a hereditary associated X-linked lymphoproliferative syndrome (XLPS) in males has been noted (379–387). It should be recognized that a small group of patients, usually males, have been reported to have a chronic mononucleosis syndrome without evidence of an immune deficiency; however, the ability to unequivocally incriminate EBV as the cause of this syndrome has been difficult in many of these patients (326,388). Similarly, some investigators have associated the chronic fatigue syndrome with EBV infection (327,389); however, there is no unequivocal evidence to support such an association.

Central Nervous System Complications of Epstein–Barr Virus

EBV has been associated with a variety of CNS complications, including meningoencephalitis, encephalitis, cerebritis, Guillain–Barré syndrome, transverse myelitis, and neuropsychiatric syndromes (390,391). The infrequency of the occurrence of neurologic manifestations of EBV infections makes it difficult to summarize existing data. It should be noted, however, that most findings of either cerebritis or encephalitic manifestations occur during the acute course of infectious mononucleosis. However, the more usual association is with Guillain–Barré syndrome, as described elsewhere in this book. It is apparent that such complications are uncommon events. The pathophysiology of CNS involvement is not clear, as noted in several reviews (346).

It has been noted that CSF examination in patients with CNS complications provides evidence of increased cell counts and elevated levels of protein (392). Abnormal neurologic findings have been defined in approximately 5% of hospitalized patients (346,393). Interestingly, when death occurs as a consequence of infectious mononucleosis, neurologic complications are considered a more frequent cause than those usually described in the literature, such as splenic rupture (394).

While the pathogenesis of infection is unknown, in those patients dying from infection, perivascular cuffing has been identified in CNS tissue along with other findings such as edema and demyelination (395,396).

In studies performed by the NIAID Collaborative Antiviral Study Group, it has been noted that several patients have been identified to have a focal encephalopathic process caused by EBV. These patients presented in a fashion similar to that of patients with HSE; however, the course of disease and outcome in the EBV patients was much less severe. Most of these individuals return to normal function following their episode of infection.

Diagnosis

Diagnosis of EBV infections is predicated on serologic response, since viral isolation is not possible in routine diagnostic laboratories. Historically, heterophile antibody responses have been used to diagnose infection, as originally described by Paul and Brunnell (397). Because of the lack of specificity of this assay, alternative diagnostic tests have been developed which utilize type-specific EBV serology. These techniques use immunofluorescence to detect either early or late antigens which appear during the replicative process of EBV. Only a very brief summary will ensue. The first antibodies to appear in the course of disease are those directed against EBV VCAs (326,327,398). As infection progresses, other routine diagnostic assays include anticomplementary antigens to nuclear proteins, identified as EBNA (399,400). Thus, antibodies directed against EBV VCAs, along with the absence of EBNA antibodies, are indicative of acute infection. In contrast, preexisting EBNA antibodies weigh against a diagnosis of primary EBV infection. Other immunofluorescence antibodies have been detected against early antigens and have been subdivided into early antigen diffuse (EA-D) and early antigen restricted (EA-R) antibody responses (326,327). The antibodies to these specific antigens are used less routinely for diagnostic purposes.

Treatment

For the most part, treatment of EBV infections is symptomatic. Thus, rest and antipyretics provide the foundation of clinical care. Corticosteroids have been employed for management of acute airway complications, notably pharyngeal edema with impending airway obstruction (401,402); however, deployment of steroids is reserved for particularly severe cases.

Thus far, no antiviral agent has been shown to be efficacious in the management of EBV infections. Control studies have evaluated the treatment of acute infectious mononucleosis and EBV-associated disorders in patients with XLPS. Irrespective of the study population, clinical benefit from treatment is not apparent (403–405). In spite of the activity of compounds such as acyclovir and ganciclovir *in vitro* (406–409), it should be noted that a recently described complication of EBV infection, namely lymphoproliferative disease in organ transplant recipients, has been cited as being amenable to acyclovir therapy (326,410).

Future Directions

CNS complications of EBV infections are very rare. As a consequence, most effort is directed toward the control of primary infection with EBV. Such efforts are directed toward the development of a vaccine and of specific and selective antiviral drugs.

CYTOMEGALOVIRUS

History

Cytomegalovirus (CMV) infections are ubiquitous, as is the case with other members of the herpesvirus family. Importantly, however, these viruses are highly species-specific, being only linked to infection of humans. Evidence of cytomegalic inclusion disease was apparent even before the causative pathogen was isolated (411). Pathologic descriptions indicate evidence of cytomegalic cells in kidney, liver, and lungs of newborn infants and in organs of newborn children dying early in life (412,413). Subsequent studies of inclusion-bearing cells indicated the commonness of such infections in young infants (414).

However, it was not until the late 1950s that three laboratories nearly simultaneously isolated CMV in cell culture systems (415–417). Subsequently, Weller coined the phrase "salivary gland virus." In all circumstances, CMV was isolated from the biological fluids or tissues obtained from children, either newborns or young children undergoing adenoidectomy.

Infectious Agent

CMV is the largest member of the herpesvirus family, being approximately 200 nm in diameter (418). The DNA of CMV is approximately 250 kb in size and has a molecular weight of 150×10^6; thus, it is approximately 50% larger than HSV. Its replicative scheme is very similar to that of HSV in that its gene replication is temporally regulated (20). Because of its size, numerous gene products are encoded during the replicative process (419).

Replication of CMV *in vitro* is dependent upon growth in cell lines of human origin; thus, human fibroblast lines are generally used to support growth (420–422). Replication is slow, and defective viral particles are common during the replicative process (420–427).

Pathology and Pathogenesis

Replication of CMV in cell culture systems is associated with the formation of cytomegalic inclusion cells with typical intranuclear inclusions. However, it can also replicate in endothelial cells and macrophages. Both *in vitro* and *in vivo* spread of CMV is cell-to-cell, with the development of both intracytoplasmic and intranuclear inclusions (420,422,425). *In vitro* evidence of enlargement of cells can occur within 6 hr after infection followed by eosinophilic cytoplasmic inclusions and within 24 hr of nuclear inclusions between 48 and 72 hr.

With cell-to-cell spread of infection, there is release of extracellular virus, leading to viremia. Clearly, impaired host defenses will lead to inability to control viremic spread of infection. Viremia is associated with seeding of other organs, particularly the kidney—resulting in viruria. Under such circumstances, evidence of cytomegalic cells can be found in the kidney, with occasional evidence for renal immune complex disease (428,429). Cytomegalic cells can be found in the collecting tubal system (430).

In addition, other organs can be involved with viremic spread of infection; these include the liver (431), lung (432,433), and CNS (433–436), among others. Involvement of the CNS in newborns will be the subject of a separate chapter. Involvement of the CNS in immuno-compromised individuals who are older children and adults will be specifically dealt with in this section.

Epidemiology

Most individuals experience CMV infection at one point or another during their lifetime. The prevalence of antibodies indicating infection increases over one's life-span (437–442). Transmission of CMV infection can be by one of many routes, including sexual, salivary, or close contact with an infected person excreting viral, parenteral (blood transfusion or organ transplantation), or transplacental infection leading to intrauterine infection (443–445). Acquisition of infection occurs early in life but is dependent upon socioeconomic status. By 1 year of age, up to 60% of populations in the Western World have acquired CMV infection. In large part, these infections are the consequence of crowded living conditions (446–450). The high prevalence of CMV infection is indicated by the frequency of viral shedding from urine of patients at varying ages. Approximately 1% of all live newborns are congenitally infected with CMV. Infection increases over the first few years of life such that 10–30% of children, according to socioeconomic status, will be found to excrete virus in the urine. Adults without evidence of disease will excrete virus at a rate of approximately 2%—except for healthy gay men, in whom excretion can occur in up to 14% (20,418,446–449,451–454). Virus has also been found in the following: cervical secretions of women, both pregnant and nonpregnant (419–421); semen (454–456); and breast milk (450,457,458).

Manifestations of infection occur in several distinct populations. The most common form of CNS infection early in life is that which is the consequence of intrauterine transmission. As noted previously, approximately 1% of newborns excrete CMV at birth, only 10% of whom will have clinical evidence of disease, including hepatosplenomegaly, a petechial/purpuric skin rash, cho-

rioretinitis, intracranial calcification, and/or ventriculomegaly. Symptomatic children with congenital CMV infection are often growth-retarded. The manifestations of CMV infection of the CNS in these children are the subject of a separate chapter.

In older individuals who are immunocompetent, a CMV mononucleosis syndrome is a common clinical presentation. These clinical manifestations include fever, myalgia, malaise, pharyngitis, splenomegaly, and adenopathy. Infection resulting in CMV mononucleosis can be acquired by sexual, parenteral, or intimate contact.

Immunocompromised patients represent a common group of patients with active CMV infection. CMV disease in these patients can be life- and sight-threatening. From large studies performed in immunocompromised organ transplant recipients, CMV is an extremely prevalent infection, occurring in the majority of individuals undergoing such procedures. Disease in these individuals has been associated with organ rejection (459–479). It is also recognized that individuals suffering from AIDS, as described elsewhere, can develop CMV pneumonitis alone or in association with *Pneumonitis carinii* pneumonia (478,480,481). Under such circumstances, pneumonitis is usually associated with a nonproductive cough, fever, dyspnea, tachypnea, and, usually, hypoxemia. In addition, immunocompromised individuals, particularly those with AIDS, are at high risk for the development of chorioretinitis (481–483), but this syndrome has been identified in renal transplant recipients as well (483). In immunocompromised patients, involvement of the gastrointestinal tract, particularly colitis, esophagitis, and gastritis, have been reported (484,485).

Central Nervous System Complications

CNS complications of CMV infection are uncommon. The most significant manifestation of CMV disease in the CNS is that which is associated with perinatal infection, which will be discussed elsewhere. Otherwise, CMV infection of the CNS can take one of three forms. The first is primary infection with concomitant involvement of the CNS resulting in an acute encephalitic episode. Such manifestations are usually associated with meningitis, encephalitis, or meningoencephalitis. Virus has been isolated from both CSF and brain tissue from normal individuals (486,487). Clinical manifestations of disease in these patients are similar to that encountered for other encephalitic and meningitic viral infections, including altered mentation, seizures, and focal or diffuse neurological findings. Neurodiagnostic evaluation usually reveals generalized slowing of the EEG with diffuse cerebral edema on CT scan. CSF examination indicates a formula of increased protein and cells. These findings are not specific for CMV infection of the CNS.

The CNS involvement in such cases is probably the

consequence of viremic spread with endothelial infection leading to perivascular cuffing and lymphocytic infiltrate in brain tissue.

A second form of CNS disease caused by CMV occurs in the immunocompromised host. This entity has been particularly well documented in organ transplant recipients, usually on postmortem examination of brain tissue (488,489). More recently, with the appearance of human immunodeficiency virus infection and AIDS, CMV has been reported as being present in the brain tissue from a variety of patients with varying stages of disease. However, clearly one of the problems in ascribing a role for CMV and disease of the brain is the known propensity of HIV to involve the CNS as well. Distinguishing between those findings associated with CMV and HIV is difficult.

Finally, CMV infection has been incriminated as the cause of Guillain–Barré syndrome. This subject has been discussed extensively in Chapter 12.

Diagnosis

The isolation of CMV from patients with disease is the gold standard for diagnosis. CMV can be isolated in cells of human origin, as noted previously. Standard cell lines for retrieval of CMV include human foreskin fibroblast and human epithelial cell lines, among others. Positive identification of CMV in these systems is confirmed by classic cytopathic effect as well as by monoclonal antibodies staining for purposes of confirmation. Further support for the diagnosis can be achieved by *in situ* hybridization.

Because of the prolonged replication cycle of CMV, it may take as long as 2–4 weeks before evidence of cytopathic effect appears in cell culture systems. As a consequence, more rapid diagnostic procedures have been developed. Two of the most promising include the shell vial technique and the polymerase chain reaction. The shell vial technique employs the inoculation of biological specimens onto cell monolayers, with the subsequent staining by a monoclonal antibody directed against immediate-early gene products. Similarly, the polymerase chain reaction has been employed on certain biological specimens, including urine, white blood cells, and tissue. These latter assays remain experimental and of unsubstantiated clinical value at the present time.

The definition of CMV as a cause of CNS disease is difficult, at best. The lack of availability of tissues for routine diagnostic purposes further magnifies the diagnostic problem. Isolation of CMV from the urine of a presumed encephalopathic patient cannot be equated with a diagnosis of CMV infection of the brain, particularly in the immunocompromised host at risk for human immunodeficiency virus infection. At the present time, the application of the polymerase chain reaction to cells obtained from the CSF for definition of CMV infection has not been evaluated. Perhaps future studies will allow for further definition of the value of such diagnostic approaches.

Serologic approaches to the diagnosis of CMV infection have been less than useful for elucidation of the etiology of acute CNS syndromes. The availability of serologic studies which detect evidence of IgM antibodies may be helpful in the future; however, these techniques currently suffer from specificity problems.

Therapy

The management of patients with CNS infections caused by CMV is complicated by inability to precisely diagnose the infection. If such infections occurred more commonly or were more readily diagnosable, then, for the most part, treatment would be reserved for life-threatening cases.

Ganciclovir, 9-hydroxyethoxymethyl guanine, has been utilized for the treatment of life- and sight-threatening CMV infections in immunocompromised individuals. Recently, this medication was licensed by the Food and Drug Administration for the treatment of CMV chorioretinitis. No data exist regarding the utility of this compound for the management of CNS infections caused by CMV. Similarly, immunoglobulin products have been used for therapy of CMV pneumonia but not for therapy of CNS infections.

Future Directions

Future efforts will focus on the development of specific and safe antiviral agents. The development of drugs without evidence of toxicity (e.g., ganciclovir), particularly bioavailable ones, is mandatory to advance the management of CMV infections in high-risk individuals. It should be noted that vaccines directed against this pathogen are in varying stages of development; however, their utility in preventing severe disease in immunocompromised hosts remains uncertain, particularly since there is evidence for exogenous reinfection in high-risk immunocompromised individuals.

B VIRUS

History

Of the nearly 35 herpesviruses reported to have been isolated from nonhuman primates, only one—B virus of Old World monkeys—is highly pathogenic for humans. In 1932, a young physician (WB) bitten by a monkey developed localized erythema at the site of the animal bite. This apparent localized infection was followed by lymphangitis, lymphadenitis, and, ultimately, transverse myelitis. The demise of WB was ascribed to respiratory failure. At the time of WB's death, tissue specimens were obtained for laboratory investigation by two independent research groups. In 1933, Gay and Holden (490) reported an ultrafilterable agent which recreated in rabbits a disease similar to that observed in WB. This virus was recovered from the neurological tissues of WB. The inoculation of this virus by either intradermal or intracranial routes was lethal in the animal model. The investigators of this laboratory thought that the virus was similar to HSV and referred to the isolate as "W." While attempts at transmission of this virus to rhesus monkeys failed, infection of cebus monkeys was successful.

Sabin and Wright (491), working independently from Gay and Holden, reported in 1934 a similar filterable agent which they identified as "B virus," named after the patient from whom it was originally isolated. Sabin and Wright (491) isolated the virus from numerous neurological tissues as well as from peripheral organs (spleen but not lymph node specimens). As with the isolate named "W," B virus also was found to result in lethal disease when inoculated by either intradermal or intracerebral routes into rabbits. It was not found to be virulent when given by these same routes to a variety of other species, including mice, dogs, and guinea pigs. Furthermore, Sabin and Wright recognized (by immunological characterization of the isolate) its relationship to HSV and pseudorabies virus (492,493). At the time when latinization of viral name was fashionable, the B virus acquired the name "herpes simiae." The name is a misnomer because nonhuman primates have yielded numerous unrelated herpesviruses. According to the present nomenclature (494), it is designated as the "cercopithecine herpesvirus 1." In this chapter the virus will be designated by its common name—that is, the B virus.

The B virus is indigenous to Old World monkeys (495–498). Most commonly, it is enzootic in rhesus (*Macaca mulatta*) and cynomolgus (*Macaca fascicularus*) monkeys, as well as in other Asiatic species of the genus *Macaca*. Most reported human cases resulted from bites by rhesus monkeys. Since the original reports of human herpes B virus infections, advances in our knowledge about human disease caused by this virus have proceeded slowly. In the world literature, approximately 24 cases of herpes B virus disease have been documented in humans (499–501), with other case reports pending.

Although B virus infection of humans is not a common public health problem, the recent diagnosis of B virus in four individuals living in Pensacola, Florida, in 1987, has refocused medical and public health attention on the neuropathogenicity of this infection (501). While two of these cases were mild, two resulted in fatal infection. More importantly, the person-to-person transmission of infection from one of the fatal cases to a relative was documented for the first time (501). More recently,

an additional case has been identified which led to infection but without evidence of life-threatening clinical disease (502). Thus, while this organism has a high propensity for mortality in the identified human cases, it is likely that a larger but unknown number of individuals have been infected by the virus but did not develop clinical evidence of disease.

Infectious Agent

Burnett et al. (503) propagated B virus on the chorioallantoic membrane of embryonated eggs. Tissue culture isolation of B virus did not occur until 1954, when it was recovered from rhesus kidney tissue which was used for preparation of poliomyelitis vaccines (504). During vaccine production it was noted that suspended cell culture systems from six kidneys elicited cytopathic effects similar to that of HSV. The resulting lesions were focal in nature and were histologically similar to those induced by HSV.

Notwithstanding numerous attempts at isolation of virus from macaques, the first report of virus isolation is that of Reissig and Melnick (505), who recovered B virus from tissue cultures of purportedly normal rhesus monkeys. Further studies led to the realization that this virus was easily propagated in monkey kidney and chick embryo cell lines (505,506). Furthermore, the virus is relatively stable in tissue culture media stored at 4°C; however, upon freezing, viral infectivity was maintained if the culture was stored at −72°C.

The replication of B virus was reported by several laboratories (493,505–516), although Reissig and Melnick (505) were the first to describe the properties of B virus in cell culture. The reproductive cycle is relatively short. The virus inhibits host cell DNA and protein synthesis during the first 4 hr after infection. Infectious virus is detectable approximately 6 hr after infection, and both extracellular and intracellular virus levels plateau approximately 24–36 hr after infection and decline thereafter (505,514). B virus causes the cells to fuse into polykaryocytes, and, like other herpesviruses, it causes the formation of Cowdry type A intranuclear inclusions in cultured cells.

Pathology and Pathogenesis

Pathology

B virus multiplies well in cell lines of simian origin (particularly primary vervet monkey), but it also multiplies well in rabbit kidney cells and other established cell lines such as BS-C-1 (517) and LLC-RK (518). The characteristic cytopathic effect is similar to that of HSV. Cells balloon, fuse into polykaryocytes, and form clusters as focal areas of infection spread through the entire cell sheet. Upon fixation and staining, Cowdry type A eosinophilic intranuclear inclusions are readily demonstrable.

Pathologic findings in humans are indicative of the target organs involved. As described below, there is little difference in the histopathologic findings encountered following either simian or human infection.

Pathogenesis of Human Infection

Disease in humans usually results from an animal bite, although disease which is the consequence of reactivation and respiratory spread has been reported (see below). Following the animal bite, as was documented in the very first case of human B virus disease, replication of virus at the local site of inoculation can be documented. Usually, there is evidence of local inflammation with mononuclear infiltrate followed by evidence of lymphangitis and subsequent lymph node involvement.

A striking characteristic of human B virus infection is the propensity to involve the CNS. As in the first case reported, transverse myelitis is a prominent neurologic finding with ultimate progression of infection to the brain. All regions of the brain can be involved by B virus without evidence of localization to any particular region. This latter observation stands in contrast to HSV of the CNS, which tends to localize in the temporal lobe. Histopathologic findings of the brain include hemorrhagic foci, necrosis, and inflammatory changes, particularly as evidenced by perivascular cuffing with mononuclear infiltrates. Edema and degeneration of motor neurons are prominent. Even with advancing disease, Cowdry type A eosinophilic intranuclear inclusions can be found in only a few cases. In addition, gliosis and astrocytosis are late histopathologic findings. Thus, there can be evidence of myelitis, encephalomyelitis, or encephalitis, or combinations thereof (519,520).

Other organs of the body can be involved, presumably as a consequence of transient viremia. These organs are usually the viscera, particularly the liver and lung. Under such circumstances, focal hemorrhagic necrosis is common.

To summarize human pathogenesis, the tissues and organs which become infected by B virus vary according to the route of inoculation. If the skin is the primary source of involvement, virus replicates in the skin; this leads to erythema and chalor at the initial site of involvement. Subsequently, lymphangitis and lymphadenitis will develop. While viremia has been documented in both rabbits and monkeys, this route of pathogenesis has not been documented for humans. Certainly, with lymphatic involvement, it is possible for the virus to spread by lymphangitic routes, particularly to abdominal viscera. Nevertheless, spread via neuronal routes must be the fundamental route of transmission of infection, as with HSV. This is likely the case because of the involve-

ment of the spinal cord and CNS. Visceral organs which are involved, including the heart, liver, spleen, lungs, kidneys, and adrenals, reflect evidence of congestion and focal necrosis; however, the degree of involvement varies from one patient to the next.

Pathogenesis of Latency

As with other herpesviruses, B virus becomes latent and can recur. As will be discussed below, prevalence of antibodies to B virus is widespread in Old World rhesus monkeys. It has been noted that rhesus monkeys captured from the wild and shipped to primate centers develop vesicular lesions of the oropharynx suggesting a pattern of virus reactivation and recrudescence of lesions similar to that encountered with HSV. Unequivocal evidence of latent infection caused by B virus in rhesus monkeys has evolved with the studies on the frequency of recovery of B virus in monkey kidney cell culture systems. Thus, Wood and Shimada (504) obtained six isolates from 650 pools of monkey kidneys, suggesting that at least 1% of rhesus monkeys contain latent virus which can be reactivated by culturing kidney cells. Virus was isolated from rhesus tissues also by Boulter and colleagues (521,522). B virus was recovered by co-cultivation from a variety of neuronal tissues (including Gasserian ganglia, trigeminal ganglia, and dorsal root ganglia) and the spinal cord (523,524). Latent virus was also isolated by co-cultivation of tissues from experimentally infected rabbits (504).

As in the case of HSV infections in humans, the most prominent factor associated with reactivation of B virus in rhesus monkeys is stress, particularly stress associated with the capture and shipping of animals from the wild to captivity. To date, nothing has been reported on the state of viral DNA during latency or on the molecular or biochemical events associated with the establishment and reactivation of latent virus.

Epidemiology of Human Infection

The epidemiology of B virus infections in humans must be considered in the context of the epidemiology of any infectious disease process, including the susceptibility of the host and quantity of virus received. It is especially important to recognize that the frequency of excretion of B virus in animals at large only averages 2–3% at the most; thus, if a human is bitten by an animal, the probability of infection is low, albeit existent. Direct contact with a source of virus—namely, an infected animal (or cells obtained from an infected animal), either actively infected or latently infected—is the means by which an infection is transmitted. Virus cannot penetrate intact skin; thus, a break in the skin is required for acquisition of infection. Sites which have been documented as becoming infected in humans include wounds, the eye, and, perhaps, the respiratory tract. Since it is well established that infected animals can excrete virus in saliva, from the eye, in vesicular fluid, and, perhaps, in the stool, these sites must be considered potential sources for human infection. Furthermore, as has been well documented in the history of the development of poliomyelitis vaccine, infected cell culture tissues can also be a source of viral infections for humans.

Person-to-person transmission of B virus has only recently been documented (501). In this instance, the wife of an animal worker, who subsequently died from B virus infection of the CNS, acquired vesicular lesions of her ring finger. She provided direct care of her husband's vesicular lesions. While she survived infection without evidence of neurologic disease, the extent of disease may have been limited by early intervention with acyclovir therapy. It should be noted that the individuals who developed B virus infection had contact either skin-to-skin or face-to-face with at least 40 other individuals during the cluster of cases in Pensacola, Florida. While these other individuals were under close surveillance, none have developed evidence of infection even a year later. Thus, casual contact can be excluded as a method of transmission of B virus infection. This is particularly important from a public health standpoint.

Nonfatal infection has not been well documented in reports of human disease (525). One recent animal bite resulted in localized viral replication but without systemic involvement (502).

Serologic assessment of humans for evidence of B virus, as a marker of subclinical infection, is confounded by cross-reactivity to HSV.

Central Nervous System Disease

Human disease caused by B virus is characterized by an ascending myelitis and/or encephalomyelitis. Disease is especially notable because of its propensity to result in increased mortality and enhanced morbidity. To date, there are a limited number of cases of human disease caused by B virus in the literature, assessed recently at 31, depending upon the criteria for case definition (491,496,498,499,501,526–533). Approximately four cases have been referred to in the literature but have not been documented, and others will soon be reported (498). An additional case report of evidence of infection without disease has recently been published (502). Regardless of the exact number of cases, the total number of patients who have experienced disease is limited. It should be emphasized that probably thousands of animal workers have been exposed to animals excreting virus but very few have developed disease. Thus, casual transmission is unlikely. Nevertheless, the lessons learned regarding the clinical manifestations of disease

in individuals exposed to B virus, as well as the necessity for methods of intervention and prevention, are reinforced by the findings of these particular patients.

Acquisition and manifestations of infection can be one of at least four findings. First, as alluded to recently, infection may be asymptomatic. It was recently reported that an animal worker exposed to a rhesus monkey with conjunctivitis was stuck by a needle which had been used for inoculations of this animal (502). The needle-stick site was subsequently biopsied and revealed evidence of multinucleated giant cells. B virus DNA was detected in the biopsy, but there was no evidence of clinical disease. This form of infection may be an underreported event for individuals exposed to B virus.

The second, and more common, route of infection is that of disease resultant from an animal bite. Following a bite of a monkey excreting B virus, a localized vesicular lesion associated with erythema and edema develops at the site of viral inoculation. Subsequently, lymphangitis with spread to regional lymph nodes occurs, along with the development of secondary lymphadenopathy. While it has not been documented in humans, transient viremia leading to seeding of viscera may ensue. These early stages of disease are generally accompanied by fever, myalgia, vomiting, cramping, meningeal irritation, and such cranial nerve signs as nystagmus and diplopia. Neurologic findings ensue very rapidly. Altered sensation, hyperesthesia, and/or paresthesia of the limbs usually precede evidence of weakness, areflexia, and flaccid paralysis. Transverse myelitis with evidence of a urinary retention syndrome may well occur. With progressive involvement of the CNS, decreased levels of consciousness, altered mentation, respiratory depression, seizures, and, ultimately, a neurologic death ensue.

Although the incubation period for B virus has been debated, the majority of cases have a relatively short incubation period of approximately 3–5 days; however, some cases have been reported to occur as late as 24 days after an animal bite. The onset of neurologic symptoms generally occurs 3–7 days after the appearance of a vesicular rash. Time to death varies from individual to individual and can occur as early as 10–14 days or much later. Improvements in intensive care for critically ill patients probably influenced these survival data. It should be emphasized that the progression of infection is probably the consequence of a variety of factors, including host immunologic status (quantity of neutralizing antibodies to herpes simplex), age of the patient, site of the bite, and quantity of virus inoculated. Prolonged incubation periods, as well as the mechanism for these prolonged incubation periods, have not been well characterized (531,532,534).

Third, two cases have been documented following presumed exposure to infected secretions by a respiratory route. Although it has been presumed that most cases of animal-to-human transmission have occurred following exposure to infected saliva by animal bite, these two cases illustrate the potential for respiratory spread. Symptoms in these individuals included those localized to the respiratory tract, including coryza, cough, laryngitis, and pharyngitis. While associated with fever, these symptoms progressed to respiratory distress, as evidenced by a radiographic picture of interstitial pneumonitis. One of these two patients had virus isolated from a vesicle. Subsequently, neurologic symptoms developed, leading ultimately to death of these patients (496,532).

The fourth manifestation of human disease is that of a recurrent infection. It has now been documented in two cases that a recurrent vesicular rash can occur as a consequence of B virus infection. In one case, infection was acquired as a consequence of person-to-person transmission (501). In another case an individual developed lesions compatible with the diagnosis of herpes zoster; however, B virus was isolated from these lesions (529). Thus, the potential for latent infection with subsequent reactivation should be recognized.

Of the total documented cases of herpes B virus infection, 20 of the 22 cases developed encephalitis, with death occurring in 75% (15 of 20) of these patients (499). Survivors of B virus infection of the CNS have been left with a broad spectrum of neurologic impairment. Of those documented in the literature, two had mild or minimal impairment, one had moderate neurologic impairment, and the remainder had severe impairment. It should be noted that the literature also includes three patients who were infected by B virus and who survived infection but did not develop encephalitis. One had severe neurologic impairment (presentation of herpes zoster), and two appeared normal on follow-up. Thus, the severity of B virus disease is evident.

Diagnosis

Clinical

It must be stressed again that the transmissibility of B virus infection is extremely limited. Thousands of animal handlers have worked with macaques, and laboratory technicians have processed monkey kidney cells not only for vaccine development but also for the isolation of other viral agents. Nevertheless, the total number of cases of B virus infection is small. The possibility of B virus infection must be considered in any individual having contact with Old World monkeys, particularly Asiatic *Macaca* species. Furthermore, because of the recent identification of person-to-person transmission, individuals having intimate contact with animal workers exposed to these animals should be considered as having B virus infection with compatible clinical findings. The suspicion of B virus infection should be reinforced in the presence of historical evidence of direct contact with a rhesus monkey either by bite or scratch or by laboratory accident. In addition, it should be emphasized that some cases have been acquired by exposure to monkey tissues; consequently, this route of transmission should not be excluded as a possibility for human infection.

Clinical evidence of disease reflects manifestations of infection previously cited. Of particular interest to the examining clinician would be the presence of a vesicular rash at a bite site with ipsiolateral regional lymphadenopathy. With a compatible incubation period, the progressive appearance of neurologic symptomatology—particularly altered sensation in extremities, weakness, hyporeflexia to areflexia, and altered mentation in the presence of the wound—should suggest the possibility of B virus infection. Progressive clinical findings of disease have been previously described.

Virus Isolation

Recovery of virus from humans suspected of having B virus infection must be attempted. Sources for retrieval of virus are those that are indicative of the pathogenesis of human disease. These include: vesicles, conjunctivae, pharyngeal swabs, and tissue biopsy material. Furthermore, retrieval of virus from the CSF should be attempted, although the yield is very low.

Specimens for virus isolation should be processed in cell lines which are susceptible to B virus. As would be expected, these would include primary vervet monkey kidney, rabbit kidney cells, or established strains such BSC1 or LLC-RK1. It should be noted that B virus will replicate in all of the cell lines listed above, in contrast to other simian viruses which have a more limited spectrum susceptible cell line (535).

Once viral isolation has been achieved, identification of virus can be accomplished using either (a) molecular methods (536,537) or (b) neutralization of isolates by serologic assays. It should be emphasized that the latter assay is cumbersome and tedious (496,538,539). Rapid identification of isolates is essential for purposes of intervention with appropriate therapeutic agents (540,541).

Serologic Evaluation

It has been previously emphasized that serologic determination of B infection is exceedingly difficult because of its cross-reactivity with HSV. Thus, attempts at absorbing out antibodies have been attempted. Nevertheless, the extensive cross-reactions of sera to simian viruses in the presence of HSV antibodies have made diagnosis difficult (496,542–544). It should be stressed that animal workers providing care for *Macaca* monkeys should be serially bled for antibody determinations. Sera should be banked for purposes of future reference.

The standard serologic assays which have been employed generally utilize either complement fixation (545) or neutralization assays. In general, complement-fixing antibody titers to HSV are higher in humans than in monkeys, whereas monkey titers against B virus are higher in *Macaca* monkeys than in humans. As previously mentioned, human sera contained higher neutralizing antibodies to HSV than to B virus. Furthermore, it has been recognized that sera derived from monkeys with B virus infection have been reported to neutralize HSV better than they could neutralize the endogenous virus (497). At the present time, no simple test exists to distinguish antibodies to HSV from antibodies to B virus. Nevertheless, a variety of new antibody assays are in the process of development to rapidly evaluate human antibody response (540,546). The advent of these newer diagnostic assays will be of value for prospectively evaluating patients exposed to B virus.

Control of B Virus Infection

As with all other infectious diseases, the principal goal is to prevent infection. Prevention has been stressed on numerous occasions by the Centers for Disease Control (CDC) as well as in reviews published over the last 15 years (496,498,499,547–550). Although a vaccine is not readily available for the prevention of B virus infections, proper laboratory and animal breeding/handling procedures will significantly decrease the risk of infection. A CDC Advisory Committee has recommended procedures for control and management of infected animals and exposed animal workers (500,548). It should be emphasized that the risk of acquisition of infection by B virus is extremely low. The reader is referred to these recommendations for further information (548). These recommendations have been provided as guidelines for the management of macaques in captivity for research purposes. Variation from these guidelines can be discussed with investigators at the CDC (Viral Exanthems and Herpesvirus Branch, Division of Viral Diseases, CDC, telephone number 404-329-1338).

Prevention and Treatment

Although vaccines have been evaluated in animal models, none have proven efficacious in humans (519,551–555). The use of hyperimmune serum or gamma globulin has not been proven effective for the treatment of human infections caused by B virus (556). Animal experimentation has revealed slight protection of rabbits following the administration of large doses of monkey gamma globulin (552), as reviewed by Hull (496). Other investigators have demonstrated protection with hyperimmune horse and rabbit sera for rabbit infec-

tion (557). The utilization of other forms of hyperimmune sera has not been proven effective.

With the advent of antiviral therapy, nucleoside analogues have been deployed for the management of B virus infection of humans. Three drugs have been examined experimentally: vidarabine, acyclovir, and ganciclovir. Each of these drugs has been reported to have varying activity. Studies with acyclovir have attracted the most attention. In cell culture systems, acyclovir has been demonstrated to be active against B virus infection. One milligram of acyclovir decreased the yield of virus by approximately 90% (558). Subsequent animal model experiments provided varying results depending upon the quantity of inoculation, delay in therapy, and duration of treatment. Overall, a beneficial effect could be achieved in animals (558). More recently, Smith et al. (559) have demonstrated that ganciclovir is extremely active against B virus at concentrations of 0.55 mg/ml or less. These concentrations are achievable in humans.

The utilization of acyclovir for therapy of human disease has been more limited. The literature includes several cases where therapy instituted early in the disease course may have slowed progression and led to a return to normal function (501,502). Two of these cases were reported in the Pensacola outbreak. The value of acyclovir under such circumstances cannot be unequivocally determined because of the small number of patients who have this disease for evaluation in controlled studies. Thus, a recommendation for acyclovir therapy is made because of the severity of disease with a uniformly near-fatal outcome. It should be administered for active infection. Therapy should be initiated intravenously for a minimum of 14 days at dosages of 10 mg/kg every 8 hr. Ganciclovir and fluro-iodo-arabinosyl cytostine may be more active *in vivo*, but the probability of toxicity must be weighed. Subsequent oral administration of acyclovir can be considered; however, there are no data regarding the value of therapy for prolonged periods of time under such circumstances.

Future Directions

B virus infection in humans should not occur. The proper deployment of control procedures among animal handlers should avoid all human infections. Regardless, the future will allow for the development of more rapid and precise diagnostic assays and the further definition of appropriate procedures for handling infected animals and humans at risk for infection.

HUMAN HERPESVIRUSES 6 AND 7

The role of human herpesvirus 6 (HHV-6) and human herpesvirus 7 (HHV-7) in CNS disease is not well identified at the present time. The isolation of HHV-6 from mononuclear cells of individuals with HIV infection in 1986 has been followed by (a) the association of HHV-6 with roseola and (b) rejection following solid organ transplantation. The relation of this virus to CNS disease is not clear at the present time. It was only in 1989 that HHV-7 was reported. The epidemiology of this infection remains to be clarified.

ACKNOWLEDGMENTS

Original studies performed by the investigators were supported by grants from the National Institute of Allergy and Infectious Diseases (NO1-AI-62554, the Division of Research Resources (RR0023) of the National Institutes of Health, and the State of Alabama.

REFERENCES

1. *Epidemic encephalitis: etiology, epidemiology, treatment.* Report of a survey by the Mathewson Commission. New York: Columbia University Press, 1929 (cited in ref. 2).
2. Smith MG, Lennette EH, Reames HR. Isolation of the virus of herpes simplex and the demonstration of intranuclear inclusions in a case of acute encephalitis. *Am J Pathol* 1941;17:55–69.
3. Meyers HM, Johnson RT, Crawford JP, et al. Central nervous system syndromes of "viral etiology: a study of 773 cases. *Am J Med* 1960;29:334–347.
4. Mettler C. *History of medicine.* Philadelphia: Blakiston, 1947;356.
5. Astruc J. *De morbis venereis libri sex.* Paris: G Cavelier, 1736;361.
6. Gruter W. Das Herpesvirus, seine atiologische und klinische Bedeutung. *Munch Med Wochenschr* 1924;71:1058.
7. Goodpasture E. The axis-cylinders of peripheral nerves as portals of entry to the central nervous system for the virus of herpes simplex in experimentally infected rabbits. *J Pathol* 1925; I(1):11–28.
8. Zarafonetis CJD, Smodel MC, Adams JW, Haymaker W. Fatal herpes simplex encephalitis in man. *Am J Pathol* 1944; 20(3):429–445.
9. Nahmias AJ, Dowdle W. Antigenic and biologic differences in herpesvirus hominis. *Prog Med Virol* 1968;10:110.
10. Corey L, Spear P. Infections with herpes simplex viruses. *N Engl J Med* 1986;314:686.
11. Nahmias AJ, Roizman B. Infection with herpes simplex viruses 1 and 2. *N Engl J Med* 1873;289:667, 719, 781.
12. Whitley RJ. Epidemiology of herpes simplex virus. In: Roizman B, ed. *The herpesviruses,* vol 3. New York: Plenum Press, 1985;144.
13. Kieff ED, Bachendheimer SL, Roizman B. Size, comparison, and structure of the DNA of subtypes 1 and 2 of herpes simplex virus. *J Virol* 1971;8:125.
14. Honess RW, Roizman B. Proteins specified by herpes simplex virus. Identification and relative molar rates of synthesis of structural and nonstructural herpesvirus polypeptides in the infected cell. *J Virol* 1973;12:1346.
15. Pereira L, Baringer JR. Use of monoclonal antibody to identify the herpes virus glycoprotein antigens. In: Nahmias AJ, Dowdle WR, Schinazi R, eds. *The human herpesviruses: an interdisciplinary perspective.* Amsterdam: Elsevier/North-Holland, 1981;642.
16. Pereira L, Cassai E, Jones RW, Roizman B, Temi M, Nahmias AJ. Variability in the structural polypeptides of herpes simplex virus-1 strains: potential application in molecular epidemiology. *Infect Immum* 1976;13:211.
17. Roizman B, Norrild B, Chan C, Pereira L. Identification of a herpes simplex virus 2 glycoprotein lacking a known type 1 counterpart. *Virology* 1984;133:242.
18. Spear PG. Glycoproteins specified by herpes simplex virus. In: Roizman B, ed. *The herpesviruses,* vol 3. New York: Plenum Press, 1984;315.
19. Honess RW, Roizman B. Regulation of herpesvirus macromolecular synthesis. Cascade regulation of the synthesis of three groups of viral proteins. *J Virol* 1974;14:8.
20. Roizman B, Furlong D. The replication of herpesviruses. In: Fraenkel-Conrat H, Wagner RR, eds. *Comprehensive virology,* vol 3. New York: Plenum Press, 1974;229.
21. Schaeffer HJ, Beauchamp PL, deMiranda P, Elion GB, Collins P. 9-(2-Hydroxyethoxymethyl)guanine activity against viruses in the herpes group. *Nature* 1978;272:583.
22. Centifanto-Fitzgerald YM, Yamaguchi T, Kaufman HE, Tognon E, Roizman B. Ocular disease pattern induced by herpes simplex virus is genetically determined by a specific region of the viral DNA. *J Exp Med* 1982;155:475.
23. Longnecker R, Chatterjee S, Whitley RJ, Roizman B. Identification of a novel herpes simplex virus 1 glycoprotein gene within a gene cluster dispensable for growth in cell culture. *Proc Natl Acad Sci USA* 1987;84:4303.
24. Boos J, Esiri MM. Sporadic encephalitis I. In: *Viral encephalitis pathology, diagnosis, and management.* Boston: Blackwell Scientific Publishers, 1986;55–93.
25. Boos J, Kim JH. Biopsy histopathology in herpes simplex encephalitis and in encephalitis of undefined etiology. *Yale J Biol Med* 1984;57:751–755.
26. Garcia JH, Colon LE, Whitley RJ, Kichara J, Holmes FJ. Diagnosis of viral encephalitis by brain biopsy. *Semin Diagn Pathol* 1984;1(2):71–80.
27. Hill TJ. Herpes simplex virus latency. In: Roizman B, ed. *The herpesviruses,* vol 3. New York: Plenum Press, 1985;175.
28. Cook ML, Stevens JG. Pathogenesis of herpetic neuritis and ganglionitis in mice: evidence of intra-axonal transport of infection. *Infect Immun* 1973;7:272–288.
29. Baringer JR. The biology of herpes simplex virus infection in humans. *Surv Ophthalmol* 1976;21(2):171.
30. Pagano JS. Diseases and mechanisms of persistent DNA virus infection: latency and cellular transformation. *J Infect Dis* 1975;132:209.
31. Roizman B. An inquiry into the mechanisms of recurrent herpes infections in man. In: Pollard M, ed. *Perspectives in virology IV.* New York: Harper & Row, 1968;283.
32. Roizman B, Sears A. Inquiring into mechanisms of herpes simplex virus latency. *Am Rev Microbiol* 1988;41:543.
33. Stevens JC. Latent herpes simplex virus and the nervous system. *Curr Top Immunol* 1975;70:31.
34. Terni M. Infection with the virus of herpes simplex—the recrudescence of the disease and the problem of latency. *J Mal Infect Parasitol* 1971;23:433.
35. Baringer JR, Swoveland P. Recovery of herpes simplex virus from human trigeminal ganglions. *N Engl J Med* 1973;288:648.
36. Bastian FO, Rabson AS, Yee CL. Herpesvirus hominis: isolation from human trigeminal ganglion. *Science* 1972;178:306.
37. Hill TJ. Mechanisms involved in recurrent herpes simplex. In: Nahmias A, Dowdle WR, Schinazi R, eds. *The human herpesvirus: an interdisciplinary perspective.* Amsterdam: Elsevier/North-Holland, 1981;241.
38. Nesburn AB, Cook ML, Stevens JG. Latent herpes simplex virus isolation from rabbit trigeminal ganglia between episodes of recurrent ocular infection. *Arch Ophthalmol* 1972;88:412.
39. Stevens JG, Cook ML. Latent herpes simplex virus in spinal ganglia. *Science* 1971;173:843.
40. Stevens JG, Cook ML. Latent herpes simplex virus in sensory ganglia. *Perspect Virol* 1974;8:171.
41. Warren KG, Brown SM, Wrobelwska Z, Gilden D, Koprowski H, Subak-Sharpe J. Isolation of latent herpes simplex virus from the superior cervical and vagus ganglions of human beings. *N Engl J Med* 1978;98:1068.
42. Cushing H. Surgical aspects of major neuralgia of trigeminal

nerve: report of 20 cases of operation upon the Gasserian ganglion with anatomic and physiologic notes on the consequence of its removal. *JAMA* 1905;4:1002.

43. Goodpasture EW. Herpetic infections with special reference to involvement of the nervous system. *Medicine* 1929;8:223.

44. Carlton CA, Kilbourne ED. Activation of latent herpes simplex by trigeminal sensory-root section. *N Engl J Med* 1952;246:172.

45. Pazin GJ, Ho M, Jannetta P. Herpes simplex reactivation after trigeminal nerve root decompression. *J Infect Dis* 1978;138:405.

46. Pazin GJ, Armstrong JA, Lam MT, Tarr GC, Jannetta PJ, Ho M. Prevention of reactivation of herpes simplex virus infection by human leukocyte interferon after operation on the trigeminal route. *N Engl J Med* 1979;301:225.

47. Ellison SA, Carlton CA, Rose HM. Studies of recurrent herpes simplex infections following section of the trigeminal nerve. *J Infect Dis* 1959;105:161.

48. Walz MA, Price RW, Norkins AL. Latent ganglionic infections with herpes simplex virus types 1 and 2: viral reactivation *in vivo* after neurectomy. *Science* 1974;184:1185.

49. Kibrick S, Gooding GW. *Pathogenesis of infection with herpes simplex virus with special reference to nervous tissue.* NINDB monograph, vol II. Washington, DC: National Institute of Neurological Diseases and Blindness, 1965;143.

50. Hill TJ, Field HJ, Roome APC. Intra-axonal location of herpes simplex virus particles. *J Gen Virol* 1972;15:253.

51. Rustigian R, Smulow JB, Tye R. Studies of latent infection of skin and oral mucosa in individuals with recurrent herpes simplex. *J Invest Dermatol* 1966;47:218.

52. Rector JT, Lausch RN, Oakes JE. Use of monoclonal antibodies for analysis of antibody-dependent immunity to ocular herpes simplex virus type 1 infection. *Infect Immun* 1982;38:168.

53. Segal AL, Katcher AH, Bringtman VJ, Miller MF. Recurrent herpes labialis, recurrent aphthous ulcers and the menstrual cycles. *J Dent Res* 1974;53:797.

54. Greenberg MS, Brightman VJ, Ship II. Clinical and laboratory differentiation of recurrent intraoral herpes simplex virus infections following fever. *J Dent Res* 1969;48:385.

55. Greenberg MS, Friedman H, Cohen SG, Oh SH, Laster L, Starr S. A comparative study of herpes simplex infections in renal transplant and leukemic patients. *J Infect Dis* 1987;156:280.

56. Baringer JR. Recovery of herpes simplex virus from human sacral ganglions. *N Engl J Med* 1974;291:828.

57. Cabrera CV, Wholenberg C, Openshaw H. Herpes simplex virus DNA sequences in the CNS of latently infected mice. *Nature* 1978;298:1068.

58. Fraser NW, Lawrence WC, Wroblewska Z, Gilden DH. Herpes simplex virus type 1 DNA in human brain tissue. *Proc Natl Acad Sci USA* 1981;78:6451.

59. Selling B, Kibrick S. An outbreak of herpes simplex among wrestlers (herpes gladiatorium). *N Engl J Med* 1964;270:982.

60. Warren KG, Gilden DH, Brown SM. Isolation of herpes simplex virus from human trigeminal ganglia, including ganglia from one patient with multiple sclerosis. *Lancet* 1977;2:637.

61. Stevens J, Wagner E, Devi-Rao O, Codi M, Seldman L. RNA complementary to a herpesvirus alpha MRNA is prominent in latently infected neurons. *Science* 1987;235:1056.

62. Croen KD, Ostrove JM, Dragovic LJ, Smialek JE, Straus SE. Latent herpes simplex virus in human trigeminal ganglia. Detection of an immediate early gene "anti-sense" transcript by *in situ* hybridization. *N Engl J Med* 1987;317:1427-1432.

63. Gordon J, 1988. Personal communication.

64. Wagner ER, 1988. Personal communication.

65. Nahmias AJ, Whitley RJ, Visintine AN, Takei Y, Alford CA Jr, the NIAID Collaborative Antiviral Study Group. Herpes simplex virus encephalitis: laboratory evaluations and their diagnostic significance. *J Infect Dis* 1982;145:829-836.

66. Whitley RJ, Lakeman AD, Nahmias A, Roizman B. DNA restriction-enzyme analysis of herpes simplex virus isolates obtained from patients with encephalitis. *N Engl J Med* 1982;307:1060-1062.

67. Johnson RT, Olson LC, Buescher EL. Herpes simplex virus infections of the nervous system. Problems in laboratory diagnosis. *Arch Neurol* 1968;18:260-264.

68. Dinn J. Transolfactory spread of virus in herpes simplex encephalitis. *Br Med J* 1980;28:1392-1392.

69. Ojeda VJ, Archer M, Robertson TA, Bucens MR. Necropsy study of the olfactory portal of entry in herpes simplex encephalitis. *Med J Aust* 1983;1:79-81.

70. Twomey JA, Barker CM, Robinson G, Howell DA. Olfactory mucosa in herpes simplex encephalitis. *J Neurol Neurosurg Psychiatry* 1979;42:983-987.

71. Whitley RJ. In: Lopez C, Roizman B, eds. *Human herpesvirus infections: pathogenesis, diagnosis, and treatment.* New York: Raven Press, 1986;153-164.

72. Schlitt M, Lakeman FD, Wilson ER, To A, Acoff R, Harsh GR, Whitley RJ. A rabbit model of focal herpes simplex encephalitis. *J Infect Dis* 1986;153:732-735.

73. Stroop WG, Schaefer DC. Production of encephalitis restricted to the temporal lobes by experimental reactivation of herpes simplex virus. *J Infect Dis* 1986;153:721-731.

74. Rock DL, Frasher NW. Detection of HSV-1 genome in the central nervous system of latently infected mice. *Nature* 1983;302:523-531.

75. Davis LE, Johnson RT. An explanation for the localization of herpes simplex encephalitis. *Ann Neurol* 1979;5:2-5.

76. Griffith JR, Kibrick S, Dodge PR, Richardson EP. Experimental herpes simplex encephalitis. Electroencephalographic, clinical, virologic, and pathologic observations in the rabbit. *Electroencephalogr Clin Neurophysiol* 1967;23:263-267.

77. Barnes DW, Whitley RJ. CNS diseases associated with varicella zoster virus and herpes simplex virus infection. In: Frank B, ed. *Neurologic clinics.* Philadelphia: WB Saunders, 1986;265-283.

78. Whitley RJ. Herpes simplex virus. In: Fields BN, Knipe DM, Chanock R, Hirsch M, Melnick J, Monath T, Roizman B, eds. *Virology,* 2nd ed. New York: Raven Press, 1990;1843-1887.

79. Fife KH, Corey L. Herpes simplex virus. In: Holmes KK, Mardh P-A, Sparling PF, Wiesner PJ, Cates W, Lemon SM, Stamm WE, eds. *Sexually transmitted diseases,* 2nd ed. New York: McGraw-Hill, 1990;941-952.

80. Black FL. Infectious diseases in primitive societies. *Science* 1975;18(7):515.

81. Glezen WP, Fernald GW, Lohr JA. Acute respiratory disease of university students with special references to the etiologic role of herpesvirus hominis. *Am J Epidemiol* 1975;101:111.

82. Burnett FM, Williams SW. Herpes simplex: new point of view. *Med J Aust* 1939;1:637.

83. Dodd K, Johnston LM, Buddingh GJ. Herpetic stomatitis. *J Pediatr* 1938;12:95.

84. Buddingh GJ, Schrum DI, Lanier JC, Guidy DJ. Studies of the natural history of herpes simplex infections. *Pediatrics* 1953;11:595.

85. Juretic M. Natural history of herpetic infection. *Helv Pediatr Acta* 1966;21:356.

86. Cesario TC, Poland JD, Wulff H, Chin TD, Wenner HA. Six years experiences with herpes simplex virus in a children's home. *Am J Epidemiol* 1969;90:416.

87. Douglas RG Jr, Couch RB. A prospective study of chronic herpes simplex virus infection and recurrent herpes labialis in humans. *J Immunol* 1970;104:289.

88. Kloene W, Bang FB, Chakroborty SM, Cooper MR, Kulemann H, Shah KV, Ota M. A two year respiratory virus survey in four villages in Weor Bengal, India. *Am J Epidemiol* 1970;92:307.

89. Komorous JM, Wheeler CE, Briggaman RA, Caro L. Intrauterine herpes simplex infections. *Arch Dermatol* 1977;113:919.

90. Lindgren KM, Douglas RG Jr, Couch RB. Significance of herpesvirus hominis in respiratory secretions of man. *N Engl J Med* 1968;276:517.

91. Overall JC Jr. Antiviral chemotherapy of oral and genital herpes simplex virus infections. In: Nahmias AJ, Dowdle WR, Schinazi RE, eds. *The human herpesviruses: an interdisciplinary perspective.* Amsterdam: Elsevier/North-Holland, 1980;447.

92. Stern H, Elek SD, Miller DM, Anderson HF. Herpetic whitlow, a form of cross-infection in hospitals. *Lancet* 1959;2:871.

93. Young SK, Rowe NH, Buchanan RA. A clinical study for the control of facial mucocutaneous herpes virus infections. I. Charac-

terization of natural history in a professional school population. *Oral Surg Oral Med Oral Pathol* 1976;41:498.

94. Scott TF, Steigman AJ, Convey JH. Acute infectious gingivostomatitis: etiology, epidemiology, and clinical pictures of a common disorder caused by the virus of herpes simplex. *JAMA* 1941;117:999.

95. Stavraky KM, Rawls WE, Chiavetta J, Donner AP, Wanklin JM. Sexual and socioeconomic factors affecting the risk of infections with herpes simplex virus type 2. *Am J Epidemiol* 1983;118:109.

96. Templeton AC. Generalized herpes simplex in malnourished children. *J Clin Pathol* 1970;23:24.

97. Rawls WE, Campione-Piccardo J. Epidemiology of herpes simplex virus type 1 and 2. In: Nahmias A, Dowdle W, Schinazi R, eds. *The human herpesviruses: an interdisciplinary perspective.* Amsterdam: Elsevier/North-Holland, 1981;137.

98. Bader C, Crumpacker CS, Schnipper LE, Ransil B, Clark JE, Arndt K, Freedberg IM. The natural history of recurrent facial-oral infection with herpes simplex virus. *J Infect Dis* 1978; 138:897.

99. Black FL, Hierholzer WJ, Pinheiro F, Evans AS, Woodall JP, Opton EM, Emmons JE, West BS, Edsall G, Downs WG, Wallace GD. Evidence for persistence of infectious agents in isolated human populations. *Am J Epidemiol* 1974;100:230.

100. Nahmias AJ, Josey WE, Naib ZM, Luce C, Duffey C. Antibodies to herpesvirus hominis type 1 and 2 in humans. I. Patients with genital herpetic infections. *Am J Epidemiol* 1970;91:539.

101. Nahmias AJ, Josey WE, Naib ZM, Luce CF, Fuest B. Antibodies to herpesvirus hominis types 1 and 2 in humans. II. Women with cervical cancer. *Am J Epidemiol* 1970;91:547.

102. Rawls WE, Tompkins WA, Melnick JL. The association of herpesvirus type 2 and carcinoma of the uterine cervix. *Am J Epidemiol* 1969;89:547.

103. Sawanabori S. Acquisition of herpes simplex virus infection in Japan. *Acta Paediatr Jpn Overseas Ed* 1973;15:16.

104. Wentworth BB, Alexander ER. Seroepidemiology of infection due to members of the herpesvirus group. *Am J Epidemiol* 1971;94:496.

105. McDonald AD, Williams MC, West R. Neutralizing antibodies to herpes virus types 1 and 2 in Montreal women. *Am J Epidemiol* 1974;100:124.

106. Smith IW, Peutherer JF, MacCallum FO. The incidence of herpesvirus hominis antibody in the population. *J Hyg* 1967;65:395.

107. Gibson JJ, Hornung CA, Alexander GR, Lee FK, Potts WA, Nahmias AJ. A cross-sectional study of herpes simplex virus types 1 and 2 in college students: occurrence and determinants of infection. *J Infect Dis* 1989;162:306–312.

108. Evans AS, Dick EC. Acute pharyngitis and tonsillitis in University of Wisconsin students. *JAMA* 1964;190:699.

109. Corey L, Adams H, Brown A, Holmes K. Genital herpes simplex virus infections: clinical manifestations, course and complications. *Ann Intern Med* 1983;98:958.

110. Kalinyak JE, Fleagle G, Docherty JJ. Incidence and distribution of herpes simplex virus types 1 and 2 from genital lesions in college women. *J Med Virol* 1977;1:173.

111. Smith IW, Peutherer JF, Robertson DH. Virological studies in genital herpes [Letter]. *Lancet* 1977;2:1089.

112. Wolontis S, Jeansson S. Correlation of herpes simplex virus types 1 and 2 with clinical features of infection. *J Infect Dis* 1977;135:28.

113. Reeves WC, Corey L, Adams HG, Vontver LA, Holmes KK. Risk of recurrence after first episodes of genital herpes: relation to HSV type and antibody response. *N Engl J Med* 1981;305:315.

114. Deardourff SL, Deture FA, Drylie DM, Centifanto Y, Kaufman H. Association between herpes virus hominis type-2 and the male genitourinary tract. *J Virol* 1974;112:126.

115. Josey WE, Nahmias AJ, Naib ZM. Genital herpes infection in the female. *Am J Obstet Gynecol* 1966;96:493.

116. Josey WE, Nahmias AJ, Naib ZM. Genital infection with type-2 herpesvirus hominis. *Am J Obstet Gynecol* 1968;101:718.

117. Josey WE, Nahmias AJ, Naib ZM. The epidemiology of type-2 (genital) herpes simplex virus infections. *Obstet Gynecol Surv [Suppl]* 1972;27:295.

118. Parker JD, Banatvala JE. Herpes genitalis: clinical and virologic studies. *Br J Vener Dis* 1967;43:212.

119. Beilby JOW, Cameron CH, Catterall RO, Davidson D. Herpesvirus hominis infection of the cervix associated with gonorrhea. *Lancet* 1968;1:1065.

120. Embil JA, Garner JB, Pereira LH, White FM, Manuel FR. Association of cytomegalovirus and herpes simplex virus infections of the cervix in four clinic populations. *Sex Transm Dis* 1985;12:224–228.

121. Nahmias AJ, Von Reyn CF, Josey WE, Naib ZM, Hutton RD. Genital herpes simplex virus infection and gonorrhea: association and analogies. *Br J Vener Dis* 1973;49:306.

122. *New vaccine development: establishing priorities.* Washington, DC: National Academy Press, Institute of Medicine, 1985;280.

123. Jeansson S, Molin L. Genital herpesvirus hominis infection: a veneral disease. *Lancet* 1970;1:1064.

124. Jeansson S, Molin L. On the occurrence of genital herpes simplex virus infection: clinical and virologic findings and relation to gonorrhea. *Arch Dermatol* 1974;54:479.

125. Corey L, Holmes K, Benedetti J, Critchlow C. Clinical course of genital herpes: implications for therapeutic trials. In: Nahmias A, Dowdle WR, Schinazi R, eds. *The human herpesviruses: an interdisciplinary perspective.* Amsterdam: Elsevier/North-Holland, 1981;496–502.

126. Magder LS, Nahmias AJ, Johnson RE, Lee FK, Brooks C, Snowden C. A seroepidemiologic survey of the prevalance of herpes simplex virus type 2 infection in the United States. *N Engl J Med.* 1989;321:7–12.

127. Vesterinen E, Purola E, Saksela E. Clinical and virological findings in patients with cytologically diagnosed gynecologic herpes simplex infections. *Acta Cytol* 1977;21:299.

128. Doerr R. Sitzungsberichte der Gesellschaft der Schweizerischen Augenartzte Diskussion. *Klin Monatsbl Augenheilkd* 1920; 65:104.

129. Kleger B, Prier JE, Rosato DJ, McGinnis AE. Herpes simplex infection of the female genital tract. I. Incidence of infection. *Am J Obstet Gynecol* 1968;102:745.

130. Naib ZM, Nahmias AJ, Josey WE, Zaki SA. Relation of cytohistopathology of genital herpesvirus infection to cervical anaplasia. *Cancer* 1973;33:1452.

131. Wolinska WA, Melamed MR. Herpes genitalis in women attending planned parenthood of New York City. *Acta Cytol* 1970;14:239.

132. Duenas A, Adam E, Melnick JL, Rawls WE. Herpes virus type-2 in a prostitute population. *Am J Epidemiol* 1972;95:483.

133. Ng ABP, Reagin JW, Yen SS. Herpes genitalis—clinical and cytopathologic experience with 256 patients. *Obstet Gynecol* 1970;36:645.

134. Ekwo E, Wong YW, Myers M. Asymptomatic cervicovaginal shedding of herpes simplex virus. *Am J Obstet Gynecol* 1979;134:102.

135. Rattray MC, Corey L, Reeves WC, Vontver LA, Holmes KK. Recurrent genital herpes among women: symptomatic versus asymptomatic viral shedding. *Br J Vener Dis* 1978;54:252.

136. Adam E, Kaufman RH, Mirkovic RR, Melnick JL. Persistence of virus shedding in asymptomatic women after recovery from herpes genitalis. *Obstet Gynecol* 1979;54:171.

137. Becker WW. The epidemiology of herpesvirus infection in three racial communities in Cape Town. *S Afr Med J* 1966;40:109.

138. Rawls WE, Adam E, Melnick JL. Geographical variation in the association of antibodies to herpesvirus type 2 and carcinoma of the cervix. In: Biggs PM, de The G, Paynes LN, eds. *Oncogenesis and herpesviruses.* Scientific Publication II. Lyon, France: International Agency for Research on Cancer, 1972;424.

139. Stagno S. Unpublished observation.

140. Lee FK, Coleman RM, Pereira L, Bailey PD, Tatsuno M, Nahmias AJ. Detection of herpes simplex virus type 2-specific antibody with glycoprotein G. *J Clin Microbiol* 1985;22:641.

141. Nahmias AJ, Josey WE, Naib ZM, Freeman MG, Fernandez RJ, Wheeler JH. Perinatal risk associated with maternal genital herpes simplex virus infection. *Am J Obstet Gynecol* 1971; 110:825.

142. Rawls WE, Gardner HL. Herpes genitalis: venereal aspects. *Clin Obstet Gynecol* 1972;15:913.

143. Rawls WE, Gardner HL, Flanders RW, Lowry SP, Kaufman RH, Melnick JL. Genital herpes in two social groups. *Am J Obstet Gynecol* 1971;110:682.

144. Rawls WE, Garfield CH, Seth P, Adam E. Serological and epidemiological considerations of the role of herpes simplex virus type 2 in cervical cancer. *Cancer Res* 1976;36:829.

145. Allen WP, Rapp F. Concept review of genital herpes vaccines. *J Infect Dis* 1982;145:413.

146. Kaufman RH, Gardner HL, Rawls WE, Dixon RE, Young RL. Clinical features of herpes genitalis. *Cancer Res* 1973;33:1446.

147. Lafferty WE, Coombs RW, Benedetti J, Critchlow C, Corey L. Recurrences after oral and genital herpes simplex virus infection. Influence of site of infection and viral type. *N Engl J Med* 1987;316:1444.

148. Nahmias AJ, Alford C, Korones S. Infection of the newborn with herpes virus hominis. *Adv Pediatr* 1970;17:185.

149. Chang TW, Fiumara NJ, Weinstein L. Genital herpes: some clinical and laboratory observations. *JAMA* 1974;229:554.

150. Choi NW, Skettigara PT, Abu-Zeid HAH, Nelson NA. Herpesvirus infection and cervical anaplasia: a seroepidemiological study. *Int J Cancer* 1977;19:167.

151. Corey L, Ashley R, Benedetti J, Selke S. The effect of prior HSV-1 infection on the subsequent natural history of genital HSV-2. Abstract No. 821, Twenty-Eighth Interscience Conference on Antimicrobial Agents and Chemotherapy, Los Angeles, California, 1988.

152. Longson M. The general nature of viral encephalitis in the United Kingdom. In: Ellis LS, ed. *Viral diseases of the central nervous system.* London: Ballière Tindall, 1975;19–31.

153. Skoldenberg B, Alestig K, Burman L, Forkman A, Lovgren K, Norby R, Stiernstedt G, Forsgren M, Bergstrom T, Dahlqvist E, Fryden A, Norlin K. Acyclovir versus vidarabine in herpes simplex encephalitis. A randomized multicentre study in consecutive Swedish patients. *Lancet* 1984;2:707–711.

154. Corey L, Spear PG. Infections with herpes simplex viruses (second of two parts). *N Engl J Med* 1986;314:749–757.

155. Straus S, Rooney JF, Sever JL, Seilding M, Nusinoff-Lehrman S, Cremer K. Herpes simplex virus infection: biology, treatment and prevention. *Ann Intern Med* 1985;103:404–419.

156. Whitley RJ, Tilles J, Linneman C, Liu C, Pazin G, Hilty M, Overall J, Visintine A, Soong SJ, Alford CA, and the NIAID Collaborative Antiviral Study Group. Herpes simplex encephalitis: clinical assessment. *JAMA* 1982;247:317–320.

157. Boston Interhospital Virus Study Group and the NIAID Sponsored Cooperative Antiviral Clinical Study (Alford, Chien, Whitley, et al.). Failure of high dose 5-iodo-2-deoxyuridine in the therapy of herpes simplex virus encephalitis. *N Engl J Med* 1975;292:600–603.

158. Longson M. Ann Microbiol Le difi des encephalitis herpetiques. *(Paris)* 1979;130:5.

159. Longson MM, Bailey AS, Klapper P. In: Waterson AT, ed. *Recent advances in clinical virology,* vol 2. Philadelphia: Churchill Livingston, 1980;147–157.

160. Whitley RJ, Soong S-J, Doline R, Galasso GJ, Chien LT, Alford CA Jr. and the Collaborative Antiviral Study Group. Adenine arabinoside therapy of biopsy-proved herpes simplex encephalitis: National Institute of Allergy and Infectious Diseases Collaborative Antiviral Study. *N Engl J Med* 1977;297:289–294.

161. Whitley RJ, Soong S-J, Hirsh MS, Karchmer AW, Dolin R, Galasso G, Dunnick JK, Alford CA Jr, and the NIAID Collaborative Antiviral Study Group. Herpes simplex encephalitis: vidarabine therapy and diagnostic problems. *N Engl J Med* 1981;304:313–318.

162. Klapper PE, Cleator GM, Longson M. Mild forms of herpes encephalitis. *J Neurol Neurosurg Psychiatry* 1984;47:1247–1250.

163. Rappel M, Dubois-Dalcq M, Sprecher S, Thiry L, Lowenthal A, Pelc S, Thys JP. Diagnosis and treatment of herpes encephalitis: a multidisciplinary approach. *J Neurol Sci* 1971;12:443–458.

164. Braun P. The clinical management of suspected herpes virus encephalitis: a decision analytic view. *Am J Med* 1980;69:895–902.

165. Braza M, Pauker SG. The decision to biopsy, treat, or wait in suspected herpes encephalitis. *Ann Intern Med* 1980;92:641–649.

166. Ch'ien LT, Boehm RM, Robinson H, Liu C, Frenkel LD. Char-

acteristic early electroencephalographic changes in herpes simplex encephalitis. *Arch Neurol* 1977;34:361–364.

167. Miller JHD, Coey A. The EEG in necrotizing encephalitis. *Electroencephalogr Clin Neurophysiol* 1959;2:582–585.

168. Radermecker J. Systématique et electrocencephalographic des encephalitis et encephalopathies. *Electroencephalogr Clin Neurophysiol* 1956;5(Suppl):239.

169. Smith JB, Westmoreland BF, Reagan TJ, Sandok BA. A distinctive clinical EEG profile in herpes simplex encephalitis. *Mayo Clin Proc* 1975;50:469–474.

170. Upton A, Grumpert J. Electroencephalography in diagnosis of herpes simplex encephalitis. *Lancet* 1970;1:650–652.

171. Enzmann DR, Ransom B, Norman D, Talberth E. Computed tomography of herpes simplex encephalitis. *Radiology* 1978;129:419–425.

172. Zimmermann RD, Russell EJ, Leeds N, Kaufman D. CT in the early diagnosis of herpes simplex encephalitis. *AJR* 1980;134:61–66.

173. Lakeman FD, Koga J, Whitley RJ. Detection of antigen to herpes simplex virus in cerebrospinal fluid from patients with herpes simplex encephalitis. *J Infect Dis* 1987;155:1172–1178.

174. Rowley A, Lakeman F, Whitley R, Wolinsky S. Diagnosis of herpes simplex encephalitis by DNA amplification of cerebrospinal fluid cells. *Lancet* 1990;335:440–441.

175. Whitley RJ, Cobbs CG, Alford CA Jr, Soong S-J, Morawetz F, Benton JW, Hirsch MS, Reichman RC, Aoki FY, Connor J, Oxman M, Corey L, Hanley DF, Wright PF, Nahmias A, Powell DA, and the NIAID Collaborative Antiviral Study Group. Diseases which mimic herpes simplex encephalitis: diagnosis, presentation, and outcome. *JAMA* 1989;262:234–239.

176. Breeden CJ, Hall TC, Tyler HR. Herpes simplex encephalitis treated with systemic 5-iodo-2' deoxyuridine. *Ann Intern Med* 1966;65:1050–1056.

177. Illis LS, Merry RTG. Treatment of herpes simplex encephalitis. *J R Coll Physicians Lond* 1972;7:34–44.

178. Nolan DC, Carruthers MM, Lerner AM. Herpesvirus hominis encephalitis in Michigan. Report of thirteen cases, including six treated with idoxuridine. *N Engl J Med* 1970;282:10–13.

179. Nolan DC, Lauter CB, Lerner AM. Idoxuridine in herpes simplex virus (type 1) encephalitis experience with 29 cases in Michigan, 1966 to 1971. *Ann Intern Med* 1973;78:243–246.

180. Rappel M, Dubois-Dalcq M, Sprecher S, Thiry L, Lowenthal A, Pelc S, Thys JP. Diagnosis and treatment of herpes simplex encephalitis: a multidisciplinary approach. *J Neurol Sci* 1971;12:443–458.

181. Sarubbi FA Jr, Sparling PF, Glezen WP. Herpesvirus hominis encephalitis virus isolation from brain biopsy in seven patients and results of therapy. *Arch Neurol* 1973;29:268–273.

182. Whitley RJ, Alford CA Jr, Hirsch MS, Schooley RT, Luby JP, Aoki FY, Hanley D, Nahmias AJ, Soong S-J, and the NIAID Collaborative Antiviral Study Group. Vidarabine versus acyclovir therapy of herpes simplex encephalitis. *N Engl J Med* 1986;314:144–149.

183. Gnann JW, Barton NH, Whitley RJ. Acyclovir—developmental aspects and clinical applications. Evaluations of new drugs. *Pharmacotherapy* 1983;3:275–283.

184. Davis LE, McLaren LC. Relapsing herpes simplex encephalitis following antiviral therapy. *Ann Neurol* 1983;13:192–195.

185. Dix RD, Baringer JR, Panitch HS, Rosenberg SH, Hagedoren J, Whaley J. Recurrent herpes simplex encephalitis: recovery of virus after ara-A treatment. *Ann Neurol* 1983;13:196–200.

186. Van Landingham KE. Relapse of herpes simplex encephalitis after conventional acyclovir therapy. *JAMA* 1988;259:1051–1053.

187. Loenig H, Rabinowitz SG, Day E, Miller V. Post-infectious encephalomyelitis after successful treatment of herpes simplex encephalitis with adenine arabinoside—ultrastructural observation. *N Engl J Med* 1979;300:1089–1093.

188. DeVita VT Jr, Young RC, Canellos GP. Combination versus single agent chemotherapy: a review of the basis for selection of drug treatment of cancer. *Cancer* 1975;35:98–110.

189. Rahal JJ. Antibiotic combinations: the clinical relevance of synergy and antagonism. *Medicine* 1978;57:179–195.

190. Ayisi NK, Gupta VS, Meldrum JB, Taneja AK, Babiuk LA. Combination chemotherapy: interaction of 5-methyoxymethylde-

oxyuridine with adenine arabinoside, 5-ethyldeoxyuridine, 5-iododeoxyuridine, and phosphenoacetic acid against herpes simplex virus types 1 and 2. *Antimicrob Agents Chemother* 1980; 17(4):558–566.

191. Biron KK, Elion GB. Effect of acyclovir combined with other antiherpetic agents on varicella zoster virus in vitro. *Am J Med* 1982;73:54–57.

192. DeClerq E, Descamps J, Verhelst G, Walker RT, Jones AS, Torrence PF, Shugar D. Comparative efficacy of antiherpes drugs against different strains of herpes simplex virus. *J Infect Dis* 1980;141:563–574.

193. Fischer PH, Leed JJ, Chen MS, Lin TS, Prusoff WH. Synergistic effect of 5'-amino-5'-deoxythymidine and 5-iodo-2' deoxyuridine against herpes simplex virus infections *in vitro*. *Biochem Pharmacol* 1979;28:3483–3486.

194. Schinazi RF, Nahmias AJ. Different *in vitro* effects of dual combinations of anti-herpes simplex virus compounds. *Am J Med* 1982;73:40–48.

195. Schinazi RF, Peters J, Williams CC, Chance D, Nahmias AJ. Effect of combinations of acyclovir with vidarabine or its 5-monophosphate on herpes simplex viruses in cell culture and in mice. *Antimicrob Agents Chemother* 1982;22:499–507.

196. Wigand R, Hassinger M. Combined antiviral effect of DNA inhibitors on herpes simplex virus multiplication. *Med Microbiol Immunol* 1980;168:179–190.

197. Barry DW, Nusinoff-Lehrman S, Ellis MN, Biron KK, Furman PA. Viral resistance. Clinical experience. *Scand J Infect Dis* 1985;47:155–164.

198. Field JH. A perspective on resistance to acyclovir in herpes simplex virus. *J Antimicrob Chemother* 1983;12:129–135.

199. Svennerholm B, Vahlne A, Lowhagen GB, Widell A, Lycke E. Sensitivity of HSV strains isolated before and after treatment with acyclovir. *Scand J Infect Dis* 1985;47:149–154.

200. Wade JC, McLaren C, Meyers JD. Frequency and significance of acyclovir-resistant herpes simplex virus isolated from marrow transplant patients receiving multiple courses of treatment with acyclovir. *J Infect Dis* 1983;148:1077–1082.

201. Gordon JE, Meader FM. The period of infectivity and serum prevention of chickenpox. *JAMA* 1929;93:2013.

202. Steiner P. Zur Inokulation der Varicellen. *Wien Med Wochenschr* 1875;25:306.

203. von Bokay J. Das Auftreten der Schafblattern unter besonderen Umstanden. *Ungar Arch Med* 1892;1:159.

204. von Bokay J. Uber den atiologischen Zusammenhang der Varizellen mit Gewissen Fallen von Herpes zoster. *Wien Klin Wochenschr* 1909;22:1323.

205. Bruusgaard E. The natural relation between zoster and varicella. *Br J Dermatol Syph* 1932;44:1.

206. Kundratiz K. Experimentelle Ubertragungen von Herpes zoster auf Menschen und die Beziehungen von Herpes zoster zu Varicellen. *Abh Kinderheilkd* 1925;39:379.

207. School Epidemics Committee of Great Britain. *Epidemics in schools*. Medical Research Council, Special Report Series, No. 227. London: His Majesty's Stationery Office, 1938.

208. Garland J. Varicella following exposure to herpes zoster. *N Engl J Med* 1943;228:336.

209. Lipschutz B. Untersuchungen uber die atiologie der krankheiten der herpesgruppe (herpes zoster, herpes genitalis, herpes febrilis). *Arch Dermatol Syph* 1921;136:428.

210. Tyzzer EE. The histology of the skin lesions in varicella. *Philippine J Sci* 1906;1:349.

211. Weller TH. The propagation *in vitro* of agents producing inclusion bodies derived from varicella and herpes zoster. *Proc Soc Exp Biol Med* 1953;83:340.

212. Weller TH. Varicella and herpes zoster. In: Lennette EH, Schmidt NJ, eds. *Diagnostic procedures for viral, rickettsial, and chlamydial infections*. Washington, DC: American Public Health Association, 1970;375.

213. Weller TH, Coons AH. Fluorescent antibody studies with agents of varicella and herpes zoster propagated *in vitro*. *Proc Soc Exp Biol Med* 1954;86:789.

214. Weller TH, Stoddard MB. Intranuclear inclusion bodies in cultures of human tissue inoculated with varicella vesicle fluid. *J Immunol* 1952;68:311.

215. Weller TH, Witton HM. The etiologic agents of varicella and herpes zoster: serologic studies with the viruses as propagated *in vitro*. *J Exp Med* 108:869–890.

216. Oakes JE, Iltis JP, Hyman R, Rapp F. Analyses by restriction enzyme cleavage of human varicella-zoster virus DNAs. *Virology* 1977;82:353.

217. Stow ND, Davison AJ. Identification of a varicella-zoster virus origin of DNA replication and its activation by herpes simplex virus type I gene products. *J Gen Virol* 1986;67:1617–1623.

218. Straus SE, Hays J, Smith H, Owens J. Genome differences among varicella-zoster virus isolates. *J Gen Virol* 1983;64:1031.

219. Straus SE, Reinhold W, Smith HA, et al. Endonuclease analysis of viral DNA from varicella and subsequent zoster infection in the same patient. *N Eng J Med* 1984;311:1362–1364.

220. Achong BC, Meurisse EV. Observations on the fine structure and replication of varicella virus in cultivated human amnion cells. *J Gen Virol* 1968;3:305.

221. Almeida JD, Howatson AF, Williams MG. Morphology of varicella (chickenpox) virus. *Virology* 1962;16:353.

222. Straus SE, Aulakh H, Ruyechan WT, Hay J, Casey TA, Vandewoude GE, Owens SJ, Smith HA. Structure of varicella-zoster virus DNA. *J Virol* 1981;40:516.

223. Hyman R. Structure and function of the varicella-zoster virus genome. In: Nahmias AJ, Dowdle WR, Schinazi RF, eds. *The human herpesviruses*. New York: Elsevier, 1981;63.

224. Iltis JP, Oakes JE, Hyman RW, Rapp F. Comparison of the DNA's of varicella-zoster viruses isolated from clinical cases of varicella and herpes zoster. *Virology* 1977;82:345.

225. Dumas AM, Geelen JL, Mares W, Van Der Noordaa J. Infectivity and molecular weight of varicella-zoster virus DNA. *J Gen Virol* 1980;47:233–235.

226. Ludwig H, Haines HG, Biswal N, Benyesh-Melnick M. The characterization of varicella-zoster virus DNA. *J Gen Virol* 1972; 14:111.

227. Plummer G, Goodheart CR, Henso D, Bowling DP. A comparative study of the DNA density and behavior in tissue cultures of fourteen different herpesviruses. *Virology* 1969;39:134.

228. Dumas AM, Geelen JL, Westrate MW, Wertheim P, Van Der Noordaa J. Xba, Pst, BgIII restriction enzyme maps of the two orientations of the varicella-zoster virus genome. *J Virol* 1981;39:390–400.

229. Straus SE, et al. Varicella-zoster virus infections. *Ann Intern Med* 1988;108:221–237.

230. Grose C, Perrotta DM, Burnell PA, Smith GC. Cell-free varicella-zoster virus in cultured human melanoma cells. *J Gen Virol* 1979;43:15.

231. Cheatham WJ, Weller TH, Dolan TF Jr, Dower JC. Varicella, report of two fatal cases with necropsy, virus isolation and serologic studies. *Am J Pathol* 1956;2:1015.

232. Cowdry EV. The problem of intranuclear inclusions in virus diseases. *Arch Pathol* 1934;18:527.

233. Gelb LD. Varicella-zoster virus. In: Fields BN, Knipe DM, Chanock R, Hirsch M, Melnick J, Monath T, Roizman B, eds. *Virology*, 2nd ed. New York: Raven Press, 1990;2011–2054.

234. Gordon JE. Chickenpox: an epidemiologic review. *Am J Med Sci* 1962;244:362.

235. Wells MW, Holla WA. Ventilation in the flow of measles and chickenpox through a community. *JAMA* 1950;142:1337.

236. Hope-Simpson RE. Infectiousness of communicable diseases in the household (measles, chickenpox, and mumps). *Lancet* 1952;2:549.

237. Yorke JA, London WP. Recurrent outbreaks of measles, chickenpox, and mumps. Systematic differences in contact rates and stochastic effects. *Am J Epidemiol* 1973;98:469.

238. Rubin D, Fusfeld RD. Muscle paralysis in herpes zoster. *Calif Med* 1965;103:261–266.

239. Hope-Simpson RE. The nature of herpes zoster: a long-term study and a new hypothesis. *Proc R Soc Med* 1965;58:9.

240. Mazur MH, Dolin R. Herpes zoster at the NIH: a 20 year experience. *Am J Med* 1978;65:738–744.

241. Applebaum E, Rachelson MH, Dolgopol VB. Varicella encephalitis. *Am J Med* 1953;15:223–230.

242. Boughton CR. Varicella-zoster in Sydney. II. Neurological complications of varicella. *Med J Aust* 1966;2:444–447.

243. Heppleston JD, Pearch KM, Yates PO. Varicella encephalitis. *Arch Dis Child* 1959;34:318–321.

244. Reuler JB, Chang MK. Herpes zoster: epidemiology, clinical features, and management. *South Med J* 1984;77:1149–1156.

245. Johnson R, Milbourn PE. Central nervous system manifestations of chickenpox. *Can Med Assoc J* 1970;102:831–834.

246. Underwood EA. The neurological complications of varicella: a clinical and epidemiological study. *Br J Child Dis* 1935;32:376–378.

247. McKendall RR, Klawans HL. Nervous system complications of varicella-zoster virus. In: Vinken PJ, Bruyn GW, eds. *Handbook of clinical neurology,* vol 34. Amsterdam: North-Holland, 1978;161–183.

248. Shope TC. Chickenpox encephalitis and encephalopathy: evidence of differing pathogenesis. *Yale J Biol Med* 1982;55:321–327.

249. Ophir O, Seigman-Igra Y, Vardinon N, et al. Herpes zoster encephalitis: isolation of virus from cerebrospinal fluid. *Isr J Med Sci* 1984;20:1189–1192.

250. Gershon A, Steinberg S, Greenberg S, et al. Varicella-zoster associated encephalitis: detection of specific antibody in cerebrospinal fluid. *J Clin Microbiol* 1980;12:764–767.

251. Peters ACB, Versteeg J, Lindeman J, et al. Varicella and acute cerebellar ataxia. *Arch Neurol* 1978;35:769–771.

252. Griffith JF, Salam MV, Adams RD. The nervous system diseases associated with varicella. *Acta Neurol Scand* 1970;46:279–300.

253. Gibbs FA, Gibbs EL, Spies HW, et al. Common types of childhood encephalitis. *Arch Neurol* 1964;10:15–25.

254. Driscoll BF, Kies MW, Alvord EC. Adoptive transfer of EAE: prevention of successful transfer by treatment of donors with myelin basic protein. *J Immunol* 1975;114:291–292.

255. Nicholaides NJ. Fatal systemic varicella: a report of three cases. *Med J Aust* 1957;2:88–91.

256. Takashima S, Becker LE. Neuropathology of fatal varicella. *Arch Pathol Lab Med* 1979;103(5):209–213.

257. Dunn M, Salter RH. Zoster encephalitis. *Br J Clin Pract* 1968;22:444–445.

258. Jemsek J, Greenberg SB, Taber L, et al. Herpes zoster-associated encephalitis: clinicopathologic report of 12 cases and review of the literature. *Medicine* 62;81–97.

259. Lidsky MD, Klass DW, McKenzie BF, et al. Herpes zoster (zona) encephalitis: case report with electroencephalographic and cerebrospinal fluid studies. *Ann Intern Med* 1962;56(5):779–784.

260. Norris FH, Leonards R, Calanchini PR, et al. Herpes-zoster meningoencephalitis. *J Infect Dis* 1970;122:335–338.

261. O'Donnell PP, Pula TP, Sellman M, et al. Recurrent herpes zoster encephalitis: a complication of systemic lupus erythematosus. *Arch Neurol* 1981;38:49–51.

262. Rose FC, Brett EM, Burston J. Zoster encephalomyelitis. *Arch Neurol* 1964;11:155–172.

263. Taber LH, Greenberg SB, Perez FI, et al. Herpes simplex encephalitis treated with vidarabine (adenine arabinoside). *Arch Neurol* 1977;34:608–610.

264. Walker RJ, Gammal TE, Allen MB. Cranial arteritis associated with herpes zoster. *Radiology* 1973;107:109–110.

265. Acers T. Herpes zoster ophthalmicus with contralateral hemiplegia. *Arch Ophthalmol* 1964;71:371–376.

266. Doyle PW, Gibson G, Dolman CL. Herpes zoster ophthalmicus with contralateral hemiplegia: identification of cause. *Ann Neurol* 1983;14:84–85.

267. Kuroiwa Y, Furukawa T. Hemispheric infarction after herpes zoster ophthalmicus: computed tomography and angiography. *Neurology* 1981;31:1030–1032.

268. Pratesi R, Freemon FR, Lowry JL. Herpes zoster ophthalmicus with contralateral hemiplegia. *Arch Neurol* 1977;34:640–641.

269. Hogan EL, Krigman MR. Herpes zoster myelitis. *Arch Neurol* 1973;29:309–313.

270. Muder RR, Lumish RM, Corsello GR. Myelopathy after herpes zoster. *Arch Neurol* 1983;50:445–446.

271. Thomas JE, Howard FM. Segmental zoster paresis: a disease profile. *Neurology* 1972;22(5):459–466.

272. Horton B, Price RW, Jimenez D. Multifocal varicella-zoster virus leukoencephalitis temporally remote from herpes zoster. *Ann Neurol* 1981;9:251–266.

273. Knox JDE, Levy R, Simpson JA. Herpes zoster and the Landry–Guillain–Barré syndrome. *J Neurol Neurosurg Psychiatry* 1961;247:167–172.

274. Meyer HM, Johnson RT, Crawford JP, et al. Central nervous system syndromes of "viral" etiology: a study of 773 cases. *Am J Med* 1960;29:334–347.

275. Reichman RC. Neurologic complications of varicella-zoster infections. In: Dolin R, ed. *Herpes zoster-varicella infections. Ann Intern Med* 1978;89:375–388.

276. Tenser RB. Herpes simplex and herpes zoster: nervous system involvement. *Neurol Clin* 1984;2(2):215–240.

277. Gold E. Serologic and virus-isolation studies of patients with varicella-zoster infection. *N Engl J Med* 1966;274:181–185.

278. Andiman WA, White-Greenwald M, Tinghitella T. Zoster encephalitis: isolation of virus and measurement of varicella-zoster specific antibodies in cerebrospinal fluid. *Am J Med* 1982;73:769–772.

279. Gold E, Robbins FC. Isolation of herpes zoster virus from spinal fluid of a patient. *Virology* 1958;6:293–295.

280. McCormich WR, Rodnitzky RL, Schochet SS, et al. Varicella-zoster encephalomyelitis: a morphologic and virologic study. *Arch Neurol* 1969;21:559–570.

281. Peterson LR, Ferguson RM. Fatal central nervous system infection with varicella-zoster virus in renal transplant recipients. *Transplantation* 1984;37:366–368.

282. Steele RW, Keeney RE, Bradsher RW, et al. Treatment of varicella-zoster meningoencephalitis with acyclovir: demonstration of virus in cerebrospinal fluid by electron microscopy. *Am J Clin Pathol* 1983;80:57–60.

283. Linnemann CC, Alvira MM. Pathogenesis of varicella-zoster angitis in the CNS. *Arch Neurol* 1980;37:239–240.

284. Ruppenthal M. Changes of the central nervous system in herpes zoster. *Acta Neuropathol* 1980;52:59–68.

285. Bieger RC, Van Scoy RE, Smith TF. Antibodies to varicella zoster in cerebrospinal fluid. *Arch Neurol* 1977;34:489–491.

286. Peters ACB, Versteeg J, Bots GTAM, et al. Nervous system complications of herpes zoster: Immunofluorescent demonstration of varicella-zoster antigen in CSF cells. *J Neurol Neurosurg Psychiatry* 1979;42:452–457.

287. Shoji H, Koya M, Ogiwara H. Meningitis associated with herpes zoster: immunofluorescent of varicella-zoster antigens in CSF cells. *J Neurol* 1976;213:269–271.

288. Blue MC, Rosenblum WL. Granulomatous angitis of the brain with herpes zoster and varicella encephalitis. *Arch Pathol Lab Med* 1983;107:126–128.

289. Nahmias AJ, Keyserling HL, Kerrick GM. Herpes simplex. In: Remington J, Klein J, eds. *Infections of the fetus and newborn infant.* Philadelphia: WB Saunders, 1983;636–678.

290. Tako J, Rado JP. Zoster meningoencephalitis in a steroid-treated patients. *Arch Neurol* 1965;12:610–612.

291. Eaglstein WH, Katz R, Brown JA. The effects of early corticosteroid therapy on the skin eruption and pain of herpes zoster. *JAMA* 1970;211:1681.

292. Elliott FA. Treatment of herpes zoster with high doses of prednisone. *Lancet* 19642:610–611.

293. Whitley RJ, Hilty M, Haynes R, Bryson Y, Connor JD, Soong SJ, Alford CA Jr, and the NIAID Collaborative Antiviral Study Group. Vidarabine therapy of varicella in immunosuppressed patients. *J Pediatr* 1982;1:125.

294. Esmann V, Kroon S, Peterslund NA, et al. Prednisolone does not prevent post-herpetic neuralgia. *Lancet* 1987;2:126–129.

295. Whitley RJ, Soong SJ, Dolin R, Betts R, Linnemann C Jr, Alford CA Jr, and the NIAID Collaborative Antiviral Study Group. Early vidarabine therapy to control the complications of herpes zoster in immunosuppressed patients. *N Engl J Med* 1982;307:971.

296. Prober DG, Kirk LE, Keeney RE. Acyclovir therapy of chickenpox in immunosuppressed children—a collaborative study. *J Pediatr* 1982;101:622.

297. Al-Nakib W, Al-Kandari S, El-Khalik DM, El-Shirbiny AM. A randomized controlled study of intravenous acyclovir (Zovirax) against placebo in adults with chickenpox. *J Infection* 1983;6:49–56.

298. Stevens DA, Merigan TC. Interferon, antibody, and other host factors, in herpes zoster. *J Clin Invest* 1972;51:1170.

299. Arvin AM, Kushner JH, Feldman S, Buchner RL, Hammond D, Merigan TC. Human leukocyte interferon for treatment of varicella in children with cancer. *N Engl J Med* 1982;306:761.

300. Arvin A, Feldman S, Merigan TC. Human leukocyte interferon in the treatment of varicella in children with cancer: a preliminary controlled trial. *Antimicrob Agents Chemother* 1978;13:605.

301. Ch'ien LT, Whitley RJ, Alford CA, Galasso GJ. Adenine arabinoside for therapy of herpes zoster in immunosuppressed patients: preliminary results of a collaborative study. *J Infect Dis* 1976;133:A184.

302. Whitley RJ, Chien LT, Dolin R, Galasso GJ, Alford CA Jr, and the Collaborative Antiviral Study Group. Adenine arabinoside therapy of herpes zoster in the immunosuppressed. *N Engl J Med* 1976;294:1193.

303. Merigan TC, Rand KH, Pollard RB. Human leukocyte interferon for the treatment of herpes zoster in patients with cancer. *N Engl J Med* 1978;298:981.

304. Balfour HH, Bean B, Laskin O, et al. Acyclovir halts progression of herpes zoster in immunocompromised patients. *N Engl J Med* 1983;308:1448–1453.

305. Shepp D, Dandliker PS, Meyers JD. Treatment of varicella-zoster virus in severely immunocompromised patients: a randomized comparison of acyclovir and vidarabine. *N Engl J Med* 1987;312:8–21.

306. Vild'e JL, Bricaire F, Leport C, Renaudie M, Burn-V'ezinet F. Comparative trial of acyclovir and vidarabine in disseminated varicella-zoster virus infections in immunocompromised patients. *J Med Virol* 1986;20:127–134.

307. Cobo LM, Foulks GN, Liesegang T, et al. Oral acyclovir in the treatment of acute herpes zoster ophthalimicus. *Ophthalmology* 1986;93:763–770.

308. Essman V, Ipens J, Peterslund NA, Seyer-Hansen K, Shonheyder H, Henning J. Therapy of acute herpes zoster with acyclovir in the nonimmunocompromised host. *Am J Med* 1982;73:320.

309. McKendrick MW, McGill JI, White JE, Wood MJ. Oral acyclovir in acute herpes zoster. *Br Med J* 1986;293:1529–1532.

310. Bean B, Braun C, Balfour HH Jr. Acyclovir therapy for acute herpes zoster. *Lancet* 1982;2:118–121.

311. Peterslund NA, Seyer-Hansen K, Ipen J, Esmann V, Schonheyder H, Juhl H. Acyclovir in herpes zoster. *Lancet* 1981;2:827–830.

312. McGill J, MacDonald DR, Fall C, McKendrick GD, Copplestone A. Intravenous acyclovir in acute herpes zoster infection. *J Infect* 1983;6:157–161.

313. Sprunt TB, Evans FA. Mononuclear leukocytosis in reaction to acute infections ("infectious mononucleosis"). *Johns Hopkins Bull* 1920;31:410.

314. Downey H, McKinlay CA. Acute lymphadenosis compared with acute lymphatic leukemia. *Arch Intern Med* 1923;32:82.

315. Burkitt D. A sarcoma involving the jaws of African children. *Br J Surg* 1958;46:218.

316. Epstein MA, Achong BG, Barr YM. Virus particles in cultured lymphoblasts from Burkitt's lymphoma. *Lancet* 1964;1:702.

317. Henle G, Henle W. Immunofluorescence in cells derived from Burkitt's lymphoma. *J Bacteriol* 1966;91:1248–1256.

318. Henle G, Henle W, Diehl V. Relation of Burkitt's tumor-associated herpes-type virus to infectious mononucleosis. *Proc Natl Acad Sci USA* 1968;59:94–101.

319. Evans AS, Niederman JC, McCollum RC. Seroepidemirologic studies of infectious mononucleosis with EB virus. *N Engl J Med* 1968;279:121–127.

320. Sawyer RN, Evans AS, Niederman JC, McCollum RW. Prospective studies of a group of Yale University freshmen. I. Occurrence of infectious mononucleosis. *J Infect Dis* 1971;123:263–269.

321. Miller G, Niederman JC, Andrews LL. Prolonged oropharyngeal excretion of EB virus following infectious mononucleosis. *N Engl J Med* 1973;288:229–231.

322. Zur Hausen H, Schulte-Holthausen H, Klein G, et al. EBV DNA in biopsies of Burkitt's tumors and anaplastic carcinoma of the nasopharynx. *Nature* 1970;228:1056–1058.

323. Purtilo DT, DeFlorio D, Hutt LM, et al. Variable phenotypic expression of an X-linked recessive lymphoproliferative syndrome. *N Engl J Med* 1977;297:1077–1081.

324. Hanto DW, Frizzera G, Gajl-Peczalska KJ, Simmons RL. Epstein–Barr virus, immunodeficiency, and B cell lymphoproliferation. *Transplantation* 1985;39:461–472.

325. Andiman W, Gradoville L, Heston L, et al. Use of cloned probes to detect Epstein–Barr viral DNA in tissues of patients with neoplastic and lymphoproliferative diseases. *J Infect Dis* 1984; 148:967–977.

326. Schooley RT, Carey RW, Miller G, et al. Chronic Epstein–Barr virus infection associated with fever and interstitial pneumonitis. Clinical and serological features and response to antiviral chemotherapy. *Ann Intern Med* 1986;104:636–643.

327. Straus SE. The chronic mononucleosis syndrome. *J Infect Dis* 1988;157:405–412.

328. Greenspan JS, Greenspan D, Lennette ET, et al. Replication of Epstein–Barr virus within the epithelial cells of oral "hairy" leukoplakia, an AIDS-associated lesion. *N Engl J Med* 1985; 313:1564–1571.

329. Swartz MN. The chronic fatigue syndrome—one entity or many? *N Engl J Med* 1988;319:1726–1728.

330. Kieff E, Liebowitz D. Epstein–Barr virus and its replication. In: Fields BN, Knipe DM, Chanock R, Hirsch M, Melnick J, Monath T, Roizman B, eds. *Virology,* 2nd ed. New York: Raven Press, 1990;1889–1920.

331. Baer R, Bankier AT, Biggin MD, et al. DNA sequence and expression of the B95-8 Epstein–Barr virus genome. *Nature* 1984;310:207–211.

332. Hummel M, Kieff E. Epstein–Barr virus RNA. VIII. Viral RNA in permissively infected B95-8 cells. *J Virol* 1982;43:262–272.

333. Dillner J, Kallin B. The Epstein–Barr virus proteins. *Adv Cancer Res* 1988;50:95–158.

334. Miller G, Enders JF, Lisco H, Kohn HL. Establishment of lines from normal human blood leukocytes by co-cultivation with a leukocyte line derived from a leukemic child. *Proc Soc Exp Biol Med* 1969;132:247–252.

335. Tanner J, Weiss J, Fearon D, Whang Y, Kieff E. Epstein–Barr virus gp350/220 binding to the B lymphocyte C3d receptor mediates adsorption, capping and endocytosis. *Cell* 1987;50:203–213.

336. Strauch B, Siegel N, Andrews L, Miller G. Oropharyngeal excretion of Epstein–Barr virus by renal transplant recipients and other patients treated with immunosuppressive drugs. *Lancet* 1974;1:234–237.

337. Young LS, Clark D, Sixbey JW, Rickinson AB. Epstein–Barr virus receptors on human pharyngeal epithelia. *Lancet* 1986; 1:240–242.

338. Sixby JW, Lomon SM, Pagano JS. A second site of Epstein–Barr virus shedding: the uterine cervix. *Lancet* 1986;2:1122–1124.

339. Jones JF, Shurin S, Ambramowsky C, et al. T cell lymphomas containing Epstein–Barr virus DNA in patients with chronic Epstein–Barr virus infections. *N Engl J Med* 1988;318:733–741.

340. Lemon SM, Hutt LM, Shaw JE, et al. Replication of EBV in epithelial cells during infectious mononucleosis. *Nature* 1977; 268:268.

341. Wolf H, Zur Hausen H, Becker V. EB viral genomes in epithelial nasopharyngeal carcinoma cells. *Nature* 1973;244:245.

342. Klein G, Giovanella BC, Lindahl T, et al. Direct evidence for the presence of Epstein–Barr virus DNA and nuclear antigen in malignant epithelial cells from patients with poorly differentiated carcinoma of the nasopharynx. *Proc Natl Acad Sci USA* 1974; 71:4737.

343. Huang DP, Ho JHC, Henle W, et al. Demonstration of EBV-associated nuclear antigen in NPC cells from fresh biopsies. *Int J Cancer* 1974;14:580.

344. Wolf H, Zur Hausen H, Klein G, et al. Attempts to detect virus-specific DNA sequences in human tumors. III. Epstein–Barr viral DNA in nonlymphoid nasopharyngeal carcinoma cells. *Med Microbiol Immunol* 1975;161:15.

345. Straus S. Epstein–Barr virus and human herpesvirus type 6. In: Galasso GJ, Whitley RJ, Merigan TC, eds. *Antiviral agents and viral diseases of man,* 3rd ed. New York: Raven Press, 1990;647–668.

346. Fleisher GR. Epstein–Barr virus. In: Belshe RB, ed. *Textbook of*

human virology. Littleton, MA: PSG Publishing Company, 1984;853–886.

347. Adams A, Lindahl T. Epstein–Barr virus genomes with properties of circular molecules in carrier cells. *Proc Natl Acad Sci USA* 1975;72:1477–1481.

348. Yates JL, Warren N, Sugden B. Stable replication of plasmids derived from Epstein–Barr virus in various mammalian cells. *Nature* 1985;313:812–815.

349. Rickinson AB, Young LS, Reive M. Influence of the Epstein–Barr virus nuclear antigen EBNA 2 on the growth phenotype of virus-transformed B cells. *J Virol* 1987;61:1310–1317.

350. Liebowitz D, Kopan R, Fuchs E, et al. An Epstein–Barr virus transforming protein associates with Vimentin in lymphocytes. *Mol Cell Biol* 1987;7:2299–2308.

351. Levy JA, Henle G. Indirect immunofluorescent tests with sera from African children and cultured Burkitt lymphoma cells. *J Bacteriol* 1966;92:275.

352. Kafuko GW, Henderson BE, Kirya BG, et al. Epstein–Barr virus antibody levels in children from the West Nile District of Uganda. *Lancet* 1972;1:706.

353. Porter DD, Wimberly I, Benyish-Melnick M. Prevalence of antibodies to EB virus and other herpesviruses. *JAMA* 1969; 208:1675.

354. Pereira MS, Blake JM, Macrae AD. EB virus antibody at different ages. *Br Med J* 1969;4:526.

355. Henle G, Henle W. Observations on childhood infections with the Epstein–Barr virus. *J Infect Dis* 1970;121:303.

356. Tallqvist H, Henle W, Klemola E, et al. Antibodies to Epstein–Barr virus at the ages of 6 to 23 months in children with congenital heart disease. *Scand J Infect Dis* 1973;5:159.

357. Fleisher G, Henle W, Henle G, et al. Primary infection with Epstein–Barr virus in infants in the United States: clinical and serological observations. *J Infect Dis* 1979;139:553.

358. Evans AS. Epidemiology of Epstein–Barr virus infection and disease. In: Nahmias AJ, Dowdle WR, Schinazi RF, eds. *The human herpesviruses.* New York: Elsevier, 1981;172.

359. University Health Physicians and PHLS Laboratories. Infectious mononucleosis and its relationship to EB virus antibody. *Br Med J* 1971;4:643.

360. Hallee TJ, Evans AS, Niederman JC, et al. Infectious mononucleosis at the United States Military Academy. *Yale Biol Med* 1974;47:182.

361. Demissie A, Svedmyr A. Age distribution of antibodies to EB virus in Swedish females as studied by indirect immunofluorescence on Burkitt cells. *Acta Pathol Microbiol Scand* 1969;75:457.

362. Lehane DE. A seroepidemiologic study of infectious mononucleosis: the development of EB virus antibody in a military population. *JAMA* 1970;212:2240.

363. Niederman JC, Evans AS, Subrahmanyan L, et al. Prevalence, incidence, and persistence of EB virus antibody in young adults. *N Engl J Med* 1970;282:361.

364. Sumaya CV, Henle W, Henle G, et al. Seroepidemiologic study of Epstein–Barr virus infections in a rural community. *J Infect Dis* 1975;131:403.

365. Fleisher G, Bolognese R. Seroepidemiology of Epstein–Barr virus in pregnancy. *J Infect Dis* 1982;145:537.

366. Penman HG. The incidence of glandular fever. *J Hyg Camb* 1966;65:457.

367. Belfrage S. Infectious mononucleosis: an epidemiological and clinical study. *Acta Med Scand* 1962;171:531.

368. Christine BW. Infectious mononucleosis. *Conn Health Bull* 1968;82:115.

369. Heath CW, Brodsky AL, Potolsky AI. Infectious mononucleosis in a general population. *Am J Epidemiol* 1972;95:46.

370. Henke CE, Kurland LT, Elveback LR. Infectious mononucleosis in Rochester, Minnesota 1950 through 1969. *Am J Epidemiol* 1973;98:483.

371. Newell KW. The reported incidence of glandular fever, and analysis of a report of the Public Health Laboratory Service. *J Clin Pathol* 1957;10:20.

372. Schooley RT, Dolin R. Epstein–Barr virus (infectious mononucleosis). In: Mandell GL, Douglas RG Jr, Bennett JE, eds. *Principles and practices of infectious diseases,* 3rd ed. New York: Churchill Livingstone, 1990;121–1184.

373. De-The G. Epidemiology of Epstein–Barr virus and associated diseases in man. In: Roizman B, ed. *The herpesvirus,* vol 1, New York: Plenum Press, 1982;25–103.

374. Erikson J, Finan J, Nowell PC, Croce CM. Translocation of immunoglobulin V_H genes in Burkitt's lymphoma. *Proc Natl Acad Sci USA* 1982;79:5611–5615.

375. Henle W, Henle G, Gunven P, et al. Patterns of antibodies to Epstein–Barr virus-induced early antigens in Burkitt's lymphoma. Comparison of dying patients with long-term survivors. *J Natl Cancer Inst* 1973;50:1163.

376. Epstein AL, Henle W, Henle G, et al. Surface marker characteristics and Epstein–Barr virus studies of two established North American Burkitt's lymphoma cell lines. *Proc Natl Acad Sci USA* 1976;73:228.

377. Nkrumah F, Henle W, Henle G, et al. Burkitt's lymphoma: its clinical course in relation to immunologic reactivities to Epstein–Barr virus and tumor related antigens. *J Natl Cancer Inst* 1976;57:1051.

378. Henle W, Henle G. Antibodies to the R component of the EBV-induced early antigens in Burkitt's lymphoma may exceed in titer antibodies to the EBV vira capsid antigen. *J Natl Cancer Inst* 1977;58:785.

379. Purtilo DT, Sakamoto K, Barnabei V, et al. Epstein–Barr virus-induced disease in boys with the X-linked lymphoproliferative syndrome (XLP). *Am J Med* 1982;73:49–56.

380. Purtilo DT. Fatal infectious mononucleosis in familial lymphohistiocytosis. *N Engl J Med* 1974;291:736.

381. Purtilo DT, Yand JPS, Allegra S, et al. The pathogenesis and hematopathology of the X-linked recessive lymphoproliferative syndrome. *Am J Med* 1977;62:225.

382. Purtilo DT, Bhawan J. Immunopathology of fatal infectious mononucleosis in a X-linked lymphoproliferative syndrome. *Lab Invest* 1978;38:31.

383. Purtilo DT, Bhawan J, DeNichola L, et al. Epstein–Barr virus infections in the X-linked recessive lymphoproliferative syndrome. *Lancet* 1978;1:798.

384. Purtilo DT, Cassel C, Yang JPS, et al. X-linked recessive progressive combined variable immunodeficiency (Duncan's disease). *Lancet* 1975;1:935.

385. Purtilo DT, Paquin LA, Defono D, et al. Immunodiagnosis and immunopathogenesis of the X-linked recessive lymphoproliferative syndrome. *Semin Hematol* 1979;16:309.

386. Sakamoto K, Fried HS, Purtilo DT. Antibody response to Epstein–Barr virus in families with X-linked lymphoproliferative syndrome. *J Immunol* 1980;125:921.

387. Sullivan JL, Byron KS, Brewster FE, et al. Deficient natural killer cell activity in X-linked lymphoproliferative syndrome. *Science* 1980;210:543.

388. Miller G, Grogan E, Rowe E, et al. Selective lack of antibody to a component of EB nuclear antigen in patients with chronic active Epstein–Barr virus infection. *J Infect Dis* 1987;156:26–35.

389. Swartz MN. The chronic fatigue syndrome—one entity or many? *N Engl J Med* 1988;319:1726–1728.

390. Bernstein TC, Wolff HG. Involvement of the nervous system in infectious mononucleosis. *Am Intern Med* 1950;33:1120.

391. McKee KT, Wright PE, Kilroy AW, et al. Herpes encephalitis after infectious mononucleosis. *South Med J* 1981;74:238.

392. Gautier-Smith PC. Neurological complications of glandular fever (infectious mononucleosis). *Brain* 1965;88:323–334.

393. Silverstain A, Steinberg G, Nathanson M. Nervous system involvement in infectious mononucleosis. *Arch Neurol* 1972; 26:353–358.

394. Penman HG. Fatal infectious mononucleosis: a critical review. *J Clin Pathol* 1970;2:765–771.

395. Ricker W, Blumberg A, Peters CH, Widerman A. The association of the Guillain–Barré syndrome with infectious mononucleosis, with a report of two fatal cases. *Blood* 1947;2:217–226.

396. Ambler M, Stoll J, Tzamaloukas A, Albala MM. Focal encephalomyelitis in infectious mononucleosis. *Ann Intern Med* 1971; 75:579–583.

397. Paul JR, Brunnell WW. The presence of heterophile antibodies in infectious mononucleosis. *Am J Med Sci* 1932;183:90–104.

398. Henle W, Henle G. Epstein–Barr virus-specific serology in immu-

nologically compromised individuals. *Cancer Res* 1981;41:4222–4225.

399. Reedman BM, Klein G. Cellular localization of an Epstein–Barr virus-associated complement-fixing antigen in producer and non-producer lymphoblastoid cell lines. *Int J Cancer* 1973; 11:499–520.

400. Henle W, Henle G, Horowitz CA. Epstein–Barr virus specific diagnostic tests in infectious mononucleosis. *Hum Pathol* 1974;5:551–565.

401. Bender CE. The value of corticosteroids in the treatment of infectious mononucleosis. *JAMA* 1967;199:529–531.

402. Bolden KJ. Corticosteroids in the treatment of infectious mononucleosis. *J R Coll Gen Pract* 1972;22:87–95.

403. Andersson J, Britton S, Ernberg I, et al. Effect of acyclovir in infectious mononucleosis: a double-blind, placebo-controlled study. *J Infect Dis* 1986;153:283–290.

404. Andersson J, Skoldenberg B, Henle W, et al. Acyclovir treatment in infectious mononucleosis: a clinical and immunological study. *Infection* 1987;15(Suppl 1):514–21.

405. Sullivan JC, Medveczky P, Forman SJ, Baker SM, Monroe JE, Mulder C. Epstein–Barr virus-induced lymphoproliferation. *N Engl J Med* 1984;311:1163–1167.

406. Colby BM, Shaw JE, Elion GB, Pagano JS. Effect of acyclovir [9-(2-hydroxyethoxymethyl) guanine] on Epstein–Barr virus DNA replication. *J Virol* 1980;34:560–568.

407. Lin JC, Smith MC, Pagano JS. Prolonged inhibitory effect of 9-(1,3-dihydroxy-2-propoxymethyl) guanine against replication of Epstein–Barr virus. *J Virol* 1984;50:50–55.

408. Lin JC, Smith MC, Pagano JS. Comparative efficacy and selectivity of some nucleoside analogs against Epstein–Barr virus. *Antimicrob Agents Chemother* 1985;27:971–973.

409. Kure S, Tada K, Wada J, Yoshie O. Inhibition of Epstein–Barr virus infection *in vitro* by recombinant human interferons α and β. *Virus Res* 1986;5:377–390.

410. Hanto DW, Frizzera G, Gail-Pexzalska KJ, et al. Epstein–Barr virus-induced B cell lymphomas after renal transplantation. Acyclovir therapy and transition from polyclonal to monoclonal B cell proliferation. *N Engl J Med* 1982;306:913–918.

411. Hanshaw JB. Cytomegalovirus. In: Gard S, Hallauer C, Meyer KF, eds. *Virology monographs.* New York: Springer-Verlag, 1968;2–23.

412. Jesionek A, Kiolemenoglou R. Uber einen Befund voc protozoenartigen Gebilden in den Organen eines heriditarluetischen Fotus. *Muench Med Wochenschr* 1904;51:1905–1907.

413. Ribbert D. Uber protozoenartige Zellen in der Niere eines syphilitischen Neugeborenen und in der Parotis von Kindern. *Zentralbl Allg Pathol* 1904;15:945–948.

414. Farber S, Wolbach SB. Intranuclear and cytoplasmic inclusions ("protozoan-like bodies") in the salivary glands and other organs of infants. *Am J Pathol Child* 1932;8:123–126.

415. Rowe WP, Hartley JW, Waterman S, Turner HC, Huebner RJ. Cytopathogenic agent resembling human salivary gland virus recovered from tissue cultures of human adenoids. *Proc Soc Exp Biol Med* 1956;92:418–424.

416. Smith MG. Propagation in tissue cultures of a cytopathogenic virus from human salivary gland virus disease. *Proc Soc Exp Biol Med* 1956;92:424–430.

417. Weller TH, Macauley JE, Craig JM, Wirth P. Isolation of intranuclear inclusion producing agents from infants with illnesses resembling cytomegalic inclusion disease. *Proc Soc Exp Biol Med* 1957;94:4–12.

418. Alford CA Jr, Britt WJ. Cytomegalovirus. In: Knipe DM, Chanock RM, Melnick JL, Roizman B, Shope RE, eds. *Virology.* New York: Raven Press, 1985;629–660.

419. Stinski MF, Thomson Dr, Wathen MW. Structure and function of the cytomegalovirus genome. In: Nahmias A, Dowdle A, Schinazi R, eds. *The human herpesviruses.* New York: Elsevier, 1981;72–84.

420. Krech U, Jung M. *Cytomegalovirus infections of man.* New York: Karger, 1971.

421. Reynolds DW, Stagno S, Alford CA. Laboratory diagnosis of cytomegalovirus infections. In: Lennette EH, Schmidt NJ, eds. *Diagnostic procedures for viral rickettsial and chlamydial infections,*

5th ed. Washington, DC: American Public Health Association, 1979;399–439.

422. Weller TH. The cytomegaloviruses: ubiquitous agents with protean clinical manifestations. *N Engl J Med* 1971;285:203–214, 267–274.

423. Furukawa T, Fiorette A, Plotkins S. Growth characteristics of cytomegalovirus in human fibroblasts with demonstration of protein synthesis early in viral replication. *J Virol* 1973;11:991–997.

424. Smith JD, DeHarven E. Herpes simplex virus and human cytomegalovirus replication in WI-38 cells. I. Sequence of viral replication. *J Virol* 1973;12:919–930.

425. Smith JD, DeHarven E. Herpes simplex virus and human cytomegalovirus replication in WI-38 cells. II. An ultrastructural study of viral penetration. *J Virol* 1974;14:945–956.

426. Kanich RE, Craighead JE. Human cytomegalovirus infection of cultured fibroblasts. I. Cytopathologic effects induced by an adapted and a wild strain. *Lab Invest* 1972;27:263–271.

427. Kanich RE, Craighead JE. Human cytomegalovirus infection of cultured fibroblasts. II. Viral replicative sequence of a wild and an adapted strain. *Lab Invest* 1972;27:273–282.

428. Ozawa T, Stewart JA. Immune-complex glomerulonephritis associated with cytomegalovirus in.ection. *Am J Clin Pathol* 1979;72:103–107.

429. Stagno S, Pass RF, Reynolds DW, Stroud R, Alford CA Jr. Immune complexes in congenital and natal cytomegalovirus infections of man. *J Clin Invest* 1977;60:838–845.

430. Fetterman GH, Sherman FE, Fabizio NS, Studnicki FM. Generalized cytomegalic inclusion disease of the newborn: localization of inclusions in the kidney. *Arch Pathol* 1968;86:86–94.

431. Bonkowsky HL, Lee RL, Klatskin G. Acute granulomatous hepatitis. Occurrence in cytomegalovirus mononucleosis. *JAMA* 1975;233:1284–1288.

432. Ho M. Pathology of cytomegalovirus infection. In: Greenough WB, Merigan TC, eds. *Biology and infection: current topics in infectious disease.* New York: Plenum Press, 1982;119–129.

433. Medearis DN Jr. Observations concerning human cytomegalovirus infection and disease. *Bull Johns Hopkins Hosp* 1964; 114:181–211.

434. McCracken GJ Jr, Shinefield HR, Cobb K, Rausen AR, Dische MR, Eichenwald HF. Congenital cytomegalic inclusion disease. A longitudinal study of 20 patients. *Am J Dis Child* 1969; 117:522–539.

435. Pass RF, Stagno S, Myers GJ, Alford CA. Outcome of symptomatic congenital CMV infection: results of long-term longitudinal follow-up. *Pediatrics* 1980;66:758–762.

436. Weller TH, Hanshaw JB. Virologic and clinical observations on cytomegalic inclusion disease. *N Engl J Med* 1964;266:1233–1244.

437. Wentworth BB, Alexander ER. Seroepidemiology of infections due to members of the herpesvirus groups. *Am J Epidemiol* 1971;94:496–507.

438. Stern H, Alexander ER. The incidence of infection with cytomegalovirus in a normal population: a serological study in greater London. *J Hyg (Camb)* 1965;63:79–87.

439. Sinha DK, Pauls PF. Cytomegalovirus complement fixation antibody response in eskimo families. *Pediatrics* 1971;48:158.

440. Lang DJ, Garruto RM, Gadjusek DC. Early acquisition of cytomegalovirus and Epstein–Barr virus antibody in several isolated Melanesian populations. *Am J Epidemiol* 1977;105:480–487.

441. Krech U. Complement-fixing antibodies against cytomegalovirus in different parts of the world. *Bull WHO* 1973;49:103–106.

442. Krech U, Tobin J. A collaborative study of cytomegalovirus antibodies in mothers and young children in 19 countries. *Bull WHO* 1981;59:605–610.

443. Onorato IM, Morens DM, Martone WJ, Stanfield SK. Epidemiology of cytomegalovirus infections: recommendations for prevention and control. *Rev Infect Dis* 1988;7:479–496.

444. Pass RF. Epidemiology and transmission of cytomegalovirus. *J Infect Dis* 1988;153:243–248.

445. Adler SP. Transfusion-associated cytomegalovirus infections. *Rev Infect Dis* 1983;5:977–993.

446. Levinsohn EM, Foy HM, Kenny GE, et al. Isolation of cytomegalovirus from a cohort of 100 infants throughout the first year of life. *Proc Soc Exp Biol Med* 1969;32:957–962.

447. Olson LC, Ketusinha R, Mansuwan P. Respiratory tract excretion of cytomegalovirus in Thai children. *J Pediatr* 1970;77:499–504.

448. Leinikki R, Heinonen K, Pettay O. Incidence of cytomegalovirus infections in early childhood. *Scand J Infect Dis* 1972;4:1–5.

449. Li F, Hanshaw JB. Cytomegalovirus among migrant children. *Am J Epidemiol* 1967;88:137–141.

450. Numazaki Y, Yano N, Marizuka T, et al. Primary infection with human cytomegalovirus: virus isolation from healthy infants and pregnant women. *Am J Epidemiol* 1970;91:410–417.

451. Larke RPB, Wheatley E, Saigal S, et al. Congenital cytomegalovirus infection in an urban Canadian community. *J Infect Dis* 1980;162:641–653.

452. Rowe WP, Hartleh JW, Cramblett MG, et al. Detection of human salivary gland virus in the mouth and urine of children. *Am J Hyg* 1958;67:57–65.

453. Stern H. Isolation of cytomegalovirus and clinical manifestations of infection at different ages. *Br Med J* 1968;1:665–669.

454. Lang DJ, Kummer JF, Hartley PD. Cytomegalovirus in semen: persistence and demonstration in extracellular fluids. *N Engl J Med* 1974;291:121–123.

455. Lang DJ, Kummer JF. Cytomegalovirus in semen: observations in selected populations. *J Infect Dis* 1975;132:472–473.

456. Embil JA, Manuel FR, Garner JB, et al. Cytomegalovirus in the semen. *Can Med Assoc J* 1982;126:391–392.

457. Hayes K, Danks DM, Gibas H, et al. Cytomegalovirus in human milk. *N Engl J Med* 1972;287:177–178.

458. Stagno S, Reynolds DW, Pass RF, et al. Breast milk and the risk of cytomegalovirus infection. *N Engl J Med* 1980;302:1073–1076.

459. Glenn J. Cytomegalovirus infections following renal transplantation. *Rev Infect Dis* 1981;3:1151–1178.

460. Winston DJ, Gale RP, Meyer DV, et al. Infectious complications of human bone marrow transplantation. *Medicine* 1979;58:1–31.

461. Stinson EB, Bieber CP, Griepp RB, et al. Infectious complications after cardiac transplantation in man. *Ann Intern Med* 1971;74:22–36.

462. Fulginita VA, Scribner R, Groth CG, et al. Infections in recipients of liver homografts. *N Engl J Med* 1968;279:619–626.

463. Duvall CP, Casazza AR, Gromley PM, et al. Recovery of cytomegalovirus from adults with neoplastic disease. *Ann Intern Med* 1966;64:531–541.

464. Dowling JN, Saslow AR, Armstrong JA, et al. Cytomegalovirus infection in patients receiving immunosuppressive therapy for rheumatologic disorders. *J Infect Dis* 1976;133:399–408.

465. Hedley-Whyte ET, Craighead JE. Generalized cytomegalic inclusion disease after renal homo-transplantation—report of a case with isolation of virus. *N Engl J Med* 1965;272:473–475.

466. Hill RB Jr, Rowlands DT, Rifkind D. Infectious pulmonary disease in patients receiving immunosuppressive therapy for organ transplantation. *N Engl J Med* 1964;271:1021–1027.

467. Craighead JE, Hanshaw JB, Carpenter CB. Cytomegalovirus infection after renal allotransplantation. *JAMA* 1967;201:725–728.

468. Andersen HK, Spencer ES. Cytomegalovirus infection among renal allograft recipients. *Acta Med Scand* 1969;186:7–19.

469. Pien RD, Smith TF, Anderson CF, et al. Herpes virus in renal transplant patients. *Transplantation* 1974;16:489–495.

470. Luby JPL, Brunett W, Hull AR. Relationship between cytomegalovirus and hepatic function abnormalities in the period after renal transplant. *J Infect Dis* 1974;129:511–518.

471. Fiala M, Payne JE, Berne TV. Epidemiology of cytomegalovirus infection after transplantation and immunosuppression. *J Infect Dis* 1975;132:421–433.

472. Naraqi S, Jackson GG, Jonasson OM, et al. Prospective study of prevalence, incidence and source of herpes virus infections in patients with renal allografts. *J Infect Dis* 1977;136:531–540.

473. Balfour HH, Slad MS, Kalis JM, et al. Viral infections in renal transplant donors and their recipients: a prospective study. *Surgery* 1977;18:487–492.

474. Chatterjee SN, Jordon GW. Prospective study of the prevalence and symptomatology of cytomegalovirus infection in renal transplant recipients. *Transplantation* 1979;28:457–460.

475. Rubin RH, Cosimi AB, Tolkoff-Rubin NE, et al. Infectious diseases syndromes attributable to cytomegalovirus and their signifi-

476. Pass RF, Long WK, Whitley RJ, et al. Productive infection with cytomegalovirus and herpes simplex virus in renal transplant recipients: role of source of kidney. *J Infect Dis* 1978;137:556–563.

477. Peterson PK, Balfour HH, Marker SC, et al. Cytomegalovirus disease in renal allograft recipients: a prospective study of the clinical features, risk factors and impact on renal transplantation. *Medicine* 1980;59:283–300.

478. Rifkind D, Goodman N, Hill RB. The clinical significance of cytomegalovirus infection in renal transplant recipients. *Ann Intern Med* 1967;66:1116–1128.

479. Whelchel JD, Pass RF, Diethelm AC, et al. Effect of primary and recurrent cytomegalovirus infections upon graft and patient survival after renal transplantation. *Transplantation* 1979;28:443–446.

480. Meyers JD, Spencer HC Jr, Watts JC, et al. Cytomegalovirus pneumonia after human marrow transplantation. *Ann Intern Med* 1975;82:181–188.

481. Jacobson MA, Mills J. Serious cytomegalovirus disease in the acquired immunodeficiency syndrome (AIDS). Clinical findings, diagnosis, and treatment. *Ann Intern Med* 1988;108:585–594.

482. Murray HW, Knox DL, Green WR, Susel RM. Cytomegalovirus retinitis in adults. A manifestation of disseminated viral infection. *Am J Med* 1977;63:574–584.

483. Pollard RB, Egbert PR, Gallagher JG, Merigan TC. Cytomegalovirus retinitis in immunosuppressed hosts. I. Natural history and effects of treatment with adenine arabinoside. *Ann Intern Med* 1980;93:655–664.

484. Henson D. Cytomegalovirus inclusion bodies in the gastrointestinal tract. *Arch Pathol* 1972;93:477–482.

485. Goodman MD, Porter DD. Cytomegalovirus vasculitis with fatal colonic hemorrhage. *Arch Pathol* 1973;96:281–284.

486. Phillips CA, Fanning WL, Gump DW, Phillips CF. CMV encephalitis in immunologically normal adults. Successful treatment with vidarabine. *JAMA* 1977;238:2299–2300.

487. Jamison RM, Hathron AW. Isolation of CMV from cerebrospinal fluid of a congenitally infected infant. *Am J Dis Child* 1978;132:63–64.

488. Schneck SA. Neuropathological features of human organ transplantation. I. Possible cytomegalovirus infection. *J Neuropathol Exp Neurol* 1965;24:415–429.

489. Schober R, Herman MM. Neuropathology of cardiac transplantation. *Lancet* 1973;1:962–967.

490. Gay FP, Holden M. The herpes encephalitis problem. II. *J Infect Dis* 1933;53:287–303.

491. Sabin AB, Wright WM. Acute ascending myelitis following a monkey bite, with the isolation of a virus capable of reproducing the disease. *J Exp Med* 1934;59:115–136.

492. Sabin AB. Studies of B virus. I. The immunological identity of a virus isolated from a human case of ascending myelitis associated with visceral necrosis. *Br J Exp Pathol* 1934;15:248–268.52.

493. Sabin AB. Studies on the B virus. II. Properties of the virus and pathogenesis of the experimental disease in rabbits. *Br J Exp Pathol* 1934;15:268.

494. Roizman B, Carmichael LE, Deinhardt F, de The G, Nahmias AJ, Plowright W, Rapp F, Sheldrick P, Takahashi M, Wolf K. Herpesviridae: definition, provisional nomenclature and taxonomy. *Intervirology* 1981;16:201–217.

495. Hartley EG. "B" virus disease in monkey and man. *Br Vet J* 1966;122:46.

496. Hull RN. The simian herpesviruses. In: Kaplan AS, ed. *The herpesviruses.* New York: Academic Press, 1973;389–425.

497. Ludwig H, Pauli G, Norrild B, Vestergaard BF, Daniel MD. Immunological characterization of a common antigen present in herpes simplex virus, bovine mammilitis virus and herpesvirus simiae (B virus). In: de The, Henle W, Rapp F, eds. *Oncogenesis and herpesviruses III,* No. 24. Lyon, France: IARC Science Publishers, 1978;235.

498. Palmer AE. B virus, herpesvirus simiae: historical perspective. *J Med Primatol* 1987;16:99–130.

499. Kaplan JE. Guidelines for prevention of herpesvirus simiae (B virus) infection in monkey handlers. *Lab Anim Sci* 1987;37:709–712.

cance among renal transplant recipients. *Transportation* 1977;24:458–464.

500. Guidelines for prevention of herpesvirus simiae (B virus) infection in monkey handlers. *MMWR* 1987;36:3493–3495.
501. Morbidity and Mortality Weekly Report. B virus infection in humans—Pensacola, Florida. *JAMA* 1987;257.
502. Benson PM, Malane SL, Banks R, Hicks CB, Hilliard J. B Virus (herpesvirus simiae) and human infection. *Arch Dermatol* 1989;125:1247–1248.
503. Burnett FM, Lush D, Jackson AV. The propagation of herpes B and pseudorabies viruses on the chorioallantois. *Aust J Exp Biol Med Sci* 1939;17:35.
504. Wood W, Shimada FT. Isolation of strains of virus B from tissue cultures of cynomolgus and rhesus kidney. *Can J Public Health* 1954;45:509–518.
505. Reissig M, Melnick JL. The cellular changes produced in tissue cultures by herpes B virus correlated with concurrent multiplication of the virus. *J Exp Med* 1955;101:341.
506. Krech U, Lewis LJ. Propagation of B virus in tissue cultures. *Proc Soc Exp Biol Med* 1954;87:174–178.
507. Benda R, Cinatl J. Isolation of two plaque variants from the prototype strain of B virus (herpesvirus simiae). *Acta Virol* 1966;10:178.
508. Bhutala BA, Mathews J. Studies on herpesvirus simiae (B virus): intracellular development. *Cornell Vet* 1963;53:494.
509. Daniel MD, Garcia FG, Melendez LV, Hunt RD, O'Connor J, Silva D. Multiple herpesvirus simiae isolation from a rhesus monkey which died of cerebral infarction. *Lab Anim Sci* 1975;25:303–308.
510. Daniel MD, Melendez LV, Hunt RD, Trum BF. In: Fiennes RNTW, ed. *The herpesvirus group. Pathology of simian primates,* Part II. Basel: Karger, 1972;592–611.
511. Espana C. Herpesvirus simiae infection in *Macaca radiata. Am J Phys Anthropol* 1973;38:447–454.
512. Falke D. Isolation of two variants with different cytopathic properties from a strain of herpes B virus. *Virology* 1961;14:492.
513. Falke D, Richter JE. Mikrokinematographische Studien uber die Enstehung von Riesenzellen durch Herpes B virus in Zellkulturen. I. Mitt: Vorgange an den Zellgrenzen und Granulabewegungen. II. Mitt: Morphologisches Verhalten und Bewegunger der Keme. *Arch Gesamte Virusforsch* 1961;11:71, 86.
514. Hilliard JK, Eberle R, Lipper SL, Monoz RM, Weiss SA. Herpesvirus simiae (B virus): replication of the virus and identification of viral polypeptides in infected cells. *Arch Virol* 1987;93:185–198.
515. Pauli G, Ludwig H, Norrild B, Daniel MD, Darai G. Differentiation of herpesvirus simiae and herpes simplex virus. *Fifth international congress of virology, Strasbourg, France, 1981;*317.
516. Roizman B, Carmichael LE, Deinhardt F, de The G, Nahmias AJ, Plowright W, Rapp F, Sheldrick P, Takahashi M, Wolf K. Herpesviridae: definition, provisional nomenclature and taxonomy. *Intervirology* 1981;16:201–217.
517. Hopps HE, Bernheim BC, Nisalak A, Tijo JH, Smadel JE. *J Immunol* 1963;91:416.
518. Hull RN, Dwyer AC, Cherry WR, Tritch OJ. *Proc Soc Exp Biol Med* 1965;118:1054.
519. Hull RN. B virus vaccines. *Lab Anim Sci* 1971;21:1068–1071.
520. Orcutt RP, Pucak GH, Foster HL, Kilcourse JT, Ferrell T. Multiple testing for the detection of B virus antibody in specially handled rhesus monkeys after capture from virgin trapping grounds. *Lab Anim Sci* 1976;26:70–74.
521. Boulter EA. The isolation of monkey B virus (herpesvirus simiae) from the trigeminal ganglia of a healthy seropositive rhesus monkey. *J Biol Stand* 1975;3:279–280.
522. Boulter EA, Grant DP. Latent infection of monkeys with B virus and prophylactic studies in a rabbit model of this disease. *J Antimicrobiol Chemother* 1977;3:107.
523. Kalter SS, Weiss SA, Heberling RL, Guajardo JE, Smith GC III. The isolation of a herpesvirus from the trigeminal ganglia of normal baboons (*Papio cynocephalus*). *Lab Anim Sci* 1978;28:705–709.
524. Vizoso AD. Recovery of herpesvirus simiae (B virus) from both primary and latent infections in rhesus monkeys. *Br J Exp Pathol* 1975;56:485–488.
525. Breen GE, Lamb SG, Otaki AT. Monkey bite encephalomyelitis: report of a case with recovery. *Br Med J* 1958;2:22–23.
526. Bryan BL, Espana CD, Emmons RW, Vijayan N, Hoeprich PD. Recovery from encephalomyelitis caused by herpesvirus simiae: report of a case. *Arch Intern Med* 1975;135:868–870.
527. Centers for Disease Control. Herpes B encephalitis—California. *MMWR* 22(40):333–334.
528. Davidson WL, Hummeler K. B virus infection in man. *Ann NY Acad Sci* 1960;85:970–979.
529. Fierer J, Bazeley P, Braude AI. Herpes B virus encephalomyelitis presenting as ophthalmic zoster. *Ann Intern Med* 1973;79:225–228.21.
530. Hummeler K, Davidson WL, Henle W, LaBoccetta AC, Rush HG. Encephalomyelitis due to infection with herpesvirus simiae (herpes B virus): a report of two fatal, laboratory acquired cases. *N Engl J Med* 1959;261:64–68.
531. Love FM, Jungherr E. Occupational infection with virus B of monkeys. *JAMA* 1962;179:160–162.
532. Nagler FP, Klotz M. A fatal B virus infection in a person subject to recurrent herpes labialis. *Can Med Assoc J* 1958;79:743–745.
533. Sabin AB. Fatal B virus encephalomyelitis in a physician working with monkeys. *J Clin Invest* 1949;28:808.
534. Pierce EC, Pierce JD, Hull RN. B virus: its current significance, description and diagnosis of a fatal human infection. *Am J Hyg* 1958;68:242–250.
535. Vizoso AD. Heterogeneity in herpes simiae (B virus) and some antigenic relationship in the herpes group. *Br J Exp Pathol* 1974;55:471.
536. Benda R, Prochazka O, Cerva L, Robin F, Dubanska H, Hronovsky V. Demonstration of B virus (herpesvirus simiae) by the direct fluorescent antibody technique. *Acta Virol* 1966;10:149.
537. Hilliard JK, Kalter SS. Development of molecular probes for simian herpesvirus detection. *Dev Biol Stand* 1985;59:79–86.
538. Kalter SS. Virus studies on the normal baboon. In: Vagtborg H, ed. *The baboon in medical research.* Austin, TX: University of Texas Press, 1965;416–417.
539. Kalter SS, Hutt R. Serodiagnosis of herpesvirus infection in primates. *Dev Biol Stand* 1978;41:235–240.
540. Heberling RL, Kalter SS. A dot-immunoblotting assay on nitrocellulose with psoralen inactivated herpesvirus simiae (B virus). *Lab Anim Sci* 1987;37:304–308.
541. Hilliard JK, Munoz RM, Lipper SL, Eberle R. Rapid identification of herpesvirus simiae (B virus) DNA from clinical isolates in nonhuman primate colonies. *J Virol Methods* 1986;13:55–62.
542. Boulter EA, Kalter SS, Heberling RL, Gualardo JE, Lester TL. A comparison of neutralization tests for the detection of antibodies to herpesvirus simiae (monkey B virus). *Lab Anim Sci* 1982;32:150–152.
543. Kalter SS, Heberling RL. Comparative virology of primates. *Bacteriol Rev* 1971;35:310.
544. Van Hoosier GL, Melnick JL. Neutralizing antibodies in human sera to herpesvirus simiae. *Texas Rep Biol Med* 1961;19:376–380.
545. Gary WG, Palmer EL. Comparative complement fixation and serum neutralization antibody titers to herpes simplex virus type 1 and herpesvirus simiae in *Macaca mulatta* and humans. *J Clin Microbiol* 1977;5:465.
546. Katz D, Hilliard JK, Eberle R, Lipper SL. ELISA for detection of group-common and virus-specific antibodies in human and simian sera induced by herpes simplex and related simian viruses. *J Virol Methods* 1986;14:99–109.
547. Hull RN. The significance of simian viruses to the monkey colony and laboratory investigator. *Ann NY Acad Sci* 1969;162:472–482.
548. Kirschstein RL, Van Hoosier GL Jr. Virus B infection of the central nervous system of monkeys used for the poliomyelitis vaccine safety test. *Am J Pathol* 1961;38:199–124.
549. McCarthy K, Tosolini FA. Hazards from simian herpes viruses: reactivation of skin lesions with virus shedding. *Lancet* 1975;1:649–650.
550. Technical Committee of Poliomyelitis Vaccine and Subcommittee on the Safety Test. The monkey safety test for poliomyelitis vaccine. *Am J Hyg* 64:119–120.
551. Buthala DA. Arusiwa on herpesvirus simiae (B virus) inactivation and attempts at vaccine production. *J Infect Dis* 1962;111:95–100.

552. MacLeod RE, Shimada FT, Walcroft JM. Experimental immunization against B virus. *Ann NY Acad Sci* 1960;85:980–989.

553. Hull RN, Nash JC. Immunization against B virus infection. I. Preparation of an experimental vaccine. *Am J Hyg* 1960;71:15–28.

554. Hull RN, Peck FB Jr. Vaccination against herpesvirus infections. *PAHO Sci Pub* 1967;147:266–275.

555. Hull RN, Peck FB Jr, Ward TG, Nash JC. Immunization against B virus infection. II. Further laboratory and clinical studies with an experimental vaccine. *Am J Hyg* 1962;76:239–251.

556. Boulter EA, Zwartouw HT, Thornton B. Postexposure immuno-prophylaxis against B virus infection [Letter]. *Br Med J* 1982;284:746.

557. Buthala DA. Hyperimmunized horse anti-B virus globulin: preparation and effectiveness. *J Infect Dis* 1962;111:101–106.

558. Boulter EA, Thornton B, Bauer EJ, Bye A. Successful treatment of experimental B virus (herpesvirus simiae) infection with acyclovir. *Br Med J* 1980;280:681.

559. Smith KO, Galloway KS, Hodges SL, Ogilvie KK, Radatus BK, Kalter SS, Heberling RL. Sensitivity of equine herpesviruses 1 and 3 *in vitro* to a new nucleoside analogue, 9-{[(2-hydroxy-1-(hydroxymethyl)ethoxy] methyl} guanine. *Am J Vet Res* 1983;44:1032–1035.

Infections of the Central Nervous System,
edited by W. M. Scheld, R. J. Whitley, and
D. T. Durack, Raven Press, Ltd., New York © 1991.

CHAPTER 5

Arthropod-Borne Encephalitides

Richard J. Whitley

This chapter will focus upon those arthropod-borne viruses (arboviruses) which cause infections of the central nervous system (CNS). Arboviruses are important causes of human disease, especially encephalitis, worldwide. Well over 20 arboviruses are capable of producing encephalitis. The most common arbovirus causes of CNS disease are summarized in Table 1. Although viruses are grouped together, they actually constitute several families and genera. The families of viruses which are arthropod-borne include Togaviridae (alphaviruses and flaviviruses), Bunyaviridae, and Reoviridae. The total number of viruses grouped in each of these genera families is immense; certainly, not all of these viruses will cause infection of the CNS. In addition to causing encephalitic syndromes, members of these genuses can result in a variety of other clinical symptoms ranging from febrile illnesses to hemorrhagic fevers. Notably, arboviruses are also important pathogens in veterinary medicine. With regard to arbovirus causes of encephalitis, these pathogens are, for the most part, geographically and seasonally restricted. Fortunately, only a few arboviruses exist in any one region. Taxonomic difficulties are encountered within each of the families; nevertheless, representative viruses from each family cause CNS disease. It should be recognized that many others—including yellow fever virus, as a prototype example—can result in significant morbidity and mortality. Nevertheless, infections caused by these viruses tend not to directly infect the CNS; thus, the brain is not the principal organ of disease.

These agents have the capability of replicating in both vertebrate and invertebrate hosts. The pathogenesis of these agents is relatively similar from one offending pathogen to another; that is, arboviruses can be inoculated subcutaneously or intravenously from infected secretions of the insect vector (mosquito or tick). Following initial replication at either a skin or muscle site, primary viremia will ensue in many instances. Primary viremia is followed by seeding of the reticuloendothelial system or direct invasion of the CNS. A secondary viremia can follow reticuloendothelial replication which, as with primary or secondary viremia, can lead to endothelial or choroid epithelial cell involvement within the CNS. A common resulting pathologic lesion is perivascular cuffing. Spread within the CNS is usually cell-to-cell. Notably, another pathogenic route for viral access to the CNS follows olfactory bulb replication of the pathogen.

This chapter will review those arboviruses commonly associated with CNS infections. The nature of the infecting organism, unique characteristics of disease pathogenesis and epidemiology, and interventive approaches will be considered.

TOGAVIRUSES

Background

Togaviruses produce a broad spectrum of clinical illness ranging from totally asymptomatic infection to life-threatening disease, including encephalitis and hemorrhagic fevers. These latter diseases are, fortunately, rare. The family Togaviridae can be subdivided into four genera: (i) *Alphavirus,* (ii) *Flavivirus,* (iii) *Rubivirus,* and (iv) *Pestivirus.* Rubella, the only member of the *Rubivirus* genus, has previously been discussed in Chapter 9. The genus *Pestivirus* has no known members which are pathogenic for humans, at least as currently recognized. The two remaining members of the family Togaviridae —alphaviruses and flaviviruses—will be considered in some detail. Alphaviruses are restricted to the New World, whereas flaviviruses are present in both Old and New Worlds. It should be noted that flaviviruses will likely be removed from this family and classified sepa-

R. J. Whitley: Departments of Pediatrics, Microbiology, and Medicine, University of Alabama, Birmingham, Alabama 35294.

TABLE 1. *Arboviruses causing encephalitis* *

Virus	Vector	Geographic location
Togaviridae		
Alphavirus		
Eastern equine	Mosquitoes (*Culiseta, Aedes*)	Eastern and Gulf coasts of United States; Caribbean; and South America
Western equine	Mosquitoes (*Culiseta, Culex*)	Western United States and Canada
Venezuelan equine	Mosquitoes (*Aedes, Culex*, etc.)	South and Central America; Florida; and southwestern United States
Flavivirus		
West Nile complex		
St. Louis	Mosquitoes (*Culex*)	Widespread in United States
Japanese	Mosquitoes (*Culex*)	Japan, China, Southeast Asia, and India
Murray Valley	Mosquitoes (*Culex*)	Australia and New Guinea
West Nile	Mosquitoes (*Culex*)	Africa and Mideast
Ilheus	Mosquitoes (*Psorophora*)	South and Central America
Rocio	Mosquitoes (?)	Brazil
Tick-borne complex		
Far Eastern	Ticks (*Ixodes*)	Eastern USSR
Central European	Ticks (*Ixodes*)	Central Europe
Kyasanur Forest	Ticks (*Haemophysalis*)	India
Louping-ill	Ticks (*Ixodes*)	England, Scotland, and Northern Ireland
Powassan	Ticks (*Ixodes*)	Canada and northern United States
Negishi	Ticks (?)	Japan
Bunyaviridae		
Bunyavirus		
California	Mosquitoes (*Aedes*)	Western United States
La Crosse	Mosquitoes (*Aedes*)	Central and eastern United States
Jamestown Canyon	Mosquitoes (*Culiseta*)	United States and Alaska
Snowshoe hare	Mosquitoes (*Culiseta*)	Canada, Alaska, and northern United States
Tahyna	Mosquitoes (*Aedes, Culiseta*)	Czechoslovakia, Yugoslavia, Italy, and southern France
Inkoo	Mosquitoes (?)	Finland
Phlebovirus		
Rift Valley	Mosquitoes (*Culex, Aedes*)	East Africa
Reoviridae		
Orbivirus		
Colorado tick fever	Ticks (*Dermacentor*)	Rocky Mountains of United States

* From Griffin DE. Viral Infections of the Central Nervous System. In: Galasso GJ, Whitley RJ, Merican TC, eds. Antiviral Agents and Viral Diseases of Man, 3rd edition, 1991.

rately, since their replication appears quite different. Alphaviruses and flaviviruses can be distinguished according to biochemical, morphological, antigenic, and biophysical properties.

Alphaviruses

Infectious Agents

The alphaviruses are small, enveloped, positive-strand RNA viruses with a particle size ranging from 50 nm to 65 nm (1,2). The RNA genome of alphaviruses is a continuous single strand with an approximate sedimentation coefficient of 42–49 S (2). Naked genomic RNA is infectious. The genome organization and replication strategy for the alphaviruses appear to be consistent features characteristic of the genus (1,2). Sequence homology of amino acid residues ranges between 30% and 90%, with greater conservation in the nonstructural proteins than in the structural ones (3). Overall, the viral particles contain nucleic acid which ranges in size from 28 nm to 49 nm.

The envelope of alphaviruses is derived from the host cell. "Surface spikes" are symmetrically arranged on the envelope and have been identified along with structural glycoproteins designated as E_1, E_2, E_3, and C. The envelope proteins are designated 1, 2, and 3 in the order of formation. The E_1 glycoprotein appears to be responsible for hemagglutinating properties of the virus, as was first described for Sindbis virus (4–6). The alphavirus E_2 glycoprotein appears to induce neutralizing antibodies, at least in the Sindbis virus system (6).

Because all alphaviruses are related, there is significant cross-reactivity between agents, utilizing classic serologic tests. Nevertheless, hemagglutination inhibition (HI) is one technique that can be used to distinguish between the six antigenic complexes or serotypes of the *Alphavirus* genus. Further identification of members within the genus requires either neutralization tests or variations in the HI test (2).

Alphaviruses replicate and produce extensive cytopathic effect in most vertebrate cell culture lines. These viruses readily form plaques on either primary or continuous cell cultures. Variation in plaque morphology can easily be identified according to the specific member of the alphavirus family. Differences in plaque size have allowed for distinctions in variants for these viruses. Alphaviruses will also replicate in invertebrate cells; however, they vary in ability to result in cytopathic effect.

Alphaviruses demonstrate a wide range of hosts which are susceptible to infection, varying from animal to arthropod species. Birds, rodents, and primates are considered the primary vertebrate species found harboring alphaviruses. No animal models exist for studying disease pathogenesis. However, the natural hosts for infection in which disease occurs have provided the basis for understanding the disease pathogenesis. Specifically, horses develop a fatal CNS infection after western equine encephalitis (WEE), eastern equine encephalitis (EEE), and Venezuelan equine encephalitis (VEE) infections. Equally relevant, newborn mice are susceptible to alphavirus infection but may require serial passage of the putative infected material from brain to brain before developing evidence of disease. As a consequence, newborn mice have been utilized for diagnostic purposes (being a marker indicative of alphavirus replication) as well as for the study of pathogenesis. Since alphaviruses are only transmitted to humans by mosquitoes, significant effort has been devoted to identifying potential disease in this arthropod. At present, it appears as though the insect vector is free of disease manifestations.

Pathology and Pathogenesis

WEE, EEE, and VEE are the three viruses which serve as prototypes for their ability to invade and replicate in the human CNS. As noted, each of these viruses can cause epidemics in equines. Notably, there are differences in the invasiveness and long-term outcome resulting from these infections. The most severe disease caused by alphaviruses results from EEE infection which, when it invades the CNS, either kills or permanently maims the host. In contrast, WEE rarely causes encephalitis except in the very young child (less than 1 year of age). The third member of the group, VEE, is more likely to cause an extreme febrile illness, with encephalitis as a coexistent complication of infection.

The characteristic pathologic findings of alphavirus infections of the CNS are relatively similar for each of these three pathogens. In general, gross examination of the brain reveals multiple punctate hemorrhages. The basal ganglia and brainstem are particularly involved with infections such as WEE (7–10). With EEE, the areas most likely involved include the globus pallidus, thalamus, pons, and cerebral cortex (9,11,12). In addition, midbrain and basal ganglia as well as cerebellar involve-

ment can be identified (13). Characteristic findings of VEE in the CNS are less amenable to definition.

Microscopic examination of brain tissue obtained following WEE, EEE, or VEE invariably reveals perivascular cuffing with lymphocytic infiltrates in the surrounding capillary endothelial cells. Thromboses of cerebral vessels are also characteristic, following any of these three infections. In addition, cellular edema, neuronal necrosis, and neuronophagia are all associated with diseases caused by these viruses.

All alphaviruses are characteristically spread by a mosquito vector. For EEE, relatively little is known about its pathogenesis in humans. It is presumed that when an adequate natural reservoir of infected birds exist and are fed upon by *Aedes* species of mosquitoes, these insects can then transmit infection to humans. In one outbreak in New Jersey the vector was identified as *Aedes solicitans,* whereas for a Michigan outbreak the vector was *Coquillettidia perturbans* (14). Presumably, after the bite of an infected insect accompanied by inoculation of saliva, viremia will occur as associated with a febrile prodrome. It is presumed that EEE has the capability of invading the CNS in approximately one in 23 cases (15). In contrast, a better understanding of the pathogenesis of WEE exists. *Culex tarsalis* and *Culiseta melanura* mosquitoes are the vector for transmission of infection between wild birds and humans (16). Humans are an incidental host for WEE, a virus which is significantly less neuroinvasive and neurovirulent than EEE. Transmission of VEE can occur by the bite of *Culex, Aedes,* or *Psorophora* species of mosquitoes. Notably, equine epizootics usually precede evidence of human illness. It should be noted that laboratory acquisition of VEE has been documented as well (17).

Eastern Equine Encephalitis

History

Eastern equine encephalitis (EEE) was first isolated in 1933 by TenBroeck and Merrill (18,19). Isolation was accomplished from the postmortem examination of brain tissue from a horse who died during an epizootic of equine encephalitis. Subsequently, in 1938, virus was isolated from a human who died during an epidemic of encephalitis (20). Over the subsequent years, EEE has been defined as a cause of severe and oftentimes fatal encephalitis occurring along the Atlantic and Gulf coasts with a few cases reported as far inland as Ontario, Michigan, and the Dakotas (2,10).

Epidemiology

Epizootics and epidemics of EEE are relatively uncommon and, furthermore, are restricted to geographically focal areas of endemicity. The *Culiseta melanura* mosquitos maintain EEE by a transmission cycle involving passerine birds which habitat swampy and forested areas. These birds have been implicated as carriers of the infection on their migrational routes (21). Because *Culiseta melanura* mosquitos do not feed on humans, it is necessary for EEE to become established in alternative species of mosquitos, such as the *Aedes,* before either human or equine infection can take place (22–26). Virus can be isolated from endemic foci. As a consequence, the phenomenon of overwintering has attracted a great deal of attention from a variety of investigators. *Culiseta melanura* overwinters as a larva in organic floating rootmat systems in the eastern United States, as summarized in refs. 2 and 27. Intensive investigations have failed to clearly define the overwintering mechanism for EEE. Certainly, information regarding this mechanism could be of benefit in preventing further outbreaks. Only a few cases occur yearly in the United States. Figure 1 summarizes the number of reported cases of EEE from 1975 to 1990.

Clinical Findings

With outbreaks of EEE, attack rates are highest in young children and the elderly. Fatality rates are also the highest in these two age groups. Illness usually begins with generalized systemic findings of malaise, fever, and vomiting. With CNS involvement, slightly altered levels of consciousness and disorientation rapidly ensue. These findings are followed quickly by the appearance of such neurologic signs as nuchal rigidity and progressive deterioration in consciousness, even to the point of coma by day 2 in the clinical illness. Mortality can occur in 50–75% of patients with CNS disease, especially if coma is present. Furthermore, survivors generally have significant neurologic sequelae, estimated to occur in 80% (28–34). Neurologic sequelae encountered in survivors include intellectual impairment, seizures, spastic paralysis, or significant personality changes. During the course of acute illness, various forms of paralysis are common.

Diagnosis

The epidemiologic association of outbreaks of EEE in equine populations with human disease is helpful in alerting the physician to the diagnosis of this infection. Laboratory findings associated with a diagnosis of EEE include initial leukopenia followed by leukocytosis. Examination of the cerebrospinal fluid (CSF) is characteristic of other findings of viral infections of the CNS, including lymphocytosis (50–100 cells per cubic millimeter) and the elevated levels of CSF protein (100–150 mg/dl) (31).

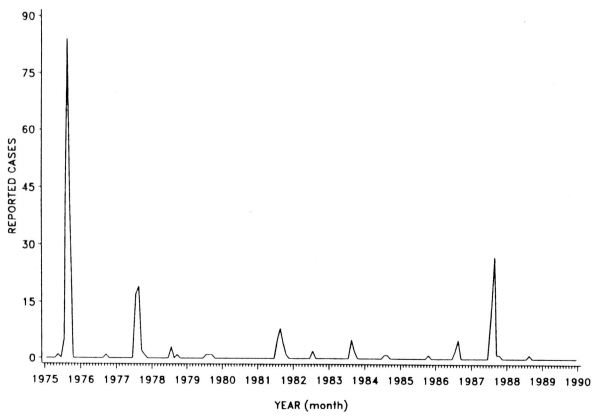

FIG. 1. Arboviral infections of the CNS. Cases due to EEE virus, by month, United States, 1975–1990. Morbid Mort Wkly Rep 1989;38:19.

Although virus can be isolated from the serum during the acute prodrome, most cases are diagnosed using routine serologic assays (35,36). Evaluation of acute and convalescent sera (obtained 2–5 weeks after the acute illness) by complement fixation (CF), HI, or neutralization assays can be useful in making a specific diagnosis. Virus can be isolated from the brain at postmortem examination.

Prevention and Treatment

There is no specific treatment other than supportive care for patients with EEE disease. While antivirals exist for the management of certain virologic infections of the CNS, there are none available for any of the diseases discussed in this chapter.

As has been noted, EEE is a relatively uncommon disease, accounting for no more than approximately five cases per year nationwide. Because of the high case fatality rate associated with this illness (50–75%), it remains a problem of public health importance (37–39). Monitoring of enzootic foci of EEE, as can be done for the breeding areas of *Culiseta melanura,* will indicate levels of activity which are higher than those normally found. Such surveillance methods may be of use in decreasing the frequency of this disease if it provides the basis for insecticide deployment.

Ultimately, as with other arboviral infections, the key to prevention of infection is its avoidance—namely, avoiding contact with mosquitoes. Appropriate avoidance of swampy areas during hot, damp months in areas of endemicity will help prevent infection.

A formalin-inactivated vaccine is available for high-risk laboratory workers (40). It should be noted that this vaccine is not routinely available for individuals at large.

Western Equine Encephalitis

History

Western equine encephalitis (WEE) was first isolated from the brain of horses during an epizootic of unknown etiology in 1930 in the San Joaquin Valley of California (41). The isolation of WEE from the brains of horses marked the first time an arbovirus was isolated in the territorial United States. Subsequently, in 1938, WEE was obtained from a child who succumbed to encephalitis (42). Although WEE causes significant mortality in horses, it appears to be somewhat less neurovirulent for humans.

Epidemiology

Disease caused by WEE occurs mainly in the western and midwestern United States. However, an antigeni-

cally related virus known as "Highlands J" (HJ) has resulted in encephalitic disease east of the Mississippi River. Other serologically related but distinct viruses include Y-62-63, Fort Morgan, Sinbis, and Avrorra viruses. In the western United States, the *Culex tarsalis* mosquito is the principal vector, with the infection being amplified in the bird population. Epidemic and epizootic activity occurs mainly during the summer months, particularly June and July, but will vary according to climate. Excellent reviews have summarized WEE activity during epidemic periods on the United States western plains and Canada (2). These studies indicate that attack rates during epidemicity ranged from 23 to 172 individuals per 100,000 cases. The case fatality rate was approximately 10% (43).

The epidemiology of the infection has changed because of the introduction of vaccines to prevent WEE in equine populations, along with decreasing populations of wild horses in the western United States. As recently as 1987, of the 148 cases of arboviral disease reported to the Centers for Disease Control, 41 cases were attributed to WEE (44). The cases of WEE reported to the Centers for Disease Control from 1975 up to 1990 are shown in Fig. 2. It should be remembered that WEE has been isolated from *Culiseta melanura* mosquitoes in eastern areas of the United States.

Clinical Findings

Clinical findings of WEE are virtually indistinguishable from those of EEE. Specifically, there are no clinically distinguishing characteristics for WEE versus EEE infection. The incubation period for WEE is 5–10 days. Notably, neurologic findings alternate between flaccid paralysis and spasticity. Disease begins with malaise, fever, and headache, often accompanied by nausea, vomiting, photophobia, and altered levels of consciousness (12,45–47). Infants and children are at greatest risk for severe infection, including fatal encephalitis and significant neurologic impairment in those who survive (48–50). In young children, most will have a seizure disorder as manifest by either focal or generalized involvement (51). Weakness of the extremities and altered reflexes (either hyporeflexia or hyperreflexia) are characteristic clinical findings. The male-to-female ratio is 1:1 in younger patients, but a male predominance occurs in older individuals.

The overall case fatality rate is approximately 10% (44). Severe disease, especially fatal encephalitis and significant neurologic impairment in survivors, is more likely in infants and young children (48–50). Distinctions between the case infection ratio for children and adults have been summarized (43). The case infection ratios for adults versus children varied from one in nearly 1200 to one in 60, respectively, for adults and

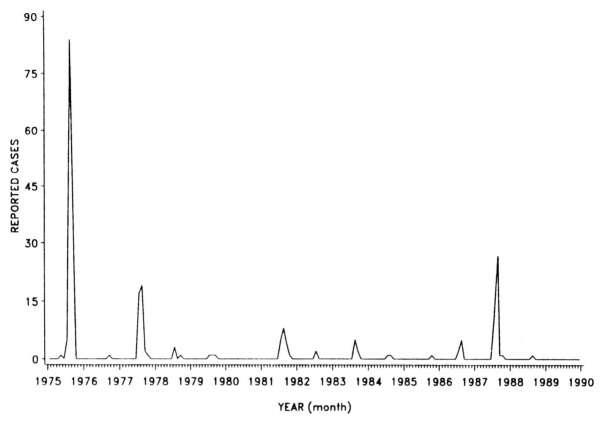

FIG. 2. Arboviral infections of the CNS. Cases due to WEE virus, by month, United States, 1975–1990. Morbid Mort Wkly Rep 1989;38:19.

children and approaches 1:1 in infants (43). *In utero* infection can occur with WEE (52,53).

Diagnosis

WEE should be suspected in an endemic area during warm, damp periods in patients with acute-onset febrile disease and CNS signs of infection. Diagnosis is usually confirmed by serologic evaluation, using HI or CF antibody assays. Early in the disease course, virus can be isolated from the CSF. In addition, WEE can be isolated from brain tissue obtained at postmortem examination.

CSF examination usually reveals pleocytosis and proteinosis with generally less than 500 cells. These findings are no different from those of other CSF formulas following viral encephalitis of arboviral etiology.

Prevention and Treatment

As with other arbovirus infections, there is no specific treatment for WEE. A major preventive effort is mosquito control, as has been developed in California (54). The success of mosquito control programs is dependent upon environmental conditions. In addition, an inactivated vaccine is also available for high-risk personnel. Inactivated vaccines can be utilized to protect equines (55).

Venezuelan Equine Encephalitis

History

Venezuelan equine encephalitis (VEE) is principally an epizootic disease of horses of South America. The virus was first isolated from the brains of dead horses in 1938 (56) and, subsequently, from humans in Colombia in 1952 (57). Currently, VEE is a prototype for a complex of related alphaviruses which includes six subtypes. These are identified as VEE, Everglades, Mucambo, Pixuna, Cabassou, and a presently unnamed subtype consisting of the representative strain AG80-663 (2). Strains of VEE capable of infecting humans and horses are amplified principally in equines. Equine disease precedes human disease. In nature, birds are not an important reservoir for VEE; the reservoir in nature remains unknown (10). Studies of disease in equines indicate a difference in the natural history associated with epizootic and enzootic viruses. These findings are characteristic in other species as well (58–60).

Enzootic strains of VEE are less pathogenic, and they are maintained in an apparent mosquito–rodent–mosquito life cycle. Mosquitoes involved in the transmission of VEE are the *Culex* species and the *Aedes aegypti*. Horses can be an amplifying host for enzootic VEE, being infected by *Culex* mosquitoes of the *Melanoconian* subgenus (61–65). As noted, rodents serve the role as being the major vertebrate counterpart for amplification of VEE infection (66). Humans living in damp, swampy forests have a high prevalence to antibodies to VEE, including soldiers stationed in such areas (67,68).

Epizootic strains of VEE are isolated mainly from the equine population, which obviously plays the major role in viral amplification (63,65,69). Outbreaks of VEE, as a consequence of epizootic strains, occur in the northern portions of South America (Venezuela, Colombia, Ecquador), as well as Peru, at regular intervals (2). In addition, cases of VEE have been identified in Central America and the southern United States (48). In humans, clinical attack rates following epizootic acquisition of VEE strains range from 10% to 60% (70–75). In South America, the attack rate in one Venezuelan study was reported to be approximately 4%, with an overall mortality rate of 0.6% (71,76).

One component of the epidemiology of VEE is aerosolized transmission. Laboratory outbreaks have been identified by this route either through handling of the virus or through laboratory accidents (17,77,78).

Clinical Findings

Most individuals experiencing VEE infection have a nonspecific febrile illness characterized by influenza-like symptoms. Regardless of the route (mosquito versus aerosol) of infection, clinical findings are indistinguishable. The average incubation period is approximately 4–6 days. Clinical illness is characterized by malaise, myalgia, anorexia, and headache, in addition to 100–105°F fever and prostration. Symptoms persist for 2–5 days, with residual malaise of clinical significance for an additional 2 weeks (2,74). Fortunately, infection is rarely associated with encephalitis. Epidemiologic investigations indicate that the probability of encephalitis as a consequence of VEE is higher in children than in adults, 4% versus 0.5% (2). The clinical findings of encephalitic involvement are no different from that associated with WEE or EEE. Specifically, altered levels of consciousness, nuchal rigidity, photophobia, and seizures are characteristic findings. More severe disease, including involvement of the reticuloendothelial system, has been reported in children (48,49,79,80).

Diagnosis

Diagnosis of infection should be suspect in the febrile individuals with flu-like symptoms who live in enzootic areas or where epizootic disease has occurred regularly. Prior evidence of VEE infection in equine populations, preceding human disease by 1–2 weeks, should increase the level of awareness for VEE. Clinical laboratory findings suggestive of VEE include altered liver function studies and a typical CSF formula of pleocytosis and proteinosis, as occurs with WEE or EEE.

Specific diagnosis of VEE is accomplished either by viral isolation or by serologic testing. Virus can be isolated from nasopharyngeal swabs early in the course of illness in some patients, or from brain tissue should death ensue. Cytopathic effect caused by replicating virus is demonstrable in a cell culture system. Evaluation of biologic specimens in suckling mice can lead to a definitive diagnosis (17,71,74,81). Acute and convalescent serologic specimens will be helpful in establishing a diagnosis as well. The late appearance of CF antibodies may be helpful for documentation of seroconversion.

Prevention and Treatment

The treatment of VEE rests on supportive care. The judicious use of antipyretics, bedrest, and supportive management is indicated to manage specific clinical findings.

Enzootic VEE can be a medical problem for humans who reside in or visit warm, moist areas where infection occurs and is transmitted. Prevention of bites by the *Culex* species of mosquitoes is indicated. On the other hand, epizootic VEE can be controlled by equine vaccination. In so doing, the amplification of VEE in equines can be prevented (82,83). A live, attenuated vaccine has been developed for use in humans and is designated TC83. It is utilized in individuals at high risk for VEE infection, especially laboratory workers (84).

Flaviviruses

Background

The genus *Flavivirus* consists of at least 66 viruses, and approximately half of these have been associated with significant human disease. The prototype flavivirus is Yellow fever virus, an agent known to be associated with a hemorrhagic fever but not directly involved in pathogenesis of CNS syndromes. During the 20th century, this family of viruses grew to include Japanese encephalitis (JE), St. Louis encephalitis (SLE), Murray Valley encephalitis (MVE), louping ill, and tick-borne encephalitis (TBE). As with members of the *Alphavirus* genus, these agents have unique properties; these include neurotropism, neurovirulence, and arthropod-borne transmission. Casals and Brown (85) were able to distinguish between flaviviruses and alphaviruses and identified them as group B and group A arboviruses, respectively. Further distinctions between flaviviruses and alphaviruses have been accomplished according to serologic response.

Infectious Agents

Flaviviruses contain single-strand RNA with a molecular weight ranging between 3.78 and 4.2×10^6. Viral particles consist of a ribonucleoprotein core surrounded by a lipoprotein envelope. Protruding from envelope, one can demonstrate a glycoprotein (E: molecular weight 50 kD) (86,87). In addition, there are two other structural proteins of flavivirions: a nucleocapsid or core protein (C: molecular weight 14 kD) and a nonglycosylated membrane protein (M: molecular weight 7 kD). The E protein of the envelope contains important antigenic determinants for hemagglutination and neutralization. The envelope of flavivirons is sensitive to lipases, chloroform, and acetone. It appears as though E-protein determinants confer type specificity unique for each virus, as do group-reactive determinants which all flaviviruses have in common (10). Utilizing neutralization and hemagglutination assays, the flaviviruses can be divided into eight subgroups, accounting for 49 members of the entire family (88).

Pathology and Pathogenesis

As with alphaviruses, flaviviruses can be transmitted by mosquito vectors; however, in addition, TBE is a flavivirus which was a tick vector. In order to understand the pathogenesis of encephalitic manifestations of flavivirus infection, the mouse model has been employed. Three alternate patterns of CNS disease have been noted (89,90): (i) rapid, progressive, fatal encephalitis, (ii) subclinical encephalitis, or (iii) inapparent infection. Host susceptibility is modified by both virus and host factors (e.g., age of the host), as reviewed recently (91).

Following the bite of an infected arthropod, local replication of the virus occurs at the site of inoculation. Local replication of virus is followed by lymphatic and bloodstream spread (92). Replication at other sites beyond the primary site of inoculation can develop and result in a secondary viremia. This secondary viremia can lead to CNS involvement. In most patients, primarily viremia is terminated primarily by a macrophage response and, subsequently, by the development of antibodies. As with alphaviruses, flaviviruses (most probably) infect endothelial cells of capillaries of the brain; however, this route of transmission has not been totally clarified. In addition, the olfactory tract may be an alternative route of spread of virus to the CNS (93), providing for a neuronal route of access to the brain (94). Flavivirus transmission can occur either by mosquitoes or by ticks. In the early 1940s, *Culex tarsalis* and *Culex pipiens* mosquitoes in California were found to transmit SLE following the bite of infected mosquitoes (16). In addition, subsequent studies identified *Culex quinquefasciatus* as a vector for transmission (95). Others identified *Culex tritaeniorhyancus* as the vector for JE (91). These studies were followed by the identification of both birds and pigs as the principal host upon which *Culex tritaeniorhyancus* fed, subsequently leading to transmission to humans (96,97). More recently, MVE has been reported to be

transmitted by *Culex annulinrostris,* being isolated from the mosquito in 1960 (98).

Vectors for TBE include, mainly, *Ixodes persulcatus* and *Ixodes ricinus.*

Pathologic Findings

Pathologic findings of human and animal disease are relatively consistent between members of the genus *Flavivirus.* The extent of CNS involvement varies from one agent to another. With JE, gross examination of the brain reveals edema, vascular congestion, and focal hemorrhages. This is in direct contrast to the SLE victim, where gross examination of the brain might only indicate apparent inflammation of the leptomeninges and parenchymal congestion.

Microscopic examination of brain tissue shows lymphocytic infiltration of both the meninges and the parenchyma, along with gliosis and microglial involvement of the parenchyma. The thalamus, substantia nigra of the midbrain, and thalamic nuclei appear to be the areas that are most involved with SLE (99,100). With JE, the histopathologic findings tend to be more extensive, with neuronal necrosis and neuronophagia involving the entire cerebral cortex, cerebellum, and spinal cord.

St. Louis Encephalitis

History

St. Louis encephalitis (SLE) was first identified as a cause of human illness after an outbreak in Paris, Illinois in 1932 and after the subsequent isolation of SLE from human brain tissue in rhesus monkeys (101). It is now recognized that SLE occurs both in endemic and epidemic form throughout the Americas, being one of the most important and common epidemic arbovirus infections in the United States. Numerous outbreaks in the United States have been reported since the early 1930s, with increased activity occurring in Texas, the Ohio–Mississippi Valley, and Florida. The history of SLE has been reviewed in detail (102). Furthermore, the current status of our knowledge of SLE, including recent advances in research on the ecology of the infectious agent, has also been reviewed (91,103).

More than 20 years after the initial isolation of the organism in brain tissue, the mosquito vectors *Culex tarsalis* and *Culex pipiens* were identified as transmitters of infection (16).

Epidemiology

Excellent and detailed reviews of the epidemiology of SLE have appeared in the literature (91,103,104). Differences in the epidemiology of SLE which distinguish disease in the western from that in the eastern and central United States have been documented. Well over 50,000 cases of SLE have been reported to the Centers for Disease Control since surveillance began in the mid-1950s. Figure 3 summarizes the reporting of SLE from 1975 up to 1990 but does not include the recent Florida and Texas outbreaks. Epidemic outbreaks appear to occur at approximately 10-year intervals, with *Culex pipiens* being the responsible mosquito (10). Outbreaks of SLE tend to be focal in nature, as illustrated by the recent occurrence of disease in southern Florida and Texas (105). Attack rates vary from approximately one to 800 cases per 100,000 individuals. Disease occurs in late summer and early fall.

Human cases of SLE have been reported in all contiguous states of the continental United States, with the exception of a series of northeastern states (Maine, Massachusetts, New Hampshire, and Rhode Island) and one Middle Atlantic state (South Carolina). In addition, disease has been reported in both Central and South America. The states most frequently involved are Florida, Texas, Mississippi, Indiana, Illinois, Tennessee, Kentucky, Alabama, and Indiana.

Disease in the central United States is generally transmitted by *Culex pipiens* and *Culex quinquefasciatus,* which tend to breed in stagnant and polluted waters. In Florida the tropical mosquito, *Culex nigripalpus,* appears to be the principal vector, whereas in the western

United States the principal vector is *Culex tarsalis,* which tends to breed in irrigated fields.

Serologic surveys demonstrate an incidence of SLE as high as 6% during epidemic periods (106). Annual incidence rates for SLE infection have been calculated at approximately 3% (107). Disease attributed to SLE appears more common in elderly individuals, particularly in studies performed in the central and eastern United States. In the elderly population the case fatality rate appears higher as well (108,109).

Clinical Findings

Three syndromes have been attributed to SLE: (i) an afebrile headache, (ii) aseptic meningitis, and (iii) encephalitis (110). Following a 3- to 4-day incubation period the onset of clinical disease is characterized by generalized illness which includes malaise, fever, myalgia, headache, nausea, and/or vomiting. These symptoms may resolve spontaneously over a period of 1–4 days or may progress to findings indicative of neurologic disease. Evidence of neurologic disease includes meningeal irritation and signs of acute encephalitis. Clinical findings of neurologic involvement attributable to SLE are indistinguishable from other arbovirus infections of the CNS. Altered levels of consciousness, abnormal reflexes, jitteriness and tremors, disorientation, and brainstem and

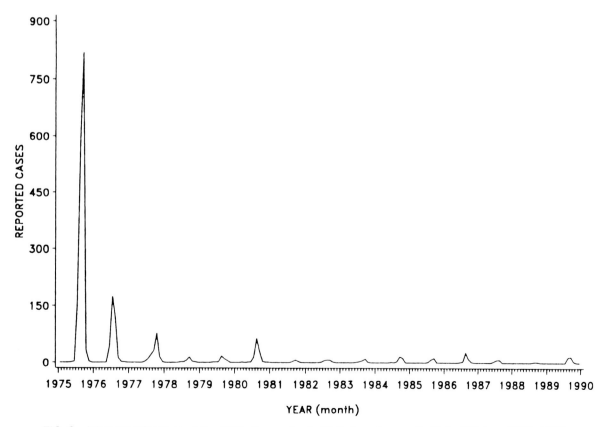

FIG. 3. Arboviral infections of the CNS. Cases due to SLE virus, by month, United States, 1975–1990. Morbid Mort Wkly Rep 1989;38:18.

cerebellar dysfunction, including ataxia and nystagmus, have all been reported as a consequence of SLE infection of the CNS. Brinker and co-workers (111,112) have identified the most common findings of patients of SLE. These include headache and nuchal rigidity in 70–80% of individuals, pathologic reflexes in 50%, cranial-nerve abnormalities in 20–30%, and coma in 11–20%. Approximately 10% of patients will have convulsions, nystagmus, paresis, and/or ataxia. It should be noted that the development of convulsions is a poor prognostic sign.

For patients who succumb, approximately 50% die within the first week after the onset of disease and nearly 80% of deaths will occur within 2 weeks of disease onset. As noted previously, mortality is higher in older individuals than in young adults (22% versus 2%) (91).

Long-term follow-up of patients who suffer from SLE indicates that approximately one-third will require a prolonged period of recovery. Findings that have been reported in the majority of surviving individuals include irritability, memory loss, and persistent headache. Nearly 25% of patients will have overt neurologic sequelae such as speech and gait disturbances as well as sensory and motor impairment (113).

Diagnosis

The diagnosis of SLE should be suspected in patients who suffer an acute-onset febrile illness with neurologic signs during late summer and early fall and who reside in an endemic area. Examination of the CSF would indicate a pleocytosis in a moderate range of 5–100 cells per cubic millimeter—with a predominance of polymorphonuclear leukocytes early in disease, followed by a lymphocytic predominance. A moderate elevation in CSF protein can be anticipated, and the CSF glucose is essentially normal.

Confirmation of SLE requires utilization of appropriate serologic tests. It should be noted that the isolation of SLE from biologic specimens (blood, urine, saliva, etc.) has been unrewarding. Nevertheless, virus can be isolated from postmortem brain tissue, as well as from other sites (114–116). More usually, the evaluation of acute and convalescent sera by both HI (group-reactive antibodies for screening) and CF are useful in the diagnosis of SLE. Unfortunately, a significant percentage of patients with SLE will fail to develop CF antibodies (117). More recently, an IgM-capture enzyme-linked immunosorbent assay (ELISA) antibody has been utilized with success for diagnostic purposes (118).

Prevention and Treatment

No treatment exists for SLE. Supportive care is essential in the management of patients infected with this virus, as with other patients suffering severe neurologic viral infections. No specific vaccine exists for the prevention of SLE. The major method for prevention is the education of individuals residing in epidemic areas during periods of disease activity. In addition, vector control following surveillance by local health authorities to detect increased levels of virus activity has proven useful.

The Centers for Disease Control has recognized that SLE is the leading cause of epidemic viral encephalitis in the United States (104,119,120). In 1975 the United States experienced the most recent large outbreak which occurred in areas along the Gulf Coast, the Mississippi Valley, and the Ohio Valley. Nearly 3000 cases were reported in this outbreak. This outbreak contributed to surveillance programs in order to detect epidemic activity of SLE. Nevertheless, rigorous surveillance has been difficult because of unrewarding cost–benefit analyses. Regardless, increasing seroprevalence in wild or sentinel avians has helped to alert communities to the potential for human infection (103,121). An example of this principle was the detection of increased sentinel flock seroconversions in Florida occurring between 1982 and 1986. In 1990 the seroconversion rates were even higher than those previously reported, indicating the possibility of viral transmission to humans during the fall months (103). In fact, these seroconversion rates predicted the recent outbreak of infection which occurred in Florida during the fall of 1990.

Japanese Encephalitis

History

Japanese encephalitis (JE) is a major medical problem in China, Southeast Asia, and India; as many as 20,000 cases per year have been reported in these areas (91,122,123). By far, JE is the most important of the arboviruses from the perspective of morbidity and mortality (123). A disease which appeared to be similar to JE, as we know it today, was recognized in horses and humans in the late 19th century, but it was not until 1935 that the virus was first isolated (10). Fortunately, with the identification of the vector and the development of a vaccine, the incidence of disease in endemic areas, where vector control and vaccination have been undertaken, has fallen significantly.

Epidemiology

The occurrence of JE infection can either be (a) endemic, as occurs in subtropical and tropical regions, which remain warm throughout the year, or (b) epidemic, as occurs in more temperate climates, where the vector population increases at regular seasonal intervals. Evidence of JE virus can be demonstrated in Japan, China, Thailand, Korea, Taiwan, the Philippines, India, and the Far Eastern Soviet Union. Because the incidence of JE infection has decreased in Japan (in large part because of vaccination and vector control), the incidence of disease in China and Southeast Asia (particularly Thailand) has remained significant over recent years. Major outbreaks continue to be reported in Thailand and China. Even in recent times, over 10,000 cases per year continue to occur. With recent outbreaks in Thailand, the attack rate has varied between 10 and 20 cases per 100,000 population (124). As with other arbovirus infections, the ratio of inapparent to apparent infection is estimated to range between 25 and 500 infections per overt case of encephalitis (125–127). On average, the ratio of inapparent to apparent infection is 200:1 to 300:1 (126). Nevertheless, when encephalitis occurs, the consequences are devastating. The associated mortality rate ranges between 20% and 50%, and significant neurologic sequelae occur in survivors. More severe disease, as evidenced by both mortality and morbidity, occurs in children less than 10 and adults over 65 years of age (128,129).

It should be remembered that JE is amplified in both bird and pig populations (97). Human infection follows several weeks after documentation of infection in amplifying hosts. As noted previously, the main epidemic vectors are *Culex* species of mosquitoes; among these, *Culex tritaeniorhynchus* is the most important. In endemic areas, sporadic cases of JE infection occur throughout the year. Infection is directly related to vector density, which is influenced by both temperature and amount of rainfall (130).

Clinical Findings

The incubation period for JE is estimated to be between 6 and 16 days, with illness beginning in a fashion very similar to that of SLE—that is, the acute onset of a nonspecific febrile illness (131). As with SLE, JE can manifest as a febrile headache syndrome, aseptic meningitis, or encephalitis. Following a 2- to 4-day nonspecific illness, the infected individual can develop progressive headache, elevated fever, rigors, and altered levels of consciousness. Some patients, particularly younger individuals, report gastrointestinal symptoms, including anorexia, nausea, vomiting, and diffuse abdominal pain. For those patients who develop encephalitis, a rapid onset and progressive downhill course can ensue. CNS findings include those previously identified for SLE and also include increased excitability, mask-like faces, paralyses of upper extremities, and, in some cases, a bulboparetic syndrome (91). Some patients will have evidence of psychosis (132). Seizures are more common in children than in adults (10,91).

After 2–4 days of illness, gradual resolution of clinical symptoms occurs; otherwise, patients proceed rapidly to death. Convalescence can be prolonged and is characterized by persistent weakness, lack of coordination, and emotional lability (131,133,134). It has been suggested that neuropsychiatric sequelae occur in a majority of survivors, especially children. Long-term prognosis for survivors of JE disease is poor (91).

Parenthetically, outcome appears to be related to the rapidity of appearance of antibodies directed against JE in the CSF (135). The rapid appearance of antibody apparently lessens the severity of clinical disease (136).

Diagnosis

The diagnosis of JE, as with other arbovirus infections, is principally by demonstrating evidence of fourfold increases in antibody concentrations in the blood. The most commonly employed assays are HI, CF, neutralization, and, more recently, the IgM-capture ELISA. This latter assay has been utilized to detect CSF antibodies in particular (135–138).

Retrieval of virus from peripheral sites during acute JE illness in uncommon. Nevertheless, virus can be retrieved from brain tissue or can be demonstrated by fluorescent antibody staining of autopsy specimens (139).

Prevention and Treatment

No specific antiviral drug exists for the treatment of JE. Strict attention to meticulous medical care, particularly the management of neurologic complications, is essential. In contrast to what is available for SLE, a vaccine exists for the prevention of human infection. Efficacy in vaccine studies ranges from 56%–90% (140,141). Persons living in endemic areas are candidates for vaccination. Although the vaccine is not licensed for administration in the United States, it has been made available under certain circumstances by efforts at the Centers of Disease Control. The vaccine was developed by the Research Foundation for Microbial Diseases (Biken) at Osaka University, Osaka, Japan. The incidence of adverse reactions to this vaccine in approximately 1% (142).

Murray Valley Encephalitis

History

Murray Valley encephalitis (MVE), first identified as "Australian X disease," was successfully isolated from a human brain following an outbreak in 1951. It was shown to be a flavivirus similar to JE virus (143,144). Since 1917, epidemics have occurred in rural areas of southeastern Australia at regular intervals (145–147). While *Culex annulirostris* was suspected to be the vector for MVE, it was not isolated from this mosquito until 1960 (98). Subsequently, the disease has also been recognized in New Guinea (148). As reports of more recent cases of clinical disease appear in the literature, MVE most closely resembles the disease of JE.

Epidemiology

As with JE and SLE infections, MVE results in a high ratio of inapparent to apparent infection, estimated to be 500–1000 infections per case of disease (149). Epidemics have occurred in defined regions of Australia, specifically the Murray Valley region of New South Wales and Victoria (150). MVE is associated with climatic conditions—namely, increased rainfall, which fosters replication of the vector. Most likely, mortality rates have decreased as medical technology has improved. Early reports of mortality were estimated to be approximately 60% but subsequently have decreased to 20% with time (10).

Seroprevalence studies during outbreaks of MVE are limited. One study in Victoria, following an outbreak in 1951, indicated seroprevalence ranging from 4.5% to 36% as determined by CF antibody evaluation (151). Other seroprevalence studies indicate a higher rate of infection in older individuals, particularly in Western Australia and the Murray Darling River Basin (138). The movement of MVE virus from the wetter endemic zones of the north to the drier south appears to be dependent upon the quantity of rainfall.

Clinical Disease

Clinical findings of MVE disease are similar to that which is the result of JE infection. After a prodrome of 2–5 days, characterized by fever, headache, myalgia, and malaise, CNS signs become prominent. Patients have been divided into three groups according to the extent of CNS involvement (152). Arbitrarily, these categories include (a) CNS involvement with no evidence of either coma or respiratory impairment, (b) severe neurologic disease, and (c) fatal cases. The appearance of coma, as a component of clinical disease, appears to be a very poor prognostic indicator. In the absence of coma, patients will recover, but some have speech disturbances or neurologic complications (10). On the other hand, patients who become comatose have a high mortality rate; survivors usually have neurologic impairment. Fatalities are often the consequence of respiratory failure or bacterial superinfection (152,153). Long-term deficits include seizure disorders, gait disturbances, intellectual impairment, and paraplegia.

Diagnosis

Residents of Australia and New Guinea with acute febrile neurologic illnesses should be considered as po-

tentially having MVE infection. Specific diagnosis is dependent upon either (a) the isolation of virus from brain tissue at postmortem examination or (b) the utilization of specific serologic tests. Serologic tests detect HI, CF, or neutralizing antibodies (154).

Prevention and Treatment

No specific treatment exists for MVE. Similarly, no vaccine is available. Surveillance efforts in areas prone to recurrent epidemics, specifically the Murray River Basin, are monitored regularly for *Culex annulirostris* breeding. If breeding activity is increased, a mass insecticide deployment program has been deployed.

Other Mosquito-Borne Flaviviruses

One other mosquito-borne flavivirus is worthy of note: Ilheus virus (ILH), isolated from Ilheus, Brazil in 1944 (155). Illness caused by ILH is usually febrile in nature and rarely produces CNS disease (156).

Tick-Borne Encephalitis

History

Tick-borne encephalitis (TBE) is a complex of agents grouped together which are antigenically related. Isolated from western and eastern Europe, including the Soviet Union, these agents are transmitted by tick vectors. Virus isolation from human brain and tick transmission were both demonstrated in the late 1930s (157). The TBE complex of agents results in a variety of different clinical entities, including central European tick-borne encephalitis, Far Eastern or Russian spring–summer encephalitis, and biphasic milk fever, among others (10,158,159). Transmission by unpasteurized goat milk has been documented for this complex of agents (160).

Epidemiology

The epidemiology of TBE is dependent upon the distribution of the Ixodid tick vectors across Europe and the Soviet Union. Virus exists in nature in a cycle alternating between Ixodid ticks and wild vertebrate hosts. Vertebrate hosts identified as amplifying vectors include shrews, moles, hedgehogs, and rodents (91,150,161). In addition, large mammals, such as goats, sheep, and cattle, can serve as hosts for ticks as well. Notably, when these animals are infected, virus can be excreted in milk.

Human disease caused by the TBE agents (tick-borne mainly) occurs in males in agricultural and rural communities, reflecting exposure of the individual to the natural habitat of the vector. In central Europe, however, both sexes can be infected equally. Under these circumstances, infection results from exposure during hiking. Incidence rates of infection from identified outbreaks have ranged between five and 20 cases per 100,000 individuals (162).

Two peaks of disease have been identified in Europe. One occurs in May through June, and the other occurs in September through October. These peaks of disease coincide with activity of adult Ixodid ticks. Smaller outbreaks often occur as a consequence of ingestion of unpasteurized milk or cheese (163). In these latter circumstances, entire families—especially, children—are involved (160). It should be noted that laboratory infection with TBE has been documented (164).

Clinical Findings

The incubation period for TBE is 8–14 days after exposure. Illness is characterized by sudden onset of fever, headache, photophobia, nausea, vomiting, and nuchal rigidity. Infection ranges from that which is totally asymptomatic to fulminant involvement of the CNS, leading to death in a significant number of cases. Disease appears more severe in children than in adults. The overall case fatality rate is approximately 20% (165). Coma and generalized seizures are characteristic of the most severe manifestations of disease. Long-term clinical follow-up has demonstrated residual paralyses in a significant number of patients (30–60%) (91,166). There does appear to be a distinction between clinical manifestations of TBE disease associated with central European encephalitis and those encountered in Russian spring–summer encephalitis. The Russian spring–summer encephalitis appears to be monophasic, whereas that associated with central Europe appears to be more biphasic (167). In the central European form, the mortality rate is lower and there is less propensity for neurologic sequelae (91,168).

Diagnosis

Epidemiologic association of tick bite and the appearance of an acute febrile neurologic syndrome is useful but not definitive for TBE, since many patients will not have a history of tick bite. Not to be casually forgotten, food intake history, particularly as it relates to unpasteurized milk products, may also be helpful. Diagnosis is dependent upon serologic confirmation of infection. Classically, HI, CF, and neutralization assays have all been employed with variable sensitivity and specificity (169). More recently, the utilization of IgM antibody assays has led to more predictable results (170). It should be remembered that serum must be obtained early in the course of disease before the appearance of antibodies (160).

Prevention and Treatment

No specific treatment exists for TBE. An inactivated vaccine for TBE is available, being produced in chick embryo cell cultures or embryonated eggs (171,172). This vaccine has been administered to individuals living in endemic areas as well as those at high risk for natural disease (157,160,173).

The avoidance of endemic areas, as well as proper preparation of food (pasteurizing milk), is of benefit in preventing disease.

Other Flavivirus Tick-Borne Encephalitides

Powassan Encephalitis

Powassan virus was isolated from a child with encephalitis in 1958 (174). It appears to be a member of the TBE complex of viruses, most likely the Russian spring–summer encephalitis group (175). Powassan virus has been isolated from a variety of *Ixodides* and *Dermacentor* ticks, including *Ixodides marxi, Ixodides cookei,* and *Dermacentor andersoni.* The life cycle of these ticks involves such wild animals as squirrels, porcupines, and groundhogs; man is an accidental host. Infected ticks can be brought into the home by domestic animals (176,177). *Ixodides spinipalpus* also has been identified as a vector for Powassan virus in the western part of the United States (178,179). It should be noted that human infections are extremely rare.

Louping Ill

Louping ill is primarily a disease of sheep in the United Kingdom. It is transmitted by *Ixodes ricinus* ticks (180–184). Disease which occurs in humans appears to be a milder form of TBE disease.

Negishi

A few cases of Negishi virus infection of the CNS have been reported (185,186). The actual frequency of CNS infection is difficult to define because of the rarity of disease. This virus is a member of the TBE family but, interestingly, appears to be more similar to JE virus (187).

BUNYAVIRUSES

Background

The Bunyaviridae family is comprised of more than 250 viruses and is divided among five genera: *Bunyavirus, Phlebovirus, Hantavirus, Nairovirus,* and *Uukuvirus* (188). In spite of different pathogenic routes and ecology for most of the five genera, these viruses share similar biochemical and structural features. Most bunyaviruses have been isolated during surveys of arthropods for infecting pathogens. A few of the bunyaviruses cause significant human disease, including the California serogroup, sandfly fever, Congo–Crimean fever, Hantaan, and Rift Valley fever viruses. This section will make no effort to discuss all *Bunyavirus* infections of insects, animals, and humans; however, it will focus on the most common ones that cause CNS disease in humans. The reader is referred to excellent reviews in the literature for more detailed considerations of these viruses (188–190).

Viruses in the Bunyaviridae family have similar morphologic and structural features. These viruses range in size between 80 and 120 nm and have a lipid envelope. Overall, they are spherical structures (191–201). The virion contains two surface glycoproteins, identified as G1 and G2, and a nucleocapsid protein. The G1 and G2 glycoproteins likely serve as hemagglutinin and neutralizing antibody targets (198,202–204). As will be noted below, they appear to be coded by one of three RNA segments. With replication, the bunyaviruses, for the most part, bud into the cytoplasm from vesicles associated with the Golgi apparatus (193,205,206). The release of progeny virions is equated with cell death.

The genome is organized into three segments, consisting of single-strand, negative-polarity RNA. These segments have been identified as large (L), medium (M), and small (S), indicating the size of the protein which is encoded (188,207). Glycoproteins G1 and G2 are coded for by the M RNA segment. Notably, there is some difference in size between genera of Bunyaviridae for G1 and G2 (188).

The S RNA segment encodes a nucleocapsid protein, which is most likely a structural antigen (198,208,209). This protein is probably the major antigen required for complement fixation (210). Those members of Bunyaviridae which are the focus of this section are identified in Table 2.

TABLE 2. *Family Bunyaviridae, genus Bunyavirus*

Bunyamwera group
Bunyamwera
Ilesha
Bwamba group
Bwamba
Pongola
California group
California encephalitis
Tahyna
Inkoo
La Crosse
Melano
Jamestown Canyon
Genus *Phlebovirus*
Rift Valley fever

Pathology and Pathogenesis

Pathology

The resultant CNS lesions caused by Bunyaviridae infections indicate a degree of similarity for each of the pathogens. For the most part, the lesions induced by bunyaviruses are typical of acute viral encephalitis, consisting of focal areas of perivascular lymphocytic infiltration, gliosis, and, infrequently, areas of focal necrosis. The most significant gross and histopathologic findings of disease are limited to the cerebral cortex. Microscopic examination of brain tissue, however, demonstrates lesions of the brainstem and medulla (188,211,212).

Pathogenesis

Pathogenesis of infections caused by the Bunyaviridae are similar to those caused by other arthropod-borne viruses. Viruses from this family infect man when humans enter the ecological niche of the pathogen. These viruses are not amplified by humans, with the possible exception of sandfly fever. Viruses in this family are considered to be transported by arthropods, most frequently mosquitoes but also sand flies, ticks, and biting midges (190). Episodes of primary viremia follow either arthropod bites or injection into capillary spaces during insect probing. Following primary viremia, there is likely a secondary viremia, with subsequent involvement of the CNS. As with similar infections, the ratio of inapparent to apparent infection is high. For the common La Crosse and Jamestown Canyon viruses (both members of the California encephalitis serogroup), members of the *Aedes* species (e.g., *Aedes triseriatus*) appear to be the most common vectors for transmission of infection to humans. For La Crosse encephalitis, *Aedes triseriatus* is amplified in chipmunks and squirrels, leading to endemic human disease. Jamestown Canyon virus is more likely amplified in the white-tailed deer.

California Serogroup Viruses

History

The California serogroup viruses is a collection of agents with similar characteristics. At present, the California serogroup includes 14 viruses transmitted by mosquitoes, and each has a very narrow host range as well as geographic distribution (188). These viruses have been isolated from tropical (Mealo), temperate (La Crosse), and arctic regions (213). The mechanism of overwintering of these viruses in temperate and arctic regions has not been defined.

The prototype of the California serogroup viruses is La Crosse virus, isolated from the brain of a child who died from encephalitis in La Crosse, Wisconsin (214). This virus is similar to that previously isolated by Reeves and Hammon (43) in the early 1940s in California (40,215). The La Crosse virus was found to be far more common across the United States and, therefore, now serves as a prototype (216). Except for epidemics of SLE, La Crosse virus infection is likely the most prevalent mosquito-borne viral infection in the United States today.

Epidemiology

As noted, La Cross virus is transmitted by *Aedes triseriatus,* being amplified in chipmunks and squirrels (216–220). Cases of La Crosse encephalitis occur mainly in the warmer months of late summer and early fall, with little year-to-year variation (107). Utilizing oligonucleotide RNA fingerprints, three subgroups has been identified; these are referred to as A, B, and C (221,222).

The greatest occurrence of human disease caused by the California serogroup viruses parallels the distribution of the *Aedes triseriatus.* Thus, the largest number of cases have been reported from Wisconsin, Ohio, Minnesota, and Illinois (190). The average number of cases reported per year is approximately 75, which most likely is underreported (216). Figure 4 summarizes the cases

reported to the Centers for Disease Control from 1975 to 1990.

Seroprevalence for the California serogroup of viruses has been ascertained mainly in the central United States. In one study performed in Indiana, seroprevalence increased with advancing years, to approximately 20% by the age of 60 (223,224). Fatality rates appear to be extremely low (0.3%) (216). The ratio of apparent to inapparent infections is approximately 1:1000.

Much of the prospectively collected data on the natural history of La Crosse virus infections has been generated in endemic areas and includes studies of seroconversion in forest workers in Wisconsin (four of 232) (225), a higher case-to-infection ratio in children (216), and a yearly seroconversion rate on an Indian reservation in North Carolina of 2.3 hospitalized children per 1000 individuals at risk each year (226). These data support an incidence of infection of 2.2% (227).

Clinical Disease

Encephalitis caused by the California serogroup viruses first appeared in the literature as anecdotal case reports (225,228,229) but was promptly supported by larger studies of patients (230–236). Each series or report

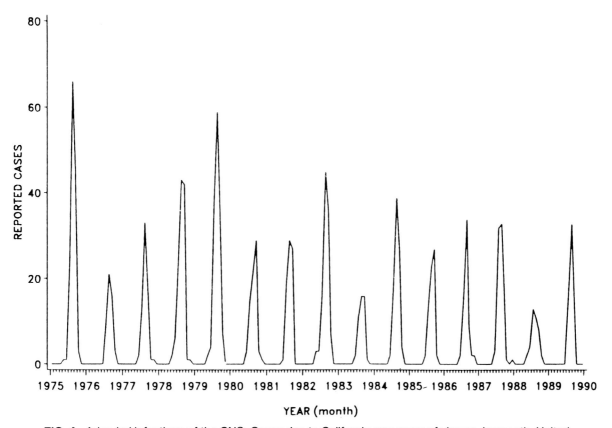

FIG. 4. Arboviral infections of the CNS. Cases due to California serogroup of viruses, by month, United States, 1975–1990. Morbid Mort Wkly Rep 1989;38:18.

identified classic clinical findings of acute encephalitis. The incubation period is presumed to be 3–7 days (211), followed by an acute neurologic syndrome characterized by photophobia, meningismus, fever, headache, lethargy, and abdominal pain. A few patients develop frank CNS findings of altered mentation and consciousness, focal seizures, and hemiparesis. These findings generally last 1–3 days.

Hospitalization is prolonged with deteriorating levels of consciousness, a not uncommon finding in the hospitalized patient with acute California serogroup virus infection of the CNS. Furthermore, in patients with more advanced disease, severe seizure disorders, hemiparesis, and other neurologic signs, including aphasia and chorea, have been reported (211). Long-term follow-up of patients with California serogroup encephalitis indicates the possibility of a persistent seizure disorder on long-term follow-up (230,233,235,237). In addition, some children will have school performance disorders, but, certainly, this is difficult to distinguish from appropriate age-matched controls (231–233,238).

Diagnosis

Laboratory evaluation of the acutely ill and febrile patient with a CNS syndrome of California serogroup virus infection is somewhat different from that of patients with other viral infections of the CNS. A large number of patients will have an increased peripheral leukocyte count, reaching values as high as 20,000 to 30,000 cells per cubic millimeter. CSF findings are no different from that reported for other viral infections of the CNS: Usual cell counts range up to 500 per cubic millimeter, accompanied by mildly elevated levels of CSF protein (<150 mg/dl). It should be noted that a few cases of California serogroup encephalitis, particularly La Crosse encephalitis, will have focal localization on both neurologic and neurodiagnostic evaluation. This is exemplified by studies performed by the NIAID Collaborative Antiviral Study Group (239), as well as other studies reported in the literature (190,211).

Specific diagnosis of California serogroup infection requires serologic confirmation utilizing either CF or HI antibody assays; neutralization assays may be of the greatest value (211,224,240,241). IgM-specific immunofluorescent assays, however, have been developed and appear to be valuable diagnostic tools (241,242).

Routine isolation of virus during the acute illness appears unrewarding.

Prevention and Treatment

At present, there is no specific treatment for the California serogroup viruses when CNS disease is the consequence. Supportive care is the optimal form of clinical management. Specific treatment of the seizure disorder with anticonvulsants is indicated. Some patients will require ventilatory support and meticulous care during episodes of acute illness. Fortunately, these infections are rarely severe or life-threatening.

Surveillance procedures are not routinely deployed for activity of California serogroup viruses.

Other Bunyaviruses

Other bunyaviruses have been associated with CNS disease, although infrequently. These include the Tahyna virus. This agent is transmitted most frequently by *Aedes vexans* and *Culiseta annulata* in Moravia, Czechoslovakia (243,244). Seroprevalence of this organism is high, and clinical disease is uncommon. Disease has been reported to range from febrile illness to evidence of significant encephalitis (245–247).

Similarly, Jamestown Canyon virus has been known to infect humans in the northern central United States, especially Michigan and New York. In these states, selected residential populations were shown to be seropositive at rates of 5–25% (248,249). During the summer of 1990, Jamestown Canyon virus was identified as the cause in several cases of encephalitis in New York State. The clinical manifestations of disease are similar to those encountered in La Crosse encephalitis.

Snowshoe hare virus is an antigenic variant of La Crosse virus and has been associated with encephalitis in a few individuals in Canada (107,250,251). These cases occur rarely and have clinical manifestations similar to those of La Crosse encephalitis.

***Phlebovirus* Genus**

One member of the *Phlebovirus* genus warrants note, specifically Rift Valley fever. During the late 1970s, there was a epizootic epidemic outbreak of Rift Valley fever in Egypt (252). The human infection rate was high and resulted in a clinical syndrome which was, for the most part, an uncomplicated clinical illness. It was characterized by abrupt onset of fever, chills, and myalgia. A few patients developed evidence of encephalitis and retinal hemorrhage (253–262). The case fatality rate was extremely low, as reiterated by the most recent Egyptian epidemic (263).

The recent addition of encephalitis to the spectrum of clinical disease should be noted. It is characterized by headache, meningeal irritation, altered levels of consciousness, and persistent fever. CSF has a characteristic elevation of lymphocytes and mild proteinosis. These findings have been described in several small clinical studies and have been summarized by Peters and others (247,258,264–266). A specific diagnosis of Rift Valley fever involving the CNS uses the demonstration of increasing quantities of antibodies, particularly IgM antibodies, in the CSF (266,267).

No specific treatment exists for Rift Valley fever. Rift Valley fever can be transmitted by *Culex pipiens.* Furthermore, it can be transmitted to humans by contact with infected tissues. Thus, there is the potential for cutaneous or aerosol exposure leading to infection (261, 268–270).

A formalin-inactivated vaccine is available to protect laboratory workers (271–274). These vaccines may be of value in laboratory workers.

ORBIVIRUSES

Background

Originally thought to be arboviruses because of vertebrate transmission, orbiviruses have been shown to be lipid-soluble. Therefore this observation, along with structural data, led to a new taxonomic category (275–277). Orbiviruses resemble reoviruses in that they lack an envelope and contain a genome of double-strand RNA. The *Orbivirus* genus was separated into its own taxonomic group as a result of these morphologic, serologic, and pathophysiologic data (278–282). Diseases caused by this family of viruses are of human and veterinary importance. The diseases of humans which warrant consideration include Colorado tick fever, Changuinola, Kamerovo, Lebombo, and Orungo. Similarly, diseases of veterinary importance include equine encephalosis, African horse sickness, and blue tongue hemorrhagic fever (282). Of these agents, only one—namely Colorado tick fever—is a cause of CNS disease. This agent will be emphasized in the subsequent discussion.

Infectious Agent

Orbiviruses, in general, are characterized as having an icosahedral symmetry and a diameter of approximately 60–80 nm, and they assume a spherical virion shape. Colorado tick fever (CTF) viruses are spherical in nature, with a diameter of 80 nm and an inner core of 50 nm (281,283,284). The viral genome of CTF consists of 12 segments—somewhat in contrast to other members of the *Orbivirus* genus, which have only 10 discrete genomic segments (282,285). At least seven polypeptides are encoded by the genome. Detailed reviews have considered these proteins (282,286–289).

California tick fever virus is relatively stable at room temperature. Electron-microscopic studies of the replication of CTF indicate intracytoplasmic maturation (281,283,284).

History

In the mid-19th century, physicians of the Rocky Mountain states identified a fever which was not possible

to distinguish from other defined clinical entities but which, in all probability, was caused by CTF virus. By 1930, the name CTF was associated with the clinical symptomatology equated with today's illness (290,291). By the mid-1940s, Florio et al. (292) were able to isolate the organism from human blood. Subsequently, Florio et al. (293) were able to demonstrate that CTF could be isolated from the tick *Dermecentor andersoni.*

Pathology and Pathogenesis

Pathology

In humans, CTF is associated with a very low case fatality rate; and therefore, descriptions of CNS pathology are uncommon. Much of the available knowledge regarding CTF has been generated from mouse model systems (294). Characteristically, in the mouse, multiple organs are involved, including the myocardium, vascular endothelium, and skeletal muscle. When the CNS is involved in the mouse model, cerebellar changes are as common as those of the cerebral cortex, indicating widespread necrosis and associated vascular endothelial infiltration.

Disease in humans is characterized, surprisingly, by leukopenia and thrombocytopenia (295).

Pathogenesis

Involvement of bone marrow precursor cells may well be indicative of the propensity of virus to be found in erythrocytes in animal model systems. This property is unique in the pathogenesis of other arthropod-borne viruses. California tick fever virus is resident in *Dermecentor andersoni* ticks; therefore, human disease parallels distribution of this vector in nature. Several characteristics of CTF involvement of *Dermecentor andersoni* should be recognized. First, and most importantly, infection with CTF produces little or no disease in the natural host, resulting in successful persistence of virus. Persistence is aided by a prolonged period of viremia (284,296–301). It is thought that this persistence intracellularly within erythrocytes, as summarized by McKee et al. (284) and others (275,302,303), contributes to persistent viremia in vertebrate species. Ground squirrels and chipmunks serve as amplifying rodents (298–300); however, other animal species can amplify CTF as well (284). Humans are considered a "dead end" host.

In contrast to other arbovirus infection, CTF has a predisposition for involvement of the bone marrow and erythrocyte precursors. Residence of virus in such a privileged site makes it impervious to normal host defense mechanisms; likely, it counts for the prolonged and persistent viremia (284,302,303). In addition, residence within erythroid precursors in red cells may account, in part, for the predisposition of the hemorrhagic and vasculatic components of human clinical disease (275).

Epidemiology

CTF is a disease associated with mountainous states, occurring at altitudes of 4,000 to 10,000 feet in the Rocky Mountains of the United States and Canada (282). The isolation of CTF virus correlates with the range of isolation of *Dermacentor andersoni* ticks. Most cases of CTF occur between March and September, with the majority of cases occurring between April and July (282).

Since CTF is not a reportable disease, most literature citations are from individual investigations. From these studies, it has been learned that most cases occur in Colorado and Idaho, as best as can be identified (304–306). Because of the lack of severity of disease, many patients never even seek medical care; therefore, cases are probably underreported.

As would be expected, individuals exposed to *Dermacentor andersoni* ticks are most likely to show evidence of infection. Thus, young adults (particularly males working in the woodlands), hikers, and campers appear to be most prone to infection.

It should also be noted that CTF can be transmitted person-to-person by transfusion (307). Furthermore, other rodents—such as woodrats and deer mice—can transmit infection.

Clinical Findings

Several reviews have summarized the clinical findings associated with CTF (282,284,305,306,308,309). It is estimated that the incubation period is approximately 3–6 days. The onset of disease is acute in nature, characterized by fever, chills, myalgia, headache, photophobia, and malaise. Nausea and vomiting are not uncommon findings.

Resolution of the acute illness can be biphasic and can last approximately 5–10 days. Persistence of the clinical symptoms of asthenia, malaise, and weakness occurs especially in children (305). Complications of infection (particularly that of the CNS) or hemorrhagic findings have been reported. When the CNS is involved, a complete spectrum from benign meningeal to severe encephalitic involvement has been identified (305, 306,309,310). The actual frequency of CNS involvement is not known but may range from 1% to 10% (309). Most children and adults recover from disease without evidence of complications.

Diagnosis

Abnormalities identified by the clinical laboratory usually include leukopenia and thrombocytopenia, par-

ticularly in patients who have hemorrhagic manifestations of disease. With evidence of CNS disease, a typical CSF formula, as found in other encephalitis cases, is encountered. The total cell count is less than 500 cells per cubic millimeter, and protein is approximately 100 mg/dl. Specific laboratory diagnosis requires isolation of virus from the blood (particularly red blood cells). This is not to be unexpected, since persistent viremia has been documented because of association of virus with erythrocytes (305,311).

As has been noted previously, serologic response to CTF virus is delayed because of erythrocyte persistence. Development of CF and neutralizing antibodies appears late after the onset of disease (282). For more complete discussions of diagnosis, the reader is referred to recent reviews (282,284).

Prevention and Treatment

At present, there is no specific treatment or prevention for CTF. Certainly, awareness of exposure to *Dermacentor andersoni* when hiking in the woods or Rocky Mountain states is indicated. Thus, health education and personal protection against tick bites are the best preventive measures, especially in high-risk endemic areas. It is unclear as to whether insecticides are helpful in disease prevention.

CONCLUSIONS

Arthropod-borne viruses represent an important cause of both human and veterinary disease. This chapter has summarized the most common causes of CNS infections mediated by arthropod-borne vectors. It must be recognized that, taxonomically, many of these viruses represent different groups of different families. Distributed widely across the world, these agents represent unique examples of vector, amplifying host, environment, and disease interactions. Future efforts must extend beyond simple identification of agents responsible for CNS infections and include methods for prevention other than education. Utilization of molecular biologic techniques for vaccine development for either the amplifying hosts, the vector, or the individuals at high risk will provide further research opportunities.

ACKNOWLEDGMENTS

Original studies performed by the investigators were supported by grants from the following sources: the National Institute of Allergy and Infectious Diseases (NO1-AI-62554); the Division of Research Resources (RR-0023) of the National Institutes of Health; and the State of Alabama.

REFERENCES

1. Schlesinger S, Schlesinger MJ. Replication of Togaviridae and Flaviviridae. In: Fields BN, Knipe DM, eds. *Virology,* 2nd ed. New York: Raven Press, 1990;697–814.
2. Peters CJ, Dalrymple JM. Alphaviruses. In: Fields BN, Knipe DM, eds. *Virology,* 2nd ed. New York: Raven Press, 1990;713–761.
3. Strauss JH, Strauss EG, Hahn CS, Rice CM. The genomes of alphaviruses and flaviviruses: organization and translation. In: Rowlands DJ, Mayo MA, Mahy BWJ, eds. *The molecular biology of the positive strand RNA viruses.* London: Academic Press, 1987;75–102.
4. Chanas AC, Gould EA, Clegg JCS, Varma MGR. Monoclonal antibodies to Sindbis virus glycoprotein E1 can neutralize, enhance infectivity, and independently inhibit haemagglutination or haemolysis. *J Gen Virol* 1982;58:37–46.
5. Dalrymple JM, Vogel SN, Teramoto AY. Antigenic components of group A arbovirus virions. *J Virol* 1973;12:1034–1041.
6. Dalrymple JM, Schlesinger S, Russell PK. Antigenic characterization of two Sindbis envelope glycoproteins seperated by isoelectric focusing. *Virology* 1976;69:93–103.
7. Bastain FO, Wende RD, Singer DB, Zeller RS. Eastern equine encephalitis. Histopathologic and ultrastructural changes with isolation of the virus in a human case. *Am J Clin Pathol* 1975;64:10–13.
8. Farber S, Hill A, Connerly MI, Dingle JH. Encephalitis in infants and children caused by the virus of the eastern variety of equine encephalitis. *JAMA* 1940;114:1725–1731.
9. Haymaker W II. Western equine encephalitis. Pathology. *Neurology* 1958;8:881.
10. Craven RB. Togaviruses. In: Belshe RB, ed. *Textbook of human virology.* Littleton, MA: PSG Publishing Co., 1984;599–648.
11. Peck R, Wust CJ, Brown A. Adoptive transfer of cross-protection among alphaviruses in mice requires allogenic stimulation. *Infect Immun* 1979;25:320–327.
12. Rozdilsky B, Robertson HE, Chorney J. Western encephalitis: report of eight fatal cases: Saskatchewan epidemic, 1965. *Can Med Assoc J* 1968;98:79–86.
13. Finley KH, Longshore WA, Palmer RJ, et al. Western equine and St. Louis encephalitis. Preliminary report of a clinical follow-up study in California. *Neurology* 1955;5:223–235.
14. McLean RG, Frier G, Parham GL, et al. Investigations of the vertebrate hosts of eastern equine encephalitis during an epidemic in Michigan, 1980. *Am J Trop Med Hyg* 1985;34:1190–1202.
15. Goldfield M, Welsh JN, Taylor BF. The 1959 outbreak of eastern encephalitis in New Jersey. 5. The inapparent infection: disease ratio. *Am J Epidemiol* 1968;87:32–38.
16. Hammon WMcD, Reeves WC, Brookman B, et al. Isolation of the viruses of western equine and St. Louis encephalitis from *Culex tarsalis* mosquitoes. *Science* 1947;94:328–330.
17. Lennette EH, Koprowski H. Human infection with Venezuelan equine encephalomyelitis virus: a report on eight cases on infection acquired in the laboratory. *JAMA* 1943;123:1088–1095.
18. TenBroeck C, Merrill MH. A serological difference between eastern and western equine encephalomyelitis virus. *Proc Soc Exp Biol Med* 1933;31:217–220.
19. Giltner LT, Shrahan MS. The 1933 outbreak of infectious equine encephalomyelitis in the eastern states. *N Am Vet* 1973;14:25–27.
20. Fothergill LD, Dingle JH, Faber S, et al. Human encephalitis caused by the virus of the eastern variety of equine encephalomyelitis. *N Engl J Med* 1938;219:411.
21. Calisher CH, Maness KSC, Lord RC, et al. Identification of two South American strains of eastern equine encephalomyelitis virus from migrant birds captured on the Mississippi Delta. *Am J Epidemiol* 1971;94:172–178.
22. Chamberlain RW. Vector relationship of the arthropod-borne encephalitides in North America. *Ann NY Acad Sci* 1958;70:312–319.
23. Crans WJ. The status of *Aedes sollicitans* as an epidemic vector of eastern equine encephalitis in New Jersey. *Mosq News* 1977;37:85–89.
24. Dalrymple JM, Young OP, Eldridge BF, Russell PK. Ecology of arboviruses in a Maryland freshwater swamp. III. Vertebrate hosts. *Am J Epidemiol* 1972;96:129–140.
25. Howard JJ, Wallis RC. Infection and transmission of eastern equine encephalomyelitis virus with colonized *Culiseta melanura* (Coquillet). *Am J Trop Med Hyg* 1974;23:522–525.
26. Kissling RE, Chamberlain RW, Sikes RK, Eidson ME. Studies on the North American arthropod-borne encephalitides. III. Eastern equine encephalitis in wild birds. *Am J Hyg* 1954;60:251–265.
27. Joseph SR, Bickley WE. *Culiseta melanura* (Coquillet) on the eastern shore of Maryland (Diptera: Culicidae). *Bull Univ MD Agricul Exp Station* 1969;A-161:1.
28. Ayers JC, Feemster RF. The sequelae of eastern equine encephalitis. *N Engl J Med* 1949;240:960–962.
29. Clarke EH. Two nonfatal human infections with the virus of eastern encephalitis. *Am J Trop Med Hyg* 1961;10:67–70.
30. Feemster FR. Outbreak of encephalitis in man due to the eastern virus of equine encephalitis. *Am J Public Health* 1938;28:1403–1410.
31. Feemster RF. Equine encephalitis in Massachusetts. *N Engl J Med* 1957;257:701–704.
32. Hart KL, Keen D, Belle EA. An outbreak of eastern equine encephalomyelitis in Jamaica, West Indies, Nov–Dec 1962. I. Description of human cases. *Am J Trop Med Hyg* 1964;13:331–334.
33. McGowan JE, Bryan JA, Gregg MB. Surveillance of arboviral encephalitis in the United States, 1955–1971. *Am J Epidemiol* 1973;97:199–207.
34. Webster H de F. Eastern equine encephalomyelitis in Massachusetts. Report of two cases, diagnosed serologically, with complete clinical recovery. *N Engl J Med* 1956;255:267–270.
35. Clarke DH. Two nonfatal human infections with the virus of eastern encephalitis. *Am J Trop Med Hyg* 1961;10:67–70.
36. Goldfield M, Taylor BF, Welsh JN. The 1959 outbreak of eastern encephalitis in New Jersey. 3. Serologic studies of clinical cases. *Am J Epidemiol* 1968;87:18–22.
37. Przelomski MM, O'Rourke E, Grady GF, Berardi VP, Markley HG. Eastern equine encephalitis in Massachusetts: a report of 16 cases: 1970–1984. *Neurology* 1988;38:736–739.
38. Bigler WJ, Lassing EB, Buff EE, et al. Endemic eastern equine encephalomyelitis in Florida: a twenty year analysis: 1955–1974. *Am J Trop Med Hyg* 1976;25:884–890.
39. Tsai TF, Monath TP. Viral diseases in North America transmitted by arthropods or from vertebrate reservoirs. In: Feigin RD, Cherry JD, eds. *Textbook of pediatric infectious diseases.* Philadelphia: WB Saunders, 1982;1417–1456.
40. Cole FE Jr. Inactivated eastern equine encephalomyelitis vaccine propagated in rolling-bottle cultures of chick embryo cells. *Appl Microbiol* 1971;22:842–845.
41. Meyer KF, Haring CM, Howitt B. The etiology of encephalomyelitis in horses in the San Joaquin Valley, 1930. *Science* 1931;74:227–228.
42. Howitt BF. Recovery of the virus of equine encephalomyelitis from the brain of a child. *Science* 1938;88:455–456.
43. Reeves WC, Hammon WMcD. Epidemiology of the arthropod-borne viral encephalitides in Kern County, California, 1943–1952. *Univ Calif Publ Public Health* 1962;4:257.
44. Centers for Disease Control. Arboviral infections of the central nervous system—United States, 1987. *MMWR* 1988;37:506–515.
45. Baker AB. II. Western equine encephalitis. Clinical features. *Neurology* 1958;8:880–881.
46. Hammon WMcD, Reeves WC, Benner SR, Brookman B. Human encephalitis in the Yakima Valley, Washington, 1942. *JAMA* 1945;128:1133–1139.
47. Sciple GW, Ray CG, Holden P, La Motte LC, Irons JV, Chin TDY. Encephalitis in the high plains of Texas. *Am J Epidemiol* 1968;87:87–98.
48. Russell PK. Alphavirus (eastern, western, and Venezuelan equine encephalitis). In: Mandell GL, Douglas RG Jr, Bennett JE, eds. *Principles and practices of infectious diseases,* 2nd ed. New York: John Wiley & Sons, 1985;917–920.
49. Griffin DE. Alphavirus pathogenesis and immunity. In: Schle-

singer S, Schlesinger MJ, eds. *The Togaviridae and Flaviviridae.* New York: Plenum Press, 1986;209–249.

50. Kokernot RH, Shinefield HR, Longshore WA. The 1952 outbreak of encephalitis in California. *Calif Med* 1953;79:73–77.

51. Finley KH. Postencephalitis manifestations of viral encephalitides. In: Fields NS, Blattner RJ, eds. *Viral encephalitis.* Springfield, IL: Charles C Thomas, 1959;69:91.

52. Copps SC, Giddings LE. Transplacental transmission of western equine encephalitis. *Pediatrics* 1959;24:31–33.

53. Shinefield HR, Townsend RE. Transplacental transmission of western equine encephalomyelitis. *J Pediatr* 1953;43:21–25.

54. Eldridge BF. Strategies for surveillance, prevention, and control of arbovirus diseases in western North America. *Am J Trop Med Hyg* 1987;37:77S–86S.

55. Hayes RO. Eastern and western encephalitis. In: Beran GW, ed. *Handbook series in zoonoses, section B: viral zoonoses,* vol 1. Boca Raton, FL: CRC Press, 1981;29–57.

56. Beck CE, Wyckoff RWG. Venezuelan equine encephalomyelitis. *Science* 1938;88:530.

57. Sanmartin-Barberi C, Groot H, Osborno-Mesa E. Human epidemic in Colombia caused the Venezuelan equine encephalomyelitis virus. *Am J Trop Med Hyg* 1954;3:283–293.

58. Gleiser CA, Gochenour WS Jr, Berge TO, Tigertt WD. The comparative pathology of experimental Venezuelan equine encephalomyelitis infection in different animal hosts. *J Infect Dis* 1961;110:80–97.

59. Johnson KM, Shelokov A, Peralta PH, Dammin GJ, Young NA. Recovery of Venezuelan equine encephalomyelitis virus in Panama. *Am J Trop Med Hyg* 1968;17:432–440.

60. Walton TW, Alverez O Jr, Buckwalter RM, Johnson KM. Experimental infection of horse with enzootic and epizootic strains of Venezuelan equine encephalomyelitis. *J Infect Dis* 1973;128:271–281.

61. Cupp EW, Scherer WF, Lok JB, Brenner RJ, Dziem GM, Ordonez JV. Entomological studies at an enzootic Venezuelan equine encephalitis virus focus in Guatemala, 1977–1980. *Am J Trop Med Hyg* 1986;35:851–859.

62. Galindo P, Grayson MA. *Culex (Melanoconion) aikenii:* natural vector in Panama of endemic Venezuelan encephalitis. *Science* 1971;172:594–595.

63. Johnson KM, Martin DH. Venezuelan equine encephalitis. *Adv Vet Sci Comp Med* 1974;18:79–116.

64. Shope RE, Woodall JP. Ecological interaction of wildlife, man, and a virus of the Venezuelan equine encephalomyelitis complex in a tropical forest. *J Wildl Dis* 1973;9:198–203.

65. Walton TE, Grayson MA. Venezuelan equine encephalomyelitis. In: Monath TP, ed. *The Arboviruses: epidemiology and ecology,* vol IV. Boca Raton, FL: CRC Press, 1988;204–231.

66. Young NA, Johnson KM, Gauld LW. Viruses of the Venezuelan equine encephalomyelitis complex. *Am J Trop Med Hyg* 1969;18:290–296.

67. Franck PT, Johnson KM. An outbreak of Venezuelan encephalitis in man in the Panama Canal Zone. *Am J Trop Med Hyg* 1970;19:860–863.

68. Sanchez JL, Lednar WM, Macaset FF, et al. Venezuelan equine encephalomyelitis: report of an outbreak associated with jungle exposure. *Milit Med* 1984;149:618–621.

69. Edelman R, Ascher MS, Oster CN, Ramsburg HH, Cole FE, Eddy GA. Evaluation of humans of a new, inactivated vaccine for Venezuelan equine encephalitis virus (C-84). *J Infect Dis* 1979;140:708–715.

70. Avilan Rovira J. Discussion. In: *Proceedings of the workshop symposium on Venezuelan encephalitis virus.* Science publication 243. Washington, DC: Pan American Health Organization, 1972;189–195.

71. Briceno Rossi AL. Rural epidemic encephalitis in Venezuela caused by a group A arbovirus (VEE). In: Melnick JL, ed. *Progress in medical virology,* vol 9. Basel: Karger, 1967;176–203.

72. Hinman AR, McGowan JE Jr, Henderson BE. Venezuelan equine encephalomyelitis: surveys of human illness during an epizootic in Guatemala and El Savador. *Am J Epidemiol* 1971;93:130–136.

73. Madalengoitia J, Palacios O, Ubiliuz JC, Alva S. An outbreak of Venezuelan encephalitis virus in man in the Tumbes department

of Peru. In: *Proceedings of the workshop symposium on Venezuelan encephalitis virus.* Science publication 243. Washington, DC: Pan American Health Organization, 1972;198–200.

74. Martin DH, Eddy GA, Sudia WD, Reeves WC, Newhouse VF, Johnson KM. An epidemiologic study of Venezuelan equine encephalomyelitis in Costa Rica, 1970. *Am J Epidemiol* 1972;95:565–578.

75. Sanmartin C. Diseased hosts: man. In: *Proceedings of the workshop symposium on Venezuelan encephalitis virus.* Science publication 243. Washington, DC: Pan American Health Organization, 1972;168–188.

76. Sellers RF, Bergold GH, Suaraez OM, Morales A. Investigations during Venezuelan equine encephalitis outbreak in Venezuela—1962–1964. *Am J Trop Med Hyg* 1965;14:460–469.

77. Casals J, Curnen EC, Thomas L. Venezuelan equine encephalomyelitis in man. *J Exp Med* 1943;77:521–530.

78. Slepushkin AN. An epidemiological study of laboratory infections with Venezuelan equine encephalitis. *Prob Virol* 1959;4:54–58.

79. de Ranitz CM, Myers RM, Varkey MJ, Isaac ZH, Carey DE. Clinical impressions of chikungunya in Vellore gained from study of adult patients. *Indian J Med Res* 1965;53:756–763.

80. Dickerman RW, Cupp EW, Groot H, et al. Venezuelan equine encephalitis virus activity in northern Colombia during April and May 1983. *PAHO Bull* 1986;20:276–283.

81. Dietz WH Jr, Peralta PH, Johnson KM. Ten clinical cases of human infection with Venezuelan equine encephalomyelitis virus, subtype I-D. *Am J Trop Med Hyg* 1979;28:329–334.

82. Aaskov JG, Ross P, Davies CEA, et al. Epidemic polyarthritis in northeastern Australia, 1978–1979. *Med J Aust* 1981;2:17–19.

83. Causey OR, Maroja OM. Mayaro virus: a new human disease agent. III. Investigation of an epidemic of acute febrile illness on the river Guama in Para, Brazil, and isolation of Mayaro virus as causative agent. *Am J Trop Med Hyg* 1957;6:1017–1023.

84. McKinney RW. Inactivated and live VEE vaccines—a review. In: *Proceedings of the workshop symposium on Venezuelan encephalitis virus.* Science publication 243. Washington, DC: Pan American Health Organization, 1972;369–389.

85. Casals J, Brown LV. Hemagglutination with arthropod-borne viruses. *J Exp Med* 1954;99:429–449.

86. Trent DW, Monath TP, Bowen GS, et al. Variation among strains of St. Louis encephalitis virus: basis for a genetic, pathogenetic, and epidemiologic classification. *Ann NY Acad Sci* 1980;354:219–237.

87. Trent DW, Qureshi AA. Structural and nonstructural proteins of Saint Louis encephalitis virus. *J Virol* 1971;7:379–388.

88. Calisher CH, Karabotsos N, Dalrymple JM, et al. Antigenic relationships among flaviviruses as determined by cross-neutralization tests with polyclonal antisera. *J Gen Virol* 1989;70:37–43.

89. Monath TP. Pathobiology of the flaviviruses. In: Schlesinger S, Schlesinger MJ, eds. *The Togaviridae and Flaviviridae.* New York: Plenum Press, 1986;375–440.

90. Nathanson N. Pathogenesis: In: Monath TP, ed. *St Louis encephalitis.* Washington, DC: APHA, 1980;201–236.

91. Monath TP. Flaviviruses. In: Fields BN, Knipe MD, eds. *Virology,* 2nd ed. New York: Raven Press, 1990;763–814.

92. Malkova D. The role of the lymphatic system in experimental infection with tick-borne encephalitis. I. The tick-borne encephalitis virus in the lymph and blood of experimentally infected sheep. *Acta Virol (Praha)* 1960;4:233.

93. Johnson RT. *Viral infections of the nervous system.* New York: Raven Press, 1982.

94. Monath TP, Cropp CB, Harrison AK. Mode of entry of a neurotropic arbovirus into the central nervous system: reinvestigation of an old controversy. *Lab Invest* 1983;48:399–410.

95. Hammon WMcD, Reeves WC, Sather GE. Western equine and St. Louis encephalitis viruses in the blood of experimentally infected wild birds and epidemiological implications of findings. *J Immunol* 1951;67:354–367.

96. Buescher EL, Scherer WF. Ecologic studies of Japanese encephalitis virus in Japan. IX. Epidemiologic correlations and conclusions. *Am J Trop Med Hyg* 1959;8:719–722.

97. Scherer WF, Buescher EL. Ecological studies of Japanese encephalitis in Japan. Parts I–IX. *Am J Trop Med Hyg* 1959;8:644–722.

98. Doherty RL, Carley JG, Mackerras MJ, et al. Studies of arthropod-borne virus infections in Queensland. III. Isolation and characterization of virus strains from wild caught mosquitoes in North Queensland. *Aust J Exp Biol Med Sci* 1963;41:17–39.
99. Brown GO, Haymaker W, Smith JE. Sequelae of the arthropod-borne encephalitides. IV. St. Louis encephalitis. *Neurology* 1958;8:883–887.
100. Shinner JJ. St. Louis virus encephalomyelitis. *Arch Pathol* 1963;75:309–322.
101. Muckenfuss RS, Armstrong C, McCordock HA. Encephalitis: studies on experimental transmission. *Public Health Rep* 1933;48:1341–1343.
102. Chamberlain RW. History. In: Monath TP, ed. *St. Louis encephalitis.* Washington, DC: APHA, 1980;3–61.
103. Monath TP, Tsai TF. St. Louis encephalitis: lessons from the last decade. *Am J Trop Med Hyg* 1987;37:40S–59S.
104. Monath TP. Epidemiology. In: Monath TO, ed. *St. Louis encephalitis.* Washington, DC: APHA, 1980;239–312.
105. Update: St. Louis encephalitis—Florida and Texas, 1990. *MMWR* 1990;39:756–759.
106. Henderson BE, Pidford CA, Work T, et al. Serologic survey for St. Louis encephalitis and other group B arbovirus antibodies in residents of Houston, Texas. *Am J Epidemiol* 1970;91:87–98.
107. Grimstad PR, Barrett CL, Humphrey RL, et al. Serologic evidence for widespread infections with LaCrosse and St. Louis encephalitis viruses in the Indiana human population. *Am J Epidemiol* 1987;119:913–930.
108. Tsai TF, Canfield MA, Reed CM, et al. Epidemiological aspects of a St. Louis encephalitis outbreak in Harris Country, Texas, 1986. *J Infect Dis* 1988;157:351–356.
109. Southern PM, Smith JW, Luby JP, Barnett JA, Sanford JP. Clinical and laboratory features of epidemic St. Louis encephalitis. *Ann Intern Med* 1969;71:681–690.
110. Burke DS, Tingpalapong M, Ward GS, et al. Intense transmission of Japanese encephalitis virus to pigs in a region free of epidemic encephalitis. *JE & HFRS Bull* 1986;1:17–26.
111. Brinker KR, Monath TP. The acute disease. In: Monath TP, ed. *St. Louis encephalitis.* Washington, DC: APHA, 1980;505–554.
112. Brinker KR, Paulson G, Monath TP, et al. St. Louis encephalitis in Ohio, September 1975, clinical and EEG studies in 16 cases. *Arch Intern Med* 1979;139:561–566.
113. Finley K, Riggs N. Convalescence and sequelae. In: Monath TP, ed. *St. Louis encephalitis.* Washington, DC: APHA, 1980;535–550.
114. Webster LT, Fite GL. A virus encountered in the study of material from cases of encephalitis in the St. Louis and Kansas City epidemic of 1933. *Science* 1933;78:463–465.
115. Luby JP, Stewart WE, Sulkin SE, et al. Interferon in human infections with St. Louis encephalitis virus. *Am J Intern Med* 1969;71:703.
116. Coleman PH, Lewis AL, Schneider NJ, et al. Isolation of St. Louis encephalitis virus from postmortem tissues of human cases in the 1962 Florida epidemic. *Am J Epidemiol* 1968;87:530.
117. Calisher CH, Poland JD. Laboratory diagnosis. In: Monath TP, ed. *St. Louis encephalitis.* Washington, DC: APHA, 1980;571–601.
118. Monath TP, Nystrom RR, Bailey RE, et al. Immunoglobulin M antibody capture enzyme-linked immunosorbent assay for diagnosis of St. Louis encephalitis. *J Clin Microbiol* 1984;20:784–790.
119. Tsai TF, Mitchell CJ. St. Louis encephalitis. In: Monath TP, ed. *The Arboviruses: epidemiology and ecology.* Boca Raton, FL: CRC Press, 1989;113–144.
120. Luby JP. St. Louis encephalitis. *Epidemiol Rev* 1979;1:55–73.
121. Monath TP. Ecology and control of mosquito-borne arbovirus diseases. In: Kurstak E, Marusyk R, eds. *Control of virus diseases.* New York: Marcel Dekker, 1984;115–134.
122. Johnson RT. The pathogenesis of acute viral encephalitis and postinfectious encephalomyelitis. *J Infect Dis* 1987;155:359–364.
123. Umenai T, Krzysko R, Bektimirov TA, Assaad FA. Japanese encephalitis: current worldwide status. *Bull WHO* 1985;63:625–631.
124. Hoke CH, Nisalak A, Sangawhipa N, et al. Protection against Japanese encephalitis by inactivated vaccines. *N Engl J Med* 1988;319:608–613.
125. Southam CM. Serological studies of encephalitis in Japan. II. Inapparent infections by Japanese B encephalitis. *J Infect Dis* 1956;99:163–169.
126. Benenson MW, Top FJ Jr, Gresso W, et al. The virulence to man of Japanese encephalitis virus in Thailand. *Am J Trop Med Hyg* 1975;24:974–980.
127. Halstead SB, Russ SB. Subclinical Japanese encephalitis. II. Antibody responses of Americans to single exposure to JE virus. *Am J Hyg* 1962;75:190–201.
128. Kono R, Kim KH. Comparative epidemiological features of Japanese encephalitis in the Republic of Korea, China (Taiwan) and Japan. *Bull WHO* 1969;40:263–277.
129. Okuno T, Tsing PT, Hsu ST, et al. Japanese encephalitis surveillance in China (Province of Taiwan) during 1968–1971. II. Age-specific incidence in connection with Japanese vaccination program. *Jpn J Med Sci Biol* 1975;28:255–267.
130. Mogi M. Relationship between number of human Japanese encephalitis cases and summer meteorological conditions in Nagasaki, Japan. *Am J Trop Med Hyg* 1983;32:170–174.
131. Dickerson RB, Newton JR, Hansen JE. Diagnosis and immediate prognosis of Japanese B encephalitis. *Am J Med* 1952;12:277–290.
132. Halstead SB, Grosz CR. Subclinical Japanese encephalitis. I. Infection of Americans with limited residence in Korea. *Am J Hyg* 1962;75:190–201.
133. Lincoln AF, Sivertson SE. Acute phase of Japanese B encephalitis. Two hundred and one cases in American soldiers, Korea. *JAMA* 1950;150:268–273.
134. Edgren DC, Polladino VS, Arnold A. Japanese B and mums encephalitis. A clinicopathologic report of simultaneous outbreaks on the island of Guam. *Am J Trop Med Hyg* 1958;7:471–480.
135. Burke DS, Nisalak A, Ussery MA, Laorakpongese T, Chantavibul S. Kinetics of IgM and IgG responses to Japanese encephalitis virus in human serum and cerebrospinal fluid. *J Infect Dis* 1985;151:1093–1099.
136. Burke DS, Lorsomrudee W, Leake CJ, et al. Fatal outcome in Japanese encephalitis. *Am J Trop Med Hyg* 1985;34:1203–1210.
137. Burke DS, Nisalak A, Gentry MK. Detection of flavivirus antibodies in human serum by epitope-blocking immunoassay. *J Med Virol* 1987;23:163–173.
138. Echuca–Melbourne Collaborative Group. Arbovirus infection in a Murray Valley community. I. Prevalence of antibodies, December, 1974. *Med J Aust* 1976;1:257–259.
139. Kimoto T, Yamada T, Ueba N. Laboratory diagnosis of Japanese encephalitis: comparison of the fluorescent antibody technique with virus isolation and serologic test. *Biken J* 1968;11:157–168.
140. Shortridge KF, Oya A, Kobayashi M, et al. Arbovirus infections in reptiles. *SE Asian J Trop Med Public Health* 1975;6:161–169.
141. Hsu TC, Hsu ST. Supplementary report. Effectiveness of Japanese encephalitis vaccine. Study in the second year following immunization. In: Hammon WMcD, Kitaoka M, Downs WG, eds. *Immunization for Japanese encephalitis.* Baltimore: Williams & Williams, 1971;266–267.
142. Oya A. Japanese encephalitis vaccine. In: Fukumi M, ed. *The vaccination.* Tokyo: International Medical Foundation of Japan, 1975.
143. French EL. Murray Valley encephalitis: isolation and characterization of the aetiological agent. *Med J Aust* 1952;1:100–103.
144. Miles JAR, Fowler MC, Haves DW. Isolation of a virus from encephalitis in South Australia: a preliminary report. *Med J Aust* 1951;1:799–800.
145. Anderson SG. Murray Valley encephalitis and Australian X disease. *J Hyg (Camb)* 1954;52:447–468.
146. Doherty RL, Carley JG, Cremer MR, et al. Murray Valley encephalitis in eastern Australia, 1971. *Med J Aust* 1972;2:1170–1173.
147. Doherty RL, Carley JG, Filippich C, et al. Murray Valley encephalitis in Australia, 1974: antibody response in cases and community. *Aust NA J Med* 1976;6:446–453.
148. French EL, Anderson SG, Price AVG, et al. Murray Valley encephalitis in New Guinea. I. Isolation of Murray Valley encephali-

tis virus from the brain of a fatal care of encephalitis occurring in a Papuan native. *Am J Trop Med Hyg* 1957;6:827–834.

149. Anderson SG. Murray Valley encephalitis: epidemiological aspects. *Med J Aust* 1952;1:97–103.

150. Marshall ID. Murray Valley and Kunjin encephalitis. In: Monath TP, ed. *The arboviruses: ecology and epidemiology,* vol III. Boca Raton, FL: CRC Press, 1988;151–190.

151. Anderson SG, Donnelley M, Stevenson WJ, et al. Murray Valley encephalitis: surveys of human and animal sera. *Med J Aust* 1952;1:110–120.

152. Bennett N McK. Murray Valley encephalitis, 1974: clinical features. *Med J Aust* 1976;2:446–450.

153. Robertson EG, McLorinan H. Murray Valley encephalitis: clinical aspects. *Med J Aust* 1952;1:103–107.

154. Wiemers MA, Stallman ND. Immunoglobulin M in Murray Valley encephalitis. *Pathology* 1975;7:187–191.

155. Theiler M, Downs WG. Group B viruses. In: *The arthropod-borne viruses of vertebrates.* New Haven: Yale University Press, 1973;153–154.

156. Spence L, Anderson CR, Downs WG. Isolation of Ilheus virus from human beings in Trinidad, West Indies. *Trans R Soc Trop Med Hyg* 1962;56:504–509.

157. Smorodintsev AA. Tick-borne spring–summer encephalitis. *Prog Med Virol* 1958;1:210–248.

158. Clarke DH. Antigenic relationships among viruses of the tick-borne encephalitis complex as studied by antibody absorption and agar gel precipitin techniques. In: Libikova H, ed. *Biology of viruses of the tick-borne encephalitis complex.* New York: Academic Press, 1962;67–75.

159. Clarke DH. Further studies on antigenic relationships among the viruses of the group B tick-borne complex. *Bull WHO* 1964;31:45–56.

160. Clarke DH, Casals J. Arboviruses: group B. In: Horsfall FL, Tamer I, eds. *Viral and rickettsial infections of man.* Philadelphia: JB Lippincott, 1965;606–658.

161. Cerny V. The role of mammals in natural foci of tick-borne encephalitis in central Europe. *Folia Parasitol (Praha)* 1976;22:271–273.

162. Blaskovic D, Pucekova G, Kubinyi L. An epidemiological study of tick-borne encephalitis in the Tribec region: 1956–1963. *Bull WHO* 1967;36:89–94.

163. Gresikova M, Sekeyova M, Stupalova S, et al. Sheep milk-borne epidemic of tick-borne encephalitis in Slovakia. *Intervirology* 1975;5:57–61.

164. Scherer WF, Eddy GA, Monath TP, et al. Laboratory safety for arboviruses and certain other viruses of vertebrates. *Am J Trop Med Hyg* 1980;29:1359–1381.

165. Gresikova M, Beran GW. Tick-borne encephalitis. In: Beran GW, ed. *CRC handbook series in zoonoses, section B: viral zoonoses,* vol 1. Boca Raton, FL: CRC Press, 1981;201–208.

166. Galant IB. Certain features of the course of contemporary Far Eastern tick-borne encephalitis. *Probl Virol* 1959;4:66–68.

167. Radsel-Medvescek A, Marolt-Gomiscek M, Gajsek-Zima M. Clinical characteristics of patients with TBE treated at the University Medical Centre Hospital for infectious diseases in Ljubljana during the years 1974 and 1977. *Zentralbl Bakteriol [Suppl]* 1980;9:277–280.

168. Radsel-Medvescek A, Marolt-Gomiscek M, Povse-Trojar M, Gajsek-Zima M. Late sequelae after tickborne meningoencephalitis in patients treated at the hospital for infectious diseases university medical centre of Ljubljana during the period 1974–1975. *Zentralbl Bakteriol [Suppl]* 1980;9:281–284.

169. Kunz C, Moritsch H. Zur serologischen diagnostik der fruhsommer-meningoencephalitis (FSME). *Arch Gesamte Virusforsch* 1961–1962;11:568–582.

170. Roggendorf M, Heinz F, Deinhardi F, et al. Serological diagnosis of acute tick-borne encephalitis by demonstration of antibodies of the IgM class. *J Med Virol* 1981;7:41–50.

171. Levkovich EN. Experimental and epidemiological bases of the specific prophylaxis of tick-borne encephalitis. In: Libikova H, ed. *Biology of the tick-borne encephalitis complex.* New York: Academic Press, 1962;317–330.

172. Kunz C, Heinz FX, Hofmann H. Immunogenicity and reactige-

nicity of a highly purified vaccine against tick-borne encephalitis. *J Med Virol* 1980;6:103–109.

173. Blaskovic D, Nosek J. The ecological approach to the study of tick-borne encephalitis. *Prog Med Virol* 1972;14:275–320.

174. McLean DM, Donohue WL. Powassan virus: isolation of virus from a fatal case of encephalitis. *Can Med Assoc J* 1959;80:708.

175. Casals J. Antigenic relationship between Powassan and Russian spring–summer encephalitis viruses. *Can Med Assoc J* 1960;82:355.

176. McLean DM, Smith PA, Livingstone SE. Powassan virus: vernal spread during 1965. *Can Med Assoc J* 1966;94:532–536.

177. Deibel R, Glanagan TD, Smith V. Central nervous system infections in New York State: etiologic and epidemiologic observations, 1974. *NY State J Med* 1975;75:2337.

178. Artsob H. Powassan encephalitis. In: Monath TP, ed. *The arboviruses: ecology and epidemiology,* vol IV. Boca Raton, FL: CRC Press, 1988;29–50.

179. Artsob H, Spence L, Surgeoner G, et al. Isolation of *Francisella tularensis* and Powassan virus from ticks (Acari: Ixodidae) in Ontario, Canada. *J Med Entomol* 1984;21:165–168.

180. Webb HE, Connolly JH, Kane FF, et al. Laboratory infections with louping ill with associated encephalitis. *Lancet* 1968;2:255–258.

181. Williams H, Thorburn H. Serum antibodies to louping ill virus. *Scott Med J* 1962;7:353–355.

182. Edward DG. Immunization against louping ill. Immunization of man. *Br J Exp Pathol* 1948;29:372–378.

183. Lawson JH, Mauderson WG, Hurst EW. Louping-ill meningoencephalitis. A further case and a serological survey. *Lancet* 1949;2:696–699.

184. Likar M, Dane DS. An illness resembling acute poliomyelitis caused by a virus of the Russian spring–summer encephalitis/louping ill group in Northern Ireland. *Lancet* 1958;1:456–468.

185. Ando K, Kuratsuka K, Arima S, et al. Studies on the viruses isolated during epidemic of Japanese B encephalitis in 1948 in Tokyo area. *Kitasato Arch Exp Med* 1952;24:49–61.

186. Okuno T, Oya A, Ho T. The identification of Negishi virus: a presumably new member of Russian spring–summer encephalitis virus family isolated in Japan. *Jpn J Med Sci Biol* 1961;14:51–59.

187. Heinz FX. Epitope mapping of flavivirus glycoproteins. *Adv Virus Res* 1986;31:103–168.

188. Gonzalez-Scarano F, Nathanson N. Bunyaviruses. In: Fields BN, Knipe DM, eds. *Virology,* 2nd ed. New York: Raven Press, 1990;1195–1228.

189. Bishop DHL. Replication of arenaviruses and bunyaviruses. In: Fields BN, Knipe DM, eds. *Virology,* 2nd ed. New York: Raven Press, 1990;1083–1110.

190. Peters CJ, LeDuc JW. Bunyaviruses, phleboviruses and related viruses. In: Belshe RB, ed. *Textbook of human virology.* Littleton, MA: PSG Publishing Co., 1984;547–598.

191. Hrzinek MC. The structure of togaviruses and bunyaviruses. *Med Biol* 1975;53:406–411.

192. Murphy FA, Whitfield SG, Coleman PH, Calisher CH. California group arboviruses: electron microscopic studies. *Exp Mol Pathol* 1968;9:44–56.

193. Murphy FA, Harrison AK, Whitfield SG. Bunyaviridae: morphologic and morphogenetic similarities of Bunyamwera serologic supergroup viruses and several other arthropod-borne viruses. *Intervirology* 1973;1:297–316.

194. Pettersson R, Kaariainen L. The ribonucleic acids of Uukuniemi virus, a noncubical tick-borne arbovirus. *Virology* 1973;56:608–619.

195. Pettersson RF, von Bonsdorff C-H. Bunyaviridae. In: Nermut MV, Steven AC, eds. *Animal virus structure.* Amsterdam: Elsevier, 1987;147–157.

196. Pettersson RF, von Bonsdorff C-H. Ribonucleoproteins of Uukuniemi virus are circular. *J Virol* 1975;15:386–392.

197. Pettersson R, Kaariainen L, von Bonsdorff C-H, Oker-Blom N. Structural components of Uukuniemi virus, a noncubical tick-borne arbovirus. *Virology* 1971;46:721–729.

198. Bishop DHL, Shope RE. Bunyaviridae. In: Fraenkel-Conrat H, Wagner RR, eds. *Comprehensive virology,* vol 14. New York: Plenum Press, 1979;1–156.

199. Smith JF, Pifat DY. Morphogenesis of sandfly fever viruses (Bunyaviridae family). *Virology* 1982;121:61-81.

200. Obijeski JF, Murphy FA. Bunyaviridae: recent biochemical developments. *J Gen Virol* 1977;37:1-14.

201. Bishop DHL. Genetic potential of bunyaviruses. In: Arber W, Falkow S, Henle W, eds. *Current topics in microbiology and immunobiology.* Berlin: Springer-Verlag, 1979;1-33.

202. Iroegbu CU, Pringle CR. Genetics of the Bunyamwera complex. In: Bishop DHL, Compans RW, eds. *The replication of negative strand viruses. Developments in cell biology,* vol 7. New York: Elsevier/North-Holland, 1981;159-172.

203. Dalrymple JM, Peters CJ, Smith JF, et al. Antigenic components of Punta Toro virus. In: Bishop DHL, Compans RW, eds. *The replication of negative strand viruses. Developments in cell biology,* vol 7. New York: Elsevier/North-Holland, 1981;167-172.

204. Gonzalez-Scarano F, Shope RE, Calisher CH, et al. Characterization of monoclonal antibodies against the G1 and N proteins of La Crosse and Tahyna, two California serogroup bunyaviruses. *Virology* 1982;120:42-53.

205. Kuismanen E, Hedman K, Saraste J, Pettersson RF. Uujuniemi virus maturation; accumulation of virus particles and viral antigens in the Golgi complex. *Mol Cell Biol* 1982;2:1444-1458.

206. Kuismanen E, Bang B, Hume M, Pettersson RF. Uukuniemi virus maturation: immunofluorescence microscopy with monoclonal glycoprotein-specific antibodies. *J Virol* 1984;51:137-146.

207. Kurogi H, Inaba Y, Takahashi E, et al. Epizootic congenital arthrogryposis–hydranencephaly syndrome in cattle: isolation of Akabana virus from affected fetuses. *Arch Virol* 1976;51:67-74.

208. Bishop DHL, Rudd E, Belloncik S, et al. Coding analyses of bunyavirus RNA species. In: Compans RW, Bishop DHL, eds. *Segmented negative strand viruses.* Orlando, FL: Academic Press, 1984;3-11.

209. Bishop DHL, Fuller F, Akashi H, et al. The use of reassortant bunyaviruses to deduce their coding and pathogenic potentials. In: Kohn A, Fuchs P, eds. *Mechanisis of virus pathogenesis.* Boston: Martinus Nijhoff, 1984;49-60.

210. Shope RE. Bunyaviruses. In: Fields BN, Knipe DM, eds. *Virology.* New York: Raven Press, 1985;1055-1082.

211. Balfour HH Jr, Siem RA, Bauer H, et al. California arbovirus (LaCrosse) infections. I. Clinical and laboratory findings in 66 children with meningoencephalitis. *Pediatrics* 1973;52:680-691.

212. Kalfayan B. Pathology of La Crosse virus infection in humans. In: Calisher CH, Thompson WH, eds. *California serogroup viruses,* vol 123. New York: Alan R Liss, 1983;179-186.

213. LeDuc JW. The ecology of California group viruses. *J Med Entomol* 1979;16:1-17.

214. Thompson WH, Kalfayan B, Anslow RO. Isolation of California encephalitis group virus from a fatal human illness. *Am J Epidemiol* 1965;81:245-253.

215. Hammon WMcD, Reeves WC. California encephalitis virus—a newly described agent. I. Evidence of natural infection in man and other animals. *Calif Med* 1952;77:303-309.

216. Kappus KD, Monath TP, Kaminski RM, et al. Reported encephalitis associated with California serogroup virus infections in the United States, 1963-1981. In: Calisher CH, Thompson WH, eds. *California serogroup viruses.* New York: Alan R Liss, 1983;31-41.

217. LeDuc JW, Suyemoto W, Keefe TJ, Burger JF, Eldridge BF, Russell PK. Ecology of California encephalitis viruses on the Del Mar Va Peninsula. I. Virus isolation from mosquitoes. *Am J Trop Med Hyg* 1975;24:118-123.

218. Turell MJ, LeDuc JW. The role of mosquitoes in the natural history of California serogroup viruses. In: Calisher CH, Thompson WH, eds. *California serogroup viruses.* New York: Alan R Liss, 1983;43-56.

219. Yuill TM. The role of mammals in the maintenance and dissemination of La Crosse virus. In: Calisher CH, Thompson WH, eds. *California serogroup viruses.* New York: Alan R Liss, 1983;77-88.

220. Calisher CH. Toxonomy, classification, and geographia distribution of California serogroup bunyaviruses. In: Calisher CH, Thompson WH, eds. *California serogroup viruses,* vol 123. New York: Alan R Liss, 1983;1-16.

221. El Said LHE, Vorndam V, Gentsch JR, et al. A comparison of La Crosse virus isolates obtained from different ecological niches and an analysis of the structural components of California encephalitis serogroup viruses and other bunyaviruses. *Am J Trop Med Hyg* 1979;28:364-386.

222. Klimas RA, Thompson WH, Calisher CH, et al. Genotypic varieties of La Crosse virus isolated from different geographic regions of the continental United States and evidence for a naturally occurring intertypic recombinant La Crosse virus. *Am J Epidemiol* 1981;114:112-131.

223. Henderson BE, Coleman Ph. The growing importance of California arboviruses in the etiology of human disease. *Prog Med Virol* 1971;13:404-461.

224. Monath TPC, Nuckolls JG, Berall J, Bauer H, Chappell WA, Coleman PH. Studies of California encephalitis in Minnesota. *Am J Epidemiol* 1970;92:40-50.

225. Thompson WH, Evans AS. California encephalitis virus studies in Wisconsin. *Am J Epidemiol* 1965;81:230-244.

226. Kappus KD, Calisher CH, Baron RC, et al. La Crosse virus infection and disease in western North Carolina. *Am J Trop Med Hyg* 1982;31:556-560.

227. Rowley WA, Wong YW, Dorsey DE, et al. California serogroup viruses in Iowa. In: Calisher CH, Thompson WH, eds. *California serogroup viruses,* vol 123. New York: Alan R Liss, 1983;237-246.

228. Young DJ. California encephalitis virus. *Ann Intern Med* 1966;65:419-428.

229. Cramblett HG, Stegmiller H, Spencer C. California encephalitis virus infections in children. *JAMA* 1966;198:128-132.

230. Gundersen CB, Brown KL. Clinical aspects of LaCrosse encephalitis: preliminary report. In: Calisher CH, Thompson WH, eds. *California serogroup viruses,* vol 123. New York: Alan R Liss, 1983;169-177.

231. Matthews CG, Chun RWM, Grabow JD, et al. Psychological sequelae in children following California arbovirus encephalitis. *Neurology* 1968;18:1023-1030.

232. Sabatino DA, Cramblett HG. Behavioral sequelae of California encephalitis virus infection in children. *Dev Med Child Neurol* 1968;10:331-337.

233. Grabow JD, Matthews CG, Chun RWM, et al. The electroencephalogram and clinical sequelae of California arbovirus encephalitis. *Neurology* 1969;19:394-404.

234. Chun RWM. Clinical aspects of La Crosse encephalitis; neurological and phychological sequelae. In: Calisher CH, Thompson WH, eds. *California serogroup viruses.* New York: Alan R Liss, 1983;193-201.

235. Chun RWM, Thompson WH, Grabow JD, et al. California arbovirus encephalitis in children. *Neurology* 1968;18:369-375.

236. Janssen RS, Nathanson N, Enders MJ, Gonzalez-Scarano F. Virulence of La Crosse virus is under polygenic control. *J Virol* 1986;59:1-7.

237. Deering WM. Neurologic aspects and treatment of La Crosse encephalitis. In: Calisher CH, Thompson WH, eds. *California serogroup viruses,* vol 123. New York: Alan R Liss, 1983;187-191.

238. Rie HE, Hilty MD, Cramblett HG. Intelligence and coordination following California encephalitis. *Am J Dis Child* 1973;125:824-827.

239. Whitley RJ, Cobbs CG, Alford CA, Soong SJ, Morawetz R, Benton JW, Hirsch MS, Reichman RC, Aoki FY, Connor J, Oxman M, Corey L, Hanley DF, Wright PF, Levin M, Nahmias A, Powell DA, and the NIAID Collaborative Antiviral Study Group. Diseases that mimic herpes simplex encephalitis: diagnosis, presentation and outcome. *JAMA* 1989;262:234-239.

240. Lindsey HS, Calisher CH, Mathews JH. Serum dilution neutralization test for California group virus identification and serology. *J Clin Microbiol* 1976;4:503-510.

241. Calisher CH, Bailey RE. Serodiagnosis of LaCrosse virus infections in humans. *J Clin Microbiol* 1981;13:344-350.

242. Beaty BJ, Jamnback TL, Hildreth SW, et al. Rapid diagnosis of La Crosse virus infections: evaluation of serologic and antigen detection techniques for the clinically relevant diagnosis of La Crosse encephalitis. In: Calisher CH, Thompson WH, eds. *Cali-*

fornia serogroup viruses, vol 123. New York: Alan R Liss, 1983;293–302.

243. Rosicky B, Malkova D, eds. *Tahyna virus natural focus in southern Moravia.* Prague: Academia Praha, 1980.

244. Bardos V, Ryba J, Hubalek Z. Isolation of Tahyna virus from filed collected *Culiseta annulata* (Schrk) larvae. *Acta Virol* 1975;19:446.

245. Bardos V, Cupkova E, Sefcovicova L. Serological study on the medical importance of Tahyna virus. In: Bardos V, eds. *Arboviruses of the California complex and the Bunyamwera group.* Bratislava: Publishing House of the Slovak Academy of Sciences, 1969;301–308.

246. Likar M, Sasals J. Isolation from man in Slovenia of a virus belonging to the California complex of arthropod-borne viruses. *Nature* 1963;197:1131.

247. Mayerova A, Hruzik J, Mayer V. Tahyna virus neutralizing antibody levels in cases of acute febrile illness. In: Bardos V, eds. *Arboviruses of the California complex and the Bunyamwera group.* Bratislava: Publishing House of the Slovak Academy of Sciences, 1969;305–308.

248. Deibel R, Srihongse S, Grayson MA, et al. Jamestown Canyon virus: the etiologic agent of an emerging human disease? In: Calisher CH, Thompson WH, eds. *California serogroup viruses.* New York: Alan R Liss, 1983;313–328.

249. Smirnova SE, Shestopalova NM, Reingold VN, Zubri GL, Chumakov MP. Experimental Hazara virus infection in mice. *Acta Virol* 1977;21:128–132.

250. Artsob H. Distribution of California serogroup viruses and virus infection in Canada. In: Calisher CH, Thompson WH, eds. *California serogroup viruses.* New York: Alan R Liss, 1983;277:292.

251. Srihongse S, Grayson MA, Deibel R. California serogroup viruses in New York State: the role of subtypes in human infections. *Am J Trop Med Hyg* 1984;33:1218–1227.

252. Meegan JM. The Rift Valley fever epizootic in Egypt 1977–78. I. Description of the epizootic and virological studies. *Trans R Soc Trop Med Hyg* 1979;73:618–623.

253. Georges AJ, Saluzzo JF, Gonzalez JP, et al. Arboviroses en Centrafrique: incidence et aspects diagnostiques chez l'homme. *Med Trop (Mars)* 1980;40:561–568.

254. Daubney R, Hudson JR, Garnham PC. Enzootic hepatitis or Rift Valley fever. An undescribed virus disease of sheep, cattle and man from East Africa. *East Afr Med J* 1933;10:2–19.

255. Peters CJ, Meegan JM. Rift Valley fever. In: Steele JH, ed. *CRC handbook series in zoonoses,* vol 1. Boca Raton, FL: CRC Press, 1981;403–420.

256. Smithburn KC, Mahaffy AF, Haddow AJ, et al. Rift Valley fever. Accidental infections among laboratory workers. *J Immunol* 1949;62:213–227.

257. Francis T Jr, Magill TP. Rift Valley fever. A report of three cases of laboratory infection and the experimental transmission of the disease to ferrets. *J Exp Med* 1935;62:433–448.

258. McIntosh BM, Russell D, Dos Santos I, et al. Rift Valley fever in humans in South Africa. *S Afr Med J* 1980;58:803–806.

259. Tomori O. Rift Valley fever virus infection in man in Nigeria. *J Med Virol* 1980;5:343–350.

260. Digoutte JP, Jacobi JC, Robin Y, et al. Infection a virus Zinga Chez L'Homme. *Bull Soc Pathol Exot Filiates* 1974;67:451–457.

261. Meegan JM, Shope RE. Emerging concepts on Rift Valley fever. *Perspect Virol* 1981;11:267–287.

262. Siam AL, Meegan JM, Gharbawi KF. Rift Valley fever ocular manifestations: observations during the 1977 epidemic in Egypt. *Br J Ophthalmol* 1980;64:366–374.

263. Laughlin LW, Meegan JM, Strausbaugh LH, Morens DM, Watten RH. Epidemic Rift Valley fever in Egypt: observations of the spectrum of human illness. *Trans R Soc Trop Med Hyg* 1979;73:630–633.

264. Van Velken DJJ, Meyer JD, Oliver J, et al. Rift Valley fever affecting humans in South Africa. A clinicopathological study. *S Afr Med J* 1977;51:867–871.

265. Boctor WM. The clinical picture of Rift Valley fever in Egypt. In: El-Kholy S, ed. *Journal of the Egyptian Public Health Association,* vol 53. Cairo: Ain Shams University Press, 1979;177–180.

266. Maar SA, Swanepoel R, Gelfand M. Rift Valley fever encephalitis. A description of a case. *Cent Afr J Med* 1979;25:8–11.

267. Meegan JM, Watten RH, Laughlin LW. Clinical experience with Rift Valley fever in humans during the 1977 Egyptian epizootic. *Contrib Epidemiol Biostat* 1981;3:114–123.

268. Chambers PG, Swanepoel R. Rift Valley fever in abattoir workers. *Cent Afr J Med* 1980;26:122–126.

269. Hoogstraal H, Meegan JM, Khalil GM, Adham FK. The Rift Valley fever epizootic in Egypt 1977–1978. 2. Ecological and entomological studies. *Trans R Soc Trop Med Hyg* 1979;73:624–629.

270. Shope RE, Peters CJ, Dives FG. The spread of Rift Valley fever and approaches to its control. *Bull WHO* 1982;60:299–304.

271. Eddy GA, Peters CJ. The extended horizons of Rift Valley fever: current and projected immunogens. In: *New developments with human and veterinary vaccines.* New York: Alan R Liss, 1980;179–191.

272. Eddy GA, Peters CJ, Meadors G, Cole FE Jr. Rift Valley fever vaccine for humans. *Contrib Epidemiol Biostat* 1981;3:124–141.

273. Kark JD, Aynor Y, Peters CJ. A Rift Valley fever vaccine trial. I. Side effects and serologic response over a six-month follow-up. *Am J Epidemiol* 1982;116:808–819.

274. Randall R, Gibbs CJ Jr, Aulisio CG, Binn LN, Harrison VR. The development of a formalin-killed Rift Valley fever virus vaccine for use in man. *J Immunol* 1962;89:660–671.

275. Casals J. Antigenic classification of arthropod-borne viruses. *Proc 6th Int Congress Trop Med Malaria* 1959;5:34–37.

276. Studdert MJ. Sensitivity of bluetongue virus to ether and sodium deoxycholate. *Proc Soc Exp Biol Med* 1965;118:1106–1009.

277. Verwoerd DW. Purification and characterization of bluetongue virus. *Virology* 1969;38:203–212.

278. Berge TO, ed. *International catalogue of Arboviruses including certain other viruses of vertebrates,* 2nd ed. DHEW publication 75:8301. Washington, DC: DHEW, 1975.

279. Borden EC, Shope RE, Murphy FA. Physicochemical and morphological relationships of some arthropod-borne viruses to bluetongue virus—a new taxonomic group: physicochemical and serological studies. *J Gen Virol* 1971;13:261–271.

280. Karabatsos N, ed. *International catalogue of arboviruses including certain other viruses of vertebrates,* 3rd ed. San Antonio, TX: The American Society of Tropical Medicine and Hygiene, 1985.

281. Murphy FA, Borden EC, Shope RE, Harrison A. Physicochemical and morphological relationships of some arthropod-borne viruses to bluetongue virus—a new taxonomic group. Electron microscopic studies. *J Gen Virol* 1971;13:273–278.

282. Knudson DL, Monath TP. Orbiviruses. In: Fields BN, Knipe DM, eds. *Virology.* New York: Raven Press, 1990;1405–1433.

283. Murphy FA, Coleman PH, Harrison AK, Gary GW Jr. Colorado tick fever virus: an electron microscopic study. *Virology* 1968;35:28–40.

284. McKee KT Jr, Peters CJ, Craven RB, Francy DB. Other viral hemorrhagic fevers and colorado tick fever. In: Belshe RB, ed. *Textbook of human virology.* Littleton, MA: PSG Publishing Co., 1984;649–677.

285. Knudson DL. Genome of Colorado tick fever. *Virology* 1981;112:361–364.

286. Barber TL, Jochim MM. Bluetongue and related orbiviruses. In: *Progress in clinical and biological research,* vol 178. New York: Alan R Liss, 1985;1–746.

287. Gorman BM, Taylor J, Walker PJ. Orbiviruses. In: Joklik WK, ed. *The Reoviridae,* New York: Plenum Press, 1983;287–357.

288. Martin SA, Zweerink HJ. Isolation and characterization of two types of bluetongue virus particles. *Virology* 1972;50:495–506.

289. Verwoerd DW, Els HJ, De Villier E, Huismans H. Structure of the bluetongue virus capsid. *J Virol* 1972;10:783–794.

290. Becker FE. Tick-borne infections in Colorado. I. The diagnosis and management of infections transmitted by the wood tick. *Colo Med* 1930;27:36.

291. Becker FE. Tick-borne infections in Colorado. II. A survey of the occurrence of infections transmitted by the wood tick. *Colo Med* 1980;27:87.

292. Florio L, Stewart MO, Mugrage ER. The experimental transmission of Colorado tick fever. *J Exp Med* 1944;80:165–188.

293. Florio L, Miller MS, Mugrage ER. Colorado tick fever. Isolation of the virus from *Dermacentor andersoni* in nature and a labora-

tory study of the transmission of the virus in the tick. *J Immunol* 1950;64:257–263.

294. Black WC, Florio L, Stewart MO. A histologic study of the reaction in the hamster spleen produced by the virus of Colorado tick fever. *Am J Pathol* 1947;23:217–224.

295. Johnson ES, Napoli VM, White WC. Colorado tick fever as a hematologic problem. *Am J Clin Pathol* 1960;34:118–124.

296. Emmons RW. Experimental Colorado tick fever virus infection in wild rodents: viremia and antibody response in active and hibernating animals. PhD Thesis, University of California, Berkeley, 1965.

297. Emmons RW. Colorado tick-fever: prolonged viremia in hibernating *Citellus lateralis. Am J Trop Med Hyg* 1966;15:428–433.

298. Burgdorfer W, Eklund CM. Studies on the ecology of Colorado tick fever virus in western Montana. *Am J Hyg* 1959;69:127–137.

299. Eklund CM, Kohls GM, Jellison WL. Isolation of Colorado tick fever virus from rodents in Colorado. *Science* 1958;128:413.

300. Burgdorfer W. Colorado tick fever. I. The behavior of CTF virus in the porcupine. *J Infect Dis* 1959;104:101–104.

301. Burgdorfer W. Colorado tick fever. II. The behavior of CTF virus in rodents. *J Infect Dis* 1960;107:384–388.

302. Emmons RW, Oshuo LS, Johnson HN, Lennette EH. Intraerythrocytic location of Colorado tick fever virus. *J Gen Virol* 1972;17:185–195.

303. Hughes LE, Casper EA, Clifford CM. Persistence of Colorado tick fever virus in red blood cells. *Am J Trop Med Hyg* 1974;23:530–532.

304. Eklund CM, Kennedy RC, Casey M. Colorado tick fever. *Rocky Mountain Med J* 1961;58:21–25.

305. Goodpasture HC, Poland JD, Francy DB, Bowen GS, Horn KA. Colorado tick fever: clinical epidemiology and laboratory aspects of 228 cases in Colorado in 1973–1974. *Ann Intern Med* 1978;88:303–310.

306. Squire KR, Chuang RY, Osburn BI, Knudson DL, Doi RH. Rapid methods for comparing the double-stranded RNA genome profiles of bluetongue virus. *Vet Microbiol* 1983;8:543–553.

307. Philip RN, Casper EA, Cory J, Whitlock J. The potential for transmission of arboviruses by blood transfusion with particular reference to Colorado tick fever. In: Greenwalt J, Janieson GA, eds. *Transmissible disease and blood transfusions.* New York: Grune & Stratton, 1975;175–196.

308. Drevets CC. Colorado tick fever. *J Kansas Med Soc* 1957;58:448–455.

309. Eklund CM, Kohls GM, Jellison WL, Burgdorfer W, Kennedy RC, Thomas L. The clinical and ecological aspects of Colorado tick fever. In: *Proceedings of the 6th international congress on tropical medicine and malaria,* September 5–13, 1958. Lisbon, Portugal: Inst. Med Trop., 1958;197–203.

310. Fraaer CH, Scheff DW. Colorado tick fever encephalitis. Report of a case. *Pediatrics* 1962;29:187–190.

311. Hughes LE, Casper EA, Clifford CM. Persistence of Colorado tick fever virus in red blood cells. *Am J Trop Med Hyg* 1974;23:530–532.

Infections of the Central Nervous System,
edited by W. M. Scheld, R. J. Whitley, and
D. T. Durack, Raven Press, Ltd., New York © 1991.

CHAPTER 6

Meningitis and Encephalitis Caused by Mumps Virus

John W. Gnann, Jr.

Mumps is a systemic human infection caused by a paramyxovirus. Mumps virus is highly transmissible and, in unimmunized populations, causes epidemics of mumps among school-aged children. Although salivary gland enlargement, especially parotitis, is the most readily recognized clinical manifestation of mumps, the infection involves many other organs, including the central nervous system (CNS). In the past, nonsuppurative parotitis was considered to be the *sine qua non* of mumps, and involvement of any other organ system was viewed as a complication. However, studies conducted over the last 50 years have made it clear that CNS involvement during mumps occurs with such high frequency that it should be considered a part of the natural history of the infection and not as an aberrant manifestation or complication. Indeed, some authors have classified the mumps virus as primarily neurotropic.

The spectrum of CNS diseases associated with mumps ranges from mild aseptic meningitis, which is very common, to fulminant and potentially fatal encephalitis, which is very rare. The literature describing CNS involvement with mumps can be difficult to critically assess because some authors have grouped together all cases of mumps neurologic disease under the label "mumps meningoencephalitis." Although this term is convenient, its use tends to obscure the fact that the clinical course and prognosis of mumps aseptic meningitis differs from that of mumps encephalitis, although there is considerable overlap between the two syndromes. It is important for the clinician to establish whether an individual patient has clear evidence of encephalitis, since

that diagnosis has important implications for management and prognosis (1).

HISTORY

Although a syndrome of epidemic febrile parotitis was recognized by Hippocrates in the 5th century B.C., Hamilton (2) was the first to describe the association between mumps and CNS symptoms in 1790. Hamilton also provided the first description of the neuropathology of a fatal case of mumps. In the early part of the 20th century, Monod (3; also see ref. 4) noted increased numbers of leukocytes in the spinal fluids of six of eight patients with mumps, thereby establishing the association between mumps and aseptic meningitis. In their series of classic studies, Johnson and Goodpasture (5) used filtrates of saliva from patients with mumps to transmit infection to monkeys, thereby establishing the viral nature of the pathogen. The discovery by Habel (6) that mumps virus could be cultivated in embryonated eggs permitted investigators to begin to characterize the virus *in vitro. In vitro* isolation was made more practical by the discovery by Henle and Deinhardt (7) that mumps virus could be cultivated in tissue culture. The role of mumps virus in CNS infection was established by experimental transmission of infection to monkeys by cerebrospinal fluid (CSF) from patients with mumps (8). Mumps virus was subsequently isolated from CSF, first in embryonated eggs (9) and later in tissue culture (10). Serodiagnosis and seroepidemiological studies became feasible in 1945 with the development of the complement-fixation antibody test by Kane and Enders (11). The modern era of mumps prevention began in 1966 with the development by Buynak and Hilleman (12) of an effective live, attenuated mumps virus vaccine.

J. W. Gnann, Jr.: Departments of Medicine and Microbiology, Division of Infectious Diseases, University of Alabama at Birmingham, Birmingham, Alabama 35294.

INFECTIOUS AGENT

Mumps virus is classified as a member of the family Paramyxoviridae in the genus *Paramyxovirus* (which also includes parainfluenza virus and Newcastle disease virus). Mumps virions are pleomorphic, irregularly spherical, enveloped particles with an average diameter of about 200 nm (13). Glycoprotein spikes project from the outer surface of the envelope, which encloses a helical nucleocapsid composed of RNA and nucleoproteins (14). The mumps virus genome is contained in a linear molecule of single-stranded, negative-sense RNA. The virus is composed of five major proteins: Nucleocapsid protein (NP) is the major structural protein; polymerase protein (P) appears to have RNA-dependent RNA-polymerase activity; matrix (M) protein is important in the assembly of virions; and two surface glycoproteins mediate hemagglutinin-neuraminidase (HN) and fusion (F) activities (15–18). The HN glycoprotein is responsible for attachment of mumps virus to the host cell, and the F glycoprotein induces the fusion of lipid membranes necessary for penetration of the virus nucleocapsid into the cell (15). There is also evidence that HN activity may modulate the neurovirulence of selected mumps isolates in animal models (19). An additional large (L) nucleocapsid-associated protein that may play a role in viral RNA synthesis has been observed by some investigators (20). There is only one serologic strain of mumps virus. The mumps complement-fixation test measures antibodies against the "viral" (V) and "soluble" (S) antigens, which are HN and NP, respectively.

Humans are the only known natural hosts for mumps virus, although infection can be experimentally induced in a wide variety of mammalian species (7,21). *In vitro,* mumps virus can be cultured in many mammalian cell lines, including monkey kidney, human embryonic kidney, BSC-1, Vero, and HeLa cells, as well as in embryonated hens' eggs. In tissue culture, the cytopathic effects caused by mumps virus are highly variable and include development of rounded cells, formation of intracytoplasmic inclusions, and fusion of cells to form syncytia (22). Guinea-pig erythrocytes will adhere to mumps-virus-infected cells, a phenomenon mediated by hemagglutinins present on the surface of infected cells. Verification of the isolate as mumps virus can be accomplished by a hemadsorption-inhibition assay, in which mumps immune serum is used to block the adherence of erythrocytes to mumps-infected epithelial cells. Direct and indirect immunofluorescence assays for detection of mumps antigens have also been developed (23).

EPIDEMIOLOGY

In unvaccinated urban populations, mumps is a disease of school-aged children (24). Mumps infrequently occurs in infants less than 1 year of age, presumably because of transplacentally acquired antibody (25). The largest number of mumps cases occurs in children between 4 and 7 years of age (24). By age 15, 92% of children have antibodies against mumps virus (26). Prior to the release of the live, attenuated mumps vaccine in the United States in 1967, mumps was an endemic disease with a seasonal peak of activity occurring between January and May (27). Mumps epidemics occurred at 2- to 5-year intervals (28). The largest number of cases reported in the United States was in 1941, when the incidence of mumps was 250 cases per 100,000 population (29). In 1968, when the live, attenuated vaccine was first entering clinical usage, the incidence of mumps was 76 cases per 100,000 population. In 1985, a total of only 2982 cases of mumps was reported, an incidence of 1.1 per 100,000 population, representing a 98% decline from the number of cases reported in 1967.

Between 1985 and 1987, the incidence of mumps in the United States increased fivefold to 5.2 cases per 100,000 population (29,30). More than one-third of the cases reported between 1985 and 1987 occurred in adolescents and young adults, reflecting the slow acceptance of universal mumps vaccination during the 1970s when this cohort of children grew up. This trend is important, since mumps generally causes a more severe disease in adults than in children. The increased incidence of mumps in susceptible young adults was most prominent in those states without comprehensive school immunization laws.

In an unimmunized population, mumps is one of the most common causes of aseptic meningitis and encephalitis. In a study conducted in Minnesota from 1950 to 1981, mumps was identified as the cause of encephalitis in six of 189 cases and the cause of aseptic meningitis in seven of 283 cases (31). In this series, mumps was the second most common cause of both encephalitis and aseptic meningitis (California virus and enteroviruses, respectively, were the most common causes). Meyer et al. (32) reviewed 713 cases of encephalitis and aseptic meningitis treated at U.S. military hospitals between 1953 and 1958. In those patients in whom a specific etiology was established, mumps was identified in 91 cases, poliomyelitis in 156, Coxsackie B virus in 80, lymphocytic choriomeningitis virus in 58, and echovirus in 53. In an analysis of 191 cases of encephalitis occurring in adults in Finland between 1967 and 1978, mumps was found to be the second most common etiology (following herpes simplex virus), accounting for 6.8% of the cases of acute encephalitis (33,34). These studies document that mumps virus can be a very important cause of aseptic meningitis and encephalitis in unvaccinated populations (35).

The frequency with which CNS manifestations occur during acute mumps has varied tremendously (from <1% to >70%) among published series (36–41). A more realistic estimate of the frequency of symptomatic CNS involvement during mumps appears to be 10–30%. Potential causes for this variability in reported incidence include the interest and skill of the observer, the population studied (e.g., school children versus military recruits, outpatients versus hospitalized patients, etc.), the case definitions used, and the frequency of use of lumbar puncture for diagnosis. Although differences in neurovirulence of mumps isolates have been noted in animal models (42,43), there is no clear evidence that differences in neurovirulence among wild-type mumps strains account for the variability in the reported incidence of CNS involvement in human mumps. Symptomatic encephalitis is observed much less frequently than aseptic meningitis, probably occurring in less than 0.1% of cases of acute mumps (1,44–46).

CSF pleocytosis occurs in 40–60% of patients with acute mumps, although only 10–30% of mumps patients will have clinical evidence of meningeal irritation. That is, about half of the mumps patients with CSF pleocytosis will not have CNS symptoms (40,47). Bang and Bang (37) performed lumbar punctures on 371 patients with mumps parotitis and found that 235 (63%) had elevated CSF white blood cell counts; of these 235 patients, 129 showed no clinical evidence of meningitis or encephalitis. Similarly, Finkelstein (48) found elevated CSF white blood cell counts in 16 of 40 patients (40%) with mumps parotitis; six of these had no clinical evidence of CNS involvement. If we accept that CSF pleocytosis occurring during acute mumps is indicative of CNS infection, then we must conclude that CNS involvement during mumps is quite common and frequently asymptomatic.

Clearly, mumps CNS disease can occur in patients without evidence of parotitis; indeed, 40–50% of patients with mumps meningitis have no evidence of salivary gland enlargement (49,50). Several authors have reported a predominance of mumps meningoencephalitis *with* parotitis occurring in the spring and a predominance of mumps meningoencephalitis *without* parotitis in the summer (11,49,51,52). Other authors have noted an increased incidence of CNS involvement with mumps during the spring and summer months, but they failed to note a seasonal association with the presence or absence of parotitis (45,53–55). In contrast, studies in Toronto established that most cases of mumps CNS disease in that city occurred between November and April (56,57).

Although males and females have the same incidence of mumps parotitis (58,59), there is a distinct male predominance (70–80%) with respect to development of CNS disease among children with mumps. In virtually every published series, the ratio of males to females is either 3:1 or 4:1 (40,45–47,54,55,60–63). This striking difference in the incidence of mumps CNS disease between the sexes has not been satisfactorily explained. Among young adults with mumps and CNS involve-

ment, the ratio of males to females is closer to 1:1 (63). The peak incidence of CNS involvement in mumps occurs at about age 7 in both sexes (46,51,63), with 60–70% of all cases occurring in children between 5 and 9 years of age (40,45,52,54,61,62).

PATHOGENESIS

Mumps is highly contagious, although some studies have suggested that it is less contagious than varicella or measles (64). This clinical observation may be skewed by the fact that up to 30% of all mumps infections are subclinical and asymptomatic (59). Over 90% of adults who give negative histories for mumps are, in fact, seropositive when tested for mumps antibodies, indicating prior subclinical infection (65).

Mumps can be experimentally transmitted to humans by inoculation of virus onto the nasal or buccal mucosa, suggesting that most natural infections result from droplet spread of upper respiratory secretions from infected to susceptible individuals. Virus can be isolated from saliva for 5–6 days prior to, and up to 5 days after, the onset of clinical symptoms, meaning that an infected individual is potentially able to transmit mumps for a period of about 10 days (66). The average incubation period for mumps is 18 days (67). During this interval, primary viral replication is thought to take place in epithelial cells of the upper respiratory tract, followed by spread of virus to regional lymph nodes and subsequent viremia with systemic dissemination (68,69).

Mumps virus disseminates readily to the CNS. Infection is transmitted to the CNS either via free plasma viremia or, more likely, by infected host mononuclear cells (70,71). Virus is thought to spread across the endothelium of the choroid plexus and to infect choroidal epithelial cells. Replication of mumps virus then takes place in the choroidal epithelium, and progeny virus is shed into the CSF. In support of this model are the observations that mumps virus can be easily recovered from CSF during the early phases of mumps meningitis (10) and that choroidal and ependymal epithelial cells containing mumps antigens can be recovered from the CSF of patients with mumps meningoencephalitis (72–74). Replication of mumps virus in the choroid plexus and ependyma (the tissue that lines the cerebral ventricles and covers the choroid plexus) has been demonstrated in rodent (70) and primate (43) models of mumps CNS infection. In instances where mumps encephalitis develops, it is presumed that virus replicating in ependymal cells spreads by direct extension into neurons within the brain parenchyma. This pattern of spread of mumps virus within the brain along neuronal pathways has been demonstrated in the hamster model of mumps encephalitis (75).

Investigators have proposed different theories to explain the pathogenesis of mumps encephalitis (76).

There has been some controversy as to whether mumps encephalitis is best described as primary destruction of neurons by mumps virus or as a postinfectious encephalitis with demyelinization. Because mumps encephalitis is rarely fatal, there have been only a small number of brains available for detailed neuropathologic studies to help resolve the issue. Recovery of mumps virus from brain tissue following a fatal case of encephalitis has been reported in only one instance (77).

Autopsy reports of patients who have died with acute encephalitis due to mumps virus have been reviewed by Donohue (78) and by Schwarz et al. (76). Many of these cases occurred prior to the availability of virologic or serologic methods for confirmation of the diagnosis, and some were likely caused by pathogens other than mumps virus. Among those cases in which mumps virus was the probable etiology of the fatal encephalitis, neuropathologic findings were quite variable (40,76,78,79). The most commonly recorded features were diffuse edema of the brain, limited mononuclear cell infiltration of the meninges, perivascular infiltration with mononuclear cells, glial cell proliferation, focal areas of neuronal cell destruction, and localized demyelinization. These histologic changes were seen in the white matter of the cerebral hemispheres and cerebellum and in the white and gray matter of the brainstem and spinal cord. Because of the pattern of perivascular demyelinization, Donohue (78) and Schwarz et al. (76) suggested that these findings were more suggestive of a postinfectious or parainfectious encephalopathy than of tissue destruction caused directly by mumps virus. Conversely, other authors have interpreted the findings of cellular destruction as being consistent with primary mumps virus cytopathic effect (80). In most cases of fatal mumps encephalitis that have been carefully studied, there has been histologic evidence of both cellular destruction (suggestive of direct virus effect) and demyelinization (suggestive of an autoimmune process). The pathogenesis of mumps encephalitis remains incompletely understood.

Investigations utilizing animal models of mumps, especially the hamster model, have made major contributions to our understanding of the pathogenesis of mumps CNS disease. CNS mumps infections have been produced experimentally by the intracerebral or intraperitoneal inoculation of newborn hamsters with a neuroadapted strain of mumps virus (70,81–84). About 9–12 days after intracerebral inoculation with mumps virus, suckling hamsters developed wasting, ruffled hair, and arched backs and usually died within 24 hr. Maximum titers of mumps virus were detected in hamster brains at 5 days, and the virus titer declined as neutralizing antibodies appeared. The clinical symptoms occurred 3–5 days after the decline in virus titers and the concurrent development of neutralizing antibody (84). During the first week after virus inoculation, the neuropathologic appearance of the brain was characterized by intense perivascular mononuclear cell infiltrates. During the second week, microglial cell proliferation and small areas of necrosis were observed. Notably, no foci of demyelinization (as has been observed in human brains) were apparent.

Immunofluorescence studies of suckling hamster brains following intracerebral inoculation with mumps virus showed that mumps virus antigens were present in endothelial cells of the choroid plexus, in ependymal cells, and in neurons of the brainstem, hippocampus, and cerebral cortex. Most of the infected neurons were morphologically normal, and there was little correlation between the major sites of neuronal infection and the observed sites of perivascular inflammation (84). The histological appearance of mumps encephalitis in suckling hamsters is more consistent with direct virus-induced pathology than with immunologically mediated pathologic changes.

Johnson and Johnson (85–87) were the first to observe a possible link between mumps virus infection and hydrocephalus. When suckling hamsters were intracerebrally inoculated with a non-neuroadapted strain of mumps virus, the animals survived the acute infection but developed aqueductal stenosis and hydrocephalus about 21 days after inoculation (86). Immunofluorescent staining of brain sections showed that mumps virus replication was limited almost entirely to the ependymal cells. Loss of ependymal cells began on day 9, and by day 11 ependymal cells had been lost from large areas of the ventricular surface (86). Hamster brains examined 21 days after inoculation showed severe stenosis or occlusion of the aqueduct of Sylvius and gross dilation of the lateral and third ventricles. When hamsters were inoculated with mumps virus plus mumps immune serum, the aqueductal stenosis failed to develop (86). The neuropathologic changes observed in this animal model system bear strong resemblances to changes observed in some human cases of aqueductal stenosis (86). Stenosis of the aqueduct of Sylvius is a common cause of human hydrocephalus that occurs most often in infancy (but is also seen in older children and adults) and that is most often considered idiopathic. Aqueductal stenosis has been noted to occur in several children 1–2 years after an episode of mumps (88–91), although it is difficult to establish with certainty a cause–effect relationship between the two events.

Intracerebral inoculation of mumps virus into adult hamsters caused acute encephalitis with ependymitis, but it did not result in the development of hydrocephalus (92). A histologic survey of 100 consecutive adult human brains showed that 65% had a benign finding known as "granular ependymitis," which had many of the characteristics seen in the focal ependymal lesions of adult rodents infected with mumps virus (92). This study suggested that granular ependymitis in humans might be residua of prior CNS mumps infection. Although no studies are available to confirm that mumps virus replicates in the ependymal cells of humans during naturally occurring infection, the proposed association of mumps with aqueductal stenosis or ependymitis appears strong.

The ability of mumps virus to establish chronic infections in tissue culture systems is well known (93,94). In the hamster model, cell-associated mumps virus can be recovered from brain explant cultures for up to 50 days after infection, well after the appearance of specific humoral immunity (70). In humans with mumps meningoencephalitis, the persistence of leukocytes and oligoclonal mumps-specific immunoglobulins in the CSF for months after the acute infection suggests the possibility of ongoing antigenic stimulation from chronic mumps CNS infection (95). A possible instance of chronic mumps encephalitis was described in the case of a 31-year-old man who recovered from severe mumps encephalomyelitis, but who at the time of his neurologic deterioration 7 years later was found to still have high titers of mumps antibody in his serum and CSF (96). Sufficient data do not yet exist to confirm or refute a potential role for mumps virus as a cause of chronic CNS infection in humans.

IMMUNE RESPONSES

Specific humoral and cell-mediated immune responses develop during the course of acute mumps infection, but the relative contributions of antibody and cellular immunity to viral clearance have not been precisely determined. Interestingly, mumps has not been demonstrated to cause unusually severe or prolonged infections in immunocompromised patients.

Mumps-specific immunoglobulin M (IgM) is detectable early in the course of infection; IgM titers begin to wane shortly after the acute illness and are usually undetectable after 6 months (97,98). A mumps-specific immunoglobulin G (IgG) response is detectable during the first week of the acute infection, peaks about 3–4 weeks after the onset of the infection, and persists for decades (99). Using the complement-fixation assay, a fourfold rise in anti-mumps IgG can usually be demonstrated within 10–14 days after the onset of the disease (51,60,100). Lifelong immunity follows natural infection. Patients who report more than one episode of mumps probably had parotitis caused by infection with a different pathogen.

Mumps-specific immunoglobulins are also detectable in CSF of patients with mumps meningoencephalitis (101–108). Using a sensitive enzyme-linked immunosorbent assay (ELISA) method, mumps-specific IgG was detected in almost all CSF specimens from patients with mumps meningitis, and mumps virus IgM was detected in about 50% of patients (107). By measuring the ratios of CSF to serum immunoglobulin and comparing this ratio with that of an index antibody (such as measles antibody), intrathecal synthesis of mumps-specific immunoglobulin was shown to occur during mumps CNS infection. There was no apparent correlation between the severity of clinical disease and the presence or absence of mumps IgM in the CSF (103). Furthermore, no correlation between the CSF leukocyte count and the titers of the CSF mumps antibody was demonstrated (103). Intrathecal production of mumps-specific IgG and IgM appears to be a common feature of mumps meningitis in children (106).

Infection with mumps virus also elicits a cell-mediated immune response. Lymphocytes that proliferate when stimulated with mumps S and V antigens can be detected in venous blood following natural infection or immunization by an in vitro blastogenesis assay (109,110). Lymphocytes recovered from the CSF of patients with mumps meningitis will also proliferate when stimulated with mumps antigens (105,111). Fryden et al. (111) reported the blastogenic response to be higher with CSF lymphocytes than with peripheral blood lymphocytes in four of five patients with mumps meningitis.

Human leukocyte antigen (HLA)-restricted cytotoxic T lymphocytes (CTLs) are also detectable in peripheral blood following mumps infection or immunization (112,113). CTL activity was exhibited by T lymphocytes isolated from CSF of patients with mumps CNS infection. Kreth et al. (114) demonstrated that T lymphocytes from CSF and from venous blood of 10 children with mumps meningitis were cytotoxic to autologous mumps-virus-infected target cells. Lymphocyte-mediated toxicity was present during the acute phase of mumps meningitis, declined over 2–3 weeks after the onset of symptoms, and was no longer apparent after 50 days (114). Fleischer and Kreth (115) cloned leukocytes directly from the CSF from a patient with mumps meningitis and demonstrated that 90% of the cells were T lymphocytes and 60% were CD8-positive suppressor/cytotoxic T cells. A high percentage of the T-cell clones showed specificity for the autologous mumps-virus-infected target cells. These findings suggest that the recruitment of CTLs into the CNS in mumps meningitis is highly antigen-specific and that mumps-specific CTLs could play a role in the immunopathologic changes observed in human brains after fatal mumps encephalitis (114–116).

Interferon levels have been measured in serum and in CSF from patients with mumps meningitis (102). In patients with self-limited mumps meningitis, the interferon disappeared within a week, whereas interferon levels remained elevated in the CSF from those patients who had persistent CSF pleocytosis (102).

Detection of complement-fixing antibodies against V antigen has previously been the routine method of determining susceptibility to mumps, but the complement-fixation assay is being replaced by sensitive and specific

ELISAs (117). The mumps skin test is not a reliable indicator of immune status.

CLINICAL COURSE AND NATURAL HISTORY

Mumps is a systemic infection, and the virus has been demonstrated to replicate in epithelial cells of multiple visceral organs. Mumps usually begins with a short prodromal phase characterized by low-grade fever, malaise, headache, and anorexia. Young children may initially complain of ear pain. The patient then develops the characteristic salivary gland enlargement and tenderness (118). The parotid glands are most commonly involved, although other salivary glands (e.g., submandibular, sublingual) may be enlarged in about 10% of cases. Parotitis may initially be unilateral, with swelling of the contralateral parotid gland occurring 2–3 days later; bilateral parotitis eventually develops in most patients with symptomatic salivary gland involvement. Painful parotid gland enlargement progresses over about 3 days, lifting the ear lobe outward and obscuring the angle of the mandible. The orifice of Stensen's duct is often edematous. Parotid gland swelling and tenderness peaks on about the third day of the illness, followed by defervescence and resolution of parotid pain and swelling within about 7 days. Long-term sequelae of parotitis are uncommon. Children with mumps are usually isolated for about 1 week after the appearance of parotitis, although this practice is of dubious benefit to classmates because the virus is known to be excreted for several days prior to the onset of clinical symptoms.

Epididymo-orchitis is rare in boys with mumps, but it occurs in 25–30% of postpubertal men with mumps infection (119). Orchitis results from replication of mumps virus in seminiferous tubules with resulting lymphocytic infiltration and edema. Orchitis is most often unilateral, but bilateral involvement occurs in 17–38% of cases. Orchitis typically develops within 1 week after the onset of parotitis, although orchitis (like mumps meningitis) can develop prior to, or even in the absence of, parotitis. Mumps orchitis is characterized by marked testicular swelling and severe pain, accompanied by fever, nausea, and headache. The pain and swelling resolve within 5–7 days, although residual testicular tenderness can persist for weeks. Testicular atrophy may follow orchitis in about 35–50% of cases, but sterility is an uncommon complication even among patients with bilateral orchitis (120).

Mumps can cause inflammation of other glandular tissues, including pancreatitis (121) and thyroiditis (122). Oophoritis and mastitis have been reported in postpubertal women with mumps (118,123). Renal function abnormalities are common in mumps, and virus can be readily isolated from urine, but significant or permanent renal damage is rare (124). Other infre-

quent manifestations of mumps include arthritis (125), myocarditis (126), and thrombocytopenia (127). Maternal mumps infection during the first trimester of pregnancy results in an increased frequency of spontaneous abortions (128), but no clear association between congenital malformations and maternal mumps has been demonstrated (129).

CNS infection is the most common extrasalivary manifestation of mumps and may precede, accompany, or follow the development of parotitis (50,130,131). There is no association between the severity of the parotitis and the occurrence or severity of meningitis (37). Most frequently, CNS symptoms will follow the onset of parotitis by about 5 days (37). In a study of 41 cases of mumps encephalitis reported by Koskiniemi et al. (46), parotitis appeared 3–14 days prior to CNS involvement in 15 patients, was coincident with encephalitis in nine patients, and occurred 1–4 days after the onset of CNS symptoms in two patients. Fifteen of the 41 patients had no evidence of salivary gland enlargement. In another series of 24 patients with mumps parotitis and meningoencephalitis, 11 patients had parotitis for 6–21 days prior to the onset of the CNS symptoms, nine patients had neurologic symptoms preceding the parotitis by 1–8 days, and four patients had parotitis and CNS symptoms that occurred simultaneously (53). Levitt (45) noted a mean interval of 2.7 days between the development of parotitis and the onset of CNS symptoms; however, the range was wide, with parotitis developing from 20 days before to 7 days after CNS disease. These data clearly indicate that the development of CNS disease in mumps is not dependent on prior development of parotitis. Indeed, approximately 50% of patients with mumps CNS disease will never develop clinical evidence of salivary gland enlargement (Table 1). The clinician examining a patient with suspected meningoencephalitis may not exclude the possibility of mumps simply because the patient does not have salivary gland involvement.

The common presenting signs and symptoms seen in patients with mumps CNS infection are summarized in Table 1. The most frequently reported presentation is a triad of fever, vomiting, and headache. Salivary gland enlargement will be present in only 50% of patients with mumps CNS disease. The fever is frequently high (39–40°C) and lasts for 72–96 hr. The headache and vomiting may also be quite severe and usually persist for about 48 hr (47,132). Defervescence is usually accompanied by overall clinical recovery, and the total duration of illness in uncomplicated cases is 7–10 days (51,53). Other frequently noted clinical findings include neck stiffness, lethargy or somnolence, and abdominal pain. The majority of mumps patients with CNS involvement will have signs of meningitis (e.g., headache, nuchal rigidity) but no evidence of cortical dysfunction.

The presence of seizures, pronounced changes in level of consciousness, or focal neurologic findings is indica-

TABLE 1. *Presenting signs and symptoms of patients with CNS mumps*

Signs and symptoms	Kravis et al. (60) (N = 74)	Murray et al. (61) (N = 50)	McLean et al. (57) (N = 39)	Azimi et al. (53) (N = 51)	Levitt et al. (45) (N = 64)
Fever	NR[a]	88%	100%	94%	100%
Vomiting	68%	76%	79%	84%	78%
Headache	47%	72%	62%	47%	88%
Parotitis[b]	53%	54%	62%	47%	53%
Neck stiffness	43%	76%	77%	71%	93%
Lethargy	28%	34%	31%	69%	NR
Abdominal pain	15%	16%	23%	14%	NR
Seizures	14%	NR	18%	18%	NR

[a] Not reported.
[b] Or swelling of other salivary glands.

tive of significant encephalitis (45). Koskiniemi et al. (46) reviewed 41 cases of mumps encephalitis occurring in Helsinki, Finland between 1968 and 1980 and reported that 83% had high fever (>39°C), 88% had vomiting, 71% had headaches, 37% had difficulty walking, 27% had nuchal rigidity, 24% had seizures, 22% had psychiatric disturbances, and 20% had significantly depressed levels of consciousness.

Mumps meningitis is a benign disease with essentially no risk of mortality or long-term morbidity. It is difficult to accurately judge the true incidence of neurologic sequelae following mumps CNS disease from published reports because of the variability in the populations studied (children versus adults, inpatients versus outpatients, etc.). Patients who develop permanent sequelae following mumps with CNS involvement are presumed to have had mumps encephalitis. However, the mortality rate for patients with mumps encephalitis is 1% or less, and permanent sequelae are rare. As with many childhood viral infections, the mortality rate for mumps appears to be substantially higher among adults than among children. Even among patients who are profoundly encephalopathic, the probability for complete recovery is high; sustained seizures and focal neurologic deficits (both of which are uncommon) may predict a less favorable outcome (46,133). In many large series of patients with mumps CNS infection, no long-term neurologic sequelae were identified (40,53,56,132). Ataxia, behavioral changes, and electroencephalographic abnormalities have been noted in children in the immediate postencephalitis period, but they usually resolve over the course of a few weeks (53).

A wide variety of neurologic complications have been observed following mumps encephalitis (134,135). Among the reported sequelae are behavioral disturbances and personality changes (46,49,60,135), seizure disorders (51,136), cranial nerve palsies (especially facial and ocular palsies) (60,137), muscle weakness [including hemiparesis (49,60) and ataxia (46)], and chronic headaches (136,138). Myelitis and polyneuritis have also been reported as sequelae of mumps (41,134,139–142).

Sensorineural hearing loss is an uncommon but well-

recognized complication of mumps that occurs with an estimated frequency of 0.5–5.0 per 100,000 cases (136,138). Deafness may be either transient or permanent and probably results from direct damage to the cochlea by the mumps virus (143). One patient with mumps meningitis developed transient ataxia and total cortical blindness that resolved completely within 6 days (144). Other rare ocular complications of mumps include keratitis, iritis, and central retinal vein occlusion (145).

DIAGNOSIS AND LABORATORY FINDINGS

The presentation of a febrile child with parotitis strongly suggests the diagnosis of mumps, particularly if the individual is known to be susceptible and has been exposed to mumps during the preceding 2–3 weeks. However, an atypical clinical presentation (e.g., meningitis or orchitis without parotitis) may require laboratory confirmation. Culturing for mumps virus is the definitive diagnostic test, but it is frequently not available. Testing of paired acute and convalescent sera should demonstrate a diagnostic fourfold rise in mumps antibody titer. Parotitis can occasionally be caused by other viruses such as influenza A, parainfluenza virus, Coxsackie virus, lymphocytic choriomeningitis virus, and bacteria such as *Staphylococcus aureus.* Noninfectious causes of parotid gland enlargement include Sjögren's syndrome, sarcoidosis, thiazide ingestion, iodine sensitivity, tumor, or salivary duct obstruction. A careful physical examination should permit parotitis to be distinguished from lymphadenitis or lymphadenopathy.

When aseptic meningitis occurs in the context of parotitis, the diagnosis of mumps is usually obvious. The etiology of the meningitis may be obscure, however, if there is no accompanying salivary gland enlargement. Mumps meningoencephalitis has been confused with nonparalytic poliomyelitis, especially when it occurs during the summer (40,146). In general, the CSF leukocyte count is higher in mumps than in poliomyelitis, and the clinical findings of neck stiffness and fever resolve more quickly in cases of mumps than in polio (40). Lennette et al. (147) reported 11 cases of encephalitis with mild local muscle weakness which were all clinically considered to be polio but which were serologically demonstrated to be caused by mumps virus.

Confirmation of CNS involvement in patients with mumps is based on examination of the CSF. CSF pleocytosis (greater than five white blood cells per cubic millimeter) occurs in 40–60% of patients with mumps parotitis (37,47). The CSF opening pressure is normal in virtually all cases (40). The CSF white blood cell count is usually in the range of 200–600 cells per cubic millimeter (Table 2), although cell counts of 1000–2000 cells per cubic millimeter are not uncommon. In the series of 45 patients with mumps meningoencephalitis reported by Wilfert (62), the CSF white blood cell count on the initial lumbar puncture was less than 100 cells per cubic millimeter in 13% of patients, 100–500 in 53%, 500–1000 in 29%, and greater than 1000 in 5%. The differential count on CSF leukocytes count demonstrates greater than 80% lymphocytes in 80–90% of patients (40,45,60,62). A small number of neutrophils are commonly seen, but neutrophil predominance in the initial CSF occurs in less than 5% of patients with mumps CNS infection (40,53,62). The CSF protein is normal in about one-half the patients and moderately elevated (<100 mg/dl) in the remainder (46,51,52,62). The CSF glucose is normal in the majority of patients, but moderate hypoglycorrhachia (glucose 20–40 mg/dl) may be present in 10–20% of patients with mumps meningitis (45,46,52,53). In the series reported by Wilfert (62), 14 of 45 patients had a CSF glucose of <40 mg/dl. Marked hypoglycorrhachia (glucose <10 mg/dl), as can be seen in pyogenic bacterial meningitis, is very uncommon in mumps meningitis. An abnormally low CSF glucose is an unusual finding in viral meningitis and has been most frequently reported in meningitis caused by mumps virus, lymphocytic choriomeningitis virus, or herpes simplex virus.

No clear association has been established between the magnitude of the CSF pleocytosis and the clinical course. The CSF white blood cell count may be higher in patients with parotitis and signs of meningitis than in patients with parotitis alone (37), but there is no correlation between the level of CSF pleocytosis and severity of illness (51). CSF findings do not differ significantly between those patients with meningitis only and those with mumps encephalitis (45). The magnitude of the CSF abnormalities is not predictive of the risk of long-term sequelae following mumps encephalitis (46).

Studies employing sequential lumbar punctures have demonstrated that the CSF white blood cell count will frequently increase during the first 2–3 days after the onset of CNS symptoms, and then begin to decline (1,49,62). Even 2 weeks after the onset of CNS symptoms, when most patients with mumps meningoencephalitis are asymptomatic or substantially improved, the CSF white blood cell count may still be in the range of 100–500 cells per cubic millimeter in some cases. Complete normalization of the spinal fluid and disappearance of CSF pleocytosis may require several weeks (40,51,148).

A definitive diagnosis depends on isolation of mumps virus or demonstration of an appropriate serologic response. Mumps virus can be isolated from saliva from virtually all patients with acute mumps parotitis (49). Virus can also be recovered from the urine for up to 2 weeks after the onset of illness (10). Green monkey kidney cells are routinely used for mumps virus isolation, but a variety of other cell lines can also be used (149). Virus can also be isolated from 30–50% of CSF samples collected early during the course of mumps CNS infection (40,56,63). Wolontis and Björvatn (150) attempted virus isolation from CSF specimens of 655 patients with mumps and CSF pleocytosis and were successful in 33% of cases. Interestingly, no significant association between the probability of viral isolation and the magnitude of the CSF pleocytosis could be demonstrated (49,150). Spi-

TABLE 2. Initial CSF findings in patients with CNS mumps

	Kilham (49) (N = 22)	Russell and Donald (1) (N = 19)	Ritter (51) (N = 30)
White blood cell count (per mm³)			
Mean	503	416	357
Range	100–2920	4–1260	15–1212
Differential count (% lymphs)			
Mean	96	69	89
Range	89–100	28–98	30–100
Protein (mg/dl)			
Mean	56	79	49
Range	17–145	20–240	17–140
Glucose (mg/dl)			
Mean	NR[a]	53	NR
Range	NR	34–69	NR

[a] Not reported.

nal fluid from six patients with early mumps parotitis and no clinical evidence of meningeal involvement was examined for mumps virus, and cultures were negative in each case (49).

Laboratory confirmation of mumps is usually based on serologic testing. A variety of assays have been developed to measure the humoral immune response to mumps virus infection. The neutralizing antibody assay has been considered the "gold standard" test, but it is technically demanding. The hemagglutination-inhibition (HAI) assay is simple and sensitive (151); however, it is less specific due to cross-reactivity with other paramyxoviruses, especially parainfluenza virus. The most widely used serologic test has been the complement-fixation assay, which detects antibodies directed against the V antigen (hemagglutinin-neuraminidase) and the S antigen (nucleocapsid). All of these assays are designed to measure a fourfold increase in mumps-specific IgG between the acute serum (collected at the time of clinical disease) and the convalescent serum (collected 2–4 weeks later). Alternatively, demonstration of mumps-specific IgM is indicative of recent infection. An IgM response is detectable early in the course of infection, and IgM titers then wane and become undetectable 2–6 months after the acute infection (152). Sensitive and specific ELISAs have now largely replaced the complement-fixation assay as the preferred method for serodiagnosis (97,98,108). In cases of mumps meningoencephalitis, involvement of the CNS can be confirmed by demonstration of elevated ratios of mumps-specific immunoglobulins in CSF.

Other routine laboratory studies are not generally helpful. The average peripheral white blood cell count in patients with mumps is 10,000–12,000 cells per cubic millimeter, with a differential of 30–40% lymphocytes (51,53,60). Approximately 30% of patients will have an elevated serum amylase, reflecting inflammation of the salivary glands or pancreas (53). During acute mumps encephalitis, the electroencephalogram characteristically shows moderate-to-severe slowing without spikes or lateralizing signs (46,153). Little information is available regarding the utility of modern imaging methods (computerized tomography, magnetic resonance imaging, etc.) in the diagnosis and management of mumps CNS infections.

THERAPY

Clinical management of the patient with mumps consists of conservative measures to provide symptomatic relief and to ensure adequate rest, hydration, and nutritional support. Therapy of orchitis includes bedrest, scrotal support, analgesics, and ice packs. Patients with clinical evidence of significant CNS involvement (altered mental status, seizures, focal neurologic findings,

etc.) will require hospitalization for observation. Supportive care for patients with mumps encephalitis includes hydration, fever control, antiemetics, and anticonvulsants as required. Lumbar puncture has been reported to relieve the headache associated with mumps meningitis in some patients. There is currently no established role for antiviral chemotherapy or passive immunotherapy in mumps. There have been anecdotal reports on the use of corticosteroids in patients with mumps encephalitis, but no benefits have been documented (51). In the series of patients with mumps meningoencephalitis reported by Ritter (51), the average duration of hospitalization was 9.1 days, with a range of 5–19 days.

PREVENTION

The cornerstone of mumps prevention is active immunization using the live, attenuated mumps vaccine. This vaccine is administered in the United States to children during the second year of life, and it produces protective antibody levels in greater than 97% of recipients (12,154). The vaccine is given subcutaneously in combination with the live measles and rubella vaccines and has virtually no side effects. Booster immunizations are not required (155).

Administration of the live mumps vaccine is relatively contraindicated in pregnant women, in persons with a history of anaphylactic reaction to eggs or neomycin (the vaccine is produced in chick-embryo cell culture), in persons who have received immunoglobulin therapy within the preceding 3 months (which might interfere with the immune response to the vaccine), or in persons with severe systemic immunosuppression. Mumps immunization is recommended for asymptomatic human immunodeficiency virus (HIV)-infected children (156).

Questions regarding prevention often arise when an individual with no history of mumps (typically an adult male) is exposed to a patient with active mumps. The immune status of the exposed individual can be determined by serologic testing, although this may involve some delay. Mumps immunoglobulin is not of proven value (64) and is no longer commercially available. Mumps vaccine can be safely administered to an individual of unknown immune status (157), although vaccine given to a susceptible individual following exposure to mumps may not provide protection. The vast majority of adults born in the United States before 1957 have been naturally infected and are therefore immune (156).

Widespread use of the mumps vaccine has had a major impact on the incidence of mumps and mumps meningoencephalitis. Through the mid-1960s, mumps was a leading cause of viral encephalitis (158). By the mid-1980s, however, mumps had been reduced to the seventh most common cause of viral encephalitis in the United States, accounting for only 0.5% of cases of viral encephalitis (159). This trend was documented in Minnesota, where mumps was the second most common cause of encephalitis between 1950 and 1981, but where no cases of mumps CNS infection were noted after 1973 (31). Similarly, mumps and measles disappeared as leading causes of encephalitis in children in Finland after the institution of a nationwide measles–mumps–rubella vaccination program in 1982 (160).

A few cases of mumps meningitis have occurred in children 1–2 months after administration of the mumps vaccine. It is not clear whether these cases represent vaccine failure or meningitis due to the vaccine strain of mumps virus (161–164). Because mumps immunization does involve administration of a live, attenuated virus, symptomatic CNS infections due to the vaccine virus is theoretically possible but is exceedingly rare, if it occurs at all.

REFERENCES

1. Russell RR, Donald JC. The neurological complications of mumps. *Br Med J* 1958;2:27–30.
2. Hamilton R. An account of a distemper, by the common people in England, vulgarly called the mumps. *London Med J* 1790;11:190–211.
3. Monod R. Reactions méningées chez l'enfant. Thèse de Paris, 1902–1903, No. 77. Cited by Wesselhoeft C. In: *Virus and rickettsial diseases.* Cambridge, MA: Harvard University Press, 1943;324.
4. Acker GN. Parotitis complicated with meningitis. *Am J Dis Child* 1917;6:399–407.
5. Johnson CD, Goodpasture EW. An investigation of the etiology of mumps. *J Exp Med* 1934;59:1–19.
6. Habel K. Cultivation of mumps virus in the developing chick embryo and its application to studies of immunity to mumps in man. *Public Health Rep* 1945;60:201–212.
7. Henle G, Deinhardt F. Propagation and primary isolation of mumps virus in tissue culture. *Proc Soc Exp Biol Med* 1955;89:556–560.
8. Swan C, Mawson J. Experimental mumps; transmission of the disease to monkeys; attempts to propagate virus in developing hens' eggs. *Med J Aust* 1943;1:411–416.
9. Henle G, McDougall CL. Mumps meningo-encephalitis. Isolation in chick embryos of virus from spinal fluid of a patient. *Proc Soc Exp Biol Med* 1947;66:209–211.
10. Utz JP, Kasel JA, Cramblett HG, Szwed CF, Parott RH. Clinical and laboratory studies of mumps. I. Laboratory diagnosis by tissue culture techniques. *N Engl J Med* 1957;257:497–502.
11. Kane LW, Enders JF. Immunity in mumps. III. The complement fixation test as an aid in the diagnosis of mumps meningoencephalitis. *J Exp Med* 1945;81:137–150.
12. Buynak EB, Hilleman MR. Live attenuated mumps virus vaccine. I. Vaccine development. *Proc Soc Exp Biol Med* 1966;123:768–775.
13. Horne RW, Waterson AP, Wildy P, Farnham AE. The structure and composition of the myxoviruses. I. Electron microscope studies of the structure of myxovirus particles by negative staining techniques. *Virology* 1960;11:79–98.
14. Hosaka Y, Shimizu K. Lengths of the nucleocapsids of Newcastle disease and mumps viruses. *J Mol Biol* 1968;35:369–373.
15. Jensik SC, Silver S. Polypeptides of mumps virus. *J Virol* 1976;17:363–373.
16. Huppertz HI, Hall WW, ter Meulen V. Polypeptide composition of mumps virus. *Med Microbiol Immunol* 1977;163:251–259.
17. Orvell C. Structural polypeptides of mumps virus. *J Gen Virol* 1978;41:527–539.
18. Herrler G, Compans RW. Synthesis of mumps virus polypeptides in infected Vero cells. *Virology* 1982;119:430–438.
19. Love A, Rydbeck R, Kristensson K, Orvell C, Norrby E. Hemagglutinin-neuraminidase glycoprotein as a determinant of pathogenicity in mumps virus hamster encephalitis: analysis of mutants selected with monoclonal antibodies. *J Virol* 1985;58:67–74.
20. McCarthy M, Johnson RT. A comparison of the structural polypeptides of five strains of mumps virus. *J Gen Virol* 1980;46:15–27.
21. Chu TH, Cheever FS, Coons AH, Daniels JB. Distribution of mumps virus in the experimentally infected monkey. *Proc Soc Exp Biol Med* 1951;76:571–574.
22. Brandt CD. Cytopathic action of myxoviruses on cultivated mammalian cells. *Virology* 1961;14:1–10.
23. Lennette DA, Emmons RW, Lennette EH. Rapid diagnosis of mumps virus infections by immunofluorescence methods. *J Clin Microbiol* 1975;2:81–84.
24. Anderson RM, Crombie JA, Grenfell BT. The epidemiology of mumps in the UK: a preliminary study of virus transmission, herd immunity and the potential impact of immunization. *Epidemiol Infect* 1987;99:65–84.
25. Hodes D, Brunell PA. Mumps antibody: placental transfer and disappearance during the first year of life. *Pediatrics* 1970;45:99–101.
26. Mortimer PP. Mumps prophylaxis in the light of a new test for antibody. *Br Med J* 1978;2:1523–1524.
27. Modlin JF, Orenstein WA, Brandling-Bennett AD. Current status of mumps in the United States. *J Infect Dis* 1975;132:106–109.
28. Centers for Disease Control. Mumps surveillance 1973. *MMWR* 1974;23:431–432.
29. Cochi SL, Preblud SR, Orenstein WA. Perspective on the relative resurgence of mumps in the United States. *Am J Dis Child* 1988;142:499–507.
30. Centers for Disease Control. Mumps—United States, 1985–1988. *MMWR* 1989;38:101–105.
31. Beghi E, Nicolosi A, Kurland LT, Mulder DW, Hauser WA, Shuster L. Encephalitis and aseptic meningitis, Olmsted County, Minnesota, 1950–1981: I. Epidemiology. *Ann Neurol* 1984;16:283–294.
32. Meyer HM, Johnson RT, Crawford IP, Dascomb HE, Rogers NG. Central nervous system syndromes of "viral" etiology. *Am J Med* 1960;29:334–347.
33. Koskiniemi M, Manninen V, Vaheri A, Sainio K, Eistola P, Karli P. Acute encephalitis: a survey of epidemiological, clinical and microbiological features covering a twelve-year period. *Acta Med Scand* 1981;209:115–120.
34. Koskiniemi ML, Vaheri A. Acute encephalitis of viral origin. *Scand J Infect Dis* 1982;14:181–187.
35. McLean DM, Larke RPB, Cobb C, Griffis ED, Hackett SMR. Mumps and enteroviral meningitis in Toronto, 1966. *Can Med Assoc J* 1967;96:1355–1361.
36. Frankland AW. Mumps meningo-encephalitis. *Br Med J* 1941;2:48–49.
37. Bang HO, Bang J. Involvement of the central nervous system in mumps. *Acta Med Scand* 1943;113:487–505.
38. Holden EM, Eagles AY, Stevens JE. Mumps involvement of the central nervous system. *JAMA* 1946;131:382–385.
39. Brown JW, Kirkland HB, Hein GE. Central nervous system involvement during mumps. *Am J Med Sci* 1948;215:434–441.
40. Bruyn HB, Sexton HM, Brainerd HD. Mumps meningoencephalitis: a clinical review of 119 cases with one death. *Calif Med* 1957;86:153–160.
41. Scheid W. Mumps virus and the central nervous system. *World Neurol* 1961;2:117–130.
42. McCarthy M, Jubelt B, Fay D, Johnson RT. Comparative studies of 5 strains of mumps virus *in vitro* and in neonatal hamsters: evaluation of growth, cytopathogenicity, and neurovirulence. *J Med Virol* 1980;5:1–15.
43. Rozina EE, Hilgenfeldt M. Comparative study on the neurovirulence of different vaccine strains of parotitis virus in monkeys. *Acta Virol* 1985;29:225–230.
44. Klemola E, Kaariainen L, Ollila O, Pettersson T, Jansson E, Haa-

panen L, Lapinleimu K, Forssell P. *Acta Med Scand* 1965;177:707–716.

45. Levitt LP, Rich TA, Kinde SW, Lewis AL, Gates EH, Bond JO. Central nervous system mumps. *Neurology* 1970;20:829–834.
46. Koskiniemi M, Donner M, Pettay O. Clinical appearance and outcome in mumps encephalitis in children. *Acta Paediatr Scand* 1983;72:603–609.
47. Bowers D, Weatherhead DSP. Mumps encephalitis. *Can Med Assoc J* 1953;69:49–55.
48. Finkelstein H. Meningoencephalitis in mumps. *JAMA* 1938;117:17–19.
49. Kilham L. Mumps meningoencephalitis with and without parotitis. *Am J Dis Child* 1949;78:324–333.
50. Eberlein WR, Lynxwiler CP. Clinical picture of mumps meningoencephalitis and report of case without parotitis. *J Pediatr* 1947;31:513–520.
51. Ritter BS. Mumps meningoencephalitis in children. *J Pediatr* 1958;52:424–432.
52. Johnstone JA, Ross CAC, Dunn M. Meningitis and encephalitis associated with mumps infection. *Arch Dis Child* 1972;47:647–651.
53. Azimi PH, Cramblett HG, Haynes RE. Mumps meningoencephalitis in children. *JAMA* 1969;207:509–512.
54. Strussberg S, Winter S, Friedman A, Benderly A, Kahana D, Freundlich E. Notes on mumps meningoencephalitis. *Clin Pediatr* 1969;8:373–377.
55. Donald PR, Burger PJ, Becker WB. Mumps meningo-encephalitis. *S Afr Med J* 1987;71:283–285.
56. McLean DM, Walker SJ, McNaughton GA. Mumps meningoencephalitis: a virological and clinical study. *Can Med Assoc J* 1960;83:148–151.
57. McLean DM, Bach RD, Larke RPB, McNaughton GA. Mumps meningoencephalitis, Toronto 1963. *Can Med Assoc J* 1964;90:458–462.
58. Centers for Disease Control. *Mumps surveillance.* Report No. 1, January 1968.
59. Levitt LP, Mahoney DH, Casey HL, Bond JO. Mumps in a general population: a sero-epidemiologic study. *Am J Dis Child* 1970;120:134–138.
60. Kravis LP, Sigel MM, Henle G. Mumps meningoencephalitis, with special reference to the use of the complement fixation test in diagnosis. *Pediatrics* 1951;8:204–214.
61. Murray HGS, Field CMB, McLeod WJ. Mumps meningo-encephalitis. *Br Med J* 1960;1:1850–1853.
62. Wilfert CM. Mumps meningoencephalitis with low cerebrospinal-fluid glucose, prolonged pleocytosis and elevation of protein. *N Engl J Med* 1969;280:855–859.
63. Björvatn N, Wolontis S. Mumps meningoencephalitis in Stockholm, November 1964–July 1971. *Scand J Infect Dis* 1973;5:253–260.
64. Reed D, Brown G, Merrick R, Sever J, Feltz E. A mumps epidemic on St. George Island, Alaska. *JAMA* 1967;199:967–971.
65. Meyer MD, Stifler WC, Joseph JM. Evaluation of mumps vaccine given after exposure to mumps, with special reference to the exposed adult. *Pediatrics* 1966;37:304–315.
66. Henle G, Henle W, Wendell KK, Rosenberg P. Isolation of mumps virus from human beings with induced apparent or inapparent infections. *J Exp Med* 1946;88:223–385.
67. Meyer MB. An epidemiologic study of mumps: its spread in schools and families. *Am J Hyg* 1962;75:259–281.
68. Overman JR. Viremia in human mumps infection. *Arch Intern Med* 1958;102:354–356.
69. Kilham L. Isolation of mumps virus from the blood of a patient. *Proc Soc Exp Biol Med* 1948;69:99–100.
70. Wolinsky JS, Klassen T, Baringer JR. Persistence of neuro-adapted mumps virus in brains of newborn hamsters after intraperitoneal inoculation. *J Infect Dis* 1976;133:260–267.
71. Fleischer B, Kreth HW. Mumps virus replication in human lymphoid cell lines and in peripheral blood lymphocytes: preference for T cells. *Infect Immun* 1982;35:25–31.
72. Boyd JF, Vince-Ribaric V. The examination of cerebrospinal fluid cells by fluorescent antibody staining to detect mumps antigen. *Scand J Infect Dis* 1973;5:7–15.

73. Herndon RM, Johnson RT, Davis LE, Descalzi LR. Ependymitis in mumps virus meningitis. *Arch Neurol* 1974;30:475–479.
74. Lindeman J, Muller WK, Versteeg J, Bots GTAM, Peters ACB. Rapid diagnosis of meningoencephalitis: immunofluorescent examination of fresh and *in vitro* cultured cerebrospinal fluid cells. *Neurology* 1974;24:143–148.
75. Wolinsky JS, Baringer JR, Margolis G, Kilham L. Ultrastructure of mumps virus replication in newborn hamster central nervous system. *Lab Invest* 1974;31:402–412.
76. Schwarz GA, Yang DC, Noone EL. Meningoencephalomyelitis with epidemic parotitis. *Arch Neurol* 1964;11:453–462.
77. deGodoy CVF, deBrito T, Tiriba ADC, deCampos CM. Fatal mumps meningoencephalitis: isolation of virus from human brain (case report). *Rev Inst Med Trop Sao Paulo* 1969;11:436–441.
78. Donohue WL. The pathology of mumps encephalitis with report of a fatal case. *J Pediatr* 1941;19:45–52.
79. Bistrian B, Phillips CA, Kaye IS. Fatal mumps meningoencephalitis. *JAMA* 1972;222:478–479.
80. Taylor FB, Toreson WE. Primary mumps meningo-encephalitis. *Arch Intern Med* 1963;112:216–221.
81. Kilham L, Overman JR. Natural pathogenicity of mumps virus for suckling hamsters on intracerebral inoculation. *J Immunol* 1953;70:147–151.
82. Overman JR, Kilham L. The inter-relation of age, immune response, and susceptibility to mumps virus in hamsters. *J Immunol* 1953;71:352–358.
83. Overman JR, Peers J, Kilham L. Pathology of mumps virus meningoencephalitis in mice and hamsters. *Arch Pathol* 1953;55:457–465.
84. Johnson RT. Mumps virus encephalitis in the hamster. *J Neuropath Exp Neurol* 1968;27:80–95.
85. Johnson RT, Johnson KP. Virus-induced hydrocephalus: development of aqueductal stenosis in hamsters after mumps infection. *Science* 1967;157:1066–1067.
86. Johnson RT, Johnson KP. Hydrocephalus following viral infection: the pathology of aqueductal stenosis developing after experimental mumps virus infection. *J Neuropathol Exp Neurol* 1968;27:591–606.
87. Johnson RT, Johnson KP. Hydrocephalus as a sequela of experimental myxovirus infections. *Exp Mol Pathol* 1969;10:68–80.
88. Timmons GD, Johnson KP. Aqueductal stenosis and hydrocephalus after mumps encephalitis. *N Engl J Med* 1962;283:1505–1507.
89. Bray PF. Mumps: a cause of hydrocephalus? *Pediatrics* 1972;49:447–449.
90. Spataro RF, Lin SR, Horner FA, Hall CB, McDonald JV. Aqueductal stenosis and hydrocephalus: a rare sequelae of mumps virus infection. *Neuroradiology* 1976;12:11–13.
91. Thompson JA. Mumps: a case of acquired aqueductal stenosis. *J Pediatr* 1979;94:923–924.
92. Johnson KP, Johnson RT. Granular ependymitis. *Am J Pathol* 1972;67:511–522.
93. Henle G, Deinhardt F, Bergs VV, Henle W. Studies on persistent infections of tissue cultures. I. General aspects of the system. *J Exp Med* 1958;108:537–560.
94. McCarthy M, Wolinsky JS, Lazzarini RA. A persistent infection of Vero cells by egg-adapted mumps virus. *Virology* 1981;114:343–356.
95. Vandvik B, Norrby E, Steen-Johnsen J, Stensvold K. Mumps meningitis: prolonged pleocytosis and occurrence of mumps virus-specific oligoclonal IgG in the cerebrospinal fluid. *Eur Neurol* 1978;17:13–22.
96. Vaheri A, Julkunen I, Koskiniemi ML. Chronic encephalomyelitis with specific increase in intrathecal mumps antibodies. *Lancet* 1982;2:685–688.
97. Nigro G, Nanni F, Midulla M. Determination of vaccine-induced and naturally acquired class-specific antibodies by two indirect ELISAs. *J Virol Methods* 1986;13:91–106.
98. Linde GA, Granstrom M, Orvell C. Immunoglobulin class and immunoglobulin G subclass enzyme-linked immunosorbent assays compared with microneutralization assay for serodiagnosis of mumps infection and determination of immunity. *J Clin Microbiol* 1987;25:1653–1658.

99. Ukkonen P, Grandstrom ML, Penttinen K. Mumps-specific immunoglobulin Mand G antibodies in natural mumps infection as measured by enzyme-linked immunosorbent assay. *J Med Virol* 1981;8:131–142.

100. Henle G, Harris S, Henle W. Reactivity of various human sera with mumps complement fixation antigens. *J Exp Med* 1948;88:133–147.

101. Fryden A, Link H, Norrby E. Cerebrospinal fluid and serum immunoglobulins and antibody titers in mumps meningitis and aseptic meningitis of other etiology. *Infect Immun* 1978;21:852–861.

102. Morishima T, Miyazu M, Ozaki T, Isomura S, Suzuki S. Local immunity in mumps meningitis. *Am J Dis Child* 1980;134:1060–1064.

103. Ukkonen P, Granstrom ML, Rasanen J, Salonen EM, Penttinen K. Local production of mumps IgG and IgM antibodies in the cerebrospinal fluid of meningitis patients. *J Med Virol* 1981;8:257–265.

104. Link H, Laurenzi MA, Fryden A. Viral antibodies in oligoclonal and polyclonal IgG synthesized within the central nervous system over the course of mumps meningitis. *J Neuroimmunol* 1981;1:287–298.

105. Reunanen M, Salonen R, Salmi A. Itrathecal immune responses in mumps meningitis patients. *Scand J Immunol* 1982;15:419–426.

106. Vandvik B, Nilsen RE, Norrby E. Mumps meningitis: specific and non-specific antibody responses in the central nervous system. *Acta Neurol Scand* 1982;65:468–487.

107. Forsberg P, Fryden A, Link H, Orvell C. Viral IgM and IgG antibody synthesis within the central nervous system in mumps meningitis. *Acta Neurol Scand* 1986;73:372–380.

108. Glikmann G, Pedersen M, Mordhorst CH. Detection of specific immunoglobulin M to mumps virus in serum and cerebrospinal fluid samples from patients with acute mumps infection, using an antibody-capture enzyme immunoassay. *Acta Pathol Microbiol Immunol Scand* 1986;94:145–156.

109. Ilonen J, Salmi A, Penttinen K. Lymphocyte blast transformation and antibody responses after vaccination with inactivated mumps virus vaccine. *Acta Pathol Microbiol Scand* 1981;89:303–309.

110. Bruserud O, Thorsby E. HLA control of the proliferative T-lymphocyte response to antigenic determination on mumps virus. *Scand J Immunol* 1985;22:509–518.

111. Fryden A, Link H, Moller E. Demonstration of cerebrospinal fluid lymphocytes sensitized against virus antigens in mumps meningitis. *Acta Neurol Scand* 1978;57:396–404.

112. Chiba Y, Tsutsumi H, Nakao T, Wakisaka A, Aizawa M. Human leukocyte antigen-linked genetic controls for T-cell-mediated cytotoxic response to mumps virus in humans. *Infect Immun* 1982;35:600–604.

113. Kress HG, Kreth HW. HLA-restriction of secondary mumps-specific cytotoxic T-lymphocytes. *J Immunol* 1982;129:844–849.

114. Kreth HW, Kress L, Kress HG, Ott HF, Eckert G. Demonstration of primary cytotoxic T cells in venous blood and cerebrospinal fluid of children with mumps meningitis. *J Immunol* 1982;128:2411–2415.

115. Fleischer B, Kreth HW. Clonal analysis of HLA-restricted virus-specific cytotoxic T lymphocytes from cerebrospinal fluid in mumps meningitis. *J Immunol* 1983;130:2187–2190.

116. Nagai H, Morishima T, Morishima Y, Isomura S, Suzuki S. Local T cell subsets in mumps meningitis. *Arch Dis Child* 1983;11:927–928.

117. Shehab ZM, Brunnell PA, Cobb E. Epidemiologic standardization of a test for susceptibility to mumps. *J Infect Dis* 1984;149:810–812.

118. Philip RN, Reinhard KR, Lackman DB. Observations on a mumps epidemic in a virgin population. *Am J Hyg* 1959;69:91–111.

119. Beard CM, Benson RC, Kelalis PP, Eveback LR, Kurland LT. The incidence and outcome of mumps orchitis in Rochester, Minnesota, 1935–1974. *Mayo Clinic Proc* 1977;52:3–7.

120. Werner CA. Mumps orchitis and testicular atrophy. II. A factor in male sterility. *Ann Intern Med* 1950;32:1075–1086.

121. Feldstein JD, Johnson FR, Kallick CA, Doolas A. Acute hemorrhagic pancreatitis and pseudocyst due to mumps. *Ann Surg* 1974;180:85–88.

122. Eyland E, Zmucky R, Sheba C. Mumps virus and subacute thyroiditis: evidence of a causal association. *Lancet* 1957;1:1062–1065.

123. Morrison JC, Givens JR, Wiser WL. Mumps oophoritis: a cause of premature menopause. *Fertil Steril* 1975;26:655–660.

124. Utz JP, Houk VN, Alling DW. Clinical and laboratory studies of mumps. IV. Viruria and abnormal renal function. *N Engl J Med* 1964;270:1283–1286.

125. Gordon SC, Lauter CB. Mumps arthritis: a review of the literature. *Rev Infect Dis* 1984;6:338–343.

126. Brown NJ, Richman SJ. Fatal mumps myocarditis in an 8-month-old child. *Br Med J* 1980;281:356–357.

127. Graham DY, Brown CH, Benrey J, et al. Thrombocytopenia: a complication of mumps. *JAMA* 1974;227:1162–1164.

128. Siegal M, Fuerst HT, Peress NS. Comparative fetal mortality in maternal virus diseases: a prospective study on rubella measles, mumps, chickenpox, and hepatitis. *N Engl J Med* 1966;274:768–771.

129. Katz M. Is there mumps embryopathy? An unanswered question. *Clin Pediatr* 1967;6:321–322.

130. Coe RPK, Lond MD. Primary mumps orchitis with meningitis. *Lancet* 1945;1:49–50.

131. Borovski M. Encephalitis preceding mumps. *Am J Dis Child* 1954;87:362.

132. Henderson W. Mumps meningo-encephalitis an outbreak in a preparatory school. *Lancet* 1952;1:386–388.

133. Mendelsberg S. Fulminating mumps meningoencephalitis with recovery. *J Pediatr* 1951;39:87–89.

134. McKaig CB, Woltman HW. Neurologic complications of epidemic parotitis. *Arch Neurol Psychiatry* 1934;31:794–808.

135. Brown EH, Dunnett WH. A retrospective survey of the complications of mumps. *J R Coll Gen Pract* 1974;24:552–556.

136. Oldfelt V. Sequelae of mumps-meningoencephalitis. *Acta Med Scand* 1949;134:405–414.

137. Beardwell A. Facial palsy due to the mumps virus. *Br J Clin Pract* 1969;23:37–38.

138. Laurence D, McGavin D. The complications of mumps. *Br Med J* 1948;1:94–97.

139. Lightwood R. Myelitis from mumps. *Br Med J* 1946;1:484–485.

140. Silverman AC. Mumps complicated by a preceding myelitis. *N Engl J Med* 1949;241:262–266.

141. Miller HG, Stanton JB, Gibbons JL. Para-infectious encephalomyelitis and related syndromes. *Q J Med* 1956;25:467–505.

142. Ghosh S. Guillain–Barré syndrome complicating mumps. *Lancet* 1967;1:895–896.

143. Smith GA, Guessen R. Inner ear pathologic features following mumps infection: report of a case in an adult. *Arch Otolaryngol* 1976;102:108–111.

144. Davis LE, Harms AC, Chin TDY. Transient cortical blindness and cerebellar ataxia associated with mumps. *Arch Ophthalmol* 1971;85:366–368.

145. Riffenburgh RS. Ocular manifestations of mumps. *Arch Ophthalmol* 1961;66:739–743.

146. Kilham L, Levens J, Enders J. Non-paralytic poliomyelitis and mumps meningoencephalitis. *JAMA* 1949;140:934–936.

147. Lennette EH, Caplan GE, Magoffin RL. Mumps virus infection simulating paralytic poliomyelitis: a report of 11 cases. *Pediatrics* 1960;25:788–797.

148. Azimi PH, Shaban S, Hilty MD, Haynes RE. Mumps meningoencephalitis: prolonged abnormality of cerebrospinal fluid. *JAMA* 1975;234:1161–1162.

149. Person DA, Smith TF, Herrmann EC. Experiences in laboratory diagnosis of mumps virus in routine medical practice. *Mayo Clin Proc* 1976;45:544–548.

150. Wolontis S, Bjorvatn B. Mumps meningoencephalitis in Stockholm, November 1964–July 1971. II. Isolation attempts from the cerebrospinal fluid in a hospitalized group. *Scand J Infect Dis* 1973;5:261–271.

151. Eckert HL, Portnoy B, Salvatore MA, Krell M. The hemagglutination inhibition and complement fixation tests in the serodiagnosis of mumps central nervous system disease. *Am J Clin Pathol* 1967;4:481–483.

152. Meurman O, Hanninen P, Krishna RV, Zeigler T. Determination of IgG- and IgM-class antibodies to mumps virus by solid-phase immunoassay. *J Virol Methods* 1982;4:249–257.

153. Gibbs FA, Gibbs EL, Spies HW, Carpenter PR. Common types of childhood encephalitis: electroencephalographic and clinical relationships. *Arch Neurol* 1964;10:1–11.

154. Hilleman MR, Buynak EB, Weibel RE, Stokes J. Live, attenuated mumps-virus vaccine. *N Engl J Med* 1968;278:227–232.

155. Weibel RE, Buynak EB, McLean AA, Roehm RR, Hilleman MR. Persistence of antibody in human subjects following administration of combined live attenuated measles, mumps, and rubella vaccines. *Proc Soc Exp Biol Med* 1980;165:260–263.

156. Advisory Committee on Immunization Practices, Centers for Disease Control. Mumps prevention. *MMWR* 1989;38:388–400.

157. Davidson WL, Buynak EB, Leagus MB, Whitman JE, Hilleman MR. Vaccination of adults with live attenuated mumps virus vaccine. *JAMA* 1967;201:995–998.

158. Rantakallio P, Leskinen M, Von Wendt L. Incidence and prognosis of central nervous system infections in a birth cohort of 12,000 children. *Scand J Infect Dis* 1986;18:287–294.

159. Centers for Disease Control. *Mumps surveillance, January 1977–December 1982.* Atlanta: U.S. Department of Health and Human Services, Public Health Service, 1984.

160. Koskiniemi M, Vaheri A. Effect of measles, mumps, rubella vaccination on pattern of encephalitis in children. *Lancet* 1989;1:31–34.

161. Gray JA, Burns SM. Mumps meningitis following measles, mumps and rubella immunization. *Lancet* 1989;2:98.

162. Thomas E. A case of mumps meningitis: a complication of vaccination? *Can Med Assoc J* 1988;138:135.

163. Cizman M, Mozetic M, Radescek-Rakar R, Pleterski-Rigler D, Susec-Michieli M. Aseptic meningitis after vaccination against measles and mumps. *Pediatr Infect Dis J* 1989;8:302–308.

164. McDonald JC, Moore DL, Quennec P. Clinical and epidemiological features of mumps meningoencephalitis and possible vaccine-related disease. *Pediatr Infect Dis J* 1989;8:751–755.

Infections of the Central Nervous System,
edited by W. M. Scheld, R. J. Whitley, and
D. T. Durack, Raven Press, Ltd., New York © 1991.

CHAPTER 7

Rabies

Richard J. Whitley and Mark Middlebrooks

Rabies infections in humans in the United States are uncommon, accounting for no more than a few cases each year. These cases are usually the consequence of exposure to animal bites which occurred outside the territorial boundaries of the United States. Nevertheless, rabies, as a disease of both animals and humans, awakens the physician's memories of historical, literary, and medical images of the horrific clinical manifestations of a disease which virtually always results in death. Ancient hieroglyphic descriptions of rabies infections, starting with the bite of a rabid dog, graphically remind the medical historian that this infection has existed for millennia. Literary citations, even in the 20th century, such as Harper Lee's description of Tim Johnson in *To Kill a Mockingbird,* elucidate the variability of disease in the rabid animal, ranging from a dog foaming at the mouth with wild, frenzied behavior to that of a paralyzed dog dragging his hind limbs or even one with a disjointed gait. The contrasting ecology of rabies infection in animal populations of developed versus third-world countries is particularly striking. The introduction of rabies control programs for domestic animals in developed countries has shifted the ecologic balance of rabies-virus-infected animals to that of wild, carnivorous or sylvatic animals, for the most part. On the other hand, rabies infection of domestic animals in third-world countries and the subsequent bites of these animals unfortunately still result in thousands of cases of human disease yearly. The image of a human with hydrophobia or frenzied behavior or of an individual with the paralytic form of involvement reinforces the devastating and painful manifestations of human disease. Furthermore, the recognition that virtually all cases of rabies are fatal reminds the biomedical investigator of the continued need to eradicate rabies from domestic urban as well as sylvatic animal populations. Lack of a specific antiviral agent to treat human or animal disease reinforces the need for the development of better methods of control. Recent and clever advances in the vaccination of wild animal populations introduces the possibility of preventing disease in targeted animal populations, which provides the hope for a decreasing incidence of human disease. These issues provide models for understanding the interactions between rabies virus infections of animals and humans, especially as it relates to the biotechnological advances which allow the possibility of inexpensive and highly efficacious vaccines for mammalian populations.

This chapter will review our knowledge of rabies infections of the human central nervous system (CNS). It will make no attempt to review the numerous epidemiologic and interventive studies performed worldwide. There are several excellent and recent reviews in the literature which are superb testimonies to the commitment of numerous investigators working in this area (1,2).

HISTORY

The history of rabies virus infections has been summarized by numerous excellent reviews (1–4). These reviews have focused on the attention that this disease has received in both animal and human populations over the ages (1–3). Well before the pre-Mosaic Eshnunni Code of Mesopotamia, which predated the Code of Hammurabi of 2300 B.C., literary reference was made to the monetary fines demanded from owners of "mad dogs" whose bites led to the death of the bitten individual (5). Interestingly, a distinction was made between a bite leading to death of a slave and that resulting in death in other members of society (6). Numerous other citations have appeared in historical documents, including those of Democritus, Aristaeus, and Artemis (3,7). However, it was Celsius in 100 A.D. who recommended a novel and, per-

R. J. Whitley and M. Middlebrooks: Departments of Pediatrics, Microbiology, and Medicine, University of Alabama, Birmingham, Alabama 35294.

haps, unconventional therapy for rabid animal bites—namely cauterization and, if possible, excision of the bite site (5,8). This latter practice of cauterizing bite wounds was practiced through the 19th century (7).

Detailed descriptions of human disease were reported in the mid-16th century by the Italian physician Fracastoro (3). Over the next several centuries, numerous reports appeared in the literature which elucidated the natural history of human disease and which provided an unequivocal association with animal rabies. This association between rabid animals and human illness led to one of the first animal control programs in history and resulted in the elimination of mammalian disease from Scandinavian countries and, subsequently, Great Britain by the early 20th century (5).

One of the most historical landmarks in our understanding of rabies infections and its control were the experiments performed by Louis Pasteur in the late 1800s. Pasteur demonstrated the transmission of rabies by inoculating homogenized spinal material from a rabid dog into the brain of a previously healthy dog. Shortly thereafter, these experiments led to the development of a vaccine for the prevention of rabies infection. This vaccine was tested initially in animals and was thought to be efficacious. However, it was only in 1885 that Pasteur (9) was pushed to administering this vaccine to a child, Joseph Meister, who was bitten by a rabid dog. The initial success of this vaccine in the prevention of rabies in several individuals immunized by Pasteur was followed by much questioning from medical experts. Nevertheless, the increased deployment of this vaccine over the next several years led to a significant decrease in the incidence of rabies, as reviewed (10). Many reviews by vaccine experts have focused on these early developments, since they provide the historical basis for subsequent vaccine development (2,11,12).

By the beginning of the 20th century, the literature was replete with cases of human and animal rabies, noting especially the clinical manifestations. For the most part, all these disease descriptions remained anecdotal. However, an important histopathologic observation was made by Negri (13) in 1903, when he identified cytoplasmic inclusion bodies—now known as "Negri bodies"—in the neuronal cells of rabid dog brains. Shortly thereafter, Babes (14) published *Traite de la Rage* in 1912. This was a compendium of cases which defined the natural history and clinical findings of human rabies. To this day, it remains one of the most complete documents available which aids our understanding of this disease.

As the 20th century has progressed, advances have been achieved in the prevention of rabies, specifically the development of vaccines for animals and the combination of vaccines and immunoglobulin for humans. Utilization of vaccines to protect domestic animals, particularly cats and dogs, has led to a significant decrease in human rabies in developed countries. Nevertheless, the absence of vaccine programs for domestic animals in developing countries still results in tens of thousands of cases of rabies worldwide each year. The nearly uniform fatality rate of rabies, as noted previously, prompts continued medical attention to the treatment and prevention of this devastating disease.

INFECTIOUS AGENT

Rabies virus belongs to the Rhabdoviridae family. "Rhabdos" is of Greek derivation, meaning *rod*. This family of viruses includes pathogens which infect a wide variety of mammals, fish, birds, and plants (15,16). As suggested by the name of the family, these viruses are bullet-like in shape. The prototype structure of a rhabdovirus is displayed in Fig. 1. The Rhabdoviridae family consists of two genera: *Lyssavirus* and *Vesiculovirus*. Members of the *Lyssavirus* genus are displayed in Table 1; this family includes rabies virus. Members of these two genera can be distinguished according to antigenic and biologic characteristics (15,17,18). As with "Rhabdos," "Lyssa" is of Greek derivation and means *rage* or *frenzy*. The morphologies of all members of this family are similar; these viruses are bullet-shaped cylinders with

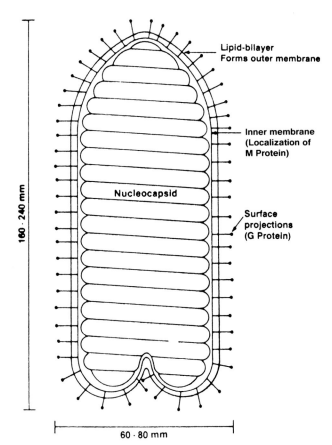

FIG. 1. Rabies virus morphology in brain tissue. Adapted from Ref. 1.

TABLE 1. *Members of the Lyssavirus genus of the Rhabdoviridae family[a]*

Virus	Source species
Rabies[b]	Mammals (dogs, cats, cattle, bats, wild carnivores, humans)
Duvenhage[b]	Bats, humans
Lagos bat	Bats
Mokola[b]	Humans, dogs, cats, shrews
Kotonkan	*Culicoides* mosquitoes
Obodhiane	*Mansonia* mosquitoes

[a] Adapted from ref. 15.
[b] Associated with human disease.

one end rounded and the other end flat, as shown in Fig. 1 (19–24).

Rabies virus consists of single-stranded RNA which has a sedimentation coefficient of 42–45 Svedberg units and a buoyant density of 1.66 g/cm. The estimated molecular weight is approximately 4.6×10^6 daltons (1,15,16,20,25,26). The single-stranded RNA makes up the nuclear capsid which also contains an RNA-dependent RNA transcriptase (16,20). The negative-sense, 12-kb RNA genome encodes five proteins: the nucleoprotein (N), a highly phosphorylated protein (NS), a matrix protein (M), the glycosylated membrane glycoprotein (G), and a large protein component of the RNA polymerase (L) (27–30).

The envelope-associated proteins, M and G, are particularly important. Both are associated with the lipid bilayer envelope. The M protein has a molecular weight of approximately 25 kD and is thought to be localized on the inner aspect of the viral envelope. This protein is thought to play a critical role in the budding process (1,31,32). The G protein is a transmembrane, fully glycosylated protein which projects in a spike-like form from the outer surface of the viral envelope. It is capable of both inducing and reacting with virus-specific neutralizing antibodies (1,33,34). It should be noted that the G protein, in conjunction with the rabies virion envelope, can generate hemagglutination activity (HA) (19,35). The envelope surrounds an infectious nucleocapsid, consisting of a series of approximately 30–35 coils.

Viral Infectivity

Rabies virus can be rapidly inactivated by exposure to ultraviolet light, sunlight, desiccation, formalin, phenol, β-propiolactone, ether, or detergents (3,36). The susceptibility of rabies virus to detergents is particularly relevant because local wound care with an agent capable of inactivating rabies is essential for disease prevention. In addition, the virus is unstable at extreme ranges of pH. Nevertheless, virion infectivity remains stable for long periods of time if the virus is properly frozen or even maintained at approximately 4°C (5,16,37).

***In Vitro* Replication**

The propagation of rabies virus either in primary cells or in continuous cell lines was not accomplished until 1958 by Kissling (38). This accomplishment was relevant in that it resulted in avoiding the necessity to produce vaccines in cells of animal origin which utilized whole neuronal cell targets, such as the brains of suckling mice. Thus, the significant complication of allergic encephalomyelitis could be avoided by cell-culture-produced vaccines. By the mid-1960s, it was possible to culture large quantities of rabies virus in primary hamster cell cultures (39). These initial observations were subsequently followed by the demonstration that virus could be passaged in continuous cell lines, particularly those of baby hamster kidney cells, BHK-21 (40).

Replication of virus *in vitro* follows a classic pathway: After an initial eclipse phase of approximately 6–8 hr, multiplication progresses to completion within 24 hr. Virion assembly is associated with budding from cytoplasmic membranes (19–21).

PATHOGENESIS AND PATHOLOGY

Pathogenesis

The pathogenesis of human rabies is inextricably linked to infections of animal populations. Rabies virus is capable of infecting most warm-blooded animal species. However, studies summarized by the World Health Organization (41) have identified a hierarchy of susceptibility to infection among different animal species. As summarized in Table 2, foxes and coyotes are extremely susceptible to acquisition of rabies virus infection. As summarized by Baer et al. (1), foxes in zootic areas do not have demonstrable antibodies, indicating uniform fatality with infection (42). These animals have the highest susceptibility to rabies infections. Yet, antibodies will appear in animals of other species, such as dogs and mongooses, if bitten by rabid animals of the same species. Dogs and nonhuman primates are considered only moderately susceptible to rabies infection, whereas opossums are the least susceptible. Hamsters, skunks, ra-

TABLE 2. *Animal susceptibility to rabies infection[a]*

Highest	High	Moderate	Low
Wolves	Hamsters	Dogs	Opossums
Foxes	Skunks	Nonhuman primates	
Coyotes	Raccoons		
Rats (kangaroo and cotton)	Domestic cats		
Field voles	Rabbits		
	Cattle		

[a] Adapted from refs. 1 and 41.

coons, cats, guinea pigs, rabbits, and cattle have a high susceptibility to infection.

The pathogenesis of rabies virus infections must be considered according to two routes of acquisition. Although most cases of human rabies occur following animal bites, it is becoming increasingly apparent that nonbite sources of rabies virus infection also account for human disease. Examples of nonbite transmission include acquisition of infection by aerosols and by person-to-person transmission following corneal transplants, among other routes. Thus, pathogenesis will be distinguished according to "bite" and "nonbite" acquisition of infection.

As noted, the most common route of acquisition of infection is that which follows the bite of a rabid animal. Thus, the hierarchy of the aforementioned susceptibility of animals is relevant when defining the risks for acquisition of disease in humans. Following the bite of a rabid animal, virus is inoculated from the saliva into local muscle tissue. As early as 1804, Zinke et al. (43) demonstrated that saliva from a rabid dog could infect a healthy dog. It is presumed that the acinar cells of salivary glands harbor infectious rabies virus (44). Parenthetically, it should be remembered that infected and rabid animals do not always continuously excrete virus in saliva, as has been well documented for the fox (45,46) and skunk (47). It is not at all unreasonable for a rabid animal to bite successively many individuals in a short period of time. This point is best illustrated by a rabid wolf who attacked 29 individuals in an Iranian village in 1954 (48). This one attack provided unequivocal evidence for the efficacy of postexposure immunoglobulin administration.

Although it was once believed that virus was initially transmitted directly to the CNS, more definitive studies have indicated that local replication of rabies virus occurs at the site of inoculation, with subsequent spread to the CNS. Murphy et al. (49) were able to demonstrate the accumulation of rabies virus antigen in muscle fibers of baby hamsters when inoculated with rabies virus intramuscularly. These studies were subsequently confirmed in skunks (50). Experimental studies provide support for these pathogenic observations. Furthermore, studies which call for limb amputation following virus inoculation demonstrate the absence of transmission of infection to the CNS (51). Taken together, these studies provide evidence of an initial phase of local replication at the inoculation site prior to transmission into the CNS.

Recently, the rate of progression of virus from local replication in muscle cells to the spinal cord has attracted a great deal of attention. A series of observations, including the localization of rabies virus antigen at subneural clefts commensurate with the distribution of acetylcholine receptors and the prevention of transmission by compounds which interfere with the nicotinic acetylcholine receptors, have contributed to developing molec-

ular hypotheses of disease pathogenesis. These data weighed in favor of receptor-mediated transmission (52–54). Furthermore, it was reported by Lentz et al. (54) that there was sequence homology between the G protein of rabies virus and the region with the greatest binding affinity for the acetylcholine receptor. However, it has not been possible to verify these experiments in more definitive studies, particularly for dose–response curves. Thus, as with the pathogenesis of many infections, there are many viral and host-specific factors at work in the transport of virus from sites in peripheral tissues to the CNS.

Once virus enters neuronal cells, potential distinctions between motor and sensory neuron uptake of rabies virus remain unclear. Regardless, virus is transmitted centrally, as proven by nerve segmentation studies (55). Once in the nervous system, virus moves by passive neuronal transit. Virions can be identified in the axonal endoplasmic reticulum and nodes of Ranvier, as noted previously. Severing the nerve tract will prevent transmission of virus from peripheral sites of inoculation to the spinal ganglia (55–59). Evidence of infection of the dorsal ganglia includes the demonstration of virions at that site by both culture and electron microscopy, as well as the demonstration of dorsal root edema (58,60). From the spinal cord, the virus can ascend extremely rapidly to the brain, at least in the animal model (55,58,61,62).

Virus reaches the brain and subsequently infects many of the lower brain structures with subsequent widespread infection (63). Infection involves the lower areas of the brain most prominently. These include the limbic system, hippocampus, brainstem, and cerebellum (62,64, 65). Clinical manifestations of disease obviously parallel the sites of involvement. Involvement of the limbic system will result in aberrant sexual behavior and loss of mechanisms of behavioral control, whereas brainstem involvement generally results in failure of body temperature control and altered patterns of respiration, leading to respiratory arrest.

An extremely important component of disease is the centrifugal spread of virus back out of the CNS to peripheral sites. Specifically, virus is transmitted back to acinar cells of the salivary and submaxillary glands, resulting in salivary excretion of virus (44,55). This transport of virus back out of the CNS can lead to infection of the head and neck. The observation of virus infection at these sites has resulted in the recognition that biopsies of the nape of the neck are extremely helpful for diagnostic purposes (66). Additionally, virus can be found in corneal cells, drawing the association between corneal smears and rapid diagnosis of rabies infection. It should be obvious that with corneal infection, corneal transplants can be a source of infection for person-to-person transmission, as has been well established (62,66–68). As is well demonstrated in animal systems, virtually all organs can become involved following natural infection, including the heart, kidney, lung, and gastrointestinal tract (69).

The pathogenesis of rabies virus infections which are the result of "nonbite" acquisition requires viral replication at the site of initial inoculation, as would be thought intuitively. Specifically, for those who acquire infection from an aerosol, such as spelunkers, replication of virus likely occurs in the olfactory epithelium with direct neuronal transmission to the brain by the olfactory tract. Somewhat surprisingly, rabies virus tends to demonstrate the same tropism following aerosol acquisition as that encountered with transmission by a bite. Similarly, with corneal acquisition of infection there is direct retrograde spread of virus from the eye to the brain.

Pathogenesis of human infection would be incomplete without raising the question of why, following infection, the incubation period can be as protracted as it is without interference by host immune defenses. The relationship between the role of cell-mediated immunity and the prevention of rabies virus propagation is not clear. In fact, current data indicate that cell-mediated immune responses probably play only a minor role in pathogenesis, as summarized by Robinson (3) and others (70–72). In contrast, with the recognized value of the administration of immunoglobulin products or the generation of humoral antibody responses by vaccine administration, circulating neutralizing antibodies certainly decrease mortality. These studies will be discussed in more detail in the section entitled "Disease Prevention."

Johnson and Mercer (73; also see ref. 74) were able to demonstrate in 1964 that replication of rabies virus occurred in perikaryon and dendritic processes of neurons. It was suggested that the long incubation period may, in large part, be related to the sequestration of virus within peripheral muscle fibers before ascending in nerves (51,74). Regardless, invasion of the CNS via peripheral neuronal pathways is well documented (74,75).

Pathology

Pathologic findings of rabies virus infection are similar to those encountered with other encephalitides; however, they are significantly less extensive, especially in light of the striking clinical symptomatology of hydrophobia, frenzied activity, and bizarre behavior. Evidence of perivascular cuffing is characteristic of rabies virus infection of the brain, although it is extremely limited. Neuronophagia and neuronal necrosis are also a component of the acute stages of disease, occurring in approximately 57% of patients (76). The areas of the brain most frequently involved include the medulla, pons, spinal column, dorsal root ganglia, cerebellum, and hippocampus (3,77).

On histopathologic examination, the pathognomonic finding of rabies is the presence of Negri bodies, which are cytoplasmic inclusions, being by-products of viral replication (16,22). These particles are composed of clusters of assembling virion nucleocapsids (19,22). Thus, Negri bodies are most commonly found in the area of viral replication, especially the hippocampus, cerebellum, and brainstem. When present, they are pathognomonic for rabies virus infection; however, the sensitivity of detection in both animal and human infected brains ranges between 70% and 90% (3,76,78).

In 1965, Dupont and Earle (76) summarized the relationship between histopathologic findings in the brain and duration of survival of humans with rabies. Death occurred most rapidly (in 31–38 days) in those patients who had either evidence of encephalitis or congestion only. When Negri bodies were present either alone or in the presence of encephalitis, survival was extended to between approximately 66 and 73 days. These findings imply that Negri bodies appear later in the course of disease.

EPIDEMIOLOGY

For the most part, the epidemiology of human rabies parallels that of rabies infections of domestic animal populations worldwide; however, the increasing prevalence of rabies in wild animal populations will pose increasing problems for humans. When efforts to control domestic rabies, particularly in the dog and cat, have succeeded, the incidence of human rabies has fallen dramatically. As a consequence, there are areas of the world designated by the World Health Organization as being rabies-free, as will be noted below. Cases of human rabies occur mainly in areas of the world where public health programs designed to control domestic rabies have not been implemented, such as India and Mexico. In these two countries alone, the current incidence of rabies ranges in the vicinity of approximately 3.3 cases per 100,000 individuals. In contrast, human rabies has declined in other areas of the world such as Cameroon, where the incidence of disease is 0.04 per 100,000 individuals (79–83). In the United States, the control of rabies in domestic animal populations has led to a significant decrease in the number of cases. Those cases recently occurring in the United States have been the consequence of individuals having been bitten by rabid dogs outside of the territorial borders of the country.

In areas where domestic rabies control programs are in effect (such as the United States, Canada, and western Europe), dogs account for very few cases of human rabies (1,84,85). In contrast, where domestic animal rabies has not been controlled, dogs account for over 90% of cases (82). Thus, for developed countries in which dog bites are excluded, the remainder of human exposures to rabies virus is the result of either (a) bites of wild animals such as foxes, skunks, bats, or bobcats, (b) bites of unimmunized domestic cats, or (c) aerosol (laboratory workers, spelunkers) or person-to-person transmission (corneal transplant). As noted previously, there is differential susceptibility of animal populations for rabies virus infection. In different areas of the world, it has been noted that there have been different wildlife sources for rabies virus infection. These include the mongoose and jackal in Africa, the fox in Europe and Arctic regions, the wolf in Asia, and the vampire bat in Latin America, as summarized by Bernard and Fishbein (84) and by Kaplan and Koprowski (86).

As shown in Fig. 2, the control of domestic rabies in the United States led to a significant decrease in the total number of cases of rabies in humans. Subsequently, in the late 1970s, it was noted that epizootic infection occurred in raccoons in mid-Atlantic states and subsequently in more southern states (87). This led to an increase in the number of cases of raccoon rabies in the early 1980s.

One important and ever-increasing source of rabies is bat populations. Over 150 human deaths have resulted from exposure to these animals (88–90). Bats account for about 10% of the rabies-infected animals in the United States today (1,91).

Other documented sources of rabies virus infection include aerosol acquisition of virus from caves in which bats lived, likely from bat stool (92).

The overall control of rabies in both domestic and wild animal populations is shown in Fig. 3. There was a progressive decrease until the late 1970s. In approximately 1979, there was an increase of rabies because of infected skunk populations in the central regions of the United States (93). Skunks now have become the most commonly reported rabid animal in the United States.

The pathologic and clinical findings of animal rabies are very similar to that encountered with human disease, resulting in either "furious" or "dumb (paralytic)" manifestations. Animals exhibiting furious behavior are known to exhibit extreme agitation, altered gait, irritability, uncontrolled nervousness, and aggressive activity toward inanimate objects. With the dumb or paralytic form of disease, there is general hind-quarter weakness and gait disturbance. When rabies occurs in bat populations, it can do so in either hematophagous or insectivorous species. When hematophagous bats are infected, rabies can be asymptomatic; with insectivorous bats, however, infection is usually associated with clinical symptoms.

Several areas of the world have been designated by the World Health Organization as being rabies-free, as noted above. To qualify for such a distinction, it must be documented that no cases of rabies could be identified in the area over a period of 2 years (81,94–96). Such countries include: Mauritius in Africa; Bermuda in North Amer-

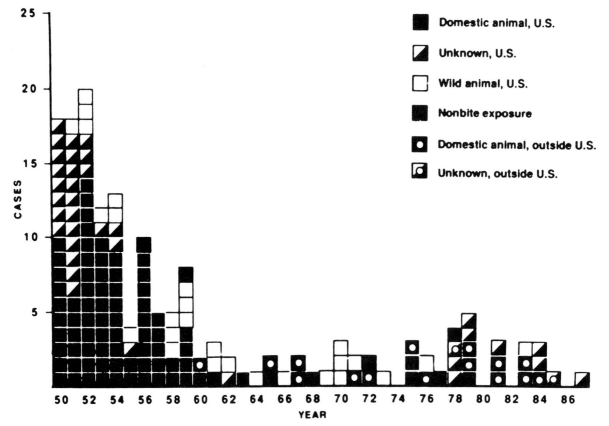

FIG. 2. Human rabies, United States, 1950–1987, with sources and location of exposure (including two Americans who died outside the United States). Adapted from Ref. 1.

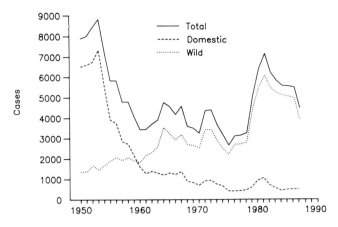

FIG. 3. Reported cases of rabies in wild and domestic animals, United States, 1953–1987.

ica; many of the islands of the Caribbean; Oman, Singapore, Taiwan, Malaysia, Kuwait, Japan, and Brunei in Asia; Uruguay in South America; Great Britain; Sweden; Portugal; Iceland; the Faeroe Islands; American Samoa; Fiji; the French Polynesian Islands; New Calendonia; and New Zealand; among others. The reader is referred to previously cited World Health Organization publications or a more detailed review (1) for a full listing of countries considered rabies-free. In 1988, the Centers for Disease Control (97) reported that one country previously identified as rabies-free, namely Australia, had cases of human rabies, presumably acquired in other countries. A similar observation was made in Finland. Furthermore, rabies was also identified in bat populations in Denmark (98,99). These identified cases of rabies in countries presumed to be rabies-free for some time should reinforce the need for continued surveillance.

Human rabies occurs most frequently in younger individuals, particularly males less than 15 years of age, accounting for nearly 50% of all cases (100). Overall, the male/female ratio indicates that the frequency in males is approximately 70–80% (83,85). Likely, the high incidence in males and younger children relates to a propensity to be outdoors and to be in frequent contact with either dogs or other wild animals. As would be expected, the times of greatest risk for exposure to rabies virus occur most frequently during the months of May through September—times when there is greater outdoor activity (101).

The World Health Organization (95) maintains a registry of cases of human rabies worldwide. Unfortunately, accurate reporting of cases worldwide does not occur. Current statistics would indicate that over 20,000 cases occur per year, with a large majority of these cases occurring in India (102). It is likely that the number of cases in India is far in excess of that actually reported. Overall, however, human cases parallel the distribution of animal cases throughout the world (103). Of great importance for international travelers is that they should be aware of endemic areas of rabies and take proper precautions for travel in these regions in order to avoid exposure. In urban populations where canine rabies is not under control, the close association between human and dog results in a high number of cases (3,83,85,103). In the United States, wild animals account for the largest number of exposures, accounting for all but 13% (85).

Other sources of exposure to virus include aerosolization, laboratory accident, and corneal transplantation with infected tissue (104–108). Nevertheless, in most of the very few cases of human rabies in the United States which have occurred, a source of exposure cannot be identified.

CLINICAL DISEASE OF HUMANS

Background

Not all humans bitten by a rabid animal develop infection. Infection is a function of a variety of factors, including: excretion of virus at the time of the bite, quantity of virus excreted, site of the bite, and whether the bite occurred through an article of clothing. Because our understanding of rabies is that infection leads to death, the relationship between the site and severity of bite (as illustrated in Table 3) is essential in the assessment of risk for the bitten subject. Utilizing a rabid dog bite as a model, mortality is directly related to the number and severity of the bites. For example, rabid-dog bites to the face which are multiple and severe are associated with a mortality of 60% in the absence of prophylactic intervention, a very similar rate for multiple, severe bites to other parts of the head. In contrast, however, severe bites to the fingers or hand are associated with significantly lower mortality rates, reflecting a lower rate of infection, being only 15%. Superficial exposures to skin or wounds with infected saliva are associated with even lower mortality rates ranging from 0% to approximately 3% (1,14,109–111). Regardless, any exposure to an infected and rabid animal should be considered as a possibility for rabies infection; therefore, appropriate control measures should be instituted.

Bites remain the most common reason for administering rabies postexposure prophylaxis, as well as the most common cause of human rabies cases worldwide (1,112). Causes of nonbite rabies in humans have been previously noted. In addition, it should be recognized that the incomplete inactivation of the Fermi vaccine resulted in 18 cases of paralytic rabies in 1960 (113). A critical issue in our understanding of rabies is whether asymptomatic infection can occur. Although this has been suggested, as indicated by the presence of low-level antibodies in veterinary and some animal workers, it has been extremely difficult to prove (1,114,115).

TABLE 3. *Representative mortality rates in nonvaccinated individuals following exposure to rabid canines*[a]

Location of exposure	Extent of exposure	Mortality (%)
Face	Bites (multiple and severe)	60
Other part of head	Bites (multiple and severe)	50
Face	Bite (single)	30
Fingers/hand	Bite (severe)	15
Face	Bites (multiple and superficial)	10
Hand	Bites (multiple and superficial)	5
Trunk/legs	Scratch	3
Hands/exposed skin	Bleeding and superficial wound	2
Skin covered by clothes	Superficial wound	0.5
Recent wound	Saliva	0.1
Wounds > 24 hr old	Saliva	0.0

[a] Adapted from refs. 1 and 14.

The progression of events following infection with rabies can be broken down into the following stages, as summarized in Table 4: (a) incubation period, (b) prodrome and early clinical symptoms, (c) acute neurologic disease, (d) coma, and (e) death or recovery. Each of these stages will be reviewed.

Incubation

The incubation period for rabies is extremely variable, being as short as a few days to as long as years (1,12). These widely discrepant incubation periods make it the most variable of all infectious diseases. The documentation of the range of incubation is well established in the literature (11,59,83,113,116–121). During the incubation period, the host is usually completely free of symptoms. For the most part, the incubation period ranges from 30 to 80 days (59,76,83,85,118,119,122,123). A recent detailed review of rabies summarized studies of human rabies totaling 2396 cases (1). These data were summarized from a variety of sources (59,85,118,119,124). In only one series of patients [a recent outbreak in Thailand reported by Wilde and Chutivongse (119)], 93% of cases (23 total cases) had an incubation period of less than 10 days. Most other studies had incubation periods in the 30- to 90-day range—with the exception of the previously noted study (119), in which the incubation period for nearly three out of every four patients was in the 10- to 30-day range. Only 55 patients in the series

TABLE 4. *Clinical progression of rabies in humans following exposure to proven rabid animals in those developing disease*

Stage	Duration	Clinical association
Incubation period	30–90 days: ~50% of cases <30 days: ~25% >90 days to 1 year: ~20% >1 year: ~5%	No clinical findings
Prodrome and early clinical symptoms	2–10 days	Paresthesia and/or pain at site of bite Fever, malaise Anorexia, nausea, vomiting Headache
Acute neurologic disease	2–7 days	"Furious rabies" (80% of cases) Hallucinations, bizarre behavior, anxiety, agitation, biting Hydrophobia Autonomic dysfunction "Paralytic rabies" (20% of cases) Flaccid paralysis Paresis and plegias Ascending paralysis
Coma	0–14 days	SIADH[a] Diabetes Insipidus Multiorgan failure Respiratory cardiac
Death or recovery (rare)	Variable	

[a] SIADH, syndrome of inappropriate secretion of antidiuretic hormone.

reviewed by Baer et al. (1) had incubation periods greater than 365 days.

The incubation period tends to be shorter in children. Furthermore, a short incubation period is also encountered in individuals with more severe exposures or those involving the head and face (11,83,92,122). As noted previously, the site of the bite varies somewhat between adults and children, with the latter more frequently experiencing bites to the head, face, and neck (125). Similarly, as was noted previously, the site of the bite as well as the extent of the exposure influences pathogenesis of disease (see section entitled "Pathogenesis"). Parenthetically, it should be noted that stress may influence the appearance of disease and decrease the incubation period (126,127).

Prodrome and Early Symptoms

The appearance of early clinical symptoms and prodrome terminates the incubation period. As noted in Table 4, initial clinical findings of disease are usually vague and nonspecific and include malaise, fever, and myalgias (76,85,122,123,128–130). In addition, chills with fever may develop in up to 50% of patients (3,85). Additional components of the nonspecific findings of the prodromal and early symptom stage include nausea, vomiting, abdominal pain, and diarrhea. Hallucinations and nightmares have also been reported during this early phase.

It is common for patients to report paresthesia and tingling as well as pain in a few circumstances at the site of the original bite.

Acute Neurologic Findings

Neurologic findings associated with rabies can be classified into one of two forms of clinical manifestations: either "furious" rabies or "paralytic" rabies. The majority of patients will suffer from a furious form of rabies, with over 80% of patients developing agitation, behavioral changes, hyperactivity, hallucinations, and extreme excitability (3,11,12,14,67,76,84,85,122,130). A varying percentage of patients have been described as having hydrophobia, consisting of episodes which last 1–5 min and which are associated with an aversion to drinking water (85,122,124,131,132).

Dr. Richard Johnson, in his textbook *Viral Infections of the Central Nervous System,* discovered a perfect description of hydrophobia from the writings of A. Trousseau at the Clinique Médical de l'Hôtel-dieu de Paris, 1865 [translated by Bloomfield in 1958 (133)]:

> Finally there appears a symptom practically constant in established rabies in man, the horror of water. The site of this liquid often suffices to bring on a general tremor; but it is, above all, when the patient wishes to bring water to

his lips that this special horror comes on, those convulsions of the face and of the entire body which make a vivid impression on those who witness an attack. The rabid man completely preserves his reason; he is thirsty; he wishes to drink, he bids his hands to carry to his lips the vessel filled with liquid, but no sooner does it touch him than the unhappy creature withdraws, terrified, sometimes he cries out that he cannot drink; his face shows agony, his eyes are fixed, his features contracted; then his limbs shake and his body quivers. The crisis lasts several seconds, gradually calm seems to return, but the least contact, even a breath of air, suffices to start a new crisis, such as the hypersensitivity of the skin. He cannot wash hands or face or comb his hair without being menaced by convulsions.

In addition, these patients may experience focal or generalized seizures, which have been associated with high mortality (76).

The alternative form of rabies is known as "paralytic" or "dumb" rabies. For patients with this form of disease, paralysis is the predominant clinical finding (14,122,129,134–138). Various forms of paralysis may develop in the afflicted patients, ranging from paralysis of one limb to quadriplegia. Combined motor and sensory involvement may occur, as might a Guillain–Barré syndrome (106,139–141). The Guillain–Barré form of disease may be present in approximately 20% of patients (11,85,106,140).

It should be noted that there can be overlap between furious and paralytic forms of rabies. The duration of either form of disease can be up to weeks.

Coma

Patients progress, with varying degrees of rapidity, to either coma or recovery. Coma can develop virtually immediately after the onset of clinical symptoms, or it can occur up to 14 days after the onset of clinical disease. Death occurs an average of 18 days after onset of illness (3,85). For those individuals who receive intensive support, survival following onset of illness averages approximately 25 days (142).

Numerous complications contribute to mortality in patients with rabies. Complications from rabies are summarized in Table 5. These have been summarized by numerous investigators (1,84). The most important of these complications relate to involvement of the CNS. Obviously, complications from rabies include multiple organs, since rabies virus can be transmitted peripherally to organs other than the CNS, as noted in the section entitled "Pathogenesis." Neurologic complications are significant and include: inappropriate secretion of antidiuretic hormone; diabetes inspidus; a hypo- or hyperventilation syndrome with involvement of the brainstem; alterations of temperature; and inability to control blood pressure (1,128,129,143).

Other organ complications include myocarditis, renal failure, and gastrointestinal involvement (128,144–147).

TABLE 5. *Clinical manifestations and complications of human rabies in different organ systems*[a]

Central nervous system
Hyperactive episodes
Hydrophobia
Seizures
Localized neurologic signs
Cerebral edema
Inappropriate secretion of antidiuretic hormone
Diabetes insipidus

Pulmonary system
Hyperventilation
Hypoxemia
Atelectasis
Pneumomediastinum
Apnea/respiratory arrest
Pneumonia
Pneumothorax

Cardiovascular system
Arrhythmia
Congestive heart failure
Hypotension
Arterial–venous thrombosis

Other
Upper gastrointestinal bleeding
Ileus
Urinary retention
Hyperthermia
Hypothermia
Renal failure

[a] Adapted from ref. 1.

To date, only three patients have recovered from rabies, all during the 1970s (107,129,148). In these three cases, all received one form of rabies vaccine: Two of the patients received either duck embryo or mouse brain vaccine, whereas the third patient worked in a laboratory with an experimental vaccine. Recovery was complete in a child, but the adults had neurologic sequelae.

DIAGNOSIS

The diagnosis of rabies is predicated on one of several parameters, including: (a) epidemiologic association with a bite or exposure to a rabid animal (bats), (b) histopathology, (c) antigen detection, (d) virus isolation, and (e) serology.

Certainly, clinical and epidemiologic findings can help suggest a diagnosis of rabies infection, particularly for individuals living in areas where rabies is endemic. Association of a dog bite with the clinical sequence of events previously described provides a strong suggestion of evidence of rabies infection. Rabies should be considered in any differential diagnosis of unexplained encephalitis.

Additional studies which may support a diagnosis of rabies in an encephalitic patient include electroencephalography or radiographic imaging of the CNS; however, the findings of either of these two neurodiagnostic procedures are nonspecific (149,150).

The utilization of the diagnostic virology laboratory is essential if a diagnosis of rabies is to be ascertained. The demonstration of rabies antigen by a fluorescent antibody technique following a full-thickness biopsy of the nape of the neck should be utilized routinely for diagnosis of rabies (151). The sensitivity of skin biopsy for diagnosis of rabies is in excess of 50% and may be as high as 90% (85,151), with a specificity of nearly 100%. Neck biopsy has replaced corneal smears as the diagnostic method of choice, since fluorescent staining of corneal cells is associated with a higher percentage of false-negative results (68,152).

Alternative approaches for diagnostic purposes include virus isolation from a putatively infected host. Rabies virus can be isolated from the saliva of infected individuals after direct intracerebral inoculation into a mouse model (76,153). The frequency of viral isolation varies according to disease duration but can be as high as 60%. The probability of viral retrieval is higher in the absence of serum-neutralizing antibodies.

Postmortem examination of tissues can yield either virus or histopathologic evidence of infection. The brain is the usual site for retrieval of rabies virus, particularly those areas of the brain usually infected by this pathogen. In addition, virus can be isolated from other visceral tissues at autopsy. Because of the peripheral excretion of rabies virus from saliva, it must be emphasized that biologic fluids from these patients can pose an environmental source for nosocomial infection (64,76,153).

Histopathologic examination of the brain will demonstrate presence of Negri bodies in nearly three out of every four patients (76,154–156). The addition of electron microscopy to the evaluation of brain specimens may increase the diagnostic yield of histopathology.

Serologic approaches to the diagnosis of rabies infection have been employed on both serum and cerebrospinal fluid specimens. A variety of antibody assays exist for determination of serologic status. These assays have been reviewed in detail (1,3,84). Of particular interest, however, is the appearance of antibodies in the cerebrospinal fluid, which is indicative of the diagnosis of rabies infection (157).

TREATMENT

At present, no specific therapy exists for rabies virus infections of humans or animals. Even in the 1990s with sophisticated technology for intensive care, it remains an untreatable infection associated with near-uniform fatality. The only specific management for patients with rabies virus infections of the CNS is superb supportive care. Attention to the medical needs of such patients in an intensive care unit setting may improve the survival rate, although the unrelenting progression of rabies virus infection in the brain does not generate optimism in the present authors.

DISEASE PREVENTION

Several components of disease prevention warrant consideration. These include: (a) evaluation of the risk for acquisition of rabies virus infection, (b) local wound cleaning, (c) administration of vaccine, and (d) the administration of rabies immunoglobulin. Each point will be considered separately.

Because of the high mortality rate associated with rabies virus infection, along with the absence of effective antiviral therapy, prevention is essential. Since humans are not the primary source of rabies virus infection but only an uncommon host as a consequence of contact with animals, interrupting the chain of events of disease progression is essential. Altering the risk of exposure can be accomplished by decreasing contact with wild or domestic rabid animals and by rapid intervention with prophylactic measures. Certainly, the control of rabies in the domestic animal population will significantly diminish the number of cases of rabies virus infection of humans; however, third-world countries still experience a large number of cases of rabies in human populations. Furthermore, in developed countries the control of rabies in wild animal populations has been of increasing relevance, as previously noted. The control of wildlife rabies still remains a practical problem for which adequate methods do not currently exist.

Pre-exposure Prophylaxis

The risk of rabies virus infection can be significantly diminished by pre-exposure prophylaxis in high-risk individuals. Pre-exposure prophylaxis should be considered for high-risk individuals with continuous exposure to rabies virus. These would include: laboratory staff who work in rabies virus research laboratories or in the production of rabies virus biologicals. These individuals would likely have continuous exposure to rabies virus. Other categories of high-risk individuals whose frequent exposure warrants immunization include: rabies diagnostic lab workers, veterinarians, animal control and wildlife workers in rabies epizootic areas, and spelunkers. Criteria for rabies pre-exposure prophylaxis have been summarized by representatives of the Centers for Disease Control (1). At present, the recommendation is administration of the preferred vaccine, namely the human diploid cell vaccine (HDCV), because of its demonstrated safety and efficacy (158–160). For individuals with frequent exposure, booster immunization is indicated, as reviewed (1). Either antibody determinations or routine boosters every 2 years have been utilized for individuals with continuous or frequent exposure to rabies virus.

It must be emphasized that preexposure prophylaxis does not substitute for postexposure treatment. Nevertheless, postexposure treatment can be greatly simplified in the preimmunized individual (reduced frequency of vaccine administration).

A standard preexposure regimen for immunization employed in the United States includes the administration of HDCV either intramuscularly or intradermally over 28 days on days 0, 7, 21, and 28. Should exposure to rabies occur, revaccination with HDCV at 1-ml dosages on two occasions (days 0 and 3) is indicated (1).

Postexposure Prophylaxis

The key element for postexposure prophylaxis is the rapid evaluation of the risk to the individual. As previously summarized in Table 3, the risk to the individual varies according to the extent of exposure and, more specifically, the site of bite and status of skin at the time of the bite. Figure 4 is an algorithm developed by the Centers for Disease Control for evaluation of risk and implementation of prophylactic strategy for individuals potentially exposed to rabies virus infection. Several observations are relevant. First, and most importantly, if a child is bitten by a healthy domestic animal, observation of this domestic animal for a period of 10 days is adequate for determination of risk of rabies virus infection. Should abnormal behavior develop in the animal, then appropriate intervention by veterinary sources to determine the presence of rabies virus infection of the animal is indicated. Under such circumstances, implementation of a postexposure prophylactic regimen is indicated. Alternatively, exposure of an individual to a wild animal, particularly one with altered behavior (such as abnormal daytime behavior for nocturnal animals or unprovoked attacks by nocturnal animals during daylight), warrants implementation of prompt and rapid postexposure prophylaxis. It is essential to assess the species of the biting animal, determine the prevalence of rabies in the area and in the afflicted animal population, ascertain the circumstances of the bite, and confirm the type of exposure. Local health department officials can be of assistance in determining risks in targeted areas. From previous discussions, wild animals most commonly infected by rabies include skunks, raccoons, foxes, coyotes, bobcats, bats, canines, and cattle in the United States. On the other hand, such rodents as squirrels, hamsters, chipmunks, rats, mice, and rabbits rarely carry rabies and, furthermore, have not been documented to transmit infection to humans. Although bites are unequivocally the most common source of rabies virus infection from wild animals to humans, it must also be remem-

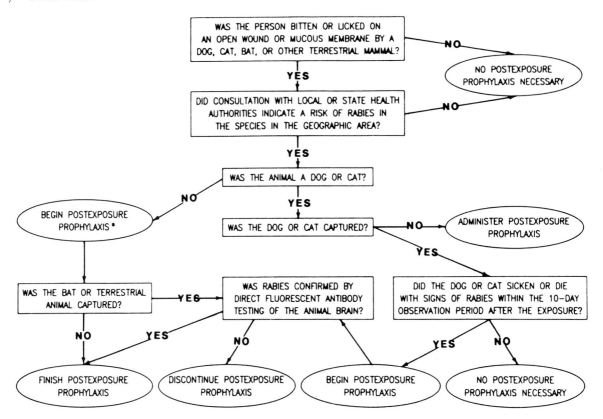

FIG. 4. Algorithm for rabies postexposure prophylaxis. *In exposures of low risk, when the animal brain is available for testing, the decision to administer postexposure prophylaxis is sometimes delayed for up to 2 days after the exposure, pending the results of fluorescent antibody testing of the animal brain. Adapted from Ref. 1.

bered that rabies virus exists in saliva and, perhaps, on the paws of animals and may be transmitted if open wounds become contaminated.

Essential to the management of an exposed individual with a documented bite is prompt local wound care. This is probably the single most effective means for preventing rabies virus infection. It has been well demonstrated that the utilization of high concentrations of soap or benzalkonium chloride greatly decreases the transmission of experimental rabies virus infection by as much as 35–95% (161–164).

Following local wound care, individuals at high risk should be given rabies immunoglobulin (RIG) and the currently available, safe, and efficacious HDCV. Human RIG is prepared by cold ethanol fractionation of plasma from immunized blood donors. Under most circumstances, RIG is given only once, but in divided dosages (20 IU per kilogram of body weight). Approximately one-half is infiltrated at the wound site, whereas the other half is administered intramuscularly in the buttock. Alternatively, horse serum obtained following hyperimmunization can be utilized as well, but it is clearly not the treatment of choice. The dose under such circumstances is 40 IU per kilogram of body weight. However, while effective, at least 40% of adults who receive horse serum will develop serum sickness, (165) particu-

larly as compared with individuals receiving efficacious material of human origin (166).

The utility of immunoglobulin products for prevention of rabies was well demonstrated by the reduced attack rate after the exposure of 29 individuals in Iran to a rabid wolf (167) and as supported by other studies (168). It should be noted that the administration of RIG does not interfere with antibody generation following vaccination; however, it should not be given at the site of vaccine administration (169–171). The safety of human RIG has been well documented (172).

Concomitant with the administration of RIG, the HDCV should be administered as soon as possible after exposure (173). The currently available and most widely utilized vaccine in the United States is that identified as HDCV which is given with RIG (174,175). Vaccine should be administered in the deltoid area as opposed to the gluteal region, which has been associated with vaccine failure (176–179). The administration schedule is five 1-ml doses intramuscularly as soon after exposure as possible and then, subsequently, on days 3, 7, 14, and 28 after the initial immunization. Infants and children should receive a similar dose of HDCV. Efficacy of the HDCV has been well established in studies done in the United States following intramuscular administration (180,181).

Many millions of doses of HDCV have been administered since being introduced in the mid-1970s. Adverse effects associated with HDCV are minimal and generally limited to systemic reactions in 0.16% of patients and include fever, headache, chills, and allergic reactions (3,182). Postvaccination encephalopathy, a commonly encountered side effect of other vaccines, as noted below, has not been reported following the administration of HDCV (183–185). Two patients with Guillain–Barré syndrome postvaccination have been identified; however, these individuals recovered completely (186,187).

When booster doses are required, especially for those individuals who received preexposure prophylaxis, side effects have been identified in varying percentages of individuals, with a range of 1–20% (56,188). However, it should be noted that these side effects do not appear to be directly related to the antigenic composition of the vaccine (189).

It is important to recognize that the HDCV vaccine is utilized primarily in the United States but that other vaccines have been utilized elsewhere in the world. As a consequence, some history regarding vaccine development is in order. Certainly, the Pasteur vaccine represented a landmark first attempt to prevent infection in humans with a vaccine. In 1882, Pasteur prepared a rabies vaccine from a viral strain isolated from a rabid cow which was subsequently passaged in rabbits. The vaccine was first used in 1885 on Joseph Meister and consisted of an injection of a suspension of material derived from desiccated, infected rabbit spinal cords. These preparations contained varying quantities of antigen (9). This vaccine was replaced in the early 1900s by the Semple vaccine, which was derived from rabies-infected rabbit brain. For this vaccine a neural tissue suspension was prepared and inactivated by exposure to formalin and phenol (190). Variations on this vaccine included its preparation in a variety of other animal species (84). The immunogenicity and the protectiveness, as well as the associated adverse effects, are significant following vaccination with the Semple vaccine. It has been estimated that encephalomyelitis and peripheral neuropathy developed as complications of vaccination in one in 200 to one in 1600 recipients of the Semple vaccine, and that approximately 14% of those individuals who suffered complications died (191–195). Nevertheless, this vaccine is still utilized in developing countries (such as those in Africa and Asia) because of its relative inexpensiveness and ease of administration (196).

The next generation of vaccine offered an attempt to avoid the occurrence of neurologic complications by eliminating the neuronal proteins which could be associated with the postvaccination complications, such as myelin basic protein. Thus, a mouse-brain-derived vaccine was developed from suckling animals in the mid 1950s (197–199). This vaccine was prepared from a brain suspension inactivated by ultraviolet light and phenol (200–202). Neurologic complications following vaccination were approximately one in 8000 (201–203). It should be noted that this vaccine is highly immunogenic, with a majority of individuals achieving antibody titers (200,204). This vaccine is still utilized in many areas of South America (200,204).

A variation of the suckling mouse brain vaccine was the duck embryo vaccine utilized in the United States until the early 1980s. This vaccine has subsequently been replaced by HDCV. The duck embryo vaccine is grown in embryonated duck eggs, and then the virus is inactivated with beta-propriolactone (181–185,205–210). Although adverse events are uncommon (namely, neurologic complications in only one in 24,000), the immunogenicity is poor. Thus, a successful vaccine series required a minimum of 23 subcutaneous injections (169,208).

Research of the early 1960s led to the contemporary HDCV, which is currently in use (181,211,212). This vaccine has established immunogenicity and efficacy (213). As noted previously, side effects to this vaccine are insignificant.

FUTURE CONSIDERATIONS

Fear of rabies leads to frequent postexposure prophylaxis through the administration of RIG and HDCV in individuals considered at risk for rabies virus infection. The current cost of the HDCV vaccine, estimated to be approximately $100 in the United States, indicates a need to develop alternative strategies for the control of rabies virus infection which are both inexpensive and efficacious (214). More recently, a vaccinia–rabies-glycoprotein recombinant virus has been constructed as a more contemporary immunogen (215). This vaccine has been shown to result in significant neutralizing antibodies which protect against lethal challenge (216). This vaccine can be administered by an oral route and offers the potential, therefore, of immunization of wild animal populations by baiting. Alternative vaccines include those prepared from the viral envelope glycoprotein, viral ribonucleoprotein, synthetic peptides, or generation of anti-idiotype antibodies (214).

It has been recognized that effective control of wildlife rabies will require immunization of sylvatic hosts whereby administration of an oral rabies vaccine may lead to acceptable animal immunization and protection rates (217–221). A clever experiment has involved the administration of live rabies virus vaccine in chicken heads across a defined area of Switzerland, resulting in a 60% immunization rate of wild foxes (220). A similar level of immunity has been achieved in other populations (222). Such an approach has attracted attention for wild animal populations in the United States (216,223,224). The duration of immunity under these circumstances and the need to achieve 100% immunity require further investigation. Nevertheless, such prospects offer significant hope for decreasing the fear associated with rabies virus infection. In addition, advances in antiviral therapy may well lead to therapeutic approaches to the control of rabies virus infection.

ACKNOWLEDGMENTS

Original studies performed by the investigators were supported by grants from the following sources: the National Institute of Allergy and Infectious Diseases (NO1-AI-62554 and PO-1-AI-24009); the Division of Research Resources (RR0023) of the National Institutes of Health; and the State of Alabama.

REFERENCES

1. Baer GM, Bellini WJ, Fishbein DB. Rhabdoviruses. In: Fields BN, Knipe DM, eds. *Virology.* 2nd ed. New York: Raven Press, 1990;883–930.
2. Baer GM. *The natural history of rabies,* vols 1 and 2. New York: Academic Press, 1975.
3. Robinson PA. Rabies virus. In: Belshie RB, ed. *Human virology.* 1984;485–511.
4. Johnson RT. Rabies. In: Johnson RT, ed. *Viral infections of the nervous system.* New York: Raven Press, 1982;159–167.
5. Tierkel ES. Rabies. *Adv Vet Sci* 1959;5:183–226.
6. Sellers TF. Rabies. In: Harrison TR, ed. *Principles of internal medicine.* New York: McGraw–Hill, 1954;1106–1109.
7. Steele JH. History of rabies. In: Baer GM, ed. *The natural history of rabies,* vol 1, Orlando, FL: Academic Press, 1975;1–29.
8. Smitheors JF. The history of some current problems in animal disease. VII. Rabies, part 2. *Vet Med* 1958;53:267–273.
9. Pasteur L. Methode pour prévenir la rage après morsure. *C R Acad Sci (Paris)* 1885;101:765.
10. Kaprowski H, Plotkin S, eds. *World's Debit to Pasteur.* New York: Alan R Liss, 1985.
11. Hattwick MAW. Human rabies. *Public Health Rev* 1974;3:229–274.
12. Kaplan C, Turner GS, Warrell DA. *Rabies: the facts.* Oxford: Oxford University Press, 1986.
13. Negri A. Zur Aetiologie der Tollwuth. Die Diagnose der Tollwuth auf Grund der neuen Befunde. *Z Hyg Infectionskr* 1903;44:519–540.
14. Babes V. *Traite de la Rage.* Paris: Ballière et Fits, 1912;81.
15. Wagner RR. Rhabdoviridae and their replication. In: Fields BN, Knipe DM, eds. *Virology,* 2nd ed. New York: Raven Press, 1990;867–881.
16. Ginsberg HS. Rhabdoviruses. In: Davis DD, Dulbecco R, Eisen HM, eds. *Microbiology.* Hagerstown, MD: Harper & Row, 1980;1167–1175.
17. Matthews REF. Fourth Report of the International Committee on Taxonomy of Viruses. Classification and nomenclature of viruses. *Intervirology* 1982;17:109.
18. Brown F, Bishop DHL, Crick J, et al. Rhabdoviridae. *Intervirology* 1979;12:1.
19. Matsumoto S. Rabies virus. *Adv Virus Res* 1979;16:257–301.
20. Howatson AF. Vesicular stomatitis and related virus. *Adv Virus Res* 1970;16:196–256.
21. Wagner RR. Reproduction of rhabdoviruses. *Comp Virol* 1975;4:1–93.
22. Ditchfield WJB. Rabies. In: Rhodes AJ, Van Rooyden eds. *Textbook of virology.* Baltimore: Williams & Wilkins, 1968;490–512.
23. Almeida JD, Howatson AF, Pinteric L, et al. Electron microscope observations on rabiesvirus by negative staining. *Virology* 1962;18:147–151.
24. Matsumoto S. Electron microscope studies of rabiesvirus in mouse brain. *Cell Biol* 1963;19:565–591.
25. Sokol F. Chemical composition and structure of rabies virus. In: Baer GM, ed. *The natural history of rabies,* vol 1. Orlando, FL: Academic Press, 1975;79–102.
26. Sokol F, Schlumberger HD, Wiktor TJ, Koprowski H. Biochemical and biophysical studies on the nucleocapsid and on the RNA of rabies virus. *Virology* 1969;38:651–665.
27. Coslett GD, Holloway BP, Obijeski JF. The structural proteins of rabies virus and evidence for their synthesis from separate monocistromic RNA species. *J Gen Virol* 1980;49:161–180.
28. Holloway BP, Obijeski JF. Rabies virus-induced RNA synthesis in BHK-21 cells. *J Gen Virol* 1980;49:181–195.
29. Tordo N, Poch O, Ermine A, Keith G, Rougeon F. Walking along the rabies genome: Is the large G–L intergenic region remnant gene? *Proc Natl Acad Sci USA* 1986;83:3914–3918.
30. Tordo N, Poch O, Ermine A, Keith G, Rougeon F. Completion of the rabies virus genome sequence determination: highly conserved domains among the L (polymerase) proteins of unsegmented negative-stranded RNA viruses. *Virology* 1988;165:656–576.
31. McSharry JJ. The lipid envelope and chemical composition of rhabdoviruses. In: Bishop DHL, ed. *Rhabdoviruses,* vol 1. Boca Raton, FL: CRC Press, 1979;107–117.
32. Dubovi EJ, Wagner RR. Spatial relationships of the proteins of vesicular stomatitis virus: induction of reversible oligomers by cleavable protein cross-linkers and oxidation. *J Virol* 1977;22:500–509.
33. Cox JH, Dietzschold B, Schneider LG. Rabies virus glycoprotein. II. Biological and serological characterization. *Infect Immun* 1977;16:754–759.
34. Dietzschold B, Cox JH, Schneider LG, Wiktor TJ, Koprowski H. Isolation and purification of a polymeric form of the glycoprotein of rabies virus. *J Gen Virol* 1978;40:131–139.
35. Halonnen PA, Murphy FA, Fields BN, Reese DR. Haemagglutinin of rabies and some other bullet-shaped viruses. *Proc Soc Exp Biol Med* 1968;127:1037–1042.
36. Johnson HN. Rabies virus. In: Horsfall FL, Tamm I, eds. *Viral and rickettsial infections of man.* Philadelphia: JB Lippincott, 1965;814.
37. Sikes RK, Larghi OP, Simpson CF, et al. Physical and chemical properties of rabies virus. International Symposium on Rabies, Telloires 1965. *Symp Series Immunobiol Standard* 1966;1:55–64.
38. Kissling RE. Growth of rabies virus in non-nervous tissue culture. *Proc Soc Trop Med Hyg* 1958;98:223–225.
39. Fenje P. A rabies vaccine from hamster kidney tissue cultures: preparation and evaluation in animals. *Can J Microbiol* 1960;6:605–609.
40. MacPherson I, Stoker M. Polyoma transformation of hamster cell clones: an investigation. *Virology* 1962;16:147–151.
41. World Health Organization. *Sixth Report of the Expert Committee on Rabies.* Technical Report Series 523. Geneva: World Health Organization, 1973.
42. Sikes RK, Tierkel ES. Wildlife rabies studies in the southeast. In: *65th Annual Proceedings of the U.S. Livestock Sanitary Association.* 1960;268–272.
43. Zinke GG, Neue Ansichten der Hundswut, ihrer Ursachen und Folgen, nebst einer sichern Behandlungsart der von tollen Thieren gebissenen Menschen. *Gabler Jena* 1804;16:212–234.
44. Dierks RE, Murphy FA, Harrison AK. Extraneural rabies virus infection. Virus development in fox salivary gland. *Am J Pathol* 1969;54:251–273.
45. Winkler WG. Fox rabies. In: Baer GM, ed. *The natural history of rabies,* vol 2, Orlando, FL: Academic Press, 1975;3–22.
46. Winkler WG, Shaddock JH, Bowman C. Rabies virus in salivary glands of raccoons *(Procyon lotor). J Wildl Dis* 1985;21:297–298.
47. Charlton KM, Casey GA, Webster WA. Rabies virus in the salivary glands and nasal mucosa of naturally infected skunks. *Can J Comp Med* 1984;48:338–339.
48. Baltazard M, Bahmanyar M, Ghodssin, et al. Essai pratique du serum antirabique chez les mordus par loups enrages. *Bull WHO* 1955;13:747.
49. Murphy FA, Bauer SP, Harrison AK, Winn WC. Comparative

pathogenesis of rabies and rabies-like viruses. Viral infection and transit from inoculation site to the central nervous system. *Lab Invest* 1973;28:361–376.

50. Charlton KM, Casey GA. Experimental rabies in skunks. Immunofluorescence light and electron microscopic studies. *Lab Invest* 1979;41:36–44.

51. Baer GM, Cleary WF. A model in mice for the pathogenesis and treatment of rabies. *J Infect Dis* 1972;125:520–527.

52. Watson HD, Tignor GH, Smith AL. Entry of rabies virus into the peripheral nerves of mice. *J Gen Virol* 1981;56:371–382.

53. Lentz TL, Burrage TG, Smith AL, Crick J, Tignor G. Is the acetylchlorine receptor a rabies virus receptor? *Science* 1982;215:182–184.

54. Lentz TL, Wilson PT, Hawrot E, Speicher DW. Amino acid sequence similarity between rabies virus glycoprotein and snake venom curraremimetic neurotoxins. *Science* 1984;226:847–848.

55. Dean DJ, Evans WM, McClure RC. Pathogenesis of rabies. *Bull WHO* 1963;29:803–811.

56. Dreesen DW, Bernard KW, Parker RA, Deutch AJ, Brown J. Immune complex-like disease in 23 persons following a booster dose of rabies human diploid cell vaccine. *Vaccine* 1986;4:45–49.

57. Baer GM, Shantha TR, Bourne GH. The pathogenesis of strep rabies virus in rats. *Bull WHO* 1968;38:119–125.

58. Baer GM, Shanthaveerappa TR, Bourne GH. Studies on the pathogenesis of fixed rabies virus in rats. *Bull WHO* 1965;33:783–794.

59. Dean DJ. Pathogenesis and prophylaxis of rabies in man. *NY State J Med* 1963;63:3507–3513.

60. Baer GM, Cleary WF, Diaz AM, Perl DF. Characteristics of 11 rabies virus isolates in mice: titers and relative invasiveness of virus, incubation period of infection, and survival of mice with sequelae. *J Infect Dis* 1977;136:336–345.

61. Murphy FA. Rabies pathogenesis—brief review. *Arch Virol* 1977;54:279–297.

62. Murphy FA, Harrison AK, Winn WC, et al. Comparative pathogenesis of rabies and rabies-like viruses. Infection of the central nervous system and centrifugal spread of virus to peripheral tissues. *Lab Invest* 1973;29:1–16.

63. Schoene WC. The nervous system. In: Robbins SL, Cotran RS, eds. *Pathologic basis of disease.* Philadelphia: WB Saunders, 1979;1530–1598.

64. Leach CN, Johnson HN. Human rabies, with special reference to virus distribution and titer. *Am J Trop Med* 1940;20:335–340.

65. Robinson PA, Shaddock J, et al. Quantitation of rabies virus isolation in a patient. Submitted for publication, 1991.

66. Kock FJ, Sagartz JW, Davidson DE, et al. Diagnosis of human rabies by the corneal test. *Am J Clin Pathol* 1975;63:509–515.

67. Centers for Disease Control: Human-to-human transmission of rabies via a corneal transplant—Thailand. *MMWR* 1981; 30:473–474.

68. Larghi OP, Gonzalez E, Held L, et al. Evaluation of the corneal test as a laboratory method for rabies diagnosis. *Appl Microbiol* 1973;25:187–189.

69. Debbie JG, Trimarchi CV. Pantropism of rabies virus in free-ranging rabid red fox (*Vulpes fulva*). *J Wildl Dis* 1970;6:500–505.

70. Turner GS. Humoral and cellular immune responses of mice to rabies and smallpox vaccines. *Nature* 1973;241:90–92.

71. Smith JS. Mouse model for abortive rabies infection of the central nervous system. *Infect Immun* 1981;31:247–308.

72. Iwasaki Y, Gerhard W, Clark HF. Role of host immune response in the development of either encephalitic or paralytic disease after experimental rabies infection in mice. *Infect Immun* 1977; 18:220–225.

73. Johnson RT, Mercer EH. The development of fixed rabies virus in mouse brain. *Aust J Exp Biol Med Sci* 1964;42:449–456.

74. Johnson RT. The pathogenesis of experimental rabies. In: Nagano Y, Davenport FM, eds. *Rabies.* Tokyo: University of Tokyo Press, 1970;59–75.

75. Murphy FA. Rabies pathogenesis. Brief review. *Arch Virol* 1977;54:279–297.

76. Dupont JR, Earle KM. Human rabies encephalitis—a study of forty-nine fatal cases with a review of the literature. *Neurology* 1965;15:1023–1034.

77. Dubos RJ. *Louis Pasteur—freelance of science.* Boston: Little, Brown, 1950.

78. Goldwasser RA, Kissling RE. Fluorescent antibody staining of street and fixed rabies virus antigens. *Proc Soc Exp Biol Med* 1958;98:219–233.

79. Acha PN. A review of rabies prevention and control status in the Americas, 1970–1980: overall status of rabies. *Bull WHO Int Epiz* 1981;93:9–52.

80. Bogel K, Motschwiller E. Incidence of rabies and post-exposure treatment in developing countries. *Bull WHO* 1986;64:883–887.

81. World Health Organization. *Guidelines for dog rabies control.* Geneva: World Health Organization, 1987;1–44.

82. Chadli A. La rage en Tunisie. Analyse des resultatas des 34 dernières années. *Arch Inst Pasteur Tunis* 1986;63:15–33.

83. Held JR, Tierkel ES, Steele JH. Rabies in man and animals in the United States, 1946–1965. *Public Health Rep* 1967;82:1009–1018.

84. Bernard KW, Fishbein DB. Rabies virus. In: *Infectious diseases and their etiologic agents.* 1291–1303.

85. Anderson LJ, Nicholson KG, Tauxe RV, Winkler WG. Human rabies in the United States, 1960–1979: epidemiology, diagnosis, and prevention. *Ann Intern Med* 1985;100:728–735.

86. Kaplan MM, Koprowski H. Rabies. *Sci Am* 1980;242:120.

87. Jenkins S, Winkler W. Descriptive epidemiology from an epizootic of racoon rabies in the Middle Atlantic states. *Am J Epidemiol* 1987;126:429–437.

88. Carini A. Sur une grandeepizootie de rage. *Ann Inst Pasteur (Paris)* 1911;25:843–846.

89. Haupt H, Rehaag H. Durch Fledermause verbreitete seuchenhafte Tollwut unter Viehbestanden in Santa Catharina (Sud Brasilien) *Z Infektionskr Hyg Haustiere* 1921;22:104–127.

90. Baer GM. Bovine paralytic rabies in the vampire bat. In: Baer GM, ed. *The natural history of rabies,* vol 2. Orlando, FL: Academic Press, 1975;155–175.

91. Centers for Disease Control. Rabies surveillance, United States, 1987. CDC surveillance summaries. *MMWR* 1988;37:1–17.

92. Constantine DG. Rabies transmission by the nonbite route. *Public Health Rep* 1962;77:287–289.

93. Centers for Disease Control. Rabies—United States, 1981. *MMWR* 1982;31:379.

94. Pan American Zoonoses Center. Epidemiological surveillance of rabies for the Americas. *Pan Am Zoonoses Center* 1988;19:1.

95. World Health Organization. *World survey of rabies XXII (for years 1984/85).* Geneva: World Health Organization, 1987:33.

96. World Health Organization and Collaborating Centre for Rabies Surveillance and Research. Rabies in Europe, 2nd quarter, 1988. *Rabies Bull Eur* 1987;12:1.

97. Centers for Disease Control. Human rabies—Australia. *MMWR* 1988;37:351–353.

98. Centers for Disease Control. Bat rabies—Europe. *MMWR* 1986;35:430.

99. Grauballe PC, Baagoe HJ, Fekadu M, Westergaard J, Zoffman N. Bat rabies in Denmark. *Lancet* 1987;1:379–380.

100. Arambulo PV, Escudero SH. Rabies in the republic of the Philippines: its epidemiology, control and eradication. *J Philipp Med Assoc* 1971;47:206–221.

101. Kappus KD. Canine rabies in the United States, 1971–1973: study of reported cases with reference to vaccination history. *Am J Epidemiol* 1976;103:242–249.

102. Sehgal S, Bhatia R. Current status of rabies in India. In: Sehgal S, Bhatia R, eds. *Rabies: current status and proposed control programmes in India.* Delhi, India: National Institute of Communicable Diseases (Directorate General of Health Service), 1985;10.

103. Turner GS. A review of the world epidemiology of rabies. *Trans R Soc Trop Med Hyg* 1976;70:175–178.

104. Winkler WG, Fashinell TR, Leffingwell L, et al. Airborne rabies transmission in a laboratory worker. *JAMA* 1973;226:1219–1221.

105. Ross E, Armentrout SA. Myocarditis associated with rabies—report of a case. *N Engl J Med* 1962;226:1087–1089.

106. Houff SA, Burtono RC, Wilson RW, et al. Human-to-human transmission of rabies virus by corneal transplant. *N Engl J Med* 1979;300:603–604.

107. Centers for Disease Control. Rabies in a laboratory worker—New York. *MMWR* 1977;26:183–184.

108. Irons JV, Eads RB, Grimes JE, et al. The public health importance of bats. *Tex Rep Biol Med* 1957;15:292–298.

109. Shah U, Jaswal GS. Victims of a rabid wolf bite in India: effect of severity and location of bites on development of rabies. *J Infect Dis* 1976;134:25–92.

110. Sitthi-Amorn C, Jiratanavattana V, Keoyoo J, et al. The diagnostic properties of laboratory tests for rabies. *Int J Epidemiol* 1987;16:602–605.

111. Veeraraghavan N. Phenolized vaccine treatment of people exposed to rabies in southern India. *Bull WHO* 1954;10:789–796.

112. McKendrick AG. A ninth analytical review of reports from Pasteur Institutes. *Bull WHO* 1940–1;9:31–78.

113. Para M. An outbreak of post-vaccinal rabies (rage de laboratoire) in Fortaleza, Brazil in 1960. *Bull WHO* 1965;33:177–182.

114. Ruegsegger JM, Black M, Sharpless GR. Primary antirabies immunization of man with HEP Flury virusvaccine. *Am J Public Health* 1961;51:706–714.

115. Black D, Wiktor TJ. Survey of raccoon hunters for rabies antibody titers: pilot study. *J Fla Med Assoc* 1986;73:517–520.

116. Phuapradit P, Manatsathit S, Warrell MJ, et al. Paralytic rabies: some unusual clinical presentation. *J Med Assoc Thai* 1985;68:105–110.

117. Warrell MJ, Looareesuwan S, Manatsathit S, et al. Rapid diagnosis of rabies and post-vaccinal encephalitides. *Clin Exp Immunol* 1988;71:229–234.

118. Wang SP. Statistical studies of human rabies in Taiwan. *J Formosan Med Assoc* 1956;55:548–554.

119. Wilde H, Chutivongse S. Rabies: current management in Southeast Asia. *Med Prog* 1988;14–24.

120. Rubin RH, Gregg MB, Sikes RK. Rabies in citizens of the United States, 1963–1968: epidemiology, treatment, and complications of treatment. *J Infect Dis* 1969;120:268.

121. Nikolitsch M. Virus concentration and incubation period. *Trop Dis Bull* 1958;55:395.

122. Warrell DA. The clinical picture of rabies in man. *Trans R Soc Trop Med Hyg* 1976;70:188–195.

123. Godwasser RA, Kissling RE, Carski RT, et al. Fluorescent antibody staining of rabies virus antigens in the salivary glands of rabid animals. *Bull WHO* 1959;20:579–588.

124. Ahuja ML, Brooks AG. Hydrophobia in India. *Indian Med Gazette* 1950;85:449–453.

125. Veeraraghavan N. *Annual report of the director 1971 and scientific report 1972. Pasteur Institute of Southern India, Coonoor, Tamil Nadu, India.* Madras: Diocesan Press, 1973;38–40.

126. Nikolitsch M. Second observation on the method of infection by neutrotropic viruses (reviewed by Spooner, etc.). *Trop Dis Bull* 1953;50:113–1134.

127. Soave OA. Reactivation of rabies virus in a guinea pig with adrenocorticotropic hormone. *J Infect Dis* 1962;110:129–131.

128. Bhatt DR, Hattwick MAW, Gerdsen R, et al. Human rabies—diagnosis complications, and management. *Am J Dis Child* 1974;127:862–869.

129. Hattwick MAW, Weis TT, Stechschulte CJ, et al. Recovery from rabies—a case report. *Ann Intern Med* 1972;76:931–942.

130. Baraff LJ, Hafkin B, Wehrle TF, et al. Human rabies. *West J Med* 1978;128:159–164.

131. Wilson JM, Hettiarachchi J, Wijesuriya IM. Presenting features and diagnosis of rabies. *Lancet* 1975;II:1139–1140.

132. Warrell DA, Davidson NM, Pope HM, et al. Pathophysiologic studies in human rabies. *Am J Med* 1976;60:180–190.

133. Bloomfield AL. *A bibliography of internal medicine—communicable diseases.* Chicago: University of Chicago Press, 1958.

134. Chopra JS, Banerjee AK, Murthy MK, et al. Paralytic rabies: a clinicopathologic study. *Brain* 1980;103:789.

135. Love SV. Paralytic rabies: review of the literature and report of a case. *J Pediatr* 1944;24:312.

136. Varma K, Maheshwari MC, Chawdhary C, et al. Acute ascending motor paralysis die to rabies: a clinical pathological report. *Eur Neurol* 1985;24:160.

137. Hemachudha TP, Phanuphak RT, Sriwanthana B. Immunologic study of human encephalitic and paralytic rabies. A preliminary study of 16 patients. *Am J Med* 1988;84:673–677.

138. Hurst EW, Pawan JL. An outbreak of rabies in Trinidad. *Lancet* 1931;II:622–628.

139. Knutti RE. Acute ascending paralysis and myelitis due to the virus of rabies. *JAMA* 1929;93:754–758.

140. Pawan JL. Paralysis as a clinical manifestation in human rabies. *Ann Trop Med Parasitol* 1939;33:21–32.

141. Turner GS. Current concepts of immunology and pathogenesis of rabies. In: Pattison JR, ed. *Rabies: a growing threat.* New York: Van Nostrand Reinhold, 1983;27–32.

142. Bell JF, Moore GJ. Allergic encephalitis, rabies antibodies, and the blood–brain barrier. *J Lab Clin Med* 1979;94:5–11.

143. Gode GR, Raju AV, Jayalakshmi TS, et al. Intensive care in rabies therapy: clinical observations. *Lancet* 1976;II:6–8.

144. Cheetham HD, Hart J, Coghill HF, et al. Rabies with myocarditis: two cases in England. *Lancet* 1970;2:921.

145. Araujo MF, Brito RD, Machada CG. Myocarditis in human rabies. *Rev Inst Med Trop Sao Paulo* 1971;13:99.

146. Gode GR, Raju AV. Intensive care in rabies therapy. *Lancet* 1976;2:6.

147. Thiodet J, Forrier A, Syergeol X. Tentatives therapeutiques de la rage déclaré chez l'homme. *Presse Med* 1963;71:172.

148. Porras C, Barboza JJ, Fuenzalida E, et al. Recovery from rabies in man. *Ann Intern Med* 1971;85:44–48.

149. Komsuoglu SS, Dora F, Kalabay O. Periodic EEG activity in human rabies encephalitis. *J Neurol Neurosurg Psychiatry* 1981;44:264–265.

150. Lumion J, Hillbom M, Roine R, et al. Human rabies of bat origin in Europe. *Lancet* 1986;1:378.

151. Blenden DC, Creech W, Torres-Anjel MJ. Use of immunofluorescence examination to detect rabies virus antigen in skin of humans with clinical encephalitis. *J Infect Dis* 1986;154:698–701.

152. Schneider LG. The cornea test: a new method for the intravitam diagnosis of rabies. *Zentralbl Veterinarmed* [B] 1969;16:24–31.

153. Helmick CG, Tauxe RV, Vernon AA. Is there a risk to contacts of patients with rabies? *Rev Infect Dis* 1987;9:511–518.

154. Assis RVC, Rosenberg S. Raiva humana. Estudio neuropatologico de trinta casos. *Rev Inst Med Trop Sao Paulo* 1984;26:346–352.

155. Miyamoto K, Matsumoto S. The nature of the Negri body. *J Cell Biol* 1965;27:677–682.

156. Tangchai P, Yenbutr D, Vejjajjva A. Central nervous system changes in human rabies: a study of twenty-four cases. *J Med Assoc Thai* 1970;53:472.

157. Warrell DA, Warrell MJ. Human rabies and its prevention: an overview. *Rev Infect Dis* 1988;10:S726–S731.

158. Centers for Disease Control. Rabies prevention. *MMWR* 1980;29:265–280.

159. Anderson LJ, Baer GM, Smith JS, et al. Rapid antibody response to human diploid rabies vaccine. *Am J Epidemiol* 1981;113:270–275.

160. Hafkin B, Hattwick MAW, Smith JS, et al. A comparison of a WI-38 and duck embryo vaccine for preexposure rabies prophylaxis. *Am J Epidemiol* 1978;107:439–443.

161. Shaughnessy HJ, Zichis J. Prevention of experimental rabies—treatment of wounds contaminated by rabies virus with fuming nitric acid, soap solution, sulfanilamide or tincture of iodine. *J Am Med Assoc* 1943;123:528–534.

162. Shaughnessy HJ, Zichis J. Treatment of wounds inflicted by rabid animals. *Bull WHO* 1954;10:805–813.

163. Kaplan MM, Cohen D, Koprowski H, et al. Studies on the local treatment of wounds for the prevention of rabies. *Bull WHO* 1962;26:765–775.

164. Dean DJ, Baer GM, Thompson WR. Studies on the local treatment of rabies-infected wounds. *Bull WHO* 1963;28:477–486.

165. II. Immunofluorescence and human viral disease. In: Kurstak E, Morisset R, eds. *Viral immunodiagnosis.* New York: Academic Press, 1974;141–179.

166. Cifuentes E, Calderon E, Bijlenga G. Rabies in a child diagnosed by a new intra-vitam method—the cornea test. *J Trop Med Hyg* 1971;74:23–25.

167. Grandien M. Evaluation of tests for rabies antibody and analysis of serum responses after administration of three different types of rabies vaccine. *J Clin Microbiol* 1977;5:263–267.

168. Louie RE, Dobkin MB, Meyer P, et al. Measurement of rabies

antibody comparison of the mouse neutralization tests (MNT) and the rapid fluorescent focus inhibition test (RFFIT). *J Biol Stand* 1975;3:365–373.

169. Hattwick MAW, Corey L, Creech WB. Clinical use of human globulin immune to rabies virus. *J Infect Dis* 1976; 133(Suppl):A266–A272.

170. Helmick CG, Johnstone C, Sumner J, et al. A clinical study of Merieux human rabies immune globulin. *J Biol Stand* 1982;10:357–367.

171. Hafkin B, Alls ME, Baer GM. Human rabies globulin and human diploid vaccine dose determinations. *Dev Biol Stand* 1978; 40:121.

172. Loofbourow JC, Cabasso VJ, Roby RE, et al. Rabies immune globulin (human): clinical trials and dose determination. *JAMA* 1971;217:1825.

173. Centers for Disease Control. Rabies prevention—United States, 1984. Recommendation of the Immunization Practices Advisory Committee (ACIP). *MMWR* 1984;33:393–402, 407–840.

174. Shill M, Baynes RD, Miller SD. Fatal rabies encephalitis despite appropriate post-exposure prophylaxis: a case report. *N Engl J Med* 1987;20:1257–1258.

175. Centers for Disease Control. Human rabies despite treatment with rabies immune globulin and human diploid cell rabies vaccine—Thailand. *MMWR* 1987;36:759–760.

176. Fishbein DB, Sawyer LA, Reid-Sanden FL, et al. Administration of human diploid cell rabies vaccine in the gluteal area [Letter]. *N Engl J Med* 1987;318:124–125.

177. Centers for Disease Control. Suboptimal responses to hepatitis B vaccine given by injection into the buttock. *MMWR* 1985;34:105–108, 113.

178. Centers for Disease Control. Rabies postexposure prophylaxis with human diploid cell rabies vaccine: lower neutralizing antibody titers with Wyeth vaccine. *MMWR* 1985;34:90–91.

179. Shaw FE, Guess HA, Colemen JP. The effect of anatomic injection site and other host factors. American Society for Microbiology Abstracts, Abstract No. 321, 1986.

180. Centers for Disease Control. Use of human diploid cell vaccine for postexposure rabies treatment—Canada. *MMWR* 1981; 30:266–267.

181. Anderson LJ, Sikes RK, Langkop CW, et al. Postexposure trial of a human diploid cell strain rabies vaccine. *J Infect Dis* 1980;142:133–138.

182. Centers for Disease Control. Adverse reactions to human diploid cell rabies vaccine. *MMWR* 1980;29:609–610.

183. Aoki FY, Tyrrell DAJ, Hill LE, et al. Immunogenicity and acceptability of the human diploid cell rabies vaccine in volunteers. *Lancet* 1975;1:660–662.

184. Costy-Berger F. Vaccination antirabique perventive par du vaccine prepare sur cellules diploides humaines. *Dev Biol Stand* 1971;40:101–104.

185. Kuwert EK, Marcus I, Hoker PG. Neutralizing and complement-fixing antibody responses in pre- and postexposure vaccines to a rabies vaccine prepared in human diploid cells. *J Biol Stand* 1976;4:249–262.

186. Boe E, Nyland H. Guillain–Barré syndrome after vaccination with human diploid cell rabies vaccine. *Scand J Infect Dis* 1980;12:231.

187. Bernard KW, Smith PW, Kader FJ, et al. Neuroparalytic illness and human diploid cell rabies vaccine. *JAMA* 1982;248:3136.

188. Centers for Disease Control. Systemic allergic reactions following immunization with human diploid cell rabies vaccine. *MMWR* 1984;33:185.

189. Anderson MC, Baer H, Frazier J, et al. The role of specific IgE and betapropiolactone in reactions resulting from booster doses of human diploid cell rabies vaccine. *J Allergy Clin Immunol* 1987;80:861–868.

190. Semple D. The preparation of a safe and efficient antirabic vaccine. *Scientific Memoranda of the Medical and Sanitation Department of India* 1911;44.

191. Abdussalem M, Bogel K. The problem of antirabies vaccination. International Conference on the Application of Vaccines Against Viral, Rickettsial, and Bacterial Diseases of Man. *PAHO Sci Publ* 1971;226:54.

192. Appelbaum E, Greenberg H, Nelson J. Neurologic complications following antirabies vaccine. *JAMA* 1953;151:188.

193. Hemachudha T, Phanuphak P, Johnson RT, et al. Neurologic complications of Semple-type rabies vaccine: clinical and immunologic studies. *Neurology (NY)* 1987;37:550–556.

194. Greenberg M, Chidress J. Vaccination against rabies with duck-embryo and Semple vaccines. *JAMA* 1960;173:333–337.

195. Pait CF, Pearson HE. Rabies vaccine encephalomyelitis in relation to incidence of animal rabies in Los Angeles. *Am J Public Health* 1940;39:875–877.

196. Plotkin SA. Rabies vaccine prepared in human cell cultures; progress and perspective. *Rev Infect Dis* 1980;2:433–448.

197. Hemachudha T, Griffin E, Giffels JJ, et al. Myelin basic protein as an encephalitogen in encephalomyelitis and polyneuritis following rabies vaccine. *N Engl J Med* 1987;316:369–374.

198. MacFarlane JO, Culbertson CG. Attempted production of allergic encephalomyelitis with duck embryo suspensions and vaccines. *Can J Public Health* 1954;45:28.

199. Patterson PY. Experimental allergic encephalomyelitis and autoimmune disease. *Adv Immunol* 1966;5:131.

200. Fuenzalida E, Palacios R, Borgono JM. Antibody response in man to vaccine made from infected suckling-mouse brain. *Bull WHO* 1964;30:431–436.

201. Toro G, Vergara I, Roman G. Neuroparalytic accidents of antibies vaccination with suckling mouse brain vaccine—clinical and pathologic study of 21 cases. *Arch Neurol* 1977;34:694–700.

202. Held JR, Adaros HL. Neurologic disease in man following administration of suckling mouse brain antirabies vaccine. *Bull WHO* 1972;42(6):321–327.

203. Kissling RE, Reese DR. Anti-rabies vaccine of tissue culture origin. *J Immunol* 1963;91:362–368.

204. Fuenzalida E. Human preexposure rabies immunization with suckling mouse brain vaccine. *Bull WHO* 1972;46:561–563.

205. Peck FB, Powell HM, Culbertson CG. Duck-embryo rabies vaccine—study of fixed virus vaccine grown in embryonated duck eggs and killed with beta-propriolactone. *JAMA* 1956;162:1373–1376.

206. Powell HM, Culbertson CG. Cultivation of fixed rabies virus in embryonated duck eggs. *Public Health Rep* 1950;65:400–401.

207. Powell HM, Culbertson CG. Recent advances in preparation of antirabies vaccine containing inactivated virus. *Bull WHO* 1954;10:815–822.

208. Rubin RH, Hattwick MAW, Jones S, et al. Adverse reactions to duck embryo rabies vaccine—range and incidence. *Ann Intern Med* 1973;78:643–649.

209. Turner GS, Aoki FY, Nicholson KG, et al. Human diploid cell strain rabies vaccine—rapid prophylactic immunization of volunteers with small doses. *Lancet* 1976;1:1379–1381.

210. Nicholson KG, Turner GS, Aoki FY. Immunization with a human diploid cell strain of rabies virus vaccine: two year results. *J Infect Dis* 1978;137:783–788.

211. Plotkin SA, Wiktor TJ. Rabies vaccine prepared in human cell cultures: progress and perspectives. *Rev Infec Dis* 1978;2:433.

212. Anderson LJ, Winkler WG, Hafkin B, et al. Clinical experience with a human diploid cell rabies vaccine. *JAMA* 1980;244:781.

213. Bahmanyar M, Faydy A, Nour-Salehi S, et al. Successful protection of humans exposed to rabies infection: post-exposure treatment with the new human diploid cell rabies vaccine and antirabies serum. *JAMA* 1976;236:2751.

214. Celis S, Rupprecht CH, Plotkin SA. New and improved vaccines against rabies. *T Cell Sci* 19;419–438.

215. Kieny MP, Lathe R, Drillien R, et al. Expression of rabies virus glycoprotein from a recombinant vaccinia virus. *Nature* 1984;312:163.

216. Wiktor TJ, Macfarlan RI, Reagan KJ, et al. Protection from rabies by a vaccinia recombinant containing the rabies virus glycoprotein. *Proc Natl Acad Sci USA* 1984;81:7194–7198.

217. Wandeler AI. Control of wildlife rabies. In: Campbell JB, Charlton KM, eds. *Rabies*. Boston: Kluwer Academic, 1988;365.

218. Baer GM, Abelseth MK, Debbie JG. Oral vaccination of foxes against rabies. *Am J Epidemiol* 1971;93:487.

219. Black JG, Lawson KF. The safety and efficacy of immunizing foxes using bait containing attenuated rabies virus vaccine. *Can J Comp Med* 1980;44:169.

220. Steck F, Wandeler A, Bichsel P, Capt S, Schneider LG. Oral immunization of foxes against rabies. *Zentralbl Veterinarmed* 1982;29:372.
221. Schneider LG. Oral immunization of wildlife against rabies. *Ann Inst Pasteur Virol* 1985;136:469.
222. Schneider LG, Cox JH. A field trial for oral immunization of foxes against rabies in the Federal Republic of Germany. *Tieraztl Umsch* 1983;38:476.
223. Wiktor TJ, MacFarlan RI, Dietschold B, Rupprecht CE, Wunner WH. Immunogenic properties of vaccinia recombinant virus expressing the rabies glycoprotein. *Ann Inst Pasteur Immunol* 1985;136:105.
224. Rupprecht CE, Dietzschold B, Koprowski H, Johnson DH. Development of an oral wildlife rabies vaccine: immunization of raccoons by a vaccinia–rabies glycoprotein recombinant virus and preliminary field baiting trials. In: Chanock RM, Lerner RA, Brown F, Ginsberg H, eds. *Vaccines 87: modern approaches to new vaccines—prevention of AIDS and other viral, bacterial, and parasitic diseases.* Cold Spring Harbor, NY: Cold Spring Harbor Laboratory, 1987;389–392.

Infections of the Central Nervous System,
edited by W. M. Scheld, R. J. Whitley, and
D. T. Durack, Raven Press, Ltd., New York © 1991.

CHAPTER 8

Slow Viral Infections of the Human Nervous System

David M. Asher

Several neurological diseases once considered to be degenerative are caused by unusual infections. The infections have long, asymptomatic incubation periods of months or years and have durations of overt clinical illness that may also be very long. Although the infectious agents may be latent in other organs of the body, pathological changes are found only in the nervous system. Several such diseases of animals were studied by Sigurdsson (1), who described them as "slow infections." Some slow infections of the human nervous system (Table 1) are caused by viruses with conventional physical properties—viruses that more often cause acute, self-limited illnesses. Other slow infections are caused by infectious agents of unknown structure (2), agents that, like viruses, are smaller than bacteria but that have an array of physical properties so unlike those of conventional viruses that some authorities have concluded that they contain no nucleic acid (3) and, thus, might not be viruses at all (4).

SLOW INFECTIONS WITH CONVENTIONAL VIRUSES

Subacute Sclerosing Panencephalitis

Epidemiology

Subacute sclerosing panencephalitis (SSPE), a slow infection with measles virus causing progressive inflammation and sclerosis of the brain (5), is a rare disease that occurs throughout the world. Data for the United States

D. M. Asher: Laboratory of CNS Studies, National Institute of Neurological Disorders and Stroke, National Institutes of Health, Bethesda, Maryland 20892.

have been compiled for more than 570 cases with onset in 1956 or later by the U.S. National SSPE Registry (6) (now maintained by Dr. Paul R. Dyken, Department of Neurology, University of South Alabama Medical Center, Mobile). The disease has been diagnosed in patients aged less than 1 year (7) to more than 30 years (8), but it primarily affects children and young adolescents. More than 85% of cases in the National Registry had onset between 5 and 15 years of age (7). The average age of onset of SSPE in cases reported before 1980 was about 10 years; between 1980 and 1984 it was almost 14 years. The risk of SSPE for boys is more than twice that for girls and is higher for rural children than for city children. SSPE was once especially common in the southeastern United States, the Ohio River Valley, and some New England states. Recently, cases have been more frequent in the western United States, especially among Hispanic children (6). Acquisition of measles before the age of 18 months seems to increase the risk of SSPE substantially (7). [Exposure to birds and other animals has been reported with abnormal frequency in histories of patients with SSPE; the reason is not clear (9).]

Mean annual incidence rates of SSPE in the United States have fallen markedly since 1960—from 0.61 cases per million persons under age 20 years to an estimated 0.06 cases in 1980 (10). Since 1982, only four or five new cases were registered each year from the entire United States. This drop roughly parallels the progressive decline in annual numbers of measles cases diagnosed since the introduction of live, attenuated measles vaccine in the United States in 1963. The risk of SSPE has been estimated at 8.5 SSPE cases per million cases of measles for a 6-year period during which the estimated risk after measles vaccination was only 0.7 cases per million doses of vaccine. Of the first 566 patients with SSPE diagnosed in the United States after 1969 and reported to the National Registry, only 14% had a history of

TABLE 1. *Slow infections of the nervous system caused by conventional viruses*

Disease	Virus	Viral group
RNA viruses		
AIDS encephalopathy (dementia, myelopathy)	HIV	Retrovirus
Kozhevnikov's epilepsy (and other chronic forms of tick-borne encephalitis)	Tick-borne encephalitis	Flavivirus
Progressive rubella panencephalitis (PRP)	Rubella	Rubivirus
Rabies	Rabies	Rhabdovirus
Subacute sclerosing panencephalitis (SSPE)	Measles	Paramyxovirus
Tropical spastic paraparesis (TSP)/ HTLV-I-associated myelopathy (HAM)	HTLV-1	Retrovirus
DNA viruses		
Cytomegalovirus (CMV) encephalitis	CMV	Herpesvirus group
Progressive multifocal leukoencephalitis (PML)	JC (?SV40)	Papovavirus
? Rasmussen's chronic encephalitis	??CMV, ??Epstein–Barr virus	Herpesvirus group

measles vaccination without also having clinically apparent measles, while a roughly equal number had no history of either acute measles illness or receiving vaccine (10). In cases occurring in vaccinated children, it has not been determined if SSPE resulted from persistent infection with the attenuated measles virus in the vaccine, from undiagnosed wild-type measles infection preceding vaccination, or from vaccine failure and subsequent undiagnosed measles. In any case, the overwhelming advantage of measles vaccination in preventing SSPE is clear. SSPE continues to occur in areas of the world where measles remains unchecked, and it may be anticipated to increase in the United States if compliance with vaccination diminishes.

Clinical Manifestations

Children with SSPE generally have a history of typical measles with full recovery several years before the onset of neurologic disease. Measles may have been either mild or severe. Some patients with SSPE had measles pneumonia, but none have had a history of typical measles encephalitis. The mean interval between measles and onset of SSPE in the United States was formerly about 7 years (10), but recently it has increased to 12 years (6). In vaccinated patients without a history of measles, the mean interval between vaccination and onset of SSPE was 5 years before 1980 (10) and 7.7 years between 1980 and 1986 (6).

The U.S. National SSPE Registry divides the clinical course of typical SSPE into four somewhat arbitrary stages marked by the onset and disappearance of myoclonic jerks and the degree of disability, and it recognizes five different patterns of progression depending on degree of chronicity and occurrence of remissions. However, the overall clinical picture of SSPE tends to be quite stereotyped; almost 70% of Registry cases were classified as either acute, subacute, or chronic progressive, and only 8% were classified as intermittent or remitting. The onset of SSPE is usually insidious, marked by subtle

changes in behavior and deterioration of school work, followed by more overtly bizarre behavior and finally by frank dementia. There is no fever, photophobia, or other findings of acute encephalitis except for occasional complaints of headache. Diffuse neurological disease becomes progressively more severe. The appearance of massive repetitive myoclonic jerks, generally symmetrical, especially involving the axial musculature and occurring at 5- to 10-sec intervals, marks the onset of the second clinical stage of SSPE. The myoclonic jerks appear to be abnormal movements rather than epileptic seizures, but true convulsions can also occur at any stage of illness. In addition to myoclonic jerks, which tend to disappear as disease progresses, a variety of other abnormal movements and dystonias have also been observed. Cerebellar ataxia may be noted as well (6,11). Retinopathy and optic atrophy may appear, sometimes even before behavioral changes (12). Dementia progresses to stupor and coma, sometimes with autonomic insufficiency. Patients may be rigid or spastic with decorticate postures or may be flaccid.

The speed of progression is highly variable, but in at least 60% of patients with SSPE the course is inexorable and relatively rapid. Total duration of illness may be as short as a few months, but most patients survive for 1–3 years after diagnosis, with a mean of about 18 months (6). Occasional patients have shown some spontaneous improvement and lived for more than 10 years. In recent years the few patients diagnosed with SSPE in the United States tended to have relatively long survival, perhaps due to improvements in chronic care. Patients with SSPE have the usual secondary complications associated with incapacitating neurological diseases—pneumonia, decubitus ulcers, and others.

Pathology

The histopathology of SSPE consists of inflammation, necrosis, and repair (6,11,13). Brain biopsy performed in the early stages of SSPE shows mild inflammation of meninges and a panencephalitis involving cortical and subcortical gray matter as well as white matter, with cuffs of plasma cells and lymphocytes around blood vessels (Fig. 1) and increased numbers of glia throughout. Neuronal loss may not be marked until later in the course of illness. Loss of myelin secondary to neuronal degeneration may be apparent. The intranuclear "Cowdry type A" inclusion bodies surrounded by clear halos noted by Dawson in his original description (5) may be seen in hematoxylin-and-eosin-stained sections (Fig. 2) within the nuclei of neurons, astrocytes, and oligodendrocytes, but they are sometimes difficult to find. By electron microscopy the inclusions are seen to contain tubular structures (14) typical of the nucleocapsids of paramyxoviruses. Measles viral antigens can be demonstrated by labeled-antibody techniques within the inclusions as well as in cells without inclusions. Lesions may be unevenly distributed throughout the brain, and biopsy is not always diagnostic, particularly if only a small sample of tissue is obtained. The same findings of inclusion-body panencephalitis are generally present in the brain at autopsy; however, late in disease it may be difficult to find typical areas of inflammation, and the main histopathological changes are necrosis and gliosis. The disease is believed to begin in the cortical gray matter, subsequently progressing to white matter and subcortical gray matter (myoclonus probably results from extrapyramidal involvement) and, finally, to lower structures (11). Although persistent infection of lymphoid tissues with measles virus has also been demonstrated (15–17), these tissues show no pathological changes.

Pathogenesis

SSPE clearly results from a persistent infection with measles virus. The genomes of strains of measles virus isolated from patients with SSPE may be somewhat larger than those isolated from typical cases of measles, and multiple mutations have been found in isolates (18). It has been proposed that some mutation may render the virus more likely to establish persistent infection; however, no consistent genomic abnormalities have been identified in strains of measles virus isolated from brains of SSPE patients, nor have clusters of SSPE cases suggestive of strains of special virulence been described. It has also been theorized that patients with SSPE have some subtle predisposing immune deficiency, or that an infection with a second virus facilitates the chronic measles encephalitis, but neither of these hypotheses has been confirmed.

Complete measles virus particles are not found in the brains of patients with SSPE, and the matrix (M) protein required for the final assembly and budding of virus from the host cells is missing, not only from brain tissues of patients but also from cells cultured from their brains; the full complement of genetic material needed to code for all proteins, including M, is present and functional, however, and when infected brain cells are cultivated together with permissive cells, complete measles virus often emerges. It has been proposed that some restriction in patients' brain cells prevents the translation of M protein, resulting in the accumulation of incomplete measles virus that cannot be cleared either by antibodies or by cell-mediated immunity (13); this hypothesis also remains unproven.

Laboratory Diagnosis

The blood is normal except for elevated titers of antibodies to measles virus; antibodies are of the immunoglobulin G (IgG) and immunoglobulin M (IgM) classes and are directed against all the component proteins of

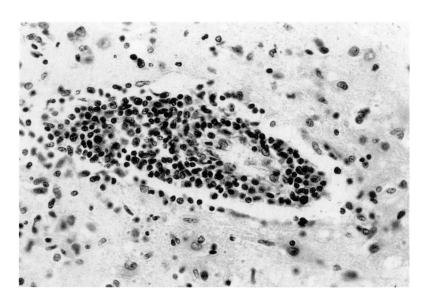

FIG. 1. A cuff of inflammatory cells surrounding a blood vessel in the cerebral cortex of a child with SSPE. (Courtesy of Dr. Peggy Swoveland, Department of Neurology, University of Maryland School of Medicine, Baltimore, Maryland.)

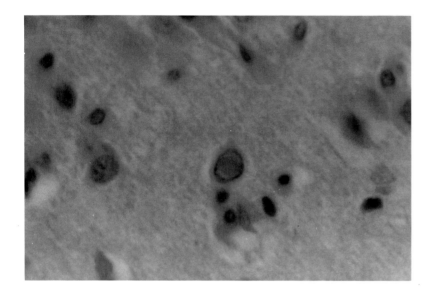

FIG. 2. An intranuclear inclusion from the same specimen as in Fig. 1. (Courtesy of Dr. Janice Stevens, National Institute of Mental Health, Washington, D.C.)

measles virus except the M protein. Examination of the cerebrospinal fluid (CSF) is most useful for establishing the diagnosis of SSPE. Cell content of the CSF is generally normal, although stained sediments have been reported to show plasma cells. Total protein content of the CSF is normal or only slightly elevated; however, the gamma-globulin fraction is greatly elevated (usually comprising at least 20% of total protein in CSF), resulting in a paretic type of colloidal gold curve. When the CSF is examined by electrophoresis or isoelectric focusing, "oligoclonal" bands of immunoglobin are often observed. IgG and IgM antibodies to measles virus, not normally found in unconcentrated CSF, make up most of the immunoglobulin, and these may often be detected in dilutions of 1:8 or higher. The complement-fixation test has been especially useful for demonstrating antibodies in CSF, but hemagglutination-inhibition, immunofluorescence, and other serologic tests, including enzyme-linked immunosorbent assay (ELISA), are also satisfactory. Serological tests for antibodies to measles virus should be performed by experienced personnel in a quality-controlled laboratory. The normal ratio of titer in serum to titer in CSF is reduced (below 200) for measles antibodies, whereas serum/CSF ratios are normal for other viral antibodies and for albumin, indicating that the increased amounts of measles antibodies in CSF of patients with SSPE result from synthesis within the nervous system and that the blood–brain barrier is normal (19).

The electroencephalogram (EEG) is also useful in supporting the diagnosis of SSPE, although early in disease it may be normal or show only moderate nonspecific slowing (20). In the myoclonic stage, most patients with SSPE have episodes of "suppression–burst" in which high-amplitude slow and sharp waves recur at intervals of 3–5 sec on a slow background; however, that pattern is not unique to SSPE (21). Later in the illness the EEG

becomes increasingly disorganized, with high-amplitude random dysrhythmic slowing; in terminal disease the amplitude may fall (6,11). (Several EEGs from patients with SSPE are presented in Fig. 3.)

Computed tomograms or magnetic resonance images of patients with SSPE may show variable cortical atrophy and ventricular enlargement, and there may be focal or multifocal low-density lesions in white matter. However, studies may be normal, especially early in the disease (22).

Brain biopsy is no longer needed to diagnose SSPE. When performed, it often shows the typical histopathological findings described above. Examination of frozen sections by the immunofluorescence technique may demonstrate the presence of measles viral antigens. Isolation of measles virus from brain tissue has been achieved by co-cultivating viable brain cells together with cells susceptible to measles virus and then propagating the mixed cultures for several serial passages. Persistence of measles virus infection in the cultures can be demonstrated by labeled-antibody techniques before complete virus appears. Even in highly experienced laboratories, many specimens failed to yield complete virus, though measles antigens could be demonstrated in cultures (23).

A modification of the polymerase chain reaction (24) detected various regions of the measles virus RNA in frozen and even paraffin-embedded brain tissues of patients with SSPE (25), and this technique may be useful for diagnosis under some circumstances (Fig. 4). Nucleic acid hybridization techniques have also been used to demonstrate the measles viral genome (17). Measles virus and viral RNA have been detected in lymphoid tissues and circulating blood lymphocytes of SSPE patients (16,17,26); it is possible that the polymerase chain reaction will identify the measles genome in blood as well, facilitating early diagnosis.

Differential Diagnosis

In the diagnosis of SSPE, as for other slow viral infections, it is most important to rule out potentially treatable illnesses, such as bacterial infections and tumors. Various cerebral storage diseases and nonstorage poliodystrophies, leukodystrophies, and demyelinating diseases of childhood can also produce progressive dementia with seizures and paralysis resembling SSPE (22). Early in the course of illness, SSPE must be distinguished from atypical acute viral encephalitides (27). Other slow viral infections, such as Creutzfeldt–Jakob disease (CJD) and progressive rubella panencephalitis, must be considered in appropriate age groups. The presence of a typical EEG pattern is suggestive of SSPE, as are unusually high levels of measles antibodies in serum. The diagnosis is practically confirmed if measles antibodies are detected in unconcentrated CSF.

Etiology

SSPE is caused by a persistent measles virus infection. It was first clearly described by Dawson (5), who also postulated its viral etiology. Bouteille et al. (14) recognized that brain cells of patients with SSPE contained tubular structures similar to those seen in cells infected with measles virus, and Connolly et al. (28) showed that patients with SSPE had (a) high levels of antibodies to measles virus in serum and CSF and (b) measles viral antigens in brain. Isolation of measles virus from brains of patients with SSPE was accomplished almost simultaneously by three groups in 1969 (29–32).

Prevention

Immunization with existing attenuated measles virus vaccines appears to prevent at least the large majority of cases of SSPE (6,10). Should cases of SSPE be convincingly attributed to vaccine strains of measles, rather than to preceding natural measles infection or to vaccination failure, then attempts to improve vaccines would be justified.

Therapy

It has been reported that treatment with inosiplex increased the number of patients with prolonged survival and might have produced some clinical improvement in degree of disability (6,33). (A study conducted through the SSPE Registry used 100 mg/kg/day in divided doses.) Other treatments have been ineffective. The use of anticonvulsants, maintenance of nutritional status, prompt treatment of secondary bacterial infections, physical therapy, and other supportive care may also prolong survival and improve the quality of life for the patient and family. Information on current therapeutic trials should be sought through the U.S. National SSPE Registry.

Precautions

The persistent measles infection in SSPE produces no complete virus particles. Patients with SSPE should pose no hazard of infecting others, and no special precautions need ordinarily be taken. If a recent report of isolation of measles virus from the blood of a patient with SSPE is confirmed, then blood precautions might be justified under special circumstances.

Progressive Rubella Panencephalitis

Progressive rubella panencephalitis (PRP) is an exceedingly rare chronic encephalitis associated with persistent rubella virus infection. PRP was first described by Lebon and Lyon (34) in 1974, and fewer than 20 cases have been reported since then. Rubella virus was first isolated from the brain of a patient with PRP by Cremer et al. (35). All patients have been males who were between the ages of 8 and 21 years at onset; most had typical stigmata of the congenital rubella syndrome, including cataracts, deafness, and mental retardation, but several had childhood rubella with full recovery (34,36–39). If the incidence of congenital and acquired rubella continues the dramatic decline that began with the advent of immunization (40), PRP should become even more rare.

The onset of PRP resembles that of SSPE (41–43), with insidious changes in behavior and deterioration in intellectual performance. Those are followed by dementia and other signs of multifocal brain disease, including seizures, cerebellar ataxia, and spastic weakness. Myoclonus and other abnormal movements may occur (41,44), but those are not as common as in SSPE. Retinopathy (similar to that of acute rubella) and optic atrophy may be found (38,41,43). The course of illness in PRP is similar to that in SSPE, progressing to coma, spasticity, brainstem involvement, and death in 2–5 years.

The peripheral blood is normal in PRP except for elevated titers of antibodies to rubella virus. The CSF shows normal or slightly elevated cell content; CSF protein is slightly elevated, with marked increase in globulin, which may make up more than 50% of total protein (39,42). Oligoclonal electrophoretic bands of globulin are found in CSF of PRP patients; the bands resemble those in SSPE but consist of antibodies to rubella-virus antigens (43). Antibodies to rubella virus are readily detectable in CSF, often at dilutions of 1:8 or higher. The complement-fixation, hemagglutination-inhibition, and ELISA techniques should be satisfactory for testing spinal fluid. Most of the rubella antibodies are IgG, al-

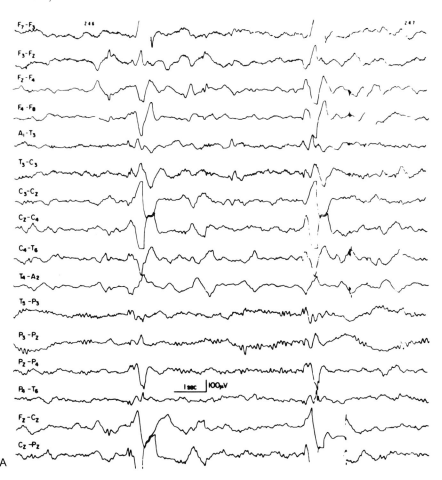

A

FIG. 3. EEGs from several patients with SSPE. (Courtesy of Drs. Ernst Niedermeyer and Eileen Vining, Department of Neurology, Johns Hopkins University School of Medicine, Baltimore, Maryland.)

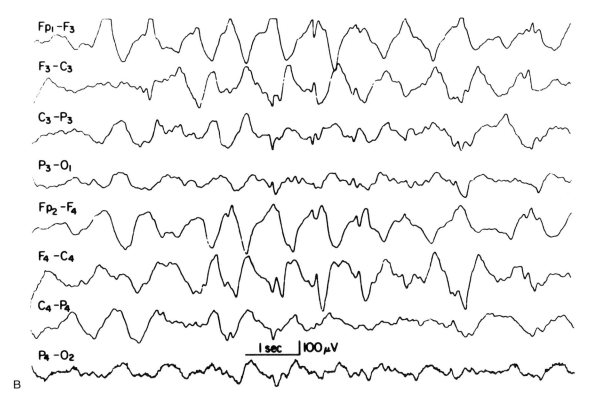

B

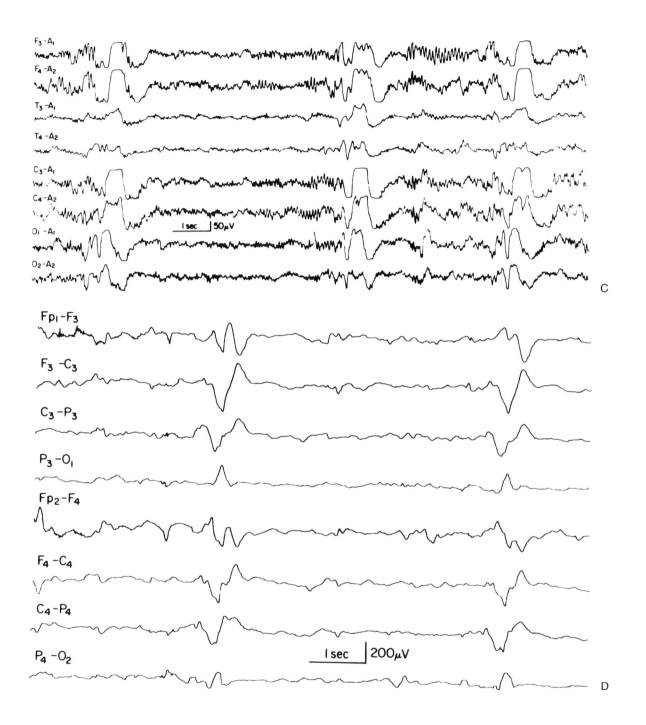

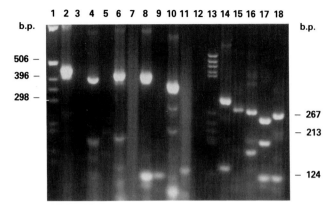

FIG. 4. Agarose gel electrophoresis, stained with ethidium bromide, showing products amplified by polymerase chain reaction with cDNA transcribed from RNA extracted from the brain of a patient with SSPE (lanes 2, 4, 6, 7, 8, and 10). RNA from the brain of a control patient (lanes 3, 5, 9, and 11) was included in the same study. Lanes 1 and 13 contain nucleic acid size markers (b.p. stands for number of base pairs). Pairs of oligonucleotide primers amplifying five regions of measles-virus genome coding for the following proteins were used: nucleoprotein (lanes 2 and 3); phosphoprotein (lanes 4 and 5); matrix protein (lanes 6 and 7); fusion protein (lanes 8 and 9); hemagglutinin (lanes 10 and 11). Digestion of the cDNA products displayed in lanes 2, 4, 6, 8, and 10 with restriction enzymes (AluI or AvaII) yielded fragments of sizes predicted for measles-virus genome (lanes 14–18), confirming identity. Lane 12 is blank. (From ref. 25, with permission.)

though some IgM antibodies have also been detected early in the course of PRP (43). The serum/CSF ratio of antibody titers to rubella virus is reduced (43), whereas ratios of titers to measles and other viruses are normal.

EEGs show generalized slowing with occasional high-voltage activity, but the suppression–burst pattern of SSPE has not been seen in PRP. Pneumoencephalo-grams show enlargement of all ventricles (especially the fourth), with prominent atrophy of the cerebellum. (Computed tomograms were not available when published cases were studied.)

Histopathologic changes in brains of patients with PRP are similar to those in SSPE, with cuffs of lympho-cytes and plasma cells around blood vessels, glial nod-ules in the cortex, some loss of neurons, and an increase in astrocytes throughout gray matter and white matter. The histopathology of PRP differs from that of SSPE in two important respects: In PRP no inclusion bodies have been recognized, and deposits of material that stains with the periodic acid–Schiff (PAS) reaction are found around vessels in subcortical white matter.

Rubella virus was isolated from brain cell cultures of one patient with PRP by co-cultivation with susceptible cells as well as by propagation of explanted cells alone (35,41). Other attempts at isolation from brain tissues were not successful (42). Rubella virus was also isolated from separated blood lymphocytes of a patient with PRP by co-cultivation with susceptible cells (39).

Differential diagnosis of PRP is the same as that of SSPE. The presence of stigmata of congenital rubella syndrome or a history of German measles in a young male with progressive neurological disease suggests PRP. Elevated levels of rubella antibodies in serum, along with the presence of rubella antibodies in the spinal fluid (and reduction of normal serum/CSF ratio for rubella anti-bodies), should establish the diagnosis of PRP. Isolation of rubella virus from blood lymphocytes may be at-tempted. Brain biopsy should not be needed to establish the diagnosis.

Patients with PRP pose no substantial risk of infection to others, although it seems reasonable to avoid exposing rubella-susceptible persons to blood of patients with PRP. Rubella virus has not been detected in urine, and secretions have apparently never been studied.

OTHER CHRONIC OR SLOW INFECTIONS OF THE NERVOUS SYSTEM WITH CONVENTIONAL VIRUSES

Chronic Tick-Borne Encephalitis

The virus of tick-borne encephalitis (TBE), a member of the flavivirus group of small enveloped RNA viruses, usually causes an acute meningoencephalomyelitis (also called "Russian spring–summer encephalitis") that may be of variable severity. A few patients—in some series as many as 20%—recover from acute encephalitis only to develop new signs of progressive neurological disease months or even years later (45). Most cases of chronic progressive TBE have been reported from the Soviet Union, but two typical patients were described in Japan. Chronic progressive TBE may have the following clinical manifestations: (a) movement or seizure disorders of which epilepsia partialis continua [Kozhevnikov's epi-lepsy (46)] is the most common; (b) paralytic disorders, often with brainstem involvement (47); and (c) mixed syndromes. The seizure and movement disorders may stabilize or remit, but the progressive paralytic syndrome is usually fatal. The CSF in one case of chronic TBE contained elevated levels of antibodies to TBE virus. Brain tissue shows panencephalitis without inclusion bodies (by light microscopy) and without virus-like structures (by electron microscopy). Isolation of TBE virus has occasionally been reported from brain tissue or CSF of patients with chronic post-TBE syndromes, but most attempts to isolate the virus have failed (48).

Rasmussen's Encephalitis

Patients with similar types of chronic encephalitis not associated with any known viral infection have been rec-ognized throughout the world. In North America a syn-drome of seizures (especially epilepsia partialis continua), spastic paralysis, and mental retardation associated with chronic encephalitis was described by Rasmussen and colleagues (49–53) in children, adolescents, and young adults. Patients had no history of preceding acute encephalitis. Computed tomograms of patients with Rasmussen's encephalitis may show cerebral cortical atrophy and ventricular dilatation, and when brain tissue is resected a panencephalitis without inclusion bodies or without virus-like particles is found. Recent reports have implicated the Epstein–Barr virus (the herpes-group virus causing infectious mononucleosis and Burkitt's lymphoma) in two cases of Rasmussen's encephalitis (54), and cytomegalovirus has been implicated in several other cases of the disease (54a); these findings remain to be confirmed. Efforts to isolate viruses from brains of patients with Rasmussen's encephalitis have been unsuccessful so far (48).

Progressive Multifocal Leukoencephalopathy (PML)

This progressive infection of oligodendroglial cells with the JC papovavirus affects immunosuppressed subjects, in whom it is almost invariably fatal. It is even more rare in children than in adults. Although PML is a well-recognized opportunistic infection complicating acquired immunodeficiency syndrome (AIDS) in adults, it has apparently not yet been described in children with that disease. (PML is described elsewhere in this volume.)

Persistent Retroviral Infections of the Nervous System

The lentivirus HIV-I (human immunodeficiency virus 1) frequently produces both an acute encephalitis at the time of primary infection and a progressive encephalopathy that is unfortunately very common in both adults and children with AIDS. Those conditions are fully described elsewhere in this volume.

The first human retrovirus to be discovered, the human T-cell leukemia/lymphoma virus I (HTLV-I), has been implicated as causing a progressive myelopathy called both "tropical spastic paraparesis" (TSP) and "HTLV-I-associated myelopathy" (HAM) (55). Limited observations suggest that HTLV-I may also cause meningoencephalitis and myositis. Fortunately, it appears that infections with HTLV-I are often completely asymptomatic, at least for very long periods of time.

SLOW INFECTIONS WITH UNCONVENTIONAL VIRUSES: THE SUBACUTE SPONGIFORM ENCEPHALOPATHIES

The subacute spongiform encephalopathies comprise a group of two or three diseases found in humans [kuru;

Creutzfeldt–Jakob disease (CJD); and CJD's clinical variant, the Gerstmann–Sträussler syndrome (GSS)] and at least four similar diseases found in animals (Table 2). These encephalopathies are all similar in clinical picture and histopathology, and all are slow infections. They take their name from one of the most striking neuropathological changes that occurs in each disease to a greater or lesser extent: spongy degeneration of the cerebral cortical gray matter (Fig. 5).

Epidemiology and Mechanisms of Transmission

Kuru once affected many children and adolescents in a restricted area of Papua New Guinea; its transmission was interrupted more than 30 years ago, and it is now found only in older adults (3). The recent dramatic decline in kuru, with the complete disappearance of this disease among young people, suggests that the practice of ritual cannibalism was the most important, if not the only, mechanism by which the infection spread in Papua New Guinea (56–58).

In major medical centers, especially those responsible for diagnosis and treatment of middle-aged patients with organic dementias, one can expect to encounter an occasional case of CJD, the most common human spongiform encephalopathy. Although CJD was formerly thought to occur only in older adults, iatrogenically transmitted cases of CJD have been recognized in adolescents and young adults. GSS, a familial spongiform encephalopathy with striking amyloid plaques and more prominent cerebellar ataxia and longer average duration than typical sporadic CJD, may be considered a variant of that disease; GSS has not been diagnosed in adolescents.

The epidemiology is more complicated for CJD and GSS than for kuru. CJD has been recognized worldwide, at rates of 0.25 to 2 cases per million population per year (59), with foci of considerably higher incidence among Libyan Jews in Israel, in isolated villages of Slovakia, and in other limited areas (3). Epidemiological surveys have investigated several hypothetical mechanisms of spread

TABLE 2. *Spongiform encephalopathies of humans and animals*

Disease	Naturally infected hosts
Creutzfeldt–Jakob disease (CJD)/ Gerstmann–Sträussler syndrome (GSS)	Humans
Kuru	Humans
Bovine spongiform encephalopathy ("mad cow" disease)	Cattle, captive ungulates, ?cats
Chronic wasting disease	American elk, mule deer
Scrapie	Sheep, goats
Transmissible mink encephalopathy	Mink

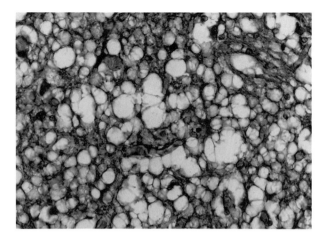

FIG. 5. Severe vacuolation (status spongiosus) in the cerebral cortex of a patient with familial CJD (hematoxylin and eosin stain).

of CJD, including (a) possible contamination of meat products with scrapie agent (60) and (b) iatrogenic spread of infection from tissues of patients (61). The striking resemblance of CJD to scrapie prompted suggestions that infected sheep tissues might be the original source and even a continuing source of spongiform encephalopathy in humans (3); thus far, epidemiological studies have not been consistent with this hypothesis. However, the recent recognition in Great Britain of bovine spongiform encephalopathy (BSE) among cattle, zoo animals (62), and, possibly, domestic cats—apparently infected by eating meat and bone meal contaminated with scrapie agent (63–67)—raised a fear that a strain of the scrapie agent, crossing one "species barrier" from sheep to cattle, may have acquired an even broader range of susceptible hosts, posing a potential danger for humans (68). Although no transmission of spongiform encephalopathy from animals to humans has even been documented, this troubling theoretical possibility has recently been the subject of concern. The degree of actual danger, if any, posed to humans by handling or eating meat contaminated with a spongiform encephalopathy agent and the frequency with which the meat supply from a given area is contaminated are unknown. However, changes in feeding of cattle and in meat-cutting-and-rendering procedures intended to prevent further spread of BSE in the United Kingdom would be expected to reduce the likelihood of human exposure there.

Iatrogenic transmission of CJD has been amply documented. More than 20 years ago a small cluster of CJD was observed in three patients who had previous neurosurgery performed in the same operating suite (69,70). Accidental transmission of CJD by transplantation of contaminated cornea (71) and by contaminated cortical electrodes used during epilepsy surgery (72) has been described. CJD has been recognized in 13 young people (seven from the United States) who had received injections of human pituitary growth hormone (73–75) in-

volving at least five contaminated lots in three countries (76); one recipient of human pituitary gonadotropin also succumbed to CJD (77). Three cases of CJD were recently diagnosed in patients who received grafts of cadaver dura mater lyophilized in large lots by one manufacturer (78–83). The danger posed to patients by pharmaceuticals and grafts derived from or contaminated with human neural tissues, particularly when obtained from unselected donors and from large pools of donors, is clear. Such products must be replaced by synthetics whenever possible, as has been done with human growth hormone in the United States. In the great majority of cases of spongiform encephalopathy, however, no definite iatrogenic events can be identified. Possible mechanisms postulated for iatrogenic transmission have included (a) ocular tonometry, (b) surgery of the head, neck, and teeth, and (c) trauma surgery; none of these has been confirmed.

Spouses and household contacts of patients seem to be at very low risk of acquiring CJD. A single conjugal case has been reported (84). It was previously stated with confidence that medical personnel had no increased risk of CJD (56,59); recent reports of CJD in histopathology technicians (85,86) (one of whom had been exposed to brains of patients with that disease), in addition to its well-documented occurrence in a neurosurgeon (87), forces a reconsideration of that issue.

The occurrence and significance of familial spongiform encephalopathies are discussed below; it must be stressed that in tissues of familial cases of spongiform encephalopathy, infectious agents with the same physical and biological properties as those found in sporadic cases are present, posing the same risk of accidental transmission.

Scrapie is a spongiform encephalopathy of sheep, less commonly of goats, that has long been recognized in Great Britain and on the European continent (88); in recent years it has increased in frequency in the United States (89). Its probable connection with BSE is discussed above. Transmissible mink encephalopathy is a similar disease (90,91) of ranch mink; it has been postulated that mink were originally infected by eating beef contaminated with a spongiform encephalopathy agent (92). A similar "wasting disease" of captive American elk and mule deer has also been described (93); it has not been recognized to occur in the wild.

Clinical Manifestations

Kuru, the first human spongiform encephalopathy recognized to be a slow infection (94,95), is a progressive degenerative disease of the cerebellum and brainstem with less obvious involvement of the cerebral cortex. The first sign of kuru is usually cerebellar ataxia followed by progressive incoordination. Typical coarse shivering tremors gave kuru its name in the Fore language. Variable abnormalities in cranial nerve function appear with frequent impairment in conjugate gaze and swallowing. Patients die of inanition and pneumonia, decubitus ulcers with septicemia, or accidental burns, usually less than a year after onset. Although changes in mentation are common, there is no frank dementia or progression to coma as in CJD. There are no signs of acute encephalitis—no fever (except during secondary infections), headaches, or convulsions.

CJD occurs throughout the world (59), affecting mainly middle-aged and older subjects (mean age in most series is 60–69 years) and occurring very rarely in older adolescents and young adults (59). Patients initially have either sensory disturbances or confusion and inappropriate behavior, with progression over weeks or months to frank dementia and ultimately coma. Some patients have cerebellar ataxia early in disease. Most patients develop myoclonic jerking movements, frequently with generalized "startle" myoclonus. GSS is a familial disease resembling CJD (57), but with more prominent cerebellar ataxia and amyloid plaques; dementia may appear only late in the course of GSS. Mean survival of patients with CJD is less than 1 year from earliest signs of illness, though about 10% live for more than 2 years (96). Patients with GSS tend to survive longer. Reports of remission have not been confirmed. In terminal illness with either CJD or GSS the usual complications secondary to any degenerative neurological disease—aspiration and pneumonia, decubitus ulcers, and thromboembolic episodes—should be anticipated.

Pathology

Definite diagnosis of kuru and CJD must be made from brain tissue. Typical changes are vacuolation and loss of neurons (Fig. 5) with hypertrophy and proliferation of glial cells (Fig. 6), most pronounced in the cerebral cortex in CJD and in the cerebellum in kuru. The pathological lesions are typically most severe in or even confined to gray matter, at least early in disease. Unusual patients with prominent white matter involvement have been described in Japan (97). Loss of myelin appears to be secondary to degeneration of neurons. There is usually no inflammation (98).

Vacuoles, the most prominent histopathological finding (Fig. 5), appear to arise by budding, first from multilaminated areas of cell membranes into the cytoplasm and later from the walls of existing vacuoles to form multiple vacuolation (99,100). A marked increase in the number and size of astrocytes is readily demonstrable by gold stain or by immunostaining of glial fibrillary acidic protein (Fig. 6).

"Amyloid" plaques (Fig. 7), staining with the periodic acid–Schiff reaction and exhibiting birefringency in polarized light when stained with Congo red, are found in brains of all patients with GSS, in at least 70% of patients with kuru, and less commonly in CJD. Amyloid plaques are most common in the cerebellum but occur elsewhere in the brain as well. The plaques contain an abnormal protein (designated here as "SAF/PrP" and described below) and react with antisera prepared against that protein (101–104), but they do not react with antisera to the amyloid "A" protein found in plaques of Alzheimer's disease (104,105); prior treatment of tissue sections with formic acid enhances immunostaining (106,107). Even in the absence of plaques, extracellular SAF/PrP has been detected by immunostaining (108,109) in brains of patients with CJD.

Tubulovesicular particles measuring about 23 nm across have often been observed in brains of patients and

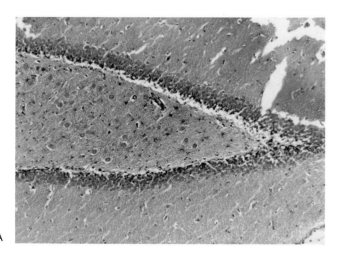
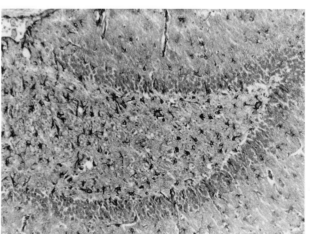

A   B

FIG. 6. Proliferation and hypertrophy of astrocytes in the dentate nucleus of a hamster with experimental scrapie (**B**) compared with that of a normal hamster (**A**). (Indirect immunoperoxidase reaction with antiserum to glial fibrillary acidic protein, stained with diaminobenzidine and counterstained with hematoxylin, kindly prepared by Ms. Jennifer Payne and Dr. Mark Godec, Laboratory of CNS Studies, National Institute of Neurological Disorders and Stroke, Bethesda, Maryland.)

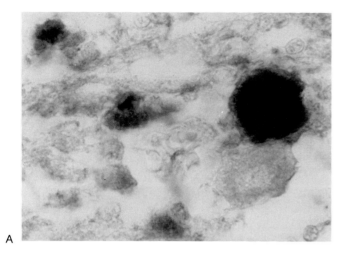

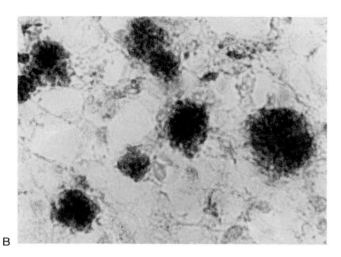

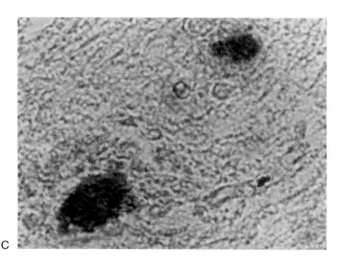

FIG. 7. "Amyloid" plaques in the cerebellum of patients with kuru (**A**), CJD (**B**) and GSS (**C**). Indirect immunoperoxidase reaction with antiserum to SAF/PrP stained with diaminobenzidine without counterstain (195). (Preparations kindly provided by Dr. Don C. Guiroy, Laboratory of CNS Studies, National Institute of Neurological Disorders and Stroke, Bethesda, Maryland.)

animals with spongiform encephalopathies (Fig. 8), particularly in postsynaptic processes of neurons (110); their origin, structure, and relationship to the infectious agents remain uncertain.

Pathogenesis

The portal of entry for the kuru agent is thought to be the integument, probably through lesions rather than intact skin and mucosa (3). The finding of scrapie agent in intestines and mesenteric lymph nodes early in the incubation period of scrapie in sheep (111) suggests that the intact intestinal tract may also be a natural portal of infection. Monkeys have been experimentally infected with the agents of scrapie, kuru, and CJD by being fed contaminated tissue (112); however, a chimpanzee carefully inoculated by gastric tube with a large amount of the kuru agent failed to develop disease (D. M. Asher, C. J. Gibbs and D. C. Gajdusek, *unpublished observation*). Whether humans can be infected with spongiform encephalopathies via the intestinal tract is not known. The first site of replication of the agents appears to be in tissues of the reticuloendothelial system (2,111). In some rodents with scrapie and CJD the agents have been detected in blood (113), and the detection of the CJD agent in human blood has been reported as well (114,115). It is not clear if "viremia" is responsible for spread of infection to the nervous system. Some evidence suggests that in mice the scrapie agent spreads to the central nervous system (CNS) by ascending peripheral nerves (2). In human kuru it is probable that the only portal of exit of the agent from the body, at least in quantities sufficient to infect others, is through exposure of infected tissues during cannibalism (3); in iatrogenically transmitted CJD there is a similar portal of exit.

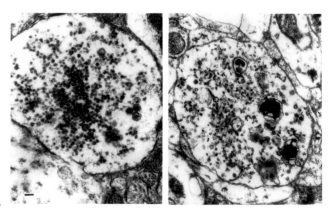

FIG. 8. Tubulovesicular particles measuring about 23 nm across in postsynaptic process of a mouse with scrapie (**A**) and a patient with CJD (**B**). Bar represents 100 nm. (Thin-section electron micrograph courtesy of Dr. Harash K. Narang, Public Health Laboratory, Newcastle-upon-Tyne, England.)

TABLE 3. *Infectivity of tissues, body fluids, and excretions from patients with Creutzfeldt–Jakob disease*

Consistently found to contain infectious agent (≥50% of attempts)	Sometimes found to contain infectious agent (4–33% of attempts)	May contain infectious agent (occasional unconfirmed reports)	Infectious agent not detected (≥3 attempts)
Brain	Cerebrospinal fluid	Blood	Adrenal gland
Eye	Kidney	Urine	Feces
Spinal cord	Liver		Myocardium
	Lung		Saliva
	Lymph node		
	Spleen		

Brain, spinal cord, and eye of patients with CJD are consistently infectious. Several other human tissues and CSF sometimes contain the agent as well (116,117) (Table 3). [A small number of studies did not find secretions or excretions from patients with CJD to be infectious. A single unconfirmed report suggested that urine contained the agent (115).]

At no time during the course of illness have antibodies or cell-mediated immunity to the infectious agents of the spongiform encephalopathies been convincingly demonstrated in either patients or animals (116). This apparent complete lack of immune response to infection is unexplained.

Laboratory Findings

Virtually all patients with CJD have abnormal electroencephalographic findings; as the disease progresses, the

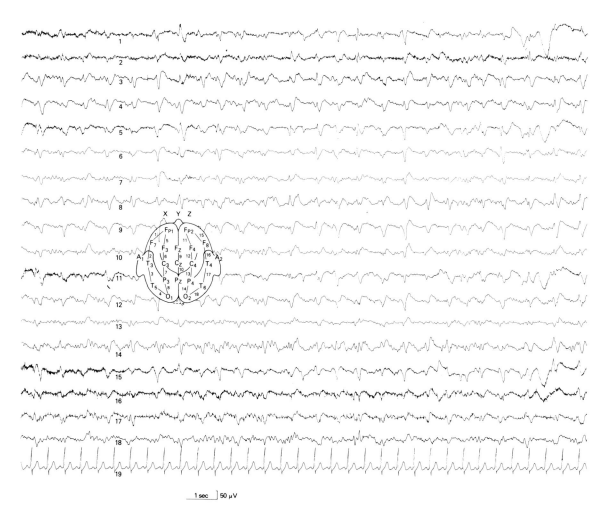

FIG. 9. EEG from a patient with CJD. Periodic high-voltage slow-wave complexes are present on a slow, poorly organized background. (Courtesy of Dr. Charles Henry, Department of Neurology, Medical College of Virginia, Richmond, Virginia.)

background becomes slow and irregular with diminished amplitude. A variety of paroxysmal discharges (slow waves, sharp waves, spike-and-wave complexes) may also appear; these may sometimes be unilateral or focal as well as bilaterally synchronous. Paroxysmal discharges may be precipitated by loud noise. Many patients with CJD have typical periodic "suppression–burst" complexes of high-voltage slow activity on EEG (Fig. 9) at some time during illness (21).

Computed tomography may show cortical atrophy and large ventricles late in the course of CJD. There may be some elevation of CSF protein. Liver function studies sometimes suggest parenchymal disease (118); the significance of this is not known. Other clinical laboratory tests are generally normal and are therefore not helpful in making the diagnosis.

One research laboratory test may ultimately be useful in establishing the diagnosis of CJD. Four abnormal protein spots were detected in the CSF of most patients with CJD (119) using a technique of gel electrophoresis in one direction and isoelectric focusing in the other (120). Two of these spots (designated "130 and 131") were found in fluids of patients with CJD, and they were also found in fluids of some patients with acute herpes simplex encephalitis. Although the source of the proteins remains unknown (they are not related to SAF/PrP), their presence in the CSF of a patient with appropriate clinical presentation strongly suggests CJD (119).

Diagnosis and Differential Diagnosis

The demonstration in detergent- and proteinase K-treated brain extracts of SAF by negative-stain electron microscopy (Fig. 10) or of PrP27-30 proteins by gel electrophoresis (Fig. 11) and immunoblotting is useful for

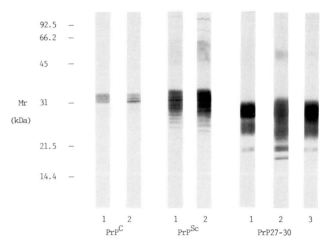

FIG. 11. Immunoblots of brain extracts with antibodies to PrP27-30. Extracts of scrapie-infected and normal brains (prepared as in Fig. 10) were fractionated by polyacrylamide gel electrophoresis and transferred to nirocellulose membranes. Strips were incubated with sera of rabbits immunized with PrP27-30 from scrapie-infected mice (lanes numbered 1) or hamsters (lanes numbered 2) or with a synthetic 15-amino-acid peptide (lane numbered 3) homologous to the N-terminus of rodent PrP27-30 (and partially homologous to human PrP27-30). Strips were stained with the indirect immunoperoxidase technique. PrP^c is a 33- to 35-kD protein encoded by the "PrP" gene (rodent equivalent of the human "PRIP" gene) prepared from the brain of a normal rodent. PrP^{Sc} is a protein of the same molecular mass and amino acid sequence (but apparently a different "isoform" resistant to digestion with proteinase K) prepared from the brain of a rodent with scrapie. PrP27-30 [also designated "SAF/PrP" or "amyloid enhancing factor" (3)] is described in the text. [Courtesy of Dr. Jiri Safar, Laboratory of CNS Studies, National Institute of Neurological Disorders and Stroke, Bethesda, Maryland, with permission of Edgell Communications, Inc. (196).]

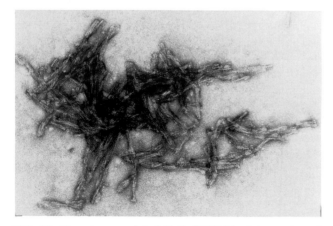

FIG. 10. Scrapie-associated fibrils (SAFs) in detergent- and protease K-treated extract of brain from a hamster with experimental scrapie. (Negative-stain electron micrograph courtesy of Mrs. Kitty L. Pomeroy, Laboratory of CNS Studies, National Institute of Neurological Disorders and Stroke, Bethesda, Maryland.)

confirming histopathological diagnosis. Transmission of disease to susceptible animals by inoculation of brain suspension must now be reserved for cases of special research interest. In our experience, chimpanzees and squirrel monkeys are the most consistently susceptible animals; animals should be observed for at least 3 years before transmission attempts are considered to be tentatively negative. Unusual cases of CJD may be difficult to distinguish from Alzheimer's disease; the finding of the 130/131 proteins in CSF (Fig. 12) strongly suggests the former. The two diseases can sometimes be distinguished only at autopsy. The plaques of CJD/GSS, where present, can be differentiated from those of Alzheimer's disease by immunostaining with specific antisera (21,104,105). Except for conventional histopathology, these are research techniques.

Although brain biopsy may be diagnostic of CJD, this procedure can be recommended only if some other potentially treatable disease remains to be excluded. Recent reports describe modified techniques successfully

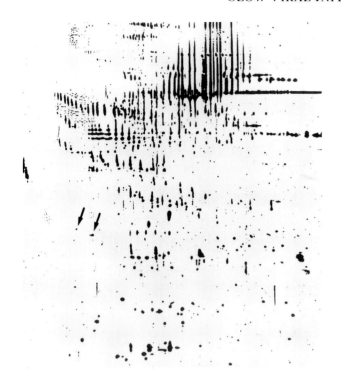

FIG. 12. Polypeptides in CSF of a patient with autopsy-confirmed CJD demonstrated by two-dimensional separation (by electrophoresis in one dimension and isoelectric focusing in the other) in gel stained with silver (120). The pair of abnormal peptides indicated by arrows, designated 130 and 131 (119), have been found in most CSF samples from patients with CJD. They are not unique to CJD (they also occur in CSF of some patients with herpes encephalitis), but they have not been identified in samples from healthy older people or in patients with Alzheimer's disease. In this figure, the image in the gel was digitized on a densitometer and processed by computer to highlight individual polypeptide spots. (Courtesy of Dr. Michael Harrington, California Institute of Technology, Pasadena, California.)

demonstrating SAF/PrP in small tissue fragments (121,122); these procedures may prove useful in evaluating biopsies. However, examination of paraffin sections of a biopsy by an experienced neuropathologist remains the diagnostic standard by which other tests must be measured.

Etiology

The spongiform encephalopathies are all slow infections transmissible to susceptible animals by inoculation of tissues from affected subjects (3). Although the infectious agents replicate in some cell cultures, they do not achieve the high titers of infectivity found in brain tissues nor do they cause recognizable cytopathic effects (123,124). Most studies of the spongiform encephalopathy agents employ *in vivo* assays in which the appearance of typical scrapie or CJD in animals is taken as evidence that the agent is present and intact. The scrapie agent has

consistently passed through filters whose pore diameter averages 50 nm or more (125,126); furthermore, titrations of infectivity of all the agents by serial dilution clearly demonstrate replication, in the sense that inoculation of the smallest amounts of infectivity present in very dilute preparations result in the accumulation in tissues of recipient animals of large amounts (in some cases of as many as a billion infectious units in a gram of brain) of an agent having the same physical and biological properties as the original agent. The pathogens transmitting spongiform encephalopathies have been generally called "viruses" (3). However, they display a spectrum of extreme resistance to inactivation by a variety of chemical and physical treatments, including heat, ultraviolet light, and ionizing radiation, not known among other viruses (127). This phenomenon stimulated hypotheses that the spongiform encephalopathy agents might not contain nucleic acid (3,4,128). The demonstration that infectivity of scrapie is substantially reduced by several treatments that denature proteins (4,129) suggested that the infectious moiety must contain, or at least be protected by, a protein. Prusiner (4) proposed that the unique infectious pathogens causing the spongiform encephalopathies are probably subviral in size, composed of protein, and devoid of nucleic acid; he suggested that they be called "prions" in recognition of their "proteinaceous" structure (4).

There remain unresolved problems with the protein hypothesis, which is not universally accepted by authorities in the field of slow infections. The unusual resistances to heat and chemical exposures of the scrapie agent seem to repose in a tiny resistant fraction, the great bulk of infectivity being destroyed with kinetics of inactivation resembling those of known viruses (130). This resistant residuum seems to be at least partially protected from inactivation by its association with host proteins and by the tendency of the infectious agents to aggregate into hydrophobic masses. These anomalies make it difficult to interpret inactivation studies as ruling out a nucleic acid component within the scrapie agent. Irradiation–inactivation kinetic studies have been reinterpreted as consistent with the hypothesis that the scrapie agent might have a nucleic acid genome of small viral size (130,131). Even the most convinced proponents of the prion theory allow for the possibility that very small amounts of nucleic acid (perhaps 45 bases of double-stranded oligonucleotide) might be present in the infectious particle (132). No published and confirmed studies have unequivocally demonstrated the complete transmissible particles to be subviral in size. Purified proteins uncontaminated with nucleic acid have not been rigorously demonstrated to retain scrapie infectivity (133,134). On the other hand, no virus-like particles have been recognized in highly infectious extracts of tissue, nor have nucleic acids unique to the spongiform encephalopathies been identified (135,136). Should the transmissible agents of the spongiform encephalopathies eventually prove to be infectious proteins, then the term "prion" might be appropriate. If, however, the spongiform encephalopathy agents ultimately prove to contain nucleic acid genomes (2), then they might more appropriately be considered atypical viruses. [Proponents of a theory that the agents are composed of a tiny unique nucleic acid surrounded and protected by components provided by the host have suggested that they be called "virinos" (137).] Until the actual structure of the pathogens is clearly determined, it seems less contentious simply to call them "agents."

Merz et al. (138–140) found specific "scrapie-associated fibrils" (SAFs) in extracts of tissues from a variety of patients and animals with spongiform encephalopathies, but not in normal tissues. SAFs (Fig. 10) resemble, but are distinguishable from, amyloid fibrils that accumulate in brains of patients with Alzheimer's disease. Prusiner and his co-workers described a group of antigenically related, low-molecular-weight proteins, ranging in mass from about 27 to 30 kD (Fig. 11), in brains of animals with scrapie (141) and patients with CJD (142) but not in brains of controls; they postulated that the abnormal proteins might be the elusive "prions," or at least a component of them, and they designated these proteins as the "prion protein 27-30" or PrP27-30 (143). PrP27-30 is clearly a component of SAF (144,145) (Fig. 13); it is found consistently in brains of patients with spongiform encephalopathies (146) and can be demonstrated in the amyloid plaques that occur in those diseases (108). SAF and PrP27-30 (henceforth designated here as "SAF/PrP") generally "copurify" with infectivity of scrapie (147,148), a finding that forms the basis of conclusions by several groups of investigators

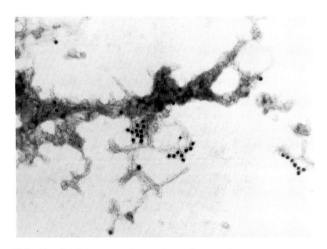

FIG. 13. SAF (prepared as in Fig. 10) reactive with antiserum to PrP27-30, demonstrated by labeling with gold particles in an indirect immunogold assay. (Immunostaining and negative-stain electron micrograph courtesy of Mrs. Kitty L. Pomeroy, Laboratory of CNS Studies, National Institute of Neurological Disorders and Stroke, Bethesda, Maryland.)

that the protein is the infectious agent or a component of it (3,149). However, other groups have claimed some success in separating infectivity from SAF/PrP (150–152), or they have found differences between the physical behavior of the infectious entity and that of SAF/PrP (134,153). So it is not yet clear whether SAF/PrP constitutes the complete infectious particle of spongiform encephalopathies (or a component of those particles) or is simply a pathological host protein not usually separated from the actual infectious entities by currently used techniques. The clear demonstration that the SAF/PrP protein is encoded by a normal host gene (154,155) and has an amino acid sequence identical to that of the normal gene product (145) seems to favor the last possibility. When spongiform encephalopathy agents of various origins were "cloned" by passage at limiting dilution and then similar numbers of infectious units were injected into inbred susceptible mice, there were substantial differences in incubation periods of disease transmitted (90,156–158) and in the presence of amyloid plaques within the brain (157); those properties appear to be determined by the agent and are usually not altered after serial passages. Changes in those properties have been observed to occur suddenly and then to remain stable on subsequent passages in animals—a phenomenon resembling mutation (156,158). It is not understood how agent-specific information can be transmitted and replicated in the absence of some genetic material independent of the host. Ingenious hypotheses have been proposed to explain how a host-coded protein, the gene for which is present and expressed in all normal subjects, might transmit pathogenic information (3,159,160). However, skeptics maintain that the agent more probably contains some unique nucleic acid of its own (2,134,161).

Whatever the relationship of SAF/PrP to the actual infectious particles, the protein must be extremely important in the pathogenesis of spongiform encephalopathies. SAF/PrP is a glycoprotein (162) consisting of some 55 amino acids (153) with attached carbohydrates, a neuraminic acid residue (162), and an inositol (163). It has the physical properties of an amyloid protein [i.e., it is birefringent in polarized light and stains with Congo red dye (142)], presumably resulting from its occurrence in β-pleated sheets. The SAF/PrP proteins of several species of animals are very similar in amino acid sequence and antigenicity but are not identical in structure (164,165). Their primary structure is clearly encoded by the host and does not appear to be influenced by the source of infectious agent provoking its formation (166). Although SAF/PrP is not related to other known proteins, it resembles aggregating proteins such as keratin and collagen in some respects (167). SAF/PrP is derived from a larger precursor protein (150) consisting of some 250 amino acids (165); this precursor protein is designated "PrP33-35" (168), "Gp35" (133), or "scrapie amyloid precursor protein" (3) by various authorities. PrP33-35 occurs both in tissues of humans and animals with spongiform encephalopathies and in normal tissues (169). The amino acid sequences of PrP33-35 extracted from normal and infected tissues are identical (155,170), but the proteins differ somewhat in physical properties: PrP33-35 from infected tissues is resistant to proteolysis with the enzyme proteinase K, whereas that from normal tissue is sensitive (168). This difference is thought to result from a post-translational change in glycosylation, the nature of which is still unknown. PrP33-35 has been detected on cell surfaces (163) as well as within Golgi apparatus and endoplasmic reticulum (104). It was first reported that PrP33-35 is synthesized almost exclusively within neurons (171). After considerable difficulty (172) it was detected in spleen and lymphoid tissues (173); it appears to be secreted into supernatant fluids of many, but not all, types of cultured cells (174). The function of PrP33-35 in normal cells is still unknown. There is a relationship between mutations in the gene coding for PrP and familial spongiform encephalopathies.

Host Genetics and Spongiform Encephalopathies

Spongiform encephalopathies sometimes run in families. In some series of CJD about 10% of cases have a family history of presenile dementia consistent with the disease (175). The pattern of occurrence roughly resembles an autosomal-dominant mode of inheritance. The clinical and histopathological findings in patients with a family history of CJD are the same as those in sporadic cases. GSS is probably always familial. Accumulating evidence indicates that the basis for familial spongiform encephalopathies lies, at least in part, in a series of mutations in the gene coding for the SAF/PrP precursor protein.

The gene coding for PrP33-35 (SAF/PrP precursor) is closely linked, if not identical, to that controlling the incubation periods of scrapie in sheep (176) and both scrapie and CJD in mice (177–179), and amino acid substitutions associated with long incubation periods have been identified (180). The gene encoding the analogous protein in humans, currently designated the "PRIP" gene, is located on the short arm of chromosome 20 (181). It has an open reading frame of some 750 nucleotides (165) in which three different mutations linked to the occurrence of spongiform encephalopathy in families have already been identified.

In several (but not all) families with GSS, an apparent genetic linkage of disease to the same mutation in the PRIP gene was present. In one family an insertion of 0.15 kb was identified in the PRIP gene of affected patients (182). In other families a point mutation (designated Leu^{102}) has been found at codon 102, where it results in the substitution of leucine for proline in the

protein product (181,183,184). Another family with GSS lacked the mutation at codon 102 but had one at codon 117 (Val^{117}), resulting in the substitution of valine for the normal alanine (184). In members of a family with familial spongiform encephalopathy diagnosed as CJD with congophilic amyloid plaques, resembling those of kuru, the Leu^{102} mutation was also found, suggesting that its presence may prove a useful criterion for diagnosis of GSS (185); interestingly, patients with kuru had neither the Leu^{102} mutation nor the insertion (186). Still another mutation, at codon 200 (Lys^{200}) in the PRIP gene, has been identified as being linked to several cases of familial CJD, resulting in a substitution of lysine for the normal glutamine in PrP (183). The Lys^{200} mutation was recently detected in several CJD patients who had no family history of spongiform encephalopathy (187), as well as in healthy relatives of CJD patients—at least one of whom was so old as to be unlikely to be in the incubation period of the disease. The same Leu^{102} mutation associated with GSS was recently recognized in a child with another obscure neurological illness (L. G. Goldfarb, *unpublished observation*), and this allele was also found in healthy relatives in one family (though it remains possible that they may ultimately succumb to spongiform encephalopathy). Two other mutations at different loci in the PRIP gene were detected in several normal subjects as well as in patients with sporadic CJD, none of whom had a family history of spongiform encephalopathy. In several families with CJD and in most patients with "sporadic" CJD, none of these mutations was identified. It has been predicted that other mutations will be found in the PRIP genes of patients in these families. For the moment, it seems wise to avoid alarming healthy subjects having miscellaneous mutations in the PRIP gene or their families, since the implications are not yet clear.

The mechanism by which the mutations act is also in dispute: Those favoring the "prion" (147) or "infectious amyloid" (3) hypothesis postulate that mutations facilitate the folding of protein into an abnormal β-pleated sheet of amyloid, whereas those who support the idea that the pathogen must contain a small nucleic acid attribute familial disease to a genetically controlled susceptibility, perhaps involving increased affinity of the receptor protein for the agent on the host cell membrane or of a host protein that protects the genome of the pathogen from inactivation, or both. Whatever the explanation, in affected families, subjects heterozygous for several mutations in the PRIP gene clearly have high probability of eventually getting spongiform encephalopathy should they live long enough.

It may be of comfort to relatives of sporadic CJD patients to know that in the United States, only about 10% of cases are familial and that, if no previous cases consistent with the diagnosis have been recognized in the family, the odds are against others coming down with a spongiform encephalopathy; in affected families, however, about 50% of siblings and children of a CJD patient may eventually get the disease (175).

Therapy

Several substances—the polyanions HPA23, carageenan, and dextran sulfate (188) and the antibiotic amphotericin B (189,190)—produced apparent interference with experimental scrapie when administered before or shortly after inoculation, but none reversed an established infection of the CNS. Remissions of human CJD after several treatments have been claimed but were not confirmed in subsequent use. Unfortunately, no therapy can be recommended for treating patients with spongiform encephalopathies. Supportive care should be provided as for other progressive fatal neurological diseases.

Prevention of Infection and Disinfection of Contaminated Materials

Brain tissues of patients with CJD are infectious, containing from a thousand to more than a million lethal doses of agent per gram of tissue when assayed in susceptible animals. CSF and non-neural tissues may sometimes contain the infectious agent (117) as well (Table 3). All materials and surfaces known to be contaminated with tissues or CSF from patients suspected of having CJD must be treated with great care. Adherence to the current policy of universal precautions for handling blood and body fluids, intended to prevent infection with hepatitis B and C viruses and human immunodeficiency virus, should also reduce the already small chance of accidental exposure to the agents of spongiform encephalopathy.

Whenever possible, contaminated instruments should be discarded by careful packaging and transport to sites of incineration. Although no method of sterilization can be relied upon to remove all infectivity from contaminated surfaces, several methods reduce titers of infectivity markedly. Contaminated tissues and biological products can probably not be completely freed of infectivity without destroying structural integrity and biological activity; medical and family histories of individual tissue donors should be carefully reviewed for dementia. The preparation of hormones from pools of unselected pituitary glands for use in humans has been discontinued in the United States.

Three treatments are currently recommended for disinfection of objects and surfaces contaminated by the infectious agents: heat, sodium hydroxide, and chlorine bleach. Heating, by incineration of disposable items or by steam autoclaving for at least 2 hr, should be employed when possible. Autoclaving at higher-than-usual

temperature (132°C instead of 121°C) and pressure would be preferable. [One study recently found that some infectivity survived even harsher conditions of heating and actually appeared to be stabilized by treatment with formaldehyde prior to heating (160).] Sodium hydroxide solutions (1 N or stronger) are highly effective in inactivating large amounts of both scrapie and CJD agents (127); we recommend that contaminated materials be exposed for at least 1 hr. Sodium hypochlorite (5.25% as fresh full-strength household bleach) had considerable inactivating potency in several experimental studies; exposure to hypochlorite for at least 1 hr is recommended where heat or sodium hydroxide cannot be used.

A recent study suggested that the same formic acid treatment used to enhance the immunostaining of amyloid in tissue sections reduced the infectivity of scrapie agent in the tissue markedly (191); such treatment might be considered by pathology laboratories. Attempts to sterilize the spongiform encephalopathy agents with ethylene oxide gas and with a variety of commercial liquid disinfectants were completely ineffective.

OTHER DEGENERATIVE DISEASES OF THE CNS CAUSED BY UNCONVENTIONAL AGENTS

It was recently claimed that two other human diseases may be caused by infections with agents similar to those causing the spongiform encephalopathies: familial Alzheimer's disease of adults (192) and Alpers' disease (a convulsive disorder with hemiatrophy and status spongiosus of the cerebral gray matter) of young children (193). These claims have not been independently substantiated (194), and accumulating evidence casts doubt upon them.

REFERENCES

1. Sigurdsson B. Observations on three slow infections of sheep. *Br Med J* 1954;110:255–270, 307–322, 341–354.
2. Kimberlin RH. Scrapie: How much do we really understand? *Neuropathol Appl Neurobiol* 1986;12:131–147.
3. Gajdusek D. Subacute spongiform encephalopathies: transmissible cerebral amyloidoses caused by unconventional viruses. In: Fields B, Knipe D, eds. *Virology.* New York: Raven Press, 1990;2289–2324.
4. Prusiner S. Novel proteinaceous particles cause scrapie. *Science* 1982;216:136–144.
5. Dawson JR. Cellular inclusions in cerebral lesions of lethargic encephalitis. *Am J Pathol* 1933;9:7–16.
6. Dyken PR, Cunningham SC, Ward LC. Changing character of subacute sclerosing panencephalitis in the United States. *Pediatr Neurol* 1989;5:339–341.
7. Modlin JF, Halsey NA, Eddins DL, et al. Epidemiology of subacute sclerosing panencephalitis. *J Pediatr* 1979;94:231–236.
8. Cape CA, Martinez AJ, Robertson JT, Hamilton R, Jabbour JT. Adult onset of subacute sclerosing panencephalitis. *Arch Neurol* 1973;28:124–127.
9. Halsey NA, Modlin JF, Jabbour JT, Dubey L, Eddins DL, Ludwig DD. Risk factors in subacute sclerosing panencephalitis: a case–control study. *Am J Epidemiol* 1980;111:415–424.

10. Centers for Disease Control. Subacute sclerosing panencephalitis surveillance—United States. *MMWR* 1982;31:585–588.
11. Dyken PR. Subacute sclerosing panencephalitis. Current status. *Neurol Clin* 1985;3:179–196.
12. Johnston HM, Wise GA, Henry JG. Visual deterioration as presentation of subacute sclerosing panencephalitis. *Arch Dis Child* 1980;55:899–901.
13. Sever JL. Persistent measles infection of the central nervous system: subacute sclerosing panencephalitis. *Rev Infect Dis* 1983; 5:467–473.
14. Bouteille M, Fontaine C, Verenne C, Delarue J. Sur un cas d'encéphalite subaiguë à inclusions. Etude anatomoclinique et ultrastructurale. *Rev Neurol* 1965;113:454–458.
15. Brown HR, Goller NL, Rudelli RD, Dymecki J, Wisniewski HM. Postmortem detection of measles virus in non-neural tissues in subacute sclerosing panencephalitis. *Ann Neurol* 1989;26:263–268.
16. Fournier JG, Tardieu M, Lebon P, et al. Detection of measles virus RNA in lymphocytes from peripheral-blood and brain perivascular infiltrates of patients with subacute sclerosing panencephalitis. *N Engl J Med* 1985;313:910–915.
17. Fournier JG, Gerfaux J, Joret AM, Lebon P, Rozenblatt S. Subacute sclerosing panencephalitis: detection of measles virus sequences in RNA extracted from circulating lymphocytes. *Br Med J* 1988;296:684.
18. Cattaneo R, Schmid A, Billeter MA, Sheppard RD, Udem SA. Multiple viral mutations rather than host factors cause defective measles virus gene expression in a subacute sclerosing panencephalitis cell line. *J Virol* 1988;62:1388–1397.
19. Tourtelotte WW, Ma BI, Brandes DB, Walsh MJ, Potvin AR. Quantitation of *de novo* central nervous system IgG measles antibody synthesis in SSPE. *Ann Neurol* 1981;9:551–556.
20. Gimenez-Roldan S, Martin M, Mateo D, Lopez-Fraile IP. Preclinical EEG abnormalities in subacute sclerosing panencephalitis. *Neurology* 1981;31:763–767.
21. Gloor P, Kalabay O, Giard N. The electroencephalogram in diffuse encephalopathies: electroencephalographic correlates of grey and white matter lesions. *Brain* 1968;91:779–801.
22. Duda EE, Huttenlocher PR, Patronas NJ. CT of subacute sclerosing panencephalitis. *Am J Neurol Res* 1980;1:35–38.
23. Katz M, Koprowski H. The significance of failure to isolate infectious viruses in cases of subacute sclerosing panencephalitis. *Arch Gesamte Virusforsch* 1973;41:390–393.
24. Saiki RK, Gelfand DH, Stoffel S, et al. Primer-directed enzymatic amplification of DNA with a thermostable DNA polymerase. *Science* 1988;239:487–491.
25. Godec MS, Asher DM, Swoveland PT, et al. Detection of measles virus genomic sequences in SSPE brain tissue. *J Med Virol* 1990;30:237–244.
26. Fournier JG, Lebon P, Bouteille M, Goutiers F, Rozenblatt S. Subacute sclerosing panencephalitis: detection of measles virus RNA in appendix lymphoid tissue before clinical signs. *Br Med J* 1986;293:523–524.
27. Whitley RJ. Viral encephalitis. *N Engl J Med* 1990;323:242–250.
28. Connolly JH, Allen IV, Hurwitz LJ. Measles-virus antibody and antigen in subacute sclerosing panencephalitis. *Lancet* 1967; i:542–544.
29. Chen TT, Watanabe I, Zeman W, Mealey J. Subacute sclerosing panencephalitis: propagation of measles virus from brain biopsy in tissue culture. *Science* 1969;163:1193–1194.
30. Horta-Barbosa L, Fuccillo DA, Sever JL, Zeman W. Subacute sclerosing panencephalitis: isolation of measles virus from a brain biopsy. *Nature* 1969;221:974.
31. Horta-Barbosa L, Fuccillo DA, London WT, Jabbour JT, Zeman W, Sever JL. Isolation of measles virus from brain cell cultures of two patients with subacute sclerosing panencephalitis. *Proc Soc Exp Biol Med* 1969;132:272–277.
32. Payne FE, Baublis JV, Itabashi HH. Isolation of measles virus from cell cultures of brain from a patient with subacute sclerosing panencephalitis. *N Engl J Med* 1969;281:585–589.
33. Dyken PR, Swift A, Durant RH. Long-term follow-up of patients with subacute sclerosing panencephalitis treated with inosiplex. *Ann Neurol* 1982;11:359–364.

34. Lebon P, Lyon G. Non-congenital rubella encephalitis. *Lancet* 1974;ii:468.
35. Cremer NE, Oshiro LS, Weil ML, Lennette EH, Itabashi HH, Carney L. Isolation of rubella virus from brain in chronic progressive panencephalitis. *J Gen Virol* 1975;29:143–153.
36. Dayras JC, Lyon G, Ponsot G, Allemon MC. Progressive chronic rubella encephalitis. Report of a personal case. *Dem Hôp Paris* 1980;56:1703–1708.
37. Meyer E, Weiss-Wichert PH, Ehrlich J, Brandeis WE, Scheffner D, ter Meulen V. Progressive rubella panencephalitis in a child with acute lymphatic leukemia. *Monatsschr Kinderheilkd* 1980;128:242–243.
38. Wolinsky JS, Berg BO, Maitland CJ. Progressive rubella panencephalitis. *Arch Neurol* 1976;33:722–723.
39. Wolinsky JS, Dau PC, Buimovici-Kleine E, et al. Progressive rubella panencephalitis: immunological studies and results of isoprinosine therapy. *Clin Exp Immunol* 1979;35:397–404.
40. Centers for Disease Control. Rubella—United States, 1979–1982. *MMWR* 1982;31:568, 573–575.
41. Weil ML, Itabashi HH, Cremer NE, Oshiro LS, Lennette EH, Carney L. Chronic progressive panencephalitis due to rubella virus simulating subacute sclerosing panencephalitis. *N Engl J Med* 1975;292:994–998.
42. Townsend JJ, Baringer JR, Wolinski JS, et al. Progressive rubella panencephalitis: late onset after congenital rubella. *N Engl J Med* 1975;292:990–993.
43. Wolinsky JS. Progressive rubella panencephalitis. In: Vinken PJ, Bruyn GW, eds. *Handbook of clinical neurology.* Amsterdam: Elsevier/North-Holland, 1978:331–341.
44. Abe T, Nukada T, Hatanaka H, Tajima M, Mirawa M, Ushijima H. Myoclonus in a case of suspected rubella panencephalitis. *Arch Neurol* 1983;40:98–100.
45. Asher DM. Chronic encephalitis. In: *Search for the cause of multiple sclerosis and other chronic diseases of the central nervous system. Proceedings of the first international symposium of the Hertie Foundation.* 1980:272–279.
46. Kozhevnikov AYa. A particular kind of cortical epilepsy (epilepsia corticalis sive partialis continua). *Med Obozren* 1894;42:97–118 (reprinted in 1952 by the State Publisher of Medical Literature, USSR).
47. Ogawa M, Okubo H, Tsuji Y, Yasui N, Someda K. Chronic progressive encephalitis occurring 13 years after Russian spring–summer encephalitis. *J Neurol Sci* 1973;19:363–373.
48. Asher DM, Gajdusek DC. Virological studies of chronic encephalitis. In: Andermann F, ed. *Chronic encephalitis.* Boston: Butterworths, 1991; in press.
49. Aguilar MJ, Rasmussen T. Role of encephalitis in pathogenesis of epilepsy. *Arch Neurol* 1960;2:663–676.
50. Rasmussen T, Olszewski J, Lloyd-Smith D. Focal seizures due to chronic localized encephalitis. *Neurology (Minneap)* 1958;8:435–445.
51. Rasmussen T, McCann W. Clinical studies of patients with focal epilepsy due to "chronic encephalitis." *Trans Am Neurol Assoc* 1968;93:89–94.
52. Rasmussen T. Further observations on the syndrome of chronic encephalitis and epilepsy. *Appl Neurophysiol* 1978;41:1–12.
53. Rasmussen T. Hemispherectomy for seizures revisited. *Can J Neurol Sci* 1983;10:89–94.
54. Walter GF, Renella RR. Epstein–Barr virus in brain and Rasmussen's encephalitis. *Lancet* 1989;i:279–280.
54a. Power C, Poland SD, Blume WD, Girvin JP, Rice GPA. Cytomegalovirus and Rasmussen's encephalitis. *Lancet* 1990;ii:1282–1284.
55. Román GC, Vernant JC, Osame M. HTLV-I and the nervous system. Neurology and Neurobiology, 1989;51:620.
56. Gajdusek DC, Gibbs CJ Jr, Asher DM, et al. Precautions in medical care of and in handling materials from patients with transmissible virus dementia (Creutzfeldt–Jakob disease). *N Engl J Med* 1977;297:1253–1258.
57. Masters CL, Gajdusek DC, Gibbs CJ Jr. Creutzfeldt–Jakob disease virus isolation from the Gerstmann–Sträussler syndrome, with an analysis of the various forms of amyloid plaque deposition in the virus-induced spongiform encephalopathies. *Brain* 1981;104:559–588.

58. Klitzman RL, Alpers MP, Gajdusek DC. The natural incubation period of kuru and the episodes of transmission in three clusters of patients. *Neuroepidemiology* 1985;3:3–20.

59. Masters CL, Harris JO, Gajdusek DC, Gibbs CJ Jr, Bernoulli C, Asher DM. Creutzfeldt–Jakob disease: patterns of world-wide occurrence and the significance of familial and sporadic clustering. *Ann Neurol* 1979;5:177–188.

60. Davanipour Z, Alter M, Sobel E, Asher DM, Gajdusek DC. Transmissible virus dementia: evaluation of a zoonotic hypothesis. *Neuroepidemiology* 1986;5:194–206.

61. Davanipour Z, Alter M, Sobel E, Asher DM, Gajdusek DC. Creutzfeldt–Jakob disease: possible medical risk factors. *Neurology* 1985;35:1483–1486.

62. Hourrigan JL. The scrapie control program in the United States. *J Am Vet Med Assoc* 1990;196:1679.

63. Fraser H, McConnell I, Wells GA, Dawson M. Transmission of bovine spongiform encephalopathy to mice. *Vet Rec* 1988; 123:472.

64. Hope J, Reekie LJ, Hunter N, et al. Fibrils from brains of cows with new cattle disease contain scrapie-associated protein. *Nature* 1988;336:390–392.

65. Wells GA, Scott AC, Johnson CT, et al. A novel progressive spongiform encephalopathy in cattle. *Vet Rec* 1987;121:419–420.

66. Wilesmith JW, Wells GA, Cranwell MP, Ryan JB. Bovine spongiform encephalopathy: epidemiological studies. *Vet Rec* 1988; 123:638–644.

67. Wilesmith JW. Epidemiology and current status of bovine spongiform encephalopathy in the United Kingdom. *J Am Vet Med Assoc* 1990;196:1674–1675.

68. Kimberlin RH. Detection of bovine spongiform encephalopathy in the United Kingdom. *J Am Vet Med Assoc* 1990;196:1675–1676.

69. Will RG, Matthews WB. Evidence for case-to-case transmission of Creutzfeldt–Jakob disease. *J Neurol Neurosurg Psychiatr* 1982;45:235–238.

70. Nevin S, McMenemy WH, Behrman D, Jones DP. Subacute spongiform encephalopathy: a subacute form of encephalopathy attributable to vascular dysfunction (spongiform cerebral atrophy). *Brain* 1960;83:519–564.

71. Duffy P, Collins G, DeVoe AG, Streeten B, Cohen D. Possible person-to-person transmission of Creutzfeldt–Jakob disease. *N Engl J Med* 1974;290:693.

72. Bernoulli C, Siegfried J, Baumgartner G, et al. Danger of accidental person-to-person transmission of Creutzfeldt–Jakob disease by surgery. *Lancet* 1977;i:478–479.

73. Brown P, Gajdusek DC, Gibbs CJ Jr, Asher DM. Potential epidemic of Creutzfeldt–Jakob disease from human growth hormone therapy. *N Engl J Med* 1985;313:728–731.

74. Brown P. The decline and fall of Creutzfeldt–Jakob disease associated with human growth hormone therapy. *Neurology* 1988;38:1135–1137.

75. Gibbs CJ Jr, Joy A, Heffner R, et al. Clinical and pathological features and laboratory confirmation of Creutzfeldt–Jakob disease in a recipient of pituitary-derived human growth hormone. *N Engl J Med* 1985;313:734–738.

76. Brown P. Iatrogenic Creutzfeldt–Jakob disease. *Aust NZ J Med* 1990;20:633–635.

77. Cochius JI, Burns RJ, Blumbergs PC, al. e. Creutzfeldt–Jakob disease in a recipient of human pituitary-derived gonadotrophin. *Aust NZ J Med* 1990;20:592–594.

78. Centers for Disease Control. Rapidly progressive dementia in a patient who received a cadaveric dura mater graft. *MMWR* 1987;36:49–50, 55.

79. Centers for Disease Control. Update: Creutzfeldt–Jakob disease in a patient receiving a cadaveric dura mater graft. *MMWR* 1987;36:324–325.

80. Centers for Disease Control. Update: Creutzfeldt–Jakob disease in a second patient who received a cadaveric dura mater graft. *MMWR* 1989;38:37–38, 43.

81. Masullo C, Pocchiari M, Macchi G, Alema G, Piazza G, Panzera MA. Transmission of Creutzfeldt–Jakob disease by dural cadaveric graft. *J Neurosurg* 1989;71:954–955.

82. Nisbet TJ, MacDonaldson I, Bishara SN. Creutzfeldt–Jakob disease in a second patient who received a cadaveric dura mater graft [Letter]. *JAMA* 1989;261:1118.

83. Thadani V, Penar PL, Partington J, et al. Creutzfeldt–Jakob disease probably acquired from a cadaveric dura mater graft. Case report. *J Neurosurg* 1988;69:766–769.

84. Jellinger K, Seitelberger F, Heiss W-D, Holczabek W. Konjugale Form der subakuten spongiöse Enzephalopatie (Jakob–Creutzfeldt Erkrankung). *Wien Klin Wochenschr.* 1972;84:245–249.

85. Miller D. Creutzfeldt–Jakob disease in histopathology technicians. *N Engl J Med* 1988;318:853–854.

86. Sitwell L, Lach B, Atack E, Atack D. Creutzfeldt–Jakob disease in histopathology technicians. *N Engl J Med* 1988;318:854.

87. Gajdusek DC, Gibbs CJ Jr, Earle K, Dammin GJ, Schoene WC, Tyler HR. Transmission of subacute spongiform encephalopathy to the chimpanzee and squirrel monkey from a patient with papulosis maligna of Köhlmeier-Degos. *Excerpta Med Int Congr Ser* 1974;319:390–392.

88. Cathala F. Scrapie in France. *J Am Vet Med Assoc* 1990; 196:1680.

89. Hadlow WJ. An overview of scrapie in the United States. *J Am Vet Med Assoc* 1990;196:1676–1677.

90. Kimberlin RH, Cole S, Walker CA. Transmissible mink encephalopathy (TME) in Chinese hamsters: identification of two strains of TME and comparisons with scrapie. *Neuropathol Appl Neurobiol* 1986;12:197–206.

91. Marsh RF, Kimberlin RH. Comparison of scrapie and transmissible mink encephalopathy in hamsters. II. Clinical signs, pathology and pathogenesis. *J Infect Dis* 1975;131:104–110.

92. Marsh RF. Bovine spongiform encephalopathy in the United States. *J Am Vet Med Assoc* 1990;196:1677.

93. Williams ES, Young S. Spongiform encephalopathy of Rocky Mountain elk. *J Wildl Dis* 1982;18:465–471.

94. Gajdusek DC, Zigas V. Degenerative disease of the central nervous system in New Guinea: epidemic occurrence of "kuru" in the native population. *N Engl J Med* 1957;257:974–978.

95. Gajdusek D, Gibbs C, Alpers M. Experimental transmission of a kuru-like syndrome in chimpanzees. *Nature* 1966;209:794–796.

96. Brown P, Rodgers-Johnson P, Cathala F, Gibbs CJ Jr, Gajdusek DC. Creutzfeldt–Jakob disease of long duration: clinicopathological characteristics, transmissibility, and differential diagnosis. *Ann Neurol* 1984;16:295–304.

97. Tateishi J, Sato Y, Ohta M. Creutzfeldt disease in humans and laboratory animals. In: Zimmerman HM, ed. *Progress in neuropathology.* New York: Raven Press, 1983;195–221.

98. Beck E, Daniel PM, Matthews WB, et al. Creutzfeldt–Jakob disease: the neuropathology of a transmission experiment. *Brain* 1969;92:699–716.

99. Beck E, Daniel PM, Davey AJ, Gajdusek DC, Gibbs CJ Jr. The pathogenesis of transmissible spongiform encephalopathy: an ultrastructural study. *Brain* 1982;105:755–786.

100. Beck E, Daniel PM, Davey AJ, Gajdusek DC, Gibbs CJ Jr. A note on membrane lamellation. *Brain* 1985;108:153–154.

101. Baron H, Baron-van Evercooren A, Brucher JM. Antiserum to scrapie-associated fibril protein reacts with amyloid plaques in familial transmissible dementia. *J Neuropathol Exper Neurol* 1988;47:158–165.

102. Kitamoto T, Tateishi J, Tashima T, et al. Amyloid plaques in Creutzfeldt–Jakob disease stain with prion protein antibodies. *Ann Neurol* 1986;20:204–208.

103. McBride PA, Bruce ME, Fraser M. Immunostaining of scrapie cerebral amyloid plaques with antisera raised to scrapie associated fibrils (SAF). *Neuropathol Appl Neurobiol* 1988;14:325–336.

104. Piccardo P, Safar J, Ceroni M, Gajdusek DC, Gibbs CJ Jr. Immunohistochemical localization of prion protein in spongiform encephalopathies and normal tissue. *Neurology* 1990;40:518–522.

105. Bobin SA, Currie JR, Merz PA, et al. The comparative immunoreactivities of brain amyloids in Alzheimer's disease and scrapie. *Acta Neuropathol (Berl)* 1987;74:313–323.

106. Kitamoto T, Ogomori K, Tateishi J, Prusiner SB. Formic acid pretreatment enhances immunostaining of cerebral and systemic amyloids. *Lab Invest* 1987;57:230–236.

107. Kitamoto T, Tateishi J. Immunohistochemical confirmation of

Creutzfeldt–Jakob disease with a long clinical course with amyloid plaque core antibodies. *Am J Pathol* 1988;131:435–443.

108. DeArmond SJ, McKinley MP, Barry RA, Braunfeld MB, McColloch JR, Prusiner SB. Identification of prion amyloid filaments in scrapie-infected brain. *Cell* 1985;41:221–235.

109. Wiley CA, Burrola PG, Buchmeier MJ, et al. Immuno-gold localization of prion filaments in scrapie-infected hamster brains. *Lab Invest* 1987;57:646–656.

110. Narang HK, Asher DM, Pomeroy KL, Gajdusek DC. Abnormal tubulovesicular particles in brains of hamsters with scrapie. *Proc Soc Exp Biol Med* 1987;184:504–509.

111. Hadlow WJ, Kennedy RC, Race RE. Natural infection of Suffolk sheep with scrapie virus. *J Infect Dis* 1982;146:657–664.

112. Gibbs CJ Jr, Amyx HL, Bacote A, Masters CL, Gajdusek DC. Oral transmission of kuru, Creutzfeldt–Jakob disease, and scrapie to nonhuman primates. *J Infect Dis* 1980;142:205–207.

113. Kuroda Y, Gibbs CJ Jr, Amyx HL, Gajdusek DC. Creutzfeldt–Jakob disease in mice: persistent viremia and preferential replication of virus in low-density lymphocytes. *Infect Immun* 1983;41:154–161.

114. Manuelidis EE, Kim JH, Mericangas JR, Manuelidis L. Transmission to animals of Creutzfeldt–Jakob disease from human blood [Letter]. *Lancet* 1985;2:896–897.

115. Tateishi J. Transmission of Creutzfeldt–Jakob disease from human blood and urine into mice [Letter]. *Lancet* 1985;2:1074.

116. Asher DM, Gibbs CJ Jr, Gajdusek DC. Pathogenesis of spongiform encephalopathies. *Ann Clin Lab Sci* 1976;6:84–103.

117. Asher DM, Gibbs CJ Jr, Gajdusek DC. Subacute spongiform encephalopathies: slow infections of the nervous system. *Clin Microbiol Newsletter* 1985;7:129–133.

118. Roos R, Gajdusek DC, Gibbs CJ Jr. The clinical characteristics of transmissible Creutzfeldt–Jakob disease. *Brain* 1973;96:1–20.

119. Harrington MG, Merril CR, Asher DM, Gajdusek DC. Abnormal proteins in the cerebrospinal fluid of patients with Creutzfeldt–Jakob disease. *N Engl J Med* 1986;315:279–283.

120. Hochstrasser DF, Harrington MG, Hochstrasser AC, Miller MJ, Merril CR. Methods for increasing the resolution of two-dimensional protein electrophoresis. *Anal Biochem* 1988;173:424–435.

121. Narang HK, Asher DM, Gajdusek DC. Tubulofilaments in negatively stained scrapie-infected brains: relationship to scrapie-associated fibrils. *Proc Natl Acad Sci USA* 1987;84:7730–7734.

122. Serban D, Taraboulos A, DeArmond SJ, Prusiner SB. Rapid detection of Creutzfeldt–Jakob disease and scrapie prion proteins. *Neurol* 1990;40:110–117.

123. Butler DA, Scott MR, Bockman JM, et al. Scrapie-infected murine neuroblastoma cells produce protease-resistant prion proteins. *J Virol* 1988;62:1558–1564.

124. Race RE, Caughey B, Graham K, Ernst D, Chesebro B. Analyses of frequency of infection, specific infectivity, and prion protein biosynthesis in scrapie-infected neuroblastoma cell clones. *J Virol* 1988;62:2845–2849.

125. Gibbs CJ Jr, Gajdusek DC, Latarjet R. Unusual resistance to ionizing radiation of the viruses of kuru, Creutzfeldt–Jakob disease and scrapie. *Proc Natl Acad Sci USA* 1978;75:6268–6270.

126. Gibbs CJ Jr. Search for infectious etiology in chronic and subacute degenerative diseases of the central nervous system. *Curr Top Microbiol Immunol* 1967;40:44–58.

127. Asher DM, Gibbs CJ Jr, Gajdusek DC. Slow viral infections: safe handling of the agents of the subacute spongiform encephalopathies. In: Miller B, Gröschel D, Richardson J, et al., eds. *Laboratory safety: principles and practice*. Washington, DC: American Society for Microbiology, 1986;59–71.

128. Gibbons RA, Hunter GD. Nature of the scrapie agent. *Nature.* 1967;215:1041–1043.

129. Cho HJ. Requirement of a protein component for scrapie infectivity. *Intervirology* 1980;14:213–216.

130. Rohwer RG. Scrapie infectious agent is virus-like in size and susceptibility to inactivation. *Nature* 1984;308:658–662.

131. Rohwer RG. Estimation of scrapie nucleic acid MW from standard curves for virus sensitivity to ionizing radiation [Letter]. *Nature* 1986;320:381.

132. Bellinger-Kawahara C, Cleaver JE, Diener TO, Prusiner SB. Puri-

fied scrapie prions resist inactivation by UV irradiation. *J Virol* 1987;61:159–166.

133. Manuelidis L, Sklaviadis T, Manuelidis EE. Evidence suggesting that PrP is not the infectious agent in Creutzfeldt–Jakob disease. *EMBO J* 1987;6:341–347.

134. Manuelidis L, Manuelidis EE. Creutzfeldt–Jakob disease and dementias. *Microb Pathogen* 1989;7:157–164.

135. Borrás T, Gibbs CJ Jr. Molecular hybridization studies with scrapie brain nucleic acids. I. Search for specific DNA sequences. *Arch Virol* 1986;88:67–78.

136. Duguid JR, Rohwer RG, Seed B. Isolation of cDNAs of scrapie-modulated RNAs by subtractive hybridization of a cDNA library. *Proc Natl Acad Sci USA* 1988;85:5738–5742.

137. Carp RI, Kascsak RJ, Wisniewski HM, et al. The nature of the unconventional slow infection agents remains a puzzle. *Alzheimer Dis Assoc Disord* 1989;3:79–99.

138. Merz PA, Somerville RA, Wisniewski HM, Iqbal K. Abnormal fibrils from scrapie-infected brain. *Acta Neuropathol (Berl)* 1981;54:63–74.

139. Merz PA, Somerville RA, Wisniewski HM, Manuelidis L, Manuelidis EE. Scrapie-associated fibrils in Creutzfeldt–Jakob disease. *Nature* 1983;306:474–476.

140. Merz PA, Rohwer RG, Kascsak R, et al. Infection-specific particles from the unconventional slow-virus diseases. *Science* 1984;225:437–440.

141. Bolton DC, McKinley MP, Prusiner SB. Identification of a protein that purifies with the scrapie prion. *Science* 1982;218:1309–1311.

142. Bockman JM, Kingsbury DT, McKinley MP, Bendheim PE, Prusiner SB. Creutzfeldt–Jakob disease prion proteins in human brains. *N Engl J Med* 1985;312:73–78.

143. McKinley MP, Bolton DC, Prusiner SB. A protease-resistant protein is a structural component of the scrapie prion. *Cell* 1983;35:57–62.

144. Barry RA, McKinley MP, Bendheim PE, Lewis GK, DeArmond SJ, Prusiner SB. Antibodies to the scrapie protein decorate prion rods. *J Immunol* 1985;135:603–613.

145. Hope J, Morton LJ, Farquhar CF, Multhaup G, Beyreuther K, Kimberlin RH. The major polypeptide of scrapie-associated fibrils (SAF) has the same size, charge distribution and N-terminal protein sequence as predicted for the normal brain protein (PrP). *EMBO J* 1986;5:2591–2597.

146. Brown P, Coker-Vann M, Pomeroy K, et al. Diagnosis of Creutzfeldt–Jakob disease by Western blot identification of marker protein in human brain tissue. *N Engl J Med* 1986;314:547–551.

147. Prusiner SB. Scrapie prions. *Annu Rev Microbiol* 1989;43:345–374.

148. Ceroni M, Piccardo P, Safar J, Gajdusek DC, Gibbs CJ Jr. Scrapie infectivity and prion protein are distributed in the same pH range in agarose isoelectric focusing. *Neurology* 1990;40:508–513.

149. Prusiner SB, Stahl N, DeArmond SJ. Novel mechanisms of degeneration of the central nervous system—prion structure and biology. In: Bock G, Marsh J, eds. Novel infectious agents and the central nervous system. Ciba Journal Symp 135, Wiley, 1988;239–256.

150. Braig HR, Diringer H. Scrapie: concept of a virus-induced amyloidosis of the brain. *EMBO J* 1985;4:2309–2312.

151. Czub M, Braig HR, Diringer H. Replication of the scrapie agent in hamsters infected intracerebrally confirms the pathogenesis of an amyloid-inducing virosis. *J Gen Virol* 1988;69:1753–1756.

152. Czub M, Braig HR, Diringer H. Pathogenesis of scrapie: study of the temporal development of clinical symptoms, of infectivity titres and scrapie-associated fibrils in brains of hamsters infected intraperitoneally. *J Gen Virol* 1986;67:2005–2009.

153. Multhaup G, Diringer H, Hilmert H, Prinz H, Heukeshoven J, Beyreuther K. The protein component of scrapie-associated fibrils is a glycosylated low molecular weight protein. *EMBO J* 1985;4:1495–1501.

154. Chesebro B, Race R, Wehrly K, et al. Identification of scrapie prion protein-specific mRNA in scrapie-infected and uninfected brain. *Nature* 1985;315:331–333.

155. Basler K, Oesch B, Scott M, et al. Scrapie and cellular PrP iso-

forms are encoded by the same chromosomal gene. *Cell* 1986;46:417–428.

156. Kimberlin RH, Cole S, Walker CA. Temporary and permanent modifications to a single strain of mouse scrapie on transmission to rats and hamsters. *J Gen Virol* 1987;68:1875–1881.

157. Bruce ME, Dickinson AG. Genetic control of amyloid plaque production and incubation period in scrapie-infected mice. *J Neuropathol Exp Neurol* 1985;44:285–294.

158. Bruce ME, Dickinson AG. Biological evidence that scrapie agent has an independent genome. *J Gen Virol* 1987;68:79–89.

159. Wills PR. Induced frameshifting mechanism of replication for an information-carrying scrapie prion. *Microb Pathogen* 1989; 6:235–249.

160. Brown P, Liberski PP, Wolff A, Gajdusek DC. Resistance of scrapie infectivity to steam autoclaving after formaldehyde fixation and limited survival after ashing at 360°C: practical and theoretical implications. *J Infect Dis* 1990;161:467–472.

161. Dees C, Wade WF, German TL, Marsh RF. Inactivation of the scrapie agent by ultraviolet irradiation in the presence of chlorpromazine. *J Gen Virol* 1985;66:845–849.

162. Bolton DC, Meyer RK, Prusiner SB. Scrapie PrP 27–30 is a sialoglycoprotein. *J Virol* 1985;53:596–606.

163. Caughey B, Race RE, Ernst D, Buchmeier MJ, Chesebro B. Prion protein biosynthesis in scrapie-infected and uninfected neuroblastoma cells. *J Virol* 1989;63:175–181.

164. Bode L, Pocchiari M, Gelderblom H, Diringer H. Characterization of antisera against scrapie-associated fibrils (SAF) from affected hamster and cross-reactivity with SAF from scrapie-affected mice and from patients with Creutzfeldt–Jakob disease. *J Gen Virol* 1985;66:2471–2478.

165. Kretzschmar HA, Stowring LE, Westaway D, Stubblebine WH, Prusiner SB, Dearmond SJ. Molecular cloning of a human prion protein cDNA. *DNA* 1986;5:315–324.

166. Bockman JM, Prusiner SB, Tateishi J, Kingsbury DT. Immunoblotting of Creutzfeldt–Jakob disease prion proteins: host species-specific epitopes. *Ann Neurol* 1987;21:589–595.

167. Locht C, Chesebro B, Race R, Keith JM. Molecular cloning and complete sequence of prion protein cDNA from mouse brain infected with the scrapie agent. *Proc Natl Acad Sci USA* 1986;83:6372–6376.

168. Meyer RK, McKinley MP, Bowman KA, Barry RA, Prusiner SB. Separation and properties of cellular and scrapie prion proteins. *Proc Natl Acad Sci USA* 1986;83:2310–2314.

169. Caughey B, Race RE, Chesebro B. Detection of prion protein mRNA in normal and scrapie-infected tissues and cell lines. *J Gen Virol* 1988;69:711–716.

170. Barry RA, Vincent MT, Kent SB, Hood LE, Prusiner SB. Characterization of prion proteins with monospecific antisera to synthetic peptides. *J Immunol* 1988;140:1188–1193.

171. Kretzschmar HA, Prusiner SB, Stowring LE, DeArmond SJ. Scrapie prion proteins are synthesized in neurons. *Am J Pathol* 1986;122:1–5.

172. Czub M, Braig HR, Blode H, Diringer H. The major protein of SAF is absent from spleen and thus not an essential part of the scrapie agent. *Arch Virol* 1986;91:383–386.

173. Doi S, Ito M, Shinagawa M, Sato G, Isomura H, Goto H. Western blot detection of scrapie-associated fibril protein in tissues outside the central nervous system from preclinical scrapie-infected mice. *J Gen Virol* 1988;69:955–960.

174. Caughey B, Race RE, Vogel M, Buchmeier MJ, Chesebro B. *In vitro* expression in eukaryotic cells of a prion protein gene cloned from scrapie-infected mouse brain. *Proc Natl Acad Sci USA* 1988;85:4657–4661.

175. Asher DM, Masters CL, Gajdusek DC, Gibbs CJ Jr. Familial spongiform encephalopathies. In: Kety S, Rowland L, Sidman R, Matthysse S, eds. *Genetics of neurological and psychiatric disorders.* New York: Raven Press, 1983;273–291.

176. Hunter N, Foster JD, Dickinson AG, Hope J. Linkage of the gene for the scrapie-associated fibril protein (PrP) to the Sip gene in Cheviot sheep. *Vet Rec* 1989;124:364–366.

177. Carlson GA, Kingsbury DT, Goodman PA, et al. Linkage of prion protein and scrapie incubation time genes. *Cell* 1986;46:503–511.

178. Hunter N, Hope J, McConnell I, Dickinson AG. Linkage of the scrapie-associated fibril protein (PrP) gene and Sinc using congenic mice and restriction fragment length polymorphism analysis. *J Gen Virol* 1987;68:2711–2716.

179. Westaway D, Goodman PA, Mirenda CA, McKinley MP, Carlson GA, Prusiner SB. Distinct prion proteins in short and long scrapie incubation period mice. *Cell* 1987;51:651–662.

180. Westaway D, Carlson GA, Prusiner SB. Unraveling prion diseases through molecular genetics. *Trends Neurosci* 1989;12:221–227.

181. Hsiao K, Baker HF, Crow TJ, et al. Linkage of a prion protein missense variant to Gerstmann–Sträussler syndrome. *Nature* 1989;338:342–345.

182. Owen F, Poulter M, Lofthouse R, et al. Insertion in prion protein gene in familial Creutzfeldt–Jakob disease [Letter]. *Lancet* 1989;1:51–52.

183. Goldgaber D, Goldfarb LG, Brown P, et al. Mutations in familial Creutzfeldt–Jakob disease and Gerstmann–Sträussler–Scheinker's syndrome. *Exp Neurol* 1989;106:204–206.

184. Doh-ura K, Tateishi J, Sasaki H, Kitamoto T, Sakaki Y. Pro-leu change at position 102 of prion protein is the most common but not the sole mutation related to Gerstmann–Sträussler syndrome. *Biochem Biophys Res Commun* 1989;163:974–979.

185. Doh-ura K, Tateishi J, Kitamoto T, Sasaki H, Sakaki Y. Creutzfeldt–Jakob disease patients with congophilic kuru plaques have a missense variant prion protein common to Gerstmann–Sträussler syndrome. *Ann Neurol* 1990;27:121–126.

186. Goldfarb LG, Brown P, Goldgaber DG, et al. Creutzfeldt-Jakob disease and kuru patients lack a mutation consistently found in the Gerstmann–Sträussler–Scheinker syndrome. *Exp Neurol* 1990;108:247–250.

187. Goldfarb LG, Brown P, Goldgaber D, et al. Identical mutation in unrelated patients with Creutzfeldt–Jakob disease. *Lancet* 1990;ii:174–175.

188. Kimberlin RH, Walker CA. Suppression of scrapie infection in mice by heteropolyanion 23, dextran sulfate, and some other polyanions. *Antimicrob Agents Chemother* 1986;30:409–413.

189. Pocchiari M, Schmittinger S, Masullo C. Amphotericin B delays the incubation period of scrapie in intracerebrally inoculated hamsters. *J Gen Virol* 1987;68:219–223.

190. Pocchiari M, Casaccia P, Ladogana A. Amphotericin B: a novel class of antiscrapie drugs. *J Infect Dis* 1989;160:795–802.

191. Brown P, Wolff A, Gajdusek DC. A simple and effective method for inactivating virus infectivity in formalin-fixed tissue samples from patients with Creutzfeldt–Jakob disease. *Neurology* 1990;40:887–890.

192. Manuelidis EE, de Figueiredo JM, Kim JH, Fritch WW, Manuelidis L. Transmission studies from blood of Alzheimer disease patients and healthy relatives. *Proc Natl Acad Sci USA* 1988;85:4898–4901.

193. Manuelidis EE, Rorke LB. Transmission of Alpers' disease (chronic progressive encephalopathy) produces experimental Creutzfeldt–Jakob disease in hamsters. *Neurology* 1989;39:615–621.

194. Goudsmit J, Morrow CH, Asher DM, et al. Evidence for and against the transmissibility of Alzheimer's disease. *Neurology (Minneap)* 1980;30:945–950.

195. Guiroy DC, Yanagihara R, Gajdusek DC. Colocalization of amyloidogenic proteins and sulfated aminoglycans in nontransmissible and transmissible cerebral amyloidoses. *Acta Neuropathol* 1991; in press.

196. Safar J, Ceroni M, Piccardo P, Gajdusek DC, Gibbs CJ Jr. Scrapie-associated precursor proteins: antigenic relationship between species and immunocytochemical localization in normal, scrapie, and Creutzfeldt–Jakob disease brains. *Neurology* 1990; 40:513–517.

Infections of the Central Nervous System,
edited by W. M. Scheld, R. J. Whitley, and
D. T. Durack, Raven Press, Ltd., New York © 1991.

CHAPTER 9

Perinatal Viral Infections

Richard J. Whitley and Sergio Stagno

Human herpesvirus infections in the perinatal period are known causes of morbidity, especially central nervous system (CNS) complications. Of all perinatal viral pathogens, herpes simplex virus (HSV) and cytomegalovirus (CMV) are notorious causes of CNS disease in the fetus and newborn. In addition, congenital rubella infection can cause significant neurologic morbidity. This chapter will review the relevant pathogenic issues surrounding HSV and CMV perinatal infections, in particular, but will provide brief reference to varicella-zoster virus (VZV), Epstein–Barr virus (EBV), and rubella infections as well. Human immunodeficiency virus (HIV) infections, which can also cause CNS disease of the newborn, are considered at length in another chapter (Chapter 10).

NEONATAL HERPES SIMPLEX VIRUS INFECTION

History

In 1941, Smith et al. (1) reported the first case of HSV infection of the CNS. This case occurred in a newborn with neonatal herpes simplex encephalitis (HSE). In 1952, Zuelzer et al. (2) reviewed eight cases of disseminated HSV infection in neonates, with involvement of most organs, including the brain in many instances. Until this time, it had been almost axiomatic that newborn infants were not susceptible to HSV infection. This latter report was the first describing visceral lesions (beyond the CNS) definitely attributable to HSV infections. These authors correctly implicated hematogenous spread of infection to multiple organs as the underlying pathogens for infection in these neonates. Furthermore,

they postulated that: (a) maternal antibodies were not completely protective; (b) infants born to mothers with genital herpetic lesions were at special risk; and (c) exposure to HSV after birth might lead to infection as well. This report was followed shortly by others indicating the association between HSV infection of the newborn and necrotizing encephalitis, including the isolation of HSV in cell cultures from brain tissue. Recognition of HSV as a cause of encephalitis in patients of all ages, but including newborns, progressed to such an extent that, in a 1960 review of CNS syndromes of viral etiology, HSV was considered the third most frequent cause of viral encephalitis (3).

Infectious Agent

For a discussion of the structure and unique biologic properties of HSV, the reader is referred to Chapter 4.

Pathology and Pathogenesis

Pathology

The general pathology of HSV infection is discussed in Chapter 4. A few pathologic characteristics appear more commonly in the newborn. Gross examination of the brain frequently reveals encephalomalacia and hydranencephaly, which are likely the consequence of extensive hemorrhagic necrosis. Porencephaly, hydranencephaly, and multicystic lesions are often sequelae in neonates who survive for several weeks or months, following neonatal HSV infection of the brain.

The microscopic appearance of the brain is characterized by a mononuclear inflammation, necrosis, and hemorrhage. Perivascular lymphocytic infiltration can be anticipated. Pictorial representation of these changes appears in Chapter 4. Mild white-matter gliosis has been

R. J. Whitley and S. Stagno: Departments of Pediatrics, Microbiology, and Medicine, University of Alabama, Birmingham, Alabama 35294.

noted frequently in one series of patients (4). These changes are not significantly different from those described for HSV encephalitis in older individuals. Nevertheless, these findings are detailed below, in the context of disease pathogenesis.

Pathogenesis

For *in utero* disease, transplacental infection results in fetal infection with involvement of skin, brain, eye, liver, and adrenals. For maternal acquisition, after direct exposure, viral replication in the newborn either is limited to the portal of entry—namely, the skin, eye, or mouth —or will progress to involve various other organs, including the brain (resulting in encephalitis), and will, under such circumstances, cause life-threatening disease. Host mechanisms responsible for control of progression of viral replication at the site of entry are unknown. For babies with encephalitis, it is possible that intraneuronal transmission of viral particles provides a privileged site that may be impervious to circulating humoral and cell-mediated defense mechanisms. Thus, transplacental maternal antibodies may be of less value in the prevention of encephalitic forms of neonatal HSV infections. In contrast, disseminated infection can be the consequence of viremia or can be secondary to extensive cell-to-cell spread, as occurs with pneumonitis after aspiration of infected secretions.

Once virus has absorbed to cell membranes and penetration has occurred, viral replication proceeds, leading to progeny viruses. The generation of progeny virus is equated with cell death. It has been noted previously that during the replication of HSV, the synthesis of cellular DNA and proteins ceases as large quantities of HSV are produced. Cell death in critical organs of the newborn, such as the brain, can obviously result in devastating consequences as reflected by long-term morbidity. The most prominent gross lesion is the appearance of small, punctate, yellow-to-gray areas of focal necrosis. Disruption of the cytoskeleton, cellular swelling, hemorrhagic necrosis, development of intranuclear inclusions, and cytolysis are all inherent, and they are recognizable events in the replicative process. When infected tissue is stained with hematoxylin–eosin or fixed in Bouin's solution and viewed by light microscopy, there is extensive evidence of hemorrhagic necrosis, clumping of nuclear chromatin, dissolution of the nucleolus, cell fusion with formation of multinucleate giant cells, and, ultimately, a lymphocytic inflammatory response (4,5). Lymphocytic perivascular cuffing is particularly prominent, especially in the CNS (1,6).

Neonatal HSV infections of the brain illustrate the two major pathogenic routes for acquisition of infection, namely hematogenous or intraneuronal. For example, hematogenous spread of virus usually occurs with disseminated disease, and diffuse involvement of the brain occurs in 60–80% of cases. In contrast, neuronal transmission probably results in the focal CNS disease encountered in babies with encephalitis only when no distal organ involvement can be documented (7).

Many factors influence disease pathogenesis; these will be discussed in the following subsections.

Times of Transmission of Infection. HSV infection of the newborn can be acquired at one of three times: *in utero*, intrapartum, or postnatally. Regardless of the time or route of acquisition, the newborn is at risk for CNS disease. Certainly, the mother is the most common source of infection for the first two of these routes of transmission of infection to the newborn. A maternal source should be suspected when herpetic lesions are discovered promptly after the birth of the child or when the baby's illness is caused by HSV-2. Each of these three times when transmission of infection occurs will be detailed.

Intrauterine infection. Information about *in utero* acquisition of infection is becoming increasingly available in the literature (8–11). Although it was originally presumed that *in utero* acquisition of infection resulted in either a totally normal baby or premature termination of gestation (12), it has become apparent that intrauterine acquisition of infection can produce clinical symptomatology similar to that of many congenital infections. Utilizing stringent diagnostic criteria, over 30 babies with symptomatic congenital HSV disease have thus far been identified in the world's literature. These babies were identified within the first 48 hr of life and, subsequently, had virologic confirmation of infection. Furthermore, other pathogens which cause similar clinical syndromes—such as congenital CMV infection, rubella, syphilis, or toxoplasmosis—were excluded. Manifestations of disease acquired *in utero* include the triad of chorioretinitis, cuteus aplasia, and hydranencephaly; the encephalomalacia complication is shown in Fig. 1.

Intrapartum infection. The overwhelmingly most common time of transmission of infection from mother to the fetus occurs intrapartum. Such transmission occurs when the infant comes in contact with infected maternal genital secretions at delivery and accounts for 80% of cases of neonatal HSV infection, as reported (13).

Acquisition of infection by intrapartum exposure to virus obviously correlates, by definition, with maternal excretion of HSV at the time of delivery. Prospective evaluations of excretion of virus in the genital tract within 48 hr of delivery indicate that shedding can occur in 0.5–1.3% of women, as reviewed elsewhere (14). Clearly, maternal primary versus recurrent infection will influence the probability of neonatal infection, as discussed below. It should be noted that with the increasing prevalence of HSV-2 infection in the population at large —estimated to be 25–40% for women of childbearing age—the likelihood of detecting HSV excretion in the genital tract at delivery should increase.

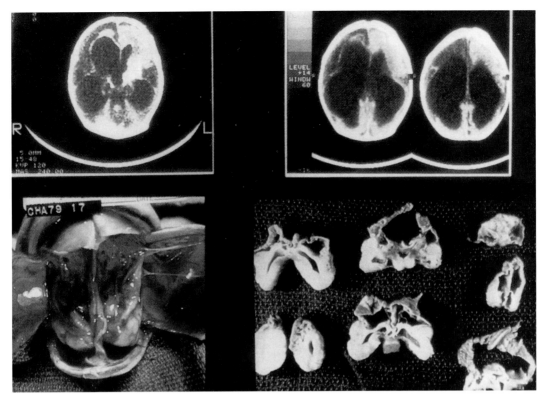

FIG. 1. Encephalomalacia resulting in *in utero* HSV infection. (From ref. 33, with permission)

Postnatal infection. The third route of transmission is postnatal acquisition (15–22). The source of virus for postnatal transmission has been inadequately studied. Documented sources for such transmission include mother-to-child (including the breast as a source of virus) (15–17), father-to-child (labial lesions) (18,19), and nosocomial transmission (nursery personnel or babies) (20–22). Even though HSV-1 has been associated with genital lesions, postnatal transmission of HSV has been increasingly suggested because 15–20% of the cases of neonatal HSV infections are caused by HSV-1 (23,24). In fact, more recent data from the NIAID Collaborative Antiviral Study Group indicate that the frequency of babies with neonatal HSV-1 infections has increased to nearly 30% (24). This observation, in light of the recognition that genital HSV-1 infections appear to account for only approximately 5–15% of all HSV infections, creates a level of concern for postnatal acquisition of infection. Regardless, at each of the three times when transmission occurs, the potential consequences for the fetus or newborn are significant. It is important to identify those factors which govern transmission in each individualized case.

Factors Which Influence Transmission of Infection to the Fetus. Risk factors associated with intrauterine transmission of infection are not precisely known; however, both primary and recurrent maternal infection can result in infection of the fetus *in utero. In utero* infection can occur as a consequence of either transplacental or ascending infection. Regarding transplacental infection, while it might be convenient to assume that only primary maternal infection is associated with transmission of HSV *in utero* to the fetus, women with recurrent maternal genital infection, not usually associated with viremia, can transmit HSV across the placenta to the fetus as well, leading to disease (10). Ascending infection which causes *in utero* disease usually occurs after prolonged rupture of membranes but can result from transmembrane infection as well.

Factors which influence the second route—namely, intrapartum acquisition of infection by the fetus—are, among others: (a) type of maternal infection (namely, primary versus recurrent) (25,26), (b) maternal antibody status (23,27,28), (c) duration of ruptured membranes (23), (d) inadvertent placement of a fetal scalp monitor in a woman excreting HSV (29,30), (e) duration of ruptured membranes, and (f) environmental sources.

Primary infection is associated with (a) larger quantities of HSV replicating in the genital tract ($>10^6$ viral particles per 0.2 ml of tissue culture inoculum) and (b) a period of viral excretion which, on average, persists for 3 weeks. In contrast, HSV is shed for an average of only 2–5 days, and at lower concentrations (approximately 10^3 per 0.2 ml of tissue culture inoculum), in women with recurrent genital infection. Because of the larger quantity of virus and the longer period of viral excretion, primary maternal infection is thought to be associated with a higher rate of transmission to the fetus—estimated to be between 20% and 30% (25,26).

Paralleling the type of maternal infection, the mother's HSV antibody status at delivery appears to be an additional factor which influences both the severity of disease in the newborn and the likelihood of transmission to the fetus. Transplacental maternal neutralizing and antibody-dependent cell-mediated cytotoxic antibodies appear to have at least an ameliorative, if not protective, effect on acquisition of infection for babies inadvertently exposed to virus (23,27,28,31).

Placement of a fetal scalp monitor in women excreting virus has been shown to lead to fetal infection. Fetal scalp monitors are one of the most common obstetrical interventions for monitoring fetal distress. Since the seroprevalence of HSV-2 is already high and increasing, a careful visual speculum examination of the cervix and genital tract at the onset of labor should help exclude lesions indicative of HSV infection. Monitor placement should be discouraged in women with a history of genital herpes or visualized lesions. Alternative methods of monitoring fetal heart rate should be sought.

The duration of ruptured membranes is reported to be an important indicator of risk for acquisition of neonatal infection. Observations by Nahmias et al. (12,23) suggested that prolonged rupture of membranes (>6 hr) increased the risk of acquisition of virus, probably the consequence of ascending infection from the cervix. Based upon this observation, as well as upon the known risk of the fetus exposed to HSV, it is recommended that women with active genital lesions at the time of labor be delivered by cesarean section, as will be discussed below.

Finally, the postnatal acquisition of infection requires exposure to an environmental source, as noted above. Many individuals symptomatically excrete HSV from the oropharynx and, theoretically, can be a source of transmission. With clinically obvious labial lesions, contact with the newborn should be avoided. Additionally, poor hygiene (handwashing), combined with lack of recognition of genital lesions, might result in postnatal transmission.

Immunity and Disease Acquisition. The relative immune-deficient state of the neonate makes this patient population particularly prone to more severe infectious diseases (32). Unlike lymphocytes from adults, unstimulated lymphocytes from neonates are permissive for HSV replication. The neonate, to a large degree, lacks the mature macrophage barrier of adults which can contain viral spread. Other differences in the neonate include a delayed T-lymphocyte proliferative response and a defect in natural killer cell responses to HSV. Furthermore, with appropriate stimuli, the newborn's lymphocyte response to interferon is depressed and its production is delayed.

As noted above, transplacental maternal antibodies do not prevent infection but appear to at least ameliorate HSV infection in the newborn (31). However, transplacental antibodies do not appear to prevent the development of CNS disease once infection has occurred (33).

Epidemiology of Maternal Infection

There is a striking paucity of data on the epidemiology and management of genital HSV infections during pregnancy. Two patterns of maternal infection can have fetal consequences. These are either disseminated maternal infection or localized primary or recurrent genital infection.

Disseminated Maternal Infection

HSV infections of pregnant women may extend beyond the usual sites of disease—namely, the oropharynx or the genital tract. As first reported by Flewett et al. (34) in 1969, dissemination can occur, leading to cutaneous or visceral disease; fortunately, this is a rare occurrence. In a limited number of cases (34–37), dissemination following primary oropharyngeal or genital infection has led to life-threatening diseases such as (a) hepatitis with or without thrombocytopenia, (b) leukopenia, (c) consumptive coagulopathy, or (d) encephalitis. Although only a small number of patients have been studied, the mortality among pregnant women with disseminated infection has been greater than 50%. Fetal deaths also occurred in more than 50% of cases, although not necessarily associated with the death of the mother. Surviving fetuses were delivered by cesarean section either during the acute illness or at term, and none had evidence of disease. This cumulative experience suggests that factors associated with pregnancy place both mother and fetus at increased risk of severe infection, possibly because of altered cell-mediated immunity (38,39).

Localized Maternal Infection

During the first 20 weeks of gestation, primary maternal genital HSV infection is associated with an increased frequency of spontaneous abortion, stillbirth, and, as noted above, congenital malformations, particularly hydranencephaly and chorioretinitis (8,10). Limited numbers of women have been followed prospectively after symptomatic primary genital infection, and spontaneous abortion occurred in 25% when the infection was acquired before 20 weeks of gestation (12). This figure is probably high because of the selection bias—namely, the very small number of women followed. Initially, it was thought that infection which occurred after 20 weeks of gestation was not associated with unusual problems, and that the children born to these women were born free of infection (40,41). More recently, however, primary maternal infection has been associated with fetal morbidity —namely, intrauterine growth retardation (42).

Asymptomatic primary infection at term can pose a high risk to the fetus and newborn. It appears as though this occurrence is not that uncommon. (R. J. Whitley, personal observation of the NIAID Collaborative Antiviral Study Group). Recurrent maternal genital infection is the most common form of HSV-2 infection during gestation. Transmission of infection to the fetus appears to be directly related to the actual prevalence of viral shedding at the time of delivery and, therefore, directly related to the risk of direct fetal contact (12). Two studies indicate that viral shedding at the time of delivery is an infrequent event: Its rate of occurrence ranges from one in 258 (0.39%) to one in 1092 (0.09%) deliveries (41,43). These studies were reported several years ago and may not describe representative populations. Studies in progress are assessing the factors associated with neonatal infection if the mother is virus-positive at delivery. These latter studies indicate viral shedding at a rate of 0.3–0.7% overall in different socioeconomic populations.

Several studies have prospectively evaluated the frequency and nature of viral shedding in pregnant women with a known history of genital herpes. In a predominantly white middle-class population, documented recurrent infection occurred in 84% of pregnant women with a prior history of infection (43). Moreover, asymptomatic viral shedding occurred in at least 12% of the recurrent episodes. Viral shedding from the cervix occurred in only 0.56% of symptomatic infections and in 0.66% of asymptomatic infections. These data are similar to those obtained in other populations (26,44–46). In asymptomatic pregnant women, an incidence of cervical shedding as high as 3% has been reported (41). However, the observed rates of shedding among pregnant women asymptomatic for genital herpes have varied more than those among nonpregnant women—from 0.2% to 7.4%, depending on the study population and the trial design (41,44–49). These data indicate that the frequency of cervical shedding is low, rendering the risk of transmission of virus to the infant low when disease is recurrent in nature (26). The frequency of shedding does not appear to vary during gestation (41,43). No increased incidence of premature onset of labor was apparent in these studies. Antepartum cultures fail to predict the risk of response to HSV at delivery (50).

More than 60% of women in various groups who give birth to infants with neonatal HSV infection report no symptoms (23,24,49,51,52). Among women without symptoms or without a history of genital herpes, a subgroup can be identified whose sexual contacts have vesicular lesions indicative of genital herpes. Yet even among these women who are especially "at risk," more than half are asymptomatic and have no history of infection. Furthermore, approximately one-third of the infected infants born to these asymptomatic women have no antibodies, which strongly suggests maternal primary infection (51,53). Thus, measures developed to identify women at risk for transmitting virus to their offspring must include late third-trimester screening, especially at the time of delivery.

Incidence and Presentation of Neonatal Infection

The incidence of neonatal HSV infections is estimated to range between one in 3000 (0.03%) and one in 5000 (0.02%) deliveries (7). Of all patients experiencing HSV infections, neonates appear to have the highest frequency of visceral and CNS infection (13,54). Overall, two-thirds of children with neonatal HSV infection will develop disease of the CNS, regardless of whether disease is localized to the brain or becomes disseminated to involve various other organs. Certainly, these children are at exceedingly high risk for death or permanent neurologic impairment. If untreated, newborns with disseminated disease have a mortality of 80%, and newborns with disease limited to the CNS have a mortality of approximately 50%.

The clinical presentation of babies with neonatal HSV infection is a direct reflection of the site and extent of viral replication. Neonatal HSV infection is almost invariably symptomatic and is (as noted) frequently lethal. Although reported cases of asymptomatic infection in the newborn exist, they are most uncommon; moreover, long-term follow-up of these children to document absence of subtle disease or neurologic sequelae has not been carefully performed.

Classification of newborns with HSV infection is mandatory for prognostic and therapeutic considerations (12,23). At the present time, babies with congenital infection, by definition, must be identified within 48 hr following birth. Those babies who are infected (either during delivery or postnatally) with HSV infection can be divided into three categories—namely, those with: (i) disease localized to the skin, eye, or mouth, (ii) encephalitis with or without skin, eye, and/or mouth involvement, and (iii) disseminated disease involving multiple organs, such as CNS, lung, liver, adrenals, skin, eye, and/or mouth. This review will focus on CNS disease predicated upon prospectively acquired data obtained through the NIAID Collaborative Antiviral Study Group. It should be remembered that *all* babies, irrespective of disease classification, should be considered at risk for CNS complications of infection. The presentation and outcome of infection (particularly prognosis after therapy) according to category varies significantly with regard to both mortality and morbidity.

Intrauterine Infection

Intrauterine infection is usually apparent at birth and is characterized by a triad of findings: (i) skin vesicles and/or scarring (cuteus aplasia), (ii) eye disease (chorio-retinitis, optic atrophy), and (iii) brain disease (microcephaly, encephalomalacia, or hydranencephaly). Serial ultrasound examination of the mothers of those babies infected *in utero* has occasionally demonstrated hydranencephaly. Chorioretinitis alone can be a presenting sign and should alert the pediatrician to the possibility of intrauterine HSV infection, although HSV infection is a less common cause of chorioretinitis when compared to other congenital infections. The frequency of occurrence of intrauterine HSV infection has been estimated to range between one in 100,000 (0.001%) and one in 200,000 (0.0005%) deliveries (8).

A small group of children will have skin vesicles or eye lesions which are present at the time of delivery. These neonates are frequently born to women who have had prolonged rupture of membranes. The babies have no other findings of invasive multiorgan involvement; specifically, there is no chorioretinitis, encephalitis, or evidence of other diseased organs. It is not uncommon for the mothers of these babies to have membranes ruptured for as long as 2 weeks prior to the onset of labor and delivery. The prognosis for successful antiviral therapy in this group of babies is obviously far better than that in the children who are born with hydranencephaly.

Disseminated Infection

Table 1 summarizes the classification of 297 babies with neonatal HSV infection from the NIAID Collabora-

tive Antiviral Study Group. Disseminated HSV infection has the worst prognosis with regard to both mortality and morbidity. Children with disseminated infection usually present to tertiary medical centers for therapy between 9 and 11 days of life; however, signs of infection are, on average, usually present 4–5 days earlier. This group of babies has historically accounted for approximately one-half to two-thirds of all babies with neonatal HSV infection.

The principal organs involved following disseminated infection are the liver, brain, and adrenals; however, infection can involve various other organs, including the larynx, trachea, lungs, esophagus, stomach, lower gastrointestinal tract, spleen, kidneys, pancreas, and heart. Constitutional signs and symptoms include irritability, seizures, respiratory distress, jaundice, bleeding diatheses, and shock, in addition to a characteristic vesicular exanthem which is often considered pathognomonic for neonatal HSV infection.

The vesicular rash, as described below, is particularly important in the diagnosis of HSV infection. Notably, over 20% of children with disseminated neonatal HSV infection will not develop skin vesicles during the course of their illness (13,23,55). In the absence of skin vesicles, the diagnosis becomes exceedingly difficult since the clinical signs are often vague and nonspecific, mimicking those of neonatal sepsis. Mortality in the absence of therapy exceeds 80%; all but a few survivors are impaired. The most common cause of death in babies with disseminated disease is either HSV pneumonitis or disseminated intravascular coagulopathy.

TABLE 1. *Demographic and clinical characteristics of infants enrolled in NIAID Collaborative Antiviral Study*

	Disease classification		
	Disseminated	Central nervous system	Skin, eye, and mouth
Number of babies	94 (32)[a]	101 (34)	102 (34)
Number of males/number of females	55/39	51/50	53/49
Race			
Number of whites/number of others	60/34	76/25	76/26
Number of premature infants (≤36 weeks)	39 (41)	24 (24)	30 (29)
Gestational age (mean weeks ± SEM)	36.5 ± 0.41	37.9 ± 0.36	37.7 ± 0.33
Enrollment age (mean days ± SEM)	11.7 ± 0.68	17.0 ± 0.79	12.0 ± 1.1
Maternal age (mean years ± SEM)	21.7 ± 0.50	23.1 ± 0.46	22.7 ± 0.52
Clinical findings (number)			
Skin lesions	67 (71)	68 (67)	87 (85)
Brain involvement	50/83[d] (60)	101 (100)	0
Pneumonia	35/82[d] (43)	0	0
Mortality at 1 year[b]	58 (62)	15 (15)	0
Neurologic impairment of survivors (number affected/total number)[c]			
Total	10/27[b] (37)	37/75[b] (49)	7/82[b] (9)
Adenine arabinoside	7/19 (37)	21/46 (46)	3/32 (9)
Acyclovir	2/6 (33)	14/26 (54)	1/43 (2)
Placebo	1/2 (50)	2/3 (67)	3/7 (43)

[a] Numbers in parentheses are percentages.
[b] Regardless of therapy.
[c] Denominators vary according to number of patients with follow-up available.
[d] Denominators vary according to number of patients evaluable.

Evaluation of the extent of disease is imperative, as with all cases of neonatal HSV infection. The clinical laboratory should be utilized to define hepatic enzyme elevation [serum glutamic-oxaloacetic transaminase (SGOT) and glutamic-glutaric transaminase (GGT)], direct hyperbilirubinemia, neutropenia, thrombocytopenia, and bleeding diatheses, among others. Unless contraindicated, examination of the cerebrospinal fluid (CSF) is imperative. In addition, chest roentgenograms, abdominal x-rays, electroencephalography (EEG), and computerized tomography (CT) [or a magnetic resonance imaging (MRI) scan] of the head can be judiciously and serially employed to determine the extent of disease. The radiographic picture of HSV lung disease is characterized by a diffuse, interstitial pattern which progresses to a hemorrhagic pneumonitis. Not infrequently, pneumatosis intestinalis can be detected when gastrointestinal disease is present.

Encephalitis is a common component of disseminated infection, occurring in about 60–70% of these newborns. Serial evaluation of the CSF and noninvasive neurodiagnostic tests, as defined below, will help assess the extent of brain disease.

Encephalitis

Infection of the CNS alone or in combination with disseminated disease presents with the findings indicative of encephalitis. Overall, nearly 90% of babies with brain infection caused by HSV have evidence of an acute neurologic syndrome. Brain infection can occur in one of two fashions: either as a component of multiorgan disseminated infection or only as encephalitis, with or without skin, eye, and mouth involvement. Nearly one-third of all babies with neonatal HSV infection have only the encephalitic component of disease. The pathogenesis of the latter type of brain infection is most likely different from that of the former type, as noted previously.

Clinical manifestations of these two types of encephalitis include seizures (both focal and generalized), lethargy, irritability, tremors, poor feeding, temperature instability, bulging fontanel, and pyramidal tract signs. Whereas babies with disseminated infection often have skin vesicles in association with brain infection, the same is not true for babies with encephalitis alone. In this latter group, only approximately 60% have skin vesicles at any time during the disease course (13,23,51,52,55). Cultures of CSF yield virus in 25–40% of all cases. Anticipated findings on CSF examination include pleocytosis and proteinosis (as high as 500–1000 mg/dl). Although a few babies with CNS infection, demonstrated by brain biopsy, have been reported to have no abnormalities of their CSF, certainly this is very uncommon. Serial CSF examinations provide a useful diagnostic approach, since the infected newborn with brain disease demon-strates progressive increases in the protein content. The importance of CSF examinations in all infants is underscored by the finding that even subtle changes have been associated with significant developmental abnormalities (56). EEG, CT, or MRI can be very useful in defining the presence of CNS abnormalities. A characteristic MRI scan is shown in Fig. 2. Death occurs in 50% of babies with localized CNS disease who are not treated, and it is usually related to involvement of the brainstem. In the absence of therapy, with rare exceptions, survivors are left with neurologic impairment in the absence of antiviral therapy (51,57).

The long-term prognosis, after either disseminated infection or encephalitis alone, is particularly poor. Up to 50% of surviving children have some degree of psychomotor retardation, often in association with microcephaly, hydranencephaly, porencephalic cysts, spasticity, blindness, chorioretinitis, or learning disabilities. It is unclear at this time whether visceral or CNS damage can be progressive after initial clearance of the viral infection, a possibility suggested by long-term assessment of children with skin, eye, or mouth disease (13,23,57) and, more recently, by study of a group of babies with more severe disease (58).

Several points warrant reiteration. Clinical manifestations of disease in children with encephalitis alone are virtually identical to those findings that occur with brain infection in disseminated cases, in spite of the presumed differences in pathogenesis. For babies with encephalitis only, approximately 60% develop evidence of a vesicular rash characteristic of HSV infection. Thus, a newborn with pleocytosis and proteinosis of the CSF but without a rash can easily be misdiagnosed as having bacterial or other viral infection unless HSV infection is carefully considered. In such circumstances, a history of genital lesions in the mother or her sexual partner may be very important in the incrimination of HSV as a cause of illness.

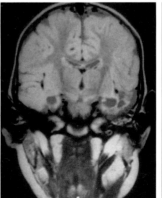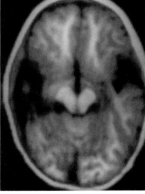

FIG. 2. MRI scans of CNS neonatal HSV infection (bitemporal disease).

Skin, Eye, and/or Mouth Infection

Infection localized to the skin, eye, and/or mouth is associated with virtually no mortality, but it can result in significant neurologic morbidity. When infection is localized to the skin, the presence of discrete vesicles remains the hallmark of disease. A characteristic vesicular rash appears in Fig. 3A and 3B. Clusters of vesicles often appear initially upon the presenting part of the body which was in direct contact with the virus during birth. With time, the rash can progress to involve other areas of the body as well. Vesicles occur in 80% of children with skin, eye, or mouth infection. Children with disease localized to the skin, eye, or mouth generally present at about 10–11 days of life. Those babies with skin lesions invariably suffer from recurrences over the first 6 months (and longer) of life, regardless of whether therapy was administered or not. Although death is not associated with disease localized to the skin, eye, and/or mouth, approximately 30% of these children eventually develop evidence of neurologic impairment in the absence of antiviral therapy (13,33,57).

The skin vesicles usually erupt from an erythematous base and generally are 1–2 mm in diameter. Vesicles can progress to larger bullous lesions greater than 1 cm in diameter. While discrete vesicles on various parts of the body are usually encountered, crops and clusters of vesicles, including satellite lesions, have also been described with regularity. For most babies with neonatal HSV infection localized to the skin, eye, and/or mouth, the vesicular skin rash involves multiple and often distant cutaneous sites; however, a limited number of babies have had infection of the skin limited to one or two vesicles, with no further evidence of cutaneous disease. This group of babies warrants careful evaluation because many have developed encephalitic involvement when antiviral ther-

apy was not administered. Failure to administer antiviral therapy usually is the consequence of the lack of clarity of the diagnosis. Other manifestations of skin lesions have included a zosteriform eruption (59).

Infections involving the eye may manifest as keratoconjunctivitis or, later, chorioretinitis. The eye can be the only site of HSV involvement in the newborn, as previously reported and as documented in our own studies (33). These children present with keratoconjunctivitis or, surprisingly, evidence of microphthalmia and retinal dysplasia. In the presence of persistent disease and no therapy, chorioretinitis can result. Chorioretinitis can be caused by either HSV-1 or HSV-2 (60–62). Keratoconjunctivitis, even in the presence of therapy, can progress to chorioretinitis, cataracts, and retinal detachment. Cataracts have been detected on long-term follow-up of proven perinatally acquired HSV infections (63).

Localized infection of the oropharyngeal cavity has been reported. Lesions of the mouth and tongue with or without systemic involvement have been described. Overall, approximately 10% of patients have evidence of HSV infection of the oropharynx. Unfortunately, many of these children did not undergo a thorough oral examination to determine the presence of lesions concomitant with excretion of virus from this site.

Long-term neurologic impairment has been encountered in children whose disease appeared localized to the skin, eye, and/or mouth. The significant findings include spastic quadriplegia, microcephaly, and blindness. Important questions regarding the pathogenesis of delayed-onset neurologic debility are raised by such clinical observations. Despite normal clinical and CSF examinations when these children complete antiviral therapy, neurologic impairment has become apparent between 6 months and 1 year of life. The clinical presentation occurs in a manner similar to that associated with congenitally acquired toxoplasmosis or syphilis.

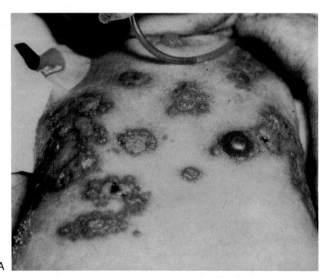
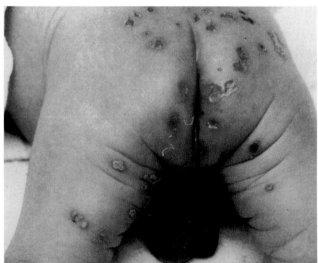

A

B

FIG. 3. **A** and **B:** Characteristic vesicular rash.

Diagnosis

The appropriate utilization of laboratory tools is essential if a diagnosis of HSV infection is to be achieved, as recently reviewed (64). Virus isolation remains the definitive diagnostic method. If skin lesions are present, a scraping of skin vesicles should be made and transferred (in appropriate virus transport media) to a diagnostic virology laboratory. Clinical specimens should be shipped on ice for prompt inoculation into cell culture systems that are susceptible for the demonstration of the cytopathic effects characteristic of HSV replication (65). It should be noted that shipping and processing of specimens should be expedited. In addition to sampling fluid within skin vesicles, other sites from which virus may be isolated include the CSF, stool, urine, throat, nasopharynx, and conjunctivae. In infants with evidence of hepatitis or other gastrointestinal abnormalities, it may also be useful to obtain duodenal aspirates for HSV isolation. The virologic results of cultures from these anatomic sites should be used in conjunction with clinical findings to define the extent of disease in the newborn. Typing of an HSV isolate may be done by one of several techniques which may not be routinely available. Since outcome with treatment does not appear to be related to the virus type, identification is only of epidemiologic and pathogenetic importance and, therefore, not usually necessary.

Every effort should be made to confirm infection by viral isolation. In the 1990s, such efforts are reasonable as well as being the expected level of care. In the absence of diagnostic virology facilities, cytologic examination of cells from the maternal cervix or from the infant's skin, mouth, conjunctivae, or corneal lesions may be useful in making a presumptive diagnosis of HSV infection. These methods only have a sensitivity of approximately 60–70% and, therefore, should not be the sole diagnostic determinant for infection in the newborn (66,67). Similar methods in adults with genital herpes have a slightly higher sensitivity and specificity (68). Cellular material obtained by scraping the periphery of the base of lesions should be smeared on a glass slide and promptly fixed in cold ethanol. The slide can be stained according to the methods of Papanicolaou, Giemsa, or Wright before examination by a trained cytologist. Deployment of Giemsa or, alternatively, Tzanck smears likely will not demonstrate the presence of intranuclear inclusions. The presence of intranuclear inclusions and multinucleated giant cells are indicative, but not diagnostic, of HSV infection. The utilization of HSV monoclonal antibodies for rapid diagnosis has gained widespread acceptance. These fluorescence studies should be performed by laboratories experienced in the procedure. More rapid diagnostic assays (10 min) are now being developed (69). Somewhat surprisingly, even electron-microscopic assays are continuing to be developed (70).

In contrast to other neonatal infections, serologic diagnosis of HSV infection is *not* of great clinical value. Therapeutic decisions *cannot* await the results of serologic studies. The inability of the commercially available serologic assays to distinguish between antibodies to HSV-1 and HSV-2, as well as to denote the presence of transplacentally acquired maternal IgG versus endogenously produced antibodies, makes the assessment of the neonate's antibody status both difficult and of little value during acute infection. Serial antibody assessments may be useful if a mother without a prior history of HSV infection has a primary infection late in gestation and, therefore, transfers little or no antibody to the fetus. The use of CT and MRI scans to define CNS disease is essential, even in the child who appears normal.

The most commonly used tests for measurement of HSV antibodies are complement fixation, passive hemagglutination, neutralization, and immunofluorescence assays, as well as the enzyme-linked immunosorbent assay (ELISA). The more recent development of type-specific antibody assays will likely replace many of the older systems. Preliminary data for DNA amplification assays offer hope for rapid, sensitive, and specific noninvasive neurodiagnostic procedures (71). These assays can detect viral DNA in clinical specimens (72).

Several aspects relating to the diagnosis of neonatal HSV should be emphasized, some of which have been noted previously but only briefly. First, the clinical diagnosis of neonatal HSV infection has become increasingly difficult because of the apparent decrease in the incidence of skin vesicles as an initial component of disease presentation. Second, alternative diagnoses must be ruled out, since a variety of infections of the newborn can resemble neonatal HSV infection. Third, virus isolation remains the definitive diagnostic method. Only in 1–2% of cases of neonatal HSV will cultures be negative from all sources sampled. If suspicion for HSE is still high when cultures are negative, brain biopsy should be performed. Brain biopsy is rarely necessary in the neonate suspected of having HSE, because (a) any positive culture in the neonate is an indication for treatment and (b) a positive culture can usually be obtained.

Finally, in contrast to other neonatal infections, serologic diagnosis of HSV infection is of no practical clinical value, as already stressed. Therapeutic decisions *cannot* await the results of serologic studies.

Prevention

Cesarean Section

There are many possibilities for intervention in the management of pregnant mothers both with and without a history of genital herpes. It is accepted practice that mothers with active herpetic lesions be delivered by cesarean section if delivery is within 4 hr of membrane rupture. Cesarean section is of unproven benefit if membranes have been ruptured for more than 4 hr. Furthermore, 76% of babies with neonatal HSV are born to mothers with no history of genital herpes. These facts underscore the need for other approaches to disease prevention (24). It must be recognized, however, that infection of the newborn has occurred in spite of delivery by cesarean section (24,73). In these circumstances, cesarean section was performed specifically to prevent neonatal infection.

Various studies are in progress to identify women at risk for HSV transmission and to devise methods for preventing disease. Current studies are evaluating the benefit of uniform screening of mothers to determine excretion of HSV at the time of delivery. The use of appropriate antibody testing to detect individuals with prior HSV-2 infections could reduce the population screened at delivery. Recent seroprevalence studies indicate that 20–40% of women of childbearing age have had prior exposure to HSV-2 (74,75). Thus, a group exists for more careful follow-up. The prophylactic use of acyclovir in women who have a history of genital herpes or antibodies to HSV-2 is another strategy yet to be evaluated. If HSV-2-seropositive women were to receive acyclovir, an average of over 1000 women would be treated to prevent disease in one baby.

It should be noted that up to 30% of newborns with HSV infection have disease caused by HSV-1; and, although some of these infections may be acquired during delivery, efforts to reduce postnatal acquisition of HSV must be employed. In family members, hospital personnel, etc., with orolabial or other mucocutaneous herpetic infections, current recommendations involve strict handwashing and, obviously, avoiding all contact the infant may have with infectious lesions. Individuals with herpetic whitlows carry an especially high risk of viral shedding, and these individuals should be removed from the care of the infant if possible. Suffice it to say that there are many strategies being evaluated to prevent neonatal acquisition of HSV, and current research should provide a rational basis for changes in practice.

Vaccination

Though various strategies for prevention of neonatal infection must be instituted, eventual control of HSV infection is most likely to be achieved through vaccination, and there is considerable research underway to design and test HSV vaccines. Several principles should be understood. First, the efficacy of the vaccine must be sufficient to prevent transmission of infection (54). It is highly unlikely that any vaccine will totally prevent infection. Second, high titers of antibody against HSV do not protect humans from reactivation with latent infection. Third, live virus vaccines tend to induce more potent and durable humoral and cellular immune responses than do subunit or purified glycoprotein vaccines (76).

Recombinant DNA technology enhances the possibility that acceptable viral or subunit vaccines can be developed (77). For example, appropriate gene deletions or mutations may abolish the transforming capability of viral DNA and may also abolish the ability of the virus to establish latency or to be reactivated from the latent state (78,79). Genetically engineered deletion mutants of HSV-1 have been shown to induce immunity and protection in mice, rabbits, guinea pigs, and monkeys, at times without establishing latency (80–82). Since significant doubt has been cast upon the oncogenic potential of HSV and because live virus vaccines induce more durable immunity, one of the live, attenuated recombinant viral vaccines (genetically engineered) may offer hope for an acceptable vaccine. This vaccine has detected putative neurovirulence and transforming genes.

Another current thrust is to prepare glycoprotein vaccines utilizing recombinant DNA techniques. At least three types of recombinant vectors containing and expressing the type gD gene are presently being studied (76). For a more complete review of HSV vaccines, the reader is referred to a recent publication (80). Several strategies are being pursued to develop an HSV vaccine. Many of these vaccines have been evaluated in animals, and some in humans. The success of research thus far provides encouraging support that an acceptable vaccine for HSV will soon be available.

Treatment

Background

Of all perinatally acquired viral infections, the one most likely to be amenable to successful therapy is that caused by HSV. Treatment has been discussed for over two decades (83). Since most babies acquire infection at the time of delivery or shortly thereafter, successful antiviral therapy should decrease mortality and improve long-term outcome. Inherent in these presumptions is the recognition that diagnosis early after the onset of clinical illness is essential for even an adequate outcome, as is the case with other perinatally acquired bacterial infections. Equally importantly, it is essential that the possibility of disease progression weigh heavily on the physician's interpretation of decisions to institute therapy. It has been documented that children presenting with disease localized to the skin, eye, and/or mouth can progress to either involvement of the CNS or disseminated infection in approximately 70% of cases (51). When such events occur, the likelihood of an adequate outcome, even with established drugs, is not optimal, since many of these children will either die or be left with significant neurologic impairment. Such factors must be considered in the development of any treatment strategy.

As in adult populations, only vidarabine and acyclovir have proven efficacy and acceptable therapeutic indices for the treatment of neonatal HSV infections. Since the initiation of studies by the NIAID Collaborative Antiviral Study Group, 291 babies with neonatal HSV infection have been entered into therapeutic trials of either vidarabine or acyclovir. Of the total, 102 babies had infection of the skin, eye, and mouth, 96 babies had encephalitis, and 93 had disseminated infection. Although the characteristics of these babies and the changing presentation of disease are reported elsewhere, a brief discussion of these therapeutic trials is in order (24,57, 83–86).

Vidarabine Trials (1973–1983). The use of vidarabine (15 mg/kg/day for 10 days) in infants with either disseminated or localized CNS disease (versus placebo recipients) was associated with a decline in mortality rate, from 75% to 30%, as shown in Fig. 4 (86). Also, the lowest mortality rate was achieved in babies with either encephalitis alone or skin, eye, and mouth infection. The mortality rate was decreased with therapy, from 90% in babies with disseminated infection to approximately 60% following vidarabine therapy (Fig. 5). For babies with encephalitis alone, the mortality rate was decreased from 50% to 15%. Approximately 30% of surviving children with either encephalitis alone or disseminated infection were reported as functioning normally at 1 year of age. Finally, with skin, eye, and mouth infection, although there were no deaths, severe neurologic impairment was decreased from 30% to 10% with therapy. Notably, there is no enhanced therapeutic benefit if mortality is used as an endpoint when the dose of vidarabine is increased to 30 mg/kg/day for 10–14 days (86). Nevertheless, the higher dose of vidarabine was asso-

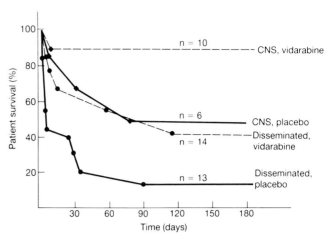

FIG. 5. Survival of newborns with either encephalitis alone or disseminated neonatal HSV infection. "Disseminated, vidarabine" versus "disseminated, placebo: $p = 0.042$. (From ref. 86, with permission.)

ciated with a decreased rate of progression to more serious disease.

Vidarabine Versus Acyclovir Trial (1983–1990). The NIAID Collaborative Antiviral Study Group has completed an evaluation of the relative value of vidarabine versus acyclovir for the treatment of neonatal HSV infection (85). Morbidity follow-up will continue for several more years. Several aspects are worthy of discussion.

First, the overall mortality rate for babies with encephalitis or disseminated infection 1 year after treatment is similar to that found in prior studies of neonatal HSV infection. There are no differences in either adverse effects or laboratory toxicity.

Second, regardless of the therapeutic employed, there has been a significant increase in the number of babies who returned to normal function. This can be accounted for largely by the introduction of therapy prior to the development of encephalitis or disseminated disease. Of the babies entered in this trial, over 48% have disease localized to the skin, eye, and mouth (85). This represents a threefold increase in the number of babies with skin, eye, and mouth involvement, when compared with that of previous studies and of historical data ($p < 0.001$). The change in spectrum of disease presentation is most likely related to earlier diagnosis. The changing spectrum of neonatal HSV infection is illustrated in Fig. 6. The number of babies with encephalitis has remained fairly constant at approximately 30%, whereas the number of babies with disseminated disease has decreased to 22%. Because of both therapy and the changing spectrum of disease, mortality and morbidity rates overall are greatly improved as shown in Figs. 7 and 8.

Third, available data indicate that therapy was initiated 3 days earlier (on average) in these studies (85). However, the mean duration of disease for all children (irrespective of disease classification) entered into these

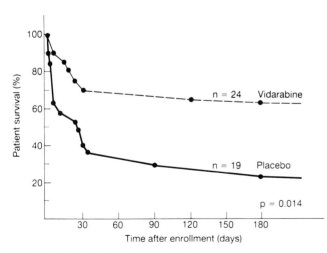

FIG. 4. Survival of newborns with either encephalitis alone or disseminated neonatal HSV infection, according to treatment regimen (vidarabine versus placebo). (From ref. 86, with permission.)

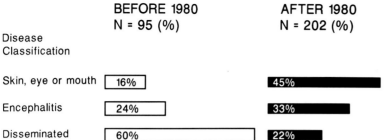

Disease Classification	BEFORE 1980 N = 95 (%)	AFTER 1980 N = 202 (%)
Skin, eye or mouth	16%	45%
Encephalitis	24%	33%
Disseminated	60%	22%

FIG. 6. Changing outcome of neonatal HSV infection.

studies was 4–5 days; therapy can, therefore, be instituted even earlier in the disease course. This "window" for earlier administration of therapy is significant if further advances in therapeutic outcome are to be achieved.

The existing database from the NIAID Collaborative Antiviral Study Group has provided an opportunity to examine those factors which influence outcome. These data are summarized in Table 2. The relative risk assessments developed from this database indicate that several factors have a major impact on the outcome of neonatal HSV infection. These include: disease classification, level of consciousness, time of initiation of therapy, virus type (for disseminated disease), and the virus type and frequency of skin recurrences for babies whose disease is localized to the skin, eye, and mouth. Our understanding of these data indicate that the limitation of disease prior to extensive multiorgan involvement or disease of the CNS is associated with the best prognosis. This information will be useful in developing future therapeutic strategies and in counseling parents of children with neonatal HSV infection.

In summary, significant progress has been made in the last 15 years in the development of antiviral therapy for neonatal HSV infection and in improving outcome, principally by earlier recognition of infection and by im-

proved treatment. Nevertheless, an ideal approach for future efforts is that of disease prevention.

CYTOMEGALOVIRUS INFECTION

History

Cytomegalovirus (CMV) infections are the most common viral infection known to be transmitted *in utero*. The ubiquitous nature of these viruses and resulting spectrum of illness in older children and adults are described in Chapter 4. The history of congenital CMV infection parallels our knowledge of its isolation in cell culture systems.

The first case of congenital CMV infection was reported in 1904 by Ribbert (87), who described cells containing intranuclear and cytoplasmic inclusions found in the kidneys of a stillborn infant with congenital syphilis. Subsequently, following the propagation of a murine CMV in explant cultures of mouse fibroblasts, two independent research groups virtually simultaneously isolated human CMV from the urine of two congenitally infected babies (88–90). Isolation of a virus from saliva and urine of babies, resulting in "megalic" cell forma-

Mortality	PRE-TREATMENT N = 361 (%)	AFTER 1980 N = 202 (%)
Overall	58%	16%
By Disease:		
SEM	0%	0%
Encephalitis	40%	11%
Disseminated	82%	54%

A

Disease Classification	(%) Mortality	
	Vidarabine N=162	Acyclovir N=116
Skin, Eye & Mouth	0/39 (0)	0/59 (0)
Encephalitis	7/60 (12)	5/38 (13)
Disseminated	37/63 (59)	11/19 (58)

B

FIG. 7. A and **B:** Changing mortality rates of neonatal HSV infection. SEM—skin, eye, and mouth.

Neurological Impairment of Survivors	BEFORE 1980 N = 361 (%)	AFTER 1980 N = 202 (%)
Overall	46%	30%
By Disease:		
SEM	43%	2%
Encephalitis	74%	49%
Disseminated	50%	35%

A

Disease Classification	(%) Patients Normal	
	Vidarabine	Acyclovir
Skin, Eye & Mouth	26/29 (90)	47/48 (98)
Encephalitis	19/39 (49)	13/30 (43)
Disseminated	10/18 (56)	5/6 (83)

B

FIG. 8. A and **B:** Changing morbidity of neonatal HSV infection.

TABLE 2. *Clinical findings in 34 newborns with congenital CMV infection, all of whom were symptomatic by 2 weeks of age*

Abnormality	Positive/total examined
Petechiae	27/34 (79%)
Hepatosplenomegaly	25/34 (74%)
Jaundice	20/32 (63%)
Microcephaly[a]	17/34 (50%)
Small for gestational age[b]	14/34 (41%)
Prematurity[c]	11/32 (34%)
Inguinal hernia	5/19 (26%)[d]
Chorioretinitis	4/34 (12%)

[a] For premature newborns, less than 10th percentile based upon Colorado Intrauterine Growth Charts; for term babies, more than 2 SD below mean based upon Nelhaus scale.
[b] Weight less than 10th percentile for gestational age.
[c] Gestational age less than 38 weeks.
[d] Males.

tion, led to the tentative names of cytomegalic inclusion disease and salivary gland virus. In 1960, Weller et al. (91) offered the term "cytomegalovirus," stating that it was less misleading.

The incidence of congenital CMV infection ranges from 0.2% to 2.2% among all live births, with no evidence of seasonal variation (92). The natural history of CMV infection during pregnancy is quite complex, and our understanding is far from complete. This chapter will only review congenital CMV infection, since it is a cause of perinatal CNS disease with the potential for long-term neurologic sequelae.

Infectious Agent

The biologic properties of CMV are described in Chapter 4.

Pathology and Pathogenesis

Pathology

The pathologic findings of CMV infections in newborns are no different from those encountered in infection of older children and adults, as described in Chapter 4.

Pathogenesis of Congenital Infection

CMV infections, as a cause of CNS disease in the newborn, can be best understood in terms of disease pathogenesis, particularly the time of acquisition of infection by the unborn child in the context of maternal infection. Congenital CMV infection appears to be the result of transmission of virus from mother to fetus, as occurs with many other infections. Many women are infected

with CMV, but only a few transmit infection to the fetus. Specifically, acquisition and reactivation of CMV infection during gestation is common; however, only a few women transmit virus to their fetuses, resulting in the potential for either acute or long-term morbidity. It should be noted that symptomatic disease or generalized infection evident in the newborn is usually the consequence of maternal primary infection, directly resulting from viremia with transplacental spread of the virus. Recurrent maternal infection can be associated with fetal damage, although this is a very uncommon occurrence (93–95). With reactivated maternal infection, it is presumed that preexisting maternal antibodies decrease the quantity of virus available in the blood for transplacental infection and spread to the fetus. As with other perinatal infections, maternal primary infection is not always associated with fetal infection, since the latter occurs in only 30–40% of cases. Thus, there must be innate host defenses (including the placenta) which protect the fetus *in utero*.

Intrauterine infection results in the highest incidence of acute disease of any population infected with CMV other than immunocompromised patients. Nevertheless, the clinical findings of intrauterine infection are significantly different from those of disease caused by postnatal infection or reactivation of CMV in the immunocompromised host. The intrauterine environment is thought to contribute significantly to clinical symptomatology.

Why some infants are severely affected and others remain free of symptoms is not entirely clear (96). Because of the low-grade virulence of CMV infection in general, it is possible that some late-appearing abnormalities may be delayed manifestations of damage that actually was initiated *in utero*. The most obvious, but not necessarily the most important, pathogenic mechanism is continuous viral replication in affected organs. Longitudinal studies have demonstrated that excretion of CMV into urine and saliva persists for years. Chronic viral replication probably also occurs at other anatomic sites that are less accessible to virologic examination (e.g., middle ear, brain, etc.) (96).

The type of maternal infection is considered to be the major pathogenic factor for congenital CMV infection. As has been noted previously, maternal primary infection is more likely to be associated with transmission to the fetus than is maternal recurrent infection (14). Intrauterine transmission following primary infection occurs in approximately 30–40% of cases; however, intrauterine infection following a recurrent reactivation of maternal CMV infection is approximately 1.5% for American populations. It is about 0.9% for women of middle and upper socioeconomic status (93,94,96,97). It should be noted that the time of primary maternal infection is thought to significantly influence clinical symptomatology. Specifically, as suggested by several studies of congenital infection, an earlier gestational age of the fetus at the time of infection is more likely to result in a poorer outcome (93).

Another factor in disease pathogenesis is vasculitis, which may occur *in utero* or after birth. Infants with congenital CMV infection who die soon after birth usually have disseminated intravascular coagulopathy. Results of preliminary studies indicate that the virulence of congenital CMV infection is not strain-dependent (98,99). Although only a few infants have been studied, viruses isolated from congenitally or perinatally infected siblings have been found to be genetically identical. In two of the pairs of siblings assessed, the first-born baby was severely affected, whereas the second-born infant was only subclinically infected (100).

Injury mediated by immunologic factors has also been evaluated. The humoral immune system of infected infants is generally intact and responds normally to antigenic stimulation (101–103). Early after birth, symptomatic congenitally infected infants have an accelerated development of IgG and IgM (101). Their specific antibody response is substantial and prolonged, regardless of the serologic assay used or the nature of the infection—symptomatic, subclinical, active, or latent (102). Unfortunately, available serologic data offer no clues that explain a propensity for symptomatic infection. At a molecular level, studies of CMV polypeptides immunoprecipitated by IgG antibodies indicated that symptomatically infected infants had a delay (until 12 months of age) in the appearance of precipitating antibodies (103). However, when a humoral immune response develops, antibodies to viral polypeptides are precipitated in greater numbers and are maintained for longer periods. This sustained humoral immune response to congenital CMV infection occurs in the presence of persistent viral replication, thereby creating the potential for the formation of immune complexes (104). During the first year of life, immune complexes circulate in a large proportion of infants with congenital infection. The molecular weight of these immune complexes is higher in symptomatic infants than in asymptomatic infants. In a few fatal symptomatic cases, deposition of immune complexes in renal glomeruli has been demonstrated.

Congenitally infected infants have also been noted to have impaired specific cell-mediated immunity (105–109). This impairment is not a reflection of a generalized disturbance, since it is restricted to a blastogenic response to CMV and is highly virus-specific. Babies infected with CMV who have antibodies to HSV, for example, have a normal blastogenic response to this virus (110). Furthermore, the number of T cells, the response to phytohemagglutinin, and the proportions of helper and suppressor subpopulations of T lymphocytes are all normal. The impairment of blastogenic response has no relation to the clinical presentation and outcome, but it

is more intense and long-lasting in babies with symptomatic CMV infection. As these children grow older, the impairment disappears, and so also does viral replication (108). It is possible that the subtle alterations of host-defense mechanisms could contribute to disease in conjunction with persistent viral replication.

The pathogenesis of CMV infections in the newborn and young infant would be incomplete without recognizing other sources and other routes of infection. These include natal acquisition of infection either from infected maternal genital secretions or from the breast milk early in life (111). While acquisition of infection by these routes does not usually result in disease, the infant becomes a source of infection. Furthermore, acquisition of infection following postnatal transfusion is also a source of CMV. These issues will be discussed in somewhat more detail below.

Epidemiology

General Epidemiology

The epidemiology of CMV infections in general is discussed in Chapter X. Those studies which specifically elucidate epidemiology of CMV infections during gestation will be briefly reiterated. Humans are the only reservoir for CMV (112). Infection is endemic in the world's populations and is without seasonal variation (113). While the prevalence of CMV infection in the world's populations increases directly with age, there are significant variations according to geographic, ethnic, and socioeconomic backgrounds (113–115). Acquisition of infection early in life, as indicated by seroprevalence of CMV, occurs earlier in populations of lower socioeconomic status and where living conditions are more crowded than in upper socioeconomic populations or more developed countries. Examples of differences in seroprevalence rates are reflected by countries such as Africa and those of the South Pacific where seropositivity among pre-school children is between 95% and 100% as contrasted to that in Great Britain and the United States where, historically, it has been approximately 20%.

Specifically, as it relates to congenital CMV infection, seroprevalence rates among women of childbearing age vary from one area of the world to another. In developed areas of the world (United States and western Europe), seropositivity rates in women of childbearing age range from 50% to 85% (115,116). In contrast, in African populations of the Ivory Coast, as well as in Japan and Chile, seroprevalence rates are in excess of 90%. It is likely that seroprevalence rates in developed countries will increase further as the epidemiology of infection in targeted populations changes.

Transmission of infection from one individual to another requires direct contact. Sources of virus include saliva, blood, vaginal secretions, semen, milk, and tears (101,117–119). Several of these sources of virus are relevant as it relates to infection of women of childbearing age. Salivary excretion of virus, particularly in association with mouthing of toys in the day-care environment, can lead to baby-to-baby transmission in the child-care setting (120–123). Thus, susceptible children can acquire infection in the day-care environment, providing a reservoir of virus for infection of susceptible family members in the home. A seronegative mother who comes in contact with infected secretions from a child attending day care is at risk for primary CMV infection. If pregnant, the consequences could be grievous for the fetus. Transmission of CMV from an infant to his mother—as well as from an infant to pregnant caretakers, with subsequent transmission to the fetus—has been documented (124,125).

Epidemiology of Maternal Infection

The natural history of CMV during pregnancy is particularly complex and has not been fully explained, although recent advances have been made. Perinatal infections such as rubella, toxoplasmosis, and syphilis cannot serve as models because, unlike what takes place in those diseases, the *in utero* transmission of CMV can occur as a consequence of reactivated infection, even in the presence of substantial humoral immunity (100). The prevalence of CMV infection in pregnant women in the United States varies according to socioeconomic background. The seropositivity rate is 50–60% for women of middle-class background, but it is 70–85% for those from lower socioeconomic sectors (126). The characteristics of CMV infection are summarized in Fig. 9.

Prospective studies in the United States, Great Britain, and Sweden have established that pregnancy itself does not increase the risk of acquiring CMV infection (94,127–133). Among susceptible women, the risk of seroconversion during pregnancy averages 2.0–2.5%, as shown in Fig. 9. However, seroconversion occurs significantly more often among women in highly immune, low-income groups than among middle-class women—a reflection of sustained higher degree of exposure to CMV (131). In primary CMV infection, as in rubella, toxoplasmosis, and syphilis, an innate barrier prevents *in utero* transmission; thus, primary maternal CMV infection leads to transmission in only about 40% of fetuses (94,97,127–133). Moreover, only 10% of infants so infected have clinical manifestations at birth (from very mild to severe), and the risk of subsequent sequelae is 15–20% overall. For the most part, gestational age, per se, has no influence on the rate of transmission of virus *in utero*; yet, the risk of neonatal disease with attendant sequelae appears to be higher when the mother has ac-

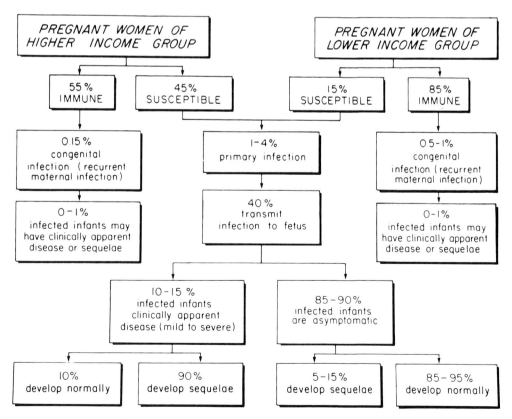

FIG. 9. Characteristics of CMV infection in pregnancy. From Baer GM, Fellini WJ, Fishbein DB. Phabdoviruses. In: BN Fields, DM Knipe, ed. *Virology,* 2nd Edition, New York: Raven Press, 1990.

quired CMV infection during the first half of pregnancy (4–24 weeks of gestation).

Primary CMV infections during pregnancy are generally asymptomatic (92,126–132). To screen women for primary infection would require the testing of all pregnant women for IgG antibodies at their first prenatal visit and retesting the seronegative women later in gestation (94,97,133–136). Detection of first-trimester primary infections would require screening of seropositive women for CMV-specific IgM antibodies (94,97,135).

Maternal immunity to CMV, unlike immunity to rubella and toxoplasmosis, does not prevent virus reactivation, nor does it control the systemic spread of virus that can produce congenital infection (94,100,133,137–139). Studies that use restriction-endonuclease analysis of viral DNA to examine the genetic relatedness between CMV strains isolated repeatedly from mother and offspring indicate reactivation of an identical latent virus rather than reinfection with an exogenous one (99). In a highly seropositive (82% of persons) urban population of low socioeconomic background in Alabama, recurrent CMV infection produced a 1.6% (13 of 835 infants) rate of congenital infection, thus indicating that most intrauterine infections in this population are due to this phenomenon (127). In contrast, the infants of immune middle-class women with a seropositivity rate of 55% had a lower rate of congenital infection (0.19%, i.e., 10 of 5242). This rate is not significantly different from that observed in Great Britain and Sweden (94,97,133). Although maternal immunity is imperfect, congenital infections that result from recurrent infection are less likely to produce fetal damage than those resulting from primary infections (127).

During pregnancy and in the immediate postpartum period, CMV can be shed at variable rates from one or more sites (127). Rates of excretion are higher in younger, nonwhite women from lower socioeconomic backgrounds. Most women who excrete virus during pregnancy do so as a result of recurrent infections (reactivation or reinfection) (99). Furthermore, it is well recognized that there is little correlation between CMV excretion from the cervix or urine during pregnancy and the later birth of a congenitally infected infant (101, 128,130). However, the presence of CMV in the maternal genital tract at delivery and in the breast milk after delivery is strongly associated with intrapartum/postpartum transmission of infection to the infant (117,119). In full-term and otherwise healthy infants, perinatal infection has little clinical importance. In some cases, the postnatal acquisition of CMV is temporally related to interstitial pneumonia (119,140,141).

Practical Epidemiologic Considerations

An average of 2% of susceptible pregnant women have a primary CMV infection during pregnancy, most of which produce no symptoms. Primary CMV infection should always be suspected in pregnant women with a heterophil-negative, mononucleosis-like syndrome. Because there is no effective drug therapy for the infection and the risk of fetal morbidity is low, several investigators have concluded that routine serologic screening of pregnant women is of limited value, particularly since it is expensive (134–136). Moreover, there are no reliable, practical ways to determine whether intrauterine transmission has occurred or to assess fetal disease. Thus, there is inadequate information to serve as a basis for recommendations regarding termination of pregnancy after maternal primary CMV infection. Similarly, there is no information regarding how long conception should be delayed after primary infection. Viral excretion is not a good marker, since virus is shed into saliva for weeks or months after infection and into urine and the cervix for months or years.

Knowledge of fetal exposure to CMV *in utero* is important for the care of the infant. The diagnosis of congenital infection is easy to confirm by viral isolation. Preexisting immunity does not prevent the virus from reactivating, nor does it control the occasional spread to the fetus effectively. However, preexisting maternal immunity may afford protection against overwhelming systemic infection of the fetus. At present, there are no techniques for identifying women who reactivate CMV and who subsequently transmit infection *in utero*. Women who are seropositive before conception do not need to be virologically or serologically tested, nor should they be excessively worried about transmitting the virus to the fetus.

Epidemiology of Other Forms of Infection

It is apparent that CMV infection can be acquired by routes other than that associated with pregnancy. Seroepidemiologic studies have indicated that female health-care workers have an occupational risk of primary infection, (142–144), whereas other studies indicate that they are at no greater risk of acquiring CMV infection than are other women (145–150). As noted, recent evidence suggests that children have a role in transmission of CMV to susceptible adults. For instance, one study demonstrated that the annual rate of seroconversion in women with at least one child living at home was more than double the rate in susceptible nursery nurses, physicians in training, and women of similar socioeconomic backgrounds who are pregnant for the first time (151).

Previously, it has been stated that children in the day-care environment can acquire CMV infection as a consequence of fomite transmission after having contact with CMV on plastic surfaces (152,153). CMVs have been found to be endemic in the day-care setting, and there is concern about the occupational risks to child-care personnel, particularly women of childbearing age

(121,154–158). The Centers for Disease Control (154) have stressed the need for strict hygienic measures—such as (a) washing hands after each contact with urine and respiratory-tract or other potentially infectious secretions and (b) careful handling and disposal of diapers and other articles known to be contaminated with urine and other secretions—in order to decrease the likelihood of transmission of infection.

Perinatal infection is a common source of infection as well. Contact of the fetus with infected maternal genital secretions, or postnatal acquisition of infection from infected breast milk, contributes to the high incidence of infection early in life. Breast milk has been reported to result in an infection rate of 63% during the perinatal period, whereas infection from the genital tract is associated with a transmission rate of 57%, as summarized elsewhere (119). Certainly, there is considerable variability in perinatal transmission of CMV throughout the world, reflecting both (a) the mother's previous exposure to CMV and (b) social acceptance for such practices as breast-feeding.

Other routes of transmission of CMV include sexual transmission from infected semen and cervical secretions (118; for review see ref. 111). Acquisition of CMV as a consequence of sexual contact has been documented both in heterosexual as well as homosexual populations.

Infection with CMV as a consequence of contact with infected blood or blood products has similarly been documented. The post-transfusion syndrome caused by CMV was suggested in 1960 (159). Subsequently, a mononucleosis syndrome following exposure to blood and blood products has been documented as being caused by CMV (160–167). It has been estimated that 2.5–12% of blood donors are capable of transmitting CMV infection. These data have been substantiated in a prospective study of seronegative children who received blood for cardiac surgery where the risk of acquisition of CMV was determined to be 2.7% (160).

As with blood products, transplanted organs (kidneys, liver, and heart) are known sources of CMV infection. Seronegative recipients from seropositive donors are at risk for primary CMV infection with subsequent evidence of CMV viremia.

Clinical Presentation of Congenital Infection

Symptomatic Infection

The abnormalities of clinical disease were first characterized by Weller and Hanshaw (168) but have been recounted by many other investigators around the world. Of the nearly 40,000 infants born with congenital CMV infection in the United States each year, only an estimated 10% are symptomatic at birth. Disease in the symptomatic newborn is characterized by hepatomeg-

aly, splenomegaly, microcephaly, direct hyperbilirubinemia, petechiae, and thrombocytopenia. Intracranial calcifications and chorioretinitis are demonstrable with regularity. The frequency of these findings appears in Table 2.

The mortality among congenitally infected infants may be as high as 20–30%. Deaths which occur early in life as a consequence of symptomatic CMV infection are usually the consequence of hepatic dysfunction, bleeding, or secondary bacterial infection. Death after the first month of life is usually the consequence of hepatic dysfunction; however, beyond the first year of life, death is usually the result of complications in the neurologically handicapped child secondary to either malnutrition, aspiration pneumonia, or overwhelming infection.

The CNS defects in these children are particularly striking. Microcephaly, as noted in studies performed at the University of Alabama at Birmingham as well as in those original case reports, occurs in at least 50% of babies with symptomatic congenital CMV infection (169,170). It has been noted that children with head circumferences smaller than those in the 5th percentile at birth may subsequently establish a normal brain growth pattern; however, the frequency at which this occurs is not well established at this time (171). Intracranial calcifications occur in approximately 20–30% of children with symptomatic congenital CMV infection. The CNS lesions of two children with intracranial calcifications evaluated by CT and MRI scans are shown in Fig. 10. If calcifications are present on neurodiagnostic evaluation, long-term neurologic impairment is unequivocal. Ocular and hearing defects are common in children with symptomatic congenital CMV infection. The principal abnormalities of the eye associated with congenital CMV infection is chorioretinitis, with optic atrophy being relatively uncommon (171). Chorioretinitis occurs in approximately 14% of infants with symptomatic congenital CMV infection from studies performed at the University of Alabama at Birmingham. Chorioretinitis in the newborn with CMV infection will usually resolve spontaneously over the first several months of life, leaving residual, characteristic pigmented scars.

More than 90% of the survivors develop late-appearing complications, such as hearing loss, mental retardation, delay in psychomotor development, chorioretinitis and optic atrophy, seizures, expressive-language delays, learning disabilities, and defects of the dentition (92,133,168–174). Table 3 compares the outcome of children with symptomatic versus asymptomatic congenital CMV infection. Of the 90% of infants with no clinical manifestations at birth, 5–15% are at risk for the development of similar abnormalities within the first 2 years of life (175–179). The single most important late-appearing sequela is sensorineural hearing loss (5–10% of cases), which is bilateral in nearly half the cases and substantial enough to interfere with learning and verbal

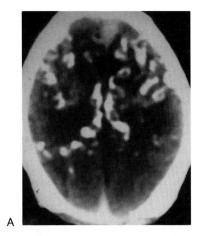

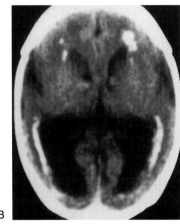

FIG. 10. A and **B:** Congenital CMV infection. These CT scans are representative of cortical atrophy and intracranial calcification.

communication. The hearing impairment may appear or become progressive only after the first year of life.

Sensorineural deafness is probably the most common handicap caused by congenital CMV infection, as first identified by Medearis (172). It is known that CMV can replicate in the inner ear as evidenced by the cytopathology of Reissner's membrane, stria vascularis, or semicircular canals or by the presence of disease in the organ of Corti. It must be emphasized that hearing impairment in the child with symptomatic congenital CMV infection can be progressive. Hearing impairment becomes signifi-

cant in infancy and early childhood. In the studies performed at the University of Alabama at Birmingham, over 60% of children evaluated for symptomatic congenital CMV infection had some degree of hearing impairment. Importantly, many of these cases did not develop or become severe until after the first year of life. Furthermore, it has been documented that in some cases it did not occur until between 4 and 14 years of life (111).

Asymptomatic Infection

Most newborns with congenital CMV infection will have no symptomatology (90%). Nevertheless, these children still are at risk for neurologic and sensorineural impairment. As shown in Table 3, up to 5% of children will have hearing loss; overall, 6% will have one or more complications directly attributable to CMV infection. These abnormalities usually become apparent within the first 2 years of life (176–180). These observations underscore the necessity for early diagnosis and intervention for CMV infection.

Diagnosis

The gold standard for the diagnosis of CMV infections is the isolation of virus in susceptible cell culture systems. Evaluation of urine specimens from the presumed infected child should lead to the prompt isolation of CMV in a short period of time following inoculation into cell lines, particularly in the case of the severely symptomatic child. More rapid and recently developed diagnostic assays, such as the shell vial technique, which utilizes monoclonal antibody to an immediate-early protein produced during viral replication, may expedite the diagnostic process. Furthermore, the application of DNA amplification by polymerase chain reaction may be of help in the future; however, it is of no established diagnostic value today.

A variety of serologic assays are available for the diagnosis of CMV infection. These include both IgG and IgM assays. These assays provide little diagnostic help for the evaluation of the newborn when culture facilities are available.

TABLE 3. *Outcome for patients presenting at birth with symptomatic or asymptomatic congenital CMV infection*

Complication	92 Symptomatic cases (%)	267 Asymptomatic cases (%)
Fatal	30	0
Microcephaly	48	4
Psychomotor retardation neuromuscular disorder	70	4
Hearing loss	59	5
Unilateral	30	64
Bilateral	70	36
Stable	43	64
Progressive	57	36
Chorioretinitis or optic atrophy	14	2
Dental defects	27	4
Serious bacterial infections	4	5
Total with one or more complications	92	6

Treatment

At present, there is no specific treatment for congenital CMV infection. Because of the severity of the disease in the symptomatic child (particularly as reflected by sensorineural hearing loss), therapeutic evaluations of ganciclovir (a nucleoside analogue licensed for the treatment of CMV infections which are life- and sight-threatening in the immunocompromised adult) are currently under evaluation in the newborn. However, at this time, it is premature to ascribe value to any therapeutic approach.

Practical Recommendations

It should be remembered that knowledge of CMV infections where transmission is likely to occur is the best approach for preventing infection. Specifically, women who work with young children and who are susceptible to infection with CMV should be aware of their potential risk of infection. Knowledge of their own risk can be ascertained through serologic assessment.

VARICELLA-ZOSTER VIRUS INFECTIONS

History

Varicella, or chickenpox, is usually a benign disease of childhood; however, it can be debilitating, particularly in immunocompromised patients or susceptible normal adults. When women, as noted below, suffer from varicella, morbidity and mortality may be enhanced because of the high risk of developing varicella pneumonia (181–183). Furthermore, it has only been since the mid-1970s that an intrauterine infection syndrome has been recognized as being caused by varicella infection of pregnant women, as reviewed elsewhere (183–200). It is these severe manifestations of varicella-zoster virus (VZV) infection during pregnancy which are particularly problematic and warrant review.

Infectious Agent

The infectious agent is described in Chapter 4.

Pathology and Pathogenesis

Pathology

The characteristic lesions of VZV infection, along with the resultant histopathologic changes of the CNS, are described in Chapter 4.

Pathogenesis

As has been previously reviewed, the naso/oropharynx is the presumed site of portal of entry and is pre-sumed to be the initial site for VZV replication; however, attempts to retrieve virus from this site have been unrewarding. Following primary replication, a period of viremia occurs, as has been documented and reviewed (187). Likely, there is a component of both primary viremia, resulting in seeding of the reticuloendothelial system, and secondary viremia, leading to skin lesions. With viremia, cutaneous lesions become the hallmark of infection with chickenpox. These lesions are characterized by coexisting erythematous, vesicular, pustular, and scabbed states in the normal host. Vesicular fluid is the usual site for virus retrieval. Virus will persist in the vesicles of the normal host with chickenpox for a relatively short period of time, usually less than 3 or 4 days. In contrast, the immunocompromised child or, in certain circumstances, the adult will have longer periods of persistent excretion of virus into newly forming vesicular lesions (188–190). Cessation of new lesion formation is paralleled by a rapid appearance of pustulation and scabbing.

The pathogenesis of disease during pregnancy is, likely, similar to that of the normal child, only with an exaggerated disease course. Necropsy analyses have indicated histopathologic findings of placentitis (191). These findings included areas of necrosis with rare giant cells. Uncommonly, decidual cells of the placenta had intranuclear inclusions. Pathologic examination of the products of conception have indicated lesions indicative of *in utero* VZV infection (192–196). Histopathologic surveys indicate that the fetal skin, lungs, and liver are sites frequently involved. Microscopically, evidence of lesions with central areas of necrosis surrounded by epithelioid and mononuclear cells have been characteristic. Furthermore, there is evidence of intranuclear inclusions. *In utero* disease of the brain of the embryo or fetus has not been considered common (191).

Progressive visceral disease in the pregnant woman has been identified (197). Demise in pregnant women has been attributed to varicella pneumonitis. It is not clear why disease is more progressive in the pregnant woman. It has been reported that varicella during pregnancy is associated with a 41% mortality rate (197) and also can result in a variety of other visceral complications (181,198). Nevertheless, the actual case-fatality rate is not known because, in all probability, cases that do not lead to significant complications remain unreported.

Epidemiology

Maternal Infection

Infection during pregnancy can pose a risk to both mother, as noted, and fetus. Primary infection (chickenpox) is estimated to occur in a minimum of one to five pregnancies per 10,000—a frequency that is probably low because of failure to report mild or subclinical cases

(184,199). Recurrent infection with herpes zoster (shingles) does not cause death, but it is a potential cause of disability. Although herpes zoster occurs during pregnancy, the actual incidence of infection cannot be adequately calculated (183,200,201). In fact, it is a disease that occurs far more often in older persons than in the childbearing population (202).

The natural histories of both chickenpox and herpes zoster in pregnancy are poorly defined. In spite of early reports of death from pneumonia in patients with varicella during pregnancy, it is likely that infection poses only a slightly greater risk to pregnant women than to other susceptible adults (192,200). Recent summaries indicate that chickenpox was benign in 86% of cases (25 of 29 women) and resulted in pneumonia in only 14%, with an overall mortality of 3% (183). These data are not strikingly different from those obtained during an analysis of 236 nonpregnant adults, among whom 11% acquired pneumonia (181).

As noted, VZV can infect the placenta and produce areas of focal necrosis (191), and fetal infection with organ damage, particularly of the skin, lungs, liver, and adrenals, as summarized by Young and Gershon (201). The frequency and effects of transmission of VZV according to trimester can only be approximated. Current evidence suggests that maternal chickenpox does not produce excessive prematurity or increased fetal death (182,199). Herpes zoster has *not* been incriminated as a cause of either fetal or maternal death during pregnancy (183).

Fetal Infection

Both *in vitro* and in vivo studies have indicated that VZV can induce chromosomal abnormalities (203). Nevertheless, the relationship between this observation and *in utero* disease is not apparent. Nevertheless, the implications are apparent. More careful studies have attempted to correlate abortion and prematurity with maternal VZV infection. Other retrospective analyses have attempted to confirm either excess prematurity or fetal death. Taken together, these studies indicate a rate of prematurity of approximately 5% (182,183,199,204). Furthermore, there was no evidence of an increased frequency of stillbirths.

Transmission of virus from mother to fetus can lead to congenital malformations, although infrequently. Overall, transmission occurs after approximately 26% of cases of maternal chickenpox (183). In a large prospective study, the frequency of congenital malformations (including psychomotor and audiologic debility) among offspring of infected mothers was about the same as that among offspring of controls. Nevertheless, since the first description of congenital anomalies after maternal chickenpox in 1947, a clinical syndrome of hypoplasia of the extremities, cortical atrophy, cicatricial skin lesions,

and ocular abnormalities has been identified (205). Maternal varicella during the first 20 weeks of pregnancy has been most often associated with this clinical syndrome, but a few cases were thought to be the consequence of herpes zoster during the same period (201). A recent study failed to demonstrate transmission of infection after herpes zoster; however, the number of patients studied was small (183).

Clinical Findings of Intrauterine Infection

Both from prospective and retrospective studies, including the associated problems with the latter, a constellation of symptoms has appeared which would indicate that VZV is a teratogen. Multiple congenital abnormalities resulting from chickenpox have been described, particularly when infection has occurred early in pregnancy (205). The most common findings in these cases included limb, CNS, and skin abnormalities. It appears as though characteristic limb findings include hypoplastic extremities (usually unilaterally, with or without hypoplastic or absent digits) and radiographic evidence of retarded bone development (205–219). CNS disease in children who acquired VZV infection *in utero* is characterized by a variety of CNS abnormalities. Cortical atrophy is among the most common of these, and it is usually associated with mental retardation and a seizure disorder (186,205,207–209,220–225). When brain tissue has been available for autopsy evaluation, focal calcifications within both the white and gray matter of the cerebrum, brainstem, and cerebellum have been identified. Furthermore, varying degrees of gliosis and inflammatory infiltrates have been diffusely identified in some children (226).

Finally, cicatricial skin scarring is a common finding in these children. These lesions usually have evidence of cuteus aplasia with or without pigmentation (208, 211–213).

Ocular findings have been identified in many children who have acquired VZV infection *in utero*. Such findings include microphthalmia, cataracts, chorioretinitis, and optic atrophy, among others. Early death has been reported in approximately one-third of the children with congenital VZV syndrome.

Neonatal VZV Infection

A more common problem has been maternal varicella in the immediate peripartum period which produces chickenpox in the immediate postpartum period. The projected attack rate for congenital varicella is 24%, a figure similar to that for *in utero* transmission (227). The time of onset of maternal lesions appears to correlate directly with the frequency and severity of neonatal disease. When the maternal rash appeared within 5 days of delivery, approximately one-third of infants became infected. After 5 days, transmission occurred in only about 18% (227). A vesicular rash that appears in the infant between 5 and 10 days of life is associated with a mortality as high as 20%; however, the overall case-fatality rate has been calculated to be 5% (192). Death probably results from the failure of the newborn to receive transplacental antibodies that are capable of ameliorating the disease. It should be noted that herpes zoster can occur early in infancy following maternal chickenpox (206).

Diagnosis

Diagnosis of fetal VZV infection is predicated on a history of maternal varicella. Since diagnosis of varicella is usually clinical, supportive laboratory evidence is not generally required. Nevertheless, isolation of VZV in susceptible cell culture systems can substantiate the diagnosis. Tissue culture isolation of virus is discussed in Chapter 4. Monoclonal antibody staining of lesion scrapings is promising.

Treatment

Treatment of VZV infections, particularly those involving the CNS in older children and adults, is discussed in Chapter 4. In general, the unique problems associated with perinatal VZV infection warrant separate consideration. Evaluation of therapeutic modalities must focus on two distinct clinical circumstances: maternal and congenital variable syndromes. For cases of maternal varicella in which pneumonitis has appeared, the utilization of acyclovir is becoming more routinely accepted, in spite of the lack of substantiating control data to indicate the efficacy of such an approach. In large part, the deployment of acyclovir under such circumstances has been predicated on both (a) the evidence indicating increased mortality in women who suffer such a disease and (b) the recognition that this drug is a useful therapeutic of VZV disease in other circumstances. Whether therapy of maternal varicella prevents transmission to the fetus *in utero* is unknown at this time.

Treatment of the newborn with evidence of congenital varicella syndrome appears to be of little clinical value. Evidence of active VZV replication at the time of birth is usually not present; therefore, the practical utility of administering an antiviral drug under such circumstances remains questionable.

Practical Recommendations for Prevention

There is no proven therapy for maternal varicella, even for cases which involve life-threatening complications such as pneumonia. Zoster immune globulin and zoster immune plasma (at a total dose of 1.25 ml) have been recommended for babies born to mothers who have chickenpox (228). However, no data indicate that these products are protective or therapeutic when administered to susceptible or infected pregnant women. Nevertheless, current recommendations support intravenous immunoglobulin administration to pregnant women. Moreover, no studies have found antiviral agents to be effective in this situation. Further efforts will be directed toward evaluation of susceptible women of childbearing age in order to develop better prophylactic procedures.

EPSTEIN–BARR VIRUS

History, Infectious Agent, and Pathology and Pathogenesis

These are presented in Chapter 4.

Epidemiology of Fetal Infection

The role of Epstein–Barr virus (EBV) infection during pregnancy and its potential effects on the fetus remain controversial (229,230). A few reports have claimed that congenital infection occurs, on the basis of findings of congenital heart disease, cataracts, or multiple fetal malformations after infectious mononucleosis in the first trimester of pregnancy (231–233). However, no case was confirmed by specific immunologic or virologic methods. At least two groups of investigators have attempted to identify congenital EBV infections by testing cord-blood lymphocytes for spontaneous transformation. Only one positive result was found among 2841 newborns examined (233–236). One of these studies also examined oropharyngeal secretions from 145 infants, and it found one specimen that was positive for spontaneous transformation indicative of EBV (236). Both these infected infants were normal at birth and subsequently developed normally.

The most convincing evidence implicating EBV as a cause of congenital infection comes from two case reports. Goldberg et al. (237) described a male infant with multiple congenital anomalies whose lymphocytes were positive for the EBV nuclear antigen. Moreover, the antigen persisted in culture for 3 months, and serologic tests confirmed the infection. Joncas et al. (238) reported on a patient with multiple congenital anomalies who had simultaneous congenital EBV and CMV infections confirmed by serologic tests, spontaneous establishment of lymphoblastoid cell lines, and molecular hybridization.

Pathogenesis of Maternal Infection

Factors that influence the pathogenicity of EBV with regard to the fetus include (a) the proportion of women of childbearing age who are susceptible, (b) the risk of acquiring infection during pregnancy, and (c) the possibility that the virus may be transmitted *in utero* after primary or reactivated infection. EBV is the most prevalent herpesvirus worldwide, and women of childbearing age are almost universally seropositive. The prevalence of antibodies to EBV, which increases with age, is influenced by socioeconomic factors. In the United States, almost all women from low socioeconomic backgrounds are seropositive by age 15, whereas women from middle-to-upper socioeconomic backgrounds continue to acquire acute primary infections until they are in their twenties. Because women in the latter group generally become pregnant at an older age, delayed acquisition of infection is of little consequence (229). Prospective studies of EBV infections during pregnancy—including more than 12,000 women in France, Canada, and the United States—reported that 1.1–4.2% of women were seronegative and that only three seroconverted (229,239–241). Congenital infection could not be documented in any of the infants born to these women, including one baby with congenital heart disease (229).

EBV appears more likely to reactivate during pregnancy than at other times, excluding reactivation induced by immune suppression (230,241–244). For instance, pregnant infected women are more likely than nonpregnant infected women to have antibodies to early antigen (55% versus 22–32%) and to excrete EBV into pharyngeal secretions (29% versus 18%) (241,244). However, reactivation of latent infection does not adversely affect the fetus, since the incidence of low birth weight, congenital anomalies, and neonatal jaundice in the offspring of women who do and do not have antibodies to early antigen is similar (243).

Practical Considerations

Because of the small number of susceptible women, primary EBV infections are rare during pregnancy. Since the virus may be transmitted to the fetus *in utero*, women with a clinical and serologic diagnosis of infectious mononucleosis should be observed carefully during pregnancy. Proof of congenital infection would require confirmation of (a) seroconversion and viral excretion or (b) spontaneous transformation of peripheral-blood lymphocytes.

RUBELLA

History

Historically, rubella has been a common cause of congenital infection and subsequent developmental delays in newborns born to mother's who experience infection early in gestation. Rubella (German measles) is characterized as a benign clinical illness occurring in young children or susceptible young adults. Characteristics of the clinical illness include fever, lymphadenopathy, and a morbilliform rash. Rubella, per se, is of little interest as a cause of CNS infections. However, rubella is one prototype for intrauterine infection, causing fetal morbidity when susceptible women acquire infection early in gestation. The potential for a chronic progressive encephalitis syndrome, as a consequence of early acquisition of rubella, can also occur. Fortunately, United States public health policy has led to the control of rubella and, more specifically, the congenital rubella syndrome. This section will review both (a) the consequences of rubella for the developing brain and (b) its subsequent prevention by mass immunization programs. Particular emphasis will be placed on progressive rubella infections of the CNS. For a more complete discussion of rubella, the reader is referred to ref. 245.

The clinical syndrome of rubella has been recognized since the early 1800s (246). It was originally called "Rotheln" by the German physicians de Bergan and Arlow. Subsequently, Veale (247) changed the name to "rubella." However, because of the continued interest by German physicians, the disease also became known as "German measles." Importantly, it was only during the middle of the 20th century, in 1941, that Dr. Norman Gregg (248) associated an epidemic of morbilliform rash, characteristic of rubella, with the appearance of cataracts in newborn children. In spite of significant skepticism, Gregg was able to confirm this association and expand the spectrum to include other congenital malformations which followed maternal rubella, as did other investigators around the world (249–253). Isolation of rubella from adults in cell culture systems was achieved in the early 1960s by Weller and Neva (254). Their initial report was subsequently followed by those from other investigators at the Walter Reed Army Institute (255) who utilized a "replication" interference technique. By the mid-1960s, worldwide epidemics of rubella peaked in the United States (256–258). In a short period of time, over 12,000,000 cases of rubella had occurred which resulted in approximately 30,000 stillbirths and 20,000 deformed infants (258). This epidemic occurrence of rubella provided the opportunity to clarify the spectrum of the congenital rubella syndrome (CRS) to include the findings of cataracts, bone lesions, heart disease, deafness, mental retardation, encephalopathy, and pneumonitis, in addition to the overt clinical findings of petechia and associated thrombocytopenia. The appearance of such a devastating disease led to the rapid development of an efficacious vaccine to prevent rubella. Vaccine rapidly became available, namely by 1969, for disease prevention (257). Utilization of this vaccine has changed the epidemiology of rubella worldwide; nevertheless, sporadic outbreaks do occur in susceptible individuals (257,259–264). A few cases of congenital rubella are reported yearly in the United States.

Infectious Agent

Rubella virus is the only member of the *Rubivirus* genus of the Togaviridae family (265). By electron-microscopic evaluation, the virus is 60–80 nm in diameter and has an electron-dense core of approximately 30 nm in diameter (266–279). The virus is composed of single-strand RNA with a molecular weight of 3×10^6 daltons (266). The RNA codes for approximately 20 virus-specific proteins (266,271–274). Surrounding the nucleocapsid, there is a single-layered envelope which contains the glycoproteins of the virus (272,275–278). It has been noted that the spikes from the envelope contain a hemagglutinin antigen (279–282).

The viral envelope contains lipids essential for infectivity (245,283–285); however, it should be remembered that naked RNA is infectious. Compounds that denature protein, alter nucleic acids (detergents), or extract lipids will all inactivate rubella virus (285). Initially, it was learned that the virus contains three distinct polypeptides, two of which are located on the viral envelope (271–281,286–288). Subsequently, however, additional polypeptides, up to 12, have been identified in rubella-infected cells. Two envelope glycoproteins have been identified as E1 and E2. Similar glycoproteins can be found in other members of the Togaviridae family. These glycoproteins project from the envelope approximately 6–8 nm. The E1 glycoprotein has a molecular weight of approximately 58,000–62,000 (for reviews see refs. 245, 272, 277, and 281). The E1 glycoprotein appears important for virus attachment to the surface of red blood cells and in initiation of viral infection (282,289,290). On the other hand, the glycoprotein E2 has a molecular weight of 42,000–54,000 (277,291). The function of E2 is not entirely clear, but it may account for strain-specific differences and for some degree of infectivity (291).

The role of the E1 glycoprotein in seroepidemiologic studies should be stressed. Antibodies directed to the E1 glycoprotein will inhibit hemagglutination and neutralize at least one epitope (279,281,289,292). This observation provides the basis for the hemagglutination-inhibition test. It should be noted that there exist a variety of other antigens for rubella virus which are useful in serologic evaluations. Among the more important antigens are those which are utilized in complement fixation (292–294), passive hemagglutination (295–297), and radioimmunoassay (298–300), among others. The utilization of these antigens in different serologic assays is well described in three excellent reviews (245,270, 301,302).

Rubella virus is capable of growing in a variety of cell culture lines of both human and animal origin (269,270,303). Peak viral replication occurs within 72 hr after the initiation of viral replication (303). Chronic infection without apparent cytopathology is characteristic of the replication of rubella in most cell systems (269,270). In fact, this observation has led to the replication interference assay by superinfection with alternative viruses, thereby allowing for the identification of rubella in cell culture systems. When interference is utilized as a mechanism of detection of rubella virus in cell systems, monkey kidney cells are usually infected and then subsequently challenged with an enterovirus challenge (269,270).

Pathology and Pathogenesis

The resulting pathology of rubella infection in the population at large is a function of the pathogenesis. Pathogenic considerations for this virus must be evaluated from two perspectives: (i) postnatal acquisition and (ii) maternal–fetal transmission.

Pathogenesis of Postnatal Infection

Rubella replicates in the oropharynx. Oropharyngeal replication provides a site for transmission, most likely by respiratory secretions (304,305). Primary replication of virus begins in nasopharyngeal epithelial cells and, perhaps, in local lymphoid tissue. Figure 11 illustrates the natural history of rubella virus infection in humans. Viral replication commences well prior to the appearance of clinical illness and is associated with viremia. Retrieval of virus can be accomplished from the numerous sites, including blood, urine, nasopharyngeal secretions, stool, tear film, synovial fluid, uterus, cervix, and lymph nodes (304–308). In general, evidence of excretion of virus from the nasopharynx begins approximately 1 week prior to the onset of clinical illness and can continue for as long as 21 days after the appearance of rash (305,309). The resulting clinical findings usually involve minimal constitutional symptoms (310). Common clinical findings include low-grade fever, postauricular lymphadenopathy, and a morbilliform rash. In older patient populations, exaggeration of clinical symptomatology can include headache, malaise, and anorexia as well as, occasionally, conjunctivitis (306,307,310). The cutaneous manifestations—lymphadenopathy and fever—have been reported by many investigators (305–307,309–313).

Adults and adolescents suffering from primary rubella infection rarely develop complications of infections; however, unique findings have been reported. These include arthritis, thrombocytopenic purpura, and, rarely, encephalitis (307,311–319). The component of arthritis has been reported to occur in up to 50% of infected adults, generally involving the proximal interphalangeal and metacarpophalangeal joints (320,321). Rubella arthritis is a self-limiting disease which does not recur. Its pathogenesis is not entirely understood.

In adults, meningoencephalitis has been reported fol-

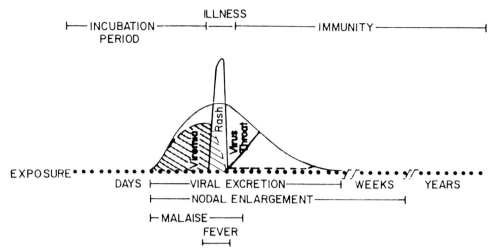

FIG. 11. Relationships between virus excretion, clinical findings, and antibody response in postnatally acquired rubella. (From ref. 301, with permission.)

lowing natural rubella. The occurrence of such a clinical syndrome is reported in approximately one in 4000 (0.03%) to one in 6000 (0.02%) adults with infection (322–326). Pathogenesis of rubella-associated infections of the CNS is unclear. The clinical manifestations of encephalitis are those that would be anticipated from other forms of encephalitis—including fever, convulsions, altered levels of consciousness, an abnormal CSF formula, and electroencephalographic findings of generalized dysrhythmia (326). Long-term follow-up of these individuals has not been well documented.

Maternal–Fetal Transmission

The pathogenesis of rubella infection in the population at large, especially young children, can be applied to susceptible women of childbearing age who are pregnant. The fetus of the pregnant woman who suffers rubella virus infection during the first trimester of gestation is at high risk for *in utero* infection. Figure 12 summarizes the pathogenesis of fetal disease. Because rubella is a systemic infection, viremia is a consistent finding of disease (308,314,327,328). This viremic phase contrib-

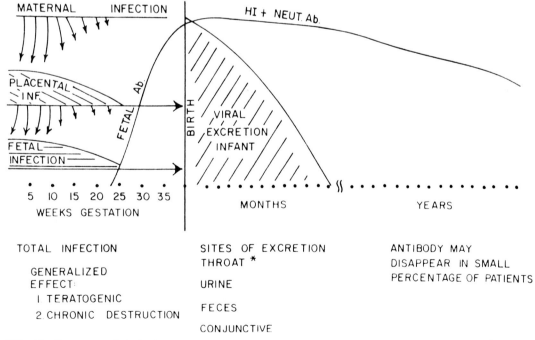

FIG. 12. Summary of virologic and serological parameters of congenitally acquired rubella. INF, infection; HI + NEUT. Ab., hemagglutination-inhibiting and neutralizing antibodies. *Common site of virus retrieval. (From ref. 301, with permission.)

utes to placental infection (329). Maternal illness with documented viremia can be either clinical or subclinical (330,331). Maternal placental infection occurs during this period of maternal viremia, whether symptomatic or not (332–334). The placenta, then, provides a source for continued release of virus to the fetus *in utero*. Histopathology of placental infection indicates scattered foci of inflammation and sometimes shows evidence of necrosis and fragmentation of endothelial cells at villus capillaries (331,335).

The mechanism by which rubella virus causes disruption of fetal growth and development is unknown at the present time. Certainly, infection during the first trimester, a time of rapid cellular differentiation, is associated with the greatest damage to the developing embryo. Whether the rubella has a direct effect on chromosomal aberrations or is a consequence of damage to vascular endothelium and subsequent blood flow to critical organs remains hypothetical at the present time.

Epidemiology

Rubella is worldwide in distribution and has a seasonal epidemicity. Rubella occurs in late winter and early spring months in temperate climates, with the number of cases reported beginning to rise in January and peaking during March, April, and May (245,336). Cycling of the virus is required in order to maintain persistence within communities (337). Characteristics of rubella epidemics were defined in the United States by outbreaks between the years 1928 and 1978 (245,338,339). Periods of increased incidence appear to occur at 6- to 9-year intervals, with major epidemics occurring at intervals of 10–30 years (245,337,339,340). The last major epidemic in the United States occurred in 1964, when nearly a half million cases were reported. Subsequent outbreaks, however, have been prevented by the introduction of a live rubella vaccine in 1969. Causes of the epidemiologic patterns of the occurrence of rubella have been the subject of considerable attention over the years; however, no clear-cut explanations exist (245,337,341). Recurrence of disease in the community is dependent upon attack rates and susceptibility of individuals at large. Factors which contribute to transmission of infection include closed populations where infection can be transmitted from one individual to another or, historically, from a congenitally infected infant (337,342–345).

Acquisition of infection is characterized by occurrence early in life. Peak years of acquisition of infection from natural infection are between the ages of 5 and 14 years (337,346). By the age of 14, following natural infection, 60% of individuals will have antibodies to rubella virus (345,347). By the time of adulthood, seroprevalence is generally in the vicinity of 85%. Notably, approximately 15% of the population remains seronegative for rubella virus (347–350). Even with current vaccine deployment, seroprevalence rates only approach 90–95%. In certain tropical areas, susceptibility to rubella infection is significantly greater than that in developed countries. Thus, a greater number of women during childbearing years are at risk for rubella infection (349,350).

The control of the rubella virus infection is mediated by humoral antibody. Several excellent reviews and primary research studies have discussed host immune response (245,301,302). Host immune response is essential for the clearance of rubella virus, particularly because of the associated viremic phases. The observation of a decrease in viremia in association with the appearance of antibody was an important recognition for vaccine development.

Congenital Rubella

Clinical Findings

The original descriptions of the congenital rubella syndrome, as described by Sir Norman Gregg, included congenital cataracts, heart defects, and low birth weight among 78 infants (248,249). The true spectrum of the congenital rubella syndrome—namely that of chronic viral infection—includes, in addition to the above, thrombocytopenia, purpura, hepatosplenomegaly, bone lesions, and pneumonitis. The incidence of congenital rubella syndrome varies between epidemic and endemic periods. During nonepidemic periods the approximate incidence is four to eight cases per 10,000 women (351); however, during the 1964 epidemic, the incidence increased to 200 cases per 10,000 women (352). More recently, the number of cases of congenital rubella has decreased significantly. Now, only approximately five per year have been reported. The largest number of cases reported recently came from an outbreak in Chicago in 1968 (353).

As it relates to chronic infection of the CNS or neurologic impairment, the most common findings for children with congenital rubella include ocular defects (reported in 50–90% of children) and evidence of mental retardation (varying between 24% and 40%) (332,353–357). In addition, cardiac defects have been reported at a frequency ranging between 37% and 74%, with frequency of hearing loss ranging between 68% and 76%. It should be noted that the range of disease in the newborn is extremely variable (301). Numerous reviews have summarized these findings (245,301,302). It should be emphasized that many of these defects are progressive as a consequence of chronic and persistent viral replication. Those defects of the CNS include encephalitis, retinopathy, cataracts, and hearing defects (either peripheral or central). Microcephaly and brain calcifications are uncommon findings in these children. An extensive review of the neurologic defects of congenital rubella has been provided by Desmond et al. (358,359) and by numerous other investigators (354–356,360–366).

The CSF findings following congenital rubella with neurologic involvement are similar to those of other CNS viral infections. Namely, one will find a CSF formula of increased protein and lymphocytosis. Virus can be isolated from the CSF in approximately 25% of cases (358). It should be noted that there have been patients who have developed what appears to be a progressive rubella encephalitis syndrome occurring much later in life (367,368).

Diagnosis

The diagnosis of congenital rubella is predicated on both (a) the proper epidemiologic identification of an outbreak of rubella in the community and (b) the classic clinical findings of rubella in the newborn. It should be remembered that babies born with the congenital rubella syndrome will appear during the late fall, since maternal infection would occur in late winter and early spring. Confirmation of diagnosis is achieved either by isolation of virus in cell culture systems or by appropriate sensitive and specific serologic assays. Viral isolation has been described on numerous occasions from throat swabs, urine, and conjunctiva (369,370). Excellent reviews describe the isolation of virus in appropriate cell culture systems (245,269,270,301,302).

In the absence of a diagnostic virology laboratory for isolation of virus, serologic assays will help confirm the infection. For diagnosis of the infection in the newborn, elevated serum IgM can be detected in most infants (370–376). Rubella-specific IgM antibody is one useful diagnostic assay (375). The utilization of differential hemagglutination versus complement-fixation assays can be employed for identifying acute infection, as discussed in several reviews (245).

Prevention

Therapy of symptomatic and congenital rubella syndrome has not been satisfactorily achieved. However, the hallmark for the management of congenital rubella is its prevention by live, attenuated vaccine. Clearly, the goal of the vaccination program is to protect the unborn fetus (377,378). The history of vaccine development for rubella has been striking. Following the isolation of virus in 1962, research attempts began immediately to develop a safe and effective vaccine. In 1966, investigators succeeded (several times) in passing rubella in monkey kidney cells, which led to the development of a vaccine identified as "high passage virus 77" or HPV_{77} (379). In order to avoid exposure of the virus to potential contaminants in tissues of monkey organ, alternative approaches included final passages in either duck embryo or dog kidney cells. These vaccines were identified as $HPV_{77}DE$ or $HPV_{77}DK$, respectively (380). An additional attenuated rubella virus vaccine is the Seddenhill vaccine, which was licensed in 1969 (381). Finally, the fourth and most active live vaccine, licensed in 1978 and the only currently available vaccine in the United States, is that identified as RA-27, which can be given subcutaneously (382). This virus was passaged in human diploid fibroblasts.

Notably, all of the vaccine viruses have the capability of infecting the human fetus *in utero* (383–386). However, they are significantly less virulent than wild-type infections. No cases of congenital rubella syndrome have been identified as a consequence of exposure to rubella virus *in utero*, particularly after exposure to RA-27/3 (387). Nevertheless, vaccination of women who are pregnant is not recommended. Termination of gestation, however, is not recommended following inadvertent rubella vaccination. It is suggested that vaccine recipients do not become pregnant for a period of 3 months following immunization (259,383). It should be noted that the intensity of immunity following vaccination is lower with the HPV and Ceddenhill vaccine strains than with RA-27/3 (387–395).

The concept of mass or herd immunity to rubella has been challenged in many circles (396,397). However, the success of the United States immunization program for the prevention of congenital rubella syndrome speaks for itself. It is unlikely that alternative approaches such as those used historically in England whereby vaccine was only given to postpartum females will occur again in the future.

Approximately 10–15% of vaccine recipients will develop reactions. Clearly, the younger the child, the less likely symptoms are to occur, although clinical illness suggestive of a mild case of rubella has been reported (398–403). Severe reactions usually occur in adults and are associated with arthritis (398,403–407). It has been suggested that peripheral neuropathy can occur after rubella immunization, but infrequently (405,408). None of these reactions should be of significant concern to be a contraindication for vaccine deployment.

Future Directions

Rubella virus infections provide a model for prevention of disease. Utilization of rubella vaccine has significantly decreased the occurrence of congenital rubella syndrome. Nevertheless, cases do occur worldwide and warrant identification. It is hoped that vaccine programs in other countries will prevent this occurrence.

ACKNOWLEDGMENTS

Original studies performed by the investigators were supported by grants from the following sources: the

National Institute of Allergy and Infectious Diseases (NO1-AI-62554); the Program Project (PO1 AI24009); the National Institute of Child Health and Human Development (HD10699); the Division of Research Resources (RR0023) of the National Institutes of Health; and the State of Alabama.

REFERENCES

1. Smith MC, Lennette EH, Reames HR. Isolation of the virus of herpes simplex and the demonstration of intranuclear inclusions in a case of acute encephalitis. *Am J Pathol* 1971;17:538.
2. Zuelzer WW, Wolf W, Stulbery CS. Herpes simplex virus as the cause of fulminating visceral disease and hepatitis in infancy. *Am J Dis Child* 1952;83:421–439.
3. Meyer MH Jr, Johnson RT, Crawford IP, Dascomb HE, Rogers NG. Central nervous system syndromes of "viral" etiology. *Am J Med* 1960;29:334–347.
4. Singer DB. Pathology of neonatal herpes simplex virus infections. In: Rosenberg HS, Bernstein J, eds. *Perspectives in pediatric pathology,* vol 6. New York: Masson, 1981;243–278.
5. Singer DB. Pathology of neonatal herpes simplex virus infection. *Perspect Pediatr Pathol* 1981;6:243.
6. McDougal RA, Beamer PR, Hellerstein S. Fatal herpes simplex hepatitis in a newborn infant. *Am J Clin Pathol* 1954;24:1250.
7. Whitley RJ. Herpes simplex virus infections of the central nervous system in children. *Semin Neurol* 1982;2:87–96.
8. Baldwin S, Benefield M, Whitley RJ. Intrauterine HSV infection. *J Teratol* 1989;39:1–10.
9. Florman AL, Gershon AA, Blackett PR, Nahmias AJ. Intrauterine infection with herpes simplex virus: resultant congenital malformations. *JAMA* 1973;225:129.
10. Hutto C, Arvin A, Jacobs R, Steele R, Stagno S, Lyrene R, Willett L, Powell D, Andersen R, Werthammer J, Ratcliff G, Nahmias A, Christy C, Whitley R. Intrauterine herpes simplex virus infections. *J Pediatr* 1987;110:97.
11. South MA, Tompkins WA, Morris CR, Rawls WE. Congenital malformation of the central nervous system associated with genital type (type 2) herpesvirus. *J Pediatr* 1969;75:8.
12. Nahmias AJ, Josey WE, Naib ZM, Freeman MG, Fernandex RJ, Wheeler JH. Perinatal risk associated with maternal genital herpes simplex virus infection. *Am J Obstet Gynecol* 1971;110:825.
13. Whitley RJ. Herpes simplex virus infections. In: Remington JS, Klein JD, eds. *Infectious diseases of the fetus and newborn infant,* 3rd ed. Philadelphia: WB Saunders, 1990;282–305.
14. Stagno S, Whitley RJ. Herpesvirus infections of pregnancy. *N Engl J Med* 1985;313:1270.
15. Dunkle LM, Schmidt RR, O'Connor DM. Neonatal herpes simplex infection possibly acquired via maternal breast milk. *Pediatrics* 1979;63:150.
16. Kibrick S. Herpes simplex virus in breast milk. *Pediatrics* 1979;64:390.
17. Sullivan-Bolyai JZ, Fife KH, Jacobs RF, Miller Z, Corey L. Disseminated neonatal herpes simplex virus type 1 from a maternal breast lesion. *Pediatrics* 1983;71:455.
18. Yeager AS, Ashley RL, Corey L. Transmission of herpes simplex virus from the father to neonate. *J Pediatr* 1983;103:905.
19. Douglas JM, Schmidt O, Corey L. Acquisition of neonatal HSV-1 infection from a paternal source contact. *J Pediatr* 1983;103:908.
20. Linnemann CC, Light IJ, Buchman TG, Ballard JL. Transmission of herpes simplex virus type 1 in a nursery for the newborn: identification of viral isolates by DNA "fingerprinting". *Lancet* 1978;1:964.
21. Light IJ. Postnatal acquisition of herpes simplex virus by the newborn infant: a review of the literature. *Pediatrics* 1979;63:480.
22. Hammerberg O, Watts J, Chernesky M, Luchsinger I, Rawls W. An outbreak of herpes simplex virus type 1 in an intensive care nursery. *Pediatr Infect Dis* 1983;2:290.
23. Nahmias AJ, Keyserling HL, Kerrick CM. Herpes simplex. In: Remington JS, Klein JO, eds. *Infectious diseases of the fetus and newborn infant.* Philadelphia: WB Saunders, 1983;636–678.
24. Whitley RJ, Corey L, Arvin A, Lakeman FD, Sumaya CV, Wright PF, Dunkle LM, Steele RW, Soong SJ, Nahmias AJ, Alford CA Jr, and the NIAID Collaborative Antiviral Study Group. Changing presentation of neonatal herpes simplex virus infection. *J Infect Dis* 1988;158:109–116.
25. Corey L. The diagnosis and treatment of genital herpes. *JAMA* 1982;248:1041.
26. Corey L, Adams HG, Brown ZA, Holmes KK. Genital herpes simplex virus infections: clinical manifestations, course and complications. *Ann Intern Med* 1983;98:958.
27. Prober CG, Sullender WM, Yasukawa LL, Au DS, Yeager AS, Arvin A. Low risk of herpes simplex virus infections in neonates exposed to the virus at the time of vaginal delivery to mothers with recurrent genital herpes simplex virus infections. *N Engl J Med* 1987;316:240–244.
28. Yeager AS, Arvin AM, Urbani LJ, Kemp JA. Relationship of antibody in outcome in neonatal herpes simplex virus infections. *Infect Immun* 1980;29:532–538.
29. Kaye EM, Dooling EC. Neonatal herpes simplex meningoencephalitis associated with fetal monitor scalp electrodes. *Neurology* 1981;31:1045–1055.
30. Parvey LS, Chien LT. Neonatal herpes simplex virus infection introduced by fetal monitor scalp electrode. *Pediatrics* 1980;65:1150–1153.
31. Kohl S, West MS, Prober CG, Sullender WM, Loo LS, Arvin AM. Neonatal antibody-dependent cellular cytoxic antibody levels are associated with the clinical presentation of neonatal herpes simplex virus infection. *J Infect Dis* 1989;160:770–776.
32. Kohl S. Herpes simplex virus immunology: problems, progress and promises. *J Infect Dis* 1985;152:435–550.
33. Whitley RJ, Hutto C. Neonatal herpes simplex virus infections. *Pediatr Rev* 1985;7:119–126.
34. Flewett TH, Parker RGF, Philip WM. Acute hepatitis due to herpes simplex virus in an adult. *J Clin Pathol* 1969;22:60–66.
35. Anderson JM, Nicholls MWN. Herpes encephalitis in pregnancy. *Br Med J* 1972;1(1):632.
36. Goyette RE, Donowho EM Jr, Hieger LR, Plunkett GD. Fulminant herpesvirus hominis hepatitis during pregnancy. *Obstet Gynecol* 1974;43:151–160.
37. Young EJ, Killam AP, Greene JF Jr. Disseminated herpesvirus infection: associated with primary genital herpes in pregnancy. *JAMA* 1976;235:2731–2733.
38. Thong YH, Steele RW, Vincent MM, Hensen SA, Bellanti JA. Impaired in vitro cell-mediated immunity to rubella virus during pregnancy. *N Engl J Med* 1973;289:604–606.
39. Petrucco OM, Seamark RF, Homes K, Forbes IJ, Symons RG. Changes in lymphocyte function during pregnancy. *Br J Obstet Gynaecol* 1976;83:245–250.
40. Grossman JH III, Wallen WC, Sever JL. Management of genital herpes simplex virus infection during pregnancy. *Obstet Gynecol* 1981;58:1–4.
41. Harger JH, Pazin GJ, Armstrong JA, Breinig MC, Ho M. Characteristics and management of pregnancy in women with genital herpes simplex virus infection. *Am J Obstet Gynecol* 1983;145:784–791.
42. Brown Z, Vontver L, Bendetti J, Critchlow C, Sells C, Berry S, Corey L. Effects on infants of first episode of genital herpes during pregnancy. *N Engl J Med* 1987;317:1246–1251.
43. Vontver LA, Hickok DE, Brown Z, Reid L, Corey L. Recurrent genital herpes simplex virus infections in pregnancy: infant outcome and frequency of asymptomatic recurrences. *Am J Obstet Gynecol* 1982;143:75–84.
44. Tejani N, Klein SW, Kaplan M. Subclinical herpes simplex genitalis infections in the perinatal period. *Am J Obstet Gynecol* 1978;135:547.
45. Bolognese RJ, Corson SL, Fuccillo DA, Traub R, Moder F, Sever JL. Herpesvirus hominis type II infections in asymptomatic pregnant women. *Obstet Gynecol* 1976;48:507–510.
46. Rattray MC, Corey L, Reeves WC, Vontver LA, Holmes KK. Recurrent genital herpes among women: symptomatic v. asymptomatic viral shedding. *Br J Vener Dis* 1978;54:262–265.
47. Adams HG, Benson EA, Alexander ER, Vontver LA, Remington MA, Holmes KK. Genital herpetic infection in men and women: clinical course and effect of topical application of adenine arabinoside. *J Infect Dis* 1976;133(Suppl):A151–A156.
48. Guinan ME, MacCalman J, Kern ER, Overall JC Jr, Spruance

SL. The course of untreated recurrent genital herpes simplex infection in 27 women. *N Engl J Med* 1981;304:759–763.

49. Jeanson S, Molin L. Genital herpesvirus hominis infection: a venereal disease? *Lancet* 1970;1:1064–1065.

50. Arvin AM, Hensleigh PA, Prober CG, Au DS, Yasukawa LL, Wittek AE, Palumbo PE, Paryani SG, Yeager AS. Failure to antipartum maternal cultures to predict the infant's risk of exposure to herpes simplex virus at delivery. *N Engl J Med* 1986;315:796–800.

51. Whitley RJ, Nahmias AJ, Visintine AM, Fleming CL, Alford CA. The natural history of herpes simplex virus infection of mother and newborn. *Pediatrics* 1980;66:489–494.

52. Yeager AS, Arvin AM. Reasons for the absence of a history of recurrent genital infections in mothers of neonates infected with herpes simplex virus. *Pediatrics* 1984;73:188–193.

53. Allen WP, Rapp F. Concept review of genital herpes vaccines. *J Infect Dis* 1982;145:413–421.

54. Corey L, Spear PG. Infections with herpes simplex viruses (second of two parts). *N Engl J Med* 1986;314:749–757.

55. Arvin AM, Yeager AS, Bruhn FW, Grossman M. Neonatal herpes simplex infection in the absence of mucocutaneous lesions. *J Pediatr* 1982;100:715.

56. Mizrahi EM, Tharp BR. A unique electroencephalogram pattern in neonatal herpes simplex virus encephalitis. *Neurology* 1981;31:164.

57. Whitley RJ, Nahmias J, Soong SJ, et al. Vidarabine therapy of neonatal herpes simplex virus infection. *Pediatrics* 1980;66:495.

58. Gutman LT, Wilfert CM, Eppes S. Herpes simplex virus encephalitis in children: analysis of cerebrospinal fluid and progressive neurodevelopmental deterioration. *J Infect Dis* 1986;154:415.

59. Musci SE, Fine EM, Togo Y. Zoster-like disease in the newborn due to herpes simplex virus. *N Engl J Med* 1971;284:24.

60. Nahmias A, Visitine A, Caldwell A, Wilson C. Eye infections. *Surv Ophthalmol* 1976;21:100.

61. Nahmias A, Hagler W. Ocular manifestations of herpes simplex in the newborn. *Int Ophthalmol Clin* 1972;12:191.

62. Reested P, Hansen B. Chorioretinitis of the newborn with herpes simplex type 1: report of a case. *Acta Ophthalmol* 1979;57:1096.

63. Cibis A, Burde RM. Herpes simplex virus induced congenital cataracts. *Arch Ophthalmol* 1971;85:220.

64. Corey L. Laboratory diagnosis of herpes simplex virus infections. Principles guiding the development of rapid diagnostic tests. *Diagn Microbiol Infect Dis* 1986;4:1115–1193.

65. Schneweis KE, Nahmias AJ. On the stability of three strains of herpes simplex virus at low temperatures. *Z Hyg Infektionskr* 1961;183:556.

66. Boehm FH, Estes W, Wright PE, Growdon JF Jr. Management of genital herpes simplex virus infection occurring during pregnancy. *Am J Obstet Gynecol* 1980;141:735.

67. Nahmias AJ, Roizman B. Infection with herpes simplex viruses 1 and 2. *N Engl J Med* 1973;289:667, 719, 781.

68. Lafferty WE, Krofft S, Remington M, Giddings R, Winter C, Cent A, Corey L. Diagnosis of herpes simplex virus by direct immunofluorescence and viral isolation from samples of external genital lesions in a high-prevalence population. *J Clin Microbiol* 1987;25:323.

69. Cleveland PH, Richman DD. Enzyme immunofiltration staining assay for immediate diagnosis of herpes simplex virus and varicella-zoster virus directly from clinical specimens. *J Clin Microbiol* 1987;25:416–420.

70. Lee FK, Nahmias AJ, Nahmias DG, McDougal JS. Demonstration of virus particles within immune complexes by electron microscopy. *J Virol Methods* 1983;7:167.

71. Rowley A, Lakeman F, Whitley R, Wolinsky S. Diagnosis of herpes simplex encephalitis by DNA amplification of cerebrospinal fluid cells. *Lancet* 1990;335:440–441.

72. Hardy DA, Arvin AM, Yasukawa LL, Bronzam RN, Lewinsohn DM, Hensleigh PA, Prober CG. Use of polymerase chain reaction for successful identification of asymptomatic genital infection with herpes simplex virus in pregnant women at delivery. *J Infect Dis* 1990;162:1031–1035.

73. Stone KM, Brooks CA, Guinan ME, Alexander ER. National surveillance for neonatal herpes simplex virus infection. *Sex Transm Dis* (in press).

74. Johnson RE, Nahmias AJ, Madger LS, Lee FK, Brooks CA, Snowden CB. A seroepidemiologic survey of the prevalence of herpes simplex virus type 2 infection in the United States. *N Engl J Med* 1989;321:7–12.

75. Nahmias AJ, Lee FK, Beckman-Nahmias S. Sero-epidemiological and sociological patterns of herpes simplex virus infection in the world. *Scand J Infect Dis [Suppl]* 1990;69:19–36.

76. Straus SE, Rooney JF, Sever JL. Herpes simplex virus infection: biology, treatment and prevention. *Ann Intern Med* 1985;103:404–419.

77. Roizman B, Jenkins FJ. Genetic engineering of novel genomes of large DNA viruses. *Science* 1985;229:1208.

78. Meignier B, Norvild B, Thuring C, Warren J, Frenkel N, Nahmias AJ, Rapp F, Roizman B. Failure to induce cervical cancer in mice by long-term frequent vaginal exposure to live or inactivated herpes simplex viruses. *Int J Cancer* 1986;38:389–394.

79. Yehiely F, Thuning C, Meignier B, Norvild B, Warren J, Nahmias AJ, Rapp F, Roizman B, Frenkel N. Analyses of transplanted murine tumors for HSV DNA sequences. *Int J Cancer* 1986;38:395–403.

80. Whitley RJ, Meignier B. Vaccines against herpes simplex infections. In: Woodrow GC, Levine MM, eds. *New generation vaccines.* New York: Marcel Dekker, 1990;825–854.

81. Meignier B, Longnecker R, Roizman B. *In vivo* behavior of genetically engineered herpes simplex virus R7017 and R7020. Construction and evaluation in rodents. *J Infect Dis* 1988;158:602–614.

82. Meignier B, Martin B, Whitley R, Roizman B. *In vivo* behavior of genetically engineered herpes simplex viruses R7017 and R7020 II. Studies in immunocompetent and immunosuppressed owl monkeys (*Aotes trivirgatus*). *J Infect Dis* 1990;162:313–321.

83. South MA, Rawls WE. Treatment of neonatal herpesvirus infection. *J Pediatr* 1970;76:497–498.

84. Whitley RJ. Neonatal herpes simplex virus infection of the central nervous system. *Am J Med* 1988;85:61–67.

85. Whitley RJ, Arvin A, Corey L, Powell D, Plotkin S, Starr S, Alford CA, Connor J, Nahmias AJ, Soong SJ, and the NIAID Collaborative Antiviral Study Group. Vidarabine versus acyclovir therapy of neonatal herpes simplex virus infection. *Proceedings of the Society of Pediatric Research*, Washington, DC, 1986; Abstract 887.

86. Whitley RJ, Yeager A, Kartus P, Bryson Y, Connor JD, Nahmias AJ, Soong SJ, and the NIAID Collaborative Antiviral Study Group. Neonatal herpes simplex virus infection: follow-up evaluation of vidarabine therapy. *Pediatrics* 1983;72:778–785.

87. Ribbert H. Uber protozoenartigen Zellen in der Nireeines syphilitischen Neugeboren und in der Parotis von Kindren. *Zentralbl Allg Pathol* 1904;15:945.

88. Smith MG. Propagation in tissue cultures of a cytopathogenic virus from human salivary gland virus (SGV) disease. *Proc Soc Exp Biol Med* 1956;92:424.

89. Rowe WP, Hartley JW, Waterman S, Turner HC, Huebner RS. Cytopathogenic agent resembling salivary gland virus recovered from tissue cultures of human adenoids. *Proc Soc Exp Biol Med* 1956;92:418.

90. Weller TH, MacCauley JC, Craig JM, Wirth P. Isolation of intranuclear inclusion-producing agents from infants with illness resembling cytomegalic inclusion disease. *Proc Soc Exp Biol Med* 1957;94:4.

91. Weller TH, Hansaw JB, Scott DE. Serologic differentiation of viruses responsible for cytomegalic inclusion disease. *Virology* 1960;12:130.

92. Stagno S, Pass RF, Dworsky ME, Alford CA. Congenital and perinatal cytomegalovirus infections. *Semin Perinatol* 1983;7:31–42.

93. Stagno S, et al. Primary cytomegalovirus infection in pregnancy: incidence, transmission to fetus and clinical outcome. *JAMA* 1986;256:1904.

94. Ahlford K, Invarsson S-A, Harris S, et al. Congenital cytomegalovirus infection and disease in Sweden and the relative importance of primary and secondary maternal infections: preliminary findings from a prospective study. *Scand J Infect Dis* 1984;16:129–137.

95. Rutter D, Griffieths P, Trompeter RS. Cytomegalic inclusion disease after recurrent maternal infection. *Lancet* 1985;2:1182.

96. Stagno S, Pass RF, Dworksy ME, Britt WJ, Alford CA. Congeni-

tal and perinatal cytomegalovirus infections: clinical characteristics and pathogenic factors. In: Plotkin SA, Michelson S, Pagno JS, Rapp F, eds. *CMV: pathogenesis and prevention of human infection. Birth defects. Original article series*, vol 20. New York: Alan R Liss, 1984;65–85.

97. Griffiths PD, Baboonian C. A prospective study of primary cytomegalovirus infection during pregnancy: final report. *Br J Obstet Gynecol* 1984;91:307.

98. Huang E-S, Kilpatrick BA, Huang Y-T, Pagano JS. Detection of human cytomegalovirus and analysis of strain variation. *Yale J Biol Med* 1976;49:29–43.

99. Huang E-S, Alford CA, Reynolds DW, Stagno S, Pass RF. Molecular epidemiology of cytomegalovirus infections in women and their infants. *N Engl J Med* 1980;303:958–962.

100. Stagno S, Reynolds DW, Huany E-S, Thames SD, Smith RJ, Alford CA Jr. Congenital cytomegalovirus infection: occurrence in an immune population. *N Engl J Med* 1977;296:1254–1358.

101. Reynolds DW, Stagno S, Hosty TS, Tiller M, Alford CA Jr. Maternal cytomegalovirus excretion and perinatal infection. *N Engl J Med* 1973;289:1–5.

102. Reynolds DW, Stagno S, Herman KL, Alford CA. Antibody response to live virus vaccines in congenital and neonatal cytomegalovirus infections. *J Pediatr* 1978;92:738–742.

103. Pereira L, Stagno S, Hoffman M, Volanakis JE. Cytomegalovirus-infected cell polypeptides immune-precipitated by sera from children with congenital and perinatal infections. *Infect Immun* 1983;39:100–108.

104. Stagno S, Volanakis JE, Reynolds DW, Stroud R, Alford CA. Immune complexes in congenital and natal cytomegalovirus infections of man. *J Clin Invest* 1977;60:838–845.

105. Reynolds DW, Dean PH, Pass RF, Alford CA. Specific cell-mediated immunity in children with congenital and neonatal cytomegalovirus infection and their mothers. *J Infect Dis* 1979;140:493–499.

106. Starr SE, Tolpin MD, Friedman HM, Paucker K, Plotkin SA. Impaired cellular immunity to cytomegalovirus in congenitally infected children and their mothers. *J Infect Dis* 1979;140:500–505.

107. Gehrz RC, Marker SC, Knorr SO, Kalis JM, Balfour HH Jr. Specific cell-mediated immune defect in active cytomegalovirus infection of young children and their mothers. *Lancet* 1977;2:844–847.

108. Pass RF, Stagno S, Britt WJ, Alford CA. Specific cell-mediated immunity and the natural history of congenital infection with cytomegalovirus. *J Infect Dis* 1983;148:953–961.

109. Okabe M, Chiba S, Tamura T, Chiba Y, Nakao T. Longitudinal studies of cytomegalovirus-specific cell mediated immunity in congenitally infected infants. *Infect Immun* 1983;41:128–131.

110. Pass RF, Dworsky ME, Whitley RJ, August AM, Stagno S, Alford CA Jr. Specific lymphocyte blastogenic responses in children with cytomegalovirus and herpes simplex virus infections acquired early in infancy. *Infect Immun* 1981;34:166–170.

111. Stagno S, Whitley RJ. Herpesvirus infection in the neonate and children. In: Holmes KK, Mardh P-A, Sparling PF, Wiesner PJ, Cates W, Lemon SM, Stamm WE, eds. *Sexually transmitted diseases*, 2nd ed. New York: McGraw–Hill, 1990;863–887.

112. Weller TH. The cytomegaloviruses: ubiquitous agents with protean clinical manifestations. *N Engl J Med* 1971;285:203.

113. Gold E, Nankervis GA. Cytomegalovirus. In: Evans AS, ed. *Viral infections of humans: epidemiology and control*. New York: Elsevier, 1976;143–161.

114. Krech U, Jung M, Jung F. *Cytomegalovirus infections of man*. Basel: Karger, 1971;28.

115. Alford CA. Epidemiology of cytomegalovirus. In: Nahmian A, Dowdle W, Schinazi R, eds. *The human herpesviruses: an interdisciplinary perspective*. New York: Elsevier, 1981;159–171.

116. Numazaki Y, Yano N, Morizuka T, Takai S, Ishida N. Primary infection with human cytomegalovirus: virus isolation from healthy infants and pregnant women. *Am J Epidemiol* 1970;91:410.

117. Hayes K, Danks DM, Gibas H, Jack I. Cytomegalovirus in human milk. *N Engl J Med* 1972;287:177.

118. Lang DJ, Krummer JF. Cytomegalovirus in semen: observations in selected populations. *J Infect Dis* 1975;132:472.

119. Stagno S, Reynolds DW, Pass RF, Alford CA. Breast milk and the risk of cytomegalovirus infection. *N Engl J Med* 1980;302:1073–1076.

120. Sarov B, Naggan L, Rosenzveig R, Katz S, Haikin H, Sarov I. Prevalence of antibodies to human cytomegalovirus in urban, kibbutz, and Bedouin children in Southern Israel. *J Med Virol* 1982;10:195.

121. Pass RF, Hutto C, Ricks R, Cloud GA. Increased rate of cytomegalovirus infection among parents of children attending day-care centers. *N Engl J Med* 1986;314:1414–1418.

122. Adler SP, Wilson MS, Lawrence LT. Cytomegalovirus transmission among children attending a day care center. *Pediatr Res* 1985;19:285A.

123. Murph JR, Bale JF Jr, Perlman S, Swack NS. The prevalence of cytomegalovirus infection in a midwest day care center. *Pediatr Res* 1985;19:205A.

124. Dworsky ME, Lakeman A, Stagno S. Cytomegalovirus transmission within a family. *Pediatr Infect Dis* 1984;3:236.

125. Spector SA, Spector DH. Molecular epidemiology of cytomegalovirus infection in premature twin infants and their mother. *Pediatr Infect Dis* 1982;1:405.

126. Alford CA, Stagno S, Pass RF. Natural history of perinatal cytomegalovirus infection. In: *Perinatal infections*. Ciba Foundation Symposium. Amsterdam: Excerpta Medica, 1980;125–147.

127. Stagno S, Pass RF, Dworsky ME, et al. Congenital cytomegalovirus infection: the relative importance of primary and recurrent maternal infection. *N Engl J Med* 1982;306:945–949.

128. Nankervis GA, Kumas ML, Cox FE, Gold E. A prospective study of maternal cytomegalovirus infection and its effect on the fetus. *Am J Obstet Gynecol* 1984;149:435–440.

129. Ahlford K, Forsgren M, Ivarsson S-A, Harris S, Svanberg L. Congenital cytomegalovirus infection: on the relation between type and time of maternal infection and infant's symptoms. *Scand J Infect Dis* 1983;15:129–138.

130. Stern H, Tucker SM. Prospective study of cytomegalovirus infection in pregnancy. *Br Med Jr* 1973;2:268–270.

131. Grant S, Edmond E, Syme J. A prospective study of cytomegalovirus infection in pregnancy. I. Laboratory evidence of congenital infection following maternal primary and reactivated infection. *J Infect Dis* 1981;3:24–31.

132. Monif GRG, Egan EH II, Held B, Eitzman DV. The correlation of maternal cytomegalovirus infection during varying stages in gestation with neonatal involvement. *J Pediatr* 1972;80:17–20.

133. Preece PM, Pearl KN, Peckham CS. Congenital cytomegalovirus infection. *Arch Dis Child* 1984;59:1120–1126.

134. Stagno S, Pass RF, Dworsky ME, Alford CA Jr. Maternal cytomegalovirus infection and perinatal transmission. *Clin Obstet Gynecol* 1982;25:563–576.

135. Peckman CS, Chin KS, Coleman JC, Henderson K, Hurley R, Preece PM. Cytomegalovirus infection in pregnancy: preliminary findings from a prospective study. *Lancet* 1983;1:325–350.

136. Hunter K, Stagno S, Capps E, Smith RJ. Prenatal screening of pregnant women for infection caused by cytomegalovirus, Epstein–Barr virus, herpesvirus, rubella, and *Toxoplasma gondii*. *Am J Obstet Gynecol* 1983;145:269–273.

137. Schopfer K, Lauber E, Krech U. Congenital cytomegalovirus infection in newborn infants of mothers infected before pregnancy. *Arch Dis Child* 1978;53:536–539.

138. Griffiths PD, Baboonian C. Intra-uterine transmission of cytomegalovirus in women known to be immune before conception. *J Hyg (Camb)* 1984;92:89–95.

139. Kamada M, Komori A, Chiba S, Nakao T. A prospective study of congenital cytomegalovirus infection in Japan. *Scand J Infect Dis* 1983;15:227–232.

140. Stagno S, Brasfield DM, Brown MB, et al. Infant pneumonitis associated with cytomegalovirus, *Chlamydia, Pneumocystis*, and *Ureaplasma*: a prospective study. *Pediatrics* 1981;68:322–329.

141. Whitley RJ, Brasfield D, Reynolds DW, Stagno S, Tiller RE, Alford CA Jr. Protracted pneumonitis in young infants associated with perinatally acquired cytomegaloviral infection. *J Pediatr* 1976;80:16–22.

142. Friedman HM, Lewis MR, Nemerofsky DM, Platkin SA. Acquisition of cytomegalovirus infection among female employees at a pediatric hospital. *Pediatr Infect Dis* 1984;3:233.

143. Yeager AS. Longitudinal, serological study of cytomegalovirus

143. infections in nurses and in personnel without patient contact. *J Clin Microbiol* 1975;2:448–452.

144. Haneberg B, Bertunes E, Haukenes G. Antibodies to cytomegalovirus among personnel at a children's hospital. *Acta Pediatr Scand* 1980;69:407–409.

145. Ahlfors K, Ivarsson S-A, Johnson T, Remmarker K. Risk of cytomegalovirus infection in nurses and congenital infection in their offspring. *Acta Pediatr Scand* 1981;70:819–823.

146. Brady MT, Demmler GJ, Anderson DC. Cytomegalovirus infection in pediatric house officers: susceptibility and risk of primary infection [Abstract]. *Pediatr Res* 1985;19:179A.

147. Adler SP, Baggett J, Wilson M, Lawrence L, McVoy M. Molecular epidemiology of cytomegalovirus in a nursery: lack of evidence for nonocomial transmission. *J Pediatr* 1986;108:117–123.

148. Demmler GJ, Yow MD, Spector SA, Brady MT, Reis EE, Anderson DC, Taber LH. Nosocomial transmission of cytomegalovirus in a children's hospital [Abstract]. *Pediatr Res* 1986;20:308A.

149. Balfour CL, Balfour HH. Cytomegalovirus is not an occupational risk for nurses in renal transplant and neonatal units. *JAMA* 1986;256:1909–1914.

150. Stagno S, Pass RF, Cloud G, Britt WJ, Henderson RE, Walton PD, Veren DA, Page F, Alford CA. Primary cytomegalovirus infection in pregnancy: incidence, transmission to the fetus and clinical outcome in two populations of different socioeconomic backgrounds. *JAMA* 1986;256:1904–1908.

151. Dworsky ME, Welch K, Cassady G, Stagno S. Occupational risk for primary cytomegalovirus infection among pediatric healthcare workers. *N Engl J Med* 1983;309:950–953.

152. Hutto C, Little A, Ricks R, Lee JD, Pass RF. Isolation of cytomegalovirus from toys and hands in a day care center. *J Infect Dis* 1986;154:527.

153. Faix RG. Survival of cytomegalovirus on environmental surfaces. *J Pediatr* 1985;106:649.

154. Centers for Disease Control. Prevalence of cytomegalovirus excretion from children in five day-care centers—Alabama. *MMWR* 1985;34:49–51.

155. Adler SP. Molecular epidemiology of cytomegalovirus: evidence for viral transmission to parents from children infected at a day care center. *Pediatr Infect Dis* 1985;106:649–652.

156. Stagno S, Cloud GA. Changes in the epidemiology of cytomegalovirus. In: Lopez C, et al., eds. *Immunobiology and prophylaxis of human herpesvirus infections.* New York: Plenum Press, 1990;93–104.

157. Adler SP. Molecular epidemiology of cytomegalovirus: viral transmission among children attending a day care center, their parents, and caretakers. *J Pediatr* 1988;112:366–372.

158. Adler SP. Molecular epidemiology of cytomegalovirus: evidence for viral transmission to parents from children infected at a day care center. *Pediatr Infect Dis* 1986;5:315–318.

159. Kreel I, Zaroff LI, Canter JW, Krasna I, Baronofsky ID. A syndrome following total body prefusion. *Surg Gynecol Obstet* 1960;111:317.

160. Adler SP. Transfusion-associated cytomegalovirus infections. *Rev Infect Dis* 1983;5:977.

161. Seaman AJ, Starr A. Febrile postcardiotomy lymphocytic splenomegaly: a new entity. *Ann Surg* 1962;156:956.

162. Onorato IM, Morens DM, Martone WJ, Stansfeild SK. Epidemiology of cytomegalovirus infections: recommendations for prevention and control. *Rev Infect Dis* 1985;7:479.

163. Armstrong JA, Tarr GC, Youngblood LA, Dowling JN, Sascow AR, Lucas JP, Ho M. Cytomegalovirus infection in children undergoing open-heart surgery. *Yale J Biol Med* 1976;49:83.

164. Prince AM, Szmuness W, Millian SJ, David DS. A serologic study of cytomegalovirus infections associated with blood transfusions. *N Engl J Med* 1971;284:1125.

165. Rinaldo CR, Black PH, Hirsch MS. Interaction of cytomegalovirus with leukocytes from patients with mononucleosis due to cytomegalovirus. *J Infect Dis* 1977;136:667.

166. Stevens DP, Baker LF, Ketcham AS, Meyer HM Jr. Asymptomatic cytomegalovirus infection following blood transfusion in tumor surgery. *JAMA* 1970;211:1341.

167. Kaariainen L, Klemola E, Paloheimo J. Rise of cytomegalovirus antibodies in an infectious mononucleosis-like syndrome after transfusion. *Br Med J* 1966;1:1270.

168. Weller TH, Hanshaw JB. Virological and clinical observations on cytomegalovirus inclusion disease. *N Engl J Med* 1964;266:1233–1244.

169. Pass RF, Stagno S, Myers GJ, Alford CA. Outcome of symptomatic congenital cytomegalovirus infection: results of long-term longitudinal follow-up. *Pediatrics* 1980;66:758–782.

170. McCracken GH Jr, Shinefield HR, Cobb K, Rausen AR, Dische MR, Eichenwald HF. Congenital cytomegalic inclusion disease: a longitudinal study of 20 patients. *Am J Dis Child* 1969;117:522–539.

171. Hanshaw JB. Congenital cytomegalovirus infection: a fifteen year perspective. *J Infect Dis* 1971;123:555–561.

172. Medearis DN Jr. Observations concerning human cytomegalovirus infection and disease. *Bull Johns Hopkins Hosp* 1964;114:181–211.

173. Berenberg W, Nankervis G. Long-term follow-up of cytomegalic inclusion disease in infancy. *Pediatrics* 1970;46:403–410.

174. Williamson WD, Desmond MM, LaFevers N, Taber LH, Catlin FI, Weaver TG. Symptomatic congenital cytomegalovirus: disorders of language, learning, and hearing. *Am J Dis Child* 1982;136:902–905.

175. Kumar ML, Nankervis GA, Jacobs IB, et al. Congenital and postnatally acquired cytomegalovirus infections: long-term follow-up. *J Pediatr* 1984;104:674–679.

176. Melish ME, Hanshaw JB. Congenital cytomegalovirus infection: developmental progress of infants detected by routine screening. *Am J Dis Child* 1973;126:190–194.

177. Reynolds DW, Stagno S, Stubbs KG, et al. Inapparent congenital cytomegalovirus infection with elevated cord IgM levels: casual relationship with auditory and mental deficiency. *N Engl J Med* 1974;290:291–296.

178. Stagno S, Reynolds DW, Amos CS, et al. Auditory and visual defects resulting from symptomatic and subclinical congenital cytomegalovirus and *Toxoplasma* infection. *Pediatrics* 1977;59:669–678.

179. Saigal S, Lunyk O, Larke RPB, Chemesky MA. The outcome in children with congenital cytomegalovirus infection: a longitudinal follow-up study. *Am J Dis Child* 1982;136:896–901.

180. Kumar ML, Nankervis GA, Gold E. Inapparent congenital cytomegalovirus infection: a follow-up study. *N Engl J Med* 1973;288:1370.

181. Harris RE, Phoades ER. Varicella pneumonia complicating pregnancy: report of a case and review of the literature. *Obstet Gynecol* 1965;23:734.

182. Siegel M, Fuerst HT, Peress NS. Comparative fetal mortality in maternal virus disease: a prospective study on rubella, measles, mumps, chickenpox, and hepatitis. *N Engl J Med* 1966;274:768.

183. Paryani SG, Arvin AM. Intrauterine infection with varicella-zoster virus after maternal varicella. *N Engl J Med* 1986;314:1542.

184. Sever J, White LR. Intrauterine viral infections. *Annu Rev Med* 1968;19:471.

185. Enders G. Varicella-zoster virus infection in pregnancy. *Prog Med Virol* 1984;29:166.

186. Seigal M. Congenital malformation following chickenpox, measles, mumps, and hepatitis. *JAMA* 1973;226:1521.

187. Gelb LD. Varicella-zoster virus. In: Fields BN, Knipe DM, Chanock RM, Hirsch MS, Melnick JL, Monath TP, Roizman B, eds. *Virology,* 2nd ed. New York: Raven Press, 1990;2100–2154.

188. Grose CH. Variation on a theme by Fenner: the pathogenesis of chickenpox. *Pediatrics* 1981;698:735.

189. Grose C. Varicella-zoster virus infections: chickenpox (varicella) and shingles (zoster). In: Glaser R, Gotleib-Stematsky T, eds. *Human herpesvirus infections. Clinical aspects.* New York: Marcel Decker, 1981;85–150.

190. Whitley RJ. Varicella-zoster virus infections. In: Galasso GJ, Whitley RJ, Merigan TC, eds. *Antiviral agents and viral diseases of man.* New York: Raven Press, 1990;235–264.

191. Garcia AGP. Fetal infection in chickenpox and alastrim, with histopathologic study of the placenta. *Pediatrics* 1963;32:895.

192. Pearson HE. Parturition varicella-zoster. *Obstet Gynecol* 1964;23:21.

193. Oppenheimer EH. Congenital chickenpox with disseminated visceral lesions. *Bull Johns Hopkins Hosp* 1944;74:240.

194. Lucchesi PE, La Boccetta AC, Peale AR. Varicella neonatorum. *Am J Dis Child* 1947;73:44.

195. Steen J, Pedersen RV. Varicella in a newborn girl. *J Oslo City Hosp* 1959;9:36.

196. Elrich RM, Turner JAP, Clarke M. Neonatal varicella. *J Pediatr* 1958;53:139.

197. Fish SA. Maternal death due to disseminated varicella. *JAMA* 1960;173:978.

198. Hackel DB. Myocarditis in association with varicella. *Am J Pathol* 1953;29:369.

199. Siegel M, Fuerst HT. Low birth weight and maternal virus disease: a prospective study of rubella, measles, mumps, chickenpox, and hepatitis. *JAMA* 1966;197:680–684.

200. Brunell PA. Varicella-zoster infections in pregnancy. *JAMA* 1967;199:315–317.

201. Young NA, Gershon AA. Chickenpox, measles and mumps. In: Remington JS, Klein JO, eds. *Infectious diseases of the fetus and newborn.* Philadelphia: WB Saunders, 1983;375–427.

202. Whitley RJ. Varicella-zoster virus. In: Mandell GL, Douglas RG, Bennett JE, eds. *Principles and practices of infectious diseases,* 3rd ed. New York: Churchill Livingstone, 1990;1153–1158.

203. Benyesh-Melnick M, Stich HF, Rapp F, et al. Viruses and mammalian chromosomes. III. Effect of herpes zoster virus on human embryonal lung cultures. *Proc Soc Exp Biol Med* 1964;117:546.

204. Fox MJ, Krumpiegel ER and Teresi JL. Maternal measles, mumps, and chickenpox as a cause of congenital anomalies. *Lancet* 1948;1:746.

205. Laforet EG, Lynch CL Jr. Multiple congenital defects following maternal varicella: report of a case. *N Engl J Med* 1947;236:534–537.

206. Brunell PA, Kotchmar GS. Zoster in infancy: failure to maintain virus latency following intrauterine infection. *J Pediatr* 1981;98:71.

207. Rinvik R. Congenital varicella encephalomyelitis in surviving newborn. *Am J Dis Child* 1969;117:231.

208. McKendry JBJ, Bailey JD. Congenital varicella associated with multiple defects. *Can Med Assoc J* 1973;108:66.

209. Savage MO, Moosa A, Gordon RR. Maternal varicella infection as a cause of fetal malformations. *Lancet* 1973;1:352.

210. Fuccillo DA. Congenital varicella. *Teratology* 1977;15:329.

211. Bai PVA, John TJ. Congenital skin ulcers following varicella in late pregnancy. *J Pediatr* 1979;94:65.

212. Borzyskowski M, Harris RF, Jones RWA. The congenital varicella syndrome. *Eur J Pediatr* 1981;137:335.

213. Dietzsch H, Rabenalt P, Trlifajova J. Varicellen-Embryopathie. Kliniche und serologische Verlaufsbeobachtungen. *Kinderarztl Prax* 1980;3:139.

214. Essex-Cater A, Heggarty H. Fetal congenital varicella syndrome. *J Infect* 1983;7:77.

215. Alfonso I, Palomino JA, DeQuesada G, et al. Picture of the month: congenital varicella syndrome. *Am J Dis Child* 1984;138:603.

216. Hajdi G, Meszner Z, Nyerges G, et al. Congenital varicella syndrome. *Infection* 1986;14:177.

217. Schlotfeldt-Schafer I, Schaefer P, Llatz S, et al. Congenitales Varicellensyndrom. *Monatsschr Kinderheilkd* 1983;131:106.

218. Kotochmar G, Grose C, Brunell PA. Complete spectrum of the varicella congenital defects syndrome in 5-year-old child. *Pediatr Infect Dis* 1984;3:142.

219. Trlifajova J, Benda R, Benes C. Effect of maternal varicella-zoster virus infection on the outcome of pregnancy and the analysis of transplacental virus transmission. *Acta Virol* 1986;30:249.

220. Srabstein JC, Morris N, Larke RPB, et al. Is there a congenital varicella syndrome? *J Pediatr* 1974;84:239.

221. Dodion-Fransen J, Dekegel D, Thiry L. Congenital varicella-zoster infection related to maternal disease in early pregnancy. *Scand J Infect Dis* 1973;5:149.

222. Pettay O. Intrauterine and perinatal viral infections. *Ann Clin Res* 1979;11:258.

223. Webster MH, Smith CS. Congenital abnormalities and maternal herpes zoster. *Br Med J* 1977;4:1193.

224. Duehr PA. Herpes zoster as a cause of congenital cataract. *Am J Ophthalmol* 1955;39:157.

225. Klauber GT, Flynn FJ, Altman BD. Congenital varicella syndrome with genitourinary anomalies. *Urology* 1976;8:153.

226. Gershon AA. Chickenpox, measles and mumps. In: Remington JS, Klein JO, eds. *Infectious diseases of the fetus and newborn infant,* 3rd ed. Philadelphia: WB Saunders, 1990:395–445.

227. Meyers JD. Congenital varicella in term infants: risk reconsidered. *J Infect Dis* 1974;129:215–217.

228. *Report of the Committee on Infectious Diseases.* Elk Grove, IL: American Academy of Pediatrics, 1990.

229. Fleisher G, Bologonese R. Epstein–Barr virus infections in pregnancy: a prospective study. *J Pediatr* 1984;104:374–379.

230. Sakamoto K, Greally J, Gilfillan RF, et al. Epstein–Barr virus in normal pregnant women. *Am J Reprod Immunol* 1982;2:217–221.

231. Belfrage S, Dahlquist E. Infectious mononucleosis: age, civil state, and pregnancy—an epidemiological study. *Scand J Infect Dis* 1969;1:57–60.

232. Miller HC, Clifford SH, Smith CA, Warkany J, Wilson JL, Yannet H. Study of the relation of congenital malformations to maternal rubella and other infections: preliminary report. *Pediatrics* 1949;3:259–270.

233. Brown ZA, Stenchever MA. Infectious mononucleosis and congenital anomalies. *Am J Obstet Gynecol* 1978;131:108–109.

234. Chang RS, Blankenship W. Spontaneous *in vitro* transformation of leukocytes from a neonate. *Proc Soc Exp Biol Med* 1983;144:337–339.

235. Chang RS, Le CT. Failure to acquire Epstein–Barr virus infection after intimate exposure to the virus. *Am J Epidemiol* 1984;119:392–395.

236. Visitine AM, Gerber P, Nahmias AJ. Leukocyte transforming agent (Epstein–Barr virus) in newborn infants and older individuals. *J Pediatr* 1976;89:571–575.

237. Goldberg GN, Fulginiti VA, Ray G, et al. *In utero* Epstein–Barr virus (infectious mononucleosis) infection. *JAMA* 1981;246:1579–1581.

238. Joncas JH, Alfieri C, Leyritz-Wills M, et al. Simultaneous congenital infection with Epstein–Barr virus and cytomegalovirus. *N Engl J Med* 1981;304:1399–1403.

239. Icart J, Didier J, Dalens M, et al. Prospective study of Epstein–Barr virus (EBV) infection during pregnancy. *Biomedicine* 1981;34:160–163.

240. Le CT, Chang RS, Lipson MH. Epstein–Barr virus infections during pregnancy: a prospective study and review of the literature. *Am J Dis Child* 1973;137:466–468.

241. Gervais F, Joncas JH. Epstein–Barr virus infection: seroepidemiology in various population groups of the greater Montreal area. *Comp Immunol Microbiol Infect Dis* 1979;2:207–212.

242. Purtilo DT, Sakamoto K. Reactivation of Epstein–Barr virus in pregnant women: social factors, and immune competence as determinants of lymphoproliferative disease—a hypothesis. *Med Hypotheses* 1982;8:401–408.

243. Fleisher G, Bolognese R. Persistent Epstein–Barr virus infection and pregnancy. *J Infect Dis* 1983;147:982–986.

244. Waterson AP. Virus infection (other than rubella) during pregnancy. *Br Med J* 1979;2:564–566.

245. Wolinsky JS, Waxham MN. Rubella. In: Fields BN, Knipe DM, Chanock RM, Hirsch MS, Melnick JL, Monath TP, Roizman B, eds. *Virology,* 2nd ed. New York: Raven Press, 1990:815–840.

246. Maton WG. Some accounts of a rash liable to be mistaken for scarlatina. *Med Tr Coll Physicians (Lond)* 1815;5:149–165.

247. Veale H. History of an epidemic of Rothelm, with observations on its pathology. *Edinburgh Med J* 1866;12:404–414.

248. Gregg NM. Congenital cataract following German measles in the mother. *Trans Ophthalmol Soc Aust (BMA)* 1942;3:35–46.

249. Gregg NM, Beavis WR, Heseltine M, et al. The occurrence of congenital defects in children following maternal rubella during pregnancy. *Med J Aust* 1945;2:122–126.

250. Erickson CA. Rubella early in pregnancy causing congenital malformation of eyes and heart. *J Pediatr* 1944;25:281–283.

251. Reese AB. Congenital cataract and other anomalies following German measles in the mother. *Am J Ophthalmol* 1944;27:483–487.

252. Hughes I. Congenital defects following rubella in pregnancy. *Proc R Soc Med* 1945;39:17–18.

253. Martin SM. Congenital defects and rubella. *Br Med J* 1945;1:855.

254. Weller TH, Neva FA. Propagation in tissue culture of cytopathic agents from patients with rubella-like illness. *Proc Soc Exp Biol Med* 1962;111:215–225.

255. Parkman PD, Hopps HE, Meyer HM. Rubella virus. Isolation, characterization and laboratory diagnosis. *Am J Dis Child* 1969;118:68–77.

256. Krugman S. Rubella Symposium. *Am J Dis Child* 1965;110:345–476.

257. Krugman S. International Conference on Rubella Immunization. *Am J Dis Child* 1969;118:2–410.

258. Centers for Disease Control. Rubella Surveillance, Report No. 1, 1969.

259. Centers for Disease Control. Rubella Surveillance, January 1976 through December 1978. Issued May 1980.

260. Polk BF, White JA, DeGirolami PC, et al. An outbreak of rubella among hospital personnel. *N Engl J Med* 1980;303:541–545.

261. Centers for Disease Control. Nosocomial rubella infection—North Dakota, Alabama, Ohio. *MMWR* 1980;29:629–631.

262. Centers for Disease Control. Rubella Surveillance, July 1973 through December 1975. Issued August 1976.

263. Centers for Disease Control. Rubella outbreak in an office building—New Jersey. *MMWR* 1980;29:517–518.

264. Centers for Disease Control. Measles and rubella at a military recruit training center—Illinois. *MMWR* 1979;28:147–148.

265. Fenner F. Classification and nomenclature of viruses. *Intervirology* 1976;7:1–115.

266. Sedwick WD, Sokol F. Nucleic acid of rubella virus and its replication in hamster kidney cells. *J Virol* 1970;5:478–489.

267. Holmes IH, Work MC, Warburton MF. Is rubella an arbovirus? II. Ultrastructural morphology and development. *Virology* 1969;37:15–25.

268. Smith KO, Hobbins TE. Physical characteristics of rubella virus. *J Immunol* 1969;102:1016–1023.

269. Herrman KL. Rubella virus. In: Lennette EH, Ballows A, Hausler WJ, Truant JP, eds. *Manual of clinical microbiology*, 3rd ed. Washington, DC: American Society for Microbiology, 1980.

270. Plotkin SA. Rubella virus. In: Lennette EH, Schmidt NJ, eds. *Diagnostic procedures for viral and rickettsial infections*, 4th ed. New York: American Public Health Association, 1969.

271. Bowden DS, Westaway EG. Rubella virus: structural and non-structural proteins. *J Gen Virol* 1984;65:933–943.

272. Oker-Blom C, Kalkkinen N, Kaariainen L, Pettersson RF. Rubella virus contains one capsid protein and three envelope glycoproteins, E1, E2a and E2b. *J Virol* 1983;46:964–973.

273. Payment P, Ajdukovic D, Pavilanis V. Le virus de la rubeole. I. Morphologie et proteines structurales. *Can J Microbiol* 1975;21:703–709.

274. Vaheri A, Hovi T. Structural proteins and subunits of rubella virus. *J Virol* 1972;9:10–16.

275. von Bonsdorff CH, Vaheri A. Growth of rubella virus in BHK21 cells: electron microscopy of morphogenesis. *J Gen Virol* 1969;5:47.

276. Toivonen V, Vainionpaa R, Salmi A, Hyypia T. Glycoproteins of rubella virus: brief report. *Arch Virol* 1983;77:91–95.

277. Pettersson RF, Oker-Blom C, Kalkkinen N, et al. Molecular and antigenic characteristics and synthesis of rubella virus structural proteins. *Rev Infect Dis* 1985;7:S140–S149.

278. Dorsett PH, Miller DC, Green KY, Byrd FI. Structure and function of the rubella virus proteins. *Rev Infect Dis* 1985;7:S150.

279. Waxham MN, Wolinsky JS. Immunochemical identification of rubella virus hemagglutinin. *Virology* 1983;126:194–203.

280. Trudel M, Ravaoarinoro M, Payment P. Reconstitution of rubella hemagglutinin on liposomes. *Can J Microbiol* 1980;26:899–904.

281. Bowden DS, Westaway EG. Changes in glycosylation of rubella virus envelope proteins during maturation. *J Gen Viro* 1985;66:201–206.

282. Ho-Terry L, Cohen A. Degradation of rubella virus envelope components. *Arch Virol* 1980;65:1–13.

283. Bardeletti G, Gautheron DC. Phospholipid and cholesterol composition of rubella virus and its host cell BHK21 grown in suspension cultures. *Arch Virol* 1978;52:19.

284. Voiland A, Bardeletti G. Fatty acid composition of rubella virus and BHK21/13S infected cells. *Arch Virol* 1980;64:319.

285. Ho-Terry L, Cohen A. Rubella virus hemagglutinin: association with a single virion glycoprotein. *Arch Virol* 1985;84:207–215.

286. Bardeletti G, Kessler N, Aymard-Henry M. Morphology, bio-chemical analysis and neuraminidase activity of rubella virus. *Arch Virol* 1975;40:175.

287. Buimovici-Kein E, Vesikari T, Santangelo CF, Cooper LZ. Study of the lymphocyte *in vitro* response to rubella antigen and phyto-hemagglutinin by a whole blood method. *Arch Virol* 1976; 52:323–331.

288. Clarke DM, Loo TW, McDonald H, Gillam S. Expression of rubella virus cDNA coding for the structural proteins. *Gene* 1988;65:23–30.

289. Gerna G, Revello MG, Dovis M, et al. Synergistic neutralization of rubella virus by monoclonal antibodies to viral haemagglutinin. *J Gen Virol* 1987;68:2007–2012.

290. Ho-Terry L, Londesborough P, Cohen A. Analysis of rubella virus complement-fixing antigens by polyacrylamide gel electrophoresis. *Arch Virol* 1986;87:219–228.

291. Green KY, Dorsett PH. Rubella virus antigens: localization of epitopes involved. *J Virol* 1986;57:893–898.

292. Vesikari T. Immune response in rubella infection. *Scand J Infect Dis* [*Suppl*] 1972;4:1.

293. Schmidt NJ, Lennette EH. Rubella complement-fixing antigens derived from the fluid and cellular phases of infected BHK-21 cells: extraction of cell-associated antigen with alkaline buffers. *J Immunol* 1966;97:815.

294. Vaheri A, Vesikari T. Small size rubella virus antigens and soluble immune complexes, analysis by the platelet aggregation technique. *Arch Gesamte Virusforsch* 1971;35:10.

295. Birch CJ, Glaun BP, Hunt V, Irving LG, Gust ID. Comparison of passive haemagglutination and haemagglutination-inhibition techniques for detection of antibodies to rubella virus. *J Clin Pathol* 1979;32:128.

296. Kilgore JM. Clinical evaluation of a rubella passive hemagglutination test system. *J Med Virol* 1979;3:231.

297. Meurman OH. Antibody responses in patients with rubella infection determined by passive hemagglutination, hemagglutination inhibition, complement fixation, and solid-phase radioimmunoassay tests. *Infect Immun* 1978;19:369.

298. Meurman OH, Viljanen MK, Granfors K. Solid-phase radioimmunoassay of rubella virus immunoglobulin M antibodies: comparison with sucrose density gradient centrifugation test. *J Clin Microbiol* 1977;5:257.

299. Ogra PL, Kerr-Grant D, Umana G, Dzierba J, Weintraub D. Antibody response in serum and nasopharynx after naturally acquired and vaccine-induced infection with rubella virus. *N Engl J Med* 1971;285:1333.

300. Sugishita C, O'Shea S, Best JM, Banatvala JE. Rubella serology by solid-phase radioimmunoassay: its potential for screening programmes. *Clin Exp Immunol* 1978;31:50.

301. Arvin AM, Alford CA Jr. Chronic intrauterine and perinatal infections. In: Galasso GJ, Whitley RJ, Merigan TC, eds. *Antiviral agents and viral diseases of man*. New York: Raven Press, 1990;497–580.

302. Lamprecht CL. Rubella virus. In: Belshe RB, ed. *Textbook of human virology*. Littleton, MA: PSG Publishing Co., 1984:679–705.

303. Fabiyi A, Sever JL, Ratner N, et al. Rubella virus: growth characteristics and stability of infectious virus and complement-fixing antigen. *Proc Soc Exp Biol Med* 1966;122:392–396.

304. Sever JL, Schiff GM, Traub RG. Rubella virus. *JAMA* 1963;182:663–671.

305. Green RH, Balsamo MR, Giles JP, et al. Studies of the natural history and prevention of rubella. *Am J Dis Child* 1965;110:348–365.

306. Schiff GM, Sever JL, Huebner RJ. Experimental rubella. Clinical and laboratory findings. *Arch Intern Med* 1965;116:537–543.

307. Phillips CA, Behbehani AM, Johnson LW, et al. Isolation of rubella virus. An epidemic characterized by rash and arthritis. *JAMA* 1965;191:615–618.

308. Alford CA, Griffiths PD. Rubella. In: Remington JS, Klein JO, eds. *Infectious diseases of the fetus and newborn infant*, 2nd ed. Philadelphia: WB Saunders, 1983;69–103.

309. Cooper LZ, Krugman S. Clinical manifestations of postnatal and congenital rubella. *Arch Ophthalmol* 1967;77:434–439.

310. Finklea JF, Sandifer SH, Moore GT. Epidemic rubella at the Citadel. *Am J Epidemiol* 1968;87:367–372.

311. Krugman S, Ward R, Jacobs KG, et al. Studies on rubella immunization. I. Determination of rubella without rash. *JAMA* 1953;151:285–288.

312. Brody JA, Sever JL, McAlister R, et al. Rubella epidemic on St. Paul Island in the Pribilofs, 1963. I. Epidemiologic, clinical, and serologic findings. *JAMA* 1965;191:619–623.

313. Anderson SG. Experimental rubella in human volunteers. *J Immunol* 1949;62:29–40.

314. Krugman S, Katz SL. Rubella (German measles). In: Krugman S, Katz SL, eds. *Infectious diseases of children,* 7th ed. St. Louis: CV Mosby, 1981;315–331.

315. Hildebrandt HM, Maassab HF. Rubella synovitis in a 1-year-old patient. *N Engl J Med* 1966;274:1428.

316. Waxham MN, Wolinsky JS. Rubella virus and its effects on the central nervous system. *Neurol Clin* 1984;2:367.

317. Judelsohn RG, Wyll SA. Rubella in Bermuda. Termination of an epidemic by mass vaccination. *JAMA* 1973;123:401–406.

318. Gross PA, Portnoy B, Mathies AW, et al. A rubella outbreak among adolescent boys. *Am J Dis Child* 1970;119:326–331.

319. Landrigan PH, Stoffels MA, Anderson E, et al. Epidemic rubella in adolescent boys. Clinical features and results of vaccination. *JAMA* 1974;227:1283–1287.

320. Johnson RE, Hall AP. Rubella arthritis. Report of cases studied by latex tests. *N Engl J Med* 1958;258:743–745.

321. Kantor TG, Tanner M. Rubella arthritis and rheumatoid arthritis. *Arthritis Rheum* 1962;5:378–383.

322. Walker JM, Nahmias AJ. Neurologic sequelae of rubella infection. *Clin Pediatr* 1966;5:699–702.

323. Sherman FE, Michaels RH, Kenny FM. Acute encephalopathy (encephalitis) complicating rubella. *JAMA* 1965;192:675–681.

324. Bell WE, McCormick WF. Rubella. In: *Neurologic infections in children.* Philadelphia: WB Saunders, 1975;262–282.

325. Mitchell W, Pampiglione G. Neurological and mental complications of rubella. *Lancet* 1954;2:1250–1253.

326. Pampiglione G, Young SE, Ramsey AM. Neurological and electroencephalographic problems of the rubella epidemic of 1962. *Br Med J* 1963;2:1300–1302.

327. Cooper LZ. Rubella. A preventable cause of birth defects. In: Bergsma D, ed. *Birth defects. Original article series,* vol 4. New York: National Foundation—March of Dimes, 1978.

328. Sever JL, Brody JA, Schiff GM, McAlister R, Cutting R. Rubella epidemic on St. Paul Island in the Pribilofs, 1963. II. Clinical and laboratory findings for the intensive study populations. *JAMA* 1965;191:88.

329. Alford CA, Neva FA, Weller TH. Virologic and serologic studies on human products of conception after maternal rubella. *N Engl J Med* 1964;271:125.

330. Avery GB, Monif GG, Sever JL, et al. Rubella syndrome after inapparent maternal illness. *Am J Dis Child* 1965;110:444–446.

331. Dudgeon JA. Congenital rubella. Pathogenesis and immunology. *Am J Dis Child* 1969;118:35–44.

332. Hortsmann DM, Banatvala JE, Riodan JT, et al. Maternal rubella and the rubella syndrome in infants. Epidemiologic, clinical and virologic observations. *Am J Dis Child* 1965;110:408–415.

333. Alford CA, Neva FA, Weller TH. Virologic and serologic studies on human products of conception after maternal rubella. *N Engl J Med* 1964;271:1275–1281.

334. Kay HE, Peppercorn ME, Porterfield JS, et al. Congenital rubella infection of human embryo. *Br Med J* 1964;2:166–167.

335. Driscoll SG. Histopathology of gestational rubella. *Am J Dis Child* 1969;118:49–53.

336. Witte JJ, Karchmer AW, Case G, et al. Epidemiology of rubella. *Am J Dis Child* 1969;118:107–111.

337. Horstmann DM. Rubella: the challenge of its control. *J Infect Dis* 1971;123:640–654.

338. Preblud SR, Serdula MK, Frank JA, et al. Current status of rubella in the United States, 1969–1979. *J Infect Dis* 1980;142:776–669.

339. Hortsmann DM. Rubella. In: Evans SA, ed. *Viral infections of humans: epidemiology and control.* New York: Plenum Medical Books, 1976;409–427.

340. Hortsmann DM. Problems in measles and rubella. *DM* 1978;24:3–52.

341. Best JM, Banatvala JE. Studies on rubella virus strain variation by kinetic hemagglutination-inhibition tests. *J Gen Virol* 1970;9:215.

342. Gremillion DH, Gengler RE, Lathrop GD. Epidemic rubella in military recruits. *South Med J* 1978;71:932.

343. Hortsmann DM. Rubella and the rubella syndrome. New epidemiologic and virologic observations. *Calif Med* 1965;102:397.

344. Hortsmann DM, Liebhaber H, LeBouvier GL, Rosenberg DA, Halstead SB. Rubella. Reinfection of vaccinated and naturally immune persons exposed in an epidemic. *N Engl J Med* 1970;283:771.

345. Wilkins J, Leedom JM, Portnoy B, Salvatore MA. Reinfection with rubella virus despite live vaccine-induced immunity. *Am J Dis Child* 1969;118:275.

346. Weller TH, Alford CA Jr, Neva FA. Changing epidemiologic concepts of rubella, with particular reference to unique characteristics of the congenital infection. *Yale J Biol Med* 1965;37:455–472.

347. Sever JL, Schiff GM, Bell JA, et al. Rubella: frequency of antibody among children and adults. *Pediatrics* 1965;25:996–998.

348. Sever JL, Schiff GM, Huebner RJ. Frequency of rubella antibody among pregnant women and other human and animal populations. *Obstet Gynecol* 1964;23:153–159.

349. Dowdle WR, Ferreira W, Gomes LFD, et al. WHO collaborative study on the sero-epidemiology of rubella in Caribbean and Middle and South American populations in 1968. *Bull WHO* 1970;42:419–422.

350. Rawls WE, Melnick JL, Bradstreet CMP, et al. WHO collaborative study on the sero-epidemiology of rubella. *Bull WHO* 1967;37:79–88.

351. White LR, Sever JL, Alepa FP. Maternal and congenital rubella before 1964: frequency, clinical features, and search for isoimmune phenomena. *J Pediatr* 1969;74:198–207.

352. Sever JL, Nelson KB, Gilkeson MR. Rubella epidemic, 1964: effect on 6,000 pregnancies. *Am J Dis Child* 1965;110:395–407.

353. Lamprecht C, Schauf V, Warren D, et al. An outbreak of rubella in Chicago. *JAMA* 1981;247:1129–1133.

354. Cooper LZ, Ziring PR, Ockerse AB, et al. Rubella: clinical manifestations and management. *Am J Dis Child* 1969;118:18–29.

355. Plotkin SA, Cochran W, Lindquist JM, et al. Congenital rubella syndrome in late infancy. *JAMA* 1967;200:435–441.

356. Forrest JM, Menser MA. Congenital rubella in school children and adolescents. *Arch Dis Child* 1970;45:64–69.

357. Cooper LZ. Congenital rubella in the United States. In: Krugman S, Gershon AA, eds. *Infections of the fetus and the newborn infant.* New York: Alan R Liss, 1975;1–22.

358. Desmond MM, Wilson GS, Melnick JL, et al. Congenital rubella encephalitis. Course and early sequelae. *J Pediatr* 1967;71:311–331.

359. Desmond MM, Montgomery JR, Melnick JL, et al. Congenital rubella encephalitis. Effect on growth and early development. *Am J Dis Child* 1969;118:30–31.

360. Hardy JB. Clinical and developmental aspects of congenital rubella. *Arch Otolaryngol* 1973;98:230–236.

361. Chess S, Fernandez P, Korn S. Behavorial consequences of congenital rubella. *J Pediatr* 1978;93:699–703.

362. Desmond MM, Fisher ES, Vorderman AL, et al. The longitudinal course of congenital rubella encephalitis in nonretarded children. *J Pediatr* 1978;93:584–591.

363. Korones SB, Ainger LE, Monif GR, et al. Congenital rubella syndrome: study of 22 infants. Myocardial damage and other new clinical aspects. *Am J Dis Child* 1965;110:434–440.

364. Rudolph AJ, Yow MD, Phillips CA, et al. Transplacental rubella infection in newly born infants. *JAMA* 1965;191:843–845.

365. Peckham CS. Clinical and laboratory study of children exposed *in utero* to maternal rubella. *Arch Dis Child* 1972;47:571–577.

366. Hardy JB, McCracken GH, Gilkeson MR, et al. Adverse fetal outcome following maternal rubella after the first trimester of pregnancy. *JAMA* 1969;207:2414–2420.

367. Townsend JJ, Baringer JR, Wolinsky JS, et al. Progressive rubella panencephalitis. Late onset after congenital rubella. *N Engl J Med* 1975;292:990–993.

368. Weil ML, Itabashi HH, Cremer NE, et al. Chronic progressive panencephalitis due to rubella virus simulating subacute sclerosing panencephalitis. *N Engl J Med* 1975;292:994–998.

369. Phillips CA, Rawls WE, Melnick JE, et al. Viral studies of a congenital rubella epidemic. *Health Lab Sci* 1966;3:118–123.

370. Bellanti JA, Artenstein MS, Olson LC, et al. Congenital rubella. Clinicopathologic, virologic, and immunologic studies. *Am J Dis Child* 1965;110:464–472.

371. Michaels RH. Immunologic aspects of congenital rubella. *Pediatrics* 1969;43:339–350.

372. Cooper LZ, Krugman S. Diagnosis and management: congenital rubella. *Pediatrics* 1966;37:335–338.

373. Alford CA. Studies on antibody in congenital rubella infections. I. Physicochemical and immunologic investigations of rubella neutralizing antibody. *Am J Dis Child* 1965;110:455–463.

374. McCracken GH, Hardy JB, Chen TC, et al. Serum immunoglobulin levels in newborn infants. II. Survey of cord and follow-up sera from 123 infants with congenital rubella. *J Pediatr* 1969;74:383–392.

375. Cradock-Watson JE, Ridehalgh MK, Chantler S. Specific immunoglobulins in infants with the congenital rubella syndrome. *J Hyg Camb* 1976;76:109–123.

376. Hayes K, Dudgeon JA, Soothill JF. Humoral immunity in congenital rubella. *Clin Exp Immunol* 1967;2:653–667.

377. Parkman PD, Hopps HE. Viral vaccines and antivirals: current use and future prospects. *J Immunol* 1964;93:595–607.

378. Meyer HM, Hopps HE, Parkman PD. Appraisal and reappraisal of viral vaccines. *Adv Intern Med* 1980;25:533.

379. Meyer HM, Parkman PD, Panos TC. Attenuated rubella virus. II. Production of an experimental live-virus vaccine and clinical trials. *N Engl J Med* 1966;275:575–580.

380. Meyer HM, Parkman PD, Hobbins TE, et al. Attenuated rubella viruses. Laboratory and clinical characteristics. *Am J Dis Child* 1969;118:155–165.

381. Prinzie A, Huygelin C, Gold J, et al. Experimental live attenuated rubella virus vaccine. Clinical evaluation of Cendehill strain. *Am J Dis Child* 1969;118:172–177.

382. Plotkin SA, Farquhar JD, Katz M, et al. Attenuation of RA 27/3 rubella virus in WI-38 human diploid cells. *Am J Dis Child* 1969;118:178–185.

383. Modlin JF, Herrmann KL, Brandling-Bennett AD, Eddins DL, Hayden GF. Risk of congenital abnormality after inadvertent rubella vaccination of pregnant women. *N Engl J Med* 1976;294:972.

384. Phillips CA, Maeck JVS, Rogers WA, Savel H. Intrauterine rubella infection following immunization with rubella vaccine. *JAMA* 1970;213:624.

385. Vaheri A, Vesikari T, Oker-Blom N, et al. Transmission of attenuated rubella vaccines to the human fetus. A preliminary report. *Am J Dis Child* 1969;118:243.

386. Preblud SR, Williams NM. Fetal risk associated with rubella vaccine: implications for vaccination of susceptible women. *Obstet Gynecol* 1985;66:121.

387. Schmidt NJ, Lennette EH. Complement-fixing and fluorescent antibody responses to an attenuated rubella virus vaccine. *Am J Epidemiol* 1970;91:351.

388. Balfour HH, Groth KE, Edelman CK. RA 27/3 rubella vaccine: a four-year follow-up. *Am J Dis Child* 1980;134:350.

389. Black FL, Lamm SH, Emmons JE, Pinheiro FP. Durability of antibody titers induced by RA 27/3 rubella virus vaccine. *J Infect Dis* 1978;137:322.

390. Grillner L. Neutralizing antibodies after rubella vaccination of newly delivered women: a comparison between three vaccines. *Scand J Infect Dis* 1975;7:169.

391. Grillner L. Immunity to intranasal challenge with rubella virus two years after vaccination: comparison of three vaccines. *J Infect Dis* 1976;133:637.

392. Heigl Z, Wasserman J, Forsgren M. *In vitro* lymphocyte reactivity to rubella antigen following vaccination. *Scand J Infect Dis* 1980;12:13.

393. LeBouvier GL, Plotkin SA. Precipitin responses to rubella vaccine RA 27/3. *J Infect Dis* 1971;123:220.

394. Liebhaber H, Ingalls TH, LeBouvier GL, Horstmann DM. Vaccination with RA 27/3 rubella vaccine. *Am J Dis Child* 1972;123:133.

395. Van Rooyen CE, Ozere RL, Perlin I, Faulkner RS. A trial of rubella RA 27/3 vaccine. *Can J Public Health* 1977;68:375.

396. Fulginiti VA. Controversies in current immunization policy and practices: one physician's viewpoint. *Curr Probl Pediatr* 1976;6:3.

397. Siegel M. Unresolved issues in the first five years of the rubella immunization program. *Am J Obstet Gynecol* 1976;124:327–332.

398. Veibel RE, Stokes J, Buynak EB, et al. Influence of age on clinical response to HPV-77 duck rubella vaccine. *JAMA* 1972;222:805–807.

399. Halstead SB, Char DF, Diwan AR. Evaluation of three rubella vaccines in adult women. *JAMA* 1970;211:991–995.

400. Horstmann DM, Liebhaber H, Kohorn EI. Postpartum vaccination of rubella-susceptible women. *Lancet* 1970;2:1003–1006.

401. Fox JP, Rainey HS, Hall CE, et al. Rubella vaccine in postpubertal women. Experience in Washington State. *JAMA* 1976;236:837–843.

402. Dudgeon JA, Marshall WC, Peckham CS. Rubella vaccine trials in adults and children. Comparison of three attenuated vaccines. *Am J Dis Child* 1969;118:237–242.

403. Weibel RE, Villarejos VM, Klein EB, et al. Clinical and laboratory studies of live attenuated RA 27/3 and HPV 77-DE rubella virus vaccines. *Proc Soc Exp Biol Med* 1980;165:44–49.

404. Weibel RE, Stokes J, Buynak EB, et al. Live rubella vaccines in adults and children. *Am J Dis Child* 1969;118:226–229.

405. Cooper LZ, Ziring PR, Weiss HJ, et al. Transient arthritis after rubella vaccination. *Am J Dis Child* 1969;118:218–225.

406. Black FL, Lamm SH, Emmons JE, et al. Reactions to rubella vaccine and persistence of antibody in virgin-soil populations after vaccination and wild-virus-induced immunization. *J Infect Dis* 1976;133:393–398.

407. Monto AS, Cavallaro JJ, Whale EH. Frequency of arthralgia in women receiving one of three rubella vaccines. *Arch Intern Med* 1970;126:635–639.

408. Kilroy AW, Schaffner W, Fleet WF. Two syndromes following rubella immunization. *JAMA* 1970;214:2287–2292.

Infections of the Central Nervous System,
edited by W. M. Scheld, R. J. Whitley, and
D. T. Durack, Raven Press, Ltd., New York © 1991.

CHAPTER 10

Neurological Manifestations of Infection with the Human Immunodeficiency Viruses

Bradley K. Evans, Diane K. Donley, and John N. Whitaker

This chapter reviews and analyzes neurological abnormalities associated with infection by human immunodeficiency viruses (HIV, previously HTLV-III, HTLV-IV, LAV, and ARV). First we review virus biology; then, infection in cell culture and in humans; and, finally, the neurological manifestations of HIV infection. Other reviews of HIV biology (1–5) and HIV-associated nervous system diseases (6–9) are available.

HUMAN IMMUNODEFICIENCY VIRUSES

A retrovirus is an RNA virus that "reverse transcribes" its genome to DNA that later integrates into cell DNA. By genome structure and antigen cross-reactivity, HIV is in the retrovirus subfamily Lentiviridae (10,11). Examples of other lentiviruses ("slow viruses") are visna, equine infectious anemia, and simian immunodeficiency viruses. Lentiviruses characteristically can be latent, cause persistent infection, be sequestered in monocytes, have antigenic variation, and seek central nervous system (CNS) sanctuary, where they may cause CNS disease (12).

Virion

The HIV virion (virus particle) contains a lipid envelope, glycosylated envelope proteins, internal proteins, and two copies (diploid) of a linear, positive-stranded, polyadenylated RNA genome (Fig. 1).

The infected cell's plasma membrane provides lipid for the envelope. The lipid envelope is delicate and easily disrupted, even by soap and water, which destroys infectivity.

The mature virion contains two noncovalently bound surface glycoproteins of molecular weights 120,000 and 41,000 daltons (gp120 and gp41), formed by the cell enzyme-induced cleavage of the parent molecule, gp160 (13). At the virion's surface, three gp120–gp41 complexes aggregate to form a protruding knob, visible by electron microscopy. gp41 is a transmembrane protein, and gp120 (derived from gp160's amino terminus) is located completely outside the lipid envelope (Fig. 1). Because gp120 is not anchored in the lipid envelope and binds noncovalently to gp41, free gp120 may be released from infected cells.

Internal virion proteins include the group-specific antigens ("gag," core, or capsid proteins: p24, p17, p9, and p7) and viral-coded enzymes (reverse transcriptase, integrase, and protease). Core proteins are the products of HIV protease action upon the primary translation product, a "polyprotein" (14–17). HIV protease is an aspartyl endopeptidase, related to pepsin, renin, and cathepsin D, except that HIV protease has twofold symmetry. HIV protease also cleaves another, larger viral polyprotein [whose translation requires ribosomal frameshifting (18)] into reverse transcriptase, integrase, and protease.

Retroviruses can mutate, recombine, and have pseudotypes (Fig. 2). HIV has frequent substitution and deletion mutations because its reverse transcriptase has poor fidelity and no proofreading mechanism (19). The viral gene most often found mutated is *env* (20), which codes for gp160. Areas within gp120's coding segment, called "hypervariable regions" (21–23), mutate most fre-

B. K. Evans and J. N. Whitaker: Department of Neurology, UAB School of Medicine, Birmingham, Alabama 35294; and Department of Neurology, Birmingham Veterans Administration Hospital, Birmingham, Alabama 35294.

D. K. Donley: Department of Pediatrics, UAB School of Medicine, Birmingham, Alabama 35294; and Sparks Center for Developmental and Learning Disabilities, Birmingham, Alabama 35294.

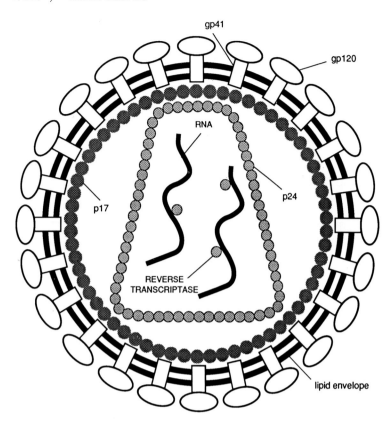

FIG. 1. Schematic diagram of the HIV virion.

quently, altering antigenic sites and causing antigenic variation (24,25). Mutations occur during HIV infection in humans (26,27). Certain mutants (e.g., noncytopathic and defective interfering types) may be important in disease pathophysiology but are not easily detectable (28). Recombination, the exchange of genetic material usually between similar nucleotide strands, is common between retroviruses. Finally, pseudotypy (a virion with the genetic material of one virus and the envelope proteins of another, possibly totally unrelated, virus) occurs (see Fig. 2).

Life Cycle

The HIV life cycle consists of the following events: binding (or attachment); fusion (or absorption); penetration; reverse transcription; nuclear transport and circularization of viral genome; integration; activation; processing; and budding (Fig. 3). Budding may not be an essential part of the life cycle, since HIV can spread by transient fusion of infected cells to neighboring cells, without budding (see Fig. 3).

gp120 binds to a normal human cell membrane protein, CD4 (cluster determinant 4) (29–33), which is the virus receptor (32,34). Next, gp41 fuses the viral lipid envelope with the cell membrane (13,35). The parent protein, gp160, cannot cause fusion. The amino terminus of gp41 is hydrophobic (36), containing a phenylalanine–X–glycine sequence (37), critical for fusion. Fusion (and therefore infection) also requires a cell surface

"fusion factor," with which gp41 interacts. Fusion is pH-independent (38,39) and happens at the plasma membrane (40). Unlike many other types of virus-induced membrane fusion, HIV fusion does not require receptor-mediated endocytosis (41). These characteristics (proteolytic cleavage required for fusion protein activation; critical hydrophobic region with Phe–X–Gly; need for a cell surface fusion factor; pH-independence; and action at the cell surface) are similar to measles-virus-induced membrane fusion (35). Because fusion happens at cell surfaces, an infected cell can fuse to adjacent cells, creating multinucleated giant cells, or syncytia (42,43). In cell culture, these giant cells die within a few days (44,45).

Inside the cell, reverse transcriptase uses a $tRNA^{Lys}$ primer (46) and Mg^{2+} to copy HIV's RNA genome into linear double-stranded DNA (47) (Fig. 4), which travels to the nucleus and circularizes. The circular, double-stranded DNA form is called an "episome." In the nuclei of HIV-infected cells, there are 10–100 episomes, compared to the 1–10 found associated with other retroviral infections. HIV episomes replicate (48,49) and may cause cytopathic effects (50). At its LTR (long terminal repeat) region, the episome inserts into cell DNA. Insertion requires viral integrase and DNA synthesis (51). The provirus (integrated viral DNA) has about 9700 base pairs, including the two LTRs, and has been sequenced (36,52–55).

Provirus expression depends upon transcription, mRNA processing, translation, and protein processing. The first step, transcription, is probably the main rate-

A

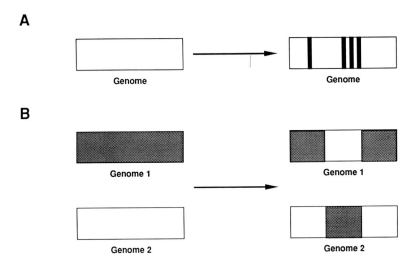

B

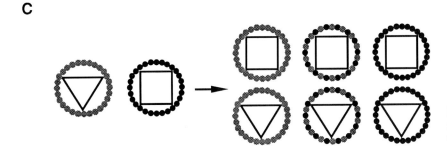

C

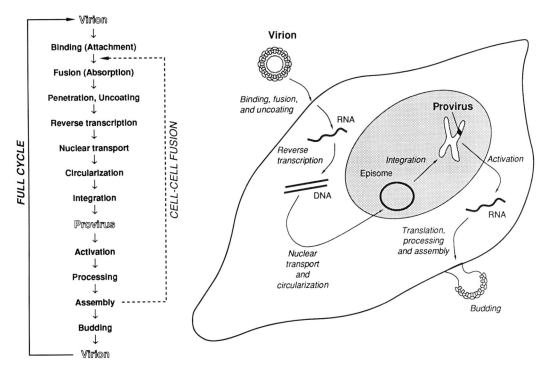

FIG. 2. Causes of retrovirus changes: (**A**) mutation, (**B**) recombination, and (**C**) pseudotypy.

FIG. 3. HIV life cycle.

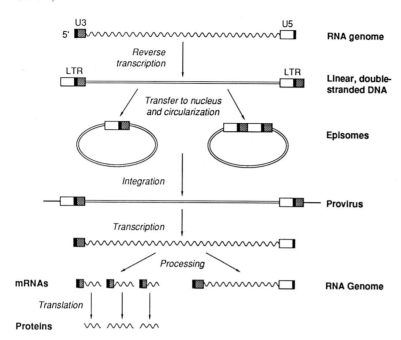

FIG. 4. HIV replication.

controlling step and is determined by HIV DNA sequences in the LTR 5′ to the viral genes (*cis*-acting regulatory elements). Provirus may be silent (latent) or actively expressing (productive). Provirus codes for regulatory proteins (tat, rev, nef, and others) (56) that affect provirus expression. Tat protein increases viral gene expression (57–60), including its own gene (positive feedback), and is necessary for provirus expression. Rev protein, also necessary for provirus expression (61), increases the proportion of full-length mRNAs coding for envelope and internal proteins (62,63). Nef, a negative regulatory protein, prevents induction, which is the transition from latent to productive infection (64,65). Not only the HIV regulatory proteins tat and rev, but also cellular factors [such as NF-κB (66–69)] and factors from other viruses [e.g., those of herpes simplex type 1, herpes zoster, adeno type 5, JC virus, and HTLV-I (70–73)], can increase provirus expression (74).

Methods of decreasing provirus expression can be developed in cell culture and may have therapeutic implications. Mutants of positive regulatory factors may block provirus activation. This has been shown for a mutant of the adenovirus-5 protein called "E1a" (75). A naturally occurring inhibitor of tat has been found by screening an expression library for proteins that bind tat (76).

CELL BIOLOGY OF HIV INFECTION (77)

Growing virus in cell culture is important in synthesizing antigens for serologic testing, screening therapeutic agents, and understanding the cellular molecular biology of infection.

HIV mainly infects cells having the CD4 cell surface protein (31,78), such as helper/inducer T lymphocytes (79), some monocytes and macrophages (80–82), Epstein–Barr virus (EBV)-transformed B lymphocytes (83), and a few other cell types (84). Normally, CD4 binds to antigen on antigen-presenting cells. This binding is important in T helper cell reactivity. CD4–gp120 binding is fairly strong ($K_d = 10^{-9}$ M) (85–87), and it interferes with CD4's antigen-recognition function (88,89). In this way, free gp120 may directly impair T helper cell function (90).

In tissue culture, agents interfering with CD4–gp120 binding prevent HIV infection. These include synthetic gp120-like peptides (91), soluble CD4 (92–97), synthetic CD4-like peptide fragments (98), and *N*-carbomethoxy-carbonyl-prolyl-phenylalanyl benzyl esters ("CBFs") (99). In addition, CD4 peptide fragments bind to infected cells having surface gp120. Toxins coupled to CD4 peptides (100–103) can be taken up by infected cells and then can kill them. These targeted toxins may be effective therapeutically; however, they can damage any cell with surface gp120, even if the cell is not infected.

HIV grows well in cultured human T cell leukemia lines, such as H9 (104). These cells are partially resistant to viral cytotoxicity and produce high-titer virus. HIV also grows in mitogen-stimulated peripheral blood leukocytes and in CD4-expressing HeLa cells. Cell types not known to have CD4 can also be infected. This may be because they express CD4 transiently or in small amounts, have fusion factor (which alone, without CD4, may be sufficient for infection), or have the Fc receptor (105), which binds to antibody-coated virus (106). In this last case, antibody–Fc-receptor binding presumably substitutes for CD4–gp120 binding in the HIV life cycle. Finally, HIV may use another virus's envelope proteins (pseudotypy) to infect cells (see above).

Virus can be latent, productive but without cytopathic effect, or cytopathic in infected cells. Cytopathic effects include altered cell function, cell-to-cell fusion, and cell death. HIV infection may change a cell's gene expression [e.g., decrease cell surface CD4 (107)] or alter cell proliferation (108). Cells with a high concentration of cell surface CD4 may die as a result of multiple virus–cell fusions (42). Syncytia formation, or cell-to-cell fusion, also kills cells (43), and there are other, presently unknown, cytotoxic mechanisms (109). Productively infected monocytes and macrophages are relatively resistant to HIV cytotoxicity (82), so these cells may be important in sequestering the virus during chronic infection. Free gp120 alone has cytopathic effects, perhaps because of its similarities to vasoactive intestinal peptide (VIP) (110) or neuroleukin (glucophosphoisomerase) (111,112), because it directly activates T cells (113), because it causes immune system attack on cells that bind it (24), or because it increases intracellular calcium (114).

TRANSMISSION AND EPIDEMIOLOGY

A detailed review of the transmission and epidemiology of HIV has been published (115). Worldwide, there are approximately 10 million HIV-infected humans. Nearly two million are in the United States. HIV spreads by sexual intercourse, inoculation of infected blood or blood products (e.g., factor VIII concentrate), and perinatal exposure (*in utero,* during delivery, or through breast milk) (116). Parent-to-child transmission due to provirus in germ cell DNA has not been reported. Persons with multiple sexual partners, intravenous drug users, recipients of blood products, persons from endemic areas such as the Caribbean and Central and West Africa, and children of HIV-infected mothers are most often infected. Living with HIV-infected persons is not a risk for infection (117,118).

HIV infection is associated with other diseases. For instance, sexually active persons may have syphilis, gonorrhea, herpes simplex, or other infections causing inflammatory genital lesions having an increased ability to transmit HIV (119,120). Many HIV-infected homosexuals also have been infected by EBV, hepatitis B, or cytomegalovirus (CMV) (121). Drug addicts may have endocarditis, polymicrobial bacteremia, or hepatitis B infection.

Although HIV is not a highly contagious virus, medical workers can become infected, mainly by needle sticks (122,123). Used needles should be discarded without resheathing (124,125). Since even "safety pins" are not always easy to close, physicians doing sensory examinations should use disposable straight pins to test pinprick

sensation or should test pain or temperature instead. For disinfection of medical equipment, the Centers for Disease Control (CDC) recommends 3% hydrogen peroxide, 0.525% sodium hypochlorite (1:10 dilution of household bleach), 70% ethanol, 70% isopropyl alcohol, or heat sterilization (125). Provided that one follows simple, practical guidelines, care of HIV-infected patients carries little or no risk for HIV transmission to healthcare workers (126,127). HIV-infected persons who are also infected with tuberculosis, herpes zoster, and CMV may transmit these organisms (126,128).

SYSTEMIC CLINICAL MANIFESTATIONS (129)

Clinical manifestations of HIV infection can be divided into early, middle, and late stages (130). Walter Reed (131) (Table 1) and University of California at San Francisco (Table 2) staging are useful.

Early Stage (Primary, Acute, Seroconversion)

One to six weeks after infection, before seroconversion, half of infected patients will have a mononucleosis-like illness with fever, night sweats, malaise, lethargy, headache, myalgias, anorexia, nausea and vomiting, diarrhea, dry cough, sore throat, and an urticarial, macular, or mixed maculopapular rash on the trunk (132–134). In addition, examination often shows conjunctivitis, palatal vesicles, pustular enanthem, nonexudative pharyngitis, tonsillar hypertrophy, and cervical, occipital, and axillary lymphadenopathy. Anti-HIV antibody tests are often negative, but serum HIV p24 antigen is usually positive (135). Later, HIV-specific immunoglobulin M (IgM) antibody is the first antibody to appear, implying that this is a primary HIV infection.

Middle Stage [Including Persistent Generalized Lymphadenopathy (PGL)]

This stage is characterized by long asymptomatic intervals. Half of patients have PGL, which is defined as enlargement of posterior and anterior cervical, submandibular, occipital, and axillary nodes, lasting more than 3 months, with no other cause found. Autoimmune diseases also occur frequently during the middle stage. Polyclonal hypergammaglobulinemia is due to T suppressor cell and EBV-infected B cell dysfunction (136). Autoreactive antibodies could be due to T suppressor and B cell dysfunction or to an immune reaction against normal cell proteins that are contained in the virion lipid envelope or matrix. Persistent, mild thrombocytopenia, due to antiplatelet antibodies (137) and HIV-infected megakaryocytes, occurs (138). Serious complications of

TABLE 1. *Walter Reed staging system for HIV disease*[a]

Stage	HIV virus or antibody	Chronic lymphadenopathy	T helper cells/mm³	Delayed hypersensitivity	Thrush	Opportunistic infections
WR0	−	−	>400	Normal	−	−
WR1	+	−	>400	Normal	−	−
WR2	+	+	>400	Normal	−	−
WR3	+	+/−	<400	Normal	−	−
WR4	+	+/−	<400	Partial	−	−
WR5	+	+/−	<400	Complete	+	−
WR6	+	+/−	<400	Complete	+	+

[a] From ref. 131.

thrombocytopenia, such as intracerebral hemorrhage, are rare. HLA-B27-positive patients may have a severe Reiter's syndrome. Cryoglobulins, rheumatoid factor, circulating immune complexes, and antineutrophil cytoplasmic antibodies may appear in serum (139,140) and persist into the late stage.

Late Stage [Acquired Immunodeficiency Syndrome (AIDS)]

AIDS diagnosis is by CDC criteria (Table 3) (141). Half of HIV-infected patients develop AIDS 5–10 years after primary infection (142,143). Some patients (e.g., children) develop AIDS earlier, and others have AIDS later, for unknown reasons. Whether all HIV-infected persons will eventually develop AIDS is not known. Patients who have a low CD4+ count (see below), low CD4:total lymphocytes ratio (see below), HIV p24 antigenemia, absent anti-p24 antibody, high serum β_2-microglobulin (part of class I MHC), high serum neopterin (a product of activated macrophages), anemia, a severe seroconversion illness, or a high plasma viral titer (see below) are most likely to develop AIDS (144–151). Median survival, before antiviral treatment was available, was about 1 year after AIDS diagnosis (152).

Clinically, patients have fevers, night sweats, fatigue, weight loss, and diarrhea. They may have adenopathy, but not as prominently as in PGL. Orofacial lesions, such as oral candidiasis, oral and perioral herpes simplex, hairy leukoplakia, Kaposi's sarcoma, non-Hodgkin's lymphoma, squamous cell carcinoma, necrotic periodontitis with purpuric gingivitis, and others, are common (153). Patients may have severe, ulcerative perirectal and genital herpes simplex infections (154, 155). *Pneumocystis carinii* and other, often unusual, lung infections are common, as are liver disease and colitis. Unusual organisms, such as *Cryptosporidium, Isospora, Microsporidia,* and CMV, are often cultured from feces. *Mycobacterium avium-intracellulare* small bowel infection is histologically similar to Whipple's disease (156,157). Adrenal insufficiency is common and, because it causes orthostatic hypotension, mimics autonomic neuropathy (158). Disseminated CMV (159), tuberculosis, histoplasmosis, and coccidioidomycosis infections, as well as treatment with ketoconazole, are particularly associated with adrenal insufficiency. Laboratory tests in AIDS patients often show anemia, leukopenia, thrombocytopenia, polyclonal hypergammaglobulinemia, hypoalbuminemia, elevated serum transaminases, skin test anergy, and disseminated CMV and *M. avium-intracellulare* infections.

TABLE 2. *University of California at San Francisco staging system for HIV disease*[a]

Stage	Clinical	T4	p24Ag	β_2-Microglobulin	Hematocrit
Acute	Mononucleosis-like illness	Normal	+	Normal	Normal
Early	Asymptomatic or persistent generalized adenopathy Aseptic meningitis Skin manifestations	>400	−	Normal	Normal
Middle	Asymptomatic or persistent generalized adenopathy Thrush, hairy leukoplakia Idiopathic thrombocytopenic purpura	200–400	+/−	Moderately high	Normal or low
Late	Opportunistic infections Malignancy Wasting Dementia	<200	+/−	High	Low

[a] From ref. 422.

TABLE 3. *CDC case definition for AIDS[a]*

Diseases diagnosed definitively, with no other causes of immunodeficiency
Candidiasis of esophagus, trachea, bronchi, or lungs
Cryptococcosis, extrapulmonary
Cryptosporidiosis, >1 month duration
CMV infection, except of liver, spleen, or lymph nodes, in patients >1 month old
HSV infection, mucocutaneous (>1 month duration) or of lungs or esophagus in patients >1 month old
Kaposi's sarcoma in patients <60 years old
Primary CNS lymphoma in patients <60 years old
Lymphoid interstitial pneumonitis or pulmonary lymphoid hyperplasia in patients <13 years old
Mycobacterium avium complex or *M. kansasii,* disseminated
Pneumocystis carinii pneumonia
Progressive multifocal leukoencephalopathy
Toxoplasmosis of the brain in patients >1 month old

Diseases diagnosed definitively, with HIV infection
Multiple or recurrent pyogenic bacterial infections in patients <13 years old
Coccidioidomycosis or histoplasmosis, disseminated
Isosporiasis, >1 month duration
Kaposi's sarcoma
Primary CNS lymphoma
Non-Hodgkin's (small, noncleaved; Burkitt, non-Burkitt, or immunoblastic sarcoma)
Mycobacterial disease other than *M. tuberculosis,* disseminated
M. tuberculosis, extrapulmonary
Salmonella septicemia, recurrent

Presumptive diagnoses with HIV infection
Candidiasis of the esophagus
Cytomegalovirus retinitis
Kaposi's sarcoma
Lymphoid interstitial pneumonitis or pulmonary lymphoid hyperplasia, patients <13 years old
Disseminated mycobacterial disease (not cultured)
Pneumocystis carinii pneumonia
Toxoplasmosis of the brain, patients >1 month old
HIV encephalopathy (ADC) or HIV wasting syndrome

[a] From ref. 141, with permission. CDC, Centers for Disease Control; AIDS, acquired immunodeficiency syndrome; CMV, cytomegalovirus; HSV, herpes simplex virus; CNS, central nervous system; HIV, human immunodeficiency virus; ADC, AIDS–dementia complex.

The hallmark of AIDS is severe immune deficiency. Although humoral immunity is severely impaired, cellular immunity is more damaged. Helper T cell function is destroyed even though 0.001–2.5% of circulating helper T cells are productively infected (1,147,148,160). There are also defects in T suppressor cell number and function, natural killer cell function, cell-mediated cytotoxicity, lymphocyte proliferative responses, and monocyte function (161). In addition to having autoreactive antibodies, serum has increased amounts of cytokines such as an unusual acid-labile α-interferon (162) and α-1 thymosin (163) that may be important in disease pathophysiology. There are impaired primary and anamnestic responses to antigens, even to T-cell-independent antigens

(164). For this reason, antibody tests have more false negatives in AIDS patients (165) and are often unreliable for diagnosis of infectious diseases.

HIV Type 2 (HIV-2)

Most infections in the United States are HIV type 1 (HIV-1). HIV-2, another lentivirus (48,49,166), can also cause AIDS (167). There have been 12 U.S. patients infected with HIV-2 (168). Most of them are West African emigrants, and three have AIDS. There is immunological cross-reactivity of HIV-1 with HIV-2; 60–90% of HIV-2-infected patients have a positive serum enzyme-linked immunosorbent assay (ELISA) for HIV-1. The Western blot, done with HIV-1 antigens, may be positive, indeterminate, or negative. Antibodies to HIV-2-specific peptides (169,170) and the polymerase chain reaction (see below) help differentiate HIV-1 from HIV-2 infections.

TESTS FOR HIV INFECTION (171)

Anti-HIV Antibody Tests (172)

These tests are designed to detect anti-HIV antibodies. The commonly used ones, ELISA and Western blot (also known as "protein blot" or "immunoblot"), use viral antigens either from purified HIV-1 grown in human cells in tissue culture or from HIV cDNA cloned in bacterial expression vectors. For ELISA, antigens bound in the wells of microtiter plates react with antibodies in serum or cerebrospinal fluid (CSF). False-positive and false-negative rates are 1–2%. False positives are often due to antibodies to human antigens, such as HLA, that are in the virion lipid envelope. Tests using antigens made from cDNA do not have this type of false positive. Positive ELISA results are checked by Western blot (WB), a more expensive and technically more difficult test. Viral proteins are separated by molecular weight on a sodium dodecyl sulfate–polyacrylamide gel, electrophoretically transferred to nitrocellulose, and reacted with serum or CSF. Procedures and interpretation of WB are not standardized. Results are negative (no bands), indeterminate, or positive. Recent criteria for a positive WB are two bands at p24, gp41, or gp120/gp160 (173). WB has about 1% false positives. The combination of positive ELISA and positive WB is only rarely a false positive; still, statistically, in an individual without risk factors, a positive ELISA and WB is frequently a false positive (174).

Viral Antigens (p24 Antigen) (171)

This test detects HIV antigens in serum or CSF. It is an enzyme immunoassay, and anti-HIV antibodies bound to wells in microtiter plates detect viral antigen, mainly p24 (175). This test is positive only when there is antigen excess. It is falsely negative if there is antibody excess. Although not yet reported, rheumatoid factor is probably capable of producing a false positive. The antigen test is useful in diagnosing early infection (since it is positive for a few weeks or months before the antibody tests become positive), in recognizing late disease, and, perhaps, as a guide to therapeutic efficacy.

Changes in Antibody and Antigen Tests During HIV Infection for Most Patients

After primary infection, anti-HIV antibodies do not appear for weeks, months, or, for a few patients, years (the "window") (176–179). p24 antigenemia is present earlier but becomes undetectable when anti-p24 antibodies appear (175). In late infection, anti-p24 antibodies often become undetectable and p24 antigens reappear (180) (Fig. 5).

Virus Culture from Lymphocytes or from Plasma (Including Plasma Viral Titer)

In these tests, one tries to grow live HIV in tissue culture, which requires special infection-control facilities. HIV grows slowly, and a positive result may require 3 or 4 weeks of culture (181). For these reasons, these tests are expensive. The patient's peripheral blood lymphocytes (from 30 ml of whole blood) or plasma are co-cultivated with mitogen-stimulated peripheral blood lymphocytes from uninfected persons (182). The cell culture supernate is tested for reverse transcriptase activity (183) (which is present with any growing retrovirus, not just HIV) or for p24 antigen. Like the serum p24 test results, virus culture may be positive before anti-HIV antibodies appear (184), but, unlike the p24 test, virus culture may be positive at any stage of illness (185). A positive plasma virus culture indicates that some provirus is activated; it also indicates that when there are circulating anti-HIV antibodies, they are not fully neutralizing (186). Virus culture has false negatives, but the percentage is not known.

Virus in plasma or in lymphocytes can be titered, or measured, using an end-point-dilution assay in which one determines the smallest dilution causing an infection of tissue culture cells. This is known as the "tissue-culture-infective dose" (TCID). Plasma viral titer measured this way correlates well with clinical stage of HIV infection and may be a useful measurement of treatment efficacy (147,148).

Polymerase Chain Reaction (PCR) (183)

PCR detects HIV provirus in peripheral blood leukocyte DNA and can be positive in seronegative HIV-infected persons (187). This test typically requires 3–5 ml of blood (188) and is expensive. Results are available in 3–4 days. HIV-specific oligonucleotides, usually from the *gag* gene, are hybridized to cell DNA, and then they are elongated by a bacterial DNA polymerase. This is repeated many times, amplifying the signal tremendously. This test theoretically detects low concentrations of HIV DNA. Sensitivity is so great that it can detect contaminating plasmids in laboratories using HIV clones. False negatives are probably rare, but therapeutic agents that inhibit the bacterial DNA polymerase might cause them if they copurify with cell DNA.

Lymphocyte Enumeration

Total CD4-positive peripheral blood lymphocytes (CD4+ cells) and CD4:CD8 and CD4:total peripheral blood lymphocyte ratios are decreased in AIDS patients (<200 cells/mm^3, 0.6, and 0.25, respectively). Decreasing values are markers for probable progression to AIDS, and increasing values may be signs of effective treatment. Other infections can cause decreased circulating CD4+ cells, so the test is not specific for HIV infection or AIDS.

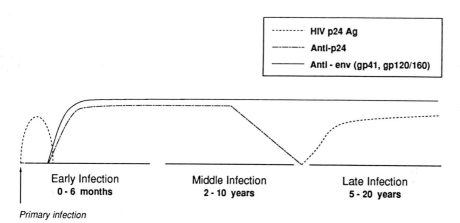

- - - - - - - HIV p24 Ag
- - - - Anti-p24
———— Anti - env (gp41, gp120/160)

Early Infection
0 - 6 months

Middle Infection
2 - 10 years

Late Infection
5 - 20 years

Primary infection

FIG. 5. Changes in antibody and antigen tests during HIV infection.

HIV-ASSOCIATED NEUROLOGICAL DISEASES

HIV and the Nervous System

HIV can infect the meninges early and persist in the CNS after the initial infection (182,189). Even so, there are usually no symptoms or signs following infection, even if one uses sophisticated neuropsychological tests (190,191). Since acute and chronic meningeal infection can be asymptomatic and HIV can infect brain even with normal CSF, CSF studies in HIV-infected patients cannot prove, or disprove, that HIV causes a particular neurological syndrome (192). HIV may enter brain by infecting nerve cells in the periphery and traveling by axonal transport to the CNS, or by direct extension through the blood–brain barrier. Since HIV does not easily infect neurons, neural spread is unlikely. HIV may pass through the blood–brain barrier either (a) through cerebral endothelial cells (either by infecting them or by passing through them in pinocytic vesicles), (b) inside infected monocytes ["Trojan horse" mechanism (193)], or (c) by infecting cells in the choroid plexus. Once in the CNS, the virus can infect brain cells. By immunohisto-chemistry (detecting HIV proteins) and *in situ* hybridization (detecting HIV RNA), the major cell types productively infected are macrophages and microglia (82,194). These cells have surface CD4 (91,195). Microglia also have Fcγ receptors (196). It is difficult to show that other cell types are not infected, since the infection may be latent or minimally productive and difficult to detect. Occasionally, endothelial cells stain for HIV antigens. Neurons and glial cells, in general, fail to show HIV antigens, except rarely in severe AIDS–dementia complex (ADC), when a few thalamic cells stain for HIV (197,198). These thalamic cells also have low levels of surface CD4 (197). In tissue culture, fetal astroglia (199) and human glioma cell lines (200) have surface CD4 and can be productively infected by some HIV isolates. Viruses isolated from CNS, compared to those from peripheral blood, are less able to infect T cells in culture, replicate better in macrophages, are less cytopathic, and have different epitopes (201).

At least 40% of all HIV-infected persons have abnormal CSF, consisting of mild lymphocytic pleocytosis (5–50 cells/mm³), increased protein (50–100 mg/dl), and normal glucose (181,182,202,203). These changes are nonspecific. Half of asymptomatic, HIV-infected patients have CSF pleocytosis or increased protein (204); in addition, 20% of CSF cultures grow HIV (202,203), often in high titer (181). Later in infection, pleocytosis tends to decrease, whereas CSF protein can increase, decrease, or be unchanged (192,205). Like peripheral blood lymphocyte ratios, the CSF CD4:CD8 ratio is low, especially late in infection (206). CSF virus titer also tends to decrease late in infection (202). These CSF changes are mild and inconsistent, and they are poor guides to disease progression and treatment efficacy.

Anti-HIV antibodies appear in CSF, often in high titer. Relative CSF and serum titers may indicate specific anti-HIV antibody synthesis within the CNS (202,207). CSF antibodies to HIV are mainly IgG, but some patients have IgA or IgM as well (208). CNS antibody synthesis is an early finding after meningeal infection (209,210). CSF oligoclonal bands also appear, are directed against HIV epitopes, and have different migration patterns compared to those in the serum (211). CSF cell counts and protein correlate poorly with anti-HIV antibody concentrations and the presence or number of oligoclonal bands (204). Patients whose CSF grows HIV usually have CSF anti-HIV antibodies and oligoclonal bands (189,202). AIDS patients, compared to asymptomatic, seropositive persons, less often have evidence for CNS synthesis of anti-HIV antibodies (202,212). CSF p24 antigen and anti-p24 antibody concentrations roughly parallel those of serum, except that the p24 antigen concentration in CSF is often much higher than that in serum (213). CSF p24 antigen concentration is highest in ADC (213), but antigen and antibody concentrations correlate poorly with clinical syndromes and are poor guides to disease progression and treatment efficacy (208,210). In HIV-infected persons, CSF has low C3 and high C4 levels (214), which may be due to changes in blood–brain barrier or to systemic conditions (214), and need not imply a pathogenic role for complement. Interleukin-2 (IL-2), β-interferon, and tumor necrosis factor α are absent from CSF of HIV-infected patients, whereas α-interferon, soluble IL-2 receptor, IL-1β, and IL-6 are frequently increased (208,215). High levels of soluble IL-2 receptor and IL-6 occur especially during opportunistic CNS infections (215), whereas high IL-1β occurs in asymptomatic, seropositive patients. There is a poor correlation between CSF cytokine levels and antibody titers (208,215). Most HIV-infected patients also have increased CSF β₂-microglobulin (205) and quinolinic acid levels (216). In one study of six HIV-infected children, there were low CSF amounts of S-adenosylmethionine, methionine, and 5-methyltetrahydrofolate, indicating impaired methylation in brain tissue (217).

Acute aseptic meningoencephalitis, ADC, and progressive encephalopathy of children are three CNS diseases that are probably a direct result of HIV infection of brain.

Acute Aseptic Meningoencephalitis

This syndrome affects 5–10% of HIV-infected patients, just before seroconversion (218) and during or after the mononucleosis-like syndrome previously described (219). Patients have headache, fever, altered mental status, and focal or generalized seizures (218). Except for a transient lower-motor-neuron facial palsy mimicking Bell's palsy, focal or lateralizing signs are uncommon. There are case reports of acute, painful myelopathy with paraparesis, normal sensation, and urinary incontinence (220) and spinal myoclonus (rhythmic abdominal contractions) (221) in early infection. CSF shows pleocytosis, slight increase in protein, and normal glucose, similar to the CSF of asymptomatic, seropositive individuals. Laboratory diagnosis of HIV infection is aided by the positive virus culture or p24 antigen in serum or CSF, or it may later be aided by seroconversion (usually 1 or 2 months later). Acute meningoencephalitis is a self-limited illness and requires symptomatic treatment only (218).

AIDS–Dementia Complex (222)

ADC—also called "HIV encephalitis," "HIV encephalopathy," "subacute encephalopathy," and other names—occurs exclusively during AIDS. It is the most common neurological disease in AIDS patients and may be the first sign of AIDS or of HIV infection (223). Early symptoms of apathy, inattention, forgetfulness, impaired concentration, mental slowing, and withdrawal are similar to those of depression. Patients may also present with acute confusion, hallucinations, or psychosis. Initially, patients usually seem normal by bedside mental status examination, but neuropsychological testing shows impaired fine and rapid motor control, diminished verbal fluency and short-term memory, impaired visual–motor and visual–spatial abilities, and deficiencies in complex problem-solving, changes that are different from those seen in depression (224). Patients have the greatest difficulties with rapid thinking and quick reactions. When dementia becomes obvious, cortical findings (such as aphasia, apraxia, and agnosia) are not prominent; for this reason, some neurologists classify ADC as a subcortical dementia, in contrast to a cortical dementia such as Alzheimer's disease. Saccadic and smooth-pursuit eye movements are often abnormal early in ADC (225). There is often an enhanced, "physiological" tremor. Patients usually have an unsteady gait that is difficult to classify as ataxic, sensory ataxic, spastic, apractic, or functional. Some patients have gait and lower-extremity neurological abnormalities associated with vacuolar myelopathy (see below). ADC may progress gradually, or stepwise with sudden deterioration, sometimes in association with a systemic illness.

ADC is a diagnosis of exclusion. Blood tests, brain imaging, and CSF studies are critical in excluding other diseases that may present as confusion, psychosis, or dementia in the AIDS patient. These diseases include not only CNS infections and tumors (see below), but also medication effects, systemic illnesses, and nutritional deficiencies. In patients with ADC, head computed tomography (CT) is normal or shows cerebral atrophy. Head magnetic resonance imaging (MRI) shows cerebral atrophy; later it shows fluffy, nonfocal white matter abnor-

malities best seen on T2-weighted images (Fig. 6). These cranial imaging abnormalities are nonspecific. Head positron emission tomography (PET) shows abnormal patterns of regional glucose metabolism. Early, there is relative thalamic and basal ganglia hypermetabolism; later, there is relative cortical and subcortical gray matter hypometabolism (226). CSF of patients with ADC may be normal or show mild pleocytosis, increased protein, and oligoclonal bands. High CSF β_2-microglobulin levels are common and correlate with ADC severity (205).

The neuropathological changes in brains of patients with ADC are unique. Almost all AIDS patients, whether symptomatic of ADC or not, show some of these changes. Grossly, there is diffuse pallor of the centrum semiovale. Microscopically, there are reactive glio-

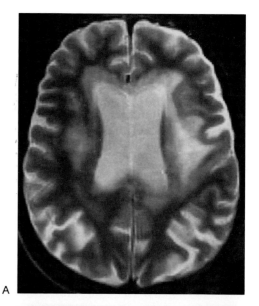

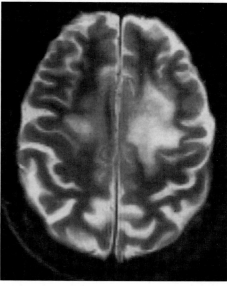

FIG. 6. A,B: T2-weighted MRI in a patient with moderate ADC, showing fluffy white matter abnormalities, slightly asymmetric in this patient. (Courtesy of Dr. Richard Price.)

sis, focal necrosis, oligodendrocytes with atypical nuclei, and demyelination. The microscopic abnormalities are worse in the cerebral white matter and subcortical gray matter (227–229). There is only mild neuronal loss. Inflammatory changes may be minor, consisting of perivascular macrophage infiltrates and microglial nodules. In severe ADC, there are multinucleated giant cells (Fig. 7) that have macrophage-type surface antigens (230) and HIV antigens (231). HIV-induced cell–cell fusion probably produces multinucleated giant cells. Almost half of patients, especially those with more severe ADC, have vacuolar myelopathy (see below). In addition to vacuolar myelopathy, the following factors also correlate with the severity of dementia: number of multinucleated cells, pallor of the centrum semiovale, and presence of HIV in brain (8,230). The neuropathological changes suggest that, with proper treatment, part or all of the syndrome may be reversible.

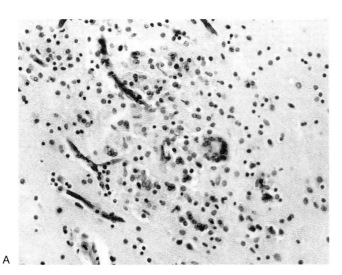

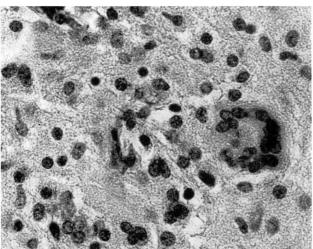

FIG. 7. Multinucleated giant cells, macrophages, and microglial nodules in white matter of a 3½-year-old boy with progressive encephalopathy. **A:** Hematoxylin and eosin, ×160. **B:** Hematoxylin and eosin, ×400. (Courtesy of Drs. Dawna Armstrong and Joel Kirkpatrick.)

The pathophysiology of ADC is poorly understood, primarily because there is no good animal model; however, there are many hypotheses. The hypotheses have to explain why ADC occurs only during late infection, why only HIV is regularly cultured from the brains of patients with ADC, and how an infection of macrophages, microglia, and multinucleated giant cells causes dementia. The first hypothesis is that HIV itself directly causes ADC. HIV infection of neurons, glia, or endothelial cells could cause dysfunction of these cells, and, consequently, ADC. Some brain cell types—for example, gliomas and fetal glia—can be infected in tissue culture (199), but if HIV does infect glia, endothelial cells, or neurons of patients with AIDS, the provirus is latent or only minimally productive, since HIV RNAs and proteins are only rarely found in these cell types at autopsy (227,229,231,232). HIV RNAs and proteins are mostly in brain macrophages, microglia, and multinucleated giant cells (194,229,233). A second hypothesis is that an HIV mutant causes ADC. In ADC, there is chronic, persistent HIV infection; during this time, HIV mutates (234). Brain isolates, compared to isolates from peripheral blood lymphocytes of the same patients, show greater ability to infect macrophages, less ability to replicate in T cells, different antigenicity, and increased ability to cause latent infection of human glioma cells in tissue culture (235). This second hypothesis does not explain how infection of macrophages and microglia causes dementia; furthermore, it predicts that patients with ADC should be capable of transmitting a virus with rapid neurotoxic effects, producing outbreaks of early, severe ADC. As yet, there is no evidence for this prediction. A third hypothesis is that infected and dying macrophages and microglia release toxins that injure neurons, glia, or endothelial cells. One neurotoxin (an "excitotoxin"), quinolinic acid (236), is increased in the CSF of patients with AIDS (216), perhaps because infected and dying macrophages increase brain endotoxin and interferon levels, both inducers of indoleamine-2,3-dioxygenase, the key enzyme of quinolinic acid synthesis (237,238). Another toxin that infected cells release is gp120. This could bind to brain cells, damaging them directly or indirectly by means of immune mechanisms. Free gp120 is neurotoxic in tissue culture (239), because of its similarities to the neurotransmitter VIP or to neuroleukin, or because it increases intracellular calcium levels (see above). There is no evidence for antibody-mediated immunopathology in ADC (240), but the CSF of patients with ADC has HIV-specific cytotoxic T cells (241) that could cause damage by cell-mediated immunity. The main problem with the quinolinic acid and gp120 neurotoxin hypotheses is that they predict neuronal death, which is not prominent in ADC. A fourth hypothesis is that there is another infectious agent, so far unidentified. This agent is activated when there is immunodeficiency. Since patients with other types of immuno-

TABLE 4. *HIV infection and CNS syndromes in children*

Diseases	Approximate percentage (clinical)
Progressive encephalopathy	50
Static encephalopathy	25
Disseminated cytomegalovirus	2–20
Primary CNS lymphoma	3
CNS toxoplasmosis	<1
Progressive multifocal leukoencephalopathy	<1
Cryptococcosis	<1

deficiency have not had ADC, if this infectious agent exists, it is intimately associated with HIV infection, much as the delta virus is associated with hepatitis B infection.

CNS Syndromes in Children (Table 4)

One-third to one-half of offspring of seropositive mothers are HIV-infected (242), but there are no clinical features of the pregnancy or newborn period differentiating infected from uninfected children (243–246). Maternal-to-child transmission causes 80% of childhood HIV infections (242).

Less than 25% of infected children have normal neurological development. One-fourth have a static encephalopathy, probably due to fetal or perinatal complications. Almost half have a progressive encephalopathy (PE) (247), clinically similar to adult ADC. Perinatally infected children may have symptoms and signs of PE from as young as 2 months old to as old as 5.5 years old,

with a mean age of onset of 18 months. The onset of the illness is usually gradual, but it may be acute. For some children, PE is the initial manifestation of HIV infection (248). Affected children have arrest or regression of intellectual and motor development. Examination shows intellectual decline, poor brain growth, and symmetric motor impairment. Early, children are inactive and apathetic; later they become demented, mute, and bedfast. Half of children with PE have acquired microcephaly (249,250). Infants initially are hypotonic and hyperreflexic, and later they develop pseudobulbar palsy and progressive spastic quadriparesis. An untreated child with PE deteriorates without improvement—either rapidly, more slowly, or stepwise. Most die within 1 year after diagnosis. As with ADC, PE is a manifestation of the late stage of HIV infection, appearing at the same time as immune deficiency. Cranial imaging in children with PE may be normal (250,251); more commonly, however, it shows diffuse brain atrophy. Head computed tomograms of children less than 5 years old may show basal ganglia and frontal white matter contrast enhancement and calcification, and these changes may be progressive (251,252) (Fig. 8). T2-weighted MRI shows increased signal intensity in the periventricular white matter (250,251). HIV-infected children usually have normal CSF cell counts, protein, and glucose. Some children with PE have mild CSF lymphocytosis (5–25 cells/mm^3) and increased protein (50–100 mg/dl). As in adults, infected children's CSF has markedly increased HIV-specific antibody titers compared to serum, suggesting antibody synthesis within the brain. Children with PE also have extremely high levels of p24 antigen in CSF (213). Serum, but not CSF, tumor necrosis factor

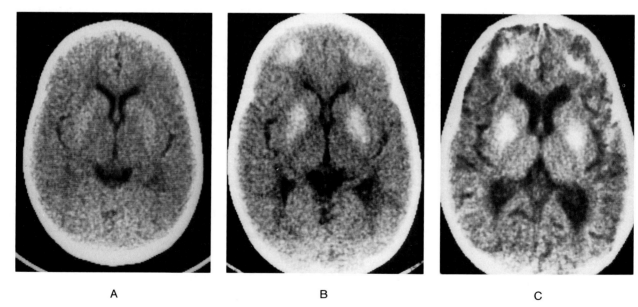

A   B   C

FIG. 8. Progressive brain calcification in a child with progressive encephalopathy (head computed tomograms without contrast). **A:** July 27, 1987. **B:** March 23, 1988. **C:** July 19, 1989. (Courtesy of Dr. Daniel Young)

(TNF) levels correlate with clinical symptoms. Three-fourths of children with PE have high serum concentrations of TNF, and 95% of HIV-infected children with increased serum TNF concentration have PE (253).

Diagnosis of HIV infection is difficult in infants. The usual anti-HIV antibody tests, ELISA and WB, are positive in both infected and uninfected babies because of transplacental transfer of IgG anti-HIV antibodies. Maternally acquired antibodies progressively decline in titer over months: 60% of uninfected children have negative antibody tests at 12 months, 80% at 15 months, and 100% at 18 months (254). Some antibody tests indicate infection, such as persistently elevated IgG antibody titers, fourfold increase in the titer of paired sera, different IgG subclasses compared to the mother, new bands on sequential WBs, and specific anti-HIV IgM or IgA antibody (neither cross the placental barrier) (243,255, 256). Unfortunately, a child can be HIV-infected and not have these antibody findings (257). A few infants have had a decline in antibody titer and signs of HIV infection (247). Tests for virus or viral material have advantages, but they also have problems. Maternal p24 antigen does not cross the placenta (258), so its presence indicates HIV infection. False-negative serum p24 tests can occur, if p24 is not in excess compared to maternally acquired antibodies. In one study, half of neonates born to infected mothers had p24-positive serum, and 80% of those positive had AIDS by age 1 year (243). The roles of virus culture and polymerase chain reaction (PCR) in early diagnosis of perinatally acquired HIV are unclear. False-negative results occur with both tests, especially in newborns and asymptomatic babies, when the amount of virus is low (259,260). Finally, approximately half of HIV-infected children have immunologic abnormalities, such as hypergammaglobulinemia and decreased circulating CD4+ cells (261,262). Presumptive diagnosis of HIV infection can be made on the basis of clinical examination and immunologic abnormalities, even if anti-HIV antibody, p24 antigen, virus culture, and PCR tests are negative.

The brains of HIV-infected children are small for age and atrophic. Microscopically, 80–90% have vascular and perivascular mineralization, most prominently in small vessels of the basal ganglia and frontal white matter (250,252). Perivascular inflammation sometimes accompanies this calcification (247,252). Other small-vessel diseases, such as fibrinoid necrosis (247) and intimal proliferation (250), occur occasionally. Despite the high frequency of blood vessel abnormalities, stroke is rare. One also finds parenchymal microglial nodules and multinucleated giant cells (especially in the basal ganglia and pons) in 75% of brains; 80% have white matter pallor and astrocytic gliosis. Loss of cerebral cortical neurons is rare (250), but their dendritic trees are abnormally shaped (263). Spinal cord involvement is common in PE. Possibly because myelin in children is different from that of adults, and myelinization is incomplete in young children, vacuolar myelopathy is rare. When reported, vacuolation affects the lateral corticospinal tracts. Two types of HIV-associated myelopathy occur in children (264): (i) a myelinopathy with poor corticospinal tract myelination but normal axons and mild cerebral white matter pallor and (ii) an axonopathy with diminished axonal numbers, poor myelination, and more severe cerebral white matter involvement. In the axonopathy type, there are prominent microglial nodules and multinucleated giant cells in the corticospinal tracts and brain. By immunohistochemistry, macrophages and giant cells stain for HIV antigens (264).

Opportunistic neurological infections occur less frequently in children with AIDS than in adults with AIDS. Disseminated CMV infection occurs in 20% (265). In contrast to adult AIDS, primary CNS lymphoma, not CNS toxoplasmosis, is the most common cause of focal and lateralizing neurological signs (266). Primary CNS lymphoma affects 3% of children with AIDS. Toxoplasmosis, cryptococcosis, and progressive multifocal leukoencephalopathy (PML) occur in <1%. CNS toxoplasmosis, when it occurs, is in older children with AIDS.

Diagnostic Approaches to CNS Diseases

About one-fifth of AIDS patients first consult a physician because of neurological symptoms (267), and 40% have neurological symptoms or signs when first diagnosed (268,269). During the course of AIDS, 70–90% have neurological symptoms or signs (270). At autopsy, 80–100% have pathological abnormalities, and half of these have more than one CNS disease (228,269,271). Although ADC is the most common CNS manifestation in AIDS patients, it is diagnosed by exclusion. Clinical features of CNS diseases in patients with AIDS are nonspecific. Diagnosis of any CNS syndrome in AIDS patients is difficult and requires a prudent, systematic approach.

CNS diseases can be divided into parenchymal diseases (having focal or lateralizing signs, abnormal cranial imaging, and definitive diagnosis by brain biopsy (272)] and meningeal diseases (focal or lateralizing signs generally limited to seizures, cranial neuropathies, and polyradiculopathies; normal cranial imaging; and diagnosis by CSF examination) (Table 5).

The common parenchymal diseases have characteristic, but not diagnostic, cranial imaging abnormalities. Toxoplasmosis, the most common parenchymal disease, causes multiple (almost never single) abscesses commonly involving the basal ganglia and having mass effect on head CT or MRI. Primary CNS lymphoma causes a single mass lesion in half of patients and multiple lesions in the other half, as detected by MRI. Lesions may be unilateral or bilateral. PML preferentially affects the

TABLE 5. *HIV infection and CNS diseases in adults*

Syndrome	Disease	Approximate percentage (clinical)	Stage
HIV-related	Acute meningitis	5–10	Early
	AIDS–dementia complex	33–67	Late
Parenchymal	CNS toxoplasmosis	3–40	Late
	Primary CNS lymphoma	2	Late
	Progressive multifocal leukoencephalopathy	2–5	Late
	Stroke	<1	Any
Either parenchymal or meningeal	Cytomegalovirus	2–20	Late
	Herpes simplex 1	?	Late
	Herpes simplex 2	?	Late
	Herpes zoster	?	Any
Meningeal	Cryptococcosis[a]	5–10	Late
	Tuberculosis[a]	2	Any
	Histoplasmosis	<1	Late
	Coccidioidomycosis	<1	Late
	Lymphoma	<1	Late
	Syphilis[a]	?	Any
	Strongyloidiasis	Case reports	Late

[a] May rarely have parenchymal manifestations.

gray–white junction and adjacent white matter. It can be single or multiple, but there is no mass effect. Other, rarer parenchymal diseases are secondary viral encephalitides, strokes, tuberculomas, fungal abscesses, bacterial brain abscesses (including those due to *Nocardia asteroides*), and metastasis from Kaposi's sarcoma, which is very rare and can cause hemorrhages.

Problems in diagnosis of parenchymal diseases arise when the patient has no focal or lateralizing findings on neurological examination and when initial cranial imaging is normal. Recognition of parenchymal disease in these cases depends upon repeating the cranial imaging studies. CSF studies are not usually valuable, except in evaluating for possible meningeal disease and for CSF myelin basic protein, which is elevated in PML and the necrotizing encephalitides (273) but normal in ADC (274,275).

Cryptococcosis is the most common cause of meningeal-type diseases in HIV-infected patients. Other causes are lymphomatous meningitis, tuberculous meningitis, syphilis, other fungal meningitides, strongyloides hyperinfection, bacterial meningitis (which is surprisingly unusual), and secondary viral meningitis. In these diseases, CSF study is critical for diagnosis. Interpretation of routine CSF tests is difficult because patients may have pleocytosis and increased protein due solely to HIV meningitis or may have a normal cell count, protein, and glucose, yet still have a meningeal infection. Diagnosis may require repeat lumbar punctures. The results of some routine CSF studies are clues that the patient has a meningeal disease that is not just HIV: CSF white cell count >100/mm^3, protein >150 mg/dl, and hypoglycorrhachia (192,276). CSF cryptococcal antigen, India ink examination, fungal culture, mycobacterial stain

and culture, and VDRL test should be done routinely. CSF anti-coccidioidomycosis antibody and cytology are also useful in certain clinical situations. Viral cultures are helpful, but, since asymptomatic patients may have positive cultures (277), virus grown from CSF may not be related to clinical disease. New tests, not yet available commercially, may be useful in recognition and diagnosis of meningeal diseases. These include (a) the CSF-soluble IL-2 receptor and IL-6 levels, which are highest in patients with opportunistic CNS infections, and (b) the new antigen tests for mycobacteria (278) and fungi.

In the following discussion of parenchymal and meningeal diseases, we emphasize manifestations and problems occurring in HIV-infected patients. Other chapters contain more complete discussions of the nature of the infectious agent, pathophysiology, diagnosis, and treatment.

Parenchymal CNS Diseases

Toxoplasmosis (279)

Toxoplasma gondii is the most common cause of a focal CNS lesion in AIDS patients. Approximately 10% of AIDS patients have CNS toxoplasmosis during the course of their illness. Most cases are due to reactivation of latent infection. Of the patients with a positive Sabin–Feldman dye test, 30% will develop CNS toxoplasmosis (280). Floridians, Haitians, Europeans, and cat owners are more likely to be seropositive. Although it is uncommon, a few patients with CNS toxoplasmosis have had negative Sabin–Feldman dye tests, so a negative test does not exclude toxoplasmosis. Diagnostic changes in titer, such as a fourfold rise in titer of paired sera, are unusual (281,282). Similarly, extracerebral involvement, such as chorioretinitis, is uncommon and unreliable in diagnosing parenchymal disease.

Brain CT or MRI is critical for diagnosis. CT commonly shows mass lesions with edema, mass effect, and contrast enhancement, often "ring enhancing" (Fig. 9). CT may be normal, although it is uncommon if one uses double-dose, delayed contrast. MRI shows multiple lesions in almost all patients. The mass lesions often involve the basal ganglia. Other diseases can show similar brain imaging abnormalities, and patients can have more than one parenchymal disease accounting for multiple lesions.

While definitive diagnosis is preferable before prescribing therapy, it is often impractical in CNS toxoplasmosis associated with HIV infection because brain biopsy has risks such as infection and hemorrhage. Diagnosis from brain biopsy specimens is difficult. Histologically, inflammation in a *Toxoplasma* abscess can mimic lymphoma. The diagnostic trophozoites (or tachyzoites), best seen by immunoperoxidase staining (283), may be hard to find. An open, rather than needle, biopsy improves the diagnostic yield, but, even with open biopsy, histology may not be definitive. Injection of brain tissue into mice or tissue culture is another way beside immunocytochemistry to diagnose toxoplasmosis.

Most patients receive a treatment trial (pyrimethamine 75–100 mg/day, sulfadiazine 1 g four times daily, and folinic acid 10 mg/day) without definitive diagnosis. Improvement, gauged by clinical and brain CT improvement, generally occurs within 10 days and is evidence that the lesions are *Toxoplasma*. Because of the mass effect of these lesions, physicians may prescribe glucocorticoids along with anti-*Toxoplasma* therapy. Gluco-

corticoids can improve many parenchymal diseases. Therefore, improvement in these cases is not evidence that the lesions are *Toxoplasma*. CNS toxoplasmosis in AIDS patients often relapses when therapy is stopped. Most patients need continual maintenance therapy.

Primary CNS Lymphoma (284,285)

Two percent of patients, during the course of AIDS, have primary CNS lymphoma. The tumor has B cell markers and is multicentric. Symptoms and signs may indicate focal or nonfocal CNS disease. Hyperventilation is common (286), and some patients have an accompanying uveocyclitis (287); these signs may be important in suspecting primary CNS lymphoma. Primary CNS lymphoma also occurs in patients immunocompromised due to causes other than AIDS. These non-AIDS patients have high anti-EBV titers and, within the tumor cells, EBV nucleic acid and proteins. In tissue culture, EBV can transform B lymphocytes. Although Koch's postulates are not fulfilled, EBV may be the cause of primary CNS lymphoma. Since EBV genome and mRNA are also present in tumor cells of patients with AIDS (288), EBV may cause primary CNS lymphoma in AIDS patients as well.

Head CT shows one or more hyper- or isodense lesions with edema, mass effect, and variable enhancement. Lesions may be unilateral or bilateral. Rarely, lesions are hypodense and do not enhance. Some lesions are "ring enhancing," mimicking toxoplasmosis. MRI is usually more sensitive than CT (Fig. 10). None of the brain imaging studies are specific. Cerebral angiography usually shows an avascular mass, although some tumors have homogeneous staining or a tumor blush. Lumbar

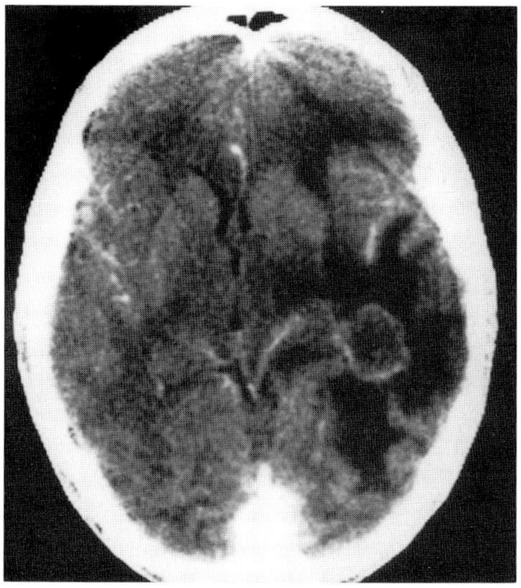

FIG. 9. Ring-enhancing lesion in a patient with AIDS and toxoplasmosis (head computed tomogram with contrast).

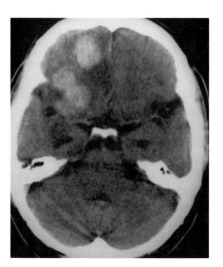

FIG. 10. Head computed tomogram, with contrast, of a patient with primary CNS lymphoma. (Courtesy of Dr. Edward Dropcho.)

puncture can be hazardous. CSF cytology shows tumor cells in only 10–25% of patients (284). Patients often have extremely high levels of CSF β_2-microglobulin, but in AIDS patients this is not specific (205). Definitive diagnosis requires brain biopsy (287). Biopsy is usually done first when there is only a single lesion seen by MRI; when there are multiple lesions, it is often delayed for an anti-*Toxoplasma* treatment trial.

Primary CNS lymphoma used to be called "reticulum cell sarcoma," "microglioma," or "perithelial sarcoma." Reticulin stains show excessive basement-membrane-like material, which is especially prominent perivascularly. Tumor cells cluster around blood vessels. AIDS-associated primary CNS lymphoma is mildly different from non-AIDS primary CNS lymphoma pathologically. AIDS-associated primary CNS lymphoma is always multicentric, always has B cell markers (never T cell), and tends to be "large cell immunoblastic" or "small cell noncleaved" (284). Non-AIDS primary CNS lymphoma sometimes is single, sometimes has T cell markers (instead of the more usual B cell markers), and is usually characterized by diffuse large or mixed cells.

Primary CNS lymphoma in AIDS shrinks markedly with steroid treatment and is radiosensitive, but median survival is still less than 2 months (284), which is worse than the 10- 18-month median survival of patients with non-AIDS primary CNS lymphoma. As yet, there is no effective chemotherapy. In contrast to other types of brain tumor, surgical decompression is harmful.

Progressive Multifocal Leukoencephalopathy

As with primary CNS lymphoma, PML can occur in patients who have abnormal immune function due to causes other than AIDS (such as in those taking glucocorticoids). Presently, 20% of PML patients have AIDS (289); however, as the number of AIDS cases increase, this percentage will rise. PML occurs in 2–5% of patients with AIDS (290,291,292). Patients commonly present with dementia or focal neurological findings (293).

Head CT shows one or more hypodense lesions without mass effect and without contrast enhancement (293). Lesions begin in the gray–white junction and subsequently involve white matter. MRI is usually more sensitive than CT (294), often showing large, multiple lesions (Fig. 11). CSF studies are unremarkable, except for an elevated myelin basic protein.

Diagnosis is made by biopsy, which shows (a) demyelination, (b) large astrocytes with bizarre, sometimes multiple, nuclei, and (c) oligodendroglia with eosinophilic intranuclear inclusions. The pathology is similar to that seen in patients with non-AIDS PML (295). JC virus, a papovavirus (296), infects glial cells, especially oligodendroglial cells (compare HIV, which infects macrophages and microglial cells). Because the abnormal as-

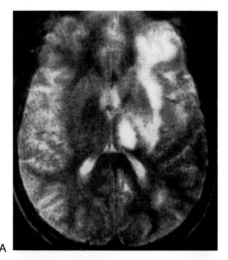

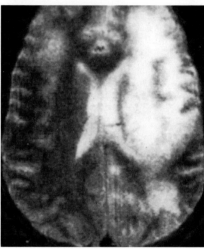

FIG. 11. A,B: T2-weighted MRI in a patient with progressive multifocal leukoencephalopathy. (Courtesy of Dr. Edward Dropcho.)

trocytes can be mistaken for a glioma and the inclusions can be mistaken for CMV, diagnosis depends upon specific detection of JC virus by immunocytochemistry. JC virus *cis*-acting regulatory elements are active in human fetal glial cells in cell culture (297), and JC virus large T antigen expression in transgenic mice causes dysmyelination (298); this suggests that JC virus probably causes PML, although it has not fulfilled Koch's postulates.

There is no good treatment. The median life expectancy is 4 months, but some AIDS patients with PML have prolonged survival (299), compared to those with non-AIDS PML.

Strokes

Hemorrhagic, thrombotic, and embolic strokes are unusual in HIV-infected patients. Hemorrhagic strokes have occurred in patients with severe thrombocytopenia [especially in hemophiliacs (228)] and in those with metastatic Kaposi's sarcoma. Thrombotic strokes have occurred in patients with angiitis. Granulomatous angiitis can occur after an attack of zoster (usually involving the head and face), but it has also occurred in HIV-infected patients who did not have zoster (300). Hepatitis B virus may also cause angiitis and strokes. A few other HIV-infected patients have thrombotic strokes with no good cause delineated. Perhaps some of these patients have "lupus anticoagulant," an anticardiolipin antibody. Clues to the presence of the lupus anticoagulant are a high partial thromboplastin time, a false-positive VDRL test, and a low platelet count. The value of the anticardiolipin antibody test in diagnosing this syndrome is not known. Embolic strokes have been reported in patients with infective endocarditis and with marantic, or nonbacterial thrombotic, endocarditis (301), which may have a particular association with Kaposi's sarcoma. There may be an association between thrombotic thrombocytopenic purpura (TTP) and AIDS (302). The full pentad of TTP (not all patients have all five) is: thrombocytopenia, microangiopathic hemolytic anemia, renal abnormalities, fever, and neurological abnormalities (usually progressive, unexplained confusion).

Herpesvirus Infections

Herpesviruses to be considered are CMV, herpes zoster virus (HZV), and herpes simplex viruses 1 and 2 (HSV-1 and HSV-2). These viruses can cause either parenchymal or meningeal diseases and, when they occur in HIV-infected patients, are termed "secondary viral encephalomyelomeningitides." Other, nonherpetic viral infections associated with immunodeficiency, such as measles inclusion body encephalitis and enterovirus encephalitis and myositis, have not been reported yet in patients with AIDS.

CMV infection has protean manifestations in HIV-infected people. A retinitis, found in 20–25% of AIDS patients, is usually due to CMV. Retinal lesions are hemorrhagic exudates in a vascular pattern and look like "crumbled cheese and ketchup" or "pizza pie." Adrenal insufficiency is common in patients with disseminated CMV disease. CMV can cause a focal, multifocal, or generalized encephalitis (288,303,304). CT and MRI may be normal. One-quarter of AIDS patients have neuropathological findings suggesting CMV infection (neuronal necrosis and eosinophilic nuclear inclusions) (305). CMV may also cause a severe motor polyradiculopathy, since, in one patient with polyradiculopathy, CMV-positive multinucleated (cytomegalic) cells were found in subpial, subependymal, and nerve root locations (306). CMV may also cause the acute polyradiculopathy syndrome (see below). Ganciclovir is effective treatment for retinitis and, perhaps, for early acute polyradiculopathy, but not for other syndromes thought to be due to CMV.

Zoster is due to reactivation of HZV and, like tuberculosis reactivation, occurs at any stage of HIV infection. AIDS patients often have disseminated zoster and postzoster neurological syndromes, including multifocal leukoencephalitis with focal or lateralizing neurological signs and mass effect and hydrocephalus by cranial imaging studies. CSF may be normal. Pathology shows ventriculitis and focal necrosis with intranuclear inclusions in ependymal cells, neurons, and glia (307,308). Cerebral granulomatous angiitis, following zoster, causes fever, confusion, and ischemic stroke. Finally, patients can have myelitis due to HZV. Treatment of the neurological manifestations of HZV requires high-dose, intravenous acyclovir.

AIDS patients frequently have severe, ulcerative skin diseases due to HSV and may be at increased risk for HSV encephalitis. HSV-2 usually causes perirectal and genital ulcers, and it may subsequently cause myelitis (309) and meningitis. The treatment of HSV neurological syndromes is intravenous acyclovir.

Meningeal Diseases

Cryptococcosis (310) and Other Fungal Infections

These infections occur mostly in patients in the late stage of HIV infection. Meningitis due to *Cryptococcus neoformans* occurs in 5–10% of AIDS patients during the course of their disease, and it is more common in New Jerseyites, intravenous drug abusers, and bird owners. Other fungal infections are rarer in AIDS patients. Disseminated histoplasmosis occurs in patients who have lived in, or visited, the Ohio River Basin, and disseminated coccidioidomycosis occurs in patients having lived in, or visited, the southwestern United States. Other fungal diseases in HIV-infected patients include aspergillosis, candidiasis, and phycomycosis (mucormycosis).

Patients with cryptococcal meningitis may have fever (65% of patients), headache or malaise (75%), stiff neck (22%), altered mental status (28%), and focal deficits or seizures (<10%). Some patients will have only fever or only headache, with a normal neurological examination.

Cranial imaging is usually normal, except in the rare patient with fungal abscesses or hydrocephalus. CSF cell count, protein, and glucose may be normal. With cryptococcal meningitis, CSF India ink preparation is positive in 72–100% of patients, CSF cryptococcal antigen test is positive in 90–100%, and serum cryptococcal antigen is positive in 95–100%. False-negative cryptococcal antigen tests occur, possibly because of the prozone phenomenon, low antigen concentrations, or infection with an unusual serotype. Rheumatoid factor can cause a false-positive test. Diagnosis of cryptococcal meningitis may require multiple lumbar punctures (311) or positive fungal culture. New antigen tests are being developed for other fungi. Many patients respond poorly or not at all to antifungal agents, and most responders require maintenance therapy.

Lymphomatous Meningitis (312)

AIDS patients frequently have non-Hodgkin's lymphoma with B cell markers. Tumor cells, like those of primary CNS lymphoma, contain EBV genomes and protein (313). The cancer is often extranodal and involves the meninges in 10–30% (312,314). Paraspinal involvement—causing, for instance, spinal cord compression—occurs in 10% (314). In the meningeal form, patients present with cranial nerve palsies, radiculopathies, or headache. The CSF shows pleocytosis, increased protein, and, occasionally, hypoglycorrhachia. Diagnosis is by CSF cytology. Treatment is combination chemotherapy and radiation.

Disseminated Tuberculosis

Tuberculosis especially occurs in poor, foreign-born, Spanish-speaking, black, and Floridian patients (315). HIV-infected, purified protein derivative (PPD)-positive patients are at high risk for having disseminated tuberculosis and should receive isoniazid prophylaxis (316). Two percent of HIV-infected patients have active tuberculosis. Active disease may occur at any stage of HIV infection (317) and is often, but not always (128), reactivation of latent infection (318). Patients have meningeal symptoms (fever, headache, and neck pain), focal signs, or altered consciousness. Patients may also have spinal cord compression due to spinal infection. There is a case report of myelopathy (319) with mycobacteria seen on spinal cord biopsy. Lastly, patients with disseminated tuberculosis may have adrenal insufficiency.

The PPD skin test is negative in 70% of AIDS patients with active tuberculosis (320). Chest radiograms may be abnormal, but they show middle- or lower-lobe infiltrates (321) instead of upper-lobe cavitation. Cerebral mass lesions (tuberculomas) may be seen on head CT or MRI. CSF shows mononuclear pleocytosis, increased protein, and, occasionally, hypoglycorrhachia. Examination of the CSF pellet shows acid-fast bacilli in 37%. CSF cultures are positive in 45–90%, but they may take 1 or 2 months to grow. Newer diagnostic techniques designed to detect mycobacterial antigens quickly are being developed (278).

The course of tuberculosis is more severe in HIV-infected patients, and treatment is probably less effective (322) and associated with more side effects. For these reasons, all patients with active tuberculosis should be tested for HIV. HIV-infected patients with acid-fast bacilli on smears or biopsies should receive antituberculous

therapy pending culture results, even though some patients will have *Mycobacterium avium-intracellulare*, not *M. tuberculosis*. HIV-infected patients with tuberculosis should receive (at least) a two-drug therapy, but the optimal treatment regimen and duration is not known.

Syphilis (323)

There is a strong epidemiologic association between syphilis and AIDS. This means that all patients with syphilis should be tested for HIV, and vice versa. Symptoms due to syphilis may occur during any stage of HIV infection. Nervous system syphilis can cause thrombotic stroke (324), lacunar stroke (325), meningitis, Bell's palsy (326), optic neuritis (327), polyradiculopathy (327), and dementia. Since probably more than 25% of HIV-infected patients with neurosyphilis will have negative serum "nonspecific" antitreponemal tests (VDRL or RPR) (328), recognition of syphilis depends on a positive specific antitreponemal test (FTA-Abs, MHA-TP, or TPHA). Both types of test detect circulating antibody, and there are probably more false negatives (329) and false positives in HIV-infected patients. The serum VDRL titer can be used to gauge treatment success in syphilitic HIV-infected patients (330). Clinicians commonly use CSF VDRL or CSF pleocytosis to diagnose neurosyphilis. Both of these tests will reveal more false positives and false negatives (331) in HIV-infected patients.

Neurosyphilis is treated with high-dose, intravenous penicillin (aqueous crystalline penicillin G, 2–4 million units every 4 hr for 10–14 days). HIV-infected patients with reactive serum FTA-Abs and CSF VDRL should be treated using this regimen. Other indications for high-dose, intravenous penicillin are not clear. There are reports of intramuscular benzathine penicillin treatment failures in treating secondary syphilis in AIDS patients (324,326). The exact indications to treatment with high-dose, intravenous penicillin are unclear.

Strongyloides Hyperinfection (332)

Stronglyoides stercoralis most often infects South Americans, although others may also be infected. Strongyloides can complete its life cycle in one host (autoinfection), especially in the immunocompromised. Autoinfection causes a hyperinfection syndrome, with diffuse pulmonary infiltrates, severe generalized abdominal pain, ileus, shock, *S. stercoralis* and gram-negative meningitis, and gram-negative sepsis. Eosinophilia is a clue to the diagnosis, but it is not always present. Diagnosis is by observing free-swimming larvae in feces, sputum, or CSF.

Spinal Cord Diseases (Table 6)

Vacuolar Myelopathy

This disease occurs exclusively in AIDS patients, affecting about 20%. Although often associated with ADC, it may occur in patients without dementia (333). Patients have gait difficulty due to a combination of spastic paraparesis and sensory ataxia. In this syndrome, examination shows hyperreflexia, spasticity, impaired vibration sensation in the lower extremities, and an abnormal Romberg test. Weeks to months later, patients have urinary incontinence. The CSF is unremarkable. Visual and brainstem auditory evoked potentials are normal. Posterior tibial nerve-evoked somatosensory evoked potentials are almost universally delayed (334), and they may be abnormal before symptoms develop (335). The differential diagnosis includes spinal cord compression (due to lymphoma or tuberculosis) and infectious myelitis, such as that due to acute HIV seroconversion, HTLV-1, or herpesviruses. At pathology (Fig. 12), there are demyelination and vacuolation in the white matter of the posterior and lateral funiculi, with rare lipid-laden macrophages. Electron microscopy indicates that the vacuoles are due to intramyelin swelling. HIV antigens are rarely found in spinal cord tissue from patients with vacuolar myelopathy. Pathological changes are most severe in the thoracic cord and are similar to those of subacute combined degeneration. Serum cobalamin concentrations are usually normal. In nitrous oxide poisoning, which causes pathological changes similar to subacute combined degeneration, patients have normal serum cobalamin concentrations. Both nitrous oxide myeloneuropathy and cobalamin deficiency interfere with cellular methylation ability (336), and this biochemical abnormality may cause the pathological changes of subacute combined degeneration. HIV may also interfere with methylation ability (217).

HTLV-1 Myeloradiculopathy

HTLV-1, like HIV, is a retrovirus and can be transmitted by sexual intercourse, inoculation of infected blood or blood products, and perinatal exposure. Not surpris-

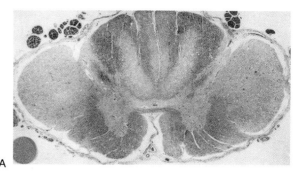
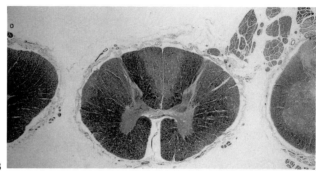

FIG. 12. Vacuolar myelopathy (luxol fast blue–PAS stain, ×2.5). There is demyelination and vacuolization in the posterior and lateral columns. **A:** Cervical cord. **B:** Thoracic cord. (Courtesy of Drs. Asao Hirano and Masayuki Shintaku.)

ingly, there is an association between HIV and HTLV-1 infection (337). Coinfected patients may have a more severe course of HIV infection (338). Neurologically, HTLV-1 can cause a myeloradiculopathy or a myopathy, or a combination of the two. The myeloradiculopathy syndrome is generally a chronic disease causing a combination of upper- and lower-motorneuron signs in the lower extremities, sensory deficits due either to cord or root damage, and urinary incontinence, with either a spastic or flaccid urinary bladder. Some cord syndromes seen in HIV-infected patients may be due to HTLV-1 coinfection (339). HTLV-1 myopathy is like polymyositis. In contrast to HTLV-1 myopathy alone, where virus is not usually found in muscle, a patient with both HIV-1 and HTLV-1 infections and polymyositis had HTLV-1 proteins in muscle fibers (340). Diagnosis is by serology, virus culture, or PCR. Some patients with HTLV-1-associated neurological syndromes improve with glucocorticoid therapy.

Cranial Neuropathies

Cranial neuropathies, most commonly isolated unilateral facial nerve palsy, occur in 10% of HIV-infected patients during the course of their disease, in association with HIV infection alone [often in the middle stage of infection (341)] or with a meningeal disease (see above). In addition, mass lesions in the orbit (e.g., lymphoma) may cause early oculomotor palsies. The lower-motor-

TABLE 6. *Spinal cord diseases and HIV infection*

Diseases	Stage
Vacuolar myelopathy	Late
Spinal cord compression	
Lymphoma	Late
Tuberculosis	Any
Myelitis	
Acute seroconversion	Early
Zoster	Late
HTLV-1	Late
Cobalamin deficiency	Any

neuron facial palsy occurring in the middle stage of infection, which is like Bell's palsy, usually recovers to the patient's satisfaction without treatment.

Neuromuscular Diseases

Approximately 30% of AIDS patients have a neuromuscular disease. Cobalamin deficiency, α-tocopherol deficiency, syphilis, thyroid dysfunction, and a side effect to drugs such as zidovudine, vincristine, or disulfiram can cause neuromuscular symptoms and signs and have specific treatments.

The five neuropathy syndromes in HIV-infected patients are: Guillain–Barré, chronic inflammatory demyelinating polyneuropathy, mononeuritis multiplex, distal sensory peripheral neuropathy, and acute polyradiculopathy (Table 7).

Guillain–Barré Syndrome (342)

This syndrome occurs mainly in the early and middle stages of infection. Like the Guillain–Barré patient who is not HIV-infected, patients present with acute weakness, sometimes requiring ventilatory support. Examination shows weakness, absent reflexes, and normal sensation. Hepatitis B antigenemia and abnormal liver function tests are common (342). The CSF frequently has a high protein. Many, but not all (343), patients have CSF pleocytosis related to HIV infection. CSF pleocytosis in a patient with Guillain–Barré syndrome should raise a suspicion of HIV infection. Nerve conduction velocities may be normal or slow with dispersion and conduction block. Electromyography shows denervation changes when the axons are involved. Nerve biopsies are normal or segmentally demyelinated. Perineurial cells may have prominent vacuolation. Inflammation is variable. There may be a CMV infection of Schwann cells, especially those of the proximal roots. The differential diagnosis includes acute spinal cord compression, toxic reaction to medication, and lymphomatous infiltration of nerve roots. Monitoring the forced vital capacity carefully is the most important thing to do in treating these patients. A decline in vital capacity to below 1 liter usually indicates incipient respiratory failure. Although untreated patients eventually improve spontaneously, therapeutic plasma exchanges probably produce more rapid and complete recovery than no treatment at all (342).

Chronic Inflammatory Demyelinating Peripheral Neuropathy (CIDP) (342)

This syndrome occurs mainly in the middle stage of infection, although AIDS patients occasionally have CIDP. Patients present with progressive or relapsing–remitting weakness. Examination shows proximal and distal weakness, normal (or only mildly abnormal) sensation, and areflexia. Often there is facial weakness. CSF shows elevated protein and often shows pleocytosis, related to HIV infection (342). Pleocytosis, the only abnormality differentiating HIV-associated CIDP from idiopathic CIDP, is not universal, but it is still a valuable clue to HIV infection. One-third of patients have increased CSF myelin basic protein (342). Correct diagnosis depends upon testing for HIV infection (342). Nerve conduction studies are slow with conduction block and dispersion, indicating segmental demyelination. The electromyogram may show denervation if the axons are involved. Nerve biopsies show demyelination with macrophage infiltration and perivascular and endoneurial inflammation. There may be prominent vacuolation of perineurial cells. HIV antigens cannot be detected in nerve biopsies (342,344). CIDP can be difficult to differentiate from Guillain–Barré syndrome, lymphomatous infiltration of nerve roots, and toxic neuropathy due to drugs (e.g., vincristine, disulfiram, isoniazid, and dapsone). CIDP responds to glucocorticoids and to plasmapheresis (345), but it may also improve spontaneously. Improvement may correlate with normalization of CSF cell count and protein (342). The cause is not known.

Mononeuropathy Multiplex

In mononeuropathy multiplex (the rarest of the four neuropathy syndromes) there are separate, abrupt lesions in individual nerves, which may include cranial nerves. The cause is usually attributed to nerve inflammation or infarction. This syndrome can be clinically difficult to differentiate from compression neuropathies in bed-bound patients, from progressive polyradiculopathy, and, when many nerves are involved, from CIDP (345).

Distal, Symmetric, Sensory Polyneuropathy (DSPN)

This is the most common neuropathy in HIV-infected patients and occurs almost exclusively in late infection (346). Thirty percent of AIDS patients have DSPN. Patients present with distal, often painful, paresthesias

TABLE 7. *Neuropathies and HIV infection*

Disease	Stage
Guillain–Barré syndrome	Early/middle
Chronic inflammatory demyelinating polyneuropathy	Middle
Mononeuritis multiplex	Late
Distal sensory peripheral polyneuropathy	Late
Acute polyradiculopathy	Late
Cobalamin deficiency	Any
Side effect of medication	Any

("burning feet"). Examination findings, often minimally abnormal compared to symptoms, are: decreased pinprick sensation in a stocking distribution, mild loss of vibration sensation distally, mild distal weakness, and absent ankle reflexes. CSF cell count and protein are usually normal (342,347), but oligoclonal bands are common (348). Nerve conduction velocities show decreased amplitude sensory nerve action potentials (349), and electromyography shows mild distal denervation. The electrophysiologic studies are consistent with a dying-back axonopathy. Symptomatic treatment is with amitriptyline or carbamazepine. Pathology shows mild dorsal root ganglia inflammation, gracile tract degeneration in the cervical cord (350), and axonal degeneration in the peripheral nerves. Epineurial and endoneurial inflammation may be present in the nerve biopsy (348). The cause and pathophysiology are not known.

Progressive Polyradiculopathy (351)

In this syndrome, patients in the late stage of infection develop acutely or subacutely progressive sensorimotor deficits and areflexia localized to the lumbosacral roots, in combination with early flaccid urinary bladder and rectal sphincter. Patients are unable to walk and have urinary retention and fecal incontinence. Patients often die within months of the onset of this syndrome. In half of patients, CSF shows marked inflammation, with an increased cell count, high protein, and low glucose. About half have positive CSF culture for CMV. Electromyograms show acute denervation (fibrillations and positive sharp waves). The differential diagnosis includes acute spinal cord compression, meningeal lymphomatosis, and neurosyphilis. At pathology, many patients have CMV infection of endoneurial and endothelial cells of spinal roots (352). Early ganciclovir treatment may reverse some symptoms and signs.

Autonomic Neuropathy

Autonomic neuropathy, usually mild, occurs in late infection and causes orthostatic hypotension (353). Both parasympathetic and sympathetic dysfunction occur (353,354). There is little correlation with other neurological disease (353). Adrenal insufficiency must be excluded.

Myopathies

Myopathies can be difficult to diagnose because many AIDS patients are ill, bed-bound, and thin. In general, patients with myopathy have proximal weakness, normal sensation, and normal tendon reflexes. Serum creatine kinase (CK) is often elevated. If the CK test is not done, elevations of other serum enzymes (lactate dehydrogenase and the aminotransferases), due to muscle disease, may be attributed to liver disease. Some patients have myoglobinuria (355). Four myopathic syndromes occur in HIV-infected patients: polymyositis-like, nemaline-like, zidovudine-induced, and HTLV-1-associated (see above for HTLV-1-associated) (Table 8). They are difficult to differentiate.

HIV-infected patients, usually those with AIDS, can have a syndrome similar, or identical (356), to polymyositis. In contrast to zidovudine-induced myopathy (see below), there is less muscle pain or tenderness and the CK is normal or only mildly elevated (357). Electromyography shows brief, low-amplitude ("myopathic") potentials and abnormal, spontaneous muscle fiber activity. Muscle biopsy shows inflammation (in 40%), microvesicular changes (358), muscle fiber necrosis, and phagocytosis (359), but no HIV antigens or mitochondrial changes. The pathogenesis is not clear.

Another myopathy is histologically similar to nemaline (or rod body) myopathy. It may occur in the middle or late stages of infection. There is proximal weakness and wasting, increased CK, myopathic potentials on electromyography, and rod bodies in type 1 fibers. Some patients have had both polymyositis and nemaline myopathy (359).

A third myopathy is seen in patients who have taken zidovudine for a prolonged time (>6 months) (360). These patients have weight loss, myalgias, proximal weakness, severe proximal atrophy, and muscle tenderness. CK is elevated, and the electromyogram shows myopathic potentials. Muscle biopsy shows ragged-red fibers, myofibril dissolution and necrosis, and slight inflammation (361,362). Ragged red fibers represent abnormal mitochondria (363), possibly due to inhibition of mitochondrial DNA polymerase γ. The number of ragged red fibers correlates with the severity of the myopathy (364). After stopping zidovudine, the patients' symptoms and strength improve, and the CK returns to normal (365). About half of patients improve with glucocorticoids, despite continuing zidovudine (364). The reason for improvement in these patients is not clear.

Treatment of HIV Infection (366,367)

Dideoxynucleotides are deoxynucleotide analogues that, after specific intracellular kinases activate them to triphosphates, inhibit reverse transcriptase and other en-

TABLE 8. *Myopathies and HIV infection*

Polymyositis
Nemaline-like
Zidovudine
HTLV-1

zymes polymerizing deoxynucleotide triphosphates into a DNA strand. Inhibiting reverse transcriptase interferes with an early step in the virion life cycle. These medications will decrease the number of newly infected cells, but they will not affect provirus expression in already infected cells (368). Enzyme activity is decreased by competitive inhibition and by premature "chain termination" of DNA synthesis (dideoxynucleotides have no 3' hydroxyl group for further polymerization). Cell DNA polymerases vary in sensitivity to these drugs. DNA polymerase α (responsible for replication) is generally resistant. DNA polymerases β (repair and recombination) and γ (mitochondrial replication) are relatively sensitive. Inhibition of these normal cell enzymes may be the cause of some side effects.

The dideoxynucleotide zidovudine (ZDV), formerly azidothymidine (AZT), decreases opportunistic infections and death, increases CD4+ cell counts, decreases p24 antigenemia, partially restores skin test responsiveness, and increases body weight in patients with AIDS (369), but therapeutic effects are transient. The reasons why ZDV loses effectiveness are not clear. Low-dose ZDV also delays transition to AIDS in asymptomatic HIV-infected patients who had a CD4+ cell count of less than 500/ml (370). Typical doses are 100 mg every 6 hr (low dose) to 200 mg every 4 hr (high dose). Pediatric dosage is 180 mg/m^2 (up to 200 mg) every 6 hr for ages 3 months to 12 years. It is available as a syrup (50 mg/5 ml) or as capsules. ZDV is glucuronidated in the liver and excreted in the urine. Probenecid prolongs drug elimination. Nonsteroidal anti-inflammatory agents, narcotics, and sulfonamides may also inhibit glucuronidation. In addition, ZDV side effects may be more prominent if the patient is also taking acetaminophen (371). The CSF ZDV concentration is about 60% of that in plasma (372). ZDV crosses the placental barrier as well (373). Reverse transcriptase mutations, especially at residues 67, 70, 215, and 219 (374), can cause ZDV resistance. Resistant isolates occur naturally, but it is not clear whether they cause clinical deterioration (375,376). ZDV-resistant isolates are usually sensitive to other dideoxynucleotides. ZDV side effects are headache, dizziness, insomnia, anorexia, nausea, vomiting, malaise, and myalgia. These symptoms often disappear with continued therapy. Megaloblastic anemia and neutropenia are dose-related and dose-limiting (377). Recombinant human erythropoietin (epoetin) decreases transfusion requirements, but it is expensive (378). High doses can cause anxiety, confusion, and tremulousness. Seizures (379) and Wernicke's encephalopathy (380) have been reported in patients taking ZDV. High-dose therapy for more than 6 months can cause a myopathy (360) (see above).

ZDV can partially reverse ADC (372,381), especially in its early stages (382), and can prevent ADC in AIDS patients without dementia (383). When studied by serial cognitive tests, ZDV-treated AIDS patients maintained normal intellectual function while placebo-treated controls did not (384). In addition, ZDV treatment improved walking. ZDV is also a promising treatment for progressive encephalopathy of children (385,386). Cognition, language, socialization, affect, coordination, and gait all improve during continuous ZDV infusion (385,386). In some cases the head CT scan shows less brain atrophy, and the PET scan shows improved cerebral cortical glucose utilization (386). These improvements begin within 1 month and persist. Since these early studies are unblinded, uncontrolled, and nonrandomized, further studies to confirm ZDV's benefits for children with progressive encephalopathy are in progress (254).

2',3'-Dideoxycytidine (DDC) and 2',3'-dideoxyinosine (DDI), like ZDV, are dideoxynucleotides and inhibit HIV replication in tissue culture (387). HIV isolates resistant to ZDV are sensitive to these nucleotides. In clinical trials, half of patients taking DDC, at doses of 0.03–0.25 mg/kg every 8 hr for 6–14 weeks, developed a painful peripheral neuropathy (388). Other side effects (e.g., maculovesicular cutaneous eruptions, aphthous ulcers, fever, and malaise) disappeared with continued therapy. DDI, at doses of 500–750 mg/day (approximately 10–20 mg/kg once or twice daily), increases CD4+ counts, decreases p24 levels, and increases body weight (389–391). HIV infections seemingly resistant to ZDV usually respond to DDI (392). Pancreatitis (6–30%) and a painful peripheral neuropathy (3–45%) are common, dose-related side effects. DDI also causes headaches, insomnia, nausea, emesis, fever, rash, confusion, dry mouth, diarrhea, hypokalemia, thrombocytopenia, and hyperuricemia. Compared to ZDV, anemia and leukopenia are rare. Further studies to determine the therapeutic efficacy and indications, optimal dose, and side effects of DDI and DDC are in progress. Their effect in treating or preventing ADC is not known.

Foscarnet (phosphonoformate) is a pyrophosphate analogue active against HIV. It is also used intravenously for CMV retinitis. Doses are 40–60 mg/kg (intravenously) for 14–21 days. Foscarnet causes renal damage, and its dose must be reduced in patients with renal insufficiency. Other side effects are malaise, nausea, vomiting, fatigue, headache, genital ulcers, seizures, hypocalcemia, hypercalcemia, hypophosphatemia, hyperphosphatemia, hypomagnesemia, anemia, proteinuria, nephrogenic diabetes insipidus, leukopenia, and abnormal liver function tests.

Based on the features and life cycle of HIV, other treatment approaches can be considered. CD4 formulations (393), gp120-like synthetic peptides (394), HIV protease (aspartyl endopeptidase) inhibitors (395,396), ribosomal frameshifting inhibitors, glycosylation inhibitors (e.g., castanospermine), α-interferon [blocks provirus expression (368,397)], acyclovir, ribavirin (398), "hammerhead" ribozymes (399), and "anti-sense" oligonucleotides (400), each affecting different steps of the viral life cycle (372,401), may also prove therapeutically useful (402). Immune-system-stimulating agents [such as diethyldithiocarbamate (403), disulfiram, inosine pranobex (404), and ampligen], inhibitors of the cytopathic effects [such as tetracycline (405)], and dideoxynucleoside potentiators [such as dipyridamole (406)] are also possible therapeutic agents.

Patients may take unproven medications [such as dextran sulfate, hydrogen peroxide, tricosanthin (GLQ223; Compound Q; or root of the Chinese cucumber, *Trichosanthes kirilowii*), and others] that have side effects. The unrefined Chinese cucumber root extract, for instance, can cause fever, thrombosis, strokes, and seizures.

Treatment of some of the complications of AIDS may necessitate prescription of medications having direct or indirect neurological side effects. AIDS patients frequently have headaches, myalgias, and mental confusion when taking medications, for unknown reasons. Perhaps HIV-infected patients will have more neurotoxic reactions to all medications. For instance, AIDS patients taking benzodiazepines and opiates have more sedation, drowsiness, amnesia, and respiratory depression than usual. Ganciclovir may cause mental confusion (407). Recombinant α-interferon (α-2a or α-2b), for HIV or for Kaposi's sarcoma, can cause headache, fatigue, depression, and myalgia. Dapsone can cause methemoglobinemia and, consequently, headaches. Patients taking disulfiram or metronidazole may have alcohol reactions. Metoclopramide (for nausea and vomiting) and haloperidol can cause a parkinsonism syndrome and dystonic reactions. Early in treatment, parenteral pentamidine can cause hypoglycemia (408), which can cause mental confusion and focal signs that mimic a stroke. AIDS patients frequently have psychotic reactions to tricyclic antidepressants (409). Thalidomide, for painful mouth ulcers, can cause a polyneuropathy (410,411), and so can dapsone, vincristine, isoniazid, disulfiram, DDI, and DDC. Amphotericin can cause hypokalemia or hypomagnesemia, leading to nervous system dysfunction.

HIV Infection and Vaccines (412,413)

In general, there are four types of virus vaccines: live, attenuated; killed; purified subunit; and recombinant. Live, attenuated HIV vaccines will probably not be used because of safety concerns. Killed vaccines produce relatively low titer antibodies, and, because there is no virus replication, there may be no antibody response at all to certain virus proteins. Subunit vaccines are purified preparations of virus protein, usually made by molecular cloning technology (414). In recombinant vaccines, part of the HIV genome is cloned into another genome (e.g.,

that of vaccinia virus), and this hybrid virus is used as vaccine (415).

There are problems with developing any vaccine, particularly ones with HIV. First, the virus has a high mutation rate, especially in the gp120 coding region (antigenic variation), and vaccine-induced immunity may not recognize altered virus proteins. Second, even if the antibodies do recognize viral proteins, antibodies may inadvertently enhance infection (101). So far, enhancement has only been shown in tissue culture (416). Finally, an unusual response to a vaccine may occur. One example occurred in persons who had received the formalin-inactivated (killed) measles vaccine. These persons, when later infected with measles, developed a severe, atypical measles. This may have been because the vaccines did not have antifusion protein antibodies, because formalin inactivation destroyed the fusion protein's immunogenicity (417). Similarly, HIV vaccines may need to induce antibodies to the fusion protein, gp41, in order to work properly.

HIV vaccines may be given either to prevent primary infection or, since late infection is associated with loss of immunity to HIV, to boost anti-HIV titers, in the hope that one thereby retards disease progression.

All HIV-infected patients should receive the influenza and pneumococcal vaccines, and they should probably receive the *Hemophilus influenzae* type b vaccine as well. Children should receive inactivated poliovirus, diphtheria–tetanus–pertussis, and measles–mumps–rubella vaccines (418). These vaccines, however, may not be immunizing (419), especially late in infection; therefore, all vaccines should be given as early as possible in HIV infection, and the immune response should be documented whenever possible. Also, there have been case reports of live vaccines causing adverse reactions in AIDS patients. For example, BCG vaccine can cause disseminated *Mycobacterium bovis* infection, and smallpox vaccine can cause disseminated vaccinia (420,421). Many HIV-infected and AIDS patients, however, have received these and other live vaccines (such as measles–mumps–rubella) without having reactions. If possible, for HIV-infected patients, one should avoid live, attenuated vaccines.

REFERENCES

1. Fauci AS. The human immunodeficiency virus: infectivity and mechanisms of pathogenesis. *Science* 1988;239:617–621.
2. Haseltine WA, Wong-Staal F. The molecular biology of the AIDS virus. *Sci Am* 1988;259:64–71.
3. Levy JA. Mysteries of HIV: challenges for therapy and prevention. *Nature* 1988;333:519–522.
4. Wong-Staal F. Human immunodeficiency virus: genetic structure and function. *Semin Hematol* 1988;25:189–196.
5. Levy JA. Human immunodeficiency viruses and the pathogenesis of AIDS. *JAMA* 1989;261:2997–3006.
6. Rosenblum ML, Levy RM, Bredesen DE. *AIDS and the nervous system*. New York: Raven Press, 1988.

7. Brew BB, Rosenblum M, Price RW. Central and peripheral nervous system complications of HIV infection and AIDS. In: DeVita VT, Hellman S, Rosenberg SA, eds. *AIDS: etiology, diagnosis, treatment, and prevention.* Philadelphia: JB Lippincott, 1988:185–197.

8. Price RW, Brew B, Sidtis J, Rosenblum M, Scheck AC, Cleary P. The brain in AIDS: central nervous system HIV-1 infection and AIDS dementia complex. *Science* 1988;239:586–591.

9. Pinching AJ. Neurological aspects of the acquired immunodeficiency syndrome. *J R Coll Physicians Lond* 1988;22:136–139.

10. Gonda MA, Wong-Staal F, Gallo RC, Clements JE, Narayan O, Gilden RV. Sequence homology and morphologic similarity of HTLV-III and visna virus, a pathogenic lentivirus. *Science* 1985;227:173–177.

11. Sonigo P, Alizon M, Staskus K, et al. Nucleotide sequence of the visna lentivirus: relationship to the AIDS virus. *Cell* 1985; 42:369–382.

12. Haase AT. Pathogenesis of lentivirus infections. *Nature* 1986; 322:130–136.

13. Kowalski M, Potz J, Basirpour L, et al. Functional regions of the envelope glycoprotein of human immunodeficiency virus type 1. *Science* 1987;237:1351–1355.

14. Navia MA, Fitzgerald PMD, McKeever BM, et al. Three-dimensional structure of aspartyl protease from human immunodeficiency virus HIV-1. *Nature* 1989;337:615–620.

15. Wlodawer A, Miller M, Jaskolski M, et al. Conserved folding in retroviral proteases: Crystal structure of a synthetic HIV-1 protease. *Science* 1989;245:616–621.

16. Blundell T, Pearl L. A second front against AIDS. *Nature* 1989;337:596–597.

17. Weber IT, Miller M, Jaskolski M, Leis J, Skalka AM, Wlodawer A. Molecular modeling of the HIV-1 protease and its substrate binding site. *Science* 1989;244:928–931.

18. Jacks T, Power MD, Masiarz FR, Luciw PA, Barr PJ, Varmus HE. Characterization of ribosomal frameshifting in HIV-1 *gag-pol* expression. *Nature* 1988;331:280–283.

19. Coffin JM. Genetic variation in AIDS viruses. *Cell* 1986;46:1–4.

20. Benn S, Rutledge R, Folks T, et al. Genomic heterogeneity of AIDS retroviral isolates from North America and Zaire. *Science* 1985;230:949–951.

21. Willey RL, Rutledge RA, Dias S, et al. Identification of conserved and divergent domains within the envelope gene of the acquired immunodeficiency syndrome retrovirus. *Proc Natl Acad Sci USA* 1986;83:5038–5042.

22. Modrow S, Hahn BH, Shaw GM, Gallo RC, Wong-Staal F, Wolf H. Computer-assisted analysis of envelope protein sequences of seven human immunodeficiency virus isolates: prediction of antigenic epitopes in conserved and variable regions. *J Virol* 1987;61:570–578.

23. Starcich BR, Hahn BH, Shaw GM, et al. Identification and characterization of conserved and variable regions in the envelope gene of HTLV-III/LAV, the retrovirus of AIDS. *Cell* 1986; 45:637–648.

24. Siliciano RF, Lawton T, Knall C, et al. Analysis of host–virus interactions in AIDS with anti-gp120 T cell clones: effect of HIV sequence variation and a mechanism for CD4+ cell depletion. *Cell* 1988;54:561–575.

25. Looney DJ, Fisher AG, Putney SD, et al. Type-restricted neutralization of molecular clones of human immunodeficiency virus. *Science* 1988;241:357–360.

26. Fisher AG, Ensoli B, Looney D, et al. Biologically diverse molecular variants within a single HIV-1 isolate. *Nature* 1988;334:444–447.

27. Saag MS, Hahn BH, Gibbons J, et al. Extensive variation of human immunodeficiency virus type-1 *in vivo. Nature* 1988; 334:440–444.

28. Weiss RA. Defective viruses to blame? *Nature* 1989;338:458.

29. Maddon PJ, Dalgleish AG, McDougal JS, Clapham PR, Weiss RA, Axel R. The T4 gene encodes the AIDS virus receptor and is expressed in the immune system and the brain. *Cell* 1986;47:333–348.

30. Lasky LA, Nakamura G, Smith DH, et al. Delineation of a region of the human immunodeficiency virus type 1 gp120 glycoprotein critical for interaction with the CD4 receptor. *Cell* 1987;50:975–985.

31. Dalgleish AG, Beverley PCL, Clapham PR, Crawford DH, Greaves MF, Weiss RA. The CD4 (T4) antigen is an essential component of the receptor for the AIDS retrovirus. *Nature* 1984;312:763–766.

32. Klatzman D, Champagne E, Chamaret S, et al. T-lymphocyte T4 molecule behaves as the receptor for human retrovirus LAV. *Nature* 1984;312:767–768.

33. McDougal JS, Kennedy MS, Sligh JM, Cort SP, Mawle A, Nicholson JKA. Binding of HTLV-III/LAV to T4+ T cells by a complex of the 110K viral protein and the T4 molecule. *Science* 1986;231:382–385.

34. Sattentau QJ, Weiss RA. The CD4 antigen: physiological ligand and HIV receptor. *Cell* 1988;52:631–633.

35. Gallaher WR. Detection of a fusion peptide sequence in the transmembrane protein of human immunodeficiency virus. *Cell* 1987;50:327–328.

36. Muesing MA, Smith DH, Cabradilla CD, Benton CV, Lasky LA, Capon DJ. Nucleic acid structure and expression of the human AIDS/lymphadenopathy retrovirus. *Nature* 1985;313:450–458.

37. Bosch ML, Earl PL, Fargnoli K, et al. Identification of the fusion peptide of primate immunodeficiency viruses. *Science* 1989; 244:694–697.

38. McClure MO, Marsh M, Weiss RA. Human immunodeficiency virus infection of CD4-bearing cells occurs by a pH-independent mechanism. *EMBO J* 1988;7:513–518.

39. Stein BS, Gowda SD, Lifson JD, Penhallow RC, Bensch KG, Engleman EG. pH-independent HIV entry into CD4-positive T cells via virus envelope fusion to the plasma membrane. *Cell* 1987;49:659–668.

40. Bedinger P, Moriaty A, von Borstel RC II, Donovan NJ, Steimer KS, Littman DR. Internalization of the human immunodeficiency virus does not require the cytoplasmic domain of CD4. *Nature* 1988;334:162–165.

41. Maddon PJ, McDougal JS, Clapham PR, et al. HIV infection does not require endocytosis of its receptor, CD4. *Cell* 1988;54:865–874.

42. Sodroski J, Goh WC, Rosen C, Campbell K, Haseltine WA. Role of HTLV-III/LAV envelope in syncytium formation and cytopathicity. *Nature* 1986;332:470–474.

43. Lifson JD, Feinberg MB, Reyes GR, et al. Induction of CD4-dependent cell fusion by the HTLV-III/LAV envelope glycoprotein. *Nature* 1986;323:725–728.

44. Lifson JD, Reyes GR, McGrath MS, Stein BS, Engleman EG. AIDS retrovirus induced cytopathology: giant cell formation and involvement of CD4 antigen. *Science* 1986;232:1123–1127.

45. Yoffe B, Lewis DE, Petrie BL, Noonan CA, Melnick JL, Hollinger FB. Fusion as a mediator of cytolysis in mixtures of uninfected CD4+ lymphocytes and cells infected by human immunodeficiency virus. *Proc Natl Acad Sci USA* 1987;84:1429–1433.

46. Rabson AB, Martin MA. Molecular organization of the AIDS retrovirus. *Cell* 1985;40:477–480.

47. Larder BA, Purifoy DJM, Powell KL, Darby G. Site-specific mutagenesis of AIDS virus reverse transcriptase. *Nature* 1987; 327:716–717.

48. Evans JA, Moreau J, Odehouri K, et al. Characterization of a noncytopathic HIV-2 strain with unusual effects on CD4 expression. *Science* 1988;240:1522–1525.

49. Kong LI, Lee S, Kappes JC, et al. West African HIV-2-related human retrovirus with attenuated cytopathicity. *Science* 1988; 240:1525–1529.

50. Levy JA, Kaminsky L, Morrow WJW, et al. Infection by the retrovirus associated with the acquired immunodeficiency syndrome. *Ann Intern Med* 1985;103:694–699.

51. Weinberg RA. Integrated genomes. *Annu Rev Biochem* 1980; 49:197–226.

52. Wain-Hobson S, Sonigo P, Danos O, Cole S, Alizon M. Nucleotide sequence of the AIDS virus, LAV. *Cell* 1985;40:9–17.

53. Sanchez-Pescador R, Power MD, Barr PJ, et al. Nucleotide sequence and expression of an AIDS-associated retrovirus (ARV-2). *Science* 1985;227:484–492.

54. Ratner L, Haseltine W, Patarca R, et al. Complete nucleotide

sequence of the AIDS virus, HTLV-III. *Nature* 1985;313:277–284.

55. Starcich B, Ratner L, Josephs SF, Okamato T, Gallo RC, Wong-Staal F. Characterization of long terminal repeat sequences of HTLV-III. *Science* 1985;227:538–540.

56. Chen ISY. Regulation of AIDS virus expression. *Cell* 1986;47:1–2.

57. Rosen CA, Sodroski JG, Goh WC, Dayton AI, Lippke J, Haseltine WA. Post-transcriptional regulation accounts for the *trans*-activation of the human T-lymphotropic virus type III. *Nature* 1986;319:555–559.

58. Rice AP, Mathews MB. Transcriptional but not translational regulation of HIV-1 by the *tat* gene product. *Nature* 1988;332:551–553.

59. Frankel AD, Bredt DS, Pabo CO. Tat protein from human immunodeficiency virus forms a metal-linked dimer. *Science* 1988;240:70–73.

60. Fisher AG, Feinberg MB, Josephs SF, et al. The *trans*-activator gene of HTLV-III is essential for virus replication. *Nature* 1986;320:367–371.

61. Terwilliger E, Burghoff R, Sia R, Sodroski J, Haseltine W, Rosen C. The *art* gene product of human immunodeficiency virus is required for replication. *J Virol* 1988;62:655–658.

62. Sadaie MR, Benter T, Wong-Staal F. Site-directed mutagenesis of two trans-regulatory genes (tat-III, trs) of HIV-1. *Science* 1988;239:910–913.

63. Malim MH, Hauber J, Le S, Maizel JV, Cullen BR. The HIV-1 *rev trans*-activator acts through a structured target sequence to activate nuclear export of unspliced viral mRNA. *Nature* 1989;338:254–256.

64. Guy B, Kieny MP, Riviere Y, et al. HIV F/3′ *orf* encodes a phosphorylated GTP-binding protein resembling an oncogene product. *Nature* 1987;330:266–269.

65. Luciw PA, Cheng-Mayer C, Lecy JA. Mutational analysis of the human immunodeficiency virus: the *orf-B* region down-regulates virus replication. *Proc Natl Acad Sci USA* 1987;84:1434–1438.

66. Nabel G, Baltimore D. An inducible transcription factor activates expression of human immunodeficiency virus in T cells. *Nature* 1987;326:711–713.

67. McDougal JS, Mawle A, Cort SP, et al. Cellular tropism of the human retrovirus HTLV-III/LAV I. Role of T cell activation and expression of the T4 antigen. *J Immunol* 1985;135:3151–3162.

68. Sen R, Baltimore D. Inducibility of κ immunoglobulin enhancer-binding protein NF-κB by a posttranslational mechanism. *Cell* 1986;47:921–928.

69. Griffin GE, Leung K, Folks TM, Kunkel S, Nabel GJ. Activation of HIV gene expression during monocyte differentiation by induction of NF-κB. *Nature* 1989;339:70–73.

70. Nabel GJ, Rice SA, Knipe DM, Baltimore D. Alternative mechanisms for activation of human immunodeficiency virus enhancer in T cells. *Nature* 1988;239:1299–1302.

71. Gendelman HE, Phelps W, Feigenbaum L, et al. Trans-activation of the human immunodeficiency virus long terminal repeat sequence by DNA viruses. *Proc Natl Acad Sci USA* 1986;83:9759–9763.

72. Siekevitz M, Josephs SF, Dukovich M, Peffer N, Wong-Staal F, Greene WC, Warner C. Activation of the HIV-1 LTR by T cell mitogens and the *trans*-activator protein of HTLV-1. *Science* 1987;238:1575–1578.

73. Zack JA, Cann AJ, Lugo JP, Chen ISY. HIV-1 production from infected peripheral blood T cells after HTLV-1 induced mitogenic stimulation. *Science* 1988;240:1026–1028.

74. Griffin GE, Leung K, Folks TM, Kunkel S, Nabel GJ. Activation of HIV gene expression during monocyte differentiation by induction of NF-κB. *Nature* 1989;339:70–73.

75. Ventura AM, Arens MQ, Srinivasan A, Chinnadurai G. Silencing of human immunodeficiency virus long terminal repeat expression by an adenovirus E1a mutant. *Proc Natl Acad Sci USA* 1990;87:1310–1314.

76. Nelbock P, Dillon PJ, Perkins A, Rosen CA. A cDNA for a protein that interacts with the human immunodeficiency virus tat transactivator. *Science* 1990;248:1650–1653.

77. Weber JN, Weiss RA. HIV infection: the cellular picture. *Sci Am* 1988;259:100–109.

78. Levy JA, Shimabukuro J, McHugh T, Casavant C, Stites D, Oshiro L. AIDS-associated retroviruses (ARV) can productively infect other cells besides human T helper cells. *Virology* 1985;147:441–448.

79. Klatzmann D, Barre-Sinoussi F, Nugeyre MT, et al. Selective tropism of lymphadenopathy associated virus (LAV) for helper-inducer T lymphocytes. *Science* 1984;225:59–63.

80. Nicholson JKA, Cross GD, Callaway CS, McDougal JS. *In vitro* infection of human monocytes with human T lymphotropic virus type III/lymphadenopathy-associated virus (HTLV-III/LAV). *J Immunol* 1986;137:323–329.

81. Ho DD, Rota TR, Hirsch MS. Infection of monocyte/macrophages by human T lymphotropic virus type III. *J Clin Invest* 1986;77:1712–1715.

82. Gartner S, Markovits P, Markovitz DM, Kaplan MH, Gallo RC, Popovic M. The role of mononuclear phagocytes in HTLV-III/LAV infection. *Science* 1986;233:215–218.

83. Montagnier L, Gruest J, Chamarct S, et al. Adaptation of lymphadenopathy-associated virus (LAV) to replication in EBV-transformed B lymphoblastoid cell lines. *Science* 1984;225:63–66.

84. Seligmann M, Pinching AJ, Rosen FS, et al. Immunology of human immunodeficiency virus infection and the acquired immunodeficiency syndrome. *Ann Intern Med* 1987;107:234–242.

85. Jameson BA, Rao PE, Kong LI, et al. Location and chemical synthesis of a binding site for HIV-1 on the CD4 protein. *Science* 1988;240:1335–1338.

86. Peterson A, Seed B. Genetic analysis of monoclonal antibody and HIV binding sites on the human lymphocyte antigen CD4. *Cell* 1988;54:65–72.

87. Lasky LA, Nakamura G, Smith DH, et al. Delineation of a region of the human immunodeficiency virus type 1 gp120 glycoprotein critical for interaction with the CD4 receptor. *Cell* 1987;50:975–985.

88. Clayton LK, Sieh M, Pious DA, Reinherz EL. Identification of human CD4 residues affecting class II MHC versus HIV-1 gp120 binding. *Nature* 1989;339:548–551.

89. Landau NR, Warton M, Littman DR. The envelope glycoprotein of the human immunodeficiency virus binds to the immunoglobulin-like domain of CD4. *Nature* 1988;334:159–162.

90. Manza F, Hebeshaw JA, Dalgleish AG. HIV envelope glycoprotein, antigen specific T-cell responses, and soluble CD4. *Lancet* 1990;335:811–815.

91. Pert CB, Hill JM, Ruff MR, et al. Octapeptides deduced from the neuropeptide receptor-like pattern of antigen T4 in brain potently inhibit human immunodeficiency virus receptor binding and T-cell infectivity. *Proc Natl Acad Sci USA* 1986;83:9254–9258.

92. Deen KC, McDougal JS, Inacker R, et al. A soluble form of CD4 (T4) protein inhibits AIDS virus infection. *Nature* 1988;331:82–84.

93. Traunecker A, Luke W, Karjalainen K. Soluble CD4 molecules neutralize human immunodeficiency virus type 1. *Nature* 1988;331:84–86.

94. Hussey RE, Richardson NE, Kowalski M, et al. A soluble CD4 protein selectively inhibits HIV replication and syncytium formation. *Nature* 1988;331:78–81.

95. Fisher RA, Bertonis JM, Meier W, et al. HIV infection is blocked *in vitro* by recombinant soluble CD4. *Nature* 1988;331:76–78.

96. Smith DH, Byrn RA, Marsters SA, Gregory T, Groopman JE, Capon DJ. Blocking of HIV-1 infectivity by a soluble, secreted form of the CD4 antigen. *Science* 1987;238:1704–1707.

97. Weiss RA. Receptor molecule blocks HIV. *Nature* 1988;331:15.

98. Lifson JD, Hwang KM, Nara PL, et al. Synthetic CD4 peptide derivatives that inhibit HIV infection and cytopathicity. *Science* 1988;241:712–716.

99. Finberg RW, Diamond DC, Mitchell DB, et al. Prevention of HIV-1 infection and preservation of CD4 function by the binding of CPFs to gp120. *Science* 1990;249:287–291.

100. Capon DJ, Chamow SM, Mordenti J, et al. Designing CD4 immunoadhesins for AIDS therapy. *Nature* 1989;337:525–531.

101. Chaudhary VK, Mizukami T, Fuerst TR, et al. Selective killing of HIV-infected cells by recombinant human CD4-*Pseudomonas* exotoxin hybrid protein. *Nature* 1988;335:369–372.

102. Traunecker A, Schneider J, Kiefer H, Karjalainen K. Highly efficient neutralization of HIV with recombinant CD4-immunoglobulin molecules. *Nature* 1989;339:68–70.

103. Zarling JM, Moran PA, Haffar O, et al. Inhibition of HIV replication by pokeweed antiviral protein targeted to CD4+ cells by monoclonal antibodies. *Nature* 1990;347:92–95.

104. Popovic M, Read-Connole E, Gallo RC. T4-positive human neoplastic cell lines susceptible to and permissive for HTLV-III. *Lancet* 1984;ii:1472–1473.

105. McKeating JA, Griffiths PD, Weiss RA. HIV susceptibility conferred to human fibroblasts by cytomegalovirus-induced Fc receptor. *Nature* 1990;343:659–661.

106. Homsy J, Meyer M, Tateno M, Clarkson S, Levy JA. The Fc and not CD4 receptor mediates antibody enhancement of HIV infection in human cells. *Nature* 1989;244:1357–1360.

107. Linette GP, Hartzman RJ, Ledbetter JA, June CH. HIV-1-infected T cells show a selective signaling defect after perturbation of CD3/antigen receptor. *Science* 1988;573–576.

108. Viscidi RP, Mayur K, Lederman HM, Frankel AD. Inhibition of antigen-induced lymphocyte proliferation by tat protein from HIV-1. *Science* 1989;246:1606–1608.

109. Somasundaran M, Robinson HL. A major mechanism of human immunodeficiency virus-induced cell killing does not involve cell fusion. *J Virol* 1987;61:3114–3119.

110. Sacerdote P, Ruff MR, Pert CB. Vasoactive intestinal peptide 1–12: a ligand for the CD4 (T4)/human immunodeficiency virus receptor. *J Neurosci Res* 1987;18:102–107.

111. Lee MR, Ho DD, Gurney ME. Functional interaction and partial homology between human immunodeficiency virus and neuroleukin. *Science* 1987;237:1047–1051.

112. Faik P, Walker JIH, Redmill AAM, Morgan MJ. Mouse glucose-6-phosphate isomerase and neuroleukin have identical 3′ sequences. *Nature* 1988;332:455–457.

113. Kornfeld H, Cruikshank WW, Pyle SW, Berman JS, Center DM. Lymphocyte activation by HIV-1 envelope glycoprotein. *Nature* 1988;335:445–448.

114. Dreyer EB, Kaiser PK, Offerman JT, Lipton SA. HIV-1 coat protein neurotoxicity prevented by calcium channel antagonists. *Science* 1990;248:364–370.

115. Heyward WL, Curran JW. The epidemiology of AIDS in the U.S. *Sci Am* 1988;259:72–81.

116. Friedland GH, Klein RS. Transmission of the human immunodeficiency virus. *N Engl J Med* 1987;317:1125–1134.

117. Friedland GH, Saltzman BR, Rogers MF, et al. Lack of transmission of HTLV-III/LAV infection to household contacts of patients with AIDS or AIDS-related complex with oral candidiasis. *New Engl J Med* 1986;314:344–349.

118. Lifson AR. Do alternative modes for transmission of human immunodeficiency virus exist? *JAMA* 1988;259:1353–1356.

119. Piot P, Laga M. Genital ulcers, other sexually transmitted diseases, and the sexual transmission of HIV. *Br Med J* 1989;298:623–624.

120. Simonsen JN, Cameron DW, Gakinya MN, et al. Human immunodeficiency virus infection among men with sexually transmitted diseases: experience from a center in Africa. *N Engl J Med* 1988;319:274–278.

121. Lerner CW, Tapper ML. Opportunistic infection complicating acquired immune deficiency syndrome: clinical features of 25 cases. *Medicine* 1984;63:155–164.

122. The Cooperative Needlestick Surveillance Group. Occupational risk of the acquired immunodeficiency syndrome among health care workers. *N Engl J Med* 1986;314:1127–1132.

123. Centers for Disease Control. Update: acquired immunodeficiency syndrome and human immunodeficiency virus infection among health-care workers. *MMWR* 1988;37:229–234.

124. Jagger J, Hunt EH, Brand-Elnaggar J, Pearson RD. Rates of needle-stick injury caused by various devices in an university hospital. *N Engl J Med* 1988;319:284–288.

125. American Academy of Neurology AIDS Task Force. Human immunodeficiency virus (HIV) infection and the nervous system. *Neurology* 1989;39:119–122.

126. Conte JE, Hadley WK, Sande M, et al. Infection-control guidelines for patients with the acquired immunodeficiency syndrome (AIDS). *N Engl J Med* 1983;309:740–744.

127. Centers for Disease Control. Recommendations for prevention of HIV transmission in health-care settings. *MMWR* 1987;36:2S–18S.

128. Braun MM, Truman BI, Maguire B, et al. Increasing incidence of tuberculosis in a prison inmate population. *JAMA* 1989;261:393–397.

129. Redfield RR, Burke DS. HIV infection: the clinical picture. *Sci Am* 1988;259:90–99.

130. Selik RM, Jaffe HW, Solomon SL, Curran JW. CDC's definition of AIDS. *N Engl J Med* 1986;315:761.

131. Redfield RR, Wright DC, Tramont EC. The Walter Reed staging classification for HTLV-III/LAV infection. *N Engl J Med* 1986;314:131–132.

132. Cooper DA, Gold J, Maclean P, et al. Acute AIDS retrovirus infection. *Lancet* 1985;i:537–540.

133. Gaines H, von Sydow M, Pehrson PO, Lundbergh P. Clinical picture of primary HIV infection presenting as a glandular-fever-like illness. *Br Med J* 1988;297:1363–1368.

134. Pedersen C, Lindhardt BO, Jensen BL, et al. Clinical course of primary HIV infection: consequences for subsequent course of infection. *Br Med J* 1989;299:154–157.

135. Wall RA, Denning DW, Amos A. HIV antigenaemia in acute HIV infection. *Lancet* 1987;i:566.

136. Birx DL, Redfield RR, Tosato G. Defective regulation of Epstein–Barr virus infection in patients with acquired immunodeficiency syndrome (AIDS) or AIDS-related disorders. *N Engl J Med* 1986;314:874–879.

137. Stricker RB, Abrams DI, Corash L, Shuman MA. Target platelet antigen in homosexual men with immune thrombocytopenia. *N Engl J Med* 1985;313:1375–1380.

138. Ratnoff OD, Menitove JE, Aster RH, Lederman MM. Coincident classic hemophilia and "idiopathic" thrombodytopenic purpura in patients under treatment with concentrates of antihemophilic factor (factor VIII). *N Engl J Med* 1983;308:439–442.

139. Case Records of the Massachusetts General Hospital. Case 11-1982: a 29 year-old man admitted because of chronic urticaria, proteinuria, and cryoglobulinemia. *N Engl J Med* 1982;306:657–668.

140. Koderisch J, Andrassy K, Rasmussen N, Hartmann M, Tilgen W. "False-positive" anti-neutrophil cytoplasmic antibodies in HIV infection [Letter to the editor]. *Lancet* 1990;335:1227–1228.

141. Centers for Disease Control. Revision of the CDC surveillance case definition for acquired immunodeficiency syndrome. *MMWR* 1987;36(Suppl 1S):3S–15S.

142. Costagliola D, Mary J, Brouard N, Laporte A, Valleron A. Incubation time for AIDS from French transfusion-associated cases. *Nature* 1989;338:768–789.

143. Bacchetti P, Moss AR. Incubation period of AIDS in San Francisco. *Nature* 1989;338:251–253.

144. Frosner GG, Erfle V, Mellert W, Hehlmann R. Diagnostic significance of quantitative determination of HIV antibody specific for envelope and core proteins. *Lancet* 1987;i:159–160.

145. Polk BF, Fox R, Brookmeyer R, et al. Predictors of the acquired immunodeficiency syndrome developing in a cohort of seropositive homosexual men. *N Engl J Med* 1987;316:61–66.

146. Ho DD, Sarngadharan MG, Hirsch MS, et al. Human immunodeficiency virus neutralizing antibodies recognize several conserved domains on the envelope glycoproteins. *J Virol* 1987;61:2024–2028.

147. Ho DD, Moudgil T, Alam M. Quantitation of human immunodeficiency virus type 1 in the blood of infected persons. *N Engl J Med* 1989;321:1621–1625.

148. Coombs, RW, Collier, AC, Allain J, et al. Plasma viremia in human immunodeficiency virus infection. *N Engl J Med* 1989;321:1626–1631.

149. Kramer A, Biggar RJ, Goedert JJ. Markers of risk in HIV-1 [Letter to the editor]. *N Engl J Med* 1990;322:1886.

150. Fahey JL, Taylor JMG, Detels R, et al. The prognostic value of cellular and serologic markers in infection with human immunodeficiency virus type 1. *N Engl J Med* 1990;322:166–172.

151. Anderson RE, Lang W, Shiboski S, Royce R, Jewell N, Winkel-

stein W Jr. Use of β_2-microglobulin level and CD4 lymphocyte count to predict development of acquired immunodeficiency syndrome in persons with human immunodeficiency virus infection. *Arch Intern Med* 1990;150:73–77.

152. Rothenberg R, Woelfel M, Stoneburner R, Milberg J, Parker R, Truman B. Survival with the acquired immunodeficiency syndrome: experience with 5833 cases in New York City. *N Engl J Med* 1987;317:1297–1302.

153. Editorial. Orofacial manifestations of HIV infection. *Lancet* 1988;i:976–977.

154. Siegal FP, Lopez C, Hammer GS, et al. Severe acquired immunodeficiency in male homosexuals, manifested by chronic perianal ulcerative herpes simplex lesions. *N Engl J Med* 1981;305:1439–1444.

155. Goodell SE, Quinn TC, Mkrtichian E, Schuffler MD, Holmes KK, Corey L. Herpes simplex virus proctitis in homosexual men: clinical, sigmoidoscopic, and histopathological features. *N Engl J Med* 1983;308:868–871.

156. Strom RL, Gruninger RP. AIDS with *Mycobacterium avium-intracellulare* lesions resembling those of Whipple's disease. *N Engl J Med* 1983;309:1323–1324.

157. Roth RI, Owen RL, Keren DF. AIDS with *Mycobacterium avium-intercellulare* lesions resembling those of Whipple's disease. *N Engl J Med* 1983;309:1324–1325.

158. Guy RJC, Turberg Y, Davidson RN, Finnerty G, MacGregor GA, Wise PH. Mineralocorticoid deficiency in HIV infection. *Br Med J* 1989;298:496–497.

159. Macher AM, Reichert CM, Straus SE, et al. Death in the AIDS patient: role of cytomegalovirus. *N Engl J Med* 1983;309:1454.

160. Harper ME, Marselle LM, Gallo RC, Wong-Staal F. Detection of lymphocytes expressing human T-lymphotropic virus type III in lymph nodes and peripheral blood from infected individuals by *in situ* hybridization. *Proc Natl Acad Sci USA* 1986;83:772–776.

161. Smith PD, Ohura K, Masur H, Lane HC, Fauci AS, Wahl SM. Monocyte function in the acquired immune deficiency syndrome: defective chemotaxis. *J Clin Invest* 1984;74:2121–2128.

162. Eyster ME, Goedert JJ, Poon M, Preble OT. Acid-labile alpha interferon: a possible preclinical marker for the acquired immunodeficiency syndrome in hemophilia. *N Engl J Med* 1983;309:583–586.

163. Seligmann M, Chess L, Fahey JL, et al. AIDS—an immunologic reevaluation. *N Engl J Med* 1984;311:1286–1292.

164. Lane HC, Masur H, Edgar LC, Whalen G, Rook AH, Fauci AS. Abnormalities of B-cell activation and immunoregulation in patients with the acquired immunodeficiency syndrome. *N Engl J Med* 1983;309:453–458.

165. Dylewski J, Chou S, Merigan TC. Absence of detectable IgM antibody in cytomegalovirus disease in patients with AIDS [Letter to the editor]. *N Engl J Med* 1983;309:493.

166. Hahn BH, Kong LI, Lee S, et al. Relation of HTLV-4 to simian and human immunodeficiency-associated viruses. *Nature* 1987;330:184–186.

167. Clavel F, Mansinho K, Chamaret S, et al. Human immunodeficiency virus type 2 infection associated with AIDS in West Africa. *N Engl J Med* 1987;316:1180–1185.

168. Centers for Disease Control. Update: HIV-2 infection—United States. *MMWR* 1989;38:572–580.

169. Norrby E, Biberfeld G, Chiodi F, et al. Discrimination between antibodies to HIV and to related retroviruses using site-directed serology. *Nature* 1987;329:248–250.

170. Gnann JW Jr, Mccormick JB, Mitchell S, Nelson JA, Oldstone MBA. Synthetic peptide immunoassay distinguishes HIV type 1 and HIV type 2 infections. *Science* 1987;237:1346–1349.

171. The Medical Letter. Diagnostic tests for AIDS. *Med Lett* 1988;30:73–74.

172. Steckelberg JM, Cockerill FR III. Serologic testing for human immunodeficiency virus antibodies. *Mayo Clin Proc* 1988;63:373–380.

173. Centers for Disease Control. Interpretation and use of the Western blot assay for serodiagnosis of human immunodeficiency virus type 1 infections. *MMWR* 1989;38(Suppl):S-7.

174. Meyer KB, Pauker SG. Screening for HIV: Can we afford the false positive rate? *N Engl J Med* 1987;317:238–241.

175. Goudsmit J, de Wolf F, Paul DA, Epstein LG, Lange JMA, et al. Expression of human immunodeficiency virus antigen (HIV-Ag) in serum and cerebrospinal fluid during acute and chronic infection. *Lancet* 1986;ii:178–180.

176. Marlink RG, Allen JS, McLane MF, Essex M, Anderson KC, Groopman JE. Low sensitivity of ELISA testing in early HIV infection. *N Engl J Med* 1986;315:1549.

177. Stramer SL, Heller JS, Coombs RW, Parry JV, Ho DD, Allain J-P. Markers of HIV infection prior to IgG antibody seropositivity. *JAMA* 1989;262:64–69.

178. Imagawa DT, Lee MH, Wolinsky SM, et al. Human immunodeficiency virus type 1 infection in homosexual men who remain seronegative for prolonged periods. *N Engl J Med* 1989;320:1458–1462.

179. Haseltine WA. Silent HIV infections [Editorial]. *N Engl J Med* 1989;320:1487–1489.

180. Allain J, Laurian Y, Paul DA, et al. Long-term evaluation of HIV antigen and antibodies to p24 and gp41 in patients with hemophilia. *N Engl J Med* 1987;317:1114–1121.

181. Levy JA, Shimabukuro J, Hollander H, Mills J, Kaminsky L. Isolation of AIDS-associated retroviruses from cerebrospinal fluid and brain of patients with neurological symptoms. *Lancet* 1985;ii:586–588.

182. Ho DD, Rota TR, Schooley RT, et al. Isolation of HTLV-III from cerebrospinal fluid and neural tissues of patients with neurologic syndromes related to the acquired immunodeficiency syndrome. *N Engl J Med* 1985;313:1493–1497.

183. Ou C, Kwok S, Mitchell SW, et al. DNA amplification for direct detection of HIV-1 in DNA of peripheral blood mononuclear cells. *Science* 1988;239:295–297.

184. Stramer SL, Heller JS, Coombs RW, Parry JV, Ho DD, Allain J. Markers of HIV infection prior to IgG antibody seropositivity. *JAMA* 1989;262:64–69.

185. Levy JA, Shimabukuro J. Recovery of AIDS-associated retroviruses from patients with AIDS or AIDS-related conditions and from clinically healthy individuals. *J Infect Dis* 1985;152:734–738.

186. Baltimore D, Feinberg MB. HIV revealed: toward a natural history of the infection [Editorial]. *N Engl J Med* 1990;321:1673–1675.

187. Pezzella M, Rossi P, Lombardi V, et al. HIV viral sequences in seronegative people at risk detected by *in situ* hybridisation and polymerase chain reaction. *Br Med J* 1989;298:713–716.

188. Laure F, Rouzioux C, et al. Detection of HIV-1 DNA in infants and children by means of the polymerase chain reaction. *Lancet* 1988;ii:538–541.

189. Resnick L, DiMarzo-Veronese F, Schupbach J, et al. Intra-blood-brain-barrier synthesis of HTLV-III-specific IgG in patients with neurologic symptoms associated with AIDS or AIDS-related complex. *N Engl J Med* 1985;313:1498–1504.

190. McArthur JC, Cohen BA, Selnes OA, et al. Low prevalence of neurological and neuropsychological abnormalities in otherwise healthy HIV-1-infected individuals: results from the multicenter AIDS cohort study. *Ann Neurol* 1989;26:601–611.

191. Janssen RS, Saykin AJ, Cannon L, et al. Neurological and neuropsychological manifestations of HIV-1 infection: association with AIDS-related complex but not asymptomatic HIV-1 infection. *Ann Neurol* 1989;26:592–600.

192. Hollander H. Cerebrospinal fluid normalities and abnormalities in individuals infected with human immunodeficiency virus. *J Infect Dis* 1988;158:855–858.

193. Peluso R, Haase A, Stowring L, Edwards M, Ventura P. A Trojan horse mechanism for the spread of visna virus in monocytes. *Virology* 1985;147:231–236.

194. Koenig S, Gendelman HE, Orenstein JM, et al. Detection of AIDS virus in macrophages in brain tissue from AIDS patients with encephalopathy. *Science* 1986;233:1089–1093.

195. Tourvieille B, Gorman SD, Field EH, Hunkapiller T, Parnes JR. Isolation and sequence of L3T4 complementary DNA clones: expression in T cells and brain. *Science* 1986;234:610–614.

196. Perry VH, Gordon S. Macrophages and microglia in the nervous system. *TINS* 1988;11:273–277.

197. Funke I, Hahn A, Rieber EP, Weiss E, Rietmuller G. The cellular receptor (CD4) of the human immunodeficiency virus is ex-

pressed on neurons and glial cells in human brain. *J Exp Med* 1987;165:1230–1235.

198. Gyorkey F, Melnick JL, Gyorkey P. Human immunodeficiency virus in brain biopsies of patients with AIDS and progressive encephalopathy. *J Infect Dis* 1987;155:870–876.

199. Cheng-Mayer C, Rutka JT, Rosenblum ML, McHugh T, Stites DP, Levy JA. Human immunodeficiency virus can productively infect cultured human glial cells. *Proc Natl Acad Sci USA* 1987;84:3526–3530.

200. Dewhurst S, Stevenson M, Volsky DJ. Expression of the T4 molecule (AIDS virus receptor) by human brain-derived cells. *FEBS Lett* 1987;213:133–137.

201. Cheng-Mayer C, Weiss C, Seto D, Levy JA. Isolates of human immunodeficiency virus type 1 from the brain may constitute a special group of the AIDS virus. *Proc Natl Acad Sci USA* 1989;86:8575–8579.

202. Resnick L, Berger JR, Shapshak P, Tourtellotte WW. Early penetration of the blood–brain-barrier by HIV. *Neurology* 1988;38:9–14.

203. Hollander H, Levy JA. Neurologic abnormalities and recovery of human immunodeficiency virus from cerebrospinal fluid. *Ann Intern Med* 1987;106:692–695.

204. Appelman ME, Marshall DW, Brey RL, et al. Cerebrospinal fluid abnormalities in patients without AIDS who are seropositive for human immunodeficiency virus. *J Infect Dis* 1988;158:193–199.

205. Brew BJ, Bhalla RB, Fleisher M, et al. Cerebrospinal fluid β_2-microglobulin in patients infected with human immunodeficiency virus. *Neurology* 1989;39:830–834.

206. McArthur JC, Sipos E, Cornblath DR, et al. Identification of mononuclear cells in CSF of patients with HIV infection. *Neurology* 1989;39:66–70.

207. Chiodi F, Norkrans G, Hagberg L, et al. Human immunodeficiency virus infection of the brain. II. Detection of intrathecally synthesized antibodies by enzyme linked immunosorbent assay and imprint immunofixation. *J Neurol Sci* 1988;87:37–48.

208. Reboul J, Schuller E, Pialoux G, et al. Immunoglobulins and complement components in 37 patients infected by HIV-1 virus: comparison of general (systemic) and intrathecal immunity. *J Neurol Sci* 1989;89:243–252.

209. Elovaara I, Iivanainen M, Valle S, Suni J, Tervo T, Lahdevirta J. CSF protein and cellular profiles in various stages of HIV infection related to neurological manifestations. *J Neurol Sci* 1987;78:331–342.

210. Kaiser R, Dorries R, Luer W, et al. Analysis of oligoclonal antibody bands against individual HIV structural proteins in the CSF of patients infected with HIV. *J Neurol* 1989;236:157–160.

211. Grimaldi LME, Castagna A, Lazzarein A, et al. Oligoclonal IgG bands in cerebrospinal fluid and serum during asymptomatic human immunodeficiency virus infection. *Ann Neurol* 1988; 24:277–279.

212. Elovaara I, Seppala I, Poutiainen E, Suni J, Valle S. Intrathecal humoral immunologic response in neurologically symptomatic and asymptomatic patients with human immunodeficiency infection. *Neurology* 1988;38:1451–1456.

213. Portegies P, Epstein LG, Hung ST, de Gans J, Goudsmit J. Human immunodeficiency virus type 1 antigen in cerebrospinal fluid: correlation with clinical neurologic status. *Arch Neurol* 1989;46:261–264.

214. Hadler NM, Gerwin RD, Frank MM, Whitaker JN, Baker M, Decker JL. The fourth component of complement in the cerebrospinal fluid in systemic lupus erythematosus. *Arthritis Rheum* 1973;16:507–520.

215. Gallo P, Frei K, Rordorf C, Lazdins J, Tavolato B, Fontana A. Human immunodeficiency virus type 1 (HIV-1) infection of the central nervous system: an evaluation of cytokines in cerebrospinal fluid. *J Neuroimmunol* 1989;23:109–116.

216. Heyes MP, Rubinow D, Lane C, Markey SP. Cerebrospinal fluid quinolinic acid concentrations are increased in acquired immune deficiency syndrome. *Ann Neurol* 1989;26:275–277.

217. Surtees R, Hyland K, Smith I. Central-nervous-system methyl-group metabolism in children with neurological complications of HIV infection. *Lancet* 1990;335:619–621.

218. Carne CA, Tedder RS, Smith A, et al. Acute encephalopathy coincident with seroconversion for anti-HTLV-III. *Lancet* 1985;ii:1206–1208.

219. Case Records of the Massachusetts General Hospital. Case 33-1989. *N Engl J Med* 1989;321:454–463.

220. Denning DW, Anderson J, Rudge P, Smith H. Acute myelopathy associated with primary infection with human immunodeficiency virus. *Br Med J* 1987;294:143–144.

221. Berger JR, Bender A, Resnick L, Perlmutter D. Spinal myoclonus associated with HTLV-III/LAV infection. *Arch Neurol* 1986; 43:1203–1204.

222. Brew BJ, Sidtis JJ, Rosenblum M, Price RW. AIDS–dementia complex. *J R Coll Physicians Lond* 1988;22:140–143.

223. Navia BA, Price RW. The acquired immunodeficiency syndrome dementia complex as the presenting or sole manifestation of human immunodeficiency virus infection. *Arch Neurol* 1987; 44:65–69.

224. Kovner R, Perecman E, Lazar W, et al. Relation of personality and attentional factors to cognitive deficits in human immunodeficiency virus-infected subjects. *Arch Neurol* 1989;46:274–277.

225. Currie J, Benson E, Ramsden B, Perdices M, Cooper D. Eye movement abnormalities as a predictor of the acquired immunodeficiency syndrome dementia complex. *Arch Neurol* 1988; 45:949–953.

226. Rottenberg DA, Moeller JR, Strother SC, et al. The metabolic pathology of the AIDS dementia complex. *Ann Neurol* 1987;22:700–706.

227. Walker DG, Itagaki S, Berry K, McGeer PL. Examination of brains of AIDS cases for human immunodeficiency virus and human cytomegalovirus nucleic acids. *J Neurol Neurosurg Psychiatry* 1989;52:583–590.

228. Lantos PL, McLaughlin JE, Scholtz CL, Berry CL, Tighe JR. Neuropathology of the brain in HIV infection. *Lancet* 1989; i:309–311.

229. Wiley CA, Schrier RD, Nelson JA, Lampert PW, Oldstone MBA. Cellular localization of the AIDS retrovirus infection within the brains of acquired immune deficiency syndrome patients. *Proc Natl Acad Sci USA* 1986;83:7089–7093.

230. de la Monte SM, Ho DD, Schooley RT, Hirsch MS, Richardson EP Jr. Subacute encephalomyelitis of AIDS and its relation to HTLV-III infection. *Neurology* 1987;37:562–569.

231. Pumarola-Sune T, Navia BA, Cordon-Cardo C, Cho E, Price RW. HIV antigen in the brains of patients with the AIDS dementia complex. *Ann Neurol* 1987;21:490–496.

232. Stoler MH, Eskin TA, Benn S, Angerer RC, Angerer LM. Human T-cell lymphotropic virus type III infection of the central nervous system. *JAMA* 1986;256:2360–2364.

233. Gabuzda DH, Ho DD, de la Monte SM, Hirsch MS, Rota TR, Sobel RA. Immunohistochemical identification of HTLV-III antigen in brains of patients with AIDS. *Ann Neurol* 1986;20:289–295.

234. Koyanagi Y, Miles S, Mitsuyasu RT, Merrill JE, Vinters HV, Chen ISY. Dual infection of the central nervous system by AIDS viruses with distinct cellular tropisms. *Science* 1987;236:819–822.

235. Cheng-Mayer C, Levy JA. Distinct biological and serological properties of human immunodeficiency viruses from the brain. *Ann Neurol* 1988;23:S58–S61.

236. Whetsell WO, Schwarcz R. Prolonged exposure to submicromolar concentrations of quinolinic acid causes excitotoxic damage in organotypic cultures of rat corticostriatal system. *Neurosci Lett* 1989;97:271–275.

237. Takikawa O, Yoshida R, Kido R, Hayaishi O. Tryptophan degradation in mice initiated by indoleamine 2,3-dioxygenase. *J Biol Chem* 1986;261:3648–3653.

238. Yoshida R, Oku T, Imanishi J, Kishida T, Hayaishi O. Interferon: a mediator of indoleamine 2,3-dioxygenase induction by lipopolysaccharide, poly(I)·poly(C), and pokeweed mitogen in mouse lung. *Arch Biochem Biophys* 1986;249:596–604.

239. Brenneman DE, Westbrook GL, Fitzgerald SP, et al. Neuronal cell killing by the envelope protein of HIV and its prevention by vasoactive intestinal peptide. *Nature* 1988;335:639–642.

240. Lenhardt TM, Wiley DA. Absence of humorally mediated dam-

age within the central nervous system of AIDS patients. *Neurology* 1989;39:278–280.

241. Sethi KK, Naher H, Stroehmann I. Phenotypic heterogeneity of cerebrospinal fluid-derived HIV-specific and HLA-restricted cytotoxic T-cell clones. *Nature* 1988;335:178–181.

242. American Academy of Pediatrics Task force on Pediatric AIDS. Perinatal human immunodeficiency virus infection. *Pediatrics* 1988;82:941–944.

243. Johnson JP, Nair P, Hines SE, et al. Natural history and serologic diagnosis of infants born to human immunodeficiency virus-infected women. *Am J Dis Child* 1989;143:1147–1153.

244. Selwyn PA, Schoenbaum EE, Davenny K, et al. Prospective study of human immunodeficiency virus infection and pregnancy outcomes in intravenous drug users. *JAMA* 1989; 261:1289–1309.

245. Blanche S, Rouzioux C, Moscato M, et al. A prospective study of infants born to women seropositive for human immunodeficiency virus type 1. *N Engl J Med* 1989;320:1643–1648.

246. Ryder RW, Nsa W, Hassig SE, et al. Perinatal transmission of the human immunodeficiency virus type 1 to infants of seropositive women in Zaire. *N Engl J Med* 1989;320:1637–1642.

247. Epstein LG, Sharer LR, Goudsmit J. Neurological and neuropathological features of human immunodeficiency virus infection in children. *Ann Neurol* 1988;23:S19–S23.

248. Davis SL, Halsted CC, Levy N, Ellis W. Acquired immune deficiency syndrome presenting as progressive infantile encephalopathy. *J Pediatr* 1987;110:884–888.

249. Rubinstein A. Background, epidemiology, and impact of HIV infection in children. *Ment Retard* 1989;27:209–211.

250. Mintz M, Epstein LG, Koenigsberger MR. Neurological manifestations of acquired immunodeficiency syndrome in children. *Int Pediatr* 1989;4:161–171.

251. Chatkupt S, Mintz M, Epstein LG, Bhansali D, Koeningsberger MR. Neuroimaging studies in children with human immunodeficiency virus type 1 infection (poster presentation). Child Neurology Society, 1989, abstract 86, p. 49.

252. Belman AL, Lantos G, Horoupian D, et al. AIDS: calcifications of the basal ganglia in infants and children. *Neurology* 1986;36:1192–1199.

253. Mintz M, Rapaport R, Oleske JM, et al. Elevated serum levels of tumor necrosis factor are associated with progressive encephalopathy in children with acquired immunodeficiency syndrome. *Am J Dis Child* 1989;143:771–774.

254. Nicholas SW, Sondheimer DL, Willoughby AD, Yaffe SJ, Katz SL. Human immunodeficiency virus infection in childhood, adolescence, and pregnancy: a status report and national research agenda. *Pediatrics* 1989;83:293–308.

255. Weiblen BJ, Lee FK, Cooper ER, et al. Early diagnosis of HIV infection in infants by detection of IgA HIV antibodies. *Lancet* 1990;335:988–990.

256. Walter EB, McKinney RE, Lane BA, Weinhold KJ, Wilfert CM. Interpretation of Western blots of specimens from children infected with human immunodeficiency virus type 1: implications for prognosis and diagnosis. *J Pediatrics* 1990;117:255–258.

257. Goetz DW, Hall SE, Harbison RW, Reid MJ. Pediatric acquired immunodeficiency syndrome with negative human immunodeficiency virus antibody response by enzyme-linked immunosorbent assay and Western blot. *Pediatrics* 1988;81:356–359.

258. Epstein LG, Boucher CAB, Morrison SH, et al. Persistent human immunodeficiency virus type 1 antigenemia in children correlates with disease progression. *Pediatrics* 1988;82:919–924.

259. Rogers MF, Ou C-Y, Rayfield M, et al. Use of the polymerase chain reaction for early detection of the proviral sequences of human immunodeficiency virus in infants born to seropositive mothers. *N Engl J Med* 1989;320:1649–1654.

260. Husson RN, Comeau AM, Huff R. Diagnosis of human immunodeficiency virus infection in infants and children. *Pediatrics* 1990;86:1–10.

261. The European Collaborative Study. Mother-to-child transmission of HIV infection. *Lancet* 1988;ii:1039–1043.

262. Nadal D, Hunziker U, Schüpbach J, et al. Immunological evaluation in the early diagnosis of prenatal or perinatal HIV infection. *Arch Dis Child* 1989;64:662–669.

263. Armstrong DD, Kirkpatrick JB. Neuropathology of pediatric AIDS. *Semin Pediatr Infect Dis* 1990;1:112–123.

264. Dickson DW, Belman AL, Kim TS, Horoupian DS, Rubinstein A. Spinal cord pathology in pediatric acquired immunodeficiency syndrome. *Neurology* 1989;39:227–235.

265. Rogers MF. AIDS in children: a review of the clinical, epidemiologic and public health aspects. *Pediatr Infect Dis* 1985;4:230–236.

266. Epstein LG, DiCarlo FJ, Joshi VV, et al. Primary lymphoma of the central nervous system in children with acquired immunodeficiency syndrome. *Pediatrics* 1988;82:355–363.

267. Berger JR, Moskowitz L, Fischl M, Kelley RE. Neurologic disease as the presenting manifestation of acquired immunodeficiency syndrome. *South Med J* 1987;80:683–686.

268. Levy RM, Bredesen DE, Rosenblum ML. Neurological manifestations of the acquired immunodeficiency syndrome (AIDS): experience at UCSF and review of the literature. *J Neurosurg* 1985;62:475–495.

269. Fischer P, Enzensberger W. Neurological complications in AIDS. *J Neurol* 1987;234:269–279.

270. Malouf R, Jacquette G, Dobkin J, Brust JCM. Neurologic disease in human immunodeficiency virus-infected drug abusers. *Arch Neurol* 1990;47:1002–1007.

271. Laskin OL, Stahl-Bayliss CM, Morgello S. Concomitant herpes simplex virus type 1 and cytomegalovirus ventriculoencephalitis in acquired immunodeficiency syndrome. *Arch Neurol* 1987; 44:843–847.

272. Jarvik JG, Hesselink JR, Kennedy C, et al. Acquired immunodeficiency syndrome: magnetic resonance patterns of brain involvement with pathologic correlation. *Arch Neurol* 1988;45:731–736.

273. Whitaker JN, Lisak RP, Bashir RM, et al. Immunoreactive myelin basic protein in the cerebrospinal fluid in neurological disorders. *Ann Neurol* 1980;7:58–64.

274. Marshall DW, Brey RL, Butzin CA. Lack of cerebrospinal fluid myelin basic protein in HIV-infected asymptomatic individuals with intrathecal synthesis. *Neurology* 1989;39:1127–1129.

275. Pfister HW, Einhaupl KM, Wick M, et al. Myelin basic protein in the cerebrospinal fluid of patients infected with HIV. *J Neurol* 1989;236:288–291.

276. Levy RM, Bredesen DE. Central nervous system dysfunction in acquired immunodeficiency syndrome. In: Rosenblum ML, Levy RM, Bredesen DE, eds. *AIDS and the nervous system.* New York: Raven Press, 1988:29–63.

277. Dix RD, Bredesen DE, Erlich KS, Mills J. Recovery of herpesviruses from cerebrospinal fluid of immunodeficient homosexual men. *Ann Neurol* 1985;18:611–614.

278. Gandy SE. Tuberculosis of the central nervous system: Recent experience and reappraisal. In: Plum F, ed. *Advances in contemporary neurology.* Philadelphia: FA Davis, 1988:153–184.

279. Navia BA, Petito CK, Gold JWM, Cho E, Jordan BD, Price RW. Cerebral toxoplasmosis complicating the acquired immune deficiency syndrome: clinical and neuropathological findings in 27 patients. *Ann Neurol* 1986;19:224–238.

280. McCabe R, Remington JS. Toxoplasmosis: the time has come. *N Engl J Med* 1988;318:313–315.

281. Horowitz SL, Bentson JR, Benson DF, Davos I, Pressman B, Gottlieb MS. CNS toxoplasmosis in acquired immunodeficiency syndrome. *Arch Neurol* 1983;40:649–652.

282. Luft BJ, Conley F, Remington JS, et al. Outbreak of central-nervous-system toxoplasmosis in western Europe and North America. *Lancet* 1983;i:781–784.

283. Luft BJ, Brooks RG, Conley FK, McCabe RE, Remington JS. Toxoplasmic encephalitis in patients with acquired immune deficiency syndrome. *JAMA* 1984;252:913–917.

284. So YT, Beckstead JH, Davis RL. Primary central nervous system lymphoma in acquired immune deficiency syndrome: a clinical and pathological study. *Ann Neurol* 1986;20:566–572.

285. O'Neill BP, Illig JJ. Primary central nervous system lymphoma. *Mayo Clin Proc* 1989;64:1005–1020.

286. Pauzner R, Mouallen M, Sadeh M, Tadmor R, Farfel Z. High incidence of primary cerebral lymphoma in tumor-induced central neurogenic hyperventilation. *Arch Neurol* 1989;46:510–512.

287. O'Neill BP, Kelly PJ, Earle JD, Scheithauer B, Banks PM. Com-

puter-assisted stereotaxic biopsy for the diagnosis of primary central nervous system lymphoma. *Neurology* 1987;37:1160–1164.

288. Rosenberg NL, Hochberg FH, Miller G, Kleinschmidt-DeMasters BK. Primary central nervous system lymphoma related to Epstein–Barr virus in a patient with acquired immune deficiency syndrome. *Ann Neurol* 1986;20:98–102.

289. Walker DL. Progressive multifocal leukoencephalopathy. In: Vinken PJ, Bruyn GW, Klawans HL, eds. *Handbook of clinical neurology. Demyelinating diseases,* vol 47. Amsterdam: Elsevier, 1985:503–524.

290. Levy RM, Bredesen DE, Rosenblum ML. Neurological manifestations of the acquired immunodeficiency syndrome (AIDS): experience at UCSF and review of the literature. *J Neurosurg* 1986;62:475–495.

291. Krupp LB, Lipton RB, Swerdlow ML, Leeds NE, Llena J. Progressive multifocal leukoencephalopathy: clinical and radiographic features. *Ann Neurol* 1985;17:107–116.

292. Snider WD, Simpson DM, Nielson S, Gold JWM, Metroka CE, Posner JB. Neurological complications of the acquired immunodeficiency syndrome: analysis of 50 patients. *Ann Neurol* 1983;14:403–418.

293. Miller JR, Barrett RE, Britton CB, et al. Progressive multifocal leukoencephalopathy in a male homosexual with T-cell immune deficiency. *N Engl J Med* 1982;307:1436–1438.

294. Levy JD, Cottingham KL, Campbell RJ, et al. Progressive multifocal leukoencephalopathy and magnetic resonance imaging. *Ann Neurol* 1986;19:399–400.

295. Aksamit AJ, Gendelman HE, Orenstein JM, Pezeshkpour GH. AIDS-associated progressive multifocal leukoencephalopathy (PML): comparison to non-AIDS PML with *in situ* hybridization and immunohistochemistry. *Neurology* 1990;40:1073–1078.

296. Aksamit AJ, Mourrain P, Sever JL, Major EO. Progressive multifocal leukoencephalopathy: investigation of three cases using *in situ* hybridization with JC virus biotinylated DNA probe. *Ann Neurol* 1985;18:490–496.

297. Kenney S, Natarajan V, Strike D, Khoury G, Salzman NP. JC virus enhancer–promoter active in human brain cells. *Science* 1984;226:1337–1339.

298. Small JA, Scangos GA, Cork L, Jay G, Khoury G. The early region of human papovavirus JC induces dysmyelination in transgenic mice. *Cell* 1986;46:13–18.

299. Berger JR, Mucke L. Prolonged survival and partial recovery in AIDS-associated progressive multifocal leukoencephalopathy. *Neurology* 1988;38:1060–1065.

300. Yankner BA, Skolnik PR, Shoukimas GM, Gabuzda DH, Sobel RA, Ho DD. Cerebral granulomatous angiitis associated with isolation of human T-lymphotropic virus type III from the central nervous system. *Ann Neurol* 1986;20:362–364.

301. Garcia I, Fainstein V, Rios A, et al. Nonbacterial thrombotic endocarditis in a male homosexual with Kaposi's sarcoma. *Arch Intern Med* 1983;143:1243–1245.

302. Leaf AN, Laubenstein LJ, Raphael B, Hochster H, Baez L, Karpatkin S. Thrombotic thrombocytopenic purpura associate with human immunodeficiency virus type 1 (HIV-1) infection. *Ann Intern Med* 1988;109:194–197.

303. Fuller GN, Guiloff RJ, Scaravilli F, Harcourt-Webster JN. Combined HIV–CMV encephalitis presenting with brainstem signs. *J Neurol Neurosurg Psychiatry* 1989;52:975–979.

304. Masdeu JC, Small CB, Weiss L, Elkin CM, Llena J, Mesa-Tejada R. Multifocal cytomegalovirus encephalitis in AIDS. *Ann Neurol* 1988;23:97–99.

305. Petito CK, Cho E, Lemann W, Navia BA, Price RW. Neuropathology of acquired immunodeficiency syndrome (AIDS): an autopsy review. *J Neuropathol Exp Neurol* 1986;45:635–646.

306. Behar R, Wiley C, McCutchan JA. Cytomegalovirus polyradiculoneuropathy in acquired immune deficiency syndrome. *Neurology* 1987;37:557–561.

307. Ryder JW, Croen K, Kleinschmidt-DeMaster BK, Ostrove JM, Straus SE, Cohn DL. Progressive encephalitis three months after resolution of cutaneous zoster in a patient with AIDS. *Ann Neurol* 1986;19:182–188.

308. Gilden DH, Murray RS, Wellish M, Kleinschmidt-DeMasters BK, Vafai A. Chronic progressive varicella-zoster virus encephalitis in an AIDS patient. *Neurology* 1988;38:1150–1153.

309. Britton CB, Mesa-Tejeda R, Fenoglio CM, Hays AP, Garvey GG, Miller JR. A new complication of AIDS: thoracic myelitis caused by herpes simplex virus. *Neurology* 1985;35:1071–1074.

310. Chuck SL, Sande MA. Infections with *Cryptococcus neoformans* in the acquired immunodeficiency syndrome. *N Engl J Med* 1989;321:794–799.

311. Berlin L, Pincus JH. Cryptococcal meningitis: false-negative antigen test results and cultures in nonimmunosuppressed patients. *Arch Neurol* 1989;46:1312–1316.

312. Kaplan LD, Abrams DI, Feigal E, et al. AIDS-associated non-Hodgkin's lymphoma in San Francisco. *JAMA* 1989;261:719–724.

313. Young L, Alfieri C, Hennessy K, et al. Expression of Epstein–Barr virus transformation-associated genes in tissues of patients with EBV lymphoproliferative disease. *N Engl J Med* 1989;321:1080–1085.

314. Ziegler JL, Beckstead JA, Volberding PA, et al. Non-hodgkin's lymphoma in 90 homosexual men. *N Engl J Med* 1984;311:565–570.

315. Centers for Disease Control. Tuberculosis and acquired immunodeficiency syndrome—Florida. *MMWR* 1986;35:587–580.

316. Pitchenik AE, Burr J, Cole CH. Tuberculin testing for persons with positive serologic studies for HTLV-III. *N Engl J Med* 1986;314:447.

317. Reider HL, Cauthen GM, Kelly GD, Bloch AB, Snider DE Jr. Tuberculosis in the United States. *JAMA* 1989;262:385–389.

318. Selwyn PA, Hartel D, Lewis VA, et al. A prospective study of the risk of tuberculosis among intravenous drug users with human immunodeficiency virus infection. *N Engl J Med* 1989;320:545–550.

319. Woolsey RM, Chambers TJ, Chung HD, McGarry JD. Mycobacterial meningomyelitis associated with human immunodeficiency virus infection. *Arch Neurol* 1988;45:691–693.

320. Pitchenik AE, Cole C, Russell BW, Fischl MA, Spira TJ, Snider DE Jr. Tuberculosis, atypical mycobacteriosis, and the acquired immunodeficiency syndrome among Haitian and non-Haitian patients in south Florida. *Ann Intern Med* 1984;101:641–645.

321. Case Record of the Massachusetts General Hospital. Case 2-1986: a 58-year-old woman with fever and nodular pulmonary infiltrates. *N Engl J Med* 1986;314:167–174.

322. Sunderam G, Mangura BT, Lombardo JM, Reichman LB. Failure of "optimal" four-drug short-course tuberculosis chemotherapy in a compliant patient with human immunodeficiency virus. *Am Rev Respir Dis* 1987;136:1475–1478.

323. Tramont EC. Syphilis in the AIDS era. *N Engl J Med* 1987;316:1600–1601.

324. Berry CD, Hooton TM, Collier AC, Lukehart SA. Neurologic relapse after benzathine penicillin therapy for secondary syphilis in a patient with HIV infection. *N Engl J Med* 1987;316:1587–1589.

325. Johns DR, Tierney M, Parker SW. Pure motor hemiplegia due to meningovascular neurosyphilis. *Arch Neurol* 1987;44:1062–1065.

326. Johns DR, Tierney M, Felsenstein D. Alteration in the natural history of neurosyphilis by concurrent infection with the human immunodeficiency virus. *N Engl J Med* 1987;316:1569–1572.

327. Lanska MJ, Lanska DJ, Schmidley JW. Syphilitic polyradiculopathy in an HIV-positive man. *Neurology* 1988;38:1297–1301.

328. Sparling PF. Diagnosis and treatment of syphilis. *N Engl J Med* 1971;284:642–653.

329. Hicks CB, Benson PM, Lupton GP, Tramont EC. Seronegative secondary syphilis in a patient infected with the human immunodeficiency virus. *Ann Intern Med* 1987;107:492–494.

330. Katz DA, Berger JR. Neurosyphilis in acquired immunodeficiency syndrome. *Arch Neurol* 1989;46:895–898.

331. Feraru ER, Aronow HA, Lipton RB. Neurosyphilis in AIDS patients: initial CSF VDRL may be negative. *Neurology* 1990;40:541–543.

332. Maagan S, Wormser GP, Widerhorn J, Sy ER, Kim YH, Ernst JA. *Strongyloides stercoralis* hyperinfection in a patient with the acquired immune deficiency syndrome. *Am J Med* 1987;83:945–948.

333. Goldstick L, Mandybur TI, Bode R. Spinal cord degeneration in AIDS. *Neurology* 1985;35:103–106.

334. Helwig-Larsen S, Jakobsen J, Boesen F, et al. Myelopathy in AIDS. A clinical and electrophysiological study of 23 Danish patients. *Acta Neurol Scand* 1988;77:64–73.

335. Jakobsen J, Smith T, Gaub J, Helweg-Larsen S, Trojaborg W. Progressive neurological dysfunction during latent HIV infection. *Br Med J* 1989;299:225–228.

336. Scott JM, Wilson P, Dinn JJ, et al. Pathogenesis of subacute combined degeneration: a result of methyl group deficiency. *Lancet* 1981;ii:334–337.

337. Cortes E, Detels R, Aboulafia D, et al. HIV-1, HIV-2, and HTLV-1 infection in high-risk groups in Brazil. *N Engl J Med* 1989;320:953–958.

338. Page JB, Lai S, Chitwood DD, Klimas NG, Smith PC, Fletcher MA. HTLV-I/II seropositivity and death from AIDS among HIV-1 seropositive intravenous drug users. *Lancet* 1990; 335:1439–1441.

339. Aboulafia DM, Saxton EH, Koga H, Diagne A, Rosenblatt JD. A patient with progressive myelopathy and antibodies to human T-cell leukemia virus type I and human immunodeficiency virus type 1 in serum and cerebrospinal fluid. *Arch Neurol* 1990; 47:477–479.

340. Wiley CA, Nerenberg M, Cros D, Soto-Aguilar MC. HTLV-I polymyositis in a patient also infected with the human immunodeficiency virus. *N Engl J Med* 1989;320:992–995.

341. Brown MM, Thompson A, Goh BT, Forster GE, Swash M. Bell's palsy and HIV infection. *J Neurol Neurosurg Psychiatry* 1988;51:425–426.

342. Cornblath DR, McArthur JC, Kennedy PGE, Witte AS, Griffin JW. Inflammatory demyelinating peripheral neuropathies associated with human T-cell lymphotropic virus type III infection. *Ann Neurol* 1987;21:32–40.

343. Riggs JE, Rogers JSI, Schochet SS, Gutmann L. AIDS-related neuropathy. *West Va Med J* 1987;83:167–169.

344. de la Monte SM, Gabuzda DH, Ho DD, et al. Peripheral neuropathy in the acquired immunodeficiency syndrome. *Ann Neurol* 1988;23:485–492.

345. Miller RG, Parry GJ, Pfaeffl W, Lang W, Lippert R, Kiprov D. The spectrum of peripheral neuropathy associated with ARC and AIDS. *Muscle Nerve* 1988;11:857–863.

346. Cornblath DR, McArthur JC. Predominantly sensory neuropathy in patients with AIDS and AIDS-related complex. *Neurology* 1988;38:794–796.

347. Charnock E, Newton N. Case report: AIDS peripheral neuropathy. *Am J Med Sci* 1989;298:256–260.

348. Bailey RO, Baltch AL, Venkatesh R, Singh JK, Bishop MB. Sensory motor neuropathy associated with AIDS. *Neurology* 1988;38:886–891.

349. So YT, Holtzman DM, Abrams DI, Olney RK. Peripheral neuropathy associated with acquired immunodeficiency syndrome. *Arch Neurol* 1988;45:945–948.

350. Rance NE, McArthur JC, Cornblath DR, Landstrom DL, Griffin JW, Price DL. Gracile tract degeneration in patients with sensory neuropathy and AIDS. *Neurology* 1988;38:265–271.

351. Miller RG, Storey JR, Greco CM. Ganciclovir in the treatment of progressive AIDS-related polyradiculopathy. *Neurology* 1990; 40:569–574.

352. Eidelberg D, Sotrel A, Vogel H, Walker P, Kleefield J, Crumpacker CS III. Progressive polyradiculopathy in acquired immune deficiency syndrome. *Neurology* 1986;36:912–916.

353. Cohen JA, Laudenslager M. Autonomic nervous system involvement in patients with human immunodeficiency virus infection. *Neurology* 1989;39:1111–1112.

354. Miller RF, Semple SJG. Autonomic neuropathy in AIDS [Letter to the editor]. *Lancet* 1987;ii:343–344.

355. Lange DJ, Britton CB, Younger DS, Hays AP. The neuromuscular manifestations of human immunodeficiency virus infections. *Arch Neurol* 1988;45:1084–1088.

356. Stern R, Gold J, DiCarlo EF. Myopathy complicating the acquired immune deficiency syndrome. *Muscle Nerve* 1987; 10:318–322.

357. Helbert M, Fletcher T, Peddle B, Harris JRW, Pinching AJ. Zidovudine-associated myopathy. *Lancet* 1988;ii:689–690.

358. Panegyres PK, Tan N, Kakulas BA, Armstrong JA, Hollings-worth P. Necrotising myopathy and zidovudine. *Lancet* 1988; i:1050–1051.

359. Simpson DM, Bender AN. Human immunodeficiency virus-associated myopathy: Analysis of 11 patients. *Ann Neurol* 1988;24:79–84.

360. Fischl MA, Richman DD, Causey DM, et al. Prolonged zidovudine therapy in patients with AIDS and advanced AIDS-related complex. *JAMA* 1989;262:2405–2410.

361. Gorard DA, Henry K, Guiloff RJ. Necrotising myopathy and zidovudine. *Lancet* 1988;i:1050.

362. Dalakas M, Pezeshkpour GH. AZT-induced destructive inflammatory myopathy with abnormal mitochondria (DIM-Mi): study of seven patients [Abstract]. *Neurology* 1989;1(Suppl):152.

363. Pezeshkpour G, Dalakas M. A comparative study of the electron microscopic findings in the muscle biopsy specimens from patients with myopathies due to AZT and human immunodeficiency virus [Abstract]. *Neurology* 1990;1(Suppl):237.

364. Dalakas MC, Illa I, Pezeshkpour GH, Laukaitis JP, Cohen B, Griffin JL. Mitochondrial myopathy caused by long-term zidovudine therapy. *N Engl J Med* 1990;322:1098–1105.

365. Bessen LJ, Greene JB, Louie E, Seitzman P, Weinberg H. Severe polymyositis-like syndrome associated with zidovudine therapy of AIDS and ARC. *N Engl J Med* 1988;318:708.

366. Yarchoan R, Mitsuya H, Broder S. AIDS therapies. *Sci Am* 1988;259:110–119.

367. Yarchoan R, Mitsuya H, Myers CE, Broder S. Clinical pharmacology of 3'-azido-2',3'-dideoxythymidine (zidovudine) and related dideoxynucleosides. *N Engl J Med* 1989;321:726–738.

368. Poli G, Orenstein JM, Kinter A, Folks TM, Fauci AS. Interferon-α but not AZT suppresses HIV expression in chronically infected cell lines. *Science* 1989;244:575–578.

369. Fischl MA, Richman DD, Grieco MH, et al. The efficacy of azidothymidine (AZT) in the treatment of patients with AIDS and AIDS-related complex. *N Engl J Med* 1987;317:185–191.

370. Volberding PA, Lagakos SW, Koch MA, et al. Zidovudine in asymptomatic human immunodeficiency virus infection: a controlled trial in persons with fewer than 500 CD4-positive cells per cubic millimeter. *N Engl J Med* 1990;322:941–949.

371. Fishman DA, Fischl MA, Grieco MH, et al. The toxicity of azidothymidine (AZT) in the treatment of patients with AIDS and AIDS-related complex. *N Engl J Med* 1987;317:192–197.

372. Yarchoan R, Broder S. Development of antiretroviral therapy for the acquired immunodeficiency syndrome and related disorders: a progress report. *N Engl J Med* 1987;316:557–564.

373. Lyman WD, Tanaka KE, Kress Y, Rashbaum WK, Rubinstein A, Soeiro R. Zidovudine concentrations in human fetal tissue: implications for perinatal AIDS [Letter to the editor]. *Lancet* 1990;335:1280–1281.

374. Larder BA, Kemp SD. Multiple mutations in HIV-1 reverse transcriptase confer high-level resistance to zidovudine (AZT). *Science* 1989;246:1155–1158.

375. Larder BA, Darby G, Richman DD. HIV with reduced sensitivity to zidovudine (AZT) isolated during prolonged therapy. *Science* 1989;243:1731–1734.

376. Boucher CAB, Tersmette M, Lange JMA, et al. Zidovudine sensitivity of human immunodeficiency viruses from high-risk, symptom-free individuals during therapy. *Lancet* 1990;336:585–590.

377. Fishman DD, Fischl MA, Grieco MH, et al. The toxicity of azidothymidine (AZT) in the treatment of patients with AIDS and AIDS-related complex. *N Engl J Med* 1987;317:192–197.

378. Fischl M, Galpin JE, Levine JD, et al. Recombinant human erythropoietin for patients with AIDS treated with zidovudine. *N Engl J Med* 1990;322:1488–1493.

379. Hagler DN, Frame PT. Azidothymidine neurotoxicity. *Lancet* 1986;2:1392.

380. Davtyan DG, Vinters HV. Wernicke's encephalopathy in AIDS patient treated with zidovudine. *Lancet* 1987;1:919–920.

381. Yarchoan R, Bewrg G, Brouwers P, et al. Response of human-immunodeficiency-virus associated neurological disease to 3'-azido-2',3'-deoxythymidine. *Lancet* 1987;i:132–135.

382. Fiala M, Cone LA, Cohen N, et al. Responses of neurologic complications of AIDS to 3'-azido-3'-deoxythymidine and 9-(1,3-dihydroxy-2-propoxymethyl)guanine. I. Clinical features. *Rev Infect Dis* 1988;10:250–256.

383. Portegies P, de Gans J, Lange JMA, et al. Declining incidence of AIDS dementia complex after introduction of zidovudine treatment. *Br Med J* 1989;299:819–821.

384. Schmitt FA, Bigley JW, McKinnis R, et al. Neuropsychological outcome of zidovudine (AZT) treatment of patients with AIDS and AIDS-related complex. *N Engl J Med* 1988;319:1573–1578.

385. Pizzo PA. Emerging concepts in the treatment of HIV infection in children. *JAMA* 1989;262:1989–1992.

386. Pizzo PA, Eddy J, et al. Effect of continuous intravenous infusion of zidovudine (AZT) in children with symptomatic HIV infection. *N Engl J Med* 1988;319:889–896.

387. Yarchoan R, Mitsuya H, Thomas RV, et al. *In vivo* activity against HIV and favorable toxicity profile of 2′,3′-dideoxyinosine. *Science* 1989;245:412–415.

388. Yarchoan R, Thomas RV, Allain J-P, et al. Phase I studies of 2′,3′-dideoxycytidine in severe human immunodeficiency virus infection as a single agent and alternating with zidovudine (AZT). *Lancet* 1988;i:76–81.

389. Lambert JS, Seidlin M, Reichman RC, et al. 2′,3′-Dideoxyinosine (ddIO in patients with the acquired immunodeficiency syndrome or AIDS-related complex: a phase I trial. *N Engl J Med* 1990;322:1333–1340.

390. Cooley TP, Kunches LM, Saunders CA, et al. Once-daily administration of 2′,3′-dideoxyinosine (ddI) in patients with the acquired immunodeficiency syndrome or AIDS-related complex: results of a phase I trial. *N Engl J Med* 1990;322:1340–1345.

391. Yarchoan R, Pluda JM, Thomas RV, et al. Long-term toxicity/activity profile of 2′,3′-dideoxyinosine in AIDS or AIDS-related complex. *Lancet* 1990;336:526–529.

392. Bach MC. Clinical response to dideoxyinosine in patients with HIV infection resistant to zidovudine [Letter to the editor]. *N Engl J Med* 1990;323:275.

393. Schooley RT, Merigan TC, Gaut P, et al. Recombinant soluble CD4 therapy in patients with the acquired immunodeficiency syndrome (AIDS) and AIDS-related complex: a phase I–II escalating dosage trial. *Ann Intern Med* 1990;112:247–253.

394. Wetterberg L, Alexius B, Saaf J, Sonnenborg A, Britton S, Pert C. Peptide T in treatment of AIDS [Letter to the editor]. *Lancet* 1987;i:159.

395. Roberts NA, Martin JA, Kinchinston D, et al. Rational design of peptide-based HIV proteinase inhibitors. *Science* 1990;248:358–361.

396. Erickson J, Neidhart DJ, VanDrie J, et al. Design, activity, and 2.8 Å crystal structure of a C2 symmetric inhibitor complexed to HIV-1 protease. *Science* 1990;249:527–532.

397. Ho DD, Hartshorn KL, Rota TR, et al. Recombinant human interferon-α suppresses HTLV-III replication *in vitro*. *Lancet* 1985;i:602–604.

398. Crumpacker C, Heagy W, Bubley G, et al. Ribavirin treatment of the acquired immunodeficiency syndrome (AIDS) and the acquired-immunodeficiency-syndrome-related complex (ARC). *Ann Intern Med* 1987;107:664–674.

399. Sarver N, Cantin EM, Chang PS, et al. Ribozymes as potential anti-HIV-1 therapeutic agents. *Science* 1990;247:1222–1225.

400. Buck HM, Koole LH, van Genderen MHP, et al. Phosphate-methylated DNA aimed at HIV-1 RNA loops and integrated DNA inhibits viral infectivity. *Science* 1990;248:208–212.

401. Mitsuya H, Broder S. Strategies for antiviral therapy in AIDS. *Nature* 1987;325:773–778.

402. Crumpacker CS II. Molecular targets of antiviral therapy. *N Engl J Med* 1989;321:163–172.

403. Reisinger EC, Kern P, Ernst M, et al. Inhibition of HIV progression by dithiocarb. *Lancet* 1990;335:679–682.

404. Pedersen C, Sandström E, Petersen CS, et al. The efficacy of inosine pranobex in preventing the acquired immunodeficiency syndrome in patients with human immunodeficiency virus infection. *N Engl J Med* 1990;322:1757–1763.

405. Lemaitre M, Guétard D, Hénin Y, Montagnier L, Zerial A. Protective activity of tetracycline analogs against the cytopathic effect of the human immunodeficiency viruses in CEM cells. *Res Virol* 1990;141:5–16.

406. Szebeni J, Wahl SM, Popovic M, et al. Dipyridamole potentiates the inhibition by 3′-azido-3′-deoxythymidine and other dideoxynucleosides of human immunodeficiency virus replication in monocyte-macrophages. *Proc Natl Acad Sci USA* 1989;86:3842–3846.

407. Laskin O, Cederberg DM, Mills J, Eron LJ, Mildvan D, Spector SA. Ganciclovir for the treatment and suppression of serious infections caused by cytomegalovirus. *Am J Med* 1987;83:201–207.

408. Waskin H, Stehr-Green JK, Helmick CG, Sattler FR. Risk factors for hypoglycemia associated with pentamidine therapy for *Pneumocystis* pneumonia. *JAMA* 1988;260:345–347.

409. Holmes VF, Fricchione GL. Hypomania in an AIDS patient receiving amitriptyline for neuropathic pain. *Neurology* 1989;39:305.

410. Wulff CH, Hoyer H, Asboe-Hansen G, Brodhagen H. Development of polyneuropathy during thalidomide therapy. *Br J Dermatol* 1985;112:475–480.

411. Youle M, Clarbour J, Farthing C, et al. Treatment of resistant aphthous ulceration with thalidomide in patients positive for HIV antibody. *Br Med J* 1989;298:432.

412. Matthews TJ, Bolognesi DP. AIDS vaccines. *Sci Am* 1988;259:120–127.

413. Schild GC, Minor PD. Human immunodeficiency virus and AIDS: challenges and progress. *Lancet* 1990;335:1081–1084.

414. Orentas RJ, Hildreth JEK, Obah E, et al. Induction of CD4+ human cytolytic T cells specific for HIV-infected cells by a gp160 subunit vaccine. *Science* 1990;248:1234–1237.

415. Karacostas V, Nagashima K, Gonda MA, Moss B. Human immunodeficiency virus-like particles produced by a vaccinia virus expression vector. *Proc Natl Acad Sci USA* 1989;86:8964–8967.

416. Bolognesi DP. Do antibodies enhance the infection of cells by HIV? *Nature* 1989;340:431–432.

417. Choppin PW, Richardson CD, Merz DC, et al. The functions and inhibition of the membrane glycoproteins of paramyxoviruses and myxoviruses and the role of the measles virus M protein in subacute sclerosing panencephalitis. *J Infect Dis* 1981;143:352.

418. Committee on Infectious Diseases. *Report of the Committee on Infectious Diseases*, 21st ed. Elk Grove Village, IL: American Academy of Pediatrics, 1988;91–115.

419. Miotti PG, Nelson KE, Dallabetta GA, et al. The influence of HIV infection on antibody responses to a two-dose regimen of influenza vaccine. *JAMA* 1989;262:779–783.

420. Halsey NA, Henderson DA. HIV infection and immunization against other agents. *N Engl J Med* 1987;316:683–685.

421. Redfield RR, Wright DC, James WD, Jones TS, Brown C, Burke DS. Disseminated vaccinia in a military recruit with human immunodeficiency virus (HIV) disease. *N Engl J Med* 1987;316:673–675.

422. Chaisson RE, Volberding PA. Clinical manifestations of HIV infection. In: Mandel GL, Douglas RG Jr, Bennett JE, eds. *Principles and practice of infectious disease*, 3rd ed. New York: Churchill Livingston, 1990;1062.

Infections of the Central Nervous System,
edited by W. M. Scheld, R. J. Whitley, and
D. T. Durack, Raven Press, Ltd., New York © 1991.

CHAPTER 11

Viral Vaccines that Protect the Central Nervous System

Mark F. Mangano and Stanley A. Plotkin

Vaccines have been a prominent force in protecting children and adults against neurological damage caused by infectious agents. In this chapter we have chosen to discuss five of the most prominent viral vaccines in use today: polio, measles, mumps, rabies, and Japanese B encephalitis. This list is by no means exhaustive. One might have also discussed either (a) the profound impact of rubella vaccine on the encephalitis of rubella syndrome or (b) the rapidly improving effects of *Hemophilus influenzae* type b vaccination on meningitis. Nevertheless, the examples we have chosen comprise three diseases in which the infection is primarily of the central nervous system (polio, rabies, and Japanese B encephalitis) and two diseases in which neurological involvement is an important complication (measles and mumps). Thus, the range and effectiveness of prevention by vaccination, as well as the differences between living and nonliving products, should be apparent.

MEASLES

History

Written records of disease processes that probably correspond to modern-day measles can be found as far back as the 10th century. In that period, a Persian physician named Rhazes described such a disease (164) and

even referred to similar work done by the Hebrew physician El Yahudi, some 300 years earlier (50). Rhazes was the first to be clinically able to distinguish between measles and smallpox (164).

Measles was first described in the United States by John Hall, who wrote of the Boston epidemic of 1657. It was noted that the frequency of U.S. epidemics increased as the population increased and as faster ships were built (which were capable of more frequent contact with the epidemics in Europe) (50).

In 1846, a Danish physician named Peter Panum first described the 14-day incubation period of measles and noted that immunity after infection lasted a lifetime (164). In 1896, Henry Koplik described the enanthem that often precedes the typical measles rash and that now bears his name. Human measles virus was first transmitted to monkeys in a set of experiments done by Goldberger and Anderson in 1911, thus demonstrating that the disease was caused by a small transmissible infectious agent (164). A U.S. physician named Harry Plotz was first able to culture the virus *in vitro* in 1938; however, it was not until the 1950s that this technique became reliable, through the use of cell culture (50). The first licensed vaccine appeared shortly thereafter, in March 1963.

Virology

Measles virus is a single-stranded (negative-sense) RNA virus of the genus *Morbillivirus,* in the Paramyxoviridae family. It is a spherical, enveloped virus, ranging from 120 to 300 nm in diameter (164). The RNA packaged in the viral particles is approximately 20,000 nucleotides in length. The viral particle is composed of six proteins: Three of these are complexed with the RNA

M. F. Mangano: Division of Infectious Diseases, The Children's Hospital of Philadelphia, Philadelphia, Pennsylvania 19104; and The Wistar Institute, Philadelphia, Pennsylvania 19104.

S. A. Plotkin: Division of Infectious Diseases, The Children's Hospital of Philadelphia, Philadelphia, Pennsylvania 19104; The Wistar Institute, Philadelphia, Pennsylvania 19104; and Departments of Pediatrics and Microbiology, The University of Pennsylvania, Philadelphia, Pennsylvania 19104.

[nucleocapsid protein (NP), large protein (L), and a phosphoprotein (P)], and three are associated with the envelope (84). The two outer envelope proteins (F protein and H protein) are glycosylated. The F protein is involved in viral-cell fusion and cell membrane penetration, and the H protein is responsible for the viral hemagglutination characteristics. The third envelope protein, the matrix (M) protein, is thought to be involved in viral particle assembly, as well as in budding from the cell membrane (50). Lack of formation of antibodies to the F protein in an infection is thought to result in "atypical" measles, and lack of antibodies to the M protein has been associated with subacute sclerosing panencephalitis (SSPE), a chronic form of measles encephalitis (164). The virus is fairly labile and can be inactivated by sunlight, heat, or extremes in pH.

Although it is possible to culture the virus *in vitro,* it is technically difficult, and a clinical diagnosis is most often confirmed on the basis of serology rather than on isolation of the virus from a clinical specimen. If one wishes to grow the virus, the best host cells for *in vitro* growth of a direct clinical isolate are primary cells (human fetal cells, infant kidney cells, or monkey kidney cells). On subsequent passages, a wider variety of cells may be used (human amnion cells, human embryonic lung cells, HeLa cells, chick embryo cells, etc.) (164). Cytopathic effects (CPEs) seen histologically from direct clinical specimens or from virus during its first passage in tissue culture consist of multinucleated syncytia formation, whereas spindle-shaped cells or stellate-shaped cells without syncytia are seen after multiple passages.

Time-course studies of *in vitro* cell infection have shown viral attachment to the host cell membrane in the first hour post-inoculation. There is next seen an "eclipse period," lasting from 6 to 12 hr, during which time no viral proteins can be detected. At about 12 hr post-inoculation, viral antigens can be seen in the perinuclear cytoplasm. These migrate through the cytoplasm over the next 12 hr, and they can be found on the cell surface by 30 hr post-inoculation (50).

Epidemiology

Measles is a highly contagious virus, with a secondary infection rate of greater than 90% of susceptible contacts (164). Just prior to the institution of vaccination programs, reported infection rates in the United States ranged from 200,000 to 600,000 cases yearly. Conditions of urban crowding improved viral spread, and widespread epidemics were seen every few years, lasting a few months at a time. The interval between epidemics decreased as crowded conditions worsened. With the institution of a measles vaccine, infection rates plummeted, dropping from 315 cases per 100,000 population per year to less than 1.5 cases per 100,000 per year (average U.S. rate, 1981–1987) (50) (Fig. 1). Prior to the institution of an immunization program, school-aged children made up the largest infected group, with the 5- to 9-year-old group accounting for 53% of all infections in 1960–1964. This pattern changed after the introduction of the vaccine in 1963, and younger children (0- to 4-year-olds) and adolescents now make up the majority of those infected (27% and 42%, respectively, 1984–1985) (164).

The virus is spread by the respiratory route via fomites. Outbreaks are most commonly seen during the late

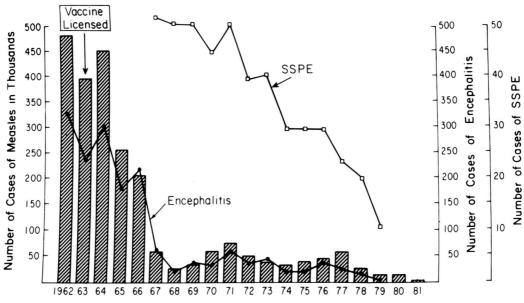

FIG. 1. Number of reported cases of measles, measles encephalitis, and subacute sclerosing panencephalitis (SSPE) in the United States, 1962–1981. (From ref. 116a, with permission.)

winter and early spring. Patients are maximally contagious during the prodromal period, a few days prior to development of the typical rash.

There is no evidence of the existence of an asymptomatic carrier state in humans (164), and although the virus can be spread to monkeys by the respiratory route (50), there is no known common animal reservoir. This would seem to imply that a total eradication of the disease should be possible with a vaccination program; however, since the virus is so contagious and ubiquitous, a large portion of the population will have to be made immune prior to eradication. Recent outbreaks have illustrated the ability of the virus to "seek out" the few susceptibles in the population and infect them (81).

Clinical Considerations

Typical Measles

Infection with the measles virus usually occurs when viral-laden fomites land on and infect epithelial cells of the conjunctiva or upper respiratory tract. Over the next 2 days, local viral replication occurs, with spread of the virus to the regional lymph nodes. A primary viremia occurs about the third day post-infection, with spread of the virus to distant locations. Multiplication continues at the sites initially infected, as well as at the secondarily infected sites, and by the fifth to the seventh day a second viremia takes place. At this point, there is seeding of the virus to the lower respiratory tract and the skin, and clinical symptoms start on the 10th to 14th day post-infection. These include a fever, which is initially mild but which progressively worsens over the next few days. In addition, a cough, coryza, and conjunctivitis are usually present. The pathognomonic enanthem which Koplik described usually appears about 2–3 days after the onset of symptoms. It appears as white patches, initially next to the molars on the buccal mucosa, but eventually it spreads to include much of the mucosa. These patches are regions of local viral replication within the epithelial cells of the mucosa. One to two days later, the typical exanthem appears. This usually coincides with the peak of the fevers and with the peak of the respiratory symptoms. It starts on the forehead and behind the ears and then progresses in a rostral-to-caudal direction, sequentially involving the neck, trunk, upper extremities, buttocks, and lower extremities, all within 3 days. The rash is erythematous, maculopapular in appearance, and nonpruritic. It can become confluent at its peak. After a day or so, it starts to fade, and this fading also progresses from head to foot. The rash initially blanches with pressure; however, after fading starts, it can appear brownish and no longer blanches. Virus can be isolated from skin and respiratory tract, and once the rash has appeared, it can also be isolated from blood. Complete resolution of

the rash, along with other symptoms, usually occurs by the 5th to 7th day after its appearance (50).

The diagnosis is usually made on the basis of the clinical presentation; however, in difficult cases, especially those modified by partial immunity, serology can be used to confirm a diagnosis. Total antibody appears a few days after the rash, peaks within 4 weeks, and then declines. Anti-measles immunoglobulin M (IgM) peaks just after the rash disappears, and is only present for about 6 weeks, whereas immunoglobulin G (IgG) can be detected at low levels for life. Enzyme-linked immunosorbent assays (ELISAs) are being used more often now in the diagnosis, and they have started to replace the older antibody detection tests (plaque neutralization, complement fixation, and hemagglutination inhibition) (164).

Atypical Measles

One of the early vaccines developed against measles consisted of a formalin-killed viral vaccine. This was administered from 1963 to 1967, and an estimated 1.8 million doses were given in the United States (164). It was later noted that this particular vaccine conferred only short-lived immunity and that patients immunized with this vaccine did not develop antibodies against the viral F protein. When these patients were exposed to the natural virus, they tended to develop a type of delayed hypersensitivity reaction that could be quite severe (164). After a 1- to 2-week incubation period, these patients experience fevers, headaches, abdominal pain (which at times can be intense), myalgias, and cough. They develop a rash over the next 2–3 days; this rash is erythematous, maculopapular, vesicular, or petechial in nature, and it starts on the extremities and spreads inwards. The rash is associated with swelling of the extremities. It can be mistaken for the rashes of Rocky Mountain spotted fever (147), meningococcemia, Henoch–Schonlein purpura, or a drug eruption. These patients often have an associated nodular pneumonia (164). No new cases of atypical measles have been reported since 1983 (59).

Modified Measles

This consists of a shortened, mild form of measles which occurs in a patient who is partially protected with anti-measles antibody. The disease can occur in patients who have been exposed to a case of typical measles and who then received immune serum globulin. It also is occasionally seen in infants who have decreasing amounts of protective maternal antibody at the time of exposure, as well as in cases of partial vaccine failure. These patients have a shorter prodrome and a milder rash than do patients with typical measles (50).

Complications

Complications from measles infection are fairly common; these can range from mild complications (such as otitis media) to severe complications with significant sequelae (such as encephalopathy). The mortality rate in measles infections is approximately 1 per 3000 reported cases in the United States (42), and it may be as high as 10% of cases in developing countries (164). Death is usually caused by pneumonia or central nervous system (CNS) involvement. Chronic CNS infection, presenting months or years after the initial infection (subacute sclerosing panencephalitis, or SSPE), does occur, although quite rarely.

Otitis media is probably the most common complication associated with typical measles infections. It occurs in approximately 7–18% of all cases (164,203). The organisms do not differ from those usually found causing otitis, and the mechanism behind its association with measles infection is not clear.

Pneumonia is found in many patients with measles. Serious pulmonary involvement can be seen in up to 6% of patients (164), whereas milder pulmonary involvement can be seen in 26–55% of patients (50,203). Pneumonia is usually seen in the more serious cases, and it is often the cause of death in these patients. It tends to be most common in infants and older adults (164).

Many studies in the past have shown a decrease in tuberculosis skin test reaction in patients with acute measles infection. Investigators have hypothesized that measles may predispose patients to tuberculosis. Recent reviews, however, reveal that there are no good data to support the hypothesis that the decreased ability to react to tuberculosis skin antigens is accompanied by more frequent or more severe infections with tuberculosis (70).

Encephalitis carries with it the highest morbidity and mortality rates of all possible complications of measles infection. In its "peri-infectious" form, encephalitis usually occurs at the time of the rash, or within 8 days after the start of the rash (50). Presenting symptoms include seizures (56%), lethargy (46%), coma (28%), and irritability (26%) (50). Studies in these patients have shown cerebrospinal fluid (CSF) ranging from normal to a mild pleocytosis with elevated protein concentrations (50). A Centers for Disease Control (CDC) study of reported cases of measles encephalopathy between 1962 and 1969 in the United States revealed a 15% mortality rate associated with this complication. The investigators found that 25% of the reported cases had severe sequelae, including mental retardation, seizures, severe behavioral disorders, deafness, hemiplegia, and paraplegia (41). The data revealed (a) a measles encephalitis death rate of 1 per 10,000 reported cases of measles and (b) 0.73 cases of encephalitis per 1000 estimated total cases of measles.

Others have reported neurological sequelae in up to 50–60% of cases of measles encephalopathy (1).

Encephalitis during or shortly after a measles infection may occur from direct viral-induced cellular damage or from an autoimmune-mediated process of tissue damage, and both of these mechanisms have been proposed. Until recently, researchers had been unable to obtain measles virus from the CNS of infected patients. However, virus has now been found in clinical specimens (50,201). This does not rule out the possibility of both mechanisms contributing to the pathology seen.

Immunocompromised Host

Measles can often be fatal in the immunocompromised patient, especially in those with impaired cell-mediated immunity. Quite frequently, these patients get a more severe form of pulmonary involvement, with pulmonary symptoms worsening over the course of the illness. This can occur in the context of the other symptoms of a normal infection (rash, enanthem, etc.), in which cases the pulmonary symptoms worsen quickly, or it may accompany vague, nonspecific symptoms, in which case the pulmonary status may worsen over weeks. Histologically, many "giant cells" are seen in the lung parenchyma in these patients (50).

Immunocompromised patients are also at risk for developing an acute progressive encephalitis, formerly called "measles inclusion body encephalitis" (MIBE). After a 5-week to 6-month incubation period, the illness begins with seizures. Hemiplegia, slurred speech, stupor, coma, and hypertonia may develop. This disorder is usually fatal, with death occurring within 1 week to 2 months after presentation of neurological findings (50). It is quite often seen in patients with neoplasia of the immune system (leukemia, lymphoma) (13). Electron-microscopic studies of brain specimens from these patients demonstrate nucleocapsid structures in the cytoplasm (Cowdry inclusion bodies); however, the viral budding that can be seen in acutely infected cells is not present. Also, most of these patients do not mount a significant immune response to the measles virus, presumably because of their underlying immunodeficiencies (13).

Subacute Sclerosing Panencephalitis

SSPE is a chronic, progressively degenerative CNS disease which occurs years after measles infection. The disease was first clinically described in the 1930s (57); it has undergone many name changes, including "lethargic encephalitis with inclusions," "subacute inclusion body encephalitis" (57), and "subacute sclerosing leukoencephalitis" (80,200). The term "SSPE" was coined in 1950 by

Greenfield (80), to stress the fact that both the white and gray areas of the brain are affected.

SSPE is clinically very similar to MIBE; however, the asymptomatic period after the acute measles infection is much longer in SSPE. In addition, SSPE patients often mount a strong immune response to most measles virus proteins, with the exception of M-protein, whereas MIBE patients respond poorly to measles antigens (11,13,60).

This measles complication usually afflicts children and young adults; the age of reported patients ranges from 1 year old (136) to 35 years old (27), with an average age of onset of about 9 years old (136). There is a 2.3:1 male-to-female prevalence ratio (136). Greater than 50% of all cases occur in patients who had their typical measles infection when they were younger than 2 years of age (27,136). In the United States, there seems to be a higher prevalence in whites and in rural (compared to urban) populations. There also seems to be a higher prevalence in the southeastern portion of the United States (136). Overall annual incidence estimates in the general population range from 1 case per million per year worldwide (27) to 0.35 cases per million per year in the United States (136), and from 0.6 to 2.2 cases of SSPE per 100,000 cases of measles worldwide (50).

SSPE first presents with subtle changes in mental status, followed by delirium, dementia, myoclonus, motor incoordination, seizures, visual and speech impairment, and, eventually, stupor, mutism, coma, and death (27,71,164,189). Jabbour established a clinical staging for the disease (100): He estimated the first stage (cerebral changes) to last 1–2 months, with the second stage (convulsive stage) lasting 2–3 months, the third stage (coma and opisthotonus) lasting 1–4 months, and the final stage (autonomic dysfunction) lasting anywhere from months to years.

Pathologically, gray matter is always affected, with occasionally extensive white matter sclerosis (71). Classically, intranuclear and intracytoplasmic inclusion bodies are seen in the affected neurons. These "Cowdry inclusion bodies" eventually were shown to contain measles virus (96).

The diagnosis of SSPE can often be made on clinical and laboratory grounds. There is a typical electroencephalographic (EEG) pattern, consisting of bilateral periodic bursts of high-voltage activity every 3–20 sec, with background suppression (189). Computed tomographic (CT) scans show atrophy involving the cerebrum, cerebellum, and brainstem; they also show diffuse white matter involvement, as well as involvement of the thalamic and lentiform nuclei (101). CSF protein is elevated, on the basis of elevated oligoclonal IgG directed against measles antigens (11,13,17).

Although the exact pathogenesis is still unknown, measles virus has now been demonstrated consistently in brain biopsy specimens from these patients, using a variety of techniques (11,13,28,72,73,84,96,149). Intranuclear and cytoplasmic inclusion bodies can be detected in the neurons, astrocytes, and oligodendrocytes, and nucleocapsid particles can be visualized in these bodies by electron microscopy (200). Electron microscopy of infected cells in an acute measles infection reveals budding of the assembled viral particles from the cell surface; however, in SSPE, while nucleocapsid particles can be seen inside the cells, they are not seen to assemble and bud out from the cell surface, leading investigators to believe that there may be a block in the formation of competent viral particles.

Inoculation of cell-free extracts of brain tissue into tissue culture does not cause infection, as assayed by CPE, hemagglutination, and fluorescent staining, again consistent with the idea of a block in the formation of free measles virus. This block seems to be reversed by the presence of non-neural cell types, since when intact brain tissue is co-cultivated with tissue culture cells (HeLa cells, Hep II cells), infection of the tissue culture cells does take place (96,149).

When monoclonal antibodies directed against the six measles virus proteins became available, investigators reported that, while all the proteins could be seen in various brain tissue specimens, all six proteins were never found simultaneously in one tissue—in contrast to what was found in tissue-culture cells infected with the virus. One protein would be missing in one sample, and another would be missing in a different sample (11–13,28,37,84). Occasionally, they found a different pattern of proteins present in different parts of the same brain specimen (37). M protein was least often present, and since this protein is known to be involved in viral assembly and budding, researchers concentrated on it. By analysis of messenger RNA in SSPE infections, they found that there is a high mutation rate in all of the viral proteins (36–38). These mutations are not seen in virus isolated during acute infections; however, it is thought that they occur with the same regularity, but are simply selected against in the acute infection. Selection pressures in nondividing neural tissues may be less than those in actively dividing tissues, and they may permit viruses with defects to survive. In fact, those with "defects" which prevent them from acutely lysing the neural cells may actually have selective advantages, in that they remain "hidden" from the immune system when they solely reside in the cells and do not bud out (37).

There have been reports suggesting that inosiplex (isoprinosine) (64,87,108) and alpha-interferon (143,154) may be effective in slowing the progression of SSPE; however, there have been no controlled studies in these areas, and more definitive work needs to be done before firm conclusions concerning efficacy can be made. There are good data suggesting that the risk of SSPE after vaccination (0.5 to 1.1 cases per million per year) is less than that after natural measles infection (5.2 to 9.7 cases per million per year) (137), and that the incidence of SSPE has fallen dramatically with the initiation of vaccination programs.

VACCINATION AGAINST MEASLES

History

The progenitor measles strain for all of today's vaccines was isolated from a patient named Edmonston. A killed vaccine (formalin-inactivated) derived from this strain was used from 1963 through 1967. This conveyed a short-term immunity against measles, and about 1.8 million doses of this vaccine were given during this period (164).

A live, attenuated form of the original strain, termed "Edmonston B," was developed, and 18.9 million doses were administered between 1963 and 1975. Protection was better with the live virus; however, side effects (fever, rash, etc.) were quite common, and immunoglobulin had to be given along with the vaccine, to strike a balance between protection and frequent complications.

A number of "further attenuated" strains were derived from the original Edmonston strain; these conferred good protection against natural disease and caused fewer side effects, thereby eliminating the need for simultaneous immunoglobulin administration. The Schwarz strain was administered primarily from 1965 through 1976, and it is still used in some parts of the world. The Moraten strain has been licensed for use in the United States since 1968, and over 160 million doses have been given since that time (42). Combination vaccines, which include mumps and rubella as well as measles (the "MMR" vaccines), have been available since 1971.

Vaccine Complications

The Centers for Disease Control (42) have been compiling data on the complications associated with the Moraten vaccine in the United States since its licensure. Between 5% and 15% of recipients develop a temperature of >39.4°C about 5–11 days post-vaccination, probably caused by vaccine viral replication. This is usually the only symptom seen in these patients. About 5% of all recipients develop a transient rash. True encephalitis or encephalopathy is seen in these patients at a rate equal to or lower than that seen in unvaccinated populations (less than one case per million), and it has not been associated with the vaccine other than temporally (42). Seizures post-vaccination have been reported in children, coinciding with the occurrence of fever. These clinically resemble "febrile seizures" and, like febrile seizures, have

been noted to occur with a higher incidence in children with a personal or family history of seizure disorders. The Committee of Infectious Diseases of the American Academy of Pediatrics has pointed out that this complication is relatively rare and self-limited, and the benefits of vaccination should not be withheld from these patients on the basis of this potential complication (4). Parental education regarding the timing of expected fevers in these patients is recommended. Antipyretic therapy is not recommended immediately post-vaccination (since fevers usually begin days after vaccination), but it may be helpful in these patients at the onset of fever (42).

The vaccine virus is grown in avian embryos, and therefore trace amounts of egg proteins may be present in the final vaccine. Patients who have demonstrated prior severe egg allergies or who have a suspicious history may be screened for the potential of moderate allergic reactions to the vaccine by skin testing with the vaccine prior to its use (79,109). Of the 160 million doses given in the United States, there have been five reported incidences of anaphylactoid reactions with associated respiratory problems (121).

Measles vaccination, like infection, is associated with a transient impairment of cell-mediated immunity, demonstrated by a blunted cutaneous delayed-hypersensitivity reaction to administered antigens (e.g., purified protein derivative of tuberculin). This is not thought to be clinically significant of itself, but it should be considered prior to skin-testing these patients. The blunted responses can last as long as 4–6 weeks post-vaccination (164).

Isolation of vaccine virus from human blood post-vaccination has never been reported, leading investigators to think that viremia either does not occur in this setting or is present transiently, at very low levels. There have been no cases reported of person-to-person spread of the vaccine virus, and there is no evidence of vaccine viral shedding (164).

Vaccine Contraindications

It is recommended not to vaccinate any woman who is pregnant or who may become so within 3 months of vaccination, in order to avoid the theoretical risk of fetal infection with the vaccine virus (42). (No cases of *in utero* infection with vaccine measles virus have yet been reported.)

Interferon induced during a severe febrile illness is thought to be able to potentially interfere with the immune response to vaccination, and therefore these patients should have vaccination deferred. However, mild febrile illnesses should not delay immunization.

Patients with severe immunodeficiencies should not be immunized with live virus, with the following exceptions: (a) human immunodeficiency virus (HIV)-

infected children who have not yet manifested the symptoms of acquired immunodeficiency syndrome (AIDS) (121,130) and (b) leukemia patients in remission whose chemotherapy was stopped at least 3 months prior (121). The incidence and severity of measles infection in these patients are thought to outweigh the theoretical risks involved in giving the vaccine (121).

Vaccination should be deferred in those who have received immunoglobulin or whole blood within 3 months, to avoid anti-measles antibody interfering with the vaccine.

Vaccine Recommendations

Although there has been a marked decrease in the overall incidence of measles in the United States since the institution of a vaccination program, over the past few years the number of cases has risen. Older children, adolescents, and college students make up a large part of the increase, and analysis has shown that most of these cases are considered "nonpreventable" by current vaccination criteria, meaning that these individuals had received the appropriate vaccination at the appropriate age (126). These data suggest that today's single-dose measles vaccination program is not adequate; therefore, both the CDC's Advisory Committee on Immunization Practices (ACIP) and the American Academy of Pediatrics Committee on Infectious Diseases (Redbook Committee) have recently revised their recommendations, and they now call for a two-dose measles immunization regimen (56). The ACIP has recommended the second dose to be given at the time of school entry (5 years of age), for ease of implementation and documentation, and the Redbook Committee has recommended the second dose to be administered at the time of middle school or junior high school entry (11 or 12 years of age), for better immunological response (56). It is hoped that the two-dose regimen will successfully protect those who did not respond to a single dose, or that it will catch those who missed immunization under a single-dose regimen.

The most current recommendations include the following:

1. Everyone born after January 1, 1957 should receive a two-dose vaccination regimen.
2. Vaccinate all children (MMR) at 15 months of age, with a second dose at 11–12 years of age (or at school entry, if legally required).
3. Vaccinate all higher-education students and medical facility staff born after January 1, 1957 who cannot document either natural measles infection or receipt of a two-dose regimen; if no prior vaccination can be documented, a single-dose can be followed in 1 or more months by the second dose.
4. Vaccinate measles-exposed children 6–12 months old within 72 hr of documented measles exposure.
5. Administer immunoglobulin to those exposed children 6–12 months old if exposure was >72 hr ago and <6 days ago.
6. Revaccinate those vaccinated prior to 1 year old, according to routine regimen (one dose at 15 months, plus one additional dose).
7. Revaccinate (two doses) those vaccinated with live virus plus immunoglobulin.
8. Revaccinate (two doses) those vaccinated with either killed vaccine or vaccine of an unknown type (56,121).

In addition, for those infants at high risk of exposure, vaccination is now recommended at 9 months, with revaccination at 15 months (plus one additional dose) (56,121).

Worldwide Measles Elimination

Studies done on the incidence of measles have shown a marked decrease since the institution of a vaccination program in Canada, China, the United Kingdom, and the United States (93,119,134,222). A drop in the incidence of SSPE has been demonstrated in the United Kingdom (134) since vaccination was begun; during this time there has also been a decrease in the incidence of measles encephalitis in the United States (93). Data collected by the World Health Organization has shown a drop in the annual worldwide reported incidence of measles, from 90 cases per 100,000 in 1976 to 70 cases in 1980 (8).

Since measles virus has no common vector for spread other than humans, it should be possible, through a worldwide vaccination program, to completely eradicate the virus. Thus far, there have been a number of problems achieving this goal.

In order to eliminate measles, a sufficient number of the world's population must be seroprotected. When enough people are resistant to infection, the virus will no longer be able to find enough susceptibles to continue spreading. Mathematical models based upon viral infectivity have suggested that no less than 94% of the world's population must be resistant to infection in order to eliminate the virus. Because the vaccines currently available are not completely effective in eliciting a protective response, approximately 97–98% of the world's population must be vaccinated to achieve a population that is 94% protected (164). While some countries have made measles elimination a priority, others have fallen behind in their immunization projects (16).

Another difficulty is that the current vaccines available are not sufficiently immunogenic to adequately protect children less than 1 year old, probably due in part to maternal IgG and in part to an immature immune system. When first introduced in the United States in 1963, measles vaccine was given to 9-month-old children. This was moved back to 12 months in 1965, and back to 15 months in 1976, based upon efficacy studies which demonstrated higher seroconversions in the older children (126). Vaccinating at this age is effective in developed countries, where the incidence of measles has become low and the exposure risk at young ages is also low. However, in developing countries, where the incidence is still high, the rate of infection in the young children is proportionally high. [Greater than 2 million children per year die in developing countries from measles, and the highest mortality rates are seen in those less than 1 year old (125).] As solutions to this problem, multidose vaccination programs have been proposed and started (43,125,222); other investigators have proposed the use of new vaccine strains that may be more effective in younger children (110,125), along with alternative means of administering the vaccine, to avoid inactivation by maternal IgG antibodies (e.g., aerosolized) (110,125,176).

Finally, the incredible infectivity of measles virus leads to another problem. Even in developed countries, where there are laws requiring routine vaccination, there will be a small segment of the population which is vaccinated properly (i.e., receives an effective vaccine at the appropriate age) but which does not seroconvert. This is a small percentage of the population, but because the virus is so contagious, it can "find" this group of susceptibles during an outbreak and infect them (81,126). It is hoped that when the population of susceptibles is made up of only true vaccine failures, the absolute number of susceptibles will be too small to sustain continued spread of the virus, and worldwide elimination will take place.

MUMPS

History

Mumps, like measles, has been a recognized disease entity for quite some time. In his "Book 1 of Epidemics," Hippocrates described mumps as a swelling around the ears, occasionally associated with a painful swelling of the testes (208). The exact derivation of the term "mumps" is not known, but may have come from the Old English for "grimace" (208). Although experiments suggesting a virus as the infectious agent causing mumps were performed as early as 1908 by Granata, it was not until 1934 that Johnson and Goodpasture (103) were able to definitively demonstrate this. By inoculating saliva from human patients into Stensen's duct in monkeys, Johnson and Goodpasture showed that mumps was caused by a transmissible agent capable of passing through the smallest filters; these monkeys became infected, and extracts from their parotid glands caused the same disease when inoculated into other monkeys. In 1942 the details of complement-fixation detection of mumps were worked out by Enders and Cohen

(66), and in 1945 both Habel (83) and Levens and Enders (123) were able to propagate the virus in chick eggs. The latter investigators discovered the hemagglutination properties of the virus, and they suggested that this could be used as a diagnostic tool. Gertrude Henle's group was first able to successfully grow the virus in tissue culture in 1954 (92), and the first vaccine was licensed in the United States in December of 1967 (53).

Prior to the 1930s, the question of whether CNS involvement occurred during mumps infection was controversial. Some investigators, as early as Monod in 1902, thought that meningeal inflammation occurred in most cases of mumps, regardless of whether symptoms of meningismus were present. However, contradictory data were presented by others during the same period (35). When symptomatic CNS involvement was documented, there were numerous theories expounded to account for the damage seen; these ranged from cerebral congestion and compression due to pressure on the jugular veins secondary to parotitis, to emboli from endocarditis. In 1898, Gallavardin first proposed that the CNS involvement was actually due to an infection of the meninges. In 1919, Casparis (35) went on to propose a direct viral infection of both the brain and meninges. In 1934, Montgomery (139) presented data that supported the idea that most cases of mumps are associated with some CNS inflammation (albeit, often without symptoms).

In 1967, when mumps vaccine was first licensed, vaccination was not considered a high priority, partly because of the relatively high cost of the vaccine (47). It was "considered" for use in children approaching puberty, as well as in adolescents and adults. In 1972, it was determined to be "of particular value" in these groups (53). The MMR vaccine was licensed in 1971, but was not routinely used until about 1977, at which time it was recommended for all children older than 1 year.

Virology

Mumps is a single-stranded (negative-sense) RNA virus of the genus *Paramyxovirus,* in the Paramyxoviridae family (30). It is a spherical enveloped virus, with particles about 150 nm in diameter. There are three proteins associated with the viral core: an RNA-dependent RNA polymerase (P protein), a matrix (M) protein, and nucleocapsid protein (N, previously termed S protein). The envelope contains two glycoproteins, a fusion protein (F protein) that has cell-membrane fusion and hemolytic properties, and a protein with both hemagglutination and neuraminidase activities (HN protein, formerly called V protein) (208).

The virus can be grown in (a) embryonated chick eggs, (b) tissue culture in chick embryo fibroblast cells, and (c) other cell types (African green monkey kidney cells, Hela cells, etc.) (30,208). It can be isolated from saliva in humans up until 7 days after the start of symptoms, from the CNS until 8–9 days, and from the urine until 2 weeks after the symptoms have started. It also has been grown from blood, human milk, and testicular biopsy specimens (208). The virus can be isolated from throat swabs as early as 48 hr before the onset of parotid swelling (30).

Epidemiology

Prior to the use of mumps vaccine, the infections tended to occur in epidemics about every 3–4 years. Infection tends to be more common during the late winter and early spring (30). Since the institution of vaccination programs, the yearly incidence in the United States has dropped, from 152,000 cases in 1968 to a low of 2982 reported cases in 1985, approximately 1.2 cases per 100,000 population (44) (Fig. 2). This has risen, however, to 7790 cases in 1986 (2.8 per 100,000) and 12,900 cases in 1987 (44). The most recent outbreaks have occurred in high school and college populations. This shift from a predominantly young-child-susceptible population to a susceptible young adult cohort may be due, in part, to the slow onset of early vaccination programs, with only partial coverage of those first few groups. Laws requiring mumps vaccination prior to school entry were slow in being passed by the various states (44,48,53), and they have still not been passed in 16 states (46). Two of these states (Illinois and Tennessee) alone accounted for more than 50% of the reported cases in the United States in 1986 (46). The incidence in these two states was almost 10 times that of the national average (23.7 and 24.4 per 100,000, respectively); in the 16 states as a whole, the incidence was 1.7 times higher than that in states requiring immunization prior to school attendance (45). Vaccine coverage in the United States did not include 50% of any specific age group until 1976, when over half of the 5- to 9-year-old group was vaccinated. It was not until 1983 that over half of the 15- to 19-year-old age group was vaccinated (53). This slow start in the vaccination program, coupled with a decline in the incidence of natural infection in the early 1970s, has left a cohort of young adults susceptible to infection, whereas today's immunization practices have made mumps in the younger age groups relatively rare. This is reflected in the recent resurgence of mumps in the young-adult age group (53).

Clinical Considerations

Mumps is thought to be fomite spread, with initial acquisition through the oral cavity. Replication is thought to begin in the upper respiratory tract and regional lymph nodes, followed by a transient viremia lasting a few days (208), with dissemination to the various target organs, including the parotid, the CNS, kidneys, pancreas, testes or ovaries, and thyroid (30). Viral replication occurs primarily in ductal epithelial cells. Spread to the CNS is thought to take place from blood-borne seeding of the choroid plexus (208). About 12–25 days after exposure (average 18 days), the prodromal symptoms start, including headache, low-grade fever, malaise, myalgias, and anorexia. Photophobia is occasionally seen, as is abdominal pain and vomiting (perhaps due to CNS and pancreatic involvement, respectively) (30). A few days after the onset of the prodrome, high fever (up to 40°C) and parotid swelling starts. The swelling is usually bilateral, but unilateral involvement is occasionally seen. Parotid inflammation peaks about 2–3 days after it starts, and it resolves in about a week. It is accompanied by an elevation in serum amylase, presumably due to viral replication in parotid and pancreatic ductal cells. Salivary excretion of the virus usually starts a few days prior to the onset of parotid swelling, and infectivity can last from a few days to a week after parotid symptoms have started (30).

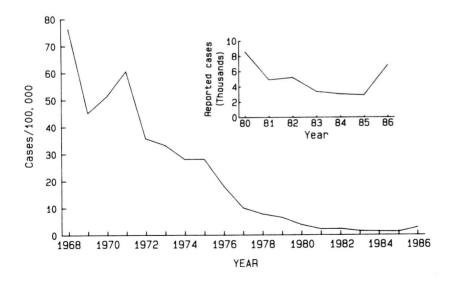

FIG. 2. Mumps incidence rates—United States, 1968–1986. *Note:* When this figure was originally published, the 1986 data were provisional. (From ref. 46, with permission.)

Although most cases are recognized by the typical parotid involvement, about 20–40% of cases confirmed serologically are without symptoms, and it is this high rate of asymptomatic infection that can make it difficult to determine both (a) the index case in an outbreak and (b) the overall prevalence of the virus. Also, other viruses (influenza, parainfluenza, and cytomegalovirus) have been noted to cause parotitis, and purulent parotitis can be caused by bacterial infection (30).

Antibodies directed against two antigens seen in mumps infection—viral-associated and soluble—can be detected by complement-fixation (CF) techniques. Antibody against the soluble antigen is transient, and it can be a sign of recent infection (30). Also, a fourfold or greater rise between acute and convalescent antibody titers is indicative of acute infection. Both CF and hemagglutination inhibition assays tend to cross-react with other paramyxoviruses (208). Tissue culture viral neutralization assays are more specific, but not as widely used. ELISA tests for mumps IgG and IgM are currently being developed (77,82).

Complications

Other than the typical fever and parotitis seen in classical disease, both epididymo-orchitis and CNS involvement are very common in mumps infections (9,44,169). Orchitis is thought to occur in about 20–30% of older males infected with mumps (17,45,158,168). It is seen most often in postpubertal males, with the highest incidence rate in the 15- to 29-year-old age group (30), although it has been reported in young children (168). In those cases in which biopsy specimens have been taken, the virus has been grown directly from testicular tissue. Involvement is usually unilateral, but it occurs bilaterally about 20% of the time (17,158). Some amount of testicular atrophy occurs in 30–50% of cases with testicular involvement, but sterility is rare (17,158,168). Testicular involvement usually starts at the end of the first week of symptoms, accompanied by persistent fever, severe pain, and swelling. It has been reported during "silent" mumps infections, without parotid involvement (17,158,168).

In addition to the above, other complications have been reported. Mastitis is common, occurring in 31% of postpubertal women (158). Pancreatitis is seen (documented by elevated amylase and abdominal tenderness) in less than 1% of cases (9,44,169). Thyroiditis, hepatitis, nephritis, and arthritis are rarer complications (9,30,44). A sensorineural hearing loss (usually unilateral) is seen in up to a few percent of cases (17,192). This is usually reversible, but it can be severe, sudden, and permanent (208). Mumps virus has been isolated from perilymph fluid a few days after the onset of mumps-associated deafness (209).

Central Nervous System

There is good evidence now that meningeal viral involvement occurs in about half of all cases of mumps infection, and that this involvement may not be reflected by clinical signs of meningismus (3,10,29,69). In 1902, Monod performed lumbar punctures on eight children with mumps who had no symptoms of CNS involvement, and he found six of them to have an elevated CSF white blood cell count (3,35). In the winter of 1937, 40 children admitted to Willard Parker Hospital in New York with a diagnosis of mumps also had CSF drawn. Sixteen of 40 (40%) had a CSF leukocytosis and protein elevation. Six of these 16 children had no CNS symptoms, whereas 10 had mild-to-severe symptoms (drowsiness, nuccal rigidity, seizures, severe headache, coma). All recovered without sequelae. Finkelstein (69) concluded that there was no correlation between CSF findings and severity of CNS involvement. In 1943, a study done on 372 patients with mumps parotitis showed 235 (63%) to have increased CSF white cell counts (10). In 1948, during an outbreak on an army base, 77 adults developed mumps (76 with parotitis, one with orchitis). Nine patients had CNS symptoms (headache, stiff neck, nausea). Twenty-six patients (34%) had a CSF pleocytosis (10).

Clinically apparent meningitis or meningoencephalitis does occur in mumps infections and can occur before, during, or more than a week after the onset of parotitis. While laboratory evidence of CNS inflammation is present in a large proportion of patients with mumps, clinical encephalitis occurs more rarely, on the order of two to eight cases per 1000 cases of mumps (44,169). Symptoms occur slightly before or during the parotid swelling in about two-thirds of all cases (21,29,107,116,139), and in these cases the symptoms are probably due to the direct effects of viral replication. Virus can be isolated from the CSF in these cases (111), and histology shows neuronal breakdown (21,199). In the late-onset "secondary" or "postinfectious" cases of CNS involvement (3,63,217), the pathology seen may be caused indirectly, perhaps through an autoimmune mechanism. Here, perivascular leukocytic infiltration and demyelination are present on histological examination of the brain (21,63,199).

In those cases that present clinically with meningitis or meningoencephalitis, there typically is a moderate elevation of the CSF white cell count, from 500 to 1000 cells/mm^3, predominantly lymphocytes. Protein content is usually normal or mildly elevated, and glucose content is normal.

Studies vary with regard to the estimates of sequelae occurring after mumps meningitis or meningoencephalitis, but sequelae are usually quoted as occurring in less than 1% of cases with CNS symptoms (17,141,196,217). When they do occur, they consist of ataxia, flaccid paralysis, incontinence, and behavioral changes (107,111, 116,124,171). Fatal cases have been reported after mumps meningoencephalitis (21,63).

VACCINATION AGAINST MUMPS

History

A formalin-killed mumps vaccine was first tested in 1950. It was noted to convey only short-term protection (less than 1 year), was found to have a low protective efficacy, and was discontinued (208). The attenuated strain used in today's vaccines was derived from a child named Jeryl Lynn; this strain was attenuated by serial passage through embryonated eggs (33). The vaccine was first licensed in the United States in December 1967, and since then over 80 million doses have been administered (53,208). Studies have shown high seroconversion rates in children and adults, with an estimated protective efficacy of 95% at 20 months post-vaccination (208). Conversion can be detected in some as early as 2 weeks, and in 90% of recipients by 4–6 weeks. Neutralizing antibody has been demonstrated to persist for at least 19 years post-administration (208). Since the first administration of the vaccine, there has been greater than a 98% decrease in the incidence of reported mumps in the United States (53). Although complications temporally related to vaccination have been reported (142,202), the frequency of neuritis, encephalitis, deafness, or other CNS problems post-vaccination is generally thought to be no higher than in unvaccinated populations (157,208).

Recommendations

Current recommendations include: (a) live, attenuated virus immunization of all children at 15 months (MMR vaccine); (b) vaccination prior to puberty of those without documentation of prior mumps vaccination or natural infection; and (c) vaccination of those older than 21 in cases known to be seronegative.

In addition, the same precautions as those taken with the measles vaccine should be taken for mumps vaccine in (a) immunocompromised patients, (b) postpubertal females with regard to possible pregnancies, (c) individuals with severe febrile illnesses, and (d) individuals with egg allergies (54).

Mumps vaccination is followed by a lag of up to a few weeks prior to the development of antibodies, and therefore it is not protective in those cases that have recently been exposed (e.g., parents of index cases) (133). However, vaccination will prevent those susceptibles from acquiring disease from future exposures. Also, there are no data to support the use of immunoglobulin in exposed susceptibles, in either preventing or ameliorating disease (54,168,208).

JAPANESE ENCEPHALITIS VIRUS

Japanese encephalitis virus (JEV) is a mosquito-borne virus capable of infecting a variety of animals, including humans. It was first reported in Japan in 1924 and was originally termed "Japanese summer encephalitis" because of its tendency to occur in epidemics during the summer months. It was also called "Japanese B encephalitis," to distinguish it from the year-round epidemic encephalitis occurring in Japan at that time (von Economo's encephalitis, or "Japanese A encephalitis") (174).

JEV is the most common cause of arthropod-borne human encephalitis in the world. Its most common vector is the mosquito *Culex tritaeniorhynchus,* and its distribution mirrors that of the insect, with epidemics occurring throughout China, in northern parts of Southeast Asia, and in areas of India and Sri Lanka (106). The prevalence of the disease has been decreasing in regions employing vaccination programs, such as Japan and Korea; however, it has been recently seen in new areas, including northern India and Nepal (40,106). Encephalitis is rare during infection, with over 90% of all cases being asymptomatic (85). However, when clinical encephalitis occurs, mortality rates can be as high as 20–50%, with over half of those surviving having neurological sequelae (85,106). JEV encephalitis mortality rates usually range between 2% and 10%, depending upon the population studied (85).

Virology

The virus was previously classified in the Togaviridae family; however, recent molecular genetic information has led to its reclassification into the family Flaviviridae, along with dengue and yellow fever viruses (174). The complete viral particle is about 50 nm in diameter, with a 25-nm core. It is a budding virus, and therefore it carries a lipid envelope (85). The particle contains linear single-stranded RNA (positive-sense) of about 13,000 nucleotides in length. Structural proteins present in the particle include an envelope protein (E protein) and a viral membrane protein (M protein) (85). The virus can be grown through intracerebral inoculation in mice, as well as in tissue culture (primary hamster kidney cells, chick embryo cells, Vero cells) (85).

Epidemiology

JEV is found in all provinces of mainland China, with the exception of the western provinces of Xizang (Tibet) and Xinjiang (Sinkiang). It extends as far west as the western portion of India, south to Indonesia, east to the Philippines and Japan, and north to China's Manchurian province and the southern part of the Soviet Union

(174). From 1978 to 1982, it spread from Nepal to northern India (Bihar, Uttar Pradesh, and the West Bengal states) (40).

In the temperate zones, JEV is seen during times of activity of its carrier mosquito, during July through September. It has been thought to be able to survive in hibernating adult mosquitos during the winter months (98). In tropical climates it can be seen throughout the year.

The major vector, *Culex tritaeniorhynchus,* feeds on large domestic animals and birds, and humans are only occasionally fed upon. Other members of the *Culex* genus, as well as those of the *Aedes* genus, have also been noted to carry the virus (85). Once infected, mosquitos undergo a 15-day incubation period. They then become infectious and carry the virus for life (85). In order for a mosquito to become infected, it must feed upon a host with the virus present in high concentrations in the blood. Although humans have a transient viremia after infection, this is rapid and not of a sufficiently high level to infect a mosquito. No evidence exists for human-to-mosquito transmission of the virus (174). Animals tend to develop a longer-lasting, high-titer viremia and tend to act as viral "amplifiers," allowing spread to mosquitos and subsequently to humans. Farm animals, especially swine and horses, are thought to be the predominant amplifier species involved in human epidemics (174). Swine usually undergo an asymptomatic infection, and they can maintain a viremia for days (85). Other animals known to be capable of infection include birds, bats, lizards, frogs, snakes, and turtles (85).

Symptomatic JEV infection accounted for up to 10 hospitalizations per 100,000 people per year in Japan between 1924 and 1961, with a yearly case fatality rate (symptomatic patients) of 24–92% (85). China has reported an average of 10,000 cases of encephalitis due to JEV per year over the past decade, with about 1000 deaths per year caused by the virus (104). Thailand reported about 1500 cases per year in the same period (104). A large portion of the survivors of these infections have been left with neurological sequelae (32,40,104). Both young children and elderly adults are more likely to develop encephalitis during infection than are young and middle-aged adults (85).

Clinical Considerations

Although only a small fraction of those infected will have symptoms, these patients very often will be severely affected and can suffer permanent CNS damage or death. Inoculation occurs during the bite of an infected mosquito. There then ensues a 4- to 14-day incubation period, during which the patient is asymptomatic. Most persons clear the infection at this point without further signs; however, symptomatic patients manifest a prodro-

mal period lasting 2–3 days, during which the patient suffers headaches, anorexia, nausea, vomiting, and abdominal pain. Low-grade fever and CNS changes, to the point of frank psychosis, can also occur during this time (85).

Next is an acute stage, lasting from 3 to 7 days. At this time, a high fever is common. Seizures are seen in about 20% of children during the acute stage, but they are only seen rarely in adults. Also seen are signs of meningismus and hyperreflexia (with hyporeflexia seen later), along with a worsening of cortical function (confusion, disorientation, delirium, and coma). Diarrhea, oliguria, and bradycardia can occur at this time. CSF examination shows a moderate pleocytosis ($100–1000$ cells/mm^3, initially with polymorphonuclear cells and later with lymphocytes), with an elevated protein. Fatal cases progress to coma and death within 10 days of the start of the acute stage (85).

Those that survive go on to a subacute stage, and later a convalescent stage. The former lasts from the second to the fourth week, with lessening of the cortical symptoms. Patients tend to develop secondary problems at this time, including pneumonia, bed sores, and urinary tract infections. Neural motor deficits exhibit themselves (spastic paralysis, fasciculation, extrapyramidal tract abnormalities), and resolution of these problems occurs slowly, if at all. During the convalescent period, from the end of the first month to the second month, there is slow resolution of weakness, lethargy, and tremors, with slow weight gain (85). Anywhere from 5% to 70% of survivors are left with permanent sequelae, including mental retardation, emotional instability, personality disturbances, and motor and speech abnormalities (86).

Adult swine are usually not affected by infection with JEV; however, infection in early pregnancy is known to cause an increase in stillbirths (49). In humans, JEV has been isolated from brain, liver, and placenta in cases of spontaneous abortion related to infection of women early in pregnancy (49). There have been cases of neurological symptoms in newborns born after first-trimester maternal infection with JEV (49).

It is not clear how much of the pathology seen in cases of encephalitis is due to direct viral replication in the CNS, and how much damage is caused by the immune response to the virus. When spider monkeys are given the virus intracerebrally, they usually show no overt symptoms unless they are given immunosuppressive agents prior to infection. In normal monkeys, there is some mild gray matter destruction seen on histological examination of the brain and spinal cord. However, in immunosuppressed monkeys, severe-to-overwhelming lesions are seen, with much neural damage. Clinically, these monkeys develop severe flaccid paralysis (144). This would argue against immune-mediated damage and in favor of direct damage of the neurons due to viral replication. This also makes sense clinically, since most deaths occur during the acute phase, when virus can still be cultured from the CSF and brain tissue (104). In human tissue examined histologically from fatal cases, severe destruction of the gray matter throughout the brain is noted, especially in the regions of the basal nuclei, the floor of the fourth ventricle, the cerebellum, and the cerebral cortex. Involvement is usually noted diffusely throughout the spinal cord in these cases (71).

Immunity is thought to be lifelong after infection; however, loss of protection with subsequent second infection in the elderly has been postulated (85). Prior infection with dengue seems to confer some protection, presumably by development of cross-reacting antibodies (85). Antigenic differences do exist between freshly isolated JEV and strains that have been passaged in tissue culture in the lab for some time, and minor antigenic drift in the wild has been noted, both across time and across geographic regions (85).

The differential diagnosis for JEV encephalitis includes leptospirosis, enterovirus, mumps meningoencephalitis, herpes encephalitis, rabies, dengue, bacterial meningitis, cysticercosis, Reye's syndrome, neoplasia, toxins, and postinfectious encephalitides (85).

A diagnosis is usually made on the basis of serology. Virus can be grown in the lab, but it is not likely to be isolated except from brain specimens in fatal cases, although it has rarely been isolated from blood and CSF (85). Viral antigens are also not easily detectable in CSF or serum, but they can be identified from tissue culture of the virus by complement fixation (85).

Because JEV is quite prevalent in some regions, and because JEV infection can often be asymptomatic, populations may have a high proportion of seropositive (IgG) individuals. This may make it difficult to distinguish a patient with clinical JEV encephalitis from one who had JEV in the past and who now presents with anti-JEV antibodies and an encephalitis of a different cause. An anti-JEV IgM serum antibody titer can distinguish between current and prior infection. Simultaneous CSF and serum IgM titers are useful in diagnosing JEV encephalitis. It has been shown that in acute JEV encephalitis, patients have a high CSF IgM titer against JEV, and the titer in these cases is usually higher in the CSF than in the serum (31,32,85). In acute, asymptomatic JEV, CSF IgM is normal or low while serum IgM is high (31).

The CSF IgM titer in cases of JEV encephalitis has been used prognostically. Those patients who present with encephalitis with high CSF IgM titers tend to have a higher survival rate than those who do not mount a good CSF immune response (106).

Therapy consists of supportive measures in treating airway obstruction, cerebral edema, seizures, and secondary infections. Theoretically, since the immune response seems to play a role in prognosis, one might think that hyperimmune gamma globulin would be useful. However, it would probably have to be given early in infection, and at this time there are no data to support its efficacy in patients with clinical CNS symptoms at presentation (85).

Vaccination

Two types of killed vaccine are commercially prepared today: one grown in mouse brains and prepared in Japan and Korea, and one grown in hamster kidney cells in tissue culture and prepared in China (58). Field tests of the Japanese vaccine showed a two-dose regimen (given 1 month apart) to yield seroconversion in 90–100% of 400,000 children tested. The protective efficacy of the vaccine was estimated to be 80% (58). The Chinese vaccine has been tested in 71,000 children and has an estimated protective efficacy of 95% (58).

Side effects of both vaccines (including fever, headache, local pain, and swelling) occurred in less than 1% of recipients, with allergic reactions occurring in less than 0.02% (58,85). No significant side effects have been noted in over 26 years of use (58).

JEV has been uncommon in Japan since 1966, most likely due to (a) widespread vaccination of children and (b) a decrease in the mosquito population as a result of insect control measures (40).

Vaccine Recommendations

In addition to childhood immunizations for those in endemic regions, vaccination against JEV is recommended for travelers who are going to an endemic region during an endemic season and who are residing in the region for at least 2 weeks (58,195). Two immunizations, separated by at least 7–14 days, are required, with a booster at 1 year after the first dose to ensure continued immunity (58).

Since the major reservoir for the virus lies in domesticated animals, programs of animal vaccination have been initiated (85). Live, attenuated vaccines have been used in swine, since killed vaccine hasn't been effective in this species in conferring immunity (85).

JEV vaccine, supplied by a Japanese manufacturer, had been available in the United States through the CDC. However, in June 1987, the manufacturer discontinued U.S. shipments when its request for release of responsibility for product liability in the United States was turned down (129). There is no legally imported vaccine currently available to U.S. citizens traveling abroad; however, attempts at remedying this situation are currently underway (CDC spokesman, *personal communication*).

POLIO

History

Poliomyelitis, a disease which is known to have occurred in ancient times, but which was not recognized until late in the 19th century (172), has been brought under control in recent years and is now a candidate for elimination by vaccination.

The fact that the agent of the disease is an infectious virus was demonstrated in 1908 by Landsteiner and Popper (118). Although much was learned by monkey experiments, it was only with the adaptation of the virus to tissue culture by Enders et al. (67) that the disease could be fully understood and that reliable vaccines could be produced.

Etiology

Poliomyelitis is caused by three different enteroviruses, called polio types 1, 2, and 3 (24). Like other enteroviruses, they are small (28 nm) RNA-containing viruses consisting of four viral polypeptides. Vp1 is particularly important immunologically, since it is exposed on the surface of the virion (135).

The polioviruses replicate in the pharynx and intestines, from which they are excreted. Intestinal replication leads to viremia, which in some cases is accompanied by invasion of the CNS. Transmission to other humans takes place by the fecal–oral route, by pharyngeal secretions, and by contamination of water with excreta.

Clinical Disease

Three forms of illness caused by polioviruses are recognized: paralysis, aseptic meningitis, and minor febrile illness. These are best understood in terms of the pathogenesis of infection (23,98). After implantation in the gastrointestinal tract, poliovirus replicates in local lymphatic glands, such as the tonsils and Peyer's patches. This replication leads to a low-level viremia, during which other lymphatic tissues and brown fat are infected. The clinical accompaniment of the primary viremia is the minor illness (fever, malaise, headache, sore throat).

A secondary viremia then develops, usually 7–14 days after infection, during which symptoms of CNS involvement develop (25,95). In some cases the involvement is only in the form of meningeal signs with fever, headache, vomiting, and evidence of meningitis, which resolve within a week. In other cases, neurons are infected and die, leading to flaccid paralysis, often asymmetric and variable in location and extent.

The distribution of cases in the above categories depends on the virulence of the poliovirus strain and the age of those infected, with adults being more likely to be paralyzed. In any epidemic, however, inapparent infection and minor illness predominate and account for at least 95% of the outcomes. Aseptic meningitis may be present in 1–2% of those infected, and paralysis may occur in only 0.1–2% (94). However, these estimates should not be taken too literally, since the paralytic rate is quite variable from one outbreak to another (122). Nevertheless, when paralysis does occur, approximately 10% will die and more than half will never fully recover (140).

Thus, paralytic poliomyelitis is the infrequent result of the viremia that usually accompanies a gastrointestinal infection with one of the three polioviruses.

Post-Polio Syndrome

Recently it became evident that individuals who had recovered from paralytic polio years ago are subject to the onset of new paralysis or muscle-wasting (105). The cause is unclear, but it is not due to persistence of infection.

Epidemiology

Until very recently, paralytic polio was a worldwide disease, with the only differences being due to climate and age at infection. In the tropics the polioviruses circulate with all of the other enteroviruses and generally infect children at early ages (152,155). Although passively acquired maternal antibodies provide some protection early in life, eventually the loss of those antibodies—together with the high exposure—leads to a significant incidence of infantile paralysis, which occurs throughout the year. Infantile paralysis was also the pattern in temperate climates before the advance of personal hygiene.

In developing countries, infantile paralysis may not be noticed because of the prevalence of other causes of death and disability, but where it has been carefully studied, the rates of endemic paralytic polio are as high in these countries as rates of polio during epidemics in Western countries.

Meanwhile, in developed countries of temperate climates the pattern has evolved during the last 100 years. At first, epidemics were noted in infants during the summer months. As hygiene improved, the age incidence also increased, since more children and young adults escaped infection in infancy, only to acquire it later in life (131). Thus, polio became a summertime scourge of Americans, in whom the incidence rose to more than 30 per 100,000 before the introduction of vaccination (39).

VACCINES AGAINST POLIO

Inactivated Polio Vaccine (IPV)

The history of polio vaccine development is full of drama and strong personalities. Before the modern era there were several attempts to produce polio vaccines, which ended in blind alleys or disasters. In the early 1950s, Jonas Salk worked out the inactivation kinetics of formalin on polioviruses that had been grown in the recently discovered monkey kidney cell culture system (185,186). Because it had been shown that antibody in the form of gamma globulin could prevent paralysis (86), it was evident that a vaccine that could induce antibody formation should protect. The large Francis field trial of 1954 (75) showed that IPV was successful, and the vaccine was licensed in the United States in 1955.

Apart from the "Cutter incident" (145,146), in which a lot of the vaccine that contained residual uninactivated virus was the source of a large outbreak of polio, IPV proved highly effective in reducing the incidence of polio (181). Nevertheless, there were some flaws in the success. To raise antibodies, three doses were necessary at 0, 1, and 6 months. Even then, protection was not 100%, and it appeared that booster inoculations would be needed at regular intervals. Moreover, primate experiments and observations in human families showed that IPV did not block replication of the virus in the alimentary tract and therefore could not be expected to eradicate polio (51,74).

In the last several years, however, cell-culture technology has come to the rescue of IPV. Microbeads in suspension serve as the attachment for primary or continuous monkey cells in which polioviruses grow. These cultures produce large amounts of virus, which can be concentrated and inactivated, leading to an enhanced-potency IPV (E-IPV) (138). The new vaccine has shown itself to be immunogenic and protective after two doses (87), and new evidence shows that it may also block excretion of poliovirus to some degree (187). This has led to a resurgence of interest in applying IPV to routine vaccination schedules in the United States. IPV has been the standard vaccine in the Scandinavian countries and in the Netherlands (183).

Oral Polio Vaccine (OPV)

Experiments with live virus vaccines actually began in the late 1940s, when Koprowski et al. (115) administered an attenuated type 2 virus to humans. In the 1950s, three sets of competing attenuated viruses were developed by Koprowski et al. (115), Cox and co-workers (34), and Sabin (178). Sabin's strains eventually won the competition, helped in part by the extensive field trials carried out in the Soviet Union.

The vaccine in use today consists of a mixture of three attenuated viruses: the LS-c 2ab type 1 strain, the P-712 type 2 strain, and the Leon 12ab type 3 strain (180). These strains are highly attenuated for monkeys when inoculated intrathalamically and intraspinally. In addition, they have certain *in vitro* markers that correlate with attenuation. The dosage of the three strains actually administered in each dose is usually between 100,000 and 1,000,000 tissue-culture infectious doses for each virus. However, different manufacturers use slightly different ratios of one virus to the other, in order to reduce interference (131).

The reason for the large amount of virus is that lower doses result in inadequate seroconversion under field conditions. Moreover, when given as a trivalent vaccine, each strain competes against the other for susceptible cells. The large amount of virus guarantees that after several administrations each type will have had a chance to replicate in the intestine and to produce local and systemic immune responses.

Thus OPV protects by two mechanisms. As it induces antibody, there is a barrier to the passage of virulent poliovirus from the intestine to the brain. In this respect it is not different from IPV. However, in addition, OPV induces local antibody responses mediated through secretory IgA which block the replication of virulent poliovirus if the vaccinee is subsequently exposed (153). This effect is thought to offer the advantage of preventing the spread of wild virus through vaccinated communities, and it is argued that the freedom of the United States from wild poliovirus is a result of the OPV-induced herd immunity (179). Another advantage claimed for OPV is that because it may spread from vaccinee to contact by the fecal–oral route, there is an augmentation of the public health effect by such vaccination by proxy (18).

Complications and Contraindications

The problems caused by OPV derive from the fact that it contains living, plastic organisms (114). Genetic analysis shows that the attenuated viruses contain a small number of point mutations that have changed their neurovirulence (148). However, these mutants can back-mutate during replication in the intestine to become more virulent (18). Although the level of virulence is still low when compared to that of wild viruses, it is sufficient to cause occasional cases of paralysis. In the United States, an estimated 1 in 2,000,000 doses causes paralytic polio, although the rate is higher for the first dose (151). In addition, if the mutated virus spreads from the original vaccinee to a contact person, polio may develop in the contact individual.

Accordingly, in the United States the paradoxical situation has arisen that there is no longer any natural polio (apparently because the vaccine is so successful), but there are about 5–10 cases per year caused by the OPV itself. These cases are due predominantly to the type 3 strain, less often to the type 2 strain, and rarely to type 1 (219).

A related point is that immunodeficient individuals are particularly at risk for vaccine-associated polio, perhaps because the viruses replicate longer in immunodeficient hosts (151). OPV is contraindicated in immunodeficient individuals or in their close contacts. It is also contraindicated as a routine vaccine for adults, who have a slightly higher risk of vaccine-associated polio. However, if an adult is going to be exposed to polio, OPV is the fastest way of producing immunity.

Table 1 lists the indications and contraindications for OPV and IPV vaccines (55).

Public Health Effects of Polio Vaccine

Both IPV and OPV have had spectacular successes, but both have also had inglorious failures. In the large industrialized countries of the temperate zones, such as the United States and the Soviet Union, OPV has apparently interrupted the circulation of wild poliovirus and has essentially eradicated polio from these nations (78,113). When one considers the ethnic diversity of the United States, combined with the constant flow of immigrants, the effectiveness of OPV is remarkable.

On the other hand, IPV has enjoyed similar success in small northern European countries, such as Sweden, Finland, and the Netherlands, where vaccine policies are easily enforced and booster vaccination is feasible (182).

In the tropics, individual OPV vaccination in the style of the industrialized countries has not been particularly successful, a fact which is generally attributed to interfer-

ence with the vaccine viruses by competing nonpolio enteroviruses (62). In contrast, limited experience with the new E-IPV showed a high degree of effectiveness even in a tropical country such as Senegal, where it was almost 90% protective (173).

Saturation vaccination with OPV, in which entire populations are vaccinated repeatedly within short periods of time, does work in tropical countries and has been used in India and Brazil (102,170).

However, troubling failures have also occurred. In 1980, an outbreak of polio was observed in Taiwan, despite an OPV vaccination rate of over 90% (112). In 1985, Finland experienced a polio epidemic despite the fact that virtually 100% of its population had received IPV (97). Although explanations have been offered for these failures, they illustrate the effect of circumstances on the success of any vaccine.

Table 2 compares and contrasts the advantages and disadvantages of OPV and IPV.

In 1987, an epidemic occurred in the Hadera district of Israel, which may underline the virtues and faults of both OPV and IPV (162). In that district for many years there had been a policy of giving OPV to both Jews and Arabs, so that the adult population had received nothing but OPV. However, in 1986 it was decided to give Jewish children IPV. Arab children, in whom the risk was thought to be greater, were given both IPV and OPV. The polio cases that occurred during the outbreak were localized in Jewish adults, but in addition, extensive circulation of wild virus was noted among the Jewish children.

Thus it appeared that OPV, probably because of the interference caused by other viruses, did not immunize all of the Jewish adults, but in the past they had been protected by the herd immunity their children derived from OPV. When the children started to receive IPV

TABLE 1. *Indications for OPV or IPV vaccine[a]*

Persons for whom OPV immunization is indicated	Persons for whom IPV immunization is indicated
Normal infants and children receiving routine immunization	Persons who have compromised immunity and who are unimmunized or partially immunized
Unimmunized or partially immunized children who are at imminent risk of exposure to poliovirus	Asymptomatic persons known to be infected with the human immunodeficiency virus (HIV)
Adults who are at future risk of exposure to poliomyelitis and who have received one or more doses of OPV or IPV[b]	Household contacts of an immunodeficient individual
Adults who are at imminent (within 4 weeks) risk of exposure to poliomyelitis and who are unimmunized[b]	Partially immunized adults in households (or other close contacts) of children to be given OPV, provided that immunization of the child can be assured
Adults who are at imminent (within 4 weeks) risk of exposure to poliomyelitis and who have had a partial or complete series with IPV[b]	Unimmunized adults at future risk of exposure to poliomyelitis
	Adults who are at future risk of exposure to poliomyelitis and who have been partially immunized with IPV or OPV[c]
	Adults who are at future risk of exposure to poliomyelitis and who have had a primary series of IPV[c]
	Individuals who refuse OPV immunization

[a] From 1988 Edition of Academy of Pediatrics Redbook.
[b] Enhanced-potency IPV immunization also is acceptable.
[c] OPV also is acceptable.

TABLE 2. *Comparison of poliomyelitis vaccines*

Characteristic	IPV	OPV
Administration	Injection	Oral
Virus excretion	None	1–6 weeks
Humoral immunity	Yes	Yes
Mucosal immunity	Variable	Yes
Gastrointestinal tract reinfection	Yes	Brief
Prevents paralysis	Yes	Yes
Rare paralytic sequelae	No	Yes
Spread to contacts	No	Yes
Duration of immunity	Uncertain	Enduring
Thermostability	Yes	No

only, they themselves were protected from viremia, but their intestines could still be infected and they could still transmit virus to their parents.

Considerations such as these have persuaded some to recommend a combined schedule of IPV and OPV for the United States (127), a strategy that has worked elsewhere (120). In this concept, two doses of E-IPV would be given in infancy to provide humoral antibodies which would protect the infant from polio caused either by wild virus or mutant attenuated viruses. Two doses of OPV would be given later in life in order to induce intestinal and herd immunity.

Elimination of Polio

Thus there are two highly successful polio vaccines available, and there are at least two roads to the elimination of polio (128,177,184). It has now become feasible to consider the elimination of poliomyelitis from the world, in a manner analogous to the smallpox campaign. Although poverty, war, and poor sanitation are formidable obstacles, and although the high rate of inapparent infection creates a troublesome reservoir of wild virus, hopes are high for success by the year 2000.

The success in the fight against polio is reflected by the sharp decrease in polio cases being reported from the Americas; this is the result of a campaign organized by the Pan American Health Organization (using OPV) and financed by American charities (131,165). Whether or not the goal of polio elimination will be reached is uncertain; but if the end result is disappointing, it will not be for lack of potent and protective vaccines.

RABIES

History

This viral disease has been known since antiquity, and a tremendous amount of both history and folklore is associated with its clinical manifestations and with attempts to cure it (194). Rabies is perhaps the only infectious disease that is virtually 100% fatal to those

infected. Although a few human cases have survived and some animals give serologic evidence of having survived rabies, only the bat under certain conditions seems to be able to live with the virus.

Louis Pasteur's name has become inextricably intertwined with the history of rabies, although he did not understand the nature of the agent and although the development of a rabies vaccine was not his greatest accomplishment. Nevertheless, the story of rabies created (for the first time) an aura of the scientist as hero (161).

It was clear to the Greeks and Romans that rabies was an infection transmitted by the bites of rabid animals. In the 19th century, Pasteur and others showed that the infecting principle was present in nervous tissue and also in the saliva. Later workers showed that it was a virus. Pasteur's initial vaccine was composed of dried rabbit spinal cords, inoculated first as a suspension in which all the virus had been inactivated, followed eventually by cord containing living virus. Evidently, the first inoculations produced enough of an immune response to allow the subsequent ones to give a booster response without (in most cases!) causing the disease itself (211). Other nervous tissue vaccines were subsequently developed in which the virus was completely inactivated (68,188). Rabies viruses grown in chick or duck embryo (156) eventually replaced nerve tissue vaccines in the United States, only to be superseded more recently by tissue culture vaccines (215), which have now become the standard of vaccination throughout the world. In these recent developments the work of Hilary Koprowski of The Wistar Institute in Philadelphia has been as preeminent as that of Pasteur 100 years ago.

Virus

The rabies virus is an RNA-containing, bullet-shaped rhabdovirus (221). The relatively simple genome codes for five proteins, of which three—the virion transcriptase (L), the nucleoprotein (N), and the nucleocapsid-associated protein (NS)—are associated with the RNA to form a coiled nucleocapsid. The fourth, the matrix (M) protein, is present within a lipoprotein envelope which also contains the glycoprotein (G). This last protein is critical to the induction of neutralizing antibody, whereas the NS protein is more important in cellular immunity.

Epidemiology

The epidemiology of rabies is completely dependent on its epizootiology, since human-to-human transmission is extremely rare (5,91). The dog is still the most important vector of rabies in terms of transmission to humans, and it is particularly important in Asia, Africa, and Latin America. The wolf and jackal are the greatest problems in the Middle East, whereas various species of fox are associated with human exposures in Europe and the Soviet Union. In Central and South America, vampire bats transmit rabies to other animals. In the Caribbean, mongooses are a local problem. Although not well publicized, the cat is a significant vector of rabies in many parts of the world. In the United States the species that most often are involved in rabies exposures of humans are the skunk, the raccoon, and the fox (220).

In fact, no one really knows the number of people who die of rabies each year, since most occur in areas with poor reporting (5). An estimate of 25,000 is a reasonable guess. During 1988, no cases of rabies were reported in the United States. However, since several cases were diagnosed at autopsy of individuals with encephalitis of unknown etiology (99), and over 4000 animals were proven to have rabies during the same year, the actual number of human cases may be higher (150). Meanwhile, hundreds of cases continue to occur in tropical countries such as India, Indonesia, Thailand, Mexico, Brazil, and Ecuador (2).

Clinical Considerations

The clinical picture of rabies is justly described as terrifying because of its inexorability and because in the early stages the patient is frequently able to fully understand what is happening.

The incubation period is quite variable, but it usually occurs 1–2 months after the exposure (90). The illness begins with a prodrome, in which pain or paresthesia at the site of inoculation is combined with manifestations of anxiety and irritability. After 2–10 days of the prodrome, frank neurological symptoms develop, including hyperactivity, nuchal rigidity, and disorientation. These symptoms usually progress to paralysis and hydrophobia (acute pharyngeal and laryngeal spasms at the sight of water), the latter of which is an exaggerated respiratory tract reflex (205,206). Despite good supportive care, death follows in all but rare cases (163,218).

The neuropathology of rabies consists of neuronal destruction and glial infiltration in the hippocampus, thalamus, basal ganglia, pons, and medulla. The Negri body, which is pathognomonic but not always present, is a collection of viral nucleocapsid in the cytoplasm of neurons (207).

Pathogenesis

Despite extensive research, the pathogenesis of rabies is not completely understood (52,65,193). By extrapolation from animal studies, the following picture emerges:

The process of virus attachment and penetration is a slow one, judging from the fact that mechanical removal of the inoculum is useful just after the bite. The virus replicates first in myocytes at the site of the bite, remaining there for variable periods of time. Probably a low degree of replication takes place in the muscle cells, with release of extracellular virus which can be neutralized if exogenous antibody is provided. The amount of virus produced up to this point is insufficient to induce an endogenous immune response. At some time (sooner if the particular area is highly innervated), rabies virus attaches to acetylcholine receptors at the neuromuscular junction. Once the virus has penetrated the nerve endings, passive movement to the neuronal body (where it replicates and spreads to other cells within the CNS), is probably inevitable. Active immunization seeks to generate antibody and (perhaps) cellular immunity, which control the infection before it reaches the CNS.

The spread of rabies to new hosts is ensured by the retrograde passage of virus down nerve endings to the salivary glands, where virus is released in the saliva that contaminates bites and scratches.

Vaccines

Although never submitted to a double-blind, placebo-controlled trial, rabies vaccines are judged to be effective by comparison to historical controls. The rate of rabies after exposure to a proven rabid animal varies with the type of animal and many other circumstantial factors, not the least of which are the amount of virus inoculated and the severity of the bite. However, rates of about 45–50% are generally accepted (88,191).

The first rabies vaccines were based on inactivated rabies virus grown in the brains of animals such as the sheep or rabbit. The need for repeated inoculations of large volumes (owing to the low antigen content), along with the occurrence of frequent neurological reactions to the myelin in the vaccine, led to the search for better vaccines. Duck eggs (156) and neonatal mouse brain (76) were used to grow rabies virus, from which less reactogenic vaccines were produced. However, immunogenicity was still low (198).

Rabies virus was adapted to growth in human diploid cell strains, from cultures of which the virus could be concentrated and inactivated (215). This provided an abundant source of antigen for the preparation of a vaccine [human diploid cell vaccine (HDCV)], which has now become the standard for pre- and postexposure vaccination (160). In the absence of controlled comparative data it is impossible to be sure that one vaccine is more protective than another. Nevertheless, the speed and height of antibody response, together with the accumulated observations, argue that HDCV is more potent than vaccines heretofore available (5,6,14,213).

HDCV can be administered intramuscularly or intradermally. The former route should always be used for postexposure prophylaxis, since it guarantees the highest responses. However, the latter route requires less vaccine and is therefore cheaper. For preexposure vaccination, either the intramuscular or intradermal routes are acceptable. As usual with killed vaccines, timing and volume of doses are important to ensure an adequate response (159,214). In the case of preexposure vaccination, inoculations are given at 0, 7, and 21 (or 28) days. The first two doses prime the immune cells and the third stimulates a secondary response, which is then remembered by the immune system. For postexposure vaccination the objective is to give a large antigenic mass during the first week (0, 3, and 7 days), followed by two boosters (14 and 28 days) (166). The five-dose regimen invariably induces an immune response, even with the simultaneous administration of rabies immune globulin (89).

Recently, other regimens have been advocated to increase the speed of response and decrease the number of visits. One of the most accepted is the 2:1:1 regimen, in which two doses are given on day 0, followed by one on day 7 and one on day 14 (204).

Inoculation in the arm is preferable to the thigh, in order to ensure an intramuscular delivery. Simultaneous medication with the antimalarial agent chloroquine may inhibit the development of antibody, and if an individual receiving chloroquine needs rabies vaccine, an intramuscular route should be used (167).

Rabies Immune Globulin

With the prescribed regimen of immunization with HDCV, a week passes before antibodies appear. In order to provide antibodies during the immediate postbite period, exogenous antibodies are given (89,132). Immune globulin is collected from volunteers immunized with HDCV, and it is then standardized to contain 150 IU (international units) per milliliter (166). This substance, called human rabies immune globulin (HRIG), should be administered as soon as possible after the exposure, at a dose of 20 IU per kilogram body weight. Up to half of the volume is infiltrated locally around the wound, the objective being to neutralize any extracellular virus that may have been inoculated or replicated in non-neural cells.

Formerly, before the availability of HRIG, animal antisera (usually equine) were given. Indeed, the only clinical efficacy trial of combined vaccine and antiserum was performed in Iran, where 18 villagers were bitten by the same rabid wolf (15). While three of five patients given standard vaccine alone died of rabies, only one of 13 recipients of both vaccine and antiserum did so. Although effective, 40% of adults developed serum sickness after equine rabies antiserum, and it is seldom used in the United States (166). Nevertheless, it is less expensive, and recent preparations are said to be less allergenic. The dose is 40 IU/kg.

Efficacy

HDCV has an excellent record of success in preventing rabies. Series have been performed in which humans were bitten by proven rabid animals, vaccinated, and then followed for the outcome. In this way, impressive data were collected on Iranians exposed to rabid dogs and wolves (14), Americans exposed to rabid skunks and raccoons (6), and Europeans exposed to rabid foxes (117).

Nevertheless, failures after HDCV vaccination have been reported (190,216). Usually, there has been an error in the management such as omission of antiserum, but sometimes the problem seems to be a short incubation period in which the virus escapes the immune response.

Complications

The chief concern with regard to reactions to rabies vaccine has been neuroparalytic reactions. HDCV and duck embryo vaccine (DEV) were developed, in part, to eliminate nervous tissue from rabies vaccines, which caused neuroparalytic reactions in approximately one per 1600 vaccines (sheep brain) to one per 8000 vaccinees (suckling mouse brain) (210).

In the more than 500,000 people who have received the vaccine, HDCV has not been associated with such reactions. However, several cases of Guillain–Barré syndrome have followed its administration (20,26). Because Guillain–Barré syndrome occurs at a certain background rate, it is difficult to say whether HDCV actually caused the reaction.

With regard to less significant complications, about 25% of HDCV recipients have local reactions at the site of the injection, whereas 20% have mild systemic reactions (including headache and nausea) (6,160). In addition, allergic reactions characterized by urticaria, arthralgia, and angioedema have followed HDCV, mainly after boosters. This type of reaction occurs in about one in 1000 primary vaccinees, but in 6% of those receiving boosters (47). The allergic reaction appears to be caused by beta-propiolactone-induced modification of the human albumin present in the vaccine, which renders it more capable of forming immune complexes (7,198). About 10% of reactions are anaphylactic in type, but fortunately none has been fatal.

In view of the importance of rabies immunization, there are no contraindications to vaccination. Reactions are treated with aspirin, antihistamines, and epinephrine but not with steroids, since steroids may potentiate rabies. In unusual circumstances it may be necessary to use the rabies vaccine developed in fetal rhesus kidney cells by the Michigan State Health Department (19).

When to Vaccinate Post-exposure

To make a decision regarding whether to vaccinate against rabies, the physician must take into account a number of factors, including the species of animal involved, the circumstances of the attack, whether the skin was broken, the status of animal rabies in that geographical area, and whether the biting animal had been vaccinated or is under surveillance (166). The table (Table 3) prepared by the Advisory Council on Immunization Practices gives an idea of how to make the decision, but the advice of experts should usually be sought. Fortunately, the low reaction rate to HDCV makes the decision much less agonizing than it was in the past.

Can Rabies Be Eliminated?

Human rabies is the product of rabies in domestic animals or in wild animals. The reservoir in wild animals may impinge on humans either directly (when there is contact—for example, with a rabid skunk) or indirectly (when wild species bite domestic animals with which humans have contact—for example, when a bat bites a cow). Thus, elimination depends on how well we can control rabies in animals.

Certain island countries, such as the United Kingdom and Australia, have eliminated rabies through quarantine and through the absence of native sylvatic rabies. In other vast areas, such as Asia and Africa, trapping and killing stray dogs and cats would drastically reduce the numbers of rabid pets, but religious ideas sometimes prevent that from happening (52). Nevertheless, licensing and vaccination of pets have had a dramatic effect on rabies in developed countries, and some day this system may be applied elsewhere.

The extension of preexposure vaccination to individuals likely to come in contact with rabid animals also could reduce human rabies. In some geographic areas this might include a significant proportion of the population, particularly children.

Two other developments could have a rapid beneficial effect on the incidence of human rabies. First is the construction of a recombinant vaccinia virus in which the gene for the rabies glycoprotein gene has been inserted (212). This recombinant virus is immunogenic and protective when given to animals by parenteral, intradermal, or oral routes (22). When placed in baits it has been taken up by wild animals such as skunks, foxes, and raccoons, which have then been immunized (175). Field trials applying the recombinant rabies vaccine to areas where enzootic rabies is present have begun with results that are already very encouraging. This invention opens the prospect of controlling sylvatic rabies by vaccination.

TABLE 3. *Rabies postexposure prophylaxis guide—1989 (CDC recommendations)[a]*

Animal species	Condition of animal at time of attack	Treatment of exposed person[b]
Dog and cat	Healthy and available for 10 days of observation	None, unless animal develops rabies
	Rabid or suspected rabid	Rabies-immune serum and HDCV or RVA
	Unknown (escaped)	Consult public health officials. If treatment is indicated, give rabies-immune serum and HDCV or RVA.
Skunk, raccoon, fox, bat, and other carnivores	Regard as rabid unless proven negative by laboratory tests[c]	Rabies-immune serum and HDCV or RVA
Livestock, rodents, and lagomorphs (rabbits and hares)	Consider individually. Local and state public health officials should be consulted on questions about the need for rabies prophylaxis. Bites of groundhogs, squirrels, hamsters, guinea pigs, gerbils, chipmunks, rats, mice, and other rodents, as well as those of rabbits and hares, almost never call for antirabies prophylaxis.	

[a] These recommendations are only a guide. In applying them, take into account the animal species involved, the circumstances of the exposure, the vaccination status of the animal, and the presence of rabies in the region. Local or state public health officials should be consulted if questions arise about the need for rabies prophylaxis.

[b] All bites and wounds should immediately be thoroughly cleansed with soap and water. If antirabies treatment is indicated, rabies-immune serum and rabies vaccine (HDCV or RVA) should be given as soon as possible, regardless of the interval from exposure. Local reactions to vaccines are common and do not contraindicate continuing treatment. Discontinue vaccine if immunofluorescence tests of the animal are negative. During the usual holding period of 10 days, begin treatment with rabies-immune serum and HDCV or RVA at first sign of rabies in a dog or cat that has bitten someone. The symptomatic animal should be killed immediately and tested. If HRIG is not available, use equine antirabies serum (ARS). Do not use more than the recommended dosage.

[c] The animal should be killed and tested as soon as possible. Holding for observation is not recommended.

The second development is the production—in the Vero cell—of a new rabies vaccine for use in humans (197). Vero is a continuous cell line derived from the kidney of an African green monkey, which can be grown on microbead carriers in suspension culture. This technology permits the growth of vast quantities of rabies virus in vat cultures, which should result in a vaccine much cheaper than HDCV. Other, less expensive cell cultures are also being used to develop rabies vaccines (210). Thus, potent rabies vaccines for human use in poor countries may be already at hand.

Although the problem of rabies in bats in the Western hemisphere does not lend itself to easy solution, human rabies is only rarely the result of exposure to bats. Elimination of rabies in domestic animals, together with control in wild mammalian species, could reduce human rabies to a rare disease in the Third World and could reduce it to an even rarer disease in affluent countries. The technologies to accomplish this end are now available.

REFERENCES

1. Aarli JA. Nervous complications of measles. *Eur Neurol* 1974;12:79–93.
2. Acha PN, Arambulo PV III. Rabies in the tropics—history and current status. In: Kuwert E, Merieux C, Koprowski H, Bogel K, eds. *Rabies in the tropics.* Berlin: Springer-Verlag, 1985;343–359.
3. Acker GN. Parotitis complicated with meningitis. *Am J Dis Child* 1913;6:399–407.
4. American Academy of Pediatrics, Committee on Infectious Diseases. Personal and family history of seizures and measles immunization. *Pediatrics* 1987;80:741.
5. Anderson LJ, Nicholson KG, Tauxe RV, Winkler WG. Human rabies in the United States, 1960 to 1979: epidemiology, diagnosis and prevention. *Ann Intern Med* 1984;100:728–735.
6. Anderson LJ, Sikes RK, Langkop CW, et al. Postexposure trial of a human diploid cell strain rabies vaccine. *J Infect Dis* 1980;142:133–138.
7. Anderson MC, Baer H, Frazier DJ, Quinnan GV. The role of specific IgE and beta-propiolactone in reactions resulting from booster doses of human diploid cell rabies vaccine. *J Allergy Clin Immunol* 1987;80:861–868.
8. Assad F. Measles: summary of worldwide impact. *Rev Infect Dis* 1983;5:452–459.
9. Association for the Study of Infectious Disease, Royal College of General Practitioners. A retrospective study of the complications of mumps. *J R Coll Gen Pract* 1974;24:552–556.
10. Azimi PH, Cramblett HG, Haynes RE. Mumps meningoencephalitis in children. *JAMA* 1969;207:509–512.
11. Baczko K, Carter MJ, Billeter M, ter Meulen V. Measles gene expression in subacute sclerosing panencephalitis. *Virus Res* 1984;1:585–595.
12. Baczko K, Liebert UG, Billeter M, Cattaneo R, Budka H, ter Meulen V. Expression of defective measles virus genes in brain tissues of patients with subacute sclerosing panencephalitis. *J Virol* 1986;59:472–478.
13. Baczko K, Liebert UG, Cattaneo R, Billeter MA, Roos RP, ter Meulen V. Restriction of measles virus gene expression in measles inclusion body encephalitis. *J Infect Dis* 1988;158:144–150.
14. Bahmanyar M, Fayaz A, Nour-Salehi S, Mohammadi M, Koprowski H. Successful protection of humans exposed to rabies infection: postexposure treatment with the new human diploid cell rabies vaccine and antirabies serum. *JAMA* 1976;236:2751–2754.
15. Baltasard M, Bahmanyar M. Essai pratique du serum antirabique chez les mordus par loups enrages. *Bull WHO* 1955;13:747–772.
16. Banatvala JE. Measles must go, and with it rubella. *Br Med J* 1987;295:2–3.
17. Beard CM, Benson RC Jr, Kelalis PP, Elveback LR, Kurland LT. The incidence and outcome of mumps orchitis in Rochester, Minnesota, 1935 to 1974. *Mayo Clin Proc* 1976;52:3–7.
18. Benyesh-Melnick M, Melnick JL, Rawls WE, et al. Studies of the immunogenicity, communicability and genetic stability of oral poliovaccine administered during the winter. *Am J Epidemiol* 1967;86:112–136.
19. Berlin BS, Mitchell JR, Burgoyne GH, Brown WE, Goswick C. Rhesus diploid rabies vaccine (adsorbed), a new rabies vaccine. II. Results of clinical studies simulating prophylactic therapy for rabies exposure. *JAMA* 1983;249:2663–2665.
20. Bernard KW, Smith PW, Kader FJ, Moran MJ. Neuroparalytic illness and human diploid cell rabies vaccine. *JAMA* 1982;248:3136–3138.
21. Bistrian B, Phillips CA, Kaye IS. Fatal mumps meningoencephalitis: isolation of virus premortem and postmortem. *JAMA* 1972;222:478–479.
22. Blancou J, Kieny MP, Lathe R, Lecocq JP, et al. Oral vaccination of the fox against rabies using a live recombinant vaccinia virus. *Nature* 1986;322:373–375.
23. Bodian D, Horstmann DM. Polioviruses. In: Horsfall FL Jr, Tamm I, eds. *Viral and rickettsial infections of man,* 4th ed. Philadelphia: JB Lippincott, 1965;430–473.
24. Bodian D, Morgan IM, Howe HA. Differentations of types of poliomyelitis viruses. III. The grouping of fourteen strains into three basic immunological types. *Am J Hyg* 1949;49:234–245.
25. Bodian D, Paffenbarger RS, Jr. Poliomyelitis infection in households; frequency of viremia and specific antibody response. *Am J Hyg* 1954;60:83–98.
26. Boe E, Nyland H. Guillain–Barré syndrome after vaccination with human diploid cell rabies vaccine. *Scand J Infect Dis* 1980;12:231–232.
27. Britt WJ. Slow virus disease. In: Feigin RD, Cherry JD, eds. *Textbook of pediatric infectious diseases.* Philadelphia: WB Saunders, 1987;1851–1854.
28. Brown HR, Goller NL, Thormar H, et al. Measles virus matrix protein gene expression in a subacute sclerosing panencephalitis patient brain and virus isolate demonstrated by cDNA hybridization and immunochemistry. *Acta Neuropathol (Berl)* 1987;75:123–130.
29. Brown JW, Kirkland HB, Hein GE. Central nervous system involvement during mumps. *Am J Med Sci* 1948;215:434–441.
30. Brunell PA. Mumps. In: Feigin RD, Cherry JD, eds. *Textbook of pediatric infectious diseases.* Philadelphia: WB Saunders, 1987;1628–1631.
31. Burke DS, Nisalak A, Lorsomrudee W, et al. Virus-specific antibody-producing cells in blood and cerebrospinal fluid in acute Japanese encephalitis. *J Med Virol* 1985;17:283–292.
32. Burke DS, Nisalak A, Ussery MA, Laorakpongse T, Chantavibul S. Kinetics of IgM and IgG responses to Japanese encephalitis virus in human serum and cerebrospinal fluid. *J Infect Dis* 1985;151:1093–1099.
33. Buynak EB, Hilleman MR. Live attenuated mumps virus vaccine. *Proc Soc Exp Biol Med* 1966;123:768–775.
34. Cabasso VJ, Jervis GA, Moyer AW, Rosca-Garcia M, Orsi EV, Cox HR. Cumulative testing experience with consecutive lots of oral poliomyelitis vaccine. *Br Med J* 1960;1:373.
35. Casparis HR. Cerebral complications in mumps. *Am J Dis Child* 1919;18:187–193.
36. Cattaneo R, Schmid A, Billeter MA, Shappard RD, Udem SA. Multiple viral mutations rather than host factors cause defective measles virus gene expression in a subacute sclerosing panencephalitis cell line. *J Virol* 1988;62:1388–1397.
37. Cattaneo R, Schmid A, Eschle D, Baczko K, ter Meulen V, Billeter MA. Biased hypermutation and other genetic changes in defective measles viruses in human brain infections. *Cell* 1988;55:255–265.
38. Cattaneo R, Schmid A, Rebmann G, et al. Accumulated measles virus mutations in a case of subacute sclerosing panencephalitis. *J Virol* 1985;56:337–340.

39. Centers for Disease Control. *Immunization against disease—1972.* Washington, DC: US Government Printing Office, 1973.
40. Centers for Disease Control. Japanese encephalitis: report of a WHO working group. *MMWR* 1984;33:119–125.
41. Centers for Disease Control. Measles encephalitis—United States, 1962–1979. *MMWR* 1981;30:362–364.
42. Centers for Disease Control. Measles prevention. *MMWR* 1987;36:409.
43. Centers for Disease Control. Measles prevention: supplementary statement. *MMWR* 1989;38:11–14.
44. Centers for Disease Control. Mumps in the workplace—Chicago. *MMWR* 1988;37:533–538.
45. Centers for Disease Control. Mumps—United States, 1984–1985. *MMWR* 1986;35:216–219.
46. Centers for Disease Control. Mumps—United States, 1985–1986. *MMWR* 1987;36:151–155.
47. Centers for Disease Control. Systemic allergic reactions following immunization with human diploid cell rabies vaccine. *MMWR* 1984;33:185–187.
48. Chaiken BP, Williams NM, Preblud JR, Parkin W, Altman R. The effect of a school entry law on mumps activity in a school district. *JAMA* 1987;257:2455–2548.
49. Chaturvedi UC, Mathur A, Chandra A, Das SK, Tandon HO, Singh UK. Transplacental infection with Japanese encephalitis virus. *J Infect Dis* 1980;141:712–715.
50. Cherry JD. Measles. In: Feigin RD, Cherry JD, eds. *Textbook of pediatric infectious diseases.* Philadelphia: WB Saunders, 1987;1607–1627.
51. Chin TDY. Immunity induced by inactivated poliovirus vaccine and excretion of virus. *Rev Infect Dis* 1984;6(Suppl 2):S369.
52. Clark HF, Prabhakar BS. Rabies. In: Olsen RG, Krakowa S, Blakeslee JR, eds. *Comparative pathobiology of viral diseases.* Boca Raton, FL: CRC Press, 1985;165–214.
53. Cochi SL, Preblud SR, Orenstein WA. Perspectives on the relative resurgence of mumps in the United States. *Am J Dis Child* 1988;142:499–507.
54. Committee on Infectious Diseases. In: Peter G, Giebink GS, Hall CB, Plotkin SA, eds. *Report of the Committee on Infectious Diseases.* Elk Grove Village, IL: American Academy of Pediatrics, 1986;248–251.
55. Committee on Infectious Diseases. *Report of the Committee on Infectious Diseases,* 20th ed. Elk Grove Village, IL: American Academy of Pediatrics, 1988;338–339.
56. Committee on Infectious Diseases (American Academy of Pediatrics). Measles: reassessment of the current immunization policy. *Pediatrics* 1989;84:1110–1113.
57. Dawson JR Jr. Cellular inclusions in cerebral lesions of lethargic encephalitis. *Am J Pathol* 1933;9:7–15.
58. Denning DW, Kaneko Y. Should travellers to Asia be vaccinated against Japanese encephalitis? *Lancet* 1987;1:853–854.
59. Dereume JL, Zech F, de Selys R, Bourlong A. Rougeole atypique. *Dermatologica* 1985;170:280–285.
60. Dhib-Jalbut S, McFarland HF, Mingioli ES, Sever JL, McFarlin DE. Humoral and cellular immune responses to matrix protein of measles virus in subacute sclerosing panencephalitis. *J Virol* 1988;62:2483–2489.
61. Dietzchold B. Oligosaccharides of the glycoprotein of rabies virus. *J Virol* 1977;23:293–296.
62. Domok I, Balayan MS, Fayinka OA, et al. Factors affecting the efficacy of live poliovirus vaccines in warm climates. *Bull WHO* 1974;51:333–347.
63. Donohue WL, Playfair FD, Whitaker L. Mumps encephalitis: pathology and pathogenesis. *J Pediatr* 1955;47:395–412.
64. Dyken PR, Swift A, Durant RH. Long term follow-up of patients with subacute sclerosing panencephalitis treated with inosiplex. *Ann Neurol* 1982;11:359–364.
65. Rupprecht C, Dietzschold B. Perspectives on rabies virus pathogenesis [Editorial]. *Lab Invest* 1987;57:603–606.
66. Enders JF, Cohen S. Detection of antibody by complement fixation in sera of man and monkey convalescent from mumps. *Proc Soc Exp Biol Med* 1942;50:180–184.
67. Enders JR, Weller TH, Robbins FC. Cultivation of the Lansing strain of poliomyelitis virus in cultures of various human embryonic tissues. *Science* 1949;109:85–87.
68. Fermi C. Uber die Immunisierung gegen Wutkrankheit. *Z Hyg Infectionskrankh* 1908;58:233–276.
69. Finkelstein H. Meningo-encephalitis in mumps. *JAMA* 1938;111:17–19.
70. Flick JA. Does measles really predispose to tuberculosis? *Am Rev Respir Dis* 1976;114:257–265.
71. Foley JM. The nervous system. In: Robbins SL, ed. *The pathologic basis of disease.* Philadelphia: WB Saunders, 1974;1499.
72. Fournier J, Gerfaux J, Joret AM, Lebon P, Rozenblatt S. Subacute sclerosing panencephalitis: detection of measles virus sequences in RNA extracted from circulating lymphocytes. *Br Med J* 1988;296:684.
73. Fournier JG, Tardieu M, Lebon P, et al. Detection of measles virus RNA in lymphocytes from peripheral-blood and brain perivascular infiltrates of patients with subacute sclerosing panencephalitis. *N Engl J Med* 1985;313:910–915.
74. Fox JP. Modes of action of poliovirus vaccines and relation to resulting immunity. *Rev Infect Dis* 1984;6(Suppl 2):S352.
75. Francis TM Jr, Korns RF, Voight RB, et al. An evaluation of the 1954 poliomyelitis vaccine trials [Summary report]. *Am J Public Health* 1955;45(5, part 2):1–63.
76. Fuenzalida E, Palacios R, Borgono JM. Anti-rabies antibody response in man to vaccine made from infected suckling-mouse brains. *Bull WHO* 1964;30:431–436.
77. Glickman G, Mordhorst CH. Serological diagnosis of mumps and parainfluenza type-1 virus infections by enzyme immunoassay, with a comparison of two different approaches for detection of mumps IgG antibodies. *Acta Pathol Microbiol Immunol Scand [C]* 1986;94:157–166.
78. Gracev VP. Long-term use of oral poliovirus vaccine from Sabin strains in the Soviet Union. *Rev Infect Dis* 1984;6(Suppl 2):S321–S322.
79. Greenberg MA, Birx DL. Safe administration of measles–mumps–rubella vaccine in egg-allergic children. *J Pediatr* 1988;113:504–506.
80. Greenfield JG. Encephalitis and encephalomyelitis in England and Wales during the last decade. *Brain* 1950;73:141–166.
81. Gustafson TL, Lievens AW, Brunnell PA, et al. Measles outbreak in a fully immunized secondary-school population. *N Engl J Med* 1987;316:771–774.
82. Gut JP, Spiess C, Schmitt S, Kirn A. Rapid diagnosis of acute mumps infection by a direct immunoglobulin-m antibody capture enzyme immunoassay with labeled antigen. *J Clin Microbiol* 1985;21:346–352.
83. Habel K. Cultivation of mumps virus in the developing chick embryo and its application to studies of immunity to mumps in man. *Public Health Rep* 1945;60:201–212.
84. Hall WW, Choppin PW. Measles-virus proteins in the brain tissue of patients with subacute sclerosing panencephalitis. *N Engl J Med* 1981;304:1152–1155.
85. Halstead SB. Arboviruses of the Pacific and Southeast Asia. In: Feigin RD, Cherry JD, eds. *Textbook of pediatric infectious diseases.* Philadelphia: WB Saunders, 1987;1502–1510.
86. Hammon W McD, Coriel LL, Wehrle PF. Evaluation of Red Cross gamma globulin as a prophylactic agent for poliomyelitis. IV. Final report of results based on clinical diagnosis. *JAMA* 1953;151:1272–1285.
87. Harbord MG, Jones T, Hicks EP, Blumberg PC. Intraventricular administration of interferon and administration of methisoprinol by mouth in the treatment of adult-onset subacute sclerosing panencephalitis. *Med J Aust* 1988;148:467–473.
88. Hattwick MA, Gregg MB. Rabies mortality rate in unvaccinated exposed persons. In: Baer GM, ed. *The natural history of rabies,* vol 2. New York: Academic Press, 1975;286.
89. Hattwick MAW, Rubin RH, Music S, Sikes RK, Smith JS, Gregg MB. Postexposure rabies prophylaxis with human rabies immune globulin. *JAMA* 1974;227:407–410.
90. Hattwick MAW. Human rabies. *Public Health Rep* 1974;3(3):229–274.
91. Helmick CG, Tauxe RV, Vernon AA. Is there a risk to contacts of patients with rabies? *Rev Infect Dis* 1987;9:511–518.
92. Henle G, Deinhardt F, Girardi A. Cytolytic effects of mumps virus in tissue cultures of epithelial cells. *Proc Soc Exp Biol Med* 1954;87:386–393.

93. Hinman AR, Orenstein WA, Bloch AB, et al. Impact of measles in the United States. *Rev Infect Dis* 1983;5:439–444.
94. Horstman DM. Clinical aspects of polio. *Am J Med* 1945;6:592–605.
95. Horstmann DM, McCollum RW, Mascola AD. Viremia in human poliomyelitis. *J Exp Med* 1954;99:355–369.
96. Horta-Barbosa L, Fuccillo DA, Sever JL. Subacute sclerosing panencephalitis: isolation of measles virus from a brain biopsy. *Nature* 1969;221:974.
97. Hovi T, Houvilainen A, Kuronen T, et al. Outbreak of paralytic poliomyelitis in Finland: widespread circulation of antigenically altered poliovirus type 3 in a vaccinated population. *Lancet* 1986;ii:1427–1432.
98. Howe HA, Bodian D. Poliomyelitis in the chimpanzee: a clinical-pathological study. *Bull Johns Hopkins Hosp* 1941;69:149–181.
99. Human rabies diagnosed 2 months postmortem. *MMWR* 1985;34:700–707.
100. Jabbour JT, Garcia JH, Lemmi H, Ragland J, Duenas DA, Sever JL. Subacute sclerosing panencephalitis: a multidisciplinary study of 8 cases. *JAMA* 1969;207:2248–2254.
101. Jayakumar PN, Taly AB, Arya By, Nagaraj D. Computed tomography in subacute sclerosing panencephalitis: report of 15 cases. *Acta Neurol Scand* 1988;77:328–330.
102. John TJ, Pandian R, Gadomski A, Steinhoff M, John M, Ray M. Control of poliomyelitis by pulse immunisation in Vellore, India. *Br Med J* 1983;286:31–32.
103. Johnson CD, Goodpasture EW. An investigation of the etiology of mumps. *J Exp Med* 1934;59:1–19.
104. Johnson RT, Burke DS, Elwell M, et al. Japanese encephalitis: immunocytochemical studies of viral antigen and inflammatory cells in fatal cases. *Ann Neurol* 1985;18:567–573.
105. Johnson RT. Late progression of poliomyelitis paralysis: discussion of pathogenesis. *Rev Infect Dis* 1984;6(Suppl):S568–S570.
106. Johnson RT. The pathogenesis of acute viral encephalitis and postinfectious encephalitis. *J Infect Dis* 1987;155:359–364.
107. Johnstone JA, Ross CA, Dunn M. Meningitis and encephalitis associated with mumps infection. *Arch Dis Child* 1972;47:647–651.
108. Jones CE, Dyken PR, Huttenlocher PR, Jabbour JT, Maxwell KW. Inosiplex therapy in subacute sclerosing panencephalitis. *Lancet* 1982;2:1034–1037.
109. Juntunen-Backman K, Peltola H, Backman A, Salo OP. Safe immunization of allergic children against measles, mumps and rubella. *Am J Dis Child* 1987;141:1103–1105.
110. Khanum S, Uddin N, Garelick H, Mann G, Tomkins A. Comparison of Edmonston–Zagreb and Schwarz strains of measles vaccine given by aerosol or subcutaneous injection. *Lancet* 1987;1:15–153.
111. Kilham L. Mumps meningoencephalitis with and without parotitis. *Am J Dis Child* 1949;78:324–333.
112. Kim-Farley RJ, Rutherford G, Lichfield P, et al. Outbreak of paralytic poliomyelitis, Taiwan. *Lancet* 1984;ii:1322–1324.
113. Kim-Farley RJ, Schonberger LB, Nkowane BM, et al. Poliomyelitis in the USA: viral elimination of disease caused by wild virus. *Lancet* 1984;ii:1315–1317.
114. Kohara M, Abe S, Kuge S, et al. An infectious cDNA clone of the poliovirus Sabin strain could be used as a stable repository and inoculum for the oral polio live vaccine. *Virology* 1986;151:21–30.
115. Koprowski H, Jervis GA, Norton TW. Immune responses in human volunteers upon oral administration of a rodent adapted strain of poliomyelitis virus. *Am J Hyg* 1952;55:108–126.
116. Koskiniemi M, Donner M, Pettay O. Clinical appearance and outcome in mumps encephalitis in children. *Acta Pediatr Scand* 1983;72:603–609.
116a. Krugman, S. Further-attenuated measles vaccine: characteristics and use. *Rev Infect Dis* 1983;5:477–481.
117. Kuwert EK, Marcus I, Werner J, Iwand A, Thraenhart O. Some experiences with human diploid cell strain (HDCS) rabies vaccine in pre- and post-exposure vaccinated humans. *Dev Biol Stand* 1978;40:79–88.
118. Landsteiner K, Popper E. Mikroscopische Präparat von einer Menschlichen- and zwei Affenruckenmarken. *Wien Clin Wochenschr* 1908;21:1830.
119. Larke RP. Impact of measles in Canada. *Rev Infect Dis* 1983;5:445–451.
120. Lasch EE, Abed Y, Gerichter ChB, et al. Results of a program successfully combining live and killed polio vaccines. *Isr J Med Sci* 1983;19:1021–1023.
121. Leads from the MMWR: measles prevention. *JAMA* 1987;258:890–895.
122. Lebrun A, Cerf J, Gelfand HM, Courtois G, Plotkin SA, Koprowski H. Vaccination with the CHAT strain of type I attenuated poliomyelitis virus in Leopoldville, Belgian Congo. I. Description of the city, its history of poliomyelitis and the plan of vaccination campaign. *Bull WHO* 1960;22:203–213.
123. Levens JH, Enders JF. The hemoagglutinative properties of amniotic fluid from embryonated eggs infected with mumps virus. *Science* 1945;102:117–120.
124. Levitt LP, Rich TA, Kinde SW, Lewis AL, Gates EH, Bond JO. Central nervous system mumps: a review of 64 cases. *Neurology* 1970;20:829–834.
125. Markowitz LE, Bernier RH. Immunization of young infants with Edmonston–Zagreb measles vaccine. *Pediatr Infect Dis J* 1987;6:809–812.
126. Markowitz LE, Preblud SR, Orenstein WA, et al. Patterns of transmission in measles outbreaks in the United States 1985–1986. *N Engl J Med* 1989;320:75–81.
127. McBean AM, Modlin JF. Rationale for the sequential use of inactivated poliovirus vaccine and live attenuated poliovirus vaccine for routine poliomyelitis immunization in the United States. *Pediatr Infect Dis J* 1987;6:881–887.
128. McBean AM, Thomas ML, Johnson RH. A comparison of the serologic responses to oral and injectable trivalent poliovirus vaccines. *Rev Infect Dis* 1984;6(Suppl 2):S552–S555.
129. McKinney WP, Barnas GP. Japanese encephalitis vaccine: an orphan product in need of adoption. *N Engl J Med* 1988;318:255–256.
130. McLaughlin M, Thomas P, Onorato I, et al. Live virus vaccines in human immunodeficiency virus-infected children: a retrospective survey. *Pediatrics* 1988;82:229–233.
131. Melnick JL. Live attenuated poliovaccines. In: Plotkin SA, Mortimer EA Jr. *Vaccines,* vol 1. Philadelphia: WB Saunders, 1988;115–157.
132. Mertz GJ, Nelson KE, Vithayasai V, Markornkawkeyoon S, et al. Antibody responses to human diploid cell vaccine for rabies with and without human rabies immune globulin. *J Infect Dis* 1982;145:720–727.
133. Meyer MB, Stifler WC, Joseph JM. Evaluation of mumps vaccine given after exposure to mumps with special reference to the exposed adult. *Pediatrics* 1966;37:304–315.
134. Miller CL. Current impact of measles in the United Kingdom. *Rev Infect Dis* 1983;5:427–432.
135. Minor PD, Schild GC, Cann AJ, et al. Studies on the molecular aspects of antigenic structure and virulence of poliovirus. *Ann Inst Pasteur Virol* 1986;137:107.
136. Modlin JF, Halsey NA, Eddins DL, et al. Epidemiology of subacute sclererosing panencephalitis. *J Pediatr* 1979;94:231–236.
137. Modlin JF, Jabbour JT, Witte JJ, Halsey NA. Epidemiologic studies of measles vaccine, and subacute sclerosing panencephalitis. *Pediatrics* 1977;59:505–512.
138. Montagnon B, Fanget B, Vincent-Falquet JC. Industrial scale production of inactivated poliovirus vaccine prepared by culture of Vero cells and microcarrier. *Rev Infect Dis* 1984;6:S341–344.
139. Montgomery JC. Mumps meningo-encephalitis. *Am J Dis Child* 1934;48:1279–1283.
140. Moore M, Katona P, Kaplan JE, et al. Poliomyelitis in the United States, 1969–1981. *J Infect Dis* 1982;146:558–563.
141. Murray HG, Field CM, McLeod WJ. Mumps meningoencephalitis. *Br Med J* 1960;1:1850–1853.
142. Nabe-Nielsen J, Walter B. Unilateral deafness as a complication of the mumps, measles and rubella vaccination. *Br Med J* 1988;297:489.
143. Nakagawa M, Michihata T, Oskioka H, Sawada T, Kusunoki T, Kishida T. Intrathecal administration of human leukocyte inter-

feron to a patient with subacute sclerosing panencephalitis. *Acta Paediatr Scand* 1985;74:309–310.

144. Nathanson N, Cole GA. Fatal Japanese encephalitis virus infection in immunosupressed spider monkeys. *Clin Exp Immunol* 1970;6:161–166.

145. Nathanson N, Langmuir AD. The Cutter incident: poliomyelitis following formaldehyde-inactivated poliovirus vaccination in the United States during the spring of 1955. I. Background. *Am J Hyg* 1963;78:16–28.

146. Nathanson N, Langmuir AD. The Cutter incident: poliomyelitis following formaldehyde-inactivated poliovirus vaccination in the United States during the spring of 1955. II. Relationship of poliomyelitis to Cutter vaccine. *Am J Hyg* 1963;78:20–60.

147. Nieburg PI, D'Angelo LJ, Herrmann KL. Measles in patients suspected of having Rocky Mountain spotted fever. *JAMA* 1980;244:808–809.

148. Nomoto A, Omata T, Toyoda H, et al. Complete nucleotide sequence of the attenuated poliovirus Sabin 1 strain genome. *Proc Natl Acad Sci USA* 2983;79:5793–5797.

149. Norrby E, Kristensson K, Brzosko WJ, Kapsenberg JG. Measles virus matrix protein detected by immune fluorescence with monoclonal antibodies in the brain of patients with subacute sclerosing panencephalitis. *J Virol* 1985;56:337–340.

150. Notifiable diseases of low frequency. *MMWR* 1988;37:774.

151. Nyowane BM, Wassilak SGF, Orenstein WA, et al. Vaccine-associated paralytic poliomyelitis. United States: 1973 through 1984. *JAMA* 1987;257:1335–1340.

152. Ofosu-Amaah S, Kratzer JH, Nicholas DD. Is poliomyelitis a serious problem in developing countries? Lameness in Ghanaian schools. *Br Med J* 1977;i:1012–1014.

153. Ogra PL. Mucosal immune response to poliovirus vaccines in childhood. *Rev Infect Dis* 1984;6(Suppl 2):S361–368.

154. Panitch HS, Gomez-Plascencia J, Norris FH, Cantell K, Smith RA. Subacute sclerosing panencephalitis: remission after treatment with intraventricular interferon. *Neurology* 1986;36:562–566.

155. Paul JR, Melnick JL, Barnett VH, Goldblum N. A survey of neutralizing antibody to poliomyelitis in Cairo, Egypt. *Am J Hyg* 1952;55:402–413.

156. Peck FB, Powell HM, Culbertson CG. Duck-embryo rabies vaccine: study of fixed virus vaccine grown in embryonated duck eggs and killed with betapropiolactone. *JAMA* 1956;162:1373–1376.

157. Peltola H, Heinonen OP. Frequency of true adverse reactions to measles–mumps–rubella vaccine. *Lancet* 1986;1:939–942.

158. Philip RN, Reinhard KR, Lackman DB. Observations on a mumps epidemic in a "virgin" population. *Am J Hyg* 1959;69:91–111.

159. Plotkin SA, Wiktor TJ, Koprowski H, Rosanoff EI, Tint H. Immunization schedules for the new human diploid cell vaccine against rabies. *Am J Epidemiol* 1976;103:75–80.

160. Plotkin SA. Rabies vaccine prepared in human cell cultures: progress and perspectives. *Rev Infect Dis* 1980;2:433–447.

161. Plotkin SL, Plotkin SA. A short history of vaccination. In: Plotkin SA, Mortimer EA Jr, eds. *Vaccine.* Philadelphia: WB Saunders, 1988;1–7.

162. Poliomyelitis—Israel. *MMWR* 1988;37:624–625.

163. Porras C, Barboza JJ, Fuenzalida E, Adards HL, et al. Recovery from rabies in man. *Ann Intern Med* 1976;85:44–48.

164. Preblud SR, Katz SL. Measles vaccine. In: Plotkin SA, Mortimer EA Jr, eds. *Vaccines.* Philadelphia: WB Saunders, 1988;182–222.

165. Progress toward eradicating poliomyelitis from the Americas. *MMWR* 1989;38:532–535.

166. Rabies prevention, United States, 1984. *MMWR* 1984;33:393–402.

167. Rabies prevention: supplementary statement on the preexposure of human diploid cell rabies vaccine by the intradermal route. *MMWR* 1986;35:767–768.

168. Reed D, Brown G, Merrick R, Sever J, Feltz E. A mumps epidemic on St. George Island, Alaska. *JAMA* 1967;199:967–971.

169. Research Unit, Royal College of General Practitioners. The incidence and complications of mumps. *J R Coll Gen Pract* 1974;24:545–551.

170. Risi JB. The control of poliomyelitis in Brazil. *Rev Infect Dis* 1984;6(Suppl 2):S400–S403.

171. Ritter BS. Mumps meningoencephalitis in children. *J Pediatr* 1958;52:424–433.

172. Robbins FC. Polio—Historical. In: Plotkin SA, Mortimer EA Jr, eds. *Vaccines,* vol 1. Philadelphia: WB Saunders, 1988;98–114.

173. Robertson SE, Drucker JA, Fabre-Teste B, et al. Clinical efficacy of a new, enhanced-potency, inactivated poliovirus vaccine. *Lancet* 1988;ii:897–899.

174. Rosen L. The natural history of Japanese encephalitis virus. *Annu Rev Microbiol* 1986;40:395–414.

175. Rupprecht CE, Wiktor TJ, Johnston DH, et al. Oral immunization and protection of raccoons (*Procyon lotor*) with a vaccinia-rabies glycoprotein recombinant virus vaccine. *Proc Natl Acad Sci USA* 1986;87:7947–7950.

176. Sabin AB, Arechiga AF, DeCastro JF, et al. Successful immunization of children with and without maternal antibody by aerosolized measles vaccine. *JAMA* 1983;249:2651–2662.

177. Sabin AB. Commentary: Is there a need for a change in poliomyelitis immunization policy? *Pediatr Infect Dis J* 1987;6:887–889.

178. Sabin AB. Immunization of champanzees and human being with avirulent strains of poliomyelitis virus. *Ann NY Acad Sci* 1955;61:1050.

179. Sabin AB. Paralytic poliomyelitis: old dogmas and new perspectives. *Rev Infect Dis* 1981;3:543–564.

180. Sabin AB. Properties and behavior of orally administered attenuated poliovirus vaccine. *JAMA* 1957;164:1216–1223.

181. Sald D. Eradication of poliomyelitis in the United States. *Rev Infect Dis* 1980;2:2343–257.

182. Salk D, Salk J. Vaccinology of poliomyelitis. *Vaccine* 1984;2:59–74.

183. Salk J, Drucker J. Noninfectious poliovirus vaccine. In: Plotkin SA, Mortimer EA Jr, eds. *Vaccines,* vol 1. Philadelphia: WB Saunders, 1988;158–181.

184. Salk J. Commentary: Poliomyelitis vaccination—choosing a wise policy. *Pediatr Infect Dis J* 1987;6:889–893.

185. Salk JE, Bennett BL, Lewis LJ, Ward EN, Youngner JS. Studies in human subjects on active immunization against poliomyelitis. I. A preliminary report of experiments in progress. *JAMA* 1953;151:1081.

186. Salk JE, Krech U, Youngner JS, Bennett BL, Lewis LJ. Formaldehyde treatment and safety testing of experimental poliomyelitis vaccines. *Am J Public Health* 1954;44:563.

187. Selvakumar R, John TJ. Intestinal immunity induced by inactivated poliovirus vaccine. *Vaccine* 1987;5:141–144.

188. Semple D. The preparation of a safe and efficient antirabic vaccine. *Sci Mem Med Sanit Dept India* 1911;44:1–32.

189. Sever JL. Persistent measles infection of the central nervous system: subacute sclerosing panencephalitis. *Rev Infect Dis* 1983;5:467–473.

190. Shill M, Baynes R, Miller S. Fatal rabies encephalitis despite appropriate post-exposure prophylaxis: a case report. *Med Intell* 1987;316:1257–1258.

191. Sitthi-Amorn C, Jiratanavattana V, Keoyoo J, Sonpunya N. The diagnostic properties of laboratory tests for rabies. *Int J Epidemiol* 1987;16:602–605.

192. Smith GA, Gussen R. Inner ear pathologic features following mumps infection. *Arch Otolaryngol* 1976;102:108–111.

193. Spriggs DR. Rabies pathogenesis: fast times at the neuromuscular junction. *J Infect Dis* 1985;152:1362–1363.

194. Steele JH. History of rabies. In: Baer GM, ed. *The natural history of rabies,* vol 1. New York: Academic Press, 1975;1–33.

195. Steffen R. Vaccinating against Japanese encephalitis. *Lancet* 1987;1:511.

196. Strussberg S, Winter S, Friedman A, et al. Notes on mumps meningoencephalitis. *Clin Pediatr* 1969;8:373–374.

197. Suntharasamai P, Warrell MJ, Warrell DA, et al. New purified vero-cell vaccine prevents rabies in patients bitten by rabid animals. *Lancet* 1986;2:129–131.

198. Swanson MC, Rosanoff E, Gurwith M, Deitch M, Schnurrenberger P, Reed CE. IgE and IgG antibodies to β-propiolactone and human serum albumin associated with urticarial reactions to rabies vaccine. *J Infect Dis* 1987;155:909–913.

199. Taylor FB, Toreson WE. Primary mumps meningoencephalitis. *Arch Intern Med* 1963;112:216–221.
200. Tellez-Nagel I, Harter DH. Subacute sclerosing leukoencephalitis. I. Clinico-pathological, electron microscopic and virological observations. *J Neuropathol Exp Neurol* 1966;25:506–581.
201. Ter Meulen V, Muller D, Kackell Y, Katz M. Isolation of infectious measles virus in measles encephalitis. *Lancet* 1972; 2:1172–1175.
202. Thomas E. A case of mumps meningitis: a complication of vaccination? *Can Med Assoc J* 1988;138:135.
203. Tidstrom B. Complications in measles with special reference to encephalitis. *Acta Med Scand* 1968;184:411–415.
204. Vodopija I, Sureau P, Lafon M, et al. An evaluation of second generation tissue culture rabies vaccines for use in man: a four-vaccine comparative immunogenicity study using a preexposure vaccination schedule and an abbreviated 2-1-1 postexposure schedule. *Vaccine* 1986;4:245–248.
205. Warrell DA, Warrell MJ. Human rabies and its prevention: an overview. *Rev Infect Dis* 1988;10:726–731.
206. Warrell DA. Clinical picture of rabies in man. *Trans R Soc Trop Med Hyg* 1976;70:188–195.
207. Warrell DA, Davidson NMcD, Pope HM, et al. Pathophysiologic studies in human rabies. *Am J Med* 1976;60:180–190.
208. Weibel RE. Mumps vaccine. In: Plotkin SA, Mortimer EA Jr, eds. *Vaccines*. Philadelphia: WB Saunders, 1988;223–234.
209. Westmore GA, Pickard BH, Stern H. Isolation of mumps virus from the inner ear after sudden deafness. *Br Med J* 1979;1:14–15.
210. Wiktor T, Plotkin SA, Koprowski H. Rabies vaccine. In: Plotkin SA, Mortimer EA Jr, eds. *Vaccine*. Philadelphia: WB Saunders, 1988;479–491.
211. Wiktor T. Historical aspects of rabies treatment. In: Koprowski H, Plotkin SA, eds. *World's debt to Pasteur*. Alan R Liss, New York: 1985;141–152.
212. Wiktor TJ, MacFarlane RI, Reagan KJ, et al. Protection from rabies by vaccinia virus recombinant containing the rabies virus glycoprotein gene. *Proc Natl Acad Sci USA* 1984;81:7194–7198.
213. Wiktor TJ, Plotkin SA, Grella DW. Human cell culture rabies vaccine. *JAMA* 1973;224:1170–1171.
214. Wiktor TJ, Plotkin SA, Koprowski H. Development and clinical trials of the new human rabies vaccine of tissue culture (human diploid cell) origin. *Dev Biol Stand* 1978;40:3–9.
215. Wiktor TJ, Sokol F, Kuwert E, Koprowski H. Immunogenicity of concentrated and purified rabies vaccine of tissue culture origin. *Proc Soc Exp Biol Med* 1969;131:799–805.
216. Wilde H, Choomkasien P, Hemachudha T, Supich C, Chutivongse S. Failure of rabies postexposure treatment in Thailand. *Vaccine* 1989;7:49–752.
217. Wilfert CM. Mumps meningoencephalitis with low cerebrospinal-fluid glucose, prolonged pleocytosis and elevation of protein. *N Engl J Med* 1969;280:855–859.
218. Winkler WG, Fashinell TR, Leffingwell L, Howard P, Conomy P. Airborne rabies transmission in a laboratory worker. *JAMA* 1973;226:1219–1221.
219. World Health Organization Consultative Group on Live Poliomyelitis Vaccine (Sabin Strains). The relation between acute persisting spinal paralysis and poliomyelitis vaccine—results of a ten-year enquiry. *Bull WHO* 1982;60:231–242.
220. World Health Organization. *World survey of rabies XXI, 1982–83*. Geneva: World Health Organization Veterinary Public Health Unit Division of Communicable Diseases, 1984.
221. Wunner WH, Dietzchold B, Wiktor TJ. Antigenic Structure of Rhabdoviruses. In: von Regenmortel MHV, Neurath AD, eds. *Immunochemistry of viruses. The basis for serodiagnosis and vaccines*. New York: Elsevier, 1985;367–388.
222. Yihao Z, Wannian S. A review of the current impact of measles in the People's Republic of China. *Rev Infect Dis* 1983;5:411–416.

Infections of the Central Nervous System,
edited by W. M. Scheld, R. J. Whitley, and
D. T. Durack, Raven Press, Ltd., New York © 1991.

CHAPTER 12

Guillain–Barré Syndrome

Gene Tenorio, Arie Ashkenasi, and John W. Benton

Guillain–Barré syndrome (GBS), or acute inflammatory demyelinating polyneuropathy (AIDP), is the most frequent cause of acute generalized paralysis. The condition is characterized by rapidly progressing symmetric weakness of the extremities which is related (in most instances) to an antecedent viral illness. Current evidence supports the concept of an acquired immune-mediated disorder.

Assigning credit for recognizing the syndrome of AIDP is difficult. Landry's description of patients with ascending flaccid paralysis of the extremities, bulbar paralysis, and death within a week is most often cited (1). In 1916, Guillain et al. (2) described two patients with a clinical syndrome consisting of motor disturbances, loss of tendon reflexes, preserved cutaneous reflexes, and increased albumin without pleocytosis in the cerebrospinal fluid (CSF). Draganesco and Claudian (3) were the first to use the eponym "Guillain–Barré syndrome," in 1927. Considerable controversy existed for several years over whether the disorder described by Landry was the same as that described by Guillain et al. Guillain insisted that fatal cases or cases with CSF protein concentrations of less than 1–2 g/dl did not qualify for his classification. It was not until a symposium on GBS in 1938 that Guillain (4) and Barré (5) agreed that GBS may end in death, be associated with lower CSF protein values, and was probably infectious in origin.

EPIDEMIOLOGY

Multiple population-based studies of GBS have been performed. The crude annual incidence rate of GBS per 100,000 people ranges from 0.4 to 2 in different populations. This wide fluctuation is at least partially accounted for by variable thoroughness of case-finding and diagnostic criteria. Most studies have revealed a male pre-

ponderance, increased incidence with age, and no major seasonal difference in frequency. Table 1 summarizes the incidence, number of cases, percentage with antecedent infections within 4 weeks, and mortality of GBS in 14 well-defined population studies (6–19).

Lesser et al. (6) reviewed the medical records and death certificates of all Olmstead County, Minnesota residents for whom a diagnostic entry consistent with GBS had been made in the years 1935 through 1968. The unique medical record retrieval system available for these residents ensures high case ascertainment and diagnostic accuracy. Twenty-nine cases were found, yielding a mean annual incidence rate of 1.6 per 100,000. Among males (18 cases) the incidence rate was 2.1, and among females (11 cases) it was 1.2. The incidence was highest between ages 40 and 59 years, though this did not reach statistical significance. Seasonal clustering was not found. Two of the 29 patients died from the disease.

Beghi et al. (8) further updated the study of GBS in Olmstead County. Forty-eight cases were identified over the 46-year period from 1935 through 1980. Features required for the diagnosis of GBS were the following criteria proposed by an ad hoc committee of the National Institute of Neurological and Communicative Disorders and Stroke (NINCDS) (20): (a) progressive motor weakness of the upper and/or lower limbs and (b) loss or marked reduction of deep tendon reflexes. In addition, the following criteria were required to support the diagnosis: (a) rapid development of symptoms and signs that peak within 1 month, (b) relative symmetry in the distribution of weakness, and (c) a high level of recovery. CSF findings of elevated protein and 10 or fewer mononuclear leukocytes per cubic millimeter were considered strongly supportive of the diagnosis; however, a normal CSF or counts of 11–50 mononuclear leukocytes per cubic millimeter did not preclude the acceptance of a case.

Patients were excluded if one of the following features were present: (a) a definite diagnosis of a disease developing into a peripheral neuropathy resembling GBS (with

G. Tenorio, A. Ashkenasi, and J. W. Benton: Department of Pediatrics, University of Alabama at Birmingham, Birmingham, Alabama 35294.

TABLE 1. *Incidence, number of cases, percentage of cases with antecedent infection within 4 weeks of onset of Guillain–Barré syndrome (GBS), and mortality of GBS in well-defined populations*

Region surveyed	Period	Average annual incidence rate per 100,000 population			Number of cases	Antecedent infection within 4 weeks of onset of GBS	Mortality
		Total	Male	Female			
Olmstead County, Minnesota (6)	34 years (1935–1968)	1.6	2.1	1.2	29	55.2%	6.8%
Olmstead County, Minnesota (7)	42 years (1935–1976)	1.7	2.3	1.2	40	70%	5%
Olmstead County Minnesota (8)	46 years (1935–1980)	1.8	2.3	1.2	48	65%	4.1%
Iceland (9)	10 years (1954–1963)	0.7	NA[a]	NA	13	NA	15%
Guam (10)	7 years (1960–1966)	1.9	2.3	1.5	5	NA	20%
Western Norway (11)	26 years (1957–1982)	1.2	1.5	0.8	109	57%	NA
Israel (12)	4 years (1969–1972)	0.75	NA	NA	89	NA	NA
San Joaquin County, California (13)	5 years (1972–1976)	1.2	1.5	1.0	18	22.2%	11.1%
Larimer County, Colorado (14)	3 years (1981–1983)	4.0	4.1	3.8	19	83%	11%
Sardinia (15)	20 years (1969–1980)	0.4	0.41	0.39	120	35.9%	21.5%
Kenya (16)	8 years (1974–1981)	NA	NA	NA	54	60%	9%
Copenhagen County, Denmark (17)	7 1/2 years (June 1977–1984)	2.0	2.1	1.9	34	58.8%	11.8%[b]
Western Australia (18)	6 years (1980–1985)	1.35	1.5	1.2	109	58%	1.8%[c]
Benghazi, Libya (19)	3 years (1983–1985)	1.7	1.6	1.8	27	25.9%	7.4%

[a] NA, not available.
[b] Three of four deaths occurred in cancer patients.
[c] Two deceased patients with diagnosis of GBS were not included in study.

special reference to toxic neuropathies, porphyria, diphtheria, poliomyelitis, and botulism) or (b) the occurrence of a purely sensory syndrome. Features contributing to the exclusion of a case were: a mononuclear leukocyte count of more than 50 per cubic millimeter; the presence of several polymorphonuclear leukocytes in the CSF; marked asymmetry of weakness; prominent sphincter impairment; a sharp sensory level; and the presence of a course suggestive of chronic relapsing polyradiculoneuritis.

The mean annual incidence rate was 1.8 per 100,000 population, with an incidence rate of 2.3 among males and 1.2 among females. No seasonal trends were discernible. Two patients died as a result of respiratory insufficiency. The rate increased with age, from 0.8 in those under 18 years to 3.2 for those 60 years and older. The rate also increased over time, from 1.2 in the interval 1935–1956 to 2.4 in the interval 1970–1980. Whether this increase is real or partially due to increased disease awareness or improved diagnostic skills is uncertain.

Larsen et al. (11) reported 109 GBS patients diagnosed in the period 1957–1982 in western Norway according to the criteria of NINCDS. The average age-adjusted incidence rate was 1.19 per 100,000 population (1.53 in males, 0.84 in females). A slight increase in incidence with increasing age was found, somewhat greater among males than among females. Most cases occurred during the colder months; however, much of the year is relatively cold in this northern country.

A 4-year nationwide study in Israel, from 1969 through 1972, revealed 89 patients with GBS (12). The average annual age-adjusted incidence was 0.75 per 100,000 population. Peaks of incidence occurred among individuals over 60 and under 4 years of age. The overall incidence was similar in Jewish groups of diverse ethnic backgrounds. Arabs had a lower overall incidence than Jews (0.46 per 100,000 population), attributed to fewer Arabs at risk among older age groups. No seasonal or geographic clustering was detected. The lower overall incidence was felt to be due to stricter diagnostic criteria, which excluded patients with common conditions (such as diabetes) which are known to produce polyneuropathies.

Nineteen cases of GBS occurred in Larimer County, Colorado (14) during the period 1981–1983. The average annual incidence during this period was 4 cases per 100,000 population, significantly higher ($p < 0.05$) than the 1.2 cases per 100,000 population in 1975–1980. No patient characteristics or predisposing events could be found to explain the increase, which the authors assumed was due to an unusual chance occurrence.

Congia et al. (15) described 120 cases of GBS in Sardinia between 1961 and 1980. The annual incidence rate was 0.4 per 100,000 population (0.41 in males, 0.39 in females). Modified NINCDS criteria were used: The classic albuminocytologic dissociation in the CSF was considered as a prerequisite. One of the NINCDS criteria is that the presence of normal CSF does not preclude the acceptance of a case. A higher incidence was found in winter and spring. A significantly higher incidence among people older than 40 was found (0.6 > 40 years, 0.3 < 40 years). The mortality rate was 21.5% and was secondary to respiratory insufficiency. The low incidence was attributed to a combination of rigid criteria and poor recognition of GBS, since increased awareness was felt to account for the higher incidence of the disease in the second decade of the study.

Fifty-four cases of GBS were seen at a tertiary care center in Kenya from 1974 through 1981 (16). NINCDS criteria were used, with the addition that there was no history of recent immunizations or exanthematous infections. An annual incidence was not given. No seasonal variation or clustering of cases was evident. Five patients (9%) died from respiratory insufficiency, and 14 patients (26%) remained severely disabled from bilateral foot drop by the end of 16 months. The overall low number of cases, together with a high incidence of poor outcome, is probably accounted for by selective patient referral: Only severe cases were referred to this tertiary hospital.

One hundred nine cases of GBS were admitted to four major teaching hospitals in Western Australia from 1980 through 1985 (18). The annual incidence rate of GBS was 1.35 per 100,000 population. The age-adjusted incidence rates were 1.49 cases per 100,000 men and 1.20 cases per 100,000 women. NINCDS criteria as outlined by Asbury (21) were used. A minor peak in the sex-adjusted incidence rate was present in the third and fourth decades, with a larger peak noted after age 50. No significant seasonal trends or patterns were discernible. The true annual incidence rate was felt to be higher than 1.35 per 100,000 population, since the study was limited to patients who were admitted to the four major teaching hospitals in Western Australia and consequently did not include milder cases who were perhaps managed at home or in a local hospital.

The incidence rates have remained relatively similar over several decades and in vastly different geographic regions. This is consistent with a hypothesis that the triggering agents responsible for GBS are widespread and multiple and that susceptibility is similar for various geographic regions.

ANTECEDENT EVENTS

A variety of minor illnesses have been associated with GBS, and most of these are secondary to viruses. The list of viruses includes measles, mumps, rubella, varicella, cytomegalovirus (CMV), Epstein–Barr virus (EBV), herpes simplex, adenovirus, ECHO, Coxsackie, and hepatitis B. Melnick and Flewett (22) identified antecedent illnesses in 36 of 52 patients. They found that 48% of cases had an upper respiratory infection within 4 weeks of onset of neurological symptoms, compared with 18% of controls. Kennedy et al. (7) reported antecedent upper respiratory infections in 38% of patients and gastrointestinal illness in 28% of patients versus 27% and 0%, respectively, of controls with Bell's palsies.

Winer et al. (23) conducted a prospective study in 100 GBS patients with age- and sex-matched controls. Upper respiratory infection occurred within 1 month of onset of neurological symptoms in 38% of patients and in 12% of controls ($p < 0.001$), and gastrointestinal illness occurred in 17% of patients and in 3% of controls ($p < 0.005$). Eight percent of patients had undergone an operation within the preceding 3 months. Serological evidence of recent infection was identified in 31% of patients. *Campylobacter jejuni* (14%) and CMV (11%) were both significantly more frequently demonstrated in patients than in controls. Serological evidence of recent infection with *Mycoplasma* (1%), EBV (1–2%), and parvovirus B19 (4%) was also identified in patients, but not more frequently than in controls. A higher proportion of those with serological evidence of *Campylobacter* infection had a poor outcome compared with the remainder ($p < 0.05$). The small number of patients with evidence of recent EBV infection may be a reflection of the age of the patients. Sixty-two of the patients were over 40 years old and only 11 were under 20 years of age, whereas primary EBV infection might be expected to be more frequent among children and young adults.

Dowling and Cook (24) used an indirect immunofluorescent technique to identify immunoglobulin M (IgM) antibody directed against CMV in the serum of 33 of 220 (15%) GBS patients. The CMV-positive patients were mainly young adults (average age 25.6 years), and only 80% had a clinically apparent antecedent illness. In a parallel study, EBV-specific IgM antibody was found in eight of 100 (8%) GBS patients. As with CMV, some EBV-infected patients had no obvious prodromal illness and others had antecedent illness not characteristic of infectious mononucleosis. Dowling and co-workers (25,26) also revealed elevated titers of CMV complement-fixing antibody in over 30% of patients in a previous large controlled serological survey of GBS. Grose et al. (27) demonstrated antibody to EBV in seven of 24 patients (29%) with GBS. In contrast to CMV and EBV, herpes simplex virus uncommonly precedes GBS. Menonna et al. (28) demonstrated IgM herpes-simplex-virus-specific antibody in only one of 75 GBS patients.

Hankey (18) identified adenovirus in seven of 109 cases (6.4%) of GBS, CMV in six cases (5.5%), parainfluenza viruses in five cases (4.6%), enteroviruses in three cases (2.8%), and *Mycoplasma pneumoniae* in five cases (4.6%). Single cases of varicella, EBV, and measles were also seen, along with two cases with herpes simplex virus. Goldschmidt et al. (29) also identified serum antibodies to *Mycoplasma pneumoniae* in five of 100 (5%) GBS patients.

GBS has been described both early (30,31) and late (32) in the course of human immunodeficiency virus (HIV) infection. Cornblath et al. (30) described nine patients who presented with progressive weakness. Two had lymphadenopathy, but all were otherwise asymptomatic. Six had chronic inflammatory demyelinating polyneuropathy (CIDP), and three had GBS. Most patients had a CSF pleocytosis (mean value: 23 cells per cubic millimeter). The authors recommended plasmapheresis for initial therapy. Berger et al. (33), however, questioned the necessity of plasmapheresis after observing an excellent recovery in 1–6 months without steroids or plasmapheresis in six HIV-seropositive patients with GBS. The neuropathy is probably immune-mediated in HIV-seropositive patients with GBS, and it is secondary to the disordered immune regulation that is characteristic of HIV infection.

Rhodes and Tattersfield (34) reported the first case of GBS following *Campylobacter* enteritis in 1982. Since then, multiple additional cases have surfaced. In fact, *Campylobacter jejuni* was the most common single identifiable pathogen in one study (35), with evidence of preceding infection found in 21 of 58 (36%) patients. In addition, a preceding *Campylobacter* infection was associated with a statistically significant, more severe form of GBS, with 90% of patients requiring mechanical ventilation (versus 40% of *Campylobacter*-negative patients). Ropper (36) and De Bont et al. (37) have also described cases of severe GBS associated with *Campylobacter*, whereas others (38–40) have described relatively mild cases. Appropriate antibiotic treatment of the enteritis is not effective in preventing the subsequent development of GBS (41). *Campylobacter jejuni* may have been responsible for two outbreaks of GBS following gastroenteritis caused by contamination of the water supply system (42,43). Occasional cases have been associated with bacterial infection such as brucellosis (44), *Yersinia* ar-

thritis (45), typhoid fever (46), tularemia (47), and listeriosis (44).

GBS has been reported following spinal or epidural anesthesia (48). Five to 10 percent of cases have occurred following intracranial, thoracic, abdominal, and orthopedic surgical procedures (14,23,49,50).

Of special interest is the association of GBS with various vaccines. In the past the only vaccines associated with GBS were former rabies vaccines containing central nervous system (CNS) tissue and the A/New Jersey/76 swine influenza vaccine. A temporary increase of GBS was reported in the United States in the period 1976–1977 after a massive A/New Jersey/76 influenza vaccination campaign (51). Arnason (52) concluded that the A/New Jersey/76 swine influenza vaccine was definitely associated with an increased risk of GBS. There were multiple flaws in this study, however (53,54). Detailed neurological examinations and follow-up evaluations were not performed on all patients. In addition, there were no uniform diagnostic criteria. Furthermore, there was a lack of variation in the number of cases of GBS in the U.S. Army based on hospital discharge diagnoses in the 6 years through 1976 (including the period in which the vaccine was widely used) (55). There was no increase in GBS in active-duty Air Force and Naval personnel, among whom 90% and 68%, respectively, had received the vaccine (53). Finally, an increased incidence of GBS was not found with earlier influenza vaccination programs, which are estimated to number about 300 million doses, including some who received this type. A reassessment determined that it was unlikely that vaccine-associated cases occurred beyond 6 weeks after vaccination (56).

An outbreak of poliomyelitis in Finland during the latter half of 1984 resulted in an intensified vaccination program with oral poliovirus vaccine (OPV) (57). Ten patients developed GBS within 10 weeks after OPV vaccination, significantly above the mean for the period (observed-to-expected ratio: 3.38). Their mean age was 43.5 years, and the mean onset occurred after 31 days. Only four patients showed symptoms of viral infection during the preceding 10 weeks, but in none of them could a specific agent be identified in throat or stool cultures. Because of the variable background frequency of GBS, the inability to rule out subclinical infections, and the small number of unexpected cases following OPV vaccination, the authors concluded that it was impossible to estimate the relative risk of this new complication of OPV. Furthermore, since the mean age in the OPV-associated GBS cases did not differ from the remaining GBS cases, if OPV is actually responsible for any GBS cases, it should not increase the risk of GBS in children, the usual population of OPV immunization (57).

Four cases of GBS have occurred after immunization with a *Hemophilus influenzae* type b conjugate vaccine composed of a capsular polysaccharide antigen, polyribosylribitol phosphate, covalently linked to diphtheria toxoid; this vaccine was called "PRP-D" (ProHIBIT, Connaught Laboratories, Inc., Swiftwater, PA) (58). Only one of three patients was tested for possible subclinical viral or bacterial infection. Approximately 6.2 million doses of PRP-D vaccine had been distributed. The authors concluded that even if a causal association between GBS and the PRP-D vaccine is proved, it would probably be very rare in view of the large number of PRP-D vaccinations administered.

Rare cases of GBS have also been reported following measles (59), smallpox (60), mumps–rubella (61), diphtheria–tetanus–pertussis (62), and polyvalent pneumococcal vaccines (63).

GBS may also occur during the postpartum period or during the latter part of pregnancy, with no effect on offspring (64,65). Clinically and pathologically typical cases of GBS have also been associated with malignancy, especially Hodgkin and non-Hodgkin lymphomas (66–68).

PATHOLOGY

The pathological hallmark of GBS consists of a perivenular mononuclear cellular infiltrate with segmental demyelination in the peripheral nervous system (PNS) (69). The pathological findings are remarkably uniform regardless of the antecedent illness or precipitating event. Perivenular infiltrates consisting of lymphocytes, transformed lymphocytes, and macrophages are seen primarily surrounding endoneural and epineural venules of the PNS (Fig. 1). Edema of nerve roots and spinal nerves noted in earlier reports (70,71) has not been noted in more recent publications (52,69). Earlier studies described the proximal portion of the PNS as the primary site of involvement. Casamajor (72) found severe changes in the anterior roots in the region where these roots emerge from the pia and where they are enclosed by arachnoid and dura. Margulis (73) found lesions to be most pronounced in the root nerves just proximal to where they are enclosed in dura. Haymaker and Kernohan (71) found the most prominent lesions where the motor and sensory roots join to form the mixed spinal nerve. Extensive involvement along the entire length of the peripheral nerves (69) and sympathetic chains and ganglia (74) has also been described. Most frequently there is no preferential involvement of anterior roots over posterior roots (52); however, some studies (69,71) have noted (a) a predominance of anterior root lesions in patients with prominent paralysis and (b) equal root involvement in patients in which profound sensory changes have accompanied the paralysis.

Small to medium-sized lymphocytes are the earliest cells to exit the venules and are found immediately outside the venules in the nerve parenchyma. Larger lymphocytes undergoing transformation along with actively phagocytic macrophages derived from blood monocytes are seen farther out from the venules. Associated with the mononuclear cellular infiltrates are areas of segmental demyelination (Fig. 2). These areas occur in zones corresponding to the areas of inflammatory infiltration (69).

Initially, lymphocytes are primarily seen. However, as lesions evolve, macrophages become the predominant cell. The earliest change noted is retraction at the node of

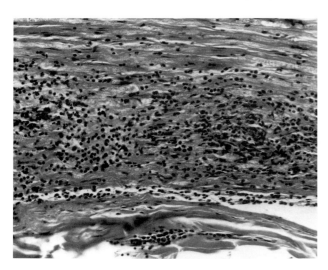

FIG. 1. Diffuse mononuclear infiltrate in peripheral nerve in GBS. (From ref. 194, with permission.)

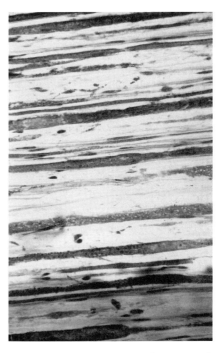

FIG. 2. Focal demyelination in GBS. (Courtesy of Dr. Shin J. Oh.)

Ranvier to produce a widened nodal gap. Signs of myelin sheath disintegration with segmentation, ovoid formation, and phagocytosis proceed from the nodal region toward the centrally located Schwann cell nucleus (52). Arstila et al. (75) demonstrated increased acid phosphatase and acid proteinase activities signifying activation of lysosomes in macrophages in areas of demyelination. Intense inflammatory lesions are associated with axonal interruption and subsequent Wallerian degeneration in addition to segmental demyelination. Polymorphonuclear leukocytes are also seen in severe lesions, probably in response to tissue necrosis (69). Arnason (52) attributes clinical progression to a summation effect as new discrete focal inflammatory deposits and focal areas of segmental demyelination continue to accumulate throughout the PNS. The mononuclear inflammatory infiltrate may persist for years following clinical recovery, as demonstrated by Asbury et al. (69) in autopsies on patients with a history of GBS who died years later of other causes.

Schwann cell proliferation, evidenced by an increase in the density of longitudinally oriented nuclei within nerve fascicles, is first seen after 8–10 days (69,71). Schwann cell proliferation occurs in association with segmental demyelination (76). A demyelinated internode is eventually replaced by several shorter, lightly myelinated ones, each new internode having its own Schwann cell. In Wallerian degeneration the internodal lengths are all uniformly shortened, and the replacement myelin is uniformly thinner. Reparative processes may proceed during ongoing myelin breakdown. Central chromatolysis (and, in some instances, dissolution) of the anterior horn cells is seen in cases with extensive Wallerian degeneration. Posterior column degeneration secondary to demyelination of dorsal roots and ganglia is seen in a minority of cases. Denervation atrophy of muscle fibers may be seen with axonal degeneration.

Electron-microscopic (EM) studies of GBS began to appear in the 1960s. Table 2 summarizes the EM findings of several studies (77–83). Finean and Woolf (77) described Wallerian degeneration with only secondary changes in myelin. Fragmentation of nerve was seen, and the authors could not be certain that this was not due to physical change.

Wisniewski et al. (78) reported EM findings in a fatal case of GBS. Various degrees of myelin sheath destruction without axonal damage was noted. Within the boundaries of the Schwann cell basement membrane, a macrophage or large mononuclear cell always appeared in association with myelin destruction (Fig. 3). Lymphocytes and plasma cells were never seen beneath the Schwann cell basement membrane of affected nerve fibers. The myelin disruption showed an unusual pattern of degeneration which was net-like or vesicular (Figs. 4 and 5). This was usually circumferential following the expected lamellar distribution. No relationship between the area of myelin destruction and the node of Ranvier could be determined. Remyelination of demyelinated axons was not seen. These authors concluded that peripheral demyelination in GBS is a primary, rather than a secondary, phenomenon.

Liu (79) described vesicular myelin alteration in the absence of cells within the basal lamina in a patient who died 17 days after the onset of symptoms. He interpreted these changes as a mode of myelin formation.

Miyakawa et al. (80) biopsied a sural nerve and also described vesicular myelin degeneration. The axoplasm of both myelinated and unmyelinated nerves were noted to contain degenerative mitochondria and vacuolar changes.

Hart et al. (81) described the EM findings in a fatal case which progressed rapidly over the course of 3 days. Characteristically, the myelin unraveled, forming coils which appeared to initiate simultaneously from the in-

TABLE 2. *Electron-microscopic findings in Guillain–Barré syndrome*

Investigators	Number of cases	Invasion of Schwann cell basal lamina by macrophages	Myelin vesiculation adjacent to invading macrophages	Myelin vesiculation in absence of cells within basal lamina	Stripping of normal myelin by macrophages	Damaged Schwann cells	Remyelination
Finean and Woolf, 1962 (77)	3	+	−	−	−	−	−
Wisniewski et al., 1969 (78)	1	+	+	−	−	−	−
Liu, 1970 (79)	1	−	−	+	−	−	−
Miyakawa et al., 1971 (80)	1	−	−	+	−	+	−
Hart et al., 1972 (81)	1	+	−	+	−	−	−
Carpenter, 1972 (82)	1	+	+	−	−	+	−
Prineas, 1972 (83)	9	+[a]	+	−	+	+	+

[a] Lymphocytes occasionally present together with macrophages.

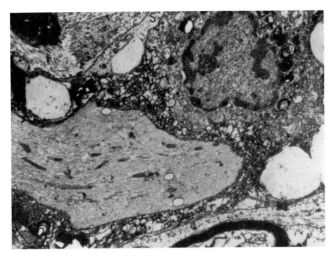

FIG. 3. Longitudinal section of myelin sheath undergoing vesicular transformation. Completely normal axis cylinder is seen within midst of severely damaged myelin. Macrophage with phagocytized myelin debris is in contact with altered myelin. Note that myelin dissolution extends far from point of contact with invading cell. Normal Schwann cell cytoplasm (S) overlies myelin and mononuclear cell. ×3300. (From ref. 78, with permission.)

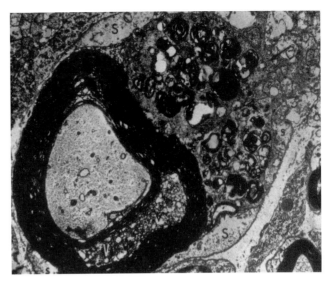

FIG. 5. Schwann-cell–macrophage relationship showing two macrophages penetrating Schwann cell basement membrane (*arrow*). Schwann cell (S) is pushed away from myelin sheath. Vesiculation (V) of myelin in middle and inner lamellae of myelin sheath is present. Several normal nerve fibers are seen in lower right field. Slit-like gaps in the thick sheath are probably artifact. ×7000. (From ref. 78, with permission.)

side and outside of the sheath, with sparing of the middle layers of the sheath until later. Less frequently seen were nerves showing uniform vesicular degeneration with axonal sparing. In a few instances, cytoplasmic extensions of macrophages appeared to dissect under the Schwann cell's basement membrane. These extensions were associated with breakage or "peeling-off" of myelin. The axons were almost always intact.

Carpenter (82) reported on a fatal case that came to

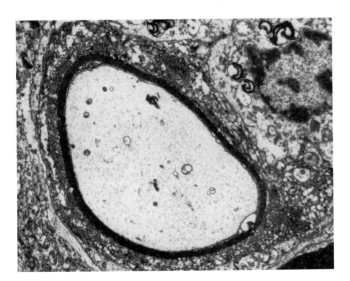

FIG. 4. Cross section of nerve fiber showing net-like and vesicular transformation of outer layers of myelin sheath. Macrophage contacts only small portion of myelin sheath surface, but myelin dissolution is visible around entire circumference of fiber. S, Schwann cell cytoplasm. ×7100. (From ref. 78, with permission.)

autopsy 18 days after the onset of weakness. He noted findings similar to those reported by Wisniewski et al.—vesicular myelin breakdown in the presence of macrophages beneath the Schwann cell basement membrane. Some of the Schwann cells appeared to be damaged. Remyelination was not seen, although the occasional occurrence of thin cytoplasmic tentacles extending out from some Schwann cells may be an early indicator of impending remyelination.

Prineas (83) found evidence of active demyelination in six of nine sural nerve biopsies. In addition to extracellular vesicular degeneration of myelin, a second and more common pattern of myelin destruction was seen. After penetrating the Schwann cell basal lamina and displacing superficial Schwann cell cytoplasm away from the intact sheath, invading macrophages inserted organelle-free processes into the sheath along minor dense lines and phagocytosed groups of intact myelin lamellae. Afterwards, the Schwann cells were noted to have a severe depletion of granular endoplasmic reticulum. Remyelination occurred with the formation of new internodes. Lymphocytes were occasionally observed together with macrophages, but never alone, within the basal lamina of affected fibers.

PATHOGENESIS AND PATHOPHYSIOLOGY

The current concept that GBS is an acquired immune-mediated disorder is based on pathological findings consisting of perivascular infiltration of mononuclear cells in association with segmental demyelination. Investigation of the pathogenesis of GBS led to the successful establishment of an animal model by Waksman and Adams (84) in 1955, which they termed "experimental allergic neuritis" (EAN). EAN is nearly identical to GBS on clinical, electrophysiological, and pathological findings. Recent advances in unraveling the pathogenesis of EAN and GBS have been summarized in an excellent review by Hartung and Toyka (85). We will discuss, in detail, new findings regarding the pathogenesis of each of these disorders.

Experimental Allergic Neuritis

Waksman and Adams (84) produced EAN by injection of homogenates of whole peripheral nerve in rabbits. The main proteins of peripheral nerve myelin consist of P0 (a glycoprotein confined to the PNS) and two basic proteins, P2 and myelin basic protein (MBP). MBP is the encephalitogen of experimental allergic encephalomyelitis. Milner et al. (86) induced EAN in Lewis rats with a purified P0 preparation. Brostoff et al. (87) and Kadlubowski and Hughes (88) induced EAN with P2 in rabbits and inbred Lewis rats, respectively.

In order to better characterize the immune response to various regions of the P2 protein during EAN, peptides generated by cyanogen bromide digestion of the protein were tested for their ability to produce circulating antibody and cell-mediated responses (89). Three peptides—CN1, CN2, and CN3—were identified. CN1-immunized rats had equal or more severe clinical and histological signs of EAN but lower antibody titers than did P2-immunized animals. CN1 elicited a greater blastogenic response in both P2- and CN1-immunized animals. CN2- and CN3-immunized rats demonstrated little clinical or histological evidence of disease and no antibody. However, they did induce lymphocyte transformation. This contrast in humoral and cellular response is in accordance with the work of other investigators (90,91) who found that T-cell determinants are less dependent on conformation than are B-cell determinants. The authors concluded that the ability of CN1 to stimulate a greater lymphoblast response than that of the intact protein and other peptides may be an indication of a cell-mediated mechanism of pathogenesis. Olee et al. (92) identified the smallest region of bovine P2 protein capable of inducing EAN as an amphipathic alpha-helical structure comprising residues 61–72.

Hughes et al. (93) passively transferred EAN with lymph node cells from rats immunized with either P2 or myelin. The absence of antibody to P2 in the serum of recipients who developed EAN makes it unlikely that the disease is caused by circulating antibody; instead, EAN is probably a cell-mediated immune response. Rostami et al. (94) and Linington et al. (95) confirmed Hughes' findings by inducing EAN in Lewis rats by injection of T

helper cells specific for P2 protein. Again, lack of anti-P2 antibody in recipients of lymphocytes suggests that the transfer of EAN was not simply a result of active immunization of the recipients by P2 bound to the cultured cells.

Further evidence for a cell-mediated pathogenesis was supplied by Brosman et al. (96). The majority of Lewis rats made T-cell-deficient by adult thymectomy and lethal irradiation were less susceptible to induction of EAN. Those T-cell-deficient rats which succumbed to EAN were found to have a significantly higher percentage of residual blood T lymphocytes than those which did not. Full susceptibility to EAN was restored by an inoculum of whole thoracic duct lymphocytes from normal rats. Hartung et al. (97) injected a monoclonal antibody to the rat interleukin-2 receptor (IL-2R) prior to, and on consecutive days after, adoptive transfer EAN. Essentially all activated T cells expose on their surface a high-affinity receptor for the growth factor interleukin-2 (IL-2) as a consequence of antigenic stimulation, whereas virtually none are displayed on resting T cells (98). Early injection of this antibody suppressed EAN, whereas treatment after the appearance of clinical signs did not.

Immunohistochemistry studies (99–101) have revealed a preponderance of CD4+ helper/inducer T cells early in the course of the disease, with an increase of CD8+ cytotoxic/suppressor T cells noted during the peak and recovery phases. Macrophages increasingly outnumber lymphocytes with progression of the disease.

The mechanism by which activated T cells cross the blood–nerve barrier has been studied. The number and extent of degranulation of mast cells in the sciatic nerve of rats sensitized for the development of EAN were determined (102). No change in the number or percentage of degranulated mast cells was observed before day 8 after sensitization. On day 8 a substantial decrease in the number of detectable mast cells was seen, followed by a marked increase in the number of degranulated cells. These changes preceded the onset of clinical symptoms, which were first noted on day 10. Evidence for mast cell degranulation preceded clinical and pathological signs of disease, suggesting that transformed lymphocytes mediate mast cell degranulation or that early alteration in blood–nerve barrier function may permit access of degranulating factors to the nerve parenchyma (103). A role for vasoactive amines in the initiation of EAN was further confirmed (104). Rats immunized for EAN were injected with reserpine immediately before, during, and after the onset of symptoms. Rats injected before or during the onset of early clinical signs experienced a considerable delay in the time of disease onset. Additional studies revealed that the onset of disease activity correlated well with the depletion and recovery of serotonin and norepinephrine in the peripheral blood.

A substantial amount of evidence implicating humoral immunity in the pathogenesis of EAN exists. EM studies of EAN have revealed demyelination in association with contact with invading macrophages (105–107).

Helper/inducer T cells can recognize antigens only in association with major histocompatibility complex (MHC) class II (Ia) antigens. Schmidt et al. (108) used serial 1-μm cryosections of ventral roots from rats with EAN for immunocytochemical identification of cell types. MHC class II antigen immunoreactivity was nearly always associated with "lean" macrophages; these contain only a few lysosomes in their cytoplasm, but not Schwann cells. Interferon-gamma has been shown to increase the severity of EAN in rats by up-regulating MHC class II antigen expression, increasing cellular influx of T cells and macrophages, and augmenting release of reactive oxygen species by macrophages (109). In addition to toxic oxygen species, macrophages also release arachidonic-acid-derived eicosanoids which contribute to clinical and pathological damage in EAN. The addition of the oxygen radical scavengers catalase or superoxide dismutase prior to the onset of clinical symptoms prevented the development of EAN in Lewis rats and markedly diminished the severity when given after the onset of clinical disease (110). Proposed mechanisms include (a) restriction of secondary cellular immigration into lesions, (b) suppression of complement-mediated amplification of inflammatory responses, and (c) the prevention of direct peroxidative injury to myelin. Treatment with blockers of arachidonic conversion, such as indomethacin or dexamethasone, was also effective in preventing or greatly diminishing the severity of EAN (111).

Depletion studies have also been performed to stress the importance of humoral immunity in the development of EAN. Silica quartz dust is selectively toxic to macrophages (112). Intraperitoneal injection of silica has been demonstrated to prevent all clinical and pathological signs of EAN (111,113). Others have concluded that macrophages are not directly involved in the early stages of EAN; instead, they act as effector cells and are responsible for producing the secondary manifestations of the disease (114).

Myelin degradation by lysosomal enzymes from activated macrophages has been demonstrated (115). Sobue et al. (116) found a 1.5- to 3.0-fold increase in acid proteinase, acid phosphatase, and beta-glucuronidase in the spinal roots (and a 1.0- to 1.5-fold increase in the sciatic nerves) in rabbits with EAN compared to controls. The topographical distribution of the increase closely corresponded to the histological distribution of EAN lesions. These observations suggested that the increased lysosomal activity originated from invading lysosome-rich macrophages.

There is also evidence for a role of complement in EAN. Cobra venom factor (CVF) depletes the C3 component of complement. Lewis rats treated with CVF had delayed onset of symptoms and less severe disease when compared to control EAN rats (117).

Guillain–Barré Syndrome

The clear pathological evidence of lymphocyte and macrophage infiltration of the PNS in GBS (69,71,77–83) has led to a vigorous search for proof of abnormal cellular immunity. Several groups have attempted to demonstrate specific T-cell sensitization to P0 protein, P2 protein, and peripheral nerve myelin.

Iqbal et al. (118), using a sensitive hemagglutination assay, failed to find antibodies to P2 in sera and CSF from five patients with GBS and three patients with chronic relapsing inflammatory polyneuritis (CRIP). Abramsky et al. (119) reported evidence of cell-mediated immunity in 18 of 30 patients with GBS. The purity of the preparation they used was poorly documented, and stimulation indices were low. Sheremata et al. (120) used a macrophage migration inhibition assay to demonstrate lymphocytic sensitivity to P2 protein in GBS patients. Other investigators (121–123) have found T-cell stimulation in only a minority of patients with GBS.

Geczy et al. (124) used a macrophage/monocyte procoagulant activity (MPCA) assay to determine cell-mediated immunity in GBS patients. This test has the advantage of being a direct correlate of the intensity of delayed skin reactivity to tuberculin and mumps antigens and is far more sensitive than blast transformation or macrophage migration inhibition assays (125). A strong and specific cell-mediated response to P2 protein occurred in 13 of 16 GBS patients tested.

T cells transiently express a surface receptor recognizing the growth factor IL-2 only after antigenic or mitogenic stimulation. Increased serum concentrations of soluble IL-2 receptors indicate the presence of circulating activated T cells. Hartung et al. (126) determined serum concentrations of soluble IL-2 receptors in 50 patients with GBS, 24 with CIDP, 54 with multiple sclerosis (MS), and 73 controls with other neurological diseases. Thirty-one of 50 GBS patients had serum-soluble IL-2 receptor concentrations that were greater than 2 standard deviations (494 ± 271 U/ml versus 216 ± 96 U/ml) above the mean of the control group. Taylor and Hughes (127) have also demonstrated that patients with GBS have a greater number of IL-2 receptors than do healthy control subjects. These activated T cells may function by inducing B cells to (a) produce antibodies against myelin constituents, (b) recruit macrophages to attack the myelin sheath, (c) activate the complement system, or (d) function as effector cells that exert cytoxic activity against myelin or Schwann cells.

In recent years, involvement of the humoral immune system in GBS has been strongly implicated because of the therapeutic effect of plasmapheresis, the ability of GBS serum to demyelinate in tissue culture, and the presence (in some patients with GBS) of serum antibodies against peripheral nerve myelin (PNM).

Hirano et al. (128) produced demyelination in dorsal

root ganglia of mice by exposing them to sera from GBS patients. Whole serum from 26 of 31 patients with GBS produced complement-dependent demyelination of fetal mouse dorsal root ganglia. Demyelination was also produced by sera from one of 11 normal subjects and from 14 of 41 patients with other neurological disorders (129).

Eleven of 27 (41%) sera from patients with GBS produced focal *in vivo* demyelination in rat peripheral nerves after intraneural injection (130). Three of 40 (7.5%) sera obtained from normal subjects and patients with other neurological diseases also caused *in vivo* demyelination, although the activity was milder in degree and was significantly less frequent. In a similar study (131), serum from 13 of 17 patients with acute GBS produced focal demyelination after injection into rat sciatic nerves. Of the four patients whose sera produced no demyelination, three had mild disease and one had Miller–Fisher syndrome. Injections of control sera from patients with other diseases and from normals produced demyelination in two of 30 cases. Intraneural injection of lymphocytes from eight patients with GBS failed to produce demyelination.

Goust et al. (132) detected immune complexes in the serum of 15 of 16 GBS patients utilizing a fluid-phase C1q assay. Although these results are consistent with the presence of immune complexes in GBS sera, false-positive results for complexes may have occurred secondary to elevation of C-reactive protein commonly seen in GBS serum (133).

Serum immunoglobulin (IgA, IgG, and IgM) levels have been shown to be higher in patients with GBS than in normal control subjects (134). Melnick (135) detected antibody to peripheral nerve in 50% of GBS patients, in contrast to 2.7% of normal controls and 6.4% of patients with other diseases. A complement fixation method that involves a differential measurement between complement activity in the control and the test proper was employed. Using this method, a test result can be taken as positive only when a substantial difference in complement activity exists, thus creating a blind zone with respect to detection of minute amounts of antigen–antibody complex. Koski et al. (136,137) detected antibody to peripheral nerve myelin in all 18 patients with acute GBS tested at their institution, as compared with normal and diseased controls. A complement component 1 (C1) fixation and transfer assay was employed, which measures fixation of C1 directly, thus eliminating the previously mentioned blind zone. In serial serum samples of seven patients with GBS, the antibody titer was always highest on admission and rapidly declined during a 1- to 3-week period. Disappearance of antibodies (or very low levels of them) correlated with cessation of progression and considerable clinical improvement as documented by increased muscular strength and pulmonary vital capacity.

Griffin et al. (138) used immunostaining to study macrophages and their expression of major histocompatibility Class II markers (Ia antigen) in six patients with chronic inflammatory neuropathy and one with GBS. Macrophages were regularly found adherent to teased blood vessels. Cells presumed to be entering the nerve were elongated and Ia-positive. After entry into nerve, the Ia-positive macrophages were adherent to both demyelinating and normal fibers. Ia positivity was often retained after penetrating into the nerve fiber and removing myelin. Presumed postphagocytic foamy macrophages were Ia-negative. Foamy macrophages adherent to blood vessels were felt to be leaving the nerve.

Additional studies have provided evidence that macrophage infiltration is necessary for myelin degradation in both Wallerian degeneration and segmental demyelination (139,140). Nerve segments kept within Millipore filters failed to undergo myelin degradation unless the pore size was large enough to allow macrophage entry.

In summary, there is convincing evidence of both humoral and cell-mediated participation in the pathogenesis and pathophysiology of GBS.

CLINICAL MANIFESTATIONS

An ad hoc committee of the National Institute of Neurological and Communicative Disorders and Stroke (NINCDS, now NINDS) proposed diagnostic criteria for GBS in 1978 (20). Asbury and Cornblath (141) reaffirmed and further elaborated on these criteria in 1990. The diagnostic criteria, along with additional comments, are summarized in the following paragraphs. Features required for diagnosis include: (a) progressive motor weakness of more than one limb and (b) areflexia, although hypoactive reflexes may be seen proximally. The weakness may precede attenuation of deep tendon reflexes by 2 or 3 days early in the course of the disease (141). The usual mode of spread is bilateral ascension from the lower extremities to involve the upper extremities, trunk, and cranial nerves (7).

Features strongly supportive of the diagnosis include: (a) *Rapid progression of motor weakness, with a plateau reached by 4 weeks.* The average time which elapsed from the beginning of weakness to its maximum was 12 days in one study, while 98% had reached their maximum weakness by 4 weeks (142). (b) *Relative symmetry.* (c) *Mild sensory symptoms.* Subjective sensory complaints commonly exceed objective sensory findings (17). When objective loss occurs, proprioception and vibration are primarily involved (143), presumably because the fibers involved in their conduction are myelinated to a greater extent than are the fibers involved in conduction of temperature, pinprick, and light touch. (d) *Cranial nerve involvement.* Data (see Table 3) compiled from nine studies revealed facial palsy (frequently

TABLE 3. Clinical symptoms in nine Guillain–Barré syndrome studies

	Markland and Riley, 1967 (145)[a]	Pleasure et al., 1968 (146)	Loffel et al., 1977 (142)	Kennedy et al., 1978 (7)	Beghi et al., 1985 (8)	Hankey, 1987 (18)	Hallas et al., 1988 (17)	Winer et al., 1988 (143)	Bahemuka, 1988 (16)	Average
Number of cases:	19	81	123	40	48	109	34	100	54	
Limb weakness:	19 (100%)	NA[b]	118 (96%)	39 (98%)	48 (100%)	108 (99%)	31 (91%)	100 (100%)	54 (100%)	98%
Upper extremity:	16 (84%)	NA	101 (82%)	NA	43 (90%)	NA	23 (67%)	NA	NA	82%
Lower extremity:	19 (100%)	NA	116 (94%)	NA	48 (100%)	108 (99%)	31 (91%)	100 (100%)	NA	97%
Sensory deficit:	11 (58%)	57 (70%)	81 (66%)	30 (75%)	37 (77%)	72 (66%)[c]	29 (85%)	[d]	[e]	70%
Hyporeflexia or areflexia:	19 (100%)	81 (100%)	123 (100%)	NA	47 (98%)	107 (98%)	29 (85%)	98 (98%)	54 (100%)	98%
Facial palsy:		51 (63%)	36 (29%)	NA	20 (42%)	62 (57%)	NA	53 (53%)	17 (32%)	46%
Extraocular muscle palsy:	6 (32%)	12 (15%)	8 (7%)	NA	2 (4%)	NA	NA	13 (13%)	3 (6%)	9%
Bulbar palsy:		NA	40 (33%)	23 (58%)	13 (27%)	NA	NA	46 (46%)	8 (15%)	36%
Respiratory failure:	1 (5%)	18 (22%)	18 (15%)	4 (10%)	6 (12%)	31 (28%)	14 (41%)	23 (23%)	8 (15%)	20%
Autonomic dysfunction:	"Some"	NA	12 (10%)	10 (25%)	11 (23%)	22 (20%)	13 (38%)	32 (32%)	13 (24%)	22%
Papilledema:	1 (5%)	8 (10%)	1 (1%)	NA	0 (0%)	2 (2%)	NA	1 (1%)	4 (7%)	3%

[a] Pediatric study.
[b] NA, not available.
[c] At "onset" of disease.
[d] Fifty-nine patients with loss of vibration, 26 patients with loss of light touch, 52 patients with loss of position, 22 patients with loss of pinprick.
[e] Nine patients with loss of deep sensation, 21 with distal sensory loss.

bilateral) in 46% of patients, extraocular muscle palsy in 9%, and bulbar palsy in 36%. (e) *Recovery.* This usually begins 2–4 weeks after the cessation of progression and may be delayed for months. Little improvement is seen after $1\frac{1}{2}$–2 years (144). Complete recovery occurs in approximately 60% of patients, with mild disability seen in 34% and significant handicap present in 6% (7,19,142,144–146). (f) *Autonomic dysfunction.* This is seen in approximately 22% of cases, although the actual figure is probably much higher (147) because minor or brief fluctuations in blood pressure and heart rate are probably unnoticed and underreported. Dysfunction may be expressed as either inadequate or excessive activity of the sympathetic and/or parasympathetic nervous system. (g) *Absence of fever at the onset of neurological symptoms.*

Clinical feature variants include: (a) *Fever at the onset of neurological symptoms.* (b) *Severe sensory loss with pain.* Ropper and Shahani (148) described pain preceding weakness by 1–5 days in four of 29 patients, whereas Mikati and DeLong (149) observed a 2-year-old female with pain preceding weakness by 19 days. (c) *Progression beyond 4 weeks or a minor relapse.* Approximately 3% of patients will have one or more relapses (52). (d) *Cessation of progression without recovery or with major permanent residual deficit occurring.* (e) *Sphincteric function is usually not impaired, although transient bladder paralysis may occur.* (f) *CNS involvement.* Although controversial, occasional GBS patients demonstrate cerebellar ataxia, dysarthria, extensor plantar responses, and ill-defined sensory levels.

CSF features strongly supportive of the diagnosis include: (a) *An elevated CSF protein.* This is seen most commonly after the first week of symptoms, and it occurs in 80–90% of patients (see Table 4). There is no obvious correlation between protein values and severity, mode of onset or progression, or outcome (7). Papilledema has been associated with higher peak protein levels (18,146) and attributed to impaired CSF absorption by

the increased protein (151), but the mechanism remains uncertain and controversial. Papilledema and increased intracranial pressure have been seen in GBS with normal CSF protein (152). (b) *Ten or fewer mononuclear leukocytes per cubic millimeter in CSF.*

CSF variants include: (a) a normal CSF protein in the period of 1–10 weeks following the onset of neurological symptoms and (b) 11–50 mononuclear leukocytes per cubic millimeter in CSF. In the presence of HIV-seropositive GBS patients, CSF pleocytosis is the norm. Cornblath et al. (30) noted a mean of 23 cells per cubic millimeter in nine patients with inflammatory demyelinating polyneuropathies.

Electrodiagnostic features strongly supportive of the diagnosis exist. Nerve conduction slowing or block is seen in approximately 80% of patients at some point during the illness. Conduction velocity is usually less than 60% of normal, but the process is patchy and not all nerves are affected. Distal latencies may be increased to as much as three times normal. Use of F-wave responses often gives good indication of slowing over proximal portions of nerve trunks and roots. Conduction studies may not become abnormal until several weeks into the illness.

Features casting doubt on the diagnosis include: (a) marked, persistent asymmetry of weakness; (b) persistent bladder or bowel dysfunction; (c) bladder or bowel dysfunction at onset; (d) more than 50 mononuclear leukocytes per cubic millimeter in CSF; (e) presence of polymorphonuclear leukocytes in CSF; and (f) sharp sensory level.

Features that rule out the diagnosis include: (a) a current history of hexacarbon abuse (volatile solvents; *n*-hexane and methyl *n*-butyl ketone); (b) abnormal porphyrin metabolism indicating a diagnosis of acute intermittent porphyria; (c) a history or finding of recent diphtheritic infection, either faucial or wound, with or without myocarditis; (d) features clinically consistent with lead neuropathy and evidence of lead intoxication;

TABLE 4. *CSF findings in seven Guillain–Barré syndrome studies[a]*

Investigators	Number of cases (with spinal tap)	Elevated CSF protein (>50 mg/dl)	CSF pleocytosis (>5 WBCs/mm³)
Lopez et al., 1973 (150)	15	12 (80%)	0
Loffel et al., 1977 (142)	117	103 (88%)[b]	15 (13%)
Kennedy et al., 1978 (7)	36	31 (86%)	7 (19%)[c]
Hogg et al., 1979 (13)	17	11 (65%)	1 (6%)
Beghi et al., 1985 (8)	42	38 (90%)[d]	7 (17%)
Hankey, 1987 (18)	103	92 (89%)[e]	11 (11%)
Winer et al., 1988 (143)	92	74 (80%)[f]	11 (12%)

[a] CSF, cerebrospinal fluid; WBCs, white blood cells.
[b] Protein concentration ≥48 mg/dl is considered elevated.
[c] WBC count >4/mm³ is considered elevated.
[d] Protein concentration ≥49 mg/dl is considered elevated.
[e] Protein concentration >45 mg/dl is considered elevated.
[f] Protein concentration >40 mg/dl is considered elevated.

(e) the occurrence of a purely sensory syndrome; and (f) a definite diagnosis of a condition such as poliomyelitis, botulism, hysterical paralysis, or toxic neuropathy (e.g., from nitrofurantoin, dapsone, or organophosphorus compounds).

ELECTROPHYSIOLOGICAL FEATURES

Recent advances in electrophysiological testing have significantly increased our understanding and improved our diagnostic accuracy in patients with GBS. Areflexia and weakness, the hallmark features of GBS, are primarily due to demyelination with conduction block (153). Earlier series employing conventional nerve conduction studies failed to detect abnormalities in 14–25% of patients (154–156). Because of the random distribution of demyelinating lesions (69), the likelihood of detecting electrophysiological abnormalities increases with the number of nerves studied (157,158).

The F-wave is a late evoked muscle response that occurs after the direct motor potential following supramaximal stimulation of a nerve. Most investigators agree that it represents a recurrent antidromic discharge of a motor neuron (159,160). The H-reflex is a late response which has longer latency and which has a threshold usually lower than that of direct compound muscle action potential (CMAP) in motor nerve conduction studies. The H-reflex study measures the latency over the monosynaptic reflex arc through the afferent Ia fibers and efferent alpha motor fibers of the S1 root (161). Significant prolongation of the minimal latencies of the F-wave and H-reflex were demonstrated at a time when conventional methods of motor and sensory conduction did not reveal an abnormality in individual patients. Lachman et al. (162) found the presence of an abnormal late response latency in 18% of patients in whom peripheral motor and sensory conduction were within normal limits. One hundred percent (11/11) of GBS patients had abnormalities present on electrodiagnostic testing combining peripheral nerve conduction studies with late response studies. Albers et al. (163) demonstrated abnormalities in 69 of 70 consecutive patients with GBS by combining late responses (F-wave, H-reflex) with electromyographic (EMG) and nerve conduction studies. Kimura (164) devised a simple equation using the F-wave to calculate the ratio between motor nerve conduction time from the spinal cord to the stimulus site and that of the remaining nerve segment to the muscle (F-ratio). A majority of the nerves tested were slowed equally in the segments above and below the stimulus site, whereas the remaining nerves were predominantly slowed in either proximal or distal segments but with equal preference between the two. This is in agreement with the histological findings of random lesions throughout the PNS (69).

Somatosensory evoked potentials (SEPs) have also been found to be of benefit in detecting abnormalities in patients suspected of having GBS (157,165). Walsh et al. (165) compared SEPs and F-waves in 17 GBS patients. SEPs provided a higher yield of evidence of abnormalities of proximal conduction than did F-waves. SEPs detected proximal conduction abnormalities in 12 of 17 patients, whereas median F-wave abnormalities were present in eight of 17 patients. In addition, SEPs were abnormal in three patients with normal median peripheral nerve conduction and F-wave studies, whereas the F-wave was abnormal in only one patient with normal SEPs and median peripheral nerve conduction studies. Ropper and Chiappa (166), however, found F-waves to be more sensitive than SEPs. They studied 30 GBS patients during the first 4 weeks of illness. Seven patients with normal SEPs had abnormal F-waves from the same nerve; none had normal F-wave latencies and abnormal SEPs. Olney and Aminoff (158) detected significant electrodiagnostic abnormalities in 95% (42/44) of nerves and in 100% (15/15) of patients with SEPs, F-wave studies, and peripheral motor and sensory nerve conduction studies. Abnormalities were detected in 70% (31/44) of nerves by F-wave studies and in 52% (23/44) by SEPs. The higher sensitivity of F-wave determinations was more prominent when multiple nerves were tested, because the sensitivity of F-wave studies increased while the sensitivity of SEPs remained unchanged. Only two patients had normal peripheral nerve conduction studies on all included nerves. Both of these patients had abnormal F-wave studies, whereas neither had an abnormal SEP. The authors concluded that the recording of SEPs is indicated for diagnosis of GBS only if peripheral nerve conduction and F-wave studies are normal.

Albers et al. (163) studied the temporal evolution of electrophysiological changes in 70 patients with GBS. During the first 5 weeks of illness, motor conduction study abnormalities were more common than sensory conduction abnormalities. The nadir of abnormality occurred during the third week for motor conduction studies and during the fourth week for sensory conduction studies. Delayed sensory abnormalities were felt to reflect, in part, secondary involvement related to increased intraneural edema accentuated by compression at sites of anatomic vulnerability. Abnormalities of conduction velocity at the 20th week after onset were similar to the impairment at week 2, despite substantial clinical improvement. The CMAP amplitude, however, improved significantly from the second week to the 20th week. The most prolonged F-wave latencies were recorded during the third to fifth weeks after onset; however, absent F-waves were common early in the course of the illness. The earliest EMG abnormality was decreased motor unit action potential (MUAP) recruitment, without abnormality of configuration or evidence of abnormal spontaneous activity. No patient had normal MUAP recruitment at the time of initial examination. MUAP recruitment scores gradually improved, but not in pace with the overall clinical improvement. Abnormal spontaneous activity appeared between the second and fourth weeks following disease onset. Proximal fibrillation potentials were maximal between the sixth and 10th weeks, with distal fibrillation potentials peaking between the 11th and 15th weeks. The earliest abnormality of MUAP configuration was an increased percentage of polyphasic MUAPs during the fourth week in both proximal and distal muscles. The percentage peaked between the ninth and 15th week of illness. Increased MUAP amplitude became apparent between the fourth and fifth weeks and peaked between the 11th and 35th weeks before subsequently returning to normal. Small, low-amplitude, highly polyphasic MUAPs were demonstrated in several patients during the second month of illness. These were felt to represent regenerating axons.

TREATMENT

The mainstay of therapy is meticulous nursing and medical care. Frequent and occasionally fatal autonomic dysfunction mandates the use of continuous monitoring of the electrocardiogram and blood pressure. Frequent positioning of patients is necessary to avoid nerve pressure palsies. Passive movements of each joint through a full range of motion aids in maintaining limb flexibility and protecting against venous thrombosis. Low-dose (5000 units twice a day) subcutaneous heparin is commonly employed for prophylaxis against deep vein thrombosis and pulmonary embolism. Active physiotherapy during the recovery period hastens the return of limb control, walking, and balance.

Infections of the urinary tract and lung have been described in almost 25% of GBS patients in intensive care units (167). Regular chest physiotherapy is essential to prevent sputum retention, bronchial obstruction, and segmental collapse. A closed urinary drainage system is also recommended, along with regular sputum and urine cultures if infection is suspected.

Respiratory failure occurs in 20% of patients (see Table 3) and necessitates careful respiratory monitoring, particularly during the acutely progressive stage of illness. Elective intubation and mechanical ventilation are indicated in the presence of a rapidly falling vital capacity, deteriorating blood gases, or clinical signs such as brow sweat, dyspnea, and tachycardia. Newton-John (168) demonstrated that early assisted ventilation (before the vital capacity fell below 21 ml/kg) was associated with less infection and pulmonary complications than was late assisted ventilation (when the vital capacity fell below 15 ml/kg). By waiting until the second week of mechanical ventilation, approximately 33% of patients can be extubated and thus will not need to receive a tracheostomy (169).

The quadriplegic patient with severe GBS is susceptible to anxiety and depression. Reassurance that the disease is self-limited and that the majority of patients have a good outcome is beneficial. Visits from former patients are also very helpful.

The only two controlled trials using steroids in the treatment of GBS have given contradictory results. Swick and McQuillen (170) randomized 16 patients with mild or moderate GBS to treatment with adrenocorticotropic hormone (ACTH; 100 units intramuscularly for 10 days) or placebo. Seriously ill patients were excluded, and most of the patients received ACTH after reaching their plateau. The initiation of steroids did not cause any apparent immediate improvement in the severity of illness in any patient. The mean duration to recovery was 4.4 months in the treated patients and 9.0 months in the nontreated patients ($p = 0.05$). However, the duration of hospitalization in the treated and nontreated patients was quite similar. In view of the shorter duration of illness in patients who received steroids, the authors concluded that steroids are of value in the treatment of GBS.

Hughes et al. (171) conducted a larger, multicenter trial of prednisolone; mild-to-severe GBS patients were all included. Twenty-one patients were treated with prednisolone (60 mg daily for 1 week, 40 mg daily for 4 days, and then 30 mg daily for 3 days), and 19 did not have steroid treatment. Reassessment at 1, 3, and 12 months consistently showed greater improvement in the control group than in the prednisolone group. The only statistically significant result was in the improvement at 3 months among patients entered into the trial within a week of onset of illness. Six prednisolone patients, as opposed to one control patient, were left with considerable disability. There were three relapses in the prednisolone group, but there were none in the control group. In the absence of more information, it seems reasonable to accept the conclusion from this larger controlled trial that steroids have little effect on GBS, and that if they do have an effect, it is detrimental rather than beneficial (172).

There have been five controlled studies employing plasma exchange (PE) in the treatment of GBS. None of the trials were blind because it was considered unethical to carry out sham PE. Greenwood et al. (173) treated 14 of 29 patients with severe GBS (unable to walk 5 meters unaided) with PE. Treatment consisted of five exchanges in 10 days (55 ml of plasma per kilogram body weight per exchange). Several patients were entered into the study who were not in the early, progressive phase of the disease. Overall, there was a minor benefit in the exchange group at 2 weeks; however, it was not significant, and it diminished with longer follow-up. A slightly greater benefit at 2 weeks was seen in the patients in the exchange group who entered the study within 2 weeks of onset of symptoms; again it was not significant, and it lessened with follow-up.

In a slightly larger study from Sweden, 18 severely affected patients were treated with PE and 20 served as controls (174). PE consisted of at least 6 kg of plasma shifted over a maximum of 10 days or 10 kg over 8 days. The average time between the onset of disease and entry into the study was half (6.7 days) that for Greenwood's study (173). Significant benefits were seen in (a) time until onset of improvement, (b) course of muscular weakness, (c) improvement in disability grades over the first 2 months, and (d) working capacity after 1 month. Cost–benefit analysis showed that the PE treatment resulted in net financial savings.

The North American study group compared PE with conventional therapy in 245 patients with severe GBS (175). A total of 200–250 ml of plasma per kilogram body weight was exchanged in 7–14 days. Statistically significant differences, favoring the PE group, were found in terms of (a) improvement at 4 weeks, (b) time to improve one clinical grade, (c) time to independent walking, and (d) outcome at 6 months. The average time that patients were on a respirator was decreased by 11 days in the PE group, and the time to make a functional recovery (walking unassisted) was decreased by an average of 32 days for all patients and by 72 days for those who had been on a respirator and received PE. Regardless of disease severity, patients receiving PE within 7 days of onset recovered more rapidly. Little benefit of PE could be shown after 14 days of symptoms. There was no significant difference in the frequency of complications, relapses, or deaths in the two groups.

Farkkila et al. (176) conducted a prospective, controlled study with quantitative measurement of hand muscle force in 26 patients with severe acute GBS. The muscle forces increased and CSF protein decreased significantly more rapidly in the PE group than in the control group, but there were no differences in hospitalization or recovery periods. The failure to demonstrate an improvement in recovery in the PE group may be due to a prolonged time (mean 15.7 days) from initial neurological symptoms to first PE. The authors concluded that socioeconomic factors, rather than the efficacy of the PE treatment per se, may have been responsible for the failure to shorten the hospital stay or to decrease the recovery time.

The French Cooperative group (177) conducted a multicenter, controlled trial with 220 GBS patients. Their objectives were to study the short-term effect of PE when applied alone within 17 days of onset of the disease and to compare diluted albumin and fresh-frozen plasma with regard to efficacy and morbidity as replacement fluids. The majority of patients had severe GBS; only 10 patients were able to walk unaided on inclusion day. Treatment consisted of four plasma exchanges of two plasma volumes each, initiated on the day of randomization and repeated on alternate days. Significant short-term benefits appeared in the PE group, as demon-

strated by (a) the reduction in the proportion of patients who required assisted ventilation after randomization, (b) the decrease in time before beginning weaning from ventilator, (c) the reduction in time to onset of motor recovery, and (d) the decrease in time to walk with and without assistance. The interval from onset to entry, longer or shorter than 7 days, did not influence the time to begin motor recovery within the exchanged group. However, for patients randomized more than 1 week after onset, the reduction in time to walk with assistance was no longer significant in the PE group. No statistically significant difference was found between the group that received albumin and the groups that received fresh-frozen plasma. Incidents during exchanges and complications related to the PE were more frequent in patients who received fresh-frozen plasma. Disease-related complications such as pneumonia or autonomic disorders were less frequent in the PE group. However, septicemias were more frequent in the PE group, perhaps secondary to repeated vascular punctures required by the treatment. There was no significant difference in the incidence of relapses between the two groups.

PE has also been used successfully in children with GBS. Khatri et al. (178) treated 11 children (mean age: 7.8 years) with PE in an uncontrolled study. The interval from disease onset to the initiation of PE therapy was less than 7 days in five patients and less than 2 weeks in the others. Improvement was seen in 10 of 11 patients by 1 week after the last PE. At subsequent examination 6 months later, all patients were ambulatory and nine of 11 had no significant neurological findings. The two children with significant disability at 6 months had findings consistent with an axonal neuropathy on electrophysiologic studies performed prior to treatment initiation, whereas the nine children without significant disability had evidence of a predominant demyelinating neuropathy. No severe complications were encountered during the 76 PE procedures.

Epstein and Sladky (179) retrospectively evaluated the treatment of GBS in children admitted to The Children's Hospital of Philadelphia between January 1984 and March 1989. Of the 30 patients identified, seven were excluded because they had mild disease. Of the remaining 23, nine underwent PE and 14 served as historic control subjects. The mean time to recover to Grade II (independent ambulation) was 24 days in the PE group and 60.2 days in the control group, a statistically significant difference.

In contrast to most studies (173–175,177) some investigators have noted an increase in the incidence of relapses with PE (180,181). Osterman et al. (180) documented a relapse within 4 weeks after completing a PE treatment in six of 23 patients. All patients improved rapidly after repeated PE treatment. Two different techniques of PE were used. With the intermittent flow technique, about 1.2 kg of plasma was removed per exchange, in five to seven sessions over 8–10 days. With the continuous-flow or membrane filtration technique, typically 2.5–3 kg of plasma was removed per exchange, in three to four sessions over 3–5 days. The results did not differ between the techniques with respect to either (a) the number of patients improved at 2 weeks or (b) the degree of improvement in the nonrelapsing responders at 2 and 4 weeks after the initial PE. However, none of the nine patients who showed improvement by the intermittent flow technique relapsed, compared with six of 14 patients treated with the rapid techniques. The authors concluded that a relationship may exist between rapid removal of large amounts of plasma and the possibility of relapse.

Ropper et al. (181) detected relapses in 10 of 94 consecutive patients with acute GBS treated with continuous flow PE. Deterioration occurred 5–42 days after the first series of exchanges, was usually mild, and responded to a second or third series of PE. The relapsing groups began and ended PE slightly earlier than did the nonrelapsing group. The timing of PE, however, differed little from that in the North American study group (175), with a mean of 11 versus 12 days to first PE and a mean of 19 versus 21 days to last PE from onset of illness. Most centers in the North American study group used intermittent-flow machines; this implies, as suggested by Osterman et al. (180), that relapses may be related to the use of continuous-flow PE machines.

Treatment with intravenous gamma globulin (IVGG) may have several therapeutic advantages over PE. IVGG has been used extensively without serious complications. IVGG is not associated with viral transmission. The cost is comparable to that of PE therapy, and IVGG may be given in any hospital without delay, unlike PE therapy. Kleyweg et al. (182) treated seven patients with severe GBS with IVGG within 2 weeks after onset of symptoms. IVGG was given at a dose of 0.4 g/kg/day for five consecutive days. Only two patients failed to improve after IVGG. Electrophysiologic studies showed that, in contrast to the other patients, these two had severe axonal degeneration. The authors have since started a randomized, multicenter trial (involving at least 200 patients) comparing IVGG treatment with PE therapy.

PROGNOSIS

Although the majority of patients with GBS have a complete recovery, up to one-third of patients will have some degree of disability. This fact has prompted a multitude of investigators to search for clinical and electrophysiological signs of prognostic significance. If, for example, a patient has early signs suggesting a severe course of illness with incomplete recovery, one may proceed to promptly initiate PE therapy. On the other hand, if a patient has early signs consistent with a mild course of illness, one may forego PE and proceed with general supportive care.

Several GBS series have failed to find a correlation between the rate of recovery or failure to recover and various clinical criteria, including sex, age, prodromal illness, degree of neurological deficit, and level of CSF protein (146,156,183). Recent studies, however, have found older age to be associated with a poorer outcome (143,184,185). In addition, several studies have demonstrated a rapid quadriparesis to correlate with a poor prognosis (142–144,186). Loffel et al. (142) found that a particularly long time span between the moment at which the initial signs reached their maximum and the moment when recovery started (plateau phase) correlated with frequent residual signs at follow-up. Winer et al. (187) demonstrated a poor prognosis in 86% of patients requiring ventilation and failing to improve within 3 weeks of reaching peak deficit. In contrast, Miller et al. (186) found neither age nor the duration of the plateau phase to be helpful in predicting outcome.

There are conflicting reports concerning the correlation between electrophysiological abnormalities and clinical status and long-term outcome. Several studies have failed to find a statistical correlation between the degree of impairment of conduction velocity and the severity of illness or the long-term prognosis (155,157,188). Eisen and Humphreys (156), however, found that patients with normal electrophysiological studies had a rapid recovery and that patients with electrophysiological abnormalities were slower to recover. Investigators agree unanimously that positive sharp waves and spontaneous fibrillations indicative of axonal degeneration are associated with a slower rate of recovery and a poor prognosis for complete recovery (153–157,184,185,189). Denervation does not begin to appear until 2–5 weeks after the onset of symptoms, and thus it is not of prognostic significance early in the course of the illness (163).

McKhann et al. (185) used multivariate analysis to identify prognostic factors and the effect of plasmapheresis in the large North American GBS study (175). Four factors were found to correlate with poorer outcomes: mean amplitude of CMAP, on distal stimulation, of 20% of normal or less; older age; time from onset of disease of 7 days or less; and need for ventilatory support. The most powerful predictor of outcome was the abnormal mean amplitude of CMAP on stimulating distally. Plasmapheresis had a beneficial effect over and above any or all of these factors. Brown and Feasby (153), along with Gruener et al. (184), have also found low amplitudes of CMAP on distal stimulation to be associated with a poor prognosis. The low amplitude is felt to reflect axonal destruction and is reduced in proportion to the number of axons damaged with a delay of 5–7 days (190).

Most investigators have found that children with GBS have a better outcome than adults (145,179,187,191).

Markland and Riley (145) noted a complete recovery in 14 of 17 children with GBS. Two other patients were having progressive improvement and only minimal residual weakness 2 months and 8 months after the acute illness. Only one patient was left with significant weakness $1\frac{1}{2}$ years after the acute illness and required crutches for ambulation.

Epstein and Sladky (179) conducted a retrospective analysis of the efficacy of PE therapy in children with GBS. The mean time to recover to Grade II (independent ambulation) was 24 days in the PE group and 60.2 days in the control group. This compares favorably to adults in the North American GBS study group (175), in whom the median time to reach Grade II was 53 days in the PE group and 85 days in the control group.

Briscoe et al. (191) found a complete clinical recovery in 100% (19/19) of children with acute GBS. The mean follow-up interval ranged from 7 to 9.7 years. Three patients with subacute presentation (clinical progression for 6 weeks or more before maximum deficit) had a protracted course or incomplete recovery.

Kleyweg et al. (192), however, found no significant differences in the severity of the disease between 18 children and 50 adults in a retrospective study. The mean hospital stay was 84 days for children versus 86 days for adults; 22% of children required mechanical ventilation for a mean of 21.5 days, whereas 30% of adults required ventilation for a mean of 32 days. Ninety-two percent of adults, as opposed to 83% of children, had a good outcome at 2 years.

Eberle et al. (193) retrospectively analyzed the data from 47 children with GBS for possible predictive indicators of recovery (or lack thereof) within 3 years. The patients had all been admitted to a rehabilitation facility, and thus they had a more severe illness than did many children with GBS who are admitted to a hospital and who make a quick and complete recovery and are sent home. The most significant early predictor of incomplete recovery was the time interval between the greatest weakness and the beginning of improvement (plateau phase). A plateau greater than 18 days had a 99% probability of incomplete recovery.

ACKNOWLEDGMENTS

The authors wish to thank Stacy Carter for her countless hours in typing and preparing this chapter.

REFERENCES

1. Landry O. Note sur la paralysie ascendante aigue. *Gaz Hebd Med Chirurg* 1859;6:472–474, 486, 488.
2. Guillain G, Barré JA, Strohl A. Sur un syndrome de radiculo-nevrite avec hyperalbuminose due liquide cephalorachidien sans reaction cellulaire: remarques sur les caracteres cliniques et graphiques des reflexes tendineux. *Bull Soc Med Hop Paris* 1916;40:1462–1470.
3. Draganesco A, Claudian J. Sur un cas de radiculo-névrite curable (syndrome de Guillain–Barré) apparue au cours d'une osteomyelite du bras. *Rev Neurol* 1927;2:517–521.
4. Guillain G. Synthese generale de la discussion. *J Belge Neurol Psychiatr* 1938;38:323–329.
5. Barré JA. Consideration diverses sur le syndrome de polyradiculonévrites avec dissociation albumino-cytologique. *J Belge Neurol Psychiat* 1938;38:314–322.
6. Lesser RP, Hauser WA, Kurland LT, et al. Epidemiologic features of the Guillain–Barré syndrome. *Neurology (Minneap)* 1973;23:1269–1272.
7. Kennedy RH, Danielson MA, Mulder DW, Kurland LT. Guillain–Barré syndrome: a 42-year epidemiologic and clinical study. *Mayo Clin Proc* 1978;53:93–99.
8. Beghi E, Kurland LT, Mulder DW, Wiederhold WC. Guillain–Barré syndrome: clinicoepidemiologic features and effect of influenza vaccine. *Arch Neurol* 1985;42:1053–1057.
9. Gudmundsson KR. Prevalence and occurrence of some rare neurological diseases in Iceland. *Acta Neurol Scand* 1969;45:114–118.
10. Chen K, Brody JA, Kurland LT. Patterns of neurologic diseases on Guam. I. Epidemiologic aspects. *Arch Neurol* 1968;19:573–578.
11. Larsen JP, Kvale G, Nyland H. Epidemiology of the Guillain–Barré syndrome in the county of Hordaland, western Norway. *Acta Neurol Scand* 1985;71:43–47.
12. Soffer D, Feldman S, Alter M. Epidemiology of Guillain–Barré syndrome. *Neurology* 1978;28:686–690.
13. Hogg JE, Kobrin DE, Schoenberg BS. The Guillain–Barré syndrome: epidemiologic and clinical features. *J Chron Dis* 1979;32:227–231.
14. Kaplan JE, Poduska PJ, McIntosh GC, et al. Guillain–Barré syndrome in Larimer County, Colorado: a high incidence area. *Neurology* 1985;35:581–584.
15. Congia S, Melis M, Carboni MA. Epidemiologic and clinical features of the Guillain–Barré syndrome in Sardinia in the 1961–1980 period. *Acta Neurol (Napoli)* 1989;11:15–20.
16. Bahemuka M. Guillain–Barré syndrome in Kenya: a clinical review of 54 patients. *J Neurol* 1988;235:418–421.
17. Hallas J, Bredkjaer C, Friis M. Guillain–Barré syndrome: diagnostic criteria, epidemiology, clinical course and prognosis. *Acta Neurol Scand* 1988;78:118–122.
18. Hankey GJ. Guillain–Barré syndrome in Western Australia, 1980–1985. *Med J Aust* 1987;146:130–133.
19. Radhakrishnan K, el-Mangoush MA, Gerryo SE. Descriptive epidemiology of selected neuromuscular disorders in Benghazi, Libya. *Acta Neurol Scand* 1987;75:95–100.
20. National Institute of Neurological and Communicative Disorders and Stroke Ad Hoc Committee. Criteria for diagnosis of Guillain–Barré syndrome. *Ann Neurol* 1978;3:565–566.
21. Asbury AK. Diagnostic considerations in Guillain–Barré syndrome. *Ann Neurol* 1981;9(Suppl):1–5.
22. Melnick SC, Flewett, TH. Role of infection in the Guillain–Barré syndrome. *J Neurol Neurosurg Psychiatry* 1964;27:385–407.
23. Winer JB, Hughes RAC, Anderson MJ, Jones DM, Kangro H, Watkins RPF. A prospective study of acute idiopathic neuropathy. II. Antecedent events. *J Neurol Neurosurg Psychiatry* 1988;51:613–618.
24. Dowling PC, Cook SD. Role of infection in Guillain–Barré syndrome: laboratory confirmation of herpes viruses in 41 cases. *Ann Neurol* 1981;9(Suppl):44–55.
25. Dowling P, Cook S. Cytomegalovirus (CMV) antibodies in Guillain–Barré syndrome (GBS) [Abstract]. *Clin Res* 1973;21:974.
26. Dowling P, Menonna J, Cook S. Cytomegalovirus complement fixation antibody in Guillain–Barré syndrome. *Neurology (Minneap)* 1977;27:1153–1156.
27. Grose C, Henle W, Henle G, et al. Primary Epstein–Barr virus infection in acute neurologic diseases. *N Engl J Med* 1975;292:392–395.
28. Menonna J, Goldschmidt B, Haidri N, et al. Herpes simplex virus

—IgM specific antibodies in Guillain–Barré syndrome and encephalitis. *Acta Neurol Scand* 1977;56:223–231.

29. Goldschmidt B, Menonna J, Fortunato J, et al. Mycoplasma antibody in Guillain–Barré syndrome and other neurological disorders. *Ann Neurol* 1980;7:108–112.

30. Cornblath DR, McArthur JC, Kennedy PG, Witte AS, Griffin JW. Inflammatory demyelinating peripheral neuropathies associated with human T-cell lymphotropic virus type III infection. *Ann Neurol* 1987;21:32–40.

31. Piette AM, Tusseau F, Visnon D, Chapman A, Parrot G, Leibowitch J, Montagnier L. Acute neuropathy coincident with seroconversion for anti-LAV/HTLV III. *Lancet* 1986;1:852.

32. Eidelberg D, Sotrel A, Vogel H, Walker P, Kleefield J, Crumpacker CS III. Progressive polyradiculopathy in acquired immune deficiency syndrome. *Neurology* 1986;36:912–916.

33. Berger JR, Difini JA, Swerdloff MA, Ayyar DR. HIV seropositivity in Guillain–Barré syndrome. *Ann Neurol* 1987;22:393–394.

34. Rhodes KM, Tattersfield AE. Guillain–Barré syndrome associated with *Campylobacter* infections. *Br Med J* 1982;285:173–174.

35. Kaldor J, Speed BR. Guillain–Barré syndrome and *Campylobacter jejuni:* a serological study. *Br Med J* 1984;288:1867–1870.

36. Ropper AH. Severe acute Guillain–Barré syndrome. *Neurology* 1986;36:429–432.

37. De Bont B, Matthews N, Abbott K, Davidson GP. Guillain–Barré syndrome associated with *Campylobacter* enteritis in a child. *J Pediatr* 1986;109:660–662.

38. Wroe SJ, Blumhardt LD. Acute polyneuritis with cranial nerve involvement following *Campylobacter jejuni* infection. *J Neurol Neurosurg Psychiatry* 1985;48:593.

39. Sovilla JY, Regli F, Francioli PB. Guillain–Barré syndrome following *Campylobacter jejuni* enteritis. *Arch Intern Med* 1988;148:739–741.

40. Pryor WM, Freiman JS, Gillies MA, Tuck RR. Guillain–Barré syndrome associated with *Campylobacter* infection. *Aust NZ J Med* 1984;14:687–688.

41. Ropper AH. *Campylobacter* diarrhea and Guillain–Barré syndrome. *Arch Neurol* 1988;45:655–656.

42. Khoury SA. Guillain–Barré syndrome: epidemiology of an outbreak. *Am J Epidemiol* 1978;107:433–438.

43. Sliman NA. Outbreak of Guillain–Barré syndrome associated with water pollution. *Br Med J* 1978;1:751–752.

44. Schaltenbrand G, Bammer H. La clinique et le traitement des polyneurites inflammatoires ou sereuses aigiies. *Rev Neurol* 1966;115:783–810.

45. Faraq SS, Gelles D. *Yersinia* arthritis and Guillain–Barré syndrome. *N Engl J Med* 1982;307:755.

46. Samantray SK. Landry–Guillain–Barré-Strohl syndrome in typhoid fever. *Aust NZ J Med* 1977;7:307–308.

47. Warembourg H, Voisin C, et al. Neuropathies peripheriques aigiies associées à la bruncellose. *Lillie Med* 1969;14:536–539.

48. Steiner I, Argov Z, Cahen C, Abramsky O. Guillain–Barré syndrome after epidural anesthesia: direct nerve root damage may trigger disease. *Neurology* 1985;35:1473–1475.

49. Wiederholt WC, Mulder DW, Lambert EH. The Landry–Guillain–Barré-Strohl syndrome: historical review, report on 97 patients, and present concepts. *Mayo Clinic Proc* 1964;30:427.

50. Arnason BG, Asbury AK. Idiopathic polyneuritis after surgery. *Arch Neurol* 1968;18:500–507.

51. Schonberger LB, Bregman DJ, Sullivan-Bolyal JZ, et al. Guillain–Barré syndrome following vaccination in the national influenza immunization program, United States, 1976–1977. *Am J Epidemiol* 1979;110:105–123.

52. Arnason BGW. Acute inflammatory demyelinating polyradiculoneuropathies. In: Dyck PJ, Thomas PK, Labert EH, Bunge R, eds. *Peripheral neuropathy*, 2nd ed. Philadelphia: WB Saunders, 1984;2050–2100.

53. Kurland LT, Wiederholt WC, Kirkpatrick JW, Potter HG, Armstrong LCP. Swine influenza vaccine and Guillain–Barré syndrome: epidemic or artifact? *Arch Neurol* 1985;42:1089–1090.

54. Poser CM. Swine influenza vaccination: truth and consequences. *Arch Neurol* 1985;42:1090–1092.

55. Johnson DE. Guillain–Barré syndrome in the U.S. Army. *Arch Neurol* 1982;39:21–24.

56. Langmuir AD, Bregman DJ, Kurland LT, et al. An epidemiologic and clinical evaluation of Guillain–Barré syndrome reported in association with the administration of swine influenza vaccines. *Am J Epidemiol* 1984;119:841–879.

57. Kinnunen E, Farkkila M, Hovi T, Juntunen J, Weckstrom P. Incidence of Guillain–Barré syndrome during a nationwide oral poliovirus vaccine campaign. *Neurology* 1989;39:1034–1036.

58. D'Cruz OF, Shapiro ED, Spiegelman KN, et al. Acute inflammatory demyelinating polyradiculoneuropathy (Guillain–Barré syndrome) after immunization with Haemophilus influenza type b conjugate vaccine. *J Pediatr* 1989;115:743–746.

59. Grose C, Spigland I. Guillain–Barré syndrome following administration of live measles vaccine. *Am J Med* 1976;60:441–443.

60. Leneman F. The Guillain–Barré syndrome: definition, etiology and review of 1,100. *Arch Intern Med* 1966;118:139–144.

61. Gunderman JR. Guillain–Barré syndrome: occurrence following combined mumps–rubella vaccine. *Am J Dis Child* 1973;125:834–835.

62. Samantray SK, Johnson SC, Mathai KV, Pulimood BM. Landry–Guillain–Barré-Strohl syndrome: a study of 302 cases. *Med J Aust* 1977;2:84–91.

63. Friedland ML, Wittels EG. An unusual neurologic reaction following polyvalent pneumococcal vaccine in a patient with hairy cell leukemia. *Am J Hematol* 1983;14:189–191.

64. Novak DJ, Johnson KP. Relapsing idiopathic polyneuritis during pregnancy. *Arch Neurol* 1973;28:219–223.

65. Sudo N, Weingold AB. Obstetric aspects of the Guillain–Barré syndrome. *Obstet Gynecol* 1975;45:39–43.

66. Klingon GH. The Guillain–Barré syndrome associated with cancer. *Cancer* 1965;18:157–163.

67. Julien J, Vital CL, Aupy G, Lagueny A, Darriet D, Brechenmacher C. Guillain–Barré syndrome and Hodgkin's disease—ultrastructural study of a peripheral nerve. *J Neurol Sci* 1980;45:23–27.

68. Moore RY, Oda Y. Malignant lymphoma with diffuse involvement of the peripheral nervous system. *Neurology* 1962;12:186.

69. Asbury AK, Arnason BG, Adams RD. The inflammatory lesion in idiopathic polyneuritis. *Medicine (Baltimore)* 1969;48:173–215.

70. Krücke W. Die primar—entzündliche Polyneuritis unbekannter Ursache. In: Lubarsch O, Henke F, Rössle G, eds. *Handbuch der speziellen pathologischen Anatomie und Histologie, vol 13, part 5. Erkrankungen der peripheren Nerven*. Berlin: Springer, 1955;164–182.

71. Haymaker W, Kernohan JW. Landry–Guillain–Barré syndrome: clinicopathologic report of 50 fatal cases and a critique of the literature. *Medicine (Baltimore)* 1949;28:59–141.

72. Casamajor L. Acute ascending paralysis. *Arch Neurol Psychiatry (Chicago)* 1919;2:605–620.

73. Margulis MS. Pathologie und pathogenesis der akuten primären infektiösen polyneuritiden. *Dtsch Z Nervenheilkd* 1927;99:165–192.

74. Matsuyama H, Haymaker W. Distribution of lesions in the Landry–Guillain–Barré syndrome, with emphasis on involvement of the sympathetic system. *Acta Neuropathol (Berl)* 1967;8:230–241.

75. Arstila AV, Riekkinen PJ, Rinne VK, Pelliniemi TT, Nevalainen T. Guillain–Barré syndrome. Neurochemical and ultrastructural study. *Eur Neurol* 1971;5:257–269.

76. Gombault A. Contribution a l'étude anatomique de la névrite parenchymateuse subäique et chronique névrite segmentaire peri-axile. *Arch Neurol* 1881;1:177.

77. Finean JB, Woolf AL. An electron microscope study of degenerative changes in human cutaneous nerve. *J Neuropathol Exp Neurol* 1962;21:105–115.

78. Wisniewski H, Terry RD, Whitaker JN, Cook SD, Dowling PC. Landry–Guillain–Barré syndrome. A primary demyelinating disease. *Arch Neurol* 1969;21:269–276.

79. Liu HM. Ultrastructure of remyelination of peripheral nerves in Landry–Guillain–Barré syndrome. *Acta Neuropathol (Berl)* 1970;16:262–265.

80. Miyakawa T, Murayama E, Sumiyoshi S, Deshimaru M, Kamano A, Miyakawa K, Tatetsu S. A biopsy case of Landry–

Guillain–Barré syndrome. *Acta Neuropathol (Berl)* 1971;17:181–187.

81. Hart MN, Hanks DT, Mackey R. Ultrastructural observations in Guillain–Barré syndrome. *Arch Pathol* 1972;93:552–555.
82. Carpenter S. An ultrastructural study of an acute fatal case of the Guillain–Barré syndrome. *J Neurol Sci* 1972;15:125–140.
83. Prineas JW. Acute idiopathic polyneuritis. An electron microscope study. *Lab Invest* 1972;26:133–146.
84. Waksman BH, Adams RD. Allergic neuritis: an experimental disease of rabbits induced by the injection of peripheral nervous tissue and adjuvants. *J Exp Med* 1955;102:213–235.
85. Hartung HP, Toyka KV. T-cell and macrophage activation in experimental autoimmune neuritis and Guillain–Barré syndrome. *Ann Neurol* 1990;27(Suppl):S57–S63.
86. Milner P, Lovelidge CA, Taylor WA, Hughes RAC. P0 myelin protein produces experimental allergic neuritis in Lewis rats. *J Neurol Sci* 1987;79:275–285.
87. Brostoff SW, Levit S, Powers JM. Induction of experimental allergic neuritis with a peptide from myelin P2 basic protein. *Nature* 1977;268:752–753.
88. Kadlubowski M, Hughes RAC. Identification of the neuritogen for experimental allergic neuritis. *Nature* 1979;277:140–141.
89. Milek DJ, Cunningham JM, Powers JM, Brostoff SW. Experimental allergic neuritis: humoral and cellular immune responses to the cyanogen bromide peptides of the P2 protein. *J Neuroimmunol* 1983;4:105–117.
90. Crumpton MJ. Protein antigens—the molecular bases of antigenicity and immunogenicity. In: Sela M, ed. *The antigens,* vol 11. New York: Academic Press, 1974;1–78.
91. Thompson K, Harris M, Benjamin E. Cellular and humoral immunity—a distinction in antigenic recognition. *Nature (New Biol)* 1972;238:20.
92. Olee T, Weise M, Powers J, Brostoff S. A T cell epitope for experimental allergic neuritis is an amphipathic alpha-helical structure. *J Neuroimmunol* 1989;21:235–240.
93. Hughes RAC, Kadlubowski CM, Gray IA, Leibowitz S. Immune responses in experimental allergic neuritis. *J Neurol Neurosurg Psychiatry* 1981;44:565–569.
94. Rostami A, Burns JB, Brown MJ, Rosen J, Zweiman B, Lisak RP, Pleasure DE. Transfer of experimental allergic neuritis with P2-reactive T-cell lines. *Cell Immunol* 1985;91:354–361.
95. Linington C, Izumo S, Suzuki M, Uyemura K, Meyermann R, Wekerle H. A permanent rat T cell line that mediates experimental allergic neuritis in the Lewis rat *in vivo. J Immunol* 1984;133:1946–1950.
96. Brosman JV, Craggs RI, King RHM, Thomas PK. Reduced susceptibility of T cell-deficient rats to induction of experimental allergic neuritis. *J Neuroimmunol* 1987;14:267–282.
97. Hartung HP, Schafer B, Diamantstein T, Fierz W, Heininger K, Toyka KV. Suppression of P2-T cell line-mediated experimental autoimmune neuritis by interleukin-2 receptor targeted monoclonal antibody ART 18. *Brain Res* 1989;489:120–128.
98. Waldmann TA. The structure, function, and expression of interleukin-2 receptors on normal and malignant lymphocytes. *Science* 1986;232:727–732.
99. Olsson T, Holmdahl R, Klareskog L, Forsum U, Kristensson K. Dynamics of Ia-expressing cells and T lymphocytes of different subsets during experimental allergic neuritis in Lewis rats. *J Neurol Sci* 1984;66:141–149.
100. Hughes RAC, Atkinson PF, Gray IA, Taylor WA. Major histocompatibility antigens and lymphocyte subsets during experimental allergic neuritis in the Lewis rat. *J Neurol* 1987;234:390–395.
101. Ota K, Irie H, Takahashi K. T cell subsets and Ia-positive cells in the sciatic nerve during the course of experimental allergic neuritis. *J Neuroimmunol* 1987;13:283–292.
102. Brosnan CF, Lyman WD, Tansey FA, Carter TH. Quantitation of mast cells in experimental allergic neuritis. *J Neuropathol Exp Neurol* 1985;44:196–203.
103. Brosnan CF, Claudio L, Tansey FA, Martiney J. Mechanisms of autoimmune neuropathies. *Ann Neurol* 1990;27(Suppl):S75–S79.
104. Brosnan CF, Tansey FA. Delayed onset of experimental allergic neuritis in rats treated with reserpine. *J Neuropathol Exp Neurol* 1984;43:83–93.
105. Lampert PW. Mechanism of demyelination in experimental allergic neuritis: electron microscopic studies. *Lab Invest* 1969;20:127–138.
106. DalCanto MC, Wisniewski HM, Johnson AB, Brostoff SW, Raine CS. Vesicular disruption of myelin in autoimmune demyelination. *J Neurol Sci* 1975;24:313–319.
107. Lampert P, Garrett R, Powell H. Demyelination in allergic and Marek's disease virus induced neuritis comparative electron microscopic studies. *Acta Neuropathol (Berl)* 1977;40:103–110.
108. Schmidt B, Stoll G, Hartung HP, Heininger K, Schäfer B, Toyka KV. Macrophages but not Schwann cells express Ia antigen in experimental autoimmune neuritis. *Ann Neurol* 1990;28:70–77.
109. Hartung HP, Schäfer B, van der Meide PH, Fierz W, Heininger K, Toyka KV. The role of interferon-gamma in the pathogenesis of experimental autoimmune disease of the peripheral nervous system. *Ann Neurol* 1990;27:247–257.
110. Hartung HP, Schäfer B, Heininger K, Toyka KV. Suppression of experimental autoimmune neuritis by the oxygen radical scavengers superoxide dismutase and catalase. *Ann Neurol* 1988;23:453–460.
111. Hartung HP, Schäfer B, Heininger K, Stoll G, Toyka KV. The role of macrophages and eicosanoids in the pathogenesis of experimental allergic neuritis. *Brain* 1988;111:1039–1059.
112. Allison AC. Fluorescence microscopy of lymphocytes and mononuclear phagocytes and the use of silica to eliminate the latter. In: Bloom BR, Davids JR, eds. *In vitro methods in cell-mediated and tumor immunity.* New York: Academic Press, 1976;395–404.
113. Heininger K, Schäfer B, Hartung HP, Fierz W, Linington C, Toyka KV. The role of macrophages in experimental autoimmune neuritis induced by a P2-specific T-cell line. *Ann Neurol* 1988;23:326–331.
114. Craggs RI, King RHM, Thomas PK. The effect of suppression of macrophage activity on the development of experimental allergic neuritis. *Acta Neuropathol (Berl)* 1984;62:316–323.
115. Trotter J, Smith ME. The role of phospholipases from inflammatory macrophages in demyelination. *Neurochem Res* 1986;11:349–361.
116. Sobue G, Yamato S, Hirayama M, Matsuoka Y, Uematsu H, Sobue I. The role of macrophages in demyelination in experimental allergic neuritis. *J Neurol Sci* 1982;56:75–87.
117. Feasby TE, Gilbert TT, Hahn AF, Neilson M. Complement depletion suppresses Lewis rat experimental allergic neuritis. *Brain Res* 1987;419:97–103.
118. Iqbal A, Oger JJ-F, Arnason BGW. Cell-mediated immunity in idiopathic polyneuritis. *Ann Neurol* 1981;9(Suppl):65–69.
119. Abramsky O, Korn-Lubetzky I, Teitelbaum D. Association of autoimmune diseases and cellular immune response to the neuritogenic protein in Guillain–Barré syndrome. *Ann Neurol* 1980;8:117.
120. Sheremata W, Colby S, Karkhanis Y, Eylar EH. Cellular hypersensitivity to basic myelin (P2) protein in the Guillain–Barré syndrome. *Can J Neurol Sci* 1975;2:87–90.
121. Hughes RAC, Gray IA, Gregson NA. Immune responses to myelin antigens in Guillain–Barré syndrome. *J Neuroimmunol* 1984;6:303–312.
122. Burns J, Krasner LJ, Rostami A, Pleasure D. Isolation of P2 protein-reactive T-cell lines from human blood. *Ann Neurol* 1986;19:391–393.
123. Winer JB, Gray IA, Gregson NA, Hughes RAC, Leibowitz S, Sheperd P, Taylor WA, Yewdall V. A prospective study of acute idiopathic neuropathy. III. Immunological studies. *J Neurol Neurosurg Psychiatry* 1988;51:619–625.
124. Geczy C, Raper R, Roberts IM, Meyer P, Bernard CCA. Macrophage procoagulant activity as a measure of cell-mediated immunity to P2 protein of peripheral nerves in the Guillain–Barré syndrome. *J Neuroimmunol* 1985;9:179–191.
125. Geczy CL, Meyer PA. Leukocyte procoagulant activity in man—an *in vitro* correlate of delayed-type hypersensitivity. *J Immunol* 1982;128:331–336.
126. Hartung HP, Hughes RAC, Taylor WA, Heininger K, Reiners K, Toyka KV. T cell activation in Guillain–Barré syndrome and in MS: elevated serum levels of soluble IL-2 receptors. *Neurology* 1990;40:215–218.
127. Taylor WA, Hughes RAC. T lymphocyte activation antigens in

278 / Chapter 12

Guillain–Barré syndrome and chronic idiopathic demyelinating polyradiculoneuropathy. *J Neuroimmunol* 1989;24:33–39.
128. Hirano A, Cook SD, Whitaker JN, Dowling PC, Murray MR. Fine structural aspects of demyelination *in vitro:* the effects of Guillain–Barré serum. *J Neuropathol Exp Neurol* 1971;30:240–265.
129. Cook SD, Dowling PC, Murray MR, Whitaker JN. Circulating demyelinating factors in acute idiopathic polyneuropathy. *Arch Neurol* 1971;24:136–144.
130. Saida T, Saida K, Lisak RP, Brown MJ, Silberberg DH, Asbury AK. *In vivo* demyelinating activity of sera from patients with Guillain–Barré syndrome. *Ann Neurol* 1982;11:69–75.
131. Feasby TE, Hahn AF, Gilbert JJ. Passive transfer studies in Guillain–Barré polyneuropathy. *Neurology* 1980;32:1159–1167.
132. Goust JM, Chinais F, Carnes JE, Hames CG, Fudenberg HH, Hogan EL. Abnormal T cell subpopulations and circulating immune complexes in the Guillain–Barré syndrome and multiple sclerosis. *Neurology* 1978;28:421–425.
133. Cook SD, Dowling PC. The role of autoantibody and immune complexes in the pathogenesis of Guillain–Barré syndrome. *Ann Neurol* 1981;9(Suppl):70–79.
134. Cook S, Dowling PC, Whitaker JN. Serum immunoglobulins in the Guillain–Barré syndrome. *Neurology (Minneap)* 1970;20:403.
135. Melnick SC. Thirty-eight cases of the Guillain–Barré syndrome: an immunological study. *Br Med J* 1963;1:368–373.
136. Koski CL, Humphrey R, Shin ML. Anti-peripheral myelin antibody in patients with demyelinating neuropathy: quantitative and kinetic determination of serum antibody by complement component 1 fixation. *Proc Natl Acad Sci USA* 1985;82:905–909.
137. Koski CL, Gratz E, Sutherland J, Mayer RF. Clinical correlation with anti-peripheral nerve myelin antibodies in Guillain–Barré syndrome. *Ann Neurol* 1986;19:573–577.
138. Griffin JW, Stoll G, Li CY, Tyor W, Corblath DR. Macrophage responses in inflammatory demyelinating neuropathies. *Ann Neurol* 1990;27(Suppl):S64–S68.
139. Beuche W, Friede RL. The role of non-resident cells in wallerian degeneration. *J Neurocytol* 1984;13:767–796.
140. Beuche W, Friede RL. Myelin phagocytosis in wallerian degeneration depends on silica-sensitive, bg/bg-negative and Fc-positive monocytes. *Brain Res* 1986;378:97–106.
141. Asbury AK, Cornblath DR. Assessment of current diagnostic criteria for Guillain–Barré syndrome. *Ann Neurol* 1990;27(Suppl):S21–S24.
142. Loffel GB, Rossi LN, Mumenthaler M, Lutschg J, Ludin HP. The Landry–Guillain–Barré syndrome: complications, prognosis, and natural history in 123 cases. *J Neurol Sci* 1977;33:71–79.
143. Winer JB, Hughes RAC, Osmond C. A prospective study of acute idiopathic neuropathy. I. Clinical features and their prognostic value. *J Neurol Neurosurg Psychiatry* 1988;51:605–612.
144. Ropper AH. Severe acute Guillain–Barré syndrome. *Neurology* 1986;36:429–432.
145. Markland LD, Riley HD. The Guillain–Barré syndrome in childhood. A comprehensive review, including observations on 19 additional cases. *Clin Pediatr* 1967;6:162–170.
146. Pleasure DE, Lovelace RE, Duvoisin RC. The prognosis of acute polyradiculoneuritis. *Neurology (Minneap)* 1968;18:1143–1148.
147. Lichtenfeld P. Autonomic dysfunction in the Guillain–Barré syndrome. *Am J Med* 1971;50:772–780.
148. Ropper AH, Shanani BT. Pain in Guillain–Barré syndrome. *Arch Neurol* 1984;41:511–514.
149. Mikati MA, DeLong GR. Childhood Guillain–Barré syndrome masquerading as a protracted pain syndrome. *Arch Neurol* 1985;42:839.
150. Lopez F, Lopez JH, Holguin J, Flewett TH. An outbreak of acute polyradiculoneuropathy in Columbia in 1968. *Am J Epidemiol* 1973;98:226–230.
151. Schaltenbrand G, Bammer H. La clinique et le traitement des polynevrites inflammatoíres ou sereuses aigues. *Rev Neurol (Paris)* 1966;115:783–810.
152. Sullivan RL, Reeves AG. Normal cerebrospinal fluid protein, increased intracranial pressure, and the Guillain–Barré syndrome. *Ann Neurol* 1977;1:108–109.

153. Brown WF, Feasby TE. Conduction block and denervation in Guillain–Barré polyneuropathy. *Brain* 1984;107:219–239.
154. Raman PT, Taori GM. Prognostic significance of electrodiagnostic studies in the Guillain–Barré syndrome. *J Neurol Neurosurg Psychiatry* 1976;39:163–170.
155. McLeod JG, Walsh JC, Prineas JW, Pollard JD. Acute idiopathic polyneuritis: a clinical and electrophysiological follow-up study. *J Neurol Sci* 1976;27:145–162.
156. Eisen A, Humphreys P. The Guillain–Barré syndrome. *Arch Neurol* 1974;30:438–443.
157. McLeod JG. Electrophysiological studies in the Guillain–Barré syndrome. *Ann Neurol* 1981;9(Suppl):20–27.
158. Olney RK, Aminoff MJ. Electrodiagnostic features of the Guillain–Barré syndrome: the relative sensitivity of different techniques. *Neurology* 1990;40:471–475.
159. Thorne J. Central responses to electrical activation of the peripheral nerves supplying the intrinsic hand muscles. *J Neurol Neurosurg Psychiatry* 1965;28:482–485.
160. McLeod JG, Wray SH. An experimental study of the F wave in the baboon. *J Neurol Neurosurg Psychiatry* 1966;29:196–200.
161. Oh SJ. *Clinical electromyography: nerve conduction studies.* Baltimore: University Park Press, 1984;27 and 58.
162. Lachman T, Shahani BT, Young RR. Late responses as aids to diagnosis in peripheral neuropathy. *J Neurol Neurosurg Psychiatry* 1980;43:156–162.
163. Albers JW, Donofrio PD, McGonagle TK. Sequential electrodiagnostic abnormalities in acute inflammatory demyelinating polyradiculoneuropathy. *Muscle Nerve* 1985;8:528–539.
164. Kimura J. Proximal versus distal slowing of motor nerve conduction velocity in the Guillain–Barré syndrome. *Ann Neurol* 1978;3:344–350.
165. Walsh JC, Yiannikas C, McLeod JG. Abnormalities of proximal conduction in acute idiopathic polyneuritis: comparison of short latency evoked potentials and F-waves. *J Neurol Neurosurg Psychiatry* 1984;47:197–200.
166. Ropper AH, Chiappa KH. Evoked potentials in Guillain–Barré syndrome. *Neurology* 1986;36:587–590.
167. Ropper AH, Shahani BT. Diagnosis and management of acute arelexic paralysis with emphasis on Guillain–Barré syndrome. In: Asbury AK, Gilliat RW, eds. *Peripheral nerve disorders. A practical approach.* London: Butterworths, 1984;46–57.
168. Newton-John J. Prevention of pulmonary complications in severe Guillain–Barré syndrome by early assisted ventilation. *Med J Aust* 1985;142:444–445.
169. Ropper AH, Kehne SM. Guillain–Barré syndrome: management of respiratory failure. *Neurology* 1985;35:1662–1665.
170. Swick HM, McQuillen MP. The use of steroids in the treatment of idiopathic polyneuritis. *Neurology (Minneap)* 1976;26:205–212.
171. Hughes RAC, Newsom-Davis JM, Perkin GD, Pierce JM. Controlled trial of prednisolone in acute polyneuropathy. *Lancet* 1978;2:750–753.
172. Hughes RAC, Kadlubowski M, Hufschmidt A. Treatment of acute inflammatory polyneuropathy. *Ann Neurol* 1981;9(Suppl):125–133.
173. Greenwood RJ, Newson-Davis J, Hughes RAC, Aslan S, Bowden AN, Chadwick DW, Gordon NS, McLellan DL, Millac P, Stott RB, Armitage P. Controlled trial of plasma exchange in acute inflammatory polyradiculoneuropathy. *Lancet* 1984;1:877–879.
174. Osterman PO, Fagius J, Lundemo G, Pihlstedt P, Pirskanen R, Siden A, Safwenberg J. Beneficial effects of plasma exchange in acute inflammatory polyradiculoneuropathy. *Lancet* 1984;2:1296–1299.
175. Guillain–Barré Syndrome Study Group. Plasmapheresis and acute Guillain–Barré syndrome. *Neurology* 1985;35:1096–1104.
176. Färkkilä M, Kinnunen E, Haapanen E, Iivanainen M. Guillain–Barré syndrome: quantitative measurement of plasma exchange therapy. *Neurology* 1987;37:837–840.
177. French Cooperative Group on Plasma Exchange in Guillain–Barré Syndrome. Efficiency of plasma exchange in Guillain–Barré syndrome: role of replacement fluids. *Ann Neurol* 1987;22:753–761.
178. Khatri BO, Flamini JR, Baruah JK, Dobyns WB, Konkol RJ.

Plasmapheresis with acute inflammatory polyneuropathy. *Pediatr Neurol* 1990;6:17–19.

179. Epstein MA, Sladky JT. The role of plasmapheresis in childhood Guillain–Barré syndrome. *Ann Neurol* 1990;28:65–69.

180. Osterman PO, Fagius J, Säfwenberg J, Wikström B. Early relapse of acute inflammatory polyradiculonuropathy after successful treatment with plasma exchange. *Acta Neurol Scand* 1988; 77:273–277.

181. Ropper AH, Albers JW, Addison R. Limited relapse in Guillain–Barré syndrome after plasma exchange. *Arch Neurol* 1988; 45:314–315.

182. Kleyweg RP, van der Meché FGA, Meulstee J. Treatment of Guillain–Barré syndrome with high-dose gammaglobulin. *Neurology* 1988;38:1639–1641.

183. McFarland HR, Heller GL. Guillain–Barré disease complex: a statement of diagnostic criteria and analysis of 100 cases. *Arch Neurol* 1966;14:196–201.

184. Gruener G, Bosch EP, Strauss RG, Klugman M, Kimura J. Prediction of early beneficial response to plasma exchange in Guillain–Barré syndrome. *Arch Neurol* 1987;44:295–298.

185. McKhann GM, Griffin JW, Cornblath DR, Mellits ED, Fisher RS, Quaskey SA, and the Guillain–Barré Syndrome Study Group. Plasmapheresis and Guillain–Barré syndrome: analysis of prognostic factors and the effect of plasmapheresis. *Ann Neurol* 1988;23:347–353.

186. Miller RG, Peterson GW, Daube JR, Albers JW. Prognostic value in electrodiagnosis in Guillain–Barré syndrome. *Muscle Nerve* 1988;11:769–774.

187. Winer JB, Hughes RAC, Greenwood RJ, Perkin GD, Healy MJR. Prognosis in Guillain–Barré syndrome. *Lancet* 1985; 1:1202–1203.

188. Hausmanova-Petrusewicz I, Emeryk B, Rowinska-Marcinoska K, Jedrzejowska H. Nerve conduction in the Guillain–Barré–Strohl syndrome. *J Neurol* 1979;220:169–184.

189. Cornblath DR, Mellits ED, Griffin JW, McKhann GM, Albers JW, Miller RG, Feasby TE, Quaskey SA, and the Guillain–Barré Syndrome Study Group. Motor conduction studies in Guillain–Barré syndrome: description and prognostic value. *Ann Neurol* 1988;23:354–359.

190. Miller RG. Injury to a peripheral motor nerve. *Muscle Nerve* 1987;10:698–710.

191. Briscoe DM, McMenamin JB, O'Donohue NV. Prognosis in Guillain–Barré syndrome. *Arch Dis Child* 1987;62:733–735.

192. Kleyweg RP, van der Meché FGA, Loonen MCB, De Jonge J, Knip B. The natural history of the Guillain–Barré syndrome in 18 children and 50 adults. *J Neurol Neurosurg Psychiatry* 1989;52:853–856.

193. Eberle E, Brink J, Azen S, White D. Early predictors of incomplete recovery in children with Guillain–Barré polyneuritis. *J Pediatr* 1975;86:356–359.

194. Oh SJ. Diagnostic usefulness and limitations of the sural nerve biopsy. *Yonsei Med J* 1990;31:1–26.

PART **II**

Mycoplasmal Infections of the CNS

Infections of the Central Nervous System,
edited by W. M. Scheld, R. J. Whitley, and
D. T. Durack, Raven Press, Ltd., New York © 1991.

CHAPTER 13

Mycoplasmal Diseases of the Central Nervous System

Wallace A. Clyde, Jr.

Mycoplasmas are the cell-wall-less bacteria comprising microbial class Mollicutes ("soft skin"). These organisms produce a wide variety of diseases among animals, birds, insects, and plants, including affections of the central nervous system (CNS) by several different pathogenetic mechanisms. The association between mycoplasmas and CNS syndromes in animals was established during the early 1930s, and in humans together with the description of the atypical pneumonia syndrome by Reimann (1) in 1938, although the common etiologic agent of atypical pneumonia, *Mycoplasma pneumoniae,* was not identified until 1962 (2).

Among animals and birds, three types of CNS syndromes have been described, as illustrated by the following examples. Rolling disease of mice is produced by a neurotoxin of *M. neurolyticum,* which causes the animal to roll over and over on its long axis involuntarily, followed by convulsions, shock, and death. Encephalopathy of turkey poults is produced by the S6 strain of *M. gallisepticum;* in this case organisms proliferate in the blood and walls of cerebral arteries, and in the brain substance there is capillary cell edema and occlusion. In birds that survive the acute encephalopathy, a chronic cerebral arteritis ensues, in which there are periarteriolar infiltrations of small lymphocytes (Fig. 1). Direct invasion of the CNS occurs in the murine mycoplasmoses caused by *M. pulmonis* and *Spiroplasma mirum* (formerly called "suckling mouse cataract agent").

In humans, a wide variety of neurological syndromes have been described as complications of respiratory tract infections with *M. pneumoniae.* Here the disease mechanisms involved are less clearly defined than in the animal and bird diseases; it is likely that several different mecha-

nisms are operative based on available information. Brain abscess due to a mouth organism (presumably *M. salivarium*) has been reported in the case of a penetrating injury with a tobacco pipestem (3). The common genital tract organism *M. hominis* also has been isolated from brain abscesses in the absence of other microbial agents (4). In neonates, both *M. hominis* and *Ureaplasma urealyticum* have been recognized as causes of "sterile" meningitis.

ETIOLOGY

Absence of the rigid cell wall typical of classic bacteria confers several unusual properties upon mycoplasmas. They are the smallest free-living parasites known, measuring no more than 0.5 μm in diameter. The bacterial cell wall is the reaction site for organic dyes such as those used in Gram's stain; hence mycoplasmas cannot be visualized by this method. In addition, there are no receptor sites for the penicillin or cephalosporin antibiotics, thus mycoplasmas are not affected by these compounds. Despite containment only by trilaminar unit membranes, many of the pathogenic species of mycoplasmas present characteristic morphologic features, such as the filamentous shape of *M. pneumoniae* and the helical morphology of the spiroplasmas. Several species also possess specialized organelles that mediate attachment to host cells and also are involved in organism motility.

Smallness also is reflected in the mycoplasma genome of 5×10^8 daltons, which is roughly one-sixth the size of that in classic bacteria. This limits the genetic information available for metabolic pathways and products, requiring the use of complex media for propagation of mycoplasmas in the laboratory and restricting ways by which their pathogenicity can be expressed. Pathogenetic mechanisms used by mycoplasmas are incom-

W. A. Clyde, Jr.: Department of Pediatrics, University of North Carolina, Chapel Hill, North Carolina 27599.

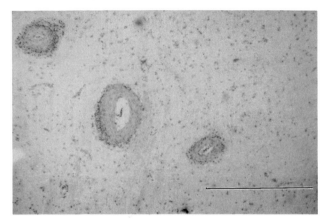

FIG. 1. Lymphocytic infiltration in cerebral vessels of a turkey poult, 30 days after inoculation with *M. gallisepticum* and partial treatment to prevent acute death. Hematoxylin and eosin; bar represents 500 μm. (From ref. 74, with permission.)

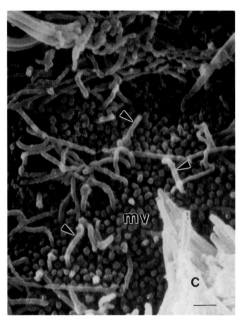

FIG. 2. Hamster trachea in organ culture infected with *M. pneumoniae*. Single, filamentous organisms (*arrowheads*) attaching between microvilli (mv) are perpendicular to the cell surface. Tufts of cilia (c) can be seen in the field. Scanning electron microscopy; bar represents 1 μm. (From ref. 75, with permission.)

pletely understood, although much new information has accrued in recent years. For example, in tracheal organ cultures *M. pneumoniae* has been shown to decrease macromolecular transport, oxygen consumption, and nucleic acid and endogenous catalase synthesis. The latter effect could enhance cell damage due to the organism's release of H_2O_2 (Fig. 2).

Taxonomically, mycoplasmas are grouped into three families containing five genera. Species associated with neurological syndromes are included in genera *Mycoplasma, Ureaplasma,* and *Spiroplasma.* In human medicine the most important pathogen is *M. pneumoniae.* This organism is filamentous in shape, measuring approximately 0.1×2 μm, with one differentiated pole which bears a cell adhesin (protein P1) and serves as the leading point for gliding motility (Fig. 3). Growth in artificial media requires the presence of serum and an extract of bakers' yeast; a variety of carbohydrates are fermented (Fig. 4).

M. hominis has a globular shape and is approximately 0.25 μm in diameter. It is less fastidious in growth requirements than is *M. pneumoniae* and does not ferment carbohydrates but hydrolyzes arginine. Depletion of this essential amino acid injures cell cultures contaminated by the mycoplasma. As the name implies, *U. urealyticum* cleaves urea with the production of ammonia, which is injurious to cells *in vitro.*

EPIDEMIOLOGY

Neurological Complications of Respiratory Mycoplasmal Disease

As early as 1889 (5) it was recognized that neurological syndromes could be seen in association with pneumonia cases, and there were further reports of such associations during the 1930s (see ref. 6). Among the 11 cases presented by Reimann (1) which first delineated the atypical pneumonia syndrome, three patients had clinical evidence of encephalitis, including one with fatal outcome. Yesnick (7) reviewed neurological complications associated with the atypical pneumonia syndrome in 1956; he estimated that these complications were rare, occurring in ≤0.1% of all cases; however, there was a 32% mortality in such cases. Because these reports were published prior to the identification of *M. pneumoniae* as the most common cause of atypical pneumonia, it is not certain that the cases were of uniform etiology, although it is likely that most were. In 1969, following definition of *M. pneumoniae*, Sterner and Biberfeld (8) estimated that 1–7% of those mycoplasmal infections severe enough to require hospitalization were associated with neurological complications. Pönkä (9) reported that 4.8% of 560 patients hospitalized for management of *M. pneumoniae* disease had neurological complications. A study by Lind et al. (10) revealed evidence of concurrent *M. pneumoniae* infections in 5–10% of patients hospitalized with acute febrile nonbacterial CNS syndromes.

Case descriptions in the literature indicate that the development of neurological findings occurs in not less than 3 days following onset of *M. pneumoniae* respiratory disease, and up to 2 weeks or longer after respiratory symptoms subside. This pattern suggests that both infectious and postinfectious mechanisms could be involved in the etiology of the CNS manifestations. The

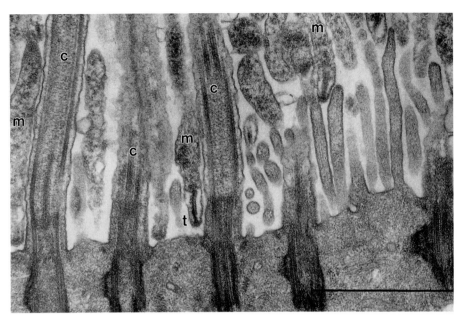

FIG. 3. Hamster trachea in organ culture infected with *M. pneumoniae*. Mycoplasmas (m) are seen among the cilia (c), attached to the epithelial cell border by a differentiated terminal organelle (t). Transmission electron microscopy; bar represents 0.5 μm. (From ref. 41, with permission.)

age distribution of these problems appears to parallel the age-related incidence of *M. pneumoniae* infections, with most occurring in school-aged children, adolescents, and young adults.

CNS Infections and Genital Tract Mycoplasmas

Mycoplasma species that have been isolated from the genitourinary tract of humans are *M. hominis, U. urealyticum, M. fermentans,* and, rarely, *M. genitalium.* The first two species have been implicated in CNS infections, particularly as a cause of neonatal meningitis.

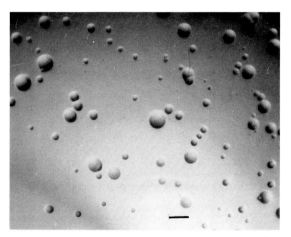

FIG. 4. Appearance of *M. pneumoniae* colonies growing on transparent mycoplasma agar medium after incubation for 1 week. The convexity of the colonies is into the agar matrix. Unstained; bar represents 0.1 mm.

Colonization of the genital tract with *M. hominis* occurs in up to 54% of women and 35% of men; the organism is sexually transmitted, and it is generally regarded as a component of the normal microflora in most instances (11). There are reports of postpartum sepsis with this organism, "sterile" pyelonephritis, arthritis, and brain abscesses (4,11). The incidence of neonatal meningitis due to *M. hominis* is unknown, although a number of case reports have appeared in the literature (12–14). Because meningitis has occurred in both term and premature infants, with or without meningomyeloceles, these infections could result from maternal sepsis with transplacental transmission to the infant or from colonization of the infant respiratory tract during the birth process. Premature infants are at special risk for intraventricular hemorrhages, offering another portal of entry into the CNS if sepsis or transient mycoplasmemia were present.

Genital tract colonization with *U. urealyticum* is somewhat greater than with *M. hominis,* occurring at a rate of up to 75% among women and 45% among men who have multiple sexual consorts. The ubiquity of these organisms has made it difficult to discern their role in genitourinary disease, but they have been implicated in nongonococcal urethritis, salpingitis, pelvic inflammatory disease, and perinatal problems such as chorioamnionitis, prematurity, stillbirth, and neonatal pneumonia (15). In addition to the potential transmission routes mentioned for *M. hominis* in connection with neonatal meningitis, ureaplasmas appear capable of penetrating intact fetal membranes and causing ascending infections before birth. While surface colonization has been demonstrated in about one-third of female infants and a smaller proportion of male infants born to colonized mothers, the frequency of invasive disease is not known.

In a prospective study of 203 young infants evaluated for possible sepsis by Likitnukul et al. (16), no genital mycoplasmas were isolated from blood or cerebrospinal fluid (CSF) cultures. In a series of similar size where only *M. hominis* was sought, Mårdh (13) also reported negative results. A more recent study by Waites et al. (17) reported eight isolates of *U. urealyticum* and five of *M. hominis* from 100 CSF samples; for the most part, these patients were preterm infants whose CSF specimens were collected both for sepsis evaluation and for treatment of hydrocephalus. These experiences suggest that premature rupture of membranes, premature labor, and fetal immaturity could represent factors contributing to the occurrence of mycoplasmal meningitis of genital origin. Current obstetrical practices, such as the placement of scalp electrodes to monitor for fetal distress during labor, could offer a portal of entry for systemic infection.

PATHOGENESIS AND PATHOPHYSIOLOGY

In human as well as animal CNS diseases associated with mycoplasmal infections there appear to be a number of possible pathogenetic mechanisms, which can be divided broadly into (a) those involving direct invasion of the CNS by mycoplasmas and (b) others where the brain and CSF are sterile. The latter category includes effects of putative mycoplasmal toxins, cerebrovascular phenomena, and autoimmunity.

Most of the reports associating CNS disease with *M. pneumoniae* infections have based the diagnosis on complement fixation serology using lipid extracts of the organism as antigen. This reaction is nonspecific to the extent that similar or identical antigens can be found in certain streptococci and in vegetables, including spinach; the test also is relatively insensitive compared to other serodiagnostic methods that have been devised. Diagnosis of *M. pneumoniae* infection by isolation of the organism from respiratory secretions bypasses the reservations about serodiagnosis; isolation from CSF specimens in cases with neurological system involvement would demonstrate more directly the association between the mycoplasma and this complication. In one experimental animal study, *M. pneumoniae* could be isolated from both lung and brain tissue following intranasal inoculation of mice (18).

Rare reports of *M. pneumoniae* recovery from CSF have appeared in the literature, although at least an equal number of negative attempts have been presented. In 1972 Fleischauer et al. (19) presented the first positive CSF culture from a patient with Guillain–Barré syndrome associated with bronchopneumonia. Other cases have been reported from Japan [associated with tremor and myoclonus (20) and meningoencephalitis (21)] and

from Israel [associated with encephalitis and cerebellar ataxia (22)]. The presence of the mycoplasma in a form precluding standard isolation methods is suggested in a single case report of pneumonia complicated by aseptic meningitis and Guillain–Barré syndrome by Bayer et al. (23). Cell cultures inoculated with CSF for virus isolation were tested by immunofluorescence using *M. pneumoniae* antiserum with positive results; at the same time, conventional mycoplasma media showed no growth. A precedent for such a "nutritionally defective" mycoplasma is provided by *M. hyorhinis,* a common cell culture contaminant which often can be propagated only in the presence of cells.

While it has been thought that *M. pneumoniae* is a mucosal surface pathogen without invasive potential, the few cases cited, together with several autopsy reports in which the organism has been recovered from blood and organs other than lung, provide evidence that spread of infection beyond the respiratory tract can occur. Further efforts to culture CSF from potential cases will be needed to estimate the frequency of this circumstance. The two Israeli cases came from a series of 125 pneumonia episodes (22); this study reported an incidence of 1.6%, which approaches the estimated frequency of neurological complications among *M. pneumoniae* illnesses severe enough to require hospitalization.

Among the animal mycoplasmoses there are several examples of CNS invasion by organisms that also cause respiratory disease, including *M. pulmonis* disease of rodents and *M. hyorhinis* and *M. hyopneumoniae* infections of swine. In the pig infection it has been reported that ependymal cells of the lateral ventricles are affected selectively by the mycoplasmas, suggesting a possible injury mechanism that could manifest a variety of neurological disturbances (24).

The possibility that *M. pneumoniae* produces a neurotoxin has been raised by several investigators, but thus far the only extracellular products of this organism that have been demonstrated are hydrogen peroxide and an inhibitor of host cell catalase. These substances may mediate injury directly to parasitized cells of the respiratory tract, but they would not be expected to act at distant sites. The best example of a mycoplasmal neurotoxin is supplied by the rodent pathogen *M. neurolyticum:* A substance present in organism-free culture filtrates, when injected intravenously into mice, reproduces the pattern of rolling disease within minutes. The exact nature of this material has not been determined, and the possibility exists that membrane fragments—rather than an extracellular product—are involved in mediation of the neurological picture.

Another pathogenetic mechanism which may mediate neurological manifestations of mycoplasmal infections relates to cerebrovascular effects, including thromboembolic phenomena. Cerebral pathology in fatal cases of *M. pneumoniae* disease and atypical pneumonia associated with meningoencephalitis frequently includes capillary thromboses and evidence of microangiopathy (6,25,26). Microinfarcts within various tissues, as well as thromboses with autoamputation of digits, have been reported. A possible model for this type of injury is provided by *M. gallisepticum*-associated encephalopathy of turkey poults. This naturally occurring disease can be reproduced experimentally by intravenous injection of cultured organisms into young birds (27,28). Ataxia, weakness and somnolence appear within 3 days, followed by coma and death in another day or two. Examination of the turkey brain reveals fibrinoid necrosis of cerebral arteries (Fig. 5); by electron microscopy, capillary endothelial swelling and occlusion are seen (29). Use of the immunofluoresence method has localized *M. gallisepticum* within the brain only in the cerebral arteries, suggesting that the capillary effects are due to toxic products of the organisms (30).

Since discovery of the cold hemagglutination phenomenon in some cases of atypical pneumonia (31), there has been interest in the role of autoimmunity with regard to many of the nonrespiratory aspects of *M. pneumoniae* disease, including the neurological complications. Cold hemagglutinins can be demonstrated in up to 70% of *M. pneumoniae* pneumonia cases, with the highest occurrence in the more severe disease. These antibodies are of the IgM class and are directed toward the I antigen of erythrocyte membranes; they appear within the first or second week of illness, peak around the third week, and disappear by about the sixth to eighth week. The possibility that these autoantibodies play a role in the thromboembolic processes occasionally seen in severe *M. pneumoniae* disease has been entertained, but it seems unlikely because the hemagglutination is temperature-dependent and is not expressed above 20°C (maximum, 4°C). Cold hemagglutinins may be seen in several other conditions, including infectious mononucleosis, adeno-

virus pneumonia, rubeola, tropical eosinophilia and collagen–vascular diseases.

Biberfeld (32) studied seven cases of *M. pneumoniae* infections associated with neurological complications (three meningitis, two meningoencephalitis, two acute psychosis) and found that all patients produced antibodies reactive with human brain tissue. The anti-brain antibodies could be absorbed from the sera using either brain tissue or *M. pneumoniae* organisms, suggesting the presence of cross-reacting antigens. However, similar antibodies could be found in patients who did not have neurological syndromes, suggesting that the antibodies were not direct mediators of these complications. Antibodies reactive with various other tissues also have been found in conjunction with *M. pneumoniae* infections, including normal lung, cardiac and skeletal muscle, and liver.

Other antibodies of the type associated with rheumatic diseases have been reported in *M. pneumoniae* infections. These include anti-smooth-muscle antibodies (33) and antibodies reactive with the mitotic spindles of dividing cells (34); these antibodies, of the IgM and IgG classes, respectively, cannot be absorbed with whole mycoplasma organisms, suggesting a different mechanism in their stimulation. However, in the case of antibodies reactive with mammalian intermediate filaments, there is evidence of shared epitopes with several mycoplasma species, including *M. pneumoniae* (35). Behan et al. (36) describe other evidence of autoimmune phenomena in five cases of mycoplasmal infections with neurological complications (hemiparesis in two, Guillain–Barré syndrome, cranial nerve palsies, polyneuritis/myelitis). Each of these patients showed evidence of circulating immune complexes and depletion of complement component C4. In the hemiparesis cases, an autopsy of one and cerebellar biopsy of the other showed changes compatible with acute disseminated encephalomyelitis, suggesting immune-complex-type vasculopathy as the damaging mechanism.

PATHOLOGY

A study of CNS pathology associated with pneumonia, together with a review of literature prior to 1945, was reported by Noran and Baker (6). Among the 10 cases they examined in detail were four considered to be compatible with the clinical descriptions of the primary atypical pneumonia syndrome, whereas the remainder were in infants younger than 4.5 months. The etiology of these cases is uncertain based on information provided, but the authors found similar brain changes in all cases and reported on the group as a whole. Gross examination showed vascular congestion, small areas of subarachnoid hemorrhage, and scattered petechiae in degrees corresponding to the clinical severity of the encephalitic picture. Extensive microscopic thrombosis of arterioles,

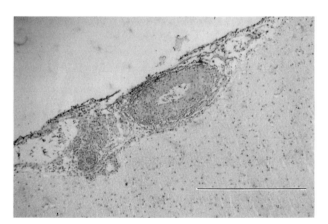

FIG. 5. Fibrinoid necrosis in the wall of a cerebral artery, 3 days after intravenous inoculation of a turkey poult with *M. gallisepticum,* strain S6. Hematoxylin and eosin; bar represents 500 μm. (From ref. 74, with permission.)

venules, and capillaries was described, and there was perivascular demyelination in some cases. These changes led the authors to speculate on the possibility that clotting disturbances or factors from injured lung tissue were involved in the pathogenesis of "pneumonic encephalitis," irrespective of the cause of pneumonia in their cases.

Published autopsy findings of fatal cases of *M. pneumoniae* disease with neurological complications are few in number. In these cases the etiologic diagnosis is based on serologic data only, including high or rising titers of cold hemagglutinins and complement fixing antibodies, providing some need for cautious interpretation (37). In a report of one fulminant case (38), *M. pneumoniae* was recovered from the brain, among other organs, but this patient had no antemortem neurological problems and the brain histology was normal. Fisher et al. (39) summarized 12 case reports while adding one new case; an additional case is supplied by Behan et al. (36).

The brain histopathology varies widely in the available reports—from no changes or cerebral or perivascular edema, to infiltrative and degenerative alterations. Only two of the cases revealed prominent microangiopathy of the type reported by Noran and Baker (6). Other findings include perivenular lymphocytic infiltrations and demyelination in perivascular locations. Similarities have been drawn between these changes and those seen in experimental allergic encephalomyelitis, suggesting that immunopathologic mechanisms may be involved in the CNS complications of *M. pneumoniae* disease (36,39).

Information on CNS pathology in some of the animal and bird mycoplasmoses has been summarized earlier. No pathologic reports on changes associated with *M. ho-*

TABLE 1. *Symptoms and signs of* Mycoplasma pneumoniae *pneumonia*[a]

Finding	Reported frequency (%)
Symptoms	
Cough	93–100
Malaise	74–89
Headache	60–84
Chills	58–78
Sore throat	53–71
Chest discomfort	42–69
Nasal symptoms	29–69
Myalgias	45
Signs	
Fever	96–100
Auscultatory changes (rales, wheezes)	80–84
Pharyngeal erythema (without exudate)	12–73
Cervical adenopathy	18–27

[a] Ranges derived from data in four different studies (57–60).

TABLE 2. *Radiographic features of* Mycoplasma pneumoniae *pneumonia*[a]

Finding	Reported frequency (%)
Location of infiltrates	
Peribronchial	34–76
Dense central	16–65
Juxtapleural	29–60
Distribution of infiltrates	
Single lesion	73–75
Lobar	0–29
Other	
Adenopathy	3–38
Septal lines	3–11
Atelectasis	5–59
Pleural changes	12–30
Punctate mottling	13–34

[a] Independent interpretations of the same radiographs (n = 97) by four different radiologists (61).

minis and *U. urealyticum* meningitis of neonates are available.

CLINICAL MANIFESTATIONS

Illnesses associated with *M. pneumoniae* infections are generally described as being influenza-like, but with more insidious onset of systemic symptoms following a 2- to 3-week incubation period after exposure (40) (Table 1). Malaise, headache, and scratchy sore throat may precede development of coughing, which is dry at first but later produces mucoid or mucopurulent sputum. The cough often has a paroxysmal quality and is more severe at night, disturbing sleep and aggravating the headache. With severe coughing the sputum may be blood-tinged and chest muscle soreness may develop, but frank hemoptysis and true pleuritic pain are unusual.

Physical findings often are minimal when patients with *M. pneumoniae* infections first present for medical attention. Other than temperature rarely exceeding 39°C and nonexudative pharyngitis, patients with tracheobronchitis (the most common clinical syndrome) seem disproportionately ill. Those with pneumonia may have rales or wheezes over involved areas, which usually are in one of the lower lobes. Pleural effusions and areas of subsegmental atelectasis occur, but generally they are too small to detect by physical examination. Bullous myringitis or sinusitis may accompany these infections, as may skin rashes of the erythema multiforme type. Rarely, extensive skin and mucus membrane involvement results in Stevens–Johnson syndrome.

In cases of mycoplasmal pneumonia the chest x-ray findings are protean and nonspecific for this diagnosis (41) (Table 2). The most frequent changes consist of peribronchial thickening, interstitial infiltration, and

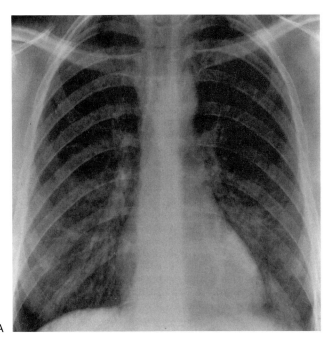 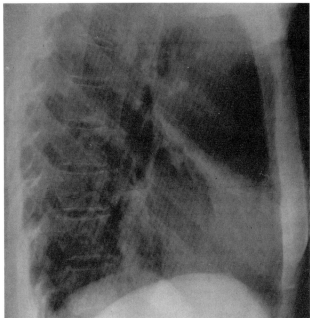

FIG. 6. Posterior–anterior (**A**) and lateral (**B**) chest x-rays of a 20-year-old patient with culture-proven *M. pneumoniae* pneumonia. Streaky, nodular densities are present in the right middle and left lower lobe areas. (From ref. 41, with permission.)

small triangular or larger "plate-like" areas of atelectasis in the involved areas (Fig. 6). At times, nodular densities, suggestive of a granulomatous process, may be seen. Hilar adenopathy is not unusual. Pleural effusions, if present, tend to be small and transient in most cases. Massive pleural effusions and lobar consolidation have been described, but such changes would suggest other etiologic diagnoses initially.

Neurological complications of *M. pneumoniae* disease have been described as beginning within 3 days of the respiratory symptomatology, and as late as 30 days afterwards. Early signs have included lethargy, stupor or

coma, agitation, psychotic behavior, aphasia, paresthesias, and cranial nerve pareses. The later findings are those of the particular neurological syndromes that have been reported; a summary of these diverse conditions is given in Table 3.

The clinical manifestations of neonatal meningitis are rather nonspecific, including hyper- or hypothermia, lethargy, poor feeding or vomiting, respiratory distress (apnea or cyanosis), seizures, irritability, and abdominal distention. Full or bulging fontanelles may be detected, but nuchal rigidity is uncommon. These findings are the same as those seen in septicemia, and evaluation generally includes blood and surface cultures as well as lumbar puncture. Male infants are involved in these processes twice as often as females; low birth weight also is a highly significant contributing risk factor.

TABLE 3. *CNS syndromes associated with* Mycoplasma pneumoniae *infections*

Condition	Key references
Aseptic meningitis	Sterner and Biberfeld (8)
Cerebellar ataxia	Steele et al. (62)
Cranial nerve palsy	Jachuck et al. (63)
Encephalitis	Pönkä (9)
Guillain–Barré syndrome	Steele et al. (64)
Hemiplegia	Vuopala et al. (65)
Meningitis	Fleischauer et al. (19)
Meningoencephalitis	Sköldenberg (66)
Meningoencephalitis, hemolytic anemia	Plotkin et al. (67)
Necrotizing myelitis	Nagaswami and Kepes (68)
Postinfectious leukoencephalitis	Fisher et al. (39)
Polyradiculitis	Holt et al. (69)
Psychosis	Sterner and Biberfeld (8)
Transverse myelitis	Nicholson (70)

DIAGNOSIS

Neurological Complications of *M. pneumoniae* Disease

The diagnosis of *M. pneumoniae* disease in conjunction with one of the syndromes listed in Table 3 might be considered in the presence of a preceding or concurrent episode of tracheobronchitis or pneumonia. These infections may occur in any season, although they are more common in the fall and early winter months in temperate climates. While any age group may be involved, the greatest incidence is between 5 and 40 years in both sexes. History of similar respiratory illnesses in a household or institutional setting is a useful epidemiologic clue.

Examination of the CSF in reported cases reveals total leukocyte counts averaging 83 per cubic millimeter (range 0–410), with polymorphonuclear cells averaging 25% (range 0–90%). Generally the glucose concentrations were normal or slightly depressed, whereas protein concentrations were normal or mildly elevated. Several patients were reported to have CSF pressure elevations. In those few cases in which *M. pneumoniae* was recovered from the specimens, changes were within the ranges given. Inadequate information is available to judge the value of computed tomographic and radionuclide scans in case evaluation (22,39,42,43).

In many of the reported neurological syndromes associated with *M. pneumoniae* disease the diagnosis was first suggested by detection of cold hemagglutinins. The reaction is nonspecific, since it may be seen in other infectious or inflammatory conditions. Nevertheless, the cold hemagglutinin test is rapid, readily available, and inexpensive, and it may suggest the value of specific tests for *M. pneumoniae* infection when positive; negative cold hemagglutinin tests do not exclude the diagnosis.

Diagnosis by isolation of *M. pneumoniae* from respiratory secretions, CSF, or tissue is a specialized process that is not offered by most diagnostic microbiology laboratories. With available techniques, 1–3 weeks or more may be required for processing and identification of isolates (44), so that results are not available to assist initial therapeutic considerations. Since organisms can remain in the respiratory tract for several weeks, even following appropriate antibiotic treatment, these factors may not preclude isolation attempts. In one study it was estimated that the sensitivity of culture was 68%, with a specificity of 97% (45).

Many procedures have been described for measurement of serum antibodies against *M. pneumoniae*. Of these, the complement fixation method has been the most popular and readily available test. With a lipid antigen derived from the organisms by chloroform–methanol extraction, sensitivity of the complement fixation test was estimated at 90%; specificity was estimated at 94% (45). Diagnostic results are ≥4-fold changes in titer between properly timed acute (as early as possible after onset of illness) and convalescent (2 or 3 weeks later) sera. In many of the published cases of neurological complications the possibility of *M. pneumoniae* infection was not considered until late in the course of illness, when antibody titers were already elevated, and no acute serum specimen was available for comparison. Since elevated complement fixation antibody titers may remain for a year or longer after infection, it is difficult to interpret the meaning of a single titer in relation to a current illness. There has been interest in testing for IgM-specific antibodies, with the rationale that these develop earlier than IgG antibodies in *M. pneumoniae* in-

fections. However, repeated infections have been documented within 18 months to 10 years, and the IgM antibodies may not be prominent except in younger children experiencing their first infections. Because of cross-reactions between the antigen used in the complement fixation test, brain and other tissues, and certain bacteria, use of this test in cases of neurological syndromes of unknown etiology without mycoplasma-compatible respiratory disease or a corroborating culture appears unwarranted (37).

A rapid diagnostic test for *M. pneumoniae* infection has been introduced that uses a radiolabeled DNA probe to detect mycoplasmal ribosomal RNA in respiratory secretions. Available test data suggest high sensitivity (100%) and specificity (98%) for this procedure, relative to a positive culture (46,47). Other studies indicate that a sharp drop in sensitivity of the probe occurs when the positive reference point is seroconversion (48). In still another comparative study the correlation between culture, serology, and probe was very good when sputum samples were the test specimen; poor results were obtained using throat swabs, which have been the recommended specimens for study (49). A theoretical shortcoming of the method is that ribosomal RNA is generated only by actively metabolizing organisms, and the content in organisms suppressed by antibiotics or antibodies may be below the level of detection. Other rapid methods now under development also appear promising, such as one based on the polymerase chain reaction which purports to detect as few as 100 organisms in respiratory secretions (50).

Neonatal Meningitis

The diagnosis of neonatal meningitis is suggested by the nonspecific clinical manifestations that have been discussed, and documentation requires lumbar or ventricular puncture. Review of the CSF findings in cases of *M. hominis* meningitis reveals total cell counts of less than 2000 per cubic millimeter, with an overall mean of 547 per cubic millimeter; 60–80% of these were polymorphonuclear cells. Slight decreases in glucose concentration, as well as slight elevations in protein concentration, have been reported. In the cases reported by Waites et al. (17), four of the five cases with isolation of *M. hominis* showed no pleocytosis. In the same series, four of the babies with *U. urealyticum* in CSF cultures had cell counts in the range of 18–5240 per cubic millimeter, whereas two showed no pleocytosis and no data were presented for two others. Some of these babies showed gradually rising protein values on repeat studies; however, since some specimens were collected as treatment for hydrocephalus, this change could be based on that problem rather than on the presence of ureaplasmas.

Specific diagnosis requires recovery of the organisms

from CSF. *M. hominis* may be isolated on standard bacterial blood agar as pinpoint colonies after 4 or more days of incubation, but it is more readily recognized on standard mycoplasma media (44). Special media formulations are required for the propagation of ureaplasmas (51), and these resources are available only in major reference diagnostic laboratories. Techniques for the serodiagnosis of genital mycoplasma infections have been described, but they remain in the province of the research laboratory at present.

Available data suggest that routine mycoplasma cultures of CSF from term infants suspected of having sepsis or meningitis would be nonproductive. Selected infants with abnormal CSF findings that are negative for classic bacteria might be considered for study, together with evaluations for viral infections. If corroborated by further experience, the study of Waites et al. (17) suggests that cultures of high-risk premature infants being evaluated for sepsis could be of more value. Media suitable for recovery of both *M. hominis* and *U. urealyticum* should be used, such as the U10C broth of Shepard (51).

TREATMENT

In selecting antibiotics for therapy of mycoplasmal infections, it should be recalled that the absence of peptidoglycan cell-wall structures confers absolute insensitivity to agents acting at this site. This includes the penicillins and cephalosporins, polymyxins, and bacitracin. Sulfonamides also are ineffective. The organisms generally are sensitive to antimicrobials which act at the ribosomal level, particularly the tetracycline family. There is variable sensitivity, by species and strains, to the macrolides, aminoglycosides, and chloramphenicol. In the case of CNS infections, selection of antimicrobials also is influenced by their ability to penetrate the blood–brain barrier.

M. pneumoniae infections are effectively treated with erythromycin or tetracycline (Table 4). Erythromycin usually is favored for children younger than 8–10 years, because of the toxic side effects of tetracyclines in this age group. It is not known how frequently *M. pneumoniae* is present in the CNS when neurological complications occur; but since direct infection has been demonstrated in some cases, tetracycline therapy may be

preferred because of superior CNS penetration. While erythromycin resistance is easily induced *in vitro,* and has been seen in mycoplasmal isolates after therapeutic courses in patients, this has not appeared to be of clinical significance in the management of respiratory infections to date. Tetracycline resistance of *M. pneumoniae* has not been reported.

Antimicrobial sensitivity of the genital mycoplasmas has been more variable, and *in vitro* studies should be obtained (if at all possible) in the management of serious infections. Most strains of *M. hominis* are sensitive to tetracycline; however, development of resistance through acquisition of the *tetM* plasmid by the mycoplasma is not uncommon. *M. hominis* is not sensitive to erythromycin, although clindamycin reportedly is effective against most strains (52,53). Since CSF concentrations of clindamycin are negligible, tetracycline appears to be the only alternative for treatment of meningitis, even in the neonate. It has been demonstrated that *M. hominis* is sensitive to ciprofloxacin *in vitro* (54). Since folic acid is not synthesized by *M. hominis,* trimethoprim-sulfamethoxazole is ineffective (53,55).

For ureaplasmal infections, erythromycin and tetracycline are usually effective. However, data from sexually transmitted disease clinics reveal that 20% (or greater) of isolates are resistant to erythromycin. Ureaplasmas also may acquire tetracycline resistance via the *tetM* plasmid. These organisms have limited susceptibility to the quinolone compounds that are now on the market, although difloxacin and ofloxacin are effective *in vitro* (54).

PREVENTION

Control measures for mycoplasmal infections have achieved only limited success (56). Several experimental vaccines for *M. pneumoniae* disease have been field-tested and have shown some effectiveness, but none are licensed for use at present. The most extensively tested preparations were killed, whole-cell injected vaccines. Seroconversion after these products ranged from 0% to 90%, and protective efficacy varied from 28% to 67%. Efforts to produce live, attenuated vaccines for respiratory mucosal application yielded materials which were effective in animal models but which produced unacceptable disease on testing in volunteers. Current research is

TABLE 4. *Treatment of* Mycoplasma pneumoniae *infections (71–73)*

Host	Antibiotic	Oral dose	Frequency	Duration
Adults	Erythromycin	0.5 g	6 hr	14 days
	Tetracycline	0.25–0.5 g	6 hr	14 days
	Doxycycline	0.1 g	12 hr	14 days
Children				
<9 years	Erythromycin	30–50 mg/kg	6 hr	14 days
>9 years	Erythromycin	30–50 mg/kg	6 hr	14 days
	Tetracycline	30–50 mg/kg	6 hr	14 days
>25 kg	Same as adult			

focused on subcellular components, with the goal of producing more concentrated and specific immunogens. A technical problem is delivery of adequate material, with sufficient duration, to the mucosal surface, since mucosal immunity is the best correlate of protective immunity.

Antibiotic prophylaxis appears to decrease clinical disease expression but does not prevent infection. The effects of appropriate antimicrobial treatment of *M. pneumoniae* respiratory infections on the prevention of associated neurological complications are unknown.

Neonatal mycoplasmal meningitis appears to be associated with maternal infection or colonization with genital mycoplasma species. Because of the rarity of this CNS infection and the high prevalence of maternal colonization, the efficacy of maternal antimicrobial treatment as a preventive measure would be difficult to assess. Since the literature suggests that meningitis may be more frequent in high-risk pregnancies and births, the general obstetrical and medical efforts being made to reduce these risks may have some preventive value.

REFERENCES

1. Reimann HA. An acute infection of the respiratory tract with atypical pneumonia. *JAMA* 1938;111:2377–2384.
2. Chanock RM, Hayflick L, Barile MF. Growth on artificial medium of an agent associated with atypical pneumonia and its identification as a pleuropneumonia-like organism. *Proc Natl Acad Sci USA* 1962;48:41–48.
3. Paine TF, Murray R, Perlmutter I, Finland M. Brain abscess and meningitis associated with a pleuropneumonia-like organism: clinical and bacteriological observations in a case with recovery. *Ann Intern Med* 1950;32:554–562.
4. Madoff S, Hooper DC. Nongenitourinary infections caused by *Mycoplasma hominis* in adults. *Rev Infect Dis* 1988;10:602–613.
5. Stephan BH. Des paralysies pneumoniques. *Rev Med Paris* 1889;9:60–77.
6. Noran HH, Baker AB. The central nervous system in pneumonia (nonsuppurative pneumonic encephalitis). II. A pathologic study. *Am J Pathol* 1946;22:579–590.
7. Yesnick L. Central nervous system complications of primary atypical pneumonia. *Arch Intern Med* 1956;97:93–98.
8. Sterner G, Biberfeld G. Central nervous system complications of *Mycoplasma pneumoniae* infections. *Scand J Infect Dis* 1969;1:203–208.
9. Pönkä A. Central nervous system manifestations associated with serologically verified *Mycoplasma pneumoniae* infection. *Scand J Infect Dis* 1980;12:175–184.
10. Lind K, Zoffman H, Larsen SO, Jessen O. *Mycoplasma pneumoniae* infection associated with affection of the central nervous system. *Acta Med Scand* 1979;205:325–332.
11. Mårdh P-A, Møller BR, McCormack WM, eds. International symposium on *Mycoplasma hominis*—a human pathogen. *Sex Transm Dis* 1983;10(4, Suppl):225–385.
12. Gewitz M, Dinwiddie L, Rees O, Volikas O, Yuille T, O'Connell B, Marshall WC. *Mycoplasma hominis.* A cause of neonatal meningitis. *Arch Dis Child* 1979;54:231–239.
13. Mårdh P-A. *Mycoplasma hominis* infection of the central nervous system in newborn infants. *Sex Transm Dis* 1983;10(4, Suppl):331–334.
14. McDonald JC, Moore DL. *Mycoplasma hominis* meningitis in a premature infant. *Pediatr Infect Dis* 1988;7:795–798.
15. Cassell GH, ed. Ureaplasmas of humans: with emphasis upon maternal and neonatal infections. *Pediatr Infect Dis* 1986;5(6, Suppl):S221–S354.
16. Likitnukul S, Kusmiesz H, Nelson JD, McCracken GH Jr. Role of genital mycoplasmas in young infants with suspected sepsis. *J Pediatr* 1986;109:971–974.
17. Waites KB, Rudd PT, Crouse DT, Canupp KC, Nelson KG, Ramsey C, Cassell GH. Chronic *Ureaplasma urealyticum* and *Mycoplasma hominis* infections of central nervous system in preterm infants. *Lancet* 1988;1:17–21.
18. Ogata S, Kitamoto O. Clinical complications of *Mycoplasma pneumoniae* disease—central nervous system. *Yale J Biol Med* 1983;56:481–486.
19. Fleischauer P, Hüben U, Mertens H, Sethi KK, Thürman D. Nachweis von *Mycoplasma pneumoniae* im liquor bei akuter polyneuritis. *Dtsch Med Wochenschr* 1972;97:678–682.
20. Suzuki K, Matsubara S, Uchikata M, Tanabe H, Okano H, Tanimoto H, Matsuoka H. A case of *Mycoplasma pneumoniae* associated with meningoencephalitis. *Yale J Biol Med* 1983;56:873–874.
21. Kasahara I, Otsubo Y, Yanase T, Oshima H, Ichimaru HA, Nakamura M. Isolation and characterization of *Mycoplasma pneumoniae* from cerebrospinal fluid of a patient with pneumonia and meningoencephalitis. *J Infect Dis* 1985;152:823–825.
22. Abramovitz P, Schvartzman P, Harel D, Lis I, Naot Y. Direct invasion of the central nervous system by *Mycoplasma pneumoniae:* a report of two cases. *J Infect Dis* 1987;155:482–487.
23. Bayer AS, Galpin JE, Theofilopoulos AN, Guze LB. Neurologic disease associated with *Mycoplasma pneumoniae* pneumonitis. Demonstration of viable *Mycoplasma pneumoniae* in cerebrospinal fluid and blood by radioisotopic and immunofluorescent tissue culture techniques. *Ann Intern Med* 1981;94:15–20.
24. Williams PP, Gallagher JE. Effects of *Mycoplasma hyopneumoniae* and *M. hyorhinis* on ependymal cells of the porcine lateral ventricles as observed by scanning and transmission electron microscopy. *Scan Electron Microsc* 1981;4:133–140.
25. Dorff B, Lind K. Two fatal cases of meningoencephalitis associated with *Mycoplasma pneumoniae* infection. *Scand J Infect Dis* 1976;8:49–51.
26. Weinblatt ME, Caplan ES. Fatal *Mycoplasma pneumoniae* encephalitis in an adult. *Arch Neurol* 1980;37:321.
27. Cordy DR, Adler HE. The pathogenesis of the encephalitis in turkey poults produced by a neurotoxic pleuropneumonia-like organism. *Avian Dis* 1957;1:235–245.
28. Thomas L, Davidson M, McCluskey RT. Studies of PPLO infection. I. The production of cerebral polyarteritis by *Mycoplasma gallisepticum* in turkeys; the neurotoxic property of the mycoplasma. *J Exp Med* 1966;123:897–912.
29. Manuelidis EE, Thomas L. Occlusion of brain capillaries by endothelial swelling in mycoplasma infections. *Proc Natl Acad Sci USA* 1973;70:706–709.
30. Clyde WA Jr, Thomas L. Tropism of *Mycoplasma gallisepticum* for arterial walls. *Proc Natl Acad Sci USA* 1973;70:1545–1549.
31. Peterson OL, Ham TH, Finland M. Cold agglutinins (autohemagglutinins) in primary atypical pneumonia. *Science* 1943;97:167.
32. Biberfeld G. Antibodies to brain and other tissues in cases of *Mycoplasma pneumoniae* infection. *Clin Exp Immunol* 1971;8:319–333.
33. Biberfeld G, Sterner G. Smooth muscle antibodies in *Mycoplasma pneumoniae* infection. *Clin Exp Immunol* 1976;24:287–291.
34. Lind K, Høier-Madsen M, Wiik A. Autoantibodies to the mitotic spindle apparatus in *Mycoplasma pneumoniae* disease. *Infect Immun* 1988;56:714–715.
35. Wise KS, Watson RK. Antigenic mimicry of mammalian intermediate filaments by mycoplasmas. *Infect Immun* 1985;48:587–591.
36. Behan PO, Feldman RG, Segerra JM, Draper IT. Neurological aspects of mycoplasmal infection. *Acta Neurol Scand* 1986;3:314–322.
37. Clyde WA Jr. Neurological syndromes and mycoplasmal infections. *Arch Neurol* 1980;37:65–66.
38. Koletsky RJ, Weinstein AJ. Fulminant *Mycoplasma pneumoniae* infection. Report of a case, and a review of the literature. *Am Rev Respir Dis* 1980;122:491–496.
39. Fisher RS, Clark AW, Wolinsky JS, Parhad IM, Moses H, Mardiney MR. Postinfectious leukoencephalitis complicating *Mycoplasma pneumoniae* infection. *Arch Neurol* 1983;40:109–113.

40. Clyde WA Jr. Mycoplasma infections. In: Braunwald E, Isselbacher K, Petersdorf R, Wilson J, Martin J, Fauci A, eds. *Harrison's principles of internal medicine,* 11th ed. New York: McGraw-Hill, 1987;758–759.

41. Clyde WA Jr. Infections of the respiratory tract due to *Mycoplasma pneumoniae.* In: Chernick V, Kendig E, eds. *Disorders of the respiratory tract in children,* 5th ed. Philadelphia: WB Saunders, 1990;403–412.

42. Decaux G, Szyper M, Ectors M, Cornil A, Franken L. Central nervous system complications of *Mycoplasma pneumoniae. J Neurol Neurosurg Psychiatry* 1980;43:883–887.

43. Hely MA, Williamson PM, Terenty TR. Neurological complications of *Mycoplasma pneumoniae* infection. *Clin Exp Neurol* 1984;20:153–160.

44. Clyde WA Jr. Mycoplasmal infections. In: Wentworth BB, ed. *Diagnostic procedures for bacterial infections,* 7th ed. Washington, DC: American Public Health Association, 1987;391–405.

45. Kenny GE, Kaiser GG, Cooney MK, Foy HM. Diagnosis of *Mycoplasma pneumoniae* pneumonia: sensitivities and specificities of serology with lipid antigen and isolation of the organism on soy peptone medium for identification of infections. *J Clin Microbiol* 1990;28:2087–2093.

46. Dular R, Kajioka R, Kasatiya S. Comparison of Gen-Probe commercial kit and culture technique for the diagnosis of *Mycoplasma pneumoniae* infection. *J Clin Microbiol* 1988;26:1068–1069.

47. Tilton RC, Dias F, Kidd H, Ryan RW. DNA probe versus culture for detection of *Mycoplasma pneumoniae* in clinical specimens. *Diagn Microbiol Infect Dis* 1988;10:109–112.

48. Harris R, Marmion BP, Varkanis G, Kok T, Lunn B, Martin J. Laboratory diagnosis of *Mycoplasma pneumoniae* disease. Comparison of methods for the direct detection of specific antigen or nucleic acid sequences in respiratory exudates. *Epidemiol Infect* 1988;101:685–694.

49. Kleemola SRM, Karjalainen JE, Räty RK. Rapid diagnosis of *Mycoplasma pneumoniae* infection: clinical evaluation of a commercial probe test. *J Infect Dis* 1990;162:70–75.

50. Bernet C, Garret M, deBarbeyrac B, Bebear C, Bonnet J. Detection of *Mycoplasma pneumoniae* by using the polymerase chain reaction. *J Clin Microbiol* 1989;27:2492–2496.

51. Shepard MC. Culture media for ureaplasmas. In: Razin S, Tully JG, eds. *Methods in mycoplasmology,* vol I. New York: Academic Press, 1983;137–146.

52. Braun P, Klein JO, Kass EH. Susceptibility of genital mycoplasmas to antimicrobial agents. *Appl Microbiol* 1970;19:62–70.

53. Bygdeman SM, Mårdh P-A. Antimicrobial susceptibility and susceptibility testing of *Mycoplasma hominis:* a review. *Sex Transm Dis* 1983;10(4, Suppl):366–370.

54. Kenny GE, Hooton TM, Roberts MC, Cartwright FD, Hoyt J. Susceptibilities of genital mycoplasmas to the newer quinolones as determined by the agar dilution method. *Antimicrob Agents Chemother* 1989;33:103–107.

55. Burman LG. The antimicrobial activities of trimethoprim and sulfonamides. *Scand J Infect Dis* 1986;18:3–13.

56. Barile MF, Bové JM, Bradbury JM, Cassell GH, Clyde WA Jr, Cottew GS, Whittlestone P. Current status on control of mycoplasmal diseases of man, animals, plants and insects. *Bull Inst Pasteur* 1985;83:339–373.

57. Foy HM, Kenny GE, McMahan R, Mansy AM, Grayston JT. *Mycoplasma pneumoniae* pneumonia in an urban setting. Five years of surveillance. *JAMA* 1970;214:1666–1672.

58. Ionno JA, Westfall RE. *Mycoplasma pneumoniae* pneumonia: clinical course and complications. *Milit Med* 1970;135:459–463.

59. Mufson MA, Manko MA, Kingston JR, Chanock RM. Eaton agent pneumonia—clinical features. *JAMA* 1961;178:369–374.

60. Alexander ER, Foy HM, Kenny GE, Kronmal RA, McMahan R, Clarke ER, MacColl WA, Grayston JT. Pneumonia due to *Mycoplasma pneumoniae.* Its incidence in the membership of a co-operative medical group. *N Engl J Med* 1966;275:131–136.

61. Foy HM, Loop J, Clarke ER, Mansy AW, Spence WF, Feigl P, Grayston JT. Radiographic study of *Mycoplasma pneumoniae* pneumonia. *Am Rev Respir Dis* 1973;108:469–474.

62. Steele JC, Gladstone RM, Thanasophon S, Fleming PC. Acute cerebellar ataxia and concomitant infection with *Mycoplasma pneumoniae. J Pediatr* 1972;80:467–469.

63. Jachuck SJ, Gardner-Thorpe C, Clark F, Foster JB. A brainstem syndrome associated with *Mycoplasma pneumoniae* infection—a report of two cases. *Postgrad Med J* 1975;51:475–477.

64. Steele JC, Gladstone RM, Thanasophon S, Fleming PC. *Mycoplasma pneumoniae* as a determinant of the Guillain–Barré syndrome. *Lancet* 1969;2:710–714.

65. Vuopala U, Juustila H, Takkunen J. Transient hemiplegia associated with *Mycoplasma pneumoniae* infection. *Ann Clin Res* 1970;2:167–170.

66. Sköldenberg B. Aseptic meningitis and meningoencephalitis in cold-agglutinin-positive infections. *Br Med J* 1965;1:100–102.

67. Plotkin GR, Slovak JP Jr, Lentz PE. *Mycoplasma* pneumonia presenting as meningoencephalitis and hemolytic anemia. *Am J Med Sci* 1979;278:235–242.

68. Nagaswami S, Kepes J. Necrotizing myelitis: a clinicopathologic report of two cases associated with *Diplococcus pneumoniae* and *Mycoplasma pneumoniae* infections. *Trans Am Neurol Assoc* 1973;98:290–292.

69. Holt S, Khan MM, Charles RG, Epstein EJ. Polyradiculoneuritis and *Mycoplasma pneumoniae* infection. *Postgrad Med J* 1977;53:416–418.

70. Nicholson G. Transverse myelitis complicating *Mycoplasma pneumoniae* infection. *Postgrad Med J* 1977;53:86–87.

71. McCracken GH Jr. Current status of antibiotic treatment for *Mycoplasma pneumoniae* infections. *Pediatr Infect Dis J* 1986;5:167–171.

72. Cherry JD. Mycoplasma and ureaplasma infections. In: Feigin RD, Cherry JD, eds. *Textbook of pediatric infectious diseases,* 2nd ed. Philadelphia: WB Saunders, 1987;1896–1924.

73. Couch RB. Mycoplasma diseases. In: Mandell GL, Douglas RG, Bennett JE, eds. *Principles and practice of infectious diseases,* 2nd ed. New York: John Wiley & Sons, 1985;1064–1080.

74. Clyde WA Jr, Thomas L. Pathogenesis studies in experimental mycoplasma disease: *M. gallisepticum* infections of turkeys. *Ann NY Acad Sci* 1973;225:413–424.

75. Muse KE, Powell DA, Collier AM. *Mycoplasma pneumoniae* in hamster tracheal organ culture studied by scanning electron microscopy. *Infect Immun* 1976;1:229–237.

PART III

Bacterial Infections of the CNS

Infections of the Central Nervous System,
edited by W. M. Scheld, R. J. Whitley, and
D. T. Durack, Raven Press, Ltd., New York © 1991.

CHAPTER 14

Pathogenesis and Pathophysiology of Bacterial Infections of the Central Nervous System

Allan R. Tunkel and W. Michael Scheld

To produce disease, bacterial pathogens must be able to gain access to the host and find a unique niche, avoid normal host protective mechanisms, multiply on or within the host, and stably infect the host or cause disease (1). These capabilities make up the so-called "pathogenic personality" of the organism. Specialized surface properties permit bacteria to colonize and invade host tissues and/or escape local and systemic host defense mechanisms. Figure 1 is a schematic of gram-negative and gram-positive bacteria, illustrating many of the important structural components of these organisms. The central nervous system (CNS) is usually protected from bacterial invasion by an intact blood–brain barrier (BBB), and bacterial species require specific virulence factors to enhance invasiveness and produce disease. Once the bacterial pathogen enters the CNS, host defense mechanisms are suboptimal to control the infection.

This chapter focuses on (a) the pathogenesis and pathophysiology of bacterial CNS infections (with emphasis on the virulence factors that mediate bacterial colonization, invasion, and survival) and (b) the host defense mechanisms that attempt to eradicate these infections. Some of the bacterial and host factors responsible for initiation and maintenance of CNS infections are listed in Table 1. Meningitis, brain abscess, and cerebrospinal fluid (CSF) shunt infection are useful examples to illustrate these concepts, and an understanding of these mechanisms may lead to the development of innovative strategies in the treatment and/or prevention of these disorders. Many of these concepts are considered in greater detail in the following chapters which specifically address these clinical entities.

A. R. Tunkel and W. M. Scheld: Department of Medicine, Division of Infectious Diseases, University of Virginia Health Sciences Center, Charlottesville, Virginia 22908.

MENINGITIS

The understanding of the pathogenesis and pathophysiology of bacterial meningitis has advanced in recent years, primarily through results obtained with experimental animal models of infection. These models differ from natural infection by the route of bacterial inoculation employed, the bacterial pathogen administered, and the animal host selected. Many studies have utilized infant rats, which develop meningitis after intranasal challenge with *Hemophilus influenzae* type b (2). This model simulates the presumed pathogenesis of *H. influenzae* meningitis in humans, with an initial nasopharyngeal focus leading to bacteremia and an age-dependent susceptibility to bacterial meningitis. The incidence of meningitis, irrespective of age, was directly related to the intensity of the bacteremia (3). Infant rats also develop meningitis after orogastric challenge with *Escherichia coli* (4). This infant rat model of experimental *H. influenzae* type b meningitis has been used primarily to study the early pathogenic sequences of bacterial meningitis, including (a) the determinants of colonization and translocation into the bloodstream, (b) intravascular survival and bacteremia, and (c) mechanisms of meningeal invasion. A major disadvantage of this model is the animal's small size permitting only small volumes of CSF (7–25 μl) to be sampled at any given time. Thus, it is an unsuitable model for the study of the pathophysiologic consequences of infection once meningitis has become established, because frequent sampling of CSF is precluded. Infant primates have also been utilized to study bacterial meningitis after the atraumatic intranasal inoculation of *H. influenzae* type b, with bacteremia and meningitis developing in 89% and 94% of animals, respectively (5). However, this expensive model is employed infrequently.

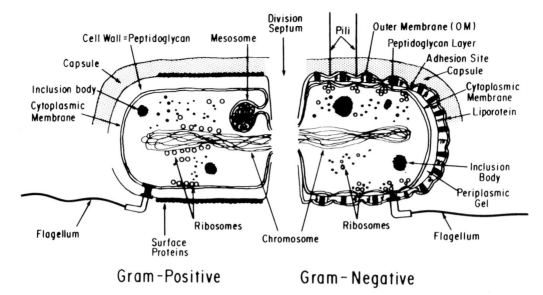

FIG. 1. Diagram of idealized typical bacterial cells. (From ref. 183, with permission.)

The pathophysiology of bacterial meningitis has been studied extensively in adult animals (predominantly rabbits or rats) following the intracisternal inoculation of microorganisms or their products to establish infection and/or CSF inflammation (6,7). These models reliably generate lethal infections after challenge with an appropriate live inoculum with a predictable time course, but they bypass the normal bacteremia–meningitis sequence, thereby creating an artificial pathogenesis. However, because of easy handling of the animals, combined with the ability to sample CSF at multiple time points, these models have proven extremely valuable in studying the consequences of bacterial meningitis once infection has been established.

The following sections review selected aspects of the pathogenesis and pathophysiology of bacterial meningitis, emphasizing the interplay between bacterial virulence factors and host defense mechanisms that are responsible for the clinical expression of disease.

TABLE 1. *Factors involved in the pathogenesis and pathophysiology of bacterial CNS infections*

Bacterial factors
Fimbriae
Capsule
Outer-membrane proteins
Lipopolysaccharide
Cell wall
Slime
Host factors
Blocking IgA antibody
Decreased CSF immunoglobulin concentrations
Decreased CSF complement concentrations
Impaired phagocytosis
Production of inflammatory cytokines (interleukin-1, tumor necrosis factor, and others)
Production of prostaglandin E_2

Bacterial Adhesion and Systemic Invasion

A critical first step in initiation of meningitis is host acquisition of a new organism by nasopharyngeal colonization through mucosal adhesion and subsequent systemic invasion. Adhesion represents a relatively stable attachment of bacteria to a surface (8). Many bacterial species have been found to express hemagglutinins or lectins on their surfaces which mediate binding to animal cells (9). These adhesive surface structures (adhesins) are ligand molecules that bind specifically to complementary receptors on host mucosal cells. Many bacteria also possess specific organelles called "fimbriae" or "pili," which mediate adhesion (10). Typically, a bacterium has 50–400 of these filaments projecting from its surface; each filament possesses a hydrophobic tip that makes contact with other cells. The same mechanisms which allow bacteria to bind to mucosal surfaces promote adherence to phagocytic cells such as neutrophils and macrophages, and lectin-mediated binding of bacteria to phagocytes can lead to stimulation, ingestion, and killing of the organism (9). The phenotypic expression of fimbriae can manifest phase variation *in vitro* and *in vivo*. Under certain cultural conditions, proportions of the bacterial population are either fimbriated or nonfimbriated (11). It has been suggested that this random, on-off switching process is a virulence trait of type 1 fimbriated *E. coli* and other fimbriated bacterial species (12–15); this trait may allow the fimbriated form to survive at phagocyte-poor sites such as mucosal surfaces, while permitting the nonfimbriated form to reach phagocyte-rich sites in deep tissues.

Many of the major meningeal pathogens possess surface characteristics that enhance mucosal adhesion. Fimbriae are important in mediating the adhesion of

Neisseria meningitidis strains to nasopharyngeal epithelial cells (16), and they have been found in 80% of primary meningococcal isolates from nasopharyngeal carriers and from the CSF of patients with meningitis (17). After attachment to the mucosal surface (Fig. 2), meningococci are transported across the nonciliated nasopharyngeal columnar epithelial cell within a phagocytic vacuole (18,19), which may be a prerequisite for subsequent hematogenous dissemination. Fimbriae also have been implicated in the adhesion of *H. influenzae* to epithelial cells in the upper respiratory tract (20,21), although fimbriae are not found on isolates from blood or CSF (20,22).

Bacterial encapsulation may also be important for nasopharyngeal colonization and systemic invasion of meningeal pathogens. There are six encapsulated types of *H. influenzae* (a through f), but greater than 95% of meningeal and systemic infections are caused by type b strains. Experiments utilizing laboratory transformants have shown that while all encapsulated strains of *H. influenzae* have the potential for systemic invasion after intraperitoneal inoculation, type b strains were the most virulent and were the only capsular types capable of systemic invasion after intranasal inoculation (23,24). Indeed, the presence of serum antibodies to the polyribosyl-ribitol phosphate capsule of type b isolates usually confers protection against invasive disease (25).

Polysaccharide capsule is also an important virulence factor for invasive *Streptococcus pneumoniae* (26). Of the 84 serotypes known, 18 are responsible for 82% of cases of bacteremic pneumococcal pneumonia (27,28),

and there is a close correlation between bacteremic subtypes and those implicated in meningitis (29–31). However, adhesion may be less important in the pathogenicity of pneumococcal infections, because low degrees of adhesion have been observed among strains isolated from patients with serious infections such as septicemia and meningitis (32). A study of *S. pneumoniae* adhesion in the nasopharynx of children showed that these organisms were more often found on desquamated cells than on cells taken from intact epithelium (33). Nasopharyngeal mucus may provide a protected nidus from which pneumococci can spread (34), but the various factors responsible for enhanced invasiveness among certain pneumococcal serotypes remain undefined.

Adhesion of microorganisms to mucosal cells may be inhibited by natural antibodies such as IgA, found predominantly in mucosal secretions. Formation of these antibodies is stimulated by colonization of organisms that share cross-reactive antigens with pathogenic strains (35). However, the presence of high concentrations of circulating IgA antibodies to *N. meningitidis* may paradoxically permit the development of invasive disease by preferentially binding to the organism and blocking the beneficial effects of IgM and IgG antibodies (36–38). In addition, many pathogenic bacteria of the genera *Neisseria*, *Hemophilus*, and *Streptococcus* produce IgA1 proteases (39) that cleave IgA in the hinge region of the immunoglobulin molecule. It has been suggested that these enzymes have a pathogenic role in allowing adhesion of bacterial strains to mucosal surfaces through local destruction of IgA (40).

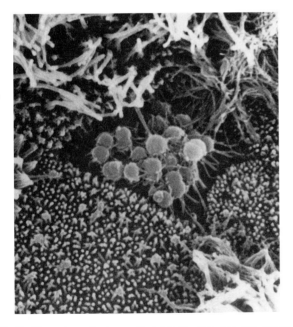

FIG. 2. Scanning electron micrograph showing the interaction of piliated *Neisseria meningitidis* (isolated from CSF) with human pharyngeal mucosa 6–8 hr after infection (×5625). (From ref. 19, with permission.)

Intravascular Survival and Meningeal Invasion

After crossing the mucosal barrier, bacteria gain access to the bloodstream and must then overcome host defense mechanisms to survive and subsequently invade the CNS. Surface encapsulation is the most important bacterial virulence factor in this regard, and the most common meningeal pathogens (*H. influenzae, N. meningitidis, S. pneumoniae, E. coli,* and *Streptococcus agalactiae*) are all encapsulated. Bacterial capsule, by effectively inhibiting phagocytosis and resisting classical complement pathway activation, may enhance bloodstream survival and facilitate production of a high-grade bacteremia.

Host defense mechanisms are available to counteract the antiphagocytic activity of bacterial capsule. Through the humoral immune response, antibodies bind to specific microbial antigens; this antigen–antibody complex can then enlist the aid of effector cells or activate the complement cascade (41). The classical and alternative pathways are the two major mechanisms of complement activation. The classical pathway is triggered by antigen–antibody complexes and proceeds through activation of the three early recognition components C1, C4, and C2, with the formation of C3 convertase. The alternative pathway, however, may be activated on the surface of many bacteria in the absence of specific antibody. Both pathways converge at C3, with the sequential activation of C5, C6, C7, C8, and C9 to form the membrane attack complex. In order to limit tissue damage, these factors must be directed against the bacterial pathogen when it is in an extracellular location. This can be accomplished through opsonization by which organisms are coated with antibody and/or specific complement fragments, thereby facilitating the phagocytic process (42,43). For example, both antipneumococcal cell-wall antibody and antipneumococcal capsular antibody promote the efficient deposition of C3b on the pneumococcal surface, although C3b deposited on the surface of the pneumococcal capsule is a more efficient opsonin *in vitro* and *in vivo* when compared to C3 deposited by anti-cell-wall antibody (44,45). The complement cascade is also activated by *H. influenzae* type b (46). Studies in C3-depleted infant rats have revealed a greater incidence and magnitude of bacteremia after intraperitoneal cobra venom factor injection when challenged with encapsulated *Hemophilus,* although the incidence of meningitis was unaffected by complement depletion (47–49).

Systemic infections with neisserial species (e.g., *N. meningitidis*) occur more commonly in complement-deficient individuals (50). Individuals with inherited deficiencies in one of the terminal complement components (C5, C6, C7, C8, and perhaps C9) have an 8000-fold greater frequency of invasive meningococcal disease, but a lower mortality rate (1.6–2.7%), than do persons with a normal complement system (19%) after invasive disease due to this organism (50–52). Therefore, the ability to assemble the membrane attack complex may contribute to mortality in patients with meningococcal infections.

The specific chemical constituents of the capsular polysaccharide may play an important role in promoting infection. Sialic acid is a prominent component of the capsular polysaccharides of type III group B streptococci, *E. coli* K1, and serogroups B and C meningococci (53). Since sialic acid is a component of host cells, these organisms do not activate the alternative complement pathway and are a poor stimulus of host antibody production. It is noteworthy that these organisms are prominent causes of neonatal and infant sepsis and meningitis.

The mechanisms by which bacterial pathogens gain entry into the CNS are largely unknown. Fimbriae may be an important virulence factor in this regard. A recent study in infant rats has shown that S fimbriae of *E. coli* specifically bind to the luminal surfaces of cerebrovascular endothelium and to the epithelium lining the choroid plexus (54), a process enhanced in neonatal animals when compared with that in adults. Phase variation to the nonfimbriated form may then be necessary for the organism to pass through the vascular endothelium (55).

Host Defense Mechanisms in the Subarachnoid Space

Once the bacterial pathogen enters the subarachnoid space (SAS), host defense mechanisms are inadequate to control the infection. Assays for complement components in CSF are usually negative or reveal only minimal concentrations (56–59). Meningeal inflammation leads to increased, although low, concentrations of complement components within CSF, and this relative complement deficiency may impede opsonization of encapsulated meningeal pathogens and preclude efficient phagocytosis. Possible explanations for the low concentrations of functional complement components in purulent CSF include insufficient traversal across the BBB, variable SAS inflammation, enhanced clearance or removal from the SAS, low production rates in the CNS, or degradation at the site of infection. Leukocyte proteases have been shown to degrade functional complement components (e.g., C3b) in CSF samples from patients with meningococcal meningitis, with the formation of nonopsonic products (e.g., C3d) (60). In addition, the intracisternal inoculation of phenyl-methyl-sulfonyl fluoride (a nonspecific protease inhibitor) into rabbits with pneumococcal meningitis led to a decline in CSF pneumococcal concentrations when compared to that of saline-inoculated controls, perhaps by influencing leukocyte-protease-mediated complement destruction in the CSF (61). Therefore, during bacterial meningitis, complement components crossing the BBB may be degraded by leukocyte proteases, resulting in inefficient opsonic activity at the site of infection.

Immunoglobulin concentrations are also low in normal CSF. Although immunoglobulin concentrations increase in the presence of bacterial meningitis, they remain lower than simultaneous serum concentrations (60,62) and, in concert with the local complement deficiency, contribute to the regional host deficiency in the CSF during bacterial meningitis.

A major consequence of SAS inflammation during bacterial meningitis is a CSF pleocytosis, predominantly neutrophilic. The exact mechanism of leukocyte traversal into the SAS is unknown, although purulent CSF is chemotactic for leukocytes *in vitro* (63,64). Experimental models of pneumococcal meningitis have identified one chemotactic substance as C5a (65,66), and the intracisternal inoculation of C5a into rabbits has been found to cause a rapid, early influx of leukocytes into CSF (67). This effect can be blocked by the CSF administration of prostaglandin E_2 (PGE$_2$), suggesting that PGE$_2$ may exert an anti-inflammatory action in meningitis. However, host defenses in the CSF remain suboptimal despite the influx of leukocytes. The lack of functional opsonic activity early in the disease course is responsible for inefficient phagocytosis, explaining the high bacterial densities in CSF characteristic of patients with bacterial meningitis (68,69). Therefore, bacterial meningitis should be considered an infection in an area of impaired host defense.

Induction and Consequences of Subarachnoid Space Inflammation

Although the most common meningeal pathogens are encapsulated, purified capsular polysaccharides do not cause SAS inflammation. Recent studies in animal models have examined (a) many of the putative bacterial virulence factors responsible for the induction of SAS inflammation and (b) the host mechanisms that maintain the inflammatory response.

Cell walls of gram-positive cocci are potent inducers of inflammation (70), and *S. pneumoniae* cell walls activate the alternative pathway of complement (71,72). The cell wall of the pneumococcus is composed of two polymers: a peptidoglycan and a ribitol phosphate teichoic acid which contains phosphorylcholine (73). Inflammatory changes are induced in the CSF of rabbits after the intracisternal inoculation of (a) both encapsulated and unencapsulated *S. pneumoniae,* (b) heat-killed unencapsulated pneumococci, or (c) pneumococcal cell walls, the most potent surface components in the induction of CSF inflammation (74). The intracisternal injection of heat-killed encapsulated strains or isolated pneumococcal capsular polysaccharides did not lead to inflammation. These findings support the concept that bacterial cell death, when accompanied by lysis and release of cell walls, could aggravate CSF inflammation. Indeed, the intracisternal inoculation of both major components of the pneumococcal cell wall, the peptidoglycan and ribitol phosphate teichoic acid, also induced CSF inflammation (75). Lysis of bacteria, which occurs after ampicillin-induced killing of pneumococci *in vivo,* is associated with a transient enhancement of the CSF inflammatory response and is correlated positively with increased concentrations of PGE_2 in CSF. This CSF inflammatory response can be partially blocked by inhibitors of the cyclooxygenase pathway of arachidonic acid metabolism (76). Inhibition of this pathway may also prevent some of the pathophysiologic consequences of SAS inflammation. A recent study has shown that the combination of either dexamethasone or oxindanac (a cyclooxygenase pathway inhibitor) with ampicillin in experimental pneumococcal meningitis led to a partial reduction in the massive influx of serum albumin and certain high- and low-molecular-weight proteins into CSF (77).

The lipopolysaccharide (LPS) of gram-negative bacteria is also known to be a potent inducer of inflammation.

The external surface of these organisms contains a lawn of LPS molecules linked tightly to outer-membrane proteins via hydrophobic interactions. The LPS molecules are composed of repeating oligosaccharide units linked to an oligosaccharide core, which is linked to lipid A via the sugar ketodeoxyoctulosonate (78). The lipid A region is responsible for virtually all of the biologic and endotoxic activity associated with LPS (79–81). Both the classical and alternative complement pathways are activated by LPS (82), although there is controversy concerning the precise role of complement in mediating the effects of LPS on the host (80). The LPS of *H. influenzae* has been characterized extensively (83), and the virulence of this organism is attenuated by altering its LPS configuration (84,85). There is also recent evidence that a family of LPS-binding proteins may participate in the host response to gram-negative bacteremia (86). The role of these LPS-binding proteins in CNS infections is not known.

Meningeal (i.e., CSF) inflammation has been induced following the intracisternal inoculation of purified *H. influenzae* type b LPS into experimental animals (87,88). The inflammatory response is attenuated by preincubation of the LPS with polymyxin B, a cationic antibiotic that binds to the lipid A region of the molecule and inactivates it (89); it is also attenuated by neutrophil acyloxyacyl hydrolase, which reduces the tissue toxicity of LPS without destroying its immunostimulatory potential. Multiple different monoclonal antibodies to the various epitopes in the oligosaccharide portion of this molecule did not reduce its inflammatory potential after injection into the CSF. Similar inflammatory changes have been observed after the intracisternal inoculation of *H. influenzae* type b outer-membrane vesicles (90,91), which may serve as relevant nonreplicating vehicles in which LPS is released into the CSF in *H. influenzae* meningitis.

Recent evidence suggests that the mechanism through which pneumococcal cell walls or *H. influenzae* LPS elicit inflammation in the CSF is by stimulation of the formation of inflammatory cytokines such as interleukin-1 (IL-1) or tumor necrosis factor (TNF) (92–96). Cytokines are proteins (or glycoproteins) that act as molecular signals permitting communication between cells and as systemic mediators of the host's response to infection. Cytokines are not stored preformed within cells, but their production requires new protein (and, in most cases, new messenger RNA) synthesis. The most important sources of inflammatory cytokines are monocytes and macrophages, although other cell types may also produce these mediators. For example, vascular endothelial cells grown in culture have been shown to produce IL-1 in response to LPS stimulation (97,98). In addition, cytokines have the capacity to enhance their own or each other's production (97–101). Both TNF and IL-1 can also induce production of prostaglandins, especially PGE_2, which, in turn, down-regulates the production of these inflammatory cytokines (102,103).

LPS and other mediators of inflammation are important factors in neutrophil emigration to extravascular sites. Neutrophil binding to specific receptors on vascular endothelial cells is a mandatory step prior to egress of these cells into the extravascular space (104,105). Neutrophil adherence to vascular endothelium is enhanced *in vitro* by pretreatment of the endothelial cells with LPS (106,107) and with either IL-1 or TNF (106,108,109), perhaps through induction of cell-surface glycoprotein molecules (integrin family) such as endothelial leukocyte adhesion molecule 1 (110).

These mechanisms may also exist in the CNS. Several recent studies have shown that the intracisternal inoculation of *H. influenzae* LPS into experimental animals leads to increased CSF concentrations of IL-1 and TNF (111,112). Further studies are needed, however, to more clearly define their role in infections of the CNS (see Chapter 16).

The consequences of SAS inflammation are responsible for many of the clinical manifestations of bacterial meningitis (Table 2). Pathologically, breakdown of the BBB occurs and is perhaps a necessary prerequisite to formation of vasogenic cerebral edema and the increased intracranial pressure observed in the advanced stages of meningitis. The BBB separates the CSF and brain from the intravascular compartment and acts as a regulatory interface with functions such as active transport, facilitated diffusion of various substances (e.g., hexoses, amino acids) aqueous secretion forming CSF, and maintenance of homeostasis within the CNS (113,114). A major site of the BBB is the cerebral capillary endothelium; furthermore, the intracisternal inoculation of various meningeal pathogens (*E. coli, S. pneumoniae,* or *H. influenzae*) into rats induced alterations in BBB permeability, manifested functionally by increased albumin permeability into the CSF and morphologically by increased numbers of pinocytotic vesicles and separation of intercellular tight junctions in the cerebral capillary endothelial cells (7). Increased permeability occurred after the intracisternal inoculation of either encapsulated or unencapsulated strains of *H. influenzae* and even in the absence of CSF leukocytes, although the presence of CSF leukocytes augmented changes in permeability late in the disease course (115). BBB injury was also observed following the intracisternal inoculation of *H. influenzae* LPS (88) and human recombinant IL-1 (116), indicating that alterations in permeability can be induced by mediators of inflammation. In addition, *H. influenzae* LPS can induce permeability changes to radioactive albumin in isolated monolayer preparations of cerebral microvascular endothelial cells grown on a semipermeable support (117), and ongoing studies will determine if LPS induces the synthesis of inflammatory mediators such as IL-1 and PGE_2 by these cells.

The parameters of brain water content (indicative of cerebral edema if elevated), CSF lactate, and CSF pressure have been measured in experimental animal models, and all three were increased following the intracisternal inoculation of *S. pneumoniae* into rabbits (118). LPS may be an important factor responsible for the production of brain edema, as has been shown in an experimental model of *E. coli* meningitis. Animals treated with cefotaxime demonstrated a marked rise in CSF LPS concentrations which was associated with an increase in brain water content (119). Cerebral edema may also result from an elevation of CSF outflow resistance by inhibition of traversal of CSF from the SAS to the major dural venous sinuses (120). CSF outflow resistance was markedly elevated in experimental models of *S. pneumoniae* and *E. coli* meningitis in rabbits.

With more precise information on the role of bacterial virulence factors and inflammatory mediators in the induction and consequences of SAS inflammation, various innovative approaches are being explored to improve the prognosis in patients with bacterial meningitis. These advancements are discussed in detail in subsequent chapters.

TABLE 2. *Pathophysiologic consequences of subarachnoid space inflammation[a]*

Increased BBB permeability
Cerebral edema (vasogenic, interstitial, cytotoxic)
Cerebral vasculitis
Increased CSF outflow resistance
Increased intracranial pressure
Decreased cerebral blood flow; loss of autoregulation of cerebral blood flow
Cerebral cortical hypoxia
CSF acidosis secondary to glucose utilization via anaerobic glycolysis
Increased CSF lactate
Decreased CSF glucose
Cranial and spinal nerve dysfunction
Encephalopathy

[a] Although many of the consequences are common during bacterial meningitis, they do not uniformly occur in all cases. BBB, blood–brain barrier; CSF, cerebrospinal fluid.

BRAIN ABSCESS

Numerous animal models of brain abscess have been developed and applied to the study of the pathogenic and pathophysiologic mechanisms operable in this disorder. These models have attempted to simulate the common mechanisms of the pathogenesis of brain abscess, namely, spread from contiguous foci of infection (e.g., from otogenic, dental, facial, or paranasal sinus infections) or as a result of hematogenous dissemination from distant sites of infection. The initial animal models of brain abscess utilized several methods to establish infection. Some models were dependent upon the direct implantation of bacteria into the brain (121–124). However, these models suffered from a lack of reproducibility, required multiple steps and an agar vehicle to initiate infection, and utilized large animals. A second method used embolization of contaminated pliable cylinders implanted into the carotid artery (123–126). These models required concomitant cerebral injury for abscess formation, and the accompanying brain infarction caused a high mortality rate even in uninfected control animals.

A better animal model, using mice or rats, utilizes a simple, one-step, easily reproducible procedure for the consistent production of brain abscesses (127,128). Infection is produced by injection of 1 μl of saline containing a fixed inoculum of bacteria through a burr hole into the frontal lobe of the brain. The advantages of this model include the following: (a) Brain abscess is achieved in one step at a specific site with the injection of bacteria alone; (b) the inoculum can be regulated in both volume and number of organisms; (c) the number of bacteria which are injected into the brain and which remain viable in the tissue at a later time can be quantified; and (d) there is precise control of the injection site, thereby reducing tissue trauma with minimal (or no) subarachnoid space infection. This model simulates human disease in several respects: The abscess is produced in the white matter at the white and gray matter junction; the abscess migrates towards the ventricle; a shift in intracranial contents occurs; there is minimal histologic evidence of meningitis; and the abscess capsule is asymmetric, more complete on the cortical than on the ventricular side of the abscess, perhaps because the increased vascularity of normal cortical gray matter allows greater fibroblast proliferation and collagen helix formation. In addition, the development of the abscess parallels clinical disease, with initial cerebritis and massive white matter edema followed by encapsulation.

These animal models have been useful in delineating the early events in brain abscess formation with respect to bacterial virulence factors and host defense mechanisms that are involved in this infection. These concepts are discussed in more detail below.

Initiation and Natural History of Infection

The usual bacterial isolates in patients with brain abscess are streptococci (especially *Streptococcus milleri* group), *Bacteroides* species, Enterobacteriaceae, and *Staphylococcus aureus* (129). There are few studies that have focused on the identification of the specific virulence factors of these organisms in the production of brain abscess. Contrary to common views, the brain itself may be more susceptible to infection than many other tissues. In comparison to skin, brain is significantly

more susceptible to appropriate bacterial challenge as shown in a rat model of experimental brain abscess (130). Using quantitative bacteriology, injections of 10^4 colony-forming units (CFU) of *S. aureus* or 10^6 CFU of *E. coli* failed to cause infection in skin, but brain tissue was susceptible to as few as 10^2 CFU of either organism with resultant abscess formation. The brain may also be more susceptible to infection by different organisms. In the rat model of experimental brain abscess, strains of *E. coli* were more virulent (i.e., abscess formation at lower inocula) than *Pseudomonas aeruginosa, S. aureus,* or *Streptococcus pyogenes* (131). In addition, strains of *E. coli* possessing the K1 antigen were more infective than K1-negative strains, indicating that certain encapsulated strains may be more virulent in the production of brain abscess. The role of capsule (or capsular type) among other bacterial species in the pathogenesis of brain abscess has not been evaluated; however, in a rat model of intra-abdominal sepsis, inoculation of encapsulated *B. fragilis* alone resulted in abscesses in most animals, whereas unencapsulated strains rarely produced this effect unless the strains were combined with another organism or purified *B. fragilis* capsular material (132). The inoculation of *B. fragilis* or aerotolerant anaerobes such as *Streptococcus intermedius* into rat brain failed to produce infection and abscess formation. This is in contrast to clinical experience where these organisms account for a high percentage of isolates from brain abscesses (131) (Chapter 19). This discrepancy may be explained by the fact that brain abscess is often a result of contiguous spread of chronic otitic or sinus infections clinically, and the synergistic infectivity of mixed populations of anaerobes plus a facultative organism may be necessary to establish the disease (133,134). In an experimental dog model of brain abscess formation, the inoculation of *B. fragilis,* in mixed culture with *Staphylococcus epidermidis,* caused a virulent reaction (135), although each organism was not tested separately. All of these experiments, however, involve direct inoculation of organisms into brain, thus bypassing the brain's normal host defense barriers. Nevertheless, they are useful in the delineation of factors responsible for brain abscess formation. The role of other bacterial virulence factors in brain abscess formation has not been evaluated. Despite extensive evidence implicating bacterial LPS in the pathophysiology of meningitis and brain injury (Chapter 16), similar studies on the effect, if any, of LPS on brain abscess formation and evolution are unavailable. *B. fragilis,* a major pathogen in brain abscess, has an LPS that is chemically distinct from the LPS of aerobic gram-negative bacilli, but the biologic function of *B. fragilis* LPS is poorly defined (136) and is unknown in the CNS.

Several animal models of brain abscess formation have been used to examine the pathologic consequences and temporal course after the initiation of infection. A canine model was utilized to define the pathologic stages of brain abscess formation after inoculation of alpha-hemolytic streptococci (137). Based on a detailed histologic evaluation, four stages of brain abscess evolution were defined (Table 3): early cerebritis (days 1–3), late cerebritis (days 4–9), early capsule formation (days 10–13), and late capsule formation (day 14 and later after initial inoculation). These stages are somewhat arbitrary but are useful in classification and comparisons of virulence between different organisms in the production of brain abscess. An acute inflammatory infiltrate with visible bacteria on Gram's stain and marked edema surrounding the lesion characterize the early cerebritis stage. During the late cerebritis stage, the center of the lesion becomes necrotic, and macrophages and fibroblasts begin to invade the periphery. With early capsule formation, the necrotic center begins to decrease in size with simultaneous development of a collagenous capsule that is less prominent on the ventricular side of the lesion. Cerebral edema starts to regress during this phase. In this canine model the collagen capsule is complete circumferentially by the end of the second week and then increases in density and thickness. Similar neuropathologic findings have been observed in experimental anaerobic brain abscess (135), although capsule formation could not be divided into early and late stages because of delayed encapsulation. Histologic evidence of a more virulent infection manifested by early ventricular rupture, and an extensive purulent encephalitis was observed in 25% of the animals. A subsequent study revealed that *S. aureus* was also more virulent than the alpha-hemolytic streptococci in brain abscess formation (138). Inoculation of similar concentrations of each organism led to a greater amount of necrosis and total area of involvement after staphylococcal challenge. In addition, the course of infection as it progressed towards resolution, the time for the abscess to reach a stable size, and the time to contain necrotic region with a collagenous capsule were all longer after inoculation of *S. aureus*. A so-called "escape" inflammation with histologic evidence of extension of inflammation, necrosis, and edema beyond the capsule was observed, similar to findings after inoculation with *B. fragilis*. It is interesting to note that capsule formation was less prominent on the ventricular surface than on the cortical surface in these studies (135,137,138), perhaps due to differences in vascularity between cortical gray and white matter allowing greater fibroblast proliferation on the cortical side of the abscess. This may explain the tendency for brain abscesses to rupture into the ventricular system rather than into the subarachnoid space. In addition, the histopathologic sequence of brain abscess formation has been examined in an experimental rat model utilizing inoculation of *E. coli* (128,139). In this model, histopathologic evaluation supported another hypothesis: Brain abscesses tended to rupture intraventricularly because the infectious process was directed along the major white matter tracts (areas of

lower tissue resistance), rather than as a result of asymmetric collagen deposition (139). This question regarding brain abscess rupture patterns requires further evaluation.

The histopathologic changes in brain abscesses that result from direct implantation are different than those produced by intracarotid embolization. Metastatic abscesses induced only transient midline displacements, inflammatory cell infiltration was reduced, and collagen formation was retarded around proliferating capsular vessels (123,124), when compared to abscesses induced from direct brain inoculation. This may have implications in patient care, since a lower degree of encapsulation contributes to patient mortality.

An additional concern is the possible development of brain abscess in patients with bacterial meningitis. Brain abscess only rarely complicates meningitis, with the exception of the high prevalence ($\sim$70%) of brain abscess formation in human neonates with meningitis due to *Citrobacter diversus* (140,141). Pathologically, cerebral necrosis and liquefaction are found, along with vasculitis of the small vessels and hemorrhagic necrosis of adjacent tissue (142). There is a propensity for contiguous inflammation in the cerebral white matter which may be due to the effects of endotoxin on the small penetrating vessels in this area. The typical abscess with capsule formation was not present in neonatal *C. diversus* meningitis. The pathogenesis of this infection was also investigated in an infant rat model. The process was initiated with a high-grade bacteremia, infiltration of the leptomeninges, and subsequent development of ventriculitis (143). Brain abscesses were found exclusively in the periventricular white matter, apparently from disruption of the ventricular ependymal lining with direct extension of the infection into the parenchyma. The virulence factors responsible for the propensity of this organism to cause brain abscess are undefined. It appears, however, that a minor outer-membrane protein (32 kD) may be a marker for strains more likely to produce ventriculitis and brain abscess (144).

Host Defense Mechanisms

The brain is usually protected from infection by an intact BBB, although once brain infection is established, immune defenses are inadequate to control the process. Since local opsonization is deficient, encapsulated bacteria such as *E. coli* and *B. fragilis* may escape efficient phagocytosis within the brain parenchyma. Several studies have shown that phagocytosis of *Bacteroides* species requires heat-labile serum factors (i.e., complement, lysozyme, or others) (145,146), and these factors are likely absent in the CNS. In addition, an outer-membrane component of *Bacteroides* species may be important in the inhibition of neutrophil chemotaxis (147), thus reducing the host response to brain abscesses associated with this organism.

The host inflammatory response following the initiation of infection has been evaluated by serial pathologic analysis in several animal models of brain abscess formation (Table 3) (135,137,138). During the early cerebritis stage, a border around the initial area of inoculation, composed of acute inflammatory cells, is observed; this is accompanied by rapid development of a perivascular infiltration of neutrophils, plasma cells, and mononuclear cells. With progression to the late cerebritis stage, the acute inflammatory cells become mixed with macrophages and fibroblasts, and reticulin formation surrounds the necrotic center. As the capsule begins to form, increased numbers of fibroblasts and macrophages infiltrate the periphery, and mature collagen is deposited to form a capsule. With further encapsulation, the necrotic center continues to decrease in size while attendant marked gliosis develops outside the capsule.

The importance of this host inflammatory response in containment of the brain abscess has been examined in immunosuppressed animals. Initial studies in the dog model of experimental brain abscess due to *S. aureus* or *Proteus mirabilis* demonstrated that the administration of dexamethasone slowed, but did not fully impair, capsule formation (122). In contrast, no evidence of encap-

sulation was found when dexamethasone was given to rabbits at the same time as inoculation of *S. pyogenes* or *S. aureus* in another study (148). In the experimental rat model of *E. coli* brain abscess, dexamethasone administration led to a reduction in the macrophage and glial response, collagen deposition, and host survival, with an increased number of viable bacteria in the brain abscess (139). It was noted, however, that rats were more sensitive than humans to the lymphoid-depleting effects of corticosteroids. Co-administration of dexamethasone also impaired the lymphocytic and fibroblastic response in a rat model of experimental *S. aureus* brain abscess (149), although it did not entirely halt the encapsulation or reduce the associated cerebral edema. Another study utilized dogs that were immunosuppressed with azathioprine and prednisone 7 days prior to the intracerebral inoculation of alpha-hemolytic streptococci (150). The immunosuppressed animals manifested a decreased inflammatory response characterized by (a) a reduction in neutrophils and macrophages in the lesion, (b) a decrease and delay in collagen deposition, and (c) persistence of viable organisms into the late capsule stage. Neutrophils, plasma cells, lymphocytes, and macrophages were markedly reduced in the areas surrounding the necrotic center of abscesses, and cerebritis was also decreased outside of the developing capsule. Gliosis, how-

TABLE 3. *Histologic findings in stages of brain abscess formation*[a]

	Early cerebritis (days 1–3)	Late cerebritis (days 4–9)	Early capsule formation (days 10–13)	Late capsule formation (day 14 and later)
Necrotic center	Acute inflammatory cells; bacteria present on Gram's stain	Enlarging necrotic center reaching maximal size	Decrease in necrotic center	Further decrease in necrotic center
Inflammatory border	Acute inflammatory cells	Inflammatory cells, macrophages, and fibroblasts	Increased numbers of fibroblasts and macrophages	Further increase in number of fibroblasts
Collagen capsule	Reticulin formation by day 3	Appearance of fibroblasts with rapid formation of reticulin	Evolution of mature collagen	Capsule completed by end of second week
Cerebritis and neovascularity	Rapid perivascular infiltration of neutrophils, plasma cells, and mononuclear cells	Maximal extent of cerebritis with rapid increase in new vessel formation	Maximal degree of neovascularity	Cerebritis restricted to outside of collagen capsule; less neovascularity
Reactive gliosis and cerebral edema	Marked cerebral edema	Prominent cerebral edema with appearance of reactive astrocytes	Regression of cerebral edema with increase in reactive astrocytes	Regression of cerebral edema; by third week there is marked gliosis outside capsule

[a] Adapted from ref. 137.

ever, was markedly increased in the area surrounding the collagen capsule in these immunosuppressed dogs. Although this decreased inflammatory response and edema formation resulted initially in less mass effect, the eventual size and area of the abscess may have become larger as a result of the less effective host response. The influence of immunosuppressive agents on the diagnosis and treatment of brain abscess in humans is discussed in Chapter 19.

CEREBROSPINAL FLUID SHUNT INFECTION

Infection of CSF shunts is a major cause of morbidity in patients with these devices (151). There are no animal models that have specifically examined the role of CSF shunts in initiation or propagation of CNS infection. Several models of foreign-body infections illustrate many of the bacterial virulence factors and host defense mechanisms operable after foreign-body placement that may be relevant to the pathogenesis and pathophysiology of CSF shunt infections. Characteristically, foreign-body infections require a low-infecting bacterial inoculum to establish disease, evolve over a protracted clinical course, do not spread beyond the vicinity of the foreign body, and require removal of the device for optimal management of the condition. Previous models of prosthetic device infection have been useful for defining the minimal dose required to establish the process and for examining the morphology of the infecting microorganism *in vivo* (152,153). However, the major disadvantages of these models include the high cost of the animals employed, the need for complicated surgical procedures, and the inability to study local host defense mechanisms.

A guinea-pig model has been developed which involves the subcutaneous implantation of a perforated polymer cylinder (154). This tissue-cage model permits (a) analysis of the natural history and pathogenicity of various microorganisms in foreign-body infections, (b) testing of different prosthetic materials, (c) study of bacterial adherence to foreign bodies, and (d) examination of the local host defense mechanisms in the area of the foreign body. Commercially available polymethylmethacrylate and polytetrafluoroethylene tubes are perforated with 1-mm holes and sealed at each end before subcutaneous implantation. During the first week after surgery, interstitial fluid accumulates inside the cage and is accessible to percutaneous aspiration for assessment of functional opsonic and overall phagocytic activity. The tissue-cage model is somewhat artificial, since the cage does not perform any mechanical function; however, this model is inexpensive, reproducible, and permits serial evaluation of the biologic characteristics of an individual infection. The following sections review the use of this and other models of foreign-body infections, and the results are extrapolated to the pathogenic and pathophysiologic mechanisms operable in CSF shunt infections.

Bacterial Virulence Factors

The vast majority of CSF shunt infections are caused by staphylococci which colonize the wound at the time of shunt replacement (151). These organisms can adhere directly to prosthetic devices and produce substances which protect them from phagocytosis and the actions of antimicrobial agents (155,156). Adhesion is an important step in the pathogenesis of foreign-body infections, although the exact mechanisms of attachment remain undefined. Some results suggest that *S. epidermidis* strains with the greatest hydrophobicity are more adherent to polymer surfaces (157), but others have found little correlation between hydrophobicity and adherence of microorganisms to biomaterials (158,159). There is also evidence that *S. epidermidis* strains, in particular, may excavate into some polymer surfaces (Fig. 3), hydrolyzing the plastic as a food source (160,161). In addition, host proteins, such as fibronectin and collagen, enhance *S. epidermidis* and *S. aureus* adhesion to foreign surfaces (162–165), although strains of *S. epidermidis* adhere quite avidly even in the absence of these plasma proteins. To determine the precise role of host-derived molecules in the pathogenesis of foreign-body infections, further study is required.

Another mechanism of attachment may involve the production of an extracellular slime substance by these microorganisms. Little is known about the chemical structure of slime except that it is water-soluble, contains 40% sugar and 27% protein, and may vary among different organisms (156). Slime production by coagulase-negative staphylococci may be important in the pathogenesis of foreign-body infections (153,166,167). In a

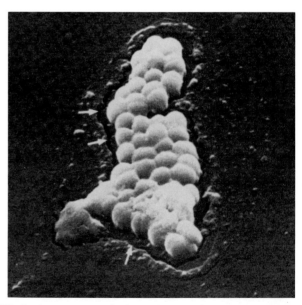

FIG. 3. Appearance of microcolonies of coagulase-negative staphylococci (strain KH 11) on the inner surface of a polyethylene catheter, showing erosion of layers of the catheter surface after incubation for 48 hr. (From ref. 160, with permission.)

study (in experimental animals) comparing two strains of *S. epidermidis* differing in slime production, the presence of slime production correlated with the ability of the organism to bind to foreign bodies (168). This concept is supported by clinical studies in which the ability of certain isolates of coagulase-negative staphylococci to produce slime was associated with a propensity to cause disease in patients with prosthetic devices (169,170). Growth of bacterial species *in vivo* occurs on both the inner and outer slime surfaces (171). However, it is unclear whether slime functions as a ligand for initial attachment or is produced after the organism has adhered to the foreign body, or both (159,160).

Slime production has also been examined in coagulase-negative staphylococcal isolates from patients with CSF shunt infections (172,173). In one study, it was determined that 88% of CSF shunt isolates were adherent to plastic tissue-culture plates and that antibiotic therapy was ineffective in patients with these adherent strains unless the colonized shunt was removed (172). However, while all slime-producing strains were adherent, not all of the adherent strains produced slime. Slime production by other organisms (e.g., *P. aeruginosa*) may also contribute to virulence in foreign-body infection, although other factors undoubtedly play an important role in the pathogenesis of CNS shunt infections (174).

Host Defense Mechanisms

The persistence of CSF shunt infections probably relates not only to specific virulence factors that establish infection, but also to the inadequacy of host defense mechanisms in the CNS. In addition, the foreign body itself may interfere with host defenses. In the tissue-cage model of foreign-body infections, complement concentrations and opsonic titers are decreased when compared to serum with presumed impairment of efficient phagocytosis within the infected site (154). However, these diminished titers do not explain the high susceptibility of tissue cages to infection because *S. aureus,* the major pathogen investigated, can still be opsonized optimally *in vivo* and *in vitro* at identical concentrations. On the other hand, granulocytes harvested from the tissue cage show diminished phagocytic activity against *S. aureus* strain Wood 46, manifested by a decreased ingestion rate, granular enzyme activity, and oxidative metabolism (154,175). The explanation for these findings are unclear, but there is evidence that contact between neutrophils and foreign bodies can lead to the release of lysosomal enzymes and oxygen free radicals, which, in turn, causes leukocyte damage and inefficient phagocytosis and killing (176). This resistance to phagocytosis may be related to the adhesion of the organism to the foreign body, because adherence of *S. aureus* to polymethylmethacrylate increases its resistance to the killing action

of neutrophils (177). Another study, however, suggested that the shunt catheter itself may interfere with phagocytosis. Neutrophils adhered poorly to the catheters, leading to inefficient ingestion of the bacteria despite maintaining qualitatively normal phagocytosis (178).

Slime from coagulase-negative staphylococci may protect organisms from host defenses by altering neutrophil function, thus impairing the inflammatory response and leading to the persistence of disease (177,179). High slime concentrations also interfere with the cellular immune system by inhibiting the lymphoproliferative response of mononuclear cells (180), inhibiting immunoglobulin synthesis (181), decreasing natural killer cell cytotoxicity, and lowering the T helper/suppressor ratio *in vitro* (181). All of the above findings in concert support removal of an infected CSF shunt as an important adjunctive measure for optimal therapy in the eradication of this infection (151,182) (Chapter 23).

SUMMARY

This review highlights important aspects of the pathogenesis and pathophysiology of bacterial infections of the CNS, in preparation for further discussions in subsequent chapters. Certain virulence factors are crucial for bacterial access to the CNS, where host defense mechanisms are often inadequate to control infection. Although antimicrobial agents have substantially decreased mortality rates from these bacterial infections, much more information is essential to further reduce fatality rates and the incidence of neurologic sequelae that occur even in the antibiotic era. Future studies of new therapeutic agents will be based on knowledge gained about the pathogenic and pathophysiologic mechanisms operating in these disorders. Vaccines against specific bacterial virulence factors (e.g., *H. influenzae* type b) have already proved efficacious in the prevention of meningitis, and vaccines or antibodies against other bacterial surface constituents may be critical in preventing initiation of infection. In addition, attenuation of the pathophysiologic consequences of infection (e.g., with anti-inflammatory agents) may reduce overall morbidity and mortality once infection has become established. These exciting areas of investigation may lead to innovative strategies in the treatment of bacterial CNS infections.

ACKNOWLEDGMENTS

This work was supported, in part, by a research grant (RO1-AI17904) and a training grant (T32-AI07046) from the National Institute of Allergy and Infectious Diseases. W. M. Scheld is an established investigator of the American Heart Association. We are indebted to

Eve Lorraine Schwartz for secretarial and editorial assistance.

REFERENCES

1. Falkow S, Small P, Isberg R, Hayes SF, Corwin D. A molecular strategy for the study of bacterial invasion. *Rev Infect Dis* 1987;9(Suppl 5):S450–S455.
2. Moxon ER, Smith AL, Averill DR, Smith DH. *Haemophilus influenzae* meningitis in infant rats after intranasal inoculation. *J Infect Dis* 1974;129:154–162.
3. Moxon ER, Ostrow PT. *Haemophilus influenzae* bacteremia in infant rats: role of bacteremia in pathogenesis of age dependent inflammatory response in cerebrospinal fluid. *J Infect Dis* 1977;135:303–307.
4. Moxon ER, Glode MP, Sutton A, Robbins JB. The infant rat as a model of bacterial meningitis. *J Infect Dis* 1977;136(Suppl):S186–S190.
5. Scheifele DW, Daum RS, Syriopoulou VP, Averill DR, Smith AL. *Haemophilus influenzae* bacteremia and meningitis in infant primates. *J Lab Clin Med* 1980;95:450–462.
6. Dacey RG Jr, Sande MA. Effect of probenecid on cerebrospinal fluid concentrations of penicillin and cephalosporin derivatives. *Antimicrob Agents Chemother* 1974;6:437–444.
7. Quagliarello VJ, Long WJ, Scheld WM. Morphologic alterations of the blood–brain barrier with experimental meningitis in the rat. Temporal sequence and role of encapsulation. *J Clin Invest* 1986;77:1084–1095.
8. Jones GW, Isaacson RE. Proteinaceous bacterial adhesins and their receptors. *Crit Rev Microbiol* 1983;10:229–260.
9. Ofek I, Sharon N. Lectinophagocytosis: a molecular mechanism of recognition between cell surface sugars and lectins in the phagocytosis of bacteria. *Infect Immun* 1988;56:539–547.
10. Beachey EH. Bacterial adherence: adhesin-receptor interactions mediating the attachment of bacteria to mucosal surfaces. *J Infect Dis* 1981;143:325–345.
11. Duguid JD, Old DC. Adhesive properties of *Enterobacteriaceae*. In: Beachey EH, ed. *Bacterial adherence,* vol 6. New York: Chapman & Hall, 1980;184–218.
12. Ofek I. Adhesin receptor interaction mediating adherence of bacteria to mucosal tissues: importance of phase transition in the expression of bacterial adhesins. In: Falcon G, ed. *Bacterial and viral inhibition and modulation of host defenses.* London: Academic Press, 1984;7–24.
13. Ofek I, Silverblatt FJ. Bacterial surface structures involved in adhesion to phagocytic and epithelial cells. In: Schlessinger D, ed. *Microbiology—1982.* Washington, DC: American Society for Microbiology, 1982;296–300.
14. Silverblatt FJ, Dreyer JS, Schauer S. Effect of pili on susceptibility of *Escherichia coli* to phagocytosis. *Infect Immun* 1979;24:218–223.
15. Silverblatt FJ, Ofek I. Influence of pili on the residence of *Proteus mirabilis* in experimental hematogenous pyelonephritis. *J Infect Dis* 1978;128:664–667.
16. Stephens DS, McGee ZA. Attachment of *Neisseria meningitidis* to human mucosal surfaces: influence of pili and type of receptor cell. *J Infect Dis* 1981;143:525–532.
17. Devoe I, Gilchrist J. Pili on meningococci from primary cultures of nasopharyngeal carriers and cerebrospinal fluid of patients with acute disease. *J Exp Med* 1975;141:297–305.
18. McGee ZA, Stephens DS, Hoffman LH, Schlech WF, Horn RG. Mechanisms of mucosal invasion by pathogenic *Neisseria. Rev Infect Dis* 1983;5(Suppl 4):S708–S714.
19. Stephens DS, Hoffman LH, McGee ZA. Interaction of *Neisseria meningitidis* with human nasopharyngeal mucosa: attachment and entry into columnar epithelial cells. *J Infect Dis* 1983;148:369–376.
20. Mason EO, Kaplan SL, Wiedermann BL, Norrod EP, Stenback WA. Frequency and properties of naturally occurring adherent piliated strains of *Haemophilus influenzae* type b. *Infect Immun* 1985;49:98–103.
21. Stull TL, Mendelman PM, Haas JL, Schoenborn MA, Mack KD,

Smith AL. Characterization of *Haemophilus influenzae* type b fimbriae. *Infect Immun* 1984;46:787–796.
22. Pichichero ME, Loeb M, Anderson P, Smith DH. Do pili play a role in pathogenicity of *Haemophilus influenzae* type b? *Lancet* 1982;2:960–962.
23. Moxon ER, Vaughn KA. The type b capsular polysaccharide as a virulence determinant of *Haemophilus influenzae:* studies using clinical isolates and laboratory transformants. *J Infect Dis* 1981;143:517–524.
24. Roberts M, Stull TL, Smith AL. Comparative virulence of *Haemophilus influenzae* with a type b or type d capsule. *Infect Immun* 1981;32:518–524.
25. Anderson P, Johnston RB, Smith DH. Human serum activities against *Haemophilus influenzae* type b. *J Clin Invest* 1972;51:31–38.
26. Robbins JB. Vaccines for the prevention of encapsulated bacterial diseases: current status, problems, and prospects for the future. *Immunochemistry* 1978;15:839–854.
27. Austrian R, Gold J. Pneumococcal bacteremia with special reference to bacteremic pneumococcal pneumonia. *Ann Intern Med* 1964;60:759–776.
28. Finland M. Excursions into epidemiology: selected studies during the past four decades at Boston City Hospital. *J Infect Dis* 1973;128:76–124.
29. Broome CV, Facklam RR, Allen JR, Fraser DW, Austrian R. Epidemiology of pneumococcal serotypes in the United States. *J Infect Dis* 1980;141:119–123.
30. Fraser DW, Geil CC, Feldman RA. Bacterial meningitis in Bernalillo County, New Mexico: a comparison with three other American populations. *Am J Epidemiol* 1974;100:29–34.
31. Gray BM, Converse GM III, Dillon HC Jr. Serotypes of *Streptococcus pneumoniae* causing disease. *J Infect Dis* 1979;140:979–983.
32. Andersson B, Eriksson B, Falsen E, et al. Adhesion of *Streptococcus pneumoniae* to human pharyngeal epithelial cells *in vitro:* differences in adhesive capacity among strains isolated from subjects with otitis media, septicemia, or meningitis or from healthy carriers. *Infect Immun* 1981;32:311–317.
33. Lundberg C, Lonnroth J, Nord CE. Adherence in the colonization of *Streptococcus pneumoniae* in the nasopharynx of children. *Infection* 1982;10:63–69.
34. Freter R. Prospects for preventing the association of harmful bacteria with host mucosal surfaces. In: Beachey EH, ed. *Bacterial adherence,* vol 6. New York: Chapman & Hall, 1980;441–459.
35. Schneerson R, Robbins JB. Induction of serum *Haemophilus influenzae* type b capsular antibodies in adult volunteers fed cross reacting *Escherichia coli* 075:K100:H5. *N Engl J Med* 1975;292:1093–1096.
36. Griffis JM. Bactericidal activity by IgA of lytic antibody in human convalescent sera. *J Immunol* 1975;114:1779–1784.
37. Griffis JM, Bertram MA. Immunoepidemiology of meningococcal disease in military recruits. II. Blocking of serum bactericidal activity by circulating IgA early in the course of invasive disease. *J Infect Dis* 1977;136:733–739.
38. Kayhty H, Jousimies-Somer H, Peltola H, Makela PH. Antibody response to capsular polysaccharides of groups A and C *Neisseria meningitidis* and *Haemophilus influenzae* type b during bacteremic disease. *J Infect Dis* 1981;143:32–41.
39. Plaut AG. The IgA1 proteases of pathogenic bacteria. *Annu Rev Microbiol* 1983;37:603–622.
40. Mulks MH, Kornfeld SJ, Frangione B, Plaut AG. Relationship between the specificity of IgA proteases and serotypes in *Haemophilus influenzae. J Infect Dis* 1982;146:266–274.
41. Frank MM, Joiner K, Hammer C. The function of antibody and complement in the lysis of bacteria. *Rev Infect Dis* 1987;9(Suppl 5):S537–S545.
42. Joiner KA, Brown EJ, Frank MM. Complement and bacteria: chemistry and biology in host defense. *Annu Rev Immunol* 1984;2:461–491.
43. Horowitz MA. Phagocytosis of microorganisms. *Rev Infect Dis* 1982;4:104–118.
44. Brown EJ, Hosea SW, Hammer CH, Burch CG, Frank MM. A quantitative analysis of the interactions of antipneumococcal an-

tibody and complement in experimental pneumococcal bacteremia. *J Clin Invest* 1982;69:85–98.

45. Brown EJ, Joiner KA, Cole RM, Berger M. Localization of complement component 3 on *Streptococcus pneumoniae:* anti-capsular antibody causes complement deposition on the pneumococcal capsule. *Infect Immun* 1983;39:403–409.

46. Quinn PH, Crosson FJ, Winkelstein JA, Moxon ER. Activation of the alternative complement pathway by *Haemophilus influenzae* type b. *Infect Immun* 1977;16:400–402.

47. Corral CJ, Winkelstein JA, Moxon ER. Participation of complement in host defense against encapsulated *Haemophilus influenzae* types a, c, and d. *Infect Immun* 1982;35:759–763.

48. Crosson FA Jr, Winkelstein JA, Moxon ER. Participation of complement in the nonimmune host defense against experimental *Haemophilus influenzae* bacteremia and meningitis. *Infect Immun* 1976;14:882–887.

49. Zwahlen A, Winkelstein JA, Moxon ER. Surface determinants of *Haemophilus influenzae* pathogenicity: comparative virulence of capsular transformants in normal and complement depleted rats. *J Infect Dis* 1983;148:385–394.

50. Ross SC, Densen P. Complement deficiency states and infection: epidemiology, pathogenesis, and consequences of neisserial and other infections in an immune deficiency. *Medicine* 1984;63:243–273.

51. Zimran A, Rudensky B, Kramer MR, et al. Hereditary complement deficiency in survivors of meningococcal disease: high prevalence of C7/C8 deficiency in Sephardic (Moroccan) Jews. *Q J Med* 1987;63:349–358.

52. Orren A, Potter PC, Cooper RC, du Toit E. Deficiency of the sixth component of complement and susceptibility to *Neisseria meningitidis* infections: studies in 10 families and five isolated cases. *Immunology* 1987;62:249–253.

53. Fearon DT, Austen KF. The alternative pathway of complement—a system for host resistance to microbial infection. *N Engl J Med* 1980;303:259–263.

54. Parkkinen J, Korhonen TK, Pere A, Hacker J, Soinila S. Binding sites in the rat brain for *Escherichia coli* S fimbriae associated with neonatal meningitis. *J Clin Invest* 1988;81:860–865.

55. Saukkonen KMJ, Nowicki B, Leinonen M. Role of type 1 and S fimbriae in the pathogenesis of *Escherichia coli* 018:K1 bacteremia and meningitis in the infant rat. *Infect Immun* 1988;56:892–897.

56. Buchanen N, McNab GS. Cerebrospinal fluid complement and immunoglobulins in meningitis and encephalitis. *S Afr Med J* 1972;46:1376–1382.

57. Rahal JJ Jr, Simberkoff MS. Host defense and antimicrobial therapy in adult gram-negative bacillary meningitis. *Ann Intern Med* 1982;96:468–474.

58. Simberkoff MS, Moldover HN, Rahal JJ Jr. Absence of detectable bactericidal and opsonic activities in normal and infected human cerebrospinal fluids. A regional host defense deficiency. *J Lab Clin Med* 1980;95:362–372.

59. Tofte RW, Peterson PK, Kim Y, Quie PG. Opsonic activity of normal human cerebrospinal fluid for selected species. *Infect Immun* 1979;26:1093–1098.

60. Whittle HC, Greenwood BM. Cerebrospinal fluid immunoglobulins and complement in meningococcal meningitis. *J Clin Pathol* 1977;30:720–722.

61. Scheld WM, Keeley JM. Effect of cerebrospinal fluid antibody-complement on the course of experimental pneumococcal meningitis. *Clin Res* 1983;31:375A.

62. Smith H, Bannister B, O'Shea MJ. Cerebrospinal fluid immunoglobulins in meningitis. *Lancet* 1973;1:591–593.

63. Greenwood BM. Chemotactic activity of cerebrospinal fluid in pyogenic meningitis. *J Clin Pathol* 1978;31:213–216.

64. Wyler DJ, Wasserman SI, Karchmer AW. Substances which modulate leukocyte migration are present in CSF during meningitis. *Ann Neurol* 1979;5:322–326.

65. Ernst JD, Hartiala KT, Goldstein IM, Sande MA. Complement (C5)-derived chemotactic activity accounts for accumulation of polymorphonuclear leukocytes in cerebrospinal fluid of rabbits with pneumococcal meningitis. *Infect Immun* 1984;46:81–86.

66. Nolan CM, Clark RA, Beaty HN. Experimental pneumococcal

meningitis. III. Chemotactic activity in cerebrospinal fluid. *Proc Soc Exp Biol Med* 1975;150:134–136.

67. Kadurugamuwa JL, Hengstler B, Bray MA, Zak O. Inhibition of complement-factor-5a-induced inflammatory reactions by prostaglandin E_2 in experimental meningitis. *J Infect Dis* 1989;160:715–719.

68. Feldman WE. Concentrations of bacteria in cerebrospinal fluid of patients with bacterial meningitis. *J Pediatr* 1976;88:549–552.

69. Feldman WE. Relation of concentrations of bacteria and bacterial antigens in cerebospinal fluid to prognosis in patients with bacterial meningitis. *N Engl J Med* 1977;296:433–435.

70. Rasanen L, Arvilommi H. Cell walls, peptidoglycans, and teichoic acids of gram-positive bacteria as polyclonal inducers and immunomodulators of proliferative and lymphokine responses of human B and T lymphocytes. *Infect Immun* 1981;34:712–717.

71. Winkelstein JA, Tomasz A. Activation of the alternative complement pathway by pneumococcal cell wall teichoic acid. *J Immunol* 1978;120:174–178.

72. Hummell DS, Berninger RW, Tomasz A, Winkelstein JA. The fixation of C3b to pneumococcal cell wall polymers as a result of activation of the alternative complement pathway. *J Immunol* 1981;127:1287–1289.

73. Mosser JL, Tomasz A. Choline-containing teichoic acid as a structural component of pneumococcal cell wall and its role in sensitivity to lysis by an autolytic enzyme. *J Biol Chem* 1970;245:287–298.

74. Tuomanen E, Tomasz A, Hengstler B, Zak O. The relative role of bacterial cell wall and capsule in the induction of inflammation in pneumococcal meningitis. *J Infect Dis* 1985;151:535–540.

75. Tuomanen E, Liu H, Hengstler B, Zak O, Tomasz A. The induction of meningeal inflammation by components of the pneumococcal cell wall. *J Infect Dis* 1985;151:859–868.

76. Tuomanen E, Hengstler B, Rich R, Bray MA, Zak O, Tomasz A. Nonsteroidal anti-inflammatory agents in the therapy for experimental pneumococcal meningitis. *J Infect Dis* 1987;155:985–990.

77. Kadurugamuwa JL, Hengstler B, Zak O. Cerebrospinal fluid protein profile in experimental pneumococcal meningitis and its alteration by ampicillin and anti-inflammatory agents. *J Infect Dis* 1989;159:26–34.

78. Ryan JL. Microbial factors in pathogenesis: lipopolysaccharides. In: Root RK, Sande MA, eds. *Septic shock*. New York: Churchill Livingstone, 1985;13–25.

79. Rietschel ET, Wollenweber H, Russa R, Brade H, Zähringer U. Concepts of the chemical structure of lipid A. *Rev Infect Dis* 1984;6:432–438.

80. Morrison DC, Ulevitch RJ. The effects of bacterial endotoxins on host mediation systems. *Am J Pathol* 1978;93:527–617.

81. Morrison DC, Ryan JL. Bacterial endotoxins and host immune function. *Adv Immunol* 1979;28:293–450.

82. Morrison DC, Kline LF. Activation of the classical and properdin pathways of complement by bacterial lipopolysaccharides. *J Immunol* 1977;118:362–368.

83. Flesher AR, Insel RA. Characterization of lipopolysaccharide of *H. influenzae. J Infect Dis* 1978;138:719–730.

84. Zwahlen A, Rubin LG, Connelly CJ, Inzana TJ, Moxon ER. Alteration of the cell wall of *Haemophilus influenzae* type b by transformation with cloned DNA: association with attenuated virulence. *J Infect Dis* 1985;152:485–492.

85. Kimura A, Hansen EJ. Antigenic and phenotypic variations of *Haemophilus influenzae* type b lipopolysaccharide and their relationship to virulence. *Infect Immun* 1986;51:69–79.

86. Tobias PS, Mathison JC, Ulevitch RJ. A family of lipopolysaccharide binding proteins involved in responses to gram-negative sepsis. *J Biol Chem* 1988;263:13479–13481.

87. Syrogiannopoulos GA, Hansen EJ, Erwin AL, Munford RS, Rutledge J, Reisch JS, McCracken GH Jr. *Haemophilus influenzae* type b lipooligosaccharide induces meningeal inflammation. *J Infect Dis* 1988;157:237–244.

88. Wispelwey B, Lesse AJ, Hansen EJ, Scheld WM. *Haemophilus influenzae* lipopolysaccharide-induced blood brain barrier permeability during experimental meningitis in the rat. *J Clin Invest* 1988;82:1339–1346.

89. Jacobs DM, Morrison DC. Inhibition of the mitogenic response

to lipopolysaccharide (LPS) in mouse spleen cells by polymyxin B. *J Immunol* 1977;118:21–27.

90. Mustafa MM, Ramilo O, Syrogiannopoulos GA, Olsen KD, McCracken GH Jr, Hansen EJ. Induction of meningeal inflammation by outer membrane vesicles of *Haemophilus influenzae* type b. *J Infect Dis* 1989;159:917–922.

91. Wispelwey B, Hansen EJ, Scheld WM. *Haemophilus influenzae* outer membrane vesicle-induced blood–brain barrier permeability during experimental meningitis. *Infect Immun* 1989;57:2559–2562.

92. Urbaschek R, Urbaschek B. Tumor necrosis factor and interleukin 1 as mediators of endotoxin-induced beneficial effects. *Rev Infect Dis* 1987;9(Suppl 5):S607–S615.

93. Beutler B, Krochin N, Milsark IW, Leudke C, Cerami A. Control of cachectin (tumor necrosis factor) synthesis: mechanisms of endotoxin resistance. *Science* 1986;232:977–980.

94. Dinarello CA. An update on human interleukin-1: from molecular biology to clinical relevance. *J Clin Immunol* 1985;5:287–297.

95. Movat HZ. Tumor necrosis factor and interleukin-1: role in acute inflammation and microvascular injury. *J Lab Clin Med* 1987;110:668–681.

96. Tracey KJ, Lowry SF, Cerami A. Cachectin: a hormone that triggers acute shock and chronic cachexia. *J Infect Dis* 1988;157:413–420.

97. Libby P, Ordovas JM, Auger KR, Robbins AH, Birinyi LK, Dinarello CA. Endotoxin and tumor necrosis factor induce interleukin 1 gene expression in adult human vascular endothelial cells. *Am J Pathol* 1986;124:179–185.

98. Miossec P, Cavender D, Ziff M. Production of interleukin 1 by human endothelial cells. *J Immunol* 1986;136:2486–2491.

99. Nawroth PP, Bank I, Handley D, Cassimeris J, Chess L, Stern D. Tumor necrosis factor/cachectin interacts with endothelial cell receptors to induce release of interleukin 1. *J Exp Med* 1986;163:1363–1375.

100. Philip RM, Epstein LB. Tumor necrosis factor as immunomodulator and mediator of monocyte cytotoxicity induced by itself, γ-interferon and interleukin-1. *Nature* 1986;323:86–89.

101. Dinarello CA, Cannon JG, Wolff SM, et al. Tumor necrosis factor (cachectin) is an endogenous pyrogen and induces production of interleukin 1. *J Exp Med* 1986;163:1433–1450.

102. Beutler B, Cerami A. Cachectin and tumor necrosis factor as two sides of the same biological coin. *Nature* 1986;320:584–588.

103. Nathan CF. Secretory products of macrophages. *J Clin Invest* 1987;79:319–326.

104. Gimbrone MA Jr, Buchanen MR. Interaction of platelets and leukocytes with vascular endothelium: *in vitro* studies. *Ann NY Acad Sci* 1982;401:171–183.

105. Harlan JM. Leukocyte–endothelial interactions. *Blood* 1985;65:513–525.

106. Schleimer RP, Rutledge BK. Cultured human vascular endothelial cells acquire adhesiveness for neutrophils after stimulation with interleukin 1, endotoxin, and tumor-promoting phorbol diesters. *J Immunol* 1986;136:649–654.

107. Thomas PD, Hampson FW, Casale JM, Hunninghake GW. Neutrophil adherence to human endothelial cells. *J Lab Clin Med* 1988;111:286–292.

108. Bevilacqua MP, Pober JS, Wheeler ME, Cotran RS, Gimbrone MA Jr. Interleukin 1 acts on cultured human vascular endothelium to increase the adhesion of polymorphonuclear leukocytes, monocytes, and related leukocyte cell lines. *J Clin Invest* 1985;76:2003–2011.

109. Varani J, Bendelow J, Sealey DE, Kunkel SL, Gannon DE, Ryan US, Ward PA. Tumor necrosis factor enhances susceptibility of vascular endothelial cells to neutrophil-mediated killing. *Lab Invest* 1988;59:292–295.

110. Bevilacqua MP, Stengelin S, Gimbrone MA Jr, Seed B. Endothelial leukocyte adhesion molecule 1: an inducible receptor for neutrophils related to complement regulatory proteins and lectins. *Science* 1989;243:1160–1165.

111. Wispelwey B, Long WJ, Castracane JM, Scheld WM. Cerebrospinal fluid interleukin-1 activity following intracisternal inoculation of *Haemophilus influenzae* lipopolysaccharide into rats. In: *Program and Abstracts of the 28th Interscience Conference on Antimicrobial Agents and Chemotherapy.* Los Angeles: American Society for Microbiology, 1988;265.

112. Mustafa MM, Ramilo O, Olsen KD, Franklin PS, Hansen EJ, Beutler B, McCracken GH Jr. Tumor necrosis factor in mediating experimental *Haemophilus influenzae* type b meningitis. *J Clin Invest* 1989;84:1253–1259.

113. Bradbury MWB. The structure and function of the blood–brain barrier. *Fed Proc* 1984;43:186–190.

114. Goldstein GW, Betz AL. The blood–brain barrier. *Sci Am* 1986;255:74–83.

115. Lesse AJ, Moxon ER, Zwahlen A, Scheld WM. Role of cerebrospinal fluid pleocytosis and *Haemophilus influenzae* type b capsule on blood brain barrier permeability during experimental meningitis in the rat. *J Clin Invest* 1988;82:102–109.

116. Quagliariello VJ, Long WJ, Scheld WM. Human interleukin-1 modulates blood–brain barrier (BBB) injury *in vivo*. In: *Program and Abstracts of the 27th Interscience Conference on Antimicrobial Agents and Chemotherapy.* New York: American Society for Microbiology, 1987;204.

117. Tunkel AR, Rosser SW, Scheld WM. *Haemophilus influenzae* lipopolysaccharide (LPS)-induced alterations in blood–brain barrier (BBB) permeability in an *in vitro* model. In: *Program and Abstracts of the 29th Interscience Conference on Antimicrobial Agents and Chemotherapy.* Houston: American Society for Microbiology, 1989;219.

118. Täuber MG, Khayam-Bashi H, Sande MA. Effects of ampicillin and corticosteroids on brain water content, cerebrospinal fluid pressure, and cerebrospinal lactate levels in experimental pneumococcal meningitis. *J Infect Dis* 1985;151:528–534.

119. Täuber MG, Shibl AM, Hackbarth CJ, Larrick JW, Sande MA. Antibiotic therapy, endotoxin concentration in cerebrospinal fluid, and brain edema in experimental *Escherichia coli* meningitis in rabbits. *J Infect Dis* 1987;156:456–462.

120. Scheld WM, Dacey RG, Winn HR, Welsh JE, Jane JA, Sande MA. Cerebrospinal fluid outflow resistance in rabbits with experimental meningitis. Alterations with penicillin and methylprednisolone. *J Clin Invest* 1980;66:243–253.

121. Falconer MA, McFarlan AM, Russell DS. Experimental brain abscess in the rabbit. *Br J Surg* 1943;30:245–260.

122. Long WD, Meacham WF. Experimental method for producing brain abscess in dogs with evaluation of the effect of dexamethasone and antibiotic therapy on the pathogenesis of intracerebral abscesses. *Surg Forum* 1968;19:437–438.

123. Wood JH, Doppman JL, Lightfoote WE II, Girton M, Ommaya AK. Role of vascular proliferation on angiographic appearance and encapsulation of experimental traumatic and metastatic brain abscesses. *J Neurosurg* 1978;48:264–273.

124. Wood JH, Lightfoote WE II, Ommaya AK. Cerebral abscesses produced by bacterial implantation and septic embolization in primates. *J Neurol Neurosurg Psychiatry* 1979;42:63–69.

125. Molinari GF, Smith L, Goldstein MN, Satran R. Pathogenesis of cerebral mycotic aneurysms. *Neurology* 1973;23:325–332.

126. Molinari GF, Smith L, Goldstein MN, Satran R. Brain abscess from septic cerebral embolism: an experimental model. *Neurology* 1973;23:1205–1210.

127. Winn HR, Rodeheaver G, Moore P, Wheeler CB. A new model for experimental brain abscess in rats and mice. *Surg Forum* 1978;29:500–502.

128. Winn HR, Mendes M, Moore P, Wheeler CB, Rodeheaver G. Production of experimental brain abscess in the rat. *J Neurosurg* 1979;51:685–690.

129. Wispelwey B, Scheld WM. Brain abscess. *Clin Neuropharmacol* 1987;6:483–510.

130. Mendes M, Moore P, Wheeler CB, Winn HR, Rodeheaver G. Susceptibility of brain and skin to bacterial challenge. *J Neurosurg* 1980;52:772–775.

131. Costello GT, Heppe R, Winn HR, Scheld WM, Rodeheaver GT. Susceptibility of brain to aerobic, anaerobic, and fungal organisms. *Infect Immun* 1983;41:535–539.

132. Onderdonk AB, Kasper DL, Cisneros RL, Bartlett JG. The capsular polysaccharide of *Bacteroides fragilis* as a virulence factor: comparison of the pathogenic potential of encapsulated and unencapsulated strains. *J Infect Dis* 1977;136:82–89.

133. Onderdonk AB, Kasper DL, Mansheim BJ, Louie TJ, Gorbach SL, Bartlett JG. Experimental animal models for anaerobic infections. Rev Infect Dis 1979;1:291–301.
134. McGowan K, Gorbach SL. Anaerobes in mixed infections. J Infect Dis 1981;144:181–186.
135. Britt RH, Enzmann DR, Placone RC Jr, Obana WG, Yeager AS. Experimental anaerobic brain abscess. Computerized tomographic and neuropathological correlations. J Neurosurg 1984;60:1148–1159.
136. Kasper DL. Chemical and biological characterization of the lipopolysaccharide of Bacteroides fragilis subspecies fragilis. J Infect Dis 1976;134:59–66.
137. Britt RH, Enzmann DR, Yeager AS. Neuropathological and computerized tomographic findings in experimental brain abscess. J Neurosurg 1981;55:590–603.
138. Enzmann DR, Britt RR, Obana WG, Stuart J, Murphy-Irwin K. Experimental Staphylococcus aureus brain abscess. AJNR 1986;7:395–402.
139. Neuwelt EA, Lawrence MS, Blank NK. Effect of gentamicin and dexamethasone on the natural history of the rat Escherichia coli brain abscess model with histopathological correlation. Neurosurgery 1984;15:475–483.
140. Graham DR, Band JD. Citrobacter diversus brain abscess and meningitis in neonates. JAMA 1981;245:1923–1925.
141. Kline MW. Citrobacter meningitis and brain abscess in infancy: epidemiology, pathogenesis, and treatment. J Pediatr 1988;113:430–434.
142. Foreman SD, Smith EE, Ryan NJ, Hogan GR. Neonatal Citrobacter meningitis: pathogenesis of cerebral abscess formation. Ann Neurol 1984;16:655–659.
143. Kline MW, Kaplan SL, Hawkins EP, Mason EO Jr. Pathogenesis of brain abscess formation in an infant rat model of Citrobacter diversus bacteremia and meningitis. J Infect Dis 1988;157:106–112.
144. Kline MW, Mason EO Jr, Kaplan SL. Characterization of Citrobacter diversus strains causing neonatal meningitis. J Infect Dis 1988;157:101–105.
145. Casciato DA, Rosenblatt JE, Goldberg LS, Bluestone R. In vitro interaction of Bacteroides fragilis with polymorphonuclear leukocytes and serum factors. Infect Immun 1975;11:337–342.
146. Ingham HR, Sisson PR, Middleton RL, Narang HK, Codd AA, Selkon JB. Phagocytosis and killing of bacteria in aerobic and anaerobic conditions. Med Microbiol 1981;14:391–399.
147. Adamu SA, Sperry JF. Polymorphonuclear neutrophil chemotaxis induced and inhibited by Bacteroides spp. Infect Immun 1981;33:806–810.
148. Quartey GRC, Johnston JA, Rozdilsky B. Decadron in the treatment of cerebral abscess. An experimental study. J Neurosurg 1976;45:301–310.
149. Yildizhan A, Pasaoglu A, Kandemir B. Effect of dexamethasone on various stages of experimental brain abscess. Acta Neurochir 1989;96:141–148.
150. Obana WG, Britt RH, Placone RC, Stuart JS, Enzmann DR. Experimental brain abscess development in the chronically immunosuppressed host. Computerized tomographic and neuropathologic correlations. J Neurosurg 1986;65:382–391.
151. Schoenbaum SC, Gardner P, Shillito J. Infections of cerebrospinal fluid shunts: epidemiology, clinical manifestations, and therapy. J Infect Dis 1975;131:543–552.
152. Grogan EL, Sande MA, Clark RE, Nolan SP. Experimental endocarditis in calf after tricuspid valve replacement. Ann Thorac Surg 1980;30:64–69.
153. Christensen GD, Simpson WA, Bisno AL, Beachey EH. Experimental foreign body infections in mice challenged with slime-producing Staphylococcus epidermidis. Infect Immun 1983;40:407–410.
154. Zimmerli W, Waldvogel FA, Vaudaux P, Nydegger UE. Pathogenesis of foreign body infection: description and characteristics of an animal model. J Infect Dis 1982;146:487–497.
155. Quie PG, Belani KK. Coagulase-negative staphylococcal adherence and persistence. J Infect Dis 1987;156:543–547.
156. Dougherty SH. Pathobiology of infection in prosthetic devices. Rev Infect Dis 1988;10:1102–1117.
157. Ludwicka A, Jansen B, Wadstrom T, Pulverer G. Attachment of staphylococci to various synthetic polymers. Zentralbl Bakteriol Mikrobiol Hyg 1984;256:479–489.
158. Hogt AH, Dankert J, Feijen J. Adhesion of Staphylococcus epidermidis and Staphylococcus saprophyticus to a hydrophobic biomaterial. J Gen Microbiol 1985;131:2485–2491.
159. Hogt AH, Dankert J, Hulstaert CE, Feijen J. Cell surface characteristics of coagulase-negative staphylococci and their adherence to fluorinated poly(ethylenepropylene). Infect Immun 1986;51:294–301.
160. Peters G, Locci R, Pulverer G. Adherence and growth of coagulase-negative staphylococci on surfaces of intravenous catheters. J Infect Dis 1982;146:479–482.
161. Franson TR, Sheth NK, Menon L, Sohnle PG. Persistent in vitro survival of coagulase-negative staphylococci adherent to intravascular catheters in the absence of conventional nutrients. J Clin Microbiol 1986;24:559–561.
162. Vaudaux P, Suzuki R, Waldvogel FA, Morgenthaler JJ, Nydegger UE. Foreign body infection: role of fibronectin as a ligand for the adherence of Staphylococcus aureus. J Infect Dis 1984;150:546–553.
163. Vaudaux P, Waldvogel FA, Morgenthaler JJ, Nydegger UE. Adsorption of fibronectin onto polymethylmethacrylate and promotion of Staphylococcus aureus adherence. Infect Immun 1984;45:768–774.
164. Maxe I, Ryden C, Wadström T, Rubin K. Specific attachment of Staphylococcus aureus to immobilized fibronectin. Infect Immun 1986;54:695–704.
165. Vaudaux P, Lew D, Waldvogel FA. Host-dependent pathogenic factors in foreign body infection: a comparison between Staphylococcus epidermidis and S. aureus. In: Pulverer G, Quie PG, Peters G, eds. Pathogenicity and clinical significance of coagulase-negative staphylococci. Stuttgart: Gustav Fisher Verlag, 1987;183–193.
166. Bayston R, Penny SR. Excessive production of mucoid substance in Staphylococcus SIIA: a possible factor in colonisation of Holter shunts. Dev Med Child Neurol [Suppl] 1972;27:25–28.
167. Christensen GD, Simpson WA, Bisno AL, Beachey EH. Adherence of slime-producing strains of Staphylococcus epidermidis to smooth surfaces. Infect Immun 1982;37:318–326.
168. Christensen GD, Baddour LM, Simpson WA. Phenotypic variation of Staphylococcus epidermidis slime production in vitro and in vivo. Infect Immun 1987;55:2870–2877.
169. Christensen GD, Parisi JT, Bisno AL, Simpson WA, Beachey EH. Characterization of clinically significant strains of coagulase-negative staphylococci. J Clin Microbiol 1983;18:258–269.
170. Davenport DS, Massanari RM, Pfaller MA, Bale MJ, Streed SA, Hierholzer WJ Jr. Usefulness of a test for slime production as a marker for clinically significant infections with coagulase-negative staphylococci. J Infect Dis 1986;153:332–339.
171. Fishman M. Microbial adherence and infection—clinical relevance. Infect Control 1986;7:181–184.
172. Younger JJ, Christensen GD, Bartley DL, Simmons JCH, Barrett FF. Coagulase-negative staphylococci isolated from cerebrospinal fluid shunts: importance of slime production, species identification, and shunt removal to clinical outcome. J Infect Dis 1987;156:548–554.
173. Diaz-Mitoma F, Harding GKM, Hoban DJ, Roberts RS, Low DE. Clinical significance of a test for slime production in ventriculoperitoneal shunt infections caused by coagulase-negative staphylococci. J Infect Dis 1987;156:555–560.
174. Pollack M. The virulence of Pseudomonas aeruginosa. Rev Infect Dis 1984;6(Suppl 3):S617–S626.
175. Zimmerli W, Lew PD, Waldvogel FA. Pathogenesis of foreign body infection: evidence for a local granulocyte defect. J Clin Invest 1984;73:1191–1200.
176. Dougherty SH, Simmons RL. Endogenous factors contributing to prosthetic device infections. Infect Dis Clin North Am 1989;3:199–209.
177. Vaudaux PE, Zulian G, Huggler E, Waldvogel FA. Attachment of Staphylococcus aureus to polymethylmethacrylate increases its resistance to phagocytosis in foreign body infections. Infect Immun 1985;50:472–477.

178. Borges LF. Cerebrospinal fluid shunts interfere with host defenses. *Neurosurgery* 1982;10:55–60.
179. Johnson GM, Lee DA, Regelmann WE, Gray ED, Peters G, Quie PG. Interference with granulocyte function by *Staphylococcus epidermidis* slime. *Infect Immun* 1986;54:13–20.
180. Gray ED, Peters G, Verstegen M, Regelmann WE. Effect of extracellular slime substance from *Staphylococcus epidermidis* on the human cellular immune response. *Lancet* 1984;1:365–367.
181. Gray ED, Regelmann WE, Peters G. Staphylococcal slime and host defenses: effects on lymphocytes and immune function. In: Pulverer G, Quie PG, Peters G, eds. *Pathogenicity and clinical significance of coagulase-negative staphylococci.* Stuttgart: Gustav Fischer Verlag, 1987;45–54.
182. Schlesinger LS, Ross SC, Schaberg DR. *Staphylococcus aureus* meningitis: a broad based epidemiologic study. *Medicine* 1987;66:148–156.
183. Wheat RW. Bacterial morphology and ultrastructure. In: Joklik WK, Willett HP, Amos DB, Wilfert CM, eds. *Zinsser microbiology,* 19th ed. Norwalk, CT: Appleton & Lange, 1988;14–24.

Infections of the Central Nervous System,
edited by W. M. Scheld, R. J. Whitley, and
D. T. Durack, Raven Press, Ltd., New York © 1991.

CHAPTER 15

Neonatal Bacterial Meningitis

Arnold L. Smith and Joel Haas

Meningitis in neonates was first described by Aschoff in 1897 (1). In this publication, he described the histopathological features and noted that *Escherichia coli* and *Staphylococcus aureus* were the most common etiology. Subsequent reports emphasized that sepsis often preceded or accompanied the infection and that group B streptococci were also an important cause. With the advent of neonatal intensive care, the causative bacteria mirrored those organisms causing nosocomial sepsis. In the early 1900s, gram-positive organisms predominated (2–5), whereas in the 1990s there is an equal distribution between gram-positive and gram-negative ones.

Sepsis in the newborn is defined as present if a blood culture yields a traditional neonatal pathogen: *S. aureus; E. coli;* group A, B, or D streptococci; *Streptococcus pneumoniae; Listeria monocytogenes; Haemophilus influenzae;* or all other gram-negative rods (6). Epidemiologists have traditionally defined the newborn period as the first 30 days of life (7). The risk for acquiring meningitis is greater in the first 30 days of life than anytime thereafter. In reality, the risk factors, diagnostic tests, and treatment may extend to infants who are several months old. The majority of these infants have been born prematurely, but term newborns with underlying disease are also included.

In the 1990s, group B streptococci and *E. coli* continue to be responsible for more than 75% of all cases of neonatal sepsis. Table 1 depicts the incidence in several geographic locations. Surprisingly, the overall incidence has not changed significantly since the preantibiotic era.

Table 2 depicts the etiology of neonatal meningitis; the data are summarized from refs. 8–10. Certain of these bacteria appear to cause disease in epidemics, and there is marked regional variation. For example, an *L.*

monocytogenes epidemic was associated with contaminated goat cheese. *S. aureus* disease was one of the most common causes in a Finnish hospital (11), whereas in Tel Aviv the *Klebsiella–Enterobacter* species were the most common (12). In addition, many bacteria have been reported as a cause of neonatal meningitis. The more common of these will be addressed separately.

EPIDEMIOLOGY

Although many factors may contribute to infection of a newborn leading to meningitis, certain key features are commonly present. The most significant of these is low birth weight. Low-birth-weight infants have meningitis at a rate three times that of those weighing more than 2500 g (7). In general, the smaller the infant, the higher the incidence of sepsis. A study of 483 infants conducted at the Boston City Hospital in 1970 (13) showed, in addition, that sepsis was most common in infants who required resuscitation at birth and who were born to mothers who had a temperature greater than 37.8°C in the immediate postpartum period. Premature rupture of the membranes is also related to the incidence of neonatal meningitis, particularly in those mothers whose membranes ruptured more than 24 hr prior to delivery (14).

Gram-Positive Organisms

Group B Streptococci

Group B streptococci (GBS) are identifiable in the vagina in 5–35% of normal women (15–23). The organisms are then acquired by the infant during delivery, producing early-onset disease, or are introduced into the infant later in the nursery by the hands of the hospital personnel, producing late-onset disease. The infant–mother concordance for acquiring organisms varies

A. L. Smith and J. Haas: Division of Infectious Diseases and Department of Pathology, Children's Hospital and Medical Center, Seattle, Washington 98105.

TABLE 1. *Incidence of bacterial meningitis (percent live births)*

Location	Period	All	<2,500 g	References
Chicago, Illinois	1928–1947	—	1.60	192
Cincinnati, Ohio	1948–1959	0.40	2.20	193
Leeds, England	1947–1960	0.50	—	194
United States	1959–1966	0.46	1.36	7
Panorama City, California	1962–1987	0.30	2.80	195
The Netherlands	1976–1982	0.23	—	196
Gottingen, Federal Republic of Germany	1975–1982	0.50	—	10, 197

from 40% to 70%. However, of the infants acquiring GBS, only 2% will develop invasive disease. Some data suggest that if the infant is colonized at multiple sites, or if the mother has high density of colonization, the likelihood of invasive disease may be greater (24). All GBS causing invasive infection are capsulated. The capsular types (namely Ia, Ib, Ic, II, and III), which are immunologically defined, occur with approximately equal frequency among infants with early-onset disease. In contrast, type III GBS cause most of the late-onset illnesses; overall, type III GBS cause two-thirds of neonatal infections.

Staphylococci

Staphylococcus epidermidis is usually acquired in the hospital, most often due to infections of intravascular cannulae. *Staphylococcus aureus* is also commonly acquired in the hospital; usually a primary focus of infection is evident.

TABLE 2. *Bacteria causing meningitis in newborns: 1971 to present[a]*

Bacteria	Percentage of total[b]
Gram-positive	
Streptococci	38.5
Group A	0.5
Group B	36
Group D	2
Listeria monocytogenes	6
Staphylococcus aureus	2
Staphylococcus epidermidis	1
Streptococcus pneumoniae	1
Gram-negative	
Escherichia coli	38
Klebsiella–Enterobacter species	6
Pseudomonas aeruginosa	2
Haemophilus influenzae	0.5
Citrobacter diversus	1
Salmonella species	2
Other miscellaneous	2

[a] Summarized from refs. 8–10, and from 10 years of experience at author's institution.
[b] Based on 263 total isolates.

Gram-Negative Organisms

Escherichia coli

The overwhelming majority of infants with *E. coli* meningitis have an *E. coli* which bears an acidic capsular polysaccharide classified immunologically as K1. The polysaccharide is an $\alpha2–\alpha8$ homopolymer of sialic acid. In a study performed in the Netherlands (10), 88% of neonatal CSF *E. coli* isolates were K1-producing. Approximately half of hospital nurses carry *E. coli* K1 in their fecal flora (25,26), whereas only 7–38% of other women in the childbearing age harbor *E. coli* K1. The high rates of carriage by hospital personnel indicate that, like GBS, *E. coli* K1 may be acquired during delivery from the mother or after delivery from the hands of hospital personnel (27).

Sarff et al. (26) examined the prevalence of *E. coli* K1, the most common capsular type associated with *E. coli* meningitis in rectal swabs of newborns from 14 different nurseries. The prevalence varied from 7% to 38%, with the overall rate being 19%. There were variations in prevalence over time, but this was not explicable on the basis of antibiotic administration or other identified nursery practices. Cultures obtained within the first 9 hr of life yielded *E. coli* K1 in only four of 101 healthy neonates. All four strains were isolated from ear canal cultures, suggesting that the infant acquired the organism during the intrapartum period. Data suggesting later acquisition of *E. coli* K1 from hospital personnel were found: 13 of 20 hospital personnel had *E. coli* K1 in their stool of identical serotypes (K, O, and H) as the infants under their care. By day 2 of life, 29% of these infants had the same *E. coli* in their stool. The incidence of acquisition from the vagina during delivery appears to be high. One-third of the neonates born to mothers who had *E. coli* K1 in the vagina acquired the organisms; of these, 88% were serologically identical (26).

Citrobacter

Citrobacter is a genus which is taxonomically related to the *Salmonella arizona* group of Enterobacteriaceae. In certain individuals, it can be a normal colonizer of the human gastrointestinal tract. *Citrobacter diversus* causes both sporadic and epidemic neonatal meningitis. A unique feature of this illness is the proclivity for multiple brain abscesses (28–35). The *Citrobacter* species causing this infection are primarily *C. diversus,* but *C. koseri* and *C. freundii* disease have also been recognized.

Enterobacter

Enterobacter species such as *E. sakazakii* can cause a necrotizing meningitis (32–38), as can *Pseudomonas aeruginosa* (39). These have in common nosocomial acquisition and severe disease with a mortality rate that approaches 50%.

Respiratory Pathogens

Bacteria normally colonizing the respiratory tract of infants, children, and adults can also cause neonatal meningitis. *S. pneumoniae, H. influenzae,* and *Neisseria meningitidis* have all been associated with neonatal meningitis. The disease is most similar to early-onset GBS infection with evidence of placentitis and chorioamnionitis. These same organisms have been isolated from vaginal secretions and/or amniotic fluid. There are no distinct clinical features identifying neonatal infections caused by these organisms until cultures uncover their identity.

PATHOGENESIS

Neonatal Factors

The normal newborn is thought to be born without bacterial flora. The infant who becomes infected can acquire the organism by transcervical passage, with or without intact membranes (40). In addition, the infant may acquire the organism from the birth canal. When a potentially pathogenic bacterium is acquired, it is most commonly recovered from the gastric aspirate, in contrast to the infant's surface (41). However, the majority of infants who acquire potentially pathogenic bacteria while within the uterus (42) or during delivery do not develop bacteremia or meningitis. This observation implies that the infant's host defense is able to protect the newborn.

For the two most common neonatal pathogens, GBS and *E. coli,* to produce an invasive infection in the newborn, the organisms must adhere to epithelial cells, penetrate or disrupt the epithelial barrier, evade local nonspecific host defenses, and multiply in the bloodstream. The infant's epithelial cells may possess ligands, which are present in decreased amounts in adults, and the mucosal surface may lack secretory IgA (43). In addition, the mucosal epithelial surfaces of the newborn may lack fibro-

nectin (44). Fibronectin may decrease bacterial adherence to mucosal surfaces (45). After surface adherence and invasion, the bacteria must evade killing by tissue phagocytes and replicate within the host.

The common neonatal pyogens, GBS and *E. coli,* are not killed by antibody and complement in the absence of phagocytes. Alveolar macrophages are absent at birth, and the peripheral pool of polymorphonuclear leukocytes (PMNs) is smaller than that in adults (46). In addition, PMNs in neonates are less able to perform chemotaxis when compared to those in adults (47); moreover, once they are at the site of infection, neonatal PMNs are not as effective as adult PMNs in killing pathogens.

In addition to diminished phagocytic function, virtually all infants with neonatal meningitis lack specific antibody directed to the capsule of the invading organism. Prior to 32 weeks of gestation, the infant's serum immunoglobulin G (IgG) concentration is less than 50% of the maternal value, whereas at term the infant's IgG concentration may exceed that of the mother (48). Thus, premature infants may not receive maternal IgG even if the mother has antibodies directed against the capsule of the invading bacteria. Even when infected, the newborn rarely makes type-specific IgG antibodies; an occasional infant will synthesize IgM but not IgG. This defect in anticapsular antibody synthesis is caused by (a) failure of differentiation of B lymphocytes into antibody-secreting plasma cells and (b) a lack of T-lymphocyte facilitation of antibody synthesis (49).

Acquisition

Amniotic fluid is inhibitory to the growth of *E. coli* and other organisms (50) as a result of the presence of lysozyme, transferrin, and certain immunoglobulins (51). Thus, organisms that gain access to the amniotic fluid may not grow and may be cleared by macrophages. These macrophages may be derived from the placenta or from the mother's systemic circulation. The amniotic fluid is no longer a hostile environment for *E. coli* if it contains meconium or vernix (52,53). In contrast, GBS grow in normal amniotic fluid. Prior to delivery, bacteria can be inoculated into the fetus during fetal monitoring (54), or by forceps during delivery. Shortly after birth, organisms can be introduced by tracheal suctioning and intubation (55). Most often, the organisms are introduced by the hands of hospital personnel caring for a sick infant (Fig. 1). Once organisms are introduced into the infant, infection can result if the infant's host response is not adequate to contain the inoculated bacteria.

Infant Metabolism

Abnormal metabolism by an infant may also predispose to infection. There are two striking metabolic features which predispose to gram-negative meningitis in

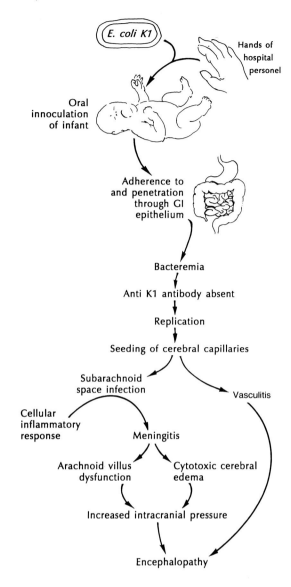

FIG. 1. Schematic of pathogenesis of *E. coli* meningitis in neonates.

serum concentration of these two compounds in galactosemic infants has not fulfilled this hypothesis.

The concentration of free iron in the serum of newborns appears to be directly related to the susceptibility of the neonate to infection. Iron added to the serum *in vitro* enhances the growth of many bacteria, whereas iron-binding proteins such as transferrin, present in serum and saliva, inhibit growth. Breast milk also contains an iron-binding protein called "lactoferrin." The newborn, however, has low serum levels of these proteins (59). In a well-intentioned experiment in Polynesia, intramuscular iron-dextran was administered prophylactically to newborns to prevent the subsequent development of iron-deficiency anemia. The incidence of sepsis in the infants receiving iron was 1.7% (60). The incidence of infants who did not receive iron was 0.3%, a rate comparable to that seen in European infants. More striking was the lack of the usual risk factors in these infants. Similar results were reported in New Zealand (61). In this study the incidence of *E. coli* meningitis was increased fivefold in infants who received parenteral iron.

Pathogenesis of Gram-Positive Meningitis

As mentioned previously, GBS are classified into five serotypes on the basis of structurally and antigenically distinct capsular polysaccharides (Table 2). Antibody directed against types II and III polysaccharides provides protection by opsonization; that is, antibody enhances phagocytic activity of, and killing by, PMNs in the presence of complement. Conversely, the type-specific capsular polysaccharide appears to be a virulence factor. A type III GBS, devoid of capsule, was derived by a single insertion of the transposon Tn 916. The LD_{50} for the acapsular mutant was $>5 \times 10^7$ colony-forming units (CFU), whereas the LD_{50} for the wild-type parent was 5×10^5 CFU (62). In addition, when the virulence of a panel of GBS which vary in the amount of capsule on the surface is examined, the greater the amount of capsule, the lower the LD_{50} in neonatal mice (63,64). The critical portion of the GBS type III capsule appears to be the terminal sialic acid (see Table 3). Mutants lacking the terminal sialic acid residue but possessing the core structure are less virulent than wild-type organisms (65). The capsular polysaccharide is both secreted and cell-associated, with high producers being more virulent in chick-embryo (63) and mouse (66) models of infection. One mechanism by which the type III carbohydrate increases virulence is via inhibition of PMN chemotaxis (66). Neutrophil chemotaxis in response to standard stimuli (fMLP or zymosan-activated serum) was decreased by type II antigen, which promoted adhesiveness of PMNs to endothelium (66) in antibody-free serum.

Most infants, whether or not they have GBS sepsis and meningitis, lack antibodies directed against GBS capsular polysaccharide (67). The level needed for protection

newborns, particularly that due to *E. coli*. Galactosemia in an infant is a risk factor for *E. coli* meningitis (56,57). In several states in which there is routine screening of newborns for galactosemia, it is found that one-third had died of *E. coli* sepsis by the time they had been identified. In almost all cases, the meningitis is due to gram-negative bacteria, particularly *E. coli*. There is no readily identifiable reason for this increased susceptibility of infants with galactosemia to *E. coli* sepsis and meningitis. It has been observed (58) that the susceptibility abates when the serum galactose concentration is corrected. Some have speculated that galactatol (reduced galactose, a known granulocyte cytotoxin) or *N*-acetylglucosamine (capable of inducing dysfunction of fixed macrophages in animal models) might play a role in this susceptibility. Inhibition of galactose metabolism results in accumulation of these metabolites. However, measurements of the

TABLE 3. *Capsular polysaccharides of* Streptococcus agalactiae

Capsular type	Structure[a]
Ia	β-D-glu (1 → 4)-β-D-gal (3 ↑ 1) β-D-NAcn-glc (4 ↑ 2) α-D-NAcNeur
Ib	β-D-glu (1 → 4)-β-D-gal (3 ↑ 1) β-D-NAcn-glc (3 ↑ 2) α-D-NAcNeur
II	β-D-NAcn-glc (1 → 3)β-D-gal(1 → 4)β-D-glu(1 → 3)β-D-glu(1 → 2)β-D-gal (6 ↑ 1) (3 ↑ 2) β-D-gal α-D-NAcNeur
III	β-D-glu(1 → 6)β-D-NAcn-glc(1 → 3)β-D-gal (4 ↑ 1) β-D-gal (6 ↑ 2) α-D-NAcNeur

[a] glu, glucose; gal, galactose; NAcn-glc, *N*-acetyldeoxyglucose; NAcNeur, *N*-acetylneuraminic acid.

against GBS infection is debated: An anti-type II IgG concentration of 1.3 μg/ml has been suggested (68); however, Baker et al. (69) found 2.0 μg/ml of anti-type III to be the minimum protective level. Infants infected with GBS lack type-specific antibody: Those with type III disease have <2.0 μg/ml, those with type Ia have <0.2 μg/ml, and those with type Ib have <0.1 μg/ml. Regardless of the magnitude of the maternal titer of IgG directed against GBS capsule(s), the infant does not receive significant amounts until after 34 weeks of gestation. Thus, the low levels of specific IgG directed against these capsular polysaccharides explains in part why prematurity is a risk factor for GBS disease.

GBS appear to adhere to and invade the placental membranes. The mechanism by which this occurs is not known. It is not clear whether it is a primary effect of GBS or a result of the inflammatory response to the organism. Once GBS enter the amniotic cavity, they can grow at rates similar to that observed *in vitro* with common bacteriologic media. This is in contrast to the above-mentioned observations with *E. coli.* Once the amniotic fluid is infected at high density, the infant apparently swallows and aspirates amniotic fluid *in utero.* This, then, permits the organism to invade the bloodstream from the lungs, or perhaps from the gastrointestinal tract. Neonatal GBS infections are most often fatal if the infant has been infected longer *in utero.* The overwhelming majority (80%) of the infants with GBS meningitis have pneumonia. Histologic examination of fatal cases shows large numbers of organisms in the airway, PMNs congesting alveolar capillaries, and, in half the cases, hyaline membranes.

GBS produce many extracellular products thought to have a role in virulence. These include hyaluronidase, proteases, nucleases, and neuraminidase (65,68,70,71). It was initially thought that the neuraminidase production was a marker for virulence; however, it has not been found in all meningeal isolates. The GBS also produces a protein identified as Ibc, which binds immunoglobulins through their Fc receptors. This would be a means by which organisms could circumvent antibody activity but bind to choroid plexus, an organ rich in Fc receptors

(72). Beta-hemolysin produced by GBS is related to streptolysin S of the group A organisms. However, hemolysin is not a virulence factor, because the generation of isogenic mutants by transposon mutagenesis has not shown that hemolysin-negative mutants are less virulent (73). The LD_{50} in infant rats less than 24 hr old was not significantly different in capsulated type III GBS whether or not they had detectable hemolysin production.

Pathogenesis of Escherichia coli Meningitis

There also appears to be a clonality in the *E. coli* K1 which cause neonatal meningitis and sepsis (74,75). It appears that there is co-segregation of K1 with certain O antigens (O2, O7, O18) and other potential virulence factors such as type 1, type s, type 1C, and type p fimbriae and hemolysin (76). The frequency distribution of the genetic distance between K1 *E. coli* causing neonatal meningitis and those isolated from the intestinal flora of healthy individuals has been compared (75). It is clear that approximately half the disease in newborns is caused by a clone present in normal gastrointestinal flora, with the other half being caused by a distinct widespread subclone. The mechanism by which *E. coli* K1 adhere to and invade gastrointestinal epithelium is not known. Some data suggest that adherence to oral pharyngeal cells is mediated by type 1 pili, with strains lacking this surface organelle being considerably less adherent and less virulent in animal model systems (77). More recent data, using isogenic mutants in which the structural gene for the subunit of type 1 pili was specifically mutated, indicate that these organelles are necessary for oropharyngeal colonization but not gastrointestinal colonization (78). In addition, it was observed that the physiological milieu in the ileum of the animals predisposed to the expression of type S pili (79); this expression would favor adherence to a sialic acid receptor on enterocytes permitting adherence and subsequent invasion. The genetic basis of *E. coli* K1 capsular polysaccharide production has begun to be deciphered. It

appears that there is a 20-kb segment of chromosomal DNA which encodes for two enzyme clusters (80–82) (Fig. 2). One cluster is responsible for the synthesis and activation of N-acetylneuraminic acid. The genes in this cluster encode for two essential proteins: A 50-kD protein is responsible for activation of N-acetylneuraminic acid to cytidine-monophosphate-N-acetylneuraminic acid, encoded by *neuA*. This precursor is then polymerized to form the linear sialic homopolymer. The second enzyme is encoded by gene *neuS*, a 45-kD protein which is thought to be sialic acid polymerase. A gene cluster adjacent to these two genes consists of five proteins whose gene products vary in molecular weight from 37 kD to 80 kD. These later genes, which are present in all K types of *E. coli*, appear to deal with (a) translocation of the polymerized carbohydrate through the cell membrane and (b) anchoring to the cell surface (80–82). It is not known whether the capsular polysaccharide and other putative virulence factors are co-regulated, but there is a quantitative relationship between the capsular content of an individual isolate and virulence (83). The strains harboring large amounts of capsule with a rough lipopolysaccharide (LPS) are not lysed by serum, whereas strains with a small amount of capsule and a rough LPS are readily lysed. Thus, at a given level of capsular polysaccharide content, the LPS phenotype is an important determinant of virulence. In addition, the low capsular polysaccharide containing rough LPS strains are readily lysed by normal serum and/or phagocytosed and killed by PMNs and macrophages. If, however, the LPS is one with extensive side-chain complexity, then the organism is resistant to these host defense mechanisms and is of increased virulence, regardless of the amount of capsule produced. The intrinsic or physiological regulation of K1 antigen production is not only important for virulence but also important in disease severity. In infants with high concentrations of K1 antigen in the cerebrospinal fluid (CSF), a fatal outcome is more likely (84). The amount of K1 capsule produced by the *E. coli* strains also appears to be related to virulence in animal models. Strains producing more K1 have a lower LD_{50} and are more likely to be isolated from a fatal

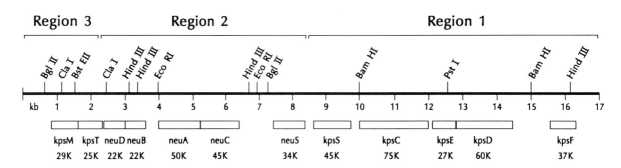

FIG. 2. Organization of the gene cluster responsible for capsulation in *E. coli*. Only *neuA* and *neuS* are specific for K1 capsule synthesis. (Courtesy of Dr. R. Silver, University of Rochester.)

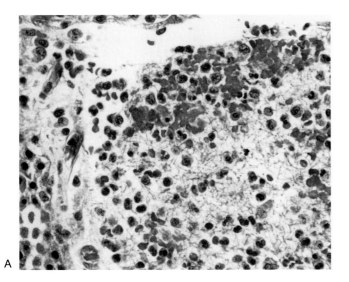

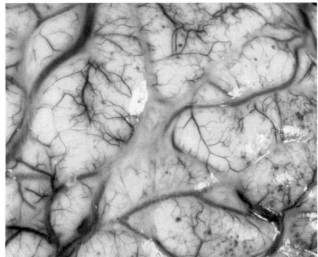

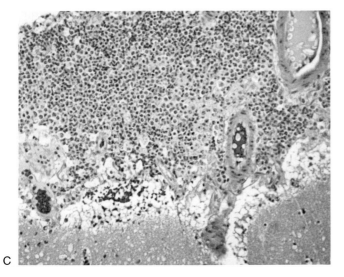

FIG. 3. A: Neutrophil leukocytes and granular debris with bacteria occupy the stroma of the choroid plexus. Cuboidal plexus epithelium is at top and the left of the figure. H&E stain, ×400. **B:** Purulent arachnoidal exudate does not obscure cerebral cortical hyperemia and hemorrhage. **C:** Acute neutrophilic exudate distends the subarachnoid space. H&E stain, ×200.

case. In contrast, strains producing less K1 antigen have a higher LD_{50}, but it is still lower than that in the non-K1 strains.

Localization in choroid plexus has been suggested to be caused by the presence of s fimbriae (85). However, not all strains isolated from ventricular CSF produce this organelle on subculture. It is not clear whether this is caused by down-regulation of the production of S fimbriae *in vitro* or by the absence of the genes for its synthesis in certain strains. Cloning experiments need to be performed before the role of this organelle in *in vivo* localization is defined.

Both GBS and K1 *E. coli* can enter the bloodstream of the infants by penetration across the gastrointestinal epithelium. This route appears to be important only in late-onset GBS disease and in *E. coli* disease. The invading organism is acquired from the hands of hospital personnel or of other caretakers, colonizes the gastrointestinal tract, penetrates the epithelium, and causes bacteremia.

Histopathology

After bacteremia is established in neonatal rat models of meningitis, the first histopathological lesion that appears to occur in the brain is choroid plexitis. There is polymorphonuclear infiltration of the choroid plexus stroma and of the lateral cerebral ventricle just external to the plexus (Fig. 3A). Bacteria subsequently enter the ventricular system and move via normal CSF flow to the arachnoid granulations. Arachnoiditis is most prominent around the base of the brain: This is a striking finding in half the neonates; in the remainder, the exudate is distributed over the cerebral cortex surface (Fig. 3B). The bacteria can be visualized in PMNs and macro-

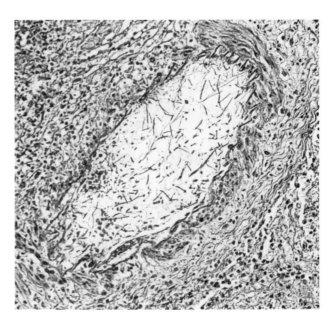

FIG. 4. Neutrophilic exudate obscures the outer layers of the wall of this basilar artery branch. H&E stain, ×225.

phages, but they are also free in the ventricular fluid. The inflammatory exudate in the subarachnoid space (Fig. 3B) surrounds the blood vessels and extends into the brain parenchyma along the Virchow–Robin space. Vasculitis is an invariable feature of neonatal meningitis (86). The inflammation involves both arterioles and veins. In the arterioles the adventitia is infiltrated by PMNs, with sparing of the intima and absence of thrombosis (Fig. 4). In contrast, phlebitis is characterized by thrombosis with complete occlusion (Fig. 5). Clusters of veins involved in phlebitis are responsible for the hemorrhagic cerebrocortical infarctions seen in neonatal meningitis (Fig. 6). These changes around the blood vessels are prominent during the very first days of meningitis. Vasculitis appears to be caused by bacterial factors in that it occurred even in early-onset GBS disease in the presence of minimal arachnoid inflammation. After bacteria enter the CSF compartment through the choroid plexus, they presumably exit through arachnoid villi, as in meningitis in older infants. One explanation for the presumed increase in severity and incidence of neonatal meningitis is the relative paucity and functional immaturity of arachnoid villi in the newborn. Thus, the egress of bacteria is slower, and it can lead to bacterial accumulation in the CSF. The inflammatory exudate in the ventricular CSF impacts on the arachnoid villi, producing dysfunction of this exit valve. Increasing intracranial pressure results from arachnoid villus dysfunction and cytotoxic cerebral edema, producing vomiting and obtundation. Choroid plexitis and the associated ventriculitis lead to ependymal epithelium being denuded and active ependymitis (87). This leads to glial tufts projecting into the ventricular lumen and subsequently leads to

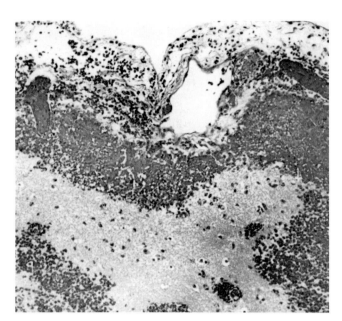

FIG. 6. Cerebral cortical hemorrhagic necrosis is a sequel of venous thrombosis. H&E stain, ×200.

glial bridges (in the second or third weeks of disease). These glial bridges can produce obstruction, particularly at the aqueduct of Sylvius, but they can also produce multiple ventricular septations (88). Both of these septations and the arachnoid villus dysfunction can lead to hydrocephalus. In postmortem studies, hydrocephalus is present in approximately half the cases. In 12 of 14 cases of neonatal meningitis with hydrocephalus (86), eight were communicating; four appeared to be due to obstruction at the aqueduct of Sylvius, whereas in two the obstruction was at the outlet of the fourth ventricle. In all probability in an individual case, there are multiple sites of potential obstruction. The histological correlates of the above pathogenic sequence readily explain the complications and sequelae of neonatal E. coli meningitis. Figure 1 schematically depicts the pathogenesis of E. coli meningitis.

DIAGNOSIS

Signs and Symptoms

Newborns who are brought to medical attention because of meningitis are separable into two groups: those with early-onset disease (i.e., those less than 48 hr old) and those with late-onset disease (i.e., those whose illness is recognized later than 14 days after birth). This separation is arbitrary but is of significance because of differences in the manifestations of the signs and symptoms of the disease, the causative organisms, and, most importantly, mortality (Table 4). Infants with early-onset disease most commonly present with the signs and symp-

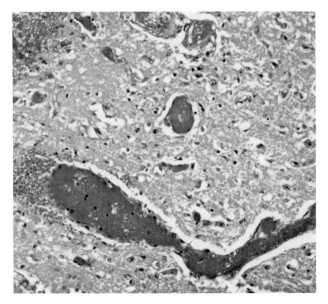

FIG. 5. Cortical venous thrombosis is accompanied by perivascular hemorrhage. H&E stain, ×200.

TABLE 4. *Differences between early-onset and late-onset neonatal meningitis*

Feature	Early	Late
Median age of onset	≤2 days	>14 days
Obstetric complications	Yes	No
Transmission	Mother → infant	Mother, other adults (hospital environment)
Prematurity	Uncommon	Often
Clinical presentation	Sepsis	CNS
Group B streptococci	Common	Common (especially type III)
Escherichia coli	Common	Uncommon
Mortality	35%	15%

toms of sepsis dominating the clinical picture: Specific symptoms referable to the central nervous system (CNS) are often not detected (Table 5) (87–90). In both groups, fever is a common manifestation. The definition of fever in a newborn has not been rigorously undertaken. Three articles address this sign (91–93) and permit some general conclusions. A portion of the reason for the lack of emphasis of fever is that the most common cause of fever in a nursery is not an infectious disease but is, instead, an error in care by the hospital personnel or the temperature serve controls on the incubators. Thus, increased incubator temperature, overswaddling, dehydration, atropine administration, etc., are far more common than infection. However, virtually all infants ultimately proven to have a bacterial infection have a core temperature of >100.1°F on more than one occasion, separated by 1 hr. Using this definition, fever is present alone in approximately 1% of all newborn infants. One study (94) suggested that there was a linear relationship between the magnitude of fever and the prevalence of a life-threatening bacterial illness. Four of 22 neonates with a rectal temperature of ≥40°C had a bacterial infection, whereas 11 of 144 with a rectal temperature between 39.1°C and

39.9°C had such an infection. It is to be emphasized that fever alone is not a reliable symptom of infection. Virtually all infants with ultimately proven bacterial meningitis have fever and some other sign and symptom. In the early-onset group, the organ system whose symptoms predominate is the gastrointestinal tract, followed by the respiratory tract (Table 5): CNS dysfunction is present in one-third. Frequency of these signs and symptoms listed in Table 5 exceed 100% because, as mentioned above, virtually all infants have more than one of these manifestations. The typical newborn with neonatal sepsis and meningitis may have fever, with subsequent temperature instability, respiratory distress, abdominal distention, vomiting, and lethargy; in addition, they may have increased serum concentration of unconjugated bilirubin.

In contrast, infants with late-onset disease have more symptoms referable to the CNS (Tables 4 and 5). Fever is more prominent, and the presence of CNS dysfunction is more striking. Seizures are reported to be present in approximately half the cases of early- and late-onset neonatal meningitis. However, others (95) have pointed out that subtle seizures may be missed.

TABLE 5. *Clinical manifestations of neonatal sepsis and meningitis[a]*

Sign or symptom	Sepsis frequency (%)	Meningitis frequency (%)
Fever	50	65
Hypothermia	15	0
Respiratory distress	33	35
Gastrointestinal dysfunction	50	50
Anorexia	28	—
Vomiting	25	—
Abdominal distention	25	—
Diarrhea	10	—
CNS dysfunction	30	90
Lethargy	25	60
Irritability	15	30
Bulging fontanelle		20
Meningismus		10
Jaundice	35	0

[a] Derived from refs. 3–5, 12, 88, and 197 (sepsis), refs. 7, 10, 88–90 (meningitis), and authors' experience.

Laboratory Tests for Bacteriological Agents

For the diagnosis of neonatal meningitis to be made, it must first be considered. Any infant with known risk factors and with the signs and symptoms listed above should have blood, CSF, urine, and other appropriate body fluids cultured. The culture that should be performed first is a blood culture. The minimum volume of blood needed to be cultured has not been precisely defined. The study by Dietzman et al. (96) suggests that 0.2 ml of blood would be sufficient to detect *E. coli* bacteremia. They found that only infants with greater than 1000 colonies per milliliter of blood had meningitis: six of 11 had that density of bacteremia (96). Although heel stick cultures have been advocated (97–99), comparative studies with peripherally obtained venous blood have not been rigorously performed.

Lumbar puncture must be performed in all infants in whom the diagnosis is suspected. Although the majority of the infants have bacteremia and/or a urinary tract infection, Visser and Hall (100) found that blood culture was sterile when the CSF yielded an organism in 15% of the neonates with bacterial meningitis. In addition to culture, CSF should ideally be tested for (a) the presence of endotoxin from gram-negative organisms and (b) antigens of GBS (see below). Because *E. coli* and GBS account for the majority of the cases, these procedures can be of high yield.

The CSF of newborn infants is routinely examined for its content of leukocytes, protein, and sugar. Interpretation of these findings is limited by the fact that there is normal CSF pleocytosis in newborns. In addition, the CSF glucose may be low because of the physiologic hypoglycemia occurring in normal newborns. Intracranial hemorrhage can also produce hypoglycorrhachia. Nelson et al. (101) found that the CSF/blood glucose ratio ranged from 0 to 0.29 in seven infants with hemorrhage: Two CSF glucose concentrations were undetectable, and the highest value observed was 24 mg/dl. Table 6 depicts CSF obtained from normal newborns. It is to be noted that the trends toward pleocytosis and an increased protein concentration are accentuated in premature newborns. A prudent approach would be to assume that any newborn (premature or term) is at risk for bacterial meningitis if their CSF contains more than 20 white blood cells per microliter, has more than five PMNs per microliter, or a CSF protein concentration of >100 mg/dl. CSF C-reactive protein (CRP) concentration was examined for its ability to define the neonate with meningitis (102). Only two of 11 infants with meningitis had abnormal amounts of CRP in the CSF (102). In contrast, the CSF leukocyte count was >30 cells per microliter in 10 of 11, and an overlapping but separate 10 of 11 had a CSF glucose concentration of <40 mg/dl (102). A limitation of the interpretation of "normal CSF studies" is the fact that there was no long-term follow-up. Infants de-

fined as normal may have a congenitally acquired nonbacterial infection which will become apparent only later. From the data of Sarff et al. (103), which show significant overlap between noninfected and infected in all CSF indices, it is clear that the most prudent action is to administer antibiotics to any infant whose CSF formula is suggestive of meningitis.

In addition to culture of CSF, this fluid can be assayed directly for the presence of GBS antigen. The group B carbohydrate can be detected, using high-titer antisera raised in animals, by countercurrent immunoelectrophoresis (CIE). In this procedure, precipitin bands are formed, permitting rapid identification. Alternatively, the antibody can be adsorbed to latex particles or can be bound to protein A of nonviable *S. aureus* with agglutination of the particles in the presence of GBS antigen. The particle agglutination procedures are more sensitive, detecting 30–60 ng of polysaccharide per milliliter and can detect antigen after therapy has been initiated; CIE is often unreactive after antibiotic therapy has been initiated (104,105). Testing CSF by particle agglutination leads to false-positives in 1.2–4.5% of the specimens; in culture-confirmed cases, however, 0–100% (mean 88%) contain antigen (106–108).

Testing of serum from infants with suspected GBS sepsis for group B antigen is not as reliable. Rabalais et al. (109) studied 25 infants with culture-proven GBS infection; 18 had antigen in one or more body fluids. In four bacteremic infants (without meningitis) the admission serum lacked GBS antigen, but specimens obtained after therapy was initiated indicated the presence of group B antigen. Urine has also been tested for the presence of group B antigen. However, it contains many false-positives as a result of (a) naturally occurring proteins reactive with antibody from other species and (b) mucosal colonization (vagina or rectum) by GBS (109,110).

TABLE 6. *Characteristics of CSF in normal newborns*[a]

Birth weight (kg)	Reference	Postnatal age (days)	n	RBCs per microliter	WBCs per microliter	PMN (%)	Protein (mg/dl)	Glucose (mg/dl)
1	198	0–7	6	335 ± 709	3 ± 3	11 ± 20	162 ± 37	70 ± 17
		8–28	17	1465 ± 4062	4 ± 4	8 ± 17	159 ± 77	68 ± 48
		29–84	15	808 ± 1843	4 ± 3	2 ± 9	137 ± 61	49 ± 22
1.0–1.5	198	0–7	8	407 ± 853	4 ± 4	4 ± 10	136 ± 35	74 ± 19
		8–28	14	1101 ± 2643	7 ± 11	10 ± 19	137 ± 46	59 ± 23
		29–84	11	661 ± 1198	8 ± 8	11 ± 19	122 ± 47	47 ± 13
	199	0–7	21		9 ± 5	0	100 ± 20	NA
0.9–2.5	200	<7–28	28	NA	8.2 ± 7.1	157 ± 15	115 ± 15	52 ± 12
≥2.5	201	1	135	9 ± 142	5 ± 20	50 ± 10	63 ± 55	51 ± 15
≥2.5	202	1	87	NA	8.2 ± 7.1	61 ± 14	90 ± 12	52 ± 36
Term	202	7	135	3 ± 26	2 ± 2	50	47 ± 13	55 ± 9
Median (range) in meningitis:		<42	64	NA	3.73 ± 3.4	1.97 ± 2.98	150 ± 30	40 ± 20

[a] Mean ± the standard deviation is depicted. CSF, cerebrospinal fluid; RBCs, red blood cells; WBCs, white blood cells; PMNs, polymorphonuclear leukocytes; NA, not available.

Blood Analysis

Leukocytes

The neutrophil number is increased in the peripheral blood in two-thirds of infants with neonatal meningitis. However, there is a wide range in the absolute value. If one examines the normal neonatal neutrophil counts in term infants (Fig. 7), then it is clear that the time after birth that neutrophil density is quantitated is very important. The presence of a normal neutrophil count does not exclude the likelihood of neonatal sepsis. One study found that 13 of 64 infants ultimately proven to have sepsis had falsely normal neutrophil indices (111). In addition, there was no difference in the prevalence of known risk factors in infants with falsely normal leukocyte counts when compared to those with infection and abnormal leukocyte counts (111). It has also been suggested that neutropenia might be an indicator of neonatal infection. When this has been examined, the positive predictive value is only approximately 50% (112). The neutropenia in such infants appears to be the result of marrow exhaustion from untreated, continuing infection. The neutrophil morphology on smears appears to be of little or no diagnostic value. The ratio of immature cells to mature cells or the presence or absence of toxic granulations and Döhle bodies does not correlate well with the presence of neonatal meningitis. Despite the relative insensitivity of the absolute immature neutrophil count, a persistent increase in the numbers of these cells, exceeding the two standard deviation lines on Fig. 7, in the peripheral blood of an infant warrants appropriate cultures.

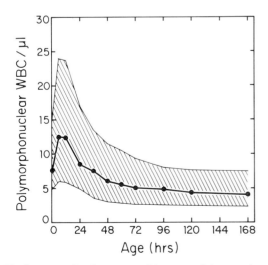

FIG. 7. Computerized tomographic scan of the cranium of a 2-week-old infant with neonatal meningitis. Ventriculitis was suspected on clinical grounds. A ventricular puncture yielded the organism.

Platelet Count

Thrombocytopenia has been observed in infants with neonatal meningitis. This diminished platelet count appears to be caused by a direct effect of the bacteria on platelets. This results in platelet aggregation, adhesion, and perhaps destruction. The thrombocytopenia appears not to be due to disseminated intravascular coagulation. However, only 10–60% of the infants with neonatal meningitis have platelet counts of <100,000 per microliter. Thus, it is seldom a useful laboratory finding in the diagnosis of meningitis.

Serum

Acute-phase reactants can be synthesized by the fetus. It has been suggested that their measurement in serum might be an indicator of a primitive, nonspecific host defense mechanism resulting from bacterial infection. Several of these "acute-phase reactants" have been evaluated. These include: C-reactive protein, fibrinogen, haptoglobin, and alpha-1 acid glycoprotein (Orosomucoid).

C-Reactive Protein

C-reactive protein (CRP) is a globulin which forms precipitates when it is mixed with the C polysaccharide of *S. pneumoniae.* It is associated with tissue injury, and its physiologic function is unknown. Thus, CRP is increased in the serum of adults with tissue infections. This has prompted its use to distinguish neonates with a viral illness from those with bacterial infection. In infants with neonatal meningitis, 50–90% will have an increased serum CRP concentration at the time of onset of symptoms. However, given this range, reliance on this test as a screen for neonatal meningitis is not possible. False-positive increases in CRP serum concentrations are seen in infants delivered from women with chorioamnionitis and premature rupture of the membranes (113–115). In addition, serum concentrations are occasionally elevated in infants with presumed viral infection (113–115). An increased CRP is also seen in infants with isolated urinary tract infection (116). Serial measurements of CRP in an infant suspected of neonatal meningitis, but in whom cultures are sterile, could be helpful. Serial measurements of CRP indicate that the serum concentration peaks 2–3 days after the onset of a bacterial infection and then begins to return to normal within 5–10 days in infants with adequately treated disease (113,117–119). As expected, in infants in whom there are relapses or complications, the CRP does not fall. Its latter use to document adequacy of treatment is probably the main clinical value of neonatal measurement of CRP.

Fibrinogen

Fibrinogen, the protein primarily responsible for alterations in the erythrocyte sedimentation rate, has been measured directly in an effort to discriminate between infants with neonatal meningitis and those without disease. There is marked overlap between values obtained in infected infants and those obtained in normals (120–123). This greatly limits the utility of this measurement for the diagnosis of neonatal meningitis. It has not been examined serially in infected infants to determine if it has a value similar to or greater than serial measurement of CRP.

Haptoglobin

Haptoglobin, an alpha-2 glycoprotein, reacts with free hemoglobin, thereby permitting removal of the latter compound from the systemic circulation by the reticuloendothelial system. Enthusiasm for the measurement of this molecule as an indicator of neonatal sepsis suggested that its concentration was increased in 35 of 38 infants with neonatal meningitis (124).

Subsequently, it was found that the test is extremely unreliable with normal values in a considerable proportion of infected infants (119,123,125). In addition, increased concentrations in healthy noninfected infants have been found.

Alpha-1 Acid Glycoprotein

This protein appears to be an integral membrane protein in leukocytes and perhaps in hepatocytes. It is liberated into the circulation with cell turnover. The normal values for serum concentrations of this protein are carefully defined (126–130), suggesting that infants with sepsis and meningitis might have increased serum concentrations resulting from increased leukocyte turnover. Unfortunately, this has not been confirmed. Falsely low values are present in 15–50% of the newborns with neonatal sepsis, particularly those infected with GBS (123,126,128,131). In addition, 10–25% of the ill infants, but without bacterial meningitis, have increased serum concentrations (129,130). Thus, the concentration of this protein in serum is of no significant predictive value. It has been suggested that it, like the CRP, might be useful in following response to therapy; however, it has a much longer half-life, suggesting that changes in serum concentrations will mirror those with CRP but will be slower in onset.

Immunoglobulin

Because the first antibody made in response to bacterial invasion is IgM and also because IgM does not cross the placenta, it has been suggested that the presence of increased serum IgM concentrations might be predictive of sepsis. This hypothesis appears to be correct, but only when the infection has been present for 7 or more days (132–134). In addition, the IgM can be directed against viruses as well as bacteria; thus, viral infections as well as minor localized bacterial infections increase the serum IgM concentration (132,133,135,136). Because of these observations, this test is not a reliable indicator for bacterial sepsis and meningitis.

Erythrocyte Sedimentation Rate

Although the erythrocyte sedimentation rate (ESR) is easy to perform and there are micromethods for its rapid determination, changes in this test can result from many nonspecific reactions to inflammation. It has been suggested that ESR might be a better index of identifying infants with neonatal sepsis and meningitis. When this has been examined (115,137–141), it has been found that the ESR ultimately increases in newborns with bacterial infection. However, at the time of diagnosis, it may be normal in 30–70% of the infected infants. In addition, once appropriate therapy has been initiated and a clinical response occurs, the ESR may not return to normal for several weeks. These factors greatly mitigate the potential usefulness of the ESR in the diagnosis of neonatal sepsis.

Sepsis Screen

Certain groups have suggested that a combination of the above laboratory tests might be used as a "sepsis screen." This usually includes performing a total leukocyte count, estimating the percentage of immature neutrophils, and measurement of the CRP and haptoglobin concentration, as well as determining the ESR. Using this "sepsis screen" (142–144), 60 of 524 infants were thought to be infected and received antibiotics. Unfortunately, three infants with subsequently proven bacterial infection were not identified, although 39% of the 60 infants did have a bacterial infection. A more recent study (145) assigned a score to (a) the total leukocyte count, (b) the ratio of immature to total leukocytes, (c) the total PMN density, (d) the density of immature cells, (e) the presence of degenerative changes in PMNs, and (f) the presence of a platelet count less than 150,000 cells per microliter. If six of these seven indices were abnormal, the positive predictive value in 27 septic neonates (of 298 evaluated) was 80% whereas the negative predictive value was 93% (145). The sepsis screen may be helpful, but it is not infallible and cannot be used to decide whether a given infant should or should not receive antibiotics.

TREATMENT

Neonates suspected of having meningitis should have prompt diagnostic evaluation and receive parenteral antibiotics. In several studies, it has been shown that 95% of neonatal infants suspected of having sepsis and meningitis are ultimately shown to have sterile cultures. Therefore, initial therapy should be efficacious but should not do the infant any harm. In most institutions, the initial therapy consists of ampicillin and an aminoglycoside (146). The exact choice of the aminoglycoside, whether it be gentamicin, kanamycin, amikacin, or tobramycin, depends on the susceptibility of the gram-negative bacteria found in the nursery housing the infant. The regimen most commonly used by directors of programs in pediatric infectious disease is ampicillin and gentamicin (147). In infants without culture-proven disease, it is not necessary to have the serum concentrations of the aminoglycosides measured unless the infant is in renal failure. The reason for this recommendation is that the majority of infants will have the antibiotic discontinued within 48–72 hr after administration was initiated. Thus, there is too little time for aminoglycoside accumulation and subsequent toxicity. The usual doses for infants suspected of sepsis and meningitis are indicated in Table 7. The route of administration of ampicillin and gentamicin, the two most common choices, can be intramuscular, but intravenous is preferred. This antibiotic combination can produce a therapeutic response. However, more potent drugs are available for specific infections. The rationale of the choice of ampicillin and gentamicin is based on the observation that the routine administration of a potent third-generation cephalosporin (such as cefotaxime) for infants suspected of having sepsis and meningitis results in emergence of Enterobacteraceae resistant to that antibiotic in that nursery (148).

If the CSF is grossly purulent when it is obtained, or if bacteria are seen on gram stain of CSF, then ampicillin and a third-generation cephalosporin should be administered until the specific microorganism is identified. Cefotaxime is preferred over other potent third-generation cephalosporins because of (a) its low protein-binding ability (a situation less likely to be associated with interference in bilirubin binding) and (b) its low rate of subsequent bilirubin neurotoxicity in a jaundiced (often acidotic) newborn. The dose of alternative agents is indicated in Table 7. Antibiotics should be administered to neonates with meningitis for at least 2 weeks after the CSF is sterile. This necessitates monitoring of CSF every 2–3 days during the first week after initiation of therapy until sterility is confirmed and there is clinical improvement. In neonates with uncomplicated gram-negative enteric meningitis, the CSF will yield the organism from 2 to 5 days after the appropriate, ultimately efficacious, antibiotic. With meningitis caused by GBS, the CSF is sterile in most cases within 48 hr. Most experts administer antibiotics to neonates with enteric gram-negative meningitis for a minimum of 3 weeks. In general, infants with GBS meningitis, which promptly responds by sterilization of the CSF in 24 hr, are treated for a total of 2 weeks. Most other neonatal meningitides are treated for 3 weeks.

SPECIFIC PATHOGENS

1. Group B Streptococci

Antibiotics

Although all GBS are intrinsically resistant to aminoglycosides, there is synergism between this class of antibiotics and beta-lactams (149). Penicillin G and ampicillin are active against all GBS isolated to date. Relapse during the treatment of GBS meningitis (150–152) resulted in a sequential increase in the dose of ampicillin or penicillin G administered for this disease. The second and third relapses have been treated with a variety of agents and are suspected to be due to penicillin tolerance (153). However, not all relapses are bacteriologically proven; in these cases, there is an increase in the pleocytosis along with fever and irritability, with sterile CSF cultures. Such infants have been treated with a variety of agents, including vancomycin and chloramphenicol. There are no data to support any one alternative regimen for the treatment of second and third relapses of GBS meningitis.

Supportive Therapy

Since Santos et al. (154) showed that modified immune serum globulin with high titers against type III GBS was protective in neonatal animals, several laboratories have confirmed the finding. Hill and co-workers (155) found that antibody levels could be increased in the neonate if they were transfused with a volume of blood equal to or greater than 40% of the infant's blood

TABLE 7. Antibiotic agents for treatment of neonatal meningitis

Age (days):	0–7	8–14	15–30
Frequency:	Every 12 hr	Every 8 hr	Every 6 hr
Antibiotic	mg/day[a]	mg/day[a]	mg/day[a]
Ampicillin	100–150	200	200
Nafcillin	100–150	200	200
Oxacillin	100–150	200	200
Cefotaxime	100	150	200
Ceftazidime	60	90	125–150
Vancomycin	20	30	40–50
Ticarcillin	150–200	200–300	300–400
Kanamycin	15–20	20–30	30–50
Gentamicin	5	7.5	7.5
Tobramycin	5	7.5	7.5
Amikacin	15–20	20–30	20–30

[a] Daily dose in milligrams per kilogram.

volume. The survival rate in infants who were transfused and who had a marked increase in their antibody titer was 50% greater than that in infants who received the transfusion but who did not exhibit an increase in their opsonic activity against an infecting strain (155). In this study, none of nine with a titer increase died, as compared to three out of six not having such an increase. Using an exchange transfusion to increase titers, the same workers subsequently found that antibody was not the critical protective factor. The authors then found, from studies in a neonatal rat model, that the protective factor was both antibody and PMNs (156). Using this approach in experimental animals, close to 1000 mg of intravenous immunoglobulin is necessary to achieve survival rates equal to or greater than 90%. This is because of the intrinsic low anti-GBS titer in most preparations. This detrimental effect can be overcome with hybridoma technology. Using an IgM monoclonal antibody directed at type III polysaccharide, there is a 90% survival with extremely low doses, 0.25 mg/kg (157). Importantly, the monoclonal antibody preparation was active, even if administration was withheld for 24 hr after the initiation of experimental infection. In the neonatal rat model, the monoclonal antibody administration prevents depletion of the granulocyte stores in GBS-infected animals (158). Clinical studies are currently in progress comparing high-titer anti-GBS antibody to standard intravenous immunoglobulin using both polyclonal and monoclonal preparations (159).

Prognosis

Edwards et al. (160) followed 51 survivors of GBS meningitis, 30% early-onset, for an average of 6 years. They found that 50% of the survivors were normal but that 21% had severe sequelae. Other studies also show a high incidence of sequelae (161).

2. *Escherichia coli* Meningitis

Antibiotics

If *E. coli* is isolated from the CSF, most experts administer a third-generation cephalosporin alone. This choice is based on the high potency of these drugs against this genus, which leads to high CSF bactericidal titers with standard CSF penetration of 5–20%. There are no data comparing ampicillin plus an aminoglycoside and currently used third-generation cephalosporins in patients. There was a comparison between ampicillin and amikacin versus moxalactam (162). However, moxalactam administration was associated with hypoprothrombinemia and bleeding in septic infants. This precludes against its routine administration to newborns. Chloramphenicol has been administered to neonates

with gram-negative meningitis (163). However, for this drug to be used safely, monitoring of the serum concentration every 2–3 days is necessary. The usual question is whether cefotaxime or ceftriaxone should be administered to an infant with *E. coli* meningitis: Favoring cefotaxime is its lack of interference with the plasma-binding protein of bilirubin and the fact that its elimination is exclusively performed by the kidney. Favoring ceftriaxone is its concentration-dependent protein binding and the fact that it needs to be administered only once daily. The former leads to high and constant serum concentrations of unbound antibiotic throughout the dosing interval. There are no data that directly compare ceftriaxone with cefotaxime in neonatal gram-negative meningitis.

Supportive Therapy

Although antibody directed against the K1 capsular polysaccharide is opsonic and protective in experimental animals, the majority of the protection is conferred by IgM (164). This protection has also been shown with a murine IgM monoclonal directed against the K1 antigen. In addition, protection of experimental animals against K1 *E. coli* infection has been achieved with an IgM monoclonal directed against the LPS side chain. Because of the presence of K1-like antigens in the human neonatal brain (165), enthusiasm for the administration of anti-K1 antibody to newborns has been dampened because of concerns of immune complex disease. Thus, if there will be adjunctive immunotherapy of neonatal *E. coli* meningitis, it is likely to be directed against non-K1 antigens.

Infections with *Klebsiella* species and *Enterobacter* species should be treated with a third-generation cephalosporin and an appropriate aminoglycoside if the organisms are susceptible. The duration of antibiotic therapy in one study was 31 ± 14 days, and aminoglycosides were co-administered for 16 ± 10 days (162). These infections are rare, and there are no data comparing alternative courses of antibiotic therapy.

3. *Citrobacter diversus* Meningitis

CNS disease caused by this *Citrobacter* species involves the meninges and the brain parenchyma. As noted previously (35), approximately one-half of the cases have concomitant brain abscess. It appears that the organism invades small penetrating vessels, leading to septic, necrotizing vasculitis which is followed by hemorrhagic infarction (35). The infarct is accompanied by extensive necrosis and liquefaction without a surrounding fibrous capsule. This histopathological finding has led some (35) to advise against surgical drainage. However, Curless (166) has pointed out that the outcome is better in those cases drained surgically. Most *Citrobacter* species are resistant to penicillin G, and aminoglycoside susceptibility varies. Antibiotics used for *Citrobacter* meningitis include ampicillin, chloramphenicol, and trimethoprin-sulfamethoxazole (167). Third-generation cephalosporins (168) have been administered for *Citrobacter* meningitis and seem to be a logical choice, but the infrequency of the disease makes acquisition of comparative data nearly impossible.

4. Monitoring Therapy

Because of the lack of specificity of signs and symptoms of the neonate with meningitis, lumbar punctures should be performed daily, after antibiotic therapy has been initiated. Any clinical deterioration at any time in the course, or a failure to sterilize the CSF with the time anticipated, requires imaging of the cranial contents. Some experts recommend routine cranial computerized tomography. Early in disease, it provides information on the presence or absence of cerebral edema, the adequacy of CSF flow, the occurrence of major infarction, and the type of associated encephalopathy. Subsequent computerized tomographic examinations will detect the degree of cerebrocortical and white-matter atrophy, hydrocephalus (prior to a detectable increase in head size), and the presence of multicystic encephalomalacia.

Lumbar punctures are not necessary at the conclusion of administration of antibiotics. When therapy has been efficacious with regard to clinical criteria, sterilization of CSF, and cranial imaging studies, little information will be gained by examination of the CSF.

5. Treatment Failure

Persistence of an organism in the CSF or clinical deterioration (or both) constitutes treatment failure. Treatment failure is far more common with gram-negative neonatal meningitis than with infections caused by gram-positives. Because antibiotic resistance can emerge during therapy of gram-negative neonatal meningitis, retesting isolates for their antibiotic susceptibility or a change in the choice of antibiotics to be administered is warranted. However, most treatment failures are not associated with antibiotic resistance. The reasons that a newborn has treatment failure are (a) presence of the infection in a site that is not accessible to the antibiotic and (b) intrinsic absence of neonatal host defense.

In infants with treatment failure, ventriculitis is an important factor. In the strictest sense, ventriculitis is present in virtually every neonate with meningitis; that is, there are acute inflammatory cells and bacteria in the ventricular CSF. Ventriculitis is of clinical importance when bacteria are isolated from the ventricular fluid and are absent from the lumbar subarachnoid space, or when the inflammatory response in the cerebral ventricles is

greater than that in CSF sampled from the lumbar space. Clinically relevant ventriculitis can be suspected when the infant's lumbar CSF appears to be improving but the infant is worsening clinically: There is persistent fever and/or apnea or bradycardia, signaling the presence of isolated ventricular infection. Contemporary imaging techniques can be very useful in documenting the presence of ventriculitis. The lateral cerebral ventricles are enlarged, and there is inflammatory exudate and necrotic debris inferiority with less dense CSF superiority. When there is persistent infection in the ventricular system, direct installation of antibiotics can be beneficial (169–175). Antibiotics instilled in the lateral cerebroventricle should be administered in concentrations which exceed those normally sought in serum. The installation is best performed through a ventriculostomy, which is either externalized or connected to a subcutaneous reservoir. The dose of antibiotics ranges from 1 to 5 mg and should lack the preservatives present in multidose vials. There is a specific formulation of gentamicin without preservative for intrathecal use. The amount to be instilled can be more accurately gauged if the ventricular volume is known. This volume of ventricular CSF can be estimated from computerized tomography of the brain using that information and a nomogram (176). Table 8 depicts commonly used intraventricular antibiotics and the concentrations sought. The frequency of intraventricular administration is unknown. Clearance of antibiotics from ventricular CSF is dependent not only on transependymal adsorption but also on bulk CSF flow, arachnoid villus function, and the efficacy of the choroid plexus pump for organic acids if the antibiotic is in that class. The best approach is to administer an antibiotic at a dose calculated to produce a concentration approximately 20 times the measured minimal bactericidal concentration. Serial measurements of CSF concentration will describe the elimination of drug from the ventricular compartment. The intraventricular dose is readministered when the CSF concentration approaches the minimal bactericidal concentration. Intraventricular therapy is invariably accompanied by systemic administration of the same agents. There is no comparative data indicating the optimal management of an infant with such a severe infection.

TABLE 8. *Intraventricular antibiotics for ventriculitis*

Antibiotic	Dose (mg)	Desired peak CSF concentration (µg/ml)
Gentamicin	1–5	80–120[a]
Vancomycin	4–5	80–100[b]
Polymyxin	1–2	Unknown
Amikacin	Unknown	Unknown

[a] Histological change in white matter seen with concentrations >150 µg/ml.

[b] CSF concentrations of 800 µg/ml seen without clinically apparent adverse events.

Because of the early presence of ventriculitis in all cases, and the association of ventriculitis with treatment failures and fatal cases, alternative strategies have been developed to treat this aspect of the infection early in the course of disease. Lumbar intrathecal antibiotic therapy is not effective in preventing this complication or in ameliorating the outcome. In a study of 117 infants, of which 82 infections were caused by *E. coli,* the daily administration of 1 mg of gentamicin intrathecally for a minimum of 3 days had no effect on case fatality rate or sequelae. Failure to demonstrate any benefit of lumbar intrathecal antibiotics may be a result of (a) poor distribution into the ventricles against the flow or (b) failure to administer the antibiotic in an adequate volume to permit distribution over cerebral convexities (177). With this background information, intraventricular therapy was studied (178). The study population, although having significant overlap with the same group of investigators, differed in that 29% of the 87 infants enrolled were from Latin America. The Latin American infants accounted for nine of the 10 infants with *Salmonella* meningitis, and they accounted for a higher incidence of ventriculitis (86%). In addition, infants up to 12 months of age were enrolled. From this study, there was no difference in those infants receiving 2.5 mg of gentamicin intraventricularly when compared to the infants receiving only parenteral ampicillin and gentamicin. In the group receiving only parenteral therapy, the CSF yielded the organism 3.9 ± 1.3 days after therapy was initiated; in the group receiving additional intraventricular therapy, the duration was 3.4 ± 1.5 days. Overall, the mortality was higher in the group receiving intraventricular therapy (12 of 28) than in those with meningitis and ventriculitis receiving paranteval therapy alone (3 of 24). It is not clear why there was a higher fatality rate, particularly in Latin American infants receiving intraventricular gentamicin. This compound can be neurotoxic (179, 180), as can amikacin (181), but the concentrations in these experimental models far exceed those predicted to be achieved and measured in infants with gram-negative neonatal meningitis; that is, toxic values appear to be in the milligram-per-milliliter concentration range. In any event, it appears that routine intraventricular administration of antibiotics for neonatal meningitis is not advisable.

Intraventricular administration of beta-lactams is not recommended. These agents, which are dispensed from the pharmacy in extremely high concentrations, require 1- to 5000-fold dilution prior to administration into the intrathecal space. This allows chance for error, because it is difficult to make such high dilutions on the wards. Inadvertent installation of high concentrations of beta-lactams can cause seizures and, occasionally, cardiorespiratory arrest. The infections for which intrathecal beta-lactams have been chosen are caused by enterococci and occasionally by other gram-positive organisms. Vancomycin is the drug of choice for these infections because of (a) its relative lack of toxicity and (b) its efficacy against gram-positive bacteria (173).

PREVENTION

Prevention of GBS Meningitis

Two major strategies for the prevention of GBS meningitis exist: immunization and chemoprophylaxis.

Immunization

The major effort has concentrated on immunizing pregnant women with low-antibody titers against capsular polysaccharide. Because two-thirds of the GBS infections are caused by type III, efforts have concentrated on that antigen. Purified type III polysaccharide elicits primarily IgG antibody after administration to pregnant women (182). In women with low "nonprotective" titers (assumed to be ≤2 µg/ml) (183), only 54–60% of immunized subjects increased their titer to ≥2 µg/ml (182). Although GBS infection can be immunogenic in adult women, immunization of women who had an infant with GBS infection resulted in the same poor rate of seroconversion (184). It appears that there is a genetic restriction of the immune response to type III polysaccharide. The G2m(n) allotype is a regulator of IgG 2 subclass antibody synthesis. Individuals with IgG2 of the G2m(n) allotype are more likely to develop antipolysaccharide antibodies after immunization (185). In order to improve immunogenicity, the type III polysaccharide is being conjugated to protein. It is not yet known whether this approach will evoke protective antibodies.

Chemoprophylaxis

GBS are inhibited by low concentrations of penicillin G. Procaine penicillin G has been administered to infants at birth, resulting in a subsequent decrease in the incidence of neonatal GBS sepsis (186). There was an increase in the incidence of serious infections and penicillin-resistant bacteria, primarily *E. coli* and *S. epidermidis.* In an attempt to make chemoprophylaxis more specific, Pyati et al. (187) administered crystalline penicillin G to half of 1186 neonates weighing ≤2 kg. They found that the attack rate of GBS disease was not significantly different (10 of 598 receiving penicillin, as compared to 14 of 598 in the controls). Although penicillin sterilized the blood in certain infants, the fatality rate was unchanged (six of 10 in the treatment group; eight of 14 in the controls). Administration of penicillin G or ampicillin to GBS-colonized parturient women reduces the rate of transmission to the infant (188). However, the GBS carriage rate may be 30% if multiple maternal sites are cultured, but the incidence of neonatal GBS disease may only be 0.2%. Thus, parenteral administration of ampicillin or penicillin to every pregnant woman would produce a life-threatening allergic reaction in one woman for each case of neonatal GBS disease that was presented, assuming the allergy rate to be one per 2000. To avoid unnecessary penicillin administration, identification of the infants at risk is necessary. One approach is to administer penicillin to women with risk factors for having a neonate with GBS disease: premature labor, rupture of membranes ≥12 hr prior to delivering, and intrapartum fever. When this was studied, 160 of 1808 women had risk factors; 85 received ampicillin (2 g initially, followed by 1 g every 4 hr until delivery) (189). GBS bacteremia occurred in none of the infants born from women receiving ampicillin, whereas it was present in five of 79 controls (189). Extending this concept, Lim et al. (190) used short-term culture and antigen detection to identify GBS carriers among women with premature rupture of the membrane. Ampicillin was administered to 20 of 49 with GBS colonization; there were no cases of neonatal GBS infection in these women, but there were two cases in infants from the 29 untreated mothers (190).

Immunoprophylaxis

Because IgG can cross the placenta after the 34th week of gestation [including antibody against GBS capsular polysaccharides (191)], administration of specific antibody might protect the infants at risk. This approach is potentially attractive because of the relatively high incidence of invasive disease in both the mother and infant. Administration of intravenous immunoglobulin with high titers of functional antibody against GBS is also feasible. Studies to date have not permitted firm conclusions regarding the efficacy of this approach (192).

REFERENCES

1. Aschoff L. *Z Ohren* 1897;31:2952–2966.
2. Dunham EC. Septicemia in the new-born. *Am J Dis Child* 1933;45:229–253.
3. Craig WS. Meningitis in the newborn. *Arch Dis Child* 1936;11:171–186.
4. Nyhan WL, Fousek MD. Septicemia of the newborn. *Pediatrics* 1958;22:268–278.
5. Freedman RM, Ingram DL, Gross I, et al. A half century of neonatal sepsis at Yale: 1928 to 1978. *Am J Dis Child* 1981;135:140–144.
6. Gladstone IG, Ehrenkranz RA, Edberg SC. A ten-year review of neonatal sepsis and comparison with the previous fifty-year experience. *Pediatr Infect Dis J* 1990;9:819–825.
7. Overall JC Jr. Neonatal bacterial meningitis. *J Pediatr* 1970;76:499–511.
8. Wilson HD, Eichenwald HF. Sepsis neonatorum. *Pediatr Clin North Am* 1974;21:571–582.
9. Yow MD, Baker CJ, Barrett FF, et al. Initial antibiotic management of bacterial meningitis. *Medicine* 1973;52:305–309.
10. Mulder CJJ, van Alphen L, Zanen HC. Neonatal meningitis caused by *Escherichia coli* in the Netherlands. *J Infect Dis* 1984;150:935–940.
11. Vesikari R, Janas M, Gronroos P, et al. Neonatal septicemia. *Arch Dis Child* 1985;60:542–546.
12. Karpuch J, Goldberg M, Kohelet D. Neonatal bacteremia: a 4-year prospective study. *Isr J Med Sci* 1983;19:963–966.
13. Braun P. Epidemiology and clinical correlates of genital mycoplasmas in pregnancy and the newborn. Personal communication.
14. Niswander KR, Gordon M. *The women and their pregnancies.* The Collaborative Perinatal Study of the National Institute of Neurological Diseases and Stroke. US Department of Health, Education and Welfare publication no. (NIH) 73-379. Washington, DC: US Government Printing Office, 1972.
15. Baker CJ, Edwards MS. Group B streptococcal infections. In: Remington JS, Klein JO, eds. *Infectious diseases of the fetus and newborn infant.* Philadelphia, WB Saunders, 1983;820.
16. Anthony BF. Carriage of Group B streptococci during pregnancy: a puzzler. *J Infect Dis* 1982;145:789.
17. Boyer KM, Gadzala CA, Kelly PD, et al. Selective intrapartum chemoprophylaxis of neonatal group B streptococcal early-onset disease. II. Predictive value of prenatal cultures. *J Infect Dis* 1983;148:802.
18. Baker CJ, Barrett FF. Transmission of group B streptococci among parturient women and their neonates. *J Pediatr* 1973;83:919–925.
19. Anthony BF, Okada DM, Hobel CJ. Epidemiology of the group B streptococcus: maternal and nosocomial sources for infant acquisitions. *J Pediatr* 1979;95:431–436.
20. Pass MA, Gray BM, Kharre S, Dillon HC Jr. Prospective studies of group B streptococcal infections in infants. *J Pediatr* 1979;95:437–443.
21. Yow MD, Leeds LJ, Thompson PK, et al. The natural history of group B streptococcal colonization in the pregnant woman and her offspring. I. Colonization studies. *Am J Obstet Gynecol* 1980;137:34–38.
22. Allardice JG, Baskett TF, Seshia MMK, et al. Perinatal group B streptococcal colonization and infection. *Am J Obstet Gynecol* 1982;142:617–620.
23. Hoogkamp-Korstanje JAA, Gerards LJ, Cats BP. Maternal carriage and neonatal acquisition of group B streptococci. *J Infect Dis* 1982;145:800–803.
24. Jones DE, Kanarek KS, Lim DV. Group B streptococcal colonization patterns in mothers and their infants. *J Clin Microbiol* 1984;20:438–440.
25. McCracken GH Jr, Sarff LD. Current status and therapy of neonatal *E. coli* meningitis. *Hosp Pract* 1974;9:57.
26. Sarff LD, McCracken GH Jr, Schiffer MS, et al. Epidemiology of *Escherichia coli* K, in healthy and diseased newborns. *Lancet* 1975;1:1099–1104.
27. Peter G, Nelson JS. Factors affecting neonatal *E. coli* K, rectal colonization. *J Pediatr* 1978;93:866–869.
28. Graham DR, Anderson RL, Ariel FE, et al. Epidemic nosocomial meningitis due to *Citrobacter diversus* in neonates. *J Infect Dis* 1981;144:203–209.
29. Gwynn CM, George RH. Neonatal *Citrobacter* meningitis. *Arch Dis Child* 1973;48:455–458.
30. Tamborlane WV, Soto EV. *Citrobacter diversus* meningitis: a case report. *Pediatrics* 1975;55:739–741.
31. Ribeiro CC, Davis P, Jones DM. *Citrobacter koseri* meningitis in a special care baby unit. *J Clin Pathol* 1976;29:1094–1096.
32. Vogel LC, Ferguson L, Gotoff SP. Citrobacter infections of the central nervous system in early infancy. *J Pediatr* 1978;93:86–88.
33. Lin FYC, Devol WF, Morrison C, et al. Outbreak of neonatal *Citrobacter diversus* meningitis in a suburban hospital. *Pediatr Infect Dis* 1987;6:50–55.
34. Williams WW, Mariano J, Spurrier M, et al. Nosocomial meningitis due to *Citrobacter diversus* in neonates: new aspects of the epidemiology. *J Infect Dis* 1984;150:229–235.
35. Foreman SD, Smith EE, Ryan NJ, et al. Neonatal *Citrobacter* meningitis; pathogenesis of cerebral abscess formation. *Ann Neurol* 1984;16:655–659.
36. Kleiman MB, Allen SD, Neal P, et al. Meningoencephalitis and

compartmentalization of the cerebral ventricles caused by *Enterobacter sakazakii. J Clin Microbiol* 1981;14:352–354.

37. Muytjens HL, Zanen HC, Sonderkamp JH, et al. Analysis of eight cases of neonatal meningitis and sepsis due to *Enterobacter sakazakii. J Clin Microbiol* 1983;18:115–120.

38. Willis J, Robinson JE. *Enterobacter sakazakii* meningitis in neonates. *Pediatr Infect Dis J* 1988;7:196–199.

39. Ghosal SP, SenGupta PC, Mukherjee AK. Noma neonatorum; its aetiopathogenesis. *Lancet* 1978;2:2889–2891.

40. Bernischke K. Routes and types of infection in the fetus and newborn. *Am J Dis Child* 1960;99:714–720.

41. Brook I, Barrett CT, Brinkman CR, et al. Aerobic and anaerobic bacterial flora of the maternal cervix and newborn gastric fluid and conjunctiva: a prospective study. *Pediatrics* 1979;63:451–455.

42. Roos PJ, Malan AF, Woods DL, et al. The bacteriological environment of preterm infants. *S Afr Med J* 1980;57:347–350.

43. Burgio GR, Lanzavecchia A, Plebani A, et al. Ontogeny of secretory immunity: levels of secretory IgA and natural antibodies in saliva. *Pediatr Res* 1980;14:1111–1114.

44. Gerdes JS, Yoder MC, Douglas DS, et al. Decreased plasma fibronectin in neonatal sepsis. *Pediatrics* 1983;72:877–881.

45. Van De Water L, Destree AT, Hynes RO. Fibronectin binds to some bacteria but does not promote their uptake by phagocytic cells. *Science* 1983;220:201–204.

46. Christensen RD, Rothstein G. Exhaustion of mature marrow neutrophils in neonates with sepsis. *J Pediatr* 1980;96:316–318.

47. Miller ME. Phagocytic function in the neonate: selected aspects. *Pediatrics* 1979;64:709–712.

48. Yeung CY, Hoffs JR. Serum γ-g-globulin levels in normal, premature, postmature, and small-for-dates newborn babies. *Lancet* 1968;1:1167–1169.

49. Nagaoki T, Mitawaki T, Ciorfaru R, et al. Maturation of B-cell differentiation ability and T-cell regulatory functions during child growth assessed in a *Nocardia* water-soluble mitogen driven system. *J Immunol* 1981;126:2015–2019.

50. Larsen B, Snyder IS, Galask RP. Bacterial growth inhibition by amniotic fluid. 1. *In vitro* evidence for bacterial growth-inhibiting activity. *Am J Obstet Gynecol* 1974;119:492–496.

51. Galask RP, Snyder IS. Antimicrobiol factors in amniotic fluid. *Am J Obstet Gynecol* 1970;106:59–65.

52. Florman AL, Teubner D. Enhancement of bacterial growth in amniotic fluid by meconium. *J Pediatr* 1969;74:111–114.

53. Kitzmiller JL, Highby S, Lucas WE. Retarded growth of *E. coli* in amniotic fluid. *Obstet Gynecol* 1973;41:38–42.

54. Cordero J Jr, Hon EH. Scalp abscess. A rare complication of fetal monitoring. *J Pediatr* 1971;78:533–536.

55. Storm W. Transient bacteremia following endotracheal suctioning in ventilated newborns. *Pediatrics* 1980;65:487.

56. Kelly S. Septicemia in galactosemia. *JAMA* 1971;216:330.

57. Levy HL, Sepe SJ, Shih VE, et al. Sepsis due to *Escherichia coli* in neonates with galactosemia. *N Engl J Med* 1977;297:823–825.

58. Shurin SB. *Escherichia coli* septicemia in neonates with galactosemia. Letter to the editor. *N Engl J Med* 1977;297:1403–1404.

59. Weinberg ED. Iron and susceptibility to infectious disease. In the resolution of the contest between invader and host, iron may be the critical determinant. *Science* 1974;184:952–956.

60. Barry DMJ, Reeve AW. Increased incidence of gram-negative neonatal sepsis with intramuscular iron administration. *Pediatrics* 1977;60:908–912.

61. Farmer K. The disadvantages of routine administration of intramuscular iron to neonates. *NZ Med J* 1976;84:286–289.

62. Rubens CE, Wessels MR, Heggen LM, et al. Transposon mutagenesis of type III group B streptococcus: correlation of capsule expression with virulence. *Proc Natl Acad Sci USA* 1987;84:7208–7212.

63. Klegerman ME, Boyer KM, Papierniak CK, et al. Type-specific capsular antigen is associated with virulence in late-onset group B streptococcal type III disease. *Infect Immun* 1984;44:124–129.

64. Yeung MK, Mattingly SJ. Biosynthetic capacity for type-specific antigen synthesis determines the virulence of serotype III strains of group B streptococci. *Infect Immun* 1984;44:217–221.

65. Wessels MR, Rubens CE, Vicente-Javier B, et al. Definition of a bacterial virulence factor: sialylation of the group B streptococcal capsule. *Proc Natl Acad Sci USA* 1989;36:8983–8987.

66. McFall TL, Zimmerman GA, Augustine NH, et al. Effect of group B streptococcal type-specific antigen and polymorphonuclear leukocyte function and polymorphonuclear leukocyte–endothelial cell interaction. *Pediatr Res* 1987;21:517–523.

67. Gray BM. Seroepidemiology of group B streptococcus type III colonization at delivery. *J Infect Dis* 1989;159:1139–1142.

68. Durham DL, Mattingly SJ, Doran TI, et al. Correlation between the production of extracellular substances by type III group B streptococcal strains and virulence in a mouse model. *Infect Immun* 1981;34:448–454.

69. Baker CJ, Edwards MS, Kasper DL. Role of antibody to native type III polysaccharide of group B streptococcus in infant infection. *Pediatrics* 1981;60:544–549.

70. Straus DC, Brown JG. Characterization of protease production by a type-III group B streptococcus. *Curr Microbiol* 1985;12:127–134.

71. Mattingly SJ. Extracellular neuraminidase production by clinical isolates of group B streptococci from infected neonates. *J Clin Microbiol* 1980;12:633–635.

72. Levine S. Choroid plexus: target for systemic disease and pathway to the brain [Editorial]. *Lab Invest* 1987;56:231–233.

73. Weiser JN, Rubens CE. Transposon mutagenesis of group B streptococcus beta-hemolysin biosynthesis. *Infect Immun* 1987;55:2314–2316.

74. Achtman M, Heuzenroeder M, Kusecek B, et al. Clonal analysis of *Escherichia coli* O2:K1 isolated from diseased humans and animals. *Infect Immun* 1986;51:268–276.

75. Selander RK, Korhonen TK, Väisänen-Rhen V, et al. Genetic relationships and clonal structure of strains *Escherichia coli* causing neonatal septicemia and meningitis. *Infect Immun* 1986;52:213–222.

76. Korhonen TK, Valtonen MV, Parkkinen J, et al. Serotypes, hemolysin production, and receptor recognition of *Escherichia coli* strains associated with neonatal sepsis and meningitis. *Infect Immun* 1985;48:486–491.

77. Guerina NG, Kessler TW, Guerina VJ, et al. The role of pili and capsule in pathogenesis of neonatal infection with *Escherichia coli* K1. *J Infect Dis* 1983;148:395–405.

78. Bloch CA, Orndorff PE. Impaired colonization by and full invasiveness of *Escherichia coli* K1 bearing a site-directed mutation in the type 1 pilin gene. *Am Soc Microbiol* 1990;58:275–278.

79. Nowicki B, Vuopio-Varkila J, Viljanen P, et al. Fimbrial phase variation and systemic *E. coli* infection studied in the mouse peritonitis model. *Microb Pathol* 1986;1:335–347.

80. Silver RP, Aaronson W, Vann WF. The K1 capsular polysaccharide of *Escherichia coli. Rev Infect Dis* 1988;10:2S:282–286.

81. Brill JA, Quinlan-Walshe C, Gottesman S. Fine-structure mapping and identification of two regulators of capsule synthesis in *Escherichia coli* K-12. *J Bacteriol* 1988;170:2599–2611.

82. Roberts IS, Mountford R, Hodge R, et al. Common organization of gene clusters for production of different capsular polysaccharides (K antigens) in *Escherichia coli. J Bacteriol* 1988;170:1305–1310.

83. Vermeulen C, Cross A, Byrne WR, et al. Quantitative relationship between capsular content and killing of K1-encapsulated *Escherichia coli. Infect Immun* 1988;56:2723–2730.

84. McCracken Jr. GH, Sarff LD, Glode MP, et al. Relation between *Escherichia coli* K1 capsular polysaccharide antigen and clinical outcome in neonatal meningitis. *Lancet* 1974;2:246–250.

85. Parkkinen J, Korhonen TK, Pere A, et al. Binding sites in the rat brain for *Escherichia coli* s fimbriae associated with neonatal meningitis. *J Clin Invest* 1988;81:860–865.

86. Berman PH, Banker BQ. Neonatal meningitis: a clinical and pathological study of 29 cases. *Pediatrics* 1966;38:6–24.

87. Hill A, Shackelford GD, Volpe JJ. *J Pediatr* 1981;99:133–136.

88. Groover RV, Sutherland JM, Landing BH. Purulent meningitis of newborn infants. *N Engl J Med* 1961;264:1115–1121.

89. Watson DG. Purulent neonatal meningitis. A study of forty-five cases. *J Pediatr* 1957;50:352–360.

90. Yu JS, Grauang A. Purulent meningitis in the neonatal period. *Arch Dis Child* 1963;38:391–396.

91. Craig WS. The early detection of pyrexia in the newborn. *Arch Dis Child* 1963;38:29–35.
92. Voora S, Srinivasan G, Lilien LD, et al. Fever in full-term newborns in the first four days of life. *Pediatrics* 1982;69:40–44.
93. Osborn LM, Bolus R. Temperature and fever in the full-term newborn. *J Fam Pract* 1985;20:261–264.
94. Bonadio WA, Romine K, Gyuro J. Relationship of fever magnitude to rate of serious bacterial infections in neonates. *J Pediatr* 1990;116:733–735.
95. Volpe JJ. *Neurology of the newborn,* 2nd ed. Philadelphia: WB Saunders, 1987;608.
96. Dietzman DE, Fischer GW, Schoenknecht FD. Neonatal *Escherichia coli* septicemia—bacterial counts in blood. *J Pediatr* 1974;85:128–130.
97. Holt RJ, Frankcombe CH, Newman RL. Capillary blood cultures. *Arch Dis Child* 1974;49:318–321.
98. Mangurten HH, LeBeau LJ. Diagnosis of neonatal bacteremia by a microblood culture technique. A preliminary report. *J Pediatr* 1977;90:990–992.
99. Knudson RP, Alden ER. Neonatal heel-stick blood culture. *Pediatrics* 1980;65:505–507.
100. Visser VE, Hall RT. Lumbar puncture in the evaluation of suspected neonatal sepsis. *J Pediatr* 1980;96:1063–1067.
101. Nelson RM, Bucciarelli, Nagel JW, et al. Hypoglycorrachia associated with intracranial hemorrhage in newborn infants. *J Pediatr* 1979;94:800–803.
102. Philip AGS, Baker CJ. Cerebrospinal fluid C-reactive protein in neonatal meningitis. *J Pediatr* 1983;102:715–717.
103. Sarff LD, Platt LH, McCracken GH Jr. Cerebrospinal fluid evaluation in neonates: comparison of high-risk infants with and without meningitis. *J Pediatr* 1976;88:473–477.
104. Edwards MS, Kasper DL, Baker CJ. Rapid diagnosis of type III group B streptococcal meningitis by latex particle agglutination. *J Pediatr* 1979;95:202–205.
105. Bromberger PI, Chandler B, Gezon H, et al. Rapid detection of neonatal group B streptococcal infections by latex agglutination. *J Pediatr* 1980;96:104–106.
106. Wilson CB, Smith AL. Rapid tests for the diagnosis of bacterial meningitis. *Curr Clin Top Infect Dis* 1986;5:134–156.
107. Friedman CA, Wender DF, Rawson JE. Rapid diagnosis of group B streptococcal infection utilizing a commercially available latex agglutination assay. *Pediatrics* 1984;73:27–30.
108. Rench MA, Metzger TG, Baker CJ. Detection of group B streptococcal antigen in body fluids by a latex-coupled monoclonal antibody assay. *J Clin Microbiol* 1984;20:852–854.
109. Rabalais GP, Bronfin DR, Daum RS. Evaluation of a commercially available latex agglutination test for rapid diagnosis of group B streptococcal infection. *Pediatr Infect Dis J* 1987;6:177–181.
110. Sanchez PJ, Siegel JD, Cushion NB, et al. Significance of a positive urine group B streptococcal latex agglutination test in neonates. *J Pediatr* 1990;116:601–606.
111. Rozycki HJ, Stahl GE, Baumgart S. Impaired sensitivity of a single early leukocyte count in screening for neonatal sepsis. *Pediatr Infect Dis J* 1987;6:440–442.
112. Monroe BL, Weinberg AG, Rosenfeld CR, et al. The neonatal blood count in health and disease. I. Reference values for neutrophilic cells. *J Pediatr* 1979;95:89–98.
113. Ainbender EC, Cabatu EE, Guzman DM, et al. Serum C-reactive protein and problems of newborn infants. *J Pediatr* 1982;101:438–440.
114. Forest JC, Lariviere F, Dolce P, et al. C-reactive protein as biochemical indicator of bacterial infection in neonates. *Clin Biochem* 1986;19:192–194.
115. Matesanz JL, Malaga S, Santos F, et al. Valor diagnostico de la proteina C reactiva en la sepsis neonatal. *An Esp Pediatr* 1980;13:671–674.
116. Sabel K-G, Wadsworth C. C-reactive protein (CRP) in early diagnosis of neonatal septicemia. *Acta Paediatr Scand* 1979;68:825–831.
117. Sabel K-G, Hanson LA. The clinical usefulness of C-reactive protein (CRP) determinations in bacterial meningitis and septicemia in infancy. *Acta Paediatr Scand* 1974;63:381–388.
118. Magny JF, Benattar C, Saby M-A, et al. C-reactive proteine et diagnostic d'infection neonatale. Etude retrospective de 242 dossiers. *Pediatrie* 1986;41:105–107.
119. Speer C, Bruns A, Gahr M. Sequential determination of CRP, alpha-1-antitrypsin and haptoglobin in neonatal septicaemia. *Acta Paediatr Scand* 1983;72:679–683.
120. de Gamarra E, Savaglio N, Moriette G, et al. Surveillance du taux de fibrinogene chez le nouveau-ne. Interet au cours de l'evolution des infections bacteriennes par contamination d'origine maternelle. *Arch Fr Pediatr* 1980;37:163–166.
121. Raichvarg D, Carre J, Relier JP, et al. Interet de la determination conjointe d'un fibrinogene et de l'orosomucoide pour le diagnostic rapide des infections neonatales. *Ann Pediatr* 1982;29:679–672.
122. Relier JP, de Gamarra E. Place du fibrinogene parmi les proteines de l'inflammation dans les infections neonatales. *Pediatrie* 1984;39:379–383.
123. Brazy JE, Grimm JK, Little VA. Neonatal manifestations of severe maternal hypertension occurring before the thirty-sixth week of pregnancy. *J Pediatr* 1982;100:265–271.
124. Salmi TT. Haptoglobin levels in the plasma of newborn infants. With special reference to infections. *Acta Paediatr Scand* 1973;241(Suppl):1–55.
125. Guttebert TJ, Haneberg B, Jorgensen T. Lactoferrin in relation to acute phase proteins in sera from newborn infants with severe infections. *Eur J Pediatr* 1984;142:37–39.
126. Boichot P, Schirrer J, Menget A, et al. L'orosomucoide a la periode neonatale. Etude chez le nouveau-ne sain et le nouveau-ne infect. *Pediatrie* 1980;35:577–581.
127. Lee SK, Thibeault W, Heiner DC. α_1-Antitrypsin and α_1-acid glycoprotein levels in the cord blood and amniotic fluid of infants with respiratory distress syndrome. *Pediatr Res* 1978;12:775–777.
128. Sann L, Bienvenu J, Lahet C, et al. Serum orosomucoid concentration in newborn infants. *Eur J Pediatr* 1981;136:181–185.
129. Bievenu J, Sann L, Bienvenu F, et al. Laser nephelometry of orosomucoid in serum of newborns: reference intervals and relation to bacterial infections. *Clin Chem* 1981;27:721–726.
130. Philip AG, Hewitt JR. Alpha 1-acid glycoprotein in the neonate with and without infection. *Biol Neonate* 1983;43:118–124.
131. Bienvenu J, Bienvenu F, Baltassat P, et al. Le profile proteique normal du nouveau-ne. *Pediatrie* 1984;39:359–363.
132. Blankenship WJ, Cassady G, Schaefer J, et al. Serum gamma-M globulin responses in acute neonatal infections and their diagnostic significance. *J Pediatr* 1969;75:1271–1281.
133. Korones SB, Roane JA, Gilkeson MR, et al. Neonatal IgM response to acute infection. *J Pediatr* 1969;75:1261–1270.
134. Rothberg RM. Immunoglobulin and specific antibody synthesis during the first weeks of life of premature infant. *J Pediatr* 1969;75:391–399.
135. Khan WN, Ali RV, Werthmann M, et al. Immunoglobulin M determinations in neonates and infants as an adjunct to the diagnosis of infection. *J Pediatr* 1969;75:1282–1286.
136. Rothberg RM. Immunoglobulin and specific antibody synthesis during the first weeks of life of premature infants. *J Pediatr* 1969;75:391–399.
137. Adler SM, Denton RL. The erythrocyte sedimentation rate in the newborn period. *J Pediatr* 1975;86:942–948.
138. Evans HE, Glass L, Mercado C. The microerythrocyte sedimentation rate in newborn infants. *J Pediatr* 1970;76:448–451.
139. Milanovich RA, Maurer HM. Use of the microerythrocyte sedimentation rate (ESR) in the diagnosis of systemic infection in infants [Abstract]. *Proc Am Pediatr Soc/Soc Pediatr Res* 1971:230.
140. Bassol FA, Gutierrez LJ, Vargas LER. Velocidad de sedimentation globular como indice de infeccion en el recien nacido. *Bol Med Hosp Infant* 1978;35:507–510.
141. Moodley GP. The micro-erythrocyte sedimentation rate in black neonates and children. Part I. Its value in suspected neonatal infection. *S Afr Med J* 1981;59:943–944.
142. Philip AG, Hewitt JR. Early diagnosis of neonatal sepsis. *Pediatrics* 1980;65:1036–1041.

143. Gerdes JS, Polin RA. Sepsis screen in neonates with evaluation of plasma fibronectin. *Pediatr Infect Dis* 1987;6:443–446.
144. Speer C, Bruns A, Gahr M. Sequential determination of CRP, alpha 1-antitrypsin and haptoglobin in neonatal septicaemia. *Acta Paediatr Scand* 1983;72:679–683.
145. Rodwell RL, Leslie AL, Tudehope DI. Early diagnosis of neonatal sepsis using a hematologic scoring system. *J Pediatr* 1988;112:761–767.
146. Starr SE. Antimicrobial therapy of bacterial sepsis in the newborn infant. *J Pediatr* 1985;106:1043–1048.
147. Word BM, Klein JO. Current therapy of bacterial sepsis and meningitis in infants and children: a poll of directors of programs in pediatric infectious diseases. *Pediatr Infect Dis* 1988;7:267–271.
148. Bryan CS, John JF, Pai MS, et al. Gentamicin vs cefotaxime for therapy of neonatal sepsis. *Am J Dis Child* 1985;139:1086–1089.
149. Schauf V, Deveikis A, Riff L, et al. Antibiotic-killing kinetics of group B streptococci. *J Pediatr* 1976;89:194–198.
150. Dorand RD, Adams G. Relapse during penicillin treatment of group B streptococcal meningitis. *J Pediatr* 1976;89:188–190.
151. Truog WE, Davis RF, Ray CG. Recurrence of group B streptococcal infection. *J Pediatr* 1976;89:185–186.
152. Walker SH, Santos AQ, Quintero BA. Recurrence of group B III streptococcal meningitis. *J Pediatr* 1976;89:187–188.
153. Allen JL, Sprunt K. Discrepancy between minimum inhibitory and minimum bactericidal concentrations of penicillin for group A and group B beta-hemolytic streptococci. *J Pediatr* 1978;93:69–71.
154. Santos JI, Shigeoka AO, Rote NS, et al. Protective efficacy of a modified immune serum globulin in experimental group B streptococcal infection. *J Pediatr* 1981;99:873–879.
155. Shigeoka AO, Hall RT, Hill HR. Blood-transfusion in group B streptococcal sepsis. *Lancet* 1978;636–638.
156. Hall RT, Shigeoka AO, Hill HR. Serum opsonic activity and peripheral neutrophil counts before and after exchange transfusion in infants with early onset group B streptococcal septicemia. *Pediatr Infect Dis* 1983;2:356–358.
157. Christensen RD, Rothstein G, Hill HR, et al. Treatment of experimental group B streptococcal infection with hybridoma antibody. *Pediatr Res* 1984;18:1093–1096.
158. Christensen RD, Rothstein G, Hill HR, et al. The effect of hybridoma antibody administration upon neutrophil kinetics during experimental type III group B streptococcal sepsis. *Pediatr Res.* 1983;17:795–799.
159. Fischer GW, Hemming VG, Hunter KW, et al. Intravenous immunoglobulin in the treatment of neonatal sepsis: therapeutic strategies and laboratory studies. *Pediatr Infect Dis.* 1986;5:S171–S175.
160. Edwards MS, Rench MA, Haffar AAM, et al. Long-term sequelae of group B streptococcal meningitis in infants. *J Pediatr* 1985;106:717–722.
161. Chin KC, Fitzhardinge PM. Sequelae of early-onset group B hemolytic streptococcal neonatal meningitis. *J Pediatr* 1985;106:819–822.
162. Kaplan SL, Patrick CC. Cefotaxime and aminoglycoside treatment of meningitis caused by gram-negative enteric organisms. *Pediatr Infect Dis* 1990;9:810–814.
163. Mulhall A, DeLouvois J, Hurley R. Efficacy of chloramphenicol in the treatment of neonatal and infantile meningitis: a study of 70 cases. *Lancet* 1983;284–287.
164. Bortolussi R. Potential for intravenous gamma-globulin use in neonatal gram-negative infection: an overview. *Pediatr Infect Dis* 1986;5:S198–S200.
165. Finne J, Leinonen M, Mäkelä PH. Antigenic similarities between brain components and bacteria causing meningitis: implications for vaccine development and pathogenesis. *Lancet* 1983;2:355–357.
166. Curless R. Neonatal intracranial abscess: two cases caused by *Citrobacter* and a literature review. *Ann Neurol* 1980;8:269–272.
167. Greene GR, Heitlinger L, Madden J. *Citrobacter* ventriculitis in a neonate responsive to trimethoprim-sulfamethoxazole. *Clin Pediatr* 1983;22:515–517.
168. Kline MW, Kaplan SL. *Citrobacter diversus* and neonatal brain abscess. *Pediatr Neurol* 1987;3:178–180.
169. Salmon JH. Ventriculitis complicating meningitis. *Am J Dis Child* 1972;124:35–39.
170. Lee EL, Robinson MJ, Thong ML, et al. Intraventricular chemotherapy in neonatal meningitis. *J Pediatr* 1977;91:991–995.
171. Corbeel L, deBoeck K, Logghen F, et al. Treatment of purulent meningitis in infants. *Lancet* 1977;1:622–624.
172. Wright PF, Kaiser AB, Bowman CM, et al. The pharmacokinetics and efficacy of an aminoglycoside administered into the cerebral ventricles in neonates: implications for further evaluation of this route of therapy in meningitis. *J Infect Dis* 1981;143:141–147.
173. Pau AK, Smego RA, Fisher MA. Intraventricular vancomycin: observations of tolerance and pharmacokinetics in two infants with ventricular shunt infections. *Pediatr Infect Dis* 1986;5:93–96.
174. Pickering LK, Ericsson CD, Ruiz-Palacios G, et al. Intraventricular and parenteral gentamicin therapy for ventriculitis in children. *Am J Dis Child* 1978;132:480–483.
175. Wirt TC, McGee ZA, Oldfield EH, et al. Complicated gram-negative meningitis and ventriculitis. *J Neurosurg* 1979;50:95–99.
176. Gooskens JM, Gielen AM, Hanlo PW. Intracranial spaces in childhood macrocephaly; comparison of length measurements and volume calculations. *Dev Med Child Neurol* 1988;30:509–519.
177. Rieselbach RE, DiChiro G, Frojreich E, et al. Subarachnoid distribution of drugs after lumbar injection. *N Engl J Med* 1962;267:1273–1278.
178. McCracken GH Jr, Mize SG, Threlkeld N. Intraventricular gentamicin therapy in gram-negative bacillary meningitis of infancy. *Lancet* 1980;787–791.
179. Watanabe I, Hodges GR, Dworzack DL, et al. Neurotoxicity of intrathecal gentamicin: a case report and experimental study. *Ann Neurol* 1978;4:564–572.
180. Hodges GR, Watanabe I, Singer P, et al. Central nervous system toxicity of intraventricularly administered gentamicin in adult rabbits. *J Infect Dis* 1981;143:148–155.
181. Hodges GR, Wantanabe IS, Worley SE. Safety of intracisternal amikacin in adult rabbits. *Curr Ther Res* 1983;34:325–331.
182. Baker CJ, Rench MA, Edwards MS, et al. Immunization of pregnant women with a polysaccharide vaccine of group B streptococcus. *N Engl J Med* 1988;319:1180–1185.
183. Baker CJ, Edwards MS, Kasper DL. Role of antibody to native type III polysaccharide of group B streptococcus in infant infection. *Pediatrics* 1981;68:544–549.
184. Baker CJ, Rench MA, Kasper DL. Response to type III polysaccharide in women whose infants have had invasive group B streptococcal infection. *N Engl J Med* 1990;322:1857–1860.
185. Pandey JP, Baker CJ, Kasper DL, et al. Two unlinked genetic loci interact to control the human immune response to type III group B streptococcal antigen. *J Immunogenet* 1984;11:159–163.
186. Siegel JD, McCracken Jr GH, Threlkeld N, et al. Single dose penicillin prophylaxis against neonatal group B streptococcal infections. *N Engl J Med* 1980;303:769–775.
187. Pyati SP, Pildes RS, Jacobs NM, et al. Penicillin in infants weighing two kilograms or less with early-onset group B streptococcal disease. *N Engl J Med* 1983;308:1383–1389.
188. Yow MD, Mason EO, Leeds LJ, et al. Ampicillin prevents intrapartum transmission of group B streptococcus. *JAMA* 1979;241:1245–1247.
189. Boyer KM, Gotoff SP. Prevention of early-onset neonatal group B streptococcal disease with selective intrapartum chemoprophylaxis. *N Engl J Med* 1986;314:1665–1669.
190. Lim DV, Morales WJ, Walsh AF. Group B strep broth and coagglutination for rapid identification of group B streptococci in preterm pregnant women. *J Clin Microbiol* 1987;25:452–453.
191. Morell A, Sidiropoulos D, Herrmann U, et al. IgG subclasses and antibodies to group B streptococci, pneumococci, and tetanus toxoid in preterm neonates after intravenous infusion of immunoglobulin to the mothers. *Pediatr Res* 1986;20:933–936.
192. Kagan GM, Hess JH, Mirman B, et al. Meningitis in premature infants. *Pediatrics* 1949;4:479–483.
193. Groover RV, Sutherland JM, Landing BH. Purulent meningitis of newborn infants. *N Engl J Med* 1961;264:1115–1121.

194. Craig WS. *Care of the newly born infant,* 2nd ed. Baltimore: Williams & Wilkins, 1962;324–338.
195. *Kaiser Foundation Hospitals Report.* Panorama City, CA: 1988.
196. Mulder CJJ, Zaven HC. Neonatal meningitis in Nederlands. *Ned Tijdschr Geneeskd* 1979;123:1832–1831.
197. Ziai M, Haggerty RJ. Neonatal meningitis. *N Engl J Med* 1958;259:314–320.
198. Rodriguez AF, Kaplan SL, Mason Jr EO. Cerebrospinal fluid values in the very low birth weight infant. *J Pediatr* 1990;116:971–974.
199. Widell, S. The CSF protein and its fractions. *Acta Paediatr* 1958;S115:15–57.
200. Sarff LD, Platt LH, McCracken GH. Cerebrospinal fluid evaluation in neonates: comparison of high risk infants with and without meningitis. *J Pediatr* 1976;88:473–477.
201. Gyllensward A, Malmstrom S. The cerebrospinal fluid in immature infants. *Acta Paediatr* 1962;S135:54–62.
202. Naidoo BT. The cerebrospinal fluid in the healthy newborn infant. *S Afr Med J* 1968;42:933–935.

Infections of the Central Nervous System,
edited by W. M. Scheld, R. J. Whitley, and
D. T. Durack, Raven Press, Ltd., New York © 1991.

CHAPTER 16

Acute Bacterial Meningitis in Children and Adults

Karen L. Roos, Allan R. Tunkel, and W. Michael Scheld

The meningitis syndrome has been recognized for centuries. Hippocrates realized the important intracranial consequences of otitic infection, and clear clinical descriptions of meningitis have been found dating from the 16th century. However, the syndrome of epidemic meningitis with a purpuric rash was not identified until 1805; Viesseux described an epidemic of "malignant purpuric fever" surrounding Geneva, Switzerland, the first clinical description of meningococcemia with meningitis. The pathologic hallmark of the condition, inflammation within the subarachnoid space (SAS), was described in autopsy reports in the French literature the following year. Danielson and Mann recorded the first observations of meningococcemia and meningitis in the United States in 1806. Many of these early descriptions were collated in a treatise by Elisha North of Connecticut in 1811 (summarized in refs. 1 and 2). Then, as now, the disease could present dramatically in a fulminant form. The epidemic nature of meningococcemia was frightening to physicians and laypersons alike. For example, Dr. Samuel Woodward, of Torrington, Connecticut, wrote the following in *The American Mercury,* Hartford, in 1807:

> The violent symptoms were great lassitude, with universal pains in the muscles, chills; heats, if any, were of short duration; unusual prostration of strength; delerium, with severe pain in the head; vomiting, with undescribable

anxiety of stomach; eyes red and watery, and rolled up, and the head drawn back with spasm; pulse quick, weak, and irregular; petechiae and vibices all over the body, and a cadaverous countenance and smell; death often closed the scene in ten or fifteen hours after the first attack . . . the body, near the fatal period, and soon after, became as spotted as an adder. . . .

Similarly, the following was written by Rev. Festus Foster of Petersham, Massachusetts as a letter to the editor of *The Worchester Spy,* dated March 6, 1810:

> I hasten to give you a sketch of the spotted fever in this place. It made its first appearance about the beginning of January last; but the instances were few and distant from each other, until last week. Although it had proved fatal in most instances, seven only had died belonging to this town, previous to the 25th of February. Since that time the disorder has come upon us like a flood of mighty waters. We have buried eight persons within the last eight days. About twelve or fifteen new cases appeared on Thursday last; many of them very sudden and violent. This was the most melancholy and alarming day ever witnessed in this place. Seven or eight physicians were continually engaged in the neighborhood north of the meeting house, and I believe not one half hour passed in the forenoon without presenting a new case. Pale fear and extreme anxiety were visible in every countenance. . . .

It is inconceivable that this fulminant form of meningococcemia had been previously unrecognized, especially given the excellent clinical descriptions of rashes in the literature from the period. One must speculate that the virulence of meningococci for humans changed in the early 19th century.

Meningococci were first isolated in 1887 by Anton Weichselbaum in Vienna; they were obtained from the cerebrospinal fluid (CSF) of six patients with meningitis and were initially named *Diplococcus intracellularis meningitidis.* All three of the major meningeal patho-

K. L. Roos: Department of Neurology, Regenstrief Health Center, Indiana University Medical Center, Indianapolis, Indiana 46202.
A. R. Tunkel: Department of Medicine, Division of Infectious Diseases, Medical College of Pennsylvania, Philadelphia, Pennsylvania 19129.
W. M. Scheld: Department of Medicine, Division of Infectious Diseases, University of Virginia Health Sciences Center, Charlottesville, Virginia 22908.

gens (*Neisseria meningitidis, Streptococcus pneumoniae,* and *Hemophilus influenzae*) were isolated and described in the last two decades of the 19th century. Quincke introduced lumbar puncture in 1891, and the major CSF alterations associated with meningitis (pleocytosis, hypoglycorrhachia, and elevated protein) were well recognized by the turn of the century.

The treatment of bacterial meningitis in the early years of this century was dominated by methods for removal of large volumes of CSF and/or direct instillation of substances (e.g., dyes, enzymes, etc.) into the SAS. After early leads from European investigators, the first truly significant therapeutic modality for this disorder on a large scale was documented by Simon Flexner in 1913, utilizing systemic and intrathecal anti-meningococcal antisera raised in horses. Although toxic, antisera therapy reduced the mortality of meningococcal meningitis (from approximately 80% to 30%) during the First World War, and for decades thereafter. The principles of serum therapy were applied by Dr. Hattie Alexander and others to meningitis due to *H. influenzae* in the 1940s.

The approach to the patient with bacterial meningitis was profoundly altered by the advent of antimicrobial therapy. The first successful account of the therapy of meningococcal meningitis with an antimicrobial agent in this country was published by Schwentker et al. (3) in 1937; nine patients survived after receiving subcutaneous and intraspinal injections of sulfanilamide, and the sole death occurred after eradication of the organism from CSF. The introduction of penicillin and other antimicrobial agents (e.g., streptomycin, chloramphenicol, etc.) ushered in the modern antimicrobial era, likened to an industrial revolution (4). These developments led to the widespread belief that serious bacterial infections were "solved." Despite the introduction of a myriad of new antimicrobial agents and the development of newer diagnostic techniques, the mortality from meningitis due to the three major bacterial pathogens has not changed appreciably in the last four decades. However, the use of the third-generation cephalosporins during the 1980s for therapy of gram-negative aerobic bacillary meningitis has substantially reduced the mortality of this condition. Recent years have revealed an explosion of new knowledge on the pathogenesis and pathophysiol-

ogy of bacterial meningitis (see below), with attendant ramifications on the use of adjunctive therapy (e.g., corticosteroids, nonsteroidal anti-inflammatory agents, monoclonal antibodies, etc.) for this disease.

EPIDEMIOLOGY

Approximately 25,000 cases of bacterial meningitis occur annually in the United States, but this disease is much more common in developing countries (see below). About 70% of cases occur in children less than 5 years of age. The relative frequency with which each of the various bacterial species cause meningitis is age-related (Table 1). Gram-negative bacilli (principally *Escherichia coli* K1), other enteric bacilli, and, much less commonly, *Pseudomonas* species and group B streptococci are the major causative agent's during the neonatal period (Chapter 15). *Hemophilus influenzae* and *Neisseria meningitidis* are the major causes among children beyond 1 month of age. Meningitis in adults is primarily due to meningococci and pneumococci, although disease due to aerobic gram-negative bacilli is increasing in frequency, especially in the elderly. *N. meningitidis* is the only major cause of epidemics of bacterial meningitis. Recent trends indicate an increase in the proportion of cases due to gram-negative bacilli and *Listeria monocytogenes.*

The development of meningitis is dependent upon a complex array of factors, including virulence properties of the organisms, the carrier state, and the host's humoral immune response. Because these factors differ among the major pathogens, the epidemiology, the carrier state, and the role of host immunity are considered separately for each of the three major etiologic agents in this section. The classification of the pathogens, putative virulence factors, and the clinical settings associated with less prevalent agents, are discussed in the section entitled "Etiology."

Hemophilus influenzae

H. influenzae type b (Hib) is the leading cause of bacterial meningitis in the United States, with an estimated

TABLE 1. *Bacterial etiology of meningitis, stratified by age*

Organism	Neonates (≤1 month), %	Children (1 month to 15 years), %	Adults (>15 years), %
H. influenzae	0–3	40–60	1–3
N. meningitidis	0–1	25–40	10–35
S. pneumoniae	0–5	10–20	30–50
Gram-negative bacilli	50–60	1–2	1–10
Streptococci	20–40[a]	2–4	5
Staphylococci	5	1–2	5–15
Listeria species	2–10	1–2	5

[a] Nearly all isolates are group B streptococci.

11,000 cases annually. Other serious infections due to Hib also occur, particularly epiglottitis. Among 333 consecutive culture-proven cases of invasive Hib disease occurring in Finland from 1985 to 1986 (5), the proportion among disease entities was as follows: meningitis, 46%; epiglottitis, 29%; other forms of invasive disease (including arthritis, septicemia, cellulitis, pneumonia, and pyelonephritis), 25%. The proportion of meningitis cases was lower than the 60% reported in an earlier Finnish study (6). This spectrum also differed from that reported from the United States (7), where the meningitis-to-nonmeningitis ratio has a range of approximately 1.5:1 to 2:1. Although these differences may reflect genetic and/or socioeconomic factors or an underreporting of epiglottitis, they are likely explained by the superior surveillance system in Finland (8). Meningitis and epiglottitis are seen more frequently in boys than in girls (59% and 65%, respectively, in boys) (5), whereas the opposite pattern is observed among children with other forms of invasive Hib disease (44% boys). Meningitis due to Hib displays an interesting bimodal seasonal pattern in northern Europe and the northern United States (5,9), with peaks in June and September through November.

The overall annual incidence of serious Hib disease differs between geographic locales and among populations. Significant interannual variations in the incidence of meningitis due to Hib have also been reported within a single geographic area over time (10), an important consideration in assessing the efficacy of Hib vaccines. The overall rate of Hib meningitis in the United States is ~60 per 100,000 children less than 5 years of age (7), greater than the figures from Finland (26 per 100,000 children less than 5 years of age) (5,8) and other countries in northern Europe. These incidence rates differ markedly among age groups (see below) and in children less than 6 years of age. The mean incidence in King County, Washington from 1977 to 1986 also confirms the predilection for Hib meningitis in boys (89.1 per 100,000) when compared with girls (37.4 per 100,000;

$p < 0.001$) (10). The age-specific incidence rate for children less than 5 years of age also differs among geographic areas within the United States (Table 2). Some of this variability is due to active versus passive case reporting. Some studies report a higher incidence in nonwhites (9,14). For example, the incidence rate for Hib meningitis for the total population of Washington State was 2.2, 3.4, and 13.5 per 100,000 for whites, blacks, and native Americans, respectively (14). In contrast, others (12) have found no differences between rates for blacks and whites less than 1 year of age.

The epidemiology of Hib meningitis reveals a striking age distribution: Nearly all cases occur in children less than 5 years of age. Prior to the availability of the current Hib vaccines, one in every 200 children developed invasive Hib disease by 5 years of age. Meningitis due to Hib in the first 2 months of life is rare, presumably due to placental transfer of protective concentrations of maternal bactericidal antibody. Most cases occur between 4 months and 2 years of age. The median age of onset in Finnish children is 1.5 years (5,8). The highest rate of illness occurs in U.S. children 6–17 months of age (Table 3); children more than 2 years old have lower incidence (5–8,10–15). Approximately 80% of cases develop in children less than 2 years old in this country, but this proportion varies by geographic locale. The proportion of cases is approximately 20% lower in this age group in northern European countries (Table 4). These differences in age distribution may directly influence the efficacy of candidate Hib vaccines. Epiglottitis occurs in older children (median age ~ 3.5 years). The age distribution is dependent on multiple factors, chiefly acquisition of the organism and the host immune status.

Nontypable strains of *H. influenzae* are commonly carried in the nasopharynx of asymptomatic individuals. Carriage of encapsulated strains (usually type b) is rare: less than 5% in children and less than 1% in adults. However, the carriage rates among household contacts of an index case are much higher: 20–25% overall and greater

TABLE 2. *Comparison of age-specific incidence of Hib meningitis in children ≤ 5 years of age—United States*[a]

Reference	Geographic area	Years of study	Mean number of cases per year	Age-specific incidence rate in children <5 years of age (per 100,000)
11	Charleston County, South Carolina	1961–1971	20	38.0
12	Baltimore City and Baltimore County, Maryland	1965–1975	25	19.3
13	Fresno County, California	1976–1978	24	46.5[b]
14	State of Washington	1977	79	31.8
10	King County, Washington	1977–1986	42	49.0
15	Bethel, Alaska	1980–1982	22[c]	68.6

[a] Adapted from ref. 10.
[b] Includes children 1–4 years old.
[c] Includes only non-natives.

TABLE 3. *Mean incidence of Hib meningitis by age group—King County, Washington, 1977–1986[a]*

Age class (months)	Mean incidence per 100,000
0–5	63.5
6–11	128.2
12–17	118.0
18–23	64.7
24–35	36.0
36–47	16.1
48–59	8.5
Overall, <60	49.6

[a] Adapted from ref. 10.

than 50% among children less than 5 years old. This varies with the clinical setting. For example, carriage rates among children ≤ 5 years old are 20% and 55% for household contacts of epiglottitis and meningitis cases, respectively. This prevalence is reflected in the increased risk of serious Hib disease among household contacts of the index case, which is age-dependent: 4% for children ≤ 2 years of age, 2% for children 2–3 years old, and 0.1% for children 4–5 years of age, respectively. The risk of Hib infection among household contacts is approximately 600-fold greater than the age-adjusted risk for the population at large and is the basis for chemoprophylaxis strategies. Carriage is usually asymptomatic and may occur despite the presence of circulating anticapsular antibodies or effective eradication of the meningitis following antibiotic therapy. The Hib carrier state may persist for weeks to months.

The occurrence of Hib meningitis is inversely proportional to the age-related concentration of type-specific anticapsular antibodies (16). Finnish studies, measuring

TABLE 4. *Age distribution of children with Hib meningitis among different populations[a]*

Country or population	Time interval	Proportion (%) of children ≤6 months	≤2 years
Finland	1976–1981	7	61
Finland	1985–1986	5	59
Sweden	1971–1980	10	54
The Netherlands	1975–1983	n.a.[b]	64
United States Michigan	1974–1977	n.a.	69
White Mountain Apaches	1973–1982	38	100
Alaskan Eskimos	1980–1982	34	91
Dallas, Texas	1982–1984	16	92
Minnesota	1982–1984	20	84
United States (estimate)	1984	19	81
Southern Israel	1981–1985	33	90
Australian aborigines	1985–1986	n.a.	100

[a] Adapted from, and summarized in, ref. 8.
[b] n.a., not analyzed.

anti-polyribosyl-ribitol phosphate (anti-PRP) antibodies by radioimmunoassay, confirm the age-related susceptibility to systemic Hib disease: 90% of children (3–12 months old) had concentrations ≤ 150 ng/ml, whereas adults had higher concentrations (17). These anti-PRP antibodies are, in concert with complement, both (a) opsonic and bactericidal against Hib *in vitro* and (b) protective *in vivo*. Antibodies to Hib outer-membrane proteins also appear protective, but only against the homologous subtype. The anti-PRP response to infection is age-related, being poor in infants; older children and adults develop higher titers. It is also dependent on PRP concentrations and clearance rates. PRP antigenemia may persist for weeks in younger children with Hib meningitis, delaying the antibody response. Approximately 80% of children with Hib meningitis develop an antibody response within 3 months. The antibody response is blunted in children with agammaglobulinemia or IgG_2 subclass deficiency, as well as in all children ≤ 24 months of age receiving the Hib PRP vaccine, since this polysaccharide is a poor immunogen in this age group (7; see below). The age-related acquisition of protective anticapsular antibodies is too rapid to be accounted for by the low incidence of carriage or disease due to Hib alone. Cross-reacting antigens from *E. coli* and other bacteria within the gut are postulated to serve as the primary immunogen.

Acquisition of Hib (nasopharyngeal carriage) and the concentration of circulating anticapsular antibody are the two main factors which determine risk for disease in most subjects. Some of these risk factors have been alluded to above (e.g., immunoglobulin or complement deficiency, household contacts of an index case, etc.). Other conditions which also may be important in increasing susceptibility to invasive Hib infection include sickle cell anemia, postsplenectomy states, CSF fistulas, chronic pulmonary infections, alcoholism, and probably lower socioeconomic status, (e.g., Eskimos and American Indians). A recent population-based matched case–control analysis of risk factors for invasive Hib disease conducted among 117 patients in Finland during 1985 and 1986 (18) confirms and extends this information. Day care outside the home and the presence of young siblings increased the risk of invasive disease, whereas breast-feeding was protective. The risk was highest for children less than 2 years old in day care but was not apparent for older children, was equally high for those in a family day-care setting or those in a professional day-care center (mean group size 4 and 12 children, respectively), and was significantly higher ($p < 0.02$) within the first month of attendance, especially among younger children (18). The risk ratio doubled with each additional sibling younger than 7 years of age and was higher in twins (18). New associations were also found suggesting that the child's previous state of health, especially a history of otitis media and/or previous hospitalization, also increased the risk of serious Hib disease. Otitis media remained significant, especially for the younger children, even after controlling for confounding variables such as day-care attendance (19). Pharyngitis and otitis media are associated with Hib meningitis in approximately one-half and two-thirds of the cases, respectively. The protective effect of breast-feeding (18,19) may explain why Finnish children with Hib disease were somewhat older, due to the more common practice and longer duration of breast-feeding in Finland when compared to the United States.

Because of the bimodal seasonal occurrence of Hib meningitis, at least in northern latitudes, it has been suggested that preceding viral upper respiratory tract infections predispose to the acquisition of Hib and subsequent disease, but this issue remains controversial (20). Recent studies comparing the attack rates of meningitis between two ethnic groups living together in one geographic area (Jews and Bedouins in the Negev region of Israel) suggested that community-acquired bacterial meningitis is associated more strongly with the type of morbidity most prevalent in the region at any given time (e.g., upper respiratory tract or gastrointestinal infections) rather than any specific type of infection (21).

The occurrence of meningitis due to Hib in children more than 6 years old should prompt efforts to exclude common accompanying conditions such as otitis media, CSF leaks, an immunodeficiency state, other parameningeal foci of infection, and alcoholism.

Neisseria meningitidis

Meningococcal infections continue to pose serious problems on all continents (Table 5). They are influenced by multiple factors, including geography, season, climate, meningococcal serogroup, and population demographics (2,22). Although worldwide in distribution, the incidence of epidemic meningococcal meningitis and/or meningococcemia exhibits high geographic variability. The meningitis belt of sub-Saharan Africa (Fig. 1) represents a classic endemic area. Although meningococcal infections were not recorded in the area until the 1880s, large outbreaks still occur regularly. Although the precise effects of climatic conditions on the incidence of meningitis are unresolved, the belt lies within the 300- and 1100-mm rainfall lines. At least 390,000 cases with 53,000 deaths occurred within the seven countries of the belt in the 10-year period 1951–1960. The average annual incidence since 1950 has been estimated as approximately 70 cases/10^5 population by the World Health Organization (22). Similarly, within a 1-month period (October 1974), 4865 patients with meningococcal meningitis were treated at the major infectious diseases hospital in Sao Paulo, Brazil. The overall mean annual incidence of meningitis due to *N.*

TABLE 5. *Countries in which epidemics of meningococcal disease occurred during the 1970s*[a]

Continent or region	Country or territory
Africa	Chad
	Ghana
	Federal Republic of Cameroon
	Nigeria
	Senegal
	Togo
	Mauritania
	Burkina Faso
Asia	Jordan
	Syrian Arab Republic
	Mongolia
	Turkey
	Vietnam
	Bahrain
	Lao People's Democratic Republic
Europe	Finland
	Norway
	Iceland
	Great Britain
	Belgium
	The Netherlands
	Spain
	Greece
	Romania
	U.S.S.R.
North America	United States
Central America	Guatemala
	Costa Rica
South America	Brazil
	Uruguay
	Argentina
Oceania	New Caledonia
	New Hebrides

[a] Modified from ref. 22.

meningitidis reached 370 cases per 100,000 population in the greater Sao Paulo area in that year (Table 6). The attack rate was 517 cases per 100,000 inhabitants during a group C epidemic in Upper Volta (now Birkina Faso) in 1979, and recent studies documented an attack rate of 400–450 per 100,000 population in the 0- to 8-year-old age group in the Faroe Islands (23). In contrast, the mean annual attack rate in the United States (1975–1980) was approximately 1.2 per 100,000 persons but was, again, age-dependent: 17.1 per 100,000 under 1 year of age, 5.2 per 100,000 in 1- to 4-year-old children, and 0.3 per 100,000 among adults. Approximately 2500 cases of meningococcal infection were reported annually in the United States between 1984 and 1986. A similar figure of approximately 2 per 100,000 population was reported from Finland for the period 1976–1980.

The peak incidence of meningococcal meningitis in industrialized nations occurs in winter through early spring in both epidemic and endemic periods. Similar seasonal trends may also occur in tropical areas. For example, both the group C and A meningococcal epi-

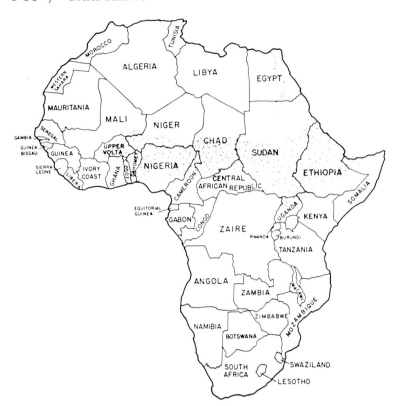

FIG. 1. The "meningitis belt" of sub-Saharan Africa; that is, areas of Africa which experience repeated epidemics of serogroup A meningococcal meningitis. (From ref. 23, with permission.)

demics in the Sao Paulo area from 1971 to 1974 began in May or June, the point of transition from the rainy to the dry season. African outbreaks occur during the dry season from December to June. Annual outbreaks in the sub-Saharan meningitis belt tend to peak in late April–early May, when the dry desert wind (harmattan) has ceased and temperatures are high throughout the day, terminating abruptly with the onset of the rainy season (22). Low humidity may alter the pharyngeal mucosal barrier, thereby predisposing it to infection. Although the introduction of a new virulent strain into a susceptible population may contribute to the epidemics, many other factors, including crowding, the presence of other respiratory pathogens, poor hygiene, and poorly defined environmental features contribute to the initiation of a meningococcal epidemic (24).

Although meningococcal meningitis may be more prevalent in males, the reports are often skewed by the inclusion of military recruits and chronic alcoholics. Meningitis due to *N. meningitidis* is primarily a disease of children and young adults (Table 1): Fewer than 10% of cases occur in patients over 45 years old. In the United States and Finland, children under 5 years of age account for approximately 55% of cases during nonepidemic conditions, whereas in Zaria, Nigeria the peak incidence occurs in 5- to 9-year-olds (23). Major epidemics are heralded by a "shift to the right" towards older age groups (i.e., adolescents instead of children), a predictive feature of epidemics in the meningitis belt identified by prospective surveillance.

Large-scale epidemics due to serogroup A meningococci have occurred at 20- to 30-year intervals throughout the world in this century and continue at approximately 8- to 12-year intervals in the African meningitis belt, where approximately 1% of the population is affected. These strains infrequently cause disease in the United States, but serious outbreaks due to serogroups A, B, or C continue in many areas (Table 6). Serogroups B and C now cause most focal outbreaks and endemic disease in many areas (see section entitled "Etiology," below).

N. meningitidis disease is exclusive to humans. No intermediate host, reservoir, or animal-to-human transmission has been proven. The nasopharynx is the natural reservoir for meningococci; transmission is facilitated by airborne droplets or close contact. Meningococcal colonization may result in an asymptomatic carrier state (which is most common) or in endemic, hyperendemic (i.e., meningitis belt between epidemics at 10–50 cases per 100,000 per year), or epidemic disease. Although there is no clear relationship between carriage rate and overt disease, the development of the carrier state and the host immune response are, as for Hib meningitis, important variables in the epidemiology of meningococcal infections.

Approximately 6% of the population develops nasopharyngeal colonization with *N. meningitidis* yearly. Nasopharyngeal carriage rates vary with age and the population under study. The carriage rate is markedly influenced by age: 0.5–1% in children 3–48 months old,

TABLE 6. *Incidence and serogroups of selected meningococcal epidemics during the 1970s[a]*

Serogroup	Location and year(s)	Maximal incidence (per 100,000 per year)	Number of cases reported
A	Brazil (Sao Paulo area), 1974	370	30,555 per year
A	Finland, 1974	15	687 per year
A	Nigeria (Zaria), 1977		1257 in 3 months
B	Norway, 1973	24	112 per year
B	Belgium, 1969–1976	5	519 per year
C	Brazil (Sao Paulo area), 1971–1972	11	2005 in 2 years
C	Vietnam, 1972–1978	20	>1000 per year

[a] Adapted from ref. 22.

approximately 5% in adolescents 14–17 years old, and 20–40% in young adults. Analogous to Hib, carriage rates are higher in close contacts of an index case. Carriage rates of meningococci of approximately 40% have been documented in close family contacts of meningococcal cases. In closed populations (e.g., military barracks during early training), carriage rates of 20–60% are commonplace and may reach 90% during epidemics of meningococcal disease. Nasopharyngeal carriage usually persists for weeks to months, similar to Hib carriage. Spread of meningococcal disease is usually carrier-mediated (i.e., not spread by case-to-case contacts) and largely accounts for the increased risk of disease (500- to 1000-fold above the background endemic rate) in household contacts of an index case. The organism is often introduced into the home environment by an adult family member, with subsequent transmission to others; infants are colonized last of all. Although uncharacterized host and environmental factors contribute to containment of infection to the nasopharynx (thereby preventing disseminated disease), host immunity also plays an important role. Nevertheless, those individuals most recently colonized with meningococci appear to be at the greatest risk of invasive disease.

Analogous to Hib disease, the age-specific incidence of meningococcal infection is inversely proportional to the presence of serum bactericidal antibodies against serogroups A, B, and C. More than 50% of infants possess bactericidal antibody at birth as a result of transplacental transfer. The specifics of the antibody response may be responsible for the occurrence of meningococcal meningitis during the neonatal period. The group B capsular polysaccharide is a polymer consisting of two to eight linked sialic acid residues but is immunologically identical to the oligosaccharides of several human glycoproteins, including brain gangliosides. Immunologic tolerance thus exists in this age group; although IgM antibody can be induced, the usual switch to IgG antibody production does not occur (23). Since IgM does not cross the placenta, IgG antibody to the serogroup B polysaccharide is lacking in neonates, contributing to the occurrence of group B meningococcal disease in this patient population (Chapter 15). In addition, group B meningo-

coccal capsular antigen is identical to the capsular polysaccharides of *E. coli* K1 and certain types of group B streptococci (Chapter 15), major causes of neonatal sepsis and meningitis. The prevalence of antimeningococcal capsular antibodies is lowest between 6 and 24 months of age, increasing to approximately 70% by early adulthood. The inverse link between occurrence of invasive disease and bactericidal antibody was first documented during an outbreak of serogroup C meningococcal meningitis among army recruits in 1968 (25). In this study, the sera of only 5.6% of the recruits who developed meningococcal disease had bactericidal activity before the onset of illness, compared with 82.2% in control sera. Notably, 5 of 13 recruits (38.5%) without bactericidal antibody developed systemic illness after colonization with the group C strain.

Although recovery from invasive meningococcal disease generally confers lifelong immunity against the homologous serogroup, this is not the major immunizing process. Nasopharyngeal colonization, particularly with serogroups B, C, or Y, may elicit the development of bactericidal activity, primarily directed against the colonizing strain but also against heterologous organisms within 5–12 days of acquisition. Colonization with nongroupable meningococci or *N. lactamica* may elicit protective immunity, especially in young children. *N. lactamica* is virtually nonpathogenic, but nasopharyngeal carriage rates of this organism are highest (4–20%) in children between 3 months and 12 years of age whereas the age-adjusted carriage rates for *N. meningitidis* are only 0.5–2%. Analogous to Hib, the carriage rates of pathogenic meningococci are too low in children to account for antibody formation, and the importance of other cross-reacting organisms has also been proposed: *Bacillus pumilis* for group A polysaccharide, and *E. coli* for group C organisms. Paradoxically, an exuberant IgA response to meningococci may actually enhance the development of systemic disease. When a large proportion of induced anticapsular antibodies are of the IgA class, complement-mediated immune bacteriolysis by IgM is blocked, thus enhancing susceptibility to invasive disease. This peculiar immunologic phenomenon is transient, lasting only a few days following asymptomatic nasopharyngeal acquisition of *N. meningitidis* or closely related organisms.

In addition to antibody, an intact complement system is also a component of host defense against invasive meningococcal disease. Recurrent or chronic neisserial infections have been associated with rare isolated deficiencies of late complement components (C5, C6, C7, or C8, and perhaps C9) occasionally in concert with failure to produce antimeningococcal antibodies. Recurrent episodes of neisserial infections may occur in these patients without an increase in susceptibility to other pathogens (26), and screening for complement defects is useful in patients with these syndromes. In addition, complement deficiency or depletion of early components (C1, C3, or C4) due to an underlying disease such as nephrotic syndrome, hepatic failure, systemic lupus erythematosis, C3 nephritic factor, or multiple myeloma may predispose to the first episode of invasive meningococcal disease. Recently, an association between homozygous C4b deficiency (present in ~3% of the population) and the development of childhood meningitis was demonstrated. Up to 30% of patients with invasive meningococcal syndromes display decreased complement function. Properdin deficiency, or dysfunction with normal concentrations, also predisposes to fulminant meningococcal infections, a defect reversible by vaccination (27). Asplenic states increase the risk of serious infections due to encapsulated organisms, especially Hib or *S. pneumoniae* but also meningococci.

Although all of the above factors (particularly recent colonization with a pathogenic strain in a nonimmune host) undoubtedly contribute to the pathogenesis of meningococcal disease, the precise determinants contributing to overt clinical illness (as opposed to the usual outcome of asymptomatic carriage) are poorly defined. Only one in 1000–5000 infected patients develops disease (23), even during epidemics. Various predisposing factors, including crowding, lower socioeconomic status, and poor general health, have been proposed to explain the increased incidence in U.S. blacks and among alcoholics in Finland or Alaska (22), but the influence of such conditions (e.g., overcrowding) has not been supported by studies in Nigeria. An antecedent viral infection has been suggested as another predisposing factor, since approximately one-third of meningococcal cases follow symptoms referable to the upper respiratory tract. An outbreak of meningococcal disease followed a large influenza epidemic in Texas in 1981, and simultaneous outbreaks of meningococcal and influenza A2 infections have been described in institutional settings. Although meningococcal pneumonia may complicate influenza (e.g., the 1918–1919 pandemic), the role of viral infections in the enhancement of meningococcal dissemination is unproven (20).

The time from nasopharyngeal acquisition to bloodstream invasion is short (usually ≤10 days). The incubation period may also be short, since "secondary" cases commonly occur within 1–4 days of the index case. Furthermore, only 20% of prospectively studied military recruits actually carried the organism within 7 days of hospitalization for meningococcal disease. Once the organism is blood-borne, over 90% of meningococcal disease is manifest as meningitis and/or meningococcemia.

Streptococcus pneumoniae

Although pneumococcal meningitis occurs in all age groups (Table 1), pneumococci remain the most common cause of bacterial meningitis in adults. Approximately 2600–6200 cases occur in the United States yearly. The annual incidence of pneumococcal meningitis has remained relatively stable in the United States for the past three decades. In seven studies analyzing data from diverse geographic areas in this country from 1959 to 1978, the annual incidence was 0.3–2.3 per 100,000 population, with a mean of 1.3 per 100,000. An identical infection rate of 1.3 per 100,000 persons per year was recorded from the Oklahoma City area in 1984 (28); higher rates of invasive pneumococcal disease were reported at the extremes of age (see below), in males, and among blacks and American Indians when compared to whites. Nearly identical incidence figures (1.2–1.4 per 100,000 population per year) were reported from the Göteborg, Sweden area for the years 1964 through 1980 (29). Pneumococcal meningitis was, again, more common in males, and most cases occurred from December through May. However, higher incidence rates have been reported from other areas. For example, surveillance studies from 1980 to 1986 among the Alaskan native population in the Yukon–Kusko–Kurin delta region of southwestern Alaska documented an extremely high frequency of invasive pneumococcal disease; the annual rate for pneumococcal meningitis was 13.2 per 100,000 persons overall (30). Perhaps more importantly, the annual incidence rate was 216 per 100,000 children under 2 years of age—18 times higher than that reported from Sweden (29), and 36- to 37-fold greater than United States rates derived from both passive and active surveillance (9,30). These rates of bacteriologically confirmed invasive pneumococcal disease are the highest reported for any population worldwide. Although the majority of the cases of invasive pneumococcal disease occurred during the Arctic summer, pneumococcal meningitis cases clustered in the winter (30), similar to other reports (9).

The risk of pneumococcal meningitis is age-dependent, with increased incidence rates occurring at the extremes of age. For example, the number of cases per 100,000 persons per year in the Göteborg, Sweden area for 1970 through 1980 were as follows: 12.0 for infants less than 12 months of age, 0.4–0.9 for children and adults 2–39 years old, 1.2–1.6 for persons 40–70 years old, and 2.2 for those over 70 years of age (29). The dramatic incidence among Alaskan native children under 2 years of age (216 per 100,000 annually) are noted above. Similarly, the annual incidence rates for all invasive pneumococcal infections (including bacteremic pneumonia) in the Oklahoma City area in 1984 were (a) 97 per 100,000 for infants less than 1 year of age and (b) 87 per 100,000 for elderly adults over age 80.

As with the other major meningeal pathogens, pneumococcal meningitis follows recent nasopharyngeal colonization by a virulent strain. The rate of asymptomatic carriage varies with age, environment, geographic locale, and the presence of an upper respiratory tract infection. Pneumococci have been isolated from the upper respiratory tract of 5–70% of normal adults; approximately 25% acquire a new strain annually. Carriage rates decline with age (30–35% for children aged 6–11 years and 18–19% in adults) and are higher in closed populations (e.g., 27–58% in schools and orphanages, 50–60% in closed military populations). The duration of pneumococcal carriage varies from weeks to months and is longer in children than in adults. Most carrier strains in the normal population are of higher-numbered capsular types and only infrequently are associated with invasive disease (see below). Carriage is prolonged in individuals with low serum antibody concentrations against the homologous capsular type before colonization. Spread of this organism within the family unit is influenced by crowding, the season (greater in fall and winter), and the presence of pneumococcal disease (particularly pneumonia and otitis media). The precise relationship between pneumococcal carriage and the development of protective immunity is poorly defined. Over 50% of children develop a rise in type-specific antibody concentrations following colonization; this is rarely observed in adults, perhaps because of the relatively high antibody concentrations already present in adults. Nevertheless, otitis media often occurs in colonized infants despite the presence of type-specific antibodies. Antibody concentrations generally decline with time despite persistent carriage of a given strain (31). In addition, antibody responses to different capsular types vary considerably and are generally poor in infants under 2 years of age. Specific antibody responses tend to be higher after repetitive periods of nasopharyngeal carriage than after continuous ones. The antibody response after pneumococcal colonization, its influence on subsequent disease, and the impact of other environmental antigens require further study.

Several factors predispose to pneumococcal meningitis (Table 7) (32). Pneumonia coexists much more commonly with pneumococcal meningitis (15–25% of patients) than with the other two major pathogens. Acute otitis media is seen in approximately 30% of patients with pneumococcal meningitis; acute sinusitis

TABLE 7. *Conditions associated with pneumococcal meningitis*

Pneumonia (~15–25% of patients)
Otitis media
Sinusitis
CSF fistulae, leak
Head injury
Alcoholism, cirrhosis
Sickle-cell disease, thalassemia major
Other asplenic states
Wiskott–Aldrich syndrome
Multiple myeloma

may also be an important antecedent event. Pneumococci are the most common cause of recurrent meningitis in the setting of CSF leaks. Recent or remote head trauma is found in about 10% of patients with pneumococcal meningitis. Alcoholism, cirrhosis, and/or spontaneous bacterial peritonitis are underlying disorders in approximately 20–35% of patients with this disease. Pneumococci are the most common cause of meningitis in children with sickle cell anemia and commonly cause meningitis in other asplenic states or in the setting of primary or acquired immunodeficiencies. *S. pneumoniae* causes 87% of pyogenic meningitis in sickle cell disease; cases in the 2- to 3-year-old group occur at a rate of 12 per 1000 patient-years. The risk of pneumococcal meningitis in this age group of children with sickle cell anemia is increased 36-fold when compared with that observed in control black children, and it is increased 314-fold over that observed in whites. Pneumococcal meningitis also occurs with increased frequency in persons with the Wiskott–Aldrich syndrome, thalassemia major, childhood nephrotic syndrome, multiple myeloma, and chronic lymphocytic leukemia. Defects in immunoglobulin concentration or function, as well as poor alternative-complement-pathway-mediated opsonization of pneumococci, are common in many of these disorders.

ETIOLOGY

The etiologic agents responsible for bacterial meningitis in four geographic areas, each representing a different continent, are listed in Table 8. Although some differences between geographic locales are apparent, the similarities are striking. Worldwide, the three major meningeal pathogens (*H. influenzae, N. meningitidis,* and *S. pneumoniae*) account for ~75–80% of cases, but the proportion due to each organism is somewhat variable. All age groups are represented in the data in Table 8, thus including pathogens of neonates such as group B streptococci and aerobic gram-negative bacilli (Chapter 15).

The most recent information from the United States (Table 8) was compiled by the National Bacterial Meningitis Surveillance Study (9). The data are based on pas-

TABLE 8. *Etiology of bacterial meningitis in four geographic areas*[a]

Organism	Percentage of total cases			
	United States 1978–1981	United Kingdom 1980–1984	Dakar, Senegal 1970–1979	Salvador, Brazil 1973–1982
H. influenzae	48	29	20	23
N. meningitidis	20	25	11	32
S. pneumoniae	13	20	29	17
Group B streptococci	3	7	4	2
L. monocytogenes	2	2	<0.5	—
Other	8	16	9	8
Unknown	6		26	19

[a] Compiled from refs. 9 and 33–36.

sive prospective reporting of 13,974 cases from 27 participating states for the years 1978 through 1981. An estimated 30–40% of all cases were actually reported for this study. *H. influenzae* was the most common etiologic agent in the United States, accounting for nearly one-half of the total number of cases. More than 30% of cases were meningococcal or pneumococcal in origin. Staphylococci and aerobic gram-negative bacilli (particularly *E. coli*) were prominent pathogens in the "other" category. From an analysis of attack rates in this study (9), underreporting obviously occurred, but the relative frequency of causative organisms was very similar to results reported in studies based on active surveillance in the United States during recent years.

The data from the United Kingdom (Table 8) were derived from a laboratory-based surveillance system for infectious diseases organized by the Public Health Laboratory Service in England, Wales, and Ireland, and is comprised of 7605 cases reported for the 5-year period 1980–1984 (33). Only culture-proven cases are shown; the proportion of cases of unknown etiology cannot be ascertained from the data provided by the Communicable Disease Surveillance Center. Although *H. influenzae* was the most common etiologic agent, it accounted for only 28.5% of cases in the United Kingdom, less than the relative frequency in the United States, whereas the percentage of cases due to meningococci and pneumococci are both higher in the British Isles. The proportion of cases due to staphylococci, streptococci, and *E. coli* were all greater in the United Kingdom when compared to those in the United States.

Little information is available on the etiology of bacterial meningitis throughout tropical Africa (34). Most data are derived from large urban centers, since cultural confirmation at rural facilities is seldom achieved. Furthermore, the relative frequency of agents is highly dependent on the geographic area, with meningococcal isolates predominating in reports from countries within the meningitis belt (Fig. 1) (34). The data in Table 8 from Dakar, Senegal (outside the meningitis belt) were compiled in one of the most recent series (2415 cases) from Africa (1970–1979) and indicate only culture-positive

results (35). The prominence of pneumococcal meningitis is apparent, and the proportion due to *H. influenzae* is similar to that of the United Kingdom. Although meningococci caused only 15% of cases in Dakar, this organism was responsible for 63–89% of cases from Burkina Faso and Chad, two countries in the meningitis belt, in the early 1970s. *Salmonella* species were more common etiologic agents among bacterial meningitis cases in Africa, accounting for 4% of cases in Dakar, whereas *L. monocytogenes* was rarely implicated (only two of 2415 cases in the Senegalese survey) (35).

Little is known of the current etiology and mortality of meningitis in less developed nations, especially in Latin America. The data from Brazil (Table 8) are derived from an analysis of cases admitted to the major isolation–fever hospital in Salvador for the decade 1973–1982 (36). During this time, 24,171 patients were admitted to Couta Maia Hospital; 6751 cases (27% of all admissions) were diagnosed as having meningitis. Of these, 4100 cases (61%) were felt to represent a bacterial etiology based on strict inclusion criteria and thus constitute one of the largest series analyzed in the past 30 years. Bacterial meningitis accounted for 17% of all admissions to the hospital during this period; 79% of cases occurred in children less than 15 years of age. Although meningococci were isolated most frequently (32% of cases; Table 8), this was largely due to sequential epidemics of serogroup C followed by serogroup A in 1975 and 1978 (36). The current annual incidence of meningococcal meningitis in Salvador is ~4 per 100,000 per year. Although pneumococcal meningitis cases remained relatively stable at ~17% of the total per year during the decade, the number of cases due to Hib more than doubled. Hib is now responsible for 43% of cases and is the most frequently isolated pathogen from meningitis patients in northeastern Brazil. Together, the three major pathogens accounted for 71.8% of all cases and 88% of all bacteriologically confirmed cases. Gram-negative bacilli were responsible for 7.9% of cases. Similar to the experience in Dakar, 44% of the Enterobacteriaceae isolates were *Salmonella* species, an infrequent cause of gram-negative bacillary meningitis in industrialized nations. Nearly all of these cases of *Salmonella* meningitis occurred in children less than 2 years of age. Meningitis due to group B streptococci, staphylococci, or *L. monocytogenes* is relatively rare in Brazil at present. Cases presumed to be bacterial in origin but in which the CSF culture and Gram's stain were negative accounted for 18% of cases.

In the following sections, each of the major meningeal pathogens is considered, including relevant classification schemes. In addition, the potential virulence characteristics of each organism are briefly discussed.

Hemophilus influenzae

Hemophilus species are small, gram-negative, pleomorphic coccobacilli. They are facultative anaerobes which grow best anaerobically with 5–10% CO_2 on blood-enriched media. *H. influenzae* requires both X factor (hematin) and V factor (NAD, NADP, or nicotinamide nucleoside) for growth under aerobic conditions and is nonhemolytic. Chocolate agar is most commonly employed for the initial isolation of *H. influenzae.*

H. influenzae strains are either encapsulated (typable) or unencapsulated (nontypable). Encapsulated strains are classified into six groups, types a through f, by specific reactions with antisera directed against epitopes on capsular antigens. Methods for grouping include: counterimmunoelectrophoresis; latex particle agglutination of culture supernatants; immunofluorescence; and the production of halos surrounding colonies on media containing antisera. Nearly all invasive *H. influenzae* infections are due to serotype b (Hib). The capsule is a repeating polymer of polyribosyl-ribitol phosphate (PRP), an important virulence determinant of this organism (see below). Hib also contains a lipo-oligosaccharide (here designated "LPS" for convenience) in the outer membrane, an additional virulence determinant. Hib strains have been further classified into subtypes based on electrophoretic mobility differences among outer-membrane proteins (OMPs). Although the pathogenic role of these OMPs is uncertain, subtype analysis is useful for epidemiologic studies. For example, in a survey of 256 invasive isolates from 22 states representing a variety of clinical settings, ~70% of cases were due to strains of three subtypes (1H, 2L, and 3L) among the 21 OMP subtypes identified. In contrast, 84% of 80 invasive isolates studied in the Netherlands had the same OMP subtype pattern (type 1, identical to subtype 3L in the Granoff classification system), and no strains of subtype 1H, 1L, or 2H were found.

It has been recently recognized, largely on the basis of multilocus enzyme electrophoretic analysis by Musser et al. (37), that the natural populations of Hib from widely divergent geographic areas are clonal as a consequence of infrequent recombination of chromosomal genes. For example, 32 distinct multilocus enzyme genotypes referred to as "electrophoretic types" (ETs) were apparent among 177 United States isolates by analysis of 16 metabolic enzymes, but 73% of invasive disease episodes were due to strains belonging to only three ETs. In the largest and most comprehensive analysis (37), 2209 encapsulated *H. influenzae* strains (including 1975 Hib) from 30 countries on six continents collected over a 40-year period were studied by multilocus electrophoresis of 17 chromosomally encoded metabolic enzymes, OMP subtyping, and the restriction-fragment-length polymorphism pattern of the cap region (the chromosome region responsible for capsular expression). On the basis of allele profiles at the enzyme loci, 280 distinct ETs in two phylogenetic divisions were identified: The population structure is definitely clonal. Currently, nearly all of the invasive disease worldwide is caused by nine clones of Hib. One genetically distinct clone complex occurs with considerable frequency worldwide, but marked geographic variation occurs for other clones or clone families. Based on an extensive analysis, it appears that this distribution of clones on an intercontinental scale is largely accounted for by the patterns of racial/ethnic composition and historical demographic movements of the human host populations (37).

Neisseria meningitidis

Neisseria species are non-spore-forming, nonmotile, oxidase-positive, gram-negative cocci (measuring ~0.8 μm $\times$ 0.6 μm) which usually appear as biscuit- or kidney-shaped diplococci on smears of infected fluids. Because other organisms (e.g., *Moraxella* species) are similar morphologically, identification rests on biochemical or immunologic techniques. All *Neisseria* species are oxidase-positive, and sugar fermentation reactions are usually sufficient for speciation within the genus. Gonococci ferment glucose (but not maltose or lactose) to acid, whereas meningococci ferment both glucose and maltose to acid. *N. lactamica,* a related organism occasionally present in throat cultures, ferments glucose, maltose, and lactose. Maltose-negative variants of meningococci have been isolated; these strains may be differentiated from gonococci by fluorescent antibody tests, coagglutination tests, or electrophoretic analysis of hexokinase isoenzymes. These strains usually acquire the ability to ferment maltose on subculture; true maltose-negative variants are rare, but this property is genetically linked to sulfadiazine resistance. Meningococci grow rapidly on blood, chocolate, gonococcal, or enriched Mueller–Hinton agar in a moist 3–10% CO_2 environment at 35–37°C. A modified Thayer–Martin medium is employed for meningococcal isolation from contaminated sites, such as detection of the carrier state. The transoral approach for obtaining specimens is more practical and is at least as sensitive as older transnasal approaches for carrier detection. Because this organism is susceptible to drying and chilling, all specimens should be inoculated promptly.

Similar to other gram-negative bacteria, the ultrastructural characteristics of meningococci are complex. The surface components include capsular polysaccharide, fimbriae or pili, LPS, and OMP; several of these structures are important virulence determinants. Meningococci are currently classified by serogroups based on structural differences among capsular polysaccharides and agglutination reactions with specific antisera, and they are further defined by serotypes based on analysis of the OMP. Capsular polysaccharide detected by positive agglutination with reference antisera is uniformly present among invasive isolates, but 20–50% or more of carrier strains are unencapsulated (nongroupable). The serogroups have important epidemiologic and prevention-related implications. Thirteen serogroups are currently recognized (23): A, B, C, D, H, I, K, L, X, Y, Z, 29E, and W135. Most meningococcal disease is caused by organisms in serogroups A, B, C, and Y, although the proportion of cases due to serogroup W135 is increasing. Although serious outbreaks of serogroup A, B, or C disease have occurred worldwide recently (Table 6), most focal outbreaks and endemic disease in many countries are due to serogroups B and C. For example, in the United States for the period 1975–1980, the distribution of serogroups among 12,980 cases was as follows: B, 56%; C, 19%; Y, 11%; W135, 10%; and A, 3%. Similar figures were reported for the period 1978–1981 (9). Serogroup W135 disease, especially among adults, is increasing in the United States and apparently also elsewhere (e.g., Senegal) since 1981. Group B organisms, especially B:15:P1.16, have recently emerged as important pathogens in northern Europe, causing serious local outbreaks peaking in the 10- to 20-year-old group. The continued high prevalence of serogroup B meningococcal disease has important implications because of the current lack of an effective vaccine against this serogroup (see section entitled "Prevention," below). An outbreak of serogroup C disease occurred in California in 1987 (38). Serious outbreaks due to serogroup A continued during the period 1983–1989 in Nepal, Saudi Arabia, Chad, and elsewhere. Approximately 40,000 cases of serogroup A disease occurred in Ethiopia in the spring of 1989, suggesting another epidemic wave currently ongoing in the meningitis belt (Fig. 1).

Serotypes within a serogroup of *N. meningitidis* are classified largely on analysis of OMP profiles in the cell envelope. At least 20 serotypes are currently recognized (39), resulting in a classification scheme which is useful in epidemiologic studies. Physicochemical characterization of the OMPs, which might be candidate antigens for vaccines, has led to the designation of five major classes.

Class 2 and 3 proteins are the major porins responsible for aqueous channels in the outer membrane. Class 5 proteins are surface-exposed and may have a role in virulence, but the function of class 1 and 4 proteins is poorly defined. The serotype designation has important epidemiologic uses and may identify virulence characteristics among meningococci. For example, serotype 2 (2a, 2b) strains are responsible for ~50% of serogroup B disease (in which 15 serotypes have been described), followed by serotypes 15 and 9; in contrast, serotypes 4 and 6 have been isolated only from carriers. Serotype 2 is also responsible for ~80% of invasive serogroup C disease and is an important marker for serogroups Y and W135 pathogenic strains as well (39). All serogroup A meningococci, in contrast, are homogeneous with respect to OMP and show no homology to serotypes within other serogroups. Serotype analysis has also been linked to certain clinical characteristics (40), but this technique is, at present, only available in research or reference laboratories. In addition, at least eight immunotypes of meningococci, classified by differences among LPS subtypes, are known to exist and may play a role in pathogenesis and disease expression. LPS immunotype analysis may also be useful in the further characterization of the epidemiology of meningococcal disease (22,23). The recent availability of monoclonal antibodies to detect variations in OMP and/or LPS will improve the resolution of these typing systems for epidemiologic analysis.

In addition to classification by serogroup, serotype, and LPS subtype, many recent reports (e.g., ref. 41) have focused on multilocus enzyme electrophoresis for the characterization of the chromosomal genome of isolates and for estimation of the genetic relatedness among strains, similar to the recent analysis of Hib (37). These studies have identified the clonal nature of *N. meningitidis* and have been useful for epidemiologic purposes. For example, electrophoretic variation (defined as less than 17% genetic distance between isolates) in seven metabolic enzymes and two OMP in 423 isolates of serogroup A strains recovered from 23 epidemics or outbreaks occurring in 38 countries on six continents over a 70-year period since 1915 identified 21 "clones" (designated A I-1 through A IV-4) containing 34 ETs (41). This technique has been useful for delineating similarities and differences among isolates from cases and carriers before, during, and after epidemics (42), as well as for tracing movements of epidemic strains geographically over time (43). For example, following an epidemic in Nepal (1983–1984), a single clonal complex of serogroup A meningococci (III-1, representing 11 closely related ETs) was introduced into Saudi Arabia in 1987 by Muslim pilgrims traveling to Mecca for the annual haj (42). The same strain was then introduced into sub-Saharan Africa following the haj, caused an explosive outbreak in Chad in 1988, and was largely responsible for the current epidemics in the meningitis belt. An analysis of 109 isolates of serogroup B meningococci in Norway (44) has also revealed differences among carriers and cases. Although 78 ETs were identified, 91% of the cases of systemic disease in 1984 were due to strains from the ET-5–ET-37 complex whereas these isolates were recovered from only 7% and 9%, respectively, of healthy carriers. The most common clonal complex found among carriers was never isolated from patients with invasive disease, suggesting a low virulence potential for these clones. Clonal analysis will undoubtedly continue to contribute important information on the epidemiology of meningococcal infection, and it may prove useful in an analysis of virulence properties.

The putative meningococcal virulence characteristics are listed in Table 9. As noted above, all isolates from invasive infections are encapsulated (serogroup-positive) but 20–90% of isolates from carriers are unencapsulated (nontypable). The capsular polysaccharide appears to be essential for meningococcal virulence, probably because of its antiphagocytic properties that allow the organism to escape host phagocytic clearance mechanisms within the bloodstream and/or CSF. Pili are protein-surface appendages composed of identical-pilin-repeating subunits. Pili from meningococci and gonococci are morphologically and chemically similar. Cross-reacting antibodies bind to a short peptide sequence (residues 69–94) of gonococcal pili which is essential for receptor-binding function. Fresh meningococcal isolates from carriers and cases contain 7–40 pili per diplococcus. Pili are important mediators of meningococcal adhesion to human nonciliated columnar nasopharyngeal epithelial cells, an important early step in the development of the carrier state. Extracellular proteases that cleave the IgA1 heavy chain in the hinge region are elaborated by pathogenic *Neisseria* species (i.e., meningococci and gonococci). Although the role of IgA proteases in the pathogenesis of disease is controversial, these enzymes are produced only by a few organisms (e.g., *N. meningitidis, N. gonorrhoeae, H. influenzae, S. pneumoniae,* and *S. sanguis*), many of which are important meningeal pathogens, and may promote invasion at the pharyngeal portal of entry. Meningococcal LPS resembles *H. influenzae* LPS by a lack of the O-antigenic polysaccharide side chains found in enteric bacilli despite a smooth phenotype and proven virulence. LPS is clearly important in the genesis of an array of the clinical manifestations of meningococcemia and/or meningitis (see below). Although the specific role for OMP in meningococcal virulence is unclear, these organisms release substantial amounts of cell-surface material (in the form of outer-membrane vesicles containing OMP and LPS) during growth *in vitro* and *in vivo* in the absence of cell lysis, a process exacerbated by antimicrobial agents. These outer-membrane vesicles, or blebs, represent relevant vehicles for central nervous system (CNS) tissue damage during meningococcal infection (see below). Tissue invasion may also be facilitated by the ability of meningococci to obtain iron from transferrin.

Streptococcus pneumoniae

Pneumococci are non-spore-forming, nonmotile, small (~0.8 μm), gram-positive streptococci that typically appear as lancet-shaped diplococci with the tapered ends in juxtaposition in clinical specimens. They tend to associate in pairs rather than in short chains, although the latter morphology is facilitated by broth culture. Pneumococci are facultative anaerobes that flourish in a variety of supplemented artificial media. Optimal growth occurs in various media supplemented with serum or blood and ≤1% glucose, at a pH of 7.8 and a temperature of 37°C in an enriched CO_2 environment. The organisms are catalase-negative and relatively fastidious. Colonies on blood agar are initially domed-shaped, but they become umbilicated with time as a result of the activity of autolytic enzymes (L-alanine muramyl amidase). Pneumococci are α-hemolytic (i.e., a greenish discoloration surrounds colonies on blood agar), although β-hemolysis occurs under anaerobic conditions. *S. pneumoniae* must be separated from other α-hemolytic streptococci in the laboratory; this is usually accomplished by the unique susceptibility of pneumococci to optochin (ethyl hydrocupreine hydrochloride) with a disk susceptibility test. Pneumococci, but not other streptococci, are also sensitive to bile or bile salts (e.g., 10% deoxycholate), but the bile solubility test is now rarely performed in hospital laboratories.

Pneumococci are classified within serotypes on the basis of antigenic differences among capsular polysaccharides. These capsular substances are complex polysaccharides that form hydrophilic gels on the surface of the organism. At present, at least 84 serotypes have been identified, classified by two systems of nomenclature (American and Danish). Capsular polysaccharides are identified by agglutination, the Neufeld quellung reaction [capsular swelling and increased refraction in the presence of antisera, also useful for identifying pneumococci in clinical specimens (e.g., CSF)], precipitation, and counterimmunoelectrophoresis. It is

TABLE 9. *Meningococcal virulence factors*

Capsular polysaccharide
Pili
IgA protease
Lipopolysaccharide (endotoxin)
Outer-membrane proteins
Outer-membrane vesicles, or blebs
Metabolic pathways (e.g., iron)

important to emphasize that cross-reactions exist between individual pneumococcal serotypes as well as with other bacteria (e.g., *E. coli*, *Klebsiella pneumoniae*, Hib, and *S. sanguis*). For example, serotype-14 pneumococcal capsular polysaccharide cross-reacts with type III group B streptococci and with certain human ABO blood group isoantigens.

Capsular polysaccharide is essential for pneumococcal virulence, and a few serotypes are associated with the majority of invasive infections. Encapsulated organisms (smooth colonies on agar) are virulent for humans and experimental animals, whereas unencapsulated (rough colonies on agar) strains are avirulent. Capsular polysaccharide enhances virulence through its antiphagocytic properties, similar to Hib and meningococci.

Of the 84 known pneumococcal serotypes, only a few (usually the lower-number types, rather than the higher-number types commonly found in the carrier state) account for the majority of invasive pneumococcal infections. The predominant capsular types were 1, 2, and 3 in the pre-antibiotic era. A different pattern has emerged in the past 40 years, and it differs between adults and children. A few capsular types cause the majority of bacteremic cases among adults: types 1, 3, 4, 7, 8, 9, 12, and 14; and, less commonly, types 6, 18, and 19. These are not listed in rank order. Approximately 66% of cases are due to eight serotypes, although no one single serotype predominates among bacteremic adults. Capsular types 14, 6, 18, 19, 23, 1, 4, and 9 cause ~85% of serious infections in children, a pattern different from those observed in adults. Perhaps more important with respect to this discussion, there is a very strong correlation between serotypes causing pneumonia (or bacteremia) and those responsible for pneumococcal meningitis (32). For example, 76–86% of blood and CSF isolates were included among the 14 serotypes represented in the original pneumococcal vaccine. However, marked geographic variations exist among pneumococcal serotypes causing invasive disease, and the serotype distribution may change over time in a given locale. Furthermore, some serotypes may be more virulent than others and are associated with less favorable outcomes, including death. Older studies of pneumococcal meningitis in the 1950s (summarized in ref. 32) noted an increased mortality with disease due to serotypes 2, 8, and 12; although type 12 caused only 2.5% of cases, it was responsible for 30.7% of the deaths. Similarly, serotype 6 was associated with four of eight deaths in a more recent survey.

The role of other cell-surface components (such as C-polysaccharide antigens, cell-wall antigens, M- or R-protein antigens, etc.) and putative toxins (such as hemolysin, neuraminidase, purpura-producing principle, etc.) in the pathogenesis and pathophysiology of pneumococcal meningitis remains poorly defined. Nevertheless, CSF inflammation is induced by pneumococcal cell wall and its constituents (particularly lipoteichoic acid) but not by purified pneumococcal capsular polysaccharide (see below).

Gram-Negative Bacilli

Approximately 84% of cases of neonatal meningitis and sepsis due to *E. coli* are caused by strains bearing the K1 capsular polysaccharide antigen (Chapter 15); this capsular type serves as a marker of neurovirulence. *E. coli* meningitis is discussed in detail in the previous chapter.

Beyond the neonatal period, aerobic gram-negative bacillary meningitis occurs in three major clinical settings: (i) head trauma, ~30% of cases, especially in conjunction with CSF rhinorrhea or otorrhea; (ii) after neurosurgical procedures, ~50% of cases; and (iii) in association with other conditions, ~20% of cases, including strongyloidiasis, gram-negative bacteremia, ruptured brain abscess, or impairment of host defense mechanisms. Many of these infections are nosocomial in origin, although community-acquired gram-negative bacillary meningitis is increasing in frequency, particularly in the elderly (over age 60) and in debilitated, alcoholic, or diabetic adults. The most common causes of gram-negative aerobic bacillary meningitis beyond the first month of life include *Klebsiella* species (~40% of cases), *E. coli* (~15–30%), and *Pseudomonas aeruginosa* (~10–20%). Meningitis due to *E. coli* K1, a common neonatal pathogen, is discussed in detail in Chapter 15.

Streptococcus agalactiae

Group B streptococci are the most common cause of invasive neonatal disease in the United States, accounting for approximately 11,000 cases of meningitis and/or bacteremia yearly. The incidence of group B streptococcal neonatal infections has remained relatively stable in this country during the past 15 years (45), but it appears to be increasing in frequency in the developing world. The morphologic and cultural characteristics, as well as the definitive identification of group B streptococci by detection of the group B cell-wall antigen common to all strains, are described in Chapter 16.

Group B streptococci are currently classified into six main serotypes (Ia, Ib/c, Ia/c, II, III, and IV) based on the expression of type-specific capsular polysaccharide antigens and various surface proteins as additional antigenic markers (46); additional candidate serotypes are under evaluation. Although all serotypes have been isolated from neonates with invasive disease, type III is responsible for the vast majority of meningeal infections, suggesting a high virulence potential and/or CNS tropism for this serotype. The chromosomal genetic diversity of *S. agalactiae* was studied recently (47), and the clonal nature of the native bacterial populations was again demonstrated. A collection of 128 isolates representing all six serotypes, including 44 type III isolates from invasive episodes (18 recovered from CSF), were subjected to multilocus enzyme electrophoresis, an analysis based on electrophoretically demonstrable allelic profiles at 11 metabolic enzyme loci all encoded at the chromosome level. Nineteen distinct ETs were identified in two primary phylogenetic divisions, each representing a multilocus clonal genotype. A single ET (ET1), comprised of 40 isolates of serotype III group B streptococci formed the first phylogenetic division. These strains produced greater amounts of neuraminidase (Chapter 16) and were more virulent than the other type III isolates found in several of the 18 ETs in the second division. This newly evolved clone (ET1) is responsible for the majority of invasive disease episodes due to group B streptococci type III in the United States (47).

In addition to the common conditions of neonatal meningitis and postpartum fever and/or bacteremia in parturient women due to group B streptococci, these organisms also cause serious infections in adults, [usually elderly (~59–68 years of age)] when bacteremia is present. Bacteremic infections in adults unrelated to pregnancy usually occur in the setting of various underlying risk factors, in approximate order of decreasing frequency, as follows: diabetes mellitus; malignancy; liver failure or history of alcoholism; neurologic impairment; renal failure; congestive heart failure; use of intravenous catheter; corticosteroid administration; asplenia; and acquired immunodeficiency syndrome (AIDS). The same underlying conditions have been represented in the ~33 adults with group B streptococcal meningitis reported in the literature (48).

Listeria monocytogenes

This organism remains an important cause of neonatal meningitis (Chapter 15), where the source is the genital tract or subclinical infection of the mother. Although *L. monocytogenes* may cause meningitis in normal adults, most patients are diabetic, alcoholic, elderly, or immunosuppressed. *L. monocytogenes* has been the major cause of bacterial meningitis among renal transplant recipients, but this appears to be decreasing in frequency as a result of the use of trimethoprim-sulfamethoxazole prophylaxis.

L. monocytogenes is widespread in nature. Although clusters of nosocomial cases and focal outbreaks are reported, most cases of human listeriosis are sporadic. The incidence of *L. monocytogenes* infections is difficult to quantitate. Many countries in northern Europe have reported annual incidence figures of ~2–3 per million per year. After a large (142 cases) food-borne outbreak in Los Angeles County, California, in 1985, mandatory reporting of *L. monocytogenes* isolates by clinical laboratories was instituted. During the first year of active

surveillance, 94 cases of listeriosis were reported (49), for an annual crude incidence rate of 11.7 per million persons, similar to figures (11.3 per million per year) reported from France in 1984. Listeriosis is undoubtedly underreported.

Approximately one-third of cases in the United States are in neonates and/or their mothers (39% in the Los Angeles survey) (49), whereas the proportion of perinatal infections in Europe is higher. Among the nonperinatal cases, various risk factors for listeriosis were identified, including: immunosuppression as a documented history of steroid ingestion or chemotherapy (35% of cases, the single most important risk factor); age ≥ 75 years; renal disease; cancer; alcoholism and/or cirrhosis; and AIDS. Nevertheless, serious *Listeria* infections, including meningitis, remain uncommon in patients with AIDS. Of the nonperinatal cases, only two of 57 had no definable underlying risk factor; 21 of 57 had meningitis (49). As stated above, *L. monocytogenes* remains a distinctly unusual cause of meningitis in developing countries.

In the nonperinatal cases, the route of transmission is often unknown. At least 1% of normal individuals excrete the organism in their stools, but contacts of symptomatic patients have much higher excretion rates (~25%). Nevertheless, the true carriage rate, its duration, and its relationship to invasive disease are poorly defined. Although often considered a zoonosis, most patients do not report animal exposure. Recent reports have emphasized food-borne transmission of *L. monocytogenes,* a route of transmission which accounts for at least 20% of sporadic cases. Many foods have been implicated, including cole slaw, Mexican-style cheese (50), raw vegetables, seafood, pasteurized milk, Swiss cheese, raw hot dogs, and undercooked chicken (51). Some studies report a higher frequency of listeriosis in summer, opposite to the seasonal pattern seen with most other forms of bacterial meningitis.

L. monocytogenes is a gram-positive, non-spore-forming, catalase-positive, aerobic rod which may be difficult to culture upon initial isolation but which, once grown, passes readily on a variety of laboratory media. The organism may appear coccoid on Gram's stains of clinical specimens, particularly CSF, and is often mistaken for pneumococci. More importantly, *L. monocytogenes* resembles diphtheroids and may thus be dismissed as a "contaminant," a grave error. The presence of β-hemolysis and a characteristic tumbling motility at room temperature are used to separate *L. monocytogenes* from similar diphtheroid-like organisms. A hemolytic and cytolytic toxin (listeriolysin 0) of 52 kD appears essential for virulence; the toxin is expressed under conditions of low pH and low iron concentration and may facilitate phagolysosomal disruption and growth within mononuclear phagocytes. At least 11 serotypes are recognized, but more than 90% of invasive infections are due to three serotypes: Ia, Ib, and IVb.

Staphylococcus epidermidis

Coagulase-negative staphylococci are very rare causes of bacterial meningitis in children and adults—except in the setting of an indwelling CSF shunt, where these organisms are the most prevalent pathogen. Therefore, this group is discussed elsewhere in this volume (Chapter 23).

Staphylococcus aureus

Meningitis due to *S. aureus* is relatively unusual; this organism was responsible for 0.8–8.8% of cases in various surveys (52,53). *S. aureus* is the second most common cause of CSF shunt infections (Chapter 23), accounting for 12–36% of cases. This organism is also frequently isolated from patients with nosocomial meningitis and is responsible for ~20% of such cases. Although secondary meningitis in the setting of infective endocarditis is an uncommon event (Chapter 22), most of these infections are due to *S. aureus.* Other important associated conditions have been recognized, including head trauma, neurosurgical procedures, various abscesses (cerebral, epidural, oral, abdominal), sinusitis, osteomyelitis, decubitus ulcers, pneumonia, cellulitis, and infected intravascular grafts or shunts. Several other predisposing factors have been proposed. In a retrospective review of 28 cases of *S. aureus* meningitis seen during the 10-year period 1972–1982 at three North Carolina teaching hospitals, 22 occurred beyond the neonatal period (53). Among the adult patients ($n = 20$) with a mean age of 52 years, 45% had an underlying condition (diabetes mellitus, malignancy, renal failure, immunosuppression), 35% followed head trauma or neurosurgery (ventriculoperitoneal shunt, craniotomy), and ~20% developed in association with endocarditis or a paraspinal infection. Mortality was high (50% in adults), especially when *S. aureus* meningitis complicated a distant extracranial focus of infection (five of the six patients with purulent meningitis during active endocarditis died) (53). The prognosis for *S. aureus* CSF shunt infections is more favorable.

Anaerobic Bacteria

Meningitis caused by anaerobic bacteria is rare, accounting for less than 1% of pyogenic cases, except following the intraventricular rupture of a brain abscess. Anaerobic meningitis may be underrecognized, because CSF is not routinely cultured anaerobically. Enriched media and proper transport of CSF to the laboratory are essential for isolation of anaerobes and are not uniformly performed. Only five cases due to strict anaerobes were reported among 18,642 patients recently analyzed by the Centers for Disease Control (9).

Anaerobic meningitis is associated with a variety of clinical conditions, including: brain abscess rupture or extension to the surface of the brain; chronic otitis, mastoiditis, or sinusitis; head trauma; neurosurgical procedures (e.g., craniotomy, laminectomy); congenital dural defects; abdominal trauma or surgery; gastrointestinal disease; head and neck cancer; suppurative pharyngitis; CSF shunts; and immunosuppression (particularly corticosteroid administration) (54). Most cases arise from spread of infection secondary to a contiguous focus of disease; anaerobic meningitis rarely complicates bacteremia from a distant extracranial focus.

A variety of bacterial species are responsible for anaerobic meningitis. Only nine cases of *Bacteroides fragilis* meningitis, unaccompanied by a brain abscess, have been reported in the modern era through 1987 (55); seven occurred in premature infants or neonates (median age 20 days), thereby complicating congenital defects or gastrointestinal disease such as necrotizing enterocolitis (56). Meningitis due to *Fusobacterium* species, usually *F. necrophorum,* usually occurs in older children (median age ~ 5 years) or adults as a complication of acute or chronic otitis media (56). A variety of anaerobic gram-positive cocci have been isolated in a few cases, particularly peptostreptococci. Meningitis caused by *Clostridium* species almost always develops following head trauma or a neurosurgical procedure. For example, in a summary of 17 cases due to *C. perfringens* (57), only three were not associated with CNS trauma or surgery. Although the disease course is highly variable, some cases of clostridial meningitis are characterized by intracranial gas formation (visible on plain skull radiographs or computerized tomography, etc.), CSF white blood cell concentrations exceeding 20,000 per cubic millimeter, and death within hours of presentation. A few cases of meningitis due to *Actinomyces* species (in the absence of brain abscess formation) and *Propionibacterium acnes* (usually subacute with a predominantly monocytic CSF pleocytosis) have also been reported. In approximately one-eighth of patients, the infection is mixed with anaerobic plus aerobic or microaerophilic organisms recovered from CSF.

Unusual Etiologic Agents

CNS infections due to higher bacteria (e.g., *Mycobacterium* species, *Nocardia* species, *Actinomyces* species), spirochetes (e.g., *Treponema pallidum, Borrelia burgdorferi, Leptospira* species), *Brucella* species, and so on, are discussed elsewhere in this volume. A plethora of bacteria have been documented as the cause of meningitis in isolated case reports or in small numbers of patients, including: group A streptococci; nonpneumococcal α-hemolytic streptococci such as *S. mitis* (58); enterococci; *S. bovis;* diphtheroids; *N. gonorrhoeae* (~30 cases reported in the past 20 years); *N. subflava;*

Gardnerella vaginalis (one case report); many members of the Enterobacteriaceae in addition to *E. coli* and *Salmonella* species; *Flavobacterium meningosepticum; Hemophilus* species other than *H. influenzae; Acinetobacter* species; and many others. Fewer than 0.5% of adult cases of bacterial meningitis are caused by group C streptococci; however, mortality is high, perhaps due to the unpredictable susceptibility of this organism to β-lactam agents.

Polymicrobial bacterial meningitis, with simultaneous recovery of two or more bacterial species from CSF, is unusual. Mixed infections account for ~1% of bacterial meningitis cases. In a review (59) of 34 series encompassing 11,281 cases of bacterial meningitis, 116 cases (1%) were mixed. This condition appears to be evolving in the antibiotic era. Prior to 1950, nearly all cases occurred in children and were caused by combinations of bacteria commonly associated with meningitis (the three major meningeal pathogens). Since 1950, the majority of cases have occurred in adults, with a wider spectrum of etiologic agents, particularly gram-negative aerobic bacilli. Approximately one-third of cases were nosocomially acquired. Common predisposing conditions in the older population affected since 1950 include: contiguous foci of infection; tumors in close proximity to the neuraxis (e.g., head and neck); rectal carcinoma; or fistulous communications with the CNS. The mortality rate is 63% for cases occurring after 1950. Several cases of meningitis caused by mixed bacterial and mycobacterial or fungal agents have also been reported.

Simultaneous isolation of viruses and bacteria from the CSF is rare; only seven well-documented cases were reported prior to 1988 (60). However, in a 1-year (1986) retrospective review from the Ohio State University (60), 5 of 176 children (2.8%) with CSF enteroviral isolates also had bacterial meningitis. Conversely, CSF samples from 5 of 105 children (4.8%) with bacterial meningitis also grew an enterovirus. All of the patients presented in late summer at the peak of the enterovirus season, and each case was due to a different bacterial pathogen. Because the CSF formula was indistinguishable from that of patients with typical bacterial meningitis, and the clinical course and response to therapy were similar to those of patients with typical bacterial meningitis, this condition may be underrecognized, since CSF viral cultures are rarely performed when bacterial meningitis is the likely diagnosis.

PATHOGENESIS AND PATHOPHYSIOLOGY

Despite the availability of effective antimicrobial therapy, bacterial meningitis continues to be a potentially fatal illness. Several investigators have examined the pathogenic and pathophysiologic mechanisms operating in meningitis (Fig. 2), with the aim of improving the

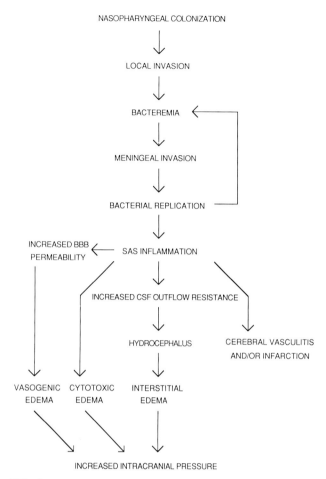

FIG. 2. Hypothetical scheme of the pathogenic and pathophysiologic mechanisms in bacterial meningitis. BBB, blood–brain barrier; SAS, subarachnoid space; CSF, cerebrospinal fluid.

outcome of patients with this disorder. Most studies have utilized animal models to investigate these mechanisms (Chapter 14), and these models have defined the bacterial virulence factors and host defense mechanisms that are relevant to the initiation, maintenance, and consequences of infection. Here we utilize the information presented in Chapter 14 to describe the pathogenesis and pathophysiology of bacterial meningitis, emphasizing principles for the development of innovative strategies in the treatment of this disorder.

Nasopharyngeal Colonization and Invasion

Initiation of bacterial meningitis usually depends upon host acquisition of a new organism by colonization of the nasopharynx. Specific bacterial virulence factors —in particular, specialized surface components—are crucial for the establishment of infection at this site. Strains of *H. influenzae* colonize the nasopharynx in most children by the age of 3 months; however, the majority of these strains are unencapsulated, and type b strains make up less than 5% of isolates (61). Studies utilizing laboratory transformants have demonstrated that after the intraperitoneal inoculation of encapsulated strains types a through f, type b strains were the most virulent and were the only strains which invaded following intranasal inoculation (62). Indeed, the presence of serum antibodies to polyribosyl-ribitol phosphate, the capsular polysaccharide of type b isolates, is protective against invasive disease. Lack of sufficient concentrations of this antibody correlates with an increased risk of invasive disease. Antibodies to type b capsule are almost uniformly detectable in humans by the age of 4 years, even in the absence of known exposure to Hib. The presence of these antibodies may relate to the ability of unencapsulated strains to produce some type b capsular material. It has been suggested that the source of bacterial capsule may be from acquisition of new DNA from organisms colonizing the gastrointestinal tract (63,64). *E. coli* K100 possesses a capsule that is immunologically nearly identical to the type b capsule of *H. influenzae,* and it may stimulate the production of cross-reacting anticapsular antibodies.

For Hib to colonize the nasopharynx, the organism(s) must first adhere to the nasopharyngeal epithelial cells via specific surface structures. Fimbriae have been implicated in this adhesion process, although these organelles are not found on isolates from blood or CSF (65,66). Acquisition and colonization of Hib may also be promoted after viral infection by a variety of respiratory viruses, including influenzae A Victoria and respiratory syncytial virus (61). Hib proliferates more when inoculated into the nasopharynx of virus-infected animals than when inoculated into that of normals.

Bacterial capsule may also be important for adhesion. It is crucial for the virulence of *S. pneumoniae;* of the 84 known serotypes of pneumococci, 18 are responsible for the majority (~82%) of bacteremic pneumococcal pneumonia, with a close correlation between bacteremic subtypes and those implicated in meningitis (67). The factors that mediate dissemination from a recently colonized site are largely unknown, but lack of specific antibody appears critical for the development of invasive pneumococcal disease.

Adhesion of *N. meningitidis* to nasopharyngeal epithelial cells occurs via fimbriae, which have been found in 80% of primary meningococcal isolates from nasopharyngeal carriers and from CSF isolates (68). Meningococci, like gonococci, possess different types of fimbriae which differ in their morphologic, antigenic, and binding properties (69). Morphologically, fimbriae can appear as aggregated bundles or aggregated single filaments. The aggregated bundles are found predominantly among disease isolates and exhibit a low degree of adherence to human buccal epithelial cells, whereas the single filaments are found primarily among carrier isolates with medium-to-high adherence. Meningococci bind to nasopharyngeal epithelial cells via a specific cell-surface receptor (70) and are then transported across nonciliated columnar nasopharyngeal cells within a phagocytic vacuole (71). These early pathogenic events result in the propensity for hematogenous dissemination with this organism.

Intravascular Survival

Once bacteria gain access to the intravascular space, they must overcome additional host defense mechanisms to survive. The virulence of the meningeal pathogens relates to the ability of the polysaccharide capsule to resist classical complement pathway bactericidal activity and inhibit neutrophil phagocytosis. For example, about 84% of cases of neonatal meningitis due to *E. coli* are caused by K1-positive strains, and, in the absence of K1-specific host antibody, these organisms are profoundly resistant to phagocytosis (72). The K1 antigen of *E. coli* shares antigenic characteristics with capsular material from other organisms such as serogroup B meningococci and type III group B streptococci. Human monoclonal antibodies with reactivity against specific epitopes on the K1 capsule of *E. coli* or on the group B polysaccharide of *N. meningitidis* may be effective in prevention and/or therapy of bacteremia due to these organisms (73), but this remains conjectural in humans.

The host possesses several defense mechanisms to counteract the antiphagocytic activity of bacterial capsule (32). For example, the capsular polysaccharides of *S. pneumoniae* activate the alternative complement pathway; this results in cleavage of C3 with subsequent attachment of C3b to the bacterial surface, thereby facilitating opsonization, phagocytosis, and intravascular clearance of the organism. Impairment of the alternative complement pathway occurs in patients with sickle-cell disease and in those who have undergone splenectomy, and these groups of patients are predisposed to the development of pneumococcal meningitis. The complement cascade is also activated by Hib. Experiments utilizing C3-depleted infant rats demonstrated a greater incidence and magnitude of bacteremia after either intravenous or intraperitoneal challenge with *H. influenzae* of varying serotypes (a, b, c, or d) (74). Although the incidence of bacteremia due to type b organisms was increased from 63% to 95% in complement-depleted rats, the incidence and severity of meningitis were unaffected.

Activation of the complement system is an essential defense mechanism in protection from invasive disease due to *N. meningitidis*. Patients with deficiencies in the terminal complement components (C5, C6, C7, C8, and perhaps C9) are particularly prone to infection with neisserial species (including *N. meningitidis*), usually with a favorable outcome (26). A recent study has shown that a qualitative relationship exists among the level of circulating meningococcal lipopolysaccharide (LPS), a fatal outcome, and the degree of complement activation (75), indicating that the prognosis is worse in patients with an intact complement system.

Meningeal Invasion

The mechanism of bacterial invasion into the SAS is largely unknown. One factor may be the concentration of organisms in the blood. The intranasal inoculation of Hib into infant rats initially led to a low-grade bacteremia [$\sim 10^2$ colony-forming units (CFU)/ml]; at this concentration, no organisms were present in CSF (76). Bacterial multiplication occurred at a rapid rate, and bacterial densities of 10^5 CFU/ml were reached at 48 hr. In addition, meningitis was induced in an age-dependent manner, with a higher incidence in 5-day-old rats than in 20-day-old rats. It is also important to note that sustained, as opposed to transient, bacteremia was found in the animals that ultimately developed meningitis. However, this high-grade bacteremia is not the only factor responsible for meningeal invasion, because many other organisms (e.g., viridans streptococci) rarely invade the CNS despite the presence of bacteremia, often continuous as during infective endocarditis.

The exact sites of CNS invasion by bacteria are unknown. Early experimental studies in the infant rat model of Hib meningitis utilized fluorescein-conjugated rabbit antiserum and suggested that the route of invasion from the bloodstream into the CSF was through the dural venous sinus system (76). However, subsequent experiments using the same model suggested that during the ensuing bacteremia, a nonspecific, sterile, focal inflammation above the cribriform plate facilitated CNS invasion at this site. Additional studies on the pathogenesis of bacterial meningitis in infant rats and primates suggested that bacteria enter the CSF via the choroid plexus, which has an exceptionally high rate of blood flow (~ 200 ml/g/min); this implies that more bacterial organisms would be delivered to this site per unit time than to most other anatomic locations in the body. In addition, if CSF compartments are sampled early in the course of bacterial meningitis, higher bacterial densities are found in the lateral ventricles than in the cisterna magna, lumbar SAS, or supracortical SAS, although there is equilibration in these other locations with time (Table 10).

Recent studies have suggested that cells in the choroid plexus and/or cerebral capillaries possess receptors for adherence of meningeal pathogens, which facilitate the movement of these pathogens into the SAS. Strains of E. coli possessing S fimbriae bind to the luminal surface of the vascular endothelium and to the epithelium lining the choroid plexus and brain ventricles, as demonstrated in cryostat sections of infant rat brain cortical slices (77). Binding was abolished by pretreatment of the brain sections with neuraminidase or the trisaccharide receptor analogue of S fimbriae. In a subsequent series of experiments, 1 hr after intraperitoneal challenge with the S-fimbriated population of E. coli, about 50% of CSF organisms were S-fimbriated and 50% were nonfimbriated (78), indicating that phase variation to the nonfimbriated form may be necessary for the bacteria to pass through the vascular endothelium.

Other microbial virulence factors may also be important for bacterial invasion into the CNS. The liberation of the LPS of N. meningitidis may contribute to the pathogenicity of this organism in invasive infections (79). However, the importance of OMPs in less clear. A recent report has suggested that H. influenzae strains with OMP subtype 1c caused more episodes of meningitis and fewer episodes of epiglottitis than strains of subtype 1 (80), perhaps as a result of the ability of each subtype to release LPS under appropriate circumstances. Additional studies are needed to examine these concepts in greater detail.

Once bacteria invade the SAS, a secondary bacteremia can result from the local suppurative process in the CNS so that the meningeal pathogen can continue to enter and leave the CSF compartment. In an experimental dog model of pneumococcal meningitis, the early transport of bacteria from CSF to blood was presumed to be transendothelial, via arachnoid villi containing pores large enough to accommodate bacteria; the bacteria would then enter the superior sagittal sinus and return to the central venous blood (81). This transport occurred only after active bacterial multiplication within the CSF, but before the height of the febrile response or CSF pleocytosis. This same phenomenon was also observed with other

TABLE 10. *Number of* H. influenzae *in CSF after intranasal inoculation of* 10^9 *CFU into five 14-day-old infant primates*[a]

Time after inoculation (days)	Lateral cerebral ventricle	Cisterna magna	Lumbar subarachnoid space	Supracortical subarachnoid space
1	3.6	3.0	2.9	2.8
3	6.9	5.6	5.9	3.7
5	8.0	8.8	7.7	8.7
7	8.6	8.5	8.3	8.7

[a] Initial densities of *H. influenzae* are highest in the lateral ventricles, with equilibration in other CSF loci after 3–5 days. Results are expressed in terms of mean $\log_{10}$ CFU/ml CSF. Adapted from ref. 76.

organisms: When Hib was inoculated into the cisterna magna, bacteremia was detected almost instantaneously (61).

Host Defense Mechanisms in the Subarachnoid Space

Once meningeal pathogens penetrate into the SAS, host defense mechanisms are inadequate. Bacterial meningitis is an infection in an area of impaired host defense. The following sections review the importance of CSF complement, antibody, and neutrophils in the SAS during bacterial meningitis.

In general, assays for the various complement components in normal CSF are usually negative or reveal only minimal concentrations. Meningeal inflammation leads to increased, although low, concentrations. A wide variety of neurologic processes, including meningococcal meningitis, tuberculous meningitis, aseptic meningitis, cerebral hemorrhage, cerebral ischemia, and seizures, increase CSF concentrations of complement. This is of little or no value in the diagnosis of these various CNS syndromes. These low complement concentrations are important because complement plays an important role in opsonization of encapsulated meningeal pathogens, a process necessary for subsequent phagocytosis. Opsonic and bactericidal activity have been shown to be absent or barely detectable in patients with various forms of meningitis (82), and these observations have also been observed in experimental animal models of bacterial meningitis. In the rabbit model, the *in vitro* opsonization of a serum-sensitive *E. coli* strain was absent when incubated with CSF from animals challenged with *E. coli* K1, although CSF from animals with *Staphylococcus aureus* meningitis was opsonically active *in vitro* against *E. coli* (83). Despite the fact that there is low functional and bactericidal activity in purulent CSF, the presence of some measurable opsonic activity may correlate with a favorable outcome, as demonstrated in concentrated CSF samples from 15 of 27 patients with bacterial meningitis (84). This suggests that although complement-mediated opsonic activity was absent in normal CSF, this activity can appear in CSF during acute bacterial meningitis, particularly in patients who recover completely.

The reasons for low concentrations of complement components in purulent CSF are unknown, although multiple factors responsible have been suggested, including: (a) variable permeability of the blood-brain barrier (BBB); (b) variable degrees of SAS inflammation; (c) enhanced clearance from the SAS; (d) low production rates in the CNS; or (e) degradation at the site of infection (32). Leukocyte proteases have been shown to degrade functional complement components (e.g., C3b), with resultant formation of nonopsonic breakdown products (e.g., C3d) supporting the last possibility as a plausible explanation for decreased opsonic activity in CSF. These C3 breakdown products have been detected in CSF samples from patients with meningococcal meningitis. In addition, the intracisternal inoculation of a nonspecific protease inhibitor (phenyl-methyl-sulfonyl-fluoride) into the CSF of rabbits with pneumococcal meningitis led to a decline of CSF concentrations of *S. pneumoniae,* perhaps by altering leukocyte-protease-mediated complement destruction *in vivo.*

Like complement, immunoglobulin concentrations are low in normal CSF. IgM is usually undetectable, whereas IgG and IgA concentrations are approximately 3.1 and 0.6 mg/dl, respectively. Normally, the average blood-to-CSF ratio of IgG is about 800:1 (32). Immunoglobulin concentrations increase in bacterial meningitis, but they remain low in comparison to simultaneous serum concentrations and appear late in the disease course. There is evidence of local antibody synthesis within the CSF in some forms of infectious meningitis which may be critical in local host defense during bacterial meningitis. The importance of antibodies in defense against bacterial meningitis was examined in a rabbit model of experimental pneumococcal meningitis. Intracisternal inoculation of type-specific antibodies against *S. pneumoniae* decreased CSF pneumococcal concentrations, but at a much slower rate than appropriate bactericidal antibiotics. Heating immune serum to 56°C for 30 min and preabsorption of the immune serum with homologous type III pneumococci at 4°C for 18 hr abolished this effect, suggesting an important role for specific antibody in this situation. The systemic administration of type-specific monoclonal antibodies has recently been examined in the rabbit model of experimental meningitis (85). Intravenous injection of a bactericidal monoclonal antibody against the polyribosyl-ribitol phosphate of Hib produced high serum concentrations (~1000–6000 ng/ml) of antibody, but the monoclonal antibody crossed the blood-brain barrier poorly (≤5.5%) even in the presence of meningeal inflammation, suggesting that systemic administration of type-specific antibodies would be suboptimal in the treatment of bacterial meningitis. It remains to be determined, however, whether the intrathecal administration of type-specific monoclonal antibodies is useful in bacterial meningitis. In the pre-antibiotic era, outcome of bacterial meningitis was improved by instillation of immune serum supplemented with complement into the CSF. This area requires additional study, although the intrathecal injection of specific antibody is unlikely to be beneficial if there are insufficient concentrations of complement components in purulent CSF.

One of the hallmarks of bacterial meningitis is the development of a neutrophilic pleocytosis. The mechanisms responsible for leukocyte traversal across the BBB are unknown. The complement component C5a has been identified as a chemotactic substance in an experimental model of pneumococcal meningitis (86), with chemotactic activity appearing 2–4 hr before the influx of neutrophils into the CSF. Chemotactic activity has been measured in the CSF of patients with pyogenic meningitis (32), and this activity correlates with total protein and C3 concentrations in purulent CSF. The precise role of C5a as a chemotactic factor was recently examined in a rabbit model in which intracisternally administered C5a caused a rapid early influx of leukocytes into CSF, peaking at 1 hr after inoculation (87). Co-administration of prostaglandin E_2 attenuated this response in a dose-dependent manner perhaps due to an inhibitory action of PGE_2 on this C5a-mediated response, suggesting an anti-inflammatory action of PGE_2 in bacterial meningitis. However, despite the entry of leukocytes into the CSF, host defenses remain suboptimal because of the lack of functional opsonic and bactericidal activity with resultant inefficient phagocytosis and attainment of huge bacterial densities in CSF.

The pathway by which neutrophils enter the SAS is unknown. Adherence of neutrophils to vascular endothelial cells may be a necessary prerequisite for this traversal, and formation of specific adhesion molecules such as endothelial leukocyte adhesion molecule 1 by endothelium can be induced by pretreatment of endothelial cells in culture with cytokines (88). It is unclear whether similar adhesion mechanisms exist between neutrophils and cerebral vascular endothelium, although a recent study in a rabbit model of experimental meningitis has suggested that the intravenous inoculation of a monoclonal antibody (IB4) against the CD18 family of receptors on leukocytes can block the accumulation of leukocytes in the SAS despite intracisternal challenge with either Hib, N. meningitidis, pneumococcal cell wall, or LPS (89). In addition, this monoclonal antibody blocked the parameters of BBB permeability (i.e., influx of serum proteins and penetration of antibiotics into CSF), and cerebral edema was absent in monoclonal-antibody-treated animals. The CSF bacterial concentrations and bactericidal response to ampicillin therapy were not affected by monoclonal antibody administration. However, animals receiving the monoclonal antibody exhibited a delay in the onset of bacteremia and an attenuated CSF inflammatory response after ampicillin-induced bacterial killing. This suggests that blockade of leukocyte-mediated damage during bacterial meningitis is feasible with this systemic monoclonal antibody approach.

The precise role of the neutrophil in host defense within the CNS is undefined. There have been conflicting studies as to whether the leukocytic response is beneficial or detrimental in bacterial meningitis. Low concentrations of CSF leukocytes are associated with increased mortality rates in experimental animal models of bacterial meningitis and in patients. In contrast, a study on survival in dogs with pneumococcal meningitis revealed that leukopenic dogs actually had an increased

survival time when compared to animals with normal peripheral leukocyte counts (62 versus 47 hr) (90). However, the small number of dogs studied precluded statistical analysis. In a rabbit model of experimental pneumococcal meningitis, animals were rendered leukopenic by the prior intravenous inoculation of nitrogen mustard. The parameters of bacterial growth rate, final bacterial concentration in CSF, and CSF protein, glucose, and lactate concentrations were no different from those in control animals despite the lack of neutrophils in the CSF (91). The magnitude of the resultant bacteremia, however, was about 100-fold higher in the leukopenic animals, suggesting that neutrophils either prevent traversal of pneumococci from CSF to blood or enhance elimination from the bloodstream at extraneural sites. Thus, the role of the neutrophilic response in bacterial meningitis is unclear. The contribution of neutrophils to the various pathophysiologic consequences of bacterial meningitis, such as BBB permeability and brain edema, is discussed in subsequent sections of this chapter.

Induction of Subarachnoid Space Inflammation

Despite the fact that bacterial capsule is crucial for intravascular and SAS survival of meningeal pathogens, capsular polysaccharides are notably noninflammatory. Recent studies have examined the bacterial virulence factors that lead to SAS inflammation and have provided many new, exciting areas of investigation.

Various surface components of S. pneumoniae have been examined to determine their roles in SAS inflammation. The CSF inflammatory response was invoked in rabbits following the intracisternal inoculation of live encapsulated and unencapsulated S. pneumoniae, heat-killed unencapsulated pneumococci, and pneumococcal cell walls (92). The inoculation of heat-killed encapsulated strains or isolated capsular polysaccharide did not induce inflammation. The most potent inducer of CSF inflammation was the pneumococcal cell wall. In addition, independent intracisternal injection of the major components of the pneumococcal cell wall, teichoic acid and peptidoglycan, also induced CSF inflammation (93). Teichoic acid had the highest specific activity of the cell-wall fractions tested, with peak SAS inflammation occurring 5 hr after instillation. Activity was markedly reduced if the teichoic acid or peptidoglycan was extensively degraded. These findings led the authors to suggest that bacterial cell-wall lytic products released during antibiotic-induced autolysis during treatment of bacterial meningitis contributed to the host inflammatory response in the SAS and resulted in significant morbidity and mortality. This CSF inflammatory response was reduced by inhibition of the cyclooxygenase pathway of arachidonic acid metabolism (94). Simultaneous treatment with methylprednisolone and oxindanac were particularly effective in decreasing inflammation induced by pneumococcal cell walls, whereas another inhibitor, diclofenac sodium, was effective at 5 and 7 hr after CSF inoculation but was not inhibitory 24 hr after cell-wall challenge (Table 11). Nordihydroguaiaretic acid, an inhibitor of the lipoxygenase pathway was ineffective in preventing cell wall-induced inflammation. When tested against natural infection after challenge with live pneumococci, cyclooxygenase inhibitors in conjunction with ampicillin also reduced inflammation associated with release of inflammatory bacterial products during ampicillin-induced bacterial lysis. There was a correlation between the CSF concentrations of the arachidonic acid metabolite PGE_2 and leukocytes after inoculation of live pneumococci or pneumococcal cell walls, and inhibition of the cyclooxygenase pathway reduced both the CSF concentrations of PGE_2 and CSF inflammation. It was suggested that the use of these anti-inflammatory agents, in conjunction with appropriate antimicrobial therapy, may improve outcome in patients with bacterial meningitis by reduction of the CSF inflammatory response.

SAS inflammation is also induced by purified Hib LPS. In an experimental rabbit model, the intracisternal inoculation of purified LPS (dose range of 2 fg to 200 ng) produced a dose-dependent increase in CSF concentrations of white blood cells and protein, whereas no inflammation was invoked after inoculation of purified Hib capsular polysaccharide (95). This inflammatory response was blocked by polymyxin B (a cationic antibiotic that binds to the lipid A region of the LPS molecule), indicating that the lipid A region of the molecule is essential for its inflammatory properties. The tissue toxicity of LPS was also attenuated by neutrophil acyloxyacyl hydrolase, which removes nonhydroxylated fatty acids from the lipid A region of the LPS. A monoclonal antibody to epitopes on the oligosaccharide portion of the LPS molecule did not reduce its inflammatory potential, adding further support to the importance of the lipid A region of LPS. Similar results were obtained in a rat model of experimental meningitis (Table 12)

following the intracisternal inoculation of *H. influenzae* LPS with the maximal degree of CSF inflammation observed 8 hr after challenge with a 20-ng dose (96). However, *H. influenzae* LPS is not in the free state in nature, but rather in the form of outer-membrane vesicles which may represent a relevant nonreplicating vehicle for the delivery of the toxic moieties of LPS to host cells. The intracisternal inoculation of *H. influenzae* type b outer-membrane vesicles induced meningeal inflammation in both rabbits and rats in a dose- and time-dependent manner (97,98). The response was blocked by polymyxin B, but not by two monoclonal antibodies directed against the surface epitopes of LPS within outer-membrane vesicles, supporting the concept that LPS carried via outer-membrane vesicles leads to induction of SAS inflammation.

The mechanisms by which LPS, and more specifically lipid A, bind to host cells to produce deleterious effects are unknown. Many investigators have suggested that mammalian cells possess specific LPS receptors, but the nonspecific binding of LPS to cells has confounded efforts to identify these receptors (99). Utilizing a radioiodinated LPS derivative which maintains the biologic functions of LPS, specific LPS-binding sites have been identified in murine lymphocytes and macrophages (100). This LPS-binding protein exhibits specificity for lipid A, is expressed on the cell membrane of lymphoid cells, and might represent a specific receptor for LPS. No studies have been performed to identify LPS-binding proteins on cells in the CNS, but future studies will determine whether specific binding is an important initial step for the biologic activity of LPS.

Recent mechanistic evidence is accumulating that pneumococcal cell wall or *H. influenzae* LPS elicits SAS inflammation through the release of inflammatory mediators such as interleukin 1 (IL-1) and/or tumor necrosis factor (TNF) within CSF. Intact pneumococci and pneumococcal cell walls or lipoteichoic acid induced large amounts of IL-1 production by human peripheral monocytes *in vitro* (101). Purified teichoicated cell wall had the highest specific activity in this regard. Chemical

TABLE 11. *Effect of cyclooxygenase and lipoxygenase inhibitors on CSF leukocyte concentrations after intracisternal inoculation of 30 µg of pneumococcal cell wall*[a]

Inhibitor (dose and route)[b]	Concentration of CSF leukocytes[c]		
	5 hr	7 hr	24 hr
Control	677 ± 34	1545 ± 90	870 ± 92
Methylprednisolone (30 mg/kg, I.M.)	50 ± 20	198 ± 30	54 ± 20
Diclofenac sodium (5 mg/kg, I.V.)	110 ± 40	433 ± 210	1183 ± 150
Indomethacin (5 mg/kg, P.O.)	115 ± 60	300 ± 50	320 ± 50
Nordihydroguaiaretic acid (5 mg/kg, P.O.)	1093 ± 500		870 ± 240
Oxindanac (5 mg/kg, P.O.)	118 ± 57	59 ± 14	500 ± 325

[a] Adapted from ref. 94.
[b] P.O., orally; I.M., intramuscularly; I.V., intravenously.
[c] Mean number of leukocytes per cubic millimeter.

TABLE 12. *CSF leukocyte concentrations after intracisternal inoculation of 20 ng of H. influenzae type b LPS[a]*

Time after inoculation (hr)	CSF leukocyte concentration (mean/mm³)	
	Control (mean ± SEM)	LPS (mean ± SEM)
2	0 ± 0	0 ± 0
3	0 ± 0	1,030 ± 345[b]
4	0 ± 0	24,294 ± 3,252[b]
6	0 ± 0	36,393 ± 3,834[b]
8	0 ± 0	42,556 ± 6,014[b]
18	10 ± 10	19,900 ± 4,682[b]

[a] Adapted from ref. 96.
[b] $p < 0.05$ compared to control.

alteration of, or antibody against, the major determinant of the teichoic acid, phosphorylcholine, dramatically reduced IL-1 production. However, pneumococcal cell wall did not induce production of TNF—in contrast to the situation with LPS, which induced production of both IL-1 and TNF (see below).

The intracisternal inoculation of Hib LPS into rats led to elevated CSF concentrations of both IL-1 and TNF within 30–120 min (102). Elevated CSF concentration of TNF have also been observed in the rabbit model following the intracisternal inoculation of *H. influenzae* LPS (103). TNF activity was detected as early as 45 min, peaked at 120 min, and was no longer detectable 5 hr after inoculation. Interestingly, simultaneous analysis of serum revealed no TNF activity, indicating that the TNF was principally produced within the CNS. The administration of intravenous dexamethasone or intracisternal anti-TNF antibodies concomitant with the inoculation of *H. influenzae* LPS resulted in a significantly decreased CSF inflammatory response. These experiments were extended in the rabbit model of experimental meningitis following the intracisternal inoculation of live Hib (Table 13) (104). The administration of ceftriaxone 6 hr after infection provoked rapid bacterial lysis followed by greatly increased CSF concentrations of LPS and TNF (peak TNF activity at 2 hr). The simultaneous administration of dexamethasone with ceftriaxone did not affect LPS release, but there was a substantial attenuation of

CSF TNF activity and the CSF inflammatory response. In addition, the increased concentrations of TNF in the CSF may be specific for bacterial meningitis—as suggested in a recent study in which TNF concentrations, measured in mice and humans with either bacterial or viral meningitis, were elevated in the CSF only during bacterial meningitis (105). Only a small sample of humans was included in this study, however.

The above findings have implications with regard to outcome in patients with bacterial meningitis. Persistence and concentrations of endotoxin in CSF (as detected by the *Limulus* lysate assay) correlated with outcome from meningitis due to gram-negative bacilli (106). A recent study in children with *H. influenzae* meningitis found that treatment with ceftriaxone induced a marked increase in CSF concentrations of LPS which correlated positively with the number of bacteria killed in the CSF (107). The initial CSF LPS concentrations correlated with the Herson–Todd clinical severity score and number of febrile hospital days, suggesting that release of free LPS with antimicrobial therapy enhanced the host inflammatory response in the SAS. Elevated concentrations of CSF IL-1β activity also correlated significantly with outcome from neonatal gram-negative bacillary meningitis (108) in which patients with concentrations ≥500 pg/ml were more likely to develop neurologic sequelae. CSF IL-1β concentrations were reduced when the patients were treated with dexamethasone, suggesting that dexamethasone may exert its anti-inflammatory effects in the SAS by inhibiting IL-1β gene expression (Table 14). Elevated CSF concentrations of TNF have also been observed in patients with bacterial meningitis (109), although there was no correlation between CSF concentrations of TNF and outcome, and concentrations were not decreased after dexamethasone treatment. The role of other inflammatory cytokines in the induction of SAS inflammation is less clear. The synthesis of interleukin 6 (IL-6) or of B-cell stimulating factor 2 is induced by IL-1, and increased serum concentrations of IL-6 correlated with outcome in patients with meningococcal septic shock (110). IL-6 activity has also been documented in the CSF of patients with bacterial meningitis, whereas activity was undetectable (<10 U/

TABLE 13. *Effects of treatment with ceftriaxone alone or ceftriaxone plus dexamethasone in rabbits with H. influenzae meningitis[a]*

Time after treatment (hr)	Control		Ceftriaxone		Ceftriaxone plus dexamethasone	
	LPS/CFU	TNF	LPS/CFU	TNF	LPS/CFU	TNF
6	0.4 ± 0.2	1.1 ± 0.7	0.5 ± 0.2	1.0 ± 0.5	0.5 ± 0.2	0.7 ± 0.6
8	0.5 ± 0.3	1.3 ± 0.3	20.3 ± 13.9	11.4 ± 1.8[b]	313.0 ± 309.0	2.0 ± 0.8[b]
10	0.4 ± 0.1	2.7 ± 0.7	4415.0 ± 2900.0[c]	11.9 ± 4.2	1029.0 ± 426.0[c]	2.6 ± 1.0

[a] LPS, lipopolysaccharide; CFU, colony-forming units; TNF, tumor necrosis factor (ng/ml); LPS/CFU, ng/ml of LPS/CFU/ml × 10^{-6}. Adapted from ref. 104.
[b] $p = 0.0184$ versus controls.
[c] $p = 0.0047$ versus controls.

TABLE 14. *CSF concentrations of IL-1β and TNF in infants and children with bacterial meningitis*[a]

Time after treatment (hr)	Cytokine concentration (mean pg/ml ± SD)			
	IL-1β		TNF	
	Control	Dexamethasone	Control	Dexamethasone
0	1040 ± 1363	828 ± 1206	774 ± 2974	841 ± 3014
18–30	225 ± 442	28 ± 74[b]	28 ± 85	12 ± 22[c]

[a] Adapted from ref. 108.
[b] $p = 0.002$ compared to control.
[c] Not significant compared to control.

ml) in CSF samples from patients with chronic headache, dementia, multiple sclerosis, subacute sclerosing panencephalitis, measles encephalitis, and various degenerative diseases of the CNS (111). Additional studies are necessary to precisely define the role of IL-6 in bacterial meningitis.

The source of these inflammatory cytokines in the CSF of patients with bacterial meningitis is unclear. Astrocytes and microglia are capable of releasing cytokines *in vitro* after stimulation with LPS (112), and vascular endothelial cells grown in culture can produce IL-1 in response to either LPS or TNF (113–115). Ongoing studies will address these issues as they pertain to bacterial meningitis and infections of the CNS.

Alterations of the Blood–Brain Barrier

Bacterial meningitis, like many other disease states, increases the permeability of the BBB. The barrier separates the brain from the intravascular compartment and maintains homeostasis within the CNS (116,117). Lipophilic substances readily diffuse across the BBB, but the transport of other nutrients (i.e., hexoses, amino acids, etc.) is regulated by active transport and facilitated diffusion. The major sites of the BBB are the arachnoid membrane, choroid plexus epithelium, and cerebral microvascular endothelium. Previous morphologic studies have demonstrated an intact arachnoid membrane in animals with bacterial meningitis (118), indicating that the increased BBB permeability seen in this disease must occur at the level of the choroid plexus epithelium or of the cerebral microvascular endothelium, or of both. The endothelial cells of the cerebral microvasculature have been the site of intensive study in bacterial meningitis.

The distinguishing features of cerebral capillaries, as opposed to other systemic capillaries, are as follows: Adjacent endothelial cells are fused together by pentalaminar tight junctions (zonulae occludens) that prevent intercellular transport; pinocytotic vesicles are rare or absent; and mitochondria are abundant. Increased permeability of the BBB at the level of the cerebral capillary endothelial cell may result from separation of intercellular tight junctions, from increased pinocytosis, from both alterations, or by processes as yet unknown.

An adult rat model of bacterial meningitis has been utilized to investigate the propensity for bacterial meningitis to induce functional and morphologic alterations in the BBB (119). Morphologic alterations of BBB integrity were assessed utilizing methods to harvest cerebral microvessels from rats by homogenization, dextran centrifugation, and collection on 53-μm nylon filters, followed by examination by transmission electron microscopy. Functional alterations were assessed by measuring the blood-to-CSF transfer of circulating radioactive albumin which is normally excluded by an intact BBB. After the intracisternal inoculation of either *E. coli, S. pneumoniae,* or *H. influenzae,* the following results were observed: (a) a uniform host response to experimental meningitis, with all three encapsulated pathogens at the level of the cerebral capillary endothelium characterized morphologically by an early and sustained increase in pinocytotic vesicle formation as well as a progressive increase in separation of intercellular tight junctions (from 4 to 18 hr post-inoculation); (b) correlation of these morphologic alterations with the functional penetration of albumin across the BBB, with highest values of albumin entry at 18 hr post-inoculation when both morphologic changes were evident; and (c) inoculation with unencapsulated *H. influenzae* (Rd strain) led to an increase in pinocytotic vesicle formation, but separation of intercellular tight junctions did not occur (Table 15). It is likely that this discrepancy between encapsulated and unencapsulated strains of *H. influenzae* occurred as a result of removal of unencapsulated organisms from the CSF by host defense mechanisms, whereas deficient opsonic mechanisms in CSF permitted sustained concentrations of encapsulated strains. Thus, encapsulation of *H. influenzae* was not essential for BBB injury but facilitated its progression by avoidance of host clearance mechanisms in the CSF and/or blood.

To define the importance of the host leukocyte response on BBB permeability, this model was modified by first rendering the animals leukopenic by the intraperitoneal injection of cyclophosphamide (120). In addition, to examine the role of encapsulation on BBB permeability, new strains of *H. influenzae* were chosen for analysis: Rd⁻/b⁺/02 was obtained by transformation of strain Rd using donor DNA from strain Eagan (type b) and Rd⁻/b⁻/02, a spontaneous, one-step, capsule-deficient mu-

TABLE 15. *Correlation of morphologic and functional alterations of the BBB in experimental rat H.* influenzae *meningitis*[a]

Time after treatment (hr)	Inoculum (n)	CSF bacterial concentration (log_{10} CFU/ml)	CSF penetration of ^{125}I-albumin (%)	Change in BBB morphology[b]
4	Saline (3)	0	0.26 ± 0.08	—
	H. influenzae Rd (3)	5.25 ± 0.35	4.12 ± 1.25[c]	↑ PV
	H. influenzae type b (4)	6.26 ± 0.34	3.80 ± 0.75[c]	↑ PV
18	Saline (4)	0	1.25 ± 0.27	—
	H. influenzae Rd (4)	3.32 ± 0.32[d]	4.64 ± 0.80[c]	↑ PV
	H. influenzae type b (4)	8.06 ± 0.35[e]	8.10 ± 1.20[c,e]	↑ PV + ↑ SJ

[a] Values given as mean ± SEM. From ref. 119, with permission.
[b] PV, pinocytotic vesicles; SJ, separated junctions; ↑, increase.
[c] $p < 0.05$ compared to control.
[d] $p < 0.05$ compared to *H. influenzae* Rd at 4 hr.
[e] $p < 0.05$ compared to *H. influenzae* type b at 4 hr and *H. influenzae* Rd at 18 hr.

tant derived from strain Rd⁻/b⁺/02. Functional increases of BBB permeability (assessed by radioactive albumin penetration from blood to CSF) were observed in both normal and leukopenic rats 18 hr following inoculation of either encapsulated or unencapsulated strains of *H. influenzae* (Fig. 3). Permeability, however, was greater after challenge with the encapsulated strain. In addition, significant increases in BBB permeability occurred in the near absence of CSF leukocytes, although the presence of CSF leukocytes augmented changes in permeability at least late (18 hr post-inoculation) in the

disease course. It appeared that type b capsule inhibited the host clearance mechanisms in the CSF, but again it was not essential for altered BBB permeability. Finally, the alterations of BBB permeability correlated with bacterial CSF concentrations late in the disease course.

With the knowledge that bacterial capsule was not essential for the increased BBB observed in bacterial meningitis, BBB permeability following the intracisternal inoculation of bacterial virulence factors that induce SAS inflammation was examined. As stated in the previous section, the intracisternal inoculation of rats with Hib

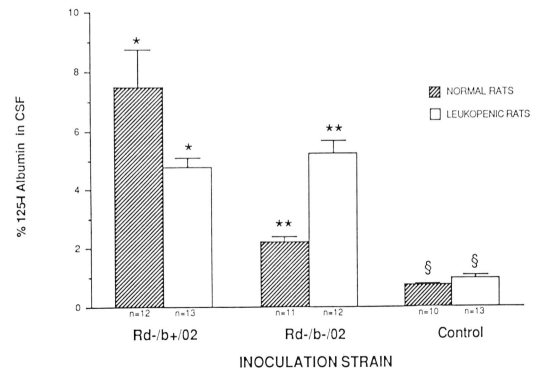

FIG. 3. BBB permeability to circulating ^{125}I-albumin 18 hr after intracisternal challenge with encapsulated (Rd⁻/b⁺/02) or unencapsulated (Rd⁻/b-/02) isogenic mutants of *H. influenzae* or saline (control). Percent BBB permeability calculated as [cpm ^{125}I-CSF/cpm ^{125}I-blood] × 100. Values represent mean ± SEM for normal and leukopenic animals. *$p = 0.04$; **$p < 0.001$; and §p = NS (Student's *t* test, unpaired). (From ref. 120, with permission.)

LPS led to dose- and time-dependent increases in SAS inflammation. Functional alterations of BBB permeability were also observed after the intracisternal inoculation of LPS (96), characterized by the following (Fig. 4): (a) dose-dependent increases of BBB permeability from 2 pg to 20 ng, with attenuation in peak response after challenge with 500 ng or 1 μg; (b) time-dependent increases in BBB permeability, with maximal alteration at 4 hr and complete reversal at 18 hr; (c) greater increases in permeability than after challenge with the live parent strain at identical LPS concentrations; (d) close correlation between CSF pleocytosis and BBB permeability at 4 hr post-inoculation; (e) the LPS effect on BBB permeability was significantly inhibited by preincubation of the LPS with polymyxin B or neutrophil acyloxylacyl hydrolase but not by monoclonal antibodies directed against the oligosaccharide portion of the molecule; and (f) no change in BBB permeability after LPS inoculation into leukopenic rats. Increased BBB permeability was also observed following the intracisternal inoculation of Hib outer-membrane vesicles (98). As with the inoculation of LPS, the increased permeability following injection of *H. influenzae* outer-membrane vesicles was blocked by preincubation with polymyxin B but not by a monoclonal antibody directed against the oligosaccharide side chain of the LPS, and no change in permeability was evident in leukopenic animals. With the knowledge that LPS induced alterations of BBB permeability in the rat model of bacterial meningitis, it was next determined if inflammatory cytokines, which mediate many of the deleterious effects of LPS, also induced permeability changes. Intracisternal inoculation of human recombinant IL-1 into rats led to a peak increase in BBB permeability at 3 hr after inoculation, prior to the peak response with LPS (121), an effect that was significantly attenuated by preincubation of the cytokine with a monoclonal antibody to IL-1 and totally abolished in leukopenic animals. No permeability changes were induced following the intracisternal inoculation of human recombinant TNF, although it appeared that IL-1 and TNF may act synergistically because inoculation with submaximal doses of IL-1 plus TNF, at concentrations that produced no changes individually, enhanced BBB permeability (102).

These changes induced by LPS and inflammatory cytokines on BBB permeability may provide a target for the prevention of subsequent vasogenic cerebral edema and increased intracranial pressure that result once the BBB is disrupted (see below). A recent study has shown that the combination of an anti-inflammatory agent (dexamethasone or oxindanac) and ampicillin was effective in preventing the massive influx of serum albumin and certain proteins of high and low molecular weight into the CSF in animals with pneumococcal meningitis (122), indicating that this combination may be useful in preventing some of the pathophysiologic consequences of bacterial meningitis.

Increased Intracranial Pressure

The major element leading to increased intracranial pressure (ICP) in bacterial meningitis is the development of cerebral edema which may be vasogenic, cytotoxic, or interstitial in origin. Vasogenic cerebral edema is primarily a consequence of increased BBB permeability (see above). Cytotoxic cerebral edema occurs secondary to swelling of the cellular elements of the brain, most likely due to release of toxic factors from neutrophils and/or bacteria. Subsequently, there is increased intracellular water content from alteration in the membranes of brain cells, resulting in potassium leakage, glucose utilization via anaerobic glycolysis, and lactate production (123). Secretion of antidiuretic hormone also contributes to the pathogenesis of cytotoxic edema by producing hypotonicity of extracellular fluid and increasing the permeability of the brain to water (124).

Interstitial edema occurs secondary to obstruction of CSF flow from SAS to blood, as in hydrocephalus. Studies in an experimental rabbit model of pneumococcal and *E. coli* meningitis have shown that the CSF outflow resistance, defined as factors that inhibit the flow of CSF from the SAS to the major dural sinuses, was markedly elevated (125). These alterations of outflow resistance remained for as long as 2 weeks despite CSF sterilization with penicillin therapy. The early administration of methylprednisolone (30 mg/kg, intramuscularly) at 16 and 20 hr after intracisternal inoculation of organisms rapidly lowered CSF outflow resistance towards control values. These results suggested that attenuation of the normal CSF absorptive mechanisms during meningitis may decrease the ability of the brain to compensate in situations of increased ICP.

Subsequent studies attempted to solidify these concepts by measuring the brain water content, which indi-

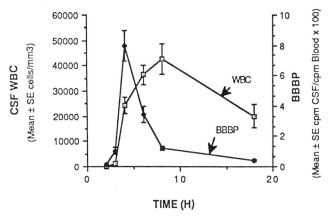

FIG. 4. Kinetics of changes in CSF white blood cell (WBC) and BBB permeability (BBBP) after inoculation of 20 ng of Hib LPS. (From ref. 96, with permission.)

TABLE 16. *Experimental parameters in animals infected with pneumococci for 24 hr and then treated for 24 hr with ampicillin[a]*

Time after infection (hr)	CSF lactate concentration (mg/dl)	Change in CSF pressure (mmHg), mean $\pm$ SD	Brain water content (g H$_2$O/100 g dry weight)
Control	16.2 $\pm$ 4.5	—	398 $\pm$ 10
24	69.5 $\pm$ 28.2[b]	+8.3 $\pm$ 3.6[b]	410 $\pm$ 11[c]
48 (24 hr after treatment)	36.8 $\pm$ 8.3[b]	0.0 $\pm$ 1.1[d]	399 $\pm$ 11[d]

[a] Adapted from ref. 126.
[b] $p < 0.005$ compared to controls.
[c] $p < 0.001$ compared to controls.
[d] Not significant compared to controls.

cates cerebral edema if elevated, CSF lactate, and CSF pressure in animals with pneumococcal meningitis (126). All three parameters were elevated in infected animals (Table 16). Antibiotic therapy normalized CSF pressure and brain edema within 24 hr, whereas CSF lactate concentrations remained elevated. However, the administration of dexamethasone reduced all three parameters, whereas methylprednisolone only reduced brain water content, suggesting that increased CSF outflow resistance is not the only determinant of increased ICP in bacterial meningitis. Indomethacin also decreased brain water content in the experimental pneumococcal meningitis model, although ICP recordings were no different than those observed in the control group. The indomethacin-induced decrease in brain water content was associated with decreased CSF concentrations of PGE$_2$ (127), suggesting again that this prostaglandin may have an important pathophysiologic role in bacterial meningitis. These parameters have also been evaluated in experimental models of Hib meningitis in which the combination of dexamethasone and ceftriaxone was compared to ceftriaxone alone (128). The corticosteroid, as well as the antibiotic and corticosteroid combination, consistently reduced brain water content, CSF pressure, and CSF lactate in infected rabbits more than in animals that received ceftriaxone alone (Table 17). However, the magnitude of reduction, as compared to the ceftriaxone-treated animals, did not reach statistical significance, and by 29 hr the values were comparable whether the animals received antibiotic alone, dexamethasone alone, or the combination. The authors

suggested that dexamethasone may be more beneficial during the early phase of antimicrobial therapy in bacterial meningitis, when there are increased numbers of viable bacteria in the SAS or release of microbial products from antibiotic-induced bacteriolysis. This question was subsequently addressed in an experimental model of *E. coli* meningitis (129). Infected animals were treated with cefotaxime or chloramphenicol. Both antibiotics were effective in reducing CSF bacterial titers. However, treatment with cefotaxime was associated with an increase in brain water content from 389 $\pm$ 8 to 405 $\pm$ 12 g per 100 g of dry weight, which correlated with elevated LPS concentrations in CSF. The increases were neutralized by polymyxin B and by a monoclonal antibody to lipid A, suggesting that antimicrobial therapy with bacteriolytic antibiotics may be important in the pathogenesis of cerebral edema in bacterial meningitis. The role of the neutrophil in this process, however, is unclear. In sterile meningitis induced by the intracisternal inoculation of *N*-formyl-methionyl-leucyl-phenylalanine (fMLP), a chemotactic peptide, both high and low doses induced a CSF pleocytosis whereas only high doses produced an increase in brain water content but without altering ICP, CSF lactate, or CSF protein (130). No increase in brain water content was observed in neutropenic animals. Similar results were seen when high doses of fMLP were injected during pneumococcal meningitis, suggesting that neutrophils may contribute to cerebral edema if adequately stimulated, although the parameters of increased ICP, CSF lactate, and CSF protein appear unrelated to the presence of neutrophils. However, this area remains

TABLE 17. *Changes in CSF pressure and brain water content in rabbits with H. influenzae type b meningitis[a]*

Groups, treatment	Changes in CSF pressure (mmHg)		Brain water content (g H$_2$O/100 g dry weight)	
	20 hr	29 hr	Pretreatment	29 hr
Uninfected rabbits	—	—	405 $\pm$ 14	—
Dexamethasone	+2.69 $\pm$ 1.83	+0.65 $\pm$ 1.00	—	404 $\pm$ 12
Dexamethasone plus ceftriaxone	+2.67 $\pm$ 1.87	+0.61 $\pm$ 1.28	—	406 $\pm$ 12
Ceftriaxone	+2.79 $\pm$ 2.94	+1.12 $\pm$ 1.48	—	411 $\pm$ 14
No therapy	+2.07 $\pm$ 1.80	+2.77 $\pm$ 3.01	—	419 $\pm$ 10

[a] Adapted from ref. 128.

controversial because neutrophils were required for the increased BBB permeability seen with bacterial products and inflammatory mediators (see above), and additional studies are required to precisely define the role of the neutrophil in the pathophysiology of bacterial meningitis.

The infusion of hypertonic mannitol to treat increased ICP has been evaluated in the rabbit model of experimental Hib meningitis (131). In all animals, mannitol consistently reduced intracisternal pressure, although the magnitude of reduction was greater in infected animals. CSF lactate concentrations were also significantly reduced after mannitol treatment in infected animals, perhaps as a result of improved cerebral blood flow and restoration of aerobic cerebral glucose metabolism. Brain water content, however, was no different in mannitol-treated animals than in untreated ones. Mannitol has been used, although infrequently, in patients with bacterial meningitis and has been effective in lowering ICP (132,133). Further studies are needed, however, to define the optimal use of mannitol in this disorder.

Cerebral Vasculitis and Alterations in Cerebral Blood Flow

Bacterial meningitis exerts profound effects on large blood vessels coursing through the SAS, with resultant vasculitis. This vasculitis leads to narrowing of cerebral blood vessels, with the propensity for ischemia and/or infarction of underlying brain (134). When arteriography was performed in children with bacterial meningitis, leakage of contrast material due to the vascular involvement was observed, but these changes reverted to normal following successful antimicrobial therapy. With involvement of the large arteries at the base of the brain, severe neurologic complications (e.g., hemiparesis and quadriparesis) with permanent sequelae may ensue (135). There may also be release of humoral factors elaborated within the CSF or blood vessel wall, with subsequent vasospasm progressing to vasodilation and organic stenosis later in the disease course (136). Phlebitis of major cortical draining vessels and/or dural sinuses may result in thrombosis with secondary brain infarction, focal neurologic deficits, and prominent seizure activity. The above changes, along with increased ICP, may result in alteration of cerebral blood flow in patients with bacterial meningitis (76). In the infant rhesus monkey model of *H. influenzae* meningitis, cerebral blood flow was measured by an autoradiographic technique utilizing [^{14}C]antipyrine. It was determined that certain areas of the cortex (postcentral, temporal, and occipital) were hypoperfused relative to the hypothalamus and midbrain while the brainstem was hyperperfused, suggesting that one of the initial physiologic changes in *H. influenzae* meningitis is cerebral cortical hypoperfusion with resultant relative cerebral anoxia.

A recent report has shown that cerebrovascular autoregulation is lost in experimental bacterial meningitis, with a parallel fluctuation between cerebral blood flow and ICP (137). Cerebral blood flow increased when blood pressure was raised and decreased when blood pressure was lowered, indicating that flow was pressure-passive. The same changes were observed with ICP (i.e., increased cerebral blood flow was associated with increased ICP). These results suggest that adequate volume status and minimization of stimuli that increase blood pressure may have important roles in the treatment of patients with bacterial meningitis, since minimal changes in blood pressure may adversely affect outcome as a result of the alterations in ICP. Cerebral blood flow has been shown to be altered in patients with bacterial meningitis. Measurement of cerebral blood flow by the xenon-133 intra-arterial injection method revealed a 30–40% reduction in average total blood flow in five patients with pneumococcal meningitis (mean age of 54 years) but not in five patients with meningococcal meningitis (mean age of 20 years). In infants with bacterial meningitis, there was an inverse correlation between cerebral blood flow velocity (measured by Doppler techniques through the anterior fontanelle) and ICP (138). These alterations were only detected in the four older infants aged 3–10 months but not in the four neonates 5–30 days old in whom no changes in cerebral blood flow velocity were observed. The importance of bacterial virulence factors or inflammatory mediators on cerebral blood flow alterations has not been defined; further studies are needed. However, blood flow alterations may lead to regional hypoxia, increased brain lactate concentration secondary to utilization of glucose by anaerobic glycolysis, and CSF acidosis (which could be a precursor to encephalopathy).

PATHOLOGY

Adams et al. (139) described the pathology of bacterial meningitis in 1948 based on examination of autopsy material from patients with *H. influenzae* meningitis. Experimental models of bacterial meningitis, knowledge of host defense mechanisms, and the pathophysiology of associated complications have subsequently allowed for a more complete understanding of the pathologic processes operating in this disorder.

Bacteria reach the meninges through one of the following pathways: (a) hematogenous dissemination from a distant site (e.g., nasopharynx, lung, skin, genitourinary tract); (b) spread from an adjacent suppurative focus of infection (e.g., otitis media, sinusitis, mastoiditis); and (c) through either a congenital or acquired structural defect (140). The mechanisms by which bacteria enter and multiply within the subarachnoid space have been discussed in the previous section.

Once bacteria gain access to the SAS, an inflammatory

process ensues. Neutrophils migrate into the SAS, producing a purulent exudate. On gross examination, the exudate has a grayish-yellow or yellowish-green appearance (Fig. 5). It is most abundant in the cisterns at the base of the brain and over the convexities of the hemispheres in the rolandic and sylvian sulci (Fig. 6) (139). The tendency for exudate to accumulate in the cisterns at the base of the brain is explained by the anatomy of the SAS. The SAS is deepest at the base of the brain. The various cisterns are expansions of the SAS, with the largest of these areas lying between the cerebellum and medulla and extending downward below the foramen magnum, the so-called cisterna magna or cerebellomedullary cistern (141). Purulent exudate accumulates in this cistern and extends into the other basal cisterns and onto the posterior surface of the spinal cord (Figs. 7 and 8). The exudate also extends into the arachnoidal sheaths of the cranial nerves and into the perivascular spaces of the cortex. A small amount of exudate may be found in the ventricular fluid and attached to the ventricular walls and choroid plexus; thus, the appearance of the ventricular fluid is usually cloudy by the end of the first week of the infection (139).

Microscopic examination of the subarachnoid exudate in the early stages of the infection demonstrates large numbers of neutrophils and bacteria (lying either free in the exudate or within neutrophils) (140). The role of the neutrophil in eradicating the infection at this stage is unknown. The presence of free-living bacteria in the exudate suggests that phagocytosis by neutrophils is in-

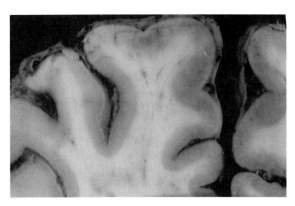

FIG. 6. Purulent exudate in the cerebral sulci.

complete as a result of deficient opsonic activity in CSF; however, low CSF leukocyte concentrations in the presence of high CSF bacterial concentrations have been associated with a poor prognosis in both experimental and human meningitis (67). These observations suggest that the neutrophils have a beneficial role in partial control of the early stages of the infection. The presence of large numbers of neutrophils in the SAS and vessel walls may, however, also be detrimental to the host as has been discussed in the previous section.

Within the first 48–72 hr of infection, there is evidence of inflammation in the walls of the small and medium-sized subarachnoid arteries (Fig. 9). The endothelial cells swell and multiply, narrowing the lumen. The adventitia is infiltrated by neutrophils, and neutrophils and lymphocytes form a layer beneath the intima (Fig. 10). Subintimal arterial infiltration by neutrophils and lymphocytes is relatively unique to infection of the meninges, and it may be related to the anatomy of the meningeal arteries. It is only rarely observed in inflammatory processes in other organs (139). The adventitia of the subarachnoid vessels, as they enter the brain parenchyma, is formed by the arachnoid membrane. As arteries and

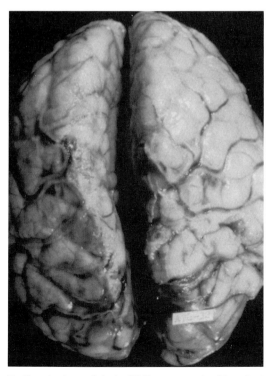

FIG. 5. Purulent exudate in SAS over cerebral hemispheres.

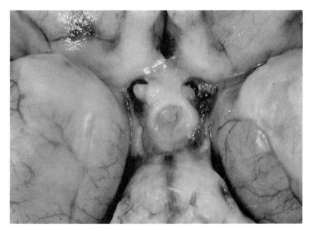

FIG. 7. Purulent exudate surrounding the temporal poles, optic chiasm, and pons.

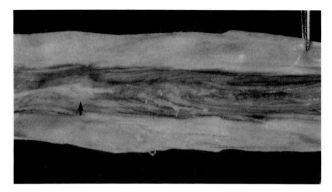

FIG. 8. Purulent exudate (*arrow*) covering spinal cord and nerve roots.

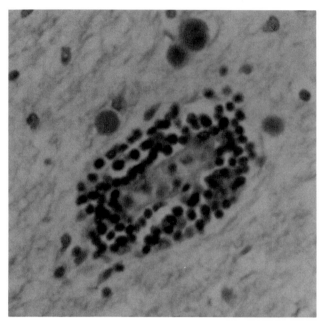

FIG. 9. Inflammatory cells in perivascular space.

veins enter the brain parenchyma, they carry with them a sleeve of arachnoid immediately surrounding the vessel and a sleeve of pia mater external to this. Between these two layers lies an extension of the SAS, known as the "perivascular space" or "Virchow–Robin space," which is filled with CSF (Fig. 11) (141). Because the vessel wall is enveloped by the arachnoid membrane, it is affected early by any inflammatory process in the meninges. However, as shown in animal models of bacterial meningitis, the arachnoid membrane generally remains intact.

The meningeal veins become distended and develop mural inflammation during bacterial meningitis. There may be focal necrosis of the vessel wall, along with mural thrombus formation in the lumen of the vein or in the dural sinus (Fig. 12) (139). Hemorrhagic cortical infarction is the result of cortical venous and dural sinus thrombosis.

Toward the end of the first week of meningeal infection, there is a change in the cellular composition of the subarachnoid exudate. Neutrophils begin to degenerate and are removed by macrophages, which are derived from meningeal histiocytes. Lymphocytes and fibroblasts proliferate in the exudate. Microscopic changes in the brain parenchyma may also be present. The nuclei of neurons and glial cells become shrunken, pyknotic, and darkly staining (Fig. 13). Rod-shaped microglial cells and astrocytes increase in number in the cerebral and

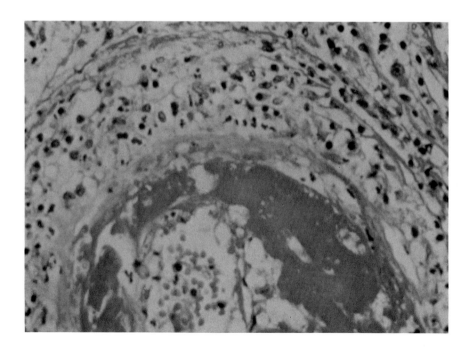

FIG. 10. Small artery with inflammatory infiltration of the vessel wall and mural thrombus.

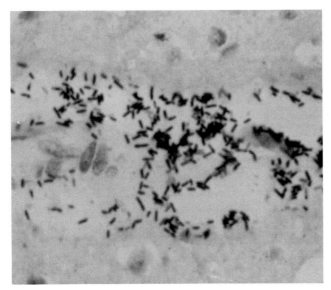

FIG. 11. Tissue Gram's stain depicting pneumococci in the Virchow–Robin space.

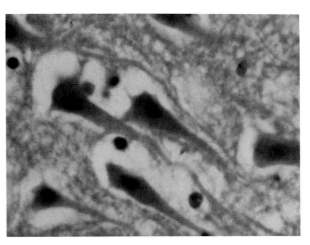

FIG. 13. Shrunken "red" neurons.

cerebellar cortex, brainstem, and spinal cord (Fig. 14). Astrocytic processes become swollen (Fig. 15). There is a loss of myelinated fibers in the subcortical white matter, cerebellum, and brainstem (139). Similar morphological changes are seen in ischemic and hypoxic cortical injury, suggesting that ischemia and/or hypoxia may contribute to the pathological changes from bacterial meningitis at this stage.

Also at the end of the first week of the infection, there is infiltration of the subependymal tissues and perivascu-

lar spaces by neutrophils and lymphocytes. The ependymal and subependymal tissues become edematous, and cells begin to die; also occurring is desquamation of the ependymal lining. Rod-shaped microglial cells and swollen astrocytes proliferate and overgrow the remnants of the ependymal lining. An inflammatory infiltrate in the walls of the subependymal arteries may occlude the vessel, leading to tissue necrosis (139).

As the infection continues, the subarachnoid exudate continues to accumulate. In some areas it may become several millimeters thick (Fig. 16). Toward the end of the second week, the exudate separates into two layers. The outer layer, just beneath the arachnoid membrane, is comprised of neutrophils and fibrin. The inner layer, which is contiguous with the pia, is composed of lymphocytes, plasma cells, and macrophages (139). As the subarachnoid exudate continues to accumulate, the flow of CSF may become obstructed.

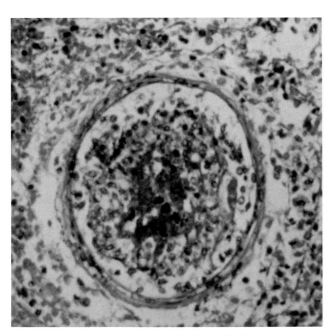

FIG. 12. Inflammatory infiltrate in the wall of a cerebral vein with thrombosis. Note inflammatory cells in thrombus.

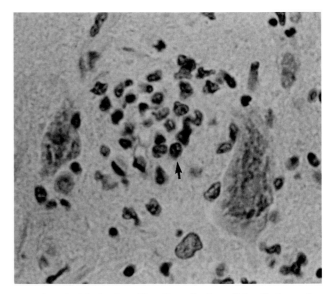

FIG. 14. Marked proliferation of microglial cells (*arrow*).

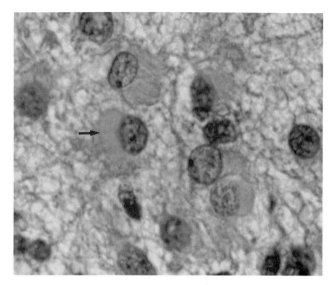

FIG. 15. Reactive "gemistocytic" astrocytes (*arrow*).

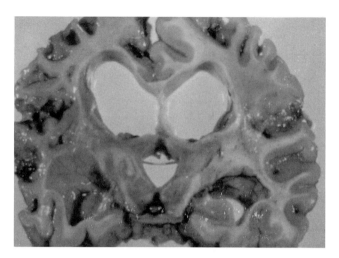

FIG. 17. Hydrocephalus.

The dynamics involved in obstruction of CSF flow are as follows. The bulk of CSF is formed by the choroid plexus in the lateral and third ventricles, and it flows through the cerebral aqueduct into the fourth ventricle. CSF leaves the fourth ventricle through the midline foramen of Magendie and the lateral foramina of Luschka to reach the SAS (141). When the foramina of Magendie and Luschka are blocked by exudate, the spinal fluid cannot circulate to the convexities of the brain where it is normally absorbed. The flow of CSF is blocked at the level of the fourth ventricle, resulting in noncommunicating or obstructive hydrocephalus (Fig. 17).

From the fourth ventricle, CSF normally flows to the SAS at the base of the brain. From here, CSF flows up over the convexity of the hemispheres, to be absorbed by the arachnoid villi in the intracranial venous sinuses (141). The presence of a fibrinopurulent exudate in the SAS interferes with the absorption of CSF by the arach-

noid villi. This obstruction to CSF resorption due to inflammatory changes in the arachnoid granulations results in communicating hydrocephalus. When the subarachnoid exudate has been present for several weeks, there is (a) marked fibrosis of the arachnoid villi and (b) pockets of exudate walled off by adhesions between the arachnoid membrane and dura (139). These fibrotic changes produce further mechanical obstruction to the resorption of CSF by the arachnoid villi. The end result is (a) transependymal movement of CSF from the ventricular system into the brain parenchyma and (b) the development of interstitial cerebral edema.

The development of diffuse cerebral edema and increased intracranial pressure further complicates the pathological changes already described. Cerebral edema is defined as an increase in the volume of the brain resulting from an increased water content (Fig. 18) (142). The cerebral edema in meningitis is a combination of vasogenic, cytotoxic, and interstitial edema (143). Vasogenic edema is a result of increased permeability of brain capillaries with the subsequent accumulation of water

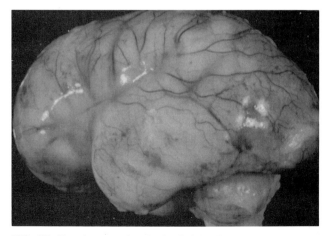

FIG. 16. Purulent exudate in the Sylvian fissure and covering the cerebellum in the brain of a premature infant with meningitis.

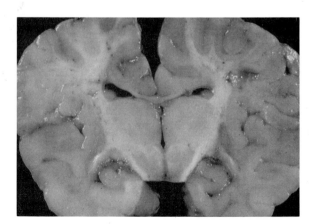

FIG. 18. Specimen demonstrating the characteristic changes of cerebral-edema-flattened gyri and narrowed ventricles.

and protein molecules in the extracellular space, mainly in the subcortical white matter. Cytotoxic edema is due to an accumulation of intracellular water and sodium with subsequent swelling of cells. Membrane polyunsaturated fatty acids and other toxic factors released from leukocytes contribute to the development of cytotoxic edema (67). Interstitial edema is a result of obstruction to CSF resorption as discussed above.

Cerebral edema leads to an increase in ICP, and increased ICP adversely affects cerebral perfusion pressure. Cerebral perfusion pressure (CPP) is defined as the difference between the systemic mean arterial pressure (MAP) and the ICP (CPP = MAP − ICP) (144). Cerebral blood flow may be maintained at normal or near-normal levels in the presence of increased ICP, provided that the CPP is maintained at a range of at least 50–60 mmHg. As ICP continues to rise or if there is a decrease in systemic arterial pressure, cerebral ischemia and infarction may result.

There is experimental evidence for loss of autoregulation of cerebral blood flow in bacterial meningitis (145) (see previous section). This is another potential contributing factor to the development of cerebral ischemia in this infection. Cerebral blood flow is normally constant within a range of mean systemic arterial pressure from 50 to 150 mmHg. When autoregulation is disturbed, systemic hypotension results in decreased cerebral blood flow and cerebral ischemia (146).

Cerebral edema may lead to herniation of brain tissue. Herniation may compress intracerebral arteries, leading to ischemia and infarction; it may also compress the surface of the brain against the dura, leading to necrosis of brain tissue. Tonsillar herniation, the downward displacement of the cerebellar tonsils through the foramen magnum, can result in apnea, hemodynamic instability, coma, and death (142,147).

The pathological lesions described above are typical of meningitis caused by bacteria, but some distinctions among lesions caused by *H. influenzae, N. meningitidis,* and *S. pneumoniae* infection have been observed. The subarachnoid exudate in *H. influenzae* meningitis is very thick and purulent with loculated pockets of pus in the basilar cisterns and cerebral sulci. In contrast, the exudate in pneumococcal meningitis tends to be more extensive over the convexities of the hemispheres than in the basilar cisterns (Fig. 19). In meningococcal meningitis, the pathological changes depend on the severity and duration of the infection. In acute fulminating meningococcemia, death may occur before pus can accumulate in the SAS. At autopsy, severe hyperemia and swelling of cerebral tissue is evident, with petechial hemorrhages in the gray and white matter (Fig. 20) and in the subependymal regions of the lateral ventricles. A hemorrhagic ependymitis is typical of severe lethal meningococcal infection (Fig. 21). The presence of pus in the SAS may only be evident by microscopic examination (147). The

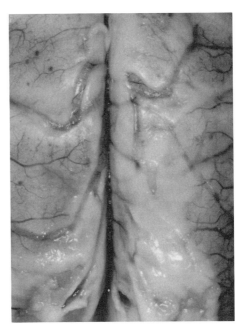

FIG. 19. Purulent exudate over the cerebral convexities from pneumococcal meningitis.

pathological changes in meningococcal meningitis of longer duration are similar to those described for meningitis caused by pyogenic organisms in general.

Cranial and spinal nerve deficits, focal neurological deficits, seizure disorders, and subdural effusions are well-recognized complications of meningitis. The cranial and spinal nerve deficits are usually transient and due to exudate in the SAS surrounding the nerves. Focal neurological deficits and seizure activity arise from cortical and subcortical ischemia and infarction (bland and hemorrhagic), which is the result of inflammation and thrombosis in arteries and veins. Subdural effusions are relatively common in the course of bacterial meningitis in children; they are due to an increase in the permeabil-

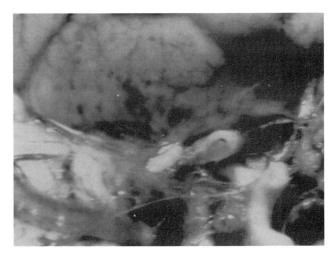

FIG. 20. Petechial hemorrhages in gray matter secondary to meningococcal meningitis.

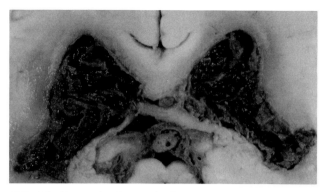

FIG. 21. Hemorrhagic ventriculitis complicating meningitis.

TABLE 18. *Symptoms and signs of bacterial meningitis by age group*

Age group	Symptoms	Signs
Child	Fever Lethargy or altered level of consciousness Headache Irritability Nausea and vomiting Respiratory symptoms Photophobia	Nuchal rigidity Purpuric or petechial rash Seizures Ataxia Focal neurological deficits, including cranial-nerve palsies
Adult	Fever Headache Lethargy, confusion, or coma Nausea and vomiting Photophobia Respiratory symptoms	Nuchal rigidity Altered level of consciousness Seizures Focal neurological deficits, including cranial-nerve palsies
Elderly	Fever Confusion or coma Headache Respiratory symptoms	Nuchal rigidity Altered level of consciousness Seizures—status epilepticus

ity of the thin-walled capillaries and veins in the inner layer of the dura, with leakage of fluid into the subdural space.

Bacteremia also contributes to the pathology of this disease. Bacteremia is present in 30–90% of cases of bacterial meningitis. It can be either (a) the primary event leading to development of meningitis or (b) a secondary event arising from the clearance of bacteria from the SAS through the arachnoid villi to the bloodstream. Pneumococcal cell walls activate the alternative complement pathway with the generation of chemotactic peptides in the systemic circulation as well as in CSF. The principal component of this activity is C5a, a highly chemotactic peptide that is the stimulus for an intense CSF accumulation of neutrophils. By this process, neutrophils also become sequestered in the pulmonary vascular bed, leading to cardiopulmonary dysfunction, neutrophil-mediated vascular damage, and the development of the adult respiratory distress syndrome, thereby contributing to the morbidity and mortality from meningitis (67).

CLINICAL MANIFESTATIONS

Children

The initial symptoms of bacterial meningitis in children may be any of the following: fever, stiff neck, headache, lethargy, irritability, nausea, vomiting, and photophobia (Table 18). Although the symptoms are nonspecific, the combination of one or more of these symptoms with signs of meningeal irritation should suggest the diagnosis of meningitis. The classic signs of meningeal irritation are nuchal rigidity and Brudzinski's and Kernig's signs. Brudzinski actually described several signs of meningeal irritation, including the nape-of-the-neck sign, the identical contralateral reflex sign, and a reciprocal contralateral reflex sign, as well as others (148,149). The nape-of-the-neck sign is Brudzinski's best-known sign and is universally recognized today as "Brudzinski's sign." The nape-of-the-neck sign is positive when passive flexion of the neck results in flexion of the hips and knees. The identical contralateral reflex sign

is elicited with the patient in the supine position by passively flexing the hip and knee on one side. This sign is positive when the contralateral leg flexes with this maneuver. The reciprocal contralateral reflex sign is positive when the leg that has flexed in response to passive flexion of the other leg begins to extend spontaneously, resembling a "little kick." The identical and reciprocal contralateral reflex signs are not elicited as often as the nape-of-the-neck sign (149). The manner in which Kernig's sign is elicited and the interpretation of the results of the maneuver as it is done today are different from those originally described by Kernig (150). The maneuver as described by Kernig was performed with the patient in a seated position while the physician attempted to passively extend the knee. In the presence of meningitis, knee extension was resisted so that a "contracture of the extremities" was maintained (149,150). Today the sign is elicited with the patient in a supine position. The thigh is flexed on the abdomen, with the knee flexed. The leg is then passively extended. When meningeal inflammation is present, the patient resists leg extension (151). Nuchal rigidity and Brudzinski's and Kernig's signs are observed in only ~50% of children with bacterial meningitis.

The possibility of bacterial meningitis should be considered in every child with fever, vomiting, nuchal rigidity, and lethargy or an altered mental status. In a review of 110 cases of culture-proven bacterial meningitis in children, fever (38.5°C or greater) was the most frequent symptom, being present in 94% of patients. The absence of fever, particularly hypothermia, is associated with a worse prognosis, perhaps relating to the slower rate of bacterial replication in CSF when elevated temperatures are present. Apart from fever, the most common symptoms were (a) vomiting (82%) and nuchal rigidity (77%) in the 1- to 4-year-old children and (b) headache (92%) in the children aged 5–12 years. Vomiting and nuchal rigidity were present in 80% of the children who were 12 months of age or older. Nuchal rigidity is a classic sign of meningitis but can be absent early in the course of this illness; therefore, the absence of nuchal rigidity should not exclude the diagnosis of bacterial meningitis (152).

In a review of 709 spinal taps done on children in an outpatient setting in which there was a concern for meningitis, the CSF was abnormal in 16% (112). There were 30 cases of bacterial meningitis, 70 of viral meningitis and 12 of unknown etiology. Lethargy was more common in the children with bacterial meningitis than in the children with viral meningitis: 50% of the children with bacterial meningitis were lethargic, and 32% of the children with viral meningitis were lethargic ($p = 0.14$). Although vomiting is a symptom of meningeal irritation, it is a nonspecific symptom in children. Vomiting occurred in 336 children, 84 of whom had bacterial or viral meningitis. Fever was present in every child with meningitis. The temperature elevations were higher in bacterial meningitis than in viral meningitis; 80% of the children with bacterial meningitis had temperatures of 38.8°C or higher. In children with viral meningitis, 40% had temperatures of 38.8°C or greater (153). The possibility of meningitis in a child who does not or cannot complain of headache or stiff neck and who does not have meningeal signs should be suspected when fever accompanies changes in behavior, changes in mental status, or new onset of seizures.

In a review of 1064 cases of bacterial meningitis in infants and children, there were no signs of meningeal irritation in 16 cases (1.5%). Eight patients were older than 2 years of age. Lumbar puncture was performed because of unexplained fever associated with an altered level of consciousness, behavioral changes, seizure activity, or petechial skin lesions. Meningitis was caused by *N. meningitidis* in seven patients, *H. influenzae* in six, *S. pneumoniae* in two, and *Salmonella enteritidis* in one. The majority of patients had a peripheral leukocytosis with a left shift. The peripheral white blood cell count was greater than 10,000 per cubic millimeter in 12 patients and greater than 20,000 per cubic millimeter in seven patients (154). The results of this review suggest that although meningitis may occasionally occur without meningeal signs, there will usually be other signs or symptoms of intracranial infection as well as a peripheral leukocytosis.

Observational data that are useful in predicting the presence of serious illness (e.g., meningitis) in a febrile child include the following: (i) quality of cry, (ii) reaction to parent stimulation, (iii) level of consciousness, (iv) color, (v) hydration, and (vi) response to social stimulation. These six items were identified as significant and independent predictors of serious illness from a list of 14 observational items, scored by pediatricians, for 312 febrile children aged 24 months or younger (155). The quality of the cry in a child with a serious illness was weak, moaning, or high-pitched. A healthy child was either not crying or had a strong cry with normal tone. Reaction to parental stimulation was judged based on the parent holding the child, talking to the child, or giving the child a bottle. The child with a serious illness did not stop crying or barely responded to stimulation by its parent. Consciousness was impaired in children with serious illnesses. They were lethargic, stuporous, or obtunded. Sick children were described as pale, cyanotic, or ashen. Signs of dehydration were present. The response to social stimulation was judged as to whether the child would smile when talked to or smiled at. Sick children did not respond to social stimulation. These six items, when used together, had a specificity of 88% and a sensitivity of 77% for the presence of serious illness. When combined with history and physical examination, the sensitivity of the six-item model increased to 92%. If all six of the observation items were normal in a child, the probability of that child having a serious illness was only 4.7% (155).

The possibility of meningitis in a febrile child may also be suggested by the tempo of the illness. The presentation of meningitis in children is either that of a subacute infection or an acute, fulminant illness. Children with a subacute presentation have fever, lethargy, and nuchal rigidity which progresses over one to several days and which is usually preceded by an upper respiratory tract infection or otitis media (156). *H. influenzae* type b is the most common etiologic agent of bacterial meningitis in children aged 6 months to 6 years. Children with meningitis due to this organism usually present with an illness that has been progressive over 24–72 hr (157); however, some children have a fulminant illness that develops over several hours.

Children with a more rapidly progressive illness will have signs and symptoms of meningeal irritation and increased ICP on initial presentation. CSF pressures exceeding 300 mmH$_2$O are common in acute bacterial meningitis, and ICPs exceeding 500–600 mmH$_2$O are not unusual (156,158). Increased ICP in bacterial meningitis in children is due, in part, to vasogenic and cytotoxic cerebral edema, altered CSF resorption, and the inappropriate secretion of antidiuretic hormone (159) (see above). The clinical manifestations of increased ICP include: (a) an altered level of consciousness; (b) dilated, poorly reactive or nonreactive pupils; (c) ocular motility abnormalities; (d) pathologically brisk lower-extremity reflexes; and (e) bradycardia and hypertension, also known as "Cushing's reflex." The development of elevated ICP should be anticipated and monitored in a child with bacterial meningitis. The absence of papilledema does not exclude the presence of increased ICP. Papilledema is rarely observed early in the course of increased ICP and is usually not evident until increased ICP has been present for at least several hours (156,158). For this reason, the presence of papilledema at the time of the initial presentation should raise suspicion of a focal intracranial process such as a brain abscess or other localized mass lesion, and it is an indication for computerized tomography (CT) prior to lumbar puncture.

Seizures occur in 30–40% of children with acute bacterial meningitis, usually during the first 3 days of illness (160). In one review of 52 cases of *H. influenzae* meningitis in children, seizures occurred in 44% (23 cases) (158). There has been a longstanding controversy about whether to do a lumbar puncture in febrile children with new-onset seizures. The vast majority of children who present with a new-onset seizure associated with fever and who have a normal neurological examination do not have meningitis. One series reviewed the results of lumbar puncture performed on 328 children presenting with their first febrile convulsion. None of the children had meningeal signs. Meningitis was diagnosed by lumbar puncture in four children (1.2%). Three of the children had viral meningitis, and one had *H. influenzae* meningitis. All four children were less than 18 months old. All of the children in this series that were over 18 months of age had unequivocal signs of meningitis (161). A similar observation was made in a review of lumbar puncture performed on 304 children for evaluation of new-onset seizures associated with fever. There were 15 cases of meningitis, and in only one case were there no meningeal signs. In that case, the child had a viral meningitis and recovered fully without treatment (162). These studies suggest that lumbar puncture should not necessarily be routinely performed in children for evaluation of simple febrile convulsions in the absence of meningeal signs.

Convulsive seizure associated with fever is a problem unique to young children. A simple febrile seizure, as defined by the Consensus Development Meeting on Long-Term Management of Febrile Seizures (1980), occurs between ages 3 months and 5 years in association with fever and is of brief duration (less than 15 min), nonfocal, nonrepetitive, and without associated neurological deficits. If the seizure fits this definition, and the child is awake and alert after the seizure, the yield of a lumbar puncture is very low. If, however, there are clinical signs of meningitis, a lumbar puncture is indicated. If the seizure has a focal onset or there is a focal neurological deficit on examination, a CT scan is indicated before lumbar puncture is performed. All children with new-onset febrile convulsions in whom lumbar puncture is not performed should be reexamined 1–4 hr after the initial examination, to be sure that serious disease is not present (163).

The presence of a diffuse erythematous maculopapular rash may be an early manifestation of meningococcemia or may represent a viral illness. The presence of a purpuric or petechial rash on the trunk and lower extremities is suggestive of meningococcemia, although petechiae are sometimes seen in echovirus type 9 meningitis, acute staphylococcal endocarditis, and, rarely, pneumococcal or *H. influenzae* meningitis (158,164). Petechiae are found in the skin, mucous membranes, or conjunctivae, but never in the nail beds, in patients with meningococcemia; they usually fade in 3 or 4 days (165). Petechiae and/or purpura occur in 50–75% of children with meningococcal meningitis. Children with fulminating meningococcal septicemia may have the Waterhouse–Friderichsen syndrome, characterized by the following: (a) sudden onset of a febrile illness, (b) large petechial hemorrhages in the skin and mucous membranes, (c) cardiovascular collapse, and (d) disseminated intravascular coagulation. Of all patients with a meningococcal infection, 10–20% have a fulminant meningococcal septicemia (166) (Color figures 1–6).

Focal neurological signs, such as cranial-nerve palsies with ocular motility abnormalities, hemiparesis, visual field defects, and ataxia, may occur early or late in the course of bacterial meningitis in approximately 15% of children (156). Cranial-nerve palsies likely develop as the nerve becomes enveloped by exudate in the arachnoidal sheath surrounding the nerve. Alternatively, cranial nerve palsies may be a sign of increased ICP. The presence of bilateral sixth-nerve palsies, manifest as weakness of lateral rectus muscles, is a well-recognized sign of increased ICP.

Hemiparesis may be due to vasculitis and cerebral infarction or may be a sign of the presence of a large subdural effusion. Subdural effusions commonly develop in the course of bacterial meningitis in children and are not usually associated with clinical symptomatology. Subdural effusions develop when the infection in the adjacent SAS leads to an increase in the permeability of the thin-walled capillaries and veins in the inner layer of the dura. The result is leakage of albumin-rich fluid into the subdural space, usually a self-limited process. When the inflammatory process subsides, fluid formation usually ceases and the fluid in the subdural space is resorbed (156). Some subdural effusions are, however, clinically significant. The development of a hemiparesis or of increased ICP may be due to an enlarging subdural effusion causing mass effect. The presence of a prolonged fever in a child with a subdural effusion suggests that the effusion has become infected.

Ataxia may be the presenting sign of bacterial meningitis in a child. This is more common in *H. influenzae* meningitis than in meningococcal or pneumococcal

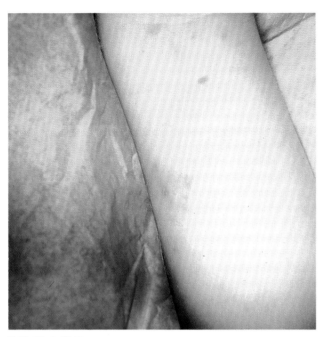

COLOR FIGURE 1. Early appearance of rash in patient with acute meningococcemia.

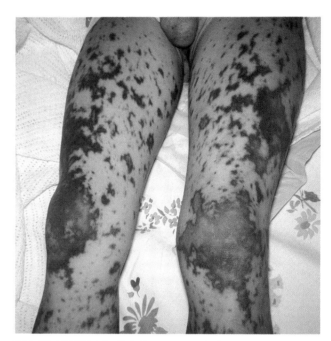

COLOR FIGURE 3. Fulminant petechial/purpuric rash in patient with meningococcemia.

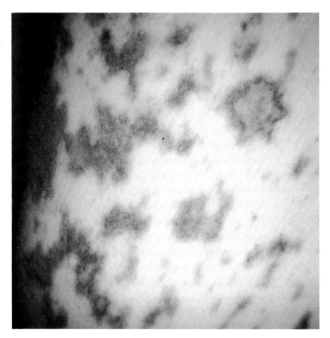

COLOR FIGURE 2. Close up of rash in patient with acute meningococcemia.

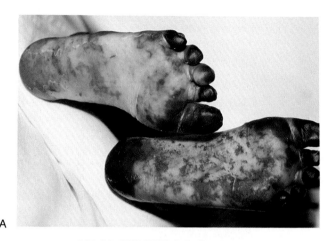
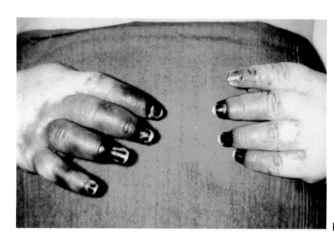

A   B

COLOR FIGURES 4 A, B. Examples of severe purpura fulminans and peripheral gangrene in two patients with acute meningococcemia.

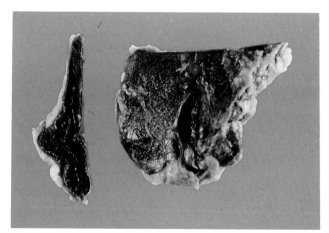

COLOR FIGURE 5. Gross pathologic specimen depicting adrenal hemorrhage in fulminant acute meningococcemia (Waterhouse-Friderichsen syndrome).

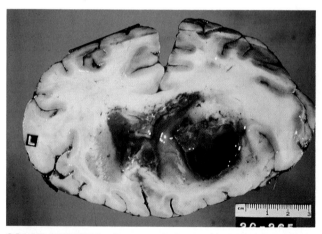

COLOR FIGURE 6. Gross pathologic specimen showing intraventricular hemorrhage from a patient with acute meningococcemia and disseminated intravascular coagulation. Note marked right-to-left herniation (fatal in this case) and periventricular white matter edema.

meningitis, although the reason for this remains obscure. Ataxia is a sign of vestibular dysfunction, and in this clinical setting it suggests the presence of labyrinthitis. In most children it is a transient symptom; however, it has implications for prognosis, since auditory and vestibular disturbances usually occur together. As such, ataxia is associated with postmeningitic hearing loss (167).

At least 50% of children with *H. influenzae* meningitis will develop hyponatremia and the syndrome of inappropriate secretion of antidiuretic hormone (SIADH) (124). The symptoms of hyponatremia and/or SIADH are lethargy, stupor, confusion, and/or seizure activity. When the following criteria are met, the diagnosis of SIADH should be considered: (a) serum sodium less than 135 mEq/liter, (b) serum osmolality less than 270 mOsm/liter, (c) urine osmolality greater than two times the serum osmolality, (d) urine sodium greater than 30 mEq/liter, and (e) no clinical evidence of hypovolemia or dehydration (168). SIADH is not the only etiology of hyponatremia in children with bacterial meningitis. Hyponatremia may also develop when fluid therapy is too aggressive. Regardless of etiology, the serum sodium should be monitored frequently in every child with bacterial meningitis. This will be discussed further in the section on therapy, below.

Ocular complications, including fundal abnormalities, cranial-nerve palsies (see above), pupillary dysfunction, and corneal or conjunctival lesions, are actually quite common during the course of bacterial meningitis in children, but only one case of transient cataract formation has been reported in association with meningococcal meningitis.

Adults

The typical presentation of bacterial meningitis in an adult is that of an upper respiratory tract infection during which a meningeal symptom, such as headache, nuchal rigidity, vomiting, or an altered level of consciousness, develops (169) (Table 18). The clinical signs and symptoms of bacterial meningitis in an adult are very similar to that in children, with a few exceptions. The most common bacterial cause of meningitis in adults is *S. pneumoniae*. The clinical presentation of meningitis caused by *S. pneumoniae* is somewhat different than meningitis caused by the meningococcus or *H. influenzae*. Adults with pneumococcal meningitis frequently have an altered mental status on admission and rapidly become stuporous or comatose. In addition, recurrent seizure activity and focal neurological deficits are more common in the early stages of pneumococcal meningitis than in meningococcal or *H. influenzae* meningitis. These and other factors may contribute to the continued high mortality rate in pneumococcal meningitis. *S.*

pneumoniae meningitis is associated with the highest mortality rate among the three major meningeal pathogens. For example, a mortality of 33% was reported in a recent series from the Netherlands (170), whereas the case fatality rate was 68% in Bahia, Brazil for cases analyzed through 1982. Death is more likely to occur in patients of advanced age, in the absence of meningismus, and in the presence of pneumonia, other extraneural complications, or a prolonged duration of illness prior to therapy (≥7 days). Nevertheless, it appears that most deaths occur later in the disease course due to cardiorespiratory insufficiency (170) and are not usually due to early overwhelming CNS damage.

A classic paper describing the clinical presentation of bacterial meningitis in adults was presented by Carpenter and Petersdorf (169) in 1962. This review included 209 cases of bacterial meningitis: 53 cases were due to meningococci, 63 were caused by pneumococci, 35 were due to *H. influenzae,* and 58 were the result of other bacterial organisms. A reliable history of the onset of symptoms was obtained in 134 patients. Thirty-six patients (27%) had sudden onset of headache, confusion, lethargy, and loss of consciousness and sought hospitalization within the first 24 hr. Only three of these 36 patients had symptoms of respiratory tract infection. In contrast, 71 of the 134 patients (53%) had more slowly progressive symptoms of meningitis for 1–7 days prior to admission. Of these, 26 patients (37%) had respiratory symptoms. In 27 of the 134 patients (20%), an infection in the respiratory tract developed 1–3 weeks before the first symptom of meningitis. The results of physical examination for meningeal signs was recorded in 199 cases. Either nuchal rigidity, Kernig's signs, or Brudzinski's signs were present in 161 patients (81%). Level of consciousness on admission was recorded in 191 cases (96%); only nine (5%) patients were alert, 48 (24%) were lethargic, 44 (22%) were confused, and the remainder were obtunded or comatose. Patients with meningococcal meningitis were most often alert, and those with pneumococcal meningitis were more often obtunded.

Geiseler et al. (171) made observations [similar to those of Carpenter and Petersdorf (169)] of altered consciousness at presentation in bacterial meningitis. They recorded level of consciousness at the time of admission in 1289 patients with community-acquired bacterial meningitis. Overall, 230 (17.8%) were alert, 672 (52.1%) were irritable or lethargic, 262 (20.3%) were stuporous or obtunded, and 125 (9.7%) were comatose and/or convulsing (171). In adults, as in children, lethargy or an altered mental status is the strongest indicator of bacterial meningitis.

Pneumonia is present on admission in 25–50% of adults with pneumococcal meningitis (169). Acute and chronic otitis media are also predisposing conditions for pneumococcal meningitis. In one series of 178 patients with pneumococcal meningitis, acute otitis media was present in 59 (33.1%) (171). When pneumonia or otitis media are not present, the possibility of a dural sinus fistula should be considered. *S. pneumoniae* is the most common causative agent in meningitis following head trauma with basilar skull fracture or when there is a structural defect (either congenital or traumatic in origin) creating a communication between the paranasal sinuses, nasopharynx, or middle ear and the SAS (172).

In adults aged 15–60 years, underlying host factors may increase the risk of meningitis while simultaneously blunting its presenting signs. Such predisposing factors include malignancy, alcoholism, sickle-cell disease, diabetes, organ transplantation, splenectomy, high-dose steroid therapy, and long-term dialysis. In this clinical setting the symptoms of meningitis may include altered sensorium, persistent headache, or new-onset seizures. Fever or nuchal rigidity may not develop (173).

Although *H. influenzae* is the most common bacterial cause of meningitis in childhood, it is relatively rare in adults. The occurrence of *H. influenzae* meningitis in an adult should prompt consideration of the presence of (a) otitis media, (b) paranasal sinusitis, (c) other parameningeal foci of infection, (d) CSF leak from previous head trauma, or (e) a concurrent pneumonia, pharyngitis, or immunodeficiency disease. The clinical presentation of *H. influenzae* meningitis in adults is typical of bacterial meningitis and includes headache, fever, altered mental status, and nuchal rigidity (174).

Elderly

Meningitis should be suspected in every elderly patient who is febrile and either disoriented, stuporous, or comatose (Table 18). In a review of 54 cases of bacterial meningitis in the elderly, confusion was present in 92% (12 of 13) of the patients with pneumococcal meningitis and in 78% (seven of nine) of those with gram-negative meningitis on initial presentation. This review compared the clinical presentation of bacterial meningitis in the elderly (patients aged 50 years and older) with that in younger patients (aged 15–49 years). On initial presentation, the incidence of more severe mental status abnormalities in the older age group with bacterial meningitis was statistically different from that of the younger group, and concurrent pneumonia was present more often in the older patients than in the younger group (175). In another review (176) of CNS infections in patients older than 65 years at the Mt. Sinai Hospital (New York) from 1970 through 1985, 28 cases of bacterial meningitis were identified. Although fever (often low grade) was uniformly present, only 57% had meningismus and only 21% complained of headache. Pneumococci were the most common etiologic agent, and these cases were often (58%) accompanied by pneumonia, sinusitis, or otitis media; the overall mortality was ~40%.

The majority of elderly patients with meningitis will have nuchal rigidity; that is, there will be resistance to passive flexion of the neck. Resistance to passive movement of the neck is a common physical finding in elderly patients because of the presence of cervical spondylosis. It is important to be able to distinguish between cervical rigidity due to cervical spondylosis and nuchal rigidity due to meningitis. In the presence of nuchal rigidity, the neck resists flexion but can be passively rotated from side to side. In the presence of rigidity due to cervical spine disease, lateral rotation, extension, and flexion of the neck are all associated with resistance. Similarly, hypertonicity of the neck muscles due to basal ganglia disease such as parkinsonism can be distinguished from true nuchal rigidity.

Specific comments should be made about the presentation of nontraumatic, spontaneous, gram-negative bacillary meningitis in the elderly or debilitated patient. In these patients, the classic signs and symptoms of meningitis may be subtle at initial presentation. They may have only low-grade fever and altered mental status without headache or nuchal rigidity; however, patients with spontaneous gram-negative bacillary meningitis tend to have a rapidly progressive fulminant course associated with bacteremia, shock, and coma (177). The elderly patient with gram-negative meningitis may rapidly become comatose after presenting with what appeared to be a minor illness. Once coma develops, nuchal rigidity may not be present, since this symptom is lost during deep coma.

Post-traumatic Meningitis

Bacterial meningitis may develop following a traumatic head injury producing a dural fistula between the SAS and the nasal cavity, paranasal sinuses, or middle ear. The infection may develop shortly after the injury or may not occur until months to years later (178). Traumatic head injury is the most common cause of recurrent meningitis in the adult (174). Conversely, congenital fistulous connections to the CNS, often via the middle ear in association with Mondini's dysplasia, are the most common underlying process in children with recurrent bacterial meningitis (179). An immunodeficiency state may also be instrumental in the development of this syndrome.

A dural fistula develops when the force of the injury is sufficient to fracture bone and tear the dura. The most frequent site for dural fistula is in the anterior cranial fossa, in the area of the cribriform plate. Here the bone is very thin and the dura is tightly adherent to the bone. A fracture in this area allows CSF to leak through torn arachnoid and dura into the nasal cavity, resulting in CSF rhinorrhea (178). There may also be loss of the sense of smell, or anosmia. CSF rhinorrhea can be distinguished from nasal secretions by testing the fluid for glucose. This should be done by chemical determination or by using a glucose-oxidase-containing strip. Because normal nasal secretions contain only a small amount of glucose, a positive reaction indicates that the fluid is CSF. Dextrostix is the test tape of choice. More sensitive glucose oxidase reagents such as Testape and Clinistix are not recommended to test nasal secretions, since they may give false-positive reactions in the absence of CSF rhinorrhea (180). It is important, however, to emphasize that this test may be falsely negative during acute bacterial meningitis, when CSF glucose is decreased.

Physical signs indicating a basilar skull fracture with the potential for development of a dural fistula and meningitis include periorbital ecchymoses, bruising behind the ear (Battle's sign), hemotympanum, and/or blood in the external auditory canal (178).

In the majority of cases, CSF rhinorrhea will cease spontaneously. Approximately one in four patients with CSF rhinorrhea will develop meningitis (178); the reported frequency ranges from 9% to 36%. Surgery is indicated in patients who develop meningitis with persistent rhinorrhea. The management of meningitis occurring in this setting and the approach to demonstration of the location of the dural fistula will be discussed later in this chapter.

Meningitis Following Neurosurgical Procedures

Meningitis complicating a neurosurgical procedure, such as a craniotomy, is usually insidious in onset and difficult to distinguish clinically from the neurological abnormalities expected in the postoperative period. Although an altered level of consciousness and signs of meningeal irritation may be expected in the postoperative period, the presence of fever or prolonged obtundation should prompt an examination of the CSF.

Approximately 60–70% of all cases of meningitis complicating a neurosurgical procedure, with the exception of a shunting procedure, are caused by gram-negative bacilli (177). In the postneurosurgical patient, *K. pneumoniae, Acinetobacter calcoaceticus,* and *E. coli* are the most common infecting gram-negative organisms. Craniotomy for trauma or for tumor represent the most common surgical procedures associated with postoperative gram-negative bacterial meningitis (181).

Although the surgical insertion of, and subsequent constant presence of, an indwelling ventriculoperitoneal (VP) or ventriculoatrial (VA) shunt catheter for decompression of hydrocephalus allow bacteria to enter the CSF space, signs of meningitis usually do not accompany these infections in the early stages. The bacteria involved in early shunt infection gain entry to the lumen of the shunt from a contaminated wound or from the patient's skin surface at the time of operation (182). The initial symptoms of shunt infection are nonspecific and include fever, nausea, vomiting, and lethargy (Chapter 23). Fever is the most common manifestation of shunt infection. Virtually all patients will have temperatures greater than 37.8°C, and the majority will have temperatures greater than or equal to 38.8°C (183). Fever is often the sole manifestation of infection in patients with VA shunts, whereas patients with infected VP shunts are more likely to present with signs of shunt malfunction and/or signs of inflammation around the shunt reservoir or along the course of the tubing (183,184). Signs of shunt malfunction are secondary to progressive hydrocephalus and, in children, include enlarging cranial circumference, tense nonpulsatile fontanelle, and papilledema. Signs of shunt malfunction may be associated with signs of meningitis. Examination of CSF from the lumbar area may be negative; therefore CSF should be obtained by aspiration from the infected shunt reservoir.

Infections of the CNS may also develop when subcutaneous CSF reservoirs, such as Ommaya and Rickham reservoirs, are placed for therapeutic purposes. These and other types of indwelling intraventricular catheters may lead to meningitis with coagulase-negative staphylococci, *S. aureus, Corynebacterium* species, or gram-negative bacilli. Infections usually occur within the first 3 months after insertion of the device and, as with infections of VP or VA shunts, are probably due to contamination by skin flora during implantation or subsequent use for therapeutic purposes. In these patients, signs of meningitis are usually not present, but most will complain of fever, lethargy, headache, or nausea and vomiting (185).

Immunosuppressed Host

The risk of an immunocompromised patient developing bacterial meningitis is dependent on a number of factors such as the underlying disease and its treatment, the duration of immunosuppression, and the type of immune abnormality. There are four major types of host defense abnormalities in the immunocompromised patient: (i) defects in T-lymphocyte–macrophage function (cell-mediated immunity); (ii) defects in humoral immunity; (iii) defects in the number and function of neutrophils; and (iv) loss of splenic function from surgery, disease, or radiotherapy, resulting in the inability to remove encapsulated bacteria. Knowledge of the type of host defense abnormality is often helpful in the prediction of the infecting organism (186,187).

Patients with defects in cell-mediated immunity include: (a) those with lymphomas, particularly Hodgkin's disease; (b) organ transplant recipients; (c) patients treated with daily corticosteroid therapy; and (d) patients with AIDS. These patients are most susceptible to CNS infection by microorganisms that are intracellular parasites, the eradication of which is dependent upon an intact T-lymphocyte–macrophage system (186). In many medical centers, *L. monocytogenes* is the most common cause of bacterial meningitis in patients with defective cell-mediated immunity (187). The clinical presentation of *L. monocytogenes* meningitis includes fever and headache, as well as an increased tendency for focal neurological deficits and seizures during the initial presentation. Meningitis due to this organism may also present with a clinical picture suggestive of an acute brainstem disorder or rhombencephalitis, with signs of ataxia, cranial-nerve deficits, and nystagmus (188).

Patients with defective humoral immunity are unable to mount an antibody response to bacterial infection, and they are therefore unable to control infection caused by encapsulated bacteria. Patients with this type of host defense abnormality include those with chronic lymphocytic leukemia, multiple myeloma, or Hodgkin's disease following chemotherapy and radiotherapy, among others. These patients are at particular risk for meningitis caused by *S. pneumoniae, H. influenzae* type b, and, less commonly, *N. meningitidis.* The presentation of meningitis in these patients is often that of a fulminant illness resulting in death in several hours. Patients with splenectomy may develop (a) overwhelming bacteremia and fulminant meningitis with the same organisms, due to loss of the filtering function of the splenic sinusoids in removing encapsulated bacteria from the bloodstream, and (b) a reduced ability to produce IgM opsonizing antibodies (186,187).

Patients with neutropenia are at particular risk for meningitis caused by *Pseudomonas aeruginosa* and members of the Enterobacteriaceae family (187). The clinical presentation of bacterial meningitis in patients with neutropenia may be subtle, consisting of low-grade fever and lethargy or a change in headache pattern (186). Signs of meningeal irritation are dependent upon the host's ability to mount an inflammatory response; therefore, in the neutropenic patient they are often minimal.

APPROACH TO DIAGNOSIS

Differential Diagnosis

Although the diagnosis of meningitis is usually made by examination of the CSF, the decision to perform a lumbar puncture is based on the clinical presentation. When the signs and symptoms suggest meningitis, and the decision is made to examine the CSF, the next step is to be certain that a focal intracranial mass lesion does not exist that may predispose to brain herniation following lumbar puncture. If the history and neurological examination suggest a focal mass lesion, then lumbar puncture should be delayed until a cranial CT scan, without and with contrast enhancement, is obtained.

Lumbar puncture is contraindicated in the presence of a focal mass lesion because of the danger of brain hernia-

tion. However, it has become common practice to delay lumbar puncture until a CT scan has been obtained despite the absence of focal neurological deficits by history or examination. The time involved in waiting for a CT scan significantly delays treatment, and delay in treatment is the most critical factor in determining morbidity and mortality in bacterial meningitis. Therefore, if a CT scan is to be performed, antimicrobial therapy should be initiated promptly, pending results. In the absence of focal neurological signs and/or papilledema, a lumbar puncture can be safely performed without first obtaining a CT scan. Focal infectious lesions that have clinical presentations similar to meningitis, and that could result in significant morbidity if lumbar puncture is unknowingly performed, include brain abscess, subdural empyema, and epidural abscess. The clinical presentation of each of these disorders has similarities and distinguishing features when compared to that of meningitis.

The most common symptom of a brain abscess is a hemicranial or generalized headache seen in over 75% of patients (189). A brain abscess presents as an expanding intracranial mass lesion, rather than as an infectious process (Chapter 19); as such, fever is present in only 45–50% of patients and usually is not prominent (190). More than 50% of patients will have focal neurological deficits, and one-third of patients present with new-onset focal or generalized seizure activity (189). The findings on neurological examination are related both to the site of the abscess and to the presence of raised ICP due to an expanding mass lesion. Hemiparesis is the most common sign of a frontoparietal lobe abscess. A disturbance of language or behavior or an upper homonymous quadrantanopsia is the sign of a temporal lobe abscess. Ataxia is the most common sign of a cerebellar abscess. Nuchal rigidity rarely occurs until the abscess has ruptured into the ventricle or until infection has spread to the SAS.

The majority of patients with a subdural empyema (Chapter 20) initially complain of headache which is localized to the side of the subdural infection. The headache becomes increasingly more severe and generalized, and it is followed by an alteration in the level of consciousness. The disturbance in consciousness is due to increasing intracranial pressure. Fever, chills, and nuchal rigidity are present in most cases. Focal neurological deficits are present in 80–90% of patients, and they include hemiparesis or hemiplegia, paralysis of horizontal gaze to the side opposite the lesion, and focal or generalized seizures (191). The presentation of a posterior fossa subdural empyema includes severe headache, vomiting, marked nuchal rigidity, cerebellar signs, cranial-nerve deficits, and pupillary abnormalities (192).

A typical presentation of an intracranial epidural abscess (Chapter 21) is an unrelenting hemicranial headache and fever that developed during or after treatment for frontal sinusitis, mastoiditis, or otitis media. If the abscess is large, mild alterations of consciousness may occur; however, focal neurological deficits, seizures, and signs of increased ICP do not develop until extension of the infection into the subdural space has occurred or until a deeper intraparenchymal complication has developed (191).

The decision to delay lumbar puncture until CT scan is obtained may be made when the patient does not appear to be seriously ill or when there is uncertainty about the findings on neurological examination. Patients with viral meningitis usually do not appear as ill as patients with bacterial meningitis and often have had symptoms for several days. When the history suggests a focal onset to the headache or a transient neurological symptom, lumbar puncture is best delayed until a CT scan is obtained.

The initial symptoms of viral meningitis (Chapter 3) are fever, headache, lethargy, myalgias, and nuchal rigidity. There are several distinguishing clinical features of viral meningitis: (a) Viral meningitis has a more insidious onset and a slower progression than does bacterial meningitis; (b) patients with viral meningitis often complain of an incapacitating headache that is not relieved by analgesics, but they are otherwise awake and alert; (c) the fever is usually higher in bacterial meningitis than in viral meningitis; and (d) although generalized malaise may be present, stupor, obtundation, and coma are rare in viral meningitis (173).

Altered level of consciousness, focal neurological deficits, and new-onset seizure activity are symptoms of a viral encephalitis, meningoencephalitis, or bacterial meningitis. The presentation of herpes simplex virus (HSV) encephalitis (Chapter 4) is often subacute and, on examination, is characterized by (a) fever, confusion, or a change in behavior, (b) new-onset seizure activity, and/or (c) focal neurological deficits. A history of hemicranial headache of several days' duration, preceding the onset of the confusional state, is a classic presentation of this illness. HSV has a predilection for the temporal and orbitofrontal areas; therefore, a change in mentation or behavior is a common finding (193).

Signs and symptoms of meningitis represent the most common neurological presentation of Lyme disease (Chapter 28). The duration and severity of the symptoms are much longer than would be expected for typical bacterial meningitis. Patients have symptoms of headache, stiff neck, nausea, vomiting, malaise, and fatigue of several weeks' duration that may alternate with several-week periods of milder symptoms. The characteristic skin lesion of Lyme disease, erythema chronicum migrans (ECM), precedes the symptoms of meningitis in approximately 80–90% of patients. Signs and symptoms of meningitis occur weeks to a few months after the initial infection, or they may be the first manifestation of the disease without antecedent ECM (194).

The presence of a rash with meningitis suggests me-

ningococcemia. As has been discussed, the classic lesions associated with fulminating meningococcal septicemia are large petechial hemorrhages in the skin and mucous membranes. Between 50% and 75% of children with meningococcal meningitis have a purpuric or petechial rash, principally on the trunk and lower extremities. Petechiae are found in the skin, mucous membranes, and conjunctiva, but not in the nail beds, in meningococcemia. Petechiae are also sometimes seen on the trunk and extremities in echovirus type 9 meningitis, acute staphylococcal endocarditis, and, rarely, pneumococcal or *H. influenzae* meningitis except in asplenic patients (158,164). Petechiae may be found in the nail beds in acute staphylococcal endocarditis. Petechial rashes should be promptly examined microscopically in the initial evaluation of meningococcemia after aspiration or after making a "touch-prep" on a glass slide; ~70% of these preparations will reveal the organisms, usually within vacuolated neutrophils. In fulminant meningococcemia, the organisms may be visualized in the peripheral blood smear. Although the sensitivity of this method is low, this simple test should always be performed in suspected meningococcemia.

Headache, fever, rash, and altered mental status are symptoms of rickettsial infections (Chapter 17) and, as such, enter into the differential diagnosis of meningitis. A petechial rash is characteristic of Rocky Mountain spotted fever (RMSF), which is caused by *Rickettsia rickettsii*. The rash of typhus is a faint macular–papular pink rash (195). The rash of RMSF consists initially of 1- to 5-mm pink macules which are often noted first on the wrist and ankles and which then spread centrally to the chest, face, and abdomen. The rash of RMSF usually does not involve the mucous membranes. Petechial lesions in the axillae and around the ankles, accompanied by lesions on the palms and soles of the feet, are characteristic of RMSF, but this classic pattern is often absent. The macules will initially blanch with pressure, but after a few days they will become fixed and turn dark red or purple. Diagnosis can be made by biopsy of the lesions and staining of the specimen with fluorescent antibodies to *R. rickettsii* (196). A negative result does not exclude RMSF, because sensitivity of this test is only 70%.

The characteristic rash caused by an enterovirus consists of erythematous macules and papules on the face, neck, trunk, and, to a lesser degree, the extremities. Rarely, the rash associated with enteroviral infection may become petechial in nature.

The rash of Lyme disease, erythema chronicum migrans, begins as a red macule or papule at the site of the tick bite that then expands centrifugally as an erythematous lesion with central clearing. This may be the only lesion, or the disease may disseminate to form multiple secondary ring-like lesions. Symptoms of meningitis may develop while the skin lesions are still present, or they may begin 1–6 months after the skin lesions have resolved (194). CSF examination during stage I Lyme disease usually reveals no abnormalities despite the presence of meningeal symptoms (Chapter 28).

Noninfectious neurological disorders that have clinical presentations similar to meningitis are subarachnoid hemorrhage, neuroleptic malignant syndrome, and posterior fossa tumors. The classic presentation of a subarachnoid hemorrhage is the sudden onset of a severe, excruciating headache or a sudden transient loss of consciousness followed by a severe headache. The majority of patients complain of vomiting. Syncope accompanies the explosive onset of headache in about 50% of cases. Nuchal rigidity develops within a few hours of the onset of a subarachnoid hemorrhage and is usually associated with a change in the level of consciousness. Low-grade fever may develop within several days. When an intracranial aneurysm ruptures into the brain parenchyma, a focal neurological deficit is usually present. A unilateral third-nerve palsy, with a dilated, nonreactive pupil, is suggestive of third-nerve compression by an aneurysm at the junction of the posterior communicating artery and the internal carotid artery. The triad of headache, neck stiffness, and vomiting should raise a suspicion of a warning leak from an aneurysm (197).

The symptoms of neuroleptic malignant syndrome (NMS) are fever, generalized lead-pipe rigidity (including cervical rigidity), fluctuating level of consciousness ranging from agitation to stupor and coma, and autonomic instability. The latter is characterized by pallor, blood-pressure instability, diaphoresis, tachycardia, and arrhythmias. A leukocytosis of 15,000–30,000 cells per cubic millimeter, with a shift to the left, is common. Liver function abnormalities are frequently seen, but the most specific laboratory abnormality in this disorder is marked elevation in the serum creatine kinase (CK) concentration, usually exceeding 10,000 IU per liter (198).

Signs of a posterior fossa tumor are stiff neck, cranial-nerve abnormalities, gait disturbance, vomiting, cerebellar deficits, and occasionally an altered level of consciousness.

A cranial CT scan and examination of the CSF will narrow the differential diagnosis. The possibility of the presence of increased ICP should be considered prior to lumbar puncture. Increased ICP is an expected complication of bacterial meningitis and is *not* a contraindication to lumbar puncture; however, lumbar puncture should be performed cautiously in patients with suspected increased ICP.

The clinical signs of increased ICP are (a) a dilated, nonreactive pupil, (b) drowsiness, (c) ocular motility abnormalities, the most common of which are due to unilateral or bilateral cranial nerve VI palsies, and (d) bradycardia and hypertension, the Cushing reflex. Pupillary dilation is usually secondary to parenchymal midbrain distortion from either raised ICP or transtentorial herniation. Drowsiness or stupor is often the first sign of

increasing ICP and is due to interference with the reticular activating system in the brainstem.

If raised ICP appears likely and a focal intracranial mass lesion has been excluded by CT scan, lumbar puncture can usually be safely performed. One suggested approach is to electively intubate and hyperventilate the patient and infuse mannitol intravenously in a bolus dose of 1 g per kilogram of body weight. Twenty minutes after the mannitol infusion, a 22-gauge needle can be used to collect the minimum amount of CSF necessary for diagnosis. An alternative approach is to use a mannitol bolus injection without prior intubation. Either approach is acceptable. The use of a larger spinal needle may result in the creation of a rent in the dura through which CSF will continue to leak. This may theoretically result in brain herniation several hours after lumbar puncture.

When the decision is made to delay lumbar puncture until a CT scan has been obtained, blood cultures should be obtained and intravenous antibiotics begun while awaiting CT scan. Intravenous antibiotics usually will not sterilize the CSF in the time it takes to obtain a CT scan and spinal fluid. Blood cultures may identify the infecting organism in 50–80% of cases of bacterial meningitis (although this frequency varies with the causative organism), and they are more often positive in patients that have not been treated with prior oral antibiotic therapy (156).

Laboratory Diagnosis

Cerebrospinal Fluid (Table 19)

Opening Pressure. The first step in examination of the CSF is measurement of the opening pressure with an air–water manometer. This step is often neglected, but knowledge of the presence of raised ICP is important in management of the patient. Normal CSF pressure, with the patient in the lateral recumbent position, is usually defined as less than 180 mmH$_2$O (199), although normal opening pressure can be as high as 250 mmH$_2$O in obese patients (200). CSF pressure should not be measured with the patient in a seated position. If the spinal needle is inserted with the patient seated, the patient should then be changed to a lateral recumbent position and the opening pressure recorded. As has been discussed, elevated CSF pressure in the 200- to 500-mmH$_2$O range is common in bacterial meningitis.

Appearance. Normal CSF is clear. The presence of greater than 200 white blood cells (WBCs) per cubic millimeter, greater than 400 red blood cells (RBCs) per cubic millimeter, bacteria ($\geq 10^5$ CFU/ml), and/or an elevated protein concentration makes the fluid appear cloudy or turbid. When the lumbar puncture is traumatic and the initial CSF sample appears bloody, the

TABLE 19. *Typical cerebrospinal fluid findings in bacterial versus aseptic meningitis[a]*

CSF parameter	Bacterial meningitis	Aseptic meningitis
Opening pressure	>180 mmH$_2$O	Normal or slightly elevated
Glucose	<40 mg/dl	>45 mg/dl
CSF/serum glucose ratio	<0.31	>0.6
Protein	>50 mg/dl	Normal or elevated
White blood cells	>10 to <10,000 white blood cells per cubic millimeter—neutrophils predominate	50–2000 white blood cells per cubic millimeter—lymphocytes predominate
Gram's stain	Positive in 70–90% of untreated cases	Negative
Lactate	≥3.8 mmol/l	Normal
C-reactive protein	>100 ng/ml	Minimal
Limulus lysate assay	Positive indicates gram-negative meningitis	Negative
Latex agglutination	Specific for antigens of *S. pneumoniae, N. meningitidis* (not serogroup B), and Hib	Negative
Coagglutination	Same as above	Negative
Counterimmunoelectrophoresis	Same as above	Negative

[a] Data from refs. 164, 199, 201, 202, 210, and 215–217.

fluid should clear as flow continues. "Xanthochromia" refers to a yellow or yellow–orange color in the supernatant of centrifuged spinal fluid. The presence of xanthochromia distinguishes CSF that is bloody secondary to subarachnoid hemorrhage from CSF that is bloody as a result of a traumatic lumbar puncture. When CSF is bloody secondary to traumatic lumbar puncture, the supernatant of the centrifuged fluid is clear. In subarachnoid hemorrhage, the supernatant is xanthochromic within 2 hr after the hemorrhage. Elevated CSF protein concentrations greater than 150 mg/dl also cause xanthochromia (199,201), and this is the usual etiology of xanthochromia in bacterial meningitis.

Glucose. The normal CSF glucose concentration is greater than 45 mg/dl. A glucose concentration less than 40 mg/dl occurs in approximately 58% of patients with bacterial meningitis (202); however, the CSF glucose may be falsely low in the presence of hypoglycemia, or it may be erroneously interpreted as normal in the presence of CNS infection when the serum glucose is elevated. An accurate interpretation of the CSF glucose concentration is done by determining the CSF/serum glucose ratio. A normal CSF/serum glucose ratio is about 0.6 (202). Values less than 0.31 are an indication of low CSF glucose, and they are observed in approximately 70% of patients with bacterial meningitis (202). A decreased CSF/serum glucose ratio is also consistent with fungal or tuberculous meningitis, carcinomatous meningitis, herpes simplex encephalitis, mumps encephalitis, subarachnoid hemorrhage in 15–20% of patients, and several other conditions (201).

Protein. Any process that disrupts the BBB results in an elevated CSF protein concentration. Values greater than 50 mg/dl in CSF obtained from the lumbar SAS, as well as ventricular CSF protein concentrations greater than 15 mg/dl, are considered abnormal. When the lumbar puncture is traumatic and there is blood in the CSF, the true protein concentration is corrected by subtracting 1 mg of protein per deciliter for every 1000 RBCs in CSF (201).

White Blood Cell Count. The CSF abnormalities characteristic of bacterial meningitis include a polymorphonuclear pleocytosis, a low glucose concentration, and an elevated protein concentration. The CSF should be examined promptly after it is obtained, because WBCs in the CSF begin to disintegrate after about 90 min. The normal WBC count in the CSF of adults and children is 0–5 mononuclear cells (lymphocytes and monocytes) per cubic millimeter; a WBC count of greater than 10 cells indicates a pathological process such as infection. Normal CSF does not contain polymorphonuclear leukocytes (PMNs); however, following centrifugation, an occasional PMN may be seen. It has been stressed that for the CSF to be considered normal, no more than a single PMN should be seen in the differential count, accompanied by a total WBC count of less than 5 per cubic millimeter (201). However, most CSF differential counts are now performed on cytocentrifuged specimens in hospital laboratories. In these preparations, a few PMNs may be seen, even in the absence of disease (203) (i.e., when minimal blood contamination is present) or in association with a high peripheral leukocyte concentration.

A traumatic puncture or an intracerebral or subarachnoid hemorrhage introduces RBCs and WBCs into the CSF. The correction factor for the WBC count in the presence of blood in the CSF is as follows: (a) If the peripheral RBC and WBC counts are normal, then 1 WBC per 700 RBCs can be subtracted from the total WBC count in CSF; and (b) in the presence of an abnormal peripheral WBC or RBC count, the following formula can be used: true WBC (CSF) = WBC actual (CSF) − WBC (blood) × RBC (CSF)/RBC (blood) (201).

Generalized seizures may induce a transient CSF pleocytosis consisting predominantly of PMNs. However, to attribute a CSF pleocytosis to seizure activity, the following criteria should be met: (a) The fluid should be clear and colorless; (b) the opening pressure should be normal; (c) the CSF glucose should be normal; (d) the WBC count should not exceed 80 cells per cubic millimeter; (e) there should be no meningeal signs or other evidence of infection; and (f) Gram's stain should be negative (204). Even if these conditions are met, patients should usually be treated with antibiotics until the results of bacterial cultures are known. There also remains the possibility that a viral meningitis or encephalitis, with a predominance of PMNs in CSF, is the etiology of the seizure activity.

In large reported series of bacterial meningitis, in 90% of cases there are greater than 100 WBCs per cubic millimeter in the CSF, and in 65–70% of cases there are greater than 1000 WBCs per cubic millimeter (169,171,205,206). The differential count usually shows a predominance of PMNs. In about 10% of cases of bacterial meningitis, there may be a predominance of lymphocytes early in the infection, especially if the total WBC concentration is less than 1000 per cubic millimeter. In one series, 32% (13 of 41) of patients with bacterial meningitis with a CSF WBC concentration of 1000 per cubic millimeter or less had a predominance of lymphocytes (207). In addition, in about 20–75% of patients with viral meningitides the CSF may initially have a predominance of PMNs, with an eventual shift (over the course of several hours) to a monocytic predominance. This has led to controversy about the necessity for repeat lumbar puncture and in what time period a repeat lumbar puncture should be obtained to demonstrate a shift in cell type. It is our feeling that a repeat lumbar puncture is usually not necessary unless there is further clinical deterioration. In the presence of a lymphocytic pleocytosis, the results of CSF chemistries, Gram's stain, and other tests (see below) suggest the diagnosis. If bacterial meningitis is suspected, even though there is a predominance of lymphocytes, the patient should be treated with antibiotics until the results of bacterial cultures are known.

Gram's Stain. Examination of CSF by Gram's stain allows for rapid, accurate identification of the infecting organism. If the CSF is cloudy, smears should be obtained from fresh, uncentrifuged fluid for Gram's stain. If the CSF is clear, smears should be obtained from the centrifuged sediment. The Gram's stain is positive in identifying the organism in 60–90% of cases of bacterial meningitis (202,208), although the probability of detecting bacteria on a gram-stained specimen is dependent on the number of organisms present. The majority of

smears will be positive when there are greater than 10^5 CFU/ml CSF. Only 25% of smears are positive when the bacterial concentration is less than 10^3 CFU/ml (156).

Acridine Orange Stain. The acridine orange stain (AOS) is a fluorochrome that stains the nucleic acids of some bacteria. When the specimen is examined under a fluorescent microscope, the bacteria appear bright red-orange and the background of cell debris and human cells appears yellow to pale green. AOS may demonstrate bacteria when the Gram's stain of CSF is negative, and it is better for identifying intracellular bacteria than the Gram's stain. When the Gram's stain is positive, the AOS provides no additional information (199). The AOS and the Wayson stain (a modified methylene blue stain) are both more sensitive than the Gram's stain in the detection of bacteria in the CSF; however, neither is routinely performed in hospital laboratories.

Culture. Culture of CSF is positive in approximately 80% of cases of bacterial meningitis usually requiring ≥48 hr for accurate identification (202). CSF cultures may be positive even when all other tests (e.g., glucose, protein, leukocyte concentration, Gram's stain, etc.) are negative, particularly in early meningococcal meningitis.

CSF Lactate. The lactic acid concentration in CSF has been reported to be useful in differentiating between bacterial and viral meningitis—especially in those patients that have been partially treated with antibiotics prior to examination of the CSF, as well as in those patients with low CSF WBC concentrations. In a recent European study, the lactic acid in CSF was measured in 50 patients with acute bacterial meningitis. In 46 patients (92%), the CSF lactate concentration was ≥3.5 mmol/liter. The investigators in this study concluded that CSF lactate was useful in the diagnosis of acute bacterial meningitis if it was ≥3.5 mmol/liter (209). Other studies have demonstrated that in the majority of cases of acute bacterial meningitis, the CSF lactate concentration is ≥3.8 mmol/liter (199). Although the CSF lactate level has a high sensitivity for bacterial meningitis, it has a low specificity.

In a review of the lactic acid concentrations in 493 samples of CSF from 434 adults with various CNS conditions, the lactate concentration was greater than 35 mg/dl in 50 cases. Only 19 of the 50 cases had infective meningitis due to either bacterial or viral pathogens. Although the lactic acid concentration was elevated in the majority of cases of bacterial meningitis in this study, the CSF samples with elevated lactic acid concentrations had cell counts and chemistries suggestive of bacterial meningitis; therefore, the elevated lactate concentration provided little additional information (210). In this review, as in others, an elevated CSF lactic acid concentration was nonspecific. Other etiologies of elevated CSF lactate concentrations include recurrent seizure activity, cerebral ischemia, hypocapnia, closed head injury, neoplasms, and craniotomy (199,210). Although the source of the CSF lactate is debated, contributions by cerebral hypoxia/ischemia, anaerobic glycolysis, vascular compromise, and metabolism of the CSF leukocytes (211) are all potentially important.

Other Tests. The CSF concentration of multiple other substances also increases in the presence of bacterial meningitis, including various enzymes (e.g., lactate dehydrogenase, creatine phosphokinase, etc.) and fibrin degradation products; however, the elevations are nonspecific. Tests for these compounds are rarely, if ever, performed in hospital laboratories.

Combinations of CSF Tests. Although many of the above tests commonly performed on CSF may suggest the diagnosis of bacterial meningitis, none is irrefutable evidence of this disease, except perhaps a positive culture and/or positive stains. Combinations of test results with clinical parameters may permit a more accurate assessment of the probability of bacterial versus viral meningitis. This approach appears to have merit, as emphasized in a recent retrospective review (212) of 422 patients with acute meningitis at Duke University. The following CSF parameters were individual predictors of bacterial meningitis with greater than 99% certainty: glucose < 1.9 mmol/liter, CSF/blood glucose ratio < 0.23, protein > 2.2 g/liter, leukocytes > 2000×10^6 per liter, or neutrophils > 1180×10^6 per liter. Although any one of these results ruled in bacterial meningitis with high probability, none could rule it out. A multiple regression model utilizing four parameters (age, month of onset, CSF/blood glucose ratio, and CSF neutrophil concentration) proved highly reliable in separating bacterial from aseptic-viral meningitis. Although the model requires further validation, a nomogram is included in the article (212) and should be consulted for more precise analysis of gram-negative cases.

Partially Treated Meningitis. The effect of oral antibiotic therapy on CSF analysis was studied in two prospective studies of 281 children with Hib meningitis. Ninety-four (33%) children had been treated with more than one dose of antibiotics within 1 week prior to admission. Compared with those in untreated children, the results of CSF analysis in children pretreated with antibiotics showed significant decreases in the percentage of neutrophils ($p < 0.03$), protein concentration ($p < 0.001$), and percentage with a positive Gram's stain or culture ($p < 0.05$). The total WBC count, glucose concentration, CSF/serum glucose ratio, percentage with a positive counterimmunoelectrophoresis (CIE) or latex agglutination test, and blood culture results were not significantly different. When adjustment was made for duration of illness before admission, only the CSF protein concentration remained significantly different ($p < 0.01$) in children who were pretreated compared with that in untreated children. The duration of illness preceding admission was significantly longer in children who had

been treated with antibiotics compared to that in untreated children. These observations suggested that the natural progression of illness in the pretreated group was less rapid than that in the untreated group and possibly accounted for the differences in numbers of WBCs and bacteria in the pretreated group, in whom infection was less fulminant (213).

Intravenous antibiotic therapy, even for as long as several days prior to initial lumbar puncture, does not markedly alter the chemical or morphological characteristics of the CSF in cases of bacterial meningitis (156). CSF was examined in 68 children with acute bacterial meningitis on admission and 44–68 hr after intravenous antibiotic therapy. Initial antibiotic therapy in all cases consisted of ampicillin (200 mg/kg/day, in six divided doses) in combination with chloramphenicol (100 mg/kg/day, in four divided doses). In those cases where meningococci, pneumococci, or group A streptococci were isolated from CSF culture, aqueous penicillin G (400,000 units/kg/day, in six divided doses) was substituted. In 65 children with meningitis caused by Hib, pneumococci, group A streptococci, and meningococci, intravenous antibiotic therapy did not significantly alter the CSF protein, glucose, or WBC concentrations. However, bacteria were not evident on smear and did not grow in culture from CSF obtained after intravenous antibiotic therapy of this duration (214).

In general, bacteria should not be seen on Gram's stain or grow in culture from CSF examined 24 hr after treatment has begun with appropriate antibiotic therapy. The CSF glucose concentration approaches normality by the third day of antibiotic therapy in 80% of patients, but it may remain low for as long as 10 days. The CSF protein concentration remains elevated for at least 10 days. The WBC count in CSF remains elevated in over 50% of cases after a standard 7- to 10-day course of antibiotic therapy, but it typically decreases when compared with the value obtained prior to therapy or early in the course of bacterial meningitis (201).

Rapid Diagnostic Tests. Several techniques are available for the rapid detection of bacterial antigens in the CSF, including the latex agglutination (LA) test, the staphylococcal or other coagglutination (CoA) tests, and CIE, among many others. These techniques use serum-containing bacterial antibodies or commercially available antisera directed against the capsular polysaccharide to detect the presence of bacterial antigens in CSF. The advantages of these tests are as follows: They are not dependent upon the presence of viable organisms to be positive, and they may give positive results in cases in which the Gram's stain and culture are negative, as may occur in partially treated meningitis (199). The LA test has a sensitivity of 81–100% for detection of Hib in CSF. It is less effective for detecting *S. pneumoniae* and *N. meningitidis* antigens in the CSF, with published series reporting sensitivities of 50–69% for detection of *S.*

pneumoniae and 30–70% for detection of *N. meningitidis.* The LA test has a specificity of 96–100% for these three bacterial antigens. The CoA test has a specificity of 96–100%, and it has a sensitivity of 71–83% for detection of Hib, 0–93% for detection of *S. pneumoniae,* and 17–100% for detection of *N. meningitidis* in the CSF. The CIE test has a sensitivity of 67–85% for Hib, 50–100% for *S. pneumoniae,* and 50–90% for *N. meningitidis.* The percentage of positive results for detection of *N. meningitidis* by CIE in published series depends on the serogroups of *N. meningitidis* causing infection, because the detection kits currently available do not detect group B meningococci (208,215,216).

Both the LA and CoA tests are highly sensitive and specific for the detection of Hib in CSF. The LA and CIE are approximately equivalent for the detection of *S. pneumoniae* antigens in the CSF. The detection of *N. meningitidis* in CSF by any of these three tests is only about 50% accurate (208,215). LA and CoA are more simple to perform than CIE, do not require specialized equipment, and can be done rapidly, even at the bedside or in the emergency room. For these reasons, LA or CoA tests have supplanted CIE for the rapid detection of bacterial antigen in CSF.

The *Limulus* amebocyte lysate test can detect minute quantities of endotoxin (e.g., ≤10 ng/ml) in the CSF. It is reported to have a sensitivity of 77–100%, with the more recent studies reporting sensitivities of 97–99% for detecting gram-negative endotoxin. It has been recommended as a useful method for the detection of gram-negative bacterial meningitis (217). It is occasionally employed in the setting of an abnormal CSF following neurosurgery or head trauma. Nevertheless, the results of the test rarely change patient management because physicians should employ antimicrobials with activity against gram-negative aerobic bacilli in this clinical setting, even if the *Limulus* lysate test is negative.

C-Reactive Protein. The C-reactive protein (CRP) is an acute-phase reactant that, when present in concentrations greater than 100 ng/ml in CSF, is quite sensitive for differentiating bacterial from viral meningitis. The CRP response is minimal in viral meningitis. CRP concentrations in CSF may be elevated in other CNS inflammatory or necrotic conditions and thus are not specific for bacterial meningitis; however, when cell counts and chemistries suggest meningitis, the CRP concentration is useful in distinguishing between bacterial meningitis and viral meningitis (218,219). In this circumstance, a negative CSF CRP result excludes bacterial meningitis with 99% certainty.

Neuroimaging

In the acute stage of bacterial meningitis, the CT scan may be normal; or it may demonstrate enhancement of the meninges and ependyma with widening of the cisterns at the base of the brain and the cortical sulci, a result of the accumulation of purulent exudate in the basal cisterns and over the convexities of the hemispheres (220). However, the presence of these abnormalities on CT scan contributes very little to the diagnosis of meningitis. The diagnosis is made by the clinical presentation and analysis of the CSF. The extent of meningeal enhancement on CT also does not influence management or prognosis. The value of CT in suspected bacterial meningitis is in the exclusion of other CNS pathologic processes and in the investigation of the complications of this infection, including: (a) prolonged fever for several days after the initiation of antibiotic therapy, (b) fever that develops after an afebrile period during therapy (secondary fever), (c) prolonged obtundation or coma, (d) new or recurrent seizure activity, (e) signs of increased ICP, and (f) focal neurological deficits.

The most common etiologies of prolonged fever in patients with bacterial meningitis are subdural effusions, drug fever, and concomitant arteritis or pneumonia. In published series, 9–13% of patients with Hib or with pneumococcal or meningococcal meningitis had fever for 10 days or longer after the initiation of appropriate antibiotic therapy. In approximately 25% of these patients, the fever was attributed to the presence of a subdural effusion. The most common etiologies of secondary fever are nosocomial infections and subdural effusions (221). Although the intracranial complications of meningitis are demonstrated well by CT scan, the results of the CT scan rarely influence management of children with meningitis and prolonged fever (222) in the absence of other clinical features suggesting CNS complications.

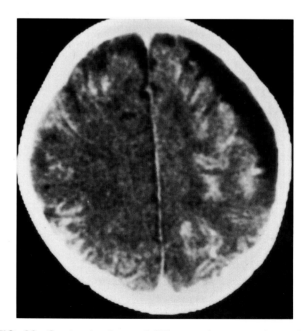

FIG. 22. Contrast-enhanced CT scan demonstrating subdural effusion.

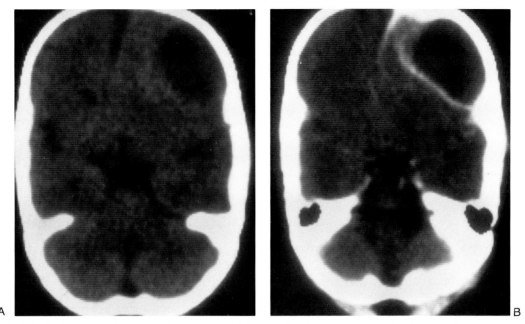

FIG. 23. A: CT scan demonstrating extra-axial fluid collection suggestive of subdural effusion as opposed to subdural empyema. **B:** After contrast administration, the medial border of the subdural fluid collection enhances; thus it is a subdural empyema.

Subdural effusions are a relatively common complication of bacterial meningitis, being reported in 20–50% of infants and children with meningitis. Only a small percentage are clinically significant (223–226). In the majority of cases, the fluid in the subdural space is sterile and is resorbed when the inflammatory process subsides; however, when a subdural effusion is demonstrated by CT in a patient with prolonged fever, the possibility of the development of a subdural empyema is raised. Subdural effusions are typically low-density collections of fluid adjacent to the inner border of the skull that are hypodense to brain and nearly isodense to spinal fluid (Fig. 22). They are often bilateral and may flatten and displace the frontal horns posteriorly. When a subdural effusion becomes purulent, its density on CT scan may appear higher than that of CSF. After the administration of an intravenous contrast agent, there is significant enhancement, when the effusion is an empyema, at the border between the extra-axial fluid collection and the underlying cortex (Fig. 23). Sterile subdural effusions do not typically demonstrate contrast enhancement of the medial border (Fig. 24) (220).

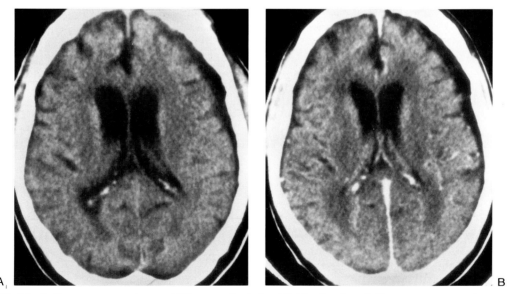

FIG. 24. A: Pre-contrast-enhanced CT scan of subdural fluid collection. **B:** Post-contrast-enhanced CT scan. The medial border of the subdural fluid collection does not enhance; therefore it is a subdural effusion.

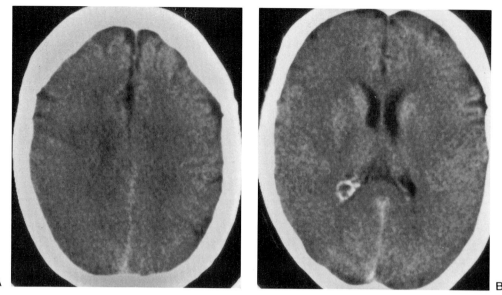

FIG. 25. A and **B:** CT scans demonstrating diffuse cerebral edema. There is loss of gray-matter–white-matter differentiation, and the sulci are markedly less prominent.

The possibility of raised ICP secondary to diffuse cerebral edema or obstructive or communicating hydrocephalus should be considered in patients with a progressive or prolonged alteration of consciousness. The CT abnormalities consistent with diffuse cerebral edema include: (a) loss of gray-matter–white-matter differentiation; (b) compression of the ventricles, giving the frontal horns a slit-like appearance; (c) loss of sulcal markings; and (d) lack of visualization of the perimesencephalic, suprasellar, or quadrigeminal cisterns (Fig. 25) (220). The CT appearance of communicating hydrocephalus is an enlargement of the entire ventricular system, including the fourth ventricle with periventricular lucencies surrounding the frontal horns (Fig. 26). The latter abnormality represents transependymal movement of CSF from the ventricular system into the brain parenchyma as a result of blockage in the normal CSF resorption pathways (220). The development of an obstructive hydrocephalus secondary to blockage of CSF flow by exudate at the foramina of Magendie and Luschka has the CT appearance of dilated lateral and third ventricles, with nonvisualization of the fourth ventricle.

The development of seizure activity and/or focal neurological symptoms and signs during the course of meningitis are clear-cut indications for CT scan. The etiology of these abnormalities may be indications for CT scan. The etiology of these abnormalities may be cerebritis, brain abscess, cortical infarction, enlarging subdural effusions, or empyema. Areas of cerebritis can easily be missed by CT scan. When they are visualized, they appear as low-density lesions on the noncontrasted scan that, after contrast administration, are surrounded by an inhomogeneous "halo." There may also be diffusion of contrast medium into the low-density center of an area of cerebritis. As the abscess matures and a capsule is formed, it becomes a low-density lesion with a sharply demarcated dense ring of contrast enhancement, surrounded by a variable hypodense region of edema (227) (Chapter 19).

Cortical infarctions complicating bacterial meningitis are the result of vasculitis. The CT appearance of a cortical infarction is that of a hypodense lesion that conforms to a vascular territory. Following the administration of contrast, cortical infarctions have a gyriform, nodular, or ring pattern of enhancement (Fig. 27) (228). Hemorrhagic infarctions are characteristically associated with hyperdense areas on noncontrasted scans and are fre-

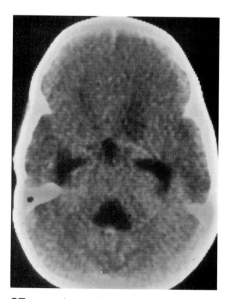

FIG. 26. CT scan demonstrating enlargement of the entire ventricular system, including the fourth ventricle, characteristic of communicating hydrocephalus.

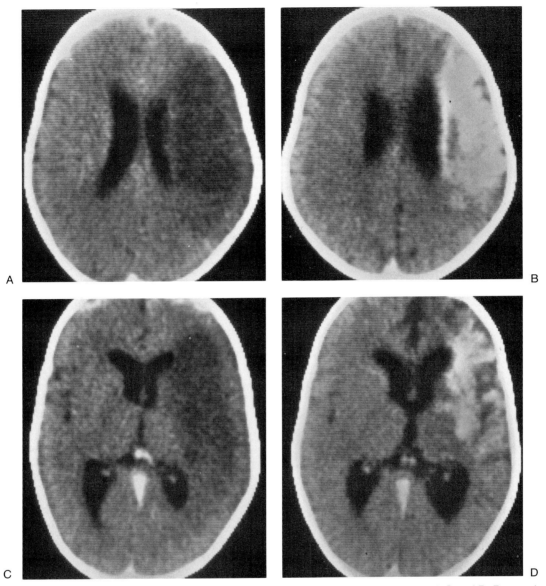

FIG. 27. A and **B:** Pre- and post-contrast-enhanced CT scan. High ventricular level. **C** and **D:** Pre- and post-contrast-enhanced CT scan. Low ventricular level. Hypodense lesion characteristic of cortical infarction in a patient with Hib meningitis. Following the administration of contrast, there is a gyriform pattern of enhancement.

quently reported as a complication of *H. influenzae* meningitis (220).

Magnetic resonance imaging (MRI), like CT, is useful for evaluating the complications of bacterial meningitis. Subdural empyemas, cortical infarctions, and areas of cerebritis are more readily imaged by MRI than by CT, but in a sick patient an MRI is more difficult to obtain than a CT scan. It is considerably more difficult to manage a critically ill patient in an isolated MRI scanner suite than in the CT scanner, thereby limiting the use of MRI in patients with bacterial meningitis.

The extent and degree of leptomeningeal enhancement from bacterial meningitis is well demonstrated by MRI after the intravenous administration of the paramagnetic

contrast agent, gadolinium (Fig. 28). Paramagnetic contrast agents produce local alterations in magnetic environments that directly affect the magnetic resonance signal obtained from protons. The image that is obtained after the administration of the contrast agent visualizes this effect on proton relaxation. The contrast agent itself is not visualized. Areas of active breakdown in the BBB are enhanced when scans are obtained after the administration of gadolinium (229). Pathological examination of animals with experimental bacterial meningitis demonstrated that areas of contrast enhancement on both CT and MRI scans correlated with inflammatory cell infiltration, and gadolinium-enhanced T1-weighted MRI scans revealed inflammatory meningeal and epen-

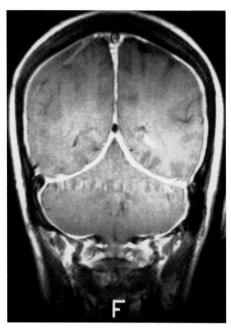

FIG. 28. Gadolinium-DTPA-enhanced T1-weighted MRI scan demonstrating diffuse meningeal enhancement in a patient with meningitis.

dymal lesions more effectively than did contrast-enhanced CT. Unenhanced T1- and T2-weighted MRI scans did not detect meningeal inflammation (230).

Subdural effusions can sometimes be distinguished from subdural empyemas by their magnetic resonance appearance. Subdural effusions are low-protein collections; therefore, they appear isointense to spinal fluid on MRI (Fig. 29). Subdural empyemas are more proteinaceous and, therefore, appear to have a higher signal in-

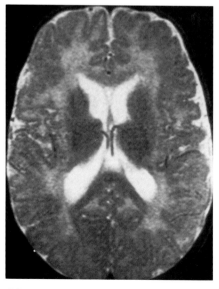

FIG. 29. T2-weighted MRI scan demonstrating subdural effusion.

tensity than CSF on T2-weighted MRI scans (231). MRI is superior to CT in detecting areas of infarction and of cerebritis. Both of these abnormalities appear as high-signal-intensity lesions on T2-weighted MRI scans.

TREATMENT

General Principles of Therapy

Bacteriologic cure of meningitis is defined as the eradication of bacteria from CSF. Effective antimicrobial therapy of bacterial meningitis is dependent on attaining adequate bactericidal activity in the CSF. Several factors, largely elucidated in experimental animal models of meningitis, determine whether bactericidal activity is achieved, including: (a) the ability of an antibiotic to penetrate the BBB, (b) the activity of the antibiotic within purulent CSF, and (c) the rate of metabolism of an antibiotic and its rate of clearance from CSF (232,233).

The BBB poses physiologic restrictions, allowing only highly lipid-soluble substances or substances transported by carrier-mediated facilitated diffusion to traverse it under normal conditions (232,234). The ability of an antibiotic to penetrate the BBB is dependent on several factors: (a) degree of lipid solubility, (b) degree of ionization at physiologic pH, (c) protein binding in serum, (d) molecular size and structure of the antibiotic, and (e) the status of the BBB. The BBB acts physiologically like a lipid bilayer. In general, the greater the lipid solubility of an antibiotic, the better its penetration into CSF. For example, chloramphenicol is a highly lipophilic substance that easily penetrates the BBB. The beta-lactam antibiotics have poor lipid solubility, limiting their entry into CSF under normal conditions (232). The un-ionized form of a drug possesses a greater lipid solubility than the ionized form. Thus, a lesser degree of ionization at the pH of serum and CSF increases entry of antibiotics into CSF by increasing their lipid solubility. Penicillin G has a high degree of ionization at the pH of plasma and CSF. This, combined with its low lipid solubility, may explain the poor penetration of penicillin G across intact meninges. The normal plasma-to-CSF pH gradient is ≤0.1 pH unit (235). The plasma-to-CSF pH gradient is altered, however, by purulent meningitis. The accumulation of lactate in CSF during bacterial meningitis decreases the pH of CSF, increases the gradient, and enhances the penetration of some antibiotics into CSF. Conversely, as metabolic acidosis develops, the pH gradient is reversed and the penetration of antibiotics into CSF is reduced (232).

Protein binding and molecular size limit the ability of an antibiotic to enter the CSF. Only the free non-protein-bound portion of an antibiotic in serum can enter the CSF; therefore, highly protein-bound antibiotics have lower CSF concentrations than do antibiotics with a lower degree of protein binding, other factors being equal. Increased binding to plasma proteins reduces the amount of antibiotic penetration into CSF; however, it is the concentration of free antibiotic in CSF in relation to its minimal bactericidal concentration (MBC) that determines its therapeutic effectiveness (234).

Although the pharmacokinetics of an antibiotic greatly influence its ability to penetrate the BBB, the most important factor appears to be the presence of meningeal inflammation. A moderate degree of meningeal inflammation results in a marked increase in the penetrability of most antibiotics. In many instances, altered BBB permeability is essential for an antibiotic to be effective in bacterial meningitis. The morphofunctional alterations of the BBB observed in an adult rat model of experimental meningitis consist of an early and sustained increase in pinocytotic vesicles with a progressive separation of intercellular tight junctions in the cerebral microvasculature (119), which may contribute to antimicrobial entry into purulent CSF.

Once the antibiotic penetrates into CSF, several factors influence its ability to eradicate the infection: (a) Sufficient concentrations of free active drug must be achieved in CSF, since this form of the antibiotic is necessary for bactericidal effect. The high protein concentrations in purulent CSF limit the concentration of free, unbound antibiotic. (b) An antibiotic must achieve concentrations in CSF, *in vivo,* exceeding the MBC of the infecting organism by 10- to 20-fold for optimal efficacy (236). (c) The bactericidal activity of an antibiotic may be diminished by the co-administration of a bacteriostatic agent. For example, chloramphenicol inhibits the bactericidal effect of aminoglycosides against gram-negative aerobic bacilli within the CSF (237). Conversely, antimicrobial combinations may exert an enhanced, synergistic improvement in the rate of bactericidal activity within the CSF *in vivo* (e.g., ampicillin plus gentamicin versus *L. monocytogenes* or *S. agalactiae*). (d) Early in the course of bacterial meningitis, there may be very large numbers of bacteria in CSF (i.e., $>10^8$ CFU/ml). Some antibiotics—in particular the beta-lactam antibiotics—demonstrate an inoculum effect *in vitro,* such that the minimal inhibitory concentration (MIC) increases dramatically as the inoculum of the test strain is increased from 10^5 to 10^7 CFU/ml under standardized *in vitro* conditions (232). The inoculum effect may explain the failure of certain antibiotics *in vivo,* as the *in vitro* activity of an antibiotic is routinely determined in standard growth media using 10^5 CFU/ml (234). (e) An antibiotic must remain physically stable in the presence of bacterial inactivating enzymes, such as beta-lactamase and chloramphenicol acetyltransferase (234).

The effectiveness of an antibiotic in eradicating bacterial meningitis is also determined by its rate of metabolism and the activity of its metabolites. For example, cephalothin is metabolized *in vivo* to desacetylcephalothin, which is less active *in vitro* than the parent compound (232). In contrast, the metabolite of cefotaxime (desacetylcefotaxime) is as active *in vitro* as the parent compound. Antibiotics are removed from CSF either by simple resorption through arachnoid villi or by an energy-dependent active transport process that removes the antibiotic from the CSF to the intravascular compartment across the epithelium of the choroid plexus. This "exit pump" is inhibited by weak organic acids, such as salicylates and probenecid, and to some extent by meningitis itself. Beta-lactam antibiotics and aminoglycosides are cleared from the CSF by this process. The third-generation cephalosporins (e.g., ceftriaxone and cefotaxime) possess decreased affinity (as compared with penicillin G) for the choroid plexus "exit pump," thus prolonging the duration they remain in CSF (234).

ANTIMICROBIAL THERAPY FOR SPECIFIC ORGANISMS

Hemophilus influenzae Type b

A combination of chloramphenicol and ampicillin has been the recommended initial therapy for Hib meningitis for over a decade. The increasing prevalence of beta-lactamase-producing strains and chloramphenicol-resistant strains has complicated the therapy of this infection and has made antimicrobial susceptibility testing a necessity. Approximately 25% of Hib strains causing meningitis in the United States are resistant to ampicillin, due to the production of beta-lactamase, although a smaller number of strains are resistant to ampicillin because of reduced affinity for penicillin-binding proteins. An increasing number of Hib strains are resistant to chloramphenicol, due to the production of chloramphenicol acetyltransferase (159). At the present time, chloramphenicol resistance is rare in the United States (<1%) but is becoming increasingly common worldwide. Greater than 50% of ampicillin-resistant *H. influenzae* CSF isolates from Spain are also chloramphenicol-resistant (238); thus, in some countries, Hib isolates resistant to both ampicillin and chloramphenicol are common (159). DNA coding for both the beta-lactamase enzyme and the chloramphenicol acetyltransferase enzyme can reside on plasmids, although chromosomal-mediated resistance [e.g., to trimethoprim (239)] has been described; therefore, any beta-lactamase-positive Hib isolate should be tested for susceptibility to chloramphenicol. When the results of antibiotic susceptibility tests are available, if the isolate is sensitive to ampicillin, chloramphenicol is discontinued. If the isolate is a beta-lactamase producer but is sensitive to chloramphenicol, chloramphenicol is continued as the single drug. Chloramphenicol has the advantage of being the only

TABLE 20. *Recommended doses of antibiotics in children[a]*

Antibiotic	Daily dose (mg/kg/day)	Dosing interval
Penicillin G	250,000–400,000 U	4–6 hr
Ampicillin	150–200	4–6 hr
Chloramphenicol	100	6 hr
Ceftriaxone	80–100	12–24 hr[b]
Cefotaxime	200	6 hr
Cefuroxime	240	8 hr
Ceftazidime	125–150	8 hr
Nafcillin	100–150	4 hr
Vancomycin	40–60	6 hr
Rifampin	20	
Gentamicin	5	8 hr
Amikacin	20	8 hr
Trimethoprim/sulfamethoxazole	10 (based on trimethoprim)	12 hr

[a] Data from refs. 52, 173, 208, 234, 260–262, 267, and 269.

[b] If a once-daily regimen is used, we recommend that on the first day an 80-mg/kg dose be given at diagnosis, at 12 and 24 hr, and then every 24 hr thereafter.

currently studied antibiotic that can be administered orally to treat bacterial meningitis. The oral form of chloramphenicol is absorbed almost entirely from the gastrointestinal tract and is equivalent in efficacy to the parenteral form in the treatment of *H. influenzae* meningitis (159). Recommended doses of ampicillin and chloramphenicol are shown in Tables 20 and 21.

We prefer the alternative of a third-generation cephalosporin (e.g., cefotaxime or ceftriaxone) for ampicillin and chloramphenicol. These antibiotics have been shown to be as efficacious as ampicillin plus chloramphenicol for the therapy of *H. influenzae* meningitis (240). The use of cefotaxime or ceftriaxone, which are the most exhaustively studied of the third-generation agents, has the following advantages: (a) It eliminates the need to monitor serum chloramphenicol concentra-

TABLE 21. *Recommended doses of antibiotics for bacterial meningitis in adults (15 years of age and older)[a]*

Antibiotic	Total daily dose (dosing interval)
Penicillin G	20–24 miU/day (every 4 hr)
Ampicillin	12 g/day (every 4 hr)
Ceftriaxone	4–6 g/day (every 12 hr)[b]
Cefotaxime	8–12 g/day (every 4 hr)
Ceftazidime	6 g/day (every 8 hr)[c]
Vancomycin	2 g/day (every 12 hr)
Nafcillin, oxacillin	9–12 g/day (every 4 hr)[d]
Chloramphenicol	4 g/day (every 6 hr)[e]
Gentamicin, tobramycin	5 mg/kg/day (every 8 hr)
Amikacin	15 mg/kg/day (every 8 hr)
Trimethoprim/ sulfamethoxazole	10 mg/kg/day (every 12 hr) (based on trimethoprim)

[a] Data from refs. 173 and 236.

[b] Actual dose studied was 50 mg/kg, every 12 hr.

[c] Not enough patients studied to make firm recommendation.

[d] Higher doses associated with leukopenia.

[e] Use 6 g/day for pneumococcal meningitis.

tions, (b) it avoids the potential toxicities of chloramphenicol, and (c) it decreases the number of daily doses of antibiotics (159). In addition, therapy with the third-generation cephalosporins may result in a more rapid sterilization of the CSF when compared to therapy with ampicillin plus chloramphenicol. Although the clinical significance of this finding on ultimate mortality and morbidity remains controversial, the American Academy of Pediatrics (241) has now endorsed the use of third-generation cephalosporins for the initial empiric therapy of bacterial meningitis in children. Third-generation cephalosporins are clearly the drugs of choice for the rare, doubly resistant (i.e., resistant to both ampicillin and chloramphenicol) Hib isolates in the United States (242) and should be considered initially in other areas where these strains are common.

The pharmacokinetics of chloramphenicol are highly variable among individuals; therefore, serum concentrations of this antibiotic must be monitored to ensure therapeutic concentrations while avoiding potential toxic concentrations, especially in infants (Chapter 15). Therapeutic serum concentrations are in the range of 15–25 μg/ml obtained 60–120 min after the completion of an intravenous or oral dose. Concentrations in excess of 30 μg/ml are associated with an increased incidence of bone marrow suppression, and levels exceeding 50–80 μg/ml may depress myocardial contractility (157). The pharmacology of chloramphenicol is altered in patients in shock or with liver disease. In either clinical situation, excessive serum concentrations of chloramphenicol could potentially decrease cardiac contractility. Chloramphenicol should therefore be avoided in patients with these conditions (157).

When chloramphenicol is used in combination with phenobarbital and phenytoin, serum concentrations of all three drugs must be monitored. Chloramphenicol inhibits hepatic microsomal enzymes and will therefore prolong the half-life of phenytoin in serum, resulting in toxic phenytoin concentrations. Phenytoin, conversely, interferes with hepatic metabolism of chloramphenicol, resulting in toxic serum concentrations. Phenobarbital induces hepatic microsomal enzymes, increases chloramphenicol metabolism, and decreases serum chloramphenicol concentrations. These drug interactions interfere with the eradication of the infection as well as with the management of seizure activity (208,243).

The long half-life of ceftriaxone allows for twice-daily (or even once-daily) administration of this antibiotic. Several studies have documented that once-daily administration of ceftriaxone is safe and efficacious for the treatment of bacterial meningitis. However, this is not yet recommended as standard therapy for adults; a twice-daily dose is preferred (236). Ceftriaxone has shown promise as once-daily therapy for completion of the therapeutic course in the home setting in stable children with meningitis following an uncomplicated hospital stay. The recommended doses of ceftriaxone and cefotaxime are listed in Tables 20 and 21.

A 10-day course of antibiotics is recommended for Hib meningitis, although current studies suggest that a 7-day course of treatment is adequate for most cases of uncomplicated meningitis due this organism in children. Some children require antibiotics for 14–17 days or longer for treatment of prolonged or recurrent fever or other complications (157).

Despite initial enthusiasm, cefuroxime, a second-generation cephalosporin, is not recommended for the treatment of Hib meningitis in children. The *in vitro* bactericidal activity of this drug has been shown to be inferior to the third-generation cephalosporins, and there have been reports of an unusually high incidence of positive Gram's stain and cultures in CSF obtained several days into treatment; in addition, there is one report of a child developing a secondary bacteremia with Hib on the 10th day of cefuroxime therapy, and there is another report of a child developing epiglottitis 17 days after a 10-day course of cefuroxime (240). In a prospective, multicenter study, 106 children with acute bacterial meningitis were randomly assigned to receive either ceftriaxone or cefuroxime. There were 62 cases of Hib meningitis. Delayed sterilization of CSF was more frequent among patients given cefuroxime (six patients) than among those given ceftriaxone (one patient) ($p = 0.112$). All seven patients in this study with delayed sterilization of CSF had Hib meningitis. Two of the six patients whose CSF cultures remained positive 24 hr after initiation of cefuroxime therapy later had severe bilateral hearing impairment. Six of 35 patients (17%) with Hib meningitis treated with cefuroxime had sensorineural hearing loss, and two of 27 patients (7%) with Hib meningitis treated with ceftriaxone had sensorineural hearing loss (244). When all children with positive CSF cultures (Hib, *N. meningitidis, S. pneumoniae, S. aga-*

lactiae) were included in the analysis, therapy with ceftriaxone resulted in: (a) more rapid sterilization of the CSF at follow-up lumbar puncture at ~24 hr (2% versus 12% positive cultures; $p = 0.11$); (b) less moderate to profound sensorineural hearing loss at the 2-month follow-up examination (4% versus 17%; $p < 0.05$); and (c) reversible biliary pseudolithiasis on serial abdominal ultrasonography (16 of 35 versus 0 of 35; $p < 0.001$) when compared with cefuroxime (244). In another comparative trial (245), ceftriaxone also led to a more rapid clinical response when compared with cefuroxime. The third-generation cephalosporins, cefotaxime and ceftriaxone, seem clearly preferable to cefuroxime in the treatment of Hib meningitis.

Neisseria meningitidis

Penicillin G (250,000 U/kg/day, intravenously, in divided doses every 4 hr) and ampicillin (300–400 mg/kg/day, in divided doses every 4 hr) are the preferred antibiotics for the treatment of meningitis caused by *N. meningitidis* (156,173,240). A 7-day course of therapy is adequate for most cases of uncomplicated meningococcal meningitis. There are reports of strains of *N. meningitidis* resistant to penicillin (246), although beta-lactamase-producing isolates are still rare (247). Penicillin - resistant strains that are not beta-lactamase-producing appear, instead, to have a reduced affinity for penicillin-binding proteins (e.g., PBP-3) and have been reported from Spain, the United Kingdom, and other countries (246–248). Meningococcal meningitis due to these strains has, however, been successfully managed with penicillin therapy, and thus the clinical significance of this partial resistance is unclear at this time (236). Nevertheless, this situation must be carefully monitored, since meningococci with relative resistance to penicillin (i.e., MICs in the 0.1- to 1.0-μg/ml range) are increasing in incidence worldwide. If an alternative agent is chosen for the therapy of meningococcal meningitis due to these relatively resistant strains, we prefer ceftriaxone based on *in vitro* susceptibility data (249); chloramphenicol is reasonable in patients with significant penicillin allergy.

Streptococcus pneumoniae

Penicillin G or ampicillin are the recommended antibiotics for meningitis due to *S. pneumoniae*. The doses are the same as those given for the treatment of meningococcal meningitis. Strains of pneumococci that are resistant to penicillin are becoming increasingly recognized. These organisms appear to be resistant to penicillin because of an alteration in the structure and molecular size of PBPs, and many patterns of altered penicillin affinity have been recognized (159,236). In view of the increasing number of strains resistant to penicillin, all CSF isolates of *S. pneumoniae* should be tested for penicillin susceptibility with a 1-μg oxacillin disk. A third-generation cephalosporin (i.e., cefotaxime or ceftriaxone) is recommended for relatively resistant strains of pneumococci (penicillin MICs of 0.1–1.0 μg/ml), since many strains are also chloramphenicol-resistant (250). For highly resistant strains (minimal inhibitory concentration $\geq$ 2 μg/ml), vancomycin (40–60 mg/kg/day, in divided doses every 6 hr) is the antimicrobial agent of choice (173,236).

Gram-Negative Bacilli

The results of clinical trials in patients with gram-negative bacillary meningitis favor the use of a third-generation cephalosporin over conventional aminoglycoside-containing regimens (173,177,251). Cefotaxime, ceftizoxime, ceftriaxone, and ceftazidime penetrate well into inflamed CSF and are highly active against gram-negative enteric bacilli (177,252). Cure rates of 78–94% have been achieved with the cephalosporins, compared to previous mortality rates of 40–90% with predominantly aminoglycoside-containing regimens (236).

In general, the above third-generation cephalosporins appear to be equally efficacious for the treatment of gram-negative bacillary meningitis, with the exception of meningitis due to *P. aeruginosa*. Ceftazidime is recommended when *P. aeruginosa* is suspected, since it is the only cephalosporin with sufficient activity against this organism in the CNS (253). Clinical trials suggest the efficacy of ceftazidime alone for *Pseudomonas* meningitis, but a combination of ceftazidime and an aminoglycoside may be used if response is delayed (236).

Although clinical experience is scant, quinolones have demonstrated efficacy in animal models of gram-negative bacillary meningitis. Intravenous pefloxacin has shown good efficacy with bacteriologic eradication from the CSF in 9 of 10 patients with gram-negative aerobic bacillary meningitis failing conventional therapy in one recent study (254). At the present time, however, the quinolones should be considered only for gram-negative bacillary meningitis caused by multiresistant strains or in patients unresponsive to standard therapies (255).

Although extended-spectrum penicillins (e.g., ticarcillin-clavulanate, temocillin, etc.) and aztreonam have proven effective in the therapy of experimental models of gram-negative bacillary meningitis in animals, their use is not recommended because the clinical experience with third-generation cephalosporins in humans is far more extensive.

Streptococcus agalactiae

A combination of penicillin G or ampicillin and an aminoglycoside has been standard therapy for neonatal meningitis due to group B streptococci (GBS) and is the recommended therapy for treatment of *S. agalactiae* meningitis in adults (256,257). The combination of these two agents is recommended because there are reports of synergy between these agents against GBS *in vitro* (258), and there appears to be an increasing number of penicillin-resistant strains of GBS (257). Infection with strains of *S. agalactiae* resistant to tetracycline, erythromycin, lincomycin, and clindamycin have been reported; therefore, the use of these penicillin substitutes in patients with GBS infections is not recommended (257).

The therapy of group B streptococcal meningitis in patients with life-threatening penicillin allergy presents a problem. If third-generation cephalosporins must be avoided, then vancomycin or teicoplanin may be tried, but clinical experience is almost nonexistent.

Listeria monocytogenes

Ampicillin is the drug of choice (often combined with gentamicin during the initial phase of treatment) for meningitis due to *L. monocytogenes*. The third-generation cephalosporins are inactive against this organism (236). For treatment of *L. monocytogenes* meningitis in patients allergic to ampicillin, intravenous trimethoprim-sulfamethoxazole (TMP-SMZ) is recommended. Initial therapy with intravenous TMP-SMZ followed by oral TMP alone has been successful in treating *Listeria* meningitis in penicillin-allergic patients; however, the duration of intravenous therapy prior to oral TMP alone has not been established (259).

Staphylococci

Meningitis due to *S. aureus* is treated with nafcillin or oxacillin, in a dose of 9–12 g/day in adults or 200–300 mg/kg daily in divided doses every 4 hr in children (52,53,260,261). Vancomycin is the drug of choice for methicillin-resistant staphylococci and for patients allergic to penicillin. The recommended intravenous dose of vancomycin for staphylococcal meningitis is 2 g/day for adults (1 g every 12 hr or 500 mg every 6 hr) and 40 mg/kg/day for children. The CSF should be monitored during therapy, and if the spinal fluid continues to yield viable organisms after 48 hr of intravenous treatment, then either intrathecal or intraventricular vancomycin, 20 mg once daily (in adults), can be added (260–262). The role of adjunctive rifampin therapy is unclear. Based on animal data and limited clinical experience, the use of TMP-SMZ for the therapy of *S. aureus* meningitis is inadvisable (53) despite *in vitro* susceptibility of *S. aureus* to this combination.

Anaerobes

A combination of chloramphenicol and penicillin G has been recommended for meningitis due to anaerobes.

Penicillin G has excellent activity against most anaerobes, with the exception of *Bacteroides fragilis.* Chloramphenicol is active against *B. fragilis.* Analogous to the experience in patients with brain abscess (Chapter 19), we prefer metronidazole for the therapy of the rare cases of anaerobic meningitis. Penicillin G should be used in addition pending culture results. Metronidazole is bactericidal against virtually all strict anaerobic organisms and penetrates into the CSF and brain well. Table 22 lists the recommended antibiotics according to microbial etiology.

EMPIRIC ANTIMICROBIAL THERAPY BY AGE GROUP AND UNDERLYING CONDITION

Children

Hib is the most common cause of bacterial meningitis in children. A third-generation cephalosporin, or a combination of chloramphenicol and ampicillin, is recommended for the treatment of Hib meningitis, as well as for the initial treatment of acute meningitis in children in whom the etiologic agent has not been identified. The empiric therapy of bacterial meningitis in children should also include coverage for *S. pneumoniae* and *N. meningitidis,* which is provided by the above two regimens. We favor the use of a third-generation cephalosporin alone, pending culture results. The recommended doses of these antibiotics are listed in Table 20.

Nevertheless, the optimal empiric regimen for meningitis in children remains controversial. In a large, randomized multicenter study conducted in Finland (263) involving 220 consecutive cases in children (Hib in 146), chloramphenicol alone was inferior to ampicillin plus chloramphenicol, cefotaxime, or ceftriaxone; the latter three regimens were therapeutically equivalent. It should be noted, however, that delayed CSF sterilization has been observed in children with meningitis receiving

newer cephalosporins (264,265), a finding associated with more frequent seizures, subdural effusions, and hemiparesis during hospitalization and neurologic sequelae among survivors (265). These, as well as other factors, are reflected in a survey of 63 program directors of pediatric infectious disease fellowships in the United States (266). When asked to indicate an empiric regimen for a 5-month-old infant with meningitis, the choices (percentage of respondents) were as follows: cefotaxime, 37%; ampicillin plus chloramphenicol, 32%; ceftriaxone, 22%; cefuroxime, 5%; ampicillin plus a third-generation cephalosporin, 5%. When compared to an earlier, similar survey in 1987, it was apparent that empiric use of ampicillin plus chloramphenicol (or cefuroxime alone) is declining for the initial therapy of meningitis in young (non-neonatal) children in the United States, whereas empiric use of third-generation cephalosporins is increasing in frequency. As stated above, we favor this latter approach in this age group (≥ 3 months and ≤ 10 years of age).

Adults (15–50 years)

S. pneumoniae and *N. meningitidis* are the causative organisms of ~85% of cases of bacterial meningitis in otherwise healthy adults (267). Empiric therapy of meningitis in adults should, therefore, be directed toward these organisms. Penicillin G (20–24 million units/day, in divided doses every 4 hr and ampicillin (12 g/day, in divided doses every 4 hr) are equally effective therapy for meningitis due to either of these organisms. Alternatively, a third-generation cephalosporin (e.g., cefotaxime or ceftriaxone) can be used. The recommended doses of these antibiotics are listed in Table 21. All CSF isolates of pneumococci or meningococci should be tested for penicillin or ampicillin resistance. A third-generation cephalosporin is recommended for relatively penicillin-resistant pneumococci, and vancomycin is suggested for

TABLE 22. *Recommended antibiotics for the treatment of bacterial meningitis*

Organism	Antibiotic
H. influenzae type b	Third-generation cephalosporin[a] or ampicillin plus chloramphenicol
N. meningitidis	Penicillin G or ampicillin
S. pneumoniae	Penicillin G or ampicillin
P. aeruginosa	Ceftazidime (plus an aminoglycoside)
S. aureus (methicillin-sensitive)	Nafcillin or oxacillin
S. aureus (methicillin-resistant)	Vancomycin
Coagulase-negative staphylococci	Vancomycin[b]
L. monocytogenes	Ampicillin (plus an aminoglycoside)
Enterobacteriaceae	Third-generation cephalosporin[a,c]
S. agalactiae	Penicillin G or ampicillin (plus an aminoglycoside)

[a] Cefotaxime or ceftriaxone.
[b] Rifampin is added when there is no improvement after 48 hr of therapy.
[c] Ceftazidime if *P. aeruginosa* is suspected or proven.

highly penicillin-resistant pneumococci (236). A third-generation cephalosporin can be used for penicillin-resistant (MIC $\leq$ 1 μg/ml) meningococci.

Older Adults

The most common organisms causing meningitis in the adults over 50 years of age are *S. pneumoniae* and enteric gram-negative bacilli; however, meningitis due to *Listeria* and *H. influenzae* are increasingly recognized. For initial therapy of meningitis in elderly patients, either ceftriaxone or cefotaxime in combination with ampicillin is recommended (173,175,208).

The recommended doses of antibiotics for meningitis in older adults are listed in Table 21.

Duration of Therapy

The standards for the duration of therapy of bacterial meningitis have been derived from clinical experience rather than rigid scientific analysis (268) and are basically empiric. Although shorter courses of therapy may be equally efficacious, we recommend the following duration of treatment as general guidelines, not rigid standards, when the etiologic agent is known: Hib, 7–10 days; *N. meningitidis,* 7 days; *S. pneumoniae,* 10–14 days; and gram-negative aerobic bacilli, 3–4 weeks. Nevertheless, it must be stressed that the patients response, as assessed by clinical and laboratory parameters, is the most important criteria in the decision to terminate therapy within this discretionary range.

Post-traumatic Meningitis

S. pneumoniae is the most common cause of meningitis following traumatic head injury in association with the formation of a dural sinus fistula (172). *H. influenzae* is a less frequent, but also important, pathogen in this setting. A third-generation cephalosporin is recommended for empiric treatment of meningitis in patients with closed-head injury. The regimen can subsequently be modified based on the results of CSF cultures.

Meningitis Following Neurosurgical Procedures

The most common organisms causing meningitis in the patient who has undergone a neurosurgical procedure, with the exception of a shunting procedure, are gram-negative bacilli (177). Initial therapy of meningitis in the postneurosurgical patient should be directed against gram-negative bacilli, but also against *P. aeruginosa* and *S. aureus* (173). A third-generation cephalosporin is recommended for the treatment of gram-negative bacillary meningitis (177,251). Ceftazidime, perhaps

with an aminoglycoside, should be used. Ceftazidime is the only cephalosporin with sufficient activity against *Pseudomonas* in the CNS (253). Vancomycin should be added until infection with staphylococci is excluded.

Coagulase-negative staphylococci and *S. aureus* are the most common pathogens causing CSF shunt infections. Vancomycin is recommended for shunt infections due to staphylococci (52,260,261), unless the organism is clearly susceptible to methicillin. Therapy of methicillin-resistant staphylococcal shunt infections should include a combination of intravenous vancomycin (2 g/day; 40 mg/kg/day in children) and either oral rifampin (1200 mg/day; 20 mg/kg/day in children) or intrashunt or intraventricular vancomycin (20 mg once daily) (Chapter 23) (261,269). Although cefuroxime may enter ventricular fluid in the presence of an infected CSF shunt, the concentrations are quite variable (270); this agent is not recommended for shunt infections.

Immunosuppressed Host

As has been discussed, the risk of an immunocompromised patient developing bacterial meningitis is dependent on a number of factors, such as (a) the underlying disease and its treatment, (b) the duration of immunosuppression, and (c) the type of immune abnormality. Knowledge of the latter helps predict the infecting organism (186,187). Patients with defects in cell-mediated immunity are most susceptible to CNS infections by microorganisms that are intracellular parasites, the eradication of which is dependent upon an intact T-lymphocyte–macrophage system. *L. monocytogenes* is the most common cause of bacterial meningitis in patients with defective cell-mediated immunity (187). Patients with defective humoral immunity are unable to mount an antibody response to a bacterial infection, and they are therefore unable to control infection caused by encapsulated bacteria. These patients are at particular risk for meningitis caused by *S. pneumoniae,* Hib, and, less commonly, *N. meningitidis.* Patients with neutropenia are at particular risk for meningitis caused by *P. aeruginosa* and by members of the Enterobacteriacae family (186). The choice of antibiotic for empiric treatment of bacterial meningitis in the immunosuppressed patient should be made based on the type of immune abnormality.

Table 22 lists the recommended antibiotics based on microbial etiology.

ADJUNCTIVE THERAPY

As has been discussed previously in this chapter, the generation of bacterial cell-wall components in CSF during treatment of meningitis with antibiotics contributes to increased inflammation in the SAS (93). The mechanism through which bacterial cell-wall components produce an inflammatory response in the SAS has not yet been defined; however, recent data suggest that bacterial cell-wall components may stimulate the release of inflammatory cytokines in the CNS, such as TNF, IL-1, and prostaglandins (236). It may be possible to reduce the inflammatory response in the SAS and thus improve the outcome of this infection by administering antiinflammatory agents in conjunction with antibiotics.

TNF is a macrophage-secreted hormone that is released in response to bacterial endotoxin. The injection of small doses of purified endotoxin into healthy volunteers causes the appearance of elevated serum concentrations of TNF within 90 min after the infusion, accompanied by symptoms of headache, fever, rigors, and myalgia (271). Endogenous TNF release has been observed in septic patients and in patients with meningococcemia. Damas et al. (272) detected very high serum concentrations of TNF (mean of 701 ± 339 pg/ml, normal 75 ± 15 pg/ml) in patients in septic shock. Waage et al. (273) found elevated serum TNF concentrations in patients with meningococcal disease. The patients with the highest concentrations (>0.1 ng/ml) died. Ming et al. (274) found elevated concentrations of TNF in CSF during bacterial meningitis in both mice and humans. None of the CSF samples from patients with viral (echo, coxsackie, or mumps) meningitis or other neurological diseases (e.g., multiple sclerosis) in this study contained measurable concentrations of TNF (274), suggesting that the presence of TNF in CSF may be specific for bacterial meningitis (236).

TNF induces IL-1 release from endothelial cells and macrophages (275). IL-1 represents a family of polypeptides that are both beneficial and detrimental to the host. The primary sources of IL-1 are monocytes and macrophages, but IL-1 is also produced by brain astrocytes and microglia as well. IL-1 is a potent chemoattractant for neutrophils, monocytes, B cells, and T cells; it has an important role in B-cell proliferation and antibody production, as well as in T-cell activation (276). IL-1 may, however, also be detrimental to the host. IL-1 released into tissue induces a proliferative response. IL-1 released by astrocytes into brain tissue may contribute to brain gliosis and scar formation (276). IL-1 increases the concentration of metabolites of arachidonic acid—most notably prostaglandin E_2 and leukotriene B_4, which are potent mediators of inflammation (275).

Possible therapeutic approaches to decrease the harmful effects of TNF and/or IL-1 might include (a) drugs or procedures to decrease their production, block their biological activity, or enhance removal from the circulation, (b) passive immunization with antibodies against TNF and IL-1, and (c) drugs which interfere with IL-1-induced arachidonic acid metabolites. Corticosteroids are highly effective in reducing IL-1 production *in vitro* and *in vivo*. Many of the biological activities of IL-1 are inflammatory; aspirin, acetaminophen, and nonsteroi-

dal anti-inflammatory agents can reduce fever, muscle PGE_2 production, leukocyte chemotaxis, and so on. Therapeutic concentrations of nonsteroidal anti-inflammatory agents and antipyretic blood levels of aspirin do not, however, reduce IL-1 production, IL-1-mediated lymphocyte activation, or IL-1 synthesis of acute-phase proteins (276).

Passive immunization with monoclonal antibodies directed against TNF and IL-1 may be a future therapeutic option. Beutler et al. (277) passively immunized mice with antiserum to murine TNF and protected them from the lethal effects of gram-negative bacteremia.

Despite aggressive supportive care and the administration of appropriate antimicrobial agents, the outcome from fulminant meningococcemia is often poor. Serum TNF concentrations correlate directly with outcome in this condition. Plasmapheresis has been attempted, although on an extremely limited scale, in these desperately ill patients and may lead to a rapid decrease in serum TNF concentrations (278) and/or improved mortality and morbidity. Despite the lack of a controlled clinical trial, this approach definitely deserves further study.

Recent clinical trials suggest a beneficial effect from dexamethasone in the treatment of bacterial meningitis in children and adults. In a prospective, randomized trial, 429 patients with bacterial meningitis were treated with either (a) dexamethasone, ampicillin, and chloramphenicol or (b) ampicillin and chloramphenicol only. Dexamethasone was administered intramuscularly with the first dose of antibiotic, at a dose of 8 mg to children younger than 12 years and 12 mg to adults every 12 hr for 3 days. There were 56 cases of Hib meningitis, 106 cases of pneumococcal meningitis, and 267 cases of meningococcal meningitis. The case fatality rate was significantly lowered in patients with pneumococcal meningitis receiving dexamethasone; only seven of 52 patients died, compared with 22 of 54 patients not receiving dexamethasone ($p < 0.01$). Dexamethasone therapy also significantly reduced the incidence of hearing loss in patients with pneumococcal meningitis. None of the 45 surviving patients in the dexamethasone-treated group developed hearing loss, whereas four of 32 patients treated with antibiotics alone became deaf ($p < 0.05$). These investigators were unable to evaluate hearing loss in children with Hib meningitis (279).

The results of a double-blind, placebo-controlled trial of 200 infants and children with bacterial meningitis demonstrated a beneficial effect of dexamethasone therapy in reducing the incidence of sensorineural hearing loss. Patients were treated with ceftriaxone or cefuroxime, with either dexamethasone (0.15 mg/kg every 6 hr for 4 days) or placebo. Thirteen of 84 patients (15.5%) in the placebo group had moderate or more severe bilateral hearing loss as compared with three of 92 (3.3%) of the dexamethasone-treated children ($p < 0.01$) (280). The beneficial effects of dexamethasone were only observed in the children receiving concurrent cefuroxime (which may be suboptimal therapy) and not in those treated with ceftriaxone, thus rendering interpretation difficult. Dexamethasone appeared to be of particular benefit in children with Hib meningitis of milder severity (280); however, the subset(s) of patients most appropriate for this form of adjunctive therapy remains unsettled at the present time.

Similar trends suggesting a beneficial effect of dexamethasone were observed in a third randomized, placebo-controlled trial by the Dallas group for children receiving cefuroxime (281). Once again, patients receiving dexamethasone became afebrile sooner, and the CSF glucose concentration rose more rapidly during the first day of therapy. Although the small sample size precluded a significant result from an analysis of hearing loss, the data combined with that of ref. 280 continued to reveal an advantage for corticosteroid therapy (282). The relative risk of hearing loss requiring hearing aids was ~13-fold greater in the placebo group when compared to those children receiving dexamethasone therapy. Nevertheless, the use of cefuroxime, a suboptimal agent (see above; also see ref. 245), in ~160 of 260 patients in these trials has led some (283) to question the routine use of dexamethasone as adjunctive therapy in children over 2 months of age. In addition, the beneficial effects of dexamethasone have only been shown in Hib meningitis, and too few patients with pneumococcal or meningococcal meningitis have been studied to assess efficacy. Furthermore, routine use may lead to unnecessary exposure of children with viral meningitis to dexamethasone because of concern over the initial CSF formula, and it may also lead to difficulty in excluding a bacterial cause; the potential risk(s) of this practice are unknown. A meta-analysis of all nine available controlled trials of corticosteroids for adjunctive therapy also suggests that only certain subgroups of patients may benefit from their use (284).

Others (285) feel that the bulk of current experimental and clinical evidence supports the routine use of corticosteroids in children with bacterial meningitis. Apparently, many of the directors of pediatric infectious disease programs agree: 17% "always" use dexamethasone, and an additional 60% "sometimes" employ this agent as adjunctive therapy in childhood meningitis (266).

To reduce the incidence of sensorineural hearing loss, it seems reasonable (on the basis of currently available data) to treat children with bacterial meningitis with a short course of dexamethasone therapy. A daily dose of 10–12 mg/m^2 (0.15 mg/kg) in four divided doses is recommended for 3–4 days (286). Children should, however, be carefully monitored for potential complications of corticosteroid use, specifically gastrointestinal hemorrhage and hyperglycemia. If corticosteroids are used, they should definitely be administered early—that is, be-

fore or simultaneously with the first dose(s) of antimicrobial agents. This is particularly important because administration of currently available bacteriolytic agents (e.g., ceftriaxone) leads to rapid release of free endotoxin from gram-negative organisms into CSF with an attendant accentuation of the host's inflammatory response (287). Dexamethasone therapy may be beneficial to adults with meningitis, as suggested by the lower fatality rate in patients with pneumococcal meningitis treated with dexamethasone in one study (279); however, clear-cut recommendations await the results of further clinical trials.

In addition to corticosteroids, several other adjunctive approaches to the therapy of bacterial meningitis have been proposed (288), including: (a) bactericidal but non-bacteriolytic antibiotics to reduce endotoxin and other injurious substance (e.g., outer-membrane vesicle) release into CSF (a theoretical but, as yet, impractical method); (b) nonsteroidal anti-inflammatory agents; (c) other prostaglandin inhibitors; (d) anti-endotoxin-binding agents; and (e) monoclonal antibodies directed against endotoxin, cytokines, or leukocyte–endothelium adhesion molecules. Although several of these interesting possibilities have proven beneficial (with different end-points) in experimental models of meningitis in animals, none has, as of this writing, been subjected to critical analysis in clinical trials in humans.

Treatment of Complications

Raised Intracranial Pressure

ICP is usually increased in bacterial meningitis; therefore, this complication should be anticipated and treated promptly. The clinical signs of increased ICP are: (a) an altered level of consciousness ranging from drowsiness to coma; (b) a dilated, poorly reactive or nonreactive pupil; (c) ocular motility abnormalities; and (d) bradycardia and hypertension, the Cushing reflex. Increasing ICP may be associated with only one or a combination of these clinical signs. Papilledema does not develop until increased ICP has been present for several hours; therefore, the absence of papilledema should not be used to exclude the presence of increased ICP. Increased ICP may lead to herniation. Signs of impending herniation include: (a) midposition, nonreactive pupils; (b) unequal or dilated, nonreactive pupils; (c) skew deviation or dysconjugate eye movements; (d) decorticate or decerebrate posturing; and (e) bradycardia and abnormal respiratory patterns.

Patients that are awake and alert can be watched clinically for signs of advancing increased ICP. Patients who are stuporous or comatose may benefit from an ICP monitoring device. ICP exceeding 20 mmHg are abnormal, and they should be treated; however, outcome may be improved if pressures greater than 15 mmHg are treated. The rationale for treating the smaller elevations in pressure is to avoid large elevations, or so-called "plateau waves," that can lead to herniation and irreversible brainstem injury (144,208). Plateau waves are sustained elevations in ICP that may occur spontaneously or as the result of small increases in cerebral blood volume from hypoxia, fever, or intratracheal suctioning. When ICP is already high, plateau waves may be reached quickly and lead to brain death (146,208). The treatment of increased ICP is outlined in Table 23.

Elevating the head of the bed 30° reduces the ICP. Turning the head to the side (particularly to the left) or hyperextending the neck may trigger an increase in ICP. Intratracheal suctioning or endotracheal intubation may increase ICP. This may be reduced by an intravenous injection of lidocaine (1.5 mg/kg) prior to suctioning or intubation (146,208,289).

Hyperventilation, by decreasing $PaCO_2$, causes cerebral vasoconstriction; this reduces cerebral blood volume, thereby decreasing ICP. Cerebral blood flow changes by approximately 2% per 1-mmHg change in $PaCO_2$ (144,208). ICP decreases within 30 sec of lowering the $PaCO_2$, and this effect is sustained for 15–20 min (146,208). The $PaCO_2$ should be maintained between 27 and 30 mmHg. If $PaCO_2$ is reduced below 20 mmHg, cerebral ischemia may occur. The effectiveness of hyperventilation decreases with time and may be minimal after 48 hr of continuous treatment; therefore, hyperventilation should be slowly discontinued 24 hr after the ICP has remained continuously below 15 mmHg, or earlier if brain edema is not likely to worsen (144,146,208).

Hyperosmolar agents, such as mannitol, decrease ICP by decreasing cerebral edema. Mannitol remains almost entirely in the extracellular intravascular space, making this compartment hyperosmolar to brain tissue. The result is movement of water from brain tissue into the intravascular space. Mannitol can be given either as a bolus intravenous injection of 1 g/kg over 10–15 min or in small frequent doses of 0.25 g/kg every 2–3 hr. A bolus injection can be repeated at 3- to 4-hr intervals in order to maintain the serum osmolality between 315 and 320 mOsm/liter (144,146,208,289).

Dexamethasone appears to be beneficial in reducing ICP and cerebral edema in animal models of bacterial meningitis (126,128), but its efficacy for reducing cerebral edema in patients with bacterial meningitis has not been established. Steroids are known to be beneficial in reducing cerebral edema surrounding tumors. In this situation, cerebral edema is largely vasogenic in origin. Steroids reduce vasogenic edema by reducing the permeability of cerebral capillary endothelial cells (290). There is experimental evidence to suggest that steroids reduce interstitial edema in meningitis (125). Cerebral edema in meningitis is a combination of vasogenic, cytoxic, and interstitial edema (143). The evidence that steroids decrease vasogenic and interstitial edema suggests a role for corticosteroids in the management of this complication, which may contribute to raised ICP.

The use of steroids to reduce cerebral edema in meningitis also has disadvantages. Steroids decrease inflammation in the meninges. As has been discussed, a moderate degree of inflammation in the meninges is required for the CSF penetration of many antibiotics. By reducing meningeal inflammation, the concentration of antibiotics in CSF is reduced. This may be most important several days into treatment when meningeal inflammation has been reduced substantially by antibiotic treatment. Steroids should, therefore, be discontinued within ~4 days of treatment (286).

High-dose barbiturate therapy is useful when hyperventilation and hyperosmolar agents have failed to control ICP. Barbiturates decrease the cerebral metabolic demand for oxygen and thus decrease cerebral blood flow. The result is a decrease in ICP. Pentobarbital is administered in an initial dose of 20–30 mg/kg, followed by a dose of 1–1.5 mg/kg/hr. This therapy requires an intracranial monitoring device or an electroencephalogram (EEG) to monitor cerebral activity, since the clinical examination is severely limited by the depressive effects of barbiturate. Pentobarbital is administered until the ICP is reduced below 20 mmHg or until the EEG demonstrates a burst–suppression pattern. Recommended serum concentrations of pentobarbital to reduce ICP are 20–40 μg/dl. A Swan–Ganz catheter should be in place to monitor cardiac output. High-dose barbiturates are associated with significant cardiac toxicity, including decreased cardiac output, decreased contractile force, arrhythmias, and hypotension. Pentobarbital is the recommended barbiturate when barbiturate coma is desired, because this drug has a relatively shorter half-

TABLE 23. *Treatment of increased intracranial pressure*[a]

1. Elevate the head of the bed 30°.
2. Hyperventilation to maintain $PaCO_2$ between 27 and 30 mmHg.
3. Mannitol
   a. Children: 0.5–2.0 g/kg infused over 30 min, and repeated as necessary.
   b. Adults: 1.0 g/kg bolus injection or 0.25 g/kg every 2–3 hr.
4. Pentobarbital
   a. Initial dose: 20–30 mg/kg
   b. Maintenance dosage: 1–2 mg/kg/hr

[a] Data from refs. 144, 146, 208, 286, and 289.

life. The half-life of pentobarbital is 24 hr, compared to the longer half-life of phenobarbital (5 days). The use of pentobarbital allows for a more rapid reversal of barbiturate coma than does the use of phenobarbital. Pentobarbital coma is maintained until the ICP has been below 20 mmHg for 24 hr. The dose of barbiturate is then slowly decreased to prevent a rebound increase in ICP (208,289,291).

Seizures

Seizures occur in 30–40% of children with acute bacterial meningitis (160), and they occur in greater than 30% of adults with pneumococcal meningitis in the first few days of illness (172). If not managed quickly and aggressively, status epilepticus may develop. Severe or prolonged seizure activity can produce permanent damage due to anoxic ischemic changes in areas of the temporal lobe, cerebellum, and thalamus (208,291). The increased energy requirements of discharging neurons cannot be met by cerebral blood flow during sustained seizure activity. The result is ischemic necrosis and loss of cortical neurons (286). Status epilepticus that is continuous for 90 min or longer can cause permanent neurological sequelae.

For early termination of seizure activity, a short-acting anticonvulsant with a rapid onset of action (such as lorazepam or diazepam) is recommended. Lorazepam is administered intravenously in 1- to 4-mg doses in adults, and in an initial dose of 0.05 mg/kg in children. Lorazepam has a duration of action three to four times longer than that of diazepam in adults (286); 4 mg of lorazepam is therapeutically equivalent to 10 mg of diazepam (292). Diazepam is administered in a dose of 0.25–0.4 mg/kg (maximum 10 mg) at a rate of 1–2 mg per minute. The 10-mg dose may be repeated up to three times at intervals of 15–20 min (293). Diazepam has a half-life of 15 min; therefore, the blood level decreases rapidly. A long-acting anticonvulsant should be administered immediately after lorazepam or diazepam. The long-acting anticonvulsant of choice in children and adults is phenytoin, administered in a dose of 18–20 mg/kg at a rate no faster than 50 mg/min. Phenytoin can prolong the Q–T interval or lead to hypotension. If either of these side effects are observed, the rate of administration is decreased. Phenytoin is very effective in controlling convulsions without depressing consciousness or respiration (208). Intravenous phenytoin reaches peak brain and blood concentrations within 15 min (294). The half-life of phenytoin following a loading dose is approximately 36 hr (292). Serum concentrations greater than 25 μg/ml are usually necessary to terminate status epilepticus. If a dose of 18–20 mg/kg of phenytoin fails to control seizure activity, an additional 500 mg of phenytoin can be given. A maintenance dose of 100 mg every 6 hr (in adults) should be started after the loading dose.

If phenytoin fails to control seizure activity, the patient should be intubated, mechanically ventilated, and treated with phenobarbital. For adults, phenobarbital is administered intravenously, at a rate of 100 mg/min until seizure activity stops or to a loading dose of 20 mg/kg (208). The loading dose of phenobarbital in children is 20 mg/kg, administered intravenously, at a rate of 30 mg/min (295). The most common adverse effects of phenobarbital loading are hypotension and respiratory depression. If these complications are managed and seizure activity continues, an additional 10 mg/kg can be given (295). The primary reason for failure to control seizures is that anticonvulsants are administered in subtherapeutic doses or that the rate of administration is too slow.

The combination of phenytoin and phenobarbital will control seizure activity in the vast majority of patients. When they fail to do so, general anesthesia with pentobarbital can be tried. The dose of pentobarbital is the same for children and adults: loading dose of 3–5 mg/kg and a maintenance dose of 1–2 mg/kg/hr (208,295). In the past, paraldehyde or a continuous intravenous diazepam drip were used to treat status epilepticus; however, paraldehyde is no longer available, and a diazepam drip is no longer recommended.

Fluid Management

A majority of children with bacterial meningitis are hyponatremic (serum sodium concentration < 135 mEq/liter) early in the course of their illness (286); ~50% of children have evidence of SIADH on admission to the hospital (124). Restriction of fluids to correct serum sodium is important, since the degree and duration of hyponatremia correlate with the development of neurologic sequelae. The initial rate of intravenous fluid administration is limited to approximately one-half of normal maintenance requirements, or about 800–1000 ml/m^2/day. A 5% dextrose solution with one-fourth to one-half normal saline and 20–40 mEq/liter potassium is recommended. The serum sodium concentration and urine specific gravity should be measured every 6–12 hr (286). The mean duration of hyponatremia in children with Hib meningitis in one study was 20 hr (range: 0–240 hr) (296). The volume of fluids administered can be gradually increased when the serum sodium concentration rises above 135 mEq/liter. In most cases, maintenance rates (1500–1700 ml/m^2/day) will be reached by 36–48 hr after admission. These recommendations do not apply to the child who is admitted in shock or who is severely dehydrated (286).

Subdural Effusion

The majority of subdural effusions do not need intervention and are associated with no permanent deficits (159). Routine subdural paracentesis should be avoided.

Only the rare effusion becomes an empyema or is large enough to have a mass effect. In either instance, serial imaging of the fluid collection by CT or MRI will allow for early detection of these complications.

PREVENTION

As stated above, bacterial meningitis continues to carry a significant morbidity and mortality despite the availability of effective antimicrobial therapy. It has become clear in recent years that the spread of several types of meningitis can be prevented by antibiotic prophylaxis of contacts of cases. In addition, vaccines have been developed that may have efficacy in decreasing the incidence of meningitis due to the three common meningeal pathogens. The following sections review the data concerning chemoprophylaxis and immunoprophylaxis against these infectious agents.

Hemophilus influenzae Chemoprophylaxis

The importance of chemoprophylaxis to prevent secondary spread of disease due to Hib was recognized as early as 1955 (297). It was suggested that close contacts (especially those in the younger age groups) of patients with Hib meningitis receive chemoprophylaxis based on several observations: Close contacts of patients with Hib meningitis were more likely to be colonized with the organism than were age-matched controls, and other sporadic associated episodes in siblings had been reported. However, despite these observations, chemoprophylaxis of household contacts was not widely practiced because secondary spread was believed to be infrequent. Subsequently, several studies documented the transmission of Hib to household contacts from patients with meningitis (298). In a summary of five studies, the risk of secondary disease was markedly age-dependent, being highest for children less than 2 years of age (Table 24). The overall risk of 0.3% was 600 times greater than the endemic risk for the general population. Seventy-five percent of the secondary cases occurred within 6 days of onset of the index case, although untreated household contacts were at increased risk of Hib disease for at least 1 month after onset in the index patient. Studies have also demonstrated that the nasopharyngeal carriage rates of Hib are significantly higher in people living in the homes of patients who have the disease than in the homes of controls (298). This colonization is also age-dependent, with rates as high as 71% in young siblings of a patient. In addition, twins have been found to be at increased risk of primary invasive Hib disease (9), since the healthy twin was more often found to carry Hib in the nasopharynx than were non-twin siblings of the patients, suggesting frequent transmission of the organism between twins.

Another risk factor for transmission of Hib is day care outside of the home (9), with the risk being equally high for both family day-care settings and professional day-care centers (whose group sizes were 4 and 12 children, respectively). The children most likely to develop secondary disease were younger than 2 years of age; in addition, Hib disease was significantly higher within the first month of attendance, especially in children less than 2 years old. However, there is controversy regarding (a) the risk of secondary disease in these high-risk children with respect to the exact magnitude of the risk, (b) whether the risk is higher than the background risk of primary Hib disease in children of that age attending day-care facilities, and (c) whether an increased risk can be decreased by chemoprophylaxis. In a review of six studies (299), three showed a risk of disease above 1%, which is approximately 25 times higher than the expected rate of primary disease in these children. Two studies, in Dallas County and Minnesota, revealed 0% attack rates (95% confidence interval: 0–1.0), but the reasons for these differences are not well-defined; there may be some geographic differences in day-care characteristics and risk of disease. This has led to disagreement concerning the recommendation for chemoprophylaxis of children in day-care facilities (see below).

The rationale for the use of chemoprophylaxis for prevention of secondary disease is eradication of nasopharyngeal carriage of Hib. Therefore, transmission of Hib to young, susceptible contacts is prevented, as is the development of disease in those already colonized. In addition, the index case must receive prophylaxis because the usual antibiotics given for invasive Hib disease do not necessarily eliminate nasopharyngeal carriage. Initial reports (298) examined several antimicrobials for efficacy in eradication of Hib carriage from the nasopharynx (Table 25). However, most studies were not placebo-controlled and involved relatively few carriers, and nearly all were performed in institutional settings. Rifampin—at a dosage of 20 mg/kg, orally, for 4 days—was the most efficacious, eradicating carriage in 96% of contacts. On the basis of these findings, the Centers for Disease Control and the American Academy of Pediatrics recommended rifampin prophylaxis (20 mg/kg for 4 days) for all individuals, including adults, in households with at least one child younger than 24 months of age or with a nonimmunized child 24–48 months of age (300,301). The index patient should also receive rifampin chemoprophylaxis. Rifampin is not recommended

TABLE 24. *Percent risk of secondary* H. influenzae *type b disease in household contacts of a patient in the first month after the index case*[a]

Age of contact (years)	Average risk (%)
≤1	4.4
2–3	1.2
4–5	0.06
≥6	0
All ages	0.3

[a] Adapted from ref. 298.

TABLE 25. *Elimination rate of nasopharyngeal carriage of* H. influenzae *type b after treatment with various drug regimens*[a]

Regimen	Rate (%) of elimination of Hib carriage
No therapy or placebo	26
Cefaclor	18
Erythromycin-sulfasoxazole	20
Trimethoprim-sulfamethoxazole	58
Ampicillin	70
Rifampin (10 mg/kg dose)	71
Rifampin (20 mg/kg dose)	96

[a] Adapted from ref. 298.

for pregnant women who are contacts of affected infants, since the effect of rifampin on the fetus has not been established.

The management of day-care contacts is less clear. The current recommendation is no chemoprophylaxis for day-care contacts 2 years of age or older, although prophylaxis is indicated if two or more cases occur in a day-care center. However, controversy exists with regard to chemoprophylaxis for contacts less than 2 years of age. The Centers for Disease Control recommends prophylaxis in day-care contacts younger than 2 years old, whereas the American Academy of Pediatrics does not recommend prophylaxis in most of these cases (301). Until further data are available, the question of whether to administer prophylaxis to this age group should be individualized and considered more strongly in day-care centers which resemble households and in which the children have prolonged contact. This issue requires further study, but certainly close surveillance of young contacts is important regardless of prophylactic measures.

Hemophilus influenzae Immunoprophylaxis

The development of a vaccine against Hib initially focused on the PRP capsule because anti-PRP antibodies possessed *in vivo* and *in vitro* protective activity against Hib (302). Beginning in 1974, a large study from Finland examined the efficacy of this PRP vaccine (17). The response to vaccination was age-dependent, with serum concentrations of >1.0 μg/ml (the level thought to be indicative of long-term protection) attained only in children 16 months of age or older. This study also prospectively followed patients 4 years after vaccination to determine protective efficacy. Approximately 49,000 children received 7.5 μg of the PRP vaccine, and no differences in the number of Hib cases were found in children aged 3–17 months whether they received the PRP or group A meningococcal vaccine (control group). Children aged 18–71 months, however, who received the PRP vaccine had a significantly decreased risk of Hib disease when compared to that of the control children

(two cases versus 10 cases; $p < 0.001$). The overall vaccine efficacy in this age group was 90%, and based on this efficacy study of these age groups in Finland as well as on safety and immunogenicity studies, several PRP vaccines were licensed in 1985 by the Food and Drug Administration (FDA) for use in older children in the United States. Vaccination was recommended for all children at 24 months of age, and at 18 months for children at high risk of Hib disease.

After licensure, additional studies were undertaken in the United States to determine the efficacy of the PRP vaccine. Five studies were reported by three groups (303–307). Four of the five studies showed moderate efficacy (41–88%), whereas the fifth study from Minnesota showed no efficacy (306). The distribution of actual point estimates in the five studies was most consistent with an overall efficacy of approximately 50%. The vaccine was most efficacious in preventing meningitis when compared with other diseases due to Hib, perhaps because higher levels of bacteremia were found in Hib meningitis than in the other disease states.

Since the PRP vaccine showed little efficacy in children less than 2 years of age, other vaccines were developed by conjugating a form of the type b capsular polysaccharide with a protein carrier, with the aim of enhancing immunogenicity and efficacy in younger children (less than 2 years of age). Presently, four Hib conjugate vaccines have proceeded to clinical trials, and several differences have been observed in comparison to the PRP vaccine (302): (a) Significantly greater amounts of antibodies are produced with the conjugate vaccine, especially in children and infants who usually do not respond to the unconjugated vaccine; (b) the conjugate vaccine exhibits a booster response (higher antibody levels attained with repeated administration), whereas the PRP vaccine does not; (c) a higher proportion of IgG antibody (as opposed to IgM antibody) is attained with the conjugate vaccine, indicating a more differentiated immune response, especially after booster doses; and (d) when the conjugate vaccine is given at the same time as (or after) vaccination with the carrier protein, further enhancement is seen as a result of carrier priming. The following section reviews the important characteristics of candidate Hib conjugate vaccines.

In the early 1980s, a PRP–diphtheria toxoid conjugate vaccine (PRP-D) was prepared. Initial immunogenicity studies revealed that anti-PRP antibody concentrations (geometric mean: 1.2 μg/ml) considered to be protective could be induced and maintained in children aged 9–15 months with two or three doses, and booster responses indicative of T-cell-dependent immunologic memory were induced (302). However, the immune responses were poorer in younger children (2–3 months of age), an important age group at risk for invasive Hib disease. A large Finnish study (308) demonstrated an overall efficacy of 94% (95% confidence interval: 82–98%) of the

PRP-D conjugate vaccine in 30,000 children less than 12 months of age (vaccinated at 3, 4, and 6 months of age). Interestingly, despite excellent efficacy, there was only a minimal increase in serum concentrations of anti-PRP antibodies (only 34% of patients reached a level of 1.0 μg/ml), suggesting the possibility that priming of T cells for a rapid booster response on subsequent exposure may have been more important for protection in this trial. These results were not confirmed in a study of this conjugate vaccine in Native Alaskan infants vaccinated at 2, 4, and 6 months of age (309) in which vaccine efficacy was only 35% (not significantly different from a 0% efficacy), although immunologic responses were low (0.18 μg/ml after third dose), similar to those observed in the Finnish study (0.42 μg/ml after third dose). These disparate findings in efficacy and the generally poor immunogenicity of the vaccine in young children led to doubts concerning the use of this vaccine in this U.S. population.

However, the vaccine was demonstrably more immunogenic than the PRP vaccine alone in children 18 months of age and older (310,311), leading to FDA licensure of the PRP-D vaccine for this age group. It is also important to note that initially after vaccination, serum concentrations of anti-PRP antibodies may be depressed. A recent study found depressed serum concentrations after immunization of 18-month-old infants with PRP-D vaccine during the first week after vaccination (312), although by day 7 all had achieved anti-PRP antibody concentrations greater than 0.15 μg/ml, suggesting that these children may be more susceptible to invasive Hib disease during the first week after vaccination.

Other conjugate vaccines have also been developed (302). A PRP–tetanus toxoid conjugate (PRP-T) has been shown to have enhanced immunogenicity in in-

TABLE 26. *Recommendations for use of the Hib conjugate vaccine*[a]

1. Vaccinate all infants at age 2, 4, and 6 months. Unvaccinated infants 7–11 months of age should receive two doses 2 months apart. Previously unvaccinated children 12–14 months of age should receive one dose; a booster dose is recommended after 15 months of age for this group.
2. Unvaccinated children 15–60 months of age should receive a single dose and do not require a booster.
3. Children older than 60 months should be vaccinated based on disease risk (asplenia, sickle-cell disease, immunosuppressive malignancy).
4. Use of the Hib vaccine does not preclude recommendations for rifampin prophylaxis of Hib contacts or timing of other vaccines.
5. Children with a history of invasive Hib disease or vaccinated at $\geq$ age 24 months with the PRP vaccine do not need revaccination.

[a] Adapted from MMWR 1990; 39:698–699 (complete ACIP statement pending.)

fants as well as a booster effect. However, a high rate of any local reaction (65%) was observed in children aged 18–24 months when compared with that of PRP (0%). The PRP–outer-membrane-protein conjugate (PRP-OMP) utilizes a carrier, which is a vesicle composed of the OMPs of *N. meningitidis* group B covalently linked via a novel thioether linkage to the type b capsular polysaccharide. This vaccine has demonstrated excellent immunogenicity (geometric mean serum concentrations: >5.0 μg/ml). A recent study in 200 children (age range: 2–53 months) revealed serum concentrations $\geq$ 0.15 μg/ml in all but one (313), suggesting that the PRP-OMP vaccine may confer protection from invasive Hib disease as early as age 2 months. The PRP-OMP vaccine has recently been licensed by the FDA for routine use in children $\geq$ 18 months of age, but it may be given to children as young as 15 months of age during a routine office visit for pediatric vaccination when it is expected that the child will not return at 18 months of age. The Hib oligosaccharide–CRM$_{197}$ mutant diphtheria toxin conjugate (Hboc) differs from the other conjugate vaccines in that a protein carrier is covalently linked directly to a short-chain ribosyl-ribitol-phosphate molecule. This vaccine also has excellent immunogenicity: After a single dose at 15–18 months of age in a U.S. study, serum concentrations were >1.0 μg/ml in nearly all recipients. This vaccine was recently licensed in the United States. General recommendations for the use of this conjugate vaccine (diptheria CRM$_{197}$ protein conjugate) are shown in Table 26.

All four of these conjugate vaccines demonstrate the induction of immunologic memory, the ability to prime for a booster response, immunogenicity greater than that of the PRP vaccine in children < 18 months of age, and elevated serum concentrations of anti-PRP antibodies for at least 6 months after immunization. Direct, randomized trials are now underway to compare the various conjugate vaccines, but some conclusions can be made (302): (a) The Hboc conjugate was more effective than PRP-D in overcoming the age-related hyporesponsiveness to polysaccharide antigens; (b) protective levels of anti-PRP antibodies were seen only after three doses of PRP-D, and even then they were significantly lower than those achieved with one dose of PRP-OMP; and (c) single doses of either PRP-OMP or Hboc led to an immunogenic response, although PRP-OMP recipients had significantly higher titers (1.04 versus 0.35 μg/ml) at 3–4 months after the first dose. Taken together, these studies indicate that PRP-D is less immunogenic than PRP-OMP or Hboc.

One final point concerns passive prophylaxis in infants less than 6 months of age with hyperimmune Hib anticapsular antibody preparations, since these infants demonstrate (a) lack of immunogenicity to the PRP vaccine and (b) poor immunogenicity to the conjugate vaccines. One study utilized bacterial polysaccharide immune globulin (BPIG) versus a saline placebo given at 2, 6, and 10 months of age (314). Protective efficacy against the development of Hib disease was 100% at 3 months and 86% at 4 months after injection. Hyperimmune globulin may be especially useful for passive immunization of high-risk populations (e.g., Native American infants), prophylaxis of contacts of cases of Hib disease, and treatment of severely ill patients with Hib disease. Clinical trials are in progress to examine these questions.

Neisseria meningitidis Chemoprophylaxis

The risk of invasive meningococcal disease among household contacts of an index case during nonepidemic periods is approximately 3 in 1000 (i.e., approximately 500-fold to more than 1000-fold higher than the background endemic rate) and is particularly increased in young children (23). Up to 10% of meningococcal meningitis cases have had contact with another known case. The secondary attack rate in households has been estimated to be as high as 0.4% overall (Meningococcal Disease Surveillance Group, 1976), but it is substantially higher for children under 5 years of age. Close contacts (e.g., household contacts or day-care center members that sleep and eat in the same dwelling, close contacts in a closed community such as a military barracks or boarding school, medical personnel performing mouth-to-mouth resuscitation) are at an increased risk of developing systemic meningococcal disease, often within 5 days of recognition of the index case. These contacts should receive chemoprophylaxis as soon as the primary case is identified, but the agent of choice remains controversial.

Oral sulfadiazine, generally at a dosage of 1.0 g every 12 hr (for a total of four doses) in adults, was widely used as a chemoprophylactic agent for more than 20 years. This strategy was highly effective in the control of epidemics in military populations as well as for mass prophylaxis in the community. Widespread sulfonamide resistance was first recognized in serogroup B meningococci in California in 1963, following failure of sulfonamide prophylaxis. Sulfonamide resistance peaked in the United States in 1970 (67% of strains were resistant) but had declined to 12% by 1980 (8% of group B, 30% of group C, 4% of group W135, and 0% of group Y were resistant). If these trends continue, and sulfonamide resistance declines to ≤10%, this class of agents may again be useful for prophylaxis against meningococci. Nevertheless, sulfonamide resistance varies widely by geographic locale and serogroup (315), and these agents cannot be recommended routinely for chemoprophylaxis at the present time.

Many antimicrobials have been evaluated in a search for a suitable replacement for the sulfonamides. Oral penicillins—including ampicillin, tetracycline, erythromycin, and nalidixic acid—have all failed to eradicate nasopharyngeal carriage. Rifampin has been studied extensively and is currently recommended (e.g., by the Centers for Disease Control) but has several shortcomings: (a) Eradication rates of meningococci from the nasopharynx are only ∼80% and transient; (b) some adverse side effects occur; (c) 2 days of administration with multiple doses are required; and (d) resistance has developed in up to 10–27% of isolates, and such resistant strains can cause invasive disease. Rifampin is given in divided doses at 12-hr intervals for 2 days as follows: adults, 600 mg; children beyond the neonatal period, 10 mg/kg; infants less than 1 month of age, 5 mg/kg. Minocycline, at a dosage of 100 mg every 12 hr for 5 days, is marginally less effective than rifampin in eradication of the carrier state, but no resistant strains have emerged. Rifampin plus minocycline simultaneously or sequentially has also been studied, but the use of minocycline is compromised by the development of undesirable vestibular toxicity in a substantial minority of patients. Furthermore, minocycline is relatively contraindicated in children, the group at highest risk for invasive disease.

Two other potential chemoprophylactic agents deserve comment. Recently, it was documented (316) that a single intramuscular injection of ceftriaxone (250 mg) eliminated the serogroup A carrier state in 97% of Saudi subjects for up to 2 weeks, but this agent requires parenteral administration. Perhaps of more importance, a single oral dose of ciprofloxacin (500 or 750 mg for adults) achieves the same result (317–319). In a large-scale prophylaxis campaign in the military setting, the eradication of carriage was 97% and 93% at 4 days and 3 months, respectively, after 500 mg ciprofloxacin orally (318). Similar results were achieved in a recent placebo-controlled, randomized, double-blind study (319) of single-dose ciprofloxacin (750 mg) in persistent *N. meningitidis* carriers; all cultures obtained from 23 subjects at 1 day post-dose were negative, and 96% of specimens remained negative at 7 and 21 days after administration. Large-scale prospective studies are needed to settle this issue, but ciprofloxacin is the only agent proven effective after a single oral dose, even for minocycline-resistant strains (319), and may be less prone to the emergence of resistance than rifampin. Although ciprofloxacin is relatively contraindicated in the highest risk group (i.e., children) because of concerns regarding arthropathy, a single dose is probably safe. Ciprofloxacin may well supplant rifampin for chemoprophylaxis, at least in adults, but is also relatively expensive. Chemoprophylaxis during pregnancy is problematic; although data are scant, ceftriaxone is probably the safest alternative among the agents discussed above. Because high-dose penicillin does not reliably eradicate meningococci from the nasopharynx in patients with systemic disease (four of 14 patients still culture-positive 1 week after concluding therapy in one study) (320), chemoprophylaxis should be given (currently rifampin; ciprofloxacin has not been tested but should be efficacious in this clinical setting) to the index patient prior to hospital discharge.

Widespread chemoprophylaxis to low-risk contacts should be strongly discouraged because of the emergence of resistance and its attendant future limitations on this approach. In addition, chemoprophylaxis must be coupled with continued surveillance and education programs to detect resistance patterns, other primary cases, and/or sources outside of the household.

Neisseria meningitidis Immunoprophylaxis

Earlier monovalent vaccines of purified serogroup A and C capsular polysaccharide antigens of N. meningitidis have been shown to be immunogenic and safe in humans. The immunogenicity of both preparations increases with increasing molecular weight. Field trials conducted in Europe and Africa with the serogroup A vaccine documented efficacy of ~85–95%, and they demonstrated utility of this treatment in the control of epidemics. Similar results with the serogroup C vaccine have been observed in military recruit populations and during an epidemic. Protection has been ~90% for at least 1 year in children older than 4 years of age and in young adults. However, the efficacy of serogroup A vaccine in African children less than 4 years old is less than 30% at 1 year (321), and studies with the serogroup C vaccine in Brazil document lack of efficacy in children less than 24 months old. Although the exact serum antibody concentration required for a protective effect is unknown (some authorities have suggested ≥2 μg/ml), the vaccines appear immunogenic in children above 2 years of age; however, younger infants and toddlers do not mount an effective response. Similar poor antibody titers have been documented with the newly licensed quadrivalent vaccine (serogroups A, C, Y, and W135) in children (322), but bactericidal antibody responses to each of the four capsular polysaccharide antigens are elicited in adults. The vaccines are safe; reactions are generally limited to local erythema at the injection site and increased irritability in young children in 4% and 6% of vaccine recipients, respectively.

In addition to the poor immunogenicity in children less than 2 years of age with the current vaccines, another major obstacle to the control of meningococcal disease is the lack of a suitable vaccine against serogroup B, the major cause of endemic infections in many areas of the world. Serogroup B is responsible for ~55% and 64% of meningococcal disease in the United States and the United Kingdom, respectively; in some northern European countries, the proportion of cases due to this serogroup is even higher. This proportion varies with age. For example, in the United Kingdom, 70% of meningococcal cases in children less than 4 years of age are caused by serogroup B, as opposed to only 50% in those over 10 years old; the absence of an effective serogroup B vaccine is, therefore, a major problem. Although it is often stated that the serogroup B capsular polysaccharide is poorly

immunogenic, it is more proper to consider the type of immune response. Most adults have antibodies to serogroup B polysaccharide, but these antibodies are not bactericidal (the property most closely correlated with protection) in the presence of human complement, although bactericidal activity against the homologous serogroup is achievable when rabbit complement is added. In addition, the antibody response to the group B polysaccharide is almost entirely IgM (323), in contrast to the diverse isotype antibody response to the other meningococcal polysaccharides.

Several approaches have been explored to overcome these difficulties, including the chemical alteration of the serogroup B polysaccharide to improve immunogenicity, the search for other cell-wall antigens that elicit bactericidal antibodies, polysaccharide–protein conjugates, and vaccines based on anti-idiotypic antibodies (324). Vaccines based on serotype OMPs appear promising because (a) most outbreaks of serogroup B disease are caused by a few serotypes (principally types 2 and 15), although geographic and temporal shifts occur; (b) invasive disease induces bactericidal antibodies to cell-surface OMPs; and (c) LPS-depleted outer-membrane vesicle preparations of OMPs appear immunogenic in animals. The immunogenicity of the protein vaccines was improved by the addition of a meningococcal capsular polysaccharide and adjuvants (e.g., aluminum hydroxide or aluminum phosphate). Recent results with this approach in adults are promising (325). The vaccine was comprised of LPS-depleted outer-membrane vesicles (i.e., OMPs) from a serotype 2b strain (3006-M2) noncovalently complexed to serogroup B capsular polysaccharide and was administered to adult volunteers at a dosage of 25 μg (each of protein and polysaccharide) twice, 6 weeks apart, intramuscularly, either in 0.9% saline or adsorbed onto aluminum hydroxide. Although mild local reactions were frequent, the vaccine induced antibodies to both serotypes 2a: P1.2 and 2b:P1.2, primarily of the IgG class, which proved bactericidal for both a serotype 2a and a serotype 2b strain. This approach, as well as the continued search for cell-surface antigens common to most serogroup B isolates and the incorporation of multiple serotype proteins into vaccine preparations, is important and holds promise for the future.

Routine immunization of the entire population against meningococcal disease is not presently recommended, because of the problems outlined above (poor immunogenicity in young children, the greatest group at risk, and the lack of an effective vaccine against serogroup B) and the low risk of disease in the absence of an outbreak. Immunization is currently recommended (generally with the quadrivalent vaccine) in several industrialized countries for certain high-risk groups, including: (a) those with terminal complement component, or with properdin deficiency or dysfunction; (b) those with asplenia; (c) those who travel to areas with hyperendemic or epidemic meningococcal disease (e.g., Nigeria); and (d) those with close contacts of the primary case as an adjunct to chemoprophylaxis, although the latter practice is controversial and of unproven efficacy. However, the major use of meningococcal vaccines is during outbreaks of disease due to the serogroup(s) represented in the preparation. Adaption of this principle to developing countries with hyperendemic conditions is difficult. The potentially susceptible population in certain areas (e.g., the meningitis belt) is huge; in addition, since protection is of short duration, millions of doses would be required annually. Furthermore, the risk–benefit analysis of multiple doses and the booster effect are incompletely defined. Selective vaccination in affected villages has met with some success (326,327) but requires an excellent surveillance system, readily available and stable vaccine, and trained vaccination teams. In addition, the immune response is affected by underlying malnutrition and parasitic infections, the age of the recipient, and other factors. Mass immunization programs within four states of northern Nigeria between 1978 and 1981 to over 7.4 million people largely eliminated the yearly epidemics in the region (328), at least temporarily; however, the cost-effectiveness of this approach remains unknown. Nevertheless, significant progress towards eradication of meningococcal disease will be dependent on immunoprophylactic strategies, not on the development of new antibiotics or diagnostic techniques. It is hoped that appropriate use of available tools (i.e., chemo- and immunoprophylaxis), the development of new reagents (i.e., a safe, immunogenic, and effective serogroup B vaccine), and novel methods of deployment will lead to better control of invasive meningococcal disease.

Streptococcus pneumoniae Immunoprophylaxis

Although controversy abounds, pneumococcal vaccine is currently recommended in several countries for the prevention of pneumococcal pneumonia and its antecedent complications (e.g., bacteremia and meningitis). The efficacy of pneumococcal vaccine against *S. pneumoniae* meningitis has never been documented. Nevertheless, it would seem prudent to offer the current 23-valent preparation (representing ~90% of serotypes isolated from blood and CSF) to certain high-risk groups over 2 years of age, including: (a) the elderly (age over 65), especially upon entering chronic-care institutions; (b) patients with diabetes, congestive heart failure, and other chronic cardiorespiratory conditions, or significant hepatic or renal disease; (c) pneumonia patients upon hospital discharge; (d) chronic alcoholics; and (e) those with a CSF fistula or leak, asplenic states, multiple myeloma, the Wiskott–Aldrich syndrome, or human immunodeficiency virus infection. The dose of 0.5 ml, intramuscularly, is generally well-tolerated. The optimal interval or actual need for booster injections is unsettled.

REFERENCES

1. Danielson L, Mann E. The first American account of cerebrospinal meningitis. [Reprinted from Adams D, ed. *Medical and agricultural register for the years 1806 and 1807*, vol. 1, no. 5. Boston: Manning & Loring]. *Rev Infect Dis* 1983;5:969–972.
2. North E. Concerning the epidemic of spotted fever in New England. Excerpts reprinted in *Rev Infect Dis* 1980;2:811–816.
3. Schwentker FF, Gelman S, Long PH. The treatment of meningococcic meningitis with sulfanilamide. *JAMA* 1937;108:1407–1408.
4. Scheld WM, Mandell GL. Sulfonamides and meningitis. *JAMA* 1984;251:791–794.
5. Takala AK, Eskola J, Peltola H, Makela PH. Epidemiology of invasive *Haemophilus influenzae* type b disease among children in Finland before vaccination with *Haemophilus influenzae* type b vaccine. *Pediatr Infect Dis J* 1989;8:297–302.
6. Peltola H, Virtanen M. Systemic *Haemophilus influenzae* infection in Finland. *Clin Pediatr* 1984;23:275–280.
7. Cochi SL, Broome CV, Hightower AW. Immunization of U.S. children with *Haemophilus influenzae* type b polysaccharide vaccine: a cost-effectiveness model of strategy assessment. *JAMA* 1985;253:521–529.
8. Takala AK. Epidemiologic characteristics and risk factors for invasive *Haemophilus influenzae* type b disease in a population with high vaccine efficacy. *Pediatr Infect Dis J* 1989;8:343–346.
9. Schlech WF III, Ward JI, Band JD, et al. Bacterial meningitis in the United States, 1978 through 1981: the national bacterial meningitis surveillance study. *JAMA* 1985;253:1749–1754.
10. Sherry B, Emanuel I, Kronmal RA, Smith AL, Char LF, Gale JL, Walkley E. Interannual variation of the incidence of *Haemophilus influenzae* type b meningitis. *JAMA* 1989;261:1924–1929.
11. Fraser DW, Darby CP, Koehler RE, et al. Risk factors in bacterial meningitis: Charleston County, South Carolina. *J Infect Dis* 1973;127:271–277.
12. Santosham M, Kallman CH, Neff JM, et al. Absence of increasing incidence of meningitis caused by *Haemophilus influenzae* type b. *J Infect Dis* 1979;140:1009–1012.
13. Granoff DM, Basden M. *Haemophilus influenzae* infections in Fresno County, California: a prospective study of effects of age, race, and contact with a case on incidence of disease. *J Infect Dis* 1980;141:40–46.
14. Ostroy PR. Bacterial meningitis in Washington State. *West J Med* 1979;131:339–343.
15. Ward JI, Lum MK, Hall DB, et al. Invasive *Haemophilus influenzae* type b disease in Alaska: background epidemiology for a vaccine trial. *J Infect Dis* 1986;153:17–26.
16. Fothergill LD, Wright J. Influenzal meningitis: relation of age incidence to bactericidal power of blood against causal organism. *J Immunol* 1933;24:273–284.
17. Peltola H, Kayhty H, Virtanen M, Mäkelä PH. Prevention of *Haemophilus influenzae* type b bacteremic infections with the capsular polysaccharide vaccine. *N Engl J Med* 1984;310:1561–1566.
18. Takala AK, Eskola J, Palmgren J, et al. Risk factors of invasive *Haemophilus influenzae* type b disease among children in Finland. *J Pediatr* 1989;115:694–701.
19. Cochi SL, Fleming DW, Hightower AW, et al. Primary invasive *Haemophilus influenzae* type b disease: a population-based assessment of risk factors. *J Pediatr* 1986;108:887–896.
20. Krasinski K, Nelson JO, Butler S. Possible association of mycoplasma and viral respiratory infections with bacterial meningitis. *Am J Epidemiol* 1987;125:499–508.
21. Rosenthal J, Dagan R, Press J, Sofer S. Differences in the epidemiology of childhood community-acquired bacterial meningitis between two ethnic populations cohabiting in one geographic area. *Pediatr Infect Dis J* 1988;7:630–633.
22. Peltola H. Meningococcal disease: still with us. *Rev Infect Dis* 1983;5:71–91.
23. Scheld WM. Meningococcal diseases. In: Warren KS, Mahmoud AAF, eds. *Tropical and geographical medicine*, 2nd ed. New York: McGraw–Hill, 1990;798–814.
24. Schwartz B, Moore PS, Broome CV. The global epidemiology of meningococcal disease. *Clin Microbiol Rev* 1989;2:S118–S124.

25. Goldschneider I, Gotschlich EC, Artenstein WA. Human immunity to the meningococcus. I. The role of humoral antibodies. *J Exp Med* 1969;129:1307–1326.

26. Ross SC, Densen P. Complement deficiency states and infection: epidemiology, pathogenesis and consequences of neisserial and other infections in an immune deficiency. *Medicine* 1984; 63:243–273.

27. Sjoholm AG, Kuijper EJ, Tijsen CC, et al. Dysfunctional properdin in a Dutch family with meningococcal disease. *N Engl J Med* 1988;319:33–37.

28. Istre GR, Tarpay M, Anderson M, Pryor A, Welch D, Pneumococcus Study Group. Invasive disease due to *Streptococcus pneumoniae* in an area with a high rate of relative penicillin resistance. *J Infect Dis* 1987;156:732–736.

29. Burman LA, Norrby R, Trollfors B. Invasive pneumococcal infections: incidence, predisposing factors, and prognosis. *Rev Infect Dis* 1985;7:133–142.

30. Davidson M, Schraer CD, Parkinson AJ, et al. Invasive pneumococcal disease in an Alaska native population, 1980 through 1986. *JAMA* 1989;261:715–718.

31. Gray BM, Dillon HC Jr. Epidemiologic studies of *Streptococcus pneumoniae* in infants: antibody to types 3, 6, 14, and 23 in the first two years of life. *J Infect Dis* 1988;158:948–955.

32. Scheld WM. Bacterial meningitis in the patient at risk: intrinsic risk factors and host defense mechanisms. *Am J Med* 1984;76(5A):193–207.

33. Noah ND. Epidemiology of bacterial meningitis: UK and USA. In: Williams JD, Burnie J, eds. *Bacterial meningitis.* London: Academic Press, 1987;93–115.

34. Greenwood BM. The epidemiology of acute bacterial meningitis in tropical Africa. In: Williams JD, Burnie J, eds. *Bacterial meningitis.* London: Academic Press, 1987;61–91.

35. Cadoz M, Denis F, Diop Mar I. Etude epidemiologique des cas de meningites purulents hospitalises à Dakar pendant la decennie 1970–1979. *Bull WHO* 1981;59:574–584.

36. Bryan JP, Rodriques de Silva H, Tavares A, Rocha H, Scheld WM. Etiology and mortality of bacterial meningitis in northeastern Brazil. *Rev Infect Dis* 1990;12:128–135.

37. Musser JM, Kroll JS, Granoff D, et al. Global genetic structure and molecular epidemiology of encapsulated *Haemophilus influenzae. Rev Infect Dis* 1990;12:75–111.

38. McCaw BR, Silva J. Meningococcal infections: an update. *Med Rounds* 1989;2:123–128.

39. Frasch CE, Zollinger WE, Poolman JT. Serotype antigens of *Neisseria meningitidis* and a proposed scheme for designation of serotypes. *Rev Infect Dis* 1985;7:504–510.

40. Spanjaard L, Bol P, de Marte S, et al. Association of meningococcal serotypes with the course of disease: serotypes 2a and 2b in the Netherlands, 1959–1981. *J Infect Dis* 1987;155:277–282.

41. Olyhoek T, Crowe BA, Achtman M. Clonal population structure of *Neisseria meningitidis* serogroup A isolated from epidemics and pandemics between 1915 and 1983. *Rev Infect Dis* 1987;9:665–692.

42. Crowe BA, Wall RA, Kusecek B, et al. Clonal and variable properties of *Neisseria meningitidis* isolated from cases and carriers during and after an epidemic in the Gambia, West Africa. *J Infect Dis* 1989;159:686–700.

43. Moore PS, Reeves MW, Schwartz B, Gellin BG, Broome CV. Intercontinental spread of an epidemic group A *Neisseria meningitidis* strain. *Lancet* 1989;2:260–263.

44. Caugant DA, Kristiansen B-E, Froholm LO, Bovre K, Selander RK. Clonal diversity of *Neisseria meningitidis* from a population of asymptomatic carriers. *Infect Immun* 1988;56:2060–2068.

45. Dillon HC Jr, Khave S, Gray BM. Group B streptococcal carriage and disease: A 6-year prospective study. *J Pediatr* 1987;110:31–36.

46. Henrichsen J, Ferrieri P, Jelinkova J, et al. Nomenclature of antigens of group B streptococci. *Int J Syst Bacteriol* 1984;34:500.

47. Musser JM, Mattingly SJ, Quentin R, Goudeau A, Selander RK. Identification of a hig-virulence clone of type III *Streptococcus agalactiae* (group B streptococcus) causing invasive neonatal disease. *Proc Natl Acad Sci USA* 1989;86:4731–4735.

48. Edwards MS, Baker CJ. *Streptococcus agalactiae* (group B streptococcus). In: Mandell GL, Douglas RG JR, Bennett JE, eds. *Principles and practice of infectious diseases,* 3rd ed. New York: Churchill Livingstone, 1990;1554–1563.

49. Mascola L, Sorvillo F, Neal J, Iwakoshik, Weaver R. Surveillance of listeriosis in Los Angeles County, 1985–1986. A first year's report. *Arch Intern Med* 1989;149:1569–1572.

50. Linnan LJ, Mascola L, Lou XD, et al. Epidemic listeriosis associated with Mexican-style cheese. *N Engl J Med* 1988;319:823–828.

51. Schwartz B, Ciesielski CA, Broome CV, Gaventa S. Association of sporadic listeriosis with consumption of uncooked hot dogs and undercooked chicken. *Lancet* 1988;2:779–782.

52. Schlesinger LS, Ross SC, Schaberg DR. *Staphylococcus aureus* meningitis: a broad-based epidemiologic study. *Medicine* 1987;66:148–156.

53. Kim JH, van der Horst C, Mulrow CD, Corey GR. *Staphylococcus aureus* meningitis: review of 28 cases. *Rev Infect Dis* 1989;11:698–706.

54. Heerema MS, Ein ME, Musher DM, Bradshaw MW, Williams TW Jr. Anaerobic bacterial meningitis. *Am J Med* 1979;67:219–227.

55. Feder HM Jr. *Bacteroides fragilis* meningitis. *Rev Infect Dis* 1987;9:783–786.

56. Tarnvik A. Anaerobic meningitis in children. *Eur J Clin Microbiol* 1986;5:271–274.

57. Long JG, Preblud SR, Keyserling HL. *Clostridium perfringens* meningitis in an infant: case report and literature review. *Pediatr Infect Dis J* 1987;6:752–754.

58. Bignardi GE, Isaacs D. Neonatal meningitis due to *Streptococcus mitis. Rev Infect Dis* 1989;11:86–88.

59. Downs NJ, Hodges GR, Taylor SA. Mixed bacterial meningitis. *Rev Infect Dis* 1987;9:693–703.

60. Sferra TJ, Pacini DL. Simultaneous recovery of bacterial and viral pathogens from cerebrospinal fluid. *Pediatr Infect Dis J* 1988;7:552–556.

61. Smith AL. Pathogenesis of *Haemophilus influenzae* meningitis. *Pediatr Infect Dis J* 1987;6:783–786.

62. Moxon ER, Vaughn KA. The type b capsular polysaccharide as a virulence determinant of *Haemophilus influenzae:* studies using clinical isolates and laboratory transformants. *J Infect Dis* 1981;143:517–524.

63. Moxon ER, Anderson P. Meningitis caused by *Haemophilus influenzae* in infant rats: protective immunity and antibody priming by gastrointestinal colonization with *Escherichia coli. J Infect Dis* 1979;140:471–478.

64. Schneerson R, Robbins JB. Induction of serum *Haemophilus influenzae* type b capsular antibodies in adult volunteers fed cross-reacting *Escherichia coli* 075:K100:H5. *N Engl J Med* 1975;292:1093–1096.

65. Mason EO, Kaplan SL, Wiedermann BL, Norrod EP, Stenback WA. Frequency and properties of naturally occurring adherent piliated strains of *Haemophilus influenzae* type b. *Infect Immun* 1985;49:98–103.

66. Stull TL, Mendelman PM, Haas JL, Schoenborn MA, Mack KD, Smith AL. Characterization of *Haemophilus influenzae* type b fimbriae. *Infect Immun* 1984;46:787–796.

67. Scheld WM. Pathogenesis and pathophysiology of pneumococcal meningitis. In: Sande MA, Smith AL, Root RK, eds. *Bacterial meningitis.* London: Churchill Livingstone, 1985;37–69.

68. Devoe I, Gilchrist J. Pili on meningococci from primary cultures of nasopharyngeal carriers and cerebrospinal fluid of patients with acute disease. *J Exp Med* 1975;141:297–305.

69. Greenblatt JJ, Floyd K, Philipps MW, Frasch CE. Morphologic differences in *Neisseria meningitidis* pili. *Infect Immun* 1988;56:2356–2362.

70. Stephens DS, McGee ZA. Attachment of *Neisseria meningitidis* to human mucosal surfaces: influence of pili and type of receptor cell. *J Infect Dis* 1981;143:525–532.

71. Stephens DS, Hoffman LH, McGee ZA. Interaction of *Neisseria meningitidis* with human nasopharyngeal mucosa: attachment and entry into columnar epithelial cells. *J Infect Dis* 1983;148:369–376.

72. Cross AS, Gemski P, Sadoff JC, Orskov F, Orskov I. The importance of the K1 capsule in invasive infections caused by *Escherichia coli. J Infect Dis* 1984;149:184–193.

73. Raff HV, Devereux D, Shuford W, Abbott-Brown D, Maloney G. Human monoclonal antibody with protective activity for *Escherichia coli* K1 and *Neisseria meningitidis* group B infections. *J Infect Dis* 1988;157:118–126.

74. Zwahlen A, Winkelstein JA, Moxon ER. Surface determinants of *Haemophilus influenzae* pathogenicity: comparative virulence of capsular transformants in normal and complement depleted rats. *J Infect Dis* 1983;148:385–394.

75. Brandtzaeg P, Mollnes TE, Kierulf P. Complement activation and endotoxin levels in systemic meningococcal disease. *J Infect Dis* 1989;160:58–65.

76. Smith AL, Daum RS, Scheifele D, Syriopolou V, Averill DR, Roberts MC, Stull TL. Pathogenesis of *Haemophilus influenzae* meningitis. In: Sell SH, Wright PF, eds. *Haemophilus influenzae: epidemiology, immunology, and prevention of disease.* New York: Elsevier, 1982;89–109.

77. Parkkinen J, Korhonen TK, Pere A, Hacker J, Soinila S. Binding sites in the rat brain for *Escherichia coli* S fimbriae associated with neonatal meningitis. *J Clin Invest* 1988;81:860–865.

78. Saukkonen KMJ, Nowicki B, Leinonen M. Role of type 1 and S fimbriae in the pathogenesis of *Escherichia coli* 018:K1 bacteremia and meningitis in the infant rat. *Infect Immun* 1988;56:892–897.

79. Andersen BM, Solberg O. Endotoxin liberation and invasivity of *Neisseria meningitidis. Scand J Infect Dis* 1984;16:247–254.

80. Takala AK, Eskola J, Bol P, van Alphen L, Palmgren J, Mäkelä PH. *Haemophilus influenzae* type b strains of outer membrane subtypes 1 and 1c cause different types of invasive disease. *Lancet* 1987;2:647–650.

81. Scheld WM, Parks TS, Dacey RG, Winn HR, Jane JA, Sande MA. Clearance of bacteria from cerebrospinal fluid to blood in experimental meningitis. *Infect Immun* 1980;24:102–106.

82. Simberkoff MS, Moldover HN, Rahal JJ Jr. Absence of detectable bactericidal and opsonic activities in normal and infected human cerebrospinal fluids. A regional host defense deficiency. *J Lab Clin Med* 1980;95:362–372.

83. Bernhardt LL, Simberkoff MS, Rahal JJ Jr. Deficient cerebrospinal fluid opsonization in experimental *Escherichia coli* meningitis. *Infect Immun* 1981;32:411–413.

84. Zwahlen A, Nydegger UE, Vaudaux P, Lambert PH, Waldvogel FA. Complement-mediated opsonic activity in normal and infected human cerebrospinal fluid: early response during bacterial meningitis. *J Infect Dis* 1982;145:635–646.

85. Gigliotti F, Lee D, Insel RA, Scheld WM. IgG penetration into the cerebrospinal fluid in a rabbit model of meningitis. *J Infect Dis* 1987;156:394–398.

86. Ernst JD, Hartiala KT, Goldstein IM, Sande MA. Complement (C5)-derived chemotactic activity accounts for accumulation of polymorphonuclear leukocytes in cerebrospinal fluid of rabbits with pneumococcal meningitis. *Infect Immun* 1984;46:81–86.

87. Kadurugamuwa JL, Hengstler B, Bray MA, Zak O. Inhibition of complement-factor-5a-induced inflammatory reactions by prostaglandin E$_2$ in experimental meningitis. *J Infect Dis* 1989;160:715–719.

88. Bevilacqua MP, Stengelin S, Gimbrone MA Jr, Seed B. Endothelial leukocyte adhesion molecule 1: an inducible receptor for neutrophils related to complement regulatory proteins and lectins. *Science* 1989;243:1160–1165.

89. Tuomanen EI, Saukkonen K, Sande S, Cioffe C, Wright SD. Reduction of inflammation, tissue damage, and mortality in bacterial meningitis in rabbits treated with monoclonal antibodies against adhesion-promoting receptors of leukocytes. *J Exp Med* 1989;170:959–968.

90. Petersdorf RG, Luttrell CN. Studies on the pathogenesis of meningitis. I. Intrathecal injection. *J Clin Invest* 1962;41:311–319.

91. Ernst JD, Decazes JM, Sande MA. Experimental pneumococcal meningitis: role of leukocytes in pathogenesis. *Infect Immun* 1988;41:275–279.

92. Tuomanen E, Tomasz A, Hengstler B, Zak O. The relative role of bacterial cell wall and capsule in the induction of inflammation in pneumococcal meningitis. *J Infect Dis* 1985;151:535–540.

93. Tuomanen E, Liu H, Hengstler B, Zak O, Tomasz A. The induction of meningeal inflammation by components of the pneumococcal cell wall. *J Infect Dis* 1985;151:859–868.

94. Tuomanen E, Hengstler B, Rich R, Bray MA, Zak O, Tomasz A. Nonsteroidal anti-inflammatory agents in the therapy for experimental pneumococcal meningitis. *J Infect Dis* 1987;155:985–990.

95. Syrogiannopoulos GA, Hansen EJ, Erwin AL, Munford RS, Rutledge J, Reisch JS, McCracken GH Jr. *Haemophilus influenzae* type b lipooligosaccharide induces meningeal inflammation. *J Infect Dis* 1988;157:237–244.

96. Wispelwey B, Lesse AJ, Hansen EJ, Scheld WM. *Haemophilus influenzae* lipopolysaccharide-induced blood brain barrier permeability during experimental meningitis in the rat. *J Clin Invest* 1988;82:1339–1346.

97. Mustafa MM, Ramilo O, Syrogiannopoulos GA, Olsen KD, McCracken GH Jr, Hansen EJ. Induction of meningeal inflammation by outer membrane vesicles of *Haemophilus influenzae* type b. *J Infect Dis* 1989;159:917–922.

98. Wispelwey B, Hansen EJ, Scheld WM. *Haemophilus influenzae* outer membrane vesicle-induced blood–brain barrier permeability during experimental meningitis. *Infect Immun* 1989;57:2559–2562.

99. Morrison DC. Nonspecific interactions of bacterial lipopolysaccharides with membranes and membrane components. In: Berry LJ, ed. *Handbook of endotoxin*, vol 3. *Cellular biology of endotoxin.* Amsterdam: Elsevier, 1985;25–55.

100. Roeder DJ, Lei MG, Morrison DC. Endotoxic-lipopolysaccharide-specific binding proteins on lymphoid cells of various animal species: association with endotoxin susceptibility. *Infect Immun* 1989;57:1054–1058.

101. Riesenfeld-Orn I, Wolpe S, Garcia-Bustos JF, Hoffmann MK, Tuomanen E. Production of interleukin-1 but not tumor necrosis factor by human monocytes stimulated with pneumococcal cell surface components. *Infect Immun* 1989;57:1890–1893.

102. Wispelwey B, Long WJ, Castracane JM, Scheld WM. Cerebrospinal fluid interleukin-1 activity following intracisternal inoculation of *Haemophilus influenzae* lipopolysaccharide into rats. In: *Program and abstracts of the 28th interscience conference on antimicrobial agents and chemotherapy.* Los Angeles: American Society for Microbiology, 1988;265.

103. Mustafa MM, Ramilo O, Olsen KD, Franklin PS, Hansen EJ, Beutler B, McCracken GH Jr. Tumor necrosis factor in mediating experimental *Haemophilus influenzae* type b meningitis. *J Clin Invest* 1989;84:1253–1259.

104. Mustafa MM, Ramilo O, Mertsola J, Risser RC, Beutler B, Hansen EJ, McCracken GH Jr. Modulation of inflammation and cachectin activity in relation to treatment of experimental *Haemophilus influenzae* type b meningitis. *J Infect Dis* 1989;160:818–825.

105. Leist TP, Frei K, Kam-Hansen S, Zinkernagel RM, Fontana A. Tumor necrosis factor α in cerebrospinal fluid during bacterial, but not viral, meningitis. Evaluation in murine model infections and in patients. *J Exp Med* 1988;167:1743–1748.

106. McCracken GH Jr, Sarff LD. Endotoxin in cerebrospinal fluid. Detection in neonates with bacterial meningitis. *JAMA* 1976;235:617–620.

107. Arditi M, Ables L, Yogev R. Cerebrospinal fluid endotoxin levels in children with *H. influenzae* meningitis before and after administration of intravenous ceftriaxone. *J Infect Dis* 1989;160:1005–1011.

108. Mustafa MM, Lebel MH, Ramilo O, Olsen KD, Reisch JS, Beutler B, McCracken GH Jr. Correlation of interleukin-1β and cachectin concentrations in cerebrospinal fluid and outcome from bacterial meningitis. *J Pediatr* 1989;115:208–213.

109. McCracken GH Jr, Mustafa MM, Ramilo O, Olsen KD, Risser RC. Cerebrospinal fluid interleukin 1-beta and tumor necrosis factor concentrations and outcome from neonatal gram-negative enteric bacillary meningitis. *Pediatr Infect Dis J* 1989;8:155–159.

110. Waage A, Brandtzaeg P, Halstensen A, Kierulf P, Espevik T. The complex pattern of cytokines in serum from patients with meningococcal septic shock. Association between interleukin 6, interleukin 1, and fatal outcome. *J Exp Med* 1989;169:333–338.

111. Houssiau FA, Bukasa K, Sindic CJM, Van Damme J, Van Snick J. Elevated levels of the 26K human hybridoma growth factor (interleukin 6) in cerebrospinal fluid of patients with acute infec-

tion of the central nervous system. *Clin Exp Immunol* 1988;71:320–323.

112. Fontana A, Kristensen F, Dubs R, Gemsa D, Weber E. Production of prostaglandin E and an interleukin-1 like factor by cultured astrocytes and C$_6$ glioma cells. *J Immunol* 1982;129:2413–2419.

113. Libby P, Ordovas JM, Auger KR, Robbins AH, Birinyi LK, Dinarello CA. Endotoxin and tumor necrosis factor induce interleukin 1 gene expression in adult human vascular endothelial cells. *Am J Pathol* 1986;124:179–185.

114. Miossec P, Cavender D, Ziff M. Production of interleukin 1 by human endothelial cells. *J Immunol* 1986;136:2486–2491.

115. Nawroth PP, Bank I, Handley D, Casimeris J, Chess L, Stern D. Tumor necrosis factor/cachectin interacts with endothelial cell receptors to induce release of interleukin 1. *J Exp Med* 1986;163:1363–1375.

116. Bradbury MWB. The structure and function of the blood–brain barrier. *Fed Proc* 1984;43:186–190.

117. Goldstein GW, Betz AL. The blood–brain barrier. *Sci Am* 1986;255:74–83.

118. Waggener JD. The pathophysiology of bacterial meningitis and cerebral abscesses: an anatomical interpretation. *Adv Neurol* 1974;6:1–17.

119. Quagliarello VJ, Long WJ, Scheld WM. Morphologic alterations of the blood–brain barrier with experimental meningitis in the rat. Temporal sequence and role of encapsulation. *J Clin Invest* 1986;77:1084–1095.

120. Lesse AJ, Moxon ER, Zwahlen A, Scheld WM. Role of cerebrospinal fluid pleocytosis and *Haemophilus influenzae* type b capsule on blood brain barrier permeability during experimental meningitis in the rat. *J Clin Invest* 1988;82:102–109.

121. Quagliarello VJ, Long WJ, Scheld WM. Human interleukin-1 modulates blood–brain barrier injury *in vivo*. In: *Program and abstracts of the 27th interscience conference on antimicrobial agents and chemotherapy*. New York: American Society for Microbiology, 1987;204.

122. Kadurugamuwa JL, Hengstler B, Zak O. Cerebrospinal fluid protein profile in experimental pneumococcal meningitis and its alteration by ampicillin and anti-inflammatory agents. *J Infect Dis* 1989;159:26–34.

123. Fishman RA. Brain edema. *N Engl J Med* 1975;293:706–711.

124. Kaplan SL, Feigin RD. The syndrome of inappropriate secretion of antidiuretic hormone in children with bacterial meningitis. *J Pediatr* 1978;92:758–761.

125. Scheld WM, Dacey RG, Winn HR, Welsh JE, Jane JA, Sande MA. Cerebrospinal fluid outflow resistance in rabbits with experimental meningitis. Alterations with penicillin and methylprednisolone. *J Clin Invest* 1980;66:243–253.

126. Täuber MG, Khayam-Bashi H, Sande MA. Effects of ampicillin and corticosteroids on brain water content, cerebrospinal fluid pressure, and cerebrospinal lactate levels in experimental pneumococcal meningitis. *J Infect Dis* 1985;151:528–534.

127. Tureen JH, Stella FB, Clyman RI, Mauray F, Sande MA. Effect of indomethacin on brain water content, cerebrospinal fluid white blood cell response and prostaglandin E$_2$ levels in cerebrospinal fluid in experimental pneumococcal meningitis in rabbits. *Pediatr Infect Dis J* 1987;6:1151–1153.

128. Syrogiannopoulos GA, Olsen KD, Reisch JS, McCracken GH Jr. Dexamethazone in the treatment of experimental *Haemophilus influenzae* type b meningitis. *J Infect Dis* 1987;155:213–219.

129. Täuber MG, Shibl AM, Hackbarth CJ, Larrick JW, Sande MA. Antibiotic therapy, endotoxin concentration in cerebrospinal fluid, and brain edema in experimental *Escherichia coli* meningitis in rabbits. *J Infect Dis* 1987;156:456–462.

130. Täuber MG, Borschberg U, Sande MA. Influence of granulocytes on brain edema, intracranial pressure, and cerebrospinal fluid concentrations of lactate and protein in experimental meningitis. *J Infect Dis* 1988;157:456–464.

131. Syrogiannopoulos GA, Olsen KD, McCracken GH Jr. Mannitol treatment in experimental *Haemophilus influenzae* type b meningitis. *Pediatr Res* 1987;22:118–122.

132. Horwitz SJ, Boxerbaum B, O'Bell J. Cerebral herniation in bacterial meningitis in childhood. *Ann Neurol* 1980;7:524–528.

133. Nugent SK, Bausher JA, Moxon ER, Rogers MC. Raised intracra-

nial pressure: its management in *Neisseria meningitidis* meningoencephalitis. *Am J Dis Child* 1979;133:260–262.

134. Raimondi AJ, DiRocco C. The physiopathogenetic basis for the angiographic diagnosis of bacterial infection of the brain and its coverings in children. I. Leptomeningitis. *Child's Brain* 1979;5:398–413.

135. Igarashi M, Gilmartin RC, Gerald B, Wilburn F, Jabbour JT. Cerebral arteritis and bacterial meningitis. *Arch Neurol* 1984;41:531–535.

136. Yamashima T, Kashihara K, Ikeda K, Kubota T, Yamamoto S. Three phases of cerebral arteriopathy in meningitis: vasospasm and vasodilatation followed by organic stenosis. *Neurosurgery* 1985;16:546–553.

137. Tureen JH, Dworkin RJ, Kennedy SL, Sachdeva M, Sande MA. Loss of cerebral autoregulation in experimental meningitis in rabbits. *J Clin Invest* 1990;85:577–581.

138. McMenamin JB, Volpe JJ. Bacterial meningitis in infancy: effects on intracranial pressure and cerebral blood flow velocity. *Neurology* 1984;34:500–504.

139. Adams RD, Kubik CS, Bonner FJ. The clinical and pathological aspects of B influenzal meningitis. *Arch Pediatr* 1948;65:408–441.

140. Escourolle R, Poirier J. Pathology of infectious diseases. In: Escourolle R, Poirier J, eds. *Manual of basic neuropathology*. Philadelphia: WB Saunders, 1978;105–120.

141. Walton J. The cerebrospinal fluid (CSF): anatomy and physiology. In: Walton J, ed. *Brain's disease of the nervous system*, vol 1, 9th ed. Oxford: Oxford University Press, 1985;64–71.

142. Miller JD, Adams JH. The pathophysiology of raised intracranial pressure. In: Adams JH, Corsellis JAN, Duchen LW, eds. *Greenfield's neuropathology*, 4th ed. New York: Wiley Medical, 1984;53–84.

143. Swartz MN. Bacterial meningitis: more involved than just the meninges. *N Engl J Med* 1984;311:912–914.

144. Dacey RG. Monitoring and treating increased intracranial pressure. *Pediatr Infect Dis J* 1987;6:1161–1163.

145. Sande MA, Scheld WM, McCracken GH. Summary of a workshop on the pathophysiology of bacterial meningitis: implications for new management strategies. *Pediatr Infect Dis J* 1987;6:1167–1171.

146. Ropper AH. Raised intracranial pressure in neurologic disease. *Semin Neurol* 1984;4:397–407.

147. Rorke LB, Pitts FW. Purulent meningitis: the pathologic basis of clinical manifestations. *Clin Pediatr* 1963;2:64–71.

148. Brudzinski J. Un signe nouveau sur les membres inferieurs dans les meningites chez les infants (signe de la nuque). *Arch Med Enfants* 1909;12:745–752.

149. Verghese A, Gallemore G. Kernig's and Brudzinski's signs revisited. *Rev Infect Dis* 1987;9:1187–1192.

150. Kernig VM. Ueber ein Krankheits Symptom der acuten Meningitis. *St. Petersburg Med Wochenschr* 1882;7:398.

151. DeMyer W. Examination of the patient who has a disorder of consciousness. In: DeMyer W, ed. *Technique of the neurologic examination*, 3rd ed. New York: McGraw-Hill, 1980;359–404.

152. Valmari P, Peltola H, Ruuskanen O, Korvenranta H. Childhood bacterial meningitis: initial symptoms and signs related to age, and reasons for consulting a physician. *Eur J Pediatr* 1987;146:515–518.

153. Gururaj VJ, Russo RM, Allen JE, Herszkowicz R. To tap or not to tap: What are the best indicators for performing a lumbar puncture in an outpatient child? *Clin Pediatr* 1973;12:488–493.

154. Geiseler PJ, Nelson KE. Bacterial meningitis without clinical signs of meningeal irritation. *South Med J* 1982;75:448–450.

155. McCarthy PL, Sharpe MR, Spiesel SZ, et al. Observation scales to identify serious illness in febrile children. *Pediatrics* 1982;70:802–809.

156. Klein JO, Feigin RD, McCracken GH. Report of the task force on diagnosis and management of meningitis. *Pediatrics* 1986;78S:959–982.

157. Kaplan SL. *Haemophilus influenzae* meningitis. In: Vinken PJ, Bruyn GW, Klawans HL, Harris AA, eds. *Handbook of clinical neurology*. Amsterdam: Elsevier, 1988;59–70.

158. Dodge PR, Swartz MN. Bacterial meningitis—a review of selected aspects II: Special neurologic problems, postmeningitic

complications and clinicopathological correlations. *N Engl J Med* 1965;272:954–1010.

159. Kaplan SL, Fishman MA. Update on bacterial meningitis. *J Child Neurol* 1988;3:82–93.

160. Dunn DW. Neurologic complications of bacterial meningitis. In: Dunn DW, Epstein LG, eds. *Decision making in child neurology.* Toronto: BC Decker, 1987;162–163.

161. Rutter N, Smales OR. Role of routine investigations in children presenting with their first febrile convulsion. *Arch Dis Child* 1977;52:188–191.

162. Lorber J, Sunderland R. Lumbar puncture in children with convulsions associated with fever. *Lancet* 1980;1:785–786.

163. Nelson KB, Ellenberg JH. Febrile seizures. In: Dreifuss FE, ed. *Pediatric epileptology.* Boston: John Wright, 1983;173–198.

164. McGee ZA, Baringer JR. Acute meningitis. In: Mandell GL, Douglas RG, Bennett JE, eds. *Principles and practice of infectious diseases,* 3rd ed. New York: Churchill Livingstone, 1990;741–755.

165. Harter DH, Jubelt B. Bacterial infections. In: Rowland LP, ed. *Merritt's textbook of neurology.* Philadelphia: Lea & Febiger, 1984;53–72.

166. Frederiks JAM. Meningococcal meningitis. In: Vinken PJ, Bruyn GW, Klawans HL, Harris AA, eds. *Handbook of clinical neurology.* Amsterdam: Elsevier, 1988;21–40.

167. Kaplan SL, Feigin RD. Clinical presentations, prognostic factors and diagnosis of bacterial meningitis. In: Sande MA, Smith AL, Root RK, eds. *Bacterial meningitis.* New York: Churchill Livingstone, 1985;83–94.

168. Kanakriyeh M, Carvajal HF, Vallone AM. Initial fluid therapy for children with meningitis with consideration of the syndrome of inappropriate anti-diuretic hormone. *Clin Pediatr* 1987;26:126–130.

169. Carpenter RR, Petersdorf RG. The clinical spectrum of bacterial meningitis. *Am J Med* 1962;33:262–275.

170. Bruyn GAW, Kremer HPH, de Marie S, Padberg GW, Hermans J, van Furth R. Clinical evaluation of pneumococcal meningitis in adults over a twelve-year period. *Eur J Clin Microbiol Infect Dis* 1989;8:695–700.

171. Geiseler PJ, Nelson KE, Levin S, Reddy KT, Moses VK. Community acquired purulent meningitis: a review of 1316 cases during the antibiotic era, 1954–1976. *Rev Infect Dis* 1980;2:725–745.

172. Sokalski SJ, Fliegelman RM. Pneumococcal meningitis. In: Vinken PJ, Bruyn GW, Klawans HL, Harris AA, eds. *Handbook of clinical neurology.* Amsterdam: Elsevier, 1988;41–57.

173. Keroack MA. The patient with suspected meningitis. *Emerg Med Clin North Am* 1987;5:807–826.

174. Spagnuolo PJ, Ellner JJ, Lerner PI, et al. *Haemophilus influenzae* meningitis: the spectrum of disease in adults. *Medicine* 1982;61:74–84.

175. Gorse GJ, Thrupp LD, Nudleman KL, Wyle FA, Hawkins B, Cesario TC. Bacterial meningitis in the elderly. *Arch Intern Med* 1984;144:1603–1607.

176. Behrman RE, Meyers BR, Mendelson MH, Sacks HS, Hirschman SZ. Central nervous system infections in the elderly. *Arch Intern Med* 1989;149:1596–1599.

177. Lefrock JL, Smith BR. Gram-negative bacillary meningitis in adults. In: Vinken PJ, Bruyn GW, Klawans HL, Harris AA, eds. *Handbook of clinical neurology.* Amsterdam: Elsevier, 1988;103–115.

178. Hirschman JV. Bacterial meningitis following closed cranial trauma. In: Sande MA, Smith AL, Root RK, eds. *Bacterial meningitis.* New York: Churchill Livingstone, 1985;95–104.

179. Kline MW. Review of recurrent bacterial meningitis. *Pediatr Infect Dis J* 1989;8:630–634.

180. Hand WL, Sanford JP. Posttraumatic bacterial meningitis. *Ann Intern Med* 1970;72:869–874.

181. Berk SL, McCabe W. Meningitis caused by gram-negative bacilli. *Ann Intern Med* 1980;93:253–260.

182. Bayston R, Lari J. A study of the sources of infection in colonised shunts. *Dev Med Child Neurol* 1974;16(Suppl 32):16–22.

183. Schoenbaum SC, Gardner P, Shillito J. Infections of cerebrospinal fluid shunts: epidemiology, clinical manifestations, and therapy. *J Infect Dis* 1975;131:543–552.

184. Forward KR, Ferver HD, Stiver HG. Cerebrospinal fluid shunt infections: a review of 35 infections in 32 patients. *J Neurosurg* 1983;59:389–394.

185. Brown MJ, Dinndorf PA, Perek D, et al. Infectious complications of intraventricular reservoirs in cancer patients. *Pediatr Infect Dis J* 1987;6:182–189.

186. Rubin RH, Hooper DC. Central nervous system infections in the compromised host. *Med Clin North Am* 1985;69:281–293.

187. Armstrong D, Wong B. Central nervous system infections in immunocompromised hosts. *Annu Rev Med* 1982;33:293–308.

188. John JF. *Listeria monocytogenes.* In: Vinken PJ, Bruyn GW, Klawans HL, Harris AA, eds. *Handbook of clinical neurology.* Amsterdam: Elsevier, 1988;89–101.

189. Kaplan K. Brain abscess. *Med Clin North Am* 1985;69:345–360.

190. Wispelwey B, Scheld WM. Brain abscess. *Clin Neuropharmacol* 1987;10:483–510.

191. Silverberg AL, DiNubile MJ. Subdural empyema and cranial epidural abscess. *Med Clin North Am* 1985;69:361–374.

192. Morgan DW, Williams B. Posterior fossa subdural empyema. *Brain* 1985;108:983–992.

193. Barnes DW, Whitley RJ. CNS diseases associated with varicella zoster virus and herpes simplex virus infection: pathogenesis and current therapy. *Neurol Clin* 1986;4:265–283.

194. Reik L. Lyme disease: the new masquerader. Presented at the American Academy of Neurology, Infectious Disease Course, April 1988.

195. Hornick RB. The typhus group. In: Wyngaarden JB, Smith LH, eds. *Cecil textbook of medicine.* Philadelphia: WB Saunders, 1988;1738–1742.

196. Hornick RB. Rocky mountain spotted fever. In: Wyngaarden JB, Smith LH, eds. *Cecil textbook of medicine.* Philadelphia: WB Saunders, 1988;1742–1743.

197. Mohr JP, Kistler JP, Zabramski JM, Spetzler RF, Barnett HJM. Intracranial aneurysms. In: Barnett HJM, Mohr JP, Stein BM, Yatsu FM, eds. *Stroke: pathophysiology, diagnosis, and management.* New York: Churchill Livingstone, 1986;643–677.

198. Guze BH, Baxter LR. Neuroleptic malignant syndrome. *N Engl J Med* 1985;313:163–166.

199. Dougherty JM, Roth RM. Cerebral spinal fluid. *Emerg Med Clin North Am* 1986;4:281–297.

200. Corbett JJ, Mehta MP. Cerebrospinal fluid pressure in normal obese subjects and patients with pseudotumor cerebri. *Neurology* 1983;33(10):1386–1388.

201. Conly JM, Ronald AR. Cerebrospinal fluid as a diagnostic body fluid. *Am J Med* 1983;75:102–107.

202. Marton KI, Gean AD. The spinal tap: a new look at an old test. *Ann Intern Med* 1986;104:840–848.

203. Hayward RA, Oye RK. Are polymorphonuclear leukocytes an abnormal finding in cerebrospinal fluid? Results from 225 normal cerebrospinal fluid specimens. *Arch Intern Med* 1988;148:1623–1624.

204. Schmidley JW, Simon RP. Postictal pleocytosis. *Ann Neurol* 1981;9:81–84.

205. Karandanis D, Shulman JA. Recent survey of infectious meningitis in adults: review of laboratory findings in bacterial, tuberculous, and aseptic meningitis. *South Med J* 1976;69:449–457.

206. Swartz MN, Dodge PR. Bacterial meningitis—a review of selected aspects: general clinical features, special problems and unusual meningeal reactions mimicking bacterial meningitis. *N Engl J Med* 1965;272:725–731.

207. Powers WJ. Cerebrospinal fluid lymphocytosis in acute bacterial meningitis. *Am J Med* 1985;79:216–220.

208. Roos KL, Scheld WM. The management of fulminant meningitis in the intensive care unit. *Crit Care Clin* 1988;4:375–392.

209. Lindquist L, Linne T, Hansson LO, Kalin M, Axelsson G. Value of cerebrospinal fluid analysis in the differential diagnosis of meningitis: a study in 710 patients with suspected central nervous system infection. *Eur J Clin Microbiol Infect Dis* 1988;7:374–380.

210. Lannigan R, MacDonald MA, Marrie TJ, Haldane EV. Evaluation of cerebrospinal fluid lactic acid levels as an aid in differential diagnosis of bacterial and viral meningitis in adults. *J Clin Microbiol* 1980;11:324–327.

211. Kolmel HW, von Maravic M. Correlation of lactic acid level, cell count and cytology in cerebrospinal fluid of patients with bacte-

rial and non-bacterial meningitis. *Acta Neurol Scand* 1988; 78:6–9.

212. Spanos A, Harell FE Jr, Durack DT. Differential diagnosis of acute meningitis. An analysis of the predictive value of initial observations. *JAMA* 1989;262:2700–2707.

213. Kaplan SL, O'Brian Smith E, Wills C, Feigin RD. Association between preadmission oral antibiotic therapy and cerebrospinal fluid findings and sequelae caused by *Haemophilus influenzae* type b meningitis. *Pediatr Infect Dis* 1986;5:626–632.

214. Blazer S, Berant M, Alon U. Bacterial meningitis: effect of antibiotic treatment on cerebrospinal fluid. *Am J Clin Pathol* 1983;80:386–387.

215. Kaplan SL. Antigen detection in cerebrospinal fluid—pros and cons. *Am J Med* 1983;75(1B):109–118.

216. Hoban DJ, Witwicki E, Hammond GW. Bacterial antigen detection in cerebrospinal fluid of patients with meningitis. *Diagn Microbiol Infect Dis* 1985;3:373–379.

217. Dwelle TL, Dunkle LM, Blair L. Correlation of cerebrospinal fluid endotoxinlike activity with clinical and laboratory variables in gram-negative bacterial meningitis in children. *J Clin Microbiol* 1987;25:856–858.

218. Gray BM, Simmons DR, Mason H, Barnum S, Volanakis JE. Quantitative levels of C-reactive protein in cerebrospinal fluid in patients with bacterial meningitis and other conditions. *J Pediatr* 1986;108:665–670.

219. Abramson JS, Hampton KD, Babu S, Wasilauskas, Marcon MJ. The use of C-reactive protein from cerebrospinal fluid for differentiating meningitis from other central nervous system diseases. *J Infect Dis* 1985;151:854–858.

220. Enzmann DR. Acute meningitis. In: Enzmann DR, eds. *Imaging of infections and inflammations of the central nervous system: computed tomography, ultrasound, and nuclear magnetic resonance.* New York: Raven Press, 1984;188–211.

221. Lin TY, Nelson JD, McCracken GH. Fever during treatment for bacterial meningitis. *Pediatr Infect Dis* 1984;3:319–322.

222. Kline MW, Kaplan SL. Computed tomography in bacterial meningitis of childhood. *Pediatr Infect Dis J* 1988;7:855–857.

223. Cabral DA, Flodmark O, Farrell K, Speert DP. Prospective study of computed tomography in acute bacterial meningitis. *J Pediatr* 1987;111:201–205.

224. Benson P, Nyhan WL, Shimizu H. The prognosis of subdural effusions complicating pyogenic meningitis. *J Pediatr* 1960; 57:670–682.

225. Syrogiannopoulos GA, Nelson JD, McCracken GH. Subdural collections of fluid in acute bacterial meningitis: a review of 136 cases. *Pediatr Infect Dis* 1986;5:343–352.

226. Goodman JM, Mealey J. Postmeningitic subdural effusion: the syndrome and its management. *J Neurosurg* 1969;30:658–663.

227. Britt RH, Enzmann DR, Yeager AS. Neuropathological and computerized tomographic findings in experimental brain abscess. *J Neurosurg* 1981;55:590–603.

228. Weisberg L. Clinical–CT correlations in intracranial suppurative (bacterial) disease. *Neurology* 1984;34:509–510.

229. McNamara MT. Paramagnetic contrast media for magnetic resonance imaging of the central nervous system. In: Brant-Zawadzki MB, Normal D, eds. *Magnetic resonance imaging of the central nervous system.* New York: Raven Press, 1987;97–105.

230. Mathews VP, Kuharik MA, Edwards MK, D'Amour PG, Azzarelli B, Dreesen RG. Gd-DTPA-enhanced MR imaging of experimental bacterial meningitis: evaluation and comparison with CT. *AJNR* 1988;9:1045–1050.

231. Sze G, Zimmerman RD. The magnetic resonance imaging of infections and inflammatory diseases. *Radiol Clin North Am* 1988;26(4):839–859.

232. Scheld WM. Theoretical and practical considerations of antibiotic therapy for bacterial meningitis. *Pediatr Infect Dis* 1985;4:74–80.

233. Tunkel AR, Scheld WM. Therapy of bacterial meningitis: principles and practice. *Infect Control Hosp Epidemiol* 1989;10:565–569.

234. Reed MD. Current concepts in clinical therapeutics: bacterial meningitis in infants and children. *Clin Pharm* 1986;5:798–809.

235. Barlow CF. Clinical aspects of the blood–brain barrier. *Annu Rev Med* 1964;15:187–205.

236. Tunkel AR, Wispelwey B, Scheld WM. Bacterial meningitis: recent advances in pathophysiology and treatment. *Ann Intern Med* 1990;112:610–623.

237. Cherubin CE, Marr JS, Sierra MF, Becker S. Listeria and gram-negative bacillary meningitis in New York City, 1972–1979. Frequent causes of meningitis in adults. *Am J Med* 1981;71:199–209.

238. Campos J, Garcia-Tornel S, Gairi JM, Fabreques I. Multiply resistant *Haemophilus influenzae* type b causing meningitis: comparative clinical and laboratory study. *J Pediatr* 1986;108:897–902.

239. Campos J, Chanyangum M, deGroot R, Smith AL, Temover FC, Reig R. Genetic relatedness of antibiotic resistance determinants in multiply resistant *Haemophilus influenzae. J Infect Dis* 1989;160:810–817.

240. McCracken GH, Nelson JD, Kaplan SL, Overturf GD, Rodriguez WJ, Steele RW. Consensus report: antimicrobial therapy for bacterial meningitis in infants and children. *Pediatr Infect Dis J* 1987;6:501–505.

241. Committee on Infectious Diseases, Academy of Pediatrics. Treatment of bacterial meningitis. *Pediatrics* 1988;81:904–907.

242. Givner LB, Abramson JS, Wasilauskas B. Meningitis due to *Haemophilus influenzae* type b resistant to ampicillin and chloramphenicol. *Rev Infect Dis* 1989;11:329–334.

243. Krasinski K, Kusmiesz H, Nelson JD. Pharmacologic interactions among chloramphenicol, phenytoin, and phenobarbital. *Pediatr Infect Dis* 1982;1:232–235.

244. Schaad UB, Suter S, Gianella-Borradori A. A comparison of ceftriaxone and cefuroxime for the treatment of bacterial meningitis in children. *N Engl J Med* 1990;322:141–147.

245. Lebel MH, Hoyt MJ, McCracken GH Jr. Comparative efficacy of ceftriaxone and cefuroxime for treatment of bacterial meningitis. *J Pediatr* 1989;114:1049–1054.

246. Van Esso D, Fontanals D, Uriz S, et al. *Neisseria meningitidis* strains with decreased susceptibility to penicillin. *Pediatr Infect Dis* 1987;6:438–439.

247. Dillon JR, Pauze M, Yeung KH. Spread of penicillinase-producing and transfer plasmids from the gonococcus to *Neisseria meningitidis. Lancet* 1983;1:779–781.

248. Sutcliffe EM, Jones DM, El-Sheikh S, Percival A. Penicillin-insensitive meningococci in the UK [Letter]. *Lancet* 1988;1:657–658.

249. Trallero EP, Garcia Arenzana JM, Ayestaran I, Barroja IM. Comparative activity *in vitro* of 16 antimicrobial agents against penicillin-susceptible meningococci and meningococci with diminished susceptibility to penicillin. *Antimicrob Agents Chemother* 1989;33:1622–1623.

250. Weingarten RD, Markewicz Z, Gilbert DN. Meningitis due to penicillin-resistant *Streptococcus pneumoniae* in adults. *Rev Infect Dis* 1990;12:118–124.

251. Landesman SH, Corrado ML, Shah PM, Armengaud M, Barza M, Cherubin CE. Past and current roles for cephalosporin antibiotics in treatment of meningitis: emphasis on use in gram-negative bacillary meningitis. *Am J Med* 1981;71:693–703.

252. Cherubin CE, Eng RHK, Norrby R, Modai J, Humbert G, Overturf G. Penetration of newer cephalosporins into cerebrospinal fluid. *Rev Infect Dis* 1989;11:526–548.

253. Norrby SR. Role of cephalosporins in the treatment of bacterial meningitis in adults. Overview with special emphasis on ceftazidime. *Am J Med* 1985;79:56–61.

254. Segev S, Barzilai A, Rosen N, Joseph G, Rubinstein E. Pefloxacin treatment of meningitis caused by gram-negative bacteria. *Arch Intern Med* 1989;149:1314–1316.

255. Scheld WM. Quinolone therapy for infections of the central nervous system. *Rev Infect Dis* 1989;11(Suppl 5):S1194–S1202.

256. Bleck TP. Streptococcal meningitis. In: Vinken PJ, Bruyn GW, Klawans HL, Harris AA, eds. *Handbook of clinical neurology.* Amsterdam: Elsevier, 1988;77–88.

257. Lerner PI, Gopalakrishna KV, Wolinsky E, McHenry MC, Tan JS, Rosenthal M. Group B streptococcus (*S. agalactiae*) bacteremia in adults: analysis of 32 cases and review of the literature. *Medicine* 1977;56:457–473.

258. Swingle HM, Bucciarelli RL, Ayoub EM. Synergy between peni-

cillins and low concentrations of gentamicin in the killing of group B streptococci. *J Infect Dis* 1985;12:515–520.

259. Gunther G, Philipson A. Oral trimethoprim as follow-up treatment of meningitis caused by *Listeria monocytogenes. Rev Infect Dis* 1988;10:53–55.

260. Roos KL, Scheld WM. Staphylococcal infections of the central nervous system. In: Klass E, White A, eds. *Handbook of infectious diseases,* vol 3, 1991;in press.

261. Everett ED, Strausbaugh LJ. Antimicrobial agents and the central nervous system. *Neurosurgery* 1980;6:691–714.

262. Gump DW. Vancomycin for treatment of bacterial meningitis. *Rev Infect Dis* 1981;3:S289–S292.

263. Peltola H, Anttila M, Renkonen O-V, Finnish Study Group. Randomized comparison of chloramphenicol, ampicillin, cefotaxime, and ceftriaxone for childhood bacterial meningitis. *Lancet* 1989;1:1281–1287.

264. Hatch DL, Overturf GD. Delayed cerebrospinal fluid sterilization in infants with *Haemophilus influenzae* type b meningitis. *J Infect Dis* 1989;160:711–719.

265. Lebel MH, McCracken GH Jr. Delayed cerebrospinal fluid sterilization and adverse outcome of bacterial meningitis in infants and children. *Pediatrics* 1989;83:161–167.

266. Word BM, Klein JO. Therapy of bacterial sepsis and meningitis in infants and children: 1989 poll of directors of programs in pediatric infectious diseases. *Pediatr Infect Dis J* 1989;8:635–637.

267. McCabe WR. Empiric therapy for bacterial meningitis. *Rev Infect Dis* 1983;5:S74–S83.

268. Radetsky M. Duration of treatment in bacterial meningitis: a historical inquiry. *Pediatr Infect Dis J* 1990;9:2–9.

269. Gardner P, Leipzig T, Phillips P. Infections of central nervous system shunts. *Med Clin North Am* 1985;69(2):297–314.

270. Edwards MS, Baker CJ, Butler KM, Mason EO Jr, Laurent JP, Cheek WR. Penetration of cefuroxime into ventricular fluid in cerebrospinal fluid shunt infections. *Antimicrob Agents Chemother* 1989;33:1108–1110.

271. Hesse DG, Tracey KJ, Fong Y, et al. Cytokine appearance in human endotoxemia and nonhuman primate bacteremia. *Surg Gynecol Obstet* 1991;in press.

272. Damas P, Reuter A, Gysen P, Demonty J, Lamy M, Franchimont P. Tumor necrosis factor and interleukin-1 serum levels during severe sepsis in humans. *Crit Care Med* 1989;17:975–978.

273. Waage A, Haltensen A, Espink T. Association between tumour necrosis factor in serum and fatal outcome in patients with meningococcal disease. *Lancet* 1987;1:355–357.

274. Ming WJ, Bersani L, Mantovani A. Tumor necrosis factor is chemotactic for monocytes and polymorphonuclear leukocytes. *J Immunol* 1987;138:1469–1474.

275. Tracey KJ, Lowry SF, Cerami A. Cachectin: a hormone that triggers acute shock and chronic cachexia. *J Infect Dis* 1988;157:413–420.

276. Dinarello CA. An update on human interleukin-1: from molecular biology to clinical relevance. *J Clin Immunol* 1985;5:287–297.

277. Beutler B, Milsark IW, Cerami A. Passive immunization against cachectin/tumor necrosis factor protects mice from lethal effect of endotoxin. *Science* 1985;229:869–871.

278. Drapkin MS, Wisch JS, Gelfand JA, Cannon JG, Dinarello CA. Plasmapheresis for fulminant meningococcemia. *Pediatr Infect Dis J* 1989;8:399–400.

279. Girgis NI, Farid Z, Mikhail IA, Farrag I, Sultan Y, Kilpatrick ME. Dexamethasone treatment for bacterial meningitis in children and adults. *Pediatr Infect Dis J* 1989;8:848–851.

280. Lebel MH, Freij BJ, Syrogiannopoulos GA, et al. Dexamethasone therapy for bacterial meningitis: results of two double-blind, placebo-controlled trials. *N Engl J Med* 1988;319:964–971.

281. Lebel MH, Hoyt J, Waagner DC, Rollins NK, Finitzo T, McCracken GH Jr. Magnetic resonance imaging and dexamethasone therapy for bacterial meningitis. *Am J Dis Child* 1989;143:301–306.

282. McCracken GH Jr, Lebel MH. Dexamethasone therapy for bacterial meningitis in infants and children. *Am J Dis Child* 1989;143:287–289.

283. Kaplan SL. Dexamethasone for children with bacterial meningitis. Should it be routine therapy? *Am J Dis Child* 1989;143:290–292.

284. Havens PL, Wendelberger KJ, Hoffman GM, Lee MB, Chusid MJ. Corticosteroids as adjunctive therapy in bacterial meningitis. A meta-analysis of clinical trials. *Am J Dis Child* 1989;143:1051–1055.

285. Täuber MG, Sande MA. Dexamethasone in bacterial meningitis: increasing evidence for a beneficial effect. *Pediatr Infect Dis J* 1989;8:842–845.

286. Kaplan SL, Fishman MA. Supportive therapy for bacterial meningitis. *Pediatr Infect Dis J* 1987;6:670–677.

287. Arditi M, Ables L, Yogev R. Cerebrospinal fluid endotoxin levels in children with *H. influenzae* meningitis before and after administration of intravenous ceftriaxone. *J Infect Dis* 1989;160:1005–1011.

288. Tuomanen E. Partner drugs: a new outlook for bacterial meningitis. *Ann Intern Med* 1988;109:690–692.

289. Marshall LF, Marshall SB. Medical management of intracranial pressure. In: Cooper PR, ed. *Head injury,* 2nd ed. Baltimore: Williams & Wilkins, 1987;177–196.

290. Fishman RA. Brain edema and disorders of intracranial pressure. In: Rowland LP, ed. *Merritt's textbook of neurology,* 8th ed. Philadelphia: Lea & Febiger, 1989:262–266.

291. Meldrum BS, Vigouroux RA, Brierley JB. Systemic factors and epileptic brain damage: prolonged seizures in paralyzed artifically ventilated baboons. *Arch Neurol* 1973;29:82–87.

292. Leppik I. Status epilepticus. Presented at the American Academy of Neurology Meeting, San Diego, April 1983.

293. Dreifuss FE. Status epilepticus. In: Dreifuss FE, ed. *Pediatric epileptology: classification and management of seizures in the child.* Boston: John Wright, 1983;221–230.

294. Treiman DM, Delgado-Escueta AV. Status epilepticus. In: Thompson RA, Green JR, eds. *Critical care of neurological and neurosurgical emergencies.* New York: Raven Press, 1980;53–99.

295. Dunn DW. Status epilepticus. In: Dunn DW, Epstein LG, eds. *Decision making in child neurology.* Toronto: BC Decker, 1987;124.

296. Kaplan SL, Mason EO, Mason SK, et al. Prospective comparative trial of moxalactam versus ampicillin or chloramphenicol for treatment of *Haemophilus influenzae* type b meningitis in children. *J Pediatr* 1984;104:447–453.

297. Rothman M, Nahil FJ. Prophylaxis in meningitis due to type b *Haemophilus influenzae. N Engl J Med* 1955;253:653.

298. Band JD. Chemoprophylaxis of *Haemophilus influenzae* type b disease: a strategy for preventing secondary cases. In: Sell SH, Wright PF, eds. *Haemophilus influenzae: epidemiology, immunology, and prevention of disease.* New York: Elsevier, 1982:309–315.

299. Broome CV, Mortimer EA, Katz SL, Fleming DW, Hightower AW. Use of chemoprophylaxis to prevent the spread of *Haemophilus influenzae* b in day-care facilities. *N Engl J Med* 1987;316:1226–1228.

300. Committee on Infectious Diseases. Revision of recommendation for use of rifampin prophylaxis of contacts of patients with *Haemophilus influenzae* infection. *Pediatrics* 1984;74:301–302.

301. Peter G. Treatment and prevention of *Haemophilus influenzae* type b meningitis. *Pediatr Infect Dis J* 1987;6:787–790.

302. Wenger JD, Ward JI, Broome CV. Prevention of *Haemophilus influenzae* type b disease: Vaccines and passive prophylaxis. In: Remington JS, Swartz MN, eds. *Current clinical topics in infectious diseases,* vol 10. Boston 1989;306–339.

303. Harrison LH, Broome CV, Hightower AW, et al. A day care-based study of the efficacy of *Haemophilus* b polysaccharide vaccine. *JAMA* 1988;260:1413–1418.

304. Black SB, Shinefield HR, Hiatt RA, Fireman BH, The Kaiser Permanente Pediatric Vaccine Study Group. Efficacy of *Haemophilus influenzae* type b capsular polysaccharide vaccine. *Pediatr Infect Dis J* 1988;7:149–156.

305. Shapiro ED, Murphy TV, Wald ER, Brady CA. The protective efficacy of *Haemophilus* b polysaccharide vaccine. *JAMA* 1988;260:1419–1422.

306. Osterholm MT, Rambeck JH, White KE, et al. Lack of efficacy of *Haemophilus* b polysaccharide vaccine in Minnesota. *JAMA* 1988;260:1423–1428.

307. Harrison LH, Broome CV, Hightower AW. The *Haemophilus* Vaccine Efficacy Study Group. *Haemophilus influenzae* type b

polysaccharide vaccine: an efficacy study. *Pediatrics* 1989; 84:255–261.

308. Eskola J, Peltola H, Takala AK, et al. Efficacy of *Haemophilus influenzae* type b polysaccharide-diphtheria toxoid conjugate vaccine in infancy. *N Engl J Med* 1987;317:717–722.

309. Ward JI, Brenneman G, Letson G, Heyward W, Alaska Vaccine Efficacy Trial Study Group. Limited protective efficacy of an *H. influenzae* type b conjugate vaccine (PRP-D) in native Alaskan infants immunized at 2, 4, and 6 months of age. In: *Program and abstracts of the 28th interscience conference on antimicrobial agents and chemotherapy.* Los Angeles: American Society for Microbiology, 1988;1127.

310. Berkowitz CD, Ward JI, Meier K, et al. Safety and immunogenicity of *Haemophilus influenzae* type b polysaccharide and polysaccharide diphtheria toxoid conjugate vaccines in children 15 to 24 months of age. *J Pediatrics* 1987;110:509–514.

311. Hendley JO, Wenzel JG, Ashe KM, Samuelson JS. Immunogenicity of *Haemophilus influenzae* type b capsular polysaccharide vaccines in 18-month-old infants. *Pediatrics* 1987;80:351–354.

312. Marchant CD, Band E, Froeschle JE, McVerry PH. Depression of anticapsular antibody after immunization with *Haemophilus influenzae* type b polysaccharide–diphtheria conjugate vaccine. *Pediatr Infect Dis J* 1989;8:508–511.

313. Shapiro ED, Capobianco LA, Berg AT, Zitt MQ. The immunogenicity of *Haemophilus influenzae* type b polysaccharide–*Neisseria meningitidis* group B outer membrane protein complex vaccine in infants and young children. *J Infect Dis* 1989; 160:1064–1066.

314. Santosham M, Reid R, Ambrosino DM, et al. Prevention of *Haemophilus influenzae* type b infections in high-risk infants treated with bacterial polysaccharide immune globulin. *N Engl J Med* 1987;317:923–929.

315. Feldman HA. The meningococcus. A twenty-year perspective. *Rev Infect Dis* 1986;8:288–294.

316. Schwartz B, Al-Rumais A, A'ashi J, et al. Comparative efficacy of ceftriaxone and rifampicin in eradicating carriage of group A *Neisseria meningitidis. Lancet* 1988;1:1239–1242.

317. Pugsley MP, Dworzack DL, Roccaforte JS, Sanders CC, Bakken JS, Sanders WE Jr. An open study of the efficacy of a single dose of ciprofloxacin in eliminating the chronic nasopharyngeal carriage of *Neisseria meningitidis. J Infect Dis* 1988;157:852–853.

318. Gaunt PN, Lambert BE. Single-dose ciprofloxacin for the eradication of pharyngeal carriage of *Neisseria meningitidis. J Antimicrob Chemother* 1988;21:489–496.

319. Dworzack DL, Sanders CC, Horowitz EA, et al. Evaluation of single-dose ciprofloxacin in the eradication of *Neisseria meningitidis* from nasopharyngeal carriers. *Antimicrob Agents Chemother* 1988;32:1740–1741.

320. Abramson JS, Spika JS. Persistence of *Neisseria meningitidis* in the upper respiratory tract after intravenous antibiotic therapy for systemic meningococcal disease. *J Infect Dis* 1985;151:370–371.

321. Reingold AL, Hightower AW, Bolan GA, et al. Age specific differences in duration of clinical protection after vaccination with meningococcal polysaccharide vaccine. *Lancet* 1985;2:114–118.

322. Lepow ML, Beeler J, Randolph M, Samuelson JS, Hankins WA. Reactogenicity and immunogenicity of a quadrivalent combined meningococcal vaccine in children. *J Infect Dis* 1986;154:1033–1036.

323. Skerakis L, Frasch CE, Zahradnik JM, Dolin R. Class-specific human bactericidal antibodies to capsular and noncapsular surface antigens of *Neisseria meningitidis. J Infect Dis* 1984; 149:387–396.

324. Westerink MAJ, Campagnari AA, Wirth MA, et al. Development and characterization of an anti-idiotype antibody to the capsular polysaccharide of *Neisseria meningitidis* serogroup C. *Infect Immun* 1988;56:1120–1127.

325. Frasch CE, Zahradnick JM, Wang LY, Mocca LF, Tsai C-M. Antibody response of adults to an aluminum hydroxide-absorbed *Neisseria meningitidis* serotype 2b protein-group B polysaccharide vaccine. *J Infect Dis* 1988;158:710–718.

326. Greenwood BM, Wai SS. Control of meningococcal infection in the African meningitis belt by selective vaccination. *Lancet* 1980;1:729–732.

327. Greenwood BM. Selective primary health care: strategies for control of disease in the developing world. XIII. Acute bacterial meningitis. *Rev Infect Dis* 1984;6:374–389.

328. Mohammed I, Obineche EW, Onyemelukue GC, et al. Control of epidemic meningococcal meningitis by mass vaccination. I. Further epidemiologic evaluation of groups A and C vaccines in northern Nigeria. *J Infect* 1984;9:190–196.

Infections of the Central Nervous System,
edited by W. M. Scheld, R. J. Whitley, and
D. T. Durack, Raven Press, Ltd., New York © 1991.

CHAPTER 17

Rickettsiae and the Central Nervous System

Jerome H. Kim and David T. Durack

The family Rickettsiaceae comprises a group of obligate intracellular bacteria which normally infect animals but which sometimes cause disease in humans. The most important rickettsial disease of humans is typhus fever. Epidemics of typhus have had major impact on the history of Western civilization, especially during times of war and social upheaval. Rickettsiae are pleomorphic coccobacilli, $0.3 \times 1.0–2.0$ μm in size, which closely resemble gram-negative bacilli in structure and physiology. The definitive hosts for most rickettsiae are rodents or other mammals, while the vectors are ticks, mites, fleas, or lice. With the exception of *Coxiella burnetii,* the causative agent of Q fever, rickettsiae cannot survive for long outside a living host. Again with the exception of *C. burnetii,* rickettsiae cause systemic, vasculitic infections characterized by microvascular injury of multiple organs, including the central nervous system (CNS). The endoangiitis caused by rickettsiae can cause CNS damage, varying in degree from trivial to fatal. In fact, the name "typhus" is derived from the Greek word "$\tau\bar{\upsilon}\phi\delta\omega$" which means smoky or hazy, referring to the delirium or confused mental state of patients with CNS manifestations of the disease.

The rickettsial diseases which affect humans are best categorized into four divisions: the spotted fever group, the typhus fever group, the scrub typhus group, and a group of heterogeneous conditions including Q fever, ehrlichiosis, and acute febrile cerebrovasculitis—a recently described disease of presumed but unproven rickettsial etiology. Some of the main features of these groups are listed in Table 1.

This chapter will begin with a general discussion of the pathogenesis and pathophysiology of rickettsial infection, followed by a more detailed description of CNS manifestations of individual rickettsial diseases.

J. H. Kim and D. T. Durack: Division of Infectious Diseases and International Health, Duke University Medical Center, Durham, North Carolina 27710.

PATHOGENESIS AND PATHOPHYSIOLOGY

Vasculitis is the pathologic common denominator of rickettsial infection. Rickettsiae are introduced into the blood by feeding ticks (Rocky Mountain spotted fever [RMSF] and boutonneuse fever), feeding mites (scrub typhus and rickettsialpox), or inoculation of infected arthropod feces by scratching (epidemic typhus and murine typhus). Once in the bloodstream, the rickettsiae enter host cells and proliferate, causing disease. *Rickettsia rickettsii* preferentially enters endothelial cells, but Walker (1) believes that this is an accidental outcome of spread via the bloodstream rather than specific receptor-mediated tropism. Certainly, other cells can be infected; for example, *R. rickettsii* also infects vascular smooth muscle cells.

Rickettsial penetration into host cells begins with an interaction at the cell surface. The appearance of the early rash of RMSF on the extremities and that of typhus on the trunk may reflect a tendency of different rickettsial species to bind to host cells preferentially at different temperatures (2). A host cell surface receptor for rickettsiae has not yet been defined. The adsorption of *R. rickettsii* and *R. prowazekii* may involve an interaction with host plasmalemmal cholesterol (3,4), although there is some evidence against this (5). Internalization requires that both the rickettsiae (6–8) and the host cell (6) be metabolically active. Internalization seems to require the participation of microfilaments (7,8) but not microtubules (6). An important role for intracellular calcium gradients in entry of rickettsiae into cells is indicated by the work of Walker (8), who used calcium ionophore. In the model of "induced phagocytosis" (7), successful entry of rickettsiae into cells requires (a) the active participation of rickettsia-induced phagocytosis and (b) subsequent escape of the pathogen from the incipient phagosome into the cytoplasm.

Virulence of some rickettsial species may be dependent upon the ability to escape from the endocytic vacu-

TABLE 1. *Summary of the major rickettsial diseases*

Disease	Organism	Vector	Vertebrate host	Means of transmission to humans	Geographic distribution
SPOTTED FEVER GROUP					
Rocky Mountain spotted fever	*Rickettsia rickettsii*	Ticks	Rodents	Tick bite	North, Central, and South America
Boutonneuse fever	R. conorii	Ticks	Rodents	Tick bite	Africa, Asia, and Mediterranean basin
North Asian tick typhus	R. sibirica	Ticks	Rodents	Tick bite	Asia
Queensland tick typhus	R. australis	Ticks	Rodents, marsupials	Tick bite	Northern Australia
Rickettsialpox	R. akari	Mite	Mouse	Mouse → mite → human	USA, USSR, possibly worldwide
Oriental spotted fever	R. japonica	Unknown	Unknown	Presumed tick bite	Japan
TYPHUS GROUP					
Epidemic typhus	R. prowazekii	Body louse	Humans, flying squirrels	Human → louse → human	Worldwide
Murine typhus	R. typhi (R. mooseri)	Rat flea	Rodents	Rat → rat flea → human	Worldwide
SCRUB TYPHUS GROUP					
Scrub typhus	R. tsutsugamushi	Larvae of mites (chiggers)	Rat, other rodents, birds	Mite → wild rodents → mite → human	Asia, Pacific islands, and Australia
OTHER GENERA					
Q fever	*Coxiella burnetii*	Tick	Cattle, goats, sheep, other mammals	Livestock → human	Worldwide
Ehrlichiosis	*Ehrlichia canis*	Presumed to be a tick	Dog	Tick bite	North America, possibly worldwide

ole (9). For both *R. rickettsii* (4) and *R. prowazekii* (10), escape from the endocytic vacuole following attachment and internalization is thought to be mediated by phospholipase A. Inhibitors of phospholipase reduced, in dose-dependent fashion, the formation of rickettsial plaques *in vitro* (5). Furthermore, free fatty acids and lysophosphatides (products of phospholipid hydrolysis) increased after infection of mouse fibroblasts by rickettsiae (10).

The next step in pathogenesis of rickettsial disease is multiplication of the intracellular organisms. Spotted fever and typhus group rickettsiae both proliferate within the cytoplasm of the host cell, but in addition the spotted fever group rickettsiae multiply within the nucleus. *C. burnetii* and *Ehrlichia canis* remain within endocytic vacuoles and proliferate there. The multiplying rickettsiae divert cellular micronutrients and energy stores to their own use. Eventually the infected cell is destroyed by the invaders; however, *R. rickettsii, R. tsutsugamushi,* and possibly *R. conorii* are capable of exit-

ing cells without cell lysis, being extruded from long cytoplasmic processes by an unknown mechanism (11,12). *R. prowazekii* proliferates intracellularly and is then released in a single lytic burst, possibly mediated by phospholipase A. Shortly before cell lysis a number of ultrastructural changes occur in host mitochondria and rough endoplasmic reticulum (13), and host cell protein synthesis ceases (14).

In the absence of effective immunity, rickettsial proliferation leads ultimately to cell death. Endothelial damage secondarily causes increased vascular permeability, formation of microthrombi, recruitment of mononuclear inflammatory cells, and, occasionally, luminal obstruction and microinfarction. These vasculitic changes can be identified in nearly all organs: cutaneous vasculitis, interstitial pneumonitis, hepatic portal triaditis, interstitial nephritis, interstitial myocarditis, and meningoencephalomyelitis.

It is likely that microvascular injury is caused directly by the presence of the parasite itself, as stated by Wolbach (15) in 1919. Patients dying of acute, fulminant RMSF have intense endothelial damage but show little evidence of an inflammatory cellular infiltrate (16–19). Pathologically, the endoangiitis of rickettsial infection is characterized by endothelial swelling, necrosis, and a mononuclear cell infiltrate; this contrasts with the polymorphonuclear-leukocyte-rich leukocytoclastic vasculitis of immune complex injury. The primary importance of rickettsia-induced vascular injury in pathogenesis is further substantiated by studies showing that immunocompromised animals are not protected from rickettsial disease (20–23) and by the observation that rickettsiae are directly cytopathic in cell culture (12).

Host cell damage caused by Q fever has two components: first rickettsial proliferation leading to endothelial cell death, then an inflammatory response dominated by macrophages and, to a lesser degree, lymphocytes and neutrophils. Together these form the granulomas seen in Q fever (24,25).

Other elements of host immunity may be involved in the pathogenesis of rickettsial infection. Specific antibody responses to rickettsiae, such as cross-reacting antibodies to Proteus antigens OX-2, OX-19 and OX-K, are associated with immune complex formation in 36% of patients with boutonneuse fever during the first week of infection, declining to 0% during the third (26). Activation of the kallikrein–bradykinin system has been proposed to account for the vasodilation seen in RMSF (27); however, normal levels of high-molecular-weight kininogen and prekallikrein were reported in all of 20 patients with boutonneuse fever (28). The release of prostaglandin E2 and prostacyclin by endothelial cell cultures infected with R. prowazekii may also participate in the pathogenesis of vascular injury, though the effects of these autacoids in vivo have not yet been determined (18).

Though thrombocytopenia is fairly common in severe rickettsial disease, true disseminated intravascular coagulation is relatively rare. In meningococcemia, sites of intravascular coagulation do not necessarily correspond to sites of infection; complete occlusion of otherwise healthy blood vessels occurs as a result of fibrin thrombi. In RMSF, however, areas of rickettsial infection and vascular injury coincide, and thrombi only rarely occlude normal blood vessels. Animal studies suggest that fibrin thrombi in RMSF are hemostatic—that is, physiologic rather than pathologic (29). Coagulation tests in patients with boutonneuse fever and RMSF show a slight rise in fibrin split products but no significant consumption of coagulation factors, consistent with the view that the increased activity of the coagulation system in acute rickettsial disease is secondary to endothelial injury rather than to disseminated intravascular coagulation (28,29).

The similarity between certain aspects of rickettsial infection and gram-negative endotoxic shock raises the possibility that endotoxin or lipopolysaccharide might contribute to the pathophysiology of rickettsial diseases. Rickettsiae appear to possess lipopolysaccharide, but it is anchored in the outer rather than the inner membrane. Lipopolysaccharide from R. prowazekii seems to be a weaker endotoxin than that from Salmonella typhi, because larger doses of rickettsial lipopolysaccharide were required to elicit a localized Schwartzmann reaction (18,30). Sera from four of six patients with RMSF tested negative for endotoxin by the Limulus lysate assay, even though three of these four patients had proven rickettsemia at the time (31). It is not clear at present whether rickettsial endotoxin or a yet undescribed exotoxin participates in the pathogenesis of rickettsial disease (18). Rickettsiae also possess a polysaccharide slime layer which has been visualized by electron microscopy but which has not yet been characterized (1,32).

The immune system of the host interacts with rickettsiae at several levels. Rickettsial infection causes mild immune suppression, primarily of delayed-type hypersensitivity. It is not clear whether this is directly attributable to infection or to some host immunomodulatory event (33). The antibody response to rickettsiae, useful though it may be diagnostically, is not an important immune defense mechanism in vivo. While there is in vitro evidence that rickettsiae pretreated with immune serum are more actively taken up and killed by "unactivated" macrophages (34–36), the passive transfer of immune sera to athymic, nude mice results in no enhancement of macrophage-dependent rickettsial killing of R. typhi, R. tsutsugamushi, R. conorii, or C. burnetii (23,34,35,37). However, immune serum does appear to have an effect on the clearance of rickettsiae in normal mice and in mice anti-mu-suppressed from birth (inhibiting B-cell development) despite the presence of intact T-cell immunity (38). There is no unifying explanation for these data; perhaps T lymphocytes are required for antibody-dependent cellular cytotoxicity (ADCC), the critical induction of helper T cells, or the generation of cytotoxic T cells (21–23,39). Interestingly, it has been shown that spleen cells from R. typhi-immune mice were cytotoxic for rickettsia-infected cells in tissue culture (40). Guinea pigs given R. typhi immune serum are partially protected from systemic infection by R. typhi, but skin lesions develop at the site of inoculation. Immune spleen cells, however, confer some protection against both systemic infection and skin lesions (41).

Activated macrophages play a significant role in the host response to rickettsiae. Tissue macrophages are important barriers to rickettsial infection; saturation of the mononuclear phagocyte system with silica abrogates resistance to experimental rickettsial infection (42). In vitro, macrophages infected by C. burnetii (37) or R. tsutsugamushi (35) readily permit intracellular proliferation of the organism; however, treatment with supernatant from antigen- or mitogen-activated lymphocytes inhibits intracellular growth. Lymphokines with molecular weights of 10 kD, 50 kD, and 130 kD appear to mediate the anti-rickettsial activation of macrophages. Interferon gamma, found in the 50-kD fraction, activates macrophages to inhibit the proliferation of *R. prowazekii* and *R. conorii* (43).

Rickettsiae of the genera *Coxiella* and *Ehrlichia* do not infect endothelial cells and therefore do not cause vasculitis. *Coxiella* is most frequently acquired by inhalation of infected aerosols after exposure to the placentas of various ungulates or fowl. Infected volunteers become rickettsemic 1–4 days prior to development of symptoms. Infection with *C. burnetii* may result, acutely, in bronchopneumonia, granulomatous hepatitis, or meningoencephalitis. A large number of infected persons are asymptomatic. The pneumonia is characterized by interstitial infiltrates of mononuclear cells with alveolar and bronchial inflammatory exudates. In the liver, granulomata caused by Q fever are distinguished by a histologic appearance described as a "doughnut hole." In the CNS, Q fever is associated with endothelial swelling and occasional capillary thrombi (44). No perivascular infiltrate is seen. The virulence factors of *C. burnetii* include lipopolysaccharides. Lipopolysaccharide I is produced by virulent strains, whereas lipopolysaccharide II is produced by some strains after serial passage in tissue culture; the chemical composition of the latter is different from that of the former (25,45). Strains producing lipopolysaccharide II are avirulent; this phase change is analogous to the smooth-to-rough variation observed among enterobacteriaciae. Q fever endocarditis has been associated with specific variations in *C. burnetii* lipopolysaccharide and in plasmid type (46–48). Host factors are felt to be necessary for the pathogenesis of Q fever; granuloma formation appears to be induced by T-cell-mediated, delayed-type hypersensitivity. Mice inoculated with killed *C. burnetii* develop granulomas even though they are not truly infected (49). Moreover, athymic mice are unaffected by *C. burnetii* infection despite the massive proliferation of organisms within reticuloendothelial organs, implicating the host cell immune response in the pathogenesis of tissue injury in this condition (50).

Rickettsiae of the genus *Ehrlichia* replicate within cytoplasmic vacuoles of leukocytes, giving rise to a cluster of organisms, called a morula. So far, little is known of the pathology or pathogenesis of this disease in humans; granuloma formation has been noted in the bone marrow of several patients (19).

RICKETTSIAL DISEASES

Rocky Mountain Spotted Fever

RMSF is an important rickettsial infection caused by *Rickettsia rickettsii*. In 1906, Howard T. Ricketts (51) traveled from Chicago to Montana to seek the etiology of

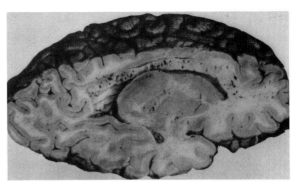

FIG. 1. Cerebral petechiae in RMSF. These lesions are commonly found in the gray matter, but in this specimen they are prominent in the white matter. (From ref. 137, with permission.)

"black measles," as spotted fever was then called in the West. He soon showed that the infectious agent was transmitted by tick bite and could be agglutinated by immune serum. His brilliant studies were cut short by his death from typhus while studying rickettsial diseases in Mexico City in 1910 (52).

The vectors for this pathogen are *Dermacentor andersoni* (the wood tick), *D. variabilis* (the common dog tick), *Amblyomma americanum* (the Lone Star tick), *Rhipicephalus sanguineus* (the brown dog tick), and *A. cajennense* (see Table 1). The disease is found throughout the Western hemisphere. It is known by various names: fiebre maculosa or Sao Paulo typhus in Brazil, fiebre manchada in Mexico, fiebre petequial in Colombia, and tick typhus in England. In the United States the greatest number of cases occurs in the South Atlantic and South Central states. After an incubation period of 2–12 days the illness begins with the sudden onset of fever, prostration, myalgias, chills, and headache which last for 2–3 weeks. The rash of spotted fever begins as a blanching, macular exanthem which progresses to petechiae and, if untreated, to ecchymoses. The classic triad of features that suggest RMSF is fever, rash, and a history of tick bite. However, all three will be present in only 3% of patients with RMSF at first presentation, and in only 60% of patients by the time the illness has run its course. In the preantibiotic era, mortality was about 20%; this rose to as high as 50% in patients over 50 years of age.

CNS manifestations are often prominent among the symptoms of RMSF. Nearly all patients have headache, which is often frontal, severe, and unresponsive to analgesics. Irritability, restlessness, insomnia, vertigo, photophobia, stiff neck, confusion, and lethargy have been reported (53–58). The neurological findings are typically nonfocal, although hyperreflexia, Babinski's signs, spasticity, hyperesthesia, athetosis, deafness, facial diplegia, gaze palsies, nystagmus, ataxia, dysphagia, and positive Kernig's and Brudzinski's signs all have been noted occasionally. Transverse myelitis, neurogenic bladder, hemiplegia, paraplegia, and quadriplegia also have been

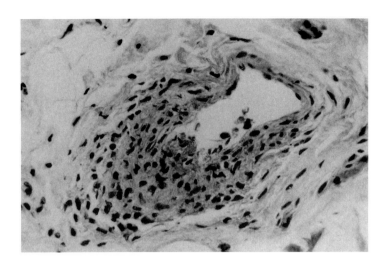

FIG. 2. A characteristic endovasculitic lesion from the skin of a patient with RMSF, showing mononuclear infiltration of the blood vessel wall with hemorrhage and thrombus formation. Similar lesions are found throughout the body, including the brain. (From ref. 19, with permission.)

recognized. In the eye, retinal vasculitis, an iris nodule, and anterior uveitis have been described (59). Stupor, delirium, or coma are relatively common in seriously ill patients; these signs of encephalitis are found in about 25% of cases (60,61). Encephalitis is associated with a poor prognosis: 86–88% of patients with encephalitis died, as opposed to 6–28% of patients without encephalitis (61,62) in the pre-antibiotic era.

Laboratory studies often show a normal or low total white blood cell count with a marked left shift, thrombocytopenia, hyponatremia, elevated liver enzyme concentrations, and increased levels of bilirubin. The syndrome of inappropriate antidiuretic hormone secretion has been reported (63). The cerebrospinal fluid (CSF) can be normal. Opening pressure and glucose are normal in most cases, but there is often a mild CSF pleocytosis; values may range from 1 to 200 white blood cells per cubic millimeter, with variable combinations of mononuclear and polymorphonuclear leukocytes. CSF protein concentration is elevated in 30–50% of cases, ranging from 19 to 236 g/dl (55,64). Computerized tomography (CT) of six cases of RMSF showed prominent white matter in one case, the others being normal (55). Magnetic resonance imaging of the brain in RMSF has not yet been reported, but this imaging modality should be more likely to demonstrate abnormalities than should a CT scan. Electroencephalography is usually abnormal but nonfocal, typically revealing diffuse slowing (53–55).

The diagnosis of RMSF usually must be made clinically, followed much later by serologic confirmation. The correct diagnosis is often delayed or missed, even in endemic areas. A rapid and specific immunofluorescence test can be performed on skin biopsies; however, it is not highly sensitive, nor is it widely available (1,65,66). The pathology of RMSF in the brain parallels the systemic lesions described earlier. Inspection of the brain from a fatal case of RMSF demonstrates a variable amount of cerebral and meningeal edema and conges-

tion; punctate hemorrhages are often seen. An endoangiitis of small and medium vessels, with a mononuclear cellular exudate, is present. Arteriolar thrombonecrosis and microinfarcts are seen predominantly in the white matter. Extra- and paravascular glial nodules are almost always present and are nearly pathognomonic of rickettsial disease. These are accumulations of enlarged endothelial cells, lymphocytes, and macrophages, 60–80 μm in size, which resemble the typhus nodule. These tend to be present after day 11 of illness. Rickettsial organisms can be demonstrated in glial nodules by immunofluorescence but are rarely visualized by histologic stains (18,19,29,53,67).

The drugs of choice for treatment of RMSF are tetracycline (20–50 mg/kg/day in children over 8 years of age or 500 mg four times daily in adults) or doxycycline (100 mg twice daily). Chloramphenicol (50 mg/kg/day in four divided doses) is recommended for children under 8 years of age because even short courses of a tetracycline can cause tooth discoloration in this age group. The use of chloramphenicol might also be considered if the patient is pregnant or azotemic, though doxycycline is less likely than other tetracyclines to exacerbate azotemia. There is no basis for the common belief that chloramphenicol is superior to tetracycline for treatment of RMSF. Ciprofloxacin, a broad-spectrum quinolone, possesses *in vitro* activity against *R. conorii* and is effective against Mediterranean spotted fever (68), but its potential value for RMSF has not yet been established. Treatment for 7–10 days is recommended (56,57); however, some argue that treatment may safely be discontinued earlier if the patient is improving and has been afebrile for 24 hr (69). Improvement is usually manifest within 36–48 hr; cases presenting with diffuse rash, edema, azotemia, profound thrombocytopenia, or obtundation may require 7–10 days before signs of improvement are seen. Supportive care is given as necessary; as for any critically ill patient, modern intensive care can be lifesaving. The use of steroids for the initial

2–3 days in critically ill patients, particularly those with encephalitis, has been recommended (53,69,70). Because this therapy is unvalidated, with no evidence of benefit for most cases (56), we do not routinely use steroids.

The prognosis for severe RMSF has improved greatly since the introduction of antirickettsial therapy. Case fatality rates vary with age; in 1986 the rate in patients over 40 years of age was 5.8%, compared with a rate of 1.9% in younger age groups (71). The case fatality rate in blacks (16%) is higher than that in whites (3%), possibly due to delayed recognition of the characteristic rash (61,72). The disease may be more severe in patients who are deficient in glucose-6-phosphate dehydrogenase (73). Other factors associated with poor prognosis include: hepatomegaly; jaundice; azotemia; stupor; absence of a history of tick exposure; presentation with symptoms other than fever, rash, and headache; and inappropriate antimicrobial therapy (61).

Other Spotted Fever Group Rickettsioses

The designation "tick typhus" comprises a collection of spotted fever group (SFG) rickettsioses which are widely distributed geographically but which share many clinical characteristics. These infections include: boutonneuse fever (Marseilles fever, Mediterranean spotted fever), East African tick typhus (Kenyan tick typhus), and South African tick-bite fever, all caused by *R. conorii;* Indian tick typhus, caused by a rickettsia similar to *R. conorii;* North Asian (Siberian) tick typhus, caused by *R. sibirica;* and Queensland tick typhus, caused by *R. australis* (Table 1). This discussion will focus on CNS manifestations of these diseases, with special attention to the differences from RMSF.

Infections caused by *R. conorii* begin with the introduction of rickettsiae into the skin of the patient by the bite of a tick. The organisms multiply in endothelial cells at the site of inoculation, leading to local inflammation and thrombosis. An erythematous papule arises. As the infection progresses, the center of the papule becomes necrotic. This lesion is the "tache noire," a raised, erythematous papule with a necrotic center. It is the hallmark of infection with *R. conorii,* even though it is not always present. From the tache noire, the infection spreads to regional lymph nodes and then into the general circulation, where a typical rickettsial endovasculitis is initiated (74,75).

Symptoms begin about 1 week after the tick bite and are dominated by fever, headache, tender lymphadenopathy, and rash. In addition to the prominent headache, patients occasionally become delirious and experience visual hallucinations. Only a small number of cases are severe enough to require hospitalization; among these, meningismus is seen in 11% of cases, and stupor in 10% (76). The rash becomes evident on days 3–5; it has both macular and papular components. The extent of the rash is directly proportional to the severity of illness. Eye involvement is uncommon, but retinal vasculitis with "typhus nodules" and retinal vein obstruction can occur with reversible vision loss (74). Laboratory studies show a normal-to-low white blood count, with a tendency toward granulocytosis in the elderly and lymphocytosis in the young. Thirty-five percent of patients have a platelet count below 150,000 per cubic millimeter. Liver function tests are mildly abnormal. Azotemia is uncommon (6%). The CSF formula in patients with *R. conorii* infection may show a lymphocytic pleocytosis, xanthrochromia, some red blood cells, and elevated protein; glucose is usually normal (77,78). CT of the head in a comatose patient showed ventriculomegaly (77). Pathological findings resemble those of RMSF: (a) cerebral and cerebellar perivascular, mononuclear infiltrates resembling typhus nodules and (b) mild mononuclear leptomeningitis. Rickettsiae were identified by immunofluorescence in all these sites (79).

The diagnosis can be made on the basis of clinical findings: fever, rash, and eschar. A specific diagnosis can be made serologically or by the use of specific immunofluorescent antibodies applied to biopsy specimens (75,79). Treatment with tetracycline or chloramphenicol usually results in clinical improvement within 24–48 hr. Ciprofloxacin or josamycin can be effective (80,81). Re-

TABLE 2. *Major neurological manifestations of different rickettsial infections*

Neurological manifestation	Typhus	Rocky Mountain spotted fever	Scrub typhus	Mediterranean spotted fever	Q fever
Headache	64%	91–93%	100%	56%	65–90%
Nausea/vomiting	29%	56–60%	28%	—	49%
Delirium–stupor	48%	16–28%	13–22%	10%	3–7%
Coma	6%	5–10%	0–7%	—	—
Meningismus	—	18%	7–14%	11%	5–11%
Seizures	—	5–8%	0–6%	—	—
Decreased hearing	4%	7%	—	—	—
Focal neurological exam	21%	2–5%	2%	1%	—
Papilledema	—	1.5%	—	—	—
Restlessness/agitation	—	—	13%	—	—

lapse of Mediterranean spotted fever following treatment with chloramphenicol has been reported (82). Recovery in patients with severe disease (those who require critical care or who are stuporous) may be slow, but it will be complete. Mortality is low, being 1.4% in hospitalized patients and even lower overall (77,83).

Infection by *R. sibirica* or by *R. australis* does not differ substantively from that by *R. conorii;* eschar, fever, headache, and rash are prominent manifestations (84–86). Occasionally, Queensland tick typhus causes a vesicular rash. An SFG rickettsia serologically similar to *R. montana* was isolated from a Japanese patient with fever, eschar, and a rash (87,88). Subsequent studies (89,90) have characterized a new rickettsia, *R. japonica* sp. nov.; so far, little is known of the pathology of the illness caused by this species (88).

Rickettsialpox is a benign SFG rickettsiosis caused by *R. akari.* In contrast to the rash of most other SFG diseases, rickettsialpox causes a maculopapular/vesicular exanthem. The vector of rickettsialpox is a mite, *Allodermanyssus sanguineus,* whose primary hosts include mice, voles, and rats. After an 8- to 14-day incubation period an eschar appears over the location of the mite bite (91–94). Fever, chills, headache, myalgias, and photophobia occur; in general these are less severe than in RMSF. The CSF in rickettsialpox is reportedly normal (94). The histology of this disease resembles that of other vasculotropic rickettsiae (19,94,95). The disease is benign; no fatalities have been recorded (93,94).

Epidemic Typhus

For many centuries, epidemic typhus has kept close and malign company with wars and natural disasters of Europe, as reflected in its many names: European typhus, ship fever, jail fever, dermatypho (Italy), tifus exanthematico (Spain), and fleckfieber (Germany). In 1909, Nicolle and associates demonstrated that the disease was transmitted by lice, providing the first effective means to control typhus epidemics. Despite this, over 200,000 people died from typhus during World War I, and about 3 million died in Russia between 1917 and 1925.

Typhus is transmitted by the inoculation of louse feces infected with *R. prowazekii* into the skin, typically by scratching. It has been thought that humans were the definitive host and reservoir of infection; recently, flying squirrels (*Glaucomys volans*) were found to harbor *R. prowazekii* (96). Human infections associated with flying squirrels (sylvatic typhus) have been reported from North Carolina, Virginia, and Texas (97).

Clinically, epidemic typhus resembles severe RMSF (16). An incubation period of about 7 days is followed by the abrupt onset of mounting, unremitting pyrexia, headache, chills, myalgias, and prostration. Roughly 5 days

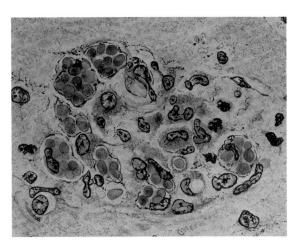

FIG. 3. A hemorrhagic lesion in the superficial cerebral cortex in a patient with epidemic typhus. Macrophages have ingested extravasated red blood cells. (From ref. 16, with permission.)

later a macular rash appears in the axillae and spreads centrifugally; it later becomes petechial and sometimes confluent. The patient has a "dusky" appearance. CNS manifestations are prominent (16,97–101) (Table 2 and Figs. 3–5). Nearly all patients have headache. Other symptoms may include spasticity, agitation, seizures, stupor, and coma. Agitated delirium is present in 86% of

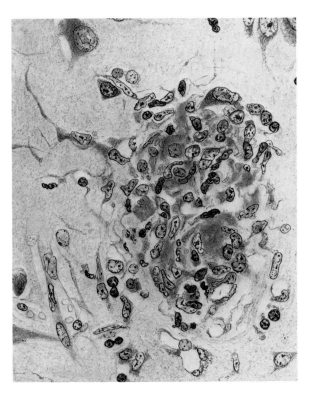

FIG. 4. Illustration of a typhus nodule of the cerebral cortex in a patient with epidemic typhus. Note the proliferative character of the lesion and the absence of necrosis. (From ref. 16, with permission.)

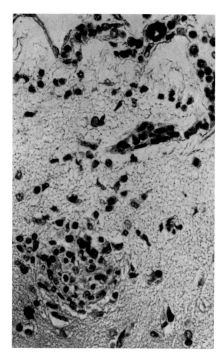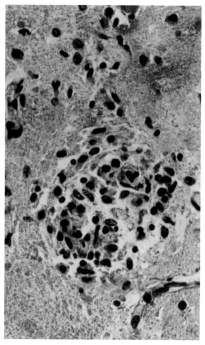

FIG. 5. Two examples of typhus nodules in the gray matter of a patient with epidemic typhus. Such lesions typically show marked inflammatory reaction with infiltrating macrophages and lymphocytes. (From ref. 19, with permission.)

untreated patients (16); this progressed to coma and death in 6% of these patients. More recently, six of 15 patients with epidemic typhus had CNS manifestations other than headache: One of 15 had meningismus, three were confused or delirious, and two were comatose (97,98). Edema and inflammation of the optic nerve is often seen, and up to 80% of patients with epidemic typhus develop small white spots (typhus nodules) on retinal vessels. These usually resolve after 8–20 days (99).

Wolbach et al. (16) reported that over 80% of patients have peripheral blood leukocyte counts of greater than 10,000 per cubic millimeter (predominantly neutrophils), with a prominent left shift—greater than 50% juvenile forms. Yeomans (102) states that the white blood cell count is reduced during the first week after infection, sometimes increasing after the appearance of the rash. Platelet counts have not been systematically reported. Of the 15 patients described above, only one had thrombocytopenia. Liver enzyme concentrations can be elevated. Findings in CSF have been reported in only a few patients; in one case the CSF examination was normal, and in another case a CSF pleocytosis was found with a leukocyte count of 85 per cubic millimeter (98% lymphocytes) and a red blood cell count of 15 per cubic millimeter (97). The pathology of typhus in the CNS resembles that of RMSF. The extent of disease in the CNS parallels the extent of skin disease. Typhus nodules, described earlier, are most frequently found in the gray matter, with the medulla being particularly affected (16,103). In fatal cases, cellular infiltrates of the pia and arachnoid are found commonly at necropsy (103).

Treatment with tetracycline (25 mg/kg/day in four doses), doxycycline (100 mg twice daily), or chloram-

phenicol (50 mg/kg/day in four doses) is curative. Mortality, which ranges from 15–20% to as high as 60% in debilitated patients in severe epidemics, can be reduced to near 0%, provided that the treatment is started prior to the development of serious complications. In louse-borne typhus, a single 200-mg dose of doxycycline may suffice; in epizootically acquired typhus, antimicrobial therapy is continued for 2–3 days after defervescence. Response to therapy is generally rapid; in untreated patients with CNS disease, recovery may be prolonged (102). Recurrent illness sometimes occurs after early treatment; it can be treated with a second course of therapy.

Brill–Zinsser Disease

In 1906, Nathan Brill reported the occurrence of typhoid-like illnesses among Europeans who had migrated to New York City, often years before. Widal-test serology remained negative. Hans Zinsser proposed in 1934 that this disease was a late recurrence of epidemic typhus, associated with waning immunity to a past infection with *R. prowazekii* (104). This was confirmed, and the infection is now known as "Brill–Zinsser disease." It is a milder than the primary disease, presenting with the sudden onset of fever, headache, and rash. Neurological complaints are much less prominent in this condition than in primary louse-borne typhus. Differentiation of primary epidemic typhus from Brill–Zinsser disease can be made by analysis of the antibody response. In primary disease the antibody is IgM; in Brill–Zinsser disease it is IgG (105). CSF studies in Brill–Zinsser disease are reportedly normal (104). The disease is treated with either tetracycline or chloramphenicol, in the same manner as for epidemic typhus.

Endemic (Murine) Typhus

Endemic or murine typhus is caused by inoculation of flea feces infected with *R. typhi* (*R. mooseri*) into the skin of the host. In many respects, murine typhus resembles epidemic typhus. The patient presents with the gradual onset of fever, myalgias, and headache 7–14 days after initial infection (106–109). The gradual onset and lack of prostration help to differentiate murine from epidemic typhus. A maculopapular rash is found in 60–80% of patients, appearing first in the axillae and becoming truncal; the extremities are seldom involved. Neurological manifestations tend also to be less severe than in epidemic typhus; "profound muttering delirium," coma, and mania are much less prominent in this condition (109). Localizing neurological findings are rare, though transient deafness and weakness may be present.

The white blood count is normal, with an unremarkable differential. Platelet counts may be reduced in severe cases but are usually normal. Elevated liver enzyme concentrations have been reported, generally in more severe cases. Woodward (109) states that the CSF is clear, with normal pressure and chemistry, though increased protein, hypoglycorrhachia, and lymphocytic pleocytosis have been reported rarely (110). Pathological data are limited because of the benign nature of this illness; CNS findings in a recent case included white matter petechiae and multifocal perivasculitis in the brain and spinal cord. Involvement of the anterior pituitary was also noted. Rickettsiae were identified by immunofluorescence in the brain and spinal cord (111). Serologic evidence of a rise in titer of specific antibody to *R. typhi* is useful diagnostically.

The prognosis for murine typhus is good; mortality is less than 1%. The condition responds rapidly to therapy with tetracycline or chloramphenicol, but several relapses after treatment with chloramphenicol have been reported (82). Therapy is continued until there is clinical improvement and the patient has been afebrile for 24 hr.

Scrub Typhus

Scrub typhus, also known as tsutsugamushi (translation: disease mite) disease, kedani (hairy mite) fever, akamushi (red mite) fever, flood fever, Japanese river fever, tropical typhus, and rural typhus, is transmitted to humans by the bite of trombiculid mite larvae, or chiggers. In ancient Japan, tsutsugamushi mites were sometimes burned in effigy to ward off this noxious bug. Tsutsugamushi fever became a major medical problem

for Allied troops in the Far East during World War II; over 16,000 cases occurred among servicemen.

The classic triad of symptoms in scrub typhus consists of fever, adenopathy, and eschar, but these are not always present. An eschar at the site of the chigger bite is present in 11–60% of patients. The disease begins gradually after 8–10 days of incubation with fever, headache, and chills. Rash is present in 30–70% of cases. The fever often reaches 40°C and is unremitting (Table 2). Headache is found in nearly all patients, myalgias in 32%, nuchal rigidity in 6%, and confusion and slurred speech in 3%. Tremors, nervousness, tinnitus, and deafness have been reported (112,113). Seizures varying from clonic to grand mal typically occur in the third week of illness (114). Focal CNS damage is rare; one patient was reported who had transient paraplegia and urinary retention (114). In the preantibiotic era a significant number of patients with scrub typhus had a coarse intention tremor, which lasted for about 8 weeks. Persistent delusions and defective judgment were also reported (114). These neurological manifestations were not found in a smaller series of patients who received antibiotic therapy.

The white blood count is usually normal, with a progressive relative lymphocytosis. Liver function tests may be elevated but show no correlation with disease severity. In reported series, 40–50% of patients with nuchal rigidity have had CSF pleocytosis (112,114). Mononuclear cells predominate in the CSF (114). CSF protein concentrations may be normal or elevated. The CNS pathology of scrub typhus is similar to that of RMSF except that there appear to be fewer capillary thrombi (19). Mononuclear cell meningitis, typhus nodules, and focal parenchymal and meningeal hemorrhages have been noted (18,115). Typhus nodules were most common in the medulla and pons.

Mortality in the preantibiotic era was 5–7%. Scrub typhus responds rapidly to oral therapy with chloramphenicol or tetracyclines; defervescence within 48 hr is the rule. Tetracycline eliminates fever more rapidly than does chloramphenicol (116). Moreover, single-dose therapy with 200 mg doxycycline is effective in scrub typhus, though occasional recurrences have been reported (71). These typically respond to a second dose.

Q Fever

Coxiella burnetii is the etiologic agent of Q fever, a disease with diverse clinical manifestations (117–121). It is most frequently a self-limited febrile illness, but it may present as atypical pneumonia, endocarditis, granulomatous hepatitis, osteomyelitis, or a variety of different neurological syndromes. Humans acquire *C. burnetii* from infected animals, probably by inhalation. A single organism may be sufficient to cause disease.

After an incubation period of about 20 days, the patient develops fever, chills, myalgias, headache, and fatigue. Rash is not typical of acute Q fever; it may appear later in chronic Q-fever endocarditis, when palpable purpura secondary to immune complex-mediated leukocytoclastic angiitis occurs. The acute illness then abates, leaving little or no memory of the primary illness (117,122). The infection may, however, become chronic, progressing to involve nearly all organ systems, though the lung, liver, and heart valves are most commonly affected. Neurological findings are frequently associated with pneumonia, hepatitis, or endocarditis but have also been described separately. Neurological abnormalities have been reported in roughly 7% of patients with Q fever (120–122) and include severe headache (65–90%), myalgias (50–60%), insomnia, nuchal rigidity, aseptic meningitis, encephalitis, extrapyramidal disease, dementia, toxic confusional states, and manic psychosis (119,123) (Table 2).

The majority of patients (89%) have a normal peripheral blood leukocyte count. Liver function tests were abnormal in 85% of patients. Specific immunofluorescence or serologic evidence of infection establishes this diagnosis. Examination of the CSF is said to be "invariably normal" (117,123); however, Spelman (117) reported mild CSF pleocytosis in two of 26 cases and an elevated CSF protein concentration in 14 of 26 cases. A case of meningoencephalitis with a CSF white blood cell count of 180 cells per cubic millimeter (87% mononuclear) and a protein of 200 mg/dl has also been described. An electroencephalographic study of a patient with encephalitis showed "diffuse encephalitic involvement"; CT of the head in this patient revealed a right frontal hypodensity (124). CT of the head in a second patient with Q-fever meningoencephalitis was normal.

Q fever is not associated with endoangiitis, unlike the vasculotropic rickettsia (19,44,125–127). During acute Q-fever pneumonia, the alveolar septa are widened by infiltrating macrophages, lymphocytes, plasma cells, and neutrophils. Alveolar exudates containing macrophages, lymphocytes, neutrophils, red blood cells, and fibrin are seen. In chronic Q fever, granulomatous inflammation occurs. Focal accumulations of mononuclear cells, giant cells, and neutrophils with a central clearing have been described in the liver and bone marrow. As might be expected, no focal perivascular infiltrates were found in the brain, though occasional capillary thromboses and endothelial swelling were observed (44). In the brain, rickettsiae were identified in neuroglial cells by Giemsa staining.

Acute Q fever is typically a self-limited illness; mortality was low even in the preantibiotic era. Functional recovery following CNS involvement is good, with few residua (53,119). Headache may, however, persist after successful treatment. Though strains of C. burnetii vary in antimicrobial susceptibility (80), tetracycline or chloramphenicol for 2 weeks is generally effective for Q-fever pneumonia, hepatitis, or CNS disease (117,119). Erythromycin, trimethoprim-sulfamethoxazole, and rifampin are also effective, though rifampin must sometimes be combined with erythromycin to achieve optimal therapeutic response. Quinolones are active in vitro (alone and in combination with other antimicrobials), but their clinical efficacy is not yet established (80,128).

Ehrlichiosis

Ehrlichia canis, an intraleukocytic rickettsia, was originally implicated as the cause of tropical canine pancytopenia, a form of aplastic anemia which in certain canine breeds causes life-threatening hemorrhage and secondary opportunistic infections 50–100 days after exposure. It has recently been implicated as a human pathogen (129–132) on the basis of serological tests. E. canis is transmitted to humans by the bite of a tick. Disease may be asymptomatic. Clinically, the disease is characterized by fever (96%), chills (70%), myalgias (74%), headache (80%), and a history of a tick bite (132). Rash is present in 20% of cases. Confusion may develop as the illness progresses. Leukopenia is found in 61% of cases, often with a left shift; lymphopenia may be prominent. Blue granules may be visible in peripheral blood leukocytes. Thrombocytopenia is present in 52% of cases. Liver enzyme concentrations are elevated. The CSF in one case (130) revealed an elevated protein concentration, a normal glucose level, and only one lymphocyte and four red blood cells per cubic millimeter. A repeat CSF several days later was normal. CSF in a second case showed leukocytosis with 56 leukocytes (80% neutrophils). The protein concentration was elevated to 1.12 g/liter, but the CSF glucose level was near normal at 3.1 mmol/liter (131). CT of the head was normal. Patients appear to respond to tetracycline or doxycycline in the same doses used for RMSF (132). The value of chloramphenicol in this illness is currently unknown. One fatality is known; the other patients appear to have recovered completely (132).

The diagnosis of E. canis infection in these cases rests on serologic studies suggesting a rise in specific antibody to E. canis and/or on electron micrographs depicting the clustered, intraleukocytic inclusion bodies (morulae) typical of this pathogen (130). It is not yet clear whether some cases of "Rocky Mountain spotless fever" are indeed caused by E. canis or some other related rickettsia (133,134).

E. sennetsu is associated with an infectious mononucleosis-like illness. Little is known of its effects on the CNS.

Acute Febrile Cerebrovasculitis

Wenzel et al. (135) have reported the occurrence of a syndrome of fever, headache, altered mental status, multifocal neurological signs, CSF pleocytosis, and abdominal pain in five patients, two of whom died. Clinically, the patients showed significant neurological impairment: decorticate/decerebrate posturing, seizures, vertical nystagmus, bilateral Babinski's reflexes, nuchal rigidity, gaze preferences, somatagnosia, somnolence, diplopia, and slurred speech. Fundoscopic examination revealed changes consistent with microvascular disease, retinitis, and vitritis. Laboratory findings include (a) normal-to-high peripheral leukocyte counts with a left shift and (b) normal platelet counts. Rickettsial serologies for *R. rickettsii, R. typhi,* and *R. prowazekii* were essentially negative. Computed tomograms of the head were normal in three of five cases and revealed diffuse edema in the other two (135) (Fig. 6). Radionuclide brain scans showed diffuse uptake in two of five cases. Electroencephalography in all five cases revealed diffuse slowing. Brain biopsy and autopsy findings showed cerebral vasculitis and perivasculitis, worse in the venules and capillaries. The thalami and brainstem had the greatest number of lesions, but lesions were present throughout the white and gray matter (135).

Four of five patients received tetracycline or chloramphenicol. A similar patient was reported by Linnemann et al. (136). They found serologic evidence of infection by either *R. typhi* or *R. canada.* The authors point out that the patient did not have an illness compatible with murine typhus, and that *R. canada* has never been associated with human disease. The similarities between this disease (symptoms, clinical findings, and pathology) and rickettsial infections are striking, but not sufficient to establish the etiology of acute febrile cerebrovasculitis.

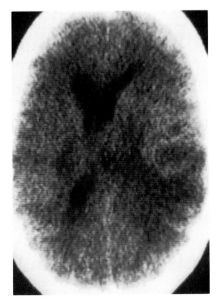

FIG. 6. Computed tomographic scan of a 41-year-old man with acute febrile cerebrovasculitis, showing marked brain edema and effacement of ventricles. (Photograph kindly provided by Dr. R. P. Wenzel.)

REFERENCES

1. Walker DH. Rocky Mountain spotted fever: a disease in need of microbiological concern. *Clin Microbiol Rev* 1989;2:227–240.
2. Rodbard D. The role of regional body temperature in the pathogenesis of disease. *N Engl J Med* 1981;305:808–814.
3. Ramm LE, Winkler HH. Identification of cholesterol in the receptor site for Rickettsiae on sheep erythrocyte membrane. *Infect Immun* 1976;13:120–126.
4. Walker DH, Firth WT, Ballard JG, Hegarty BC. Role of phospholipase-associated penetration mechanism in cell injury by *Rickettsia rickettsii. Infect Immun* 1983;40:840–842.
5. Austin FE, Winkler HH. Relationship of rickettsial physiology and composition to the rickettsia–host cell relationship. In: Walker DH, ed. *Biology of rickettsial diseases.* Boca Raton, FL: CRC Press, 1988;29–44.
6. Cohn ZA MD, Bozeman FM, Campbell JM, Humphries JW, Sawyer TE. Study on growth of Rickettsiae. V. Penetration of *Rickettsia tsutsugamushi* into mammalian cells *in vitro. Growth of Rickettsiae* 5:271–292.
7. Walker TS, Winkler HH. Penetration of cultured mouse fibroblasts (L cells) by *Rickettsia prowazekii. Infect Immun* 1978;22:200–208.
8. Walker TS. Rickettsial interactions with human endothelial cells *in vitro:* adherence and entry. *Infect Immun* 1984;44:205–210.
9. Gambrill MR, Wisseman CL Jr. Mechanisms of immunity in typhus infections. II. Multiplication of typhus Rickettsiae in human macrophage cell cultures in the nonimmune system: influence of virulence of rickettsial strains and chloramphenicol. *Infect Immun* 1973;8:519–527.
10. Winkler HH, Miller ET. Phospholipase A and the interaction of *Rickettsia prowazekii* and mouse fibroblasts (L-929 cells). *Infect Immun* 1982;38:109–113.
11. Schaechter M, Bozeman FM, Smadel JE. Study on growth of Rickettsiae. II. Morphologic observations of living Rickettsiae in tissue culture cells. *Virology* 1957;3:160–172.
12. Walker DH MD, Cain BG. The rickettsial plaque. Evidence for direct cytopathic effect of *Rickettsia rickettsii. Lab Invest* 1980;43:388–396.
13. Silverman DJ, Wisseman CL Jr, Waddell A. *In vitro* studies of rickettsia–host cell interactions: ultrastructural study of *Rickettsia prowazekii*-infected chicken embryo fibroblasts. *Infect Immun* 1980;29:778–790.
14. Weiss E, Newman LW, Grays R, Green AE. Metabolism of *Rickettsia typhi* and *Rickettsia akari* in irradiated L cells. *Infect Immun* 1972;6:50–57.
15. Wolbach SB. Studies on Rocky Mountain spotted fever. *J Med Res* 1919;41(1):1–197.
16. Wolbach SB, Todd JL, Polfrey FW. *The etiology and pathology of typhus.* Cambridge, MA: Harvard University Press, 1922.
17. Walker DH, Hawkins HK, Hudson P. Fulminant Rocky Mountain spotted fever. Its pathological characteristics associated with glucose-6-phosphate dehydrogenase deficiency. *Arch Pathol Lab Med* 1983;107:121–125.
18. Walker DH. Pathology and pathogenesis of the vasculotropic rickettsioses. In: Walker DH, ed. *Biology of the rickettsial diseases,* vol I. Boca Raton, FL: CRC Press, 1988;115–138.
19. Walker DH. Rickettsial and chlamydial diseases. In: Kissane JM, ed. *Anderson's pathology,* vol I, 9th ed. St. Louis: CV Mosby, 1990;348–361.
20. Walker DH, Henderson FW. Effect of immunosuppression on *Rickettsia rickettsii* infection in guinea pigs. *Infect Immun* 1978;20:221–227.
21. Shiral A, Catanzaro PJ, Phillips SM, Osterman JV. Host defenses in experimental scrub typhus: role of cellular immunity in heterologous protection. *Infect Immun* 1976;14:39–46.
22. Kenyon RH, Pedersen CE Jr. Immune responses to *Rickettsia akari* infection on congenitally athymic mice. *Infect Immun* 1980;28:310–313.
23. Kokorin IN, Kabanova EA, Shirokova EA, Abrosimova GE, Rybkina NN, Pushkareva VL. Role of T-lymphocytes in *Rickettsia conorii* infection. *Acta Virol* 1982;26:91–97.
24. Khavkin T. Experimental studies of the infectious process in Q fever. In: Marrie TJ, ed. Boca Raton, FL: CRC Press, 1990;71–106.

25. Waag DM. Immune response to *Coxiella burnetii* infection. In: Marrie TJ, ed. Boca Raton, FL: CRC Press, 1990;107–123.
26. Tringali G, Mansueto S. Circulating immune complexes in fievre boutonneuse. *Ann Trop Med Parasitol* 1985;79:275–279.
27. Yamada T, Harber P, Pettit GW, Wing DA, Oster CN. Activation of the kallikrein–kinin system in Rocky Mountain spotted fever. *Ann Intern Med* 1978;88:764–768.
28. Vincente V, Alegre A, Ruiz R, Herrero JI, Portugal J, Alberca I. Kinin–prekallikrein system in Mediterranean spotted fever. *J Infect Dis* 1986;154:541.
29. Walker DH, Bradford WD. Rocky Mountain spotted fever in childhood. *Perspect Pediatr Pathol* 1981;6:35–61.
30. Schramek S, Brezina R, Tarasevich IV. Isolation of a lipopolysaccharide antigen from *Rickettsia* species. *Acta Virol* 1976;270.
31. Kaplowitz LG, Lange JV, Fischer JJ, Walker DH. Correlation of rickettsial titers, circulating endotoxin, and clinical features in Rocky Mountain spotted fever. *Arch Intern Med* 1983;143:1149–1151.
32. Silverman DJ, Wisseman CL Jr, Waddell AD, Jones M. External layers of *Rickettsia prowazekii* and *Rickettsia rickettsii:* occurrence of a slime layer. *Infect Immun* 1978;22:233–246.
33. Oster CN, Kenyon RH, Pedersen CE Jr. Suppression of cellular immune responses in guinea pigs infected with spotted fever group Rickettsiae. *Infect Immun* 1978;22:411–417.
34. Gambrill MR, Wisseman CL. Mechanisms of immunity in typhus infections; III. Influence of human immune serum and complement on the fate of Rickettsia mooseri within human macrophages. *Infect Immune* 1973;8:631–640.
35. Nacy CA, Osterman JV. Host defenses in experimental scrub typhus: role of normal and activated macrophages. *Infect Immun* 1979;26:744–750.
36. Osterman JV. Rickettsiae and hosts. *Acta Virol* 1985;29:166–173.
37. Hinrichs DJ, Jerrells TR. In vitro evaluation of immunity to *Coxiella burnetii*. *J Immunol* 1976;3:996–1003.
38. Jerrells TR. Mechanisms of immunity to *Rickettsia* species and *Coxiella burnetii*. In: Walker DH, ed. *Biology of rickettsial diseases.* Boca Raton, FL: CRC Press, 1988;79–100.
39. Jerrells TR, Eisemann CS. Role of T-lymphocytes in production of antibody to antigens of *Rickettsia tsutsugamushi* and other *Rickettsia* species. *Infect Immun* 1983;41:666–675.
40. Rollwagen FM, Dasch GA, Jerrells TR. Mechanisms of immunity to rickettsial infection: characterization of a cytotoxic effector cell. *J Immunol* 1986;4:1418–1421.
41. Murphy JR, Wisseman CL, Fiset P. Mechanisms of immunity in typhus infection: analysis of immunity to *Rickettsia mooseri* infection of guinea pigs. *Infect Immun* 1980;27:730–738.
42. Jerrells TR, Osterman JV. Role of macrophages in innate and acquired host resistance to experimental scrub typhus infection of inbred mice. *Infect Immun* 1982;37:1066–1073.
43. Jerrells TR, Turco J, Winkler HH, Spitalny GI. Neutralization of lymphokine-mediated antirickettsial activity of fibroblasts and macrophages with monoclonal antibody specific for murine interferon gamma. *Infect Immun* 1986;51:355–359.
44. Whittick JW. Necropsy findings in a case of Q fever in Britain. *Br Med J* 1950;979–980.
45. Amano K, Williams JC. Chemical and immunological characterization of lipopolysaccharides from phase I and phase II *Coxiella burnetii*. *J Bacteriol* 1984;160:994–1002.
46. Hackstadt T, Peacock MG, Hitchcock PJ, Cole RL. Lipopolysaccharide variation in *Coxiella burnetii:* intrastrain heterogeneity in structure and antigenicity. *Infect Immun* 1985;48(2):359–365.
47. Hackstadt T. Antigenic variation in the phase 1 lipopolysaccharide of *Coxiella burnetii* isolates. *Infect Immun* 1986;52(1):337–340.
48. Samuel JE, Frazier ME, Mallavia LP. Correlation of plasmid type and disease caused by *Coxiella burnetii*. *Infect Immun* 1985;49(3):775–779.
49. Williams JC, Cantrell JL. Biological and immunological properties of *Coxiella burnetii* vaccines in C57BL/10ScN endotoxin-nonresponder mice. *Infect Immun* 1982;35(3):1091–1102.
50. Kishimoto RA, Rozmiarek H, Larson EW. Experimental Q fever infection in congenitally athymic nude mice. *Infect Immun* 1978;22(1):69–71.
51. Ricketts HT. The transmission of Rocky Mountain spotted fever by the bite of the wood tick (*Dermaceutor occidentalis*). *JAMA* 1906;47:358–358.
52. Weiss E. History of rickettsiology. In: Walker DH, ed. *Biology of rickettsial diseases,* vol I. Boca Raton, FL: CRC Press, 1988;15–32.
53. Harrell GT. Rickettsial involvement of the nervous system. *Med Clin North Am* 1953;395–421.
54. Miller JQ, Price TR. The nervous system in Rocky Mountain spotted fever. *Neurology* 1972;22:561–566.
55. Massey EW, Thames T, Coffey CE, Gallis HA. Neurologic complications of Rocky Mountain spotted fever. *South Med J* 1985;78(11):1288–1290.
56. Walker DH, Lane TW. Rocky Mountain spotted fever: clinical signs, symptoms, and pathophysiology. In: Walker DH, ed. *Biology of rickettsial diseases.* Boca Raton, FL: CRC Press, 1988;63–78.
57. Kamper CA, Chessman KH, Phelps SJ. Rocky Mountain spotted fever. *Clin Pharm* 1988;7:109–116.
58. Kirk JL, Fine DP, Sexton DJ, Muchmore HG. Rocky Mountain spotted fever: a clinical review based on 48 confirmed cases, 1943–1986. *Medicine* 1990;69:35–45.
59. Duffey RJ, Hammer ME. The ocular manifestations of Rocky Mountain spotted fever. *Ann Ophthalmol* 1987;19:301–306.
60. Kaplowitz LG, Fischer JJ, Sparling PF. Rocky Mountain spotted fever: a clinical dilemma. *Curr Clin Top Infect Dis* 1981;2:89–108.
61. Helmick CG, Bernard KW, D'Angelo LJ. Rocky Mountain spotted fever: clinical, laboratory, and epidemiological features of 262 cases. *J Infect Dis* 1984;150:480–488.
62. Hattwick MAW, O'Brien RJ, Hanson BF. Rocky Mountain spotted fever: epidemiology of an increasing problem. *Ann Intern Med* 1976;84:732–739.
63. Sexton DJ, Clapp J. Inappropriate antidiuretic hormone secretion. *Arch Intern Med* 1977;137:362–363.
64. Petersdorf RG, Pelletier LL, Durack DT. Some observations on experimental endocarditis. *Yale J Biol Med* 1977;50:67–75.
65. Walker DH, Cain BG, Olmstead PM. Laboratory diagnosis of Rocky Mountain spotted fever by immunofluorescent demonstration of *Rickettsia rickettsii* in cutaneous lesions. *Am J Clin Pathol* 1978;69:619–623.
66. Walker DH, Burday MS, Folds JD. Laboratory diagnosis of Rocky Mountain spotted fever. *South Med J* 1980;73:1443–1449.
67. Lillie RD. Pathology of Rocky Mountain spotted fever. *NIH Bull* 1941;177:1–27.
68. Raoult D, Roussellier P, Galicher V, Perez R, Tamalet J. In vitro susceptibility of *Rickettsia conorii* to ciprofloxacin as determined by suppressing lethality in chicken embryos and by plaque assay. *Antimicrob Agents Chemother* 1986;29:424–425.
69. Woodward TE. Rocky Mountain spotted fever and typhus fever. In: Gear JHS, ed. *Handbook of viral and rickettsial hemorrhagic fevers.* Boca Raton, FL: CRC Press, 1988;210–214.
70. Woodward TE. Rocky Mountain spotted fever: epidemiological and early clinical signs are keys to treatment and reduced mortality. *J Infect Dis* 1984;150:465–468.
71. Brown GW, Saunders JP, Singh S, Huxsoll DL, Shirai A. Single dose doxycycline therapy for scrub typhus. *R Soc Trop Med Hyg* 1978;72:412–415.
72. Centers for Disease Control. Rocky Mountain spotted fever—United States, 1985. *MMWR* 1986;35:247–249.
73. Walker DH, Kirkman HN. Rocky Mountain spotted fever and deficiency in glucose-6-phosphate dehydrogenase. *J Infect Dis* 1980;142:771–777.
74. Gear JHS. Other spotted fever group rickettsioses: clinical signs, symptoms, and pathophysiology. In: Walker DH, ed. *Biology of rickettsial disease,* vol 1. Boca Raton, FL: CRC Press, 1988;101–109.
75. Montenegro MR, Mansueto S, Hegarty BC, Walker DH. The histology of "taches noires" of boutonneuse fever and demonstration of *Rickettsia conorii* in them by immunofluorescence. *Pathol Anat* 1983;400:309–317.
76. Raoult D, Weiller PJ, Chagnon A, Chaudet H, Gallis H, Casanova P. Mediterrean spotted fever: clinical, laboratory and epide-

miological features of 199 cases. *J Trop Med Hyg* 1986;35:851–859.

77. Raoult D, Zuchelli P, Weiller PJ, et al. Incidence, clinical observations and risk factors in the severe form of Mediterranean spotted fever among patients admitted to hospital in Marseilles 1983–1984. *J Infect* 1986;12:111–116.

78. Gear JHS, Miller GB, Martins H, Swanepoel R, Wolstenholme B, Coppin A. Tick-bite fever in South Africa. *S Afr Med J* 1983;63:807–810.

79. Gear JHS, Walker DH. Correlation of the distribution of *Rickettsia conorii*, microscopic lesions, and clinical features in South African tick bite fever. *Am J Trop Med Hyg* 1985;34:361–371.

80. Gudiol F, Pallares R, Carratala J, et al. Randomized double-blind evaluation of ciprofloxacin and doxycycline for Mediterranean spotted fever. *Antimicrob Agents Chemother* 1989;33:987–988.

81. Bella F, Font B, Uriz S, et al. Randomized trial of doxycycline versus Josamycin for Mediterranean spotted fever. *Antimicrob Agents Chemother* 1990;34:937–937.

82. Shaked Y, Samra Y, Maier MK, Rubinstein E. Relapse of rickettsial Mediterranean spotted fever and murine typhus after treatment with chloramphenicol. *J Infect* 1989;18:35–37.

83. Segura-Porta F, Font-Creus B, Espejo-Arenas E, Bella-Cueto F. New trends in Mediterranean spotted fever. *Eur J Epidemiol* 1989;5:438–443.

84. Ming-Yuan F, Walker DH, Qing-Huai L, et al. Rickettsial and serologic evidence for prevalent spotted fever rickettsiosis in inner Mongolia. *Am J Trop Med Hyg* 1987;36:615–620.

85. Ming-Yuan F, Walker DH, Shu-Rong Y, Qing-Huai L. Epidemiology and ecology of rickettsial diseases in the People's Republic of China. *Rev Infect Dis* 1987;9:823–840.

86. Andrew R, Bonnin JM, Williams S. Tick typhus in North Queensland. *Med J Aust* 1946;8:253–258.

87. Uchida T, Tashiro F, Funato T, Kitamura Y. Isolation of a spotted fever group rickettsia from a patient with febrile exanthematous in Shikoku, Japan. *Microbiol Immunol* 1986;30:1323–1326.

88. Kawamura A Jr, Tanaka H. Rickettsiosis in Japan. *J Exp Med* 1988;58:169–184.

89. Uchida T, Yu X, Uchiyama T, Walker D. Identification of a unique spotted fever group rickettsia from humans in Japan. *J Infect Dis* 1989;159:1122–1126.

90. Okada T, Tange Y, Kobayashi Y. Causative agent of spotted fever group rickettsiosis in Japan. *Infect Immun* 1990;58:887–892.

91. Greenberg M, Pellitteri O, Klein IF, Huebner RJ. Rickettsialpox —a newly recognized rickettsial disease. *JAMA* 1947;133:901–906.

92. Barker LP. Rickettsialpox. *JAMA* 1949;141:1119–1122.

93. Lackman DB. A review of information in rickettsialpox in the United States. *Clin Pediatr* 1963;2:296–301.

94. Brettman LR, Lewin S, Holzman RS, et al. Rickettsialpox: report of an outbreak and a contemporary review. *Medicine* 1981;60:363–372.

95. Dolgopol VB. Histologic changes in rickettsialpox. *Am J Pathol* 1948;24:119–133.

96. Sonenshine DE, Bozeman FM, Williams MS, et al. Epizootiology of epidemic typhus (*Rickettsia prowazekii*) in flying squirrels. *Am J Trop Med Hyg* 1978;27:339–349.

97. Duma RJ, Sonenshine DE, Bozeman FM, et al. Epidemic typhus in the United States associated with flying squirrels. *JAMA* 1981;245:2318–2323.

98. McDade JE, Shepard CC, Redus MA, Newhouse VF, Smith JD. Evidence of *Rickettsia prowazekii* infections in the United States. *J Trop Med Hyg* 1980;277–284.

99. Karsner HT. Pathology of epidemic typhus. *Arch Pathology* 1953;56:397–435.

100. Devaux A. Nervous complications of exanthematic typhus. *Lancet* 1919;1:567–569.

101. Kinnier Wilson SA. *Neurology*. Baltimore: Williams & Wilkins, 1940.

102. Yeomans A. The symptomatology, clinical course, and management of louse-borne typhus fever. In: Moulton FR, ed. *Rickettsial diseases of man*. Washington, DC: American Association for the Advancement of Science, 1948;126–133.

103. Lillie RD, Smith DE, Black BK. Pathology of epidemic typhus. *Arch Pathol* 1953;56:512–553.

104. Murray ES, Baehr G, Shwartzman G, et al. Brill's disease. *JAMA* 1950;142:1059–1066.

105. Ormsbee R, Peacock M, Philip R, et al. Serologic diagnosis of epidemic typhus fever. *Am J Epidemiol* 1977;105:261–271.

106. Maxcy KF. Clinical observations in endemic typhus (Brill's disease) in southern United States. *Public Health Rep* 1926;25:1213–1220.

107. Stuart BM, Pullen RL. Endemic (murine) typhus fever: clinical observations of 180 cases. *Ann Intern Med* 1945;23:520–536.

108. Woodward TE. Endemic (murine) typhus fever: symptomatology. In: Moulton FR, ed. *Rickettsial diseases of man*. Washington, DC: American Association for the Advancement of Science, 1948;134–138.

109. Woodward TE. Murine typhus fever: its clinical and biologic similarity to epidemic typhus. In: Walker DH, ed. *Biology of rickettsial diseases*, vol 1. Boca Raton, FL: CRC Press, 1988;79–92.

110. Gastel B. Murine typhus. *John Hopkins Med J* 1977;141:303–314.

111. Walker DH, Parks FM, Betz TG, Taylor JP, Muehlberger JW. Histopathology and immunohistologic demonstration of the distribution of *Rickettsia typhi* in fatal murine typhus. *Am J Clin Pathol* 1989;91:720–724.

112. Berman SJ, Kundin WD. Scrub typhus in South Vietnam. *Ann Intern Med* 1973;79:26–30.

113. Brown GW. Scrub typhus: pathogenesis and clinical syndrome. In: Walker DH, ed. *Biology of rickettsial diseases*, vol 1. Boca Raton, FL: CRC Press, 1988;93–100.

114. Sayen JJ, Pond HS, Forrester JS, Wood FC. Scrub typhus in Assam and Burma. *Medicine* 1946;25:155–214.

115. Allen AC, Spitz S. A comparative study of the pathology of scrub typhus (Tsutsugamushi disease) and other rickettsial diseases. *Am J Pathol* 1945;21:603–681.

116. Sheehy TW, Hazlett D, Turk RE. Scrub typhus. *Arch Intern Med* 1973;132:77–80.

117. Spelman DW. Q fever—a study of 111 consecutive cases. *Med J Aust* 1982;1:547–553.

118. Sawyer LA, Fishbein DB, McDade JE. Q fever: current concepts. *Rev Infect Dis* 1987;9:935–946.

119. Marrie TJ. Pneumonia and meningo-encephalitis due to *Coxiella burnetii*. *J Infect* 1985;II:59–61.

120. Powell O. "Q" fever: clinical features in 72 cases. *Aust Ann Med* 1960;9:214–223.

121. Marrie TJ. Acute Q fever. In: Marrie TJ, ed. *Q fever, vol 1: The disease*. Boca Raton, FL: CRC Press, 1990;125–160.

122. Clark WH, Lennette EH, Railsback OC, Romer MS. Q fever in California. *Arch Intern Med* 1949;155–167.

123. Robbins FC. Q fever, clinical features. In: Moulton FR, ed. *The rickettsial diseases of man*. Washington, DC: American Association for the Advancement of Science, 1948;160–168.

124. Rodrequez AN, Morens JW, Gomez AF, Diaz JP, Acebol MR, Cortes LL. Computed tomographic brain scan findings in Q fever encephalitis. *Neuroradiology* 1984;26:329–331.

125. Perrin TL. Histopathologic observations in a fatal case of Q fever. *Arch Pathol* 1949;47:361–365.

126. Ferguson IC, Craik JE, Grist NR. Clinical, virological, and pathological findings in a fatal case of Q fever endocarditis. *J Clin Pathol* 1962;15:235–241.

127. Walker DH. Pathology of Q fever. In: Walker DH, ed. *Biology of rickettsial diseases*, vol II. Boca Raton, FL: CRC Press, 1988;18–27.

128. Yeaman MR, Mitscher LA, Baca OG. *In vitro* susceptibility of *Coxiella burnetii* to antibiotics, including several quinolones. *Antimicrob Agents Chemother* 1987;31:1079–1084.

129. Fishbein DB, Sawyer LA, Holland CJ, et al. Unexplained febrile illnesses after exposure to ticks—infection with an Ehrlichia? *JAMA* 1987;257:3100–3104.

130. Maeda K, Markowitz N, Hawkey RC, Ristic M, Cox D, McDade JE. Human infection with *Ehrlichia canis*, a leukocytic rickettsia. *N Engl J Med* 1987;316:853–856.

131. Dimmitt DC, Fishbein DB, Dawson JE. Human ehrlichiosis as-

sociated with cerebrospinal fluid pleocytosis: a case report. *Am J Med* 1989;87:677–678.

132. Centers for Disease Control. Human ehrlichiosis—United States. *MMWR* 1988;37:270–277.

133. Ewing SA, Johnson EM, Kocan KM. Human infection with *Ehrlichia canis* [Letter]. *N Engl J Med* 1987;317:899.

134. Maeda K, Markowitz N, Hawley RC, Ristic M, McDade JE. Human infection with *Ehrlichia canis* [Letter]. *N Engl J Med* 1987;317:899–900.

135. Wenzel RP, Hayden FG, Groschel DHM, et al. Acute febrile cerebrovasculitis: a syndrome of unknown, perhaps rickettsial, cause. *Ann Intern Med* 1986;104:606–615.

136. Linnemann CC Jr, Pretzman CI, Peterson ED. Acute febrile cerebrovasculitis. *Arch Intern Med* 1989;149:1682–1685.

137. Pinkerton H, Strano AJ. Diseases caused by rickettsia. In: Binford CH, Connor DH, eds. *Pathology of tropical and extraordinary diseases,* 1st ed. Washington, DC: Armed Forces Institute of Pathology, 1976.

Infections of the Central Nervous System,
edited by W. M. Scheld, R. J. Whitley, and
D. T. Durack, Raven Press, Ltd., New York © 1991.

CHAPTER 18

Tuberculosis of the Central Nervous System

Abigail Zuger and Franklin D. Lowy

> Some morbid matter bred in the blood . . . and not carried off by any of the excretories, disagreeably affecting the nerves, as often as it comes into contact with them; or forming obstructions in the small vessels and producing different symptoms, according to the parts it attacks.
>
> Sir Robert Whytt, 1762 (1)

Despite worldwide infection control programs and powerful antibiotics, tuberculosis of the central nervous system (CNS) is more than a historical relic. In developing countries, it remains a prominent cause of sickness and death; in wealthier nations, pockets of indigenous poverty and large-scale immigration from endemic countries have contributed to its overall persistence. In the United States, recent data confirm its place among infections of the CNS. National rates of tuberculosis are no longer declining at the steep rates of 20 years ago. The increasing prominence of extrapulmonary infection, the troubling prevalence of drug-resistant mycobacteria, and the recent association of the acquired immunodeficiency syndrome (AIDS) epidemic with tuberculosis all suggest that CNS tuberculosis will remain a significant clinical entity in coming years.

An enormous literature of elegant clinical studies, some decades old, may well gain renewed importance as future clinicians confront this disease. At the same time, however, the changing epidemiology of the disease and the impact of newer diagnostic and therapeutic strategies on its management must be integrated into this venerable background. This discussion will include (a) a synopsis of the present understanding of CNS tuberculosis (with particular emphasis on recent epidemiologic and clinical changes in the spectrum of the disease) and (b) recent advances in diagnosis and clinical management. The following topics will be considered separately: (a)

intracranial tuberculomas and spinal cord infections, (b) infections caused by nontuberculous mycobacteria, and (c) CNS tuberculosis in the particular context of AIDS.

HISTORY

The Scottish physiologist Robert Whytt (1) has been credited with the first clinical descriptions of tuberculous meningitis in the late 18th century, in a monograph describing acute hydrocephalus in children. During the 19th century the pathology of the disease was elucidated in some detail: The term "arachnitis tuberculosa" was coined in 1830, and the arteritis associated with tuberculous meningitis was described in 1881 (2). Meanwhile, the rapidly growing appreciation of the infectious nature of tuberculosis culminated in Robert Koch's isolation of *Mycobacterium tuberculosis* in 1882 (3). When Quincke (4) introduced the lumbar puncture into clinical medicine in 1891, a synthesis between the clinical and microbiologic conceptions of the disease became possible. However, it was not until 40 years later that the pathogenesis of the disease was fully elucidated by Rich and McCordock (5), at which time a full appreciation of the importance of the immune system in its pathogenesis was established.

The modern scientific understanding of the pathogenesis of CNS tuberculosis is barely 50 years old. In the years immediately following Koch's discovery of the tubercle bacillus, most authorities assumed that the disease developed in a manner analogous to that of other bacterial meningitides, whereby an inoculum of blood-borne organisms seeds the meninges and simultaneously causes disease (6). The frequent coincidence of meningeal and miliary tuberculosis was cited in support of this theory, as was the frequency with which the cerebral vasculature was involved in the disease.

Despite this widely held assumption, a considerable amount of experimental data rapidly accumulated to

A. Zuger and F. D. Lowy: Division of Infectious Diseases, Department of Medicine, Montefiore Medical Center and the Albert Einstein College of Medicine, Bronx, New York 10467.

contradict it. Researchers were repeatedly unable to produce tuberculous meningitis in experimental animals by intravascular injections of organisms. Even massive inocula of mycobacteria introduced directly into the carotid artery failed to cause meningitis, although animals frequently succumbed to a miliary infection instead. On the other hand, meningitis could be easily produced with injections of organisms directly into the subarachnoid space, even when relatively scanty inocula were used (5). The importance of immunologic mechanisms in the pathogenesis of the disease was, in addition, becoming increasingly clear: In 1932, Burn and Finley (7) demonstrated that experimental infection of the meninges caused far more significant disease in tubercular animals than in animals without preexisting tuberculosis. In fact, much of the characteristic pathology of tuberculous meningitis in tubercular animals could be re-created with subarachnoid injections of tubercular protein alone, without infectious particles.

In 1933, Rich and McCordock (5) transformed these independent observations into a coherent pathophysiologic theory. Autopsy studies convinced them that in patients with coincident miliary and meningeal disease the tuberculous changes in the CNS were seldom the same age as the tubercles disseminated through the viscera. In some cases the visceral tubercles were clearly older, while in others a chronic fibrous meningitis coexisted with minute, fresh tubercles in the viscera. Furthermore, a close study of the cerebral vasculature involved in tuberculous meningitis revealed that the vessel adventitia was invariably more significantly involved than were the inner layers, implying that the infectious process proceeded from the exterior of the vessel inwards. Only dissemination of infection from a preexisting focus within the brain or meninges could explain these observations. Dissecting 82 tubercular brains with meticulous technique, these investigators confirmed the presence of minute caseous tubercles within the brain or meninges, discharging bacilli in the vast majority of cases. These tubercles, known as "Rich foci," are now agreed to be fundamental to our present understanding of the pathogenesis of CNS tuberculosis.

EPIDEMIOLOGY

In the first half of the 20th century, CNS tuberculosis, like all forms of tuberculosis, was common. Such personages as the Italian artist Amadeo Modigliani in 1920, as well as the American author Thomas Wolfe in 1938, succumbed to tuberculous meningitis. Although detailed epidemiologic studies from this period are lacking, large-scale autopsy series can be used to provide accurate estimates of disease rates, since CNS disease was virtually always fatal. Of 13,000 unselected autopsies done in Leeds, England, between 1910 and 1931, 3.4% revealed tuberculous meningitis or intracranial tuberculous mass lesions (8). Additional data are available from the United States: Of 2333 autopsies performed in New York on individuals dying of tuberculosis, 4.6% had meningitis (9); of 3549 similar autopsies performed in Philadelphia between 1935 and 1954, 7.5% were found to have CNS involvement (10). These and other statistics have led some authorities to generalize that 5–15% of individuals exposed to tuberculosis will develop symptomatic disease; of this number, 5–10% will ultimately develop CNS involvement (11).

As characterized in the pre-antibiotic era, CNS tuberculosis was a disease of childhood. In one autopsy series, it occurred more than three times as frequently in individuals below the age of 20 as in adults (10). Conversely, in a series of 1000 children with active tuberculosis followed in New York City between 1930 and 1940, almost 15% developed tuberculous meningitis and died from it (12). The disease occurred most commonly between 6 months and 5 years of age—as a complication of primary tuberculous infection—and constituted the single greatest cause of death of all forms of tuberculosis in the pediatric population.

In the second half of the 20th century, worldwide epidemiologic patterns of tuberculosis in general—and, as a result, of CNS tuberculosis—have diverged (13). In some countries, tuberculosis still remains a widely prevalent infection: In 1972, for instance, an estimated 40% of children in India had been exposed to tuberculosis by age 14, whereas in other Asian countries the estimated prevalence by age 14 ranged to 80% (14). A similar prevalence was documented in many parts of Africa and Oceana. In the wealthier parts of the world, on the other hand, tuberculosis had become an uncommon disease by 1972, defeated by sanitation and antimicrobial therapy (15). In no country in the Americas or Europe did prevalence of exposure exceed 20–25% in 1972; the overall prevalence of tuberculosis exposure in the United States for that year has been estimated at approximately 8% (16).

Thus, tuberculous infections of the CNS are no longer distributed uniformly around the world. In less developed countries, particularly India and some parts of Africa, the disease remains common, especially among children. For instance, in Bombay in the early 1970s, nearly 45% of the patients admitted to a referral hospital for children with tuberculosis suffered from CNS disease (2). Although the availability of treatment has changed the clinical course of the disease in these settings, the impact of prevention and treatment on its frequency is generally not yet evident: The epidemiology of the disease remains much as it was in the early years of this century.

On the other hand, in the United States, as in other developed countries, the epidemiologic patterns of CNS tuberculosis have undergone complex changes. Overall, case rates of tuberculosis in the United States steadily fell following the institution of nationwide reporting in 1930; the rate of decline steepened in 1950 with the development of antituberculous chemotherapy. Over the last 20 years, however, the decline has been confined to cases of pulmonary tuberculosis: Rates of extrapulmonary infection have remained constant at approximately 4000 cases per year. Rates of CNS infection have been similarly constant, representing between 5% and 10% of extrapulmonary cases reported—that is, an overall estimated case rate of 0.11 per 100,000 population for the years 1969–1973 (17,18).

These statistics have had a significant effect on the profile of CNS tuberculosis in the United States. No longer closely associated with primary childhood infection, almost 75% of reported cases now occur in adults, rather than children, with approximately equal case rates from age 20 to over 65. Although the absolute number of infections is quite small, the disease remains a stable clinical presence and, in fact, accounts for an increasing percentage of all tuberculous infections reported in this country.

Recent epidemiologic data in the United States have ominous implications for the morbidity to be expected from CNS tuberculosis in the future. Despite the overall low case rate of tuberculosis in this country, it has become clear that in selected populations the disease remains a more significant presence than is often appreciated. Separate investigations have reported that the prevalence rates in homeless populations are up to 300 times higher than nationwide rates (19). Similarly disproportionate rates have been seen in non-white Americans, including blacks, native American populations,

and Pacific Islanders (20,21). Significant spread of infection has been demonstrated among long-term residents of nursing homes: A declining nationwide prevalence of disease has left clusters of elderly Americans vulnerable to the acquisition of clinically significant infection at an advanced age (22). Whether, within these pockets of prevalent tuberculosis, significant increases will be seen in the case rates of CNS disease has yet to be established.

The advent of AIDS has had an additional impact on the recent epidemiology of tuberculosis in this country. In 1986, the Centers for Disease Control (23) reported a nationwide increase in the number of reported cases of tuberculosis (Fig. 1), an increase which could be ascribed neither to changes in reporting criteria nor to large influxes of immigrants from areas endemic for tuberculosis. Instead, the data strongly associated the increased case rates with the young, predominantly urban adults at risk for AIDS. Other, equally strong epidemiologic connections have developed between the causative agent of AIDS, the human immunodeficiency virus (HIV), and newly diagnosed cases of tuberculosis. Between 5% and 10% of patients with AIDS in New York City and Miami have active tuberculosis, thought to represent reactivation of previously acquired disease (24,25). Similar reactivation may be occurring among AIDS patients in Africa (26). CNS complications have been prominent in cases of conjoint HIV and tuberculous infection, occurring in as many as 4–19% of cases (see Table 10), and will be discussed in more detail subsequently. Epidemiologically, the association between these diseases has troubling worldwide implications: Unlike the other opportunistic pathogens associated with AIDS, *M. tuberculosis* causes disease in the absence of immune compromise. HIV-infected individuals with reactivated disease may

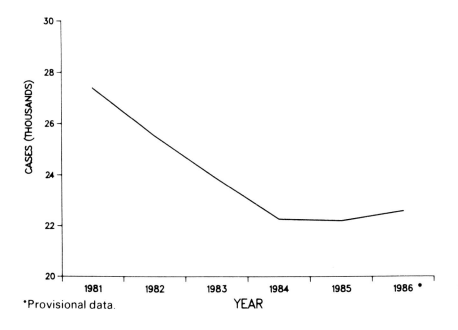

FIG. 1. Nationwide cases of tuberculosis reported to the Centers for Disease Control, 1981–1986. (From ref. 264, with permission.)

*Provisional data.

thus come to serve as reservoirs for the spread of primary tuberculous infections into the non-HIV-infected community.

ETIOLOGY AND PATHOGENESIS

Virtually all tuberculous infections of the CNS are caused by the human tubercle bacillus, *M. tuberculosis.* Infections caused by *M. bovis,* acquired from the ingestion of contaminated milk, are now quite rare, as are infections caused by other nontuberculous mycobacteria pathogenic for humans.

M. tuberculosis is a nonmotile bacillus, an obligate aerobic parasite whose only natural reservoir is man. The organisms grow slowly: Their generation time of 15–20 hr contrasts markedly with those of the pyogenic bacteria, which are usually less than 1 hr. Visible colonies are formed on media only after 2 or more weeks of incubation. The thick cell wall of the mycobacteria, invisible on Gram stain, can be demonstrated on Ziehl–Neelsen, Kinyoun, or fluorochrome staining (27). The complex antigenic structure of the cell wall includes polysaccharides, proteins, peptides, lipids, and glycolipids with specific immunologic properties. In addition, other antigens are contained within the cytoplasm: These molecules between them largely determine the characteristic immune response to tuberculous infection and its resultant pathology (28,29).

Like all other forms of tuberculosis, CNS infection begins with inhalation of infectious particles. Airborne droplet nuclei, each containing generally fewer than five organisms, reach the alveoli and multiply either within the alveolar spaces or within alveolar macrophages and macrophages derived from the circulation. For the first 2–4 weeks following infection, virtually no immune response to the infection occurs. At this initial stage of infection, hematogenous dissemination of the organisms is believed to occur in every case. Organisms are spread throughout the body, although to different degrees in different organs: Lungs, liver, spleen, and bone marrow filter many organisms from the blood, whereas organs not belonging to the reticuloendothelial system, such as the brain and meninges, trap relatively few (30).

Two to four weeks following infection, cell-mediated immunity to the organism develops. T-lymphocytes are stimulated by bacterial antigens to produce lymphokines, which, in turn, attract and activate mononuclear phagocytes from the bloodstream. Within these activated macrophages, organisms may be killed; at the same time, many of the macrophages are themselves killed by the organisms or by their toxic antigenic products. A tubercle forms, consisting of macrophages, lymphocytes, and other cells surrounding a necrotic, caseous center.

The fate of these tubercles and the subsequent course of infection are a function of both (a) the immunologic capacity of the host and (b) other, incompletely understood genetic factors. At best, minute caseous foci may be produced, only to be completely eliminated by surrounding macrophages, leaving no residua of infection but a positive tuberculin skin test. Less efficient but still effective host response will result in larger caseous foci, which, despite fibrous encapsulation, continue to shelter viable bacilli which may cause reactivated disease if the host's immune vigilance lessens. And in the presence of profoundly impaired immunity, the primary tubercles will continue to grow, the caseous centers may liquefy, organisms will proliferate, and the lesion will ultimately rupture, discharging organisms and their antigenically potent products into the surrounding tissues (31).

When these events occur within the CNS, tuberculous meningitis results. Rarely, the source of organisms is an adjacent focus of extraneural infection in the vertebrae, inner ears, or mastoid sinuses (32,33). Most often, however, the source is an intracerebral tubercle formed during the silent hematogenous dissemination of the organism, as identified by Rich and McCordock (5). If formed during primary infection of a relatively immunoincompetent host (an infant or child less than 5 years old, for instance), its rupture may complicate primary infection, resulting in coincident meningeal and pulmonary or meningeal and miliary infections. If an initially successful encapsulation of the infection subsequently wanes (in old age, for instance, or from another form of immunocompromise), meningitis may occur in the absence of other organ involvement, may accompany coincident reactivation of other dormant visceral sites of infection, or may itself result in a secondary hematogenous dissemination of the infection.

The specific CNS syndromes associated with infection are themselves a function of the original location of the infecting tubercle. Foci located on the surface of the brain or the ependyma will rupture into the subarachnoid space or the ventricular system to cause meningitis. Those deep within the brain or spinal cord parenchyma will enlarge to form tuberculomas or, more rarely, tuberculous abscesses (10,30). The pathology of these space-occupying lesions will subsequently be considered in more detail.

PATHOLOGY AND PATHOPHYSIOLOGY OF TUBERCULOUS MENINGITIS

Tuberculous meningitis is more correctly characterized as a meningoencephalitis, since its pathology encompasses not only the meninges but the parenchyma and the vasculature of the brain as well. The primary pathologic event is the formation of a thick exudate within the subarachnoid space (Fig. 2). Occasionally this exudate is localized to the immediate vicinity of the rup-

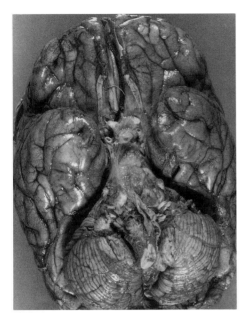

FIG. 2. Thick exudate covering the base of the brain in a confirmed case of tuberculous meningitis.

tured tubercle. More commonly, however, it is diffuse; in addition, it is particularly prominent at the base of the brain, irrespective of the location of the discharging focus. It centers around the interpeduncular fossa, enveloping the optic nerves at the chiasm and extending over the pons and cerebellum, often into the Sylvian fissures and rarely up along the cerebral hemispheres. Within the lateral ventricles a similar exudate often covers the choroid plexus. In appearance, the exudate is gelatinous and frequently nodular. Microscopically, it consists of polymorphonuclear leukocytes, red blood cells, macrophages, and lymphocytes within a fibrin network. As the disease progresses, lymphocytes come to predominate; later, fibroblasts and elements of connective tissue are present as well. Typical tubercles may develop within the exudate; occasionally, large zones of caseation necrosis are formed. The number of mycobacteria within the exudate is highly variable: In some cases none may be found; in others they are present in enormous numbers (2,5,34).

Accompanying the tuberculous exudate is a characteristic inflammation affecting the blood vessels traversing it. Most commonly, small and medium-sized arteries are involved, although capillaries and veins also may be affected. Microscopically, the adventitial layer of the vessels develops changes identical to those of the adjacent tuberculous exudate: Similar cells, tubercles, and caseation necrosis may be found therein, occasionally with clumps of tubercle bacilli as well. The intimal layers of the vessels may subsequently be similarly transformed, or they may be eroded by a fibrinoid–hyaline degeneration. A reactive subendothelial cellular proliferation follows, which may be so exuberant as to completely oc-

clude the lumen of the vessel. Ischemic cerebral infarction resulting from vascular occlusion is thus a common sequela of tuberculous arteritis, most often in the distributions of the middle cerebral artery (reflecting the presence of tuberculous exudate within the Sylvian fissure) and the lateral striate arteries, affected as they penetrate the base of the brain (35,36).

The third characteristic pathologic feature of tuberculous meningitis is the hydrocephalus that results from the profound disturbances created in the circulation of the cerebrospinal fluid (CSF). More often seen in children than adults, hydrocephalus is a frequent accompaniment of chronic infection. Occasionally an obstructive hydrocephalus is induced by exudate blocking the spinal aqueduct or the foramina of Luschka; edema of surrounding brain parenchyma may effectively block these draining channels as well. More often, the hydrocephalus is of the communicating type. Isotope cisternoventriculography with iodine-labeled human albumin has been used to confirm that this condition results from exudate blocking the basal cisterns and impeding the resorption of CSF (37). When exudate prevents the circulation of CSF within the spinal subarachnoid space, a clinically significant spinal block may occur.

Exudate, vasculitis, and hydrocephalus each exerts its own effect on the brain parenchyma in tuberculous meningitis. "Border-zone encephalitis" describes a tissue reaction frequently seen in brain tissue adjacent to zones of thick, adherent exudate: The brain tissue softens and astrocytic, microglial, and diffuse inflammatory reactions can be seen. Thrombosed vessels within the exudate frequently result in zones of hemorrhage and infarction in adjacent brain. Chronic hydrocephalus, untreated, leads to atrophy of both gray and white matter. And finally, an entity of tuberculous encephalopathy has been reported which is apparently independent of other pathology. It consists of cerebral edema, occasionally with perivascular demyelination or hemorrhagic leukencephalopathy; these changes have been observed deep in the white matter of the brain, at a distance from vascular abnormalities or exudate. Although systematic immunopathologic studies of this entity are lacking, some observers have hypothesized that it is a purely "allergic" phenomenon, mediated by tissue hypersensitivity either to bacillary antigens or to a possibly myelin-related antigen of brain tissue itself (38).

The effects of antimycobacterial chemotherapy on the pathology of tuberculous meningitis are of considerable clinical importance. This subject received much attention during the early years of streptomycin use, when it became evident that the disease retained considerable morbidity and mortality despite treatment. In brains of patients dying after streptomycin treatment, a marked tendency towards granulation, organization, and fibrosis of the basilar exudate was seen. When periods of treatment approached 2 years, most of the exudate was re-

TABLE 1. *Clinical staging of patients with tuberculous meningitis*[a]

Stage I (early):	Nonspecific symptoms and signs
	No clouding of consciousness
	No neurologic deficits
Stage II (intermediate):	Lethargy or alteration in behavior
	Meningeal irritation
	Minor neurologic deficits (cranial nerve palsies)
Stage III (advanced):	Abnormal movements
	Convulsions
	Stupor or coma
	Severe neurologic deficits (pareses)

[a] Data were taken from ref. 39.

placed with hyalinized connective tissue. A concomitant fibrosis of the intima of involved vessels was seen as well. Hydrocephalus invariably accompanied these changes (34,39). These observations confirmed that tissue damage initiated by the infection persisted despite bacterial eradication. They form the basis for the persistent interest in steroids and other forms of anti-inflammatory therapy in tuberculous meningitis.

CLINICAL PRESENTATION

The clinical picture of tuberculous meningitis is quite variable, with substantial differences among patients of different ages. In an effort to systematize the spectrum to some degree, a staging system was introduced in 1947, which has since been widely adopted in the initial assessments of these patients (Table 1). According to this schema, patients in the first stage of disease are those with only nonspecific manifestations of infection without neurologic symptoms or signs. In stage II, patients have signs and symptoms of meningeal irritation, with cranial nerve palsies but no other neurologic defects and no clouding of consciousness; in stage III, patients are severely ill, with gross neurologic defects, stupor, or coma (39). Although this staging system has been valuable in the structuring and interpretation of treatment trials for the disease, the smooth continuum of disease progression it implies is not always evident in individual patients.

Among children, the most commonly reported symptoms on presentation include nausea, vomiting, and behavioral changes (Table 2); headache is generally reported in less than 25% of children in large series, and it is virtually never identified in patients under 3 years of age (40). Abdominal pain and constipation have been commonly cited complaints among children, as is anorexia (41). Seizures are an infrequent presenting complaint, reported in 10–20% of children prior to hospitalization, although more than 50% may develop seizures during their initial hospitalization (42). Seizures are generally more frequent in younger children (40).

The medical history of children with tuberculous meningitis is often unrevealing: Even in early series, only slightly more than half had a prior diagnosis of tuberculosis (40). A history of exposure to active adult cases of tuberculosis within the household has been similarly unreliable, generally obtained in only 40–60% of pediatric cases (39,40,42,43). Early investigators noted an association between the onset of illness and a variety of precipitating factors, including measles, pertussis, routine immunizations, surgical procedures, and head trauma (40,44). These associations have not been reconfirmed in more recent series. In most children with tuberculous meningitis the disease process is relatively rapid, with a duration of illness prior to medical attention almost uniformly less than 3 weeks (41,44,45).

Among adults, the disease typically presents in a somewhat more indolent fashion. Although symptoms may prompt medical evaluation within days, median duration of symptoms is generally 2–3 weeks, with some adults describing several months of illness before seeking medical attention; the occasional patient will describe symptoms that have been present for years (46–49). A history of prior clinical tuberculosis is extremely infrequent among adult patients, generally elicited in fewer than 20% of cases (48,49,50). Precipitating factors for the onset of disease have not been satisfactorily identified.

As among children (39), no successful correlation has been established between duration of symptoms and severity of disease at presentation among adults (46). Still, symptoms among adult patients are frequently, although not invariably, more specifically neurologic than among children (Table 2). Headache is a prominent complaint,

TABLE 2. *Clinical presentation of patients with tuberculous meningitis*

Feature	Percentage of children with feature (refs.)[a]	Percentage of adults with feature (refs.)[b]
Headache	20–50% (41,43,54)	50–60% (47,51)
Nausea/vomiting	50–75% (41,43,44)	8–40% (47–49)
Apathy/behavioral changes	30–70% (43,44,54)	30–70% (47,51,55)
Seizures	10–20% (41,43,44)	0–13% (47,48)
Prior history of tuberculosis	55% (40)	8–12% (47–49)

[a] Data from series with >85% children.
[b] Data from series with >85% adults.

usually occurring in 50–75% of patients (49,51,52). Nausea is generally less frequent; behavioral changes consisting of apathy, confusion, or bizarre behavior are reported in large series with widely varying frequency, from the minority to the majority of patients (52,53). As among children, seizures are an unusual early manifestation of disease, occurring in approximately 10–15% of adult patients.

On examination, adults and children present more uniform findings, although considerable variation still occurs (Table 3). Fever is an inconstant presence among patients of all ages: Noted in 98% of pediatric patients by Edith Lincoln (44), it was present in less than 50% of children in a more recent series (54); it is identified with similar inconsistency among adults, from the vast majority (48,50,53,55) to the distinct minority (52). Meningismus and signs of meningeal irritation are similarly not uniform findings: They were an "invariable" concomitant of infection among 167 children with tuberculous meningitis in 1947, but in subsequent series they have been absent in 25–40% of children and adults (36,41,51, 54,56).

Focal neurologic signs, diagnostic of stage II disease, most frequently consist of unilateral or, less commonly, bilateral cranial nerve palsies. Up to 30% of patients may display these signs on presentation. Most frequently affected is the sixth cranial nerve, followed by the third and fourth, the seventh, and, less commonly, the second, eighth, tenth, eleventh, and twelfth (44,47). An equally common neurologic deficit in some series is hemiparesis, the result of ischemic infarction in the anterior cerebral circulation, most commonly in the territory of the middle cerebral artery (36). Less frequently seen neurologic signs include a variety of abnormal movements: Chorea, hemiballismus, athetosis, myoclonus, and cerebellar ataxia have all been observed in tuberculous meningitis, generally more frequently among children than among adults. Finally, neurologic signs directly referable to space-occupying tuberculous masses in the brain or spinal cord may precede the onset of tuberculous meningitis or may emerge during evaluation or therapy; these clinical entities will be discussed separately.

Examination of the optic fundus may occasionally offer specific clues to the presence of a tuberculous infection. The presence of visible tubercles in the choroid was once thought to correlate strongly with tuberculous meningitis. These retinal lesions occur singly or in groups of up to 20 near the optic disk. Usually one-fourth to one-half the disk diameter in size, they are initially yellow with indistinct borders, becoming strongly pigmented at the periphery with age. Clinicians now realize that choroidal tubercles, while present in more than 50% of cases of miliary tuberculosis, are far less frequent in tuberculous meningitis, generally present in only about 10% of cases of meningitis not associated with miliary disease (41,44,57). In an individual with meningitis, their presence points strongly to a tuberculous etiology for the infection, although their absence militates very little against the diagnosis.

The finding of papilledema on fundoscopic exam may similarly provide a diagnostic clue to the presence of increased intracranial pressure before more precise radiologic studies are available. Hydrocephalus in tuberculous meningitis has generally correlated well with duration of infection (40). It is present in the minority of affected patients on first evaluation, although among children that minority is sometimes as substantial as 40% (58). It often develops in the majority during the course of the disease. In infants, bulging fontanelles and increasing cranial circumference may be noted, whereas in adults the typical symptomatology of increased intracranial pressure will develop, including drowsiness, diplopia, and blurry vision (59). Severe hydrocephalus due to tuberculous meningitis may cause coma in both children and adults. In addition, a variety of focal neurologic signs, including hemiparesis and blindness, have been associated with hydrocephalus, ascribed to ventricular dilation with stretching of vessels, circulatory compromise, and local ischemia. These signs have resolved, even after weeks, when hydrocephalus is relieved (60).

Because of the nonspecific clinical presentation of patients with tuberculous meningitis, the initial differential diagnosis is wide. Their early clinical course is compatible with most other bacterial, viral, or fungal infections of the CNS, as well as with noninfectious inflammatory diseases of the meninges (such as sarcoidosis and sys-

TABLE 3. *Admission evaluation of patients with tuberculous meningitis*

Feature	Percentage of children with feature (refs.)[a]	Percentage of adults with feature (refs.)[b]
Fever	50–100% (41,43,44,54)	60–100% (49,51,55)
Meningismus	70–100% (36,40,41,54)	60–70% (47–49)
Cranial nerve palsy	15–30% (41,43,54)	15–40% (51,55)
Coma	30–45% (41,44,45)	20–30% (47,49)
PPD-positive[c]	85–90% (42,43,54)	40–65% (49,55,61)

[a] Data from series with >85% children.
[b] Data from series with >85% adults.
[c] PPD, purified protein derivative (of tuberculin).

temic lupus erythematosis) and with intracranial malignancy. In a recent series of patients with proven or probable tuberculous meningitis, another diagnosis was initially considered in 30% of cases, including bacterial sepsis, bacterial meningitis, viral meningitis, miliary tuberculosis, and brain abscess (49).

DIAGNOSTIC TESTS

Routine laboratory studies are often not helpful in cases of CNS tuberculosis. Many of the usual laboratory correlates of systemic infection may be absent: The erythrocyte sedimentation rate, for instance, is often mildly elevated, but not invariably so; in one study the median sedimentation rate among 12 adults with culture-proven tuberculous meningitis was 57 mm/hr, with a range of 18–90 mm/hr (61). The peripheral white blood cell count is similarly variable: Leukopenia as well as leukocytosis can be seen in tuberculous meningitis, with relatively normal counts identified in the majority of patients in many series (48,52,53). Differential counts of peripheral white blood cells follow no characteristic pattern.

A syndrome of inappropriate antidiuretic hormone secretion caused by tuberculous meningitis has been suggested in many cases by the presence of hyponatremia and hypochloremia on routine blood chemistry analysis. In some cases, this diagnosis has been confirmed by serum and urine osmolality determinations and the presence of high circulating levels of antidiuretic hormone (62). Superimposed electrolyte disorders caused by chronic vomiting and anorexia may occur as well. The frequency of electrolyte abnormalities on initial evaluation varies enormously between series, ranging from 25% to 92% of patients, with no clear distinctions between children and adults (42,46).

Chest X-Ray

The frequency and nature of abnormalities on chest radiograph accompanying CNS tuberculosis vary considerably with the age of the patient. Among adults, abnormalities consistent with current or remote tuberculous infection are seen in 25–50% of patients (47,61,63), whereas among children these changes are considerably more common. In 1960, Lincoln et al. (44) reported that 90% of 241 children with tuberculous meningitis had radiographs with evidence of primary or calcified primary disease. Other series have confirmed this observation in 50–80% of cases (41,42,45,54). Abnormalities have usually reflected primary tuberculosis, occasionally with superimposed calcification or with miliary spread. Miliary disease alone is less frequent, and remote calcified infection is the least frequent of all—present in less than 10% of all pediatric cases (64). Among adults, the

adenopathy and dense infiltrates of primary tuberculosis are only infrequently found. Radiologic changes range from subtle apical scarring to calcified Ghon complexes to nodular upper-lobe disease (49,51).

Miliary disease accompanying tuberculous meningitis is often diagnosed on chest radiograph. In the past, the combination of miliary and meningeal infection was extremely frequent: Up to 80% of patients dying of meningitis prior to the availability of chemotherapy had evidence of miliary disease (50,58). Now, although early intervention with antimicrobial therapy may have weakened this association to some degree, miliary and meningeal disease still frequently coexist. Miliary disease has been documented radiologically in 25–50% of cases of tuberculous meningitis among adults (49,55,63), as well as in 15–25% of children (41,45,64). Conversely, 21 of 69 patients with miliary disease (30%) were found to have meningeal involvement (65).

Delayed Hypersensitivity

The utility of the tuberculin test in the diagnosis of active tuberculous infection in the individual patient has been the subject of some recent critical analysis; its use in the diagnosis of tuberculous meningitis is no exception (66). In individual series of patients, positive tuberculin tests are the rule. Series of children generally have rates of 85–90% positivity; approximately 10% of these reactions may be to a second-strength tuberculin test alone (41,42,44,54). In one series, all children who were initially purified protein derivative (PPD)-negative became PPD-positive during convalescence (43). In later series, which consist primarily of adult patients in countries in which tuberculosis is no longer endemic, tuberculin positivity is a less reliable concomitant of infection. Approximately 35–60% of individuals thought to have tuberculous meningitis have not reacted to first- or second-strength tuberculin testing (48,49,55,61). These data must be interpreted with the caveat that in some series a clinical syndrome compatible with tuberculous meningitis has been presumed tuberculous on the basis of a positive tuberculin test; the actual rate of tuberculin reactivity in cases of tuberculous meningitis may thus be somewhat lower than reported.

Factors postulated to be responsible for these negative reactions are thought to include malnutrition, debilitation, and general immunosuppression associated with severe systemic disease, as well as a selective, generally transient inability to recognize tuberculous antigen occasionally seen with overwhelming tuberculosis (67). Improper storage or administration of the antigen and improper reading of the results may contribute as well. Finally, the interpretation of a tuberculin test in an individual with a clinical syndrome consistent with tuberculosis must also take into account the prevalence of tuberculosis in the community as well as that of atypical mycobacteria, which may cause false-positive tuberculin reactions. The prior tuberculin status of the individual patient is also of importance (68). While all these factors significantly affect the predictive power of a single tuberculin test, a coherent means of addressing them in the individual case of meningitis has yet to be established. In its absence, tuberculin testing may remain more useful as an epidemiologic tool than as a clinical one.

Extraneural Cultures

The frequency with which tuberculous meningitis coexists with other active sites of tuberculosis is often a boon to the clinician seeking a microbiologic confirmation of the disease. When meningitis is accompanied by active pulmonary or miliary disease, sputum and gastric washings frequently grow *M. tuberculosis.* In the absence of evident extraneural disease, urine cultures may occasionally be positive as well (49,51). Positive cultures from organs such as lymph node, marrow, and liver—as well as, rarely, cultures from pleura or synovium—have been used to diagnose meningitis in the presence of miliary disease. These reports are infrequent enough that frequencies of coexistent infection cannot be well established. Most investigators are content to caution that the absence of evident extraneural tuberculosis should not be used to rule out the diagnosis of tuberculous meningitis (69). The presence of extraneural tuberculosis, on the other hand, in a patient with a clinical picture compatible with tuberculous meningitis, is frequently considered to confirm the diagnosis even in the absence of confirmatory CSF microbiology.

Cerebrospinal Fluid Analysis

CSF abnormalities traditionally accompany tuberculous meningitis, although in fact these changes can be quite nonspecific. Typically, the fluid is clear or slightly opalescent. Rarely, hemorrhagic CSF has been reported in association with tuberculous meningitis, ascribed to a severe accompanying vasculitis (70). When allowed to stand for a short time at room temperature or in the refrigerator, a cobweb-like skin may form on top of the specimen, "which appears to be suspended from the surface of the fluid, and which waves to and fro as the tube is moved" (71). This web is the classic "pellicle" of tuberculous meningitis—a characteristic, although by no means invariable, presence. It results from the high fibrinogen concentration in the fluid along with the presence of inflammatory cells. Its importance lies not so much in its appearance, which is suggestive but not pathognomonic of tuberculous meningitis, as in the dictum that tubercle bacilli may become entangled in the skein of the pellicle and, thus, become more easily lo-

cated by smear or culture therein than elsewhere in tuberculous CSF (72).

Opening pressure at initial lumbar puncture is significantly elevated in a variable percentage of patients, ranging from 40% to 75% in series of children (36,73) and reported to be approximately 50% among adults (49). Opening pressure is not completely reliable in gauging the patency of the CSF circulatory pathways: The presence of spinal block in severe cases of disease may artifactually lower the opening pressure of the lumbar fluid even in the presence of hydrocephalus.

Moderate depression in CSF glucose and elevation in CSF protein are characteristic accompaniments of tuberculous meningitis (Table 4). The median glucose concentration in most series is approximately 40 mg%, with a wide range of observed values. Hypoglycorrhachia has correlated with more advanced stages of clinical disease (44); in addition, sequential CSF samples from the same patient may show a progressive gradual reduction in glucose in the absence of therapy (74). When CSF glucose values from patients with culture-proven tuberculous meningitis are contrasted with those from patients with presumed tuberculous meningitis without culture confirmation, median values have been lower in culture-confirmed cases (47,49).

CSF protein content is elevated in the majority of patients with tuberculous meningitis: Most series cite median CSF protein values of 150–200 mg%, with the observation that protein values tend to rise in sequential samples from untreated patients (44). Occasional CSF protein values in excess of 1–2 g are reported, usually in conjunction with spinal block (50,75). When CSF protein values from patients with culture-proven tuberculous meningitis are contrasted with those from patients without microbiologic confirmation of disease, no differences have been observed (47,49).

Low CSF chloride, once felt to be associated with tuberculous meningitis, is now discounted as a diagnostic tool for this disease. Generally reflecting the coexistent hypochloremia often seen in meningitis, it has been proven unhelpful in discriminating between bacterial, viral, and tuberculous infections (76).

A moderate pleocytosis in the CSF is characteristic of tuberculous meningitis, although it is not an invariable finding (Table 4). In most clinical series, 90–100% of cases have more than five white cells per cubic millimeter of CSF, and the number of cells seldom exceeds 300 per cubic millimeter; however, there have occasionally been counts of 1000 per cubic millimeter, and, exceptionally, counts of 3000–4000 per cubic millimeter have been reported (75). Differential counts can be quite variable: Initially, both lymphocytic and polymorphonuclear predominance can be seen. Sequential CSF specimens obtained from both treated and untreated patients have documented the rapid conversion of polymorphonuclear predominance, when it occurs, into a lym-

TABLE 4. *Cerebrospinal fluid findings in recent series of patients with definite or presumed tuberculous meningitis*

Author (ref.)	Number of patients	Median CSF glucose value, mg% (range)	Median CSF protein value, mg% (range)	CSF WBC/mm³ median (range)
Barrett-Connor (48)	18	18 (7–66)	206 (84–1340)	283 (29–1030)
Haas et al. (55)	19	45 (20–145)	158 (51–1000)	177 (8–900)
Traub et al. (47)	16	40 (13–108)	190 (55–950)	63 (9–520)
Klein et al. (51)	19	40 (11–146)	159 (20–980)	200 (0–960)
Ogawa et al. (49)	45	35 (7–189)	151 (35–2900)	162 (0–8600)

phocytic picture over several weeks (12,77). In most treated cases, in addition, a population of plasma cells evolved in the CSF during the course of therapy, as did a CSF eosinophilia as high as 23% in one case.

Microbiology

The identification of tuberculous organisms in the CSF has posed difficulties for decades. Implicit in the pathogenesis of tuberculous meningitis is the fact that the population of organisms in the CSF may be quite small. Accordingly, the frequency with which acid-fast bacilli are evident on stained specimens of CSF can be quite low. In many clinical series, less than 25% of specimens were smear-positive (42,46,51,53); however, in occasional series, smear-positivity was reported in less than 10% of samples (47,49,56). Even among specimens from which *M. tuberculosis* was ultimately cultured, the number with evidence of the organism on smear has been low (Table 5) (78). A variety of techniques proposed to increase the yield of CSF smears have included staining the pellicle, if present, as well as layering the centrifuged sediment of large volumes of CSF onto a single slide with repeated applications until the entire pellet can be stained at once (79). Similarly, subjecting second and third samples of CSF to careful microscopy may dramatically improve chances of identifying acid-fast organisms. Kennedy and Fallon (52) reported an 87% rate of positive smears when up to four separate specimens were examined for each patient. This rate of success has not been duplicated in the literature. In addition, the use of auramine–rhodamine (fluorochrome) staining in lieu of the more traditional Kinyoun stain may increase sensitivity in detection of acid-fast organisms in some hands, as

well as enabling a more rapid and efficient screening of multiple smears.

Proof of tuberculous meningitis requires the isolation of the organism in culture. Nonetheless, although culture is formally the gold standard of diagnosis in this disease, it is fallible. In many clinical series, mycobacteria were isolated from less than 50% of patients clinically presumed to have the disease by virtue of other criteria (Table 6). False-negative CSF culture results are so common that a diagnosis of tuberculous meningitis is generally assumed if a consistent clinical syndrome is accompanied by a consistent CSF profile, evidence of tuberculosis elsewhere in the body, a positive PPD, or response to specific antimycobacterial therapy in the absence of evidence for other diagnoses (36,45,47–49,54). Higher yields from mycobacterial cultures may be gained by processing multiple specimens for each patient, although even with as many as four CSF specimens obtained prior to or early in the course of therapy, almost 20% of patients with a clinical diagnosis have had negative CSF cultures (52). Compounding this uncertainty is the minimum incubation time of several weeks necessary for mycobacterial cultures to be formally declared positive or negative. The clinical imperative for early treatment renders this delay particularly unfortunate for the practicing clinician.

SEROUS (STERILE) TUBERCULOUS MENINGITIS

The rare condition of "serous" or sterile tuberculous meningitis has remained an infrequently seen but intriguing pathologic entity (12,80). It is distinguished from ordinary tuberculous meningitis by its distinctive CSF pro-

TABLE 5. *Frequency of positive cerebrospinal fluid smears in culture-proven tuberculous meningitis*

Author (ref.)	Number of culture-proven cases	Number of smear-positive (%)
Clark et al. (61)	12	1 (8%)
Haas et al. (55)	9	2 (22%)
Kennedy and Fallon (52)	43	37 (86%)[a]
Klein et al. (51)	19	2 (11%)
Ogawa et al. (49)	18	3 (17%)
Sumaya et al. (42)	24	7 (29%)

[a] Four specimens of CSF were examined for each patient.

TABLE 6. *Frequency of positive cerebrospinal fluid cultures in clinically diagnosed tuberculous meningitis*

Author (ref.)	Number of clinically diagnosed cases[a]	Number of culture-confirmed cases (%)
Alvarez and McCabe (50)	13	9 (70%)
Barrett-Connor (48)	18	7 (39%)
Lincoln and Sewell (12)	237	84 (35%)
Ogawa et al. (49)	45	18 (40%)
Sumaya et al. (42)	57	24 (42%)
Traub et al. (47)	16	4 (25%)

[a] Diagnostic criteria included the following: compatible clinical picture with or without evidence of extraneural tuberculosis; response to antituberculous therapy; and autopsy diagnoses.

file and good clinical prognosis. Serous meningitis is thought to result when a tubercle rupturing into the meninges releases few or no viable mycobacteria, but enough tuberculoprotein to provoke an immunologic reaction identical to that seen with a larger bacterial seeding (75). CSF analysis is generally consistent with an aseptic meningitis accompanied by elevated opening pressure, elevated cell count, and elevated protein but normal sugar levels. In a large series of children with serous meningitis from Bellevue Hospital in New York City, tubercle bacilli were never isolated from the CSF of these patients (12,81). Clinically, however, these patients could not be distinguished on presentation from those with more usual disease, although systemic signs of infection generally predominated over focal neurologic signs. In the absence of specific treatment, complete clinical recovery was the rule, generally within days to weeks. Some patients ultimately developed, and died of, typical tuberculous meningitis or nonmeningeal tuberculosis; others remained well with follow-up periods in excess of 10 years. In those patients dying of nonneurologic causes, postmortem examination revealed only areas of healed, focal meningitis, with fibrous adhesions between the dura and underlying arachnoid.

NEWER DIAGNOSTIC TECHNIQUES

The deficiencies of most ordinary diagnostic tests for tuberculous meningitis have kindled great interest in the development of clinically useful alternatives. An ideal test would be rapid and sensitive in discriminating between bacterial, viral, fungal, and mycobacterial infections. It would also be highly specific because, as pointed out by Daniel (82), a test with a high false-positive rate, causing clinicians to curtail broad-spectrum therapy and diagnostic work-ups prematurely, would be particularly injurious in this disease. Over the last 40 years a variety of alternatives have been proposed to fit these qualifications, all promising in some respects and disappointing in others (Table 7).

The newer diagnostic modalities fall into two subgroups: (i) immunologic tests that detect mycobacterial antigen or antibody in the CSF and (ii) other biochemical assays measuring some other feature of the organism or the host response to it. Of the latter, the most venerable is the bromide partition test, first conceived in the late 1920s as a means of quantitating the interruption of the blood–brain barrier by infection. It was found that the normal serum/CSF ratio of bromide following an administered dose was generally greater than 3, whereas the ratio was much lower in tuberculous meningitis. In the 1950s, several investigators confirmed the utility of this test in distinguishing tuberculous from other lymphocytic meningitides, in which the barrier was comparatively well preserved (83). However, the method of determining bromide concentrations used in these early series was cumbersome, and the test sank into obscurity until it was revived with the use of radioisotopes.

Most protocols now use an oral or intravenous dose of

TABLE 7. *Newer diagnostic tests for tuberculous meningitis*

Test (refs.)	Sensitivity	Specificity	Time required
Radiolabeled bromide partition ratio (85,86,96)	90–94%	88–96%	48 hr
CSF adenosine deaminase level (86,93,96)	73–100%	71–99%	<24 hr
CSF tuberculostearic acid level (100)	95%	99%	<24 hr
CSF mycobacterial antigen (106–108)	79–94%	95–100%	<24 hr
CSF mycobacterial antibody (96,102,103)	27–100%	94–100%	<24 hr
CSF polymerase chain reaction (108a)	83%	100%	<24 hr

[^{82}Br]ammonium bromide, with determination of simultaneous serum and CSF concentrations of radioisotope in a gamma counter after 1 or 2 days of equilibration. When a ratio of 1.6 or less is taken to be characteristic of tuberculous meningitis, most series demonstrate sensitivity and specificity rates for identifying the infection in the range of 90% (84–86). False-positive results have been reported in herpes simplex and other viral encephalitides, as well as in *Listeria* meningoencephalitis and CNS lymphoma (87,88). In addition, the ability of the test to distinguish tuberculous meningitis from neurosyphilis, originally also distinguished by its low bromide partition ratio, has not been addressed to date in the recent literature.

Determination of adenosine deaminase (ADA) in the CSF is another, newer method of assessing a biochemical parameter of the host's response in tuberculous meningitis. The enzyme is associated primarily with T lymphocytes in humans (89): Elevated plasma concentrations have been found in systemic infections which elicit significant cell-mediated immunity; and elevated pleural, pericardial, and peritoneal concentrations have been documented in tuberculous infections of these cavities (90–92). The assay for the enzyme involves a colorimetric assay for the ammonia cleaved from an adenosine substrate. Assaying CSF enzyme concentrations in patients with a variety of neurologic diagnoses including bacterial, viral, and neoplastic disorders, Ribera et al. (93) reported a sensitivity of 100% and a specifity of 99% in identifying 21 individuals with tuberculous meningitis. Markedly elevated enzyme concentrations persisted in CSF assayed through the third week of antituberculous therapy. Other studies have used the same assay but have had less successful results (94–96), with particular difficulty in distinguishing tuberculous meningitis from bacterial and viral meningitis among children. More recently, ADA elevations have been reported in a few individuals with tuberculous meningitis and AIDS, despite these patients' significant T-cell depletion (97).

Other specific chemicals detected in the CSF of individuals with tuberculous meningitis have not been studied in extensive clinical trials. 3-(2′-Ketohexyl)indoline, a substance of unknown source distantly related to serotonin, was identified in the CSF of 12 patients with untreated tuberculous meningitis by electron-capture gas–liquid chromotography, but it was not found in patients with aseptic or cryptococcal meningitis (98). A follow-up study confirmed the presence of the compound in only approximately 60% of culture-proven cases of tuberculous meningitis (99). Tuberculostearic acid, a component of the cell wall of *M. tuberculosis,* was identified with similar methodology in the CSF of 21 of 22 patients with proven or suspected tuberculous meningitis, with a sensitivity of 95% and a specificity of 99% (100). The complexity and expense of these techniques may undermine their clinical utility, particularly in the less developed areas of the world.

The possibility of detecting specific mycobacterial antigen or antibody in the CSF has generated considerable research. Hemagglutinating antibodies against crude extracts of tuberculin were reported in the serum of tuberculosis patients at the turn of the century; they were, however, sought with mixed results in the CSF through the early 1970s (101). However, the development of more sensitive and reproducible serodiagnostic techniques, particularly the enzyme-linked immunosorbent assay (ELISA), has aided these efforts in recent years.

Hernandez et al. (102) used an ELISA to detect both IgG and IgM antibodies against avirulent *M. bovis* (BCG), which shares surface antigens with *M. tuberculosis.* They found the test to be 100% sensitive and 100% specific in distinguishing between (a) a group of 20 CSF samples from patients with tuberculous meningitis and (b) 70 specimens from patients with other CNS infection or no infection at all. In a preliminary report, Kalish et al. (103) measured IgG antibody against PPD in three patients with culture-proven tuberculous meningitis and in 33 controls, with similarly good results. More recently, however, Watt et al. (104) used a similar technique in a larger trial but had less success, finding a sensitivity of only 24% for tuberculous meningitis among 127 samples. With an ELISA measuring antibody against *M. tuberculosis* antigen 5, a highly purified, well-characterized protein antigen of the organism, Coovadia et al. (96) found a similarly low sensitivity in identifying samples belonging to patients with presumed tuberculous meningitis. Although the specificity of the assay could be tuned to 100% with high values set for a positive titer, the sensitivity of the test at these levels was significantly compromised. Low circulating levels of antimycobacterial antibodies have been found in the serum of many individuals, irrespective of PPD status; their presence may be reflected in the finding of CSF antibody in individuals not suffering from tuberculous meningitis and may handicap the specificity of antibody testing at all but the highest cutoff levels (105).

Detection of soluble tuberculous antigens in the CSF of patients with presumed tuberculous meningitis is the newest immunodiagnostic technique to be explored; at present, however, it is useful only for preliminary clinical studies. In 1983, Sada et al. (106) reported the results of an ELISA for antigen in CSF using rabbit IgG raised against BCG; 13 of 16 CSF samples from patients with proven or presumed tuberculous meningitis were positive by this assay, whereas only one of 22 control samples was positive, from a patient with cryptococcal meningitis. Krambovits et al. (107) developed a latex agglutination test based on a rabbit immunoglobulin against a plasma membrane antigen from *M. tuberculosis.* All CSF specimens from 18 children with a clinical diagnosis of tuberculous meningitis were identified with this assay; 133 of 134 control samples were negative, with the one false positive belonging to a child with *H. influenzae* meningitis. A sensitive biotin–avidin radioimmunoassay against mycobacterial surface antigens developed by Kadival et al. (108) in 1987 demonstrated antigen in 15 of 19 individuals with untreated, clinically diagnosed tuberculous meningitis. Antigen detection by this method declined rapidly following the onset of treatment, suggesting that the assay might be used to monitor response to treatment as well as to diagnose the infection. Finally, in an effort to combine the strengths of antigen and antibody ELISAs in a single population, Watt et al. (104) evaluated the use of both in a group of 127 samples. The tests combined could identify CSF samples culture-positive for *M. tuberculosis* with a sensitivity of only 52%. An overall specificity of 96% was achieved with both tests, with the false-positive tests, again, occurring in patients with bacterial meningitis.

Immunodiagnostic techniques, then, hold some promise for rapid and sensitive diagnosis of tuberculous meningitis, although the presence of cross-reacting antibody against nonpathogenic mycobacteria, as well as the presence of bacterial or fungal antigenic moieties, may compromise their specificity. The newly developed technique of polymerase chain reaction (PCR) for detecting fragments of mycobacterial DNA in CSF appears to be an equally promising rapid diagnostic tool in preliminary trials (108a). Large-scale confirmatory studies of these techniques, as well as of their practicability in areas endemic for tuberculous meningitis, are not yet available. In addition, it must be remembered that the difficulty of confirming a diagnosis of tuberculous meningitis with more traditional laboratory evaluations renders a realistic evaluation of these new tests quite difficult (109). In the end, all premortem means of diagnosing the infection must be assumed to be fallible, and all—including the newest—must be considered in a complete clinical context.

RADIOLOGY

None of the radiologic changes seen in tuberculous meningitis are pathognomonic for the disease. Still, some are characteristic enough to raise the clinician's index of suspicion if the diagnosis is uncertain. In addition, the newer imaging techniques have proved invaluable in diagnosing and monitoring neurologic complications which may occur during treatment.

Plain radiographs of the skull are unlikely to show significant changes, particularly early in the course of disease. Rarely, the infection may extend from the subarachnoid space to destroy a paranasal sinus, the calvarium, or the base of the skull. In infants with active infection, spreading of the cranial sutures may be seen, reflecting increased intracranial pressure. During or after treatment of the infection, calcification may be identified in the basal meninges, near the pituitary fossa, or, less frequently, within the brain parenchyma (110). In large series, intracranial calcifications have been identi-

fied in 25–45% of children with long-term follow-up after treatment (111–113).

Similarly, abnormalities on radioisotope brain scans are infrequently reported. In one study, three patients with severe disease were found to have strikingly increased supra- and parasellar uptake of radionuclide, thought to reflect a particularly extensive inflammation of the basilar leptomeninges (114).

Angiographic evaluations of patients with tuberculous meningitis have been more revealing. A constellation of characteristic findings, dubbed the "angiographic triad" of tuberculous meningitis, was described by Lehrer (115) in 1966. Composing the triad are (i) a hydrocephalic pattern to the vessels, (ii) narrowing of the vessels at the base of the brain, and (iii) narrowed or occluded small and medium-sized vessels with scanty collaterals. A beaded pattern may be seen in involved vessels (Fig. 3), and aneurysms may arise from the damaged arteries (116). These changes are not invariably present: In a study of 48 children with angiography performed for hemiparesis, focal neurologic signs, or focal seizures prior to therapy, 13 patients had evidence of hydrocephalus on angiography. In 10 patients, narrowing or occlusion of some part of the carotid system could be seen, most commonly the supraclinoid portion of the internal carotid artery and the proximal portions of the anterior and middle cerebral arteries. In most patients, however, a collateral

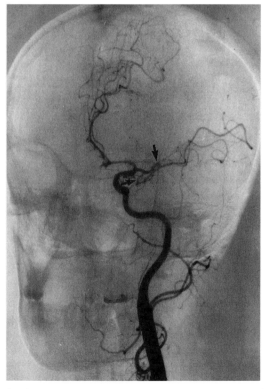

FIG. 3. Cerebral arteriogram demonstrating the type of vasculitis encountered in tuberculous meningitis. Beading of the inferior branch of the middle cerebral artery (*lower arrow*) and occlusion of a more distal branch (*upper arrow*) are demonstrated.

circulation was evident; in some cases this consisted of a weblike cluster of thin vessels at the base of the brain, and in others it consisted of transdural external–internal carotid anastomoses (117).

With the advent of computerized axial tomography (CAT), the pathologic abnormalities of the brain parenchyma, vasculature, and meninges induced by tuberculous meningitis have been made visible (Fig. 4). Hydrocephalus, a routinely described finding on CAT scan, is frequently present at diagnosis, or develops during the course of infection (118,119). With intravenous contrast administration, an enhancement of the basal cisterns results, with widening and blurring of the basilar arterial structures (120). In some cases, this enhancement may extend over the cortical surfaces, into the hemispheric fissures and cortical sinuses. Periventricular lucencies may be evident, thought to reflect the presence of periventricular tuberculous exudate and tubercle formation adjacent to the ependyma and the choroid (121). Finally, large low-density, nonenhancing areas may be seen, representing ischemic infarction in the areas of involved vessels (122).

In a study of 34 CAT scans performed on patients with tuberculous meningitis during the first month of illness, only eight scans were normal (121); 26 patients had ventricular enlargement, 22 had periventricular lucencies, and 11 had lucencies within the basal ganglia consistent with edema or infarction. Enhancement of the basal meninges was seen in nine of 14 patients given intravenous contrast. It must be emphasized that none of these CAT findings is specific for tuberculosis; in particular, hydrocephalus and the extensive basilar enhancement seen have been reported in other granulomatous CNS disease such as sarcoidosis, as well as in fungal and bacterial meningitis (123,124).

Experience is minimal with regard to the role of magnetic resonance imaging (MRI) in the radiology of tuberculous meningitis. Even without the use of intravenous contrast material, the MRI may identify basilar meningeal inflammation; when gadolinium–DTPA contrast material is used, the MRI has been reported to localize meningeal thickening, inflammation, and small tuberculoma formation with even greater precision than the CAT scan (Fig. 5), since the artifact from adjacent bone is eliminated (125,126). Large-scale studies are as yet unavailable because this technology is generally scarce in areas of high endemicity.

CENTRAL NERVOUS SYSTEM TUBERCULOMA

The pathogenesis of CNS tuberculoma is identical to that of tuberculous meningitis. Organisms lodge in the CNS during the silent hematogenous dissemination of primary infection; when cell-mediated immunity develops, small tubercles are formed. However, instead of rupturing into the subarachnoid space, the initial tubercles continue to grow, walled off from the brain parenchyma and the meninges by a dense fibrous capsule. Grossly, the lesions are gray, well-circumscribed masses whose size may vary from less than 1 cm in diameter to the size of a small orange (127). Microscopically, within the capsule the histologic changes are characteristic of tuberculosis: A caseous necrotic core is surrounded by epithelioid cells, lymphocytes, and Langhans giant cells. Occasionally, tuberculomas may develop from the enlargement of one or more meningeal tubercles, leading to a distinctive flat, adherent mass dubbed "tuberculoma en plaque" by early pathologists (128). Other pathologic variants of tuberculoma have been reported, in-

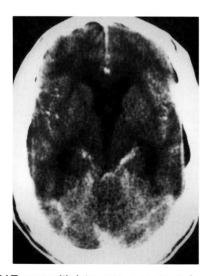

FIG. 4. CAT scan with intravenous contrast demonstrating enhancement of the basal meninges typical of tuberculous meningitis.

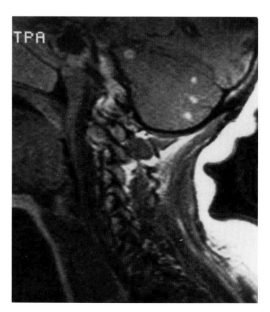

FIG. 5. Magnetic resonance imaging scan with gadolinium–DTPA enhancement demonstrating small tuberculomas in the brainstem and cerebellum in a case of tuberculous meningitis. Enhancement of the basal meninges may be seen as well.

cluding cystic tuberculomas, tuberculous brain abscesses, and an entity alternately dubbed "irregular tuberculomatosis" or "focal tuberculous meningoencephalitis"; these consist of an unencapsulated cluster of small tubercles and granulomas without caseation and are thought to represent an early stage in the development of a tuberculoma (129,130).

The epidemiology of tuberculomas parallels that of tuberculous meningitis. In the early 20th century the lesions were widely prevalent, constituting 34% of all intracranial tumors identified at autopsy in Leeds, England, from 1910 to 1931; these were seen primarily in children (8). This epidemiologic pattern persists in undeveloped countries, where tuberculoma continues to account for 15–50% of intracranial tumors seen (131). In the developed world, tuberculomas have become relatively uncommon but nonetheless persistent entities, accounting for less than 0.2% of all biopsied brain tumors seen at the Neurologic Institute in New York City between 1955 and 1980 (132).

Despite their pathogenetic and epidemiologic similarities, tuberculous meningitis and CNS tuberculoma are clinically quite separate diseases. Infrequently, tuberculomas develop during or after a course of treatment for tuberculous meningitis (133,134); similarly, tuberculous meningitis may follow the identification of a tuberculoma or may complicate its treatment (135). Largely, however, the two do not coexist: In most large clinical series of tuberculomas, tuberculous meningitis is present in less than 10% of cases (136–138). Only in older autopsy series have a majority of CNS tuberculomas been complicated by tuberculous meningitis, implying that meningitis may be a frequent terminal event in untreated cases (8).

The clinical sequelae of CNS tuberculomas are those of single or multiple intracranial mass lesions. In large series the number of identified lesions per patient has ranged from 1 to 12: Generally the majority of patients in clinical series present with single lesions; however, in those series based on autopsy data or sophisticated radiologic imaging, the proportion of patients with multiple lesions is higher, up to 70% of the total (8,139). Tuberculomas can be seen throughout the cerebral hemispheres, the basal ganglia, the cerebellum, and the brainstem. Children are said to develop infratentorial tumors more commonly than adults (136), although the determination of precise patterns of localization according to race, age, and sex has not been possible.

Symptoms are often limited to seizures and other correlates of increased intracranial pressure. Papilledema is seen in most cases, accompanied by neurologic deficits reflecting the location of the lesions (136,140,141). Fever and signs of systemic infection are rarely present, and patients generally appear quite well (142). Symptoms are frequently, although not always, chronic and slowly progressive: Mean duration of symptoms in most series is measured in weeks or months (141,143), although dura-

tion as short as 10 days and as long as 9 years have been reported (140). Some observers note that the patient's symptoms are less dramatic than would be expected from the radiologic or surgical size of the lesion, a finding they feel is pathognomonic for tuberculoma among mass lesions of the CNS (144).

Like their presentation, the laboratory evaluation of tuberculoma patients is usually quite nonspecific. Most standard clinical laboratory tests, including erythrocyte sedimentation rate, are unable to distinguish between tuberculomas and CNS neoplasm (126,136). CSF analysis is generally unavailable in these patients because lumbar puncture cannot safely be performed. When obtained, CSF may show an elevated protein concentration but is usually otherwise unremarkable (141). Search for evidence of prior or concurrent tuberculosis may be more fruitful for diagnosis: Recent series have documented tuberculin positivity in 50–85% of patients diagnosed from both endemic and nonendemic areas (138,144,145). Between 33% and 80% of individuals with tuberculoma may have chest radiographic evidence of tuberculosis (126,138,139), although a history of previously diagnosed tuberculosis is usually available in less than 50% of patients.

Until the advent of CAT scanning, the radiologic evaluation of tuberculomas was also quite nonspecific. Calcification of the lesions is agreed to be rare, usually noted in considerably less than 20% of cases (126,137,138); however, it is perhaps more frequent in chronic, "healing" lesions (143). Changes seen on plain skull radiographs are thus usually limited to those associated with elevated intracranial pressure. Angiography may demonstrate an avascular tumor with focal vessel narrowing, with or without a tumor blush; enlarged meningeal vessels or displacement of the other cerebral vessels may simulate a meningioma (142,146,147). Isotope brain scans will often, although not always, reflect the tumor as an area of markedly abnormal isotope uptake (137,148).

On CAT scanning, the appearance of the lesions is more characteristic, although still variable. The tuberculoma may appear as an isodense or hypodense area with uniform contrast enhancement; more typically, with high-resolution scanning, a thick ring of contrast enhancement may surround a characteristic punctate central clearing, signaling the presence of caseation within the lesion (Fig. 6) (149). Older lesions may calcify into high-attenuation areas with little enhancement. Surrounding edema may or may not be present. None of these patterns is sufficient to distinguish tuberculomas from other neoplastic or infectious space-occupying lesions. The little clinical experience with the MRI scanner in tuberculoma indicates that this technology may be similarly nonspecific in this infection: A tuberculoma has appeared as a discrete area of increased signal on MRI, consistent with a glioma (150).

As in tuberculous meningitis, the gold standard of diagnosis for tuberculoma remains histologic. Bacterio-

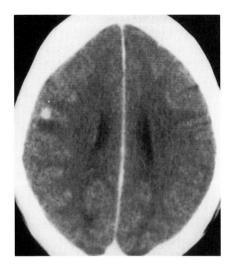

FIG. 6. CAT scan with intravenous contrast in a patient with tuberculous meningitis demonstrating a small enhancing tuberculoma in the left parietal region.

logic confirmation of the infection is often absent. Approximately 60% of tissue specimens from tuberculomas have been smear-positive for acid-fast bacilli, and generally 50–60% of specimens will grow the organism in culture. The presence of caseating granulomata and consistent cellular morphology, on the other hand, is invariable and is usually considered firm evidence of the presence of the infection.

Before effective antituberculous chemotherapy was available, the only possible treatment of tuberculoma was surgical. Mortality rates of both decompression and resection procedures generally exceeded 50%, with the bulk of postoperative deaths being caused by tuberculous meningitis (136,140,141). Powerful chemotherapy has given surgical intervention a decreasing role in the management of these infections. High-dose steroids have been used successfully to reduce the symptoms of increased intracranial pressure, with no reported incidence of overwhelming tuberculous infection. Unlike malignant tumors of the CNS, tuberculomas appear to grow without permanently destroying the surrounding neural tissue, thus enabling a good clinical recovery. In a recent study, patients treated with medical treatment alone tended to achieve significantly better functional recoveries than did those in whom surgical exploration preceded the institution of antituberculous therapy (144). Surgical exploration may be useful to establish the diagnosis and rule out concomitant bacterial infection (138). However, with good clinical and radiologic response to antimicrobial therapy (sequential studies have demonstrated a CAT resolution of lesions as early as 12 weeks after the beginning of treatment), surgery is no longer required (145).

Tuberculous Brain Abscess

When the caseous core of a tuberculoma liquefies, a tuberculous abscess will result. These lesions are rare: Of

201 tuberculomas surgically explored by Arseni (136) over a 16-year period, only one contained pus; a relatively recent survey identified only 17 cases of confirmed tuberculous brain abscesses in the medical literature through 1978 (151). Clinically, these patients are considerably more toxic than patients with tuberculomas. The duration of their symptoms is generally less than 1 week. They present with fever, headaches, and focal neurologic deficits. Of the cases reported in the literature, 35% of patients were ultimately found to have multiple intracranial abscesses (up to 100 in one individual) identified at surgery or autopsy. As in cases of tuberculoma, radiologic and other diagnostic tests are unable to distinguish definitively between these and bacterial brain abscesses (152). The treatment of tuberculous abscesses has not been as clearly addressed as that of tuberculoma. Of the 17 cases in the literature, the only survivors were those who received both medical and surgical treatment, even though the incidence of postoperative tuberculous meningitis was high and often a cause of death.

SPINAL CORD DISEASE

The spectrum of tuberculous spinal cord disease has been elucidated relatively recently. Although intraspinal tuberculoma was reported in the 18th century (152a) in 1830 and spinal block was a frequently recognized complication of intracranial infection, it was not until the late 1940s that investigators began to recognize that the same pathology seen within the cranium was occasionally re-created exclusively within the parenchyma and meninges of the cord. As in intracranial disease, the lesions described have fallen into two categories: (i) space-occupying lesions of the cord or spinal meninges and (ii) more diffuse inflammatory arachnoiditis analogous to typical intracranial meningitis.

The inflammatory spinal disease caused by *M. tuberculosis* has been variously called "spinal meningitis," "spinal arachnoiditis," and "spinal radiculomyelitis" over the last 40 years. Its first clinical description was contained in a 1947 report, by Ransome and Montiero (153), of four adults who presented with urinary retention, flaccid paresis of the legs, and rising sensory deficits before developing a more typical clinical picture of tuberculous meningitis. At autopsy the brains of the patients showed findings typical for tuberculous meningitis, while the spinal cords "looked as if a yellow jelly had been poured into the subarachnoid spaces and allowed to set" (153). This graphic pathologic entity had not previously been reported in standard reference works up to that time.

Subsequent investigations made it clear that this spinal pathology could complicate the course of treatment of tuberculous meningitis, could precede it, or could occur alone in the absence of overt intracranial disease. The reasons for its delayed recognition remains unclear; many factors have been cited, primarily the change in the natural history of tuberculous meningitis from a rapidly fatal to a chronic and curable disease. The role of intrathecal streptomycin as a cause of diffuse subarachnoid inflammation, once thought responsible for a great deal of this pathology, is now generally discounted.

Most investigators have agreed that the pathophysiology of spinal meningitis is analogous to that of tuberculous meningitis: A submeningeal tubercle formed during primary infection ruptures into the subarachnoid space and elicits all the mediators of delayed hypersensitivity. As in intracranial disease, a thick tuberculous exudate fills the subarachnoid space, frequently extending into the subdural space as well. The exudate characteristically extends over many segments of the cord: One report (154) stated that it was "so plentiful that in effect the cord and its membranes formed a structure almost solid throughout its length." Although generally circumferential, the exudate is occasionally noted to be particularly prominent posteriorly, a phenomenon some observers have ascribed to gravitational pull in a patient supine for a long period of time (155). As in intracranial disease, its microscopic appearance consists of granulomatous inflammation, areas of caseation, and tubercles, with the development of fibrous tissue in chronic or treated disease. Calcification within the exudate has not been reported. Acid-fast organisms are almost invariably absent from biopsy and autopsy specimens, possibly the result of prior antituberculous therapy. Diagnosis is generally based on the characteristic tuberculous histologic patterns alone.

Accompanying the extensive spinal exudate are characteristic vasculitic changes, as well as secondary effects on the cord parenchyma. As in tuberculous meningitis, vessels traversing the exudate are subject to medial and subintimal tuberculous changes, with fibrosis and thrombotic occlusion. The vasculitis may be limited or extensive; it has been reported to be less prominent in arteries than in veins. In contrast to intracranial disease, sudden arterial obstruction with spinal cord infarction, although reported, is uncommon (156); its rarity is thought to reflect the extensive anastomotic network present in the spinal circulation (154). The damage to the cord parenchyma, however, is no less extensive than that seen in the brain. Changes include: an edematous sponginess of the white matter (especially in the lateral columns), thought to be secondary to venous congestion; zones of demyelination with degeneration of axons and honeycombing of the parenchyma; circumscribed central necrosis secondary to an ischemic myelomalacia; and, ultimately, a withering away of the cord tissue, with glial cell replacement. The nerve roots, although grossly compressed, are usually not infiltrated by exudate (155).

In the few clinical reports available, the presentation of spinal radiculomyelopathy is variable. In a series of 80 patients with tuberculous meningitis, Brooks et al. (154) reported 11 episodes of a transverse myelitis syndrome in 10 patients. In eight of them the development of a spinal block preceded the syndrome, diagnosed by a persistently absent Queckenstedt's sign and a Froin's syndrome (xanthochromia, elevated protein content, and absence of cells) documented in multiple CSF samples. The paralysis was generally flaccid, developing in most patients over hours to days. Motor findings exceeded sensory ones; root pain was present in only 50% of cases. These patients had a significantly lower survival than did patients in this series in whom spinal cord involvement was not documented. In 18 similar patients reported by Wadia and Dastur (157), clinical evidence of cord disease followed a diagnosis of tuberculous meningitis by 1 week to 8 years. Motor deficits were again prominent in these patients; root pain was absent. Most patients had evidence of spinal block on sequential lumbar punctures. Clinical findings suggested a lesion of the thoracic cord in 10 patients, the upper lumbar cord in seven, and the cervical cord in one.

The clinical course of spinal tuberculosis in the absence of tuberculous meningitis has been characterized most fully by Wadia and Dastur (155,157) in 33 individuals with an initial diagnosis of "idiopathic radiculomyelitis." Nineteen of them ultimately had biopsy or autopsy results consistent with a tuberculous process; in the rest the diagnosis was presumptive. The major clinical features, each present in approximately two-thirds of the patients, were root pain, paresthesias, and motor weakness with mixed upper- and lower-motoneuron signs. In some patients the onset of the syndrome was sudden; in others a slower, ascending paralysis progressed over months to years. Fever and systemic malaise were seen in less than 50% of patients, usually in those with a rapid onset of symptoms. Sensory levels were seen in 21 of 33 patients, most commonly in a thoracic dermatome.

No CSF could be obtained by lumbar puncture in 6 of 33 patients. In the others an elevated protein was uniformly seen, exceeding 1000 mg% in 50% of patients. Hypoglycorrhachia was present in only 33% of specimens. A lymphocytic pleocytosis was present in approximately 50%. Myelography performed in all cases revealed a partial spinal block in 6 of 31 cases and a complete block in the rest. The edge of the block was ragged or tapered in appearance, with filling defects extending over as many as 14 vertebral segments. The extensive disease demonstrated on myelogram, often clinically unsuspected, rendered surgical intervention difficult to orchestrate: The site for optimal decompression of the cord was often unclear, and, in fact, after several attempts the authors became convinced that even with localized disease, effective decompression was impossible because of extensive arachnoid adhesions. Nonetheless, the difficulty of establishing a diagnosis without tissue made surgical exploration and biopsy necessary for management in many cases.

Systemic steroid therapy and a prolonged course of antimycobacterial treatment led to marked symptomatic improvement in 7 of 13 patients. The best response was generally seen in those with a rapid onset of relatively localized disease, in whom therapy was begun soon after diagnosis. Similar responses to medical therapy have been reported in subsequent series. Anecdotal reports have suggested the utility of adding steroids to the treatment regimen when the syndrome develops during a course of antituberculous therapy for meningitis. Nonetheless, no controlled study has conclusively supported the use of steroid therapy in this syndrome (156,158).

Space-Occupying Lesions in the Spinal Canal

As in the brain, tubercles seeded through the cord or its membranes may enlarge to cause clinically significant disease. Tuberculomas occur both within the cord parenchyma and within the dural space. In addition, epidural tuberculous granulomas encasing and compressing the cord may develop, either in conjunction with tuberculous osteomyelitis of a vertebral body (Fig. 7) or as isolated disease (156).

Of these space-occupying lesions, the most common are the intramedullary tuberculomas of the cord, yet even these are rare. In large autopsy series, spinal tuberculomas are estimated to be 15–50 times less common than those occurring within the cranium (159). Slightly over 100 cases have been reported in the literature (160). As in the brain, these tumors are well-encapsulated, with clinical symptoms identical to those of other spinal cord tumors. In many cases pulmonary tuberculosis accompanies the lesion, while in others no sign of prior or current tuberculosis can be found. Plain spine films are negative. Myelography was necessary for diagnosis until the onset of the newer imaging techniques: MRI scanning has recently been demonstrated to be useful in identifying two cervical tuberculomas with markedly low intensity signal relative to spinal cord (161).

Surgical resection has been the treatment of choice for these tumors; no experience is available with medical treatment alone. In some cases the tuberculoma is easily enucleated, while in others which are adherent to the cord, subtotal resection followed by antimycobacterial treatment for a year has resulted in almost complete recovery (162).

TREATMENT

Until 1945, tuberculous meningitis was a fatal disease. Occasional reports of spontaneous cure were invariably associated with the atypical serous meningitis (see above). In 1945, streptomycin was introduced into clinical practice, initiating two decades of rapid progress in the successful chemotherapy of the disease. However, as one powerful antituberculous agent after another became available, worldwide approaches to therapy diverged into a tangle of therapeutic alternatives that still persists. Today, although the spectacular reduction achieved in the morbidity and mortality of tuberculous meningitis ranks among the triumphs of the antibiotic era, there remains no consensus as to the best treatment regimen for this disease. Optimal drugs, doses and routes of administration, optimal duration of treatment, and indications for adjuvant agents all remain undefined. Meanwhile, the relative rarity of the disease in developed countries generally precludes the expensive large-scale studies that would be necessary to resolve these questions.

Chemotherapy

In modern clinical practice, the principles guiding the treatment of tuberculous meningitis do not differ greatly from those for other forms of tuberculosis. Chemotherapy must be directed against both intracellular and extracellular organisms; use of multiple drugs is necessary

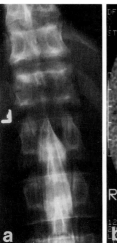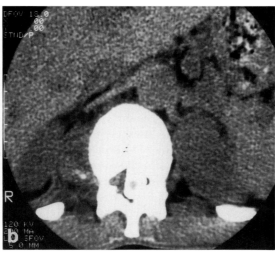

FIG. 7. (a) Myelogram demonstrating complete epidural block at T12 in a patient with tuberculous osteomyelitis of the thoracolumbar spine. (b) On CAT scan, vertebral and paraspinal foci of infections are evident, as is a large epidural mass compressing the thoracic spinal cord. Histologic section of the resected epidural mass revealed caseating granulomas and acid-fast bacilli.

to prevent the otherwise inevitable emergence of resistance. Available drugs are divided on the basis of efficacy and toxicity into first-line and second-line agents, as for other forms of the disease. Nonetheless, it should be remembered that the enormous load of mycobacteria present in cavitary lesions often has no equivalent in CNS disease. In the lung, therapy must eradicate large numbers of extracellular mycobacteria in pulmonary cavities; in the CNS, however, antimycobacterial agents must penetrate the blood–brain barrier in concentrations sufficient to eliminate smaller numbers of intracellular and extracellular organisms (Table 8).

First-Line Drugs

Isoniazid

After being introduced in 1952, isoniazid (INH) quickly became the mainstay of chemotherapy for all forms of tuberculous infection. It is active against both intracellular and extracellular organisms, in both actively growing and resting stages. Most strains of *M. tuberculosis* are inhibited *in vitro* by 0.025–0.05 μg/ml of the drug, whereas peak plasma concentrations after an oral dose generally range from 3 to 5 μg/ml (163). CNS penetration of INH is good: When the meninges are not inflamed, CSF concentrations are 15–25% of simultaneous plasma concentrations; however, in the presence of tuberculous meningitis, CSF concentrations equaling 90% of serum concentrations have been documented (164,165).

INH is well-absorbed orally, although a parenteral preparation is available. The recommended dose for children is 10 mg/kg daily, whereas adults generally receive 300 mg daily. In the presence of CNS disease, the same dose recommendations generally apply, although some clinicians are accustomed to administering 10 mg/kg/day to severely ill adult patients during the initial phase of treatment. Side effects consist most commonly of hepatotoxicity which runs the gamut from asymptomatic enzyme elevations to fulminant hepatic necrosis. Neurotoxicity is a less frequent occurrence. Peripheral neuropathy may occur during INH therapy if pyridoxine

is not administered with the drug; in addition, INH overdose is manifested by confusion, seizures, and coma. Furthermore, INH interacts with diphenylhydantoin. In patients receiving both, serum concentrations of both are elevated, often resulting in dilantin toxicity (166).

Rifampin

Rifampin was introduced into clinical use in the early 1970s. It is bactericidal against both intracellular and extracellular organisms, with minimum inhibitory concentrations ranging from 0.005 to 0.2 μg/ml. Peak serum concentration after an oral dose of 600 mg in an adult is approximately 7 μg/ml, with considerable variation among individuals (167). In the presence of meningeal inflammation, CSF concentrations approaching 20% of serum concentrations have been achieved (168). As inflammation resolves, however, CSF concentrations appear to decline, and the drug may not be evident in the CSF in the presence of normal meninges (169).

Rifampin is well-absorbed orally; an intravenous form of the drug can be obtained as well. A dose of 10–20 mg/kg/day is recommended for children, whereas adults generally receive 10 mg/kg to a maximum of 600 mg daily. No dosage adjustments are necessary for CNS disease. Side effects of rifampin are generally infrequent, consisting of renal, hepatic, and hematologic toxicities as well as a flu-like syndrome and hypersensitivity reactions seen most commonly with intermittent treatment regimens. In addition, several series have noted that up to one-third of patients with tuberculous meningitis receiving INH- and rifampin-containing regimens developed presumedly drug-related hepatotoxicity (47,170, 171), a rate nearly 10 times the frequency of hepatotoxicity seen in other patients. In most cases, the reaction subsided when rifampin was stopped. The mechanism behind these observations has not been clarified.

Pyrazinamide

Originally regarded as second-line therapy because of significant hepatotoxicity at higher doses, pyrazinamide at lower doses has become a first-line agent over the last

TABLE 8. *Penetration of antimycobacterial agents into the CSF*

Agent (refs.)	Usual daily dose	Range of mean peak concentrations (μg/ml)		
		Serum	CSF, normal meninges	CSF, inflamed meninges
Isoniazid (163–165)	5–10 mg/kg/day	3.0–5.0	0.6–1.6	2.0
Rifampin (165,167–169)	10–20 mg/kg/day	0.4–12.0	0	0.4–1.0
Ethambutol (174–176)	15–25 mg/kg/day	1.0–7.7	0	0.5–2.5
Pyrazinamide (165)	20–35 mg/kg/day	45–50		50[a]
Streptomycin (163,165,179)	15–40 mg/kg/day	25–50	Trace	9

[a] Following a dose of 50 mg/kg.

10 years. Active only at a slightly acid pH, it completely inhibits the growth of organisms contained within the cytoplasm of phagocytes, although it is inactive against extracellular organisms. A 1-g oral dose produces plasma concentrations of approximately 45 μg/ml; a concentration of 12.5 μg/ml is bactericidal against intracellular organisms (163). Penetration into the CSF is excellent, with concentrations equaling serum concentrations in the presence of meningeal inflammation (165).

The doses originally in clinical use, up to 50 mg/kg/day, produced hepatic toxicity in approximately 15% of recipients. With the presently recommended doses of 20–35 mg/kg/day, the incidence of hepatotoxicity is considerably lower. Although only limited data are available, there appears to be little additive hepatotoxicity when pyrazinamide is added to a regimen of INH and rifampin for tuberculous meningitis, even if the three drugs are continued together for up to 1 year (172).

Ethambutol

Ethambutol, a tuberculostatic drug developed in the early 1960s, has become a widely used addition to otherwise tuberculocidal regimens. Of tested strains of *M. tuberculosis,* approximately 70% are inhibited by concentrations of 1 μg/ml of the drug, with the remainder being inhibited by concentrations of 5 μg/ml (173). Following a dose of 25 mg/kg, peak serum concentrations range from 1 to 8 μg/ml, with a mean of 4 μg/ml; with a dose of 15 mg/kg, average serum concentrations are 1.8–1.9 μg/ml. CSF penetration of the drug in the presence of meningeal inflammation is good, with concentrations ranging from 10% to 50% of simultaneous serum concentrations, most over 1 μg/ml (174). In the absence of meningeal inflammation, the penetration of ethambutol into the CSF appears minimal (175,176).

Ethambutol is administered orally, at doses of 15 or 25 mg/kg/day. At the higher dose, approximately 5% of patients will develop an optic neuritis, heralded by diminished visual acuity and loss of color perception; at the lower dose, the incidence of this important side effect of the drug is approximately 1%. Some clinicians have thus chosen to reserve the higher dose of the drug for the first few months of therapy of tuberculous meningitis, completing the course of treatment with the lower dose, with acceptable clinical results (177).

Streptomycin

Although this pioneering drug has been supplanted to a large extent by more efficacious, less toxic therapy, streptomycin retains a role in the treatment of tuberculous meningitis. Whereas *in vitro* this drug is bactericidal against *M. tuberculosis, in vivo* it appears to be bacteriostatic, with activity against extracellular organisms only. Most strains are inhibited by concentrations of 10 μg/ml

or less. Serum concentrations following an intramuscular dose of 1 g in an adult persist above 20 μg/ml for a 24-hr period (178). Penetration of the drug into the CSF in the absence of meningeal inflammation is minimal; however, in the presence of meningitis, CSF concentrations may approach 25% of blood concentrations (179,180).

Streptomycin must be administered parenterally; children receive 20–40 mg/kg/day, whereas the usual adult dose is 1 g daily. Ototoxicity is the most prominent side effect, more commonly manifesting as vestibular disturbances than as deafness. Both total dose of drug and excessively high serum concentrations appear to be risk factors for the development of vestibular toxicity; although children may be able to compensate almost fully for vestibular dysfunction, older individuals are more prone to develop this irreversible toxicity from streptomycin, and less able to compensate for it, than children. In most antituberculous regimens the drug is administered daily during the first weeks of therapy; the frequency of administration is then reduced to two or three times a week, allowing for closely monitored outpatient treatment regimens. Intrathecal administration of streptomycin, once an integral part of most antituberculous chemotherapeutic regimens, is now an outmoded form of therapy.

Second-Line Drugs

A number of drugs with antituberculous activity have been consigned to second-line status by virtue of toxicity, limited efficacy, or difficulty of administration. Although treatment regimens for tuberculous meningitis can generally be constructed from first-line alternatives, multiply resistant organisms or intolerance to multiple antibiotics will occasionally necessitate the use of these agents. As with first-line agents, the ability of these drugs to penetrate the CNS varies. Para-aminosalicylic acid (PAS), once widely used in the treatment of tuberculous meningitis, does not achieve concentrations in the CSF in the presence of uninflamed meninges (181). Ethionamide penetrates the CSF well both in the presence and absence of inflammation, with concentrations approximating blood concentrations (182). Cycloserine penetrates equally well, although its considerable neurotoxicity generally precludes its use in infections of the CNS. Kanamycin and amikacin, both aminoglycoside antibiotics with antimycobacterial activity, reach minimal CSF concentrations in the absence of meningeal inflammation; however, in the presence of inflammation, CSF concentrations may be somewhat higher (178).

Treatment Regimens

A variety of chemotherapeutic regimens have been proposed for tuberculous meningitis, generally extrapolated from treatment of other forms of tuberculosis (Table 9). In all modern regimens, isoniazid and rifampin are the mainstays of treatment. In addition, more recent regimens have taken advantage of the newly appreciated merits of pyrazinamide for intracellular microbicidal action. The American Thoracic Society (183) now recommends the following treatment for all forms of tuberculosis, including meningitis: a 6-month regimen consisting of 2 months of INH, rifampin, and pyrazinamide, followed by 4 months of INH and rifampin daily or twice weekly. If pyrazinamide cannot be used as a third drug in cases of CNS disease, some authorities would substitute ethambutol or streptomycin for at least the first several months of therapy (184,185). Others would use all four drugs at the onset of treatment, particularly in cases of suspected drug resistance (69). Other variations include continuing INH alone for several months following 6 or 9 months of combined chemotherapy (186), or continuing INH and rifampin for a total of 12 months (69). The increased efficacy of these therapeutic variations is unproven. Finally, in 1982 Dutt et al. (187) demonstrated that INH and rifampin administered alone for a "short course" of 9 months' treatment was successful in more than 300 patients with a variety of forms of extrapulmonary tuberculosis. Eighteen cases of meningitis were included in this series, receiving daily treatment with the two drugs for the first month, followed by twice-weekly treatment for the following 8 months. Although some early deaths due to tuberculous meningitis occurred on this regimen, no late failures or

TABLE 9. *Chemotherapeutic options for tuberculous meningitis in adults*

Drug	Dose	Frequency	Duration
Low probability of drug resistance (183,185,187)			
A. Isoniazid	300 mg	Daily	6 months
Rifampin	600 mg	Daily	6 months
Pyrazinamide	15–30 mg/kg	Daily	2 months
B. Isoniazid	300 mg	Daily	9 months
Rifampin	600 mg	Daily	9 months
Ethambutol or	25 mg/kg	Daily	2 months
Streptomycin	1 g	Daily	2 months
C. Isoniazid	300 mg	Daily	1 month
	900 mg	Twice weekly	8 months
Rifampin	600 mg	Daily	1 month
	600 mg	Twice weekly	8 months
High probability of drug resistance (69)			
A. Isoniazid	300 mg	Daily	1 year
Rifampin	600 mg	Daily	1 year
Pyrazinamide	15–30 mg/kg	Daily	2 months
Ethambutol or	25 mg/kg	Daily	2 months
Streptomycin	1 g	Daily	2 months

B. In cases of documented drug resistance, chemotherapy must be tailored to demonstrated sensitivities.

relapses were seen. Many clinicians, nonetheless, are unwilling to initiate treatment of CNS disease with only two drugs, particularly in the setting of profound neurologic compromise or the possibility of drug resistance.

Drug-Resistant Organisms

Primary drug resistance in isolates of *M. tuberculosis* has been recognized for decades: Among large populations of organisms, approximately 1 of every 10^5 to 10^6 organisms will be resistant to individual antituberculous drugs prior to chemotherapy. Secondary drug resistance may thus develop on chemotherapy, if compliance with a multiple drug regimen is poor. When resistant organisms infect another individual, clinical disease with primarily drug-resistant organisms may result. Although relatively rare in the United States (occurring in fewer than 5% of primary isolates), clinical disease with resistant organisms occurs with higher frequency among certain populations. Among them are: immigrants from countries in Asia, Africa, and the Americas with a high prevalence of drug resistance; known contacts of drug-resistant cases; homeless and impoverished individuals; and residents of certain geographic areas in the United States, particularly those adjacent to the Mexican border (188).

Among series of patients with tuberculous meningitis, occasional cases of drug-resistant disease have been identified. In 1973, Steiner and Portugaleza (43) reported three cases of INH and/or streptomycin resistance among 25 children with tuberculous meningitis in Brooklyn, New York. Of these three, two died despite treatment and one survived after a regimen composed of first- and second-line drugs. In areas of high prevalence of resistance, then, anticipation of this phenomenon in cases of tuberculous meningitis may be lifesaving. Therapy with four bactericidal drugs is widely recommended until sensitivity testing allows therapy to be more finely tailored, with continuation of at least two agents to which the organism is demonstrated sensitive. A full 18–24 months of treatment is often advocated (188).

Mortality and Prognosis

Most available data on the course and prognosis of treated tuberculous meningitis derives from series of patients treated from 1946 through 1970. Although today's specific treatment regimens are different, the patterns previously identified in the course of response to treatment remain valid. A rapid reduction in mortality was documented during the years spanning the introductions of streptomycin and INH. With regimens containing streptomycin alone, most studies reported long-term survival in from 25–50% of cases (39,189–191), with varying rates of relapse. With the introduction of PAS, rates of survival often climbed to 50% or more (190,192), whereas the INH-containing regimens in routine use since 1952 yielded overall survival rates which usually exceeded 70% (192,193). Survival rates of 70–80% are observed in the most recent clinical studies.

Despite these trends related to chemotherapy, it was evident from the earliest studies of response to treatment that certain prognostic factors exerted powerful influences on outcome of individual cases. These have endured despite changing details of treatment. The most firmly established of these has been the clinical stage of disease at the start of treatment, as first defined by the British Medical Research Council (39) in 1948. This group documented a twofold increase in mortality when treatment was initiated in the advanced stage, as opposed to the early stage, of the disease. This correlation between neurologic compromise at the initiation of treatment and mortality has been redocumented repeatedly in patients of all ages.

Other prognostic factors correlating with poor response to treatment in tuberculous meningitis and enduring over the last 30 years have included extremes of youth or old age (44,53,189,191,193–195) and coexistence of miliary disease (189,190,193). In several studies, race has been a significant predictor of outcome: In some, black patients appeared to respond considerably better to treatment than did whites (192,194), whereas in others the reverse was true (196). No clear-cut conclusions can be drawn from these disparate results. Some clinicians have noted that tuberculous meningitis developing in pregnancy or during the puerperium may have a particularly bad outcome (197–199). Diagnostic parameters correlating with response to treatment in some (but not all) studies have included markedly elevated protein in the CNS, spinal block (195), and markedly decreased CSF glucose (190). None of these prognostic factors has been formally established as an independent predictor of mortality.

Course of Treated Disease

The early treatment studies also provided insight into the expected course of successfully treated tuberculous meningitis. A characteristic worsening in CSF parameters was noted by many clinicians immediately following the institution of antituberculous drugs, with the appearance of bacilli on previously negative CSF smears and a rise in CSF protein. This paradoxical response was felt to be so characteristic of tuberculous meningitis that some felt serious doubt was cast on the diagnosis when it failed to appear (200,201). An analogous phenomenon has been described in the medical treatment of cerebral tuberculoma, with enlargement of the lesion documented on sequential CAT scanning prior to ultimate clinical cure (202).

Clinical parameters were similarly often slow to respond to chemotherapy: Weight gain and improvement in well-being were often initial signs of recovery, although spiking fever often persisted for a month or more following initiation of ultimately successful treatment. Lepper and Spies (193) first documented the usual pattern of CSF recovery in successfully treated cases: In their series, among patients treated with INH, CSF glucose returned to normal in about 50% of treated patients within 2 months and in the vast majority by 6 months; CSF leukocytosis took over 6 months to resolve in more than 25% of patients, whereas CSF protein was slowest to return to normal, remaining elevated in 40% of patients for more than 6 months. This pattern of resolution of tuberculous infection has been consistently redocumented in subsequent studies (48).

Sequelae

The steep decline in mortality from tuberculous meningitis has been paralleled by a steep rise in the number of survivors with varying neurologic sequelae. In an early series of children treated without INH, only 64% of survivors were completely "normal"; the others were left with mild-to-marked neurologic damage (21%) or eighth-nerve damage thought to be caused by streptomycin (15%) (189). Like mortality, occurrence of sequelae appeared to correlate with stage of disease at presentation: Patients with early disease were five times more likely to recover completely than those with advanced disease. In a subsequent series which included survivors of INH-containing regimens, 77% were subjectively normal (111). The age at which meningitis occurred appeared an important prognosticator of sequelae in this series, with the most severe neurologic sequelae occurring in children who became ill at less than 2 years of age. Other series of tuberculous meningitis among children have documented moderate-to-severe neurologic sequelae in more than 50% of long-term survivors (42).

Among adults, percentage of neurologic handicaps varies similarly from 0% to more than 50% of survivors (46,48,49,55,192). As in pediatric patients, advanced stage of infection prior to treatment appears to correlate with a higher incidence of neurologic sequelae. Age and use of an INH-containing treatment regimen appear irrelevant to incidence of sequelae among adults.

The nature of the sequelae of tuberculous meningitis has been described to encompass both the neurologic and the psychiatric. Children may sustain various degrees of intellectual and emotional impairment, ranging from mild to profound and possibly related to long periods of hospitalization rather than to the disease itself (111,112,203). Among the neurologic sequelae, most common in children is generally a spastic hemiparesis, followed by seizure disorders, ataxia and mild incoordination, and, rarely, persistent cranial nerve palsies (113,191). It has been estimated that slightly more than 50% of children with seizures during the course of meningitis will be left with a seizure disorder (200).

Adult survivors most frequently are left with a chronic organic brain syndrome, followed by cranial nerve palsies (usually of the sixth nerve), paraplegia, and hemiparesis (49,192). Atrophy of the optic nerve, leading to degrees of visual impairment and complete blindness in some cases, has been seen in both children and adults (204,205). Disturbances of eighth-nerve function, once the single most common neurologic sequela of tuberculous meningitis, has decreased considerably in frequency as streptomycin has been supplanted by alternative agents (206). Finally, a variety of endocrinologic abnormalities have been documented in survivors of tuberculous meningitis, including diabetes insipidus (207), chronic hypothermia (208), and both delayed and precocious sexual development (111,112), all thought to result from arteritis or late calcification and subsequent infarction in close proximity to the hypothalamus and the pituitary gland.

Steroids and Other Adjuvants

Interest in treating CNS tuberculosis by maneuvering the immune response to the infection predated the development of antituberculous drugs by many years (209). The persistent morbidity and mortality despite the development of effective antibacterial chemotherapy has only intensified the search for additional treatment agents. Whereas bacterial growth may be halted with adequate chemotherapy, inflammation often continues at the base of the brain, with organization of necrotic tissue and exudate, fibroblastic proliferation, and formation of dense fibrocollagenous tissue compressing adjacent structures and impeding spinal fluid circulation. Similar destructive healing may take place in major cerebral blood vessels. These events, rather than the active infection itself, are often responsible for mortality during treatment as well as for the permanent neurologic sequelae of the disease.

Numerous substances have been employed as adjuvant chemotherapy in tuberculous meningitis over the years. Some provoked only brief clinical interest before prohibitive side effects or clear lack of efficacy curtailed their further use: In the 1950s heparin, streptokinase, streptodornase, and pancreatic ribonuclease were all tried and discarded as potential adjuvants (210–212). Other agents have continued to receive intermittent attention: Recently, hyaluronidase, an enzyme that breaks down the glucosaminidic bonds of hyaluronic acid in ground substance, was administered to 15 patients with hydrocephalus or optochiasmatic arachnoiditis from tuberculous meningitis, with results superior to those of shunt surgery (213). The most persistently advocated adjuvants are adrenal corticosteroids and various forms of tuberculoprotein. Both have inspired fervent advocacy among some investigators and scorn among others; neither has been proven efficacious in definitive trials.

Work with PPD as adjuvant therapy in tuberculous meningitis was pioneered by investigators at the Radcliffe Infirmary in Oxford, England, after two "hopeless" cases of meningitis recovered with this therapy and after autopsy in others showed virtually complete absence of the expected basilar exudate. The "intrathecal tuberculin reaction" provoked by intrathecally administered PPD, with its outpouring of immune mediators into the CSF and meninges, was felt to hasten the resolution of exudate and to facilitate the penetration of antituberculous drugs into the CSF. The extreme clinical symptomatology evoked by this intervention—fever, headache, and systemic toxity—was felt to be worth the price of ultimate therapeutic efficacy (191,214). No convincing animal experiments were available to support this theory, however, and no controlled clinical trials were ever done. Nonetheless, a large series of cases refractory to other forms of treatment, and apparently salvaged by the administration of intrathecal PPD, accumulated over the years. Although intrathecal PPD is now dismissed as being unnecessarily complicated and dangerous (as well as being outdated by potent chemotherapy), its utility in averting or resolving serious neurologic sequelae of disease has never been definitively disproved.

Adrenal corticosteroids were first proposed for use in tuberculous meningitis in the early 1950s on a diametrically opposed theoretical basis (215). The ability of steroids to curtail host defenses in tuberculosis had been proven in animal models (216). It was reasoned that in conjunction with specific antibacterial therapy, both overwhelming tuberculous infection and the deleterious clinical effects of cell-mediated immunity might be avoided. And, in fact, rabbits with established tuberculous meningitis treated with both INH and cortisone showed a marked decrease in leptomeningeal inflammation when compared to animals treated with antituberculous drugs alone, with resolution of all exudative subarachnoid block (217). In humans, improved survival and neurologic function, particularly in advanced cases, was the hoped-for analogy.

Despite a substantial literature accumulated over the past 30 years, the place of steroids in the treatment of tuberculous meningitis remains unclear. Case reports and small clinical trials can be found to support any result claimed for them, from an ability to work miracles (218–220) to uselessness and potential toxicity (193–195,221). The most coherent and best-controlled studies can be interpreted to indicate that in certain defined circumstances, steroids may have a place in treatment of CNS tuberculosis, although not without a potential price.

Certain points regarding the use of steroids in tuberculous meningitis are established. Their ability to abrogate signs and symptoms of the disease, even in the face of persistent infection, has been repeatedly demonstrated. Patients frequently defervesce, with clearing of sensorium and improvement in well-being, after only a few doses. Equally well documented is the existence of a steroid-withdrawal phenomenon, in which all the initial symptomatology of the disease returns after a course of steroids is stopped, even in the face of continued antituberculous therapy and a carefully tapered steroid dose. If steroids are not reinstituted, months may elapse before the patient regains the clinical status originally achieved with a few days of steroid treatment (219,222).

CSF parameters shown to be significantly affected by steroid treatment include opening pressure, protein content, and leukocyte count; these indices also may worsen when steroids are discontinued. Decreased penetration of some antituberculous agents as meningeal inflammation subsides is a frequently cited potential hazard of steroid treatment, although clinical data on this issue are lacking. A finite incidence of extrameningeal bacterial infection and gastrointestinal blood loss has accompanied the use of steroids in tuberculous meningitis, although no certain cause-and-effect relationship has been demonstrated. Occasional cases of worsening of concomitant pulmonary tuberculosis have been reported as well (218).

The effects of these phenomena on morbidity and mortality in the disease are less clear. A number of studies have suggested that the primary value of steroids may be in their ability to treat or avert the development of spinal block, possibly by lowering the protein content of the CSF (223). An improvement in overall mortality has been ascribed to their specific impact on this poor prognostic sign (222). Other investigators have documented a significant lowering of mortality when steroids were used in a particularly ill population of children (224). Repeatedly, however, even when steroids are documented to reduce mortality, a concomitant, almost compensatory, increase has been seen in survivors with significant neurologic sequelae (190,225). Efficacy in averting death, then, may result in increased neurologic impairment among survivors. Many authorities now tentatively advocate the use of steroids in tuberculous meningitis in selected cases with extreme neurologic compromise, elevated intracranial pressure, impending herniation, or impending or established spinal block. Intrathecal steroid administration appears unnecessary; a dose of 1 mg/kg/day of prednisone tapered within 1 month is often recommended, although varying doses of dexamethasone or hydrocortisone have been used as well, for variable time periods. In individual cases, profound neurologic damage may be averted by the use of steroids; the paradoxical caveat persists, however, that in the desperately ill patient, survival may be achieved at the price of neurologic damage.

Surgery

Surgical intervention in tuberculous meningitis is primarily directed at relief of hydrocephalus. Although attempts have been made at surgically resecting meningeal adhesions (particularly around the optic chiasm or spinal cord), these have not been reliably successful (157,204,226). Ventricular drainage, on the other hand, is often dramatically successful in relieving hydrocephalus and its associated neurologic compromise. Generally, only patients whose hydrocephalus is refractory to medical therapy consisting of steroids or osmotic agents are considered for these procedures: In one series, 17 of 28 patients with hydrocephalus due to tuberculous meningitis fell into this category (73).

Clinical response to ventriculoatrial shunt placement has ranged between 66% and 100% in small series of children (60,227). Less experience exists with regard to shunting in adult patients, although generally good results have been documented (73,228). Bacterial meningitis has been the most commonly reported side effect of indwelling shunts. Other potential complications—such as (a) clogging of the catheter from the high protein content of the CSF and (b) dissemination of *M. tuberculosis* into the systemic circulation—have not been well documented, and it is generally felt that shunts can be safely inserted despite active CNS disease. The use of temporary external ventricular drains, in conjunction with prophylactic antibacterial agents, has recently been advocated as a safer and more convenient alternative to indwelling shunts in tuberculous meningitis (229). An intensive pressure-reducing regimen with daily lumbar punctures and acetazolamide therapy, an alternative to surgery, has proven successful in decreasing intracranial pressure and inducing clinical improvement in 22 of 24 children with communicating hydrocephalus due to tuberculous meningitis (230).

CENTRAL NERVOUS SYSTEM INFECTIONS WITH OTHER MYCOBACTERIA

In the past, the bovine variant of *M. tuberculosis, M. bovis,* was a common contaminant of milk and a frequent etiologic agent of all forms of human tuberculosis. In older series, this organism was responsible for 1–50% of culture-proven cases of tuberculous meningitis (231). Occasional cases of human disease from *M. bovis,* including meningitis, still occur. In some case reports, the pathogenesis of the infection is obscure (232); in others, iatrogenic infection has been clearly documented from vaccination with the attenuated and theoretically avirulent strain of *M. bovis,* BCG.

Both immunocompromised and fully immunocompetent individuals have developed BCG meningitis after vaccination. In three recently reported cases in previously healthy patients, the clinical presentation in all was typical of tuberculous meningitis. Clinical symptoms developed 1–6 months after BCG inoculation. CSF chemistries and cell counts were consistent with parameters usually seen in tuberculous meningitis, and the typical complications of hydrocephalus and cranial nerve palsies often developed. In one case an intracranial tuberculoma was identified during the course of therapy. All cases responded well to standard antituberculous treatment (233,234).

In contrast to *M. tuberculosis* and *M. bovis,* the nontuberculous or atypical mycobacteria are relatively recently recognized human pathogens. Omnipresent in the environment, they were originally distinguished from the tuberculous mycobacteria as well as from each other by rapidity of growth, colony appearance, and biochemical reactions into four major groups (Runyon groups I–IV). They can now be far more precisely typed with both serologic and molecular biologic techniques. The extent of their role in human disease and its exact pathogenesis is still the subject of active investigation. Certain members of the four groups are clearly associated with cutaneous, pulmonary, and lymph node infection in humans; disseminated disease occurs in patients with AIDS as well as in other immunocompromised and occasionally immunocompetent individuals (235).

These organisms have caused very few reported cases of CNS infection, even in the presence of widely disseminated disease. In a recent literature review of disseminated *M. avium-intracellulare* infections from 1940 to 1984, meningitis complicated only one of 37 reviewed cases (236). Other case reports of meningitis caused by a variety of nontuberculous organisms vary in the completeness with which the clinical and microbiologic details support the presumed etiology of these infections. In some, single isolates of organisms from the CSF in the absence of compatible clinical disease has not excluded contamination of cultures by environmental organisms (235,237,238). In others, repeated CSF isolates and heavy growth of organism in culture have been accepted to fulfill the usual criteria for infection caused by these organisms.

Isolated cases of CNS infection with atypical organisms have occurred in both immunocompromised and immunocompetent individuals of all ages. *M. avium-intracellulare* meningitis was reported in an adult with chronic myelogenous leukemia in blast crisis (51), as well as in a 13-year-old boy with disseminated disease and autopsy-confirmed granulomatous meningitis (235). *M. flavescens* was reported to have caused meningitis in an adult diabetic male (239). *M. kansasii* meningitis was seen in a child and in a pregnant woman with disseminated disease (238,240). *M. scrofulaceum* was isolated from the CSF of a child with *M. scrofulaceum* lymphadenitis (238). *M. gordonae* meningitis developed in a child with hydrocephalus and a ventriculoperitoneal shunt (241). CNS infection in these cases was presumably a result of hematogenous dissemination of the organism. Clinical presentation, spinal fluid profiles, and response to treatment were frequently not specified in these reports.

In addition, the atypical mycobacteria have been isolated from occasional cases in conjunction with more conventional CNS pathogens. Cases of coexistent spinal fluid isolation of *M. avium-intracellulare* and *M. tuberculosis* (51), *M. kansasii* and *M. tuberculosis* (242), and *M. avium-intracellulare* and *Cryptococcus neoformans* (243) have been reported. In these cases, the significance of the nontuberculous organism in the pathogenesis of infection has been virtually impossible to ascertain.

AIDS AND CENTRAL NERVOUS SYSTEM TUBERCULOSIS

A coherent biological explanation underlies the firm epidemiologic association between AIDS and tuberculosis. HIV paralyzes precisely those cellular immune defenses essential for maintaining resistance against this organism. A high prevalence of active tuberculosis would thus be expected, and has in fact been detected, in HIV-infected populations. In 1987 a revision in the clinical diagnostic criteria for AIDS formalized this association, establishing extrapulmonary tuberculosis developing in an HIV-infected individual as an infection diagnostic of AIDS (244).

The exact pathogenesis of tuberculosis among HIV-infected individuals has not been fully defined. While in theory these individuals might be expected to acquire and to reactivate disease at high rates, the data suggest that the bulk of tuberculosis in this population represents reactivated, rather than primary, disease. Evidence for this conclusion includes (a) the particularly high incidence rates of tuberculosis observed in immigrant HIV-infected populations from areas endemic for tuberculosis, such as Haitian immigrants to Florida (245), (b) the increased rate at which active tuberculosis develops among HIV-infected, compared to noninfected, tuberculin reactors (246), and (c) the pronounced tendency for tuberculosis to occur early in the course of HIV infection, generally before other opportunistic infections have been diagnosed. *M. tuberculosis,* unlike most of the other organisms responsible for opportunistic infection in AIDS, is a virulent human pathogen: In the waning stages of cellular immunity preceding full-blown AIDS, latent tuberculosis would be expected to reactivate before other opportunistic infections supervene. Were newly acquired disease responsible for most HIV-associated tuberculosis, high incidence rates should be observed in the last stages of HIV infection as well (247).

Although much expectant attention was focused on atypical extrapulmonary manifestations of tuberculosis in HIV-infected individuals during the early years of the AIDS epidemic, subsequent data have indicated that the disease is frequently typical in presentation. The majority of cases are pulmonary, although extrapulmonary disease is detected in 25–70% of cases, rates which enormously exceed those of extrapulmonary disease in the general population. Rates of tuberculin reactivity in active disease are low but not negligible, usually between 33% and 50%. Most series agree that response to standard courses of therapy among these patients is often good (248).

CNS tuberculosis in HIV-infected patients appears to be relatively less common than other extrapulmonary manifestations, which most often consist of lymphatic, miliary, or urogenital disease. Reported rates show enormous geographic variation, and they vary among risk groups for HIV infection as well: Intravenous drug users and Haitians with HIV infection appear to have higher rates of tuberculosis and of CNS tuberculosis (Table 10) (245,249–252). A series of 10 cases of CNS tuberculosis among intravenous drug users in New Jersey was noteworthy for the large proportion of mass lesions observed (249). Eight of 10 patients had space-occupying lesions on head CAT, consisting of tuberculomas or tuberculous brain abscesses, with coincident meningitis in three cases. Whether this observation indicates that tuberculous mass lesions are in fact more common than usual in the context of HIV infection has not yet been confirmed. In other particulars, CNS disease appears to be fairly orthodox in presentation among these patients. Spinal fluid parameters in this series as well as in other case reports have been consistent with those reported for other patients (253). As in other patients, chest radiographs may be negative, and evidence of tuberculosis elsewhere may be difficult to establish.

The predilection of HIV-infected individuals to become infected with the atypical or nontuberculous mycobacteria may extend to CNS disease as well. In cases of AIDS with disseminated *M. avium-intracellulare* or other atypical mycobacteria, organisms have been cultured from brain or spinal fluid; autopsies in some of these cases have revealed a diffuse, noncaseating, granulomatous inflammation of the brain, with numerous intracellular acid-fast organisms (254,255). The frequency with which atypical organisms cause clinically significant neurologic disease in these patients is not yet clear: Although occasional cases of meningitis or abscess have been diagnosed pre-mortem, details of clinical presentation and diagnostic confirmation have been scanty (256,257). Better documented are a handful of cases of disseminated or meningeal *M. bovis* infections that have clearly resulted from the administration of BCG vaccine to HIV-infected children or adults (258,259).

The efficacy of antituberculous chemotherapy in erad-

icating CNS disease due to mycobacteria in AIDS has not yet been formally assessed. Follow-up in most reports has been poor, and patients may succumb to other AIDS-related opportunistic infections during the course of therapy. Therapy of atypical mycobacterial infections in these patients is generally unsuccessful, and CNS disease is unlikely to prove an exception to this rule. Disease caused by *M. tuberculosis,* however, may be easier to treat. Most pulmonary and extrapulmonary disease in the HIV-infected population appears to respond well to ordinary two- or three-drug regimens, with few relapses if the course is terminated at approximately 9 months. Nonetheless, some clinicians feel that longer or lifetime treatment with at least one agent is warranted. Failure of CNS mycobacterial disease to respond to routine therapy has generally been associated with drug-resistant organisms (248).

The utility of corticosteroids in CNS tuberculosis is unclear in patients with AIDS. Long-term corticosteroid treatment, generally felt to be a perilous therapy in this population, is not absolutely contraindicated in the face of potential benefit. However, the repeatedly documented occurrence of simultaneous infection with *M. tuberculosis* and other CNS opportunists such as *Toxoplasma gondii* in patients with AIDS (249,260) implies that firm etiologic diagnosis should precede this intervention in these patients.

PREVENTION

Prevention of CNS tuberculosis is linked to the wider issue of worldwide tuberculosis control. As in other aspects of the infection, the dimensions of this challenge differ in different parts of the world. In the United States and other developed countries, the elimination of tuberculosis appears to be a realistic goal. Most of the necessary components of an effective prevention strategy are in place, including mechanisms for case reporting and contact identification, means of early diagnosis of infection, and widely available prophylactic therapy for infection and curative therapy for disease. Citing these tools, the Centers for Disease Control (261) has recently issued a detailed policy and planning document anticipating the eradication of tuberculosis from the United States by the year 2010.

TABLE 10. *Prevalence of tuberculosis and tuberculous central nervous system involvement in AIDS*

Location (ref.)	Year	Cases of active tuberculosis/cases of AIDS (%)	Cases of tuberculosis with CNS disease (%)
Florida (245)	1984	27/45 (60%)	2 of 27 (7%)
New Jersey (249)	1986	52/420 (12%)	10 of 52 (19%)
New York City (250)	1986	24/280 (9%)	1 of 24 (4%)
San Francisco (251)	1987	35/1705 (2%)	2 of 35 (6%)
Barcelona, Spain (252)	1988	Not available	5 of 65 (8%)

In less developed areas of the world, where tuberculosis remains rampant, strategies for disease prevention are less easily identified. The merits of BCG vaccine in these areas continue to be debated. Large-scale trials of the vaccine have yielded contradictory results, although its efficacy in protecting very young children from disease appears to be established (262). Thus, BCG vaccination should be able to prevent some of the most serious complications of childhood tuberculosis, with tuberculous meningitis being foremost among them. A recent retrospective case–control study from Brazil has supported this conclusion: Children who were not vaccinated with BCG had three to seven times the risk of developing tuberculous meningitis when compared to that of matched controls (263).

Despite this promising finding, BCG vaccination cannot stand alone as a means of controlling tuberculous meningitis in less developed countries. The provision of adequate nutrition, housing, and basic health care to the world's destitute populations is an essential component of disease control programs as well. All these social issues must be addressed on a worldwide level before tuberculosis and its CNS complications can be overcome.

ACKNOWLEDGMENTS

The assistance of Dr. Josefina Llena, Department of Pathology, Montefiore Medical Center, as well as that of Drs. Frank Moser and Lisa Tartaglino, Department of Radiology, Montefiore Medical Center, is gratefully acknowledged.

REFERENCES

1. Whytt R. Observations on the nature, causes and cure of those Disorders which are commonly called nervous, hypochondriac or hysteric. In: Robinson DN, ed. *Significant contributions to the history of psychiatry.* Washington, DC: University Publications of America, 1978;551.
2. Dastur DK, Lalitha VS. The many facets of neurotuberculosis: an epitome of neuropathology. In: Zimmerman HM, ed. *Progress in neuropathology* vol 2. New York: Grune & Stratton, 1973;351–408.
3. Koch R. The etiology of tuberculosis. *Rev Infect Dis* 1982;4:1270–1274.
4. Quincke H. Die Lumbarpunktion des Hydrocephalus. *Klin Wochenschr* 1891;28:929–933, 965–968.
5. Rich AR, McCordock HA. The pathogenesis of tuberculous meningitis. *Bull Johns Hopkins Hosp* 1933;52:5–37.
6. Adami JG, Nicholls AG. *The principles of pathology,* vol 2. New York: Lea & Febiger, 1909;546.
7. Burn CG, Finley KH. The role of hypersensitivity in the production of experimental meningitis. I. experimental meningitis in tuberculous animals. *J Exp Med* 1932;56:203–21.
8. Garland HG, Armitage G. Intracranial tuberculoma. *J Pathol Bacteriol* 1933;37:461–471.
9. Auerbach O. Tuberculous meningitis: correlation of therapeutic results with the pathogenesis and pathologic changes, part 1. *Am Rev Tuberc* 1951;64:408–418.
10. Riggs HE, Rupp C, Ray H. Clinicopathologic study of tuberculous meningitis in adults. *Am Rev Tuberc* 1956;74:830–834.
11. Bell WE, Sachs AL. Bacterial meningitis. In: Baker AB, Baker LH, eds. *Clinical neurology,* vol 2 (Joynt RT, series ed.) Philadelphia: JB Lippincott, 1988;58–66.
12. Lincoln EM, Sewell EM. *Tuberculosis in children.* New York: McGraw-Hill, 1963.
13. Gracey DR. Tuberculosis in the world today. *Mayo Clin Proc* 1988;63:1251–1255.
14. World Health Organization. *World Health Stat Rep* 1977;30:2–37.
15. Caldwell M. *The last crusade: the war on consumption 1862–1954.* New York: Atheneum, 1988.
16. Comstock GW. Tuberculosis. In: Evans AS, Feldman HH, eds. *Bacterial infections of humans: epidemiology and control.* New York: Plenum Medical Books, 1982;605–632.
17. Snider DE. Extrapulmonary tuberculosis in Oklahoma, 1965 to 1973. *Am Rev Respir Dis* 1985;111:641–646.
18. Farer LS, Lowell AM, Meador MP. Extrapulmonary tuberculosis in the United States. *Am J Epidemiol* 1979;109:205–217.
19. Centers for Disease Control. Tuberculosis control among homeless populations. *MMWR* 1987;36:257–260.
20. Centers for Disease Control. Tuberculosis in minorities—United States. *MMWR* 1987;36:77–80.
21. Centers for Disease Control. Tuberculosis in blacks—United States. *MMWR* 1987;36:212–220.
22. Stead WW, Lofgren JP, Warren E, Thomas C. Tuberculosis as an endemic and nosocomial infection among the elderly in nursing homes. *N Engl J Med* 1985;312:1483–1487.
23. Centers for Disease Control. Tuberculosis, final data—United States, 1986. *MMWR* 1988;36:817–820.
24. Centers for Disease Control. Tuberculosis and acquired immunodeficiency syndrome—New York City. *MMWR* 1987;36:785–790.
25. Centers for Disease Control. Tuberculosis and acquired immunodeficiency syndrome—Florida. *MMWR* 1986;35:587–590.
26. Quinn TC. Interactions of the human immunodeficiency virus and tuberculosis and the implications for BCG vaccination. *Rev Infect Dis* 1989;11(Suppl 2):S379–S384.
27. Des Prez RM, Goodwin RA. Mycobacterium tuberculosis. In: Mandell GL, Douglas RG, Bennett JE, eds. *Principles and practice of infectious diseases,* 2nd ed. New York: John Wiley & Sons, 1985;1383–1406.
28. Edwards D, Kirkpatrick CH. The immunology of mycobacterial diseases. *Am Rev Respir Dis* 1986;134:1062–1071.
29. Kaufman SHE. *In vitro* analysis of the cellular mechanisms involved in immunity to tuberculosis. *Rev Infect Dis* 1989;11(Suppl 2):S448–S454.
30. Rich AR. *The pathogenesis of tuberculosis.* Springfield, IL: Charles C Thomas, 1946.
31. Dannenberg AM. Immune mechanisms in the pathogenesis of pulmonary tuberculosis. *Rev Infect Dis* 1989;11(Suppl 2):S369–S378.
32. Skolnik PR, Nadol JB, Baker AS. Tuberculosis of the middle ear: review of the literature with an instructive case report. *Rev Infect Dis* 1986;8:403–410.
33. Samuel J, Fernandes CM. Tuberculous mastoiditis. *Ann Otol Rhinol Laryngol* 1986;95:264–266.
34. Auerbach O. Tuberculous meningitis: correlation of therapeutic results with the pathogenesis and pathologic changes. Part II: pathologic changes in untreated and treated cases. *Am Rev Tuberc* 1951;64:419–429.
35. Winkelman NW, Moore MT. Meningeal blood vessels in tuberculous meningitis. *Am Rev Tuberc* 1940;42:315–333.
36. Leiguarda R, Berthier M, Starkstein S, Nogues M, Lylyk P. Ischemic infarction in 25 children with tuberculous meningitis. *Stroke* 1988;19:200–204.
37. Tandon PN, Rao MA, Banerji AK, Pathak SN, Dhar J. Isotope scanning of the cerebrospinal fluid pathways in tuberculous meningitis. *J Neurol Sci* 1975;25:401–413.
38. Udani PM, Dastur DK. Tuberculous encephalopathy with and without meningitis: clinical features and pathological correlations. *J Neurol Sci* 1970;10:541–561.
39. British Medical Research Council. Streptomycin treatment of tuberculous meningitis. *Lancet* 1948;1:582–596.
40. Lincoln EM. Tuberculous meningitis in children with special ref-

erence to serous meningitis. I. Tuberculous meningitis. *Am Rev Tuberc* 1947;56:75–94.

41. Smith AL. Tuberculous meningitis in childhood. *Med J Aust* 1975;1:57–60.

42. Sumaya CV, Simek M, Smith MHD, Seidemann MF, Ferriss GS, Rubin W. Tuberculous meningitis in children during the isoniazid era. *J Pediatr* 1975;87:43–49.

43. Steiner P, Portugaleza C. Tuberculous meningitis in children. *Am Rev Respir Dis* 1973;107:22–29.

44. Lincoln EM, Sordillo SVR, Davies PA. Tuberculous meningitis in children. A review of 167 untreated and 74 treated patients with special reference to early diagnosis. *J Pediatrics* 1960;57:807–823.

45. Delage G, Dusseault M. Tuberculous meningitis in children: a retrospective study of 79 patients, with an analysis of prognostic factors. *J Can Med Assoc* 1979;120:305–309.

46. Bateman DE, Newman PK, Foster JB. A retrospective survey of proven cases of tuberculous meningitis in the Northern region, 1970–1980. *J R Coll Physicians Lond* 1983;17:106–110.

47. Traub M, Colchester ACF, Kingsley DPE, Swash M. Tuberculosis of the central nervous system. *Q J Med* 1984;53:81–100.

48. Barrett-Connor E. Tuberculous meningitis in adults. *South Med J* 1967;60:1061–1067.

49. Ogawa SK, Smith MA, Brennessel DJ, Lowy FD. Tuberculous meningitis in an urban medical center. *Medicine* 1987;66:317–326.

50. Alvarez S, McCabe WR. Extrapulmonary tuberculosis revisited: a review of experience at Boston City and other hospitals. *Medicine* 1984;63:25–54.

51. Klein NC, Damsker B, Hirschman SZ. Mycobacterial meningitis: retrospective analysis from 1970–1983. *Am J Med* 1985;79:29–34.

52. Kennedy DH, Fallon RJ. Tuberculous meningitis. *JAMA* 1979;241:264–268.

53. Hinman AR. Tuberculous meningitis at Cleveland Metropolitan General Hospital. *Am Rev Respir Dis* 1967;95:670–673.

54. Idriss ZH, Sinno AA, Kronfol NM. Tuberculous meningitis in childhood. *Am J Dis Child* 1976;130:364–367.

55. Haas EJ, Madhavan T, Quinn EL, Cox F, Fisher E, Burch K. Tuberculous meningitis in an urban general hospital. *Arch Intern Med* 1977;137:1518–1521.

56. Naughten E, Weindling AM, Newton R, Bower BD. Tuberculous meningitis in children. *Lancet* 1981;2:973–975.

57. Illingworth RS, Lorber J. Tubercles of the choroid. *Arch Dis Child* 1956;31:467–469.

58. Illingworth RS. Miliary and meningeal tuberculosis: difficulties in diagnosis. *Lancet* 1956;2:646–649.

59. Newman PK, Cumming WJK, Foster JB. Hydrocephalus and tuberculous meningitis in adults. *J Neurol Neurosurg Psychiatry* 1980;43:188–190.

60. Bhagwati SN. Ventriculoatrial shunt in tuberculous meningitis with hydrocephalus. *J Neurosurg* 1971;35:309–313.

61. Clark WC, Metcalf JC, Muhlbauer MS, Dohan FC, Robertson JH. *Mycobacterium tuberculosis* meningitis: a report of twelve cases and a literature review. *Neurosurgery* 1986;18:604–610.

62. Smith J, Godwin-Austen R. Hypersecretion of anti-diuretic hormone due to tuberculous meningitis. *Postgrad Med J* 1980;56:41–44.

63. Stockstill MT, Kauffman CA. Comparison of cryptococcal and tuberculous meningitis. *Arch Neurol* 1983;40:81–85.

64. Zarabi M, Sane S, Girdany BR. The chest roentgenogram in the early diagnosis of tuberculous meningitis in children. *Am J Dis Child* 1971;121:389–392.

65. Munt PW. Miliary tuberculosis in the chemotherapy era with a clinical review in 69 American adults. *Medicine* 1971;51:139–155.

66. Holden M, Dubin MR, Diamond PH. Frequency of negative intermediate strength tuberculin sensitivity in patients with active tuberculosis. *N Engl J Med* 1971;285:1506–1509.

67. El-Naggar AK, Higashi GI. *In vivo* and *in vitro* cell-mediated immunity in tuberculous meningitis. *J Clin Lab Immunol* 1982;8:37–42.

68. Snider DE. The tuberculin skin test. *Am Rev Respir Dis* 1982;125(Suppl 1):108–118.

69. Sheller JR, Des Prez RM. CNS tuberculosis. *Neurol Clin* 1986;4:143–158.

70. Fishman RA. *Cerebrospinal fluid in diseases of the nervous system.* Philadelphia: WB Saunders, 1980;266.

71. Boyd W. *Physiology and pathology of the cerebrospinal fluid.* New York: Macmillan, 1920;101.

72. Holt LE, Howland J. *The diseases of infancy and childhood,* 9th ed. New York: D Appleton, 1926;618.

73. Singhal BS, Bhagwati SN, Syed AH, Laud GW. Raised intracranial pressure in tuberculous meningitis. *Neurology (India)* 1975;23:32–39.

74. Weinstein L. Bacterial meningitis. *Med Clin North Am* 1985;69:219–229.

75. Karandanis D, Shulman JA. Recent survey of infectious meningitis in adults: review of laboratory findings in bacterial, tuberculous and aseptic meningitis. *South Med J* 1976;69:449–457.

76. Ramkissoon A, Coovadia HM. Chloride levels in meningitis. *S Afr Med J* 1988;73:522–523.

77. Jeren T, Beus I. Characteristics of cerebrospinal fluid in tuberculous meningitis. *Acta Cytol* 1982;26:678–680.

78. Lipsky BA, Gates J, Tenover FC, Plorde JJ. Factors affecting the clinical value of microscopy for acid-fast bacilli. *Rev Infect Dis* 1984;6:214–222.

79. Stewart SM. The bacteriologic diagnosis of tuberculous meningitis. *J Clin Pathol* 1953;6:241–242.

80. Lincoln EM. Tuberculous meningitis in children with special reference to serous meningitis. II. Serous tuberculous meningitis. *Am Rev Tuberc* 1947;56:95–109.

81. Emond RTD, McKendrick GDW. Tuberculosis as a cause of transient aseptic meningitis. *Lancet* 1973;2:234–236.

82. Daniel TM. New approaches to the rapid diagnosis of tuberculous meningitis. *J Infect Dis* 1987;155:599–602.

83. Smith HV, Taylor LM, Hunter G. The blood–cerebrospinal fluid barrier in tuberculous meningitis and allied conditions. *J Neurol Neurosurg Psychiatry* 1955;18:237–249.

84. Mandal BK, Evans DIK, Ironside AG, Pullan BR. Radioactive bromide partition test in differential diagnosis of tuberculous meningitis. *Br Med J* 1972;4:413–415.

85. Wiggelinkhuizen M, Mann M. The radioactive bromide partition test in the diagnosis of tuberculous meningitis in children. *J Pediatr* 1980;97:843–847.

86. Mann MD, Macfarlane CM, Verburg CJ, Wiggelinkhuizen J. The bromide partition test and CSF adenosine deaminase activity in the diagnosis of tuberculous meningitis in children. *S Afr Med J* 1982;62:431–433.

87. Weinberg JR, Coppack SP. Positive bromide partition test in the absence of tuberculous meningitis. *J Neurol Neurosurg Psychiatry* 1985;48:278–280.

88. Smith GW. False positive bromide partition test in lymphomatous meningitis [Letter]. *J Clin Pathol* 1989;42:113–114.

89. Sullivan JL, Osborne WRA, Wedgwood RJ. Adenosine deaminase activity in lymphocytes. *Br J Haematol* 1977;37:157–158.

90. Ocana I, Martinez-Vazquez JM, Segura RM, Fernandez de Sevilla T, Capdevila JA. Adenosine deaminase in pleural fluids. Test for diagnosis of tuberculous pleural effusion. *Chest* 1983;84:51–53.

91. Voigt MD, Kalvaria I, Trey C, Berman P, Lombard C, Kirsch RE. Diagnostic value of ascites adenosine deaminase in tuberculous peritonitis. *Lancet* 1989;1:751–753.

92. Martinez-Vazquez JM, Ribera E, Ocana I, Segura RM, Serrat R, Sagrista J. Adenosine deaminase activity in tuberculous pericarditis. *Thorax* 1986;41:888–889.

93. Ribera E, Martinez-Vazquez JM, Ocana I, Segura RM, Pascual C. Activity of adenosine deaminase in cerebrospinal fluid for the diagnosis and follow-up of tuberculous meningitis in adults. *J Infect Dis* 1987;155:603–607.

94. Donald PR, Malan C, Schoeman JF. Adenosine deaminase activity as a diagnostic aid in tuberculous meningitis. *J Infect Dis* 1987;156:1040–1041.

95. Donald PR, Malan C, van der Walt A, Schoeman JF. The simultaneous determination of cerebrospinal fluid and plasma adenosine deaminase activity as a diagnostic aid in tuberculous meningitis. *S Afr Med J* 1986;69:505–507.

96. Coovadia YM, Dawood A, Ellis ME, Coovadia HM, Daniel TM.

Evaluation of adenosine deaminase activity and antibody to *Mycobacterium tuberculosis* antigen 5 in cerebrospinal fluid and the radioactive bromide partition test for the early diagnosis of tuberculous meningitis. *Arch Dis Child* 1986;61:428–435.

97. Ena J, Crespo MJ, Valls V, de Salmanca RE. Adenosine deaminase activity in cerebrospinal fluid: a useful test for meningeal tuberculosis, even in patients with AIDS. *J Infect Dis* 1988;158:896.

98. Brooks JB, Choudhary G, Craven RB, Alley CC, Liddle JA, Edman DC, Converse JD. Electron capture gas chromotography detection and mass spectrum identification of 3-(2′-ketohexyl)indoline in spinal fluids of patients with tuberculous meningitis. *J Clin Microbiol* 1977;5:625–628.

99. Brooks JB, Edman DC, Alley CC, Craven RB, Girgis NI. Frequency-pulsed electron capture gas-liquid chromatography and the tryptophan color test for rapid diagnosis of tuberculous and other forms of lymphocytic meningitis. *J Clin Microbiol* 1980;12:208–215.

100. French GL, Teoh R, Chan CY, Humphries MJ, Cheung SW, O'Mahony G. Diagnosis of tuberculous meningitis by detection of tuberculostearic acid in cerebrospinal fluid. *Lancet* 1987;2:117–119.

101. Kuo C. The diagnosis of tuberculous meningitis by immunologic reaction of cerebrospinal fluid. *Am Rev Respir Dis* 1969; 100:565–568.

102. Hernandez R, Munoz O, Guiscafre H. Sensitive enzyme immunoassay for early diagnosis of tuberculous meningitis. *J Clin Microbiol* 1984;20:533–535.

103. Kalish SB, Radin RC, Levitz D, Zeiss R, Phair JP. The enzyme-linked immunosorbent assay method for IgG antibody to purified protein derivative in cerebrospinal fluid of patients with tuberculous meningitis. *Ann Intern Med* 1983;99:630–633.

104. Watt G, Zaraspe G, Bautista S, Laughlin LW. Rapid diagnosis of tuberculous meningitis by using an enzyme-linked immunosorbent assay to detect mycobacterial antigen and antibody in cerebrospinal fluid. *J Infect Dis* 1988;158:681–686.

105. Daniel TM, Debanne SM. The serodiagnosis of tuberculosis and other mycobacterial diseases by enzyme-linked immunosorbent assay. *Am Rev Respir Dis* 1987;135:1137–1151.

106. Sada E, Ruiz-Palacios GM, Lopez-Vidal Y, Ponce de Leon S. Detection of mycobacterial antigens in cerebrospinal fluid of patients with tuberculous meningitis by enzyme-linked immunosorbent assay. *Lancet* 1983;2:651–652.

107. Krambovitis E, McIllmurray MB, Lock PE, Hendrickse W, Holzel H. Rapid diagnosis of tuberculous meningitis by latex particle agglutination. *Lancet* 1984;2:1229–1231.

108. Kadival GV, Samuel AM, Mazarelo TBMS, Chaparas SD. Radioimmunoassay for detecting *Mycobacterium tuberculosis* antigen in cerebrospinal fluids of patients with tuberculous meningitis. *J Infect Dis* 1987;155:608–611.

108a. Kaneko K, Onodera O, Miyatake T, Tsuji S. Rapid diagnosis of tuberculous meningitis by polymerase chain reaction (PCR). Neurology 1990;40:1617–1618.

109. Chandramuki A. Rapid diagnosis of tuberculous meningitis by ELISA to detect mycobacterial antigen and antibody in the cerebrospinal fluid. *J Infect Dis* 1989;160:343–344.

110. Chambers AA, Lukin RR, Tomsick TA. Cranial and Intracranial Tuberculosis. *Semin Roentgenol* 1979;14:319–324.

111. Lorber J. Long-term follow-up of 100 children who recovered from tuberculous meningitis. *Pediatrics* 1961;28:778–791.

112. Todd RM, Neville JG. The sequelae of tuberculous meningitis. *Arch Dis Child* 1964;39:213–225.

113. Donner M, Wasz-Hockert O. Late neurologic sequelae of tuberculous meningitis. *Acta Paediatr* 1962;51(Suppl 141):34–42.

114. Maroon JC, Jones R, Mishkin FS. Tuberculous meningitis diagnosed by brain scan. *Radiology* 1972;104:333–335.

115. Lehrer H. The angiographic triad of tuberculous meningitis: a radiographic and clinicopathologic correlation. *Radiology* 1966;87:829–835.

116. Suwanwela C, Suwanwela N, Charuchinda S, Hongsaprabhas C. Intracranial mycotic aneurysms of extravascular origin. *J Neurosurg* 1972;36:552–559.

117. Mathew NT, Abraham J, Chandy J. Cerebral angiographic features in tuberculous meningitis. *Neurology* 1970;20:1015–23.

118. Price HI, Danziger A. Computed Tomography in cranial tuberculosis. *AJR* 1978;130:769–771.

119. Stevens DL, Everett ED. Sequential computerized axial tomography in tuberculous meningitis. *JAMA* 1978;239:642.

120. Chu N. Tuberculous meningitis: computerized tomographic manifestations. *Arch Neurol* 1980;37:458–460.

121. Bullock MRR, Welchman JM. Diagnostic and prognostic features of tuberculous meningitis on CT scanning. *J Neurol Neurosurg Psychiatry* 1982;45:1098–1101.

122. Witrack BJ, Ellis GT. Intracranial tuberculosis: manifestations on computerized tomography. *South Med J* 1985;78:386–392.

123. Enzmann DR, Norman D, Mani J, Newton JH. Computed tomography of granulomatous basal arachnoiditis. *Radiology* 1976;120:341–344.

124. Cockrill H, Dreisbach J, Lowe B, Yamauchi T. CT in leptomeningeal infections. *AJR* 1978;130:511–515.

125. Sze G, Zimmerman RD. The magnetic resonance imaging of infections and inflammatory diseases. *Radiol Clin North Am* 1988;26:839–859.

126. Davidson HD, Steiner RE. Magnetic resonance imaging in infections of the central nervous system. *AJNR* 1985;6:499–504.

127. Dastur HM, Desai AD. A comparative study of brain tuberculomas and gliomas based upon 107 case records of each. *Brain* 1965;88:375–386.

128. Pardee I, Knox LC. Tuberculoma en plaque. *Arch Neurol Psychiatry* 1927;17:231–238.

129. Trautmann M, Lindner O, Haase C, Bruckner O. Focal tuberculous meningoencephalitis. *Eur Neurol* 1983;22:417–420.

130. Sinh G, Pandya SK, Dastur DK. Pathogenesis of unusual intracranial tuberculomas and tuberculous space-occupying lesions. *J Neurosurg* 1968;29:149–159.

131. Ramamurthi B. Intracranial tumors in India: incidence and variations. *Int Surg* 1973;58:542–547.

132. DeAngelis LM. Intracranial tuberculoma: case report and review of the literature. *Neurology* 1981;31:1133–1136.

133. Lees AJ, MacLeod AF, Marshall J. Cerebral tuberculomas developing during treatment of tuberculous meningitis. *Lancet* 1980;1:1208–1211.

134. Shepard WE, Field ML, James DH. Transient appearance of intracranial tuberculoma during treatment of tuberculous meningitis. *Pediatr Infect Dis* 1986;5:599–601.

135. Chang CM, Chan FL, Yu Yl, Huang CY, Woo E. Tuberculous meningitis associated with meningeal tuberculoma. *J R Soc Med* 1986;79:486–487.

136. Arseni C. Two hundred and one cases of intracranial tuberculoma treated surgically. *J Neurol Neurosurg Psychiatry* 1958;21:308–311.

137. Anderson JM, Macmillan JJ. Intracranial tuberculoma—an increasing problem in Britain. *J Neurol Neurosurg Psychiatry* 1975;38:194–201.

138. Mayers MM, Kaufman DM, Miller MH. Recent cases of intracranial tuberculomas. *Neurology* 1978;28:256–260.

139. Loizou LA, Anderson M. Intracranial tuberculomas: correlation of computerized tomography with clinicopathological findings. *Q J Med* 1982;51:104–114.

140. Asenjo A, Valladares H, Fierro J. Tuberculomas of the brain: report of one hundred and fifty-nine cases. *Arch Neurol Psychiatry* 1951;65:146–160.

141. Sibley WA, O'Brien JL. Intracranial tuberculomas: a review of clinical features and treatment. *Neurology* 1956;6:157–165.

142. Ramamurthi B, Varadarajan MG. Diagnosis of tuberculomas of the brain: clinical and radiologic correlation. *J Neurosurg* 1961;18:1–7.

143. Armstrong FB, Edwards AM. Intracranial tuberculoma in native races of Canada: with special reference to symptomatic epilepsy and neurologic features. *Can Med Assoc J* 1963;89:56–65.

144. Harder E, Al-Kawi MZ, Carney P. Intracranial tuberculoma: conservative management. *Am J Med* 1983;74:570–576.

145. Bagga A, Kaira V, Ghai OP. Intracranial tuberculoma: evaluation and treatment. *Clin Pediatr* 1988;27:487–490.

146. Damergis JA, Leftwich EI, Curtin JA, Witorsch P. Tuberculoma of the brain. *JAMA* 1978;239:413–435.

147. Elisevich K, Arpin EJ. Tuberculoma masquerading as a meningioma. *J Neurosurg* 1982;56:435–438.

148. Thrush DC, Barwick DD. Three patients with intracranial tuberculomas with unusual features. *J Neurol Neurosurg Psychiatry* 1974;37:566–569.
149. Whelan MA, Stern J. Intracranial tuberculoma. *Radiology* 1981;138:75–81.
150. O'Brien NC, van Eys J, Baram TZ, Starke JR. Intracranial tuberculoma in children: a new look at an old problem. *South Med J* 1988;81:1239–1244.
151. Whitener DR. Tuberculous brain abscess: report of a case and review of the literature. *Arch Neurol* 1978;35:148–155.
152. Reichentral E, Cohen ML, Schujman E, Eynan N, Shalit M. Tuberculous brain abscess and its appearance on computerized tomography. *J Neurosurg* 1982;56:597–600.
152a. Datsur HM. Diagnosis and neurosurgical treatment of tuberculous disease of the CNS. *Neurosurg Rev* 1983;6:111–117.
153. Ransome GA, Montiero ES. A rare form of tuberculous meningitis. *Br Med J* 1947;1:413–414.
154. Brooks WDW, Fletcher AP, Wilson RR. Spinal cord complications of tuberculous meningitis. *Q J Med* 1954;23:275–290.
155. Dastur DK, Wadia NH. Spinal meningitides with radiculomyelopathy: part 2. Pathology and pathogenesis. *J Neurol Sci* 1969;8:261–293.
156. Kocen RS, Parsons M. Neurological complications of tuberculosis: some unusual manifestations. *Q J Med* 1970;39:17–30.
157. Wadia NH, Dastur DK. Spinal meningitides with radiculomyelopathy. Part 1. *J Neurol Sci* 1969;8:239–260.
158. Frelich D, Swash M. Diagnosis and management of tuberculous paraplegia with special reference to tuberculous radiculomyelitis. *J Neurol Neurosurg Psychiatry* 1979;42:12–18.
159. Bucy PC, Oberhill HR. Intradural spinal granulomas. *J Neurosurg* 1950;7:1–12.
160. Lin, TH. Intramedullary tuberculoma of the spinal cord. *J Neurosurg* 1960;17:497–499.
161. Rhoton EL, Ballinger WE, Quisling R, Sypert GW. Intramedullary spinal tuberculoma. *Neurosurgery* 1988;22:733–736.
162. Gokalp HZ, Ozkal E. Intradural tuberculomas of the spinal cord. *J Neurosurg* 1981;55:289–292.
163. Mandell GL, Sande MA. Drugs used in the chemotherapy of tuberculosis and leprosy. In: Gilman AG, Goodman LS, Rall TW, Murad F, eds. *The pharmacological basis of therapeutics* 7th ed. New York: Macmillan, 1985;1199–1218.
164. Des Prez R, Boone IU. Metabolism of C14-isoniazid in humans. *Am Rev Respir Dis* 1961;84:42–51.
165. Forgan-Smith R, Ellard GA, Newton D, Mitchison DA. Pyrazinamide and other drugs in tuberculous meningitis. *Lancet* 1973;2:374.
166. Kutt H, Brennan R, Dehejia H, Verebely K. Diphenylhydantoin intoxication. A complication of isoniazid therapy. *Am Rev Respir Dis* 1970;101:377–384.
167. Verbist L, Gyselen A. Antituberculous activity of rifampin *in vitro* and *in vivo* and the concentrations attained in human blood. *Am Rev Respir Dis* 1968;98:923–932.
168. D'Oliveira JJG. Cerebrospinal fluid concentrations of rifampin in meningeal tuberculosis. *Am Rev Respir Dis* 1972;106:432–437.
169. Sippel JE, Mikhail IA, Girgis NI. Rifampin concentrations in cerebrospinal fluid of patients with tuberculous meningitis. *Am Rev Respir Dis* 1974;109:579–580.
170. Visudhiphan P, Chiemchanya S. Evaluation of rifampicin in the treatment of tuberculous meningitis in children. *J Pediatr* 1975;87:983–986.
171. Rahajoe NN, Rahajoe N, Boediman I, Said M, Lazuardi S. The treatment of tuberculous meningitis in children with a combination of isoniazid, rifampicin and streptomycin—preliminary report. *Tubercle* 1979;60:245–250.
172. Pauranik A, Behari M, Maheshwari MC. Pyrazinamide in treatment of tuberculous meningitis [Letter]. *Arch Neurol* 1986;43:982.
173. Karlson AG. The in vitro activity of ethambutol against tubercle bacilli and other microorganisms. *Am Rev Respir Dis* 1961;84:905–906.
174. Bobrowitz ED. Ethambutol in tuberculous meningitis. *Chest* 1972;61:629–632.
175. Place VA, Pyle MM, de la Huerga J. Ethambutol in tuberculous meningitis. *Am Rev Respir Dis* 1969;99:783–785.
176. Pilheu JA, Maglio F, Cetrangolo R, Pleus AD. Concentrations of ethambutol in the cerebrospinal fluid after oral administration. *Tubercle* 1971;52:117–122.
177. Girgis NI, Yassin MW, Sippel JE, Sorensen K, Hassan A, Miner WF, Farid Z, Abu el Ella A. The value of ethambutol in the treatment of tuberculous meningitis. *J Trop Med Hyg* 1976;79:14–17.
178. Kucers A, Bennett NM. *The use of antibiotics*, 4th ed. Philadelphia: JB Lippincott, 1987.
179. Zintel HA, Flippin HF, Nichols AC, Wiley MM, Rhoads JE. Studies on streptomycin in man. I. Absorption, distribution, excretion and toxicity. *Am J Med Sci* 1945;210:421–430.
180. Buggs CW, Pilling MA, Bronstein B, Hirshfeld JW. The absorption, distribution and excretion of streptomycin in man. *J Clin Invest* 1946;25:94–102.
181. Spector R, Lorenzo AV. The active transport of para-amino salicylic acid from the cerebrospinal fluid. *J Pharmacol Exp Ther* 1973;185:642–648.
182. Hughes IE, Smith H, Kane PO. Ethionamide: its passage into the cerebrospinal fluid in man. *Lancet* 1962;1:616–617.
183. American Thoracic Society. Treatment of tuberculosis and tuberculosis infection in adults and children. *Am Rev Respir Dis* 1986;134:355–363.
184. Molavi A, LeFrock JL. Tuberculous Meningitis. *Med Clin North Am* 1985;69:315–331.
185. National Consensus Conference on Tuberculosis. Standard therapy for tuberculosis 1985. *Chest* 1985;87(Suppl):117S–124S.
186. Editorial. Treatment of tuberculous meningitis. *Lancet* 1976;1:787–788.
187. Dutt AK, Moers D, Stead WW. Short-course chemotherapy for extrapulmonary tuberculosis. *Ann Intern Med* 1986;104:7–12.
188. Alford RH, Manian FA. Current antimicrobial management of tuberculosis. In: Remington JS, Swartz MN, eds. *Current clinical topics in infectious diseases 8*. New York: McGraw-Hill, 1987;204–226.
189. Lorber J. The results of treatment of 549 cases of tuberculous meningitis. *Am Rev Tuberc* 1954;69:13–25.
190. Wasz-Hockert O, Donner M. Results of the treatment of 191 children with tuberculous meningitis in the years 1949–1954. *Acta Paediatr* 1962;51(Suppl 141):7–25.
191. Smith HV, Vollum RL. The treatment of tuberculous meningitis. *Tubercle* 1956;37:301–320.
192. Falk A. U.S. Veterans administration-armed forces cooperative study on the chemotherapy of tuberculosis. XIII. Tuberculous meningitis in adults, with special reference to survival, neurologic residuals, and work status. *Am Rev Respir Dis* 1962;91:823–831.
193. Lepper MH, Spies HW. The present status of the treatment of tuberculosis of the central nervous system. *Ann NY Acad Sci* 1963;106:106–123.
194. Weiss W, Flippin HF. The prognosis of tuberculous meningitis in the isoniazid era. *Am J Med Sci* 1961;242:423–430.
195. Weiss W, Flippin HF. The changing incidence and prognosis of tuberculous meningitis. *Am J Med Sci* 1965;250:46–59.
196. Weinstein L, Meade RH. The treatment of tuberculous meningitis. *Med Clin North Am* 1955;39:1331–1349.
197. D'Cruz IA, Dandekar AC. Tuberculous meningitis in pregnant and puerperal women. *Obstet Gynecol* 1968;31:775–778.
198. Stephanopoulos C. The development of tuberculous meningitis during pregnancy. *Am Rev Tuberc* 1957;76:1079–1087.
199. Kingdom JC, Kennedy DH. Tuberculous meningitis in pregnancy. *Br J Obstet Gynecol* 1989;96:233–235.
200. Parsons M. *Tuberculous meningitis: a handbook for clinicians*. New York: Oxford University Press, 1979.
201. Smith H. Tuberculous meningitis. *Int J Neurol* 1964;4:134–157.
202. Chambers ST, Hendrickse WA, Record C, Rudge P, Smith H. Paradoxical expansion of intracranial tuberculomas during chemotherapy. *Lancet* 1984;2:181–184.
203. Pentti R, Donner M, Valanne E, Wasz-Hockert O. Late psychological and psychiatric sequelae of tuberculous meningitis. *Acta Paediatr* 1962;51(Suppl 141):65–77.
204. Mooney AJ. Some ocular sequelae of tuberculous meningitis. *Am J Ophthalmol* 1956;41:753–768.
205. Miettinen P, Wasz-Hockert O. Late ophthalmological sequelae of tuberculous meningitis. *Acta Paediatr* 1962;51(Suppl 141):43–49.

206. Ranta J, Wasz-Hockert O. Late otological sequelae of tuberculous meningitis. *Acta Paediatr* 1962;51(Suppl 141):50–64.

207. Lorber J. Diabetes insipidus following tuberculous meningitis. *Arch Dis Child* 1958;33:315–319.

208. Dick DJ, Sanders GL, Saunders M, et al. Chronic hypothermia following tuberculous meningitis. *J Neurol Neurosurg Psychiatry* 1981;44:255–257.

209. Don A. Case of tuberculous meningitis in boy treated with tuberculin: recovery, recurrence and death. *Br Med J* 1907;1:1360–1362.

210. Cathie IAB, MacFarlane JCW. Adjuvants to streptomycin in treating tuberculous meningitis in children. *Lancet* 1950;2:784–789.

211. Lorber J. Fibrinolytic agents in the treatment of tuberculous meningitis. *J Clin Pathol* 1964;17:353–354.

212. Johnson AJ, Ayvazian JH, Tillett WS. Crystalline pancreatic desoxyribonuclease as an adjunct to the treatment of pneumococcal meningitis. *N Engl J Med* 1959;260:893–900.

213. Gourie-Devi M, Satish P. Hyaluronidase as a adjuvant in the treatment of cranial arachnoiditis (hydrocephalus and optochiasmatic arachnoiditis) complicating tuberculous meningitis. *Acta Neurol Scand* 1980;62:368–381.

214. Fitzsimmons JM, Smith HV. Tuberculous meningitis: special features of treatment. *Tubercle* 1963;44:103–111.

215. Kinsell LW. The clinical application of pituitary adrenocorticotropic and adrenal steroid hormones. *Ann Intern Med* 1951;35:615–651.

216. Ebert RH. In vivo observations on the effect of cortisone on experimental tuberculosis using the rabbit ear chamber technique. *Am Rev Tuberc* 1952;65:64–74.

217. Feldman S, Behar AJ, Weber D. Experimental tuberculous meningitis in rabbits. I. Results of treatment with antituberculous drugs separately and in combination with cortisone. *Arch Pathol* 1958;65:343–354.

218. Kendig EL, Choy SH, Johnson WH. Observations on the effect of cortisone in the treatment of tuberculous meningitis. *Am Rev Tuberc* 1956;73:99–109.

219. Johnson JR, Furstenberg NE, Patterson R, Schoch HK, Davey WN. Corticotropin and adrenal steroids as adjuncts to the treatment of tuberculous meningitis. *Ann Intern Med* 1957;46:316–331.

220. Ashby M, Grant H. Tuberculous meningitis treated with cortisone. *Lancet* 1955;1:65–66.

221. Hockaday JM, Smith HMV. Corticosteroids as an adjuvant to the chemotherapy of tuberculous meningitis. *Tubercle* 1966;47:75–83.

222. O'Toole RD, Thornton GF, Mukherjee MK, Nath RL. Dexamethasone in tuberculous meningitis; relationship of cerebrospinal fluid effects to therapeutic efficacy. *Ann Intern Med* 1969;70:39–48.

223. Voljavec BF and Corpe RF. The influence of corticosteroid hormones in the treatment of tuberculous meningitis in Negroes. *Am Rev Respir Dis* 1960;81:539–545.

224. Escobar JA, Belsey MA, Duenas A, Medina P. Mortality from tuberculous meningitis reduced by steroid therapy. *Pediatrics* 1975;56:1050–1055.

225. Freiman I, Geefhuysen J. Evaluation of intrathecal therapy with streptomycin and hydrocortisone in tuberculous meningitis. *J Pediatr* 1970;76:895–901.

226. Scott RM, Sonntag VKH, Wilcox LM, et al. Visual loss from optochiasmatic arachnoiditis after tuberculous meningitis. *J Neurosurg* 1977;46:524–526.

227. Chitale VR, Kasaliwal GT. Our experience of ventriculoatrial shunt using Upadhyaya valve in cases of hydrocephalus associated with tuberculous meningitis. *Prog Pediatr Surg* 1982;15:223–336.

228. Murray HW, Brandstetter BD, Lavyne MH. Ventriculoatrial shunting for hydrocephalus complicating tuberculous meningitis. *Am J Med* 1981;70:895–898.

229. Chan KH, Mann KS. Prolonged therapeutic external ventricular drainage: a prospective study. *Neurosurgery* 1988;23:436–438.

230. Visudhiphan P, Chiemchanya S. Hydrocephalus in tuberculous meningitis in children: treatment with acetazolamide and repeated lumbar puncture. *J Pediatr* 1979;95:657–660.

231. Novick N. The incidence of bovine infection in tuberculous meningitis. *J Med Res* 1920;41:239–246.

232. Jones PG, Silva J. *M. bovis* meningitis. *JAMA* 1982;247:2270–2271.

233. Tardieu M, Truffot-Pernot C, Carriere JP, Dupic Y, Landrieu P. Tuberculous meningitis due to BCG in two previously healthy children. *Lancet* 1988;1:440–441.

234. Morrison WL, Webb WJS, Aldred J, Rubenstein D. Meningitis after BCG vaccination [Letter]. *Lancet* 1988;1:654–655.

235. Wolinsky, E. Nontuberculous mycobacteria and associated diseases. *Am Rev Respir Dis* 1979;119:107–159.

236. Horsburgh CR, Mason UG, Farhi DC, Iseman MD. Disseminated infection with *Mycobacterium avium-intracellulare*. A report of 13 cases and a review of the literature. *Medicine* 1985;64:36–48.

237. Yamamoto M, Sudo K, Taga M, Hibino S. A study of diseases caused by atypical mycobacteria in Japan. *Am Rev Respir Dis* 1967;96:779–787.

238. Lincoln EM, Gilbert LA. Disease in children due to mycobacteria other than *Mycobacterium tuberculosis*. *Am Rev Respir Dis* 105:683–714.

239. Virmani V, Rangan G, Shriniwas G. A study of the cerebrospinal fluid in atypical presentations of tuberculous meningitis. *J Neurol Sci* 1975;26:587–592.

240. Wood LE, Buhler VB, Pollak A. Human infection with the "yellow" acid-fast bacillus: a report of fifteen additional cases. *Am Rev Tuberc* 1956;73:917–929.

241. Gonzales EP, Crosby RMN, Walker SH. *Mycobacterium aquae* infection in a hydrocephalic child (*M. aquae* meningitis). *Pediatrics* 1971;48:974–977.

242. Huempfner HR, Kingsolver WR, Deuschle KW. Tuberculous meningitis caused by both *M. tuberculosis* and atypical mycobacteria. *Am Rev Respir Dis* 1966;94:612–614.

243. Gentry RH, Farrar WE, Mahvi TA, Prevost AE, Gionis TA. Simultaneous infection of the central nervous system with *C. neoformans* and *M. intracellulare*. *South Med J* 1977;70:865–868.

244. Centers for Disease Control. Revision of the CDC surveillance case definition for acquired immunodeficiency syndrome. *MMWR* 1987;36(Suppl):1S–15S.

245. Pitchenik AE, Cole C, Russell BW, Fischl MA, Spira TJ, Snider DE. Tuberculosis, atypical mycobacteriosis and the acquired immunodeficiency syndrome among Haitian and non-Haitian patients in South Florida. *Ann Intern Med* 1984;101:641–645.

246. Selwyn PA, Hartel D, Lewis VA, et al. A prospective study of the risk of tuberculosis among intravenous drug users with human immunodeficiency virus infection. *N Engl J Med* 1989;320:545–550.

247. Rieder HL, Cauthen GM, Bloch AB, Cole CH, Holtzman D, Snider DE, Bigler WJ, Witte JJ. Tuberculosis and acquired immunodeficiency syndrome—Florida. *Arch Intern Med* 1989;149:1268–1273.

248. Chaisson RE, Slutkin G. Tuberculosis and human immunodeficiency virus infection. *Rev Infect Dis* 1989;159:96–100.

249. Bishburg E, Sunderam G, Reichman LB, Kapila R. Central nervous system tuberculosis with the acquired immunodeficiency syndrome and its related complex. *Ann Intern Med* 1986;105:210–213.

250. Louie E, Rice LB, Holzman RS. Tuberculosis in non-Haitian patients with acquired immunodeficiency syndrome. *Chest* 1986;90:542–545.

251. Chaisson RE, Schecter GF, Theuer CP, Rutherford GW, Echenberg DF, Hopewell PC. Tuberculosis in patients with the acquired immunodeficiency syndrome. *Am Rev Respir Dis* 1987;136:570–574.

252. Soriano E, Mallolas J, Gatell JM, et al. Characteristics of tuberculosis in HIV-infected patients: a case–control study. *AIDS* 1988;2:429–432.

253. Isaksson B, Albert J, Chiodi F, Furucrona A, Krook A, Putkonen P. AIDS two months after primary human immunodeficiency virus infection. *J Infect Dis* 1988;158:866–868.

254. Hawkins CC, Gold JWM, Whimbey E, Kiehn TE, Brannon P, Cammarata R, Brown AE, Armstrong D. *Mycobacterium avium* complex infections in patients with the acquired immunodeficiency syndrome. *Ann Intern Med* 1986;105:184–188.

255. Zakowski P, Fligiel S, Berlin GW, Johnson BL. Disseminated *Mycobacterium avium-intracellulare* infection in homosexual men dying of acquired immunodeficiency. *JAMA* 1982; 248:2980–2982.

256. Greene JB, Sidhu GS, Lewin S, et al. *Mycobacterium avium-intracellulare:* a cause of disseminated life-threatening infection in homosexuals and drug abusers. *Ann Intern Med* 1982;97:539–547.

257. Maayan S, Wormser GP, Hewlett D, Miller S, Duncanson FP, Rodriguez A, Perla EN, Koppel B, Rieber EE. Acquired immunodeficiency syndrome (AIDS) in an economically disadvantaged population. *Arch Intern Med* 1985;145:1607–1612.

258. Ninane J, Grymonprez A, Burtonboy G, Francois A, Cornu G. Disseminated BCG in HIV infection. *Arch Dis Child* 1988;63:1268–1269.

259. Houde C, Dery P. *Mycobacterium bovis* sepsis in an infant with human immunodeficiency virus infection. *Pediatr Infect Dis J* 1988;7:810–812.

260. Fischl M, Pitchenik AE, Spira TJ. Tuberculous brain abscess and toxoplasma encephalitis in a patient with the acquired immunodeficiency syndrome. *JAMA* 1985;253:3428–3430.

261. Centers for Disease Control. A strategic plan for the elimination of tuberculosis in the United States. *MMWR* 1989;38(Suppl S-3):1–25.

262. Luelmo F. BCG vaccination. *Am Rev Respir Dis* 1982;125(Suppl 1):70–72.

263. Camargos PAM, Guimaraes MDC, Antunes CMF. Risk assessment for acquiring meningitis tuberculosis among children not vaccinated with BCG: a case–control study. *Int J Epidemiol* 1988;17:193–197.

264. Centers for Disease Control. Tuberculosis provisional data—United States, 1986. *MMWR* 1987;36:254–255.

Infections of the Central Nervous System,
edited by W. M. Scheld, R. J. Whitley, and
D. T. Durack, Raven Press, Ltd., New York © 1991.

CHAPTER 19

Brain Abscess

Brian Wispelwey, Ralph G. Dacey, Jr., and W. Michael Scheld

Brain abscess is a focal suppurative process within the brain parenchyma which continues to be a diagnostic and therapeutic challenge to the clinician. Paradoxically, the mortality and morbidity from a brain abscess has remained high until relatively recently despite the presence of potent, specific antimicrobial therapy and advances in neurosurgical technique.

The first reference to a brain abscess is attributed to Hippocrates in 460 B.C. In commenting on a syndrome of purulent otorrhea and fever associated with cerebral symptoms, he stated the following: "We need to pay attention in acute ear pain accompanied by fever because the patient can become delirious and in a short time die" (1,2). It can be argued, however, that he believed that the intracranial infection was primary and that involvement of the ear was secondary, being a conduit for drainage of focal suppuration of the brain. He astutely noted that as long as otorrhea persisted, the prognosis was better. A description of the disease, along with a therapeutic proposal, was found in an article dating back to the 16th century (3). In this article, Morand described the first successful drainage of a nontraumatic brain abscess. Another successfully managed case was described by Roux in 1821. In 1814, Farre was the first person to associate brain abscess with cyanotic congenital heart disease (CCHD) (4). A series of reports followed in the latter half of the 19th century describing newer surgical approaches to this problem, including the utility of dural incision associated with abscess aspiration or excision (3). These practices have remained the mainstay in the neurosurgical management of brain abscess. These new surgical ap-

proaches coincided with, and were made possible by, Lister's description of antiseptic principles in the practice of surgery in 1867. In 1893, MacEwen (5) reported the remarkable figure of 80% (8 of 10) survival following surgical drainage of temporal lobe abscesses, despite the observation that six of these patients were unconscious at the time of surgery. This publication established MacEwen as the "father" of modern brain abscess management.

In the 20th century, surgical techniques continued to be refined and antibiotics were introduced, but diagnostic delay continued to be the major obstacle in the success of therapeutic intervention. Significant improvements in the mortality and morbidity rates associated with brain abscess have only occurred in the last 10–15 years. Advances in noninvasive diagnostic techniques are largely responsible for this change. These modalities allow for both earlier diagnosis and more precise localization of abscesses before either the mass effect or uncontrolled infection leads to irreversible brain damage or death. The relative contributions of medical or surgical approaches to the individual patient with a brain abscess continues to be refined. The lack of prospective randomized trials evaluating various treatment approaches, along with the difficulty in achieving adequate numbers of truly comparable patients, contributes to some continued uncertainties regarding optimal management of any given brain abscess patient.

EPIDEMIOLOGY

The incidence of brain abscess has remained relatively stable in the antibiotic era (5–8). It is estimated that brain abscess accounts for approximately one of every 10,000 general hospital admissions, and 4–10 cases are seen yearly on active neurosurgical services in hospitals of developed countries (9,10). Some series have noted a slightly increased incidence of brain abscesses recently

B. Wispelwey: Department of Medicine, Division of Infectious Diseases, University of Virginia Health Sciences Center, Charlottesville, Virginia 22908.
R. G. Dacey, Jr.: Department of Neurosurgery, Washington University School of Medicine, St. Louis, Missouri 63110.
W. M. Scheld: Departments of Medicine and Neurosurgery, Division of Infectious Diseases, University of Virginia Health Sciences Center, Charlottesville, Virginia 22908.

(11–13). In a series of 42 brain abscesses observed from 1961 to 1971 in Texas (13), 11 were discovered between 1961 and 1965 and 31 were detected between 1966 and 1971. This increase was observed despite constant admission and autopsy rates at the monitored hospitals. However, this series also included nine cases of posttraumatic abscesses, which are often either excluded from other reports or seen less frequently in other non-military-based series. A more recent study (12) suggests that the observed increased incidence in brain abscess may represent a bias of more sensitive diagnostic techniques. These authors reported on 45 cases of brain abscess observed in Louisville, Kentucky from 1970 to 1983 and noted that the number of cases of brain abscess increased from 1.5 per year during 1970–1975 to 4.6 per year during 1977–1983. This increase coincided with the introduction of computerized tomographic (CT) scanning at the participating institutions. In contrast, the authors of a series reporting 868 brain abscesses in Hungary (1936–1984) noted a progressive decline in the incidence of brain abscess through 1960 (14). They attributed this decline to the extensive use of antibiotics beginning in 1950. This decline was followed by a more recent increase in the number of cases, with an associated increase in the recovery of antimicrobial-resistant bacteria from these lesions.

Brain abscess remains a significant problem in the developing world. Two recent publications from South Africa (15,16) report a continued high frequency of central nervous system (CNS) complications associated with inadequately treated middle ear disease, particularly in the lower socioeconomic regions in this country. At present, it is uncertain whether the increased utilization (in developed countries) of intravascular catheters and other invasive procedures, including neurosurgical intervention or the increasing average age and disease severity in hospitalized patients, will influence the incidence of brain abscess in the future (17). The advent of the acquired immunodeficiency syndrome (AIDS) has led to increased numbers of individuals with focal intracranial infections encountered in many hospital settings. For example, estimates of the prevalence of *Toxoplasma gondii* encephalitis in patients with AIDS have ranged from 2.6% to 30.8% (18).

The pathogenesis and incidence of brain abscess varies among different geographic locales. In China, 65% of brain abscesses were observed to be secondary to otitis media, but only 0.5% were found to be secondary to paranasal sinusitis (19). This is contrasted to 20–40% of brain abscesses occurring secondary to otitis media and 15–25% secondary to sinusitis in series from Northern European countries (20,21). Several authors (8,11,13) have reported a male predominance (3:1) among patients with a brain abscess; more recently, a series of 45 patients revealed a male-to-female ratio of 2.7:1 (12). In another series of 257 patients (1973–1977) the ratio was

only 1.2:1 (22,23). The median age of patients with a brain abscess is 30–40 years (19,24,25); however, the predominant age may vary somewhat by etiology. In some series, brain abscess due to otitis media displays a bimodal age distribution, with peaks in the pediatric age group and after 40 years of age (26), whereas abscess secondary to paranasal sinusitis more commonly occurs between 10 and 30 years of age (26,27). The average age, prevalence of male patients, and peak incidence in the second and third decades of life in a recently published series of brain abscesses (12) are comparable to data from other reports published over the last 30 years. Approximately 25% of all brain abscesses occur in children less than 15 years of age (11), with the peak incidence between ages 4 and 7 (28). A male predominance (2:1) has again been observed in most pediatric series (2). CCHD and contiguous ear, nose, and throat infections have been responsible for the majority of cases in almost equal percentages (29). Brain abscess prior to age 2 appears to be rare (2), but when it occurs it is most frequently associated with gram-negative bacillary meningitis (30). A recent series from Paris (30) described a marked increase in neonatal brain abscesses at the Hôpital des Enfants Malades. In 30 cases seen between 1973 and 1985, 28 were observed after 1978 and 23 after 1982. This increased incidence was largely attributed to improved diagnostic techniques, suggesting that many brain abscesses in this age group may have formerly been incorrectly diagnosed as bacterial meningitis alone. This observation may partially explain the high mortality observed in earlier series of neonatal gram-negative bacillary meningitis.

ETIOLOGY

In the preantibiotic era, analysis of intracranial pus revealed *Staphylococcus aureus* in 25–30% of cases, streptococci in 30%, coliforms in 12%, and no growth in approximately 50% (22,23). With proper attention to techniques, the role of anaerobic agents in brain abscess has become apparent. In one earlier study (31), 14 of 18 abscesses grew anaerobes on culture—predominantly streptococci in 66%, with *Bacteroides* species in 60%. Series from the United Kingdom have stressed the role of anaerobic bacteria in brain abscesses, especially of otic origin (22,23,32). In addition, some reports suggest that the proportion of abscesses due to staphylococci are decreasing in frequency, whereas members of the Enterobacteriaceae are now more prevalent (6,11). Additionally, the location of a given brain abscess or its predisposing cause often suggests the most likely etiologic agent(s) (Table 1). Several series have noted that frontal lobe abscesses resulting from a preexisting sinusitis often yield one of the *Streptococcus milleri* group of organisms in pure culture (22,23,33). Of note, brain ab-

TABLE 1. *Brain abscess: predisposing conditions, site of abscess, and microbiology*

Predisposing conditions	Site of abscess	Usual isolate(s) from abscess
Contiguous site or primary infection		
Otitis media and mastoiditis	Temporal lobe or cerebellar hemisphere	Streptococci (anaerobic or aerobic), *Bacteroides fragilis*, Enterobacteriaceae
Frontoethmoidal sinusitis	Frontal lobe	Predominantly streptococci, *Bacteroides*, Enterobacteriaceae, *Staphylococcus aureus*, and *Haemophilus* species
Sphenoidal sinusitis	Frontal or temporal lobe	Same as in frontoethmoidal sinusitis
Dental sepsis	Frontal lobe	Mixed *Fusobacterium*, *Bacteroides*, and *Streptococcus* species
Penetrating cranial trauma or postsurgical infection	Related to wound	*S. aureus*, streptococci, Enterobacteriaceae, *Clostridium sp*
Distant site of primary infection		
Congenital heart disease	Multiple abscess cavities, middle cerebral artery distribution common but may occur at any site	Viridans, anaerobic, and microaerophilic streptococci; *Haemophilus* species
Lung abscess, empyema, bronchiectases	Same as in congenital heart disease	*Fusobacterium*, *Actinomyces*, *Bacteroides*, streptococci, *Nocardia asteroides*
Bacterial endocarditis	Same as in congenital heart disease	*S. aureus*, streptococci
Compromised host (immunosuppressive therapy or malignancy)	Same as in congenital heart disease	*Toxoplasma*, fungi, Enterobacteriaceae, *Nocardia*

scess in association with chronic sinusitis is often a mixed infection, with an anaerobe-to-aerobe ratio of 1:1.5 reported in two series (34). Post-traumatic abscesses are usually caused by staphylococci. Temporal lobe abscesses are often a complication of otitis media and almost always have multiple agents isolated, including streptococci, *Bacteroides* species, and gram-negative aerobic bacilli (22,23,32,33). Some authors have noted that ~33% of chronically infected ears yield anaerobes on culture (34). In a study of 28 patients with cholesteatoma, bacteria were cultured from 24 at surgery. A total of 74 isolates were present: 40 were aerobes and 34 were anaerobes. In contrast to acute otitis in which *Streptococcus pneumoniae, Hemophilus influenzae, Moraxella catarrhalis,* and other streptococci predominate, gram-negative aerobes (i.e., *Pseudomonas aeruginosa, Proteus* species, *Klebsiella pneumoniae*), anaerobic cocci, and *Bacteroides* species were the most common isolates (35).

The current pattern of microbial isolates from brain abscesses is shown in Table 2 (11–13,22,25,36–42). These data represent a summary of 12 separate series of brain abscesses but do not include patients with AIDS, and they represent both children and adults. The organisms and their frequency of isolation in exclusively pediatric-based series of brain abscess are similar to these figures except in the neonatal setting (43). An organism's isolation frequency is expressed as a percentage of the total number of organisms that were isolated. Sterile abscesses were encountered in 0–43% of the cases, with the frequency of occurrence correlating (to some degree) with prior antibiotic use. Aerobic streptococci represented 31% of the isolates. This percentage may actually

be higher, because the microaerophilic streptococci may occasionally be classified as anaerobic streptococci in some series. Based on information from several of these series (13,22,36,40–42), aerobic or microaerophilic streptococci are isolated from as many as 70% of brain abscesses. The difference in these percentages (31% versus 70%) is related to the frequent occurrence of mixed infections (30–60% of cases), and thus the total number of organisms isolated is greater than the number of abscesses in a given series. The streptococci represent a diverse group of organisms; however, those most frequently isolated belong to the *Streptococcus milleri* group (*S. anginosus, S. constellatus, S. intermedius*), which has a recognized predilection for causing focal suppurative disease (44–46). In a survey of United States clinical isolates of viridans streptococci (1969–1975), Facklam (47) reported 28 strains from brain abscesses 23 (82%) of which belonged to the *S. milleri* group. In two other series (22,48), these organisms were isolated in 14 of 35 and 13 of 16 brain abscesses. The organism's striking association with focal suppurative disease and brain abscess remains incompletely understood. These organisms are often microaerophilic but yield aerobic patterns by gas–liquid chromotographic analysis (22,23). Most of the *S. milleri* group are placed in Lancefield group F and possess Ottens and Winklers type O III antigen. This observation of type predominance has not been confirmed by others (44). Suggested virulence factors to explain this organism's proclivity to cause suppurative disease have included its polysaccharide capsule, its ability to produce an immunodepressant, and its capacity to produce certain tissue-damaging toxins (44). Only the presence of a capsule has been correlated with capacity

TABLE 2. *Microbiologic etiology of brain abscess*

Organisms	Ref. 11 (n = 200)	Ref. 25 (n = 60)	Ref. 13 (n = 42)	Ref. 12 (n = 45)	Ref. 38 (n = 54)	Ref. 39 (n = 74)	Ref. 42 (n = 16)	Ref. 41 (n = 18)	Ref. 40 (n = 15)	Ref. 37 (n = 44)	Ref. 15 (n = 46)	Ref. 36 (n = 42)	Total (%)
Aerobes													420 (61.2)
Staphylococcus aureus	33	7	11	1	10	14	1	0	3	4	6	2	92 (13.4)
Gram-negative bacilli	15	18	10	5	3	14	3	3	2	13	7	15	108 (15.7)
Streptococci	29	22	8	16	14	34	9	11	6	23	25	23	220 (32.1)
Anaerobes													220 (32.1)
Streptococci	18	10	5	8	2	3	6	0	0	2	2	10	66 (9.6)
Bacteroides species	0	4	5	3	0	7	3	3	0	15	10	24	74 (10.8)
Others	0	8	0	6	4	1	3	4	4	27	0	23	80 (11.7)
Miscellaneous	4	4	0	3	5	10	2	4	2	8	0	4	46 (6.7)
												Grand total:	686

to induce infection in experimental animals (44). *Streptococcus pneumoniae,* despite being one of the three most common species causing bacterial meningitis, is infrequently (2–3%) isolated from brain abscesses (12). *Staphylococcus aureus* represented 12.5% of the isolates and is present in 10–15% of brain abscesses, often in pure culture. It remains the most common pathogen in abscesses that follow trauma. Aerobic gram-negative bacilli are found, usually in mixed culture in 23–33% of cases (22,23,49), and represented 15.8% of the isolates. *Proteus* species are the most frequently isolated organism of this group and exhibit a particular association with otogenic disease (23) and neonatal brain abscess (30). *Escherichia coli, Klebsiella-Enterobacter* species, and *Pseudomonas* species are the next most frequently isolated. Recently, *Pseudomonas aeruginosa* was isolated from 67% of middle ear cultures from children with chronic otitis media (50), suggesting that therapy for this organism should be included in treatment for suspected otogenic brain abscess. A polymicrobial brain abscess whose flora included *Pseudomonas paucimobilis* following a lawn dart injury was recently reported (51). *Haemophilus* species are isolated in 5–10% of cases (12), with *H. aphrophilus* being the most frequently isolated (28). Brain abscess secondary to *H. influenzae* is rare despite its status as the most frequent cause of bacterial meningitis. *Salmonella* brain abscess is also uncommon. This disease is most likely to occur in adults with certain predisposing factors: meningitis, trauma, and intracranial hematoma. The most common serotypes are *S. typhi, S. typhimurium,* and *S. enteritidis* (52). *Streptobacillus moniliformis,* the cause of the streptobacillary form of rat-bite fever, is a rare cause of brain abscess (53). *Brucella* species have been implicated in CNS infections, especially meningitis and meningoencephalitis, but brain abscess is an unusual complication. A case of multiple brain abscesses due to *B. melitensis* was recently reported (54). *Citrobacter* species, especially *C. diversus,* are frequently implicated in brain abscesses that arise as a complication of neonatal meningitis (2,30,55,56). Several cases of brain abscess due to *Eikenella corrodens* have been described (57,58); the majority of cases appear to be either dental, sinus, or otic in origin. Anaerobes are isolated in 40–100% (12) of cases and represented 32.2% of the total isolates. *Bacteroides* species, including *B. fragilis,* are isolated in 20–40% of cases of brain abscess and represented 10.8% of the isolates. They are often found in mixed culture (22,23,32,33). Many other anaerobes have been isolated, including anaerobic streptococci (9.7% of the isolates), *Clostridium* species, *Fusobacterium* species, *Actinomyces* species, and others (10,22,23, 59–61). *Proprionobacterium acnes,* an anaerobic gram-positive rod, has recently been observed as a cause of brain abscess, especially in the post-trauma or neurosurgery patient (62). *Bacillus cereus,* an aerobic gram-positive rod, has been implicated in at least three cases of

brain abscess in immunocompromised hosts (63). Several reports of brain abscesses due to *Listeria monocytogenes* or *Nocardia asteroides* have been published, again showing a predilection for the compromised host (64–66); although up to 48% of individuals with nocardial infections may have no obvious immunocompromising condition (12). *Nocardia asteroides* infections of the brain frequently have an associated pulmonary portal of entry. It has been observed that 18–44% of patients with nocardial infection have CNS involvement with this organism. *Nocardia* usually produces single CNS lesions, but cases of multiple abscesses have been described (67). Invasion of the CNS by *Mycobacterium tuberculosis* accounts for ≤0.5% of cases of tuberculosis in the United States. Space-occupying lesions due to *M. tuberculosis* were thought to be rare, but since the advent of CT scanning, focal lesions (tuberculomas) have been observed in a substantial minority of cases of tuberculous meningitis (68). This infection is also somewhat geographically dependent. In a series of 121 consecutive CNS infections in Saudi Arabia, 14 of the 25 focal intracranial infections were due to *Mycobacterium tuberculosis* and only eight of the remaining 11 were classified as typical brain abscess (69). Additionally, tuberculosis accounted for 11% of focal intracranial infections in Mexico (10).

Yeasts and dimorphic fungi have assumed an increasing role as the etiologic agents of focal intracranial infections. Most cases occur in immunocompromised patients, and mortality remains extremely high (70). Several cases of focal CNS infections due to *Aspergillus* species have been reported, but long-term survival has been documented in only five instances (71). An occipital lobe abscess due to *Aspergillus* was recently successfully treated with combined stereotactic aspiration and amphotericin B (71). Agents of zygomycosis can also invade the CNS. In addition to the rhinocerebral form of zygomycosis found in diabetics with ketoacidosis or in neutropenic hosts, cerebral zygomycosis with abscess formation also occurs in parenteral drug abusers. *Pseudallescheria boydii,* a cause of mycetoma, has received increased attention as a potential cause of CNS infection. A recent review (72) reported on the 21 previously described cases of CNS infection by *P. boydii.* Thirteen of these infections were brain abscesses. In only three of the 21 cases could no predisposing condition be found. In addition to illnesses leading to immunosuppression, four of the patients experienced a near-drowning episode as their presumed risk factor. Fifteen of the 18 patients diagnosed while still alive subsequently died. Candidiasis is the fungal infection most frequently observed at autopsy involving the CNS. Cases of diffuse cerebritis with miliary microabscesses, along with large parenchymal abscesses due to *Candida* species, have been described (73). *Cryptococcus neoformans* usually causes meningitis when it invades the CNS, but mass lesions due to this organism have been observed. *Xylohypha*

TABLE 3. *Brain abscess in the compromised host*

Abnormal cell-mediated immunity	Neutropenia or neutrophil defects
Toxoplasma gondii	Aerobic gram-negative bacteria
Nocardia asteroides	*Aspergillus* species
Cryptococcus neoformans	*Zygomycetes*
Listeria monocytogenes	*Candida* species
Mycobacterium species	

bantianum (*Cladosporium trichoides* or *bantianum*) is the most common cause of cerebral phaeohyphomycosis, accounting for 28 of the 53 reported cases (74). Other agents of phaeohyphomycosis (i.e., *Bipolaris* species, *Curvularia* species, *Wangiella* species) have been described as causes of focal CNS infections. The first cases of brain abscesses due to *Ramichloridium obovoideum* were recently reported from Saudi Arabia (75). Other fungal etiologies of brain abscess include agents of chromoblastomycosis, *Blastomyces dermatitidis*, *Coccidioides immitis*, and, rarely, *Histoplasma capsulatum*.

Various protozoa and helminths may cause brain abscesses, their incidence varying with geographic location. Toxoplasmosis is one of the most common parasitic infections of the brain, in the setting of AIDS (76) (see below). *Strongyloides stercoralis* may disseminate to the CNS from its usual site in the gastrointestinal tract in the immunosuppressed patient. A concomitant gram-negative bacillary meningitis and brain abscess can occur as a result of either (a) bacteria carried in the gut of the migrating larvae or (b) a simultaneous bacteremia (77,78). Of the pathogenic amebae, *Entamoeba histolytica* is the organism most likely to cause a brain abscess. In an autopsy study from Mexico City, 210 cases of amebiasis were documented, 17 (8.1%) of which involved the CNS. The lesions are usually multiple and are most often associated with another focal site of infection, usually hepatic (78). Of the three major species of *Schistosoma*, *S. japonicum* is the one most likely, although rarely, to cause focal involvement of the brain (78). Cysticercosis due to *T. solium* larvae (Chapter 35) is a major cause of brain lesions in the developing world. For example, cysticercosis accounted for 85% of all brain infections in Mexico City, whereas only 3% were pyogenic abscesses (10). Other helminthic infections which can occasionally lead to focal intracranial lesions include echinococcosis, paragonimiasis, and trichinosis (78).

The patient's immune system is an important determinant of the microbiology of a brain abscess (Table 3). The infecting organism can be predicted with some degree of certainty, and the differential diagnosis can be narrowed significantly by knowledge of the nature of the immune defect (79). One difficulty with any scheme relating organisms to host defects is that most patients present multiple immune abnormalities—namely, those of the underlying disease state, complicating its treatment (i.e., cancer chemotherapy or transplant immunosuppression) or resulting from a generalized deterioration in clinical status (i.e., malnutrition). Patients with T-lymphocyte or mononuclear phagocyte defects are commonly encountered in most hospital settings. Causes of this abnormality include AIDS (see below), lymphoma, lymphocytic leukemias, treatment regimens for these malignancies, chronic steroid therapy, and organ or bone marrow transplantation (with their attendant immunosuppressive regimen). Common causes of brain abscess in this patient group are *Toxoplasma gondii* and *Nocardia asteroides*. Less common but possible etiologies include *Cryptococcus neoformans* (which usually causes meningitis), *Listeria monocytogenes* (which usually causes a meningoencephalitis), or *Mycobacterium* species (79,80). Neutrophil defects are most often due to chemotherapy-induced neutropenia. Less commonly encountered are congenital defects in neutrophil function, such as chronic granulomatous disease or myeloperoxidase deficiency. An increased incidence of brain abscess secondary to the presence of *Pseudomonas aeruginosa* and members of the Enterobacteriaceae family is seen paralleling their increased presence as a cause of meningitis in this group of patients (67). Neutropenia also leads to an increased occurrence of CNS fungal disease. As noted in the preceding discussion, multiple fungal agents have been observed; prominent among these are infections with *Aspergillus* species, agents of zygomycosis, and *Candida* species. A fungal brain abscess should be strongly considered in a hospitalized patient who has been neutropenic for more than 1 week and has been receiving intravenous hyperalimentation and broad-spectrum antibiotics (80) in the appropriate clinical/radiologic setting.

AIDS has become one of the most important risk factors for the development of an intracranial infection (Table 4). Focal CNS infections of diverse etiologies have been described, and multiple pathogenic processes may coexist (81). In a recent autopsy series of patients with

TABLE 4. *Differential diagnosis of focal CNS lesions in patients with AIDS*

Toxoplasmosis	*Candida* species
Primary CNS lymphoma	*Listeria monocytogenes*
Mycobacterium tuberculosis	*Nocardia asteroides*
Mycobacterium avium-intracellulare	*Salmonella* group B
Progressive multifocal leukoencephalopathy	*Aspergillus* species
Cryptococcus neoformans	

human immunodeficiency virus (HIV) infection, 11 of 26 brains were affected by more than one disease process (82). Toxoplasmosis is the most common cause of focal disease, occurring in 103 of 366 (28%) AIDS patients with CNS complications (83). Multiple lesions are documented in the majority of cases but are otherwise difficult to distinguish from pyogenic lesions by CT. Serologic studies can be confusing; rarely, cases of CNS toxoplasmosis have been documented, even in serologically negative patients (81). This infection has been reported nearly three times more frequently in AIDS patients from Florida than in those from the rest of the United States (18). Primary CNS lymphoma is the next most common cause of focal disease in AIDS. Multiple lesions are not uncommon, especially when magnetic resonance imaging (MRI) is used for diagnosis (84). Progressive multifocal leukoencephalopathy, caused by a papovavirus, occurs in a significant minority of AIDS patients. The lack of mass effect, surrounding edema, contrast enhancement, and the confinement of these lesions to white matter are useful in differentiating this process from toxoplasmosis or lymphoma. Numerous other pathogens have been described as causes of mass lesions in patients with AIDS, including *Mycobacterium tuberculosis* (85), *Mycobacterium avium-intracellulare, C. neoformans, Candida* species, *Aspergillus* species, *Coccidiodes immitis* (86), *Nocardia asteroides, Listeria monocytogenes,* and *Salmonella* group B (81,87).

Despite the relative predictability of the etiologic agent, brain abscess in the compromised host may be difficult to detect by CT scan (67). Mass effect may be the only finding, and contrast enhancement may be decreased by steroids (88) and/or by the diminished inflammatory reaction caused by certain fungal agents (67). Negative CT scans with documented CNS toxoplasmosis are well described in AIDS patients; these lesions are often detectable by MRI.

PATHOGENESIS AND PATHOPHYSIOLOGY

A more complete understanding regarding the pathogenetic and pathophysiologic mechanisms responsible for brain abscess formation has come from careful observation of patients with this infection, supported by information derived from numerous animal models of experimental brain abscess. These animal models are discussed in detail in Chapter 14.

Brain abscesses occur most commonly in association with one of three distinct clinical settings: (i) a contiguous focus of infection; (ii) hematogenous spread from a distant focus; or (iii) cranial trauma. No predisposing factors are recognized in approximately 15–20% of reported cases.

The majority of patients with brain abscess demonstrate a contiguous focus of infection, usually sinusitis or otitis. Data compiled from 19 series of brain abscesses from 1927 to the present (12,14,19) have revealed that abscesses related to contiguous infections accounted for 47% of more than 3500 cases. Otogenic infection was the most common contiguous process associated with brain abscess and was present in more than one-third of the total cases. Metastatic or hematogenous abscesses accounted for 25% and no predisposing factor could be determined in ~14%. More recent series suggest that otogenic brain abscesses appear to be decreasing in relative frequency. In a series of 54 patients with brain abscess from Sweden (1973–1985), otogenic infections accounted for only 7.4% of the cases (38). Similarly, a review of 102 cases (1970–1986) from San Francisco included only 19 patients with any contiguous infection as a predisposing factor. These 19 cases were due to either sinusitis, otitis, or dental infections. AIDS patients with neurologic complications were not included in this series (89). However, in areas where otitis media continues to be neglected or where therapy is delayed, intracranial complications of this process still present a serious threat (15,16). In a series by Samuel et al. (15) spanning only 6 years (1978–1983) in South Africa, 335 patients with complicated otogenic infections were recognized in which an intracranial complication developed in 224. Seventy-four percent of the cases occurred in children less than 15 years of age. Meningitis was the most common complication, accounting for 37% of the cases; brain abscesses accounted for 24%, or 53 cases. However, the complication of brain abscess resulted in an overall mortality of 36%, as opposed to an 8% mortality in the cases of meningitis. A second series of 130 patients with acute and chronic mastoiditis was recently published from the same country (16). Of the 74 individuals with documented cholesteatoma, 33 developed an intracranial complication, 27 of which were brain abscesses. In the 56 remaining patients without cholesteatoma, only three brain abscesses were observed. Other series have also noted a 60% or greater frequency of associated cholesteatoma in otogenic brain abscesses (36,89). This observation stands in marked contrast to the report by Samuel et al. (15) where cholesteatomas could be documented in only 38% of the 53 brain abscesses. Chronic mucosal disease accounted for the majority of cases in this series but accounted for only 38% of cases in another report (90). Of note, prior mastoid surgery was not found to preclude later intracranial complications (90). Therefore, a cholesteatoma is not a necessary prerequisite for the development of an intracranial complication in the setting of an otitic focus of infection. In addition, an intact tympanic membrane or normal otoscopic examination is not totally reassuring, since several cases of otogenic brain abscess have been reported despite normal or unimpressive findings (90–92). Overall, chronic otitis media and/or mastoiditis leads to intracranial extension four to eight times more frequently than does acute disease. However, as emphasized in a recent publication

(93), complications of acute mastoiditis can occur frequently. Thirty children with acute mastoiditis were identified. Forty-two percent had received oral antibiotics within 2 weeks of presentation. Six children (20%) developed a neurologic complication, one of which was a brain abscess. Of note, all four children who did not have swelling over the mastoid area presented with a neurologic complication. Prior to the advent of antibiotic therapy, ~3–6% of patients with otogenic infections developed an intracranial complication, with approximately 15% of those presenting as a brain abscess (2,89). Current risk estimates are more difficult to assess; however, recent epidemiologic data from Scotland suggests that only one of 3500 cases of chronic otitis media are complicated by an intracranial abscess (90). As noted by several authors, frequent but inadequate courses of antimicrobial therapy may disguise or alter the natural history of the disease, resulting in more subtle presentations (90–92). The majority of otogenic brain abscesses (55–75%) are located in the temporal lobe. The cerebellum is the next most commonly affected area (20–30%), and it has been observed that 85–99% of cerebellar abscesses are secondary to otogenic infections. Cases of frontal lobe and rare brainstem abscesses arising from an otic focus have been reported. Most otogenic brain abscesses are solitary lesions (6–11,13,25).

Brain abscess secondary to paranasal sinusitis also appears to be decreasing in incidence; however, sinusitis continues to be the major predisposing condition leading to subdural empyema (Chapter 20). In a series from Great Britain (27), sinusitis was encountered almost as frequently as otitis media as a cause of brain abscess and accounted for 15% of brain abscesses over a 30-year period. The majority of patients were young and otherwise healthy, with peak occurrence in the 10- to 30-year age group. As in patients with otitis media, many were treated with antibiotics in the weeks preceding diagnosis. This is again thought to modify the disease process, often making the presentation less dramatic. Similarly, a review of 47 rhinogenic abscesses from Hungary (14) noted a peak incidence in the second and third decades. Rhinogenic abscesses are believed to be rare in children less than 10 years of age and in adults greater than 60 years of age. Only three of the 47 cases were observed in these age groups in this series. The frontal lobe is almost exclusively involved as a complication of sinusitis reflecting the distribution of the associated sinusitis. The majority of cases are in the setting of frontoethmoidal disease followed by maxillary disease (12,14,27). Sphenoid sinusitis, despite its relative rarity, has seemingly more frequent and severe complications. In the preantibiotic era, the sphenoids were involved in 15–30% of cases of sinusitis, but a recent review from Boston noted that sphenoid sinusitis accounted for only 3% of all documented sinusitis cases (94). Teed (95), in 1938, emphasized the high incidence of complications and mortality associated with this infection. He demonstrated a pituitary abscess in 16 of 126 patients with sphenoid sinusitis. A more recent review of 30 cases (94) also documented a high incidence of intracerebral complications (meningitis, cavernous sinus thrombosis, pituitary infarction), but no cases of brain abscess were observed. The diagnosis of sphenoid sinusitis is often missed on presentation, resulting in delay in the initiation of appropriately aggressive antimicrobial therapy. One of the predisposing factors to sphenoid sinusitis in this series was cocaine inhalation. Sinusitis and cranial osteitis are recognized complications of frequent inhalation of cocaine, and recently a case of a brain abscess as a complication of cocaine inhalation was reported (96).

Dental infection is less frequently documented as a predisposing cause of a brain abscess. Given the frequency of dental infections, intracranial complications of this process must be rare. Cavernous sinus thrombosis, subdural empyema, and meningitis all complicate odontogenic infections more frequently than does a brain abscess (97). One recent series reported six odontogenic brain abscesses out of 45 observed cases (13%), an unusually high frequency (12). Another report noted a dental source in five of 81 cases of intracranial suppuration (26). In other large series of brain abscesses, odontogenic infections were infrequently reported as the source of a brain abscess. The majority of odontogenic intracranial infections appear to be a sequel of acute, rather than chronic, infection (98). However, many cases of cryptogenic brain abscess are believed to be secondary to asymptomatic dental foci of infection. This statement is difficult to prove. Brain abscess is more likely to appear following infection of molar teeth, since the infection can spread between the muscles of mastication along facial planes to the base of the skull. Anterior dental infections have direct drainage access to the oral cavity. A large majority of intracranial infections in this setting follow a recent tooth extraction or dental manipulation. The site of an associated brain abscess is most commonly frontal, but temporal lobe localization can also occur by direct extension. (97).

Facial and scalp infections are also important because they may lead to cavernous sinus thrombosis and attendant intracranial suppuration. Brain abscess is a well-known but rare complication of cavernous sinus thrombosis. In a review of 60 cases of cavernous sinus thrombosis, additional intracranial complications were observed in 38 instances, but only five were brain abscesses (99). Some authors suggest that in most instances, development of a brain abscess is a coexisting event rather than a direct consequence of cavernous sinus thrombosis. Importantly, *Staphylococcus aureus* is involved in two-thirds of reported cases (100).

Brain abscess rarely complicates meningitis; however, it should be strongly considered as an associated possibility in the neonate with meningitis, particularly when meningitis is due to gram-negative organisms. Brain abscesses in neonates are caused by enteric gram-negative pathogens, including *Salmonella* group B in the majority of cases; however, cases due to *Hemophilus influenzae* and *Streptococcus pneumoniae* have been observed (43). Of note, the vast majority of neonatal brain abscesses complicate meningitis due to *Proteus mirabilis* or *Citrobacter diversus*. In a recent series (30), despite the fact that *Proteus mirabilis* accounts for only 0.2–4% of neonatal meningitis cases (101), 27 of 30 neonatal brain abscesses diagnosed over a 12-year period were due to this organism. Additionally, abscess formation has been associated with more than 70% of cases of *Citrobacter diversus* meningitis in the infant (101). Therefore, it is argued that any infant in whom these organisms are isolated from either the cerebrospinal fluid (CSF) or the blood should undergo head CT scanning. The increased propensity for these two organisms to cause a brain abscess is incompletely understood. Previous studies suggest that endotoxemia may play a significant role, since cerebral necrosis secondary to neonatal meningitis appears to only occur with endotoxin-containing organisms (2,102). The virulence factors of *Citrobacter diversus* have only recently been studied in detail. A minor 32-kD outer-membrane protein appears to be a marker for strains that are likely to cause meningitis or brain abscess. Fourteen of 17 strains (82%) of *C. diversus* isolated from the CSF, but only two of 21 (10%) strains isolated from other body sites, expressed this protein. This observation may have important epidemiological implications (103).

Brain abscess is the least common intracranial complication of either traumatic injury to the brain or neurosurgery. Clean neurosurgery (craniotomies or laminectomies not involving trauma) are complicated by CNS complications in 0.6–1.7% of cases. Meningitis accounts for 90% of these infections, whereas brain abscess accounts for the remaining 10% (104). CNS infections appear to be more common following transphenoidal pituitary surgery; early series reported the incidence of postoperative meningitis to be as high as 10%. Brain abscess appears to be rare in this setting. However, because of the previously noted decreased frequency of brain abscess as a complication of other processes, intracranial surgery may account for a significant percentage of brain abscesses in more recent series. In a study of 54 adults with brain abscess (1973–1983), 37% occurred following brain or skull surgery (38). The risk of a brain abscess is increased in the setting of a penetrating cranial injury. A brain abscess complicated 37 of 1221 (3%) such injuries from a series of military personnel in Vietnam, with a resultant mortality of 54% in this subset (105). Previous combat series observed an incidence of brain abscess of 3–17% (105,106). As might be expected, the more severe the injury, the greater the likelihood of a complicating brain abscess. The risk of a brain abscess was three times as great after gunshot wounds, five times as great in the setting of a multilobe injury, and eight times as great in individuals with wound complications (such as a hema-

toma, fluid collections, wound infections, and CSF fistula) when compared with those without these risk factors (104). Retained bone fragments appear to be a particularly important associated risk factor. Several series have noted the role of head trauma as the cause of brain abscess in civilians, with incidence ranging from 2.5% to 11% (43,107,108). A variety of types of cranial trauma have been implicated, including compound depressed skull fractures (108), dog bites (109,110), injuries due to rooster pecking (111), and cranial penetration with lawn darts or pencil tips (51,112–117). Several cases of brain abscess as a complication of cervical traction halo immobilization have been described. Associated pin-site cellulitis is usually observed; however, a symptomatic brain abscess may not develop for several months to a few years following the removal of the traction device (118).

Hematogenous brain abscesses often share the following characteristics: (a) a distant focus of infection, most often within the chest; (b) location in the distribution of the middle cerebral artery (Fig. 1); (c) initial location at the gray-matter–white-matter junction; (d) poor encapsulation; and (e) high mortality. These abscesses are more commonly multiple and multiloculated as compared with those that have an origin in foci of contiguous infection (6–11,13,25,57,119). As noted previously, hematogenous abscesses account for approximately 25% of cases in most series (12,14,19). Chronic pyogenic lung diseases, especially lung abscess and bronchiectasis, are important diagnostic considerations (9–11) and may account for 7–17% of total brain abscess cases, or approximately one-half of all hematogenous abscesses (120). Cystic fibrosis is, surprisingly, infrequently complicated by a brain abscess (121); when observed, it most often occurs in older adolescents or adults. In seven described cases, all the patients were 17 years of age or older and had advanced pulmonary disease. The organisms cultured from the sputum matched those cultured from the brain abscess in only two of the seven cases. Associated sinus disease was found in three of the patients; however, the fact that multiple brain abscesses were noted in six of the seven cases, coupled with the fact that the abscesses were usually distant from the sinus, suggests a hematogenous etiology. Other distant foci of infection may be associated with brain abscess and have included wound and skin infections, osteomyelitis, pelvic infection, cholecystitis, and other forms of intra-abdominal sepsis. More recently, brain abscess has been described as an unusual complication of esophageal dilatation of caustic strictures and endoscopic sclerosis of varices (12,122,123). Transient bacteremia is variably observed following both of these procedures. Despite this, brain abscess rarely develops following bacteremia in the setting of a normal blood–brain barrier. Thus, brain abscess is rare in the setting of bacterial endocarditis, despite the presence of persistent bacteremia (Chapter 22). In most series, bacterial endocarditis accounts for 1–5% of cases of

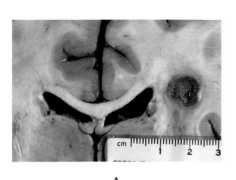 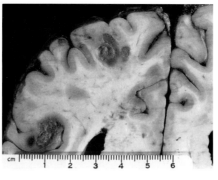 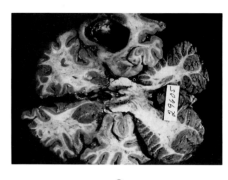

A   B   C

FIG. 1. A: Deep white-matter abscess adjacent to the body of the lateral ventricle. **B:** Multiple brain abscesses at the junction between gray and white matter. **C:** Gross photograph of a large, chronic temporal lobe abscess. The location of this abscess is immediately above the petrous temporal bone.

brain abscess. The development of a brain abscess depends on the level and duration of the bacteremia, the virulence of the organism, and the occurrence of preceding emboli. A greater incidence of brain abscess or meningitis is observed in cases of acute, rather than subacute, bacterial endocarditis. In one series, 62% of cases of acute versus 4% of cases of subacute bacterial endocarditis were complicated by a brain abscess; however, in many instances these abscesses were only seen at autopsy (124). Of 218 patients with infective endocarditis in another series, only nine cases of brain abscess were noted (125). In eight of these cases the brain abscesses were smaller than 1 cm³, and in all cases multiple lesions were found. Additionally, only four of 148 brain abscesses in two large series were due to endocarditis (8,25). Hereditary hemorrhagic telangiectasia is complicated by brain abscess, with striking regularity. A brain abscess may eventually develop in ∼1–6% of these patients, most often in the third to fifth decade of life (126,127). In a review of 31 such cases, pulmonary arteriovenous malformations could be documented in all but two instances. Cyanosis, clubbing, polycythemia, and hypoxemia were also observed in those patients most likely to develop a brain abscess and may be a necessary substrate (126). Hereditary hemorrhagic telangiectasia may be an underrecognized cause of brain abscess, since three of 36 recently described cases of brain abscess were observed in patients with this condition (127).

CCHD is found in 3.4–13.5% of brain abscess cases (128). Some pediatric series suggest that CCHD is the most common cause of brain abscess in children. As many as 25% of all brain abscesses are attributed to CCHD in this age group. The presence of a right-to-left shunt appears to be a critical abnormality. Between 2% and 6% of children with CCHD develop a brain abscess. Tetralogy of Fallot is consistently the most commonly cited, accounting for 52% of 25 recently described cases (128). Patent foramen ovale, ventricular septal defects, and transposition of the great vessels are the next most frequently observed associated disorders. Multiple abscesses have been observed in up to 20% of cases (1,2,11,128–130).

The final common pathway for brain abscess development in the above conditions appears to require a compromised area of brain. Experimental data suggest that infection is extremely difficult to establish in normal brain tissue (131). Brain abscess may develop from a contiguous infection via two major mechanisms: (i) direct extension through areas of associated osteitis or osteomyelitis and (ii) retrograde thrombophlebitic spread via diploic or emissary veins into the intracranial compartment. Additional possibilities in the case of otogenic infection include spread through preexisting channels (the internal auditory canal, cochlear and vestibular aqueducts, or between temporal suture lines). Hematogenous dissemination is occasionally implicated with contiguous foci, particularly in cases of sinus or odontogenic origin (9,10,98,119,132). None of these hypotheses explain the relative rarity of intracranial infection with sinusitis or otitis, how bacteria traverse an intact dura, or what determines the form of intracranial complication that eventually evolves (i.e., meningitis, epidural abscess, subdural empyema, or brain abscess) in the individual with the same predisposing condition.

The development of a brain abscess in the setting of neonatal meningitis deserves special comment. The pathogenesis appears to follow the initiation of a necrotizing vasculitis (particularly in the small penetrating vessels), leading to subsequent hemorrhagic necrosis and liquefaction of the subcortical white matter, an area highly susceptible to changes in cerebral perfusion (2,102). Others disagree with this formulation, contending that the evidence favors an initial ventriculitis followed by ependymal disruption and subsequent direct extension of the infection into the brain parenchyma. Similar findings have been noted in an infant rat model of *C. diversus* meningitis and brain abscess (103) and support the latter hypothesis.

In hematogenous cases, the polycythemia and systemic hypoxia observed in CCHD and hereditary hemorrhagic telangiectasia increase blood viscosity, with an associated reduction in brain capillary flow, perhaps leading to microinfarction and reduced tissue oxygenation in the brain. In both instances, right-to-left shunts are usually observed which allow microemboli to pass by or through the pulmonary circulation, avoiding the normal pulmonary capillary filter and thereby affording them direct access to the cerebral circulation. The underlying damage to the brain may facilitate seeding of certain loci during bacteremic episodes and might explain the predisposition of these patients to brain abscess.

PATHOLOGY

In approximate decreasing order of frequency, a solitary abscess may involve these various brain regions: frontal ≈ temporal > frontoparietal > parietal > cerebellar > occipital (11) (Fig. 1). This distribution reflects the associated, often contiguous, foci of infection. Intrasellar, brainstem, basal ganglia, and thalamic abscesses are rare. Intrasellar abscesses are most common in the setting of preexisting pituitary adenomata; however, cases have occurred in their absence. Some studies have noted one pituitary abscess per 200 autopsied cases. As noted previously, sphenoid sinusitis is a very important predisposing condition for an intrasellar abscess, but cases have been reported in the setting of acute otitis media, mastoiditis, peritonsillar abscess, and a variety of distant foci of infection (133). The anterior lobe of the pituitary is more likely to be involved following hematogenous dissemination. Besides infection by pyogenic bacteria, pituitary infections have been caused by *Treponema pallidum, M. tuberculosis,* and a variety of fungi, including *Histoplasma capsulatum, Blastomyces dermatitidis, Sporothrix schenkii, Candida* species, and *Aspergillus* species (133). Brainstem abscesses arise most often from hematogenous spread from a distant focus of infection; rare cases occur in association with a contiguous infection. In one-third of 48 reported cases, no source was identified. These abscesses are often fusiform and extend over several levels of the brainstem; therefore, the clinical findings can be confusing. Prior to 1974, brainstem abscesses were uniformly fatal, but recent improvements in diagnosis and the ability of neurosurgeons to drain these lesions have led to an occasional survival (134). Inflammatory lesions (especially when solitary) of the thalamus and basal ganglia are also somewhat unusual. One recent series reported five such solitary thalamic abscesses among a total of 135 cases. Most often they are hematogenous in origin (134). The incidence of multiple brain abscesses was only 1–15% in older series; however, with the advent of CT scanning, the frequency of multiple lesions has increased to 10–50% (135). Prior to more recent therapeutic modalities, the mortality from multiple brain abscesses approached 100%.

Once infection is established in the brain, acute inflammatory cells are recruited and local vascular permeability is altered. The evolution of an abscess includes four histopathologic stages (136). This staging process, described in animal models of brain abscess, correlates well with human brain abscess evolution (137). An important feature of this description is the correlation with CT findings, which has direct implications for subsequent therapy.

The first stage is an early cerebritis (days 1–3 following intracerebral inoculation in animals), which progresses to a perivascular inflammatory response surrounding the developing necrotic center by the third day. Profound edema in the surrounding white matter develops concurrently (Fig. 2).

In the second stage of late cerebritis (days 4–9), development of a well-formed necrotic center reaches its maximum size. Additionally, fibroblasts appear, setting the stage for capsule formation and a marked increase in neovascularity at the periphery of the necrotic zone. These newly formed capillaries frequently lack tight junctions and leak proteinaceous fluid (138). Surrounding this is the beginning of a reactive astrocyte response, along with persistent white matter edema.

The third stage, early capsule formation (days 10–13), is characterized by a slight decrease in the size of the necrotic center (Fig. 3). At this point there is a well-developed layer of fibroblasts, with significantly more reticulin deposition on the cortical side of the lesion than on the ventricular side. Outside this developing capsule is a region of persistent cerebritis and neovascularity, with a further increase in reactive astrocytes.

These processes continue in the fourth and final stage, late capsule formation (day 14 and later). The capsule continues to thicken with an abundance of reactive collagen present by the third week. Recent work has criticized the above model's utility in describing a uniform mode of brain abscess evolution (139). These authors, utilizing the same dog model and inoculum, were unable to detect viable organisms in the brain lesions after 3 days, and in all animals the lesions spontaneously resolved. Further work is necessary to reconcile this debate. Two other experimental models of brain abscess using organisms other than alpha-hemolytic streptococci also indicate that this view of abscess evolution is either overly stereotyped or affected by inadequate growth of the microorganisms. In a model of *Bacteroides fragilis* (inoculated with *Staphylococcus epidermidis*) brain abscess (140), the same stages of evolution were observed; however, the early and late capsule stages could not be differentiated, due to a delay in encapsulation when compared to abscesses following streptococcal challenge. These abscesses enlarged more quickly, were prone to

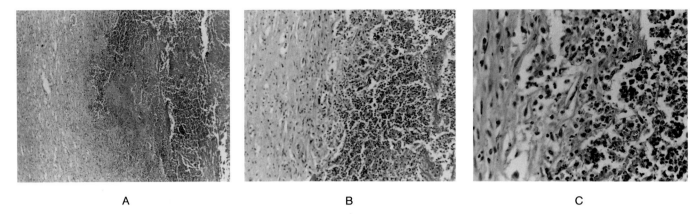

FIG. 2. A: Wall of brain abscess. Normal white matter is seen to the left, and there is an intermediate area of edematous brain adjacent to the abscess wall. **B:** Higher magnification showing periabscess inflammatory exudate. There is relatively little encapsulation at this early stage. **C:** Higher magnification of abscess wall. Note combination of increased gliosis and inflammatory cells adjacent to the abscess.

early ventricular rupture (25%), and exhibited incomplete encapsulation. This suggests the extreme virulence of *B. fragilis,* an important pathogen in brain abscess, in brain tissue when part of a mixed infection. In a model using *Staphylococcus aureus* (141), there were quantitative and qualitative differences in abscess evolution when compared with an alpha-streptococci inoculation.

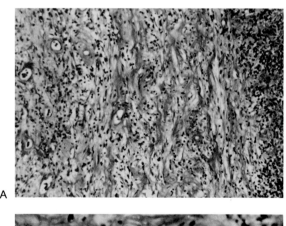

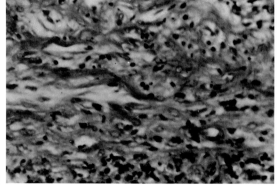

FIG. 3. A: Photomicrograph of abscess wall during a later stage of abscess development. Thick collagen fibers are seen within the capsule wall. **B:** Trichrome stain photomicrogaph of abscess wall. Thick collagen fibers are seen above the inflammatory mass.

S. aureus inoculation resulted in larger lesions, earlier ependymitis, and delayed progress toward healing, with longer periods required for the infection to reach a stable size. The same approximate stages were present, but their separation was also not as distinct as previously described. The white matter appeared more susceptible to destruction than the gray matter, and the spread of infection was more centrifugal rather than along particular white matter tracts. In contradistinction, a model of *Escherichia coli* brain abscess exhibited expansion of the abscess along white matter tracts (142). In addition, the *S. aureus* experimental model raised some questions regarding the previously held assumption that the capsule serves to contain infection. The abscess reached its maximum size in the late cerebritis stage, before any significant capsule formation had taken place, suggesting that the host was able to contain the infection prior to capsule formation. Also, even in the late capsule stage, inflammation, necrosis, and edema extended well beyond the well-formed capsule. This sequence of events is also altered in the immunocompromised host. For example, dogs immunosuppressed by azathioprine and prednisone therapy showed a decreased early inflammatory response and edema formation, followed by a delayed increase in abscess size, when compared to normal controls (143).

Two repeated observations regarding encapsulation deserve special attention: (i) Capsule formation is frequently more complete on the cortical side of the abscess than on the ventricular side (119,136), and (ii) encapsulation is less extensive in abscesses resulting from hematogenous spread than in those arising from a contiguous focus of infection (144). These observations may be related to the fact that oxygen is necessary for pro-alpha chains of collagen to form triple-helix strands (145). Normal cortical gray matter is more vascular than adjacent white matter, perhaps allowing greater fibroblast proliferation and collagen helix formation. This discrepancy probably explains the propensity for abscesses to rupture medially rather than into the subarachnoid space. Similarly, the infarct from a septic embolus might impede optimal collagen formation by fibroblasts (136).

Therefore, brain abscess formation is a continuum from cerebritis to a collagen-encapsulated necrotic focus; however, its maturity is dependent on many factors, including local oxygen concentration, the offending organism (5), and the host's immune response.

CLINICAL MANIFESTATIONS

The clinical manifestations of a brain abscess (Table 5) can vary greatly among patients and depend on several interdependent factors. These factors include the relative virulence of the infecting organism (5), the host's immune status (143), the abscess location, the number of lesions, and the presence or absence of associated meningitis or ventricular rupture. Additionally, symptoms of the primary site of infection (i.e., otitis, sinusitis, or distant suppurative foci) may predominate. The evolution of symptoms of a brain abscess may range from indolent to fulminant; in ~75% the duration of symptoms is ≤2 weeks (13). A recent series of 101 brain abscesses in children (6 days to 15 years of age) noted a duration of symptoms before diagnosis ranging from 3 to 120 days, with a median of 13.3 days (43). Similarly, in a series of 45 brain abscesses, chiefly in adults, symptoms were described from hours to up to 6 weeks before diagnosis, but the average duration was again only 11 days (12). The classic triad of fever, headache, and a focal neurologic deficit is present in less than 50% of patients and was only observed in 28 of the 101 children with a brain abscess described above (43). In most cases, the prominent clinical manifestations of brain abscess are due to an expanding intracerebral mass rather than being signs of infection. For example, fever may be present in only ~50% of patients overall, although it is more commonly observed in children. A temperature of ≥38°C was found in nearly 80% of children from one recent series (43). A moderate-to-severe headache is the most common symptom and is encountered in nearly three-quarters of patients (8,9,13,31). This frequency has been confirmed in three more recent series in which the occur-

rence of headache on presentation was described in 52–76% of patients (12,43,107). The headache may be generalized, suggesting raised intracranial—or, more commonly, hemicranial—pressure (3). A change in mental status, ranging from lethargy to frank coma, occurs in the majority of patients (8,11,13). In a recent review from San Francisco (107), the patients were graded on a five-point scale ranging from fully alert with no deficits to comatose. Eighty-six of the 102 patients were in the better neurologic grades on presentation (grades 0–2). Additionally, the neurologic grade correlated with the patient's year of presentation. Only 68% of patients were represented in grades 0–2 between 1970 and 1974, as opposed to 85–91% of patients who presented from 1975 to 1986. This observation coincided with the introduction of CT scanning at this institution. Similarly, only 12% of patients in another recent series presented in coma (12). Nausea and vomiting are observed in 22–50% of patients, frequently correlating with the presence of raised intracranial pressure (12,38,107). Seizures are consistently observed in 25–45% of patients by the time of presentation. They are most commonly generalized in character (80% of the seizures in one series) (12,39,43,107) and are more common with frontal lobe lesions (9,13,43). Papilledema is observed with varying frequency (5–35%) (9–13,24,38,43); however, the true incidence is difficult to assess, because it is not always documented in retrospective series. Papilledema did not correlate with the size of the abscess, but it was closely associated with the presence of headache and vomiting in one series (43). The presence of nuchal rigidity is also variable (~25% of patients) and tends to be more commonly observed in those patients with a shorter duration of illness (12). On occasion, the clinical presentation of a patient with brain abscess may closely mimic pyogenic meningitis. Focal neurologic findings are present in ~50% of cases and are dependent on the location and size of the lesion and concurrent surrounding edema (6–11,13). Hemiplegia appears to be the most commonly observed abnormality and was present in 33% of 518 patients in one review (3). Hemianopsias also account for a significant percentage of the focal defects observed in supratentorial lesions (3,12). Cranial nerve abnormalities were observed in 15–30% of patients from two recent series (12,43). Abscesses of the cerebellar hemispheres (10–18% of intracranial abscesses) often produce nystagmus, ataxia, vomiting, and dysmetria (146,147). The clinical presentation of frontal lobe abscesses is often dominated by headache, drowsiness, inattention, and a generalized deterioration in mental function. Hemiparesis with unilateral motor signs and a motor speech disorder are the most common focal findings. A temporal lobe abscess may present with early ipsilateral headache. If the abscess is in the dominant hemisphere, an aphasia or dysphasia may be present. An upper homonymous hemianopsia may also be demon-

TABLE 5. Clinical manifestations of brain abscess

Symptom/sign[a]	Percent
Headache	70
Fever	40–50
Focal neurologic deficit	~50
Triad of fever, headache, focal deficit	<50
Nausea/vomiting	22–50
Seizures	25–45
Nuchal rigidity	~25
Papilledema	~25

[a] Other symptoms/signs are dependent on location.

strated and may be the only sign of a right temporal lobe abscess (148). Intrasellar abscesses often simulate a pituitary tumor, presenting with headache, visual field defects, and various endocrine disturbances (133,149). Brainstem abscesses most frequently present with facial weakness, fever, headache, hemiparesis, dysphagia, and vomiting (134). Neurologic findings, however subtle, in a patient with any of the predisposing conditions previously discussed, mandate investigation of the CNS to exclude brain abscess or other intracranial complications of these disorders.

Because of their nonspecific presentation and frequent lack of fever, brain abscesses can be confused with several other processes. The differential diagnosis may include other infectious diseases, including meningitis, subdural empyema and epidural abscess, cranial osteomyelitis, viral encephalitis (especially due to herpes simplex virus), or mycotic aneurysms in the setting of infective endocarditis. Cerebrovascular diseases such as migraines, intracerebral or subarachnoid hemorrhage, cerebral venous sinus thrombosis or cerebral infarctions, and primary or metastatic malignancies of the CNS may also be confused with a brain abscess, both symptomatically and occasionally radiographically.

APPROACH TO A DIAGNOSIS

Examination of the blood or urine is rarely helpful in the diagnosis of a brain abscess. A moderate peripheral blood leukocytosis may be present in patients with brain abscesses but exceeds 20,000 cells/mm^3 in ~10% of patients, whereas 40% display a completely normal leukocyte count (8,11,59). In a recent series of 102 patients, a leukocytosis greater than 11,000 cells per cubic millimeter was observed in only 31 (30.4%) patients. This is in contrast to a pediatric series of 101 patients in which the peripheral white blood cell (WBC) count exceeded 10,000 cells per cubic millimeter in 83% (43). The erythrocyte sedimentation rate (ESR) is usually only moderately elevated, with a median of 45–55 mm/hr. Values less than 40 mm/hr were observed in 72% of patients in one recent series. In another report, eight of the 10 patients with CCHD had a normal ESR, whereas 90% of those without CCHD had an elevated ESR (107). Serum C-reactive protein, an acute-phase protein produced in the liver, has recently been evaluated in the differential diagnosis between brain abscess and neoplasm. The serum C-reactive protein was elevated in seven of nine brain abscess patients, compared to none of 11 patients with a final diagnosis of brain tumor (150). Similarly, in a second evaluation, only three of 23 patients with a brain abscess had a normal C-reactive protein level (38). Of note, the serum C-reactive protein level did not correlate closely with the ESR. Blood cultures are infrequently positive (~10%) at the time of presentation

(12,43,107). Hyponatremia may be observed as a reflection of the syndrome of inappropriate antidiuretic hormone secretion.

Lumbar puncture is contraindicated in patients with suspected or proven brain abscess, because the diagnostic yield is poor and the procedure is dangerous in this setting. The CSF profile from a patient with a brain abscess is nonspecific. Data from several older series revealed hypoglycorrhachia in 25%, elevated protein in 67–81%, and pleocytosis (usually <500 cells per cubic millimeter and predominantly mononuclear) in 60–70% of cases (8–11,13). In two more recent evaluations, the CSF was entirely normal in 11% and 19% of patients with brain abscess. A polymorphonuclear cell predominance was observed in 42% and 50% of cases, especially when the total leukocyte count exceeded 100 cells per cubic millimeter (12,43). An opening pressure of >250 mm H_2O was observed in only 25% of cases in an older report (3). Less than 10% of CSF cultures are positive, only increasing to 20% following ventricular rupture (12). Rapid deterioration, presumably due to brain herniation, may occur in 20% of patients undergoing lumbar puncture with this disease. In one series (6), 41 of 140 patients subjected to lumbar puncture deteriorated clinically in less than 48 hr; 25 of these 41 patients died (11 of these were fully alert or only mildly drowsy at the time of the procedure). Similarly, seven of 44 patients deteriorated in less than 24 hr after lumbar puncture, and six died (64). In the analysis of Samson and Clark (13), 22 of 44 patients with brain abscesses underwent lumbar puncture; five of the 22 developed signs of midbrain compression within 2 hr of the procedure. These sobering figures have been recently confirmed in a series of patients observed from 1970 to 1983. Sixty percent (27 of 45) of these patients were subjected to a lumbar puncture, and four of these 27 patients died within 24 hr of the procedure (12). The poor diagnostic yield and significant morbidity of lumbar puncture in brain abscess has been confirmed by two more recent series (38,43). For these reasons, a lumbar puncture should be delayed in patients with a febrile CNS disorder with focal neurologic signs. However, if pyogenic meningitis is also a strong consideration, blood cultures should be obtained and appropriate antibiotics started parenterally before obtaining the CT scan. In this case, if the CT scan findings are negative, a lumbar puncture should be performed promptly.

The skull roentgenogram is usually normal in patients with brain abscesses, but it may show a pineal shift, signs of raised intracranial pressure, effacement of the dorsum sellae (with intrasellar abscess), or pathognomonic collections of air within a cavity (6–11,13,24).

The electroencephalogram (EEG) is usually abnormal in patients with a brain abscess and often lateralizes to the side of the lesion; however, the overall accuracy of localization is frequently less than 50%. Low-frequency delta waves with phase reversal have been suggested to indicate a brain abscess (8,11,13,24,59).

Arteriography and ventriculography are rarely necessary in the evaluation of patients with suspected brain abscesses since the introduction of CT scan technology. Arteriograms are abnormal in about 80% of brain abscess patients and may show a "ring shadow" in 20–40%; the usual pattern is an avascular mass with surrounding hyperemia (6–11,13,151). The absence of neovascularity may be helpful in excluding a necrotic tumor. Arteriography is essential if mycotic aneurysms due to endocarditis are suspected.

A technetium-99 brain scan is a very sensitive test for the detection of a brain abscess and remains the procedure of choice in areas where CT scanning or MRI are unavailable. The results are abnormal in more than 95% of patients, and a doughnut lesion is detected in 25–35% (152). Unfortunately, this radiographic appearance is also compatible with two other important lesions: necrotic tumor or infarction. The results of some series suggest that the brain scan is more sensitive than CT in the early cerebritis stage of brain abscess formation; however, this comparison was made with older-generation CT scanners and may no longer be valid (153). Compared with CT, localization is not as accurate, posterior fossa lesions are more difficult to visualize, and postoperative uptake may obscure the recognition of persistent or recurrent abscesses (154). However, a technetium or MRI scan should be performed when a brain abscess or cerebritis is suspected and CT findings are negative.

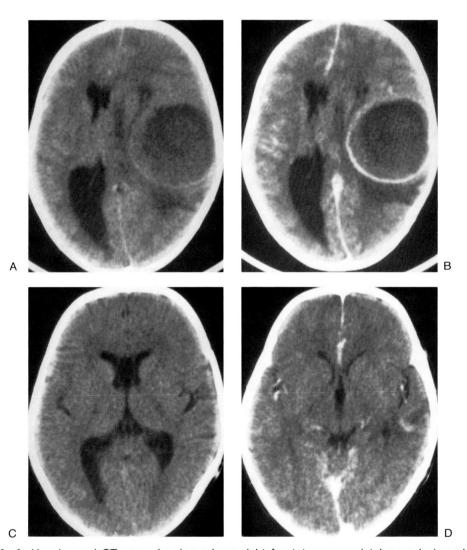

FIG. 4. A: Unenhanced CT scan showing a large right frontotemporoparietal mass lesion which is causing marked right-to-left shift of midline structures and effacement of the ipsilateral lateral ventricle. **B:** Contrast-enhanced CT scan showing a thin-rimmed, homogeneous enhancement surrounding an area of decreased attenuation within the center of the abscess. **C:** Unenhanced CT scan, performed 6 weeks after surgical aspiration of the abscess and antibiotic therapy, showing resolution of the mass effect. **D:** Enhanced scan showing minimal contrast enhancement in the temporal lobe.

The introduction of CT revolutionized the diagnostic and therapeutic approach to brain abscess. CT is far superior to previous radiologic procedures for the evaluation of the paranasal sinuses, mastoids, and the middle ear; CT scans of these areas should be obtained, along with chest roentgenograms, in all patients with suspected brain abscess (155). This technique is more sensitive (95–99%) than traditional brain scans beyond the cerebritis stage and yields more anatomic information—namely, the extent of surrounding edema and the presence of a midline shift, hydrocephalus, or imminent ventricular rupture (156,157). The characteristic appearance of a brain abscess on CT scan is a hypodense center (which contains leukocytes and necrotic debris) with an outlying uniform ring enhancement surrounded by a

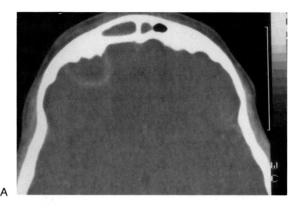

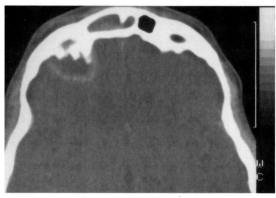

FIG. 6. A: Right anterior inferior frontal brain abscess immediately contiguous to an opacified right frontal sinus. **B:** Thin, homogeneous contrast enhancement is characteristic in this example. Direct spread of the infection from the contiguous frontal sinus, probably by thrombosed emissary veins, is the presumed route of entry of the pathogen into brain in cases such as this.

variable hypodense region of brain edema. (Figs. 4–8). Contrast enhancement is usually always seen. In a recent study of 100 consecutive brain abscesses (158) managed in the CT era, 73 cases revealed ring-enhancing lesions surrounded by a variable zone of edema; these findings,

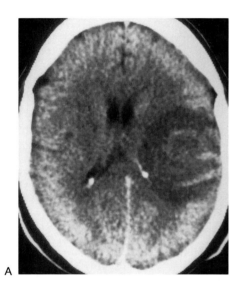

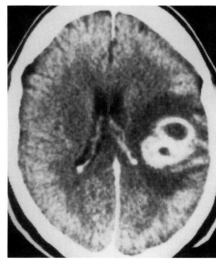

FIG. 5. A: Unenhanced axial CT scan showing irregular areas of high and low attenuation producing effacement of the sylvian cistern and ipsilateral lateral ventricle on the left. **B:** After contrast enhancement, somewhat thick, irregular, ring-enhancing lesions with multiple loculi are surrounded by an area of decreased attenuation, indicating cerebral edema.

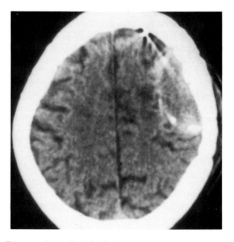

FIG. 7. Ring-enhancing lesion around an area of increased attenuation in a patient with brain abscess subsequent to penetrating intracranial injury.

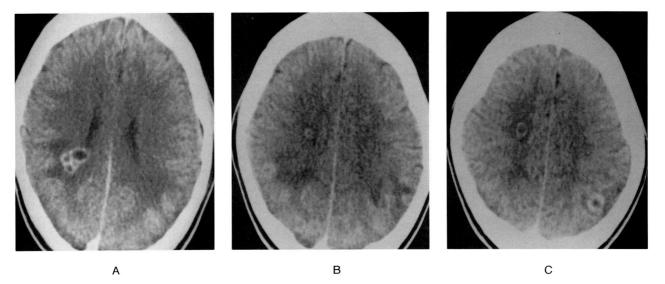

FIG. 8. Multiple cerebral abscesses presumably due to hematogenous spread of *Staphylococcus aureus* in a patient with septicemia. Lesions are seen in periventricular locations (**A**), in the centrum semiovale (**B**), and at the junction between gray and white matter (**C**).

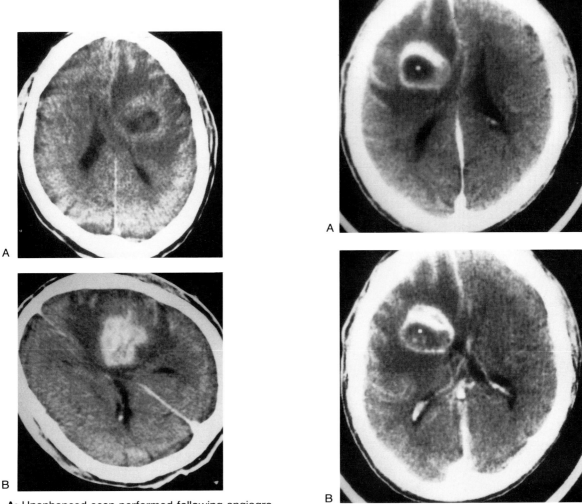

FIG. 9. A: Unenhanced scan performed following angiography shows minimal contrast enhancement around a central area of decreased attenuation producing mass effect on the ipsilateral lateral ventricle with surrounding edema. **B:** Thick, irregular contrast enhancement without a prominent ring-enhancing pattern might suggest a primary or metastatic malignancy in this patient who was found to have a brain abscess.

FIG. 10. A: Right posterior frontal abscess with irregular but homogenous ring contrast enhancement around an area of decreased attenuation. **B:** Slightly lower axial-level irregular contrast enhancement is seen in a "target" pattern. These scans demonstrate that contrast enhancement may be irregular around an abscess and that the thinnest portion of the capsule is usually adjacent to the ventricle.

when combined with the clinical data, strongly supported a diagnosis of an abscess. Eighteen cases revealed a ring-enhancing lesion that suggested either tumor or abscess. Eight scans were abnormal but nondiagnostic. Four of these eight revealed only an area of low density (no contrast was utilized), and one study revealed only diffuse swelling. One scan was interpreted as a postoperative fluid collection, whereas another was interpreted as a hematoma. Only one of the 100 scans was considered normal initially. Therefore, the initial scan strongly suggested the possibility of a brain abscess in 91 of 100 cases and would have had even higher predictive value if contrast had been used in all instances. As noted in this series, however, the impressive sensitivity of CT for brain abscess is not paralleled by an equivalent specificity; a similar appearance is occasionally seen with neoplasms, granulomas, cerebral infarction, or resolving hematoma (159,160). A recent report (161) emphasizes these points. Two patients presented with contrast CT scans that revealed frontal lobe masses with ring enhancement, and both were felt to have brain abscesses. Subsequent surgery and pathologic evaluation revealed hemorrhage in the setting of arteriovenous malformations. A previous study by Zimmerman et al. (162) examined 58

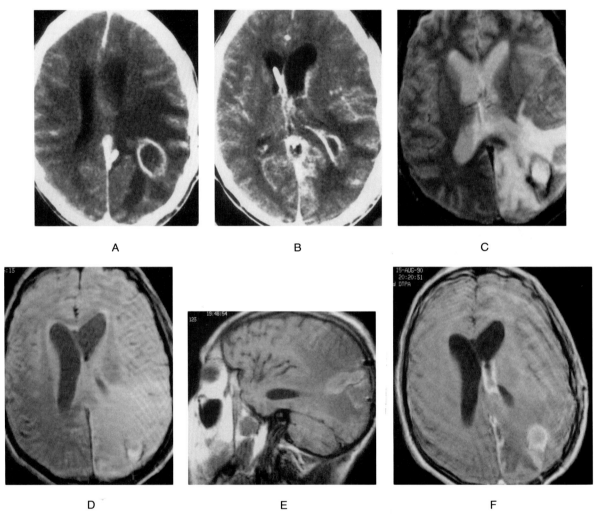

A   B   C

D   E   F

FIG. 11. A: Left parietal brain abscess with thin right enhancements surrounded by edematous white matter causing midline shift and effacement of the lateral ventricle. **B:** Despite aspiration and antibiotic treatment, the abscess ruptured into the ventricle, producing contrast enhancement of the ependymal surface. (A ventriculostomy catheter has been placed in the anterior horn of the right lateral ventricle.) **C:** T2-weighted image showing symmetrical venticular enlargement. The marked edema in the parieto-occipital region surrounds the abscess. Regions of decreased signal intensity in the abscess wall are due to paramagnetic hemoglobin degradation products in the area immediately around the wall. **D:** Proton density images of the parieto-occipital abscess. **E:** Parasagittal images of the left parietal abscess showing the lesion tracking toward the trigone of the lateral ventricle. **F:** Gadolinium-enhanced T1-weighted image showing enhancement around the abscess and the ependymal surface of the body of the lateral ventricle.

patients with proven intracerebral hematoma. Only one had a ring-enhancing lesion on initial CT examination; however, six of 13 follow-up examinations demonstrated a ring blush. Additionally, the effect of corticosteroids on the CT scan appearance of a brain abscess must be emphasized. These agents cause a decrease in enhancement and ring formation such that these signs may be present in only 40–60% of brain abscess patients in this setting (161). In addition, the characteristic ring enhancement may be lost after ventricular rupture. Features thought to discriminate abscesses from malignant tumors (thinner, more regular contrast-enhancing rim and homogeneous enhancement of the capsule after infusion of contrast medium) do not always permit a precise diagnosis (Figs. 9 and 10). Ependymal enhance-

ment, when present, is an indication of an associated ventriculitis and favors the diagnosis of brain abscess (11) (Fig. 11). Holtas et al. (163) reported a series of 26 patients with brain abscesses wherein the CT and clinical findings in eight were interpreted as representing a malignant tumor instead of abscess. As noted above, in 18% of CT scans on 100 patients eventually confirmed to have brain abscess, the diagnosis suggested was either tumor or abscess (158). In an effort to improve the diagnostic accuracy of CT, Coulam et al. (164) selected six parameters that could be used to differentiate between abscess and tumor, including patient age, ring thickness variability, outside ring diameter, lesion-to-ring ratio, maximum ring thickness, and CT mean value in the ring center. The overall classification in this study, while

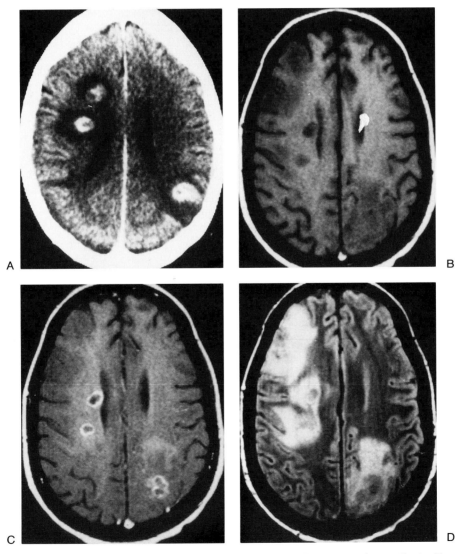

FIG. 12. A: Axial CT scan showing multiple areas of contrast enhancement in a patient with acquired immunodeficiency syndrome and cerebral toxoplasmosis. **B:** T1-weighted images showing periventricular and gray-white junction lesions consistent with hematogenous dissemination. **C:** After gadolinium administration, contrast enhancement is seen on the T1-weighted image corresponding to that in Fig. 9B. **D:** Axial T2-weighted image showing edema surrounding multiple cortical and subcortical lesions.

good, was still only 86% (84% for abscess, 96% for tumors).

A diagnostic modality that may prove complementary to CT is indium-111-labeled leukocyte scintigraphy, which has been useful in the diagnosis of occult abscesses elsewhere in the body and has been recently evaluated in the diagnosis of brain abscess. Radiolabeled leukocytes migrate to, and accumulate in, a focus of active inflammation, thus differentiating a brain abscess from other causes of mass lesions in the brain. In a study of 16 patients where CT was felt to be inconclusive in the differentiation between tumor and abscess, leukocyte scintigraphy correctly predicted tumor in 10 of 11 patients and abscess in four of five patients, for an overall diagnostic accuracy of 88% (165). A second study with this technique in 20 patients yielded a sensitivity of 100%, a specificity of 94%, and an overall accuracy of 96% in making this differentiation (166). Three other reports, totaling 17 additional patients, confirm this high degree of diagnostic accuracy (167); however, potential problems with this technique are as follows: (a) Necrotic tumors can occasionally yield a false-positive result and (b) concomitant use of steroids may produce a false-negative scan in patients with an abscess.

Encouraging experience in the utility of MRI in the diagnosis of brain abscess continues to accumulate (Fig. 12). The distinctive features that contribute to the value of MRI of the brain include: multiplanar imaging, the ability of MRI to provide high contrast between gray and white matter, the lack of bony artifacts, and the variety of imaging techniques available to elucidate pathologic changes. MRI is more sensitive than CT in the early detection of cerebritis as well as in detecting cerebral edema in normal brain tissue adjacent to a cerebritic focus (168–170). This increased sensitivity may be of limited clinical usefulness, because there is already an obvious CT lesion when most brain abscess patients present. However, MRI may detect early satellite lesions which could influence therapeutic decisions. Additionally, MRI is more accurate than CT in differentiating the central liquefactive necrosis of a brain abscess from other fluid accumulations. On CT, the central region is isodense with CSF, whereas on MRI it is usually hyperintense relative to the CSF. Also, concentric rings of intensity, or target appearance, have been observed frequently in the necrotic center with MRI, which appears to be specific for abscess rather than for necrotic or cystic malignancies (171). Contrast-enhanced MRI scans utilizing the paramagnetic agent gadolinium (Gd-DTPA) increase the information obtained with MRI even further. This agent crosses a damaged blood–brain barrier and enhances proton relaxation, which, in turn, increases T_1 signal intensity at the site of its accumulation. Gd-DTPA yields consistently increased enhancement of lesions relative to that seen with enhanced CT scans. It differentiates with greater accuracy the three regions within the abscess: (i) the central abscess, (ii) the surrounding enhancing rim, and (iii) cerebral edema around the abscess (169,170). The potential devastating complication of extraparenchymal extension of a brain abscess (such as ventricular rupture) is more easily detected by MRI, because the abscess fluid will again appear hyperintense relative to the CSF. Finally, MRI also may prove superior in the evaluation of the success of brain abscess therapy. CT enhancement may persist for more than 9 months in successfully treated abscesses; however, unenhanced MRI scans can detect a decrease in the rim hypointensity of the lesion by 2 months, suggesting it to be a more sensitive monitor of response to therapy (171,172). Therefore, MRI's lack of ionizing radiation, greater tissue characterization, lack of bone artifact (which improves sensitivity in posterior fossa lesions), and increased sensitivity in follow-up evaluations, combined with the lack of toxicity of Gd-DTPA compared to CT contrast agents, make MRI the procedure of choice in the evaluation of a brain abscess.

ANTIMICROBIAL THERAPY

The blood–brain barrier (BBB) largely resides at the level of the cerebral capillary endothelial cell and results from the presence of pentalaminar tight junctions between these cells and a number of enzymes and transport systems. This BBB serves to limit the entry of numerous substances into the CNS, including antibiotics, but several points require emphasis. Inflammation of the BBB (as in meningitis) results in disruption of these tight junctions, which, in turn, leads to increased CSF penetration of various drugs; that is, the penetration of several beta-lactam antibiotics into CSF increases 5- to 10-fold. Other major factors regulating antimicrobial agent penetration of the BBB include molecular weight, lipid solubility, protein binding, and degree of ionization at physiologic pH. For some antibiotics such as ceftriaxone, an active transport mechanism into the CSF may exist (173). Previous studies have suggested that the BBB and blood–CSF barrier are not identical and conclude that drug penetration into the CSF differs from that into the brain (174); therefore, results of CSF drug penetration may not apply directly to brain abscess therapy. Additionally, the directional flow of CSF may affect the local concentration of antibiotics. It has been suggested that abscess collections have a low surface area/volume ratio reducing the expected abscess fluid antibiotic concentration for any given serum drug concentration (175). Additional therapeutic concerns include (a) the effect of the abscess environment on the activity of the antibiotic and (b) the possibility of negative drug interactions when multiple agents are administered. For example, the activity of aminoglycosides is reduced in the acid environment of an abscess, and certain antibiotics (i.e., penicillin and chloramphenicol) may be inactivated by abscess pus (174). Additionally, chloramphenicol may antagonize the effects of penicillin and gentamicin (as noted in experimental meningitis models), resulting in an increased mortality (176). Most of these concerns are theoretical, however, and few studies have addressed these issues in the therapy of brain abscess.

An early study (177) examined brain tissue, CSF, and serum antibiotic concentrations in 27 patients subjected to a prefrontal lobotomy, presumably with an intact BBB. After collection at various intervals after dosing, tetracycline was detectable in both CSF and the brain, but penicillin was not present at either site, perhaps reflecting the low dose (600,000 units) and serum concentrations attained ($0.06-2.0$ μg/ml) 4 hr later when brain samples were analyzed. In patients undergoing excision of an intracranial neoplasm, a parenteral bolus of 2 g led to the following brain–blood ratios: chloramphenicol, 9:1; cephalothin, 1:10; penicillin 1:23; ampicillin 1:56 (178). On the basis of this evidence and activity against anaerobic bacteria, chloramphenicol has often been included in recommended regimens for the treatment of brain abscess.

Black et al. (179) analyzed antibiotic concentrations in brain abscess pus from six patients. Chloramphenicol, methicillin, and penicillin were detectable in the pus after standard dosages, whereas nafcillin was not. All six patients deteriorated clinically during medical treatment and all cultures were still positive at surgery, thus indicating the need for surgical intervention. De Louvois et al. (180) examined antibiotic concentrations in brain abscess pus obtained from 32 patients. Penicillin G was detectable consistently if the dose exceeded 24 million units daily (adults); however, the drug was $\geq$90% inactivated after incubation in pus for 1 hr *in vitro* (181) in four of 22 specimens. Fusidic acid entered the brain abscess readily, but concentrations of various cephalosporins and cloxacillin were low. CSF and brain concentrations of clindamycin are low after conventional dosages (182); however, potentially therapeutic concentrations in abscess fluid may be attainable (181). Metronidazole attains high concentrations ($\sim$35–45 μg/ml) in brain abscess pus (31), often exceeding serum concentrations after a dose of 400–800 mg every 8 hr. Because of these results and the bactericidal activity of metronidazole against strict anaerobes, this agent is often a component of antimicrobial regimens for brain abscesses (183).

Trimethoprim-sulfamethoxazole, often effective in cerebral nocardiosis (184,185) and gram-negative aerobic bacillary meningitis (186), may have a role where susceptible organisms are present. In two studies, this drug combination attained adequate brain abscess pus concentrations for the isolated organisms (*Proteus mirabilis* and *Nocardia asteroides*) and yielded successful results when combined with surgery (185,187). In a recent report (188), vancomycin also attained acceptable concentrations (for aerobic streptococci and staphylococci) in the single brain abscess studied.

Little information is currently available on the penetration of the newer antimicrobial agents into brain abscesses or on the clinical efficacy of these agents in this infection. Cefotaxime, ceftizoxime, ceftriaxone, ceftazidime, and moxalactam have been shown to penetrate the CSF in therapeutic concentrations, but, as noted above, this does not necessarily predict activity in a brain abscess. One report demonstrated good penetration of moxalactam into brain abscess fluid (189), and this agent has been used successfully in the treatment of neonates with brain abscesses (190); however, this agent is not recommended, because increased bleeding complications are associated with its use. Aztreonam, a new monobactam derivative, has been shown to be effective in the treatment of experimental cerebritis (191); however, its penetration into human brain tissue has not been evaluated, and experience with its use in human brain abscess is lacking. A single case report details a successful outcome in the treatment of a polymicrobial brain abscess with imipenem-cilastatin (192). A concentration in the abscess greater than the minimal inhibitory concentration for the various organisms involved was attained with a dose of 2.0 g/day. A major concern, however, is that the use of imipenem may be associated with an increased incidence of seizures, which may limit its use in brain abscess patients who are already seizure-prone (193).

Any study evaluating antibiotic penetration into the CNS must be interpreted cautiously. Considerable variation in tissue concentrations among different patients is often present, and frequently there are conflicting results between studies. A single tissue concentration may not represent the dynamics of antibiotic movement into the brain in the presence of inflammation. In the setting of meningitis, the *in vitro* susceptibility does not always correlate with the clinical outcome (194,195). In experimental animal models of gram-negative meningitis, CSF concentrations of aminoglycosides of 10–30 times the minimal bactericidal concentration were required for efficacy. Similar observations were made in a rabbit model of pneumococcal meningitis utilizing various beta-lactam antibiotics, including penicillin (196). The relevance of brain and abscess pus concentrations or the necessity of bactericidal activity at the site of the brain abscess remains unknown. In addition, the role of osmotic manipulation of the BBB in order to increase the penetration of various antibiotics into a brain abscess, while promising in experimental animal models, is uncertain (196).

The antimicrobial regimens commonly recommended for the therapy of brain abscess are empiric and reflect the considerations already noted, and they also reflect the *in vitro* activity of the component agent(s) against the usual pathogens. No controlled trials on the relative efficacy of various regimens have been performed. Interpretation of the success or failure of a given regimen is further confused by the various surgical procedures which may be used concomitantly.

Since the early 1960s a combination of penicillin G (20–24 million units per day, intravenously) plus chloramphenicol (1.0–1.5 g every 6 hr, intravenously) has been advocated in adults. The role of continuous infusion versus intermittent bolus injection of penicillin in the therapy of a brain abscess has not been directly evaluated. In meningitis models, both forms of delivery appear to be equivalent with regard to ultimate outcome, although more rapid bacterial killing may occur with high doses of penicillin given by frequent intermittent bolus injection (197). Penicillin remains a mainstay of therapy because of its excellent activity against streptococci *in vitro* and also because of favorable results obtained in experimental models of brain abscess (198). The introduction of penicillin in the 1940s may have been instrumental in reducing brain abscess mortality from 50–80% to 20–30% by 1950 (199–202). Because of the important role of streptococci (especially the *S. milleri* group) in brain abscesses (streptococci complicate contiguous foci of infection) and in pyogenic lung disease, penicillin should be employed in all such cases. Most anaerobes encountered in brain abscesses are also susceptible to penicillin, with the notable exception of the *B. fragilis* group. Chloramphenicol has often been administered concurrently with penicillin in the past because its high lipid solubility results in brain tissue concentrations often exceeding those in serum, and because it has good activity against anaerobic bacteria. The use of metronidazole in regimens for the therapy of brain abscess has increased greatly in recent years, for the following reasons: (a) Metronidazole is bactericidal against *B. fragilis*, whereas chloramphenicol may be bacteriostatic; (b) metronidazole also attains reproducibly excellent concentrations in brain abscess pus (31); (c) metronidazole's entry into brain abscess pus is not affected by concomitant steroid treatment, in contrast to several other antibiotics (202); (d) chloramphenicol may be degraded by desacetylation in pus, as shown in experimental intraabdominal abscess; and (e) metronidazole may have a salutary effect on mortality, as suggested by retrospective experience (181). Metronidazole, when substituted for chloramphenicol, may lead to more rapid healing and lower mortality (158,181,183,203); however, these two agents have never been compared in a prospective, randomized trial. Additionally, as noted previously, chloramphenicol may antagonize the effect of penicillin or gentamicin (176). Metronidazole may, however, cause CNS side effects—including vertigo, drowsiness, and peripheral neuropathy, which are difficult to differentiate from clinical deterioration in brain abscess patients. Both metronidazole and chloramphenicol offer the additional advantage of oral formulations with almost total absorption, thereby improving convenience and decreasing the cost of therapy. Each of these agents attains brain abscess concentrations higher than serum concentrations, and therefore this approach should be equally efficacious; however, data supporting this approach is lacking. An antianaerobic agent such as metronidazole or chloramphenicol is indicated for treatment of brain abscesses complicating otitis media, mastoiditis, or pyogenic lung disease because anaerobes, particularly *B. fragilis*, are often present. These agents may not be a necessary addition to penicillin in abscesses secondary to frontoethmoidal sinusitis, since *B. fragilis* is an uncommon isolate; however, empiric therapy with at least two agents is mandatory prior to culture confirmation.

When staphylococci are proven or suspected in posttrauma or post-neurosurgical abscesses, nafcillin (2 g every 4 hr, intravenously) is indicated. Vancomycin should be substituted if the patient is allergic to penicillin or if a methacillin-resistant strain is isolated. European investigators prefer fusidic acid for this indication, but this agent is not available in the United States. The frequent isolation of members of the Enterobacteriaceae family in brain abscesses of otic origin prompts many authorities to add a third-generation cephalosporin or trimethoprin-sulfomethoxazole to the regimen, pending culture results. Given the increased isolation frequency of *P. aeruginosa* in the setting of chronic middle ear disease, ceftazidime is a logical empiric choice. Instillation of antibiotics into the abscess cavity during aspiration (usually bacitracin or penicillin) has frequently been employed, but the efficacy of this practice has never been established. Antibiotics given in this manner may diffuse into surrounding brain tissue in high concentrations, causing seizures (23,179,200,204). In one small study (205), two groups of patients were compared in which the only therapeutic difference was repeated instillation of antibiotics into the abscess cavity. The group without local instillation had a mortality of 56%, whereas those receiving local instillation had a mortality of only 7%. Potential problems with this study are (a) the lack of a prospective, randomized design, (b) the small numbers of patients in each group (16 versus 13), and (c) the excessive mortality, by current standards, in the group receiving systemic antimicrobials alone, suggesting that other differences between the groups may have been present. Therefore, the efficacy of local antibiotic therapy remains controversial. In cases where *P. aeruginosa* is implicated, direct instillation of specific antibiotics may be warranted because adequate local antibiotic concentrations for this organism are difficult to attain after systemic administration, with the possible exception of ceftazidime or aztreonam. Finally, the optimal duration of therapy with any of the regimens remains unknown. It is often affected by the type of surgical procedure performed (see below).

SURGICAL THERAPY

Although some patients with brain abscess respond to prolonged medical therapy alone, most require surgery for optimal management. The timing of surgery and type of surgical procedure selected remain controversial. Since the first report of successful operative management of a brain abscess in 1768, at least six different surgical methods for treating brain abscesses have been described. As late as 1940, it was apparent in a statement by Bucy and Haverfield (cited in ref. 206) that no consensus among neurosurgeons had been reached: "Each neurosurgeon has his own special technique for dealing with abscesses of the brain." The methods used by various surgeons included tube drainage, marsupialization, the migration method of Kahn, tapping, aspiration, and excision. Today only aspiration and excision are used. It would be inappropriate, based on currently available data, to proclaim the superiority of either method. No prospective, randomized trial comparing these two procedures has ever been performed. In reviewing the available literature, one author noted a mortality of 38% in 941 patients treated by aspiration, as opposed to a 19% mortality in 1505 patients treated by excision (206); however, the majority of these cases were reported in the pre-CT era. Of note, patients considered for excision are more often in a satisfactory neurologic condition, whereas aspiration is more often performed in the deteriorating, neurologically compromised patient or for the drainage of inaccessible lesions (brainstem, thalamus, basal ganglia, etc.) where mortality is significant (10). A recent study (207) concluded that the results for excision are "apparently better than for aspiration or antibiotic treatment." The 35 brain abscess patients were not randomized into different groups; instead, management depended on the size, location, and multiplicity of abscesses as well as on the "inclination of the treating neurosurgeon." Therefore, the authors' conclusions are difficult to justify on the basis of data. Others have also recommended immediate primary excision as the therapy of choice whenever possible, despite the fact that most recent series show little overall difference in outcome between the two methods (6–8,13). Taylor (208) recently reported just three deaths in 50 patients treated by excision alone (1974–1986). These excellent results were achieved despite grade 3 or 4 coma on presentation in 16 of his patients, a prognostic factor which has historically been associated with a mortality in excess of 80%. In contrast, however, Rousseaux et al. (209) recently noted in a small series that patients treated with excision did worse than those treated with aspiration or antibiotics. Another, more recent study (42) supported Rousseaux et al.'s observations. These authors performed aspiration in 18 consecutive patients and only experienced one death. One or two aspirations were all that were required in the majority of patients.

It is clear, therefore, that this debate has not yet been settled. Evaluation of only those patients treated in the post-CT era is essential to more valid comparisons. However, certain principles can be summarized based on the available, albeit incomplete, data. The procedure employed must be individualized in each case and is dependent on the clinical course, size, and location of the abscesses, CT scan appearance, and other factors. Emergency surgery is mandatory when neurologic signs progress. Some authors advocate that abscesses exhibiting gas by CT or plain film should be completely excised (210). In a review of five such patients, three of whom had undergone failed aspiration procedures, total excision was required, and a persistent extracranial communication was discovered in each. As noted above, coma in a patient with brain abscess carries a poor prognosis regardless of the form of treatment (8,211). Surgery is indicated before the stage of coma. Fluid reaccumulation and incomplete drainage of a multiloculated abscess are the major disadvantages of aspiration in older series, and they are the reasons why reoperation is required more frequently after this procedure (9). Repeat aspirations may increase the likelihood of further tissue trauma and, some suggest, lead to longer hospitalization. Excision is currently the method of choice for posterior fossa lesions. Excision is also indicated for fungal brain abscesses because available drug treatment is unsatisfactory; however, one recent case report detailed a successful outcome of an *Aspergillus* brain abscess treated by aspiration (71). The incidence of postoperative seizures or other deficits following excision is not clearly different from that following aspiration (10,212). Since the advent of CT, the data may favor more conservative surgical procedures (i.e., aspiration) (209), but this conclusion still is not final.

Aspiration may now be accomplished under stereotactic CT guidance (213,214). This procedure affords the surgeon rapid, accurate (within 1 mm), and safe access to virtually any intracranial point. In a review of its use in 80 patients, recovery of tissue sufficient to establish a histologic diagnosis or to establish the etiologic factor related to the disease process was realized in 94% of cases. There was no associated mortality and only a 4% transient morbidity. The diagnoses included 20 cases of infection, six of which were pyogenic brain abscesses. In most instances the choice of antimicrobial therapy was significantly altered by the findings. In addition, this procedure permitted successful drainage of two cases with multicompartmental abscesses, previously felt to be untreatable by aspiration alone (213). A series of 102 patients (215) documented a diagnostic yield of 96% by this technique. There was no mortality and a 5.9% transient morbidity. The five abscesses that were encountered were definitively drained. In 38 cases in which the preoperative diagnosis was felt to be secure, stereotactic biopsy results led to a change in diagnosis in four patients, one of whom had a brain abscess. Several recent evaluations confirm the efficacy and low morbidity of this procedure (216–218). Two issues deserve comment. As noted previously, the incidence of multiple abscesses can be as high as 50%, and prior to the availability of CT, the mortality could approach 100%. With the advent of CT-guided stereotactic surgery, multiple, deep-seated lesions can now be successfully managed with a resultant significant reduction in mortality to 0–8% (219). Secondly, brainstem abscesses also resulted in an almost uniformly fatal outcome previously, and open operative procedures were associated with an unacceptably high morbidity. Several cases of successful drainage of brainstem abscesses by CT-guided aspiration have now been reported, suggesting that this is the therapy of choice for these lesions (216,220). The risks of stereotactic aspiration are probably less than the risks of incorrect diagnosis and choice of antibiotics; therefore, the decision to use empirical therapy alone should be made with great caution.

GENERAL MANAGEMENT

No general management guidelines can be formulated to ensure optimal results in the individual patient with a brain abscess. However, a rational approach to therapy can be outlined based on the principles previously discussed. Essential to the successful management of a brain abscess is the availability of CT and/or MRI, because these imaging techniques have dramatically altered the diagnosis and treatment of brain abscess. Studies in animal models with brain abscesses, and subsequently in humans, suggest that focal bacterial infections of the brain parenchyma may be staged by sequential CT scans (137,221) (Table 6).

Early cerebritis is characterized by an irregular area of low density on the precontrast scan which may or may not enhance following administration of contrast. Late cerebritis reveals a larger area of low density (precontrast), with the appearance of typical ring enhancement (often thick and diffuse) on the contrast-enhanced scan. The contrast enhancement does not decay on delayed scans (60 min later), but diffusion of the contrast material into the hypodense center is observed. In contrast, encapsulation is characterized by (a) a faint ring on the unenhanced scan and (b) ring enhancement that decays in the delayed scan without any diffusion into the center of the lesion. These parameters may prove useful in planning the combined medical–surgical approach.

Since 1971, it has been recognized that early antibiotic therapy alone could cure cerebritis without the later development of an encapsulated abscess (222). Since that time, nonsurgical therapy of brain abscesses has been attempted with seeming success. Between 1975 and 1985, at least 67 cases of presumably established brain abscesses were reported to be cured by medical therapy alone (223). These studies share many of the following features: (a) The initial diagnosis and resolution of brain abscesses were documented by serial CT scans, (b) prolonged courses of high-dose antibiotic therapy for 8 weeks or longer were administered, and (c) there was no surgical or histopathologic evidence of encapsulation (10,209,224–229). Rosenblum et al. (223) reviewed data from five large series in which it could be assumed—based on CT findings, presence of symptoms for greater than 2 weeks, or subsequent pathologic evaluation—that the lesions were encapsulated. Medical therapy alone was deemed successful in 74% of 50 such cases, and deaths occurred in only 4% of patients. Careful studies in animal models of brain abscess (136,230), as well as clinical observations (137,160,221,231), have clearly shown that ring enhancement on the CT scan may be observed in the cerebritis stage. Thus, it is possible that some of these results with antimicrobial therapy alone represent successful resolution of bacterial cerebritis rather than a well-encapsulated abscess. Nonetheless, it appears certain that some brain abscesses may be cured without surgical intervention. Therefore, we propose the following management guidelines. If the CT scan suggests the presence of cerebritis and the patient is neurologically stable, antibiotic therapy [penicillin and metronidazole (or chloramphenicol) and perhaps a third agent, depending on the setting and location of the lesions] can be started and the patient can be observed. If the patient remains stable and the abscess is accessible, aspiration (CT-guided, if possible) is desirable to make a specific bacteriologic diagnosis and narrow the antimicrobial regimen. Although this delay may render cultures negative, aspiration during the cerebritis stage may be associated with an increased likelihood of hemorrhage, especially in children (231). Previously, the criteria for nonoperative management also included the following: (a) medical conditions that greatly increase the risk of surgery; (b) the presence of multiple lesions, especially remote from one another; (c) abscesses in deep dominant locations; (d) concomitant meningitis or ependymitis; (e) early abscess reduction and clinical improvement attributable to antibiotic therapy; and (f) abscess diameter size under 3 cm (26,107,159,229,230). As noted above, many of these criteria become obsolete with the availability of stereotactic CT-guided aspiration. Aspiration will allow for a definitive diagnosis as well as an accurate assessment of the

TABLE 6. *"Staging" of brain abscess with computerized tomography*

Stage[a]	Precontrast	Contrast enhancement at 10 min	Contrast enhancement at 60 min
Cerebritis	Low density	Ring enhancement	No decay
Abscess	Capsule characterized by faint ring around low density	Ring enhancement	Decay in contrast enhancement

[a] Both lesions may be surrounded by low-density area of edema.

etiologic agent(s). It may be done under local anesthesia, minimizing the risk to even the most seriously ill patient. Therefore, operative therapy should remain the definitive approach for most brain abscesses.

If the lesion appears encapsulated by CT scan criteria, antibiotic treatment can be started and aspiration for diagnosis and drainage can be performed without delay (136,224). Subsequent management is dependent on clinical and imaging assessment; repeat aspiration may be required. Later neurologic deterioration, as well as failure of the abscess to decrease in size as detected by CT or MRI, is an indication for further surgery (often excision), if feasible. The duration of antimicrobial therapy remains unsettled. Lesions treated by complete excision appear to require shorter courses of antibiotics for successful therapy than do those treated by antibiotics or aspiration only. Many authorities treat parenterally for 4–6 weeks, often followed by prolonged (2–6 months) oral therapy if a suitable agent is available against the isolated pathogens. It must be stressed that such regimens are empirical and may be unnecessarily long. A cured brain abscess may continue to exhibit contrast enhancement on CT scans for 4–10 weeks to up to 6–9 months (137,159,160,171) after completion of successful therapy. The management of the HIV-infected patient with a focal CNS lesion remains somewhat controversial. Despite the numerous potential etiologies in these patients, toxoplasmosis is the most common etiology of a focal lesion, especially when multiple enhancing lesions are observed by CT or MRI (Fig. 12). Therefore, empirical therapy with pyrimethamine and sulfadiazine is reasonable and frequently recommended in this setting. For toxoplasmic encephalitis, one would expect a clinical response within 10 days—and a radiographic response within 14 days—of initiation of therapy (232). Immediate biopsy should be considered in (a) the patient with a negative *Toxoplasma* serology, (b) patients with CT findings atypical for toxoplasmosis, or (c) those who have evidence of a disseminated process due to a different pathogen.

Corticosteroids are often employed as adjunctive treatment during management of a brain abscess, but their role remains controversial. The potential drawbacks of these agents are: (a) reduced antibiotic entry into the CNS (232,233); (b) decreased collagen formation and glial response (142); and (c) alteration of the CT scan appearance of ring enhancement as inflammation subsides (80,234), which may obscure information from sequential studies for assessment of cure. Two recent studies in experimental animal models of brain abscess, however, noted no increase or decrease in mortality in those animals receiving dexamethasone (235,236). Of course, steroids could prove lifesaving in a patient with rapid neurologic deterioration due to raised intracranial pressure. In this circumstance, intracranial pressure monitoring is advisable, and elevations should be con-

trolled with steroids, hyperventilation, or mannitol. Anticonvulsants are frequently started empirically.

PROGNOSIS (TABLE 7)

The mortality of brain abscess was 40–80% in the preantibiotic era; some series report a decline after the introduction of penicillin (6–8,10,11,13,25,59,199,202). An adverse prognosis previously was associated with: (a) delayed or missed diagnosis; (b) poor localization; (c) multiple, deep, or multiloculated lesions; (d) ventricular rupture (80–100% mortality); (e) coma; (f) fungal etiology; and (g) inappropriate antibiotics (10,11,211). Additional negative factors often cited are extremes of age, large abscesses, and presence of metastatic abscesses (12). Since the introduction of CT scanning, a decreased mortality ranging between 0% and 24% has been reported in numerous series (25,154,181,237). The mortality of brain abscess in one recent series (89) declined from 40.9% to 4.3% following the introduction of CT. This improvement could be partially accounted for by a number of missed diagnoses in the pre-CT period.

The incidence of neurologic sequelae ranges between 30% and 55% (12). Most sequelae are mild, but up to 17% of patients may be incapacitated, with the severity of sequelae correlating more often with the patient's neurologic condition on admission than with the form of treatment employed (12,13,130,156). A follow-up evaluation of 32 children treated for brain abscess noted that intellectual impairment was more common in those less than 5 years of age at the time of diagnosis, but that behavioral abnormalities predominated in older children (238). This disturbing effect on mental function was confirmed in a second study of neonatal brain abscess (30). Only 24% of children were considered to be at a normal intellectual level 2 years following therapy. The likelihood of seizures is variable, ranging from 35% to more than 90%; these differences may relate to the length of follow-up. Anticonvulsant therapy appears to reduce the frequency of seizures (239,240). There is some recent suggestion that lesions treated conservatively with antibiotics and/or aspiration have a lower incidence of post-treatment sequelae, correlating with less visible abnormalities on follow-up CT scans (209).

TABLE 7. *Brain abscess: influence of preoperative mental status on mortality*

Mental status	Number of patients	Mortality (%)
Grade I (fully alert)	33	0
Grade II (drowsy)	55	4
Grade III (response to pain only)	61	59
Grade IV (coma; no pain response)	51	82

[a] Adapted from ref. 11.

Earlier diagnosis, refinements in technology, and an aggressive medical–surgical approach remain essential for the successful management of this otherwise unforgiving CNS infection.

REFERENCES

1. Theophilo F, Markakis E, Theophilo L, Dietz H. Brain abscess in childhood. *Childs Nerv Syst* 1985;1:324–328.
2. Spires JR, Smith RJH, Catlin FI. Brain abscesses in the young. *Otolaryngol Head Neck Surg* 1985;93:468–474.
3. Garfield J. Brain abscess and focal suppurative infections. In: Vinken PJ, Bruyn GW, eds. *Infections of the nervous system, part 1. Handbook of clinical neurology.* Amsterdam: North-Holland, 1979;33:107.
4. Shu-yuan Y. Brain abscess associated with congenital heart disease. *Surg Neurol* 1989;31:129–132.
5. MacEwen W. *Pyogenic infective diseases of the brain and spinal cord.* Glasgow: James MacLehose & Sons, 1893.
6. Garfield J. Management of supratentorial intracranial abscess: A review of 200 cases. *Br Med J* 1969;2:7–11.
7. Beller AJ, Sahar A, Praiss I. Brain abscess. Review of 89 cases over 30 years. *J Neurol Neurosurg Psychiatry* 1973;36:757–768.
8. Morgan H, Wood M, Murphy F. Experience with 88 consecutive cases of brain abscess. *J Neurosurg* 1973;38:698–704.
9. Garvey G. Current concepts of bacterial infections of the central nervous system. Bacterial meningitis and bacterial brain abscess. *J Neurosurg* 1983;59:735–744.
10. Carey ME. Brain abscesses. *Contemp Neurosurg* 1982;3:1.
11. Nielsen H, Gyldensted C, Harmsen A. Cerebral abscess. Etiology and pathogenesis, symptoms, diagnosis and treatment. *Acta Neurol Scand* 1982;65:609–622.
12. Chun CH, Johnson JD, Hofstetter M, Raff MJ. Brain abscess. A study of 45 consecutive cases. *Medicine* 1986;65:415–431.
13. Samson DS, Clark K. A current review of brain abscess. *Am J Med* 1973;54:201–210.
14. Arseni C, Civrea AV. Cerebral abscesses secondary to otorhinolaryngological infections. A study of 386 cases. *Zentrabl Neurochir* 1988;49:22–36.
15. Samuel J, Fernandes CMC, Steinberg JL. Intracranial otogenic complications: a persisting problem. *Laryngoscope* 1986;272–8.
16. Mathews TJ, Marcus G. Otogenic intradural complications: a review of 37 patients. *J Laryngol Otol* 1988;102:121–124.
17. Behrman RE, Meyers BR, Mendelson MH, Sacks HS, Hirschman SZ. Central nervous system infections in the elderly. *Arch Intern Med* 1989;149:1596–1599.
18. Levy RM, Janssen RS, Bush TJ, Rosenblum ML. Neuroepidemiology of the acquired immunodeficiency syndrome. *J Acquired Immun Defic Syndr* 1988;1:31–40.
19. Yang SH. Brain abscess. A review of 400 cases. *J Neurosurg* 1981;55:794–799.
20. Bradley PJ, Shaw MDM. Three decades of brain abscess in Merseyside. *J R Coll Surg Edinb* 1983;28:223–228.
21. Van Alphen HAM, Driessen JJR. Brain abscess and subdural empyema. *J Neurol Neurosurg Psychiatry* 1976;39:481–490.
22. de Louvois J, Gortvai P, Hurley R. Bacteriology of abscesses of the central nervous system. A multicentre prospective study. *Br Med J* 1977;2:981–984.
23. de Louvois J. The bacteriology and chemotherapy of brain abscess. *J Antimicrob Chemother* 1978;4:395–413.
24. Harrison MJG. The clinical presentation of intracranial abscesses. *Q J Med* 1982;51:461–468.
25. Brewer NS, MacCarty CS, Wellman WE. Brain abscess: a review of recent experience. *Ann Intern Med* 1975;82:571–576.
26. Small M, Dale BAB. Intracranial suppuration 1968–1982—a 15-year review. *Clin Otolaryngol* 1984;9:315–321.
27. Bradley PJ, Manning KP, Shaw MDM. Brain abscess secondary to paranasal sinusitis. *J Laryngol Otol* 1984;98:719–725.
28. Kaplan K. Brain abscess. *Med Clin North Am* 1985;69:345–360.
29. Patrick CC, Kaplan SL. Current concepts in the pathogenesis and management of brain abscesses in children. *Pediatr Clin North Am* 1988;35:625–637.
30. Renier D, Flaudin C, Hirsch E, Hirsch J-F. Brain abscesses in neonates. A study of 30 cases. *J Neurosurg* 1988;69:877–882.
31. Heinnemann HS, Braude AI. Anaerobic infection of the brain. Observations on eighteen consecutive cases of brain abscess. *Am J Med* 1963;35:682–697.
32. Ingham HR, Selkon JB, Roxby CM. Bacteriological study of otogenic cerebral abscesses: chemotherapeutic role of metronidazole *Br Med J* 1977;2:991–993.
33. de Louvois J. Antimicrobial chemotherapy in the treatment of brain abscess. *J Antimicrob Chemother* 1983;11:205–207.
34. Tabaqchali S. Anaerobic infection in the head and neck region. *Scand J Infect Dis (Suppl)* 1988;57:24–34.
35. Brook I. Aerobic and anaerobic bacteriology of cholesteatoma. *Laryngoscope* 1981;91:250–253.
36. Ariza J, Casanova A, Viladrich PF, et al. Etiologic agent and primary source of infection in 42 cases of focal intracranial suppuration. *J Clin Microbiol* 1986;24:899–902.
37. Giller GR, Garner JE, Brenner DA. Antimicrobial management of intracranial abscess. *Aust NZ J Surg* 1984;54:253–255.
38. Schliamser SE, Backman K, Norrby SR. Intracranial abscesses in adults: an analysis of 54 consecutive cases. *Scand J Infect Dis* 1988;20:1–9.
39. Jadavji T, Humphreys RP, Prober CG. Brain abscesses in infants and children. *Pediatr Infect Dis J* 1985;4:394–398.
40. Harris LF, Maccubbin DA, Triplett JN, Haws FP. Brain abscess: recent experience at a community hospital. *South Med J* 1985;78:704–707.
41. Mathisen GE, Meyer RD, George WL, Ditron DM, Finegold SM. Brain abscess and cerebritis. *Rev Infect Dis* 1984;6(Suppl 1):S101–S106.
42. Stroobandt G, Zech F, Thauvoy C, Mathurin P, de Nijs C, Gilliard C. Treatment by aspiration of brain abscesses. *Acta Neurochir* 1987;85:138–147.
43. Saez-Llorens XJ, Umann MA, Odio CM, McCracken GH, Nelson JD. Brain abscess in infants and children. *Pediatr Infect Dis J* 1989;8:449–458.
44. Gossling J. Occurrence and pathogenicity of the *Streptococcus milleri* group. *Rev Infect Dis* 1988;10:257–285.
45. Murray HW, Gross KC, Masur H, Roberts R. Serious infections caused by *Streptococcus milleri*. *Am J Med* 1978;64:759–764.
46. Shlaes DM, Lerner PM, Wolinsky E, Gopalakrishna KV. Infections due to Lancefield group F and related streptococci (*S. milleri, S. anginosus*). *Medicine* 1981;60:197–207.
47. Facklam RR. Physiologic differentiation of viridans streptococci. *J Clin Microbiol* 1977;5:184–201.
48. Parker MT, Ball LC. Streptococci and aerococci associated with systemic infection in man. *J Med Microbiol* 1976;9:275–302.
49. Shaw MDM, Russell JA. Cerebellar abscess—a review of 47 cases. *J Neurol Neurosurg Psychiatry* 1975;38:429–435.
50. Kenna MA, Bluestone CD. Microbiology of chronic suppurative otitis media. *Pediatr Infect Dis J* 1986;5:223–225.
51. Tiffany KK, Kline MW. Mixed flora brain abscess with *Pseudomonas paucimobilis* after a penetrating lawn dart injury. *Pediatr Infect Dis J* 1988;7:667–669.
52. Rodriquez RE, Valero V, Watanakunakorn C. *Salmonella* focal intracranial infections: review of the world literature (1884–1984) and report of an unusual case. *Rev Infect Dis* 1986;8:31–41.
53. Dijkmans BAC, Thomeer RTWM, Vielvoye GJ, Lampe AS, Mattie H. Brain abscess due to *Streptobacillus moniliformis* and *Actinobacterium meyerii*. *Infection* 1984;12:262–264.
54. Guvene H, Korabay K, Okten A, Bektas S. Brucellosis in a child complicated with multiple brain abscesses. *Scand J Infect Dis* 1989;21:333–336.
55. Curless RG. Neonatal intracranial abscess: two cases caused by *Citrobacter* and a literature review. *Ann Neurol* 1980;8:269–272.
56. Levy RL, Saunders RL. *Citrobacter* meningitis and cerebral abscess in early infancy: cure by moxalactam. *Neurology* 1981;31:1575–1577.
57. Bronitsky R, Heim CR, McGee ZA. Multifocal brain abscesses: combined medical and neurosurgical therapy. *South Med J* 1982;75:1261–1263.

58. Cheng AF, South JR, French GL. *Eikenella corrodens* as a cause of brain abscess. *Scand J Infect Dis* 1988;20:667–671.

59. Carey ME, Chou SN, French LA. Experience with brain abscesses. *J Neurosurg* 1972;36:1–9.

60. Brook I. Bacteriology of intracranial abscess in children. *J Neurosurg* 1981;54:484–488.

61. de Louvois J. Bacteriological examination of pus from abscesses of the central nervous system. *J Clin Pathol* 1980;33:66–71.

62. Berensen CS, Bia FJ. Proprionobacterium acnes causes postoperative brain abscesses unassociated with foreign bodies: case reports. *Neurosurgery* 1989;25:130–134.

63. Jensen HB, Levy SR, Duncan C, McIntosh S. Treatment of multiple brain abscesses caused by *Bacillus cereus. Pediatr Infect Dis J* 1989;8:795–798.

64. Lechtenberg R, Sierra MF, Pringle GF, Shucart WA, Butt KMH. *Listeria monocytogenes:* brain abscess or meningoencephalitis? *Neurology* 1979;29:86–90.

65. Nieman RE, Lorber B. Listeriosis in adults: a changing pattern. Report of eight cases and review of literature. *Rev Infect Dis* 1980;2:207–227.

66. Norden CW, Ruben FL, Selker R. Nonsurgical treatment of cerebral nocardiosis. *Arch Neurol* 1983;40:594–5.

67. Hooper DC, Pruitt AA, Rubin RH. Central nervous system infection in the chronically immunosuppressed. *Medicine* 1982;61:166–188.

68. Sheller JR, DesPrez RM. CNS tuberculosis. *Neurol Clin* 1986;4:143–157.

69. Bahemuka M, Babiker MA, Wright G, Ovainey AL, Obeid T. The pattern of infection of the nervous system in Riyadh: a review of 121 cases. *Q J Med* 1988;68:S17–S24.

70. Chernik NL, Armstrong D, Posner JB. Central nervous system infections in patients with cancer. *Medicine (Baltimore)* 1973;52:563–581.

71. Goodman ML, Coffey RJ. Stereotactic drainage of *Aspergillus* brain abscess with long-term survival: case report and review. *Neurosurgery* 1989;24:96–99.

72. Berenguer J, Diaz-Media villa J, Urra D, Munoz P. Central nervous system infection caused by *Pseudallescheria boydii:* case report and review. *Rev Infect Dis* 1989;11:890–896.

73. Smego RA, Perfect JR, Durack DT. Combined therapy with amphotericin B and 5-flucytosine for *Candida* meningitis. *Rev Infect Dis* 1984;6:791–801.

74. Heney C, Song E, Kellen A, Raal F, Miller SD, Davis V. Cerebral phaeohyphomycoses caused by *Xylohypha bantiana. Eur J Clin Microbiol Infect Dis* 1989;8:984–8.

75. Rahman N, Mahgoub E, Chagla AH. Fatal brain abscesses caused by *Ramichloridium obovoideum:* report of three cases. *Acta Neurochir* 1988;93:92–95.

76. Horowitz SL, Bentson JR, Benson F, Davos I, Pressman B, Gottlieb MS. CNS toxoplasmosis in acquired immunodeficiency syndrome. *Arch Neurol* 1983;40:649–652.

77. Masdeu JC, Tantulavanich S, Gorelick PP, et al. Brain abscess caused by *Strongyloides stercoralis. Arch Neurol* 1982;39:62–63.

78. Bia FJ, Barry M. Parasitic infections of the central nervous system. *Neurol Clin* 1986;4:171–206.

79. Armstrong D. Central nervous system infections in the immunocompromised host. *Infection* 1984;12(Suppl 1):S58–S64.

80. Stamm SM, Dismukes WE, Simmons BP, Cobbs GG, Elliot A, Budrich P, Harmon J. Listeriosis in renal transplant recipients: report of an outbreak and review of 102 cases. *Rev Infect Dis* 1982;4:589–619.

81. McArthur JC. Neurologic manifestations of AIDS. *Medicine* 1987;66:407.

82. Lantos PL, McLaughlin JE, Scholtz CL, Berry CI, Tighe JR. Neuropathology of the brain in HIV infection. *Lancet* 1989;1:309–311.

83. Levy RM, Bredesen DE, Rosenblum ML. Neurological manifestations of the acquired immunodeficiency syndrome (AIDS): experience at UCSF and review of the literature. *J Neurosurg* 1985;62:475.

84. Levy RM, Bredesen DE. Central nervous system dysfunction in acquired immunodeficiency syndrome. *J Acquired Immun Defic Syndr* 1988;1:41–64.

85. Bishburg E, Sunderan EG, Reichman LB, et al. Central nervous

86. Jarvik JG, Hessenlink JR, Wiley C, Mercer S, Robbins B, Higginbottom P. Coccidiomycotic brain abscess in an HIV-infected man. *West Med J* 1988;149:83–86.

87. Helweg-Larsen S, Jakobsen J, Boesen F, et al. Neurological complications and concomitants of AIDS. *Acta Neurol Scand* 1986;74:467.

88. Enzmann DR, Rritt RH, Placone RC Jr, Obana WG, Lyons B, Yeager AS. The effect of short-term corticosteroid treatment on the CT appearance of experimental brain abscesses. *Radiology* 1982;145:79–84.

89. Gower D, McGuirt WF. Intracranial complications of acute and chronic infectious ear disease: a problem still with us. *Laryngoscope* 1983;93:1028–1033.

90. Browning GG. The unsafeness of safe ears. *J Laryngol Otol* 1984;98:23–26.

91. Bradley PJ, Manning KP, Shaw MDM. Brain abscess secondary to otitis media. *J Laryngol Otol* 1984;98:1185–1191.

92. Samuel J, Fernandes CMC. Otogenic complications with an intact tympanic membrane. *Laryngoscope* 1985;95:1387–1390.

93. Ogle JW, Laver BA. Acute mastoiditis. *Am J Dis Child* 1986;140:1178–1182.

94. Lew D, Southwick FS, Montogomery WW, Weber AL, Baker AS. Sphenoid sinusitis. A review of 30 cases. *N Engl J Med* 1983;309:1149–1154.

95. Teed RW. Meningitis from the sphenoid sinus. *Arch Otolaryngol* 1938;28:589–619.

96. Rao AN. Brain abscess: a complication of cocaine inhalation. *NY State J Med* 1988;88:548–550.

97. Zachariades N, Vairaktaris E, Metzitis M, Triantafyllou D, Papavassiliou D. Cerebral abscess and meningitis complicated by residual mandibular ankylosis. *J Oral Med* 1986;41:14–20.

98. Hollin SA, Hayashi H, Gross SW. Intracranial abscesses of odontogenic origin. *Oral Surg* 1967;23:277–293.

99. Shaw RE. Cavernous sinus thrombosis—a review. *Br J Surg* 1952;40:40–48.

100. DiNubile MJ. Cavernous sinus thrombosis—a review. *Arch Neurol* 1988;45:567–572.

101. Herras JA, Ciria L, Henales V, Lopez P, dela Fuente A, Del Valle JM. Nonsurgical management of neonatal multiple brain abscesses due to *Proteus mirabilis. Helv Paediatr Acta* 1987;42:451–456.

102. Foreman SD, Smith EE, Ryan NJ, Hogan GR. Neonatal *Citrobacter* meningitis: pathogenesis of cerebral abscess formation. *Ann Neurol* 1984;16:655–659.

103. Kline MW. *Citrobacter* meningitis and brain abscess in infancy: epidemiology, pathogenesis and treatment. *J Pediatr* 1988;113:430–433.

104. Tenney JH. Bacterial infections of the central nervous system in neurosurgery. *Neurol Clin* 1986;4:91–114.

105. Rish BL, Careness WF, Dillon JD, Kistler JP, Mohr JP, Weiss GH. Analysis of brain abscess after penetrating craniocerebral injuries in Vietnam. *Neurosurgery* 1981;9:535–541.

106. Cairns H, Calvert CA, Daniel P, Northcroft GB. Complications of head wounds with special reference to infection. *Br J Surg* 1947;(Suppl 1):34:198–241.

107. Mampalam TJ, Rosenblum ML. Trends in the management of bacterial brain abscess: a review of 102 cases over 17 years. *Neurosurgery* 1988;23:451–458.

108. Jennett B, Miller JD. Infection after depressed fracture of the skull. Implications for management of nonmissile injuries. *J Neurosurg* 1972;36:333–339.

109. Klein DM, Cohen ME. *Pasturella multocida* brain abscess following perforating cranial dog bite. *J Pediatr* 1978;92:588–9.

110. Alpert G, Sutton LN. Brain abscess following cranial dog bite. *Clin Pediatr* 1984;23:580.

111. Berkowitz FE, Jacobs DWC. Fatal case of brain abscess caused by rooster pecking. *Pediatr Infect Dis J* 1987;6:941–942.

112. Duffy GP, Bhandari YS. Intercranial complications following transorbital penetrating injuries. *Br J Surg* 1969;56:685–688.

113. Dujovny M, Osgood CP, Maroon JC, Janett PJ. Penetrating intracranial foreign bodies in children. *J Trauma* 1975;15:981–986.

114. Fanning WL, Willett LR, Phillips CF, Wallman. Puncture

wound of the eyelid causing brain abscess. *J Trauma* 1976;16:919–920.

115. Foy P, Schair M. Cerebral abscesses in children after pencil tip injuries. *Lancet* 1980;2:662–663.

116. Miller CF, Brodkey JS, Colonibi BJ. The danger of intracranial wood. *Surg Neurol* 1977;7:95–103.

117. Tay JS, Garland JS. Serious head injuries from lawn darts. *Pediatrics* 1987;79:261–263.

118. Celli P, Palatinsky E. Brain abscess as a complication of cranial traction. *Surg Neurol* 1985;23:594–596.

119. Waggener JD. The pathophysiology of bacterial meningitis and cerebral abscesses: an anatomical interpretation. *Adv Neurol* 1974;6:1–17.

120. Overturf GD. Pyogenic bacterial infections of the CNS. *Neurol Clin* 1986;4:69–90.

121. Kline MW. Brain abscess in a patient with cystic fibrosis. *Pediatr Infect Dis J* 1985;4:72–73.

122. Schlitt M, Mitchem L, Zorn G, Dismukes W, Morawetz RB. Brain abscess after esophageal dilation for caustic stricture: report of three cases. *Neurosurgery* 1985;17:947–951.

123. Cohen FL, Koerne RS, Taub SJ. Solitary brain abscess following endoscopic injection sclerosis of esophageal varices. *Gastrointest Endosc* 1985;31:331–333.

124. Lerner PJ. Neurologic complications of infective endocarditis. *Med Clin North Am* 1985;69:385–399.

125. Pruitt AA, Rubin RHJ, Karchmer AW, Duncan GW. Neurologic complications of bacterial endocarditis. *Medicine* 1978;57:329–343.

126. Press OW, Ramsey PG. Central nervous system infections associated with hereditary hemorrhagic telangiectasia. *Am J Med* 1984;77:86–92.

127. Gelfand MS, Stephens DS, Howell EI, Alford RH, Kaiser AB. Brain abscess: association with pulmonary arteriovenous fistula and hereditary hemorrhagic telangiectasia: report of three cases. *Am J Med* 1988;85:718–720.

128. Yang SY. Brain abscess associated with congenital heart disease. *Surg Neurol* 1989;31:129–132.

129. Fischbein CA, Rosenthal A, Fischer EG, Nadas AS, Welch K. Risk factors for brain abscess in patients with congenital heart disease. *Am J Cardiol* 1974;34:94–102.

130. Fischer EG, McLennan JE, Suzuki Y. Cerebral abscess in children. *Am J Dis Child* 1981;135:746–769.

131. Molinari GF, Smith L, Goldstein MN, Satran R. Brain abscess from septic cerebral embolism: an experimental model. *Neurology* 1973;23:1205–1210.

132. Brand B, Caparosa RJ, Lubic LG. Otorhinological brain abscess therapy—past and present. *Laryngoscope* 1984;94:483–487.

133. Berger SA, Edberg SC, David G. Infectious disease of the sella turcica. *Rev Infect Dis* 1986;8:747–755.

134. Dake MD, McMurdo SK, Rosenblum ML, Brant-Zawadzki M. Pyogenic abscess of the medulla oblongata. *Neurosurgery* 1986;18:370–372.

135. Rousseaux M, Lesoin F, Destee A, Jomin M, Petit H. Developments in the treatment and prognosis of multiple cerebral abscesses. *Neurosurgery* 1985;16:304–308.

136. Britt RH, Enzmann DR, Yeager AS. Neuropathological and computerized tomographic findings in experimental brain abscess. *J Neurosurg* 1981;55:590–603.

137. Britt RH, Enzmann DR. Clinical stages of human brain abscesses on serial CT scans after contrast infusion. Computerized tomographic, neuropathological, and clinical correlations. *J Neurosurg* 1983;59:972–89.

138. Schoefl GI. Studies on inflammation. III. Growing capillaries: their structure and permeability. *Virchow's Arch [A]* 1963;337:97–141.

139. Kurzydlowski H, Wollenschlager C, Venezie FR, Ghobrial M, Soriano MM, Reichman OH. Reevaluation of an experimental streptococcal canine brain abscess model. *J Neurosurg* 1987;67:717–720.

140. Britt RH, Enzmann DH, Placone RC, Obana WG, Yeager AS. Experimental anaerobic brain abscess. *J Neurosurg* 1984;60:1148–1159.

141. Enzmann DR, Britt RH, Obana WG, Stuart J, Murphy-Owen K. Experimental *Staphylococcus aureus* brain abscess. *AJNR* 1986;7:395–402.

142. Neuwelt EA, Lawrence MS, Blank NK. Effect of gentamicin and dexamethasone on the natural history of the rat *Escherichia coli* brain abscess model with histopathologic correlation. *Neurosurgery* 1984;15:475–483.

143. Obana WG, Britt RH, Placone RC, Stuart JS, Enzmann DR. Experimental brain abscess development in the chronically immunosuppressed host. Computerized tomographic and neuropathological correlations. *J Neurosurg* 1986;65:382–391.

144. Wood JH, Doppman JL, Lightfoote WE. Role of vascular proliferation on angiographic appearance and encapsulation of experimental traumatic and metastatic brain abscesses. *J Neurosurg* 1978;48:264–273.

145. Prockop DJ, Kivirikko KI, Tuderman L, Guzman WA. The biosynthesis of collagen and its disorders: part I. *N Engl J Med* 1979;301:13–23.

146. Arseni C, Ciurea AV. Cerebellar abscesses. A report on 119 cases. *Zentralbl Neurochir* 1982;43:359–370.

147. Shaw MDM, Russell JA. Cerebellar abscess—a review of 47 cases. *J Neurol Neurosurg Psychiatry* 1975;38:429–435.

148. Adams RD, Victor M. Nonviral infections of the nervous system. In: Adams RD, Victor M, eds. *Principles of neurology.* New York: McGraw-Hill, 1985:552–556.

149. Domingue JN, Wilson CB. Pituitary abscesses. Report of seven cases and review of the literature. *J Neurosurg* 1977;46:601–608.

150. Hirschberg H, Bosnes V. C-reactive protein levels in the differential diagnosis of brain abscesses. *J Neurosurg* 1987;67:358–360.

151. Nielsen H, Halaburt H. Cerebral abscess with special reference to the angiographic changes. *Neuroradiology* 1976;12:73.

152. Crocker EF, McLaughlin AF, Morris JG, et al. Technetium brain scanning in the diagnosis and management of cerebral abscess. *Am J Med* 1974;56:192.

153. Masucci EF, Sauerbrunn BJL. The evolution of a brain abscess. The complementary roles of radionuclide and computed tomography scans. *Clin Nucl Med* 1982;7:166.

154. Rosenblum ML, Hoff JT, Norman D, et al. Decreased mortality from brain abscesses since advent of computerized tomography. *J Neurosurg* 1978;49:658.

155. Potter DG, ed. CT of the ear, nose and throat. *Radiol Clin North Am* 1984;22:1.

156. New PFJ, Davis KR, Ballantine HT Jr. Computed tomography in cerebral abscess. *Radiology* 1976;121:641–646.

157. Whelan MA, Hilal SK. Computed tomography as a guide in the diagnosis and follow-up of brain abscesses. *Radiology* 1980;135:663–671.

158. Miller ES, Psrilal SD, Uttley D. CT scanning in the management of intracranial abscess: a review of 100 cases. *Br J Neurosurg* 1988;2:439–446.

159. Weisberg L. Clinical–CT correlations in intracranial suppurative (bacterial) disease. *Neurology* 1984;34:509–510.

160. Dobkin JF, Healton EB, Dickinson T, Brust JCM. Nonspecificity of ring enhancement in medically cured brain abscess. *Neurology* 1984;34:139–144.

161. Salzman C, Tuazon CU. Value of the ring enhancing sign in differentiating intracerebral hematomas and brain abscesses. *Arch Intern Med* 1987;147:951–957.

162. Zimmerman RD, Leeds NE, Naidrich TP. Ring blush associated with intracerebral hematoma. *Radiology* 1977;122:707–711.

163. Holtas S, Tornquist C, Cronqvist S. Diagnostic difficulties in computed tomography of brain abscesses. *J Comput Assist Tomogr* 1982;6:683–688.

164. Coulam CM, Seshul M, Donaldson J. Intracranial ring lesions: Can we differentiate by computed tomography? *Invest Radiol* 1980;15:103–112.

165. Rehncrona S, Brismar J, Holtas S. Diagnosis of brain abscesses with indium-111 labeled leukocytes. *Neurosurgery* 1985;16:23–36.

166. Bellotti C, Aragno MG, Medina M, et al. Differential diagnosis of CT-hypodense cranial lesions with indium-111-oxine-labeled leukocytes. *J Neurosurg* 1986;64:750–753.

167. Kock-Jensen C, Anderson B, Sogaard I. Leucocyte scanning: a valuable tool in diagnosing cerebral abscess—a survey. *Acta Neurochir* 1986;83:121–124.

168. Brant-Zawadzki M, Enzmann DR, Placone RC, et al. NMR imaging of experimental brain abscess: comparison with CT. *AJNR* 1983;4:250–253.

169. Runge VM, Clanton JA, Price AC, et al. Evaluation of contrast-enhanced MR imaging in a brain-abscess model. *AJNR* 1985;6:139–147.

170. Grossman RI, Joseph PM, Wolf G, et al. Experimental intracranial septic infarction: magnetic resonance enhancement. *Radiology* 1985;155:649–653.

171. Zimmerman RD, Haimes AB. The role of MR imaging in the diagnosis of infections of the central nervous system. In: Remington JS, Swartz MN, eds. *Current clinical topics in infectious diseases.* Boston: Blackwell Scientific Publications, 1989;82–108.

172. Davidson MD, Steiner RE. Magnetic resonance imaging in infections of the central nervous system. *AJNR* 1985;6:499–504.

173. Spector R. Ceftriaxone transport through the blood–brain barrier. *J Infect Dis* 1987;156:209.

174. Gortvai P, DeLouvois J, Hurley R. The bacteriology and chemotherapy of acute pyogenic brain abscess. *Br J Neurosurg* 1987;1:189–203.

175. Ryan DM, Cars O, Hoffstedt B. The use of antibiotic serum levels to predict concentration in tissue. *Scand J Infect Dis* 1986;18:381–388.

176. Tunkel AR, Scheld WM. Therapy of bacterial meningitis: principles and practice. *Infect Control Hosp Epidemiol* 1989;10:565–571.

177. Wellman WE, Dodge HW, Heilmann FR, Peterson MG. Concentration of antibiotics in the brain. *J Lab Clin Med* 1954;43:275–279.

178. Kramer PW, Griffith RS, Campbell RI. Antibiotic penetration of the brain. A comparative study. *J Neurosurg* 1969;31:295–302.

179. Black P, Graybill JR, Charache P. Penetration of brain abscess by systemically administered antibiotics. *J Neurosurg* 1973;38:705–709.

180. de Louvois J, Gortvai P, Hurley R. Antibiotic treatment of abscesses of the central nervous system. *Br Med J* 1977;2:985–987.

181. de Louvois J, Hurley R. Inactivation of penicillin by purulent exudates. *Br Med J* 1977;1:998–1000.

182. Picardi JL, Lewis HP, Tan JS, Phair JP. Clindamycin concentrations in the central nervous system of primates before and after head trauma. *J Neurosurg* 1975;43:717.

183. Alderson D, Strong AJ, Ingham HR, Selkon JB. Fifteen year review of the mortality of brain abscess. *Neurosurgery* 1981;8:1–6.

184. Smego R, Moeller MS, Gallis HA. Trimethoprim-sulfamethoxazole therapy for *Nocardia* infections. *Arch Intern Med* 1983;143:711–718.

185. Maderazo EG, Quintiliani R. Treatment of nocardial infection with trimethoprim and sulfamethoxazole. *Am J Med* 1974;57:671–675.

186. Levitz R, Quintiliani R. Trimethoprim-sulfamethoxazole for bacterial meningitis. *Ann Intern Med* 1984;100:881–890.

187. Greene BM, Thomas FE Jr, Alford RH. Trimethoprim-sulfamethoxazole and brain abscess. *Ann Intern Med* 1975;82:812–813.

188. Levy RM, Gutin PH, Baskin DS, Pons VG. Vancomycin penetration of a brain abscess: case report and review of literature. *Neurosurgery* 1986;18:633–636.

189. Preheim LC, McCracken GH, Jubeliver DP. Moxalactam penetration into brain abscess. Program and Abstracts, 21st Interscience Conference on Antimicrobial Agents and Chemotherapy, Abstract 738, 1981.

190. Marcus MG, Atluru VI, Epstein N, Leggiadro RJ. Conservative management of *Citrobacter diverus* meningitis with brain abscess. *NY State J Med* 1984;84:252–254.

191. Scheld WM, Brodeur JP, Foresman PA, Gratz JC, Rodeheaver GT. Comparative evaluation of aztreonam in therapy for experimental bacterial meningitis and cerebritis. *Rev Infect Dis* 1985;7(Suppl 4):S635–S647.

192. Carton JA, Perry F, Maradona JA, Meadey FJ. Successful treatment of recurrent cerebral empyema and brain abscesses with imipenem. *Eur J Clin Microbiol* 1989;6:578–580.

193. Rice LB, Eliopoulos GM. Imipenem and aztreonam: current role in antimicrobial therapy. In: Remington JS, Swartz MN, eds. *Current clinical topics in infectious diseases.* Boston: Blackwell Scientific Publications, 1989;109–139.

194. Neu HC. Uses of antimicrobial agents in brain abscesses. In: Nelson JD, Grassi C, eds. *Current chemotherapy and infectious disease,* vol I. Washington, DC: American Society for Microbiology, 1980;41–42.

195. Norrby R. A review of the penetration of antibiotics into CSF and its clinical significance. *Scand J Infect Dis* 1978;14(Suppl):296–309.

196. Neuwelt EA, Enzmann DR, Pagel MA, Miller G. Bacterial and fungal brain abscess and the blood–brain barrier. In: Neuwelt EA, ed. *Implications of the blood–brain barrier and its manipulation.* New York: Plenum Press, 1989;263–305.

197. Sande MA, Korzenwioski OM, Allegro GM, et al. Intermittent or continuous therapy of experimental meningitis due to *Streptococcus pneumoniae* in rabbits: preliminary observations on the post antibiotic effect *in vivo. Rev Infect Dis* 1981;3:98.

198. Haley EC Jr, Costello GI, Rodeheaver GT, Winn HR, Scheld WM. Treatment of experimental brain abscess with penicillin and chloramphenicol. *J Infect Dis* 1983;148:737–744.

199. Ballantine HJ, White JC. Brain abscess. Influence of the antibiotic on therapy and morbidity. *N Engl J Med* 1953;248:14–19.

200. Jooma OV, Pennybacker JB, Tutton GT. Brain abscess: aspiration, drainage or excision? *J Neurol Neurosurg Psychiatry* 1951;14:308–313.

201. Tutton GK. Cerebral abscess. The present position. *Ann R Coll Surg Engl* 1953;13:281–311.

202. Holm S, Kourtopoulos H. Penetration of antibiotics into brain tissue and brain abscesses. An experimental study in steroid treated rats. *Scand J Infect Dis* 1985;44(Suppl):68–70.

203. Warner J, Perkins RL, Cordero L. Metronidazole therapy of anaerobic bacteremia, meningitis, and brain abscess. *Arch Intern Med* 1979;139:167–169.

204. LeBeau J, Creissard P, Harispe L, Redondo A. Surgical treatment of brain abscess and subdural empyema. *J Neurosurg* 1973;38:198–203.

205. Kourtopoulos H, Holm SE, West KA. The management of intracranial abscesses: comparative study between two materials with different rates of mortality. *Acta Neurochir* 1981;56:127–128.

206. Stepanov S. Surgical treatment of brain abscess. *Neurosurgery* 1988;22:724–730.

207. Westcombe DS, Dorsch NWC, Teo C. Management of cerebral abscess in adolescents and adults. *Acta Neurochir* 1988;95:85–89.

208. Taylor JC. The case of excision in the treatment of brain abscess. *Br J Neurosurg* 1987;1:173–178.

209. Rousseaux M, Lesoin F, Destee A, Jomin M, Petit H. Long term sequelae of hemispheric abscesses as a function of the treatment. *Acta Neurochir* 1985;74:61–67.

210. Young RF, Frazee J. Gas within intracranial abscess cavities: an indication for surgical excision. *Ann Neurol* 1984;16:35–39.

211. Karandanis D, Shulman JA. Factors associated with mortality in brain abscess. *Arch Intern Med* 1975;135:1145–1150.

212. Ohaegbulam SC, Saddeqi NU. Experience with brain abscesses treated by simple aspiration. *Surg Neurol* 1980;13:289–291.

213. Lunsford LD, Nelson PB. Stereotactic aspiration of a brain abscess using the therapeutic CT scanner. *Acta Neurochir* 1982;62:25–29.

214. Apuzzo MLJ, Sabshin JK. Computed tomographic guidance stereotaxis in the management of intracranial mass lesions. *Neurosurgery* 1983;12:277–285.

215. Lunsford D, Martinez AJ. Stereotactic exploration of the brain in the era of computed tomography. *Surg Neurol* 1984;22:222–230.

216. Nauta HJW, Conteras FI, Weiner RI, et al. Brain stem abscess managed with computed tomography-guided stereotactic aspiration. *Neurosurgery* 1987;20:476.

217. Itakurg T, Yokote H, Ozaki F, et al. Stereotactic operation for brain abscess. *Surg Neurol* 1987;28:196.

218. Hall WA, Martinex AJ, Dummer JS, et al. Nocardial brain abscess: diagnostic and therapeutic use of stereotactic aspiration. *Surg Neurol* 1987;28:114.

219. Dyste GN, Hitchon PW, Menezes AH, VanGilder JC, Groene GM. Stereotaxic surgery in the treatment of multiple brain abscesses. *J Neurosurg* 1988;69:188–194.

220. Rossitch E, Alexander E, Schiff SJ, Ballard DE. The use of computed tomography-guided stereotactic techniques in the treatment of brain stem abscesses. *Clin Neurol Neurosurg* 1988;90:365–368.

221. Enzmann DR, Britt RH, Placone R. Staging of human brain abscess by computed tomography. *Radiology* 1983;146:703–708.

222. Heinnemann HS, Braude AI, Osterholm JL. Intracranial suppurative disease. Early presumptive diagnosis and successful treatment without surgery. *JAMA* 1971;218:1542–1547.
223. Rosenblum ML, Manpalam TJ, Pons VG. Controversies in the management of brain abscesses. *Clin Neurosurg* 1986;33:603.
224. Berg B, Franklin G, Cuneo R, Boldrey E, Strimling B. Nonsurgical cure of brain abscess: early diagnosis and follow-up with computerized tomography. *Ann Neurol* 1978;3:474–478.
225. Rotheram EB Jr, Kessler LA. Use of computerized tomography in nonsurgical management of brain abscess. *Arch Neurol* 1979;36:25–26.
226. Rosenblum ML, Hoff JT, Norman D, Edwards MS, Berg BO. Nonoperative treatment of brain abscesses in selected high-risk patients. *J Neurosurg* 1980;52:217–225.
227. Boom WH, Tuazon CU. Successful treatment of multiple brain abscesses with antibiotics alone. *Rev Infect Dis* 1985;7:189–199.
228. Daniels SR, Price JK, Towbin RB, McLaurin R. Nonsurgical cure of brain abscess in a neonate. *Childs Nerv Syst* 1985;1:346–348.
229. Keren G, Tyrrell DLJ. Nonsurgical treatment of brain abscesses: report of two cases. *Pediatr Infect Dis J* 1984;3:331–334.
230. Enzmann DR, Britt RH, Yeager AS. Experimental brain abscess evolution: computed tomographic and neuropathologic correlation. *Radiology* 1979;133:113–122.
231. Epstein F, Whelan M. Cerebritis masquerading as brain abscess: case report. *Neurosurgery* 1982;10:757–759.
232. Luft BJ, Remington JS. Toxoplasmic encephalitis. *J Infect Dis* 1988;157:106.
233. Scheld WM, Brodeur JP. Effect of methylprednisolone on entry of ampicillin and gentamicin into the cerebrospinal fluid in experimental pneumococcal and *E. coli* meningitis. *Antimicrob Agents Chemother* 1983;23:108–112.
234. Kourtopoulos H, Holm SE, Norrby SR. The influence of steroids on the penetration of antibiotics into brain tissue and brain abscesses. An experimental study in rats. *J Antimicrob Chemother* 1983;11:245–249.
235. Black KL, Farhat SM. Cerebral abscess: loss of computed tomographic enhancement with steroids. *Neurosurgery* 1984;14:215–217.
236. Schroeder KA, McKeever PE, Schaberg DR, Hoff JT. Effect of dexamothasone on experimental brain abscess. *J Neurosurg* 1987;66:264–269.
237. Yildizhan A, Pasoglu A, Kandemir B. Effect of dexamethasone on various stages of experimental brain abscess. *Acta Neurochir* 1989;96:141–148.
238. Gruszkiewicz J, Doron Y, Peyser E, Borovich B, Schachter J, Front D. Brain abscess and its surgical management. *Surg Neurol* 1982;18:7–17.
239. Buonagnio A, Colangelo M, Daniele B, Cantone G, Ambrosio A. Neurological and behavioral sequelae in children operated on for brain abscess. *Childs Nerv Syst* 1989;5:153–155.
240. Calliauw WL, dePraetere P, Verbeke L. Postoperative epilepsy in subdural suppurations. *Acta Neurochir* 1984;71:217–223.

Infections of the Central Nervous System,
edited by W. M. Scheld, R. J. Whitley, and
D. T. Durack, Raven Press, Ltd., New York © 1991.

CHAPTER 20

Subdural Empyema

David C. Helfgott, Karen Weingarten, and Barry J. Hartman

Subdural empyema is an important form of intracranial suppuration, accounting for 15–25% of pyogenic intracranial infections (1–3). It represents an infectious process which occupies the space between the dura mater and arachnoid surrounding the brain. Left undiagnosed and untreated, subdural empyema is rapidly fatal; hence, early recognition is critical. In children and adults, subdural empyema is most often a complication of otorhinologic infection (1,4–15). Subdural empyema may also occur as a result of head trauma or surgery, osteomyelitis of the skull, or bacteremic spread from a distant focus of infection. In infants, leptomeningitis is the most common predisposing cause of subdural empyema (11,16,17). Males predominate over females by about 3:1, and about 70% of patients are in their second or third decade of life (3–5,7–10,12,13,15,18–22). Patients will present with fever and headache in more than 90% of cases, and many will have associated neurologic abnormalities (1,3–9,12,13,15,17,19,20,22–25). The diagnosis of subdural empyema is confirmed using computerized tomography (CT) or magnetic resonance imaging (MRI) scanning techniques. However, a strong clinical suspicion despite the lack of evidence for subdural empyema on scans warrants more invasive investigation. Definitive therapy consists of surgical drainage and systemic antibiotics, yet mortality remains as high as 40% in some series (14,17). Spinal subdural empyema also has been described; however, it is quite rare, with less than 20 cases reported in the literature (26). This condition is addressed briefly at the end of this chapter.

HISTORICAL PERSPECTIVE

The first comprehensive clinicopathologic descriptions of subdural empyema as a distinct entity were published in the 1940s, although the first definitive report of subdural empyema dates back to 1861 (27,28). This initial report was followed by several more around the turn of the century, with a compilation of 44 cases by Blegvad in 1910 (27). Early names for this disease included "pachymeningitis interna," "purulent pachymeningitis," "pia–arachnoid abscess," "phlegmonous meningitis," and "subdural abscess," but these were rejected by Kubik and Adams in favor of subdural empyema (8,27). Interestingly, the early publications reported a preponderance of subdural empyema secondary to otogenic infections (27). However, since the compilation of 42 confirmed cases resulting from frontal sinusitis by Courville (28), it has become clear that paranasal sinusitis is the most important causative factor in the development of subdural empyema in older children and adults.

Over the past 50 years, much has changed in the areas of therapy and diagnosis of subdural empyema. Prior to the development of antibiotics, subdural empyema was almost always fatal (27,28). Antibiotics, improved diagnosis, and newer surgical techniques have combined to lower the mortality rate to 10–40% (1,4,5,7–15,17,18,20,24,25). Physicians depended upon their clinical skills and plain roentgenograms of the sinuses and skull to direct their attention to the possibility of intracranial suppuration, until the development of cerebral angiography in the early 1960s, which proved to be an extremely sensitive method of detecting a subdural collection (13,29). The emergence of CT in the 1970s provided a noninvasive, rapid means of visualizing the cranial contents; and its reliability, safety, and ease of

D. C. Helfgott: Department of Medicine, Division of Infectious Diseases, Cornell University Medical College, New York, New York 10021; and The Rockefeller University, New York, New York 10021.

K. Weingarten: Department of Radiology, Division of Neuroradiology, Cornell University Medical College, New York, New York 10021.

B. J. Hartman: Department of Medicine, Division of Infectious Diseases, Cornell University Medical College, New York, New York 10021.

operation made it the first choice for diagnosis of suspected subdural empyema (2,10,22,30). Recently, MRI has proven to be even more sensitive than CT (31).

PATHOGENESIS AND ANATOMIC CONSIDERATIONS

The clinical features of subdural empyema are easily understood if one considers the anatomy of the subdural space with respect to its surrounding structures (Fig. 1). The subdural space is normally a potential space rather than an actual space, since the dura mater follows the contours of the skull and lies adjacent to the arachnoid and pia mater (32). The ability to form an actual space with fluid collection is greater around the convexities of the cerebral hemispheres, where the brain does not approximate the skull as closely as it does around the basal areas (15,18,28). Posteriorly, the tentorium cerebelli is a reflection of dura separating the cerebellum from the cerebral cortex (33). It is an effective barrier to the passage of subdural collection infratentorially, except at its free anterior margin where fluid may seep into the subdural space of the posterior fossa. Only about 10% of subdural empyemas are infratentorial (15,34,35). Medially, the falx cerebri is a reflection of dura extending the length of the cerebrum which separates the cerebral hemispheres (33). Subdural fluid which accumulates between the falx and the arachnoid are known as "parasaggital," "interhemispheric," or "parafalcine" subdural empyemas and are usually secondary to surface subdural collections, but rarely may be primary (36–38). A subdural empyema may communicate with the contralateral side via the inferior free margin of the falx.

Infection usually spreads to the dura via venous drainage from the sinuses, middle ear, face, or scalp. Within the dura mater are seven paired venous sinuses and five unpaired sinuses, all of which are spaces between two layers of dura. They collect blood from the veins of the brain, skull, and face, and they empty into the internal jugular veins (33). Emissary (perforating) veins allow the passage of blood from the larger veins of the face and scalp into the dural venous sinuses, serving as a potential communication for more superficial infection of the head with the venous system of the brain (32). The venous system of the head and brain is valveless, allowing retrograde spread of thrombophlebitis from infected venous sinuses into dural and cortical venous channels (17,32).

It therefore follows that infections or trauma of the head are the usual causes of subdural empyema. Table 1 reviews the conditions predisposing to subdural empyema in series reported over the past two decades (excluding series of only infants). Paranasal sinusitis overwhelmingly predominates as the precipitating factor for the development of subdural empyema. The sinusitis almost always involves a frontal sinus, often with other sinuses affected as well. The incidence of subdural empyema following frontal sinusitis is 1–2% (39). The frontal and sphenoid sinuses are intimately associated with the dura mater, separated from the dura only by a thin plate of bone. These sinuses communicate with the maxillary and ethmoid sinuses, which are more anteriorly placed. Because of its supratentorial position, the frontal sinus is almost always involved in infection which spreads to the subdural space. In addition, the growing posterior wall of the frontal sinus in boys between the ages of 9 and 20 has been offered as a possible explanation for the striking sex and age susceptibility for the development of subdural empyema (7,22).

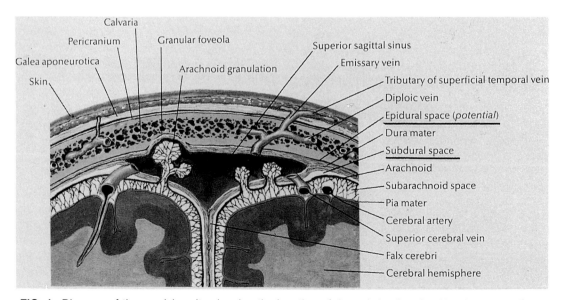

FIG. 1. Diagram of the cranial cavity showing the location of the subdural and epidural spaces. (From ref. 66, adapted and reproduced with permission from *Atlas of Human Anatomy* by Frank H. Netter, M.D. All rights reserved.)

TABLE 1. *Predisposing causes of subdural empyema*

Number of patients	Sinusitis (%)	Otogenic (%)	Head trauma/surgery (%)	Hematogenous (%)	Other[a] (%)	Reference
47	55	13	4	4	23[b]	1
37	59	12	15	0	15	4
23	35	30	26	4	4	5
8	88	0	0	0	12	6
4	100	0	0	0	0	7
15	40	7	27	13	13	8
42	74	12	0	2	12	9
49	41	2	31	2	23	10
25	32	12	28	4	24[b]	11
66	68	21	3	3	5	12
17	41	6	24	6	24[b]	13
37	43	0	16	0	41[b]	14
37	54	32	5	3	5	15
Total: 407	54	13	13	3	16	
Range:	32–100	0–32	0–31	0–13	0–41	

[a] Includes facial infections, local osteomyelitis, unknown.
[b] Includes infants with meningitis.

Two modes of extension have been proposed for the spread of infection from a frontal sinus to the subdural space—direct and indirect (28). Direct extension involves erosion of the posterior bony wall of the frontal sinus by infection, with further erosion of the underlying dura mater (28). However, pathologic studies rarely report evidence of this mechanism of spread (28). The more likely route is indirect, with extension of infection and associated thrombophlebitis through the mucosal veins of the sinus to the emissary veins which link the facial and dural venous systems (15,28,40). From the dural sinuses the infection establishes itself in the subdural space at the frontal pole and may spread posteriorly over the convexity, medially into the interhemispheric region, and contralaterally. This extension may create significant pressure on a large area of underlying brain tissue (15,18,41). As stated previously, it is unusual but possible for the empyema to spread infratentorially (15). Further retrograde thrombophlebitis often occurs, involving the valveless, deeper veins of the cerebrum, which, in turn, may lead to necrosis and infection of brain tissue (10,13,27,28).

Subdural empyema secondary to an otogenic source of infection differs only in the site at which pus enters the subdural space. The tympanic cavity is bounded superiorly by the tegmen tympani, a thin plate of bone forming part of the temporal bone of the skull, separating the tympanic cavity from the brain (32). It is through this plate of bone that perforating veins pass to communicate with the superior petrosal sinus of the dura (32). In addition, mastoid air cells within the temporal bone surrounding the middle ear communicate with the tympanic cavity and may lie very close to the posterior cranial fossa, separated from the dura by slivers of bone (32). Otitis or mastoiditis may therefore extend directly into the subdural space via erosion of the tegmen tympani or bone adjacent to the air cells and dura mater, or spread infection indirectly by way of a progressive thrombophlebitis of the perforating veins (23,27). Since the sinuses into which the veins from the middle ear and mastoid bone drain are within or beneath the tentorium (33), otogenic infection may result in posterior fossa subdural empyema (23). As opposed to subdural empyema secondary to frontal sinusitis, otitis-induced subdural empyema is initially localized posteriorly or on the tentorium (42).

In adults, the extension of a subdural empyema to acute purulent meningitis is very unusual. Although there is a subarachnoid inflammatory exudate, the arachnoid is fairly impermeable to the bacterial process occurring adjacent to it (18). Similarly, bacterial meningitis in adults is a very unusual cause of subdural empyema (17). However, in infants, meningitis is an important predisposing condition for the development of a subdural empyema (11,16,17). Subdural empyema occurs in about 2% of infants with bacterial meningitis (43). The pathogenesis is presumably infection of an initially sterile subdural effusion (13,16,17). Such sterile effusions are variably reported as occurring in 12–32% of infants with meningitis (13,16).

CLINICAL FEATURES

A high clinical suspicion and rapid diagnosis of subdural empyema are critical for a successful outcome. Certainly, an adult with a recent history of sinusitis and a new presentation suggestive of central nervous system (CNS) infection warrants an investigation to exclude subdural empyema. However, in some cases the anteced-

TABLE 2. *Sex predilection of subdural empyema*

Number of males/total	Percentage	Reference
6/6	100	3
79/102	77	4
18/23	78	5
11/14	79	7
11/15	73	8
28/42	67	9
28/49	57	10
44/66	67	12
14/17	82	13
26/37	70	15
13/22	59	18
3/6	50	19
10/14	71	20
4/4	100	21
13/17	76	22
Total: 308/434	71	
Range:	50–100	

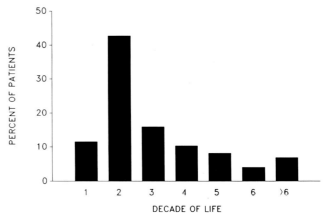

FIG. 2. Age distribution of patients reported with subdural empyema.

ent infection is subtle enough to be unrecognized. In others, the concurrent complication of a sinusitis with a subdural empyema delays the diagnosis of the latter because symptoms are attributed to the sinusitis. In other cases, the subdural empyema is not suspected because the precipitating cause for the subdural empyema is unknown or arises from a distant focus of infection. Although the clinical presentation may vary, there are key clinical features of subdural empyema which, if present, should result in its inclusion in one's initial differential diagnosis.

The sex and age distributions of patients with subdural empyema are striking. Table 2 shows the overrepresentation of males reported in series of patients (mostly adults) with subdural empyema published over the last two decades. In those which report only children, males also predominate. However, in infants this sex discrepancy may not be so marked (17,43). Figure 2 displays the age distribution of patients reported in series of consecutive patients with subdural empyema. It is clear that most cases occur during the second and third decades of life. As stated earlier, the growth of the frontal sinus in

pubertal boys has been proposed as an explanation for the uneven sex and age distribution (7,22). However, confirmatory analyses comparing patients' sex, age, and source of infection have not been reported.

The clinical features of adults with subdural empyema are presented in Table 3. Generally, patients have a nonspecific illness for a few days to a few weeks prior to presentation to the hospital acutely ill (1,5,12,13). However, if the infection is a result of head trauma or surgery, the symptoms may be milder and present more subacutely (10,19,44,45). The most common symptoms and signs are headache, fever, neurologic deficit, and stiff neck. Vomiting and malaise are often reported as well (8,15). Seizures, papilledema, and altered level of consciousness ranging from drowsiness and disorientation to coma also occur frequently. These neurologic changes may be presenting signs or, as is often the case, may develop during the course of the illness (6,7,15,24).

Diffuse neurologic signs such as altered level of consciousness, papilledema, and generalized seizures are a result of increased intracranial pressure (28,46). Focal neurologic abnormalities such as hemiparesis, jacksonian seizures, dysphasia, and cranial neuropathies may be secondary to local pressure on the underlying cortex by

TABLE 3. *Clinical signs of subdural empyema*

Sign/symptom	Number of patients[a]	Percentage	References
Fever	260	88	3, 4, 6–9, 13, 15, 17, 19, 22, 23
Headache	307	75	3–9, 13, 15, 17, 19, 20, 22, 23
Hemiparesis	330	75	3–5, 7–9, 13, 17, 19, 20, 22, 24
Altered consciousness	395	74	1, 3–9, 12, 13, 15, 17, 19, 23
Nuchal rigidity	225	69	4, 6–8, 13, 15, 17, 19, 20, 22, 23, 25
Seizures	416	53	4–9, 13, 15, 17, 19, 20, 22, 24, 25
Papilledema	179	39	6–9, 13, 15, 17, 20, 22, 23
Altered speech	332	22	3–6, 8, 9, 15, 20, 22, 24
Other focal deficits[b]	223	46	5–9, 13, 15, 20, 22, 24

[a] Total number of patients in whom finding was assessed.
[b] Includes cranial neuropathies, hemianopsia, other.

the subdural process (17,23,27,28,36,41,47) and may be precipitated by cortical venous thrombosis with accompanying brain inflammation and infarction (17,18,46). Such focal neurologic signs may help to localize the empyema. This is particularly true in cases of infratentorial subdural empyema which occur infrequently but which is easily suspected if cerebellar signs such as ataxia and nystagmus are present (23). Interhemispheric (parasagittal, parafalcine) subdural empyema, usually associated with disease over the convexities but uncommonly occurring alone (38), characteristically produces contralateral leg symptoms, including weakness and focal seizures (36,38,41,47). As the interhemispheric suppuration extends backward over the tentorium and below the occipital lobes, homonymous hemianopsia may result (41,47). Subdural empyema overlying one or both convexities yields the most nonspecific neurologic signs. Clues to the involved areas can be (a) contralateral paresis or seizures, (b) aphasia or dysphasia associated with left-sided infection, or (c) cranial neuropathies (27,28,41).

The clinical signs of subdural empyema in infants are similar to those in adults. In addition, a bulging anterior fontanelle is a common finding in infants (11,16,43).

DIFFERENTIAL DIAGNOSIS

The cardinal features of headache, fever, stiff neck, and neurologic signs are not specific for subdural empyema. The differential diagnosis also includes brain abscess, epidural abscess, meningitis, meningoencephalitis, subdural hematoma, and intracerebral thrombophlebitis (17,40). Of these, the presence of focal neurologic signs makes meningitis much less likely. The presence of nuchal rigidity is unusual in brain abscess and subdural hematoma. Unfortunately, clinical grounds alone do not allow the exclusion of most of these possibilities. Therefore, more specific testing should be undertaken as soon as the diagnosis of subdural empyema is suspected.

DIAGNOSTIC STUDIES

Routine studies such as blood tests and plain roentgenograms are of very little value in patients with suspected subdural empyema. Most patients are found to have a peripheral blood leukocytosis (3,11,13,23,28). Plain films of the skull are not useful except to demonstrate a sinusitis or mastoiditis, or to show widened sutures in infants (17).

Prior to the development of CT, cerebral arteriography, with a diagnostic accuracy of 80–90%, was the procedure of choice to diagnose subdural empyema (13,15,17,23). Although nearly perfect for the detection of hemispheric and parafalcine subdural collections, the sensitivity of carotid angiograms for posterior fossa sub-

dural empyema was not as great (23). Presently, the safety, ease of application, and reliability of CT and MRI make them the modality of choice to diagnose subdural empyema.

Computed Tomography and Magnetic Resonance Imaging

The radiologic evaluation of patients with subdural and epidural empyemas has been revolutionized by the advent of CT in 1972 and of MRI in 1984. The introduc-

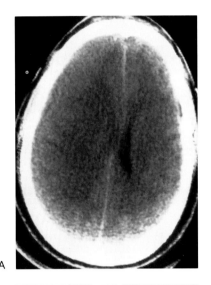
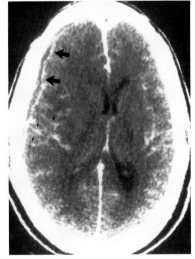

FIG. 3. Subdural and epidural empyemas due to paranasal sinus inflammatory disease. A: Noncontrast CT of the brain demonstrating right hemispheric edema with compression of the right lateral ventricle. No definite empyema is seen. B: Contrast CT demonstrating a right convexity subdural empyema with a thin rim of marginal enhancement (*large arrows*) and gyral enhancement (*small arrows*). Note the disproportionate degree of mass effect on the underlying brain with ventricular compression when compared to the size of the empyema.

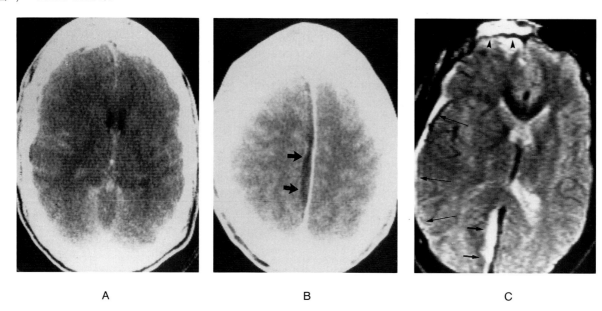

A   B   C

FIG. 4. Otorhinologically induced subdural empyema. **A:** Contrast CT demonstrating subtle right hemispheric empyema. **B:** Interhemispheric subdural empyema (*arrows*) delineated by the falx medially and with early membrane formation laterally. **C:** T2-weighted MRI the same day. Note the improved visualization of the right convexity compared to that of Fig. 4A (*long arrows*); also note the interhemispheric subdural empyema (*short arrows*) and the inflammatory disease in the frontal sinus (*arrowheads*).

tion of CT has had a major impact on the management and prognosis of subdural and epidural empyemas, because CT allows (in a noninvasive manner) earlier and more accurate detection, delineation, and characterization of these extra-axial (extraparenchymal) inflammatory lesions and their associated intra-axial (parenchymal) sequelae when compared to carotid arteriography (10). In addition, CT provides an important adjunct to standard clinical parameters in the assessment of the adequacy of patient response to therapy.

The CT findings during the early stages of development of a subdural empyema may be subtle and easily overlooked (10). Noncontrast CT typically demonstrates a crescent-shaped hypodense collection over one or both cerebral convexities and/or around the interhemispheric tissue (Fig. 3A). Contrast-enhanced CT increases the conspicuity of the collections, which represent active inflammatory disease either in the leptomeninges or in the subjacent cerebral cortex (Fig. 3B). Thick, irregular enhancement of the falx in association with a spindle-shaped collection is seen in interhemispheric subdural empyemas (38) (Fig. 4A and 4B). Parenchymal changes at this early stage include thickening and hyperdensity of the underlying cortical gray matter and hypodensity of the white matter on noncontrast CT; these changes indicate the presence of edema, hyperemia, and ischemia (10). Additionally, gyral enhancement subjacent to an extra-axial empyema on contrast CT is a frequent finding, indicative of meningitis, cerebritis, and/or venous thrombosis (Fig. 3B). Extensive mass effect on the ipsilateral cerebral hemisphere which is out of proportion to

the small size of the extra-axial collection is invariably present (Fig. 3B), and it is manifested as ventricular compression, sulcal effacement, and midline shift. It is important to examine the paranasal sinuses, middle ear cavity, and orbits for the presence of inflammation, which may reflect the origin and extent of the intracranial abnormalities (22,25) (Figs. 5 and 6A). Unrecognized and untreated, the subdural empyema rapidly increases in size and develops loculations, and the parenchymal abnormalities progress to cortical infarction and abscess formation.

MRI is proving to have a greater sensitivity and specificity in the work-up of patients with an extra-axial empyema; this is attributed to several inherent advantages of MRI over CT (31,48,49). MRI uses several standard pulse sequences referred to as "T1-weighted," "proton-

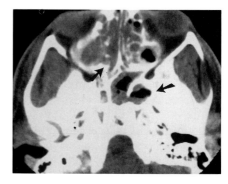

FIG. 5. Contrast-enhanced CT of the paranasal sinuses demonstrating extensive maxillary, ethmoid, and sphenoid sinus inflammation (*arrows*).

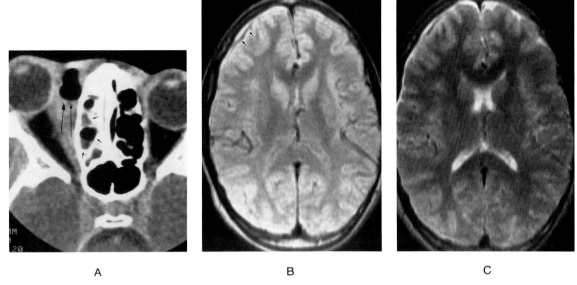

A   B   C

FIG. 6. Subdural empyema in the setting of orbital and paranasal sinus inflammatory disease. **A:** Contrast CT demonstrating a right orbital abscess (*long arrows*) and ethmoid sinusitis (*short arrows*). **B** and **C:** Proton-density MRI (**B**) and T2-weighted MRI (**C**) the same day as for part A, demonstrating a small right convexity subdural collection (*arrows*) which is brighter than CSF in Fig. 6B and which is therefore not a sterile effusion or hygroma. Note that the conspicuity of the empyema on MRI is greater than that on CT.

density-weighted," and "T2-weighted" (50). These pulse sequences are obtained by varying the values of two independent, user-selectable imaging parameters—namely, the repetition time and the echo time (50). T1-weighted images emphasize contrast between the brain and cerebrospinal fluid (CSF), and proton-density-weighted and T2-weighted images emphasize contrast between brain and pathological processes (50) (Fig. 6B and 6C).

MRI has been found to have six inherent advantages over CT. First, MRI permits excellent visualization of superficial brain anatomy, precise localization of extra-axial empyemas (Fig. 4C), and more definitive separation of extra-axial collections from their associated intra-axial complications such as edema, cerebritis, and venous thrombosis, which are more readily visualized on MRI than on CT (31). Second, streak artifacts from the bony calvarium, which are particularly problematic on CT, are not limitations on MRI. Third, MRI is superior to CT in differentiating noninfected subdural effusions and hygromas from infected empyemas. As with other proteinaceous fluids, the T1 and T2 values of purulent collections are smaller than that of CSF. These collections are therefore mildly hyperintense to CSF on T1-weighted images and markedly hyperintense to CSF on T2-weighted images (31). Fourth, the unprecedented sensitivity of MRI to subtle changes in tissue water content is uniquely suited to the goal of early detection of the parenchymal abnormalities which can occur secondary to a subdural empyema. Fifth, MRI is more specific than CT in differentiating a subdural from an epidural empyema (31). A hypodense medial rim, representing in-

flamed, displaced dura, is seen on MRI of an epidural empyema, but not on that of a subdural empyema. Lastly, the delineation of extra-axial inflammatory disease, leptomeningeal disease, and parenchymal abnormalities is undergoing further improvements with the recent introduction of an MRI contrast agent, gadolinium diethylenetriamine pentaacetic acid (Gd-DTPA) (51).

CT and MRI play a role in the follow-up of patients with extra-axial empyemas (10,31,48). Residual or recurrent collections, which may necessitate re-exploration, are particularly prone to occur in the parafalcine or subtemporal regions. These locations are well-imaged on MRI, because of its ability to obtain direct coronal sections of the brain. Long-term follow-up CT or MRI examinations frequently demonstrate cortical atrophy adjacent to a previous extra-axial empyema.

Lumbar Puncture

Lumbar puncture is often performed in patients who are subsequently diagnosed with subdural empyema, but it is neither sensitive nor specific for this disease. It is rare to recover a causative organism in the CSF, except in infants in whom meningitis preceded the development of the subdural empyema (11,16,17,43). The CSF formula in children and adults with subdural empyema is unpredictable, as shown in Table 4. Typically the white blood cell (WBC) count is elevated; however, many series report patients with 0–5 CSF leukocytes per cubic

TABLE 4. *Cerebrospinal fluid findings in subdural empyema*

CSF parameter[a]	Number of lumbar punctures with parameter reported	Number of patients	References
<5 WBCs	84	10 (12%)	6–8, 13, 17, 19, 21–23, 25, 46, 65
6–499 WBCs	70	46 (66%)	8, 13, 17, 19, 21–23, 25, 46, 65
500–999 WBCs	70	6 (9%)	8, 13, 17, 19, 21–23, 25, 46, 65
>1,000 WBCs	70	11[b] (16%)	8, 13, 17, 19, 21–23, 25, 46, 65
>50% polymorphonuclear cells	51	35 (69%)	8, 13, 17, 19, 21–23, 25, 46, 65
Elevated protein[c]	69	57 (83%)	7, 8, 13, 19, 21–23, 25, 46, 65
Normal glucose[d]	72	66[e] (92%)	7, 8, 13, 17, 19, 21, 22, 25, 46, 65
Positive Gram's stain	34	2 (6%)	6–8, 21, 23, 65
Positive CSF culture	78	6[b] (8%)	6–8, 13, 17, 19, 21–23, 25, 65

[a] From series with more than three lumbar punctures reported.
[b] Three with preceding bacterial meningitis.
[c] Reported as "elevated" or >50 mg/100 ml.
[d] Reported as "normal" or >50 mg/100 ml.
[e] Four of six patients had decreased glucose with bacterial meningitis or preceding neurosurgery.

millimeter (13,21,22,25). The differential cell count on the CSF is highly variable: Although a polymorphonuclear pleocytosis is more common, the mononuclear cell predominates in close to 40% of cases. A normal protein concentration suggests the absence of a subdural empyema, since there is an inflammatory response by the arachnoid to the overlying subdural process. However, because the arachnoid is generally impermeable to the infectious agent, CSF Gram's stain and culture almost never demonstrate the bacterial cause of the subdural empyema and are therefore not helpful in choosing antibiotic therapy.

In addition to providing no valuable diagnostic information, lumbar puncture is a potentially dangerous procedure in patients with signs of increased intracranial pressure (52). Several deaths from cerebral herniation have been reported in patients with subdural empyema shortly after undergoing lumbar puncture (13,21,22,35). Certainly, patients with papilledema or a focal neurologic abnormality, or patients with suspected increased intracranial pressure, should not undergo a lumbar puncture.

BACTERIOLOGY

The microbiologic etiology of subdural empyema is established by Gram's stain and culture of evacuated pus from the subdural space. Unfortunately, cultures of subdural pus are sterile in about one-third of cases (21), because patients are almost always receiving antibiotics preoperatively. It has been suggested that the high number of negative cultures is also related to the lack of proper handling and culture for anaerobes (21). In one study in which sinus cultures and subdural cultures were compared, three of the four sinus isolates did not correlate with the subdural isolates (22). Blood cultures may provide additional diagnostic information in cases in which the subdural fluid is sterile (11,17,22).

The organisms cultured most often from subdural infections are aerobic and anaerobic streptococci. Staphylococci are cultured less frequently, followed by aerobic gram-negative bacilli and nonstreptococcal anaerobes (Table 5). In the majority of cases a single organism is responsible for subdural empyema. However, several series have included cases in which multiple organisms have been cultured (3,5,7,17,18,21,23).

Generally, the causative organism is predictable based upon the anatomic focus from which the infection originated (3,5,8,13,39,44,45). Otorhinogenic subdural empyemas are most often due to aerobic and anaerobic streptococci and are less often due to coagulase-positive staphylococci and other anaerobes. Infections secondary to head trauma, surgery, or an indwelling foreign device are caused by coagulase-positive and coagulase-negative staphylococci and gram-negative bacilli. Subdural empyemas originating from distant foci of infection are caused by a variety of organisms. In infants with leptomeningitis, subdural empyema is caused by the same

TABLE 5. *Microbiology of adult subdural empyema*

Organism	Incidence[a] (%)
Streptococci	
Aerobic[b]	32
Anaerobic	16
Staphylococci	
Coagulase-positive	11
Coagulase-negative	5
Aerobic gram-negative bacilli[c]	8
Other anaerobes	5
Sterile	34

[a] Over 200 evaluable cases from refs. 3–5, 7, 8, 12, 13, 17–19, and 21–23; total greater than 100% because of multiple isolates from single cases.
[b] Includes alpha-hemolytic, beta-hemolytic, and nonhemolytic.
[c] Mostly enteric bacilli.

organism responsible for the meningitis, usually *Streptococcus pneumoniae* or *Hemophilus influenzae* (17,43).

Many organisms other than those mentioned have been reported to cause subdural empyema. These include *Salmonella* species (53,54), *Campylobacter fetus* (55), *Serratia marsescens* (56), *Neisseria meningitidis* (57), *Pasteurella multocida* (58,59), *Actinomyces israelii,* and *Actinobacillus actinomycetemcomitans* (60).

TREATMENT AND OUTCOME

The clinical suspicion of subdural empyema requires the immediate institution of parenteral antibiotic therapy. Antibiotics should be chosen based on the suspected source of the infection and on the organisms known to commonly cause subdural empyema. Although no prospective comparisons of antibiotic regimens for subdural empyema have been conducted, the generally accepted empiric therapy includes at least penicillin G and chloramphenicol. If staphylococci are suspected, a beta-lactamase-stable penicillin or vancomycin (depending on the prevalence of methicillin-resistant *Staphylococcus aureus* or the likelihood of coagulase-negative staphylococci) should also be used. Although there is no consensus, some advocate irrigation of the subdural space with antibiotics (2,8,9,12,14,41). There are no data to support a specific duration of antibiotic therapy; however, most patients are treated for 3–4 weeks after drainage (17). Empiric therapy for seizure prophylaxis has been advocated (8,13,24,39), and the use of steroids and mannitol have been used successfully to decrease intracranial pressure in individual cases (5,13,20).

Although anecdotal cases have been successfully treated with antibiotics alone (61,62), surgical drainage of a subdural empyema is imperative. There is disagreement, however, as to the optimal mode of surgery. The comparative efficacy of multiple burr holes versus craniotomy is complicated by clinical factors which may contribute to outcome. Several parameters have been suggested to be important in predicting patient mortality, including age of patient (12), source of infection (12), microbiology (12), time from presentation to surgery (13), management of the primary source of infection (1), extent of spread of empyema (4), level of consciousness at presentation (1,4,7–9,12,23), and surgical technique (4,5,7–9,12,14,18,20,23). Of these, only the latter two have correlated with outcome in several studies. Table 6 compares patient mortality with level of consciousness at presentation. Those patients presenting awake and alert (grade I) have the greatest chance of survival, and those presenting unresponsive to pain (grade IV) are least likely to survive. Patients who are drowsy and disoriented (grade II) or responsive only to painful stimuli (grade III) have intermediate survival statistics. Of the survivors, decreased level of consciousness at presentation correlates with more severe neurologic sequelae (4,7,8).

Several groups have advocated craniotomy over burr hole drainage, citing increased survival in the group treated by craniotomy (4,5,7–9,12,14,18,20,23) (Table 7). The advantage of craniotomy is considered to be related to the greater ease of evacuating pus from a larger area. Few investigators, however, have considered the level of consciousness of the patients when evaluating mortality of the surgical groups. In several studies in which both the patients' level of consciousness and mode of surgery are established, it is notable that patients with grades III and IV coma were more likely to undergo burr hole drainage (5,7,18,23). In fact, Mauser et al. (4) reports a higher death rate in the craniotomy group when patients presenting with grade III and IV consciousness are considered, but lower mortality in the craniotomy group among grade I and II patients. Hence, the increased survival with craniotomy may be related, in part,

TABLE 6. *Association of level of consciousness with mortality in subdural empyema*[a]

Grade I		Grade II		Grade III		Grade IV		
Number of patients	Number of deaths	Number of patients	Number of deaths	Number of patients	Number of deaths	Number of patients	Number of deaths	Reference
20	0	18	9	0	0	5	5	1
16	1	36	5	22	6	24	10	4
0	0	5	0	7	0	2	2	7
2	0	8	0	4	1	1	1	8
7	1	22	1	0	0	13	5	9
22	2	30	10	6	1	8	6	12
1	1	4	1	0	0	2	2	23
Total: 68	5	123	26	39	8	55	31	
Percentage mortality: 7%		21%		21%		56%		

[a] Grade I, awake and alert; Grade II, drowsy and disoriented; Grade III, responsive to painful stimuli; Grade IV, unresponsive to pain.

TABLE 7. *Comparative survival rates for surgical approaches to subdural empyemas*

Burr holes			Craniotomy			
Number of patients	Number of deaths	Percentage	Number of patients	Number of deaths	Percentage	Reference
46	11	24	47	10	21	4
18	4	22	4	1	25	5
11	1	9	2	0	0	7
9	1	11	5	1	20	8
22	6	27	20	1	5	9
15	7	47	24	2	8	12
11	8	73	26	6	23	14
11	2	18	7	0	0	18
2	0	0	12	2	17	20
3	3	100	4	1	25	23
Total: 148	43	29	151	24	16	
Range:		0–100			0–25	

to its more frequent use in a patient population starting with a better prognosis.

The overall mortality of subdural empyema and the extent of neurologic sequelae reported in survivors are summarized in Table 8. The potential extent of neuro-anatomic sequelae is illustrated by necropsy studies (28). Venous sinus thrombosis is a common finding in patients with subdural empyema, since the route of infection to the subdural space is generally via these venous sinuses. Aided by the absence of valves in the venous system of the brain, thrombophlebitis may extend to the cortical and subcortical veins of the cerebrum. Thrombosis of these vessels results in venous stasis and subsequent congestion and softening of adjacent brain tissue. Brain infarction and necrosis (Fig. 7A and 7B), with or without abscess formation, may ensue. Therefore, clinical neurologic sequelae may be a consequence of brain abscess(es)

or brain infarction secondary to increased intracranial pressure or venous thrombosis. More than 10% of patients with subdural empyema develop venous sinus thrombosis or brain abscess (13,28,39).

SPINAL SUBDURAL EMPYEMA

Spinal subdural empyema is a rare condition, with fewer than 20 cases reported in the literature. Signs and symptoms include fever, back pain, and subsequent signs of spinal cord compression. It can be distinguished from spinal epidural abscess by the absence of tenderness to palpation in most cases of spinal subdural empyema (63,64). Therefore, the clinical presentation may be difficult to differentiate from acute transverse myelitis. Spinal subdural empyema arises as a result of hematoge-

TABLE 8. *Mortality and neurologic sequelae of subdural empyema*

Total cases	Mortality (%)	Sequelae in survivors (%)			Reference
		Severe[a]	Mild/moderate[b]	Seizures	
47	32	—	—	—	1
102	26	18	18	29	4
23	17	5	11	37	5
14	14	—	—	—	7
15	15	15	31	46	8
42	17	—	—	—	9
49	12	—	—	—	10
22	1	—	—	—	11
66	29	—	—	—	12
17	35	—	—	—	13
37	40	—	—	—	14
37	34	16	32	—	15
17	41	0	33	11	17
22	14	25	48	8	18
14	14	8	42	37	20
89	27	0	23	34	24
23	22	—	—	—	25

[a] Disabling hemiparesis or aphasia.
[b] Sequelae not inhibiting activity.

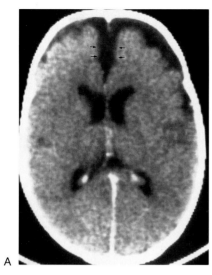

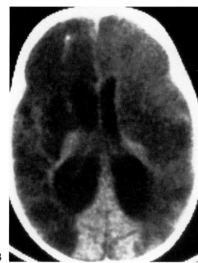

FIG. 7. Two-year-old child with *Hemophilus influenzae* meningitis. **A:** Contrast CT demonstrating extra-axial collections over both frontal convexities and in the anterior aspect of the interhemispheric fissure (*arrows*). Note the similarity of these collections to the CSF in the ventricular system, making it difficult to distinguish them from sterile effusions and prominent subarachnoid spaces. Spinal tap revealed purulent meningitis. **B:** Follow-up CT 2 months later, demonstrating extensive zones of infarction and hydrocephalus.

nous spread of infection to the spinal subdural space, with *Staphylococcus aureus* being the most common etiologic agent (63). Diagnosis is best accomplished by metrizamide spinal CT. Treatment consists of empiric antibiotic therapy initially directed against *Staphylococcus aureus,* streptococci, and gram-negative enteric bacilli, in association with laminectomy for drainage of the empyema. Antibiotics can then be adjusted based on specific culture results for a duration of 2–4 weeks.

REFERENCES

1. Bradley PJ, Shaw MDM. Subdural empyema management of the primary source. *Br J Clin Med* 1984;38:85–88.
2. Joubert MJ, Stephanov S. Computed tomography and surgical treatment in intracranial suppuration. *J Neurosurg* 1977;47:73–78.
3. Harris LF, Haws FP, Triplett JN, Maccubbin DA. Subdural empyema and epidural abscess: recent experience in a community hospital. *South Med J* 1987;80:1254–1258.
4. Mauser HW, Van Houwelingen HC, Tulleken CA. Factors affecting the outcome in subdural empyema. *J Neurol Neurosurg Psychiatry* 1987;50:1136–1141.
5. Miller ES, Dias PS, Uttley D. Management of subdural empyema: a series of 24 cases. *J Neurol Neurosurg Psychiatry* 1987;50:1415–1418.
6. Weisberg L. Subdural empyema: clinical and computed tomographic correlations. *Arch Neurol* 1986;43:497–500.
7. Hodges J, Anslow P, Gillett G. Subdural empyema—continuing diagnostic problem in the CT scan era. *Q J Med* 1986;59:387–393.
8. Khan M, Griebel R. Subdural empyema: a retrospective study of 15 patients. *Can J Surg* 1984;27:283–288.
9. Hockley AD, Williams B. Surgical management of subdural empyema. *Child's Brain* 1983;10:294–300.
10. Zimmerman RD, Leeds NE, Danziger A. Subdural empyema: CT findings. *Radiology* 1984;150:417–422.
11. Smith HP, Hendrick EB. Subdural empyema and epidural abscess in children. *J Neurosurg* 1983;58:392–397.
12. Bannister G, Williams B, Smith S. Treatment of subdural empyema. *J Neurosurg* 1981;55:82–88.
13. Kaufman DM, Miller MM, Steigbigel NH. Subdural empyema: analysis of 17 recent cases and review of the literature. *Medicine* 1975;54:485–498.
14. Le Beau J, Creissard P, Harispe L, Redondo A. Surgical treatment of brain abscess and subdural empyema. *J Neurosurg* 1973;38:198–203.
15. Bhandari YS, Sarkari NBS. Subdural empyema: a review of 37 cases. *J Neurosurg* 1970;32:35–39.
16. Curless RG. Subdural empyema in infant meningitis: diagnosis, therapy, and prognosis. *Childs Nerv Syst* 1985;1:211–214.
17. Farmer TW, Wise GR. Subdural empyema in infants, children and adults. *Neurology* 1973;23:254–261.
18. Feuerman T, Wackym PA, Gade GF, Dubrow T. Craniotomy improves outcome in subdural empyema. *Surg Neurol* 1989;32:105–110.
19. Luken MG, Whelan MA. Recent diagnostic experience with subdural empyema. *J Neurosurg* 1980;52:764–771.
20. Borzone M, Capuzzo T, Rivano C, Tortori-Donati P. Subdural empyema: fourteen cases surgically treated. *Surg Neurol* 1980;13:449–452.
21. Yoshikawa TT, Chow AW, Guze LB. Role of anaerobic bacteria in subdural empyema: report of four cases and review of 327 cases from the English literature. *Am J Med* 1975;58:99–104.
22. Kaufman DM, Litman N, Miller MM. Sinusitis: induced subdural empyema. *Neurology* 1983;33:123–132.
23. Morgan DW, Williams B. Posterior fossa subdural empyema. *Brain* 1985;108:983–992.
24. Cowie R, Williams B. Late seizures and morbidity after subdural empyema. *J Neurosurg* 1983;58:569–573.
25. Renaudin JW, Frazee J. Subdural empyema—importance of early diagnosis. *Neurosurgery* 1980;7:447–479.
26. Knudsen LL, Voldby B, Stagaard M. Computed tomographic myelography in spinal subdural empyema. *Neuroradiology* 1987;29:99.
27. Kubik CS, Adams RD. Subdural empyema. *Brain* 1943;66:18–42.
28. Courville CB. Subdural empyema secondary to purulent frontal sinusitis. *Arch Otolaryngol* 1944;39:211–230.
29. Kim KS, Weinberg PE, Magidson M. Angiographic features of subdural empyema. *Radiology* 1976;118:621–625.
30. Kaufman DM, Leeds NE. Computed tomography (CT) in the diagnosis of intracranial abscesses. *Neurology* 1977;27:1069–1073.
31. Weingarten K, Zimmerman RD, Becker RD, Heier LA, Haimes AB, Deck MDF. Subdural and epidural empyemas: MR imaging. *Am J Neuroradiol* 1987;10:81–87.
32. Warwick R, Williams PL, eds. *Gray's anatomy,* 35th ed. Philadelphia: WB Saunders, 1973.
33. Clemente CD. *Anatomy: a regional atlas of the human body,* 2nd ed. Baltimore: Urban & Schwarzenberg, 1981.

34. Weinman D, Samarasinghe HHR. Subdural empyema. *Aust NZ J Surg* 1972;41:324–330.
35. van Alphen HAM, Dreissen JJR. Brain abscess and subdural empyema: factors influencing mortality and results of various surgical techniques. *J Neurol Neurosurg Psychiatry* 1976;39:481–490.
36. Van Dellen JR, Boles DM, Van Der Heever CM. Interhemispheral subdural empyema. *S Afr Med J* 1977;52:266–269.
37. Stephanov S, Joubert MJ, Welchman JM. Combined convexity and parafalx subdural empyema. *Surg Neurol* 1979;11:147–151.
38. Holtzman RNN, Tepperberg J, Schwartz O. Parasagittal subdural empyema: a case report with computerized tomographic scan documentation. *Mt Sinai J Med* 1980;47:62–67.
39. Rosenbaum GS, Cunha BA. Subdural empyema complicating frontal and ethmoid sinusitis. *Heart Lung* 1989;18:199–202.
40. Layon J, McCulley D. Subdural empyema and Group C *Streptococcus. South Med J* 1985;78:64–66.
41. Osgood CP, Dujovny M, Holm E, Postic B. Delayed post-traumatic subdural empyema. *J Trauma* 1975;15:916–921.
42. Hadj-Djilani M, Calliauw L. A contribution to the rapid diagnosis of subdural empyema. *Acta Neurochir* 1982;61:187–199.
43. Jacobson PL, Farmer TW. Subdural empyema complicating meningitis in infants: improved prognosis. *Neurology* 1981;31:190–193.
44. Hardy TL, Minor F, Phinney ES. Chronic subdural empyema. *Surg Neurol* 1981;16:154–156.
45. Post EM, Modesti LM. "Subacute" postoperative subdural empyema. *J Neurosurg* 1981;55:761–765.
46. Sadhu VK, Handel SF, Pinto RS, Glass TF. Neuroradiologic diagnosis of subdural empyema and CT limitations. *Am J Neuroradiol* 1980;1:39–44.
47. List CF. Diagnosis and treatment of acute subdural empyema. *Neurology* 1955;5:663–670.
48. Zimmerman RD, Weingarten K. Evaluation of intracranial inflammatory disease by CT and MRI. In: Theodore WH, eds. *Clinical neuroimaging.* New York: Alan R Liss, 1988;75–100.
49. Sze G, Zimmerman RD. The magnetic resonance imaging of infections and inflammatory diseases. *Radiol Clin North Am* 1988;26:839–860.
50. Wehrli FW. Principles of magnetic resonance imaging. In: Stark DD, Bradley WG, eds. *Magnetic resonance imaging.* St. Louis: CV Mosby, 1988;3–23.
51. Bydder GM. Clinical applicability of gadolinium-DTPA. In: Stark DD, Bradley WG, eds. *Magnetic resonance imaging.* St. Louis: CV Mosby, 1988;182–200.
52. Duffy GP. Lumbar puncture in the presence of raised intracranial pressure. *Br Med J* 1969;1:407–409.
53. Okudera H, Yasutuki T, Kyoshima K. Bilateral subdural empyema due to *Salmonella enteritidis* in an infant. *Child's Nerv Syst* 1989;5:45–46.
54. Grosinger L, Lauter CB. *Salmonella* subdural empyema in a patient with brain metastasis. *Rev Infect Dis* 1986;8:830–831.
55. Mendelson MH, Nicholas P, Malowany M, Lewin S. Subdural empyema caused by *Campylobacter fetus* ssp. *Fetus J Infect Dis* 1986;153:1183–1184.
56. Safani MM, Ehrensaft DV. Successful treatment of subdural empyema due to *Serratia marcescens. Drug Intell Clin Pharm* 1982;16:777–779.
57. Edwards MS, Baker CJ. Subdural empyema: an unusual complication of meningococcal meningitis. *South Med J* 1982;75:68–69.
58. Stern J, Bernstein CA, Whelan MA, Neu HC. *Pasteurella multocida* subdural empyema. *J Neurosurg* 1981;54:550–552.
59. Khan MI, Chan R. *Pasteurella multocida* subdural empyema: a case report. *Can J Neurol Sci* 1981;8:163–165.
60. Louie JA, Kusske JA, Rush JL, Pribram HW. Actinomycotic subdural empyema: case report. *J Neurosurg* 1979;51:852–855.
61. Mauser HW, Ravijst RAP, Elderson A, Van Gijn J, Tulleken CAF. Nonsurgical treatment of subdural empyema: case report. *J Neurosurg* 1985;63:128–130.
62. Rosazza A, de Tribolet N, Deonna T. Nonsurgical treatment of interhemispheric subdural empyemas. *Helv Paediatr Acta* 1979;34:577–581.
63. Dacey RG, Winn R, Jane JA, Butler AB. Spinal subdural empyema: report of two cases. *Neurosurgery* 1978;3:400–403.
64. Theodotou B, Woosley RE, Whaley RA. Spinal subdural empyema: diagnosis by spinal computed tomography. *Surg Neurol* 1984;21:610–612.
65. Farkas AG, Marks JC. Subdural empyema: an important diagnosis not to miss. *Br Med J* 1986;293:118–119.
66. Netter FH. *Atlas of human anatomy.* Basel: Ciba–Geigy, 1989;96.

Infections of the Central Nervous System,
edited by W. M. Scheld, R. J. Whitley, and
D. T. Durack, Raven Press, Ltd., New York © 1991.

CHAPTER 21

Epidural Abscess

Bruce G. Gellin, Karen Weingarten, Francis W. Gamache, Jr.,
and Barry J. Hartman

An epidural abscess, first described by Morgagni (1) in the 18th century, is a suppurative infection in the epidural space. This space surrounds both the spinal cord and brain, being located between the dura and the overlying bone. Despite similar embryonic origins, the configuration of the epidural space below the foramen magnum differs from that of the intracranial epidural space. For this reason, infection of these spaces results in two distinct clinical entities—spinal and intracranial epidural abscesses.

Epidural abscesses are both medical and surgical emergencies, requiring prompt and accurate diagnosis and treatment to prevent irreversible spinal cord dysfunction, paralysis, and death (2–9). The introduction of antibiotics in the middle of this century had a significant impact on the outcome of these infections, which had been universally progressive and often fatal (10,11). Nevertheless, despite increasingly accurate diagnostic techniques and effective therapy, morbidity and mortality remain excessive, primarily due to delays in diagnosis (6,12,13).

SPINAL EPIDURAL ABSCESS

Epidemiology

Spinal epidural infections are uncommon. Incidence rates of spinal epidural abscesses have not been calculated from population-based data but are estimated from

B. G. Gellin and B. J. Hartman: Department of Medicine, Division of Infectious Diseases, Cornell University Medical College, New York, New York 10021.
K. Weingarten: Department of Radiology, Division of Neuroradiology, Cornell University Medical College, New York, New York 10021.
F. W. Gamache, Jr.: Department of Surgery, Cornell University Medical College, New York, New York 10021.

case series which have documented 0.2–1.2 cases per 10,000 admissions to large tertiary-care centers (2,14). A more recent case series, however, noted a significantly higher incidence rate since the mid-1970s—approximately 2.8 cases per 10,000 admissions (3).

Over the half-century that these case series have been compiled, no seasonal trends have been observed and the male-to-female ratio has remained about 1:1 (2–4,11,13,15). A broad age range of patients with spinal epidural abscess has been reported—from 3 months old (16) to 81 years old (3,17). However, over the past 50 years the average age of patients diagnosed with spinal epidural abscesses has increased from 37 years old (13) to 57 years old (3). In contrast, intravenous drug users who develop spinal epidural abscesses tend to be younger, with the average age being approximately 35 years old (17,18).

Pathogenesis and Pathophysiology

Below the foramen magnum the epidural space extends the length of the spine and should be considered as being composed of two compartments: (i) a true space posterior and lateral to the spinal cord, containing a cushioning layer of fat embedded with penetrating arteries and an extensive venous plexus, and (ii) a potential anterior space where the dura adheres to the posterior surface of the vertebral body (19,20) (Fig. 1). The epidural space is circumferential around the spinal cord distal to the second sacral segment, the terminal point of attachment anteriorly.

Given these anatomic considerations, it is not surprising that spinal epidural abscesses are located posteriorly in over 70% of cases (2,14,21). However, a recent series has reported that nearly half of the abscesses were located anteriorly (3). This was attributed to the high percentage of lumbar abscesses included in that series; the

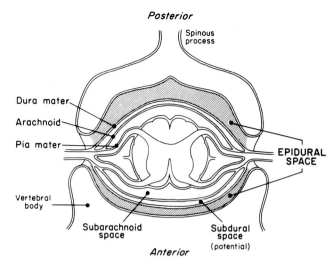

FIG. 1. Transverse section of a vertebral body showing the locations of the epidural and subdural spaces. Reprinted by permission of the New England Journal of Medicine 1975:293;467.

spinal epidural space enlarges anteriorly distal to L1 (15).

In addition to the boundary imposed by the anterior attachment to the vertebral canal, the dimensions of the epidural space vary from segment to segment. In the cervical region where the epidural space is smallest (0.1 cm) and is nearly obliterated by the spinal cord (22), epidural abscesses occur less frequently than thoracic or lumbar spinal epidural abscesses (23–25). Spinal epidural abscesses in the sacral region are much less common (26) (Table 1). While the rich circulation assures ample blood supply to the spinal cord, it also may act as a conduit along which infection may spread. Infection tracking along these pathways is the likely explanation for the longitudinal extension of spinal epidural abscesses which usually affect multiple adjacent spinal segments (27). On average, three to six spinal cord segments are involved (2,3); however, an infection of the entire length of the spinal epidural space has been reported (2).

Infection may be introduced into the epidural space by direct extension from a contiguous infection or by hematogenous or lymphatic seeding from a remote site (Table 2). Contiguous infections include: vertebral os-

TABLE 1. Location of spinal epidural abscesses[a]

Location	Number of patients
Cervical	20 (14%)
Thoracic	71 (51%)
Lumbar	48 (35%)
Total:	139 (100%)
Anterior	28 (21%)
Posterior	105 (79%)
Total:	133 (100%)

[a] Mean number of involved segments = 3.8 (range: 1–26). Adapted from Table 4 in ref. 3, with permission.

TABLE 2. Source of infection of spinal epidural abscesses[a]

Source	Number of patients
Skin and soft tissue	28 (21%)
Bone or joint	18 (13%)
Spinal surgery or procedures	14 (10%)
Abdomen	5 (4%)
Upper respiratory tract	8 (6%)
Urinary tract	3 (2%)
Intravenous drug abuse	6 (4%)
No source identified	54 (40%)
Total:	136 (100%)

[a] Adapted from Table 2 in ref. 3, with permission.

teomyelitis (24,27–29); retropharyngeal, perinephric, or psoas abscesses (30–32); decubitus ulcers (2); and persistent dermal sinus tracts (33). Local invasion from superficial infections can also occur following either (a) penetrating injuries, including prior surgery (34,35), or (b) epidural catheterization, including lumbar puncture (26,36–41). Metastatic seeding may result from any bacteremic infection. Skin and soft tissue infections are identified as the source in 20–40% of cases (2,3,13,42), but sources have also included endocarditis (43–46) respiratory tract infection (2,3,47), urinary tract infection (3), dental abscesses (2,13), and deep abdominal infection (17,48,49). However, a primary source of infection is not apparent in up to 40% of cases (2,3).

A history of trauma, either recent or remote, is elicited from 15–35% of patients with epidural abscess (2,50,51). This observation has led to the speculation that a small hematoma or area of damaged tissue may provide a fertile area for subsequent hematogenous seeding (13). Whether antecedent trauma is indeed a true risk factor for the subsequent development of a spinal epidural abscess has not been systematically examined.

Underlying medical conditions that have been associated with spinal epidural abscesses include degenerative joint disease (2,3,52), diabetes (2,9,53,54), chronic granulomatous disease (55), cirrhosis (56), malignancy (2), renal failure (57), alcoholism (3,49), and intravenous drug abuse (2,3,9,18). The few cases of epidural abscess which have been reported in acquired immunodeficiency syndrome (AIDS) patients have been in intravenous drug abusers with episodes of bacteremia (18). Although a recent study commented that steroid use was a poor prognostic factor (3), there is no evidence that steroids, per se, predispose to or aggravate spinal epidural abscess formation. Rather, steroids may reflect underlying medical conditions such as arthritis, chronic obstructive pulmonary disease (COPD), or malignancy which may be associated with spinal deformities, trauma, or higher rates of bacteremia.

Compared with the damage produced by spinal tumors and cysts, the damage produced by bacterial spinal epidural abscesses is often out of proportion to the size of the inflammatory mass (2,13,58). This important feature may be due to many factors, including: thrombosis and thrombophlebitis of veins draining the spinal cord with resultant edema and venous infarction (2,11,13); compression of the arterial supply to adjacent cord segments with local ischemia and infarction; focal areas of vasculitis induced by the adjacent inflammatory mass; or bacterial exotoxin production, especially by *Staphylococcus aureus*. Because *Staphylococcus aureus* is the predominant pathogen of spinal epidural abscesses, this hypothesis may be specific to staphylococcal infections rather than to bacterial epidural abscesses in general.

A rabbit model of a spinal epidural abscess has demonstrated that the damage to the spinal cord is more consistent with mechanical compression than with ischemia or infarction (59). This model, using a clinical isolate of *Staphylococcus aureus*, also demonstrated many of the clinical, laboratory, and pathological features seen in spinal epidural abscess in man: concurrent osteomyelitis; toxic softening of the cord; histopathologic changes (vacuolization and liquefaction, myelin degeneration, and axonal swelling); and similar cerebrospinal fluid (CSF) chemistries and cell counts (13,50,59). The model did not, however, specifically address the question of the excessive damage to the cord relative to the size of the infectious mass, leaving unanswered the possible contribution of bacterial toxin to the pathological picture.

Microbiology (Table 3)

In all series, *Staphylococcus aureus* is the most common etiologic agent of spinal epidural abscess in children and adults, being responsible for 52–95% of bacterial abscesses (2,3,6,16,17,60). However, more recent surveys have documented an increasing incidence of (a) gram-negative aerobic bacilli (especially *Escherichia coli* and *Pseudomonas* species) in 9–37% (2,44), (b) aerobic streptococci (alpha- and beta-hemolytic) in 8–15% (61), and (c) anaerobes in 7% (2,3). The increasing prevalence of

TABLE 3. *Bacteriology of spinal epidural abscesses*

Types of culture	Number of patients/total
Positive abscess cultures	96/107 (90%)
Positive blood cultures	36/60 (60%)
Positive CSF cultures	15/88 (17%)

Organism	Number of patients
Staphylococcus aureus	103 (62%)
Staphylococcus epidermidis	4 (2%)
Aerobic streptococci	14 (8%)
Aerobic gram-negative bacilli	30 (18%)
Anaerobes	3 (2%)
Others	2 (1%)
Unknown	10 (6%)
Total:	166 (100%)

ª Adapted from Table 3 in ref. 3, with permission.

gram-negative organisms may parallel the changing spectrum of bacterial infections (62,63). *Pseudomonas aeruginosa* accounted for 4% of known bacterial isolates and up to 30% of the gram-negative aerobic isolates (2,3,17,18,34,64). Multiple organisms may be found in 10% of cases (2). In a recent series, *Mycobacterium tuberculosis* accounted for 25% of all spinal epidural abscesses (17,65–70). Other, less commonly reported bacteria include: *Proteus* species (28), *Salmonella* (71–73), *Staphylococcus epidermidis* (2), *Streptococcus pneumoniae* (13,45,74), *Streptococcus sanguis* (34), *Streptococcus milleri* (61), *Enterococcus* sp. (17,25), *Actinomyces israelii* (75–78), *Serratia marcescens* (17), *Enterobacter cloacae* (17), *Enterobacter aerogenes* (3), *Morganella morganii* (3), *Listeria monocytogenes* (56), *Brucella* species (79,80), *Haemophilus aphrophilus* (81), *Actinobacillus actinomycetemcomitans* (46), *Nocardia* (82–84), *Bacillus* species (3), and anaerobic bacteria, including *Fusobacterium* species (85,86) and *Bacteroides* species (34).

Fungal etiologies of spinal epidural abscesses (55,87,88) include: blastomycosis (75), coccidiodomycosis (89), *Cryptococcus neoformans* (90,91), mucormycosis (92,93), *Aspergillus* species (94–100), and *Pseudoallescheria boydii* (101). Parasitic causes of epidural abscess have also been reported, including *Echinococcus* (102) and guinea worm (103).

Clinical Manifestations

The initial signs and symptoms of a spinal epidural abscess may be subtle. Characteristically, they include fever, back pain, and malaise (2,3,13). Early signs and symptoms may be ascribed to the "flu," and a short course of oral antibiotics may provide temporary relief until symptoms recur and progress. The duration of symptoms is variable; they may be present for just a few days or up to several months before the patient presents for evaluation (2,3,50).

The four-stage clinical progression of a spinal epidural abscess was first described by Rankin and Flothow (104) almost 50 years ago. In addition to fever and malaise, the first localizing symptoms are backache and focal vertebral pain and tenderness on examination. This is followed by "root pain" manifested by radiculopathy and/or parasthesias which often may be described as "electric shocks." Spinal cord dysfunction, the third stage, is characterized by motor and sensory deficits or by bladder or bowel dysfunction. This is followed by the final stage of complete paralysis (Table 4).

Whereas symptoms of backache may be present for weeks to months, back pain usually progresses to root pain in 3–4 days followed 4–5 days later with the onset of early signs of spinal cord dysfunction. Although neurological deficits at this stage are usually reversible, rapid surgical intervention may be crucial because progression

TABLE 4. *Spinal epidural abscess: clinical progression*

1. Back pain and tenderness
2. Nerve root pain—radiculopathy
   Deep tendon reflex changes
3. Motor paresis
   Sensory deficits
4. Paralysis

from spinal cord dysfunction to complete paralysis may occur in less than 2 hr regardless of the chronicity of the process up to this point (58).

Specific neurological signs will depend on the level of spinal cord involvement and may also influence the differential diagnosis at the time of presentation (48,53,64,65,105–108).

The presentation of a spinal epidural abscess has been described as "acute" (symptoms persisting for less than 2 weeks at the time of presentation) or "chronic" (symptoms for more than 2 weeks at the time of presentation) (2,3). The rate of progression of the initial stages often may suggest the route of infection: Acute presentations represent hematogenous seeding and rapid expansion of the inflammatory mass, whereas chronic presentations are more likely the result of a gradually expanding contiguous infection.

Patients with acute presentations generally have higher peripheral leukocyte counts (range: 12,000–15,000) and higher temperatures when compared to those of patients with long-standing symptoms who may have only mild elevations in these two parameters (2,3,17). The erythrocyte sedimentation rate (ESR) is generally elevated (>25 mm/hr), but the range of observed ESRs does not differ significantly between these two groups (3).

CSF examination is usually consistent with a parameningeal focus of infection and is remarkable for elevated protein and increased leukocytes. The CSF leukocyte count generally does not exceed 150 white blood cells (WBCs) per cubic millimeter unless there is coexisting meningitis (2,14,44). The cells usually are mixed polymorphonuclear leukocytes and lymphocytes or are predominantly polymorphonuclear leukocytes (2,3). Extremely elevated WBC counts in the CSF may indicate that the spinal needle has entered a lumbar epidural abscess (2,3,14,17). Patients with a chronic presentation of an epidural abscess generally have a lower CSF leukocyte count (average of 20 WBCs per cubic millimeter) than do those with acute presentations (average of 100 WBCs per cubic millimeter) (2,3). Markedly elevated CSF protein (greater than 350 mg/dl) may be associated with a complete block of the spinal canal; however, up to 28% of patients with elevated CSF protein, but less than 350 mg/dl, may also have a spinal block (3). The degree of protein elevation does not usually correlate with the chronicity of the symptoms (2). CSF glucose is usually normal, except in cases of accompanying meningitis when it may be low (2).

Similar to other parameningeal infections, CSF Gram's stains rarely demonstrate organisms and spinal fluid cultures are negative in 75–80% of cases except when there is concomitant meningitis (3,13,17). Blood cultures may be positive in 60–70% of cases (2,3). When the abscess is due to *Staphylococcus aureus*, blood cultures will be positive in up to 95% of the cases (3). Overall, intraoperative cultures of the abscess have the highest chance of yielding a microbiologic diagnosis, being positive in 54–89% of all cases (2,3) (Table 3). However, when a patient has been receiving antibiotics for more than 1 week prior to culture, diagnostic cultures are unlikely (3).

Differential Diagnosis

Signs of fever and back pain should raise suspicion of a spinal epidural abscess, especially when spinal tenderness or peripheral neurological abnormalities are demonstrated on physical exam. However, these signs and symptoms may not always be present and clearly lack specificity for this diagnosis.

Reviewers have repeatedly noted that the diagnosis of spinal epidural abscess is not included in the differential diagnosis on admission to the hospital in 75–80% of cases (2,3,13). Whereas the initial diagnosis may include "spinal problems" in two-thirds of the cases, the signs and symptoms of spinal epidural abscess are usually attributed to musculoskeletal pain from a recent strain or minor trauma (2,3,13), degenerative or inflammatory disk disease (2,14,17,52,107), or vertebral osteomyelitis, including tuberculosis of the spine (2,3,24,29,67,69, 109,110). Spinal epidural abscesses have also been initially misdiagnosed as meningitis (2,13), herpes zoster (2,3), infectious polyneuritis (2,3,13,15), transverse myelitis (31,111), acute abdomen [including cholecystitis, pyelonephritis (2,48), and pancreatitis (14)], viral syndrome (2,3), fibrositis (15), myocardial infarction (2), benign prostatic hypertrophy (3), drug fever (3), cerebrovascular accident (3,15), and hysteria (2,13), with the latter occurring particularly in patients experiencing the "electric shock" root pains or in patients with alcohol- or drug-dependency disorders (9,18). In the human immunodeficiency virus (HIV)-infected patient the clinical presentation of spinal epidural abscess may be attributed to HIV-related peripheral neuropathy or associated opportunistic infections such as cytomegalovirus (CMV), herpes zoster, or herpes simplex (112). In patients with a history of cancer, the signs and symptoms may initially be attributed to the development of metastatic disease involving the spine (3). Lymphoma may involve the epidural space in up to 5% of cases (113), and other tumors which may directly involve the epidural space include prostate, lung, kidney, and gastrointestinal tract malignancies (14). In addition to neoplasms, disorders which have been mistaken for, or which have caused a delay in the diagnosis of, spinal epidural abscess also include lipomatosis (114) and pregnancy (2,106).

Approach to Diagnosis

The radiologic evaluation of spinal epidural infection frequently involves a multimodality approach, utilizing plain films, computerized tomography (CT), myelography, postmyelography CT, and magnetic resonance imaging (MRI) (115). The specific radiographic examinations performed, and the order in which they are performed, should be tailored to each individual clinical situation.

Plain films of the spine will not directly visualize the spinal epidural abscess but may demonstrate certain findings which can be an indication of the presence of infection in the spinal canal (116,117). These findings include (a) intervertebral disk space narrowing in diskitis and (b) loss of definition or destruction of both the inferior cortical margin of one vertebral body and the superior cortical margin of the contiguous vertebral body in osteomyelitis (Fig. 2A). Rarefaction and loss of bony trabeculae can also be seen. In advanced or rapidly progressive cases, vertebral body collapse (or dissolution) and gibbus formation may be seen on plain films. In general, osteomyelitis most commonly occurs in the lumbar spine, and the body of the vertebrae are affected more frequently than the posterior elements. Helpful ancillary plain film findings include (a) mass effect or displacement of the larynx in a retropharyngeal abscess and (b) scoliosis and displacement of bowel loops in a lumbar paraspinal abscess. Normal plain films do not exclude the presence of a spinal epidural abscess, particularly in acute presentations. In this setting, additional radiographic examinations are almost always needed for further evaluation.

Myelography, which will not directly visualize a spinal epidural abscess, will demonstrate the associated mass effect on the spinal cord, thecal sac, or nerve roots (22,116). A spinal epidural abscess can result in a complete extradural obstructive block to the flow of water-soluble contrast (Fig. 3A, and 3B). However, in patients with a prominent ventral epidural space in the lower lumbar spine due to abundant epidural fat, an epidural abscess may not be detected on myelography if it causes indentation or obliteration of the epidural fat without indenting the opacified thecal sac.

A spinal epidural abscess is seen on noncontrast CT as an isodense or hypodense (compared to adjacent musculature) soft tissue mass (118). Associated findings include: (a) obliteration of the epidural fat surrounding the thecal sac or nerve roots and (b) a mass effect on these neural elements (119). A variable-sized paravertebral soft tissue component is frequently seen. Narrowing of an intervertebral disk or destruction of a vertebral body is observed in the setting of diskitis or osteomyelitis, respectively, though disk space narrowing may be difficult to recognize on CT without reformatted images in the sagittal plane. Infrequently, gas within bone or within

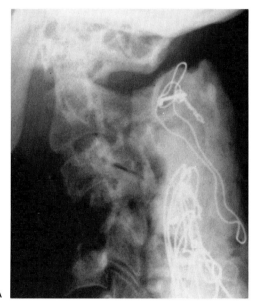 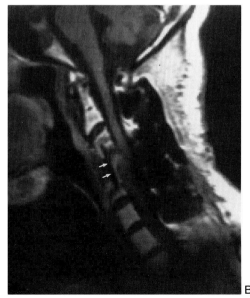

A   B

FIG. 2. Status of a 62-year-old female following surgery and radiation therapy to the cervical spine for metastatic disease 1 year ago. She presents now with diskitis, osteomyelitis, and epidural abscess at C5–C6. **A:** Plain film of the cervical spine demonstrates extensive postoperative changes with almost complete resection of the C4 and C5 vertebral bodies. **B:** Sagittal T1-weighted MRI scan obtained at the same time as part A demonstrates a soft tissue mass (*arrows*) posterior to the resected vertebrae, causing a severe degree of cord compression. Surgery revealed osteomyelitis and an epidural abscess secondary to *Staphylococcus aureus*.

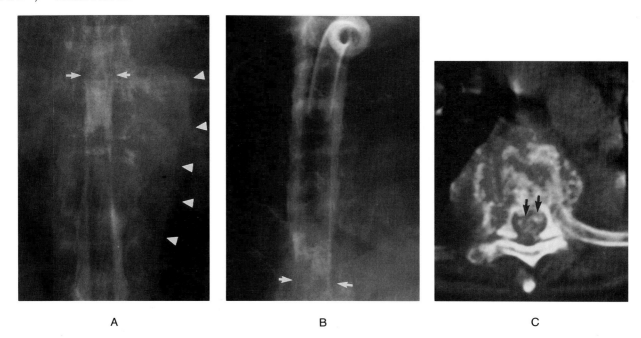

A   B   C

FIG. 3. A 45-year-old female with methicillin-resistant *Staphylococcus aureus* epidural abscess. **A:** Frontal myelography film performed via lumbar puncture reveals an epidural block to the cephalad flow of contrast in the midthoracic spine (*arrows*) Note the paraspinal soft tissue mass (*arrowheads*). **B:** Frontal myelography film performed via cervical puncture demonstrates an epidural block to the caudad flow of contrast in the midthoracic spine (*arrows*). **C:** Postmyelography CT scan demonstrates extensive osseous destruction of T7 with a large epidural soft tissue mass completely obliterating the outline of the thoracic cord (*arrows*).

intervertebral disk, or an intraspinal or paraspinal abscess, is seen on CT. The presence of an epidural mass centered on an intervertebral disk is a helpful CT characteristic indicating an infectious, rather than a neoplastic, etiology of the lesion (120). However, noncontrast CT can be limited by low soft-tissue contrast resolution. In these cases, intrathecal administration of contrast followed by CT may be needed (Fig. 3C). However, this invasive procedure carries with it the inherent risk of iatrogenic spread of infection.

Both CT and MRI can directly visualize an epidural inflammatory mass (121). As is true in the neuroimaging of many diseases of the brain and spinal canal, MRI is proving to be superior to CT for evaluation of patients with epidural abscesses. MRI obviates the need for myelography and CT in many cases (119,121). The advantages of MRI include: its ability to image long segments of the spinal canal in multiple planes, thereby enabling precise delineation of all loculations of inflammatory tissue; its ability to image all compartments around the spinal canal into which an inflammatory process might extend; its ability to directly visualize the neural elements with high-contrast resolution without the need for intrathecal contrast; and its noninvasiveness, which is a particular advantage over myelography because of the desire to avoid inadvertent puncture of the abscess or iatrogenic spread of infection from the epidural to the subarachnoid space following introduction of a needle

into the spinal canal. Furthermore, with MRI, patient follow-up is facilitated and assessment of response to therapy is readily performed. In a recent study, MRI was found to be more sensitive than plain films or CT, and at least as accurate and as sensitive as nuclear medicine studies, in the diagnosis of diskitis and osteomyelitis (122). The ability of MRI to distinguish active inflammatory tissue from chronic granulation tissue is expected to be further enhanced with the recent introduction of a paramagnetic MRI contrast agent, gadolinium diethylenetriamine pentaacetic acid (Gd-DTPA). MRI demonstrates epidural inflammatory disease to be a soft tissue mass which, compared to the spinal cord, is isointense on T1-weighted images (Fig. 2B) and hyperintense on T2-weighted images (122,123). The extradural location of disease and the associated mass effect on the thecal sac, spinal cord, or cauda equina are generally readily appreciated on MRI, as is the extradural location of disease and the associated mass effect on the thecal sac. The presence of concomitant paraspinal abscesses is easily identified (123). In the presence of diskitis, a characteristic finding on MRI is abnormal high signal intensity in the disk on T2-weighted images (122). This is in contradistinction to degenerative disk disease, which demonstrates low signal intensity. Vertebral osteomyelitis is seen as low signal intensity on T1-weighted images in the involved marrow cavity, with high signal intensity on T2-weighted images. These osseous changes are usually observed in conjunction with inflammatory disease of the subjacent intervertebral disk as described above.

Treatment (Table 5)

Therapy for spinal epidural abscess consists of antibiotics to eradicate the microbial component combined with surgery to eliminate the mechanical component that may lead to neurological deficits. Antibiotics are often selected empirically to cover those organisms that are most likely involved. Because *Staphylococcus aureus* is the most common pathogen, spinal epidural abscesses must always be treated with either (a) an antistaphylococcal penicillin, (b) a cephalosporin, or (c) vancomycin. If the infection has followed a neurosurgical procedure, an antistaphylococcal penicillin should be combined with a broad-spectrum gram-negative bacillary agent such as a third-generation cephalosporin with antipseu-

domonal activity or an aminoglycoside. In institutions where methicillin-resistant *Staphylococcus aureus* (MRSA) is a frequent nosocomial pathogen, vancomycin should be used as the antistaphylococcal agent in any antibiotic regimen. Once a specific organism(s) has been isolated, the antibiotic regimen may be modified based on the antibiotic sensitivity pattern of the pathogen.

The duration of antibiotic treatment is usually 3–4 weeks. If osteomyelitis accompanies the epidural abscess, 6–8 weeks of antibiotic treatment is recommended (2).

In the absence of frank neurologic dysfunction, the goals of surgery are to decompress the expanding mass by the removal of purulent material and inflammatory granulation tissue and to establish a microbiologic diagnosis which will guide antibiotic therapy. In the presence of neurologic dysfunction, urgent laminectomy for decompression, drainage, and diagnosis is imperative. A delay in the diagnosis of epidural abscess following the

TABLE 5. *Etiology, bacteriology, and antibiotic therapy of spinal epidural abscesses*

Etiology	Bacteriology	Empiric antibiotic therapy
Hematogenous spread	*Staphylococcus aureus* Aerobic and anaerobic streptococci	Penicillinase-resistant penicillin or First-generation cephalosporin or Vancomycin
	+ Gram-negative bacilli	+ Third-generation cephalosporin or Aminoglycoside
Penetrating injuries	*Staphylococcus aureus*	Penicillinase-reistant penicillin or First-generation cephalosporin or Vancomycin
	+ Gram-negative bacilli	+ Third-generation cephalosporin or Aminoglycoside
Local extension from adjacent infection (paraspinal abscess, ducubitus ulcer)	*Staphylococcus aureus*	Penicillinase-resistant penicillin or First-generation cephalosporin or Vancomycin
	+ Gram-negative bacilli	+ Third generation cephalosporin or Aminoglycoside
	± Anaerobes	± Metronidazole or clindamycin
Neurosurgical (lumbar puncture)	*Staphylococcus aureus*	Penicillinase-resistant penicillin or First-generation cephalosporin or Vancomycin
	+ Gram-negative bacilli	+ Third-generation cephalosporin or Aminoglycoside

development of neurologic dysfunction appears to be largely responsible for the poor outcome associated with spinal epidural abscess (13,70,124–126). Patients with subacute or chronic clinical symptoms are more likely to have inflammatory tissue rather than frank pus. In these instances, stains of the inflammatory tissue for bacteria, mycobacteria, and fungi may prove useful in establishing the microbiologic diagnosis of infection. A wound drain has been recommended at the time of primary drainage of the epidural abscess because recurrence of the extradural collection may be more frequent when a drain is omitted (127).

In general, nonsurgical therapy in spinal epidural infections should be considered only for patients without any neurologic deficits at the time of diagnosis (11,12,128–131). Because marked neurologic deterioration may occur in a matter of hours, patients treated without surgery must be monitored closely while receiving antibiotic therapy. In a recent review of patients treated with intravenous antibiotic therapy alone, it was suggested that patients who have had symptoms for less than 2 weeks and who have myelographic evidence of significant spinal cord compression in the cervical or thoracic region may be at increased risk for developing neurologic dysfunction. These patients may benefit from surgery even if their neurologic examination is normal (128). In addition, careful follow-up after being discharged from the hospital is also important because recurrences may follow abbreviated courses of antibiotic therapy.

The appropriate surgical approach depends upon the anatomic location of the lesion—that is, anterior versus posterior. When osteomyelitis is present, consideration is also given to avoiding procedures which might destabilize the spine. Persistence or recurrence of symptoms may herald the recurrence of epidural abscess or the development of subsequent diskitis which may not have been present during the acute illness. CT-guided needle biopsy and/or open surgical biopsy may be required to establish a diagnosis of recurrent infection (116). Other modalities and approaches have been used in the therapy of spinal epidural abscesses; however, not all have been universally accepted. These include: hyperbaric oxygen treatment (54), irrigation–suction techniques (132,133), and antibiotics plus bracing (7,60,131).

Prognosis (Table 6)

The outcome of a spinal epidural abscess seems to be directly related to several independent variables. When the diagnosis is made early in the course of their illness and prior to the development of significant neurologic deficit, patients fare better than when a delay in diagnosis has occurred (3). Complete recovery with the return of full neurologic function is most likely to occur in pa-

TABLE 6. *Outcome of spinal epidural abscesses*[a]

Outcome	Number of patients
Complete recovery	74 (39%)
Weakness	49 (26%)
Paralysis	41 (22%)
Death	24 (13%)
Total:	188 (100%)

[a] Adapted from Table 5 in ref. 3, with permission.

tients without a neurologic deficit at the time of diagnosis and treatment or when neurologic signs are present for less than 24 hr (2). Chances for full recovery diminish with progressive neurologic impairment (3). If weakness or paralysis exists for more than 36–48 hr, complete recovery is less likely (3). In addition, patients with cervical epidural abscesses may have more profound sequelae (24), and patients with posterior spinal epidural abscesses may have a more limited recovery rate when compared to that of patients with anterior abscesses (3). However, other parameters such as age, sex, underlying disease, and extent of spinal blockage may also affect overall outcome (3). The benefit of steroid treatment is controversial. At present, there is no proof that steroids either improve, worsen, or predispose to spinal epidural abscess formation.

TUBERCULOUS SPINAL EPIDURAL ABSCESS

During the first half of this century, spinal epidural abscesses were divided into two categories: tuberculous and nontuberculous (13). With the decline of tuberculosis in recent decades, more attention has been focused on the array of nontubercular abscesses. However, even as recently as a hospital-based series from 1968–1978, 25% of all spinal epidural abscesses were due to *Mycobacterium tuberculosis* (17). In contrast to patients with nontuberculous spinal epidural abscesses described above, patients with tuberculous spinal epidural abscesses are generally younger, with an average age of 41 years (17,18,67,134). With the recent increase in tuberculosis in the United States (135) and the observation of the numerous extrapulmonary manifestations of tuberculosis in the HIV-infected population, it is likely that this disorder will be more common in the future.

Pathogenesis and Pathophysiology

A tuberculous spinal epidural abscess usually results from local extension of tuberculous vertebral osteomyelitis or tuberculous spondylitis, since the spine is the most common site of extrapulmonary osseous involvement (65,69,110,134,136,137) (Fig. 4). Spinal abscesses can occur in up to 46% of cases of spinal tuberculosis (134). However, cases of primary mycobacterial abscesses of the epidural space have been reported without concomitant disk, bone, or pulmonary involvement,

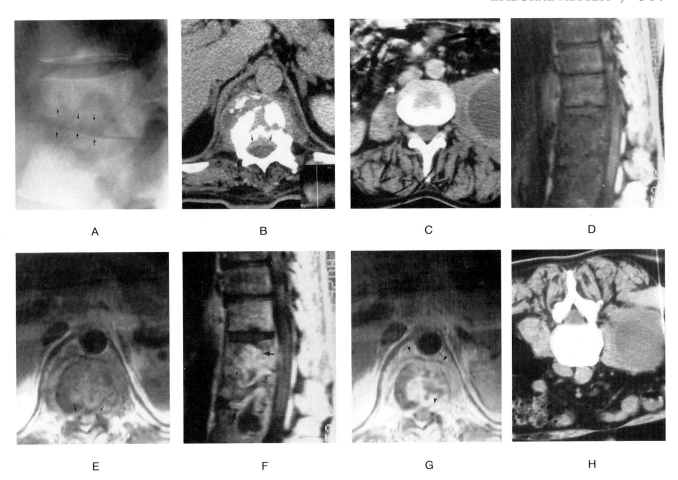

FIG. 4. Tuberculous diskitis, osteomyelitis, and epidural abscess. **A:** Plain film in the lateral projection of the thoracolumbar junction demonstrates narrowing of the disk space, rarefaction and erosion of the cortical margins of the subjacent vertebrae (*arrows*), and early gibbus formation. **B** and **C:** CT scan at the level of T12 (**B**) and L4 (**C**) after intravenous contrast demonstrates osseous destruction of T12 with an associated paraspinal and epidural (*arrows*) abscess causing compression of the thecal sac. Note the left-sided psoas abscess in part C. **D** and **E:** Sagittal (**D**) and axial (**E**) T1-weighted MRI scans 3 days later demonstrate near-complete dissolution of the T11–T12 disk space, extensive osseous destruction, and paraspinal and epidural (*arrows*) inflammatory disease. **F** and **G:** Sagittal (**F**) and axial (**G**) T1-weighted MRI scans after intravenous administration of Gd-DTPA demonstrate abnormal enhancement in the T11–T12 disk space (*small arrows*), in the subjacent vertebrae (*large arrows*), and in the paraspinal and epidural compartment (*arrowheads*), indicative of active inflammatory disease. **H:** CT-guided percutaneous aspiration of the psoas abscess with the patient in the prone position. Cultures yielded *Mycobacterium tuberculosis.*

suggesting hematogenous spread from a distant site or extension from a locally involved lymph node (67,110,134,138). The intervertebral disk may be the first tissue infected, with subsequent extension along longitudinal ligaments or via adjacent marrow spaces resulting in multiple vertebral segment involvement (66,68). The growing mass may result in neurologic dysfunction ("Pott's paraplegia") caused by direct pressure on the spinal cord or ischemic changes (66,138).

Clinical Manifestations

In contrast to patients with other bacterial spinal epidural abscesses, those with tuberculous spinal epidural abscesses may have back pain for more than 3 months. A range of 3 weeks to 8 months has been reported (17). Fever and leukocytosis are usually absent (17). Skin tests are positive in more than 70% of these patients (17). Fewer than 30% of these patients have evidence of pulmonary tuberculosis on chest x-ray (17). Cultures from material removed at surgery are positive for *Mycobacterium tuberculosis* in more than 70% of cases; caseating necrosis and granulomas with acid-fast bacilli are usually found on microscopic examination. Tuberculous spinal epidural abscesses may occur anywhere along the spine but are most common in the mid- and lower-thoracic and lumbar spine, followed by the sacroiliac and cervical spine paralleling the distribution of vertebral tuberculosis (17,68,69,110,134). Given the apparent susceptibility of the disk space, the chronicity of symptoms, and the lack of fever or leukocytosis, it is not surprising that tuberculous spinal epidural abscesses are usually diagnosed initially as noninfectious disk disease (65).

Treatment

An uncomplicated tuberculous spinal epidural abscess may be managed medically without surgical intervention (70,110,138). Antituberculous chemotherapy should include at least two agents active against the organism, usually isoniazid (INH) and rifampin. The need for additional antibiotics depends upon clinical considerations such as (a) progression of the process, (b) the antibiotic sensitivities of the organism, and (c) tolerance of the regimen by the patient.

Antituberculous chemotherapy has diminished the need for surgical intervention, except when stabilization of the spine is required (110,139,140). Because bony changes may progress radiographically for an average of 4 months following the initiation of chemotherapy, it has been emphasized that clinical parameters rather than x-ray changes should be followed to monitor therapy during the early stages of treatment (134). However, if neurologic signs and symptoms develop, decompression of a tuberculous spinal epidural abscess may be required in order to prevent permanent neurologic deficits. Furthermore, in contrast to other bacterial abscesses, paraspinal tuberculous abscesses do not necessarily require drainage unless they encroach on the spinal cord (134,138).

Controlled trials to determine the optimal chemotherapeutic regimen for tuberculous spinal epidural abscesses have not been conducted, and no firm recommendations regarding the duration of therapy have been prescribed. While some have proposed shortened courses for extrapulmonary tuberculosis (141), others have recommended prolonged treatment of up to 24 months with an INH-based regimen, particularly in cases with concomitant bone involvement (138). While bed rest is no longer considered of added benefit for patients with skeletal tuberculosis, it may be recommended for patients with large abscess formations (134).

INTRACRANIAL EPIDURAL ABSCESS

Epidemiology

The true incidence of intracranial epidural abscesses is not known. However, in a recent hospital-based series, it was found to be the third most common localized intracranial infection, following brain abscesses and subdural empyemas (34). Intracranial epidural abscesses account for about 10% of all epidural abscesses (34). Unlike intracranial subdural empyemas, uncomplicated intracranial

epidural abscesses are rare in young children and have been reported in a wide age range—from 12 to 68 years of age (34,60,142).

Pathogenesis and Pathophysiology

Above the foramen magnum where the dura is essentially the adherent inner lining of the skull, the epidural space represents only a potential space which is created when it is violated by an encroaching mass (tumor, adjacent infection, or hematoma), or as a result of trauma. As a consequence, infections of the intracranial epidural space primarily result from the extension of contiguous infections (143,144): paranasal sinusitis (60,145); frontal sinusitis (34,146–149); mastoiditis (60); orbital cellulitis (150,151); rhinocerebral mucormycosis (93); or the result of a cranial defect caused by either (a) a skull fracture (152,153), (b) a neurosurgical procedure (60,149,154–156), or (c) a complication of fetal monitoring (142). The abscess expands as the pressure generated by the growing inflammatory mass dissects the dura away from the skull. As a result, an intracranial epidural abscess is a slowly growing mass, the property that accounts for its insidious clinical presentation. Intracranial abscesses rarely dissect beyond the base of the skull, because there the dura is even more tightly laminated (155).

Microbiology

The organisms responsible for intracranial epidural abscesses are usually those associated with the primary process (156): (a) hemolytic and microaerophilic streptococci with infections of the paranasal sinuses (60) and (b) *Staphylococcus aureus* and *Staphylococcus epidermidis* associated with cranial trauma. Other organisms isolated from localized intracranial epidural abscesses without concomitant subdural empyemas included *Salmonella* (73), *Eikenella corrodens* (151), *Enterobacter cloacae* (34), *Aspergillus fumigatus* (55), and *Rhizopus* (mucormycosis) (93).

Clinical Manifestations

The slow-growing intracranial epidural abscess may cause few symptoms other than fever, localized skull tenderness, dull headache, nausea, vomiting, and lethargy (60). Papilledema may develop with increasing intracranial pressure. When cranial osteomyelitis is present, edema and cellulitis of the face and scalp also may develop (157). Thus while attention is focused on a primary process such as sinusitis, cellulitis, or skull fracture, a developing intracranial abscess may remain undetected. Symptoms may be present for several weeks or months before the diagnosis is made (60).

Depending on the location of the abscess, focal neurologic signs may develop as a result of continued expansion of the inflammatory mass. Involvement of the apex of the petrous temporal bone and cranial nerves V and VI may lead to unilateral facial pain and lateral rectus weakness called "Gradenigo's syndrome" (158). While the gradually expanding intracranial abscess may remain localized, more often the dura cannot contain the expanding epidural abscess. This may result from the development of thrombosis of the valveless emissary veins which run between the skull and meninges, or it may result from direct penetration through the necrotic dura. When this occurs the intracranial epidural abscess may be complicated by subdural empyema, brain abscess, or meningitis. The process may be further complicated by venous sinus thrombosis which, though less common, is more severe (34,149,155). Because the uncomplicated epidural abscess grows slowly, it is often the striking manifestations of the complications—meningismus, seizures, alternating mental status, or coma—which may be the first indication of an intracranial process. It is in this way that the process is similar to a meningioma or acoustic neuroma.

Approach to Diagnosis

An intracranial epidural abscess is seen on CT as a focal lentiform hypodense extra-axial collection interposed between the superior sagittal sinus and falx posteriorly and the calvarium anteriorly (159–162). Contrast CT in epidural abscesses reveals a thick medial rim enhancement, which represents inflamed, displaced dura. The degree of rim enhancement is usually thicker and more irregular in an epidural abscess than in subdural empyema (159). Calvarial osteomyelitis, subgaleal or subperiosteal abscesses, and frontal sinus inflammatory disease (Fig. 5A) are frequently associated with intracranial epidural abscesses. Large epidural abscesses can cause mass effect on the underlying brain; however, in contradistinction to the clinically more significant subdural empyema, an intracranial epidural abscess rarely demonstrates parenchymal abnormalities on CT (Fig. 5B). As noted above, it is important to appreciate that an intracranial epidural abscess frequently coexists with a subdural empyema; presence of the former should prompt a careful search for the latter (163).

Postoperative and post-traumatic extra-axial abscesses are rare (152,156,164,165). Patients with these lesions often present months to years following surgery or head trauma, respectively. These patients may have signs of local wound infection, but they generally show neither systemic signs of infection nor neurologic changes. Patients with postoperative and post-traumatic abscesses usually have underlying structural brain lesions which may lead to the persistence or the reaccumu-

lation of these collections. Postoperative abscesses occupy the cavity created by the craniotomy defect, whereas post-traumatic abscesses are often an iatrogenic complication of evacuation of a preexisting subdural or epidural hematoma. Both postoperative and post-traumatic abscesses are visualized as hypodense, extra-axial collections with medial rim enhancement on CT. Edema and mass effect on the underlying brain are usually minimal, and parenchymal abnormalities are rare (163). The indolent clinical course and the relatively benign radiographic findings compared to those of otorhinologically induced abscesses are due to the presence of a discrete limiting membrane from prior surgery or trauma, which serves to shield the underlying cerebral cortex. Abscesses in these two clinical circumstances can be very difficult, if not impossible, to differentiate from noninfected sterile effusions or chronic extra-axial hematomas. A change in density of these collections on serial CT scans, associated with subtle mass effect on adjacent brain, may be the first indication of an intracranial infection.

The morphology of post-traumatic intracranial epidural abscesses on MRI corresponds to that seen on CT—that is, lentiform or crescentic collections overlying a cerebral convexity and/or in the interhemispheric fissure (Figs. 5C and 6). MRI offers several advantages over CT in the evaluation of patients with intracranial epidural abscesses. Specifically, in otorhinologically induced abscesses, MRI can accurately identify and delineate the collections (including small loculations) early in the stage of disease, when the findings on CT can be subtle (166). This ability of MRI is attributable to the inherent high degree of contrast between the purulent collections and the subjacent calvarium, brain, and CSF, combined with the absence of streak artifacts from bone. In postoperative and post-traumatic abscesses, MRI can readily differentiate these collections from sterile effusions and chronic extra-axial hematomas based on signal intensity differences, a distinction that is usually subtle or undetectable on CT. Intracranial abscesses are usually mildly hyperintense to CSF on T1-weighted images and more markedly hyperintense to CSF on T2-weighted images (Figs. 5C and 6). In contrast, sterile effusions are isointense to CSF (166,167). Post-traumatic abscesses are hypointense on both T1-weighted and T2-weighted images, in contrast to most chronic hematomas (166–168).

Treatment

Therapy for intracranial epidural abscesses, as with spinal epidural abscesses, consists of appropriate antibiotic therapy combined with neurosurgical drainage and decompression. While antibiotics are often initiated on the basis of a primary infection elsewhere prior to the

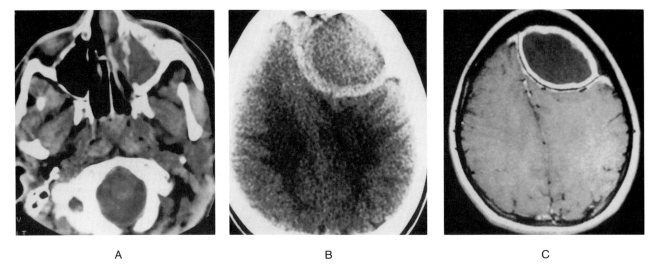

A   B   C

FIG. 5. A 19-year-old female with chronic intracranial epidural abscess. The patient had a history of acute sinusitus followed by recurrent episodes of mild headache and intermittent fevers responsive to oral antibiotics over a 4-year period. Left frontal craniotomy revealed a purulent collection which was negative by Gram's stain and culture. **A:** Noncontrast CT scan demonstrates left maxillary sinus inflammatory disease. Note thickening of the bony walls of this sinus compared to the right maxillary sinus, indicative of the chronicity of the disease process. **B:** Noncontrast CT section of the brain obtained at the same time as part A demonstrates a hypodense mass overlying the left frontal lobe associated with edema and mass effect. The hyperdense rim represents calcification, indicative of the long-standing nature of the inflammatory process. **C:** T1-weighted MRI scan obtained after the intravenous administration of Gd-DTPA demonstrates a hypointense mass with a thick enhancing rim.

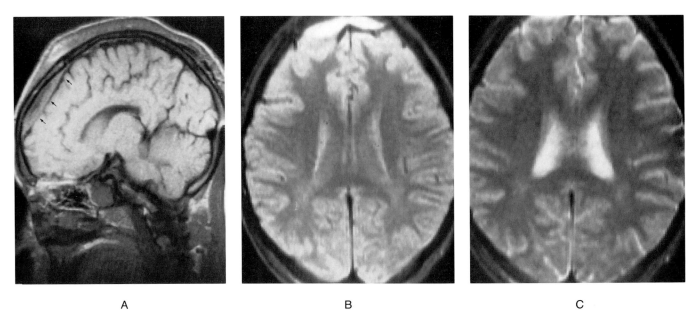

A   B   C

FIG. 6. Epidural abscess secondary to paranasal sinus inflammatory disease. **A:** Sagittal T1-weighted MRI scan demonstrates a frontal extra-axial collection with a medial hypointense rim (*arrows*), indicative of its location in the epidural space. **B** and **C:** Proton-density (**B**) and T2-weighted (**C**) MRI scans demonstrate the bifrontal epidural abscess interposed between the falx and calvarium. Note that the collection is hyperintense to CSF in Part B, indicative of its proteinaceous character. At surgery, extensive osteomyelitis of the frontal bone was found.

radiologic diagnosis of an intracranial epidural abscess, Grams stains and cultures (aerobic and anaerobic) should always be performed at the time of surgery, to guide subsequent therapy. When suspected, mycobacterial and fungal stains and cultures should also be performed. When the abscess is the presenting infection, empiric antibiotic therapy must be initiated based on the most likely pathogenic organisms. In children, empiric therapy should include antibiotics that are used for meningitis, such as the newer cephalosporins cefotaxime, ceftriaxone, or cefuroxime (or the combination of ampicillin plus chloramphenicol). When cranial defects are involved, an antistaphylococcal agent, such as penicillinase-resistant penicillin or vancomycin, should be added. In adults, since 60–90% of intracranial epidural abscesses are the result of direct extension of paranasal sinusitis or mastoiditis, empiric antibiotics should be directed against aerobic streptococci, aerobic staphylococci (155,156), and anaerobes.

The surgical therapy of intracranial epidural abscess is primarily aimed at drainage of the collection to prevent further accumulation and neurologic damage while simultaneously obtaining material for culture (169). Burr holes may suffice, but craniotomy or craniectomy may be required—particularly if overlying bone is involved (60,143,155).

Because the dura is generally not destroyed, simple débridement is usually satisfactory unless the dura has been thinned out or frankly penetrated. In this situation, dural (i.e., fascial) grafting may be necessary. Drainage for up to 1–3 days may be prudent, although it is generally not necessary if the primary site has been removed and pus in the epidural space has been drained. When there is a communication between the sinus cavity and the epidural space, closure of this communication and patching with pericranium will prevent reaccumulation of the purulent collection.

Prognosis

In contrast to the 25% mortality rate among patients with subdural empyemas (see Chapter 20), the combination of medical and surgical management of uncomplicated epidural abscesses has generally resulted in favorable outcomes. In recent series, no fatalities were reported and no evidence of long-term neurologic sequelae were documented (34,55,60). While it may be difficult to improve on this record, the increasing availability of ever more sensitive diagnostic modalities such as CT and MRI should continue to facilitate early intervention and further reduce the morbidity associated with this infection.

REFERENCES

1. Morgagni GB. De sedibus et causis morborum per anatomen indagatis. *Epist X Art* 13 (Translated by B Alexander).
2. Baker AS, Ojemann RG, Swartz MN, et al. Spinal epidural abscess. *N Engl J Med* 1975;293:463–468.
3. Danner RL, Hartman BJ. Update of spinal epidural abscess: 35 cases and review of the literature. *Rev Infect Dis* 1987;9:265–274.
4. Mooney RP, Hockberger RS. Spinal epidural abscess: a rapidly progressive disease. *Ann Emerg Med* 1987;16:1168–1170.
5. Peterson JA, Paris P, Williams AC. Acute epidural abscess. *J Emerg Med* 1987;5:287–290.
6. Russell NA, Vaughan R, Morley TP. Spinal epidural infection. *Can J Neurol Sci* 1979;6:325–328.
7. Engberg RN, Kaplan RJ. Spinal epidural abscess in children: early diagnosis and immediate surgical drainage is necessary to forestall paralysis. *Clin Pediatr* 1974;13:247–253.
8. Rockney R, Ryan R, Knuckey N. Spinal epidural abscess: an infectious emergency. Case report and review. *Clin Pediatr* 1989;28:332–334.
9. Siao P, Yagnik P. Spinal epidural abscess. *J Emerg Med* 1988;6:391–396.
10. Dandy WE. Abscesses and inflammatory tumors in the spinal epidural space (so-called pachymeningitis externa). *Arch Surg* 1926;13:477–494.
11. Hulme A, Dott NM. Spinal epidural abscess. *Br Med J* 1954;1:64–65.
12. Statham P, Gentleman D. Importance of early diagnosis of acute extradural abscess. *J R Soc Med* 1989;82:584–587.
13. Heusner AP. Nontuberculous spinal epidural infections. *Engl J Med* 1948;239:845–854.
14. Verner EF, Musher DM. Spinal epidural abscess. *Med Clin North Am* 1985;69:375–384.
15. Hakin RN, Burt AA, Cook JB. Acute spinal epidural abscess. *Paraplegia* 1979;17:330–336.
16. Fischer EG, Greene CS Jr, Winston KR. Spinal epidural abscess in children. *Neurosurg* 1981;9:257–260.
17. Kaufman DM, Kaplan JG, Litman N. Infectious agents in spinal epidural abscesses. *Neurology* 1980;30:844–850.
18. Koppel BS, Tuchman AJ, Mangiardi JR, et al. Epidural spinal infection in intravenous drug abusers. *Arch Neurol* 1988;45:1331–1337.
19. Batson OV. The function of vertebral veins and their role in the spread of metastases. *Ann Surg* 1940;112:138–149.
20. Gillilan LA. Veins of the spinal cord. *Neurology* 1970;20:860–868.
21. Esposito DP, Gulick TA, Sullivan MB Jr. Acute anterior spinal epidural abscess. *South Med J* 1984;77:1171–1172.
22. Shapiro R. *Myelography.* Chicago: Year Book Medical Publishers, 1968.
23. Durity F, Thompson GB. Localized cervical extradural abscess: case report. *J Neurosurg* 1968;28:387–390.
24. Hutton PW. Acute osteomyelitis of cervical spine with epidural abscess. *Br Med J* 1956;1:153–154.
25. Lasker BR, Harter DH. Cervical epidural abscess. *Neurology* 1987;37:1747–1753.
26. Rustin MH, Flynn MD, Coomes EN. Acute sacral epidural abscess following local anaesthetic injection. *Postgrad Med J* 1983;59:399–400.
27. Browder J, Meyers R. Pyogenic infection of the spinal epidural space: a consideration of the anatomic and physiologic pathology. *Surgery* 1941;10:296–308.
28. Ross PM, Fleming JL. Vertebral body osteomyelitis. *Clin Orthop* 1976;118:190–198.
29. Abramowitz JN, Batson RA, Yablon JS. Vertebral osteomyelitis: the surgical management of neurologic complications. *Spine* 1986;11:418–420.
30. Koopmann CF Jr, Miller RW, Coulthard SW. Retropharyngeal abscess associated with progressive quadriplegia, an epidural abscess, renal failure and jaundice. *Otolaryngol Head Neck Surg* 1984;92:114–118.
31. Heilbronn YD, Tori F, Hirsch M, et al. Transverse cervical myelopathy: an unusual complication of retropharyngeal abscess. *Head Neck Surg* 1984;6:1051–1053.
32. Atkinson L, Deambrosis W, Sheehy J, et al. A spinal epidural abscess complicating an intrauterine contraceptive device. *Aust NZ J Obstet Gynecol* 1978;18:272–273.
33. Wright RL. Congenital dermal sinuses. *Prog Neurol Surg* 1971;4:175–191.
34. Harris LF, Haws FP, Triplett JN Jr. Subdural empyema and epi-

dural abscess: recent experience in a community hospital. *South Med J* 1987;80:1254–1258.

35. Watters DA, Moussa SA, Buyukpamukcu N. Epidural abscess following Swenson procedure: a case report and a reviewing of the literature. *J Pediatr Surg* 1984;19:218–220.

36. Fine PG, Hare BD, Zahniser JC. Epidural abscess following epidural catheterization in a chronic pain patient: a diagnostic dilemma. *Anesthesiology* 1988;69:422–424.

37. Loarie DJ, Fairley HB. Epidural abscess following spinal anesthesia. *Anesth Analg* 1978;57:351–353.

38. Ferguson JF, Kirsh WM. Epidural empyema following thoracic extradural block. *J Neurosurg* 1974;41:762.

39. Sollman WP, Gaab HR, Panning B. Lumbar epidural hematoma and spinal abscess following peridural anesthesia. *Reg Anaesth* 1987;10:121–124.

40. Chan ST, Leung S. Spinal epidural abscess following steroid injection for sciatica. *Spine* 1989;14:106–108.

41. Bergman I, Wald ER, Meyer JD, et al. Epidural abscess and vertebral osteomyelitis following serial lumbar punctures. *Pediatrics* 1983;72:476–480.

42. Wayne DA, Muizelaar JP. Acute lumbosacral epidural abscess after percutaneous translumonal angioplasty. *Am J Med* 1989;87:478.

43. Elian D, Hassin D, Tomer A, et al. Spinal epidural abscess: an unusual complication of bacterial endocarditis. *Infection* 1984;12:258–259.

44. Jabbari B, Pierce JF. Spinal cord compression due to pseudomonas in a heroin addict. *Neurology* 1977;27:1034–1037.

45. Clark R, Carlisle JT, Valainis GT. *Streptococcus pneumoniae* endocarditis presenting as an epidural abscess. *Rev Infect Dis* 1989;11:338–340.

46. Brisseau JM, Derriennic M, Fritz A, et al. Septicemia due to *Actinobacillus actinomycetemcomitans* with endocarditis and spinal epidural abscess. *J Infection* 1988;17:131–134.

47. Yang SY. Spinal epidural abscess. *NZ Med J* 1982;95:302–304.

48. Tyson GW, Grant A, Strachan WE. Spinal epidural abscess presenting as acute abdomen in a child. *Br J Surg* 1979;66:3–4.

49. Schlossberg D, Shulman JA. Spinal epidural abscess. *South Med J* 1988;70:669–673.

50. Hancock DO. A study of 49 patients with acute spinal extradural abscess. *Paraplegia* 1973;10:285–288.

51. Pehrson PO, Rotmil P. Small wounds and poor friends you shouldn't dismiss, or: spinal epidural abscess as a complication of a wasp sting. *Lakartidningen* 1981;78:2612–2613.

52. Yu L, Emans JB. Epidural abscess associated with spondylolysis. A case report. *J Bone Joint Surg [Am]* 1988;70:444–447.

53. Baldwin N, Scott AR, Heller SR, et al. Vertebral and paravertebral sepsis in diabetes: an easily missed cause of backache. *Diabetic Med* 1985;2:395–397.

54. Ravicovitch MA, Spallone A. Spinal epidural abscess: surgical and parasurgical management. *Eur Neurol* 1982;21:347–357.

55. Pollack IF, Pang D, Schuit KE. Chronic granulomatous disease with fungal osteomyelitis and epidural abscess. *J Neurosurg* 1987;67:132–136.

56. Kendall MJ, Clarke SW, Smith WT. Spinal abscess due to *Listeria monocytogenes* in a patient with hepatic cirrhosis. *J Pathol* 1972;107:9–11.

57. Kolmos HJ. Spinal epidural abscess in patients on maintenance hemodialysis. Presentation of two cases. *Int Urol Nephrol* 1979;11:249–253.

58. Phillips GE, Jefferson A. Acute spinal epidural abscess. Observations from fourteen cases. *Postrad Med J* 1979;55:712–715.

59. Feldenzer JA, McKeever PE, Schaberg DR, et al. Experimental spinal epidural abscesses: a pathophysiological model in the rabbit. *Neurosurg* 1987;20:859–867.

60. Smith HP, Hendrick EB. Subdural empyema and epidural abscess in children. *J Neurosurg* 1983;58:392–397.

61. Ghosh K, Duncan L, Kennedy PG. Acute spinal epidural abscess caused by *Streptococcus milleri* [Letter]. *J Infect* 1988;16:303–304.

62. Finland M, Jones WFJ, Barnes NW. Occurrence of serious bacterial infections since introduction of antibacterial agents. *JAMA* 1959;170:2188–2197.

63. Kreger BE, Craven DE, Carling PC, et al. Gram-negative bacteremia: part III. Reassessment of etiology, epidemiology, and ecology in 612 patients. *Am J Med* 1980;68:332–343.

64. Chappel R, Verhelst A, Nagler JM, et al. Epidural abscess causing tetraparesis: case report. *Paraplegia* 1986;24:364–369.

65. Decker HG, Shapiro SW, Porter HR. Epidural tuberculous abscess simulating herniated lumbar intervertebral disc: a case report. *Ann Surg* 1959;149:294–296.

66. Ginsburg S, Gross E, Feizing EH, et al. The neurological complication of tuberculous spondylitis. Pott's paraplegia. *Arch Neurol* 1967;16:265–276.

67. Berger SA, Mayer I, Nelson S. Tuberculous epidural abscess without osteomyelitis. *Arch Neurol* 1978;35:397.

68. Cohn BNE. Tuberculous spondylitis: a histologic study. *Arch Pathol* 1941;32:641–650.

69. Tuli SM. *Tuberculosis of the spine.* Washington, DC: National Library of Medicine, 1975;1–153.

70. Griffiths DL: Tuberculosis of the spine: a review. *Adv Tuberc Res* 1980;20:92–110.

71. Rana PV, Raghunath D, Parakkal KU, et al. Spinal epidural abscess due to *Salmonella* group C monophasic 1,5. *J Neurosurg* 1985;62:942–943.

72. Herbert DA, Rushkin J. *Salmonella typhi* epidural abscess occurring 47 years after typhoid fever. *J Neurosurg* 1982;57:719–721.

73. Rodriguez RE, Valero V, Watanakunakorn C. Salmonella focal intracranial infection: review of the world literature and report of an unusual case. *Rev Infect Dis* 1986;8:31–41.

74. Marks WA, Bodensteiner JB. Anterior cervical epidural abscess with pneumococcus in an infant. *J Child Neurol* 1988;3:25–29.

75. Baylin GJ, Wear JM. Blastomycosis and actinomycosis of the spine. *AJR* 1953;69:395.

76. Krumdieck N, Stevenson L. Spinal epidural abscess associated with actinomycosis. *Arch Pathol* 1940;30:1223–1226.

77. Kannangara DW, Tanaka T, Thadepalli H. Spinal epidural abscess due to *Actinomyces israelii. Neurology* 1981;31:202–204.

78. Lane T, Goings S, Fraser DW, et al. Disseminated actinomycosis with spinal cord compression: report of two cases. *Neurology* 1979;29:890–893.

79. Sumner JW. Epidural abscess secondary to brucellosis ("Brucellosis suis"). *US Armed Forces Med J* 1950;1:218.

80. Ganado W, Craig AJ, Malta V. Brucellosis myelopathy. *J Bone Joint Surg [Am]* 1958;40:1380–1388.

81. Gaudin P, Zagala A, Juvin R, et al. *Haemophilus aphrophilus* epidural abscess studied by nuclear magnetic resonance [Letter]. *Ann Med Interne (Paris)* 1989;140:68–69.

82. Peterson JM, Awad I, Ahmad M, et al. Nocardia osteomyelitis and epidural abscess in the nonimmunosuppressed host. *Cleve Clin Q* 1983;50:453–459.

83. Siao P, McCabe P, Yagnick P. Nocardial spinal epidural abscess. *Neurology* 1989;39:996.

84. Epstein S, Holden M, Feldshuh J, et al. Unusual case of spinal cord compression: nocardiosis. *NY State J Med* 1963;63:3244–3247.

85. Guerrero IC, Slap GB, McGregor RR, et al. Anaerobic spinal epidural abscess. *J Neurosurg* 1978;48:465–469.

86. Ragnaud JM, Loste P, Aubertin J. Epidural abscess from *Fusobacterium* [Letter]. *Nouv Presse Med* 1980;9:1902.

87. Eismant FJ, Bohlmann H, Soni PL, et al. Pyogenic and fungal vertebral osteomyelitis. *J Bone Joint Surg* 1983;65A:19–29.

88. Meyer M, Gill MB. Mycosis of the vertebral column. A review of the literature. *Bone Joint Surg* 1935;17:857.

89. Rand CW. Coccidioidal granuloma: report of two cases simulating tumor of the spinal cord. *Arch Neurol Psychiatry* 1930;23:502–511.

90. Bryan CS. Vertebral osteomyelitis due to *Cryptococcus neoformans. J Bone Joint Surg* 1977;59A:275–276.

91. Litvinoff J, Nelson M. Extradural lumbar cryptococcosis: case report. *J Neurosurg* 1978;49:921–923.

92. Buruma OJ, Craane H, Kunst MW. Vertebral osteomyelitis and epidural abscess due to mucormycosis, a case report. *Clin Neurol Neurosurg* 1979;81:39–44.

93. Muresan A. A case of cerebral mucormycosis diagnosed in life with eventual recovery. *J Clin Pathol* 1960;13:34–36.

94. Polatty RC, Cooper KR, Kerkering TM. Spinal cord compression due to an aspergilloma. *South Med J* 1984;77:645–648.

95. Ingwer I, McLeish KR, Tight RR, et al. *Aspergillus fumigatus* epidural abscess in a renal transplant recipient. *Arch Intern Med* 1978;138:153–154.

96. Sheth NK, Varkey B, Wagner DK. Spinal cord *Aspergillus* inva-

sion: complication of an aspergilloma. *Am J Clin Pathol* 1985;84:763–769.

97. Wagner DK, Varkey B, Sheth NK, et al. Epidural abscess, vertebral destruction, and paraplegia caused by extending infection from an aspergilloma. *Am J Med* 1985;78:518–522.

98. Byrd BF III, Weiner MH, McGee ZA. *Aspergillus* spinal epidural abscess. *JAMA* 1982;248:3138–3139.

99. Seves JL, Hirohisa O, Benner EJ. Aspergillosis presenting as a spinal cord compression. Case report. *J Neurosurg* 1972;36:221–224.

100. Chee YC, Poh SC. *Aspergillus* epidural abscess in a patient with obstructive artery disease. *Posgrad Med J* 1983;59:43–45.

101. Selby R. Pachymeningitis secondary to *Allescheria boydii.* Case report. *J Neurosurg* 1972;36:225–227.

102. Rayport M, Wisoff HS, Zaiman H. Vertebral echinococcosis. *J Neurosurg* 1964;21:647–659.

103. Khwaja MS, Dossetor JFB, Lawrie JH. Extradural guinea worm abscess; report of two cases. *J Neurosurg* 1975;43:627.

104. Rankin RM, Flothow PG. Pyogenic infection of the spinal epidural space. *West J Surg Obstet Gynecol* 1946;54:320–323.

105. Liveson JA, Zimmer AE. A localizing symptom in thoracic myelopathy: a variation of Lhermitte's sign. *Ann Intern Med* 1972;76:769–771.

106. Hunter JC, Ryan MD, Taylor TK, et al. Spinal epidural abscess in pregnancy. *Aust NZ J Surg* 1977;47(5):672–674.

107. Keon-Cohen BT. Epidural abscess simulating disc hernia. *J Bone Joint Surg* 1968;50B:128–130.

108. Donowitz LG, Cole WQ, Lohr JA. Acute spinal epidural abscess presenting as hip pain. *Pediatr Infect Dis* 1983;244–245.

109. Roberts WA. Pyogenic vertabral osteomyelitis of a lumbar facet joint with associated epidural abscess. A case report and review of the literature. *Spine* 1988;13:948–952.

110. Waldvogel FA, Medoff G, Swartz MN. Osteomyelitis: a review of clinical features, therapeutic considerations, and unusual aspects. *N Engl J Med* 1970;282:198–206, 260–266, 316–322.

111. Altrocchi PH. Acute spinal epidural abscess vs. acute transverse myelopathy. *Arch Neurol* 1963;111–119.

112. Snider WD, Simpson DM, Nielsen S, et al. Neurological complications of the acquired immune deficiency syndrome. Analysis of 50 patients. *Ann Neurol* 1983;14:403–418.

113. Mullins GM, Flynn JPG, El-Mahdi AM, et al. Malignant lymphoma of the spinal epidural space. *Ann Intern Med* 1971;74:416–423.

114. Haid RW Jr., Kaufman HH, Schochet SS, et al. Epidural lipomatosis simulating an epidural abscess: case report and literature review. *Neurosurg* 1987;21:744–747.

115. Enzmann DR. Extracerebral infection. In: Enzmann DR, ed. *Imaging of infections of the central nervous system: computed tomography, ultrasound, and nuclear magnetic resonance.* New York: Raven Press, 1984;234–249.

116. McGahan JP, Dublin AB. Evaluation of spinal infections by plain radiographs, computed tomography, intrathecal metrizamide, and CT-guided biopsy. *Diagn Imag Clin Med* 1985;54:11.

117. Carey ME. Infections of the spine and spinal cord. In: Youmans JR, ed. *Neurological surgery,* 3rd ed. Philadelphia: WB Saunders, 1990;3749–3781.

118. Whelan MA, Schonfeld S, Post JD, et al. Computed tomography of nontuberculous spinal infection. *J Comput Assist Tomogr* 1983;9:280–287.

119. Burke DB, Brant-Zawadzkim M. CT of pyogenic spine infection. *Neuroradiology* 1985;27:131–137.

120. Lom KJV, Kellerhouse LE, Pathria MN, et al. Infections versus tumor in the spine: criteria for distinction with CT. *Radiology* 1988;166:851–855.

121. Angtauco EJC, McConnell JR, Chadduck WM, et al. MR imaging of spinal epidural sepsis. *ANJR* 1987;8:879–883.

122. Masaryk TJ, Modic MT. Lumbar spine. In: Stark DD, Bradley WG Jr, eds. *Magnetic resonance imaging.* St. Louis: CV Mosby, 1988;666–682.

123. Post MJ, Quncer RM, Montalvo BM, et al. Spinal infection: evaluation with MR imaging and intraoperative US. *Radiology* 1988;169:765–771.

124. Firsching R, Frowein RA, Nittner K. Acute spinal epidural empyema. Observations from seven cases. *Acta Neurochir* 1985;74:68–71.

125. Renaudin JW, Frazee J. Subdural empyema: importance of early diagnosis. *Neurosurgery* 1980;7:477–479.

126. Mauser HW, Houweligen HCV, Tulleken CAF. Factors affecting the outcome in subdural empyema. *J Neurol Neurosurg Psychiatry* 1987;50:1136–1141.

127. Bannister G, Williams B, Smith S. Treatment of subdural empyema. *J Neurosurg* 1981;55:82–88.

128. Mampalam TJ, Rosegay H, Andrews BT, et al. Nonoperative treatment of spinal epidural infections. *J Neurosurg* 1989;71:208–210.

129. Leys D, Lesoin F, Viaud C, et al. Decreased morbidity from acute bacterial spinal epidural abscess using computed tomography and nonsurgical treatment in selected patients. *Ann Neurol* 1985;17:350–355.

130. Leys D, Petit H. Spinal epidural abscess: surgery or conservative treatment. *Clinc Neurol Neurosurg* 1988;90:181–182.

131. Messer HD, Lenchner GS, Brust JCM, et al. Lumbar spinal abscess managed conservatively. *J Neurosurg* 1977;46:825–829.

132. Garrido E, Rosenwasser RH. Experience with the suction–irrigation technique in the management of spinal epidural infection. *Neurosurgery* 1983;12:678–679.

133. Anderson LD, Horn LG. Irrigation–suction in the treatment of acute hematogenous osteomyelitis, chronic osteomyelitis and acute and chronic joint infections. *South Med J* 1970;63:745–754.

134. Fancourt GJ, Ebden P, Garner P, et al. Bone tuberculosis: results and experience in Leicestershire. *Br J Dis Chest* 1986;80:265–272.

135. Update: Tuberculosis elimination—United States. *MMWR* 1990;39:153–157.

136. Hodgson AR. A clinical study of 100 consecutive cases of Pott's paraplegia. *Clin Orthop* 1964;36:128.

137. Gorse GJ, Paris J, Smith B, et al. Tuberculous spondylitis: a report of six cases and a review of the literature. *Medicine* 1983;62:178.

138. Des Prez RM, Heim CR: *Mycobacterium tuberculosis.* In: Mandell GL, Douglas GR Jr, Bennett JE, eds. *Principles and practices of infectious diseases,* 3rd ed. New York: Churchill Livingstone, 1990;1877–1906.

139. Chofnas I, Surrett NE, Love RW. Healing of Pott's disease with antimicrobial therapy. *Am Rev Respir Dis* 1965;93:816–817.

140. Chofnas I, Surrett NE, Severn HD. Pott's disease treated without spinal fusion. *Am Rev Respir Dis* 1964;90:888–898.

141. Dutt AK, Moers D, Steap WW. Short course chemotherapy for extrapulmonary tuberculosis. *Ann Intern Med* 1986;104:7–12.

142. Listinsky JL, Wood BP, Ekholm SE. Parietal osteomyelitis and epidural abscess: a delayed complication of fetal monitoring. *Pediatr Radiol* 1986;16:150–151.

143. Kaplan RJ. Neurological complications of infection of the head and neck. *Otololaryngol Clin North Am* 1976;9:729–749.

144. Yoshikawa TT, Quinn W. The aching head. Intracranial suppuration due to head and neck infections. *Infect Dis Clin North Am* 1988;2:265–277.

145. Kaufman DM, Litman N, Miller MH. Sinusitis-induced subdural empyema. *Neurology* 1983;33:123–132.

146. Tudor RB, Carson JP, Pulliam MW, et al. Pott's puffy tumor, frontal sinusitis, frontal bone osteomyelitis, and epidural abscess secondary to a wrestling injury. *Am J Sports Med* 1981;9:390–391.

147. Raiput MB, Rozdilsky B. Extradural hematoma following frontal sinusitis. *Arch Otol* 1971;94:83–86.

148. Gil-Carcedo LM, Izquierdo JM, Gonzalez M. Intracranial complications of frontal sinusitis. *J Laryngol Otol* 1984;98:941–945.

149. Remmler D, Boles R. Intracranial complications of frontal sinusitis. *Laryngoscope* 1980;90:1814–1824.

150. Zimmerman RA, Bilanovic LT. CT of orbital infection and its cerebral complications. *AJR* 1980;134:45–50.

151. Akhtar MJ, Chandler JR. Periorbital, subgaleal, and epidural empyema secondary to *Eikenella* sinusitis. *Ear Nose Throat J* 1979;58:358–361.

152. Larrabee WF Jr, Travis LW, Tabb HG. Frontal sinus fractures—their suppurative complications and surgical management. *Laryngoscope* 1980;90:1810–1813.

153. Opal SM, Saxon JR: Intracranial infection by *Vibrio alginolyticus* following injury in salt water. *J Clin Micro* 1986;23:373–374.

154. Mohr RM, Nelson LR. Frontal sinus ablation for frontal osteomyelitis. *Laryngoscope* 1982;92:1006–1015.

155. Silverberg AL, DiNubile MJ. Subdural empyema and cranial epidural abscess. *Med Clin North Am* 1985;90:361–374.

156. Ariza J, Casanova A, Fernandez VP. Etiological agent and primary source of infection in 42 cases of focal intracranial suppuration. *J Clin Microbiol* 1986;24:899–902.

157. Greelee JE. Epidural abscess. In: Mandell GL, Douglas GR Jr, Bennett JE, eds. *Principles and practices of infectious diseases,* 3rd ed. New York: Churchill Livingstone, 1990;791–793.

158. Lott T, Gammal T, Dasilva R, et al. Evaluation of brain and epidural abscess by computed tomography. *Radiology* 1977; 122:371–376.

159. Lee SH. Infectious diseases. In: Lee SH, Rao KCVG, eds. *Cranial computed tomography and MRI.* New York: McGraw–Hill, 1987;557–606.

160. Williams AL. Infectious diseases. In: Williams AL, Haughton VM, eds. *Cranial computed tomography.* Princeton: CV Mosby, 1985;269–315.

161. Stephanov S, Joubert MJ, Welchman JM. Combined convexity and parafalx subdural empyema. *Surg Neurol* 1979;11:147–151.

162. Moseley IF, Kendall BE. Radiology of intracranial empyemas, with special reference to computed tomography. *Neuroradiology* 1989;26:333–345.

163. Zimmerman RD, Leeds NE, Danziger A. Subdural empyema: CT findings. *Radiology* 1984;150:417–422.

164. Bhandari YS, Sarkari NB. Subdural empyemas. A review of 37 cases. *J Neurosurg* 1970;32:35–39.

165. Wright RL. *Septic complication of neurological procedures.* Springfield, IL: Charles C Thomas, 1970.

166. Weingarten K, Zimmerman RD, Becker RD, et al. Subdural and epidural empyemas: MR imaging. *AJNR* 1987;10:81–87.

167. Zimmerman RD, Weingarten K. Evaluation of intracranial inflammatory disease by CT and MRI. In: Theodore WH, ed. *Clinical neuroimaging.* New York: Alan R Liss, 1988;75–100.

168. Sze G, Zimmerman RD. The magnetic resonance imaging of infections and inflammatory diseases. *Radiol Clin North Am* 1988;26:839–860.

169. LeBeau J, Crissad P, Harispe L, et al. Surgical treatment of brain abscesses and subdural empyemas. *J Neurosurg* 1973;38:198–203.

Infections of the Central Nervous System,
edited by W. M. Scheld, R. J. Whitley, and
D. T. Durack, Raven Press, Ltd., New York © 1991.

CHAPTER 22

Central Nervous System Complications of Infective Endocarditis

Patrick Francioli

OVERVIEW OF INFECTIVE ENDOCARDITIS

Infective endocarditis (IE) was probably recognized as early as 1646 by Rivière (1), but this entity was fully described only during the 19th century. Bouillaud in France introduced the term "endocarditis" in 1830. Virchow in Germany described the pathology of the valvular vegetations in 1846, and he was the first to recognize the existence of emboli in cases of IE. Moreover, he noted the destruction of the vascular wall at embolic sites. Kirkes in 1852 and Church in 1870 associated rupture of intracranial aneurysms with bacterial endocarditis and speculated that vegetations detached from diseased valves had embolized and caused aneurysms, by lodging in the cerebral arteries. The bacterial etiology of IE was independently demonstrated by Winge and Heiberg in the 1870s (1), and Goodhart postulated than an infectious process was also playing a role in the formation of bacterial aneurysms. The full clinical spectrum of "malignant endocarditis" was first comprehensively covered by Sir William Osler (2–4) in his three Goulstonian lectures at the Royal College of Physicians in London in 1885. From his great personal experience (more than 200 cases) he not only described "the different modes of onset, and the extraordinary diversity of symptoms which may arise," but also carefully analyzed the pathophysiology of distant complications, particularly of central nervous system (CNS) manifestations such as meningitis: "The meningeal complications of endocarditis have not received much attention, considering the frequency with which it has occurred . . . somewhat over 12 per cent. In the majority of these cases it occurred in

connexion with pneumonia" (2–4). He also related IE and mycotic aneurysms to a common infectious etiology. Moreover, he emphasized the still valid principles of IE diagnosis: "With careful blood-cultures one should now be able to determine the presence of septicemia. . . . The blood-culture and the presence of the painful erythematous nodules and the occurrence of embolism furnish the most important aids (to diagnosis)" (5).

At the same time, the first experimental models of endocarditis were developed (6) which allowed a better comprehension of the pathogenesis of IE.

When the nature of the organisms causing endocarditis was more precisely recognized, it became clear that "bacterial" endocarditis was too restrictive a term; thus the term "infective endocarditis" was proposed by Thayer (7) in 1931, to take into account infection of valves by agents such as rickettsiae or fungi.

Epidemiology

In developed countries, the reported incidence of IE is 1.6–4.3 per 100,000 per year (8–13). There is little geographical variation (Table 1). Incidence is lower in children (9). IE accounts for 0.38–1.24 per 1000 admissions in general hospitals (14–20) (Table 2). This rate may be higher in specialized institutions (14). Some (17,18), but not all (16), studies have shown an increasing rate over time. More remarkable, the mortality rate has remained fairly constant during the same period, ranging from 20% to 40% despite the advent of antibiotics (8,19).

In the absence of other life-threatening underlying disease, stable mortality and incidence rates mask the evolving spectrum of IE and the great differences which exist between various types of IE. For instance, subacute IE due to viridans streptococci has an early mortality

P. Francioli: Division of Hospital Preventive Medicine and Department of Internal Medicine, Division of Infectious Disease, Centre Hospitalier Universitaire Vaudois, Lausanne, Switzerland.

TABLE 1. *Incidence of IE in various countries and at different times*

Investigators	Period	Population	IE	IE per 100,000 per year	Geographic area
Griffin et al. (8)	1950–1959	0.5×10^5	20	4.3	Olmstead county, Minnesota (USA)
	1960–1969		21	3.3	Olmstead county, Minnesota (USA)
	1970–1981	0.9×10^5	37	3.9	Olmstead county, Minnesota (USA)
Scholin et al. (9)	1970–1980	Children	66	0.4	Sweden
Rossi et al. (10)	1975–1984	3.9×10^6	629	1.6	Veneto (Italy)
Goulet et al. (11)	1982	54×10^6	970	1.8	France
Skehan et al. (12)	1982–1984	3.4×10^6	185	2.3	North East Thames (UK)
King et al. (13)	1985	4.5×10^6	75	1.7	Lousiana (USA)

rate of 5–15%, whereas acute prosthetic valve endocarditis (PVE) in an elderly patient with congestive heart failure can be fatal in up to 70% of cases (21).

Thus the apparent stability in incidence and mortality is a consequence of a decrease of certain predisposing factors such as rheumatic heart disease (22,23), which is counterbalanced by (a) the appearance of new predisposing conditions (24) such as prosthetic valves (25,26) or other intravascular devices (27), (b) drug abuse (28,29), and (c) degenerative heart diseases related to age (21,30).

The demographic patterns have changed considerably (31). The mean age, which ranged from 34 to 43 years in the early antibiotic period (1950s to 1960s) (16,32,33), has increased to 52–55 years (24,34,35), and even over 60 years in particular series (14,36). The sex ratio of men to women is presently 2:1 (8,19,31). This represents an increase of the proportion of men, probably in relation to the changing pattern of underlying predisposing factors.

Although the clinical distinction between "acute IE" and "subacute IE" has been widely used (37–39), classifications of IE according to the etiologic agent and according to the underlying conditions such as native versus prosthetic valve is more useful for the purpose of therapy and prognosis (19,21).

Predisposing Factors

There are cardiac and noncardiac conditions associated with a higher risk of IE. Their identification is important because they have a major influence on the epidemiology, clinical presentation, therapy, and prophylaxis of IE.

In the past, rheumatic heart disease (RHD) was the predominant underlying cardiac abnormality, present in 75–90% of the cases (40). There has been a continuous decline of RHD over the past decades (24); this condition is nowadays present in less than 25% of patients with IE (41), and even <10% in recent series (22,23).

Congenital heart diseases are the underlying condition in 6–20% of cases of IE (41,42). The most frequent are: ventricular septal defect, bicuspid aortic valve, ductus arteriosus, tetralogy of Fallot, coarctation of the aorta, Marfan's syndrome, and pulmonary stenosis (15,43). They account for two-thirds of IE cases in children. Congenital defects with low flow turbulence, such as atrial septal defect of the ostium secundum type, are at lower or no risk (21). A bicuspid aortic valve is also an important underlying predisposing factor in elderly persons, in whom it may be present in up to 20% of IE cases, probably because of the superimposed valvular sclerosis (44).

TABLE 2. *Incidence of IE in various hospitals and at different times*

Investigators	Period	Hospital admissions	IE	IE per 1000 hospital admissions	Hospital
Cherubin and Neu (16)	1938–1947			1.24[a]	Presbyterian Hospital (New York, USA)
	1948–1957			0.85[a]	Presbyterian Hospital (New York, USA)
	1958–1967			0.40[a]	Presbyterian Hospital (New York, USA)
Grossman et al. (17)	1951–1960	158,174	61	0.39	Chaim Sheba Medical Center (Tel Aviv, Israel)
	1970–1979	370,251	176	0.45	Chaim Sheba Medical Center (Tel Aviv, Israel)
Svanbom and Strandell (14)	1967–1971	13,580	41	3.02[b]	Roslagstull Hospital (Stockholm, Sweden)
	1967–1971	225,400	86	0.38	Five General Hospitals (Stockholm, Sweden)
Kim et al. (18)	1975–1978			0.18	Straub Hospital (Honolulu, Hawaii, USA)
	1979–1982			0.41	Straub Hospital (Honolulu, Hawaii, USA)
	1983–1987			0.71	Straub Hospital (Honolulu, Hawaii, USA)
Shaw et al. (19)	1984	23,000	15	0.65	St-Vincent Hospital (Sydney, Australia)
Francioli et al. (177)	1985–1989	129,724	63	0.49	University Hospital (Lausanne, Switzerland)

[a] Data adapted.
[b] Reference hospital for infectious diseases.

Idiopathic hypertrophic subaortic stenosis (IHSS) also predisposes to IE, occurring in about 5% of the patients suffering from that disorder (42,45,46).

Degenerative heart diseases with calcified atheromatous deposits on the valves are responsible for a proportion of cases which increases with age, and these may be the predisposing factor in up to 50% of the IE cases in elderly patients (16,30). It should be mentioned that patients with calcified mitral annulus alone do not seem to be at increased risk (47).

Mitral valve prolapse (MVP) is another recognized risk factor for IE. It is found in 10–30% of IE cases (23,48,49). However, given the high incidence of MVP (5%) in the general population (50), the risk is low and is estimated to be 0.0175% per year (one in 3480 to one in 9415)(51). Recently, it was shown that MVP was a significant risk factor for IE only when associated with a systolic heart murmur, thus being related to a certain degree of mitral valve dysfunction (52–55). Moreover, when these patients were analyzed according to the result of echocardiography, a higher risk of IE was found in those with leaflet thickening or redundancy (56).

Prosthetic valves account for 10–34% of the cases, and this proportion will depend on the referral patterns of the various centers (57–60). In patients with prosthetic valves, the occurrence of IE ranges from 0.98% to 4.4%, and the annual incidence is approximately 1% (26,57,61). Early PVE, defined as an infection occurring within 2 months of operation, represents one-third of the cases. It is predominantly due to staphylococci (40–45%) (with *Staphylococcus epidermidis* being responsible for two-thirds of staphylococcal cases), generally have an acute course and a mortality rate of 40–75%. Late PVE generally has a more subacute course, and the spectrum of etiologic agents resembles that of native valve IE. The mortality rate is 20–45% (26,60). IE associated with other intracardiac devices, such as Swan–Ganz catheters (62) or pacemakers (63), are well described but are infrequent.

Noncardiac predisposing conditions are of increasing importance. In patients at risk, nosocomial IE (27) associated with iatrogenic valvular lesions caused by catheters or hyperalimentation lines, or associated with bacteremias induced by various diagnostic or therapeutic procedures, may represent as many as 30% of the cases in certain series (24), particularly in elderly patients (27). IE is reported in 2–6% of chronic hemodialysis patients (64). The prognosis of nosocomial IE is poor, partly because the diagnosis may be obscured by the underlying diseases (27).

Drug abusers are at high risk for IE. The relative frequency of intravenous drug abusers among IE cases varies according to the geographical area (19,21). *Staphylococcus aureus* accounts for more than 50% of the cases (65), but in some areas other bacteria such as *Pseudomonas aeruginosa,* enterococci, or *Serratia* species may predominate (66,67). The microbiological spectrum may change over time in the same area (28). Fungi (5–10%) and a polymicrobial etiology are not rare (68–70). Right-sided valvular infections, especially of the tricuspid valve, occur in more than 50% of cases (70,71). Recently, IE has been associated with cocaine sniffing, probably in relation to intranasal lesions serving as a portal of entry for microorganisms (29).

Pathogenesis

In his final discussion on the pathology of malignant endocarditis, Osler speculated in a visionary fashion the precise sequence of events known today to lead to IE (72):

> Whether or not, in a given case, endocarditis will arise, depends greatly on the condition of the valve tissue. In a case of pneumonia or other disease, such as pyaemia, in which we may suppose microbes circulating in the blood, the endothelium of normal valves may be able to resist their invasion, or even if they do lodge and penetrate, the condition may be not favourable for their growth; but where an individual is debilitated, or the tissue tone lowered, or if as so often seems the case, the valves are diseased, then the micrococci find a suitable nidus, and excite, by their growth, an endocarditis which might be of the malignant type.

These postulated mechanisms are now supported by numerous and careful experimental studies, which have further expanded our understanding of the pathogenesis and pathophysiology of endocarditis (Fig. 1). The recent studies were made possible by the development of a simple animal model by Garrison and Freedman (73); this model was subsequently modified by Durack and Beeson (74,75). These studies have shown that the most important prerequisite for the development of IE is a lesion of the endothelium of the valve or of the heart cavities. In the animal, this lesion is produced by an intravascular polyethylene catheter placed across the aortic or the tricuspid valve. This will induce the deposition of platelets and fibrin and lead to the formation of a nonbacterial thrombotic endocarditis (NBTE) (74,75).

Many factors can induce endothelial lesions and promote the formation of NBTE. The most important are valvular organic lesions with perturbations of the normal blood flow (76), prosthetic valves and other intracardiac devices (25,26), hypercoagulation states [e.g., malignancies (77)], and immune injuries (78). Even microscopic lesions are prone to infection by circulating bacteria (79), so that it is not surprising that up to 50% of patients with IE have no known predisposing heart condition at the time of diagnosis (27,35).

NBTE constitutes a nidus to which circulating bacteria may attach. This attachment process is probably mediated on the host side by receptor-like structures such as fibronectin (80), fibrinogen, laminin, or collagen (81).

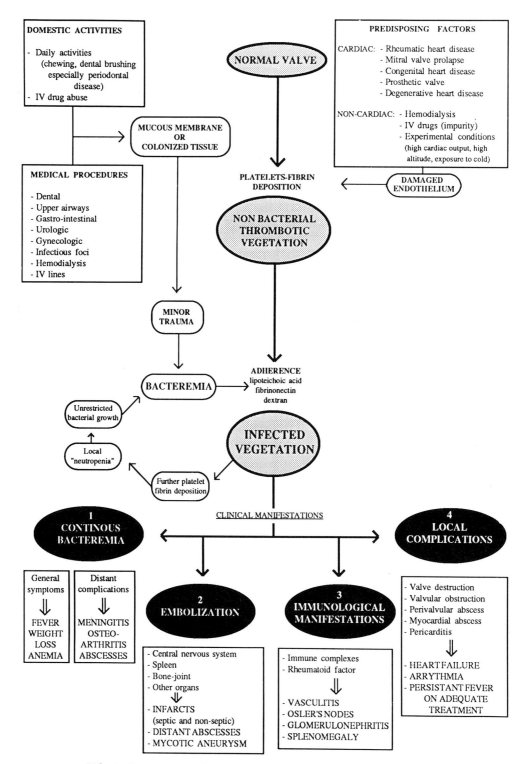

FIG. 1. Pathogenesis and pathophysiology of infective endocarditis.

The route by which the bacteria reach preexisting NBTE is the bloodstream, except for the cases acquired during open heart surgery. Transient bacteremia occurs quite frequently, and it may follow minor mucosal trauma induced by daily domestic activities such as chewing or teeth-brushing. Bacteremia may also be triggered by various iatrogenic procedures (82,83). The level of bacteremia appears to be directly related to the importance of the trauma and the number of microorganisms inhabiting the mucosal surface (83).

Among the many bacterial species that can be recovered during transient bacteremia, streptococci account for the vast majority of IE cases. In some species this is probably related to the adherence properties of their surface, conferred by the extracellular production of dextran (84,85). Indeed, it has been observed experimentally that after extraction of periodontally diseased teeth, it is not the magnitude of the bacteremia of a given species that best predicts the occurrence of IE, but instead the *in vitro* adhesiveness of the bacteria to platelet–fibrin clots mimicking NBTE (86,87).

Once microorganisms have attached to NBTE, they start to multiply, and further deposition of fibrin and platelets, possibly promoted by the bacteria themselves through the activation of tissue factors (88), will result in the deep embedding of the bacteria within the vegetation (89), where they will be protected from circulating neutrophils. This has led to the concept of an infection developing in an era of "localized agranulocytosis" (15). With regard to local host defense mechanisms, there seem to be differences between the two sides of the heart. In experimental right-sided endocarditis, infection of tricuspid valve vegetations by streptococci healed spontaneously in some normal rabbits, whereas this was prevented with treatment with dexamethasone (90) or made granulopenic with nitrogen mustard (91). This evolution toward healing in normal rabbits was not seen in left-sided endocarditis (90). Bacteria deeply seated in the vegetation are metabolically inactive (75) and may, to a certain extent, be protected from the penetration of antibiotics. This combination of factors helps to explain why cure of bacterial endocarditis requires the prolonged administration of bactericidal antibiotics (92).

Because the infection is located within the bloodstream, bacteria are constantly released, and persistent bacteremia is a hallmark of bacterial endocarditis, permitting the diagnosis through blood cultures in almost all cases (19). Moreover, further deposition of platelets, fibrin, and circulating bacteria (90) will compensate for the fragmentation, embolism, and/or resorption of the vegetation by the inflammatory response, in a delicate and complex balance.

IE also induces the stimulation of an immunological response, which may result both in elevated concentrations of nonspecific humoral antibodies, including rheumatoid factor and cryoglobulins (93), and in the appearance of circulating immune complexes. These findings tend to be found more commonly in patients with longer duration of infection (94). Circulating immune complexes may contribute to some manifestations found in IE cases thought to be related to vasculitis, such as purpura, Osler's nodes, Roth's spots, myalgia, arthralgia, and diffuse proliferative glomerulonephritis (95–97).

Etiologic Agents

The list of microorganisms recovered in IE includes almost all described human pathogenic bacteria, as well as rickettsia, chlamydia (98), fungi (21,99,100), and per-

haps viruses. However, gram-positive cocci largely predominate. The pattern of distribution of these etiologic agents differs profoundly, according to the underlying risk factors (Table 3).

In native valve endocarditis (NVE), streptococci were responsible for 70–90% of IE in the pre-antibiotic era (101). This prevalence has declined somewhat but is still around 60%, and streptococci of the viridans group account for the majority of streptococcal IE (30–60%) (34,102). They are alpha-hemolytic and are generally nontypable in the Lancefield system. They include the following species, in decreasing order of frequency: *Streptococcus sanguis, Streptococcus mutans, Streptococcus mitis,* and *Streptococcus salivarius* (103,104). The clinical course is generally subacute, and an underlying cardiac condition is often present. The prognosis is generally good, with an overall 15% mortality rate (105). *Streptococcus milleri,* a related nonhemolytic streptococcus, occasionally causes IE. It has the peculiar propensity to cause distant abscesses and local perivalvular invasion (106). Group D streptococci, normally inhabitants of the digestive tract, account for 7–10% of the cases of IE. *Enterococcus faecalis* is the most frequently encountered species in this group. It can present with an acute or subacute course. Because *E. faecalis* is particularly resistant to the bactericidal activity of antibiotics, treatment requires the use of a combination of agents, including an aminoglycoside. High-level resistance to streptomycin and gentamicin has emerged (107). It can be acquired nosocomially and tends to affect elderly persons, with a high mortality rate (108,109). It should be distinguished from another group D streptococcus commonly causing IE: *Streptococcus bovis. S. bovis* IE is often observed in association with digestive neoplasia, of which it may be the first manifestation (110,111). In contrast to *E. faecalis, S. bovis* is usually sensitive to the bactericidal activity of beta-lactams, including penicillin. *Streptococcus pneumoniae,* once a frequent cause of IE, has become very uncommon since the advent of antibiotics (112,113). Group A and other streptococci of the Lancefield groups (e.g., B, G, etc.) occasionally cause endocarditis (114,115).

S. aureus is responsible for an increasing number of IE cases, accounting for 20–30% (102). Valves with no apparent preexisting lesions are involved in up to 30% of cases. The course of the disease is generally acute, with a high propensity for local complications (myocardial abscess, valvular leaflet perforation, sinus of Valsalva thrombosis) and other complications such as embolization and abscess formation (116). The overall mortality is 40% (117).

Numerous other bacteria are classic (but less common) causes of native valve IE, particularly *Coxiella burnetii* and bacteria of the "HACEK" group (*Haemophilus* species, *Actinobacillus actinomycetemcomitans, Cardiobacterium hominis, Eikenella corrodens, Kingella*

TABLE 3. *Relevant features of the most frequent types of IE*

Organism	Predisposing factors	Particular clinical features	Treatment	Comments
Streptococci (60–80%) (non-enterococci)	Underlying cardiac disease generally present		Penicillin G 4 × 3 million units/day	For PVE, medical treatment alone is frequently sufficient
Viridans streptococci (30–40%)	Follows dental procedure in about 20% of cases	Subacute course	4 weeks 2 weeks +[a] +	Alternative: ceftriaxone 2 g/day for 4 weeks
S. bovis (5%)	Often first manifestation of a neoplastic digestive disease	Purulent complications are rare	gentamicin 3 × 1 mg/kg/day for 2 weeks	
Enterococci (5–18%) (E. faecalis, E. faecium)	About 30% nosocomially acquired; often associated with digestive disease	Acute or subacute course	Amoxicillin 6 × 2 g/day for 4 weeks (or ampicillin 6 × 2 g/day for 4 weeks) + gentamicin 3 × 1 mg/kg/day for 4 weeks	Alternative: vancomycin 2 × 15 mg/kg/day + gentamicin 3 × 1 mg/kg/day
Staphylococci (20–35%) S. aureus (10–25%)	Often on "normal" valve; drug abuse; PVE	Generally acute course; often affects tricuspid valve in drug addicts; frequent emboli; frequent local complications	Oxacillin 6 × 2 g/day for 6 weeks[b] + gentamicin 3 × 1 mg/kg/day for 1 week	For PVEs, surgery is required in most cases
Coagulase-negative staphylococci (1–5%)	60% of early PVE; 30% of late PVE; rarely on normal valves	Acute or subacute course	Oxacillin[b] + rifampin for > 6 weeks + gentamicin for 2 weeks	
Gram-negative bacilli (2–10%)	Often nosocomially acquired; PVE; drug abuse	Symptoms often masked by the underlying pathology	Beta-lactam for 6 weeks + gentamicin for 4–6 weeks	For PVE, surgery is often required; polymicrobial in 5% of drug abuse cases
Fungi (1–5%)	PVE; drug abuse; immunosuppression	Major emboli	Amphotericin B + 5-flucytosine[c]	Treatment is successful only when associated with valve replacement
Culture-negative (5–15%) Miscellaneous	Prior antibiotics; fastidious microorganisms; HACEK group[d]; fungi; Q fever	Often subacute course; often major emboli	All efforts should tend to obtain a microbiological documentation before starting empiric treatment (ampicillin + aminoglycoside unless suspected microorganisms likely to be resistant)	Consider surgery if there is no response to medical treatment (also for diagnostic purpose)

[a] The combined regimen should be used for strains with minimum inhibitory concentrations > 0.1 μg/ml.

[b] For penicillin-sensitive strains, penicillin can be used. For methicillin-resistant strains and penicillin-allergic patients, vancomycin 2 × 15 mg/kg/day is required.

[c] For *Candida* species.

[d] *Haemophilus* species, *Actinobacillus* species, *Cardiobacterium* species, *Eikenella* species, *Kingella* species.

species) (118–121). In certain countries such as Spain and Saudi Arabia, *Brucella* species can be responsible for up to 10% of IE cases (122). Gonococci have become a rare cause of IE (123).

In PVE, coagulase-negative staphylococci are responsible for 30% of the cases overall, but they are more frequently isolated in early PVE (>40%) (26,60). This is related to intraoperative contamination (124). Cases occurring in patients with native valves are rare but have been described in patients with MVP (53) or with bicuspid aortic valves (125). *S. aureus* accounts for 10–14% of the cases of PVE, and viridans streptococci are responsible for approximately 30% of late PVE. The incidence of gram-negative bacilli (120) (10–20%), diphtheroids (126), and fungi (5–10%) is higher in PVE than in native valve IE (26,60). These microorganisms are important causes of early PVE (26,61).

Drug addicts are particularly at risk for the development of IE (28). There are important geographic variations in the distribution of the etiologic agents responsible for drug-abuse-associated IE (21). Overall, *S. aureus* is the most frequent etiologic agent (60%) (28,65), probably because of its importance in local infections at the injection site (cellulitis, abscesses, suppurative thrombophlebitis) (127). In some areas, cases due to methicillin-resistant staphylococci may predominate (29). Other etiologic agents include: streptococci 15–20%, viridans streptococci (8–10%), enterococci (5–10%), gram-negative bacilli such as *P. aeruginosa* (28) or *Serratia* species (128) (10–15%), multiple microorganisms (5%), fungi (5%), and anaerobic bacteria (129) (5%). IE affects the tricuspid valve in 40–70% of the cases in intravenous drug users (71,130). The mortality rate is lower than 10% in such cases (70,71).

Patients with a clinical presentation suggestive of IE but with negative blood cultures account for 5–10% of the cases in recent series (24,131). The most common cause for culture-negative IE is prior administration of antibiotics (132,133). A single dose of 250 mg of penicillin V can lead to negative blood cultures for up to 3 weeks (19). However, in the absence of prior antibiotic administration and with appropriate blood culture media (134), most of the bacteria will eventually grow but may require repeated blood culture and prolonged incubation periods (132). Some microorganisms, such as *Aspergillus* species, *Coxiella burnetii* (135), or *Legionella pneumophilia* (136), usually cannot be recovered from the blood. In cases of *Aspergillus* IE, diagnosis is generally made on the histology and culture of the valve or of embolic material (137). The diagnosis of *C. burnetii* IE relies on the demonstration of phase I antibodies (21,135). IE with negative blood cultures has also been described in association with subacute or chronic right-sided endocarditis, uremia, and mural endocarditis (138), but the importance of these factors with recent blood culture techniques is not well established (134,139).

Clinical Manifestations

As noted by Osler (2–4) in 1885, the signs and symptoms of IE are extremely variable, owing to the diversity of the etiologic agents and of the various organs involved. Patients may have fever or be afebrile, may or may not have evidence or history of preexisting heart disease, may have a very acute or a rather chronic course, and may have specific signs or vague symptoms. Fever with a heart murmur is the most frequent clinical presentation; it may be the only clue to the diagnosis, especially early during the course of the disease and with microorganisms of low virulence. When the heart murmur is new or changing, a high level of suspicion should be maintained. More than one-half of patients will have some degree of congestive heart failure (101,140). Distant complications such as major emboli, lumbar pain, seizures, or rupture of a mycotic aneurysm may be the first presenting manifestations of IE.

Clinical manifestations of established IE may be classified into four main categories according to the principal pathophysiological mechanisms (Fig. 1):

1. Congestive heart failure is the most common cardiac complication, occurring in 50–70% of cases (36,141). It is mainly caused by valvular incompetence due to destruction. The infection can spread to other heart structures and produce myocarditis, myocardial abscesses, rhythm disturbance, or purulent pericarditis (142). Persistance of fever despite appropriate antibiotic treatment should raise the suspicion of such local complications (143).

2. Embolic phenomena are due to the fragmentation of the vegetation and occur in 30–40% of the cases. Depending on the size and on the number of emboli, this may lead to the obstruction of major vessels or may result in numerous diffuse microemboli (36,144). They affect the CNS in 50% of the cases, the abdominal viscera (spleen, hepatic, kidney, digestive structure) in 40% of the cases, and bone and limbs in less than 10% of the cases (19,145). Janeway lesions are found on the palms or soles in about 10% of IE. They are the result of small emboli with some degree of hemorrhage. Emboli are particularly frequent in *S. aureus* IE (92).

3. Bacteremia is responsible for the general symptoms such as fever, loss of appetite, anemia, splenomegaly, and distant metastatic infections (30,112).

4. Immunological stimulation results in hyperproduction of gamma-globulins and the formation of circulating immune complexes. Positive rheumatoid reaction may be present (19,146). The longer the course of IE, the higher the titers of these immune complexes (94,146, 147). This can result in petechiae, Osler and Roth spots lesions, arthritis, and glomerulonephritis (97,147). Osler nodes occur in 10–25% of IE cases. They are small, painful, nodular lesions on the pads of fingers or toes, as well as on thenar or hypothenar eminences. They are due to

an allergic vasculitis and are not specific for IE (92,95, 148). Roth spots are retinal hemorrhagic lesions, with a white center (149).

Diagnosis

Blood culture is the most important diagnostic procedure in patients with suspected IE. In some cases, diagnosis is made by culture and/or histology of the valve or of embolic material. For the main etiologic agents, the first two blood cultures will be positive in more than 90% of cases, even higher for streptococci. However, certain microorganisms may be difficult to isolate (150). Variables affecting isolation include the volume of blood cultured, the number of blood cultures obtained, prior antimicrobial therapy, the type of microorganism involved, and blood culture technique (134). The volume of blood cultured is one of the major factors (151): For each culture, at least 10 ml of blood (in adults) should be obtained and distributed in a two-bottle system, for incubation in aerobic and anaerobic conditions. Two (possibly three) separated cultures should be done, over a 24-hr period (151). In patients who have recently received antibiotics, it may be necessary to obtain additional blood cultures and, when appropriate, to use media supplemented with beta-lactamase (152,153). If the first blood cultures remain negative, additional blood cultures must be collected and special culture systems used. One should make sure that the microbiologic media are appropriate for the suspected agents. Since some agents require special or "supplemented" media, it is important that the clinicians give adequate information to the microbiology laboratory (132,154). Lysis–concentration systems are effective for the recovery of mycobacteria and fungi, and they may also improve the yield in culture-negative cases of IE (155). In addition, longer incubation times of 7–21 days are useful for isolation of fastidious microorganisms (134,153).

Routine laboratory parameters are often abnormal, but they are nonspecific. The erythrocyte sedimentation rate (ESR) is elevated in 90–100% of IE cases, with a mean value of 57 mm/hr (156). A normal ESR has a good negative prognostic value in the absence of renal or congestive heart failure or embolic manifestations (21). Mild anemia is common (70–90% of cases) and has the characteristics of anemia of chronic disease: normocytic, normochromic indices; low serum iron concentration; and low iron-binding capacity. Thrombocytopenia is uncommon (5–15% of cases). Leukocytosis is present in only 20–30% of the cases, and it is uncommon in the subacute form. Leukopenia may exist. Hypergammaglobulinemia occurs in 20–30% of cases. Urinalysis shows abnormalities in 20–30% of cases, mainly proteinuria or microscopic hematuria. Circulating immune complexes may be detected, but they are nondiagnostic and can also

be found in 40% of septicemia without IE, in 40% of drug addicts, and in 10% of healthy controls (157). Titers have been shown to decline under appropriate antibiotic therapy (94,158). Conversely, increased titers have been correlated with treatment failure (146). Except for *C. burnetii*, serology is seldom helpful (159).

Although the diagnosis of IE relies primarily on clinical and microbiological data, echocardiography is now an important diagnostic procedure in the evaluation of patients with IE. It may allow the visualization of vegetations and of other cardiac lesions, and it permits the assessment of valvular and cardiac function (160). Vegetations are detected by echocardiography in about 60% of the cases with the use of M-mode alone, in 73–77% with the combined use of M-mode and two-dimensional echocardiography, and in up to 96% when the transesophageal echocardiography approach is used (160,161). The latter approach provides an increased detection rate of perivalvular abscesses (162), and it also allows a better evaluation of mechanical prosthetic valvular IE (160). Correlations between echocardiographic findings and prognosis of IE remain controversial, but most reports indicate that vegetations greater than 10 mm in diameter are associated with a higher incidence of embolic episodes (160,163,163a). Sequential echocardiograms performed during the treatment of IE can assist in making decisions on the necessity and timing of surgery (140,164). Patients with mural vegetations might be at greater risk for embolization (160).

Cardiovascular studies involving radionuclides have received attention because they are relatively noninvasive (165). The radiopharmacological gallium-67 citrate has been used with some success in demonstrating IE (166), but the technique is limited by low sensitivity (167). Platelets and leukocytes could be labeled with indium-111 in a manner that would maintain cellular function and that would allow external imaging with conventional scintillation cameras (165). Indium-111-labeled platelets are able to identify aortic valve endocarditis in the rabbit model (168). Indium-111-labeled leukocytes have been used in humans; however, they have not been convincingly successful in detecting vegetations, probably because too few leukocytes localize at the site of endocarditis. However, this method has been helpful in detecting purulent pericarditis, myocarditis, and myocardial abscesses (169). Moreover, perivalvular abscesses in prosthetic and native valve endocarditis could be detected very early in the evolution of the disease, at a time when the complication was clinically asymptomatic. These results suggest that this technique could be a valuable noninvasive method for identifying patients who need surgery early in the course of their infection, before the development of hemodynamic failure and/or destruction of the valve annulus (170).

Imaging techniques such as computerized tomography (CT) or nuclear magnetic resonance (NMR) may be useful for the detection and assessment of distant complications of IE (171).

Cardiac catheterization provides important hemodynamic information for optimal medical and surgical management (172,173) in selected patients.

Treatment

Once the diagnosis of IE is made (or if there is a high level of suspicion), antibiotic treatment should be started promptly in order to eradicate the infecting microorganisms as soon as possible. It is well known that a prolonged course of antibiotics may be needed for cure, even if the microorganisms are highly sensitive to the drug(s) used. The location of the infection in an area of impaired host defenses in the platelet–fibrin matrix, along with the high count of microorganisms present in the vegetation and the reduced metabolic activity of certain subpopulations of bacteria (74,75), may explain the difficulties encountered in achieving eradication of the infective agents (92). The antibiotic agent(s) must be bactericidal and should be administered for a period of 2–6 weeks. Parenteral administration of a combination of antibiotics provides higher bactericidal activity and is recommended for certain microorganisms (21,140). The use of combinations may allow shorter courses of treatment for certain IE due to viridans streptococci (174). A portal of entry should be sought in all cases of IE and, if indicated, should be addressed (teeth, gums, skin, urinary and gastrointestinal tract pathology) (19). Some of the recommended regimens are shown in Table 3.

IE due to viridans streptococci and *S. bovis* can generally be treated with penicillin for 4 weeks (175), with or without a 2-week course of aminoglycosides (174). A 2-week course of penicillin with an aminoglycoside is also appropriate for viridans streptococci, except if caused by nutritionally variant species or if the course of IE has lasted more than 3 months (176). Ceftriaxone (2.0 g/day) for 4 weeks is also appropriate and may allow ambulatory treatment of some patients (177). IE caused by enterococci must be treated with a combination of antibiotics, generally penicillin or ampicillin (or vancomycin) plus gentamicin for at least 4 weeks (174).

IE caused by *S. aureus* requires administration of oxacillin or nafcillin (about 90% of the strains are resistant to penicillin) for 4–6 weeks. The addition of an aminoglycoside has been shown *in vitro* to have a synergistic effect against most strains of *S. aureus,* and it has been recommended during the first week of treatment. In drug addicts with right-sided IE, a 2-week course of parenteral oxacillin alone, followed by 2 weeks of therapy by mouth, has been shown to be effective (178). Conversely, a 2-week course of nafcillin plus tobramycin may also be used (179). IE caused by methicillin-resistant *S. aureus* can be treated with vancomycin alone for 4–6 weeks (180). Combination therapy for PVE caused by *S. aur-*

eus seems prudent. Oxacillin or vancomycin combined with rifampin and gentamicin is recommended, but surgical therapy is often necessary and, when indicated, should not be delayed (174). Treatment of coagulase-negative staphylococcal IE is governed by the same principles, but methicillin-resistant strains are more frequent (174).

In the treatment of IE due to gram-negative bacilli, the combination of a semisynthetic penicillin (or a cephalosporin) with an aminoglycoside is usually recommended (21).

In fungal IE, the use of antifungal agents alone has been almost universally associated with failure, and a combined medical–surgical approach should be undertaken (21,181–183).

For culture-negative IE, broad-spectrum antibiotic coverage should be initiated. In NVE, a combination of penicillin (or ampicillin) plus an aminoglycoside is generally recommended, unless a particular microorganism not sensitive to that regimen is suspected. In PVE, the combination of vancomycin plus an aminoglycoside and rifampin is effective against the most frequent infective agents. The response to treatment within a week appears to be correlated with survival. Surgical removal of the valve for subsequent microbiological and histological examinations may be necessary (140).

Careful clinical observation is essential for monitoring adequacy of therapy in order to detect failures or complications. Blood cultures should be performed after the end of antibiotic treatment (184). For the majority of the etiologic agents, adequate bactericidal titers may be anticipated with the use of the widely recommended regimens (based on experimental studies and clinical experience), making these tests not necessary (174). Measurement of SBT (serum bactericidal titer) is likely to be clinically helpful only when unusual organisms are treated, when unusual antibiotic regimens are used, or when treatment appears to be failing (174). Levels of SBT of at least 1:8 to 1:16 would be desirable (185).

Surgery has an important role in the management of IE, and an optimal therapeutic approach often requires operative intervention during medical treatment (186). An algorithm is shown in Fig. 2. Early surgical intervention may improve survival. If indicated, the intervention should be carried out without delay, even if antibiotics have just been started (140,187). Hemodynamic deterioration (often due to valvular regurgitation), local complications, and uncontrolled infectious process are the major indications for surgery (182,188,189). In most cases of PVE and fungal IE, combined medical and surgical treatment appears to be warranted (190,191).

Prevention of IE

The purpose of prophylaxis is to prevent the development of IE in patients with known underlying predispos-

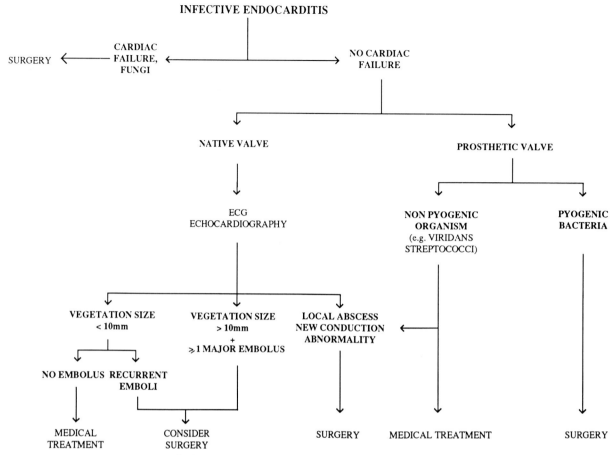

FIG. 2. Surgical management of infective endocarditis.

ing factors and who undergo a procedure which may result in bacteremia. Although the risk of infection has not been quantified, several hundred cases of streptococcal endocarditis following certain medical procedures have been reported (dental, upper airway, digestive and genitourinary tract), and thus a causal relationship may be regarded as established (83,140,192,193). In these patients, it is recommended practice to administer antimicrobial agents prophylactically for (a) procedures during which transient bacteremia may occur and (b) procedures that have been associated with IE (194–196).

Because prospective clinicals trials of antibiotic prophylaxis of IE cannot be conducted in humans for ethical as well as for statistical reasons, the questions of which antibiotics, what dosage, and for how long are a matter of controversy. However, case–control studies have suggested that antibiotic prophylaxis is efficacious in preventing PVE in humans (197,198). Moreover, experimental animal data, clinical experience, and *in vitro* studies have afforded some understanding of the conditions necessary for successful IE prophylaxis (194,199), and recommendations for humans are based on this indirect information (194,200,201).

The cardiac lesions predisposing to IE are categorized into those at high risk (PVE, previous IE) and those at

moderate risk (most congenital heart conditions; prior valvular surgery; rheumatic or acquired valvular disease; MVP with valvular incompetence or leaflet thickening/redundancy). Patients with a transvenous pacemaker seem to be at very low risk for IE (201,202). The most common indications for prophylaxis are (a) dental procedures that are likely to induce bleeding and (b) oral or upper airway procedures such as tonsillectomy/adenectomy, surgery or biopsy of respiratory tract, or endoscopy with a rigid bronchoscope. For genitourinary and lower gastrointestinal procedures, prophylaxis can be limited to a few indications such as (a) genitourinary instrumentation in the presence of infection and (b) colonoscopy with biopsy. For incision and drainage of infected tissues, antibiotics should be administered for both prophylaxis and treatment (e.g., *S. aureus*) (201,202).

The choice of recommended regimens is governed by the following principles: (a) The agent(s) must be appropriate for the likely offending organisms (streptococci, enterococci); (b) the agent(s) used must be in the bloodstream at the time of the procedure, although recent experimental data suggest that antibiotics administered shortly after the bacteremia phase might also prevent IE (203); (c) the agent(s) must be taken only shortly before the onset of the bacteremia, to avoid the emergence of resistant flora; (d) a high loading dose must be used; and (e) additional dose(s) of antibiotics following the procedure are expected to increase the effectiveness of prophylaxis (204).

An oral dose of 3 g of amoxicillin (1–2 hr before the procedure), followed by one additional dose of 750 mg (6 hr later), provides a unified regimen for both streptococcal and enterococcal prophylaxis in nonallergic patients at moderate risk. Several additional doses of 750 mg may confer an increased protection to patients at very high risk. In patients allergic to amoxicillin, alternative regimens depend on the site of the procedure. For dental or upper respiratory tract procedures (viridans streptococci), clindamycin or erythromycin may be used, whereas intravenous vancomycin is the only alternative to amoxicillin for genitourinary, gastrointestinal, or gyneco-obstetric procedures (enterococci). Parenteral administration of amoxicillin or vancomycin is indicated for hospitalized patients not able to take oral medications (201,202) and perhaps for patients with prosthetic valves.

CENTRAL NERVOUS SYSTEM COMPLICATIONS OF INFECTIVE ENDOCARDITIS

General Considerations

Incidence

Among the various manifestations of IE, the neurologic complications are of particular importance for three main reasons: (i) They occur frequently; (ii) they may be the first and/or the predominant manifestation of the disease; and (iii) they are often severe and have become a leading cause of death from IE since the advent of cardiac valve replacement. The reported overall incidence of CNS complications of IE varies greatly, and figures ranging from 9% (205) to 80% (206) have been noted. In most series, however, the incidence of CNS involvement during the course of IE ranges between 20% and 40%, with an average of 30% (Table 4). Surprisingly, the incidence has not changed much over time, despite (a) wide differences in the diagnostic criteria employed in the various studies and (b) the changes which have occurred during the past decades in many different aspects of IE (see section entitled "Overview of Infective Endocarditis"). Among 743 patients pooled from seven series published before the advent of antibiotics, 176 (24%) were noted to have neurologic manifestations (2,207–212). Among 1455 patients from six studies reported between 1947 and 1967, 335 (23%) had such complications (38,213–218). And among 796 episodes of native valve IE from seven series published between 1977 and 1989, 282 (35%) were accompanied by neurologic manifestations (24,156,219–223) (Table 4). The slight increase in incidence observed in the recent studies is likely to be due to more intensive diagnostic attention to reported neurologic manifestations in recent years, particularly imaging studies. The reported incidence is also higher in studies devoted primarily to the neurologic aspects of IE and in those based on necropsies, because brain damage often causes or contributes to death in IE

TABLE 4. *Incidence of neurological complications in IE at different times, 1885–1989*

General reviews of IE					Studies on CNS complications of IE				
Investigators	Year	Number of cases	N	%	Investigators	Year	Number of cases	N	%
Osler (2–5)	1885	200	23	12%	De Jong (209)	1937	68	17	25%
Horder (207)	1908	150	40	27%	Fetterman and Aske (210)	1938	40	18	45%
Blumer (208)	1923	150	30	20%	Krinsky and Merritt (211)	1938	100	31	31%
		500	**93**	**19%**	Toone (212)	1941	34	17	50%
Hickie (213)	1961	279	39	14%			**243**	**83**	**34%**
Pankey (214, 215)	1961–1962	240	71	30%	Harrison and Hampton (217)	1967	116	37	32%
Cooper et al. (216)	1966	159	58	36%	Jones et al. (218)	1969	385	110	29%
Lerner and Weinstein (38)	1966	100	20	20%			**501**	**147**	**29%**
		778	**188**	**24%**	Pruitt et al. (221)	1978	218	84	39%
Pelletier and Petersdorf (156)	1977	125	38	30%	Bush et al. (222)	1985	58	32	55%
Crittin and Waldvogel (220)	1977	71	12	17%	Salgado et al. (223)	1989	113	40	35%
Von Reyn et al. (24)	1981	104	39	38%	Gransden et al. (242)	1989	178	59	33%
Terpenning et al. (27)	1987	154	57	37%			**567**	**215**	**38%**
		454	**146**	**32%**					

(101,214,215,224–226). In one autopsy series of 69 cases of IE, cerebral emboli were found in up to two-thirds of the young adults and in 46% of the total cases (227). Moreover, areas of encephalomalacia due to proven or presumed cerebral embolism were found in 93% of the cases (227). Incidence also tends to be higher in series gathered from referral centers (221) or from specialized units: For example, among 86 patients with IE hospitalized in two intensive care units, 48 (56%) presented neurologic complications (228). This referral bias would alter not only the number but also the type and severity of the complications, because referral is often motivated by CNS involvement. Interestingly, the mean duration of prodromal symptoms prior to diagnosis was found to be similar in patients with and without neurologic complications (223).

Age and Sex

In many studies on adults with IE, the age of the patients did not appear to greatly influence the overall frequency of CNS complications. In a recent series, however, major neurologic events were recorded in 22%, 28%, and 34% of patients aged <40, 40–60, and >60 years old, respectively (27). Incidence as high as 80% has been noted in a small series of 10 elderly patients (206). In the elderly patients, neurologic manifestations tend to be more common as a presenting clinical sign of IE (229); as many as one-quarter to one-third of them may present with neurologic signs (36,230), as compared with 5–17% in the general population (231,232). If disorientation is included, the figure can be as high as 45% (232). Neurologic complications may be less frequent in children. In a series of 118 pediatric cases, only eight were found to have cerebral lesions (233). Because major neurologic events are infrequent in children or young adults, everyone should recall Jochman's dictum (234): "In hemiplegia in young adults or children, always think of subacute endocarditis."

Generally, the sex distribution of the patients with or without neurologic complications appears to be similar in both men and women (221,225). A higher proportion of either men (219) or women (223) has been reported. In the latter study, it was felt that the difference was most likely reflecting local referral patterns. Moreover, neurologic complications by valve involvement showed no statistically significant difference in either sex (223).

Location of IE in the Heart

Neurologic complications are a hallmark of left-sided IE. This was noted even before IE was recognized as a clinical entity (235). The incidence of complications is markedly lower in isolated right-sided IE. In a series of 40 intravenous drug users with *S. aureus* tricuspid IE, none presented cerebral manifestations, whereas two out of five of those with left-sided involvement had cerebral septic emboli (28). In another series of 48 drug addicts with IE, 16 neurologic complications (33%) were observed, but only one occurred among the 16 patients with only right-sided IE (236). Of 97 episodes of IE in drug addicts, none of the nine major CNS events present on initial evaluation occurred in the 32 cases which involved the right side of the heart (237), although the infection was caused by highly virulent organisms such as *S. aureus*. When neurologic manifestations occur in right-sided IE, they present as meningitis, cerebral abscesses, or encephalopathy and are related to highly virulent microorganisms, such as *S. aureus* or *S. pneumoniae* (238). Systemic embolization is rare in right-sided IE but can occur, either from septic thrombi found in the pulmonary veins (68,239) or via paradoxical embolization through a patent foramen ovale (227,240) as is found in 18% of the normal population (71,241).

In left-sided IE, the localization of the infection has been found to influence the occurrence of neurologic complications in some (219,221,228), but not all (223,242), studies. In the study from the Massachusetts General Hospital in Boston, only 28% of the patients with aortic valve involvement presented neurologic complications, compared to 52% of those with mitral valve infection (221); emboli accounted for this difference. In another study, neurologic complications were present in 76% of the patients with mitral valve infection, compared to 37% in other cases (228). In contrast, in a series from the Columbia Presbyterian Medical Center in New York City, patients with aortic valve infection, especially when caused by staphylococci and associated with congestive heart failure, were at increased risk for emboli (219). In a more recent study comparing 64 patients with neurologic complications with 111 patients without such complications, the proportion of infection of the aortic valve (59% and 59%, respectively), of the mitral valve (34% and 31%), and of the aortic and mitral valves combined (6% versus 9%) was similar in both groups (223).

Prosthetic Valve Endocarditis

Neurologic complications in the context of PVE are of special concern because of the threat of superimposed intracerebral hemorrhage secondary to anticoagulation. Most of the published data are derived from PVE complicating mechanical prosthetic valves. The overall incidence of focal neurologic events associated with PVE varies from 11% to 44% (25,243–250,250a), which is considerably higher than the overall thromboembolic rate of 1–4%/year observed for anticoagulated patients with uninfected prosthetic valves (251).

The incidence of CNS complications in PVE is influenced by anticoagulant therapy. In patients insufficiently anticoagulated, CNS complication rates of 38–

71% were noted (219,244,248), compared to only 8–10% in patients on appropriate anticoagulant therapy (244, 248), but when anticoagulated patients develop neurologic complications, they are at high risk for major hemorrhagic manifestations (221,243,250). However, in one recent series of 61 patients, there was no difference in the rate of embolism or risk of bleeding between patients receiving no or subtherapeutic anticoagulation and those adequately anticoagulated (250a).

Incidence may be affected by the time of onset of infection in relation to the placement of the prosthetic valve: CNS embolic episodes have been reported in 0–11% of patients with early PVE and in 23–28% of those with late PVE (57,249,250,252). This is also suggested by another study, in which peripheral manifestations occurred in 10% of early PVE compared to 34% in late PVE (58). In an earlier study, in which patients with PVE were not anticoagulated, the incidence of embolic events was approximately 50% for both early and late PVE (219).

Studies comparing the incidence of CNS complications between NVE and PVE have given conflicting results: In one study, 11 of 82 (13%) patients with NVE, compared to six of 18 (33%) with PVE, presented such complications (245); however, another study reported 40 of 113 (35%) for patients with NVE and 24 of 62 (39%) for those with PVE (223). An autopsy series comparing organ infarcts in NVE and PVE showed similar rates, when adjusted for the valve involved (mitral valve —77% and 71%, respectively; aortic valve—66% and 60%, respectively), but emboli to the CNS were not specifically analyzed (253).

The type of prosthetic valve may influence the rate of CNS manifestations. Of 33 patients with bioprosthetic valve IE gathered from three studies, four (12%) had neurologic events (245,250,254), a figure lower than that with mechanical valves. However, in another study of 62 patients with PVE, there was no statistical difference when the type of prosthetic valve involved was compared among patients with and without neurologic complications (223).

In summary, patients with PVE do not appear to be at a much higher risk for CNS complications than do patients with NVE, provided that anticoagulation is maintained and carefully controlled for complications associated with mechanical valves. However, those presenting a CNS complication are particularly threatened by massive cerebral hemorrhage (221,244,250) (see section on specific management of patients with emboli, below).

Intravenous-Drug Abuse

In intravenous (I.V.)-drug users with IE, the frequency of cerebral manifestations is dependent on the side of the heart involved. Therefore, the reported incidence of neu-

rologic complications will depend on the proportion of patients with or without isolated right-sided involvement. Isolated right-sided involvement in IE has been reported in 9–72% in series of endocarditis in addicts (236). Among 28 addicts with tricuspid valve endocarditis, only one had neurologic involvement (255). In a study comparing the clinical manifestations of S. aureus IE in addicts and nonaddicts, neurologic involvement was found in 51% of the nonaddicts compared to only 9% of the addicts. Although neurologic complications were not categorized according to the side of the heart involved, 76% of the addicts had an IE restricted to the tricuspid valve as compared to 9% in the nonaddict population (179), suggesting that the side of the heart involved plays an important role in the occurrence of neurologic complications. The frequency of neurologic complications in I.V.-drug users with left-sided endocarditis appears to be higher than that in the nonaddict population, and it has ranged from 45% to 58% (65,236,256). The higher complication rate may partly be due to the failure of some of the addicts to undergo a full antibiotic course, or it may be due, in part, to a different distribution of the etiologic agents. In drug abusers, neurologic complications may also be related to other mechanisms: Transverse myelitis, neuropathy, and various acute and chronic brain disorders have been described in the absence of IE (257).

Pathogenesis

Neurologic complications of IE relate to several main mechanisms: (a) occlusion of large or small cerebral arteries secondary to emboli, infected or not, derived from the endocardial vegetations; (b) infection of the meninges, of the brain, or of the wall of the cerebral arteries, secondary to septic emboli or bacteremia; and (c) "toxic" and possibly immune-mediated injuries. These events may result in a variety of secondary lesions such as (a) bland or hemorrhagic infarcts, (b) intracerebral, subarachnoid, or subdural hemorrhages, (c) expanding processes such as abscesses or mycotic aneurysms, or (d) brain dysfunction due to multiple factors.

When embolization is the ultimate cause of the neurologic involvement, the lesions may either (a) affect a single vessel and give focal signs or (b) affect multiple vessels and produce multifocal signs. Depending on whether or not ischemia is reversed before permanent changes occur, the clinical picture may be that of a transient ischemic attack (258) or of a longer-lasting obstruction resulting in brain damage. Since emboli of untreated or partially treated IE contain bacteria, the lesion produced may be that of ischemia or suppuration, or both (231). This may result in either (a) septic or aseptic meningitis, (b) brain abscess or microabscesses, or (c) meningoencephalitis. If the wall of an artery or its vasa vasorum is involved, a mycotic aneurysm may develop.

Arterial rupture in the absence of a detectable intracranial mycotic aneurysm (ICMA) formation can also occur (259,260). Critical factors that may determine whether a septic embolus results in a simple infarct, a mycotic aneurysm, or an abscess include the site where the embolus lodges, the virulence of the microorganism, and the timing between the event and the initiation of antibiotic therapy. Multiple other factors can cause or contribute to the neurologic manifestations of IE, such as hypoxia, metabolic disturbances, drug toxicity, and toxic phenomena secondary to the systemic infection. Immune injury to small arteries is also likely to be involved (261), and proliferative endarteritis in the absence of local infection or embolization has been described (262). Although immune complexes have been identified in the choroid plexus of a patient with IE (263), the exact significance of this finding remains to be determined.

Sustained bacteremia in tricuspid valve endocarditis, even with virulent organisms, does not result in intracranial hemorrhage, supporting the hypothesis that embolic fragments are necessary (259).

Microbiology

An important factor in determining the rate, the type, and the severity of the neurologic complications is the nature of the microorganism causing the IE. This may account for some of the differences in the incidence noted between the various studies (Table 5). In general reviews which have correlated the incidence of neurologic complications with the infectious agent causing IE, the frequency of CNS involvement ranged from 53% to 71% for *S. aureus* and was significantly higher than that observed with some other bacteria—particularly that of group D and non-group D streptococci, which ranged from 30% to 47% (219,221,223,228). Rates of 51–56% were also found in series only or predominantly due to left-sided *S. aureus* IE (130,264,265). In a series of 26 addicts with *S. aureus* with IE, neurologic symptoms were present in 50% of them, although 12 had IE restricted to the tricuspid valve and were therefore less likely to contribute to the total number of patients with complications (266). Bacteria other than *S. aureus*, such as Enterobacteriaceae or anaerobic bacteria, have been associated with a high rate of neurologic complications (221,267). Moreover, certain microorganisms are prone to a high rate of certain types of neurologic involvement. For example, although *S. pneumoniae* has become a rare cause of IE, being responsible for only 1–3% of the cases (113), associated meningitis is extremely frequent and is observed in 57–91% of the cases (113,268–271). Purulent complications are also frequently encountered with *S. aureus* IE, either as meningitis or as brain abscess (264). Certain bacteria such as *Haemophilus* species (120,121,272–274), nutritionally variant streptococci (275), or fastidious organisms (276) have been associated with high rates of large emboli; these emboli may occlude major vessels, including cerebral arteries. Of 27 patients with *Haemophilus* endocarditis reviewed by Parker et al. (121), 66% presented cerebral emboli. In patients with culture-negative IE, major embolic phenomena, including those to the brain, were noted twice as often as in patients with culture-positive IE (131). IE due to fungi are also associated with large vegetations and a high rate of embolic phenomena (277,278). Of 27 patients with IE caused by *Aspergillus* species, a total of 14 neurologic manifestations secondary to emboli were recorded in 11 (41%) patients (279). In one study, all five patients with fungal PVE had major systemic and cerebral emboli (278). Among 21 patients with *Candida* species IE, eight had large arterial emboli (277). In contrast, the rate of CNS complications in IE caused by some other bacteria, such as viridans streptococci or coagulase-negative staphylococci, appears to be particularly low. Of 21 patients with IE due to the latter bacteria, only five (24%) developed neurologic manifestations (223), a rate substantially lower than that with other bacteria.

TABLE 5. *Microbiology of IE in patients with and without CNS complications*

Organism	Pruitt et al., 1978 (221)		Salgado et al., 1989 (223)		Gransden et al., 1989 (242)	
	Number of cases	Number with CNS complications	Number of cases	Number with CNS complications	Number of cases	Number with CNS complications
Staphylococcus aureus	49	26 (53%)	20	13 (65%)	42	23 (55%)
Staphylococcus coagulase-negative	7	1 (14%)	21	5 (24%)	8	4 (50%)
Viridans streptococci	51	14 (27%)	49	20 (41%)	83	14 (17%)
Streptococcus group D	37	11 (30%)	52	15 (29%)	19	5 (26%)
Streptococcus pneumoniae	8	6 (75%)	—	— —	8	7 (88%)
Other streptococci	34	12 (35%)	7	4 (57%)	4	2 (50%)
Other	34	16 (47%)	26	9 (35%)	14	4 (29%)
	220	**86**	**175**[a]	**66**	**178**	**59**

[a] Native valve, 113; prosthetic valve, 62.

Clinical Presentation

Neurologic manifestations of IE may be the presenting symptoms of IE in 16–23% of the cases (217,219, 221,228). However, there are often other clues to the diagnosis of IE. For example, of 218 patients with IE and 84 with neurologic complications, neurologic complaints were the first overt evidence of IE in 36. In 24 of them, the neurologic problem provided an important clue to the diagnosis, but in only five were there no other hints as to the underlying IE (221). When neurologic complications manifest as presenting symptoms, major cerebral emboli constitute approximately two-thirds of the cases, but all other possible manifestations (such as seizure; meningismus; subarachnoid, intracerebral, or subdural hemorrhage; personality changes; visual disturbances; or weakness of the extremities) can occur in some cases (221). Amnesia has also been reported (280).

Neurologic complications can also occur after the initiation of antibiotic treatment in up to 30% of the cases (223). In the majority of these cases, the neurologic events tend to occur early after treatment has been started, usually within the first 2 weeks (223). However, cerebral emboli or rupture of ICMA can occur from several months to up to 2 years after the completion of successful treatment (101,281). More than one complica-tion is frequently observed in a given patient; thus, a total of 160 neurologic manifestations were recorded among 84 patients studied by Pruitt et al. (221). The neurologic complications of IE include a large variety of disorders (Tables 6 and 7) and can mimic many neurologic diseases of other etiologies.

Stroke is the most common presentation and accounts for one-half to two-thirds of the neurologic manifestations (221,223). The majority of these cases are due to cerebral emboli with infarction, but some are also due to intracerebral hemorrhage (218) or even abscesses (282). Stroke usually presents as hemiplegia with or without sensory loss, aphasia, or coma; isolated sensory loss, ataxia, or other dyskinesias can also occur (283). Brainstem lesion—accompanied by nausea, vomiting, or hiccup—has occasionally been described (282).

Meningitis (septic or aseptic) is found in less than 10% of the cases with neurologic complications reported in most general reviews, although a rate of 37% has recently been reported (242). Since it is more common in IE due to virulent bacteria such as *S. pneumoniae* and *S. aureus* (242), studies addressing IE due to these types of microorganisms report higher rates. For these bacteria, meningitis may be the most frequent neurologic complication (38,242). Meningismus may be related to the direct invasion of the meninges by the microorganism, or it may be

TABLE 6. *Neurologic syndromes in patients with IE*

Syndrome	Mechanisms	Main clinical presentation
Stroke	Emboli with bland or hemorrhagic infarction Intracranial hemorrhage due to mycotic aneurysm and necrotizing arteritis Brain abscess	Hemiplegia, aphasia
Meningitis	Multiple causes: microabscesses Bacterial seeding of the meninges Brain abscess	Meningitis with or without focal signs
"Toxic" encephalopathy	Microemboli, microabscesses, cerebritis, CNS hypertension, drug toxicity, metabolic disturbances, vasculitis, other organic CNS complications	Decreased level of consciousness
Psychiatric abnormalities	Same as "toxic" encephalopathy Reactive to conditions surrounding the diagnosis of infective endocarditis	Behavioral disorders (elderly patients)
Seizures	Any of the underlying CNS lesions Drug toxicity, metabolic imbalance, hypoxia	Focal or generalized seizures
Brainstem	Emboli in the vertebrobasilar territory	Nausea, vomiting, hiccup, dyskinesia, tremor
Cranial nerves	Emboli, space-occupying lesions	Visual disturbances, disorders of eye movements, palsies, sensory impairment
Spinal cord and peripheral disorders	Emboli, metastatic abscesses, immune injury	Para- or tetraplegia, mononeuropathy
Severe headache	Mycotic aneurysms or other CNS lesions	Severe, often localized headache
Subarachnoid hemorrhage	Infectious arteritis with or without detectable mycotic aneurysm	Meningismus with or without decreased level of consciousness

TABLE 7. Neurologic complications of IE in five series

	Jones et al., 1969 (218)	Pruitt et al., 1978 (221)	Bush et al., 1985 (222)	Salgado et al., 1989 (223)	Gransden et al., 1989 (242)	
Number of IE:	385	218	58	175	178	1014 (100%)
Patients with CNS complications:	110	84[a]	32	64	59	349 (34%)

						Proportion of CNS complications
Emboli						
Major:	44	38	15	27[b]	12	20–47%
Multiple:	—	23	—	—	—	27%
Hemorrhage:	8	15	8	5[b]	—	7–25%
Mycotic aneurysm:	3	4	5	3	—	3–16%
Meningitis:	7 (2)[c]	33 (11)[c]	7 (6)[c]	2[b] (6)[c]	22 (7)[c]	6–39%
Abscess:	—	9	5	5	—	9–16%
Encephalopathy:	21	14	—	15	15	17–25%
Seizure:	4	24	6	1	—	2–29%
Headache:	14	—	8	6	10	9–25%

[a] One patient may have more than one complication.
[b] Slightly adapted.
[c] Numbers inside parentheses denote cases with positive CSF culture.
[d] Including macroabscesses and microabscesses.

secondary to other underlying processes such as abscesses, leaking mycotic aneurysm, subarachnoid hemorrhage, cerebral infarction, or vasculitis. Meningeal symptoms or signs were encounted in 35 of 84 patients (42%) with neurologic complications reported by Pruitt et al. (221). On examination, the CSF was purulent in 16, aseptic in eight, normal in eight, and hemorrhagic in two. This variety in the CSF findings is a reflection of the several underlying conditions that may cause meningismus.

Decreased level of consciousness can be seen in association with embolism or hemorrhage. It can also occur without any other obvious cause and is often referred to as "toxic encephalopathy" or "acute brain syndrome." A mild-to-severe degree of stiff neck may be present. These cases may be caused by multiple and often combined neurologic and non-neurologic mechanisms, such as microabscesses, microemboli, hypoxia, metabolic imbalance, bacterial toxins, or drug toxicity. The patients may present with symptoms of varying severity, including impaired concentration, irritability, drowsiness, vertigo, or lethargy. The CSF is normal in approximately 50% of these cases (218,223) or may present a slightly elevated cell count of either lymphocytes, polymorphonuclear cells, or both. The maximal count in one study reporting six such patients was 45 cells per cubic millimeter (218).

Seizures are not rare, being reported in 1.5–15% of the patients with neurologic manifestations (217,221,223). In a study of 141 children with IE, seizures were the most common neurologic manifestation, occurring in 10% (284). When seizures occur, they are often part of the presenting complex of symptoms (217,221). Of 110 patients with IE and CNS complications, generalized seizures occurred as the only neurologic symptom in four (218). Three of these four patients also had focal components to the seizure activity. Focal seizures are usually the consequence of cerebral infarction. Generalized seizures can be the result of any of the organic lesions complicating IE and may be associated with other predisposing factors, such as hypoxia, metabolic disorders, or drug toxicity, especially when renal failure is present (221).

Mild, intermittent, diffuse headache is a frequent complaint in IE and can be found in 25–43% of the patients with IE (222,285). However, severe headache or localized headache is found in only about 3% of IE patients (218,285), and it may be the symptom leading to the diagnosis of IE (218) or may indicate a disastrous complication. Indeed, three of 14 patients with IE and severe headache in one series (218), as well as four of seven patients in another study (285), had intracranial mycotic aneurysms. Conversely, six of eight patients with ICMA in the latter study had severe localized headache, which should therefore prompt further investigation. This is also suggested by another study, in which eight of 58 patients with IE complained of headache; a neurologic complication occurred in seven of these eight (222).

A wide variety of psychiatric abnormalities, from minor personality changes to major psychiatric syndromes, have been described in association with IE. There are many case reports of patients whose symptoms led to an initial psychiatric diagnosis (283). This might be more frequent in elderly patients (36) or in patients with other underlying diseases, such as drug abuse or alcoholism (216,229,286). These psychiatric abnormalities may be caused by the same mechanisms that caused the toxic encephalopathy, or they may only be reactive to the conditions surrounding the diagnosis of IE. In these cases, the neurologic examination and the CSF might be entirely normal (283), and fever and a cardiac murmur may be the only clue to the diagnosis of IE.

Various types of dyskinesias have been described, the most common being tremor, parkinsonism, ataxia, myoclonus, and convulsions (283). Cases of chorea in the absence of evidence of rheumatic activity have been described (283).

Visual disturbance is a frequent manifestation of IE and may be due to retinal emboli or involvement of the peripheral or central pathways of cranial nerves II, III, IV, and VI. This may result in impairment in eye movements and varying degrees of visual loss (283). Iridocyclitis and panophthalmitis have also been described, especially in drug addicts (65). Other cranial-nerve disorders can occur, and pseudobulbar palsy has been described (287).

Spinal cord involvement, mainly in relation with ischemic lesions but also secondary to extramedullary compression by metastatic abscesses, can be observed, and it may result in girdle pain and paraplegia (65,288).

Peripheral-nerve involvement as a result of embolic or immunologic lesions may account for cases of localized pain or mononeuropathy (289,290).

Diagnostic Procedures

Cerebrospinal Fluid Examination

Lumbar puncture in patients with IE has been performed because of the presence of various neurologic signs or symptoms, including meningismus, disorientation or altered level of consciousness, focal deficit, seizure, or isolated headache. Despite similar rates of neurologic complications, the percentage of patients having had a lumbar puncture varied from 32% to 82% in four large series (218,221,223,242), the most recent studies reporting the lowest rates. This is probably related to the availability of CT scan in recent years, which obviates the necessity for invasive procedures in many cases. Hence, there has been a decreasing number of lumbar punctures performed to investigate focal deficits in the more recent studies cited above.

The largest and most detailed study on cerebrospinal fluid (CSF) in patients with neurologic complications of IE comes from the Massachussetts General Hospital (221). CSF examination was performed in 69 of 84 (82%) such patients. "Purulent CSF" was defined as a predominantly polymorphonuclear leukocyte pleocytosis, accompanied by reduced glucose and elevated protein concentrations. "Aseptic CSF" was defined as a pre-

dominantly lymphocytic pleocytosis, accompanied by normal glucose and normal or only slightly elevated protein concentrations. A CSF was considered as hemorrhagic if it contained more than 200 red blood cells per cubic millimeter. Among 35 patients who had a lumbar puncture (LP) because of nuchal rigidity and/or disorientation, the CSF was purulent in 16, aseptic in eight, hemorrhagic in two, and normal in nine. Among 25 patients who underwent a lumbar puncture because of the development of new focal deficit, CSF was normal in eight, aseptic in eight, hemorrhagic in six, purulent in two, and both hemorrhagic and purulent in one. In the nine cases with seizures, the CSF was normal in five, aseptic in one, hemorrhagic in one, and under increased pressure in one. Of the 41 LPs performed because of cerebral emboli, 18 were normal, seven were purulent, 13 were aseptic, three were hemorrhagic, and one had isolated increased pressure. Of the seven LPs performed because of cerebral abscess, three were normal, one was purulent, and three were aseptic. Of the nine hemorrhagic CSF, there were six proven or suspected intracranial mycotic aneurysms and three hemorrhagic transformations of cerebral infarcts. Eleven of the 19 patients with purulent CSF formula had meningitis due to virulent bacteria, but seven had embolism and three had brain abscesses (221). Thus, neither the clinical setting nor any of the neurologic events were associated with a specific CSF formula, except for finding a purulent CSF more frequently in patients with meningeal signs. However, there was a good correlation between the CSF findings and the nature of the infecting microorganisms, in that virulent bacteria such as *S. aureus,* enteric gram-negative bacilli, and *S. pneumoniae* were frequently associated with purulent CSF, whereas relatively avirulent bacteria such as viridans streptococci were usually associated with a normal or aseptic CSF. Positive culture of the CSF was found in only 11 of these 69 patients and was associated with purulent formula in all cases. There were eight cases of *S. aureus* and one case each of *S. pneumoniae, Proteus mirabilis,* and viridans streptococci. The findings of this series are similar to those of other studies (218,223). Occasionally, a CSF with an aseptic pattern will yield a pathogen, such as a viridans streptococcus (291,292). Conversely, purulent meningitis may be seen with organisms of low virulence, such as *Cardiobacterium hominis* (293).

Before the advent of the CT scan, CSF examination was useful to detect the presence of hemorrhage. This is still the case if high-quality CT is not available or if motion artifact precludes adequate study (294). However, it should be noted that CSF may be normal in the presence of an intracerebral hematoma (218).

The utility of CSF findings depends upon the circumstances which surround the lumbar puncture. When an LP is obtained on admission in a patient with stroke and fever, an abnormal CSF may be the first clue leading to the diagnosis of IE. Although some authors suggest that LP should be part of the routine evaluation of patients with suspected cerebral embolism of cardiac origin (295,296), others do not recommend it because the yield would be less than 0.25% (294,297). Moreover, it should be remembered that patients with septic cerebral infarcts or even brain abscess may have normal CSF (221). On the other hand, in a patient with suspected IE and neurologic manifestations (e.g., those under age 40, known drug abusers, those with prosthetic valves), CSF examination may help in deciding whether or not to start empiric treatment before the result of blood cultures. For the appropriate management of patients, the clinical course of the patient and careful use of the CT scan are better guides than the CSF findings (221).

Radiological Imaging

CT scan is very useful for the diagnosis and management of CNS disorders associated with IE. Of 51 CT scans performed in 64 patients with neurologic complications of IE, 25 were abnormal. Focal lesions were discovered in five patients who presented with no focal signs, but encephalopathy or headache as present. It was most helpful to establish the nature of the focal lesions (223). CT scan also appears promising for selecting patients with neurologic manifestations for whom angiography should be performed to exclude ICMAs. In a study comparing CT scan and angiography in 34 patients with IE and neurologic signs or symptoms, no mycotic aneurysm was found among 14 patients with a normal CT scan, whereas ICMAs were found in 11 of the 20 patients with abnormal findings (298). The exact place of CT scan for this indication awaits further prospective study.

Magnetic resonance imaging (MRI) appears promising for the diagnosis of encephalopathy due to multiple microinfarcts and microabscesses which cannot be visualized with the CT scan (171).

Overall Outcome

The overall mortality of patients with IE has decreased over the past 30 years, mostly due to the development of valve replacement. However, the mortality of patients with IE and neurologic complications has not changed appreciably, ranging from 41% to 67% (35,156, 217,218,221,299). Two recent large studies report lower rates of only 20% (24,223). A mortality rate of 83% has been reported in patients with IE referred to an intensive care unit (ICU) (228). Patients with IE who develop CNS complications have a higher overall mortality rate than do those without such complications, although this has not been found in all series (223). In series which have compared rates in patients with native valve IE, mortality occurred in 41–86% of patients with CNS involve-

ment, a rate significantly higher than the 8–32% observed in those without CNS complications (156,221, 228,299,300). Surgical treatment of IE does not appear to increase the CNS-related mortality of IE: Of 108 consecutive patients with native valve IE who underwent valve replacement, discriminant regression analysis did not reveal CNS emboli prior to surgery to be a predictor of an increased mortality (301). In patients with PVE, the overall mortality was affected by the presence of neurologic complications in some studies (243,248) but not in others (25,302). When present, CNS complications are thought to be the direct cause of death in a percentage of cases which varies greatly, and figures as low as 22% (221) and as high as 75% have been reported (228). In one study, only one of 28 deaths among 175 patients with IE was considered to be directly related to the neurologic complication (223). This variation is most likely due to referral bias [e.g., in studies from ICUs (228)] or to criteria used for definition. When only major cerebral events are considered, they are found to be the direct cause (and often the only cause) of death in over 50% of the cases who die, both in native valve and in prosthetic valve IE (25,156,218,228,243,248). In a number of cases, death is multifactorial. Neurologic complications were directly responsible for 8–20% of the deaths in patients with native valve IE (24,35,156,221) and for 10–40% in those with prosthetic valve IE (25,243–245,247). In one series, neurologic death accounted for 33% of the deaths in late PVE but accounted for only 8% of those in early PVE (25). The type of microorganism involved appears to play an important role in the outcome of patients with IE and neurologic complications, with *S. aureus*, Enterobacteriaceae, and fungi being associated with a higher mortality (221,223,278,279). Obviously, some neurologic complications such as major emboli, intracranial hemorrhage, or purulent meningitis are associated with higher mortality rates than are the less severe manifestations (217). Sequelae have been noted in up to 34% of the patients with neurologic complications who survived (222).

Cerebral Emboli

Incidence

Cardiogenic emboli are responsible for 11–23% of the strokes observed in the general population (303,304). Emboli secondary to IE account for only a small proportion of these episodes. Among 130 patients with cerebral embolism seen between 1952 and 1963, six (4.6%) were found to have IE (305). In another study, IE accounted for only 3% of cerebral emboli (306). In the stroke registry of the Cerebral Embolism Study Group, IE was the cause of ischemic stroke in less than 1% of the cases (294). The rate of CNS embolism due to IE is higher in autopsy series: For example, IE was found in 69 of 4558 autopsies (1.5%) but was present in 32 of the 126 (25%) patients with cardiogenic cerebral emboli (227). Occlusion of cerebral arteries by emboli is the most common neurologic complication of IE and accounts for approximately half of these complications. It is observed in 6–31% of patients with IE (36,218,221,223,283,307). Approximately half of the patients who present with major or minor cerebral embolism have emboli that are clinically identifiable to other organs as well (221). In contrast, evidence of systemic emboli was found in only 2% of unselected patients with stroke (308). In patients with IE and systemic emboli, cerebral emboli were also found in 40% of them (221). It has been observed that the incidence of cerebral emboli associated with IE of the mitral valve was higher than when the aortic valve was involved, despite a similar rate of peripheral emboli elsewhere (221). Except for the rare occurrence of paradoxical embolism (240,288), emboli are associated with lesions of the left side of the heart. Although some studies have shown a high frequency of emboli in patients with PVE, no significant difference in the incidence of cerebral emboli has been noted in a recent series which has compared native (15%) versus prosthetic (20%) valve IE (223).

Pathogenesis

Most emboli related to IE are a result of (a) the disruption of cardiac vegetations into fragments and (b) the subsequent lodgment of these fragments into peripheral vessels of various diameters, depending on size. Occasionally, emboli may be related to other concomitant disorders, such as atrial arrythmias. Vegetations are the result of complex interactions between various host components (such as fibrin, platelets, fibroblasts, and inflammatory cells) and microbial factors (such as growth rate, adhesion, and production of extracellular proteases). These interactions influence the growth of the vegetation and the frequency of embolic episodes (80). Experimentally, the proteolytic capacity of the infecting organism was shown to influence the size of the vegetations and the course of the disease. In rabbits with IE induced with 10 different strains of *E. faecalis,* proteolytic strains caused smaller vegetations with a soft and friable appearance, as well as an increased frequency of renal emboli, when compared to nonproteolytic strains (309). In humans, IE due to virulent microorganisms, particularly *S. aureus,* is associated with an increased frequency of systemic (16) and cerebral emboli (221,223), as compared to less virulent bacteria such as viridans streptococci. In a study of 52 patients with PVE, the calculated rate of stroke during uncontrolled infection ranged from 1% per day for nonvirulent streptococci to 9% per day for *S. aureus* (254). Pathologic examination provides some explanation for this difference: The valvular vegetations of

IE due to virulent bacteria are friable with no histological evidence of healing, whereas in subacute disease, lesions progress more slowly with evidence of fibrotic reaction and early healing (226). In addition, certain microorganisms have been noted to produce large and mobile vegetations and are associated with an increased propensity to be complicated by major systemic and cerebral embolism. This has been described in IE due to microorganisms such as *Haemophilus* species (121) or other slow-growing, fastidious gram-negative rods (276), nutritionally variant viridans streptococci (58,202), group B beta-hemolytic streptococci (310), and fungi (especially *Aspergillus* species) (279). Occlusion of vessels by fragments of vegetations results in various degrees of ischemia and infarction depending on the vessels involved and the collateral blood flow. In addition, emboli occurring before the initiation or the completion of a successful antibiotic treatment may contain microorganisms capable of producing secondary infectious complications, such as abscesses of variable sizes, meningitis, artcritis, or mycotic aneurysms. In about 20% of the cerebrovascular episodes, hemorrhagic complications are observed (218). They may be due to the infarction itself, or to the erosion of the artery by the bacteria present in the emboli, with or without formation of a detectable mycotic aneurysm (259). Concomitant anticoagulation appears to increase the risk of developing major hemorrhages at the sites of infarction (221). However, in patients with PVE, withholding anticoagulation has resulted in high rates of thromboembolic phenomena (219,244), and adequate anticoagulation has been shown to reduce the incidence of major CNS events (244).

As previously mentioned, macroscopic and microscopic cerebral emboli occurred with greater frequency in patients with mitral valve infection as opposed to those with aortic valve involvement in two studies (221,228), but this was not found in another large series (223). Pathologic examination of operative or autopsy material shows that vegetations are not always found in patients who had an embolic episode: Of 76 valves examined, a valvular vegetation was found in only 57% of patients with neurologic complications. Moreover, vegetations were found in 61% of the patients without such complications (223).

Thus, although emboli may be observed in any case of IE, they tend to be more frequent or larger with certain microorganisms. This will determine the rate, the type, and the severity of the distant complications, including those of the CNS.

Clinical Presentation

Cerebral embolism associated with IE may present with protean clinical manifestations. One important determinant of the symptomatology is the number and the size of the emboli. Some patients may present with embolic occlusion of a single major cerebral artery, with symptomatology related to the territory involved. Other patients may have multiple microemboli, with a more diverse clinical presentation. In many patients, these two forms of emboli coexist (221).

Major cerebral embolism was the presenting symptom and the first overt manifestation of IE in 22 of 218 patients (10%) (221), and in 12 of 86 patients (14%) (228) in two large series. Cerebral emboli occurring early in the course of IE tend to be associated with infection due to virulent organisms, particularly *S. aureus* (221). Because of the more subacute presentation of IE due to streptococci, emboli occur later in the course of the disease (221). The majority of the cerebral emboli occur before the initiation of antibiotic treatment or during the first weeks of therapy, at a time when the blood cultures are still positive (221,310a). Thus, among 30 episodes of stroke observed in 175 patients with IE, 12 occurred after the initiation of antibiotic treatment; the median time interval from onset of antibiotic treatment to development of neurologic complications was 4 days, with a range of 1–21 days (223). Two studies on the value of echocardiography in 105 and 77 consecutive patients with IE reported that 48–88% of embolic episodes, respectively, occurred after the procedure was performed, and therefore while the patients were presumably on antibiotic treatment (160,311). Embolization after the completion of successful antibiotic treatment is rare, but it has been described and can possibly occur up to 2 years later (221). More than 90% of the large cerebral emboli affect the middle cerebral arteries and their branches, leading mainly to contralateral hemiparesis and/or hemisensory deficit. It may also produce parietal lobe signs of sensory loss, neglect, dyspraxia, hemianopia, and, when the dominant hemisphere is involved, aphasia (231). Occlusion of anterior or posterior cerebral arteries may also produce similar symptoms, especially those involving the lower extremities (231). Posterior cerebral artery occlusion may produce homonymous hemianopia. Retinal artery emboli may cause unilateral blindness. When the vascular supply of the basal ganglia is affected, patients may develop tremor, parkinsonism, or chorea (231,283). The vertebral basilar system was affected in six of 10 and four of 84 patients with CNS complications of IE in two series (218,221). Brainstem lesions can cause dysphagia, hiccups, or vomiting (231). Emboli in the vascular supply of the spinal cord or peripheral nerves may also occur (288).

Transient ischemic attacks (TIAs) are occasionally noted and may be the presenting manifestation of IE. Such episodes were recorded in 15 of 55 patients (27%) with strokes associated with IE (218). Most of the TIA episodes occurred within hours or days before the final stroke, which was an infarct in 12 cases and a hemorrhage in three cases. Multiple episodes can occur (258).

In a study of 12 patients with IE and TIAs, seven ultimately developed permanent lesions. It should be noted that the initial TIA predicted the site of the subsequent permanent lesions in only three of the seven cases. Four of the 12 patients sustained a fatal intracerebral hemorrhage (258). In a patient with TIA, the presence of fever or of any other nonspecific signs of infection should raise the possibility of IE. Some of these patients may present with fluctuating neurologic signs, presumably from emboli that disintegrate after initial lodgment, and autopsy may reveal multiple small or microscopic infarcts (258).

Multiple cerebral microemboli are not infrequent. Of 45 patients autopsied because of a fatal neurologic complication, 38 had major embolism, but 23 were found to also have microscopic cerebral infarcts, presumably due to embolic occlusion of small vessels. Six also had microabscesses. These findings correlated with seizures or fluctuating neurologic signs in four patients and were clinically silent in four others. In 14 patients, multiple microscopic infarcts manifested as an altered level of consciousness not adequately explained by other abnormalities (221). Similarly, symptoms of acute or toxic encephalopathy (also called "acute brain syndrome") were reported in 21 of 110 patients of another series (218) and were the second most common neurologic manifestations of IE. They were the initial or presenting manifestations of IE in nine of these patients (218). Decreased level of consciousness, fluctuating confusion, disorientation, apathy, irritability, delirium, hallucinations, and paranoid ideation were the most common findings and were severe enough in a few patients to lead to direct psychiatric admission (218). In elderly patients, confusion, often without fever, was the presenting sign of IE in 26% of the patients in one recent series (36). It is likely, at least in some of these patients, that the basic pathophysiological mechanism was multiple microemboli, resulting in multifocal microinfarcts, sometimes associated with microabscesses (300). Thus, microabscesses were found in six of 23 patients with multiple microinfarcts at autopsy (221), demonstrating that a continuum exists between the ischemic cerebrovascular and infective complications of IE (300).

Thus, emboli may cause a wide variety of CNS symptoms and signs, ranging from hemiplegia to diffuse and fluctuating neurologic dysfunction, depending on their size, location, and number. Most emboli occur before or soon after the initiation of therapy (223).

Diagnostic Procedures

Cerebral CT scan is the most useful diagnostic procedure when emboli are suspected. It is helpful both in the differential diagnosis with other disorders and in the distinction between nonhemorrhagic and hemorrhagic infarcts (Fig. 3). It also provides a baseline in monitoring

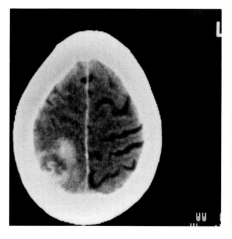 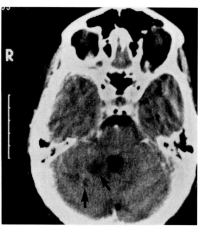

FIG. 3. Head CT scan of a patient with *S. mitis* aortic endocarditis. Right parietal hemorrhagic infarct and multiple nonhemorrhagic infarcts of the right cerebellar hemisphere (*arrows*). (Courtesy of Antoine Uske, M.D.)

for the development of ICMA which may arise at the site of a previous embolus. Follow-up studies are also indicated when the secondary formation of an abscess is suspected.

If not contraindicated by the result of the CT-scan examination or for other reasons, a lumbar puncture may be performed. If IE has already been recognized, the CSF examination may be useful in excluding an associated septic meningitis, but these findings are not likely to alter the management of the patient. In contrast, a CSF leukocytosis may be the first hint suggesting the possibility of IE in certain patients with stroke, particularly if predisposing factors for endocarditis are present. However, this does not appear to justify routine CSF examination in unselected patients with stroke, because the yield might not be greater than 0.25% (294). Moreover, normal CSF values do not exclude that CNS emboli originating from IE. Of 69 patients (including 42 with emboli) with LP performed in the context of neurologic complications of IE, 21 had normal CSF values, 18 of which had embolism. Conversely, among 42 LPs performed for embolism, 18 were normal, 13 were aseptic, seven were purulent, three were hemorrhagic, and one had increased pressure (221). In another study, 16 patients with cerebral infarcts had an examination of the CSF. The spinal fluid was normal in three, and in 13 patients there were slight elevations in protein (but up to 750 mg/liter) and in cell counts (less than 300 per cubic millimeter for either lymphocytes or polymorphonuclear cells) (218). This indicates that CSF findings usually do not help in confirming or excluding a cerebral embolism related to IE.

In order to exclude hemorrhagic transformation of a cerebral infarct, high-quality CT is a better procedure than CSF examination: Some patients with such a complication on CT may have normal CSF (312) or CSF with only a few red blood cells (RBCs) (313). Furthermore, a few RBCs are often present in the CSF in nonhemorrhagic infarcts due to traumatic taps. RBC counts of more than 500 per cubic millimeter appear to have a greater specificity for hemorrhagic infarct, but the exact timing of appearance of RBCs in the CSF is not established (297). Moreover, CT allows us to judge on the extent of the hemorrhagic transformation and on the potential indication for surgery. In anticoagulated patients, LP carries the risk of complications, deemed major in 6% of one series, with spinal hematoma and paresis occurring in 0.6–1.5% of the patients (312). However, if high-quality CT is not available or motion artifact precludes adequate study, CSF examination may be considered in these patients.

The role of MRI is not yet fully determined, but it is likely that it will be helpful in establishing the presence of microinfarcts or microabscesses in patients with signs of encephalopathy, thus allowing differential diagnosis from other causes (171).

Specific Management

Cardiac Surgery

In the management of patients with IE and cerebral emboli, several aspects should be considered—namely, the primary prevention of emboli, the prevention of new episodes, the optimal therapeutical strategy for the already established lesions, and the detection of secondary complications (Fig. 4).

The role of cardiac surgery in the prevention of embolism in IE is ill-defined, although many would accept recurrent embolism as an indication for valvular replacement.

There is no specific therapy for the already established lesions. Efforts should be directed at adequate control of arterial blood pressure and supportive care. Patients should be carefully followed clinically for the occurrence of secondary hemorrhage, and CT should be performed promptly if the patient's condition deteriorates. CT scan and angiography are recomended 1–2 weeks after the embolic episode in order to exclude the secondary for-

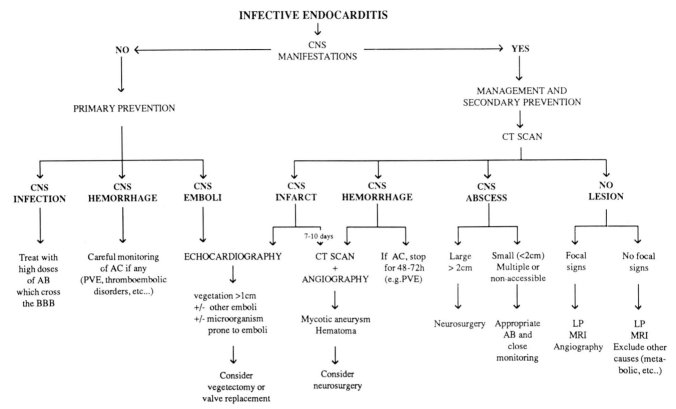

FIG. 4. Prevention and management of CNS complications of infective endocarditis. AB: antibiotics; AC: anticoagulation; BBB: blood brain barrier; PVE: prosthetic valve endocarditis; LP: lumbar puncture; MRI: magnetic resonance imaging.

mation of an abscess or an ICMA (282). A recent study comparing CT scan and angiography suggests that ICMA is unlikely to be present when the CT scan is normal (298).

Types of IE due to certain microorganisms are known for complication by embolism, but only fungal IE and some forms of PVE constitute a recognized indication for surgery even in the absence of emboli or other complications. This is not so much to prevent embolism but to avoid the high failure rate associated with medical therapy alone (279,314). The appropriate use of valvular replacement in patients who have sustained a single embolic event and/or who have a large vegetation demonstrated by echocardiography is not clear. Recurrent emboli are infrequent in patients who survive a first embolic episode and who are receiving appropriate antibiotics. Indeed, among seven survivors of 37 patients with major cerebral embolic infarction reported from the Massachusetts General Hospital, none suffered recurrent embolization after completion of therapy (221). Of 110 patients with neurologic complications reported from the Mayo Clinic, only two experienced temporally and anatomically distinct cerebrovascular accidents (218). In a more recent series of 113 patients with native valve IE and 62 with PVE, only two recurrent events were noted. In both cases a TIA preceded a stroke, and

this occurred before the patient had been started on antibiotic treatment. Both had mechanical valves and were anticoagulated (223). Thus, recurrent ischemic episodes during acute illness are rare when the patient is on appropriate antibiotic therapy. Although late embolic events after a cured episode of native valve IE have been reported (221,223,281,315), they appear to be rare, to occur late, and to be best explained by factors other than the past episode of IE (223). When considering surgery solely for prevention of recurrent emboli, both the operative and the late risks associated with prosthetic valves should be carefully balanced against the potential benefit. Vegetation excision without valve replacement deserves further investigation in patients with embolic complications (275,316,317).

Patients undergoing open heart surgery after a recent CNS complication pose a difficult management problem. There is always a risk that cardiopulmonary bypass and heparinization may exacerbate the neurologic injury (318–321). On the other hand, delay in surgery can have serious CNS consequences depending on the surgical indication: Worsening neurologic symptoms can result from hypotension, hypoxemia, low cardiac output, and renal failure. Moreover, further embolization may occur, especially with microorganisms such as *S. aureus,* gram-negative bacilli, or fungi. In a recent study, 15 patients (14 with IE) who underwent open heart surgery following a recent neurologic injury were analyzed. Before operation, 12 had focal neurologic deficits (among whom three were comatose), whereas three patients had no focal signs (the three were comatose). Twelve of the patients had embolic cerebral infarctions, and two had evidence of intracranial hemorrhage. They were operated on 2–28 days (mean 12.7 days) after the neurologic injury. None had worsening of their neurologic symptoms postoperatively. Six improved and eight had complete neurologic recovery, whereas one died 7 days after surgery from sepsis and multisystem organ failure. The authors concluded that although there is always a risk of infarct extension secondary to hemorrhage, early surgery may be safely performed in a high percentage of patients. This may even contribute to the improvement of the neurologic symptoms by improving the hemodynamic situation (322). Similar favorable experience has been reported by others (323,324). Moreover, among 108 cases of IE treated surgically, preoperative stroke was not found to be a predictor of hospital mortality (187).

Thus, when there is a clear indication for valvular surgery, the presence of a neurologic event does not appear to justify postponement of the procedure. However, because anticoagulation may precipitate hemorrhagic transformation of cerebral infarcts if administered during the first few hours after the episode (325), it would appear reasonable to postpone the operation for 48–72 hours if feasible.

Echocardiography

The value of echocardiography in assessing the degree of valvular change and the status of left ventricular function is well established (188). However, the role of this technique in predicting the risk of embolization is controversial. Moreover, most of the studies do not address the specific problem of embolism to the brain. As already mentioned, vegetations of a size that can be visualized by precordial echocardiography are detected in about 60% of cases of IE by M-mode and in 70–80% of the cases when using combined M-mode and two-dimensional imaging. Transesophageal echocardiogram has been reported as detecting vegetations in up to 96% of cases of proven IE (160,161,326). In addition, the latter technique allows a better visualization of vegetations in patients with PVE. However, false-positive diagnosis can occur with both precordial and transesophageal echocardiography. Thus, nodular thickening, rupture of a valve leaflet, or rupture of chordae tendineae can simulate a valvular vegetation. Many reports suggest that in patients with IE, vegetations detected by precordial M-mode and cross-sectional echocardiography are associated with a higher risk of embolization (163,327–330). In a composite of 11 studies, the risk was 36% with echo-

cardiographically demonstrated vegetations and 15% when echocardiograms were normal (311). However, no significant difference in the overall incidence of embolism was found in a study of 77 patients, in which chart compilation and echocardiography readings were performed by separate investigators who had no knowledge of each others' findings (311). This negative result was not related to the timing of echocardiography, because the embolic episode occurred *after* the procedure in all but two patients (one with vegetations and one without them). However, patients with vegetations larger than 10 mm had a rate of embolism of 53%, compared to 16% for those with vegetations smaller than 10 mm—a difference which is statistically significant, although not mentioned by the authors (311). In a more recent study specifically addressing the problem of neurologic complications of IE, vegetations seen on echocardiography were present in 37% of the patients with neurologic complications and in 28% of those without neurologic complications—a difference which was not statistically significant. However, in patients developing neurologic complications after initiation of antibiotic therapy, vegetations were seen on initial echography in 56%. Therefore, in some cases presenting with neurologic complications, it is possible that vegetations were not seen because of embolization prior to echocardiography (223)—a well-documented phenomenon (331). In a recent study which has used both transthoracic and transesophageal echocardiography, patients with large vegetations (>10 mm) had a significantly higher incidence of embolic events (47%) than did those with small or no vegetations (19%). Because an embolic event may reduce the size of vegetations, the analysis was also made after exclusion of the patients who had echocardiography after the embolic episode; the rate of new embolism was 36% in patients with large vegetations, compared to 6% in those with small vegetations—a difference which was also significant. The average size of the vegetations of the patients who presented with an embolic episode following echocardiography was larger than that of patients without embolism. Patients with "mobile" vegetations had a significantly higher incidence of embolic episodes than did patients with "sessile" vegetations; however, this was not an independent variable, because most of the patients with large vegetations also had mobile vegetations. In contrast, mobile vegetations were seen in less than 50% of those with small vegetations. Patients with large vegetations of the mitral valve were at a significantly higher risk of embolism (160). Mural vegetations might be at increased risk of embolization (164).

Overall, most (but not all) studies suggest that vegetations seen on echocardiography, especially those larger than 10 mm (160,163a,311) are associated with a higher risk of embolism. However, many patients with vegetations, even of large size, do not manifest clinically detectable emboli, and vegetations may persist on echocardiography after successful medical therapy. Moreover, recurrent emboli to the brain are rare. On the other hand, the presence of a vegetation on echocardiography has also been correlated with an increased risk of congestive heart failure (327), particularly large vegetations involving the aortic valve (332). Thus, many patients with large vegetations may actually be operated upon for a combination of indications; moreover, the natural course of patients with large vegetations can only be partially assessed, because patients may undergo surgery before a potential embolic event. Further prospective data are required before management decisions can be based on the presence and size of vegetations. Given the operative and postoperative risk of prosthetic valves, it seems reasonable not to operate on a patient solely because of the presence of a large vegetation. This point of view might change with the advent of valve repair surgery, which does not carry the long-term risk of prosthetic valves.

Anticoagulants

Because of the critical role played by the platelet–fibrin thrombus in the formation of the vegetations, antiplatelet agents may have a role in preventing subsequent embolization, but thus far there has been no clinical study which has addressed this issue.

The proper use of anticoagulants has given rise to much controversy. Soon after the advent of sulfonamides in the 1930s and antibiotics in the 1940s, simultaneous treatment with heparin was tried with the idea that prevention of further deposition of platelet–fibrin thrombi on infected valves would favor antibiotic penetration (333) and would possibly prevent further emboli (334). It soon became apparent that antibiotics alone were able to cure IE, and that there was no evidence that anticoagulants were a useful adjunct for the efficacy of antibiotic therapy (334). Moreover, cerebral hemorrhages were observed with a distressing frequency in anticoagulated patients (335–337), and major emboli were not prevented (334). It should be noted, however, that the antibiotic therapy was inadequate according to presently recommended regimens. In a more recent series, seven patients with cerebral emboli were subjected to anticoagulation before or within 24 hr of embolization. Three of them (43%) developed major intracranial hemorrhages at the sites of infarction. In contrast, intracranial hemorrhage was observed in only 10 of 211 patients (4.7%) not treated with anticoagulants (221). This deleterious effect of anticoagulants is also supported by experimental evidence. In an animal model of septic brain embolism, anticoagulation was associated with an increased risk of hemorrhage (338). In experimental endocarditis, animals simultaneously treated with antibiotics and anticoagulants had a worse course than those who received only antibiotics (339,340). Therefore, it is generally believed that the routine use of anticoagulants is not recommended in the course of native valve IE because clinical and experimental data indicate that the rate of hemorrhagic CNS complications is high, and because there is no proven benefit with regard to the course of the disease (303,304,341). However, some authors recently stated that "they have used anticoagulant agents cautiously and successfully to prevent recurrent emboli in patients with IE" (342). Moreover, in some patients with special indications, such as mitral valve disease and atrial fibrillation of recent onset, appropriate anticoagulant therapy should probably not be withheld (343).

The issue of anticoagulant therapy in patients with PVE should be considered separately. With the exception of those patients with bioprostheses and normal sinus rhythm, patients with prosthetic valves are at constant risk of thromboembolism and there are important reasons not to interrupt anticoagulant therapy. Patients who develop PVE are at high risk of presenting both thromboembolic and hemorrhagic complications, and the indication for the maintenance or interruption of the anticoagulation therapy should be carefully balanced. In patients with PVE and not taking an anticoagulant, the incidence of CNS thromboembolic phenomena has ranged from approximately 50% to 71% (219,244,344). An incidence of CNS hemorrhage as high as 36% has been reported in a series of patients with PVE treated with anticoagulants (245). In another study, 12 of 42 patients with late PVE and receiving anticoagulants developed major CNS events, and eight died. Five of these deaths were the direct result of massive intracerebral hemorrhage or hemorrhagic infarcts. However, in three of these five patients, the prothrombin time exceeded twice the normal value at the time of the CNS event (243). In a recent study of 20 patients with late PVE, eight (40%) presented neurologic complications, three of which were fatal intracranial hemorrhage. The prothrombin times at the time of the intracranial hemorrhage were 2.2, 1.5, and 1.3 times control in these three patients (250). In a study of 48 patients with PVE, 15 (31%) had clinical evidence of neurologic complications, which was consistent with emboli in 14. All were receiving warfarin sodium at the time of the neurologic event, but prothrombin times did not correlate with the amount of hemorrhage associated with embolic lesions (25). In a series comparing patients with PVE and receiving or not receiving anticoagulants, major CNS complications occurred in three of 38 patients (8%) who received adequate anticoagulant therapy, as compared to 10 of 14 (71%) of those who received either inadequate or no anticoagulation. Mortality was 47% among the patients with adequate anticoagulants and 57% among those without. Among the patients treated adequately with anticoagulants, three deaths occurred; all were due to the CNS injury, but only one was attributed directly to the anticoagulant therapy. Among the patients without adequate anticoagulation, eight deaths were recorded, and CNS complications were thought to be the primary cause of death in five of them. Three of these patients were found to have massive intracerebral bleeding caused by thromboembolism (244). In another rather disturbing study, 30 patients who were initially anticoagulated (with prosthetic valves in 29), were analyzed. Among the 20 who had their anticoagulation continued, seven developed a stroke (six bland infarct, one hematoma); anticoagulation was continued in four of them without further complication. In contrast, only one stroke was observed in the 10 patients in whom anticoagulation was stopped (223).

Based on these various conflicting data, most authors suggest that closely monitored anticoagulant therapy should be cautiously continued in patients with IE of mechanical prosthetic valves (58,244,248,250,343,345). Although coumarin drugs are generally used, favorable experience with heparin has recently been reported (248). If the patient develops a CNS complication, the use of anticoagulants should be temporarily discontinued; in addition, the patient should be evaluated for evidence of intracranial hemorrhage. If there is no evidence of hemorrhage or hemorrhagic infarct, carefully controlled anticoagulation may be reinstituted (244). In one of the above studies, the onset of CNS complications occurred only 7–23 days (mean 17 days) after the discontinuation of anticoagulants (244), and thus a short interruption does not appear to carry a great risk of thromboembolism. Since hemorrhagic transformation of an infarct has been associated with early initiation of anticoagulant therapy after cardioembolic stroke (<12 hr) (325), a delay of 48–72 hr between the neurologic event and the reintroduction of anticoagulant therapy seems reasonable (244).

Outcome

The mortality rate of patients with IE and CNS emboli, when specifically reported, ranges from 33% to 81%. A large proportion of these deaths are directly related to the neurologic injury (217,218,221,228,307). The mortality is particularly high in the case of hemorrhagic transformation, since it may occur in patients who are anticoagulated at the time of the embolic episode (221,223,243,244). However, in the absence of emboli, most authors feel that this should not preclude the use of adequate anticoagulation in patients with mechanical PVE, because of the high risk of embolization if anticoagulant therapy is stopped.

Conclusion

In conclusion, cerebral emboli are one of the major complications of IE, especially when caused by certain microorganisms such as *S. aureus*. Emboli may cause further complications such as meningitis, abscesses, hemorrhages, and mycotic aneurysm. In order to detect these secondary complications, CT scan and possibly angiography should be performed after the embolic episode. For these complications to be detectable, investigations are best carried out 7–10 days after the embolic event. Although large vegetations seen on echocardiography seem to be associated with an increased risk of emboli, the precise role of valvular surgery for this indication is not yet determined, except for a few situations such as fungal IE or recurrent emboli where surgery appears to be clearly indicated.

In patients with PVE, anticoagulation should not be interrupted but must be carefully monitored. Should a CNS embolic episode occur, the anticoagulant therapy should be interrupted and reintroduced 48–72 hr later if there is no evidence of hemorrhage.

Intracranial Hemorrhage

Intracranial hemorrhage (ICH) occurs in 3–6% of cases of IE (218,221,223). In selected populations of patients with IE, such as those hospitalized in an ICU, a rate of 18% for ICH has been reported (228). Although the criteria and type of investigations used in these studies are often variable and ill-defined, the rates usually refer to clinically significant episodes. In a study in which ICH was defined by CT scan and CSF findings, 17 of 209 patients (8%) with IE were found to have ICH (259). The hemorrhage usually diffuses into the cerebral substance or into the subarachnoid space (346). Rarely, the subdural space may also be involved (347).

ICH complicating IE may be the result of different mechanisms. ICH have often been attributed to ruptured ICMA, even when no aneurysms were demonstrable (218,221). In addition to ruptured ICMA, it has recently been recognized that ICH in IE can also result from the septic erosion of the arterial wall without a well-delineated aneurysm (259,348). Moreover, hemorrhagic transformation of ischemic brain infarcts can also result in ICH, particularly in anticoagulated patients (221,325). Thus, three of seven anticoagulated patients with IE and emboli developed major ICH, as compared to only 10 of 211 patients with IE but not receiving anticoagulants (221).

The proportion of ICH attributable to each mechanism varies among studies. Of the 17 patients with ICH studied by Hart et al. (259), four presented a hemorrhagic infarct and 13 had a primary hemorrhage which could be attributed to a ruptured ICMA in only two cases and to a necrotic arteritis in four cases. In five other cases, an ICMA was excluded by arteriography or autopsy, and the exact cause of ICH was not determined. In four other studies the proportion of ICH due to ICMA ranged from 26% to 40% (218,221,223,228). Thus, only a third of ICH in IE are attributable to ruptured ICMA. Septic necrosis of the arterial wall and hemorrhagic transformation of cerebral infarcts each account for another third of the cases (221,223,259). Whatever mechanism is involved in the pathogenesis of ICH, the prognosis is poor, with a mortality of 35–87% (228,259).

ICH Due to Cerebral Emboli

Aseptic cardioembolic strokes may undergo some degree of spontaneous hemorrhagic transformation, even in the absence of anticoagulation; pathologic examination reveals that this occurs in the majority of the episodes (349,350). This results from multifocal extravasations of confluent petechiae and is usually not associated with recognized clinical worsening. About 5% of the patients with embolic stroke who are not receiving anticoagulants have hemorrhagic infarcts visible on initial, early CT scan, with an additional 10–20% developing late, usually asymptomatic, hemorrhagic transformation (325). The likelihood of developing spontaneous hemorrhagic transformation appears to be directly related to infarct size (351,352). Although exact figures are not available, hemorrhagic transformation seems to occur in 6–24% of cerebral infarcts associated with NVE (218,221,228) and in 8–36% of those with PVE (243–245,250). Hemorrhage can be massive in patients receiving anticoagulant therapy for arrythmia or for a mechanical prosthetic valve (221,223,243–245,250,259). Experimental evidence suggests that the worsening role of anticoagulants may be particularly pronounced when the cerebral embolus is septic (338).

ICH Due to Acute Necrotizing Arteritis or Due to ICMA

The spectrum of arterial injury leading to ICH can range from acute, pyogenic necrosis to large, aseptic aneurysms that may rupture weeks to months after bacteriological cure. The extremes of this continuum appear to represent different clinical syndromes, although the term "mycotic aneurysm" has usually been applied to both processes (259). For the purpose of clarity, true ICMA will be considered separately (see below).

Septic emboli appear to be necessary for the occurrence of septic arteritis and ICH, although clinically recognized embolism precedes ICH in only a fraction of the patients. Sustained bacteremia in tricuspid valve IE, even with virulent bacteria, does not result in ICH, supporting the necessity of systemic embolic fragments (259). The precise sequence of events leading to ICH was demonstrated in a patient who died from a massive subarachnoid hemorrhage secondary to an erosive arteritis which developed at the site of a septic embolus visualized both at autopsy and on an arteriogram performed a few days before death (353).

Most ICHs due to acute erosive arteritis tend to occur early in the course of the disease and are often already present on admission. They are more likely to occur in *S. aureus* IE (228,259,341), although this microorganism can also be associated with the development of true ICMA at a later stage (221,351,354,355). ICH may also complicate IE due to *S. epidermidis, Streptococcus* species, or other bacteria (259,346). Most of these patients have an acute form of IE of only a few days' duration and present severe and rapidly evolving neurologic signs which are related to the site of the intracerebral or subarachnoid hemorrhage (259). ICH may be the presenting manifestation of IE (259,346). Some patients have a preceding episode of clinical embolus or of TIA (258,259). For example, four of 12 patients with IE and TIA subsequently sustained a fatal ICH (258).

CT scan obviously plays a central role in the evaluation and management of these patients (Figs. 4 and 5). Arteriography allows the precise location of the arterial rupture, and it also allows the visualization of associated ICMA and of the anatomy of the intracranial vessels. This may be particularly helpful in patients for whom surgery is considered. Surgical treatment is difficult, requiring sacrifice of the involved artery, sometimes with microvascular pedicle/bypass surgery, since there is not a well-delineated aneurysmal neck that can be readily clipped (259). Mortality may be as high as 87% (228).

Intracranial Mycotic Aneurysm

A "mycotic" aneurysm is a dilatation of the arterial wall due to an infective arteritis which can be caused by almost any microorganism. In order to obviate the confusion with aneurysms of true fungal etiology, some authors have recently suggested that all types of aneurysms due to an infectious agent be grouped under the heading of "infectious aneurysms" (356). Since most of the published literature still uses the term "mycotic" first introduced by William Osler (2–4), this designation is retained in this chapter.

Incidence

ICMAs are uncommon. Although they represented 12–32% of all intracranial aneurysms before the advent of antibiotics (357–359), they appear to constitute only 2.6–6.4% in more recent series (360–363). More than 80% of all ICMAs occur as a complication of IE (363–365). In a review of 85 cases of documented ICMA reported from 1954 to 1977, 72 (85%) were due to IE (365). In patients with IE, the incidence of recognized ICMA ranges from 1.2–5.4% in recent series (221,223,285, 363,366). In older series, incidence rates close to 10% were noted (212,214,215). Since it has been documented that some patients with IE develop intracranial aneurysms which remain asymptomatic and undergo healing under appropriate antibiotic therapy (354,367,368), the

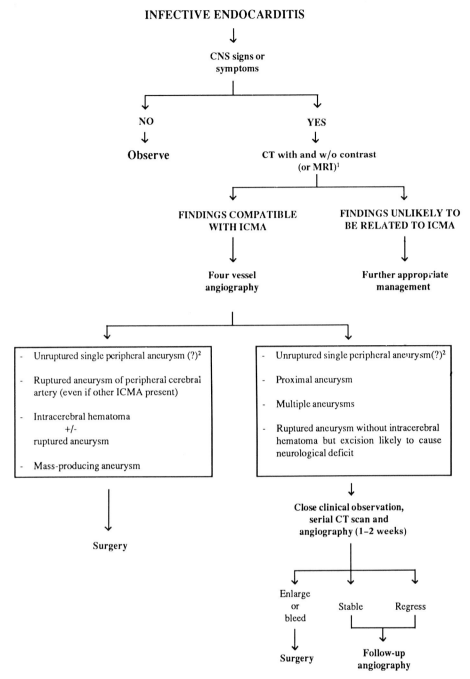

FIG. 5. Management of intracranial mycotic aneurysm. 1) Excepted if acute suarachnoid hemorrhage is suspected. 2) Divergent opinions.

true incidence of mycotic aneurysm certainly exceeds the number of cases diagnosed. This is also suggested by a recent study in which systematic CT scan and four-vessel angiography were performed in patients with endocarditis and neurologic manifestations: 11 of 35 (31%) were found to have ICMA (298).

Multiple aneurysms have been documented in about 20% of the patients with ICMA, but the true figure is unknown because only a few of the reported patients have had full angiography analysis to show all the intracranial vessels (356). In the study just mentioned, five of 11 patients had multiple ICMAs (298).

ICMAs can occur at any age. Almost all reported cases of ICMA linked to IE were observed in patients with native valve infection, but ICMAs clearly also occur in those with PVE (156).

Pathogenesis

ICMAs may develop by a variety of mechanisms. When they occur in the context of IE, they result from septic embolization to the vasa vasorum or to the intraluminal space of the vessel itself. Early observations on mycotic aneurysms indicated that the inflammation affected the adventitia first and then spread inward (369). In experimental studies, ICMAs could be produced in dogs by the injection in the carotid arteries of silicone rubber emboli coated with bacteria. Pathology showed aneurysmal dilatation of the portion of the vessel immediately adjacent to the emboli; microscopically, the vasa vasorum were packed with inflammatory cells and the inflammatory response started first on the adventitial surface, penetrated the muscularis layer, and, in ruptured aneurysms, destroyed the internal elastic membrane and the intima (370). However, peripheral arteries such as those frequently involved in ICMAs are devoid of vasa vasorum, and it was also suggested that bacteria may reach the adventitia via direct penetration through the wall (370,371). Moreover, there have been cases of ICMA developing at the site of a previously documented embolic occlusion (363,372). Thus, both microemboli to the vasa vasorum and direct penetration through the wall of the arteries appear to be possible routes of infection which may result in the formation of a mycotic aneurysm. Interestingly, treatment with an antibiotic to which the bacteria were sensitive did not prevent the development of an aneurysm but prevented early rupture in the experimental dog model (370). This parallels the observation made in humans who might develop ICMA while on appropriate antibiotic therapy (373,374). The arterial wall may rupture at various stages of dilation, depending on the severity of the necrosis, which, in turn, is presumably related to the virulence of the infectious agent. Restoration of the blood flow through the damaged segment by recanalization of the initial septic embolus may contribute to the rupture by increasing the intravascular pressure (375). Infected emboli, not just circulating bacteria, appear to be necessary for the formation of ICMAs, as suggested by the extreme rarity of this complication following a bacteremia not caused by left-sided IE.

Besides septic emboli, other pathogenic mechanisms may sometimes play a role in the occurrence of ICMA. Injury secondary to deposition of immune complexes with subsequent bacterial seeding has also been suggested as a possible pathogenic mechanism (261,376). ICMAs may also result from a thrombophlebitis of the cavernous sinus (365,377,378). Rarely, ICMAs may be of extravascular origin and may be secondary to penetrating head trauma, otitis media, or tuberculous, syphilitic, fungal, or purulent meningitis (364,365,379–383). In the latter situation, the destruction of the vessel appears to be due to the direct extension of the infectious process from the inflamed meninges (384). Superinfection of congenital aneurysm during the course of IE or during transient bacteremia has also been reported (385). This usually involves the vessels of the circle of Willis in elderly individuals (386).

The microbiologic spectrum of ICMAs of intravascular origin reflects that of IE. Alpha-hemolytic and non-hemolytic streptococci as well as staphylococci account for the vast majority of cases, being responsible for 89% of those with positive blood cultures during the period 1954–1977 reviewed by Bohmfalk et al. (365). The rest of the cases are due to various microorganisms such as *Haemophilus* species, *C. hominis, Corynebacterium* species, *Pseudomonas aeruginosa,* bacteria of the HACEK group, or other bacteria (66,367,387,388). Among 10 narcotic addicts with *P. aeruginosa* endocarditis, two had cerebral mycotic aneuryms (28). In some cases, no organisms can be recovered from the blood, as a result of the use of antibiotics. In earlier days, pneumococci were also found and syphilitic aneurysms accounted for 5% of all intracranial aneurysms before the advent of antibiotics. Polymicrobial ICMAs have been reported in drug addicts (389). *S. aureus* appears to be the most common offender in ICMAs associated with thrombophlebitis of the cavernous sinus. ICMAs have been associated with bacterial meningitis due to *S. pneumoniae, N. meningitidis, M. tuberculosis,* and other less common causes of meningitis (384,390–392). True fungal ICMAs have been described either as the result of a concomitant IE or of direct or hematogenous spread from a sinusitis. Most of them were caused by *Aspergillus* species (371,393–396). Cases associated with *Candida* species have been described (397). A unique case of "phytotic" ICMA, due to an "awn" of a grass inflorescence of the genus *Horedum,* has been reported (398).

Pathology

Mycotic aneurysm complicating IE may occur in any artery and at any location. The proportion of mycotic aneurysms which are located in the CNS ranges from 15% to 54%, according to various series (285,364,366, 399,400). After the aorta, it is one of the most common locations (285,364,399).

ICMAs are usually small and may be saccular or fusiform. Most are peripheral to the first bifurcation of a major cerebral artery (401) and affect the middle cerebral artery in approximately 75% of the cases (363). This contrasts with congenital aneurysms, which are usually located near the circle of Willis. Vessel branchings are often affected, probably because they favor the impaction of emboli (285). This has been clearly documented in some cases by serial angiography showing the formation of an ICMA at the site of a previous embolus (363,372). Multiple intracranial sites are involved in approximately 20% of the cases but may not occur simultaneously (365). Although it is conceivable that ICMAs and mycotic aneurysms located elsewhere may develop in the same patient, it was not found in the one study which specifically investigated this possibility (221).

Histologically, mycotic aneurysms are characterized

by (a) the destruction of the normal architecture of the arterial wall, (b) focal areas of necrosis, and (c) infiltration by inflammatory cells. Strictly speaking, mycotic aneurysms are pseudoaneurysms, because they result from destruction of the muscular layer. In acute lesions, polymorphonuclear cells are predominant and microabscesses are not uncommon (285). In more chronic lesions or when rupture has not occurred, polymorphonuclear cells are mixed with lymphocytes and plasmocytes in fibroblastic granulation tissue. The fibrotic reaction may contribute to the resistance of the wall and prevent rupture. Adhesions may form between the arachnoid and the brain in the region of the ICMA. With rupture of the aneurysm, these adhesions may prevent free escape of the blood into the subarachnoid space. Bleeding therefore tends to occur into the brain substance or into the subdural space (402). Since ICMAs are small and usually affect peripheral branches of cerebral arteries, they may be easily overlooked at autopsy. When ruptured, the partially destroyed sacs may be obscured by hemorrhage, making their identification equally difficult (375).

Clinical Presentation

Most ICMAs occur in patients with IE. In many of the reported cases, ICMA is described as presenting with a sudden, often fatal, subarachnoid or intracerebral hemorrhage without recognized warning signs (365). Among 58 patients with ICMA reviewed by Bohmfalk et al. (365), 33 already presented with major neurologic manifestations on admission, which were due to a subarachnoid hemorrhage in 19 cases. IE may not even be suspected before the rupture (361). Moreover, rupture can occur while the patient is already on antibiotics (373,403,404) or after treatment has been completed (261,374).

Some authors have called attention to the fact that early neurologic signs are often present before the rupture. For example, the presence of severe, localized headache in a patient with IE should raise the suspicion of an ICMA. Among 213 patients with IE seen at the Mayo Clinic from 1975 to 1979, seven complained of severe localized headache and four had a proven ICMA. The other three also had an ICH, but ICMA could not be demonstrated (285). Focal neurologic events, such as seizures, ischemic deficit, or cranial-nerve abnormality (283), may often precede the development and the rupture of ICMA and should be regarded as serious warning signs prompting further investigations (363,365,368). In 16 patients with ruptured ICMA reported by Pruitt et al. (221), eight had a history suggesting embolization prior to the hemorrhage. At angiography, an occluded vessel was often found in association with the aneurysm. Among 81 cases of ICMA reviewed by Ojemann and Crowell (356), 65 were reported with enough clinical information to determine the initial neurologic event that led to angiography. This was a definite or probable hemorrhage in 42, an infarction in 16, an infarction followed by a hemorrhage in five, and headache without hemorrhage in two. Four of the eight patients with ICMA reported by Wilson et al. (285) presented with homonymous hemianopsia. The occurrence of a TIA may also precede subsequent rupture of an ICMA (258).

Although premonitory signs or symptoms may precede a catastrophic hemorrhage only by a few hours, the delay is generally of several days. Among 13 patients reported by Frazee, the median delay was 6 days, with a range of 6 hr to 35 days (363). Some aneurysms may leak slowly before rupture and produce a mild meningeal irritation; the CSF is sterile but shows an initial neutrophilic reaction and a moderate amount of RBC (231,285,368).

Overall, hemorrhage has been documented from LP, surgery, or autopsies in 65% of the cases of ICMA gathered from the literature by Bohmfalk et al. (365). In approximately half of the cases, hemorrhage occurred before the hospitalization. In patients with diagnosed IE, recent reports suggest that an aggressive diagnostic approach in patients with neurologic manifestations may allow diagnosis before massive hemorrhage in a substantial number of patients (285,363). When rupture of ICMA occurs, it almost always causes either a subarachnoid or an intracerebral hemorrhage (365). Subdural hematomas have also been described (347). In some cases, ICMA may present as a space-occupying lesion or may be accompanied by a cerebral abscess (405,406). Finally, it has been documented that ICMAs may remain totally asymptomatic and resolve under antibiotic therapy (80,354,368).

As already mentioned, ICMAs may become symptomatic or may even develop after appropriate antibiotic therapy for IE has been initiated (80,285,361, 365,372,373,407) or completed (285,365,374). Delay of several months and up to 2 years has been reported (259,281,294), and a high level of suspicion should be maintained in patients with a previous history of IE. Cases of ruptured ICMA during the postoperative period of cardiac valve replacement for IE have been reported, and full systemic anticoagulation may constitute an aggravating factor (408).

In ICMA of extravascular origin, the clinical presentation is dominated by the underlying disorder such as meningitis or thrombophlebitis of the cavernous sinus, in which case ICMA is often discovered casually on angiography (378,409), but they may occasionally be associated with hemorrhage (410,411).

Diagnosis

Since some ICMAs may benefit from surgical treatment, it is of utmost importance to maintain a high level of suspicion of ICMA in patients with active or treated IE who develop neurologic manifestations, and to initiate appropriate diagnostic procedures. CT scan should be done with and without contrast enhancement. It may localize ICMA either directly or by demonstrating adjacent hematoma. CT is of considerable value in assessing the extent of intracerebral or intraventricular bleeding and may also show edema, infarction, abscess, and hydrocephalus (356). In a systematic study comparing CT scan and angiography in 34 patients with IE and neurologic manifestations, no mycotic aneurysm was detected in the 14 patients with normal CT scan whereas 11 cases with one or more ICMAs were diagnosed at angiography in the 20 patients who had an abnormal CT scan (298). This suggests that ICMA is unlikely to be present when the CT scan is normal. Although CT-scan abnormalities may be suggestive of an ICMA, they are rarely diagnostic; therefore, angiography should be performed when ICMA is considered (285,298).

The exact value of MRI in this setting is not yet determined. MRI is not useful in demonstrating acute (less than 24–48 hr) subarachnoid hemorrhage, because the acute blood loss causes little change in the signal characteristics of the CSF (412). However, the formation of methemoglobin in subacute clot results in a high signal on both short and long spin–echo sequences, and MRI may be valuable in confirming that bleeding has occurred and in determining its site of origin (413). This may be particularly helpful when multiple aneurysms are present. Because not all episodes of subarachnoid hemorrhage result in a residual focal clot, MRI may fail to localize the source of bleeding; the exact role of this technique remains to be explored. In the future, the development of MRI angiography might allow the noninvasive demonstration of ICMA. This might be particularly valuable when serial examinations are indicated.

At the present time, angiography is the only reliable means to establish the diagnosis and to outline the location of the aneurysm and its relationship to the parent vessel (Fig. 6A). Since multiple aneurysms are common, examination of all four vessels is recommended (298). Some authors have suggested that all patients with IE, even those without neurologic manifestations, should undergo complete cerebral angiography, possibly on repeated occasions during and after treatment (365, 367,403). In view of the relatively low incidence of symptomatic ICMA in patients with IE, other authors would limit the indication to patients with abnormal CT scan and/or some neurologic abnormality (285). Given the potential complications of cerebral angiography and the relative rarity of symptomatic ICMA, the latter approach appears to be more appropriate.

If meningitis is suspected, an examination of the CSF is indicated after the CT scan has been done. Because some aneurysms may leak slowly before rupture, a mild meningeal irritation may be present: The CSF is sterile but shows a few hundred RBCs and leukocytes, with a mild protein elevation.

In patients in whom evidence of ICMA is the first manifestation of their illness, all efforts should be made to identify the exact underlying disease and to isolate the causative microorganism by blood and other pertinent cultures.

Specific Management

Optimal management of ICMA should include appropriate medical and surgical treatment, as well as adequate surveillance (Figs. 4 and 5).

Antimicrobial therapy should be initiated as soon as possible. Although few data exist for ICMA, it is gener-

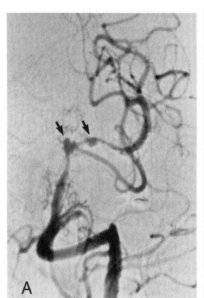
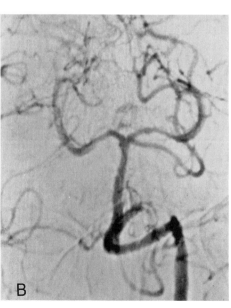

FIG. 6. Frontal view of a left vertebral arteriogram of a patient with *S. mitis* endocarditis. **A:** Mycotic aneurysms of the basilar tip and left posterior cerebral artery. Spasm of the basiliar artery (April 16, 1985). **B:** Resolution of the aneurysms on antibiotic therapy (May 8, 1985). Occlusion of the right superior cerebellar artery. (Courtesy of Antoine Uske, M.D.)

ally accepted that the regimen should be chosen according to the same principles and guidelines applied for patients with IE (see Table 3) (174,285); however, it has been recommended that the duration of administration be extended to 6–8 weeks, even if the ICMA is resected surgically (21). Supportive measures such as control of the arterial pressure by antihypertensive agents, steroids, and avoidance of anticoagulation should be carefully considered. Until recently, it was believed that the majority of ICMAs would rupture if not resected (285). Although the true natural course of ICMA on appropriate antibiotics is not known, it has become increasingly apparent that a certain proportion of unruptured ICMAs may resolve with medical treatment alone (356,367,368) (Fig. 6A and 6B). Among 27 patients reviewed by Ojemann and Crowell (356) in whom follow-up angiography was performed during antibiotic therapy, complete disappearance of the lesions was observed in eight cases and there was a decrease in size in five cases. The lesions were unchanged in four cases and larger in six. In four patients, a new ICMA was found. Bingham (367) found that small ICMAs disappeared or regressed in size during antibiotic therapy in 17 of 21 patients.

This variable and unpredictable outcome with medical treatment alone has given rise to controversies with regard to the optimal therapeutic strategy. Bingham (367) analyzed the mortality of 45 patients with ICMA: Among 20 patients receiving only antibiotics, three died from hemorrhage while under treatment, compared to six deaths among the 25 cases who had combined surgical and medical treatment; however, most of the latter deaths were observed in poor-risk patients. Mortality associated with surgical procedure for ICMA located on distal arterial branches was quite low in the absence of major cardiac or other medical problems. This was also noted by Bohmfalk et al. (365), who recorded no deaths in their review of 17 patients who had surgical removal of ICMA of distal arterial branches. Ojemann and Crowell (356) reviewed the treatment and outcome of 81 patients with ICMA detectable on angiography. Of 30 patients treated with antibiotics, 13 died. Elective surgery was done in 29 patients; two died but both had recovered from surgery and experienced a second fatal hemorrhage from an unrecognized ICMA. Among the 14 patients who underwent emergency surgery, six deaths were recorded, mostly because of the serious neurologic deficit caused by intracerebral hematoma. When surgery is contemplated, it should be realized that standard techniques usually include the ligation of the involved arterial segment (in areas uninvolved by the suppurative process) followed by the excision of the necrotic aneurysm and adjacent vessel wall (414). This may result in permanent neurologic sequelae. In only some cases is the fibrotic process generated by the infection sufficiently developed so as to allow successful aneurysm clipping without sacrifice of the parent vessel. In some cases, the parent vessel may already be occluded by the embolus presumably responsible for the formation of the ICMA (415). When surgical treatment is required for aneurysms located on proximal arteries or on important peripheral arteries, extracranial–intracranial bypass has been successfully attempted (414).

Although there is no rationale for treatment plans based on controlled series, the suggested principles of management of IE patients with proven or suspected ICMA are outlined in Fig. 5, based on the proposals of several authors (285,354,363,365,384). Patients with focal CNS signs or with localized or severe headache should have a CT scan with and without contrast enhancement. If the CT scan is normal, further investigations will depend on the type and evolution of the CNS manifestations. For instance, in the presence of severe and persistent localized headache [a presentation highly suggestive of ICMA (285)], cerebral angiography should be performed even if the CT scan is normal. If the CT scan is abnormal but not diagnostic for disorders other than ICMA, four-vessel angiography should be performed, especially if the findings are compatible with an ICMA, such as presence of hematoma, subarachnoid hemorrhage, or punctiform contrast enhancement (298). If the initial event is an embolic episode, angiography should be done only 5–7 days later, in order to detect a forming ICMA.

Surgery should be performed for ruptured aneurysm of the peripheral cerebral arteries, if the patient's medical condition is stable. Surgery is also indicated when intracerebral hematoma or mass-producing aneurysms are present. When the aneurysm is located at a site where excision is likely to cause a new neurologic deficit, the indication for surgery should be carefully weighed, and close follow-up may aid in the decision regarding surgical intervention. It is important to take into consideration that administration of antibiotics during a certain period prior to surgery may facilitate arteritis resolution with subsequent development of fibrosis in the wall of the aneurysm and of the parent vessels. The lesion could then be handled more safely at surgery (361).

For unruptured peripheral ICMAs, it has become increasingly apparent that a rather large proportion of them resolve under antibiotic therapy alone (356). Medical cures with appropriate antimicrobial therapy alone have also been reported for proximal ICMAs (365,367,372,407) and for aneurysms of the cavernous sinus (365,378,409). Therefore, close clinical follow-up associated with serial CT scan and angiography is advocated for unruptured ICMAs by certain authors (285,356,365,367,386,416). How often these repeated investigations should be performed has not been established, but an interval of 7–14 days is generally recommended (356,363). If the aneurysm does not disappear after antibiotic treatment or enlarges or bleeds at any time, excision should be performed if feasible. An aggressive surgical approach is favored by others (363), especially for easily accessible peripheral ICMAs (282, 363,365,368,400,417).

Multiple aneurysms may present a complex problem. A review of 15 cases of multiple ICMAs due to all causes, including meningitis, revealed that 11 were treated nonsurgically and that none died as a direct result (363). In another series of 10 patients with multiple aneurysms related to IE, seven were treated by antibiotics alone and there was only one death (356). Therefore, it seems appropriate to analyze each individual case along the same guidelines as those for single ICMA. If one or more of the aneurysms enlarge or bleed, prompt surgical excision should be attempted. The excision of the other aneurysms during the same operation will depend on their accessibility (356,363).

If a patient with a suspected or proven ICMA requires urgent cardiac valve replacement, the operation may be performed before the repair of ICMA, unless the patient is threatened by a mass effect due to intracerebral hematoma or abscess. Despite the heparinization necessary for cardiopulmonary bypass, there have been no ruptures of ICMA during the perioperative period among patients with ICMA who underwent valve replacement (278). In patients with ICMA suspected or identified preoperatively, a bioprosthetic valve is preferred, to obviate the need for postoperative anticoagulation (354). However, in patients without neurologic symptoms who have successfully completed an appropriate course of parenteral antibiotics, the long-term risk of subarachnoid hemorrhage is very low, and anticoagulation can be safely initiated without cerebral angiography (260).

Outcome

The mortality of recognized ICMA is high. Among the 85 cases reviewed by Bohmfalk et al. (365) the figures for patients hospitalized for IE before neurologic symptoms occurred show a true mortality of 80% for aneurysms that ruptured and of 30% if the aneurysm remained intact. The overall mortality was 46%. The analysis of outcome according to whether the patients were treated with antibiotics alone or with antibiotics plus surgery shows conflicting results. Mortality ranged from 13% to 75% for patients treated with antibiotics alone and from 0% to 42% for patients who benefited from combined antibiotics and surgery (285,356,363,365,367). Based on these figures, some authors recommend surgical excision whenever possible (363) whereas others favor a conservative approach in the management of patients with unruptured ICMA (367). Since most case descriptions do not specify the reasons for choosing one therapeutic approach over another, the differences in outcome can be attributed to many factors such as the patient's general and neurologic condition, time of diagnosis relative to antibiotic administration, size and location of the ICMA, frequency of serial angiography, or indications for surgical intervention.

Metastatic Infections

Infection of the CNS secondary to IE may present as meningitis, meningoencephalitis, cerebral micro- or macroabscesses, parameningeal abscesses, or infectious arteritis (see sections entitled "Intracranial Hemorrhage" and "Intracranial Mycotic Aneurysm," above).

Incidence of Meningitis

Meningitis may occur either as a septic process or as a sterile inflammatory reaction to infection, ischemia, or hemorrhage within the brain. Before the advent of antibiotics, clinical meningitis was one of the more frequent neurologic complications of IE, accounting for up to two-thirds of these complications in some studies (212). In more recent reviews of IE, meningitis was recorded in 1–16% of patients with IE and in 5–41% of those with CNS manifestations of IE (16,24,156,217,218,221–223,242,288). The great variability of these percentages is partly due to the fact that some authors include all meningeal reactions whatever the underlying process, whereas others restrict the diagnosis to cases presumably due to true bacterial meningitis. Referral bias and a changing spectrum of IE may also account for some differences.

Although meningitis may be the presenting symptom of IE (218,221), IE is an infrequent cause of bacterial meningitis in general. Thus, in two large studies, two of 207 (1%) and 13 of 209 (6%) consecutive cases of meningitis were associated with IE (418,419). Of these 15 cases, six were due to S. pneumoniae, five were caused by S. aureus, three were a result of gram-negative bacilli, one was due to H. influenzae, and one was caused by nonhemolytic streptococci. Thus, all but one of the microorganisms recovered in these cases were either virulent or had a known tropism for the meninges, or both. When meningitis is due to agents other than the ones commonly causing that disease, the proportion of cases associated with IE is high, especially when virulent. In one study, five of 15 (33%) cases of S. aureus meningitis not related to neurosurgery were associated with IE (420). In another review of 33 patients with S. aureus meningitis seen between 1976 and 1984, seven (21%) had concomitant IE (421). This association was high in drug abusers, since five of six intravenous drug users with S. aureus meningitis had IE (421). In a study of 10 adult patients with meningitis caused by streptococci, five had concomitant IE (291).

Conversely, IE due to virulent microorganisms is more often complicated by meningitis (156,221). In S.

aureus IE, meningitis has been observed in 27–67% (61,130,242,264). In pneumococcal endocarditis, meningitis has been recorded in as many as 71–87% of the cases in recent series (113,242). In *P. aeruginosa* IE, meningitis was diagnosed clinically in six of 17 cases gathered from the literature (422). Meningitis is not unusual in IE due to enterococci or due to enteric gram-negative bacilli (221). In IE due to less virulent microorganisms, meningitis occurs only rarely. Thus meningitis was noted in only one of 60 cases of subacute IE in one series (214), whereas during the same period, acute purulent meningitis was the most common presenting feature in cases of staphylococcal IE with CNS involvement (215). However, culture-positive viridans streptococcal meningitis developing during the course of IE has been described (291). Purulent meningitis with positive CSF cultures has also been associated with IE due to bacteria of very low virulence, such as *C. hominis* (293). Chronic forms of meningitis have been described in IE caused by certain fungi, such as *Candida* species and *Histoplasma capsulatum* (423,424).

Incidence of Brain Abscess

Brain abscesses associated with IE are uncommon. In a series of 218 patients with IE, eight (3.6%) developed abscesses (221). In other large series, rates of 1–8.6% were recorded (38,218,222,223). Older studies have documented the presence of brain abscess in 18–24% of patients with IE due to virulent bacteria (215,397), and in 40% of those who were autopsied (215). In one series published before the advent of antibiotics, nine of 10 cases with acute IE had multiple cerebral abscesses (224).

In large series of brain abscesses, IE is not a common cause. A recent review of 102 patients with brain abscess mentions no patients with the diagnosis of IE, although some of the 17 patients with congenital heart disease might have had IE (425). Among 314 patients with brain abscess collected from six different series, 13 (4%) had IE (426–431). This reveals that IE should always be suspected in the presence of brain abscess when there is no other obvious source. This suspicion must be particularly high when multiple abscesses are present (Fig. 7). Thus, IE was responsible for two of five cases who presented with multiple abscesses in a series of 41 patients with brain abscesses observed in our institution from 1977 to 1989 (431). Similar findings were made by others (428). In studies of IE reporting brain abscesses, multiple locations were noted in the majority of the cases (218,221–223,236,288). Drug addicts with IE might be especially predisposed to cerebral abscesses: In a series of 46 episodes of IE, 16 had neurologic manifestations, among which there were four cases of microabscesses and one case of macroabscess (236).

Obviously, the incidence and the size of brain ab-

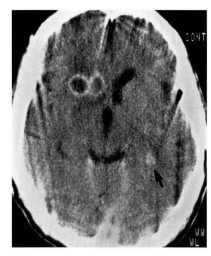

FIG. 7. Head CT scan of a patient with *S. aureus* endocarditis. Abscesses of the deep right frontal lobe and area of cerebritis of the temporal lobe (*arrow*). (Courtesy of Antoine Uske, M.D.)

scesses associated with IE will depend upon the type of imaging techniques used and upon whether or not the study includes pathologic examination. In a series of IE patients from the Massachusetts General Hospital, nine of 218 had evidence of brain abscess, all cases of which were diagnosed at autopsy. In eight of the patients, the abscesses were less than 1 cm³, were mainly microscopic in nature, and were not sufficient in size to create a mass effect. In six of these eight patients, multiple microscopic abscesses were present, usually in association with microabscesses in other organs. These patients also had multiple microscopic infarcts, demonstrating the interrelationship between vascular and infectious complications of IE. Seven of the eight patients had an acute IE (four cases of which were due to *S. aureus*), and one had subacute IE due to viridans streptococci. Only one patient in this series had a large abscess, which was probably caused by the direct extension from *S. aureus* otitis media and mastoiditis and not by bacterial seeding from the bloodstream (221). Other series have confirmed that large abscesses are uncommon in IE, occurring in 1–2% of the cases (218,222,223).

Because areas of cerebritis (Fig. 8A) or cerebral abscesses of small size (Fig. 8B) may resolve with appropriate antibiotic therapy alone (425,427,431,432), it is likely that the true incidence of these lesions is underestimated, even in recent studies which have benefited from CT. Thus, among 64 patients with neurologic complications of IE, abscesses were diagnosed in only two of the 51 patients who had a head CT scan (223). It is noteworthy that among these 51 patients, 15 presented with encephalopathy, a clinical presentation which is often associated with multiple microabscesses and/or microinfarcts (221,300). None of these 15 patients had CT findings consistent with abscesses, although one had mi-

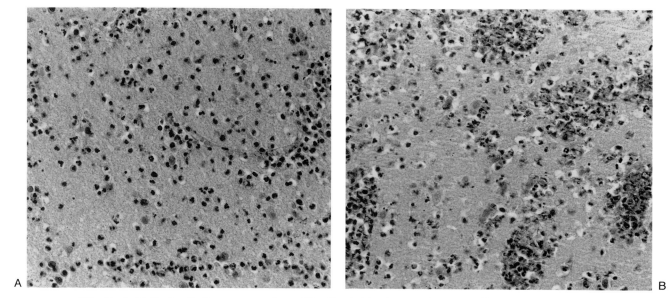

FIG. 8. A: Patient with *S. aureus* endocarditis. Cerebritis characterized by diffuse infiltration of brain parenchyma by polymorphonuclear cells. **B:** Microabscesses with focal infiltration of brain parenchyma by polymorphonuclear cells. (Original magnification 250×, hematoxylin–eosin; courtesy of Robert Janzer, M.D.)

croabscesses at autopsy (223). Likewise, 11 of these 51 had a focal deficit with a normal CT scan, and some of them may have had undetected cerebritis (223). This suggests that small abscesses or cerebritis may be beyond the level of detection of the CT scan (433). MRI has been shown experimentally to be superior to CT in the detection of early cerebritis (434,435). Recently, two patients with IE and "toxic" encephalopathy were described who had a normal CT scan but an MRI scan showing multiple lesions suggesting microembolization and/or microabscesses (171). Reports of abnormalities seen on MRI but undetected by CT have also included small infarcts (436,437). Thus, it is likely that cerebritis, cerebral microinfarcts, and microabscesses associated with IE will be diagnosed with increased frequency if MRI is performed, especially in patients with toxic encephalopathy or focal deficit with normal CT scan.

Brain scan with technetium-99 is a very sensitive test for the detection of brain abscess or cerebritis, and it should be performed if CT is negative and MRI is not available (438).

Pathogenesis

Clinical signs of meningitis may be associated with multiplication of the causative microorganism in the subarachnoid space or may be a reflection of various parameningeal lesions, such as brain micro- and macroabscesses, septic or nonseptic cerebral micro- or macroemboli, leaking mycotic aneurysms, subarachnoid hemorrhage, or immune-mediated arteritis. Several

of these mechanisms can occur simultaneously or sequentially (127,221). Except for the immunological arterial lesions, all these complications ultimately relate to embolization of infected material to cerebral or meningeal vessels. Critical factors that may determine whether a septic embolus results in a simple infarct, a mycotic aneurysm, meningitis, cerebritis, an abscess, or a combination of these lesions include the size of the embolus, the site in which the embolus lodges, the virulence of the microorganism, and the defenses of the host, including the timing and adequacy of antibacterial therapy (236). This is illustrated by cases of intracerebral mycotic aneurysms associated with brain abscesses (405,406). As already mentioned, neurologic complications are characteristic of left-sided IE, indicating that emboli play a major role in the pathogenesis of cerebral manifestations, including meningitis and abscesses (221). Although these emboli may be clinically silent, the development of macroscopic brain abscess 1–3 weeks after a contralateral hemiplegic stroke due to embolism has been well documented (228). However, with certain bacteria, meningitis can occur in the context of isolated right-sided IE, indicating that the mere presence of certain bacteria in the blood can cause meningeal seeding. This has been described with *S. pneumoniae;* this is not surprising, given the well-known propensity of this bacteria to cause hematogenous meningitis (113,238). In right-sided *S. aureus* IE, meningitis has also been described, but it occurred in only two of 53 of such episodes. The CSF showed an "aseptic" formula (29). When *S. aureus* bacteremia is caused by IE, the incidence of CNS involvement is higher (29–54%) than in the absence of endocardial involvement (3–10%) (61,439). In a recent study of 81 episodes of *S. aureus* IE, 22 neurologic complications were recorded. All but one occurred in the 42 patients with left-sided involvement; there were five brain abscesses and two cases of meningitis (179).

Thus, the occurrence of CNS infectious complications of IE depends on two major factors: (i) the virulence characteristics of the microorganism and (ii) the side of the heart involved. The fact that right-sided and left-sided IE are both characterized by persistent bacteremia but are very much different with respect to the incidence of CNS infectious complications suggests that emboli associated with bacteria are more capable of disrupting the normal blood–brain barrier.

Clinical Presentation

Meningitis, which can be the first manifestation of IE, occurred in three of 218 cases in the series from the Massachusetts General Hospital (221), as well as in seven of 385 patients in the series from the Mayo Clinic (218). There is a continuum in the clinical presentation of meningitis, meningoencephalitis, and microscopic and macroscopic brain abscesses.

Patients may display a typical clinical presentation of primary meningitis. Meningoencephalitis characterized by confusion, decreased level of consciousness, stiff neck, and headache, associated with normal or slightly abnormal CSF (minimal pleocytosis, normal glucose concentration, normal or slightly elevated protein concentration, and sterile culture), has been termed "acute brain syndrome," "acute encephalopathy," or "toxic encephalopathy" (218,226). Psychiatric manifestations may predominate, including personality change, disorientation, drowsiness, irritability, or even hallucinations (300). This may account for the frequent presence of confusion in elderly patients with IE, in the absence of fever or metabolic abnormalities (36). This presentation is related to multiple microemboli and microinfarcts, with or without microabscesses (221). This mode of presentation accounts for 17–21% of the neurologic manifestations of IE (218,221).

The clinical presentation of brain abscesses depend on the stage, the size, the number, and the location of the lesions. This may result in clinical manifestations of a focal deficit, a space-occupying lesion, toxic encephalopathy, or meningitis. The accompanying meningitis will usually be sterile unless the abscess ruptures into the subarachnoid space. Headache, confusion, increased intracranial pressure, and focal signs, often developing slowly over several days, are noted with abscess of large size (226).

Parameningeal abscess is another metastatic infection of IE which may cause osteoarticular and neurologic

manifestation. Back pain may be a preeminent symptom of IE and may be the first manifestation of the disease. It has been noted in up to 10% of the patients with IE. Some of these cases are due to vertebral osteomyelitis (440–442). Although vertebral osteomyelitis is well known for its potential to result in epidural abscess, this has rarely been described. Of 39 patients with epidural abscess, none was found to be associated with IE (443), but case reports have been related to IE caused by pyogenic and virulent organisms, such as *S. aureus* or *S. pneumoniae* (444–446).

Management

The treatment of IE-associated meningitis is covered by the antibiotic regimens recommended for the underlying IE, provided that high doses of bactericidal antibiotics that cross the blood–brain barrier are used. In this regard, it should be remembered that first- and second-generation cephalosporins do not penetrate into the CSF in sufficient concentration.

For brain abscesses, the size, the number, and the location of the lesion(s) should be carefully considered when therapy is planned (Fig. 4). A large abscess can be refractory to antibiotic treatment alone. "Two centimeters" appears to be the critical diameter size beyond which surgery is strongly indicated (425). Most patients have small and multiple microabscesses, and surgery is generally neither feasible nor desirable. In patients with cerebritis, early therapy alone could also be curative, but surgery should be considered in case of neurologic deterioration (438). For CNS suppurative complications of IE, it is generally recommended that the duration of antimicrobial therapy be extended to 6–8 weeks (221,226).

Since cerebral abscess (as well as ICMA) may develop within 1–2 weeks after an embolic event, a CT scan is indicated in the follow-up of these patients (Fig. 9). Epi-

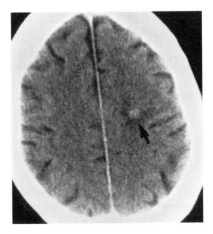

FIG. 9. Head CT of a patient with streptococcal endocarditis. Left frontal cerebritis with early abscess formation. (Courtesy of Antoine Uske, M.D.)

dural abscess requires surgical drainage, which should be performed as an emergency in the presence of signs of spinal cord compression (443).

Outcome

Neurologic metastatic infectious complications of IE are associated with a very poor prognosis. Acute suppurative meningitis has been associated with a mortality rate of over 80% (113,218,221,228). The mortality is also high (approximately 50%) in toxic encephalopathy (218, 221) and in cerebral abscesses (over 80%) (221,228).

Various Disorders

Spinal Cord

Lesion of the spinal cord may be due to external compression by a parameningeal abscess or may be the consequence of emboli to the vascular supply. Despite the frequency of embolic phenomena in IE, there have been only rare case reports of embolic infarction of the spinal cord (65,288), and no cases are reported in the major series of IE.

Cranial and Peripheral Nerves

In two large series of patients with neurologic manifestation of IE, mononeuropathies have been reported in five of 110 and five of 84 patients (218,221). Five of these patients were reported in detail (289). Viridans streptococci were the responsible microorganisms in all of them. All had an elevated ESR. In four, neuropathy was the initial manifestation of IE. The nerves involved were ulnar (three), peroneal (two), and facial, median, and sciatic (one each). Three had concomitant involvement of multiple nerves, emphasizing the need to consider IE in the differential diagnosis of mononeuritis multiplex. All patients improved after treatment, and only two of the eight nerves involved presented minimal residual deficit (300). Because of the temporal and spatial association with cutaneous emboli, embolic occlusion of the vasa vasorum was the postulated physiopathological mechanism (289). This was also suggested by a case of polyneuropathy associated with *S. aureus* IE in which histology of the peripheral nerves disclosed an acute microabscess and features compatible with septic microinfarcts (447). Immune-complex-mediated vasculitis in the peripheral nerves is another possible mechanism.

Cerebral emboli or compression may affect the cranial nerves, causing paralysis of the face, palate, tongue, and larynx; pseudobulbar palsy has also been described (211,283).

Although immune complexes have been identified in the choroid plexus of a patient with IE (263), the exact significance of this finding remains to be determined.

Ocular Manifestations of IE

Ocular manifestations of IE are not infrequent: They have been reported in 2–25% of cases, depending on their type (16,21,140). They may be the first or the predominant manifestation of IE in certain cases (221), or they may be asymptomatic findings at funduscopy which may help in establishing the diagnosis of IE. They may involve the eye structures, the cranial nerves, or the optical pathways, and they can be caused by emboli, infection, immunological mechanisms, or mass effect (283,369).

Acute embolic occlusion of either the central retinal artery or one of its main branches is one of the most dramatic complications of IE; it will result in sudden loss of vision, which may be transient (300) or permanent (300,448). In a large series reported before the antibiotic era, an incidence of 2.5% was recorded (208). In a recent series, the incidence was 2.8% (223). Funduscopic examination will reveal a milky-white retina, with the macula appearing as a cherry-red spot. There is usually no retinal hemorrhage (449). Emboli to the middle and posterior cerebral arteries may also result in optic pathway involvement (hemianopia, scotoma) (283) or cortical blindness (221). Similar manifestations may be caused by other mechanisms, such as CNS compression or hemorrhage.

Involvement of cranial nerves III, IV, and VI, as well as involvement of their central pathways, are possible complications of IE (450) and may result in strabismus, diplopia, and conjugate deviation of the eyes, as well as nystagmus and unequal pupils (283,451).

Abnormalities seen on funduscopic examination have been reported in 10–25% of patients with IE (21,452), and they have been observed in 35% of those with neurologic complications (218). It should be noted that these lesions are nonspecific (448).

Papilledema was observed in nine of 39 patients examined in a series of 110 cases of IE with CNS complications (218). It was probably related to various degrees of intracranial hypertension, due to space-occupying lesions (448).

Retinal hemorrhages are found in 10–25% of IE cases. They are thought to be the consequence of small emboli (140). Those with a white center are described as Roth spots (453) and occur in 2–9% of IE cases (24,36,112,156). They are probably due to a hypersensitivity reaction and not to emboli (144,149). Microscopically, they consist of lymphocytes surrounded by edema and hemorrhage in the nerve fiber layer of the retina (454,455).

In fungemia with or without associated endocarditis, funduscopic examination may reveal multiple white, cotton-like, circumscribed exudates with filamentous borders located in the chorioretina and extending into the vitreous cavity. They may be an important clue to the diagnosis, because blood cultures are often negative (112). They may initially be confused with Roth spots (456), but they may proceed to vitreous abscess and endophthalmitis (65,277,314).

Endophthalmitis associated with IE due to other microorganisms has also been described (450). It may be caused by pyogenic bacteria, such as pneumococci (36), but has also been observed with microorganisms of low virulence, such as viridans streptococci (457,458) or *A. actinomycetemcomitans* (459). The incidence of endophthalmitis may be higher in drug addicts; this has been observed in three of 28 cases in one series (65). Although systemic and local antibiotics may clear the infection, partial or complete loss of vision is often observed. Enucleation of the eye is sometimes necessary (453).

ACKNOWLEDGMENTS

We wish to thank the following individuals: Philippe Eggimann, M.D., for his invaluable help in review of the manuscript; Mario Franciolli, M.D., and Michel-Pierre Glauser, M.D., for their encouragement and comments; and Ms. Hanny Muller, for gathering the literature.

REFERENCES

1. Major RH. Notes on the history of endocarditis. *Bull Hist Med* 1945;17:351.
2. Osler W. Gulstonian lectures on malignant endocarditis. Lecture I. *Lancet* 1885;1:415–418.
3. Osler W. Gulstonian lectures on malignant endocarditis. Lecture II. *Lancet* 1885;1:459–464.
4. Osler W. Gulstonian lectures on malignant endocarditis. Lecture III. *Lancet* 1885;1:505–508.
5. Osler W. On some points in the etiology and pathology of ulcerative endocarditis. *Q J Med* 1909;2:219–230.
6. Weichselbaum A. Zur Aetiologie des akuten Endocarditis. *Wien Med Wochenschr* 1885;11:717–719.
7. Thayer WS. Bacterial or infective endocarditis. *Edinburgh Med J* 1931;38:237–265.
8. Griffin MR, Wilson WR, Edwards WD. Infective endocarditis. Olmsted Country, Minnesota, 1950 through 1981. *JAMA* 1985;254:1199–202.
9. Schollin J, Bjarke B, Wesstrom G. Infective endocarditis in Swedish children. I. Incidence, etiology, underlying factors and port of entry of infection. *Acta Paediatr Scnad* 1986;75:993–998.
10. Rossi L, Castello C, Franceschini L, et al. Clinico-epidemiological aspects of infectious endocarditis in a present-day Italian population. *G Ital Cardiol* 1986;16:30–37.
11. Goulet V, Etienne J, Fleurette J, Netter R. Infective endocarditis in France. Epidemiological characteristics. *Presse Med* 1986;15:1855–1858.
12. Skehan JD, Murray M, Mills PG. Infective endocarditis: incidence and mortality in the North East Thames Region. *Br Heart J* 1988;59:62–68.
13. King JW, Nguyen VQ, Conrad SA. Result of a prospective study statewide reporting system for infective endocarditis. *Am J Med Sci* 1988;295:517–527.
14. Svanbom M, Strandell T. Bacterial endocarditis. I. A prospective study of etiology, underlying factors and foci of infection. *Scand J Infect Dis* 1978;10:193–202.
15. Freedman LR. *Infective endocarditis and other intravascular infections.* New York: Plenum Medical Books, 1982.
16. Cherubin CE, Neu HC. Infective endocarditis at the Presbyterian Hospital in New York City from 1938–1967. *Am J Med* 1971;51:83–96.
17. Grosmann E, Holtzman T, Rosenthal T, Semesh E, Samra Y, Michaeli D. A comparative study of infective endocarditis. *Isr J Med Sci* 1984;20:389–393.
18. Kim EL, Ching DL, Pien FD. Bacterial endocarditis at a small community hospital. *Am J Med Sci* 1990;299:87–93.
19. Shaw J, Bochner F, Brooks PM, Moulds RFW, Ravenscroft PJ, Smith AJ. Infective endocarditis in the 1980s. Part 1. Aetiology and diagnosis. *Med J Aust* 1986;144:536–540.
20. Eggimann P, Francioli P. Infective endocarditis at the Centre Hospitalier Universitaire Vaudois 1985–1989. *Rev Med Suisse Romande* 1991;in press.
21. Scheld WM, Sande MA. Endocarditis and intravascular infections. In: Mandell GL, Douglas RG, Benett JE, eds. *Principles and practice of infectious disease,* 3rd ed. New York: Churchill Livingstone, 1990;670–706.
22. Kaye D. Changing pattern of infective endocarditis. *Am J Med* 1985;78(Suppl 6B):157–162.
23. McKinsey DS, Ratts TE, Bisno AL. Underlying cardiac lesions in adults with infective endocarditis. The changing spectrum. *Am J Med* 1987;82:681–688.
24. Von Reyn CF, Levy BS, Arbeit RD, Friedland G, Crumpacker CS. Infective endocarditis: an analysis based on strict case definition. *Ann Intern Med* 1981;94:505–518.
25. Masur H, Johnson WD. Prosthetic valve endocarditis. *J Thorac Cardiovasc Surg* 1980;80:31–37.
26. Heimberger TS, Duma RJ. Infections of prosthetic heart valves and cardiac pacemakers. *Infect Dis Clin North Am* 1989;3:221–245.
27. Terpenning MS, Buggy BP, Kaufman CA. Hospital-acquired infective endocarditis. *Arch Intern Med* 1988;148:1601–1603.
28. Levine DP, Crane LR, Zervos MJ. Bacteremia in narcotic addicts at the Detroit Medical Center II. Infectious endocarditis: a prospective comparative study. *Rev Infect Dis* 1986;8:374–396.
29. Chambers HF, Morris DL, Tauber MG, Modin BS. Cocaine use and the risk for endocarditis in intravenous drug users. *Ann Intern Med* 1987;106:833–836.
30. Lowes JA, Hamer J, Williams G, et al. 10 years of infective endocarditis at St. Bartholomew's Hospital: analysis of clinical features and treatment in relation to prognosis and mortality. *Lancet* 1980;1:133–136.
31. Petersdorf RG, Goldman P. Changes in the natural history of bacterial endocarditis. *J Chronic Dis* 1979;32:287–291.
32. Vogler WR, Dorney ER, Bridges HA. Bacterial endocarditis. A review of 148 cases. *Am J Med* 1962;32:910–921.
33. Rabinovich S, Evans J, Smith IM, January LE. A long-term view of bacterial endocarditis, 337 cases 1924 to 1963. *Ann Intern Med* 1965;63:185–198.
34. Bayliss R, Clark C, Oakley CM. The microbiology and pathogenesis of infective endocarditis. *Br Heart J* 1983;50:513–519.
35. Lien EA, Solberg CO, Kalager T. Infective endocarditis 1973–1984 at the Bergen University Hospital: clinical feature, treatment and prognosis. *Scand J Infect Dis* 1988;20:239–246.
36. Terpenning MS, Buggy BP, Kauffman CA. Infective endocarditis: clinical features in young and elderly patients. *Am J Med* 1987;83:626–634.
37. Thayer WS. Studies on bacterial (infective) endocarditis. *Johns Hopkins Hosp Rep* 1926;22:1–10.
38. Lerner PI, Weinstein L. Infective endocarditis in the antibiotic era. Part I. *N Engl J Med* 1966;274:199–206.
39. Kaye D. Infective endocarditis. In: Wyngaarden JB, Smith AL Jr, eds. *Cecil textbook of medicine,* 16th ed. Philadelphia: WB Saunders, 1982;1457–1466.
40. Kerr A Jr, Pullen RL. *Subacute bacterial endocarditis.* Springfield, IL: Charles C Thomas, 1955.

41. Bayliss R, Clark C, Oakley CM, Somerville W, Whitfield AG. The teeth and infective endocarditis. *Br Heart J* 1983;50:506–512.

42. Geva T, Frand M. Infective endocarditis in children with congenital heart disease: the changing spectrum 1965–1985. *Eur Heart J* 1988;9:1244–1249.

43. Kaye D. Definitions and demographic characteristics. In: Kaye D, ed. *Infective endocarditis.* Baltimore: University Park Press, 1976;1–10.

44. Delahaye JP, Loire R, Milon H. Infective endocarditis on stenotic aortic valves. *Eur Heart J* 1988;9(Suppl E):43–49.

45. Chagnac A, Rudniki C, Loebel H, Zahari I. Infectious endocarditis in idiopathic hypertrophic sub-aortic stenosis. *Chest* 1982;81:346–349.

46. Stulz P, Zimmerli W, Mihatsch J, Gardel E. Recurrent infective endocarditis in idiopathic hypertrophic subaortic stenosis. *Thorac Cardiovasc Surg* 1989;37:103–104.

47. Fulkerson PK, Beaver BM, Avseon JC. Calcification of the mitral annulus: etiology, clinical associations, complications and therapy. *Am J Med* 1979;66:967–977.

48. Corrigan D, Bolen J, Handcock EW. Mitral valve prolapse and infective endocarditis. *Am J Med* 1977;63:215–222.

49. Clemens JD, Horwitz RI, Jaffe CC, Feinstein AR, Stanton BF. A controlled evaluation of the risk of bacterial endocarditis in person with mitral-valve prolapse. *N Engl J Med* 1982;307:776–781.

50. Savage DD, Garrison RJ, Devereux RB, et al. Mitral valve prolapse in the general population. I. Epidemiology features: the Framingham study. *Am Heart J* 1983;106:571–576.

51. MacMahon SW, Roberts JK, Kramer-Fox R, Zucker DM, Roberts RB, Devereux RB. Mitral valve prolapse and infective endocarditis. *Medicine* 1987;113:1291–1298.

52. Nishimura RA, McGoon MD, Shub C, Miller FA, Ilstrup DM, Tajik AJ. Echocardiographically documented mitral-valve prolapse. Long term follow up 237 patients. *N Engl J Med* 1985;313:1305–1309.

53. Baddour LM, Bisno AL. Infective endocarditis complicating mitral valve prolapse: epidemiologic, clinical and microbiologic agents. *Rev Infect Dis* 1986;8:117–137.

54. Schatz IJ. Mitral valve prolapse: the unresolved question. *Hosp Pract* 1987;30.3:39–56.

55. Danchin N, Voiriot P, Briancon S, et al. Mitral valve prolapse as risk factor for infective endocarditis. *Lancet* 1989;i:743–745.

56. Marks AR, Choong CY, Chir MBB, Sanfilippo AJ, Ferre M, Weyman AE. Identification of high-risk and low-risk subgroups of patients with mitral-valve prolapse. *N Engl J Med* 1989;320:1031–1036.

57. Wilson WR. Prosthetic valve endocarditis: Incidence, anatomic location, cause, morbidity and mortality. In: Duma RJ, ed. *Infections of prosthetic heart valves and vascular grafts.* Baltimore: University Park Press, 1977;3–16.

58. Wilson WR, Danielson GK, Giuliani ER, Geraci JE. Prosthetic valve endocarditis. *Mayo Clin Proc* 1982;57:155–161.

59. McClung JA, Stein JH, Ambrose JA, Herman MV, Reed GE. Prosthetic heart valves: a review. *Progress Cardiovasc Dis* 1983;26:237–270.

60. Threlkeld MC, Cobbs CG. Infectious disorders of prosthetic valves and intravascular devices. In: Mandell GL, Douglas RG, Benett JE, eds. *Principles and practice of infectious diseases,* 3rd ed. New York: Churchill Livingstone, 1990;706–717.

61. Watanakunakorn C. Prosthetic valve endocarditis. *Prog Cardiovasc Dis* 1979;22:181–192.

62. Rowley KM, Clubb KS, Smith JW, Cabin HS. Right-sided infective endocarditis as consequence of flow-directed pulmonary-artery catheterization. *N Engl J Med* 1984;311:1152–1156.

63. Wade JC, Cobbs CG. Infections in cardiac pacemakers. *Curr Clin Top Infect Dis* 1988;9:44–61.

64. Cross AS, Steigbigel RT. Infective endocarditis and access site infection in patients on hemodialysis. *Medicine* 1977;55:453–466.

65. Dreyer NP, Fields BN. Heroin-associated infective endocarditis. A report of 28 cases. *Ann Intern Med* 1973;78:699–702.

66. Reyes MP, Palutke WA, Wylin RF, Werner AM. *Pseudomonas* endocarditis in the Detroit Medical Center 1969–1972. *Medicine* 1973;52:173–194.

67. Reiner NE, Gopalakrishna KV, Lerner PI. Enterococcal endocarditis in heroin addicts. *JAMA* 1976;235:1861–1863.

68. Menda KB, Gorbach SL. Favorable experience with bacterial endocarditis in heroin addicts. *Ann Intern Med* 1973;78:25–32.

69. Lange M, Salaki JS, Middleton JR, et al. Infective endocarditis in heroin addicts: epidemiological observations and some unusual cases. *Am Heart J* 1978;96:144–152.

70. Reisberg BE. Infective endocarditis in the narcotic addict. *Prog Cardiovasc Dis* 1979;22:193–204.

71. Chan P, Ogilby JD, Segal BL. Tricuspid valve endocarditis. *Medicine* 1989;117:1140–1146.

72. Golden RL, Horrocks TA. William Osler's view on malignant endocarditis from an "unknown" report. *Am J Cardiol* 1989;63:241–244.

73. Garrison PK, Freedman LR. Experimental endocarditis. I. Staphylococcal endocarditis in rabbits resulting from placement of a polyethylene catheter in the right side of the heart. *Yale J Biol Med* 1970;42:394–410.

74. Durack DT, Beeson PB. Experimental bacterial endocarditis. I. Colonization of a sterile vegetation. *Br J Exp Pathol* 1972;53:44–49.

75. Durack DT, Beeson PB. Experimental endocarditis. II. Survival of bacteria in endocardial vegetations. *Br J Exp Pathol* 1972;53:50–53.

76. Angrist AA, Oka M, Nakao K. Vegetative endocarditis. *Pathol Ann* 1967;2:155.

77. Bryan CS. Nonbacterial thrombotic endocarditis in patients with malignant tumors. *Am J Med* 1969;46:787–793.

78. Sande MA. Experimental endocarditis. In: Kaye D, ed. *Infective endocarditis.* Baltimore: University Park Press, 1976;11–28.

79. Durack DT. Experimental endocarditis. IV. Structure and evolution of very early lesions. *J Pathol* 1975;115:81–89.

80. Scheld WM, Strunk RW, Balian G. Microbial adhesion to fibronectin *in vitro* correlates with production of endocarditis in rabbits. *Proc Soc Exp Biol Med* 1985;180:474–482.

81. Becker RC, DiBello PM, Lucas FV. Bacterial tissue tropism: an *in vitro* model for infective endocarditis. *Cardiovasc Res* 1987;21:813–820.

82. Okell CC, Elliott SD. Bacteraemia and oral sepsis with special reference to the aetiology of subacute endocarditis. *Lancet* 1935;ii:869–872.

83. Everett ED, Hirschmann JV. Transient bacteremia and endocarditis prophylaxis: a review. *Medicine* 1977;56:61–77.

84. Scheld WM, Valone JA, Sande MA. Bacterial adherence in the pathogenesis of endocarditis. Interaction of bacterial dextran, platelets and fibrin. *J Clin Invest* 1978;61:1394–1404.

85. Crawford I, Russel C. Comparative adhesion of seven species of streptococci isolated from the blood of patients with subacute bacterial endocarditis to fibrin-platelet clot *in vitro*. *J Appl Bacteriol* 1986;60:127–133.

86. Overholser CD, Moreillon P, Glauser MP. Experimental bacterial endocarditis after dental extractions in rats with peritonitis. *J Infect Dis* 1987;155:107–112.

87. Moreillon P, Overholser CD, Malinverni R, Glauser MP. Predictors of endocarditis in isolates from cultures of blood following dental extractions in rats with periodontal disease. *J Infect Dis* 1988;157:990–995.

88. Clawson CC, Rao Gunda HR, White JG. Platelet interaction with bacteria. IV. Stimulation of the release reaction. *Am J Pathol* 1975;81:411–420.

89. Clawson CC. Role of platelets in the pathogenesis of endocarditis. In: Kaplan EL, ed. *Infective endocarditis.* Dallas, TX: American Heart Association, 1977;22–24.

90. Francioli P, Freedman LR. Streptococcal infection of endocardial and other intravascular vegetations in rabbits: natural history and effect of dexamethasone. *Infect Immun* 1979;24:483–491.

91. Yersin B, Glauser MP, Freedman LR. Effect on nitrogen mustard on natural history of right-sided streptoccal endocarditis: role of cellular host defences. *Infect Immun* 1982;35:320.

92. Sande MA, Strausbaugh LJ. Infective endocarditis. In: Mandell GL, Gwaltney JM, Sande MA, eds. *Current concepts of infectious diseases.* New York: John Wiley & Sons, 1977;55–68.

93. Mason PD, Lockwood CM. SBE presenting with type III cryoglobulinemia. *J Clin Lab Immunol* 1985;18:199–201.

94. Bayer AS, Theofilopoulos AN. Circulating immune complexes in infective endocarditis. *N Engl J Med* 1976;295:1500–1505.
95. Alpert JS, Krous HF, Dalen JE. Pathogenesis of Osler's nodes. *Ann Intern Med* 1976;85:471–473.
96. Inman RD, Redecha PB, Knechtle SJ. Identification of bacterial antigens in circulating immune complexes of infective endocarditis. *J Clin Invest* 1982;70:271.
97. Neugarten J, Baldwin DS. Glomerulonephritis in bacterial endocarditis. *Am J Med* 1984;77:197–303.
98. Marrie TJ, Harczy M, Mann OE, et al. Culture-negative endocarditis probably due to *Chlamydia pneumoniae*. *J Infect Dis* 1990;161:127–129.
99. Lerner PI. Infective endocarditis. A review of selected topics. *Med Clin North Am* 1974;58:605–622.
100. Hammann KP, Henkel B, Erbel R, Kramer G. Hemichorea associated with varicella-zoster reinfection and endocarditis. A case report. *Eur Arch Psychiatry Neurol Sci* 1985;234:404–407.
101. Cates JE, Christie RV. Subacute bacterial endocarditis. *Q J Med* 1951;20:93–130.
102. Barry J, Gump DW. Endocarditis: an overview. *Heart Lung* 1982;11:138–143.
103. Parker MT, Ball LC. Streptococci and aerococci associated with systemic infection in man. *J Med Microbiol* 1976;9:275–302.
104. Sussman JI, Baron EJ, Tenenbaum MJ, et al. Viridans streptococcal endocarditis: clinical, microbiological, and echocardiographic correlations. *J Infect Dis* 1986;154:597–603.
105. Hayward GW. Infective endocarditis: a changing disease. *Br Med J* 1973;2:706–709.
106. Gossling J. Occurrence and pathogenicity of *Streptococcus milleri* group. *Rev Infect Dis* 1988;10:257–285.
107. George RC, Uttley AHC. Susceptibility of enterococci and epidemiology of enterococcal infection in the 1980s. *Epidemiol Infect* 1989;103:403–413.
108. Wilkowske CJ. Enterococcal endocarditis. *Mayo Clin Proc* 1982;57:101–105.
109. Maki DG, Agger WA. Enterococcal bacteremia: clinical features, the risk of endocarditis, and management. *Medicine* 1988;67:248–69.
110. Watanakunakorn C. *Streptococcus bovis* endocarditis associated with villous adenoma following colonoscopy. *Am Heart J* 1988;116:1115–1116.
111. Henderson S, Rowald B, Harvey C. *Streptococcus bovis* endocarditis and carcinoma of the colon. *Br J Hosp Med* 1989;41:85–85.
112. Weinstein L, Rubin RH. Infective endocarditis. *Prog Cardiovasc Dis* 1973;16:239–274.
113. Powderly WG, Stanley SL, Medoff G. Pneumococcal endocarditis: report of a series and review of the literature. *Rev Infect Dis* 1986;8:786–791.
114. Stein DS, Panwalker AP. Group C streptococcal endocarditis: case report and review of the literature. *Infection* 1985;13:282–285.
115. Scully BE, Spriggs D, Neu HC. *Streptococcus agalactiae* (group B) endocarditis—a description of twelve cases and review of the literature. *Infection* 1987;15:169–176.
116. Bayer AS. Staphylococcal bacteremia and endocarditis. *Arch Intern Med* 1982;142:1169–1177.
117. Thompson RL. Staphylococcal infective endocarditis. *Mayo Clin Proc* 1982;57:106–114.
118. Jemsek JG, Greenberg SB, Centry LO, Welton DE, Mattox KL. Hemophilus parainfluenzae endocarditis. Two cases and review of the literature in the past decade. *Am J Med* 1979;66:51–59.
119. Geraci JE, Wilson WR, Washington JA II. Infective endocarditis caused by *Actinobacillus actinomycetemcomitans*. *Mayo Clin Proc* 1980;55:415–419.
120. Geraci JE, Wilson WR. Endocarditis due to gram-negative bacteria. Report of 56 cases. *Mayo Clin Proc* 1982;57:145–148.
121. Parker SW, Apicella MA, Fuller CM. *Hemophilus* endocarditis. Two patients with complications. *Arch Intern Med* 1983;143:48–51.
122. Madkour MM. Cardiovascular complications. In: Madkour MM, ed. *Brucellosis.* London: Butterworths, 1989;116–130.
123. Wall TC, Peyton RB, Corey GC. Gonococcal endocarditis: a new look at an old disease. *Medicine* 1989;68:375–380.
124. Kluge RM, Calia FM, McLaughlin JS. Source of contamination in open heart surgery. *JAMA* 1974;230:1415–1419.
125. Caputo GM, Archer GL, Calderwood SB. Native valve endocarditis due to coagulase negative staphylococci. Clinical and microbiologic features. *Am J Med* 1987;83:619–625.
126. Murray BE, Karchmer AW, Moellering RC. Diphtheroid prosthetic valve endocarditis: a study of clinical features and infecting organisms. *Am J Med* 1980;69:838–848.
127. Durack DT, Hoeprich PD. Infective endocarditis. In: Hoeprich PD, Jordan MC, eds. *Infectious disease. A modern treatise of infectious processes,* 4th ed. Philadelphia: JB Lippincott, 1989;1237–1253.
128. Cooper R, Mills J. Serratia endocarditis. A follow-up report. *Arch Intern Med* 1980;140:199–202.
129. Jackson RT, Dopp AC. *Bacteroides fragilis* endocarditis. *South Med J* 1988;81:781–782.
130. Chambers HF, Korzeniowski OM, Sande MA. *Staphylococcus aureus* endocarditis: clinical manifestations in addicts and non-addicts. *Medicine* 1983;62:170–177.
131. Pesanti EL, Smith IM. Infective endocarditis with negative blood cultures. *Am J Med* 1979;66:43–50.
132. Van Scoy RE. Culture-negative endocarditis. *Mayo Clin Proc* 1982;57:149–154.
133. Walterspiel JN, Kaplan EL. Incidence and clinical characteristics of "culture negative" infective endocarditis in a pediatric population. *Pediatr Infect Dis* 1986;5:328–332.
134. Washington JA II. The microbiological diagnosis of infective endocarditis. *J Antimicrob Chemother* 1987;20(Suppl A):29–39.
135. Fernandez-Guerrero ML, Muelas JM, Aquado JM. Q fever endocarditis on porcine bioprosthetic valves. Clinicopathologic features and microbiologic findings in three patients treated with doxycyclin, cotrimoxazole, and valve replacement. *Ann Intern Med* 1988;108:209–213.
136. Tompkins LS, Roessler BJ, Redd SC, Markowitz LE, Cohen ML. Legionella prosthetic-valve endocarditis. *N Engl J Med* 1988;318:530–535.
137. Carrizosa J, Levison ME, Lawrence T. Cure of *Aspergillus ustus* endocarditis of prosthetic valve. *Arch Intern Med* 1974;133:486–490.
138. Cannady PB, Sanford JP. Negative blood cultures in infective endocarditis: a review. *South Med J* 1976;69:1420–1424.
139. Abraham AK, MacCulloch D, Neutze JM, Connere B. Culture-negative infective endocarditis. *Aust NZ J Med* 1984;14:223–226.
140. Durack DT. Infective and noninfective endocarditis. In: Hurst JW, Schlant RC, eds. *The heart, arteries and veins,* 7th ed. New York: McGraw-Hill, 1989;1230–1255.
141. Mills J, Utley JR, Abbott J. Heart failure in infective endocarditis: predisposing factors, course and treatment. *Chest* 1974;66:151–157.
142. Roberts WC. Characteristics and consequences of infective endocarditis (active or healed or both) learned from morphologic studies. In: Rahimtoola SH, ed. *Infective endocarditis.* New York: Grune & Stratton, 1978;55.
143. Douglas A, More-Gilleron J, Eykyn SJ. Fever during treatment of infective endocarditis. *Lancet* 1986;ii:1341–1443.
144. Heffner JE. Extracardiac manifestations of bacterial endocarditis. *West J Med* 1979;131:85–91.
145. Infective endocarditis [Editorial]. *Lancet* 1984;i:603–604.
146. Kauffman RH, Thompson J, Valentin RM. The clinical implications and pathogenetic significance of circulating immune complexes in infective endocarditis. *Am J Med* 1981;71:17–25.
147. Bayer AS, Theofilopoulos AN. Immunopathogenetic aspects of infective endocarditis. *Chest* 1990;97:204–212.
148. Yee J, MacAllister K. The utility of Osler's nodes in the diagnosis of infective endocarditis. *Chest* 1987;92:751–752.
149. Jarrett WH, Christy JH. Retinal hole formation. From septic embolization in acute bacterial endocarditis. *Am J Ophthalmol* 1967;64:472–474.
150. Washington JA II. The role of the microbiology laboratory in the diagnosis and antimicrobial treatment of infective endocarditis. *Mayo Clin Proc* 1982;57:22–32.
151. Washington JA II, Ilstrup DM. Blood cultures: issues and controversies. *Rev Infect Dis* 1986;8:792–802.
152. Washington JA II. Controversies in the diagnosis and management of infectious diseases. Session II: Diagnosis. Summary and discussion. *Rev Infect Dis* 1986;8:825–827.

153. Washington JA II. Bacteria, fungi, and parasites. In: Mandell GL, Douglas RG, Benett JE, eds. *Principles and practice of infectious diseases,* 3rd ed. New York: Churchill Livingstone, 1990;160–193.

154. Aronson MD, Bor DH. Blood cultures. *Ann Intern Med* 1987;106:246–253.

155. Washington JA II, Reller LB, Murray PR, MacLowry JD. Blood cultures II. *CUMITECH (Am Soc Microbiol)* 1982;1A:1–10.

156. Pelletier LL, Petersdorf RG. Infective endocarditis. A review of 125 cases from the University of Washington Hospitals. *Medicine* 1977;56:287–312.

157. Williams RC, Kunkel HG. Rheumatoid factors and their disappearance following therapy in patients with SBE. *Arthritis Rheum* 1962;5:126–131.

158. Cabane J, Godeau P, Herreman G, Acar J, Didegon M, Bach JF. Fate of circulating immune complexes in infective endocarditis. *Am J Med* 1979;66:277–282.

159. Roberts-Johnson PJ, Koh LY, Kenedy A, Smith MD, Neoh S, Turmidge J. Serological investigations in the diagnosis and management of infective endocarditis. *Aust NZ J Med* 1986;16:761–765.

160. Mugge A, Daniel WG, Frank G, Lichtlen PR. Echocardiography in infective endocarditis: reassessement of prognostic implications of vegetation size determined by the transthoracic and transoesophageal approach. *J Am Coll Cardiol* 1989;14:631–638.

161. Erbel R, Rohmann S, Drexler M. Improved diagnostic value of echocardiography in patients with infective endocarditis by transesophageal approach: a prospective study. *Eur Heart J* 1988;1:43–53.

162. Cormier B, Starkam C, Kulas A, Grimberg D, Enriquez L, Acar J. Transesophageal echography. Value of the technic apropos of a preliminary experiment in 320 patients (385 examinations). *Ann Med Interne* 1989;140:561–565.

163. Davis RS, Strom JA, Frishman W. The demonstration of vegetations by echocardiography in bacterial endocarditis. An indication for early surgical intervention. *Am J Med* 1980;69:57–63.

163a.Jaffe WM, Morgan DE, Pearlman AS, Otto CM. Infective Endocarditis, 1983–1988: Echocardiographic Findings and Factors Influencing Morbidity and Mortality. *J Am Coll Cardiol* 1990;15:1227–1233.

164. Kim JH, Weisman A, Kisslo J, Durack DT. Echocardiographic detection and clinical significance of left atrial vegetations in active infective endocarditis. *Am J Cardiol* 1989;64:950–952.

165. Berger HJ, Zaret BL. Use of radionuclides to evaluate myocardial structure and function. *Adv Intern Med* 1980;25:239–275.

166. Wiseman J, Rouleau J, Rigo P, Strauss HW, Pitt B. Gallium-67 myocardial imaging for the detection of bacterial endocarditis. *Radiology* 1976;120:135–138.

167. Miller MH, Casey JI. Infective endocarditis: new diagnostic techniques. *Am Heart J* 1978;96:123–128.

168. Riba AL, Thakur ML, Gottschalk A, Andriole VT, Zaret BL. Imaging experimental infective endocarditis with indium-111 labeled blood cellular components. *Circulation* 1979;59:336–343.

169. Oates E, Sarno RC. Detection of a prosthetic aortic valvular abscess with indium-111 labeled leucocytes. *Chest* 1988;94:872–874.

170. Cerqueira MD, Jacobson AF. Indium-111 leucocyte scintigraphic detection of myocardial abscess formation in patients with endocarditis. *J Nucl Med* 1989;30:703–706.

171. Bertorini TE, Laster RE, Thompson BF, Ford P. Magnetic resonance imaging of the brain in bacterial endocarditis. *Arch Intern Med* 1989;149:815–817.

172. Utley JR, Mills J, Mobin-Uddin K, Dillon ML, Bryant LR, Roe BB. Hemodynamic selection of patients with bacterial endocarditis for valve replacement. *Bull Soc Int Chir* 1974;33:269–277.

173. Mills J, Abbott J, Utley JR. Role of cardiac catheterization in infective endocarditis. *Chest* 1977;72:576–582.

174. Bisno AL, Dismukes WE, Durack DT, et al. Antimicrobial treatment of infective endocarditis due to viridans streptococci, enterococci, and staphylococci. *JAMA* 1989;261:1471–1477.

175. Tuazon CU, Gill V, Gill F. Streptococcal endocarditis: single vs combination antibiotic therapy and role of various species. *Rev Infect Dis* 1986;8:54–60.

176. Starinsky R, Wald U, Michowitz SD, Lahat E, Schiffer J. Dermoids of the posterior fossa. Case reports and review. *Clin Pediatr (Phila)* 1988;27:579–582.

177. Francioli P, and the Bacterial Endocarditis Study Group. Ceftriaxone as single daily dose for 4 weeks in the treatment of bacterial endocarditis. In: *Fifth International Congress for Infectious Diseases, Rio de Janeiro, Brazil, 1988* (Abstract 480). 1990.

178. Parker RH, Fossieck BE Jr. Intravenous followed by oral therapy for staphylococcal endocarditis. *Ann Intern Med* 1980;93:832–834.

179. Chambers HF, Miller RT, Newman MD. Right-sided *Staphylococcus aureus* endocarditis in intravenous drug abusers: two weeks combination therapy. *Ann Intern Med* 1988;109:619–624.

180. Eykyn SJ. The treatment of staphylococcal endocarditis. *J Antimicrob Chemother* 1987;20(Suppl A):161–167.

181. Rubenstein E, Noriega ER, Simberkoff MS. Fungal endocarditis: analysis of 24 cases and review of the literature. *Medicine* 1975;54:331–344.

182. Ernst JD, Rusmak M, Sande MA. Combination antifungal chemotherapy for experimental disseminated candidiasis. Lack of correlation between *in vitro* and *in vivo* observations with amphotericin B plus rifampin. *Rev Infect Dis* 1983;3(Suppl):626–630.

183. Maderazo EG, Hickingbotham N, Cooper D, Murcia A. Aspergillus endocarditis: cure without surgical valve replacement. *South Med J* 1990;83:351–352.

184. Shaw J, Bochner F, Brooks PM, Moulds RFW, Ravenscroft PJ, Smith AJ. Infective endocarditis in the 1980s. Part 2. Treatment and management. *Med J Aust* 1986;144:588–594.

185. Stratton CW. The role of the microbiology laboratory in the treatment of infective endocarditis. *J Antimicrob Chemother* 1987;20(Suppl A):41–49.

186. Freeman R, Hall R. Infective endocarditis. In: Juilian D, Camm AJ, Fox KM, Hall RJC, Poole-Wilson PA, eds. *Diseases of the heart.* London: Ballière & Tindall, 1989;853–876.

187. Mullany CJ, McIssacs AI, Rowe MH, Hale GS. The surgical treatment of infective endocarditis. *World J Surg* 1989;13:132–136.

188. Alsip SG, Blackstone EH, Kirklin JW, Coobs CG. Indications for cardiac surgery in patients with active infective endocarditis. *Am J Med* 1985;78(Suppl 6B):138–148.

189. Cohn LH, Doty DB, McElvein RB. *Decision making in cardiothoracic surgery.* Toronto: BC Decker 1987.

190. Dinubile MJ. Surgery in active endocarditis. *Ann Intern Med* 1982;96:650–659.

191. Defraigne JD, Dalem AM, Demoulin JC, Limet R. Surgical management of left heart endocarditis. *Acta Chir Belg* 1989;89:247–252.

192. Sullivan NM, Sutter VL, Mims MM. Clinical aspects of bacteremia after manipulation of the genitourinary tract. *J Infect Dis* 1973;127:49–55.

193. Shorvon PJ, Eykyn SJ, Cotton PB. Gastrointestinal instrumentation, bacteria and endocarditis. *Gut* 1983;24:1078–1093.

194. Shulman ST, Bisno AL, Amren DP, Dajani AS, Durack DT. Prevention of bacterial endocarditis. A statement for health professionals by the Committee on Rheumatic Fever and Infective Endocarditis of the Council on Cardiovascular Disease in the Young. *Circulation* 1984;70(Suppl A):1123–1127.

195. Prevention of bacterial endocarditis. *Med Lett* 1984;26:4–6.

196. Oakley CM. Controversies in the prophylaxis of infective endocarditis: a cardiological view. *J Antimicrob Chemother* 1987;20(Suppl A):99–104.

197. Horstkotte D, Friedrichs W, Pippert H, Bricks W, Loogen F. Nutzen der Endokarditisprophylaxe bei Patienten mit prothetischen Herzklappen. *Z Kardiol* 1986;75:8–11.

198. Imperiale TF, Horwitz RI. Does prophylaxis prevent postdental infective endocarditis? A controlled evaluation of protective efficacy. *Am J Med* 1990;88:131–136.

199. Glauser MP, Francioli P. Relevance of animal models to the prophylaxis of infective endocarditis. *J Antimicrob Chemother* 1987;20(Suppl A):87–93.

200. Prophylaxe der bakteriellen endokarditis. Empfehlungen des Schweizerischen Arbeitsgruppe für Endokarditisprophylaxe. *Schweiz Med Wochenschr* 1984;114:1246–1252.

201. Antibiotic prophylaxis of infective endocarditis. *Lancet* 1990;335:88–89.

202. Shulman ST. Prevention of infective endocarditis: the view from the United States. *J Antimicrob Chemother* 1987;20(Suppl A):111–118.

203. Berney P, Francioli P. Successful prophylaxis of experimental

streptococcal endocarditis with single dose amoxicillin administered after bacterial challenge. *J Infect Dis* 1990;161:281–285.

204. Moreillon P, Francioli P, Overholser CD, Meylan P, Glauser MP. Mechanisms of successful amoxicillin prophylaxis of experimental endocarditis due to *Streptococcus intermedius. J Infect Dis* 1986;154:801–807.

205. Tompsett R. Bacterial endocarditis: changes in the clinical spectrum. *Arch Intern Med* 1967;119:329–332.

206. Price EC, Headley RN, Sawyer CG. Bacterial endocarditis: its behavior in the elderly. *NC Med J* 1962;23:284–290.

207. Horder TJ. Infective endocarditis with an analysis of 150 cases and with special reference to the chronic form of the disease. *Q J Med* 1908;2:289–324.

208. Blumer G. Subacute bacterial endocarditis. *Medicine* 1923;2: 105–170.

209. DeJong RN. Central nervous system complications in subacute bacterial endocarditis. *J Nerv Ment Dis* 1937;85:397–410.

210. Fetterman GL, Aske WF. Cerebral debut of certain cases of cardiac disease. *Ohio M J* 1938;34:1354–1358.

211. Krinsky CM, Merritt HH. Neurological manifestations of subacute bacterial endocarditis. *N Engl J Med* 1938;218:563–566.

212. Toone EC. Cerebral manifestations of bacterial endocarditis. *Ann Intern Med* 1941;14:1551–1574.

213. Hickie J. Bacterial endocarditis in Sydney 1950–1959. *Med J Aust* 1961;1:929–934.

214. Pankey GA. Subacute bacterial endocarditis at University of Minnesota Hospitals 1939–1959. *Ann Intern Med* 1961;55:550–561.

215. Pankey GA. Acute bacterial endocarditis at the University of Minnesota Hospitals. *Am Heart J* 1962;64:583–591.

216. Cooper ES, Cooper JW, Schnabel TG. Pitfalls in the diagnosis of bacterial endocarditis. *Arch Intern Med* 1966;118:55–61.

217. Harrison MJ, Hampton JR. Neurological presentation of bacterial endocarditis. *Br Med J* 1967;2:148–151.

218. Jones HR Jr, Siekert RG, Geraci JE. Neurologic manifestations of bacterial endocarditis. *Ann Intern Med* 1969;71:21–28.

219. Garvey GJ, Neu HC. Infective endocarditis—an evolving disease. *Medicine* 1978;57:105–127.

220. Crittin J, Waldvogel FA. Bacterial endocarditis: clinical and bacteriological aspects and prognostic factors. *Schweiz Med Wochenschr* 1977;5:1–26.

221. Pruitt AA, Rubin RH, Karchmer AW, Duncan GW. Neurologic complications of bacterial endocarditis. *Medicine (Baltimore)* 1978;57:329–343.

222. Bush M, Masferrer R, Teitel R, Pittman HW. Neurologic complications of infectious endocarditis. *BNI Q* 1985;1:13–18.

223. Salgado AV, Furlan AJ, Keys TF, Nichols TR, Beck GJ. Neurologic complications of endocarditis: a 12-year experience. *Neurology* 1989;39:173–178.

224. Kernhoan GW, Woltman HW, Barnes AR. Involvement of the nervous system associated with endocarditis. *J Nerv Ment Dis* 1937;85:397.

225. Lerner PI. Neurologic complications of infective endocarditis safety of NMR [Editorial]. *Lancet* 1985;1:913–914.

226. Lerner PI. Neurologic complications of infective endocarditis. *Med Clin North Am* 1985;69:385–398.

227. Kane WC, Aronson SM. Cardiac disorders predisposing to embolic stroke. *Stroke* 1970;1:164–172.

228. Le Cam B, Guivarch G, Boles JM, Garre M, Cartier F. Neurologic complications in a group of 86 bacterial endocarditis. *Eur Heart J* 1984;5:97–100.

229. Cantrell M, Yoshikawa TT. Aging and infective endocarditis. *J Am Geriatr Soc* 1983;31:216–222.

230. Robbins N, DeMaria A, Miller MH. Infective endocarditis in the elderly. *South Med J* 1980;73:1335–1338.

231. Greenlee JE, Mandell GL. Neurological manifestations of infective endocarditis: a review. *Stroke* 1973;4:958–963.

232. Appelfeld MA, Hornick RB. Infective endocarditis in patients over age 60. *Am J Med* 1974;88:90–94.

233. Naganuma M. Infective endocarditis in children. *Jpn Circ J* 1985;49:545–552.

234. Nocht B, Paschen E, Hegler C. *Jochmann's Lehrbuch der Infectionskrankheiten.* Berlin: Springer, 1924;144–148.

235. Kirkes WS. Principal effects resulting from detachment of fibrin-

236. Openshaw H. Neurological complications of endocarditis in persons taking drugs intravenously. *West J Med* 1976;124:276–281.

237. Hubbel G, Cheitlin MD, Rapaport E. Presentation, management, and follow-up evaluation of infective endocarditis in drug addicts. *Am Heart J* 1981;102:85–94.

238. Roberts WC, Buchbinder NA. Right-sided valvular infective endocarditis. A clinicopathologic study of twelve necropsy patients. *Am J Med* 1972;53:7–19.

239. Olsson RA, Romansky MJ. Staphylococcal tricuspid endocarditis in heroin addicts. *Ann Intern Med* 1962;57:755–762.

240. Jones HR, Caplan LR, Come PC, Swinton NW, Breslin DJ. Cerebral emboli of paradoxical origin. *Ann Neurol* 1983;13:314–319.

241. Shenoy MM, Greif E, Friedman SA, Leibowitz I. Paradoxical embolism secondary to tricuspid valve endocarditis. *Am J Cardiol* 1984;54:1374–1375.

242. Gransden WR, Eykyn SJ, Leach RM. Neurological presentations of native valve endocarditis. *Q J Med* 1989;73:1135–1142.

243. Karchmer AW, Dismukes WE, Buckley MJ, Austen WG. Late prosthetic valve endocarditis: clinical features influencing therapy. *Am J Med* 1978;64:199–206.

244. Wilson WR, Geraci JE, Danielson GK, et al. Anticoagulant therapy and central nervous system complications in patients with prosthetic valve endocarditis. *Circulation* 1978;57:1004–1007.

245. Carpenter JL, McAllister CK. Anticoagulation in prosthetic valve endocarditis. *South Med J* 1983;76:1372–1375.

246. Quenzer RW, Edwards LD, Levin S. A comparative study of 48 host valve and 24 prosthetic valve endocarditis cases. *Am Heart J* 1976;92:15–22.

247. Madison J, Wang K, Gobel FL, Edwards JE. Prosthetic aortic valvular endocarditis. *Circulation* 1975;51:940–949.

248. Leport C, Vilde JL, Bricaire F, et al. Fifty cases of late prosthetic valve endocarditis: improvement in prognosis over a 15 year period. *Br Heart J* 1987;58:66–71.

249. Dismukes WE, Karchmer AW. The diagnosis of infected prosthetic heart valves: bacteremia versus endocarditis. In: Duma RJ ed. *Infections of prosthetic heart valves and vascular grafts, prevention, diagnosis, and treatment.* Baltimore: University Park Press, 1977;61–80.

250. Keyser DL, Diller J, Coffman TT, Adams HP Jr. Neurologic complications of late prosthetic valve endocarditis. *Stroke* 1990;21:472–475.

250a. Davenport J, Hart RG. Prosthetic valve endocarditis. Antibiotics, Anticoagulation, and Stroke. *Stroke* 1990;21:993–999.

251. Schoen FJ. Cardiac valve protheses: review of clinical status and contemporary biomaterials issues. *J Biomed Materials Res* 1987;21:91–117.

252. Dismukes WE, Karchmer AW, Buckley MJ, Austen WG, Swartz MN. Prosthetic valve endocarditis. *Circulation* 1973;63:365–377.

253. Arnett EN, Roberts WC. Prosthetic valve endocarditis. Clinicopathologic analysis of 22 patients with comparison of observations in 74 necropsy patients with active infective endocarditis involving natural left-sided cardiac valves. *Am J Cardiol* 1976;38:281–292.

254. Davenport J, Foster J, Hart R. Prosthetic valve endocarditis (PVE): antibiotics, anticoagulation and stroke [Abstract 66]. *Stroke* 1988;19:145–145.

255. Ramsey RG, Gunnar RM, Tobin JR Jr. Endocarditis in the drug addicts. *Am J Cardiol* 1970;25:608–618.

256. Louria DB. Infectious complications of nonalcoholic drug abuse. *Annu Rev Med* 1974;25:219–231.

257. Richter RW, Baden MM. Neurological complications of heroin addiction. *Trans Am Neurol Assoc* 1969;94:330–332.

258. Siekert RG, Jones HR Jr. Transient cerebral ischemic attacks associated with subacute bacterial endocarditis. *Stroke* 1970;1: 178–193.

259. Hart RG, Kagan Hallet K, Joerns SE. Mechanisms of intracranial hemorrhage in infective endocarditis. *Stroke* 1987;18:1048–1056.

260. Salgado AV, Furlan AJ, Keys TF. Mycotic aneurysm, subarachnoid hemorrhage, and indications for cerebral angiography in infective endocarditis. *Stroke* 1987;18:1057–1060.

261. Venger BH, Aldama AE. Mycotic vasculitis with repeated intra-

cranial aneurysmal hemorrhage case report. *J Neurosurg* 1988;69:775–779.

262. Winkelman NW, Eckel JL. The brain in bacterial endocarditis. *Arch Neurol Psychiatry* 1930;23:1161–1182.

263. Davis WA, Kane JG, Garagusi VF. Human Aeromonas infections: a review of the literature and a case report of endocarditis. *Medicine (Baltimore)* 1978;57:267–277.

264. Watanakunakorn C, Tan JS, Phair JP. Some salient features of *Staphylococcus aureus* endocarditis. *Am J Med* 1973;54:473–481.

265. Epersen F, Frimodt-Moller N. *Staphylococcus aureus* endocarditis. A review of 119 cases. *Arch Intern Med* 1986;146:1118–1121.

266. Ogbuawa O, Fam WM. Comparison of staphylococcal and nonstaphylococcal endocarditis in narcotic addicts. *Am J Med* 1979;1157–1163.

267. Felner JM, Dowell VR Jr. Anaerobic bacterial endocarditis. *N Engl J Med* 1970;283:1188–1192.

268. Preble HB. Pneumococcal endocarditis. *Am J Med Sci* 1904;128:782–797.

269. Straus AL, Hamburger M. Pneumococcal endocarditis in the antibiotic era. *Arch Intern Med* 1966;118:190–198.

270. Ruegsegger JM. Pneumococcal endocarditis. *Am Heart J* 1958;66:867–877.

271. Austrian R. Pneumococcal endocarditis, meningitis, and rupture of the aortic valve. *Arch Intern Med* 1957;99:539–544.

272. Elster SK, Mattes LM, Meyers BR, Jurado RA. Hemophilus aphrophilus endocarditis: review of 23 cases. *Am J Cardiol* 1975;35:72–79.

273. Johnson RH, Kennedy RP, Marton KI, Thornsberry C. Hemophilus endocarditis: new cases, literature review and recommendations for management. *South Med J* 1977;70:1098–1102.

274. Bamrah VS. Hemophilus parainfluenza mitral valve vegetation with hemodynamic abnormality: demonstration by angiography and serial echocardiography. *Am J Med* 1979;66:543–546.

275. Wilson WR, Giuliani ER, Danielson GK, Geraci JE. Management of complications of infective endocarditis. *Mayo Clin Proc* 1982;57:162–170.

276. Ellner PD. Endocarditis due to group L *Streptococcus. Ann Intern Med* 1970;72:547–548.

277. Andriole VT, Kravetz HM, Roberts WC, Utz JP. *Candida* endocarditis. *Medicine* 1962;32:251–285.

278. Richardson JV, Karp RB, Kirklin JW, Dismukes WE. Treatment of infective endocarditis: a 10-year comparative analysis. *Circulation* 1978;58:589–597.

279. Woods GL, Wood RP, Shaw BW. Aspergillus endocarditis in patients without prior cardiovascular surgery: report of a case in a liver transplant recipient and review. *Rev Infect Dis* 1989;11:263–272.

280. Grillo RA Jr, Olson NH. Amnesia as a presenting symptom in subacute bacterial endocarditis. *J Clin Psychiatry* 1986;47:383–384.

281. Alajouanine T, Castaigne P, Lhermitte F, Cambier J. L'artérite cérébrale de la maladie d'Osler et ses complications tardives. *Semin Hop Paris* 1959;15:202–207.

282. Coobs CG, Livingston WK. Special problems in the management of infective endocarditis. In: Bisno AL, ed. *Treatment of infective endocarditis.* New York: Grune & Stratton, 1981;147–166.

283. Ziment I. Nervous system complications in bacterial endocarditis. *Am J Med* 1969;47:593–607.

284. Johnson DH, Rosenthal A, Nadas AS. Bacterial endocarditis in children under 2 years of age. *Am J Dis Child* 1975;129:183–186.

285. Wilson WR, Lie JT, Wayne Houser O, Piepgras DG, Geraci JE. The management of patients with mycotic aneurysm. *Curr Clin Top Infect Dis* 1981;2:151–183.

286. Gleckler WJ. Diagnostic aspects of subacute bacterial endocarditis in the elderly. *Arch Intern Med* 1958;102:761–765.

287. Shafar J. Bacterial endocarditis presenting as pseudobulbar palsy. *Br Med J* 1967;4:338–338.

288. Bademosi O, Falase AO, Jaiyesimi F, Bademosi A. Neuropsychiatric manifestations of infective endocarditis: a study of 95 patients at Ibadan, Nigeria. *J Neurol Neurosurg Psychiatry* 1976;39:325–329.

289. Jones HR Jr, Siekert RG. Embolic mononeuropathy and bacterial endocarditis. *Arch Neurol* 1968;19:535–537.

290. Pamphlett R, Walsh J. Infective endocarditis with inflammatory lesions in the peripheral nervous system. *Acta Neuropathol (Berl)* 1989;78:101–104.

291. Lerner PI. Meningitis caused by *Streptococcus* in adults. *J Infect Dis* 1975;131:9–16.

292. Kerr KG. Low back pain as the only presenting symptom in *Streptococcus sanguis* endocarditis. *Rev Infect Dis* 1989;11:836–837.

293. Francioli PB, Roussianos D, Glauser MP. *Cardiobacterium hominis* endocarditis manifesting as bacterial meningitis. *Arch Intern Med* 1983;143:1483–1484.

294. Hart RG, Foster JW. Should lumbar puncture be part of the routine evaluation of patients with cerebral ischemia? *Stroke* 1986;17:333–333.

295. Powers WJ. Should lumbar puncture be part of the routine evaluation of patients with cerebral ischemia? *Stroke* 1985;16:737–737.

296. Powers WJ. Should lumbar puncture be part of the routine evaluation of patients with cerebral ischemia? *Stroke* 1986;17:332–333.

297. Hart RG. Should lumbar puncture be part of the routine evaluation of patients with cerebral ischemia? *Stroke* 1985;16:737.

298. Stilhart B, Aboulker J, Khouadja F, Robine D, Ouahes O, Redondo A. Should the aneurysms of Osler's disease be investigated and operated on prior to hemorrhage? *Neurochirurgie* 1986;32:410–417.

299. Chateau R, Groslambert R, Boucharlat J, Chatelain R. Hemiplegia during slow malignant endocarditis: 2 cases. *Lyon Med* 1969;221:325–329.

300. Jones HR, Siekert RG. Neurological manifestations of infective endocarditis. Review of clinical and therapeutic challenges. *Brain* 1989;112:1295–1315.

301. D'Agostino RS, Miller DC, Stinson EB, Mitchell RS, Oyer PE, Jamieson SW. Valve replacement in patients with native valve endocarditis: What really determines operative outcome? *Ann Thorac Surg* 1985;40:429–438.

302. Ben Ismail M, Hannachi N, Abid F, Kaabar Z, Rouge JF. Prosthetic valve endocarditis. A survey. *Br Heart J* 1987;58:72–77.

303. Sherman DG, Dyken ML, Fisher M, Harrison MJG, Hart RG. Cerebral embolism. *Chest* 1986;89(Suppl 2):82–98.

304. Sherman DG, Dyken ML, Fisher M, Harrison MJ, Hart RG (Cerebral Embolism Task Force). Cardiogenic brain embolism. *Arch Neurol* 1986;43:71–84.

305. Carter AB. Prognosis of cerebral embolism. *Lancet* 1965;2:514–519.

306. McDevitt E. Treatment of cerebral embolism. *Mod Treat* 1965;2:52–63.

307. McGivern D, Ispahani P, Banks D. Factors influencing mortality from infective endocarditis in two distinct general hospitals. *Postgrad Med J* 1987;63:345–349.

308. Mohr JP, Caplan LR, Melski JW, et al. The Harvard cooperative stroke registry: a prospective registry. *Neurology* 1978;28:754–762.

309. Gutschik E, Moller S, Christensen N. Experimental endocarditis in rabbits. 3. Significance of the proteolytic capacity of the infecting strains of Streptococcus faecalis. *Acta Pathol Microbiol Scand* 1979;87:353–357.

310. Lerner PI, Gopalakrishna KV, Wolinsky E, McHenry MC, Tan JS, Rosenthal M. Group B streptococcus (*S. agalactiae*) bacteremia in adults: analysis of 32 cases and review of the literature. *Medicine (Baltimore)* 1977;56:457–473.

310a.Paschalis C, Pugsley W, Jdiu R, Harrison MJG. Rate of Cerebral Embolic Events in Relation to Antibiotic and Anticoagulant Therapy in Patients with Bacterial Endocarditis. *Eur Neurol* 1990;30:87–89.

311. Lutas EM, Roberts RB, Devreux RB, Prieto LM. Relation between the presence of echocardiographic vegetations and the complication rate in infective endocarditis. *Am Heart J* 1986;112:107–113.

312. Ruff RL, Dougherty JH. Evaluation of acute cerebral ischemia for anticoagulant therapy: computed tomography or lumbar puncture? *Neurology* 1981;31:736–740.

313. Lee MC, Heaney LM, Jacobsen RL, Klassen AC. CSF in cerebral hemorrhage and infarction. *Stroke* 1975;6:638–642.

314. Sobel JD. *Candida* infections in the intensive care unit. *Crit Care Clin* 1989;4:325–344.
315. Morgan WL, Bland EF. Bacterial endocarditis in the antibiotic era, with special reference to the later complications. *Circulation* 1959;19:753–765.
316. Jagger JD, MacCaughan BC, Pawsey CGK. Tricuspid valve endocarditis cured by excision of a single vegetation. *South Med J* 1986;79:626–627.
317. Hughes CF, Noble N. Vegectomy: an alternative surgical treatment for infective endocarditis of the atrioventricular valves in drug addicts. *J Thorac Cardiovasc Surg* 1988;95:857–861.
318. Bruetman ME, Fields WS, Crawford ES, Debakey ME. Central hemorrhage in carotid artery surgery. *Arch Neurol* 1963;9:458–467.
319. Wylie EJ, Hein MF, Adams JE. Intracranial hemorrhage following surgical revascularization for treatment of acute strokes. *J Neurosurg* 1964;21:212–215.
320. Furlan AJ, Breuer AC. Central nervous system complications of open heart surgery. *Stroke* 1984;15:912–915.
321. Gilman S. Cerebral disorders after open-heart operations. *N Engl J Med* 1965;272:489–498.
322. Zisbrod Z, Rose DM, Jacobowitz IJ, Kramer M, Acinapura AJ, Cunningham JN Jr. Results of open heart surgery in patients with recent cardiogenic embolic stroke and central nervous system dysfunction. *Circulation* 1987;76(Suppl V):109–112.
323. Nelson RJ, Harley DP, French WJ, Bayer AS. Favorable ten-year experience with valve procedures for active endocarditis. *J Thorac Cardiovasc Surg* 1984;87:493–502.
324. Jara FM, Lewis JF Jr, Magilligan DJ Jr. Operative experience with infective endocarditis and intracerebral mycotic aneurysm. *J Thorac Cardiovasc Surg* 1980;80:28–30.
325. Cerebral Embolism Study Group. Cardioembolic stroke, early anticoagulation, and brain hemorrhage. *Arch Intern Med* 1987;147:636–640.
326. Daniel WG, Schroder E, Mugge A, Lichtlen PR. Transesophageal echocardiography in infective endocarditis. *Am J Cardiac Imaging* 1988;2:78–85.
327. Stewart JA, Silmperi D, Harris P, Wise NK, Fraker TD, Kisslo JA. Echocardiographic documentation of vegetative lesions in infective endocarditis: clinical implications. *Circulation* 1980;61:374–380.
328. Buda AJ, Zotz RJ, LeMire MS, Bach DS. Prognostic significance of vegetations detected by two-dimensional echocardiography in infective endocarditis. *Am Heart J* 1986;112:1291–1296.
329. O'Brien JT, Geiser EA. Infective endocarditis and echocardiography. *Am Heart J* 1984;108:386–394.
330. Hickey AJ, Wolfers J, Wilcken DEL. Reliability and clinical relevance of detection of vegetations by echocardiography in bacterial endocarditis. *Br Heart J* 1981;46:624–628.
331. Sharma S, Desai A, Kumar A, Hansoti RC. Two dimensional echocardiographic documentation of disappearance of mobile vegetations following fatal embolization. *Indian Heart J* 1983;35:247–249.
332. Wong D, Chandraratna AN, Wishnow RM, Dusitnanond V, Nimalasuriya A. Clinical implications of large vegetations in infectious endocarditis. *Arch Intern Med* 1983;143:1874–1877.
333. Friedman M, Hamburger WW, Katz LN. Use of heparin in subacute bacterial endocarditis. *JAMA* 1939;113:1702–1703.
334. Priest WS, Smith JM, McGee CJ. The effect of anticoagulants on the penicillin therapy and the pathologic lesion of subacute bacterial endocarditis. *N Engl J Med* 1946;235:699–706.
335. McLean J, Meyer BBM, Griffith JM. Heparin in subacute bacterial endocarditis. *JAMA* 1941;117:1870–1875.
336. Katz LN, Elek SR. Combined heparin and chemotherapy in subacute bacterial endocarditis. *JAMA* 1944;124:149–152.
337. Thill CJ, Meyer OO. Experiences with penicillin and dicumarol in the treatment of subacute bacterial endocarditis. *Am J Med Sci* 1947;213:300–307.
338. Foote RA, Reagan TJ, Sandok BA. Effects of anticoagulants in an animal model of septic cerebral embolization. *Stroke* 1978;9:573–579.
339. Hook EW III, Sande MA. Role of the vegetation in experimental *Streptococcus viridans* endocarditis. *Infect Immun* 1974;10:1433–1438.
340. Thompson J, Fulderink F, Lemkes H, Furth R. Effect of warfarin on the induction and course of experimental endocarditis. *Infect Immun* 1976;14:1284–1289.
341. Weinstein L. Life-threatening complications of infective endocarditis and their management. *Arch Intern Med* 1986;146:953–957.
342. Naggar CZ and Forgacs P. Infective endocarditis: a challenging disease. *Med Clin North Am* 1986;70:1279–1294.
343. Levine HJ, Pauker SG, Salzman EW. Antithrombotic therapy in valvular heart disease. *Chest* 1989;95(Suppl 2):98–106.
344. Block PC, DeSanctis RW, Weinberg AN. Prosthetic valves endocarditis. *J Thorac Cardiovasc Surg* 1970;60:540–548.
345. Mayer KH, Schoenbaum SC. Evaluation and management of prosthetic valve endocarditis. *Prog Cardiovasc Dis* 1982;25:43–54.
346. Vincent FM, Zimmerman JE, Auer TC, Martin DB. Subarachnoid hemorrhage—the initial manifestation of bacterial endocarditis. Report of a case with negative arteriography and computed tomography. *Neurosurgery* 1980;7:488–490.
347. King AB. Successful surgical treatment of an intracranial mycotic aneurysm complicated by a subdural hematoma. *J Neurosurg* 1960;17:788–791.
348. Siekert RG. Neurologic manifestations of infective endocarditis. In: Vinken RG, Bruyen GW, eds. *Handbook of clinical neurology,* vol 43. Amsterdam: Elsevier, 1980;469–477.
349. Fisher CM, Adams RD. Observation on brain emboli. *J Neuropathol Exp Neurol* 1951;10:92–93.
350. Jorgensen L, Torvik A. Ischaemic cerebrovascular diseases in an autopsy series. Part 2. Prevalence, location, pathogenesis, and clinical course of cerebral infarcts. *J Neurol Sci* 1969;9:285–320.
351. Cerebral Embolism Study Group. Immediate anticoagulation of embolic stroke: brain hemorrhage and management options. *Stroke* 1984;15:779–789.
352. Looder J. CT-detected hemorrhagic infarction: relation with the size of the infarct, and the presence of midline shift. *Acta Neurol Scand* 1984;70:329–335.
353. Yock DH Jr. Septic saddle embolus causing basilar artery rupture without mycotic aneurysm. *AJNR* 1984;5:822–824.
354. Morawetz RB, Karp RB. Evolution and resolution of intracranial bacterial (mycotic) aneurysms. *Neurosurgery* 1984;15:43–49.
355. Leipzig TJ, Brown FD. Treatment of mycotic aneurysms. *Surg Neurol* 1985;23:403–407.
356. Ojemann J, Crowell RM. Infectious intracranial aneurysms. In: Ojeman RG, ed. *Surgical management of cerebrovascular disease.* Baltimore: Williams & Wilkins, 1983;225–263.
357. Fearnsides EG. Intracranial aneurysms. *Brain* 1916;39:224–296.
358. McDonald CA, Korb M. Intracranial aneurysm. *Arch Neurol Psychiatry* 1939;42:298–328.
359. Mitchell N, Angrist A. Intracranial aneurysms—a report of thirty-six cases. *Ann Intern Med* 1943;19:909–923.
360. Housepian EM, Lawrence Pool J. A systematic analysis of intracranial aneurysms from the autopsy file of the Presbyterian Hospital. *J Neuropathol Exp Neurol* 1958;17:409–423.
361. Roach MR, Drake CG. Ruptured cerebral aneurysms caused by micro-organisms. *N Engl J Med* 1965;273:240–244.
362. Bequet D, Martini L, Jacquin Cotton L, Ndiaye IP, Diop Mar I. Infectious intracranial aneurysms. Apropos of 5 cases seen in Senegal. *Dakar Med* 1979;24:197–211.
363. Case records of the Massachusetts General Hospital. Case 27-1980. *N Engl J Med* 1980;303:92–100.
364. Stengel A, Wolferth CC. Mycotic (bacterial) aneurysms of intravascular origin. *Arch Intern Med* 1923;31:527–554.
365. Bohmfalk GL, Story JL, Wissinger JP, Brown WE. Bacterial intracranial aneurysm. *J Neurosurg* 1978;48:369–382.
366. Mansur AJ, Grinberg M, Leao PP, Chung CV, Stolf NAG. Extracranial mycotic aneurysms in infective endocarditis. *Clin Cardiol* 1986;9:65–72.
367. Bingham WF. Treatment of mycotic intracranial aneurysms. *J Neurosurg* 1977;46:428–437.
368. Moskowitz MA, Rosenbaum AE, Tyler HR. Angiographically monitored resolution of cerebral mycotic aneurysms. *Neurology* 1974;24:1103–1108.
369. Eppinger H. Pathogenesis (Histogenesis und Actiologie) der An-

eurysmen einschliesslich des Aneurysma equi veminosum. *Pathol Anat Stud Arch Klin Chir* 1887;35:1.

370. Molinari GF, Smith L, Goldstein MN, Satran R. Pathogenesis of cerebral mycotic aneurysms. *Neurology* 1973;23:325–332.

371. Horten BC, Gerald FA, Robert SP. Fungal aneurysms of intracranial vessels. *Arch Neurol* 1976;33:577–579.

372. Katz RI, Goldberg HI, Selzer ME. Mycotic aneurysm. Case report with novel sequential angiographic findings. *Arch Intern Med* 1974;134:939–942.

373. Schold C, Earnest MP. Cerebral hemorrhage from a mycotic aneurysm developing during appropriate antibiotic therapy. *Stroke* 1978;9:267–268.

374. Bamford J, Hodges J, Warlow C. Late rupture of a mycotic aneurysm after "cure" of bacterial endocarditis. *J Neurol* 1986; 233:51–53.

375. Ghatak NR. Pathology of cerebral embolization caused by nonthrombotic agents. *Hum Pathol* 1975;6:599–610.

376. Weinstein L, Schlesinger JJ. Pathoanatomic, pathophysiologic and clinical correlations in endocarditis (second of two parts). *N Engl J Med* 1974;291:1122–1126.

377. Shibuya S, Igaraschi S, Amo T. Mycotic aneurysms of the internal carotid artery. Case report. *J Neurosurg* 1976;44:105–108.

378. Suwanwela C. Intracranial mycotic aneurysms of extravascular origin. *J Neurosurg* 1972;36:552–559.

379. Adams RD, Kubik CS, Bonner FJ. The clinical and pathological aspects of influenzal meningitis. *Arch Pediatr* 1948;65:354–376.

380. Davis DO, Dilenge D, Schlaepfer W. Arterial dilatation in purulent meningitis: case report. *J Neurosurg* 1970;32:112–115.

381. Greitz T. Angiography in tuberculous meningitis. *Acta Radiol [Diagn] (Stockh)* 1964;2:369–378.

382. Wadia NH. Vascular changes in tuberculous meningitis: an arteriographic study in 33 patients. *Proc Aust Assoc Neurol* 1968;5:623–629.

383. Hadley MN, Martin NA, Spetzler RF, Johnson PC. Multiple intracranial aneurysms due to *Coccidioides immitis* infection. Case report. *J Neurosurg* 1987;66:453–456.

384. Ojemann RG. Intracranial aneurysms associated with bacterial meningitis. *Neurology* 1966;16:1222–1226.

385. Ray H, Wahal KM. Subarchnoid hemorrhage in subacute bacterial endocarditis. *Neurology* 1957;7:265–269.

386. Bullock R, Van Dellen JR. Rupture of bacterial intracranial aneurysms following replacement of cardiac valves. *Surg Neurol* 1981;17:9–10.

387. AhFat LNC, Pickens S. *Actinobacillus actinomycetemcomitans* endocarditis in hypertrophic obstructive cardiomyopathy. *J Infect* 1983;6:81–84.

388. Laguna J, Derby BM, Chase R. *Cardiobacterium hominis* endocarditis with cerebral mycotic aneurysm. *Arch Neurol* 1975;32:438–439.

389. Gilroy J, Andaya L, Thomas VJ. Intracranial mycotic aneurysms and subacute bacterial endocarditis in heroin addiction. *Neurology* 1973;23:1193–1198.

390. Hanneson B, Sachs E. Mycotic aneurysms following purulent meningitis. *Acta Neurochir (Wien)* 1971;24:305–313.

391. Sypert GW, Young HF. Ruptured mycotic pericallosal aneurysms with meningitis due to *Neisseria meningitidis* infection. *J Neurosurg* 1972;37:467–469.

392. Heidelberger KP, Layton WM, Fischer RG. Multiple cerebral mycotic aneurysms complicating posttraumatic *Pseudomonas* meningitis. *J Neurosurg* 1968;29:631–635.

393. Davidson P, Robertson DM. A true mycotic (*Aspergillus*) aneurysm leading to fatal subarachnoid hemorrhage in a patient with hereditary hemorrhagic telangiectasia. *J Neurosurg* 1971;35:71–76.

394. Visudhipan P, Bunyaratave JS, Khantanaphar S. Cerebral aspergillosis. Report of three cases. *J Neurosurg* 1973;38:472–476.

395. Collins GJ, Rich NM, Hobson RW, Andersen CA, Green D. Multiple mycotic aneurysms due to *Candida* endocarditis. *Ann Surg* 1977;186:136–139.

396. Morris FH Jr, Spock A. Intracranial aneurysm secondary to mycotic orbital and sinus infection. Report of a case implicating *Penicillium* as an opportunistic fungus. *Am J Dis Child* 1970;119:357–362.

397. Meade RH. Staphylococcal bacteremia and endocarditis. *Circulation* 1959;10:440–457.

398. Steele JJ, Kilburn HL, Leech RW. Phytotic (mycotic) intracranial aneurysm with an unusual pathogenesis: a case report. *Pediatrics* 1972;50:936–939.

399. Shnider IB, Cotsonas NJ Jr. Embolic mycotic aneurysms, a complication of bacterial endocarditis. *Am J Med* 1954;16:246–255.

400. Dean RH, Waterhouse G, Meacham PW, Weaver FA, O'Neil JA. Mycotic embolism and embolomycotic aneurysms. *Ann Surg* 1986;204:300–307.

401. Pailloncy M, Francois MA, Georget AM, Heiligenstein D, Vaudey F, Gras H. Intracranial aneurysms of bacterial endocarditis. Apropos of 4 cases. *Arch Mal Coeur* 1982;75:1077–1084.

402. Allcock G. *Radiology of the skull and brain angiography.* St. Louis: CV Mosby, 1974;435–442, 489.

403. Hourihane JB. Ruptured mycotic intracranial aneurysm. A report of three cases. *Vasc Surg* 1970;4:21–29.

404. Holzman RNN, Dickinson PCT, Hughes JEO, and Brust JCM. Cerebral mycotic aneurysm: presentation and outcome. *Ann Neurol* 1988;124:129–129.

405. Sato T, Sakuta Y, Suzuki J, Takaku A. Successful surgical treatment of intracranial mycotic aneurysm with brain abscess. Report of a case. *Acta Neurochir (Wien)* 1979;47:53–61.

406. Pozzati E, Tognetti F, Padovani R, Gaist G. Association of cerebral mycotic aneurysm and brain abscess. *Neurochirurgia (Stuttg)* 1983;26:18–20.

407. Cantu RC, LeMay M, Wilkinson HA. The importance of repeated angiography in the treatment of mycotic–embolic intracranial aneurysms. *J Neurosurg* 1966;25:189–193.

408. Bullock R, Van Dellen JR. Rupture of bacterial intracranial aneurysms following replacement of cardiac valves. *Surg Neurol* 1982;17:9–11.

409. Devadiga KV, Mathai KV, Chandy J. Spontaneous cure of intracavernous aneurysm of the internal carotid artery in a 14-month-old child: case report. *J Neurosurg* 1969;30:165–168.

410. Barker WF. Mycotic aneurysms. *Ann Surg* 1954;139:84–89.

411. Hansmann GH, Schenken JR. Melitensis meningo-encephalitis: mycotic aneurysm due to *Brucella melitensis* var. porcine. *Am J Pathol* 1932;8:435–444.

412. Bradley WG Jr, Schmidt PG. Effect of methemoglobin formation on the MR appearance of subarachnoid hemorrhage. *Radiology* 1985;156:99–103.

413. Hackney DB, Lesnick JE, Zimmerman RA, Grossman RI, Goldberg HI, Bilaniuk LT. MR identification of bleeding site in subarachnoid hemorrhage with multiple intracranial aneurysms. *J Comput Assist Tomogr* 1986;10:878–880.

414. Day AL. Extracranial–intracranial bypass grafting in the surgical treatment of bacterial aneurysms: report of two cases. *Neurosurgery* 1981;9:583–588.

415. McNeel D, Evans RA, Ory EM. Angiography of cerebral mycotic aneurysms. *Acta Radiol [Diagn] (Stockh)* 1969;9:407–412.

416. Rodesch G, Noterman J, Thys JP, Flament Durand J, Hermanus N. Treatment of intracranial mycotic aneurysm: surgery or not. A case report. *Acta Neurochir (Wien)* 1987;85:63–68.

417. Pecker J, Vallee B, Camuzet JP, Faivre J, Javalet A. Cerebral aneurysms complicating bacterial endocarditis. Seven cases. *Semin Hop Paris* 1980;56:1671–1676.

418. Schwartz MN, Dodge PR. Bacterial meningitidis—a review of selected subjects. *N Engl J Med* 1965;272:779–783.

419. Carpenter RR, Petersdorf RG. The clinical spectrum of bacterial meningitidis. *Am J Med* 1962;33:262–275.

420. Fong IW, Ranalli P. *Staphylococcus aureus* meningitis. *Q J Med* 1984;53:289–299.

421. Schlessinger LS, Ross SC, Schaberg DR. *Staphylococcus aureus* meningitidis: a broad-based epidemiology study. *Medicine* 1987;66:148–156.

422. Carruthers MM, Kanokvechayant R. *Pseudomonas aeruginosa* endocarditis. Report of a case, with review of the literature. *Am J Med* 1973;55:811–818.

423. Pasternack JG. Subacute *Monilia* endocarditis. A new clinical and pathologic entity. *Am J Clin Pathol* 1942;12:496–505.

424. Gerber HJ, Schoonmaker FW, Vazquez MD. Chronic meningitis associated with *Histoplasma* endocarditis. *N Engl J Med* 1966;275:74–76.

425. Mampalam TJ, Rosenblum ML. Trends in the management of bacterial brain abscesses: a review of 102 cases over 17 years. *Neurosurgery* 1988;23:451–458.

426. Chin Hak Chun, Johnson JD, Hofstetter M, Raff MJ. Brain abscess. A study of 45 consecutive cases. *Medicine* 1986;65:415–431.
427. Rosenblum ML, Hoff JT, Nordman D, Weinstein PR, Pitts L. Decreased mortality from brain abscesses since the advent of computerized tomography. *J Neurosurg* 1978;49:658–668.
428. Brewer NS, MacCarty CS, Wellman WE. Brain abscess: a review of recent experience. *Ann Intern Med* 1975;82:571–576.
429. Morgan H, Wood MW, Murphey F. Experience with 88 consecutive cases of brain abscess. *J Neurosurg* 1973;38:698–704.
430. Mathisen GE, Meyer RD, George WL, Citron DM, Finrgold SM. Brain abscess and cerebritis. *Rev Infect Dis* 1984;6(Suppl 1):101–106.
431. Seydoux P, Francioli P. Brain abscess: factors influencing mortality and sequelae. Submitted for publication, 1991.
432. Berg B, Franklin G, Cuneo R, Boldrey E, Strimling B. Nonsurgical cure of brain abscess: early diagnosis and follow-up with computerized tomography. *Ann Neurol* 1978;3:474–478.
433. Sawar M, Falkoff G, Naseem M. Radiologic techniques in the diagnosis of CNS infections. *Neurol Clin* 1986;4:41–68.
434. Brant-Zawadzki M, Enzmann DR, Placone RC. NMR imaging of experimental brain abscess: comparison with CT. *AJNR* 1983;4:250–253.
435. Runge VM, Clanton JA, Price AC. Evaluation of contrast enhanced MR imaging in a brain-abscess model. *AJNR* 1985;6:139–147.
436. DeWitt LD, Buonanno FS, Kistler JP, et al. Nuclear magnetic resonance imaging in evaluation of clinical stroke syndromes. *Ann Neurol* 1984;16:535–545.
437. Aisen AM, Gabrielsen TO, McCune WJ. MR imaging in systemic lupus erythematosus involving the brain. *AJR* 1985;144:1027–1031.
438. Wispelwey B, Scheld WM. Brain abscess. *Clin Neuropharmacol* 1987;10:483–510.
439. Wilson R, Hamburger M. Fifteen years' experience with *Staphylococcus* septicemia in a large city hospital. *Am J Med* 1957;22:437–457.
440. Allen SL, Salomon JE, Roberts RB. *Streptococcus bovis* endocarditis presenting as acute vertebral osteomyelitis. *Arthritis Rheum* 1981;24:1211–1212.
441. Meyers OL, Commerford PJ. Musculoskeletal manifestations of bacterial endocarditis. *Ann Rheum Dis* 1977;36:517–519.
442. Churchill MA Jr, Geraci JE, Hunder GG. Musculoskeletal manifestations of bacterial endocarditis. *Ann Intern Med* 1977;87:754–759.
443. Baker AS, Ojemann RG, Schwartz MN. Spinal epidural abscess. *N Engl J Med* 1975;293:463–467.
444. Clark R, Carlisle JT, Valainis GT. *Streptococcus pneumoniae* endocarditis presenting as an epidural abscess. *Rev Infect Dis* 1989;11:338–340.
445. Case records of the Massachusetts General Hospital. Case 35-1968. *N Engl J Med* 1969;281:492–499.
446. Case records of the Massachusetts General Hospital. Case 7-1988. *N Engl J Med* 1988;318:427–440.
447. Ochiai C, Takakura K, Basugi N, Machida T, Araki T, Iio M. Visualization of cerebellopontine angle diseases by nuclear magnetic resonance imaging. *No To Shinkei* 1983;35:1191–1198.
448. Hermans PE. The clinical manifestations of infective endocarditis. *Mayo Clin Proc* 1982;57:15–21.
449. Richards RD. Simultaneous occlusion of the central retinal artery and vein. *Trans Am Ophthalmol Soc* 1979;77:191–209.
450. Sigal SL, Smith GJ. Fever, rash, and blindness in a previously healthy young male. *Yale J Biol Med* 1983;56:219–229.
451. Case records of the Massachusetts General Hospital. Case 35-1966. *N Engl J Med* 1966;275:325–331.
452. Dienst EC, Gartner S. Pathologic changes in the eye associated with subacute bacterial endocarditis: report of five cases with autopsy. *Arch Ophthalmol* 1944;31:198–206.
453. McDonnel PJ, Green WR. Endophthalmitis. In: Mandell GL, Douglas RG, Benett JE, eds. *Principles and practice of infectious diseases,* 3rd ed. New York: Churchill Livingstone, 1990;987–995.
454. Kennedy JE, Wise GN. Clinicopathological correlation of retinal lesions. Subacute bacterial endocarditis. *Arch Ophthalmol* 1965;74:658–662.
455. Silverberg HH. Roth spots. *Mt Sinai J Med (NY)* 1970;37:77–79.
456. Edwards JE, Foos RY, Montgomerie JZ, Guze LB. Occular manifestations of candida septicemia: review of seventy-six cases of hematogenous *Candida* endophthalmitis. *Medicine* 1974;53:47–75.
457. McCue JD, Dreher RJ. Bilateral endophthalmitis with *Streptococcus viridans* endocarditis. *J Maine Med Assoc* 1979;70:463–465.
458. Treister G, Rothkoff L, Yalon M, Thaler M, Kaplinsky N, Frankl O. Bilateral blindness following panophthalmitis in a case of bacterial endocarditis. *Ann Ophthalmol* 1982;14:663–664.
459. Donzis PB, Rappazzo JA. Endogenous *Actinobacillus actinomycetemcomitans* endophthalmitis. *Ann Ophthalmol* 1984;16:858–860.

Infections of the Central Nervous System,
edited by W. M. Scheld, R. J. Whitley, and
D. T. Durack, Raven Press, Ltd., New York © 1991.

CHAPTER 23

Infections of Cerebrospinal Fluid Shunts

Bruce A. Kaufman and David G. McLone

Modern treatment of many central nervous system (CNS) diseases utilizes multiple methods of accessing the CNS and cerebrospinal fluid (CSF) spaces. The various indications for such access can be classified as: access, diversion, drainage, and monitoring. Table 1 summarizes the types and uses of devices used for these purposes. The CSF may require continuous diversion, or be intermittently utilized for repetitive sampling, drug infusion, or drainage. The CNS may be entered for monitoring purposes, such as the placement of intracranial pressure (ICP) measuring devices or electrodes for the detection of seizures.

All of these uses involve prosthetic implants, of either a temporary or permanent nature. In addition, these devices may be completely internal or "externalized," brought from within the CNS to a terminus outside the body. For example, most ICP monitors are placed in the epidural, subarachnoid, and intraventricular spaces and then brought to transducing devices outside the patient. There are also completely internalized telesensor ICP monitors. CSF reservoirs are implanted beneath the skin or scalp and can then be used for intermittent percutaneous access. They are commonly used for drainage in premature infants suffering from intraventricular hemorrhage and hydrocephalus, who are too small to tolerate a more permanent CSF diversion technique. The reservoir can also be used for intermittent pressure determinations. The intermittent infusion of medication—such as morphine for pain control, or any of a variety of antibacterial agents and antifungal, antiviral, or antineoplastic medications—overcomes the protected state of the CNS imposed by the blood–brain barrier (1–4). By far the

most common procedure involving the implantation of a device is for continuous CSF diversion, or "shunting," in the treatment of hydrocephalus.

HISTORY

Davidoff (5), Pudenz (6), and Scarff (7) have provided excellent reviews of the early history of the treatment of hydrocephalus. Hydrocephalus was recognized in ancient times by Hippocrates, and it has been documented by many observers through the ensuing centuries. Although "treatments" were proposed and carried out in the early 1700s, only since the late 19th century has therapy based on physiologic concepts been attempted. The modern era of treatment began with the advent of antisepsis, and it led to the refinement of surgical techniques in the early 20th century. Today's treatment of hydrocephalus has dramatically improved the patient's life, but it merely involves technical refinements of procedures proposed and attempted nearly 100 years ago.

The treatment of hydrocephalus has focused on three areas: reducing the production of CSF, diverting CSF around an obstruction, or diverting CSF outside the CNS for absorption. Attempts to reduce the production of CSF included reduction of blood flow to the choroid plexus which was proposed by Stiles in 1898 and performed by Fraser and Dott in 1922, by ligation of the carotid arteries bilaterally (5). Ablation of the choroid plexus by surgical resection or cauterization was proposed and performed by Dandy in the 1920s (7). These procedures had significant technical problems, not to mention a tremendous operative morbidity and mortality, and achieved equivocal success at best.

In the 1920s a number of surgical procedures were introduced to bypass obstructions to CSF flow at the level of the third or fourth ventricles. Recannulation of the cerebral aqueduct was reported in 1920 by Dandy; this procedure continues to be used, although infre-

B. A. Kaufman: Department of Neurosurgery, St. Louis Children's Hospital, Washington University, St. Louis, Missouri 63110.

D. G. McLone: Children's Memorial Hospital, Department of Neurosurgery, Northwestern University, Chicago, Illinois 60611.

TABLE 1. *CNS prosthetic devices*

Internalized (for long-term or permanent use)		Externalized (for temporary use)	
Diversion (shunts)	Access (reservoirs)	Drainage	Monitoring
Ventriculoperitoneal	Ventricular	Ventriculostomy	ICP monitoring
Ventriculovenous	Lumbar	Lumbar drain	Epidural
Lumboperitoneal		Externalized shunt	Subdural
			Intraparenchymal
			Intraventricular[a]

[a] Includes ventriculostomy for drainage.

quently (6,8). Ventriculocisternostomy, introduced by Torkildsen in 1939, was used intermittently into the 1960s (6,7). Both of these procedures had significant morbidity, and they carried a mortality of 20–30%. Third ventriculostomy, fenestration of the third ventricle into the subarachnoid space, has been performed with better success. As early as 1908, von Bramann attempted transcallosal fenestration, and in 1932 Dandy used a subfrontal, and subsequently a subtemporal, approach to fenestrate the base of the third ventricle (7). With the addition of radiographic and stereotactic methodology, this procedure continues to have a role in the management of selected patients (9).

For the vast majority of patients with hydrocephalus, effective treatment of this condition has only been available since the 1950s and involves diversion of the CSF to another part of the body for absorption—that is, shunting. Nulsen and Spitz (10) created the first competent one-way valved shunt in 1949. Prior to that, shunting of CSF from the ventricles to the intracranial venous sinuses depended on the presumed pressure differential between the compartments, or it depended on the natural valves in the venous portions of the systems used. In the last 30 years, shunt diversion to every conceivable compartment has been attempted. This has included drainage to the thoracic duct, salivary gland ducts, bone marrow, various intra-abdominal locations (gallbladder, stomach, ileum, ureters, omental bursa, fallopian tube),

extracerebral spaces (subdural space, dural venous sinuses, cisterna magna, cervical subarachnoid space), the mastoid sinuses, and the subgaleal space (6,11). Shunts terminating in the gallbladder, dural venous sinuses, cisterna magna, and cervical subarachnoid spaces function well, but they are technically more difficult to construct. An inability to adequately handle the large volumes of CSF produced daily, or an unacceptably high infection rate, led to the abandonment of the other sites. Refinements in materials [with the introduction of medical silicone (Silastic)], along with the evolution of surgical techniques, have led to effective drainage into the central venous system, or into peritoneal or pleural spaces, on a routine basis. At the present time, most neurosurgeons prefer the peritoneal cavity as the terminus of a shunt [ventriculoperitoneal (VP) shunt] over the central venous shunt [ventriculoatrial (VA) shunt]. VP shunts have been reported to require fewer revisions; they are easier to place and revise and have fewer serious complications, particularly when compared to those involving the cardiopulmonary and vascular systems (12–15). Ventriculoatrial and ventriculopleural shunts are still frequently utilized, particularly when peritoneal or vascular access, respectively, is not possible (16).

The typical CSF shunt has only a few basic components. The "proximal" portion of the system enters the CSF space. Although usually consisting of a catheter into one of the cerebral ventricles (ventricular catheter), a

FIG. 1. Common CSF shunt types. The most common shunt types are illustrated here. Any of these systems can be varied by the addition or deletion of various types of reservoirs, valves, connectors, and devices. Only one style is illustrated here. Any of them may be "externalized" by directing the distal end of the shunt through a skin incision and then collecting the CSF outside the patient. These would then be referred to as an "externalized ventriculostomy" or a "lumbar drain," depending on the proximal catheter origin. A: Ventriculoperitoneal (VP) shunt. A catheter within the ventricular system diverts the CSF outside the skull, through a reservoir (R) and a pressure-regulating valve (V) and through the distal tubing; all are placed in the subcutaneous tissues. The distal catheter is inserted into the peritoneal cavity. B: Ventriculoatrial (VA) or ventriculovenous shunt. Similar to the VP shunt, but the distal catheter is inserted into a vein in the neck and is then advanced so that the catheter tip is in the vena cava at the level of the atrium. C: Ventriculopleural (VPL) shunt. The proximal components remain the same as the VA and VP shunts, but the distal catheter is inserted into the pleural cavity through a small intercostal incision. D: Lumboperitoneal (LP) shunt. The proximal end of the system collects CSF from the lumbar subarachnoid space. The catheter is brought out dorsally, tunneled subcutaneously to the ventral aspect of the abdomen, and inserted into the peritoneal cavity (as with the VP shunt). The pressure is regulated by a valve incorporated into the peritoneal tip of the tubing, or it may be inserted into the system anywhere between open-ended proximal and distal catheters.

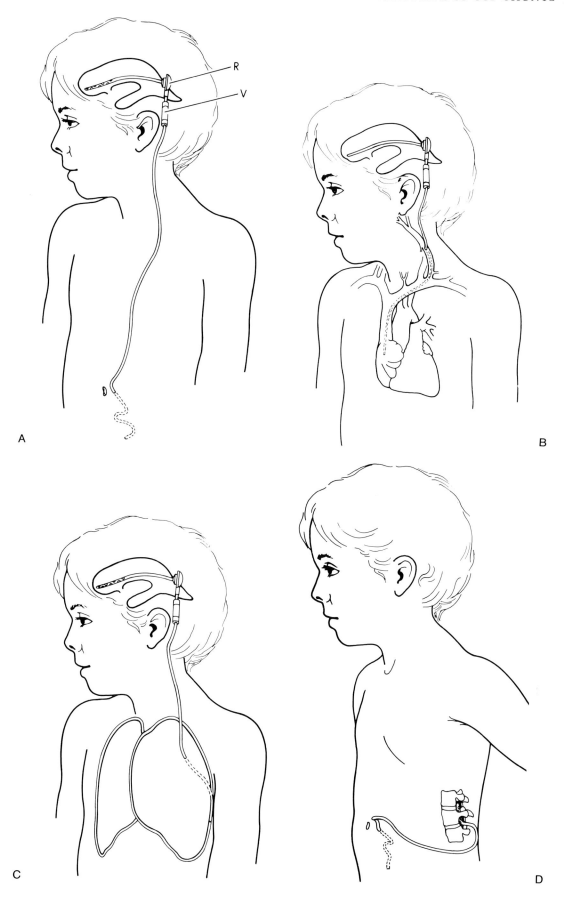

A

B

C

D

catheter placed into an intracranial cyst or into the lumbar subarachnoid space may represent the proximal portion. The rest of the shunt is the "distal" portion, whether terminating in the peritoneal, pleural, or vascular space or externalized from the patient. A pressure-regulating valve is part of the system, as a separate component usually placed just outside the skull or as an integral part of the distal tubing. Reservoirs for intermittent percutaneous access can be added to the system or incorporated into the valve assembly. Additional hardware includes (a) antisiphon valves and (b) various connectors allowing interconnection of more than one catheter or device. Figure 1 illustrates the most common shunt types.

Externalized devices are most commonly used in the treatment of infected shunts, but they may also be used for ICP monitoring or for the temporary diversion of CSF from an obstructed ventricular system ("external ventriculostomy"). Some ICP monitors are, in fact, external ventriculostomies, and CSF drainage through the monitor is then possible. Others are placed directly into the brain parenchyma or into the subdural or epidural space.

As with any procedure, the placement of these devices is not without some associated morbidity. The complications may be directly related to the placement of the device (hemorrhage), its malfunction (recrudescence of the original symptoms and their sequelae), or its repair (and the attendant risks of the operative procedure). The risk of infection, however, has been and continues to be a major source of concern in these procedures.

When a shunt infection occurs, permanent adverse outcome may result from the deleterious effects of the CNS infection (17,18). Given the frequency with which these procedures are performed, even a low rate of infection leads to a large number of cases. Therefore, the neurosurgical community has undertaken a significant effort to quickly and effectively treat, as well as to prevent, these infections. The areas of significant controversy—such as the origin of these infections, the best methods of treatment, and the best methods of prophylaxis—will be discussed below. We will review the epidemiology, clinical manifestations, diagnosis, treatment, and prophylaxis of shunt infections in particular, but we will also address infections of all CNS prosthetic devices when pertinent.

EPIDEMIOLOGY

When defining the incidence of shunt infections, a distinction between the "case infection rate" and the "operative infection rate" must be made. The "case infection rate" refers to the occurrence of infection per given patient, whereas the "operative infection rate" describes the occurrence of infection per procedure. This difference is particularly important in considering the group of neurosurgical patients with shunts. They almost always require shunting for life; and because those with benign diseases survive for several decades and beyond, they will require several revisions of their shunts for noninfectious reasons. Even if the operative infection rate were to remain constant, the case infection rate should continue to increase as the patients grow older, have more revisions, and are followed longer. In several large studies since 1971, the case incidence of shunt infection has ranged from 8% to 40%, and the operative incidence has ranged from 4.5% to 14% (13,19–26). As expected, those studies with longer follow-up had the higher case incidences of infection (Table 2). Other series report a similar, although variable, range of infection rates, from 2% to 40% (12,15,27–36).

Obviously, if the operative infection rate were to increase with succeeding revisions rather than remain constant, a larger increase in the case incidence would occur. Two studies reported an increased risk of infection for each subsequent revision (20,21). Odio et al. (21) actually demonstrated an increasing case incidence, where those with infections had undergone more revisions than those without infection. George et al. (20), however, showed that the operative incidence of infection in a patient undergoing a third (or greater) revision was significantly greater than that in one undergoing a first or second revision. Two other large series demonstrated no

TABLE 2. *Shunt infection review articles*

Authors (reference)	Year	Number of procedures	Follow-up (years)	Infection rate Case (%)	Operative (%)
Shurtleff et al. (25)	1971	299	12[a]	41	9
Schoenbaum et al. (23)	1975	743	2–11	27	13
Keucher and Mealey (13)	1979	754	5–7	22	7
George et al. (20)	1979	840	4[a]	27	14
Odio et al. (21)	1984	516	1[a]	17	11
Renier et al. (22)	1984	1174	—	—	8
Shurtleff et al. (26)	1985	1201	1[a]	8	4
Shapiro et al. (24)	1988	505	—	—	4
Ersahin et al. (19)	1989	2538	3[a]	10	5

[a] Average.

change in the operative incidence for those patients undergoing subsequent revisions (13,22). Keucher and Mealey (13) noted that the actual case infection rates for their study population were the same as would be predicted from a constant operative infection rate for each revision. Spanu et al. (35) had a slightly lower operative infection rate for revisions.

Interestingly, over the past 15 years a gradual decrease in the incidence of shunt infections has been noted (12,13,19–21,23,25,26,35). Within several studies that examined the incidence of infection over time, the operative rate was noted to decrease significantly (20,23, 26,35).

As previously mentioned, the type of shunting procedure used has changed over the years. Recent patients have received VP shunts more frequently, but this does not fully explain the decline in reported incidence. The same studies reporting declining rates of infection showed no significant difference between VA and VP infection rates (13,15,23,26). The difference, however, between ventriculo- and lumboperitoneal shunting infection rates does seem significant, with lumboperitoneal infection rates ranging from 0.8% to 4% (23,37).

Many diverse factors have been invoked to account for these variations in the incidence of shunt infections. Some of these have been inferred, whereas others have been observed during studies of shunt infection, although most studies utilize a retrospective analysis. Changes in the manufacture of the shunt materials have gradually taken place, and today nearly all shunting components are sterilely pre-packaged (23,26). This has only been inferred to reduce shunt infections. The decline in pre-shunting invasive studies such as lumbar punctures and pneumoencephalography with ventricular punctures has been inferred in the reduction of infection by some, and not associated with infection by others (22,26,38). Improvement in operating room facilities has also been inferred as a factor in the reduction of the infection rate. Better detection of some infected shunts preoperatively has also been considered in the apparent reduction of infection rates.

"Operative technique" covers several factors—such as operative time, fewer people traversing the operating theatre, experience of the surgeon, patient preparative techniques, and variations in the shunt insertion. All these have been felt to have direct implications for shunt infection. Although the experience of the surgeon has been felt to be a definite factor in two large studies where infection rates varied from 2% to 50%, and has been considered to be a possible factor in the experience of others, several other studies have not found any variation (20–25,39–42). The length of the shunt procedure has been directly correlated with increasing risk of infection, although in clean neurosurgical procedures this has not necessarily been the case (28,42–44). In VA shunting, position of the atrial catheter below T7 has been asso-

ciated with an increased rate of infection (40,45). This was felt to reflect the presence of foreign-body irritation on the tricuspid valve, with thrombus formation and subsequent infection during bacteremia.

Patient skin preparation and exposure of large areas of the patient's skin during the procedure have been considered as sources of infection (36,46). This is reinforced by the findings of Reneir et al. (22) and Spanu et al. (35) associating increased infection with poor skin condition and ventricular (i.e., scalp) revisions. The differences between the rate of infection of ventricular and of lumbar shunts might be explained by this association also.

The underlying cause of the patient's hydrocephalus has not been consistently associated with the frequency of shunt infections. Although a trend towards more shunt infections in the myelomeningocele population has been reported, this may more reasonably reflect the factors of frequent revisions and their often young age at the time of shunting (see section entitled "Pathogenesis," below) (36). In several large studies, no association between this diagnosis and infection has been found, regardless of either (a) shunt type or (b) relationship to time of neural tube closure (12,22,25,35,38,47).

The rate of externalized device infection has been reported to range from 0% to 15%, but it is probably consistently in the 5–7% range (48–56). The most commonly reported factor associated with an increased risk of infection is prolonged externalization. With ICP monitoring, most authors suggest that the risk of infection rises consistently and significantly after 72 hr (48–51,53,57). The risk may be significantly less for those devices that do not penetrate the ventricles or that do not require a fluid column for function (50,51,53,58,59).

The authors have experienced an extremely high rate of infection (nearing 40%) in the group of premature neonates with intraventricular hemorrhage treated with external ventriculostomy. This was felt to represent a combination of factors, including the physical status of the patients, their prematurity, and an extended time on externalized drainage. By utilizing a subcutaneous CSF reservoir and intermittent percutaneous punctures in place of the ventriculostomy, the infection rate has been reduced to approximately 5%, the rate seen with shunts in that age group (60).

Implanted CSF reservoirs represent a situation somewhere between standard shunts and externalized devices. The reservoirs are true internal devices, but they are repeatedly punctured percutaneously. The reported incidence of infection is 3%–15% (61). The majority of infections occur within the first month of implantation. Since this is also the time of greatest use, the mechanisms of infection are less clear, but colonization at the time of surgery and introduction of infection with subsequent taps are most likely.

Several studies have demonstrated a significantly increased risk of infection in those patients undergoing revision after treatment for an infected shunt, with an operative incidence of approximately 12–20% (19,22,25, 35,62). In these infections, the same organism was cultured at least 50% of the time. This suggests that failure to accurately determine the efficacy of treatment, or inadequate treatment, is involved in this higher rate of infection.

Shunt infections have been noted to occur with a bimodal distribution from the time of last shunt surgery (13,63). By 6 months postoperatively, 70–80% of the infections have presented. The second peak of infection occurs after 12 months (13,20,21,23,30,32,39,63–65). Attempts to explain this clustering of early infections have focused on (a) the infecting organisms and (b) what they imply regarding the etiology of the infection.

ETIOLOGY

A summary of the etiologic agents usually responsible for shunt infections is presented in Table 3. Greater than two-thirds of all shunt infections are caused by staphylococcal species (19,20–24,35,46,62–67). *Staphylococcus epidermidis* is the most frequently isolated of these organisms, being responsible for 47–64% of the infections. *Staphylococcus aureus* is the next most common organism, occurring in 12–29% of infections. Gram-negative enteric organisms, usually *Escherichia coli* and *Klebsiella* species, are responsible for the next most frequent group of infections, having an incidence ranging from 6% to 20%. *Proteus* and *Pseudomonas* species also are not infrequently isolated. Streptococcal species are found in 8–10% of infections. The traditional meningitis pathogens (e.g., *Haemophilus influenzae*, *Streptococcus pneumoniae*, *Neisseria meningitidis*) have been described in approximately 5% of shunt infections, and

there has been some suggestion that shunted patients are more susceptible to these organisms (23,62,67–70). A variety of much less common organisms make up the remainder of the infections, including fungi and other commensal microbes. In approximately 10–15% of shunt infections, a culture with more than one organism is obtained, and one of the organisms isolated is usually a staphylococcal species or *E. coli* (20,21,24,62,63).

There does not seem to be a significant difference in the distribution of organisms isolated from those infections classified as "acute" presentations and those presenting "delayed." George et al. (20) noted no variation between the organisms isolated from infections diagnosed at less than 30 days versus beyond 30 days. Although Odio et al. (21) had a slightly larger number of *S. aureus* infections in the "acute" group, and a slightly greater number of gram-negative infections in the "delayed" group, this may be an artifact of their definition of "acute" as less than 2 weeks. When Sells et al. (65) examined a group of gram-negative shunt infections, they found that 80% had presented before 5 months (usually within the first few weeks) and that the "delayed" gram-negative infections presented, on average, at 24 months post-procedure.

It has been suggested that shunt systems with a peritoneal end are at greater risk of infection with the gram-negative organisms more common to the gut (21,63,71). The only identifiable association between peritoneal shunts and infectious agents has been when the catheter has perforated a hollow viscus, usually resulting in a mixed infection with multiple gram-negative organisms (24,63). In comparing the organisms isolated from infections of different shunt types (i.e., VA versus VP), Walters et al. (46) noted a slight prevalence of gram-negative infections in those shunts with peritoneal terminations. Schoenbaum et al. (23), however, demonstrated no difference in the spectrum of infections between VA and VP shunts. Lumboperitoneal shunts, despite having the previously mentioned lower overall infection rate, have similar distributions of infecting organisms (23,46).

The pathogens isolated from infected CSF reservoirs are typical of standard shunt infections, with staphylococcal species accounting for up to 75% of the infections. The distribution of pathogens isolated from infected externalized devices, however, reflects a slightly higher incidence of gram-negative organisms than is seen in most shunt infections. Coagulase-negative staphylococci and *S. aureus* account for nearly 50% of the infections, with *Klebsiella*, *E. coli*, and other gram-negatives comprising another 25% (61).

One significant change in the pattern of infection in recent years has been an increasing prevalence of diphtheroid infections (24,63,67,72), up to 50% in the series reported by Rekate et al. (73). It is possible that the incidence of this infection is not actually increasing, but that previously the diagnosis was not made as often. Positive-

TABLE 3. *Etiologic agents*[a]

Agent	Incidence (%)
Staphylococcal species	65–85
S. epidermidis	47–64
S. aureus	12–29
Others	2–6
Gram-negative species	6–20
E. coli	8–10
Klebsiella	3–8
Proteus/Pseudomonas	2–8
Streptococcal species	8–10
Traditional meningitides	2–8
H. influenzae	
S. pneumoniae	
N. meningitidis	
Diphtheroids	1–14
Anaerobes	6
Mixed cultures	10–15

[a] Table derived from refs. 19, 21, 23, 24, 46, 62–64, and 67

culture results with these organisms may have been ignored, interpreted as culture contaminants, particularly when associated with an "asymptomatic" patient (see section entitled "Diagnosis," below). Poor culture techniques, such as failure to routinely plant in thioglycolate, anaerobically maintain, or observe for up to 14 days, would also limit their discovery (46,71,73). Rekate et al. (73) have postulated that a true increase in incidence may be related to prophylactic antibiotics given to these patients. When certain antibiotics reduce the staphylococcal populations, the growth of the more fastidious diphtheroids may no longer be suppressed, and they are then able to propagate to a level that causes infection.

Although fungal infections of shunts have been rare, the number of these infections can be expected to increase, primarily due to an increasing number of "susceptible" patients (74). Those factors or situations that put patients at risk include prior use of broad-spectrum antibiotics, hyperalimentation, leukemia, lymphoma, diabetes mellitus, steroid use (particularly as seen in renal and heart transplant patients), and immunecompromised states (i.e., AIDS, post-chemotherapy) (75,76).

PATHOGENESIS

Four mechanisms may be postulated by which shunts become infected: (i) "retrograde" infection from the distal end, (ii) wound or skin breakdown, (iii) hematogenous seeding, and (iv) colonization at the time of surgery. These pathways have been derived from observations of the infection, from the various factors seen in association with infected shunts, and from the experiences of other surgical specialties.

"Retrograde" infection is frequently a function of the time of diagnosis of a shunt infection. A patient presenting with ventriculitis, found to have the source of the infection at the distal end, may be referred to as having a retrograde infection. Holt (45) constructed a closed artificial shunt system and demonstrated that retrograde progression of infection could occur in the presence of a one-way valve and with proximal-to-distal CSF flow. Bayston (77), however, repeated this experiment on several shunt systems. Using physiologic flow rates and careful bacteriological monitoring, he found no retrograde passage of infecting organisms past competent one-way valves.

Retrograde infection was felt to occur frequently in ureteral shunts (23,78). Schoenbaum et al. (23) noted that the spectrum of infection was different for ureteral shunts. Gram-negative organisms accounted for 35% of the ureteral shunt infections, but for only 6% of the remainder. In addition, they found that S. epidermidis accounted for only 10% of ureteral shunt infections, but for a majority of the other shunt infections. Based on these bacteriologic differences and the radiographic demonstration of urinary reflux into a ureteral shunt, Gardner et al. (78) invoked a retrograde progression of infection similar to that which occurs in peritoneal shunts when bowel perforation leads to distal catheter contamination (79).

A vascular shunt infected by contamination of the distal end is more appropriately called a "hematogenous infection." With peritoneal shunts, perforation of a hollow viscus at the time of surgery would best be classified with colonization at the time of surgery. Delayed perforation of the bowel by the distal catheter could be classified with retrograde infection, and infection of the distal end by transluminal passage of bacteria without perforation should be considered a retrograde infection.

Retrograde infection is the most likely mechanism involving infection of externalized devices. Organisms may track from the exit site alongside the device, or, in the case of devices that drain CSF, gain entry into the fluid column and ascend into the CNS. Some of the devices require intermittent "flushing," the injection of small aliquots through the tubing to maintain function. This is another obvious possible portal of entry for infection.

Breakdown of the surgical wounds or of the skin overlying the shunt hardware allows direct access of microbes to the shunt. This may be surgically acquired, where the incision created by the surgeon fails to heal for intrinsic reasons (nutrition, improper closure), or because an impaired patient picks at or scratches open the wound (often seen with infants and small children) (80,81). In the debilitated or immobile patient, a decubitus ulcer may develop over the shunt, particularly in the scalp where the high-profile hardware is between thin skin and bone (40). Those infections caused by direct extension from infected tissues adjacent to the shunt should also be included in this category. This is most often seen after infection of nearby wounds (i.e., tracheostomy site), at the intravenous access site, or with severe spontaneous skin infections (acne, boils, cellulitis) (82).

With the exception of distal vascular shunt infections, direct hematogenous seeding and infection of CSF shunts is a possible occurrence but is probably not a frequent one. Infection of venous shunts should be considered separately, because these devices place a foreign body in the vascular system continuously and are therefore at continuous risk of infection from bacteremia (25,40,45). Nulsen and Becker (40) recognized this potential with vascular shunts, noting an increase in their infection rate with placement of the venous catheter below the level of the seventh vertebral body by chest x-ray. They felt that the lower placement increased the risk of thrombus formation and endocarditis, placing the patient at greater susceptibility for infection due to bacteremia.

The susceptibility of shunts to hematogenously spread infection is less clear. Several reports of H. influenzae infections in patients with CSF shunts note their late onset relative to shunt surgery, the presence of an obvious extra-CNS source for the infection, and the frequency of positive blood cultures (out of proportion to that seen with shunt infections in general). This has been interpreted as shunt infection secondary to hematogenous spread. The relatively increased frequency of these infections in the shunted population only suggests that the shunt plays a role in susceptibility. These may not represent true shunt infections but may represent, instead, direct hematogenous CNS infections with secondary infection of the shunt (23,26,68 70,83).

The Orthopedic literature has a number of references which infer that late infection of prosthetic joints is secondary to hematogenous spread from a distant infection. These infections represent only a small percentage of their total infectious complications. Although Irvine et al. (84) associated bacteruria with deep hip prosthesis infections, most other authors (85–88) felt that only a sustained bacteremia was associated with these infections. Charnley (89) argues against bacteremia as a cause of prosthetic device infection, even in the presence of a fresh wound or hematoma. He bases this conclusion on an extensive experience in Orthopedics, but in wounds and injuries not involving a prosthetic device. Sells et al. (65) noted one shunt infection associated temporally with a prolonged orthopedic procedure, and they only inferred bacteremia as a potential cause. Spanu et al. (35) noted a slightly greater rate of infection for those patients recently treated for distant non-shunt infections.

Transient or asymptomatic bacteremia has not been definitively associated with infections of shunts or of orthopedic prosthetic devices. It is probably impossible to identify those infections secondary to transient bacteremia, if in fact they do exist (86). From these observations and reports, it would appear that simple bacteremia is not sufficient to cause a shunt infection. A sustained bacteremia—with the shunt acting as a foreign body, or a recent shunt revision presenting the foreign body in a wound of devitalized tissue, serum, and hematoma—is probably necessary. Even so, such an infection appears to be an infrequent occurrence.

Colonization at the time of surgery is probably the most frequent cause of CNS shunt infections. This is suggested in particular by the timing of most shunt infections, and by the organisms isolated from these infections. As noted above, the majority of shunt infections occur within several weeks of a shunt operation. At operation, direct exposure and handling of the shunt can allow bacterial contamination. Bayston and Lari (28) performed quantitative wound pad cultures in 100 shunt procedures; 58% of these were found to be positive, usually with a staphylococcal species. The actual incidence of true shunt infections is much lower, so obviously not every colony-forming bacterial unit contaminating the wound leads to infection.

Since the majority of organisms isolated from infected shunts are commensal skin organisms, introduction of these at the time of surgery has long been surmised. Multiple studies utilizing surveillance culturing techniques have found, however, that less that 50% of the organisms cultured from the wound or from the infected shunt can be traced directly to the patient (24,28,45,80,81,90). Also, many of those isolates traced to the patient were not present in the operative field (24,28). Obviously, there are numerous and interrelated factors affecting the colonization and subsequent infection of CSF shunts.

It has been demonstrated repeatedly that the mere presence of any foreign body increases the risk of infection. It is estimated that in a clean surgical wound without a foreign body, approximately 10^6 staphylococci would be required to cause a subcutaneous infection (81). The presence of even a simple foreign body such as a suture may reduce that infective dose by as much as 10^4 to 10^6 times. The dose may decrease further when wound or host factors are introduced (81).

Foreign bodies, such as shunt devices, may directly affect the occurrence of infection through one of several mechanisms. Bacterial growth may be impeded, or promoted, by the foreign body. The foreign material can also directly interfere with natural host defense mechanisms, such as chemotaxis, phagocytosis, or the inflammatory process in general (91–94). In the typical surgically associated infection, the surgery and bacteria cause local tissue injury and subsequently lead to an inflammatory response. The vascular portion of the response, mediated by histamine, the kinin system, prostaglandins, and other vasoactive substances derived from the bacteria or injured cells, allows plasma proteins and leukocytes to permeate the area. The combined effect of antibody and complement activation, by any of several pathways, leads to chemotactic substance release, directing the cellular response that results in phagocytosis with destruction of the bacteria. Shunt catheters have been shown *in vitro* to decrease the mobility of neutrophils, hindering their ability to phagocytose bacteria in effective numbers. There is also a suggestion that neutrophils in the presence of shunt tubing are induced to degranulate extracellularly and therefore decrease their bactericidal abilities (95).

The colonization of intradermal sutures is well known. Even monofilament nylons and steel staples are capable of harboring bacterial colonies. Although not usually responsible for overt infections, the bacteria appear to remain in a relatively protected state until suture removal occurs. Obviously, from this opportunistic site of colonization, local extension and infection of a subjacent shunt may occur (96). This colonization involves the adhesion and glycocalyx production by the infecting agent, seen also in the attachment of organisms to a shunting device.

Attachment of bacteria to the shunt must be an initial step in colonization and infection. At first this may be a reversible nonspecific adherence related to the general physical characteristics of the artificial material, the bacterium, and the milieu. Molecular charge, hydrophobic interactions, and binding sites are just a few of the factors involved (97–99). Any proteinaceous material coating the prosthesis will affect these adhesions, usually making them stronger. Such fluid would be derived from the serum and tissues around the shunt and would contain fibrin, fibrinogen, collagen, and other proteins that might enhance bacterial binding. For instance, *S. aureus* has discrete binding sites for collagen, fibronectin, and other plasma proteins (100).

Initial bacterial adherence to shunt catheters can be quite strong, with flow rates of >200 ml/hr unable to completely clear a catheter inoculated with bacteria for only 30 min (101). Once adhered to a catheter, bacteria are not easily removed by exposure to detergents or antibiotics (102). The range of adherence varies between bacterial species and among differing strains, perhaps relating to each's specific pathogenicity. Modification and breakdown of the prosthetic device by the host over time can also affect the ability of organisms to adhere. Surface irregularities may be produced or enhanced, or additional binding sites might be created (100,101,103,104).

Subsequently, an "irreversible adhesion" occurs. The bacteria can be found in microcolonies, surrounded by a mucoid "slime" which binds the bacteria together and which adheres the collection to the shunt material (Fig. 2). The mechanism of adherence involves several factors: ionic and van der Waals forces, and receptor–ligand interactions (96). This "slime" or glycocalyx was identified in staphylococcal infections *in vitro* by Bayston and Penny (105). Others (100,101,106,107) have noted that such slime producers account for 60–80% of the coagu-

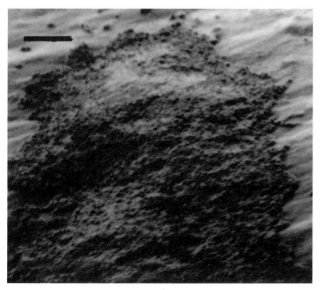

FIG. 2. Scanning electron micrograph of slime producing *S. epidermidis* on a vascular catheter. A large number of indistinct bacteria are enmeshed in the glycocalyx and are firmly attached to the catheter. Bar represents 10 μm. (From ref. 198, with permission.)

lase-negative staphylococci isolated from shunt or biomaterial infections.

Slime is not merely a fibrin aggregation of bacteria; instead, it is composed of a range of high- and low-molecular-weight polysaccharides, associated loosely and mostly through ionic interactions. It incorporates microcolonies of bacteria and may affect the clinical manifestations of an infection. Slime has been found to culture bacteria that were not able to be cultured *in vivo;* moreover, several different bacteria may be observed incorporated into the glycocalyx, whereas only one type may be cultured by traditional *in vitro* techniques (96). The glycocalyx may function to interfere with phagocytosis or to influence antibody response, and it may act as an ion-exchange resin for enhanced nutrition of the colony (100,105,108). *In vitro* tests have shown bacteria adherent to biomaterials to have a much greater minimum inhibitory concentration (MIC) than the same bacteria in free suspension (103). The apparent difficulties of treating such infections *in situ* may be manifestations of these effects, and they may account in part for the high incidence of repeat infections after treatment for an infected shunt (106,107).

There are also host factors that affect the pathogenesis of shunt infections. The status of the wound has always been important in surgery, where minimizing the amount of devitalized tissue and hematoma maximized wound healing, led to an appropriate inflammatory response, and allowed delivery of phagocytic cells where needed (80). The relatively immune-privileged state of the CNS also affects the ability to keep an operative inoculum of bacteria from producing an infection; this is merely a manifestation of the body's inability to deliver anti-infective agents to the site (91,109).

The most significant host factor for shunt infections is the age of the patient. Several series have shown greatly increased rates of infections for children less than 6 months of age at the time of surgery (21,22,46,62,110). This factor appears to be independent of the presence of myelomeningocele, or independent of the proximity to its closure (22). In neonates, a relative deficiency of the immune response to bacteria has been suggested to account for these findings. This includes (a) the low level of complement activity and (b) the lack of IgM and its effects on both gram-negative infections and control of primary bacterial infections (22).

The group of patients less than 1 year old accounted for more than 30% of the infections described by Ersahin et al. (19); however, when the operative incidence of shunt infection is calculated from the raw data, no significant difference in infection rate is seen between the various age groups.

CLINICAL MANIFESTATIONS

The presentation of a shunt infection can be quite variable, being affected by the mechanism of infection, the virulence of the infecting organism, and the type of shunt in place (20,23,46,111). The classic symptoms of infection, fever, and pain are not uniformly present in shunt infection. Although fever is usually the most common symptom, it has been reported in as few as 14% and as many as 92% of shunt infections (21,23,46,61,63,78). Therefore, its absence cannot be interpreted as a factor against infection. Pain is often related to infection at the peritoneal or the pleural endings of a shunt, or at a wound. It may be absent, however, in up to 60% of infections (63). The most frequent symptoms are the result of shunt malfunction secondary to the infection—headache, nausea, lethargy, or change in mental status (21,23,111).

Clinical presentations of shunt infections related to the surgical wounds or to the subcutaneous track of the shunt are the most easily distinguished (21). Infections with wound dehiscence, as well as drainage of purulent material, are obvious. The intact infected wound, or cellulitis along the shunt, is accompanied by varying degrees of erythema and pain. Because these infections are focal, fever is an inconsistent finding.

In considering the varied manifestations of shunt infections, it is useful to consider the shunt as being composed of a "proximal" and a "distal" portion, with symptoms and signs relatively specific to each. Other presentations can be related to surgical wounds, or to the condition of the shunt between the origin and terminus (see Table 4). Because infection of one portion of a shunt invariably leads to contamination of the remainder, a given shunt infection may present with any combination of symptoms and signs referable to the proximal or distal portions (45,112,113).

Proximal manifestations of infection are also easily recognized and are often the most acutely threatening to the health of the patient (17,114). The proximal infection may cause shunt obstruction or decreased function, appearing with all of the symptoms of shunt failure. Obviously, the proximal catheter is within a CSF space, and infection results in a meningitis or ventriculitis about 30% of the time (21,23,63). With ventricular shunts, however, meningeal symptoms should not be expected. There is usually an absence of communication between the infected ventricles and the CSF in contact with the meninges. This may be due to the original reason for shunting, or it may be developed from aqueductal stenosis acquired after ventricular shunting of communicating hydrocephalus (115,116). Walters et al. (46) found meningeal signs in three times as many infected lumbar-puncture shunts as in infected VP shunts. Although intracranial empyemas and abscesses are possible, they are rarely seen (20,117–119). They may occur either (a) secondary to a poorly treated infection, (b) in the presence of retained hardware, or (c) with externalized monitors (53).

Infections presenting with symptoms referable to the distal end are more specific to the terminus location. Infected vascular shunts invariably have bacteremia, either from the infected CSF that is being diverted into the circulation, from an infected thrombus at the end of the vascular catheter, or from true subacute bacterial endocarditis (21,40,72). In the early years of venous shunting, there was a significant morbidity and mortality attributable to bacteremia leading to sepsis (15,40,41). The patient would be acutely ill, with fever and symptoms of septicemia. Attention to this possible complication, combined with the refinement of operative and treatment techniques, makes this a rare occurrence now. The more usual presentation of an infected venous shunt is much less virulent and more nonspecific, with fever and lethargy being the most common symptoms (21). Again, some symptoms of shunt dysfunction or proximal infection may be present.

One unique complication of a chronic vascular shunt infection is the development of shunt nephritis (23,116,120,121). Only a small fraction of patients with infected vascular shunts will develop this syndrome— less than 4% in the series of Schoenbaum et al. (23). Renal dysfunction is always preceded by symptoms or signs of infection, although it is often subtle (23,120, 121). The majority of the bacteria isolated from these patients are staphylococcal species (usually coagulase-negative ones), but diphtheroid species and other less common shunt pathogens have also been associated with the syndrome (120). The pathogenesis seems similar to that seen with subacute bacterial endocarditis. With the chronic bacteremia accompanying these infections, IgM and IgG antigen–antibody immune complexes are formed and deposited in the renal glomeruli. Immunofluorescence staining has revealed IgM, IgG, and C3 staining at the basement membrane. The complement system is activated, with subsequent depletion of circulating complement factors C3 and C4. Thickening of the glomerular basement membrane, accompanied by mesangial cell proliferation, leads to a nephrotic syndrome. Although the specific immune complexes that can be identified vary between cases, the clinical presentation is similar. The patient has febrile episodes, an elevated sedimentation rate, and often has hepato-

TABLE 4. *Clinical manifestations of shunt infections*

Proximal	
Cranial:	Ventriculitis; empyema; abscess
Spinal:	Meningitis
Distal	
Vascular:	Bacteremia; subacute bacterial endocarditis; shunt nephritis
Peritoneal:	Decreased absorption; encystment; peritonitis
Pleural:	Decreased absorption; pleuritis
Wound	Cellulitis; dehiscence
Insidious	Shunt dysfunction; fluid along shunt; asymptomatic

splenomegaly, and the urine shows proteinuria with macro- or microscopic hematuria. Failure to detect this condition can lead to permanent renal failure. Treatment of the underlying shunt infection usually, but not always, leads to resolution of the renal dysfunction. With resolution, the serum complement levels return towards normal (120,121).

Shunts that terminate in the pleural or peritoneal spaces have similar mechanisms of CSF absorption, and they show evidence of infection in a similar fashion. The infection will initially cause the development of inflammation in the absorbing tissue, with subsequent failure of CSF absorption. A rather benign presentation with symptoms of a poorly functioning shunt may occur if the inflammation remains mild, and absorption failure is the only symptom (122,123). In the peritoneal cavity, the body will attempt to limit the infection. This often results in the encystment of the shunt catheter, fluid buildup within the cyst, and, not uncommonly, loculation of other pockets of fluid within the abdomen. The "CSF-oma" that forms can grow quite large, since CSF is deposited there by the shunt but is not absorbed by the peritoneal cavity. Particularly in infants, it may become palpable on physical examination and may present as an abdominal mass, sometimes interfering with feeding or bowel function (116).

Symptoms of peritonitis appear as the peritoneal inflammation grows more severe. Fever and anorexia are common, in conjunction with the abdominal tenderness. The tenderness and pain may be quite focal, with the location not necessarily related to the peritoneal catheter tip location (113). It can mimic the acute surgical abdomen of other intra-abdominal conditions unrelated to the shunt, such as appendicitis or a perforated viscus (112,113,124).

Some shunt infections are insidious, causing few or no symptoms; they may go undetected for weeks or months, while the patient has only an intermittent low-grade fever or a general malaise. The unexplained occlusion of an open-ended peritoneal catheter, or failure of peritoneal CSF absorption, has been associated with occult infection in the experience of the authors and others (125). The clinical picture may be further clouded by concurrent and unrelated infections of the urinary tract and middle ear. It becomes a particularly troublesome situation when the patient has received antibiotics for these or other infections, confounding any subsequent culture results or partially treating the shunt infection. This is the situation seen frequently in the myelodysplastic children presenting to the hospital for evaluation of fever (40,111,126).

The low-grade infection of a vascular shunt may present in such a subtle manner as to avoid detection for many months, particularly if the diagnosis is not suspected. When the infection is strictly limited to the distal portion of the shunt, there will be no ventriculitis, no CSF pleocytosis, and negative CSF cultures. Lethargy may be the only outward symptom in these cases, with bacteremia found on careful examination. S. epidermidis is usually responsible for the infection, and its isolation from blood should not be interpreted as a contaminant (23,25).

Infection with diphtheroid species can also be insidious and difficult to diagnose. They have been identified in many occult ventriculoperitoneal shunt infections, but they may infect any device. Again, symptoms may be absent or mild, with intermittent fever or lethargy (73). If the CSF is infected, a mild pleocytosis [less than several hundred white blood cells (WBCs)] and variable chemistry changes may be found (72,73). With infected peritoneal shunts, failure of absorption may be the only symptom or sign. Because of their fastidious nature, cultures for diphtheroids must be done aerobically and anaerobically, and held for at least 14 days. Care must be taken not to interpret positive culture of diphtheroids as a result of contamination (72,73).

Fungal infections usually present as a meningoencephalitis or a subacute-to-chronic meningitis. Fever, headache, change in mental status, or cranial-nerve findings may be manifestations of infection (74,75,127). Obstruction of the shunt, however, may be the only sign (74).

External devices can manifest infection in only a few ways: (a) infection of the wounds or (b) infection of the proximal end with ventriculitis, meningitis, and rarely an abscess (50,53,57). Wound infections are more frequent with external devices than with shunts. The changes in mental status occurring with ventriculitis or meningitis may not be apparent, however, because many of these patients have an impaired level of consciousness due to their underlying disease (128,129). The evaluation of fever, the most common symptom of these infections, may be complicated by other sources of infection or by concurrent antibiotic use (116). Therefore, close observation of the wounds (and frequent culture of CSF, if possible) is often the only way to diagnose these infections.

DIAGNOSIS

Shunt infections are not uncommon, and they are highly variable in presentation. Therefore, an important attitude in dealing with shunts is to have a high degree of suspicion for infection. The possibility should be considered during evaluation and treatment of any shunt patient with a fever, although only occasionally is a fever in these patients related to the shunt. Diagnosing a shunt infection requires the correlation of presentation with factors such as recency of shunt surgery and shunt type; most importantly, however, it requires appropriate bacteriologic cultures (23,63,78,130).

There are a number of diagnostic tests that may be obtained in an attempt to define a shunt infection. Blood counts, abdominal ultrasounds, and computerized tomographic (CT) scans of the head or abdomen are nonspecific studies that would only show signs of shunt dysfunction or that would indirectly indicate infection. The direct culturing of the shunt, or of fluid from within or around it, is the diagnostic procedure of choice. In VA shunts, this would include blood culturing.

The peripheral WBC count is frequently obtained during the evaluation of fever, or in preparation for surgery, but is of limited value in diagnosing a shunt infection. Whereas one-third of patients with shunt infections exhibit a WBC count greater than 20,000, up to one-quarter will have no elevation in the count (23,50,112).

Blood cultures have a similarly poor ability to reveal an infected shunt, with the exception of infected vascular shunts. As mentioned before, bacteremia is present almost invariably with infected VA shunts, and blood cultures in this situation are positive more than 90% of the time. With other shunts, however, the incidence of negative blood culture in the presence of shunt infection approaches 80% (23,61,63).

CT scans of the head or abdomen do not identify infection per se; however, they may show evidence of shunt dysfunction, an indirect indication of some infections. A CT scan of the head is always indicated for symptoms or signs suggesting a mass lesion or increased ICP. Although identification of a subdural empyema or brain abscess is unlikely, in rare situations it may be the first manifestation of an infection. Abdominal ultrasound or CT scan can be used in an attempt to identify CSF loculations. Although some *free* fluid in the pleural or peritoneal cavities is normal, it should not be confused with the larger volumes and cysts seen with infection. Such a "CSF-oma," particularly when incorporating a peritoneal catheter, strongly suggests infection.

Direct culturing of the shunt, or of any fluid in contact with it, is the most accurate diagnostic test for infection (63,73,78,111,112,114,131). Culturing a shunt wound, or sampling blood from a patient with a vascular shunt, is a self-evident method, but getting CSF from within or around a shunt is more specific to the shunt type. Lumboperitoneal shunts typically have the proximal catheter entering the lumbar subarachnoid space near the L2–L3 interspace. If the location of catheter entry can be ascertained, a lumbar puncture can be done safely to obtain CSF. The fluid sampled is in contact with the proximal portion of the shunt. Ventricular shunts, however, require the presence of a reservoir that can be tapped in order to obtain CSF. The reservoir is an integral part of the implanted system. In these cases, for the reasons mentioned earlier, sampling the lumbar CSF may not reflect the state of the ventricular fluid or may not reveal the presence of infection.

The so-called "shunt tap" has the benefits of checking the shunt function as well as investigating for the presence of infection. The shunt reservoir is typically located in an easily accessible subcutaneous location. After sterile preparation of the area, the reservoir is percutaneously punctured with a small needle. Introducing infection into the system is the only apparent risk of the procedure. In patients undergoing repetitive, frequent taps of implanted reservoirs, the incidence of infection has been reported to be as high as 12% (61). The risk for a single diagnostic tap has not been well defined by prospective or retrospective studies, but it appears to be low (23,111,114).

The fluid obtained from a tap is sent for chemistries (glucose and protein), differential cell counts, Gram's stain, and culture. The glucose determination is the least helpful, often being within normal ranges in spite of obvious infection (63,111,131). A high WBC count in the CSF is highly correlated with the presence of infection, but infection may still be present in spite of normal counts (23,50,63,111). Occasionally, the cell count is obscured by a recent surgery that may have spilled blood into the CSF or that may have caused an inflammatory reaction. A negative Gram's stain similarly does not exclude an infection with any degree of certainty.

Yogev (71) compared the CSF of those patients with shunts infected with gram-negative and with gram-positive bacteria. The gram-negative infections had significantly increased protein, decreased glucose, and increased WBCs with a predominance of neutrophils in their CSF, when compared to the gram-positive infections. Only a small percentage of the gram-positive infections were detected by Gram's stain, whereas 90% of the gram-negative infections were identified. Also, the patients with gram-negative infections were more severely ill, and they had abdominal complaints more frequently.

Culture of the tapped fluid is by far the most important test. In the vast majority of shunt infections, the culture is positive, even when there is no pleocytosis or chemistry changes (111). Unfortunately, several days to several weeks are required before the culture may be definitively read as negative, and the results can be confounded by prior treatment of the patient with antibiotics (111,126).

When only the distal portion of a VP shunt is infected, the diagnosis may be difficult. Such an infection may present with some degree of peritoneal signs, ranging from mild discomfort to an "acute abdomen," and no evidence of shunt dysfunction. A shunt tap may be completely normal, and the culture may remain negative if no retrograde progression of the infection has taken place from the abdomen (126). Even so, it is not permissible in the face of an acute abdomen to wait several days to make a diagnosis on the basis of cultures. Such cases may require the removal of a catheter from the peritoneal space ("externalizing" the shunt). Any fluid that can be aspirated from the distal end prior to removal, and from the catheter tip itself, is cultured. When a peritoneal shunt infection is present, there is usually quick resolution (within 6–12 hr) of the peritoneal symptoms after removal of the peritoneal catheter (112,113, 124,126,132).

The VP shunt that presents with evidence for distal occlusion, and without any of the symptoms or signs of infection, should still be carefully investigated for infection at the time of revision. This should include Gram's stain and culture of the distal tubing, with particular emphasis on culturing for low-grade pathogens such as coagulase-negative staphylococci and diphtheroids (15,46,73,116,133).

The shunt that is tapped for evaluation of function, with no indication or suspicion of infection, and is found to be culture-positive presents another difficult situation. Contamination of the tap or the culture, as opposed to colonization of the shunt and true infection, must be considered. Re-tapping the shunt is undertaken, and a continued positive culture with the same organism is considered and treated as a true infection. An asymptomatic patient with a culture-positive shunt may be considered to be "colonized," but we feel that he or she should be treated as a patient with an "infected" shunt.

In all cases, the correlation of the clinical situation, symptoms, laboratory findings, and cultures must be made to diagnose a shunt infection. Regardless of the reason for a shunt tap, a culture should always be obtained. Because of the often-benign presentation of shunt infections, all positive cultures must be considered in a serious light.

TREATMENT

The three main goals in the treatment of any CNS prosthetic device infection are: (i) minimizing the mortality and morbidity of the infection and its treatment, (ii) maintaining a functioning device if it is still needed, and (iii) resolving the infection. One must consider the duration of hospitalization and the associated costs as part of the morbidity of treatment, and he or she must attempt to minimize them. The treatment to be used must also take into account the need for a functioning device during or after treatment. Some devices (i.e., electrodes, ICP monitors) may be discontinued without sequelae, but most shunts can only be removed for brief periods (if at all) without risk of neurological injury.

Many methods of treating shunt infections have been reported, but no prospective, randomized studies have been done. Interpretation between studies must be done cautiously. The reports often have similar treatment protocols, but rarely are they exactly the same. Significant factors—such as the timing of hardware removal or replacement, and the duration of therapy—are frequently different. Not all authors define "infection" or "cure"

the same. Yogev (71) notes that false-positive cultures that are treated can give the impression that a treatment mode is working; similarly, false-negative cultures from a partially treated or suppressed infection will also skew the results (46,134).

Not all types of shunt infections are necessarily the same, yet in the various reports they may be grouped together. Certainly, the cellulitis or wound infection without CSF infection is not the same as the infection with severe ventriculitis (125). Factors such as bacterial virulence, gram-positive versus gram-negative organisms, or early- versus late-onset infections may vary greatly in how easily they are treated. We will attempt to review the salient points regarding the various methods of treatment that have been used. The protocols that we have found the most effective, and the reasons behind them, will then be presented.

The antibiotic chosen to treat a specific shunt infection needs to have not only bactericidal activity against the infecting organism, but also an ability to penetrate into the CNS. This is because of the relative "immune vacuum" that exists in the CNS, where cellular mechanisms of infection control are nearly absent (91,109). Since ventricular shunts penetrate the brain, a proximal infection might be expected to have some component of cerebritis or parenchymal infection. We have seen CT contrast enhancement of the parenchyma several days after removal of an infected ventriculostomy. This probably represents cerebritis, if not infected brain. Therefore, CNS penetration of a suitable drug might require penetration into the parenchyma as well as into the CSF; these two are not necessarily the same (91,135). The structure of an antibiotic, its lipid solubility, and the presence or absence of meningeal irritation are the most important factors determining CSF penetration. A brief list of the relative penetration into the CSF of several antibiotics is presented in Table 5.

Oftentimes, antibiotic treatment must begin before an organism can be isolated by culture. Coverage is selected for the most likely organisms, with due consideration to the clinical presentation and the results of a Gram's stain. As noted previously, the majority of infections are due to staphylococcal species, and appropriate antistaphylococcal treatment will initially be undertaken. A not insignificant number of infections are due to aerobic gram-negative organisms; and when indicated by Gram's stain or a more severe clinical illness, coverage of these organisms must be started. The culture results and sensitivities will subsequently allow the treatment to be specifically narrowed.

The primary drugs used for staphylococcal coverage are nafcillin and vancomycin. Nafcillin is capable of attaining detectable CSF levels, sometimes above bactericidal levels (136–139). It can also penetrate into brain tissue, especially inflamed tissue, to attain levels greater than those of the MICs of many staphylococci (137).

TABLE 5. *Antibiotic access to CSF*

Good without inflammation	Good with inflammation	Fair to poor with inflammation
Third-generation cephalosporins	Penicillins	Aminoglycosides
Ceftriaxone	Penicillin	Gentamicin
Cefotaxime	Ampicillin	Tobramycin
	Nafcillin	Amikacin
Chloramphenicol	Vancomycin	Vancomycin
Metronidazole	Rifampin	Clindamycin
	Trimethoprim/sulfa	First-generation cephalosporins

Methicillin, which will not enter the CSF without inflammation and which has more drug-induced reactions than does nafcillin, does not appear to be as good a choice (71,136,139). Clindamycin has been used for its coverage of gram-positive and anaerobic organisms. There are very little data on its CNS penetration; one study in monkeys subjected to cerebral trauma noted variable parenchymal levels (140).

Vancomycin is indicated as the first choice for staphylococcal coverage in an institution with a high incidence (5–10%) of staphylococcal species resistant to methicillin/nafcillin (71). Although vancomycin penetrates into the CSF poorly in the absence of inflammation, studies have shown levels of up to 10% of serum levels in the presence of meningeal inflammation (136,141). Clinically, it has been effective in the medical treatment of shunt infections (39).

The treatment of staphylococci (both coagulase-negative and coagulase-positive) can be augmented by combining oral rifampin with either nafcillin or vancomycin. The majority of the gram-positive organisms are exquisitely sensitive to rifampin, but they will quickly develop a resistance to it if used alone. This is prevented by concurrent use of another antibiotic. Significant CSF levels, up to 1000 times the MICs, are obtainable with only minimal meningeal irritation (136,142). When added to the treatment of shunt infections, it has effected cure without resorting to additional therapies, such as intraventricular antibiotic instillation (142,143). Bactericidal titers in the CSF have been achieved clinically without the development of resistance (32,144).

Although first-generation cephalosporins have been used in the treatment of soft-tissue staphylococcal infections, they have no indications for use in CNS infections (136,145). Animal studies of their CSF penetration, along with the results of clinical trials, confirm that even with meningeal inflammation these agents do not penetrate the CSF in effective amounts (138). Moreover, there is a high rate of staphylococcal resistance to these drugs.

Antibiotic coverage for aerobic gram-negative infections has classically utilized an aminoglycoside. Gentamicin is a potent bactericidal agent against gramnegative organisms. With some activity against staphylococcal species, it is sometimes used in combination with nafcil-

lin or vancomycin. Even with inflammation, however, gentamicin and tobramycin have only fair and erratic CSF penetration, and some organisms have developed resistance to them (136,146). To cover resistant strains, amikacin has been used increasingly. It, too, has a variable CSF penetration (71,136,138,147). All the aminoglycosides can cause oto- and nephrotoxicity.

Chloramphenicol, although concentrated in brain tissue and having activity against many gram-negative organisms, has limited value for shunt infections. Its use can lead to emergence of resistant organisms (134). Medications which are metabolized in the liver and which are frequently used by neurosurgery patients, such as phenobarbital and Dilantin, can seriously and unpredicatably affect the levels of chloramphenicol. The toxic reactions seen in neonates (gray syndrome), the blood dyscrasia it can produce, and a lack of CNS efficacy preclude its use.

The third-generation cephalosporins, which include cefotaxime and ceftriaxone, have good anti-gram-negative coverage, with the notable exception of *Pseudomonas* species. Ceftazidine, a third-generation cephalosporin with anti-pseudomonal coverage but less activity against gram-positive organisms, has also been recently used. The treatment for pseudomonal infections still requires the combination of an anti-pseudomonal penicillin with an aminoglycoside.

The third-generation cephalosporins penetrate inflamed meninges relatively well, achieving bactericidal levels (91). Their ability to penetrate the CSF seems to be inversely related to the degree of binding to serum proteins. The kinetics of CSF penetration reveal the usual correlation with inflammation. The concentration of drug in CSF increases during the initial period of treatment, and it declines as the inflammation is reduced and the blood–brain/CSF barrier is reestablished (145). This decline in antibiotic penetration of the CNS during treatment is seen with most antibiotics (148).

Instillation of antibiotics directly into the ventricles has been used to overcome the problem of poor CSF penetration after intravenous administration. The antibiotics can be injected through an external ventriculostomy, through a shunt reservoir, or by direct transcortical injection. The latter is associated with subsequent development of porencephaly, so it is rarely used. The most commonly used intraventricular antibiotic is vancomycin, because of its coverage of gram-positive organisms—in particular the methicillin-resistant staphylococci. Others have been used, including gentamicin, nafcillin, chloramphenicol, and cephalothin.

The pharmacokinetics of intraventricular antibiotic use in shunt infections have not been well studied. In the absence of compartmentalization, medication injected into one lateral ventricle quickly and evenly distributes throughout the ventricular system (149,150). Antibiotic clearance generally follows first-order kinetics, if there is no CSF drainage by shunt or external ventriculostomy. The rate of clearance is slow enough to allow once-daily dosing (138,149–152). With an external ventriculostomy, temporary occlusion for 30–60 min after antibiotic instillation may be required to achieve appropriate CSF levels. When temporary occlusion is not possible or is ineffective, increased frequency of dosing can be used.

The dosages recommended for intraventricular use have been determined empirically (see Table 6). Dosage calculations based on body surface area, weight, age, or even approximations of ventricular volume have not given reliable and predictable levels (138,152–154). Most authors recommend starting with an empiric dosage, and then adjusting the dose or dosing interval to achieve adequate CSF levels (138,150,152,154,155). The concentration of the antibiotic in the CNS and the MIC for the suspected infecting organism can be related by the "inhibitory quotient" defined as measured level divided by the MIC). In theory, the inhibitory quotient should exceed 10–20 before the cultures will consistently be sterile. The titer of CSF bactericidal activity also can be determined in establishing the adequacy of treatment. A titer greater than 1:8 gives clinical results similar to those of an inhibitory quotient of ≥10 (156).

There is both clinical and experimental evidence of neurotoxicity after the use of intraventricular antibiotics (157,158). In levels 50 times greater than those used clinically, gentamicin was felt to be directly neurotoxic (157). CSF irrigations with cephalothin and penicillin G were noted to cause ventriculitis, transient neurological deficits, and perivascular infiltration (158). Intraventricular vancomycin has not been proven to have toxic effects in clinical use (151,153,155). No untoward effects were identified in patients inadvertently given extremely large doses of intraventricular vancomycin (151,159). Pleocytosis, due to a transient ventriculitis from preservative-containing solutions associated with higher doses of gentamicin and vancomycin, has been observed (B. A. Kaufman and D. G. McLone, *unpublished data*).

Many of the early attempts to treat shunt infections used intravenous antibiotics exclusively. There was a desire to avoid additional operations, and to maintain the CSF diversion during treatment. In addition, because the vast majority of the early shunts were vascular, maintenance of the vascular access (or, rather, not losing one of the few vascular portals with shunt removal) was im-

TABLE 6. *Intraventricular antimicrobial dosages*

Antimicrobial	Dose (per day)	Reference
Cephalothin	25–100 mg	153
	1–2 mg/kg	138,154
Methicillin	100 mg	153
	1–2 mg/kg	138,154
Nafcillin	75 mg	153
	1–4 mg/kg	66
Chloramphenicol	25–50 mg	39,150
Gentamicin	2–4 mg	39
	1–8 mg	153
Vancomycin	8–10 mg	152
	4–5 mg	151
Amphotericin B	0.25–0.5 mg[a]	75
	(0.1-mg test dose)	
Miconazole	20 mg	75

[a] Diluted in 5 ml of CSF or distilled water, given every other day.

portant (39,71,116,125,160). The rate of successful treatment by this method was low (approximately 24%), with a high mortality (24%) (see Fig. 3).

The high failure rate of intravenous treatment may be attributed to many factors. Antibiotic penetration into the CNS is variable and unpredictable, particularly because the meningeal inflammation that increases drug penetration is frequently absent in shunt infection (116,138,153,154). Combined poor antibiotic penetration, development of secondary bacterial resistance, and bacterial colonization of the shunt material can result in a high rate of treatment failure, or in the suppression of infection followed by relapse (78,116).

Instillation of antibiotics into the CSF in conjunction with parenteral antibiotics increased the successful treatment rate to approximately 40% (29,67,71,78,116,138, 154). The lengthy hospitalizations needed for this treatment, the high failure rate, and the additional treatments needed for the cure of those failures caused significant morbidity (29,67,78,161–163). For these reasons, most authors do not recommend such treatment regimens (23, 31,34,65–67,71,78,91,138,160–164). These techniques may be required, however, when the patient is unable to undergo the surgical components of therapy, or in the initial treatment of retained or irremovable hardware.

Combining the removal of presumably colonized shunt hardware with immediate shunt replacement might be expected to cause an improvement in the rate of successful treatment (36,116,160,162). This concept is supported by retrospective analyses that compared the treatment course, outcome, and the ability of the infecting agents to produce a glycocalyx or slime (106,107). When the shunts were not replaced, infections by slime-producing staphylococci appeared to take longer to treat and were associated with more treatment failures (106). Also, over three-quarters of the infections cured with only *in situ* antibiotic treatment were caused by non-

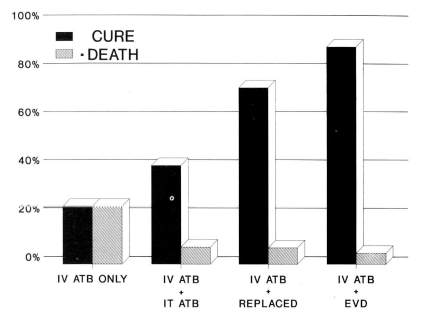

FIG. 3. Results of therapies for shunt infections. The morbidity and mortality of various treatments for shunt infections are shown. The groups received intravenous antibiotics only (IV ATB ONLY), intravenous and intrathecal antibiotics (IV ATB + IT ATB), intravenous antibiotics with shunt replacement (IV ATB + REPLACED), or intravenous antibiotics with externalization (IV ATB + EVD). The group treated with externalization not only had the lowest mortality, but also demonstrated the greatest success in initial treatment of shunt infections. This chart was derived from the following references: IV ATB ONLY—21, 23, 31, 32, 34, 46, 63, 65, 107, 161, 163; IV ATB + IT ATB—46, 65, 66, 67, 153, 162, 163, 165, 166; IV ATB + REPLACED—23, 31, 36, 46, 65, 66, 67, 167, 168; IV ATB + EVD—21, 23, 31, 32, 46, 63, 66.

slime-producing organisms (107). Thus, immediate replacement would remove the densely adherent bacteria that are otherwise protected from the antibiotic by their glycocalyx. It would also allow continued control of the hydrocephalus—and, if needed, placement of a reservoir for antibiotic injection into the CSF. In fact, when parenteral antibiotics are combined with this approach, roughly 75% of the infections can be cured (see Fig. 3).

The failure and reinfection rates still remain quite significant with this technique (13,31). Difficulties with shunt replacement (particularly at the ventricular end) can add to the morbidity, and the treatment time remains quite long (67,153). In addition, there is the possibility that the replacement hardware may become colonized by the bacteria under treatment. To obviate this possibility, hardware replacement has been delayed until several days after the institution of parenteral antibiotics or until completion of antibiotic therapy. Delayed replacement does seem to improve the cure rate, but it may also be associated with increased morbidity and mortality (46,63,167).

Antibiotic use with some component of external drainage appears to be the most effective treatment (Fig. 3) (21,23,31,46,63,67,71). The ventriculitis of shunt infections appears to clear more quickly with external drainage (67,71). Drainage may be accomplished by externalization of the distal end of the shunt, or by replacement of the entire shunt with a new ventriculostomy. It allows continued treatment of the underlying hydrocephalus and avoids the complications that might ensue with only shunt removal (13,30,66,67,78,112,138,169). With the predominance of peritoneal shunts, the loss of a vascular access site with externalization is rarely a concern. The status of the infection can be monitored by regularly collected routine CSF studies. If needed, there is also easy access for intraventricular antibiotic administration (154). With externalization, treatment success is usually greater than 90% (Fig. 3). The length of treatment consequently averages less than with the other methods (67).

As with shunt replacement, there may be difficulties associated with removing the proximal portion of the shunt and replacing the ventriculostomy. Certainly the care of the patient is complicated somewhat: The external device requires additional nursing attention, and it must be protected from accidental disconnection or removal by the unaware infant (30,91,116,153). Particularly in infants, the fluids, electrolytes, and protein lost in the ventricular drainage must be carefully monitored, and replacement may be needed.

The most significant risk with external shunts is that of secondary infection (30,41,54,57,129). Attention to maintaining a sterile, closed system, avoiding injections into the system, and repeated surveillance of the draining CSF will keep this risk minimal, probably less than 5%. For periods of extended treatment, or for treatment of a secondary infection, replacement of the external ventricular drain (EVD) may be necessary.

Our approach to the treatment of shunt infections is based on several concepts:

1. We do not attempt *in situ* treatment. All components of an infected shunt are removed at the beginning of treatment, and an external ventriculostomy is placed. The ability of many organisms to adhere to the prostheses and to survive antibiotic therapy precludes effective treatment *in situ*. The propensity for the entire shunt to become contaminated when one portion becomes infected argues against partial revisions.

2. All contaminations of shunts are treated as infections, with hardware removal and externalization. It is the "extent" of infection, determined by factors such as the physiologic response to infection and the frequency of positive cultures, that defines the length of therapy.

3. We are routinely placing a reservoir in our shunting systems to allow CSF sampling. This allows evaluation of CSF for signs of infection in those cases where the diagnosis is unclear.

Our diagnostic paradigm is presented in Fig. 4. The results of the Gram's stain are often sufficient to determine the initial therapy. It has been our experience that infections due to gram-negative organisms are almost always detected at the time of presentation. The patients are more seriously ill, the CSF studies are abnormal, and there is frequently a positive Gram's stain (71). In those cases, appropriate therapy for gram-negative organisms would be started pending the culture results.

If no organisms are seen on Gram's stain, attention is turned to the CSF studies and the clinical state of the patient. Abnormal CSF studies result in at least anti-

staphylococcal treatment, with coverage of gram-negative infections in those patients who are clinically very ill. In those patients with distal symptoms, we attempt to aspirate fluid from the distal end for Gram's stain and separate culture, and we also obtain a culture from the distal catheter tip. Only a presentation of proximal shunt dysfunction, with no outward signs of infection, a negative Gram's stain, and normal CSF cell counts, will result in a full revision and no antibiotic treatment. If the operative cultures were subsequently positive, then infection would be diagnosed and treated. Coverage of gram-negative organisms can be added to any arm of the protocol when clinically indicated. In all cases, when the culture results become available, the antibiotics are adjusted according to the organism isolated and its sensitivities.

Treatment is begun with complete removal of the infected shunt and placement of an EVD. The EVD is usually placed at the same cranial site unless there is an open wound or obvious infection at the site. In those infrequent cases where the presentation is a distal cellulitis or a peritonitis, and the CSF is completely normal,

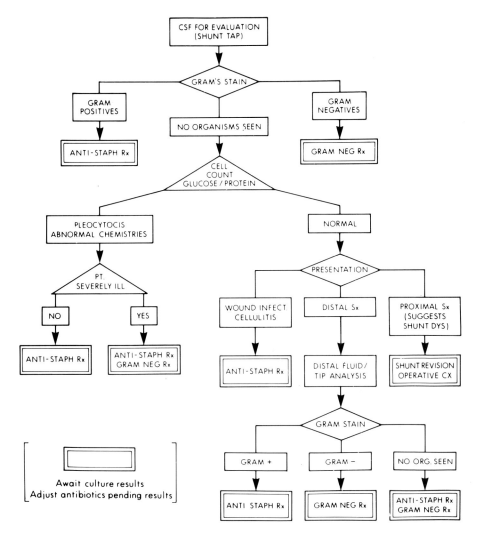

FIG. 4. Diagnostic paradigm. Our approach to determining initial antibiotic treatment for a presumed shunt infection, based on the clinical and laboratory findings, is outlined in this flow chart. In all cases, after the initial treatment has begun (denoted by double-bordered boxes), further treatment is adjusted based on subsequent culture and sensitivity results. See text for further discussion. Sx, symptoms; Rx, treatment; Cx, cultured.

externalization of the distal end may be done initially. This can be done under local anesthesia and may allow distinguishing a peritoneal shunt infection from other intra-abdominal processes without necessitating an immediate shunt surgery. When the distal infection is fully treated, the entire shunt would still require removal, because it is considered to be colonized after externalization. If a positive CSF culture is returned during externalization, the externalized shunt is replaced with a formal external ventriculostomy. Our preference is to remove the entire shunt initially, regardless of the type of infection.

The duration of therapy is dependent on the organism isolated, the extent of infection as determined by cultures obtained after externalization, and to some extent the CSF findings. A summary of therapy is presented in Table 7.

Coagulase-negative staphylococci that are cultured only from pre-externalization samples and associated with normal CSF findings are felt to represent colonization of the hardware. The absence of positive CSF cultures for 48 hr after externalization confirms that removal of the hardware effected a cure, and the patient may be reshunted on the third day. If there are signs of infection (pleocytosis, abnormal chemistries) in the CSF, then a true infection is present and a full course of treatment is necessary. When additional cultures are found to be positive, a more virulent or well-ensconced infection is felt to be present, and treatment is continued until the cultures remain negative for 10 consecutive days. There are, however, no objective data that suggest whether staphylococcal infections need more than 7 days of culture-negative therapy. Because of the difficulty in treating these infections, a 3-day period off antibiotics is observed before reshunting. This allows the detection of an infection that has been suppressed rather than cured.

Three days off antibiotics allows at least 48 hr of culture incubation before replacement is performed.

S. aureus and gram-negative organisms are treated in the same manner because of their virulence and potential for abscess formation. Also, regardless of contamination or infection, a full course of treatment is undertaken. The 10-day length of treatment was chosen based on the treatment of non-CNS gram-negative infections, and the *S. aureus* treatment period was made to match for simplicity. Again, an antibiotic hiatus is used to verify clearance of the infection.

We have observed that the vast majority of positive CSF cultures revert to negative within 2 days after EVD placement and antibiotic therapy. When the cultures remain positive, either the treatment may be inadequate or the EVD system may have become colonized. If the laboratory signs of ventriculitis (cell count, protein, glucose) are resolving, we replace the EVD, presuming it to be colonized. This will usually resolve difficulties resulting from colonization of the hardware. Failure of the CSF chemistries and cell counts to show a return toward normal values, or continued positive cultures after ventriculostomy replacement, would be evidence of ineffective therapy, and bactericidal titers are performed on the CSF. Effective treatment would be expected with growth inhibition at dilutions greater than 1:8. If the titers are at least 1:8, and the patient is not deteriorating, the same treatment will be continued for several days. This allows for those cases where the bacterial clearance is slow, seen especially with gram-negative infections. If the titers are low, then the antibiotic regimen is adjusted. The antibiotic may be changed, the dosage may be increased, or rifampin therapy may be added (for gram-positive infections only). Intraventricular antibiotics are rarely used.

For severe infections, or those that are difficult to eradicate, we have used a technique of ventricular irrigation

TABLE 7. *Duration of antibiotic therapy for shunt infections*

Organism isolated	Time of isolation	CSF findings	Therapy
Coagulase-negative staphylococcus (includes *S. epidermidis*)	OR[a] culture only	Normal	1. Three days ATB[b] 2. Reshunt
	OR culture only	Abnormal	1. Seven days ATB 2. Reshunt
	OR culture and at least one subsequent culture positive	Normal or abnormal	1. Ten days ATB 2. Three days off ATB 3. Then if cultures still negative, reshunt
Other bacteria includes *S. aureus*, gram-negatives)	OR culture only, or OR culture and subsequent culture	Normal or abnormal	1. Ten days ATB 2. Three days off ATB 3. Then if cultures still negative, reshunt

[a] OR, operating room.
[b] ATB, antibiotics.

with an antibiotic solution. An amikacin solution of 30 μg/ml, or a gentamicin solution (without perservatives) of 15 μg/ml, is introduced into the ventriculostomy. If a second ventriculostomy is present, and communication between the two can be demonstrated, a continuous flow at a low rate (<20 ml/hr) is established. If a single ventriculostomy or loculations are present, aliquots of 10–20 ml are introduced and then drained after 30 min. In both situations, care must be taken to maintain a functioning ventriculostomy and to avoid an increase in ICP from too fast or too much infusion. This technique allows delivery of intraventricular antibiotic at a concentration that is known, and it prevents antibiotic accumulation to toxic levels.

The treatment of an infection caused by an external device, or the treatment of a secondary infection caused by an EVD, is straightforward. The device, other than a ventriculostomy, is removed, and a course of treatment appropriate for the organism is begun. If the continued use of the device is required, such as the need for ICP measurement, another device at a new location is placed. For a ventriculostomy, whatever its use, the hardware is replaced, and the appropriate treatment protocol is followed, just as if it were a standard shunt infection (128).

Portions of shunting equipment that become lost in the intracranial, intrathoracic, or intra-abdominal compartments present a complicating factor in the treatment of shunt infections. There is usually no way to determine the exposure to infecting organisms of such retained hardware. We consider this equipment to be contaminated, and we make some attempt to remove it at the time of shunt externalization. The diagnostic and treatment protocols are still followed; however, if the retained hardware cannot be removed, the treatment is essentially a form of *in situ* therapy, and recurrent infection is more likely. We are more inclined to use intraventricular antibiotics in an attempt to sterilize the retained hardware. Extra vigilance for recurrent infection is maintained. If reinfection occurs, or if the treatment is unable to effect negative CSF cultures, retrieval of the lost pieces must be undertaken.

Our approach to fungal shunt infections is similar to our treatment of bacterial shunt infections. In addition to the appropriate intravenous antifungal therapy, the infected shunt should be removed, and an external ventriculostomy should be placed. As with bacteria, both *Cryptococcus neoformans* and *Candida albicans* have been found embedded in a biofilm attached to shunt material (74,76). For this reason, treatment should involve removal of the shunt (without or with immediate replacement) in addition to standard antifungal therapy (74–76). *In situ* treatment has been reported; however, we feel that this is not the best treatment, for the same reasons as mentioned above (127). External drainage allows continued treatment of the underlying hydrocephalic condition, drainage of purulent material, and intra-

ventricular administration of antifungal agents as needed. When the infection has been cleared, the shunt may be internalized. The duration of intrathecal therapy should be based on the clinical symptoms and signs of fungal infection, whereas systemic therapy should continue for the usual extended time periods.

The most widely used antifungal drug is amphotericin B, a polyene antibiotic. It has only a fair penetration into the CSF when given parenterally. In addition, it has significant systemic toxicity, primarily nephrotoxicity; it also has immediate reactions to administration, including fever, nausea, and vomiting. In the absence of a shunt, intrathecal administration is usually reserved for cases of coccidioidal meningitis and those infections that fail to respond to intravenously given drug. Intrathecal medication is warranted as part of the treatment when a prosthetic device is present. The initial intrathecal test dose should be 0.1 mg; if tolerated, this dose should be increased to 0.25–0.5 mg, given every other day. Amphotericin B given intrathecally can be absorbed through the arachnoid villi, and it may then contribute to systemic side effects (75).

A fluorinated pyrimidine derivative, 5-fluorocytosine, can achieve CSF levels of 50–70% of serum levels when given parenterally. Its use is limited, however, by the large number of resistant species or the quick development of resistance if used alone. When used, 5-fluorocytosine should be combined with amphotericin B; this combination can result in enhanced effectiveness, even if *in vitro* testing reveals resistance. Miconazole, an imidazole derivative, has been used increasingly for those infections resistant to amphotericin B. It also has poor CSF penetration when given parenterally, and it requires intrathecal administration at a dose of 20 mg/day to effectively treat CNS infections (75).

PREVENTION/PROPHYLAXIS

With the large number of shunt procedures performed each year, an operative incidence of shunt infections in the range of 5–10% results in a sizable number of infections. Given the significant morbidity and the occasional mortality associated with these infections and their treatment, effective prevention would be highly beneficial. Preventive measures can be undertaken in several areas in an attempt to reduce the incidence of infection. Alterations in the hardware, as well as changes in operating techniques, have been suggested. Certainly, the most discussed method involves prophylactic use of antibiotics.

Incorporation of antibiotics into the polymers used in shunt hardware has been attempted (77,170,171). The goal is for a relatively slow release of antibiotics from the compound during the early postoperative period ("period of risk"), thus preventing the establishment of infection (77). The feasibility of this approach was established by Bayston and Milner (170), but others have demonstrated untoward results (169). Impregnating shunt tubing with bacitracin A actually led to a 600% increase in bacterial binding, probably as a result of receptor–ligand binding of the bacteria with the incorporated bacitracin molecule (172).

Seeking the mechanisms of bacterial binding that lead to the establishment of infection, investigators turned to the molecular and atomic level of interactions at the shunt surfaces. If the bacterial binding sites on the artificial material can be reduced, establishment of infection should also decrease. In a similar fashion, increasing the degree of normal tissue integration with the material would prevent bacterial binding by covering those same sites of interaction (100,173).

Attention to operative techniques used during shunt surgery can also result in a decline in the rate of infection, either by reducing the potential for inoculating organisms or by reducing the size of the inoculum. Methods of skin preparation which reduce the total number of bacteria and which maintain that reduction (i.e., long-acting iodinated compounds) would accomplish this (77,174). Exclusion of the skin from the operative field, with adhesive plastic draping on the skin or covering the skin incision edges, may have the same effect (36,38). Standard operative techniques that minimize the milieu for infection—including decreased skin manipulation, incisions planned with good blood supply, and less use of nonabsorbable suture material—should also help (36,38,125,175).

Topically applied antibiotics have been widely used in neurosurgery for the prevention of infection, but their benefit has not been rigorously substantiated (176). The effect of commonly used topical antibiotics during brief exposures has been studied in the laboratory, quantified as a bactericidal or "kill" percentage. Bacitracin A, at a concentration of 200 U/ml (and vancomycin, at 100 μg/ml), demonstrated greater than 90% kill after 1 hr of exposure (177). Even at 50 U/ml, bacitracin showed a 50% kill after only 1 min of exposure to susceptible bacteria (178). Gentamicin was much less effective. One neurosurgeon changed his shunting technique only by using topical antibiotics (oxacillin irrigating solution combined with soaking the shunt hardware in an oxacillin solution) and had a drop in infection rate from 15% to 5% (179).

If bacterial adherence could be reduced, then infection should be reduced. Since bacteria bind mainly through ionic interactions and van der Waals forces, disruption of these bonds should reduce bacterial adherence (79,172,180). Experimentally, this can be done with any number of detergent compounds. Utilizing the detergent properties of bacitracin A, a similar reduction of 54% in bacterial adherence after only a 30-min exposure to bacitracin was documented (172). Obviously, the use of bacitracin A in shunt surgery can easily combine the effects

of bacterial killing and reduced adherence, and thus reduce infection. Clinically, there is some support for this (36). However, the effect on bacteria already adherent is not nearly as great: Only a 25% reduction in established bacterial colonization was effected *in vitro* by bacitracin at a concentration of 750 U/ml (102).

The prophylactic use of parenteral antibiotics in reducing infections associated with vascular and orthopedic prosthetic implants has been advocated and clinically supported (174,181–183). Such prophylactic antibiotic use, however, cannot be extrapolated to CNS implants. As mentioned, the CNS presents a unique environment for the evolution of infection, and the materials used in CSF shunts are often quite different from those used in vascular or orthopedic surgery.

In general neurosurgery, the use of parenteral antibiotics to prevent infections has been extensively described (184). While most of these studies are retrospective or uncontrolled, it appears likely that their use results in a three- to fivefold reduction in infection (44,185–189). From these studies, several general concepts of antibiotic prophylaxis can be summarized (184):

1. The chosen antibiotic(s) must have appropriate coverage for the likely infecting organisms.

2. The chosen antibiotic(s) must be given shortly before the start of the operation, and administration must be repeated as necessary to achieve and maintain maximal tissue levels during surgery.

3. The effectiveness of the chosen antibiotic(s) does not require continuance beyond the operative period.

4. The development of antibiotic-resistant organisms has not been detected using these methods.

The results from the large number of studies on parenteral antibiotic use in shunt surgery are less clear. Some authors have reported very low infection rates without antibiotic use, and they attribute this low rate to good surgical techniques (175). Others have interpreted from their results that there is no benefit from antibiotic prophylaxis (130,189–194). Still others have demonstrated often dramatic drops in infection rates with parenteral antibiotic use, despite using nearly identical protocols (36,71,179,195,196). In general, all the studies have been statistically weak, using a retrospective or sequential analysis of cases; in addition, they have suffered from small sample sizes.

Even less clear is the use of parenteral antibiotic prophylaxis with externalized systems. Poppen (52) in 1943 had no infections with 500 ventriculostomies and no prophylaxis. Other studies report a "low" rate of infection (2–10%) attributable to antibiotic prophylaxis (54,57,129,197). As mentioned previously, variations in the use of the externalized systems can markedly affect their rate of infection (i.e., duration of therapy, injections into the system) and thus confound any effects of antibiotic use.

We use a multifaceted approach to the prevention of shunt infections, based on the facts mentioned above. An occlusive plastic drape is applied to the exposed skin after preparation, to prevent inadvertent skin contact with the shunt. Anti-staphylococcal antibiotics are given intravenously just after induction of anesthesia and before incision, and they are continued only intraoperatively. We do not use vancomycin for prophylaxis, for fear of developing resistant bacteria and losing our most effective antibiotic against methicillin-resistant strains. The shunt equipment is soaked in bacitracin A solution (200 U/ml) prior to its use, and the same solution is used for intraoperative irrigation. Although its benefit has not been proven, we also give antibiotics for the duration of use with externalized hardware. When able, we routinely monitor the CSF from the externalized systems for evidence of infection, and we treat any such infection as stated. We have not detected the development of resistant organisms in these cases.

SUMMARY

Because of their frequency and associated morbidity, infections of CNS prostheses and shunts remain a significant problem in neurosurgery. Certainly, early detection and aggressive treatment to clear these infections reduce morbidity. Prevention, however, will ultimately result in the greatest decrease in morbidity. Investigation and development of techniques based on preventing the establishment of infection at the molecular level holds the most promise for effecting this reduction.

REFERENCES

1. Diamond RD, Bennett JE. A subcutaneous reservoir for intrathecal therapy of fungal meningitis. *N Engl J Med* 1973;288:186–188.
2. Machado M, Salcman M, Kaplan RS, Montgomery E. Expanded role of the cerebrospinal fluid reservoir in neurooncology: indications, causes of revision, and complications. *Neurosurgery* 1985;17:600–603.
3. Ratcheson RA, Ommaya AK. Experience with the subcutaneous cerebrospinal-fluid reservoir: preliminary report of 60 cases. *N Eng J Med* 1968;279:1025–1031.
4. Shetter AG, Hadley MN, Wilkinson E. Administration of intraspinal morphine sulfate for the treatment of intractable cancer pain. *Neurosurgery* 1986;18(6):740–747.
5. Davidoff LM. Treatment of hydrocephalus—historical review and description of a new method. *Arch Surg* 1929;18:1737–1762.
6. Pudenz RH. The surgical treatment of hydrocephalus—an historical review. *Surg Neurol* 1981;15(1):15–26.
7. Scarff JE. Treatment of hydrocephalus: an historical and critical review of methods and results. *J Neurol Neurosurg Psychiatry* 1963;26(1):1–26.
8. Lapras C, Bret P, Patet JD, Huppert J, Honorato D. Hydrocephalus and aqueductal stenosis. Direct surgical treatment by interventriculostomy (aqueductal cannulation). *J Neurosurg Sci* 1986;30:71–76.
9. Hoffman HJ, Harwood-Nash D, Gilday DL. Percutaneous third ventriculostomy in the management of non-communicating hydrocephalus. *Neurosurgery* 1980;7:313–321.
10. Nulsen FE, Spitz EB. Treatment of hydrocephalus by direct shunt from ventricle to jugular vein. *Surg Forum* 1951;1:399–403.
11. Ransohoff J, Shulman K, Fishman RA. Hydrocephalus—a review of etiology and treatment. *J Pediatr* 1960;56:399–411.
12. Anderson FM. Ventriculocardiac shunts: identification and control of practical problems in 143 cases. *J Pediatr* 1973;82(2):222–227.
13. Keucher TR, Mealey J. Long term results after ventriculoatrial and ventriculoperitoneal shunting for infantile hydrocephalus. *J Neurosurg* 1979;50:179–186.
14. Little JR, Rhoton AL, Mellinger JF. Comparison of ventriculoperitoneal and ventriculoatrial shunts for hydrocephalus in children. *Mayo Clin Proc* 1972;47:396–401.
15. Olsen L, Frykberg T. Complications in the treatment of hydrocephalus in children. *Acta Paediatr Scand* 1983;72:385–390.
16. Hoffman HJ, Hendrick EB, Humphreys RP. Experience with ventriculo-pleural shunts. *Child's Brain* 1983;10:404–413.
17. McLone DG, Czyzewski D, Raimondi AJ, Sommers RC. Central nervous system infections as a limiting factor in the intelligence of children with myelomeningocoele. *Pediatrics* 1982;70(3):338–342.
18. Storrs BB. Ventricular size and intelligence in myelodysplastic children. *Concepts Pediatr Neurosurg* 1988;8:51–56.
19. Ersahin Y, McLone DG, Storrs BB, Yogev R. Review of 3017 procedures for the management of hydrocephalus in children. *Concepts Pediatr Neurosurg* 1989;9:21–28.
20. George R, Leibrock L, Epstein M. Long-term analysis of cerebrospinal fluid shunt infections—a 25 year experience. *J Neurosurg* 1979;51:804–811.
21. Odio C, McCracken GH, Nelson JD. CSF shunt infections in pediatrics. *Am J Dis Child* 1984;138:1103–1108.
22. Renier D, Lacombe J, Pierre-Kahn A, Sainte-Rose C, Hirsch JF. Factors causing acute shunt infection—computer analysis of 1174 operations. *J Neurosurg* 1984;61:1072–1078.
23. Schoenbaum SC, Gardner P, Shillito J. Infections of cerebrospinal fluid shunts: epidemiology, clinical manifestations, and therapy. *J Infect Dis* 1975;131(5):543–552.
24. Shapiro S, Boaz J, Kleiman M, Kalsbeck J, Mealey J. Origin of organisms infecting ventricular shunts. *Neurosurgery* 1988;22:868–872.
25. Shurtleff DB, Christie D, Foltz EL. Ventriculoauriculostomy-associated infection—a 12 year study. *J Neurosurg* 1971;35:686–694.
26. Shurtleff DB, Stuntz JT, Hayden PW. Experience with 1201 cerebrospinal fluid shunt procedures. *Pediatr Neurosci* 1985–1986;12:49–57.
27. Ajir F, Levin AB, Duff TA. Effect of prophylactic methicillin on cerebrospinal fluid shunt infections in children. *Neurosurgery* 1981;9:6–8.
28. Bayston R, Lari J. A study of the sources of infection in colonised shunts. *Dev Med Child Neurol* 1974;16(Suppl 32):16–22.
29. McLaurin RL. Treatment of infected ventricular shunts. *Child's Brain* 1975;1:306–310.
30. Mori K, Raimondi AJ. An analysis of external ventricular drainage as a treatment for infected shunts. *Child's Brain* 1975;1:243–250.
31. Morrice JJ, Young DG. Bacterial colonisation of Holter valves: a ten year survey. *Dev Med Child Neurol* 1974;16(Suppl 32):85–90.
32. Nelson JD. Cerebrospinal fluid shunt infections. *Pediatr Infect Dis* 1984;3(Suppl):30–32.
33. Overton MC, Snodgrass SR. Ventriculo-venous shunts for infantile Hydrocephalus—a review of five years' experience with this method. *J Neurosurg* 1965;23:517–521.
34. Schimke RT, Black PH, Mark VH, Swartz MN. Indolent *Staphylococcus albus* or *aureus* bacteremia after ventriculoatriostomy. *N Engl J Med* 1961;264(6):264–270.
35. Spanu G, Karussos G, Adinolfi D, Bonfanti N. An analysis of cerebrospinal fluid shunt infections in adults. A clinical experience of twelve years. *Acta Neurochir* 1986;80:79–82.
36. Venes JL. Control of shunt infections—report of 150 consecutive cases. *J Neurosurg* 1976;45:311–314.
37. Selman WR, Spetzler RF, Wilson CB, Grollmus JW. Percutane-

ous lumboperitoneal shunt: review of 130 cases. *Neurosurgery* 1980;6:255–257.

38. McCullough DC, Kane JG, Presper JH, Wells M. Antibiotic prophylaxis in ventricular shunt surgery. I. Reduction of operative infection rates with methicillin. *Child's Brain* 1980;7:182–189.

39. McLaurin RL. Infected cerebrospinal fluid shunts. *Surg Neurol* 1973;1:191–195.

40. Nulsen FE, Becker DP. Control of hydrocephalus by valve-regulated shunt: infections and their prevention. *Clin Neurosurg* 1966;14:256–273.

41. Sayers MP. Shunt complications. *Clin Neurosurg* 1976;23:393–400.

42. Yogev R, Davis AT. Neurosurgical shunt infections—a review. *Child's Brain* 1980;6:74–81.

43. Forrest DM, Cooper DGW. Complications of ventriculo-atrial shunts: a review of 455 cases. *J Neurosurg* 1968;29:506–512.

44. Mollman HD, Haines SJ. Risk factors for postoperative neurosurgical wound infection—a case–control study. *J Neurosurg* 1986;64:902–906.

45. Holt RJ. Bacteriological studies on colonized ventriculoatrial shunts. *Dev Med Child Neurol* 1970;12(Suppl 22):83–87.

46. Walters BC, Hoffman HJ, Hendrick EB, Humphreys RP. Cerebrospinal fluid shunt infection: influences on initial management and subsequent outcome. *J Neurosurg* 1984;60:1014–1021.

47. Hoffman HJ, Hendrick ED, Humphreys RP. Management of hydrocephalus. *Monogr Neural Sci* 1982;8:21–25.

48. Clark WC, Munibauer MS, Heartman MS, Ray MW, Robertson JT, Watridge CB. Complications of ICP monitoring in trauma patients [Abstract]. *Neurosurgery* 1987;21:117.

49. Constantini S, Cotev S, Rappaport ZH, Pomeranz S, Shalit MN. Intracranial pressure monitoring after elective intracranial surgery—a retrospective study of 514 consecutive patients. *J Neurosurg* 1988;69:540–544.

50. Mayhall CG, Archer NH, Lamb VA, et al. Ventriculostomy related infections—a prospective epidemiologic study. *N Engl J Med* 1984;310(9):553–559.

51. North B, Reilly P. Comparison among three methods of intracranial pressure recording. *Neurosurgery* 1986;18(6):730–732.

52. Poppen JL. Ventricular drainage as a valuable procedure in neurosurgery—report of a satisfactory method. *Arch Neurol Psychiatry* 1943;50:587–589.

53. Rosner MJ, Becker DP. ICP monitoring: complications and associated factors. *Clin Neurosurg* 1973;23:494–519.

54. Smith RW, Alksne JF. Infections complicating the use of external ventriculostomy. *J Neurosurg* 1976;44:567–570.

55. Sundbarg G, Kjallquist A, Lundberg N, Ponten U. Complications due to prolonged ventricular fluid pressure recording in clinical practice. In: Brock M, Dietz H, eds. *Intracranial pressure: experimental and clinical aspects.* New York: Springer-Verlag, 1972;348–356.

56. Venes J. Intracranial pressure monitoring in perspective. *Child's Brain* 1980;7:236–251.

57. James HE, Langfitt TW, Kumar VS, Ghostine SY. Treatment of intracranial hypertension—analysis of 105 consecutive, continuous recordings of intracranial pressure. *Acta Neurochir* 1977;36:189–200.

58. Ostrup RC, Luerssen TG, Marshall LF, Zornow MH. Continuous monitoring of intracranial pressure with a miniaturized fiberoptic device. *J Neurosurg* 1987;67:206–209.

59. Smith KA. Head trauma: comparison of infection rates for different methods of intracranial pressure monitoring. *J Neurosci Nurs* 1987;19:310–314.

60. Hahn YS, McLone DG, Raimondi AJ, Frisbie CL. Surgical outcome of preterm newborns with severe peri-ventricular–intraventricular hemorrhage and post-hemorrhagic hydrocephalus. *Concepts Pediatr Neurosurg* 1983;4:66–80.

61. Siegal T, Pfeffer R, Steiner I. Antibiotic therapy for infected Ommaya reservoir systems. *Neurosurgery* 1988;22(1):97–100.

62. Meirovitch J, Kitai-Cohen Y, Keren G, Fiendler G, Rubenstein E. Cerebrospinal fluid shunt infections in children. *Pediatr Infect Dis J* 1987;6:921–924.

63. Forward KR, Fewer HD, Stiver HG. Cerebrospinal fluid shunt infections—a review of 35 infections in 32 patients. *J Neurosurg* 1983;59:389–394.

64. Raimondi AJ, Robinson JS, Kuwamura K. Complications of ventriculo-peritoneal shunting and a critical comparison of the three-piece and one-piece systems. *Child's Brain* 1977;3:321–342.

65. Sells CJ, Shurtleff DB, Loeser JD. Gram-negative cerebrospinal fluid shunt-associated infections. *Pediatrics* 1977;59(4):614–618.

66. James HE, Walsh JW, Wilson HD, Connor JD. The management of cerebrospinal fluid shunt infections—a clinical experience. *Acta Neurochir* 1981;59:157–166.

67. James HE, Walsh JW, Wilson HD, Connor JD, Bean JR, Tibbs PA. Prospective randomized study of therapy in cerebrospinal fluid shunt infection. *Neurosurgery* 1980;7:459–463.

68. Lerman SJ. *Haemophilus influenzae*-infections of cerebrospinal fluid shunts. *J Neurosurg* 1981;54:261–263.

69. Patriarca PA, Lauer BA. Ventriculoperitoneal shunt-associated infection due to *Haemophilus influenzae. Pediatrics* 1980;65(5):1007–1009.

70. Rennels MB, Wald ER. Treatment of *Haemophilus influenzae*-type b meningitis in children with cerebrospinal fluid shunts. *J Pediatr* 1980;97:424–426.

71. Yogev R. Cerebrospinal fluid shunt infections: a personal view. *Pediatr Infect Dis* 1985;4(2):113–118.

72. Everett ED, Eickhoff TC, Simon RH. Cerebrospinal fluid shunt infections with anaerobic diphtheroids (*Propionibacterium* species). *J Neurosurg* 1976;44:580–584.

73. Rekate HL, Ruch T, Nulsen FE. Diphtheroid infections of cerebrospinal fluid shunts—the changing pattern of shunt infection in Cleveland. *J Neurosurg* 1980;52:553–556.

74. Walsh TJ, Schlegel R, Moody MM, Costerton JW, Salcman M. Ventriculoatrial shunt infection due to *Cryptococcus neoformans:* an ultrastructural and quantitative microbiological study. *Neurosurgery* 1986;18:373–375.

75. Bell WH. Treatment of fungal infections of the central nervous system. *Ann Neurol* 1981;9:417–422.

76. Gower DJ, Crone K, Alexander E, Kelly DL. *Candida albicans* shunt infection: report of two cases. *Neurosurgery* 1986;19(1):111–113.

77. Bayston R. Microbial colonization of cerebrospinal fluid shunts. *Med Lab Sci* 1981;38:259–267.

78. Gardner P, Leipzig T, Phillips P. Infections of central nervous system shunts. Symposium on infections of the central nervous system. *Med Clin North Am* 1985;69:297–314.

79. Schoenberg H. Vesicoureteral reflux after subarachnoid ureterostomy. *J Urol* 1959;82:474–475.

80. Alexander JW. Surgical infections and choice of antibiotics. In: Sabiston DC, ed. *Textbook of surgery: the biological basis of modern surgical practice,* 13th ed. Philadelphia: WB Saunders, 1986;259–283.

81. Todd JC. Wound infection: etiology, prevention, and management—including selection of antibiotics. *Surg Clin North Am* 1968;48(4):787–798.

82. Kaufman BA, Likavec MJ. *Branhamella catarrhalis* cellulitis around a cerebrospinal fluid shunt: case report. *J Hosp Infect* 1985;6:323–325.

83. Stern S, Bayston R, Hayward RJ. *Haemophilus influenzae* meningitis in the presence of cerebrospinal fluid shunts. *Child's Nerv Syst* 1988;4:164–165.

84. Irvine R, Johnson BL, Amstutz HC. The relationship of genitourinary tract procedures and deep sepsis after total hip replacements. *Surg Gynecol Obstet* 1974;139:701–706.

85. Cruess RL, Bickel WS, von Kessler KLC. Infections in total hips secondary to a primary source elsewhere. *Clin Orthop* 1975;106:99–101.

86. D'Ambrosia RD, Shoji H, Heater R. Secondarily infected total joint replacements by hematogenous spread. *J Bone Joint Surg* 1976;58A:450–453.

87. Downes EM. Late infection after total hip replacement. *J Bone Joint Surg* 1977;59B:42–44.

88. Stinchfield FE, Bigliani LU, Neu HC, Goss TP, Foster CR. Late hematogenous infection of total joint replacement. *J Bone Joint Surg* 1980;62A:1345–1350.

89. Charnley J. Postoperative infection after total hip replacement with special reference to air contamination in the operating room. *Clin Orthop* 1972;87:167–187.

90. Yount RA, Boaz J, Kleiman M, Kalsbeck JE. The origin of organisms infecting ventricular shunts. Paper 30, AANS Annual Meeting, San Francisco, April 8–12, 1984.
91. Garvey G. Current concepts of bacterial infections of the central nervous system—bacterial meningitis and bacterial brain abscess. *J Neurosurg* 1983;59:735–744.
92. Nicastro JF, Shoji H, Rovere GD, Gristina AG. Effects of methylmethacrylate on *S. aureus* growth and rabbit alveolar macrophage phagocytosis and glucose metabolism. *Surg Forum* 1975;26:501–503.
93. Sugarman B. Infections and prosthetic devices. *Am J Med* 1986;81(Suppl 1A):78–84.
94. Zimmerli W, Waldvogel FA, Vaudaux P, Nydegger UE. Pathogenesis of foreign body infection: description and characteristics of an animal model. *J Infect Dis* 1982;146:487–497.
95. Borges LF. Cerebrospinal fluid shunts interfere with host defenses. *Neurosurgery* 1982;10(1):55–60.
96. Gristina AG, Price JL, Hobgood CD, Webb LX, Costerton JW. Bacterial colonization of percutaneous sutures. *Surgery* 1985;98(1):12–19.
97. Ashkenazi S. Bacterial adherence to plastics. *Lancet* 1984; 1:1075–1076.
98. Barrett SP. Protein-mediated adhesion of *Staphylococcus aureus* to silicone implant polymer. *J Med Microbiol* 1985;20:249–253.
99. Hogt AH, Dankert J, DeVries JA, Feijen J. Adhesion of coagulase-negative staphylococci to biomaterials. *J Gen Microbiol* 1983;129:2959–2968.
100. Gristina AG. Biomaterial-centered infection: microbial adhesion versus tissue integration. *Science* 1987;237:1588–1595.
101. Guevara JA, Zuccaro G, Trevisan BS, Denoya CD. Bacterial adhesion to cerebrospinal fluid shunts. *J Neurosurg* 1987;67:438–445.
102. Gower DJ, Gower VC, McWhorter JM, Richardson SH. Removal of adherent bacteria from shunt tubing. *Surg Forum* 1987;38:520–522.
103. Gristina AG, Hobgood CD, Webb LX, Myrvik QN. Adhesive colonization of biomaterials and antibiotic resistance. *Biomaterials* 1987;8:423–426.
104. Gristina AG, Costerton JW. Bacterial adherence to biomaterials and tissue. *J Bone Joint Surg* 1985;67A:264–273.
105. Bayston R, Penny SR. Excessive production of mucoid substance in *Staphylococcus* SIIA: a possible factor in colonisation of Holter shunts. *Dev Med Child Neurol* 1972;14(Suppl 27):25–28.
106. Diaz-Mitoma F, Harding GKM, Hoban DJ, Roberts RS, Low DE. Clinical significance of a test for slime production in ventriculoperitoneal shunt infections caused by coagulase-negative staphylococci. *J Infect Dis* 1987;156:555–560.
107. Younger JJ, Christensen GD, Bartley DL, Simmons JCH, Barrett FF. Coagulase-negative staphylococci isolated from cerebrospinal fluid shunts: importance of slime production, species identification, and shunt removal to clinical outcome. *J Infect Dis* 1987;156(4):548–554.
108. Costerton JW, Geesey GG, Cheng KJ. How bacteria stick. *Sci Am* 1978;238:86–95.
109. Simberkoff MS, Moldover NH, Rahal JJ. Absence of detectable bactericidal and opsonic activities in normal and infected human cerebrospinal fluids—a regional host defense deficiency. *J Lab Clin Med* 1980;95:362–372.
110. Pezotta S, Locatelli D, Bonfanti N, Sfogliarini R, Bruschi L, Rondini G. Shunt in high-risk newborns. *Child's Nerv Syst* 1987;3:114–116.
111. Myers MG, Schoenbaum SC. Shunt fluid aspiration. *Am J Dis Child* 1975;129:220–222.
112. Hubschmann OR, Countee RW. Acute abdomen in children with infected ventriculoperitoneal shunts. *Arch Surg* 1980;115:305–307.
113. Reynolds M, Sherman JO, McLone DG. Ventriculoperitoneal shunt infection masquerading as an acute surgical abdomen. *J Pediatr Surg* 1983;18(6):951–954.
114. Noetzel MJ, Baker RP. Shunt fluid examination: risks and benefits in the evaluation of shunt malfunction and infection. *J Neurosurg* 1984;61:328–332.
115. Foltz EL, Shurtleff DB. Conversion of communicating hydrocephalus to stenosis or occlusion of the aqueduct during ventricular shunt. *J Neurosurg* 1965;24:520–529.
116. James HE. Infections associated with cerebrospinal fluid prosthetic devices. In: Sugarman B, Young EJ, eds. *Infections associated with prosthetic devices.* Chicago: CRC Press, 1984;23–42.
117. Fischer G, Goebel H, Latta E. Penetration of the colon by a ventriculo-peritoneal drain resulting in an intracerebral abscess. *Z Neurochir* 1983;44:155–160.
118. Korosue K, Tamaki N, Matsumoto S, Ohi Y. Intracranial granuloma as an unusual complication of subdural peritoneal shunt: case report. *J Neurosurg* 1981;55:136–138.
119. Sharma BS, Kak VK. Multiple subdural abscesses following colonic perforation—a rare complication of a ventriculoperitoneal shunt. *Pediatr Radiol* 1988;18:407–408.
120. Arze RS, Rashid H, Morley R, Ward MK, Kerr DNS. Shunt nephritis: report of two cases and review of the literature. *Clin Nephrol* 1983;19(1):48–53.
121. Finney HL, Roberts TS. Nephritis secondary to chronic cerebrospinal fluid–vascular shunt infection: 'shunt nephritis'. *Child's Brain* 1980;6:189–193.
122. Goodman GM, Gourley GR. Ascites complicating ventriculoperitoneal shunts. *J Pediatr Gastroenterol Nutr* 1988;7:780–782.
123. Noh JM, Reddy MG, Brodner RA. Cerebrospinal fluid ascites following ventriculoperitoneal shunt. Report of a case and review of the literature. *Mt Sinai J Med* 1979;46(5):475–477.
124. Rekate HL, Yonas H, White RJ, Nulsen FE. The acute abdomen in patients with ventriculoperitoneal shunts. *Surg Neurol* 1979;11:442–445.
125. O'Brien M, Parent A, Davis B. Management of ventricular shunt infections. *Child's Brain* 1979;5:304–309.
126. Younger JJ, Simmons JCH, Barrett FF. Occult distal ventriculoperitoneal shunt infections. *Pediatr Infect Dis* 1985;4(5):557–558.
127. Yadav SS, Perfect J, Friedman AH. Successful treatment of cryptococcal ventriculoatrial shunt infection with systemic therapy alone. *Neurosurgery* 1988;23:372–373.
128. Gerner-Smidt P, Stenager E, Kock-Jensen C. Treatment of ventriculostomy-related infections. *Acta Neurochir* 1988;91:47–49.
129. Lundberg N. Continuous recording and control of ventricular fluid pressure in neurosurgical practice. *Acta Psychiatr Scand* [*Suppl*] 1960;149:1–193.
130. Haines SJ, Taylor F. Prophylactic methicillin for shunt operations: effects on incidence of shunt malfunction and infection. *Child's Brain* 1982;9:10–22.
131. Finn S, Kosnik EJ. Predictive value of cerebrospinal fluid cytochemistry in shunt infection. Poster 40, AANS Annual Meeting, San Francisco, April 8–12, 1984.
132. Hadani M, Findler G, Muggia-Sullam M, Sahar A. Acute appendicitis in children with a ventriculoperitoneal shunt. *Surg Neurol* 1982;18:69–71.
133. Fokes EC. Occult infections of ventricular shunts. *J Neurosurg* 1970;33:517–523.
134. Chapman PH, Borges LF. Shunt infections: prevention and treatment. *Clin Neurosurg* 1985;32:652–664.
135. Kramer PW, Griffith RS, Campbell RL. Antibiotic penetration of the brain: a comparative study. *J Neurosurg* 1969;31:295–302.
136. Everett ED, Strausbaugh LJ. Antimicrobial agents and the central nervous system. *Neurosurgery* 1980;6(6):691–714.
137. Frame PT, Watanakunakorn C, McLaurin RL, Khodadad G. Penetration of nafcillin, methicillin, and cefazolin into human brain tissue. *Neurosurgery* 1983;12:142–147.
138. James HE, Wilson HD, Connor JD, Walsh JW. Intraventricular cerebrospinal fluid antibiotic concentrations in patients with intraventricular infections. *Neurosurgery* 1982;10:50–54.
139. Kane JG, Parker RH, Jordan GW, Hoeprich PD. Nafcillin concentration in cerebrospinal fluid during treatment of staphylococcal infections. *Ann Intern Med* 1977;87:309–311.
140. Picardi JL, Lewis HP, Tan JS, Phair JP. Clindamycin concentrations in the central nervous system of primates before and after head trauma. *J Neurosurg* 1975;43:717–720.
141. Gump DW. Vancomycin for treatment of bacterial meningitis. *Rev Infect Dis* 1981;3(Suppl):S289–S292.
142. Ring JC, Cates KL, Belani KK, Gaston TL, Sveum RJ, Marker

SC. Rifampin for CSF shunt infections caused by coagulase negative staphylococci. *J Pediatr* 1979;95(2):317–319.

143. Gombert ME, Landesman SH, Corrado ML, Stein SC, Melvin ET, Cummings M. Vancomycin and rifampin therapy for *Staphylococcus epidermidis* meningitis associated with CSF shunts. *J Neurosurg* 1981;55:633–636.

144. Archer GL, Tenenbaum MJ, Haywood HB. Rifampin therapy of *Staphylococcus epidermidis*. *JAMA* 1978;240(8):751–753.

145. Norrby SR. Role of cephalosporins in the treatment of bacterial meningitis in adults—overview with special emphasis on ceftazidime. *Am J Med* 1985;79(Suppl 2A):56–61.

146. Kaiser AB, McGee ZA. Aminoglycoside therapy of gram-negative bacillary meningitis. *N Engl J Med* 1975;293:1215–1220.

147. Strausbaugh LJ, Mandaleris CD, Sande MA. Comparison of four aminoglycoside antibiotics in the therapy of experimental *E. coli* meningitis. *J Lab Clin Med* 1977;89:692–701.

148. Barling RWA, Selkon JB. The penetration of antibiotics into cerebrospinal fluid and brain tissue. *J Antimicrob Chemother* 1978;4:203–227.

149. Howard MA, Grady MS, Park TS, Scheld WM. Pharmacokinetics of intraventricular vancomycin in hydrocephalic rats. *Neurosurgery* 1986;18:725–729.

150. Salmon JH. Intraventricular chloramphenicol. *Child's Brain* 1978;4:114–119.

151. Pau AK, Smego RA, Fisher MA. Intraventricular vancomycin: observations of tolerance and pharmacokinetics in two infants with ventricular shunt infections. *Pediatr Infect Dis* 1986;5(1):93–96.

152. Reesor C, Chow AW, Kureishi A, Jewesson PJ. Kinetics of intraventricular vancomycin in infections of cerebrospinal fluid shunts. *J Infect Dis* 1988;158(5):1142–1143.

153. Wald SL, McLaurin RL. Cerebrospinal fluid antibiotic levels during treatment of shunt infections. *J Neurosurg* 1980;52:41–46.

154. Wilson HD, Bean JR, James HE, Pendley MM. Cerebrospinal fluid antibiotic concentrations in ventricular shunt infections. *Child's Brain* 1978;4:74–82.

155. Bayston R, Hart CA, Barnicot M. Intraventricular vancomycin in the treatment of ventriculitis associated with cerebrospinal fluid shunting and drainage. *J Neurol Neurosurg Psychiatry* 1987;50:1419–1423.

156. Yogev R. A strategy for evaluating which of the new cephalosporins to use. *Pediatr Ann* 1986;15:470–477.

157. Watanabe I, Hodges GR, Dworzack DL, Kepes JJ, Duensing GF. Neurotoxicity of intrathecal gentamicin: a case report and experimental study. *Ann Neurol* 1978;4:564–572.

158. Weiss MH, Kurze T, Nulsen FE. Antibiotic neurotoxicity: laboratory and clinical study. *J Neurosurg* 1974;41:486–489.

159. Congeni BL, Tan J, Salstrom SJ, Weinstein L. Kinetics of vancomycin after intraventricular and intravenous administration. *Pediatr Res* 1977;13:459.

160. Perrin JCS, McLaurin RL. Infected ventriculoatrial shunts—a method of treatment. *J Neurosurg* 1967;27:21–26.

161. Callaghan RP, Cohen SJ, Stewart GT. Septicaemia due to colonization of Spitz–Holter valves by staphylococci. *Br Med J,* March 25, 1961, p860–863.

162. Luthardt T. Bacterial infections in ventriculo-auricular shunt systems. *Dev Med Child Neurol* 1970;12(Suppl 22):105–109.

163. Shurtleff DB, Foltz EL, Weeks RD, Loeser J. Therapy of *Staphylococcus epidermidis:* infections associated with cerebrospinal fluid shunts. *Pediatrics* 1974;53(1):55–62.

164. Bayston R. Hydrocephalus shunt infections and their treatment. *J Antimicrob Chemother* 1985;15:259–261.

165. Mates S, Glaser J, Shapiro K. Treatment of cerebrospinal fluid shunt infections with medical therapy alone. *Neurosurgery* 1982;11:781–783.

166. Frame PT, McLaurin RL. Treatment of CSF shunt infections with intrashunt plus oral antibiotic therapy. *J Neurosurg* 1984;60:354–360.

167. Nicholas JL, Kamal IM, Eckstein HB. Immediate shunt replacement in the treatment of bacterial colonisation of Holter valves. *Dev Med Child Neurol* 1970;12(Suppl 22):110–113.

168. Salmon JH. Adult hydrocephalus: evaluation of shunt therapy in 80 patients. *J Neurosurg* 1972;37:423–428.

169. Scarff TB, Nelson PB, Reigel DH. External drainage for ventricular infection following cerebrospinal fluid shunts. *Child's Brain* 1978;4:129–136.

170. Bayston R, Milner RDG. Antimicrobial activity of silicone rubber used in hydrocephalus shunts, after impregnation with antimicrobial substances. *J Clin Pathol* 1981;134:1057–1062.

171. Webb LX, Myers RT, Cordell AR, Hobgood CD, Costerton JW, Gristina AG. Inhibition of bacterial adhesion by antibacterial surface pretreatment of vascular prostheses. *J Vasc Surg* 1986;4:16–21.

172. Gower DJ, Gower VC, Richardson SH, Kelly DL. Reduced bacterial adherence to silicone plastic neurosurgical prosthesis. *Pediat Neurosci* 1985–1986;12:127–133.

173. Gristina AG, Dobbins JJ, Giammara B, Lewis JC, DeVries WC. Biomaterial-centered sepsis and the total artificial heart—microbial adhesion vs tissue integration. *JAMA* 1988;259(6):870–874.

174. Kaiser AB, Clayson KR, Mulherin JL, et al. Antibiotic prophylaxis in vascular surgery. *Ann Surg* 1978;188:283–289.

175. Gardner BP, Gordon DS. Postoperative infection in shunts for hydrocephalus: Are prophylactic antibiotics necessary? *Br Med J* 1982;284:1914–1915.

176. Haines SJ. Topical antibiotic prophylaxis in neurosurgery. *Neurosurgery* 1982;11:250–253.

177. Fischer PR, Gooch WM, Walker ML, Storrs B. Bactericidal activities of five antibiotics during short-term exposure to coagulase-negative staphylococci. *Antimicrob Agents Chemother* 1984;25(4):502–503.

178. Scherr DD, Dodd T, Buckingham WW. Prophylactic use of topical antibiotic irrigation in uninfected surgical wounds—a microbiological evaluation. *J Bone Jt Surg* 1972;54A:634–640.

179. Klein DM. Comparison of antibiotic methods in the prophylaxis of operative shunt infections. *Concepts Pediatr Neurosurg* 1983;4:131–141.

180. Absolom DR, Lamberti FV, Policova Z, Zingg W, van Oss CJ, Neumann AW. Surface thermodynamics of bacterial adhesion. *Appl Environ Microbiol* 1983;46:90–97.

181. Ericson C, Lidgren L, Lindberg L. Cloxacillin in the prophylaxis of postoperative infections of the hip. *J Bone Joint Surg* 1973;55A:808–813.

182. Guglielmo BJ, Hohn DC, Koo PJ, Hunt TK, Sweet RL, Conte JE. Antibiotic prophylaxis in surgical procedures—a critical analysis of the literature. *Arch Surg* 1983;118:943–955.

183. Hill C, Flamant R, Mazas F, Evrard J. Prophylactic cefazolin versus placebo in total hip replacement. *Lancet* 1981;1:795–797.

184. Haines SJ. Efficacy of antibiotic prophylaxis in clean neurosurgical operations. *Neurosurgery* 1989;24:401–405.

185. Blomstedt GC, Kytta J. Results of a randomized trial of vancomycin prophylaxis in craniotomy. *J Neurosurg* 1988;69:216–220.

186. Bullock R, vanDellen JR, Ketelbey W, Reinach SG. A double-blind placebo-controlled trial of perioperative prophylactic antibiotics for elective neurosurgery. *J Neurosurg* 1988;69:687–691.

187. Geraghty J, Feely M. Antibiotic prophylaxis in neurosurgery—a randomized controlled trial. *J Neurosurg* 1984;60:724–726.

188. Shapiro M, Wald U, Simchen E, et al. Randomized clinical trial of intra-operative antimicrobial prophylaxis of infection after neurosurgical procedures. *J Hosp Infect* 1986;8:283–295.

189. Young RF, Lawner PM. Perioperative antibiotic prophylaxis for prevention of postoperative neurosurgical infections—a randomized clinical trial. *J Neurosurg* 1987;66:701–705.

190. Bayston R. Antibiotic prophylaxis in shunt surgery. *Dev Med Child Neurol* 1975;17(Suppl 35):99–103.

191. Rieder MJ, Frewen TC, Del Maestro RF, Coyle A, Lovell S. The effect of cephalothin prophylaxis on postoperative ventriculoperitoneal shunt infections. *Can Med Assoc J* 1987;136:935–938.

192. Schmidt K, Gjerris F, Osgaard O, et al. Antibiotic prophylaxis in cerebrospinal fluid shunting: a prospective randomized trial in 152 hydrocephalic patients. *Neurosurgery* 1985;17:1–5.

193. Wang EEL, Prober CG, Hendrick BE, Hoffman HJ, Humphreys

RP. Prophylactic sulfamethoxazole and trimethoprim in ventriculoperitoneal shunt surgery—a double blind, randomized, placebo-controlled trial. *JAMA* 1984;251(9):1174–1177.

194. Weiss SR, Raskind R. Further experience with the ventriculoperitoneal shunt. *Int Surg* 1970;53:300–303.

195. Blomstedt GC. Results of trimethoprim-sulfamethoxazole prophylaxis in ventriculostomy and shunting procedures: a double-blind randomized trial. *J Neurosurg* 1985;62:694–697.

196. Yu HC, Patterson RH. Prophylactic antimicrobial agents after ventriculoatriostomy for hydrocephalus. *J Pediatr Surg* 1973; 8(6):881–885.

197. Wyler AR, Kelly WA. Use of antibiotics with external ventriculostomies. *J Neurosurg* 1972;37:185–187.

198. Christensen GD, Simpson WA, Bisno AL, Beachey EH. Adherence of slime-producing strains of *Staphylococcus epidermidis* to smooth surfaces. *Infect Immun* 1982;37:318.

PART **IV**

CNS Syndromes Mediated by Bacterial Toxins

Infections of the Central Nervous System,
edited by W. M. Scheld, R. J. Whitley, and
D. T. Durack, Raven Press, Ltd., New York © 1991.

CHAPTER 24

Botulism

James M. Hughes

Botulism is a rare but serious disease. The name of the disease is derived from the Latin word *botulus*, meaning sausage, a food that was responsible for many early outbreaks of the disease (1). Four clinical types of botulism occur in humans (2). Each type has different epidemiologic characteristics and pathogenetic mechanisms (Table 1).

Foodborne botulism represents a public health emergency. Although outbreaks of "sausage poisoning" were recognized in Europe during the 18th and 19th centuries (3), foodborne botulism was first clearly described by van Ermengem following his careful investigation of a large outbreak in Ellezelles, Belgium, which occurred in 1895. This outbreak, traced to inadequately cured uncooked ham, caused 23 cases and three deaths among 24 musicians (4,5). The first recognized case in the United States, caused by a beef tamale, occurred in 1899 (3,6). In November 1913, an outbreak involving 12 persons occurred following a sorority party at Stanford University. Investigation implicated a salad containing string beans and mayonnaise which had been prepared in accord with methods recommended by the U.S. Department of Agriculture (3). Follow-up studies indicated that recommended procedures would not eliminate *Clostridium botulinum* from raw vegetables, because spores were shown to survive boiling for 2 hr, resulting in recognition of the need for a new public educational campaign (3).

Wound botulism was first described in the United States in 1943 (7). Infant botulism was first described in 1976 (8,9). Botulism in adults of unknown source (adult infectious botulism, "hidden form" of botulism, botulinal autointoxication), caused by toxin production *in vivo* in the gastrointestinal tract, was first described in 1986 (10).

The toxins causing these diseases are among the most potent bioactive substances known (11,12); the oral lethal dose for humans has been calculated to be between 0.05 and 0.1 μg for toxin produced by proteolytic strains and between 0.1 and 0.5 μg for toxin produced by nonproteolytic strains (12).

EPIDEMIOLOGY

Foodborne Botulism

Foodborne botulism outbreaks are most often associated with the ingestion of low-acid (pH > 4.6) foods. High-risk foods in the United States include home-canned or home-processed low-acid fruits and vegetables, fish and fish products, and condiments such as relish and chili peppers. In other countries, different foods are more common vehicles. In Canada, Japan, and the Scandinavian countries, most outbreaks are associated with fish products, whereas in Germany, Italy, France, and Poland, meats such as home-cured hams are the most commonly implicated foods (12). Occasional outbreaks associated with commercial food products are recognized (13–15).

Foodborne botulism is most often caused by types A, B, and E toxins. Type A botulism is most common west of the Mississippi River, type B is most common in the eastern states, and type E outbreaks are most common in the Great Lakes Region (16) and Alaska (17,18). This distribution corresponds to the distribution of *C. botulinum* spores in soil (19–21). Between 1976 and 1984, 60% of reported cases in the United States were caused by type A toxin, 30% by type B toxin, and 10% by type E toxin (22). Fish and fish products are particularly likely to be associated with outbreaks of type E botulism. Type F botulism has been confirmed in California (23) and Florida (24). Recent outbreaks of foodborne botulism

J. M. Hughes: Center for Infectious Diseases, Centers for Disease Control, Public Health Service, U.S. Department of Health and Human Services, Atlanta, Georgia 30333.

TABLE 1. *Characteristics of clinical types of botulism*

Type	Age group	Reported cases per year[a]	Pathogenesis
Foodborne	Adults	15–50	Ingestion of preformed toxin
Wound	Children, adolescents, adults	1–3	Contamination of wound by spores, followed by toxin production in wound
Infant	Infants	30–100	Ingestion of spores, followed by toxin production in gastrointestinal tract
"Infectious"	Adults	3–6	Ingestion of spores, followed by toxin production in gastrointestinal tract

[a] Range in the United States.

have been traced to unusual food vehicles such as baked potatoes used in potato salad, sauteed onions, and chopped garlic in soybean oil (25–32). Several large outbreaks have been traced to food served in restaurants (25–27,31–35); one of these outbreaks resulted in the occurrence of cases in residents of three countries (27).

From 1976 to 1984, 124 outbreaks of known toxin type involving 308 cases were reported to the Centers for Disease Control (CDC) (22). Outbreaks were most frequent during the summer and fall. Home-canned foods were responsible for the vast majority of outbreaks in which the food was identified. The mean number of cases per outbreak was 2.7. Although most outbreaks involved only one (68%) or two (20%) cases, four large restaurant-associated outbreaks that occurred during this period accounted for 42% of the total cases. Twenty-three deaths occurred; the case fatality rate was 7.5%. From 1985 to 1987, 50 outbreaks involving 78 cases were reported. Seven deaths occurred; the case fatality rate during this period was 9.0% (36).

Wound Botulism

The typical patient with wound botulism is a young, previously healthy adult male who sustains severe trauma with an open fracture contaminated by soil (22,37,38). However, one case associated with a wooden splinter has been reported (39). All reported cases in which the toxin type was identified have been caused by infection with type A or type B organisms. In one case, both types were responsible (22).

Between 1976 and 1984, a total of 16 cases were reported to the CDC (22). Patients ranged in age from 7 to 41 years; the mean age was 22 years. Eleven of the patients were male. Two patients died; the case fatality rate was 13%. Toxin or organisms of type A were identified in 11 cases, toxin or organisms of type B were identified in four cases, and both types were identified in one case. Two confirmed cases occurred in parenteral drug abusers (40). An additional case associated with maxillary sinusitis following intranasal cocaine abuse has been reported (41).

Infant Botulism

Patients range in age from 1 week to 9 months; however, onset of illness is most common during the second and third months of life (42), and approximately 95% of patients have onset by 6 months of age (43). Honey ingestion has been identified as a risk factor in type B botulism and may also be associated with type A disease (44,45); however, in recent years, less than 20% of infants with botulism have eaten honey (46,47).

Epidemiologic studies have found that birth weights of hospitalized infants with the disease are higher than those in the general population and that mothers of case infants tend to be older and better educated than those in the general population (48). The disease occurs in both formula-fed and breast-fed infants. In one series, formula-fed infants were younger at onset of disease than were breast-fed infants (49). A more recent investigation of cases outside California found that risk factors varied by age. For infants less than 2 months of age, living in a rural area was a risk factor. For infants 2 months of age or older, having less than one bowel movement per day, breast-feeding, and ingestion of corn syrup were risk factors (46). A study of cases in Utah found that disruption of soil by construction or agricultural activities, dusty and windy conditions, a high water table, and alkaline soil were present in the home environment of children with the disease (50). An investigation of three cases in a small town in Colorado found environmental contamination with *C. botulinum* in the home environment of the case patients (51).

Type A cases of infant botulism are more often reported from the western United States, and type B cases are more often reported from the eastern United States; however, in the western part of the country the ratio of type A to type B cases is lower than that for foodborne botulism (48). One type F case caused by *C. baratii* has been reported from New Mexico (52–54), and two type E cases caused by *C. butyricum* (55,56) have been reported. One case caused by a strain producing both type B and type F toxin has also been reported (48).

Between 1975, when the syndrome was first recognized, and 1983, 395 cases were reported to the CDC from 36 states. The majority of cases of infant botulism have been reported from California, Utah, and Pennsylvania (57), reflecting in part the intensive level of surveillance for infant botulism in these states. Although infant botulism is most commonly reported in the United States, two cases have been reported in the United Kingdom (58,59), and the disease has been reported from Australia, continental Europe, and South America (43). Recent cases acquired in Yemen and Japan caused by types B and C toxins, respectively, have also been reported (60,60a).

Infant botulism has been implicated in some cases of sudden infant death syndrome (SIDS) (61), particularly in infants who were formula-fed (62). In one series, 10 (4.7%) of 212 infants with SIDS had postmortem stool cultures positive for *C. botulinum;* botulinum toxin was detected in specimens from two of the infants (61).

Adult Infectious Botulism of Unknown Source

In some instances, careful case investigations have failed to identify a contaminated food as a source of botulism (63). Investigations of such cases have identified (a) *C. botulinum* organisms and toxin in the intestinal tract of patients and (b) *C. botulinum* but not toxin in suspected food vehicles. Many of these patients have had a history of abdominal surgery or other abnormalities of the gastrointestinal tract, suggesting that spores had germinated and produced toxin *in vivo* (10,64–66).

From 1976 to 1984, 31 cases of botulism in which no food vehicle could be identified were reported in adults (22). The mean age of patients was 42 years, and 18 (58%) were male. Type A toxin was found in 24 patients, type B toxin was found in six patients, and type F toxin in one patient (22). Nine deaths occurred; the case fatality rate was 29% (22).

ETIOLOGY

Clostridium botulinum are gram-positive, heat-resistant anaerobic sporeforming bacilli with subterminal spores that do not produce catalase, peroxidase, or cytochrome oxidase (67). *C. botulinum* organisms can be divided into four groups (Table 2) based on metabolic characteristics and type of toxin produced (67). Group I includes the proteolytic strains producing toxins A, B, or F. Group II includes nonproteolytic strains producing toxins B, E, or F. Group III includes those strains producing toxins C and D. Group IV includes strains that produce type G toxin; these strains are sometimes known as *C. argentinense* (68,69). All toxigenic strains of *C. botulinum* except those producing type G toxin are lipase-positive (67). Group I and II strains cause nearly all cases of human botulism.

C. botulinum is commonly found in soil samples and aquatic sediments (67). Strains of *C. botulinum* produce one of seven antigenically distinct protein neurotoxins designated A, B, C, D, E, F, and G. The vast majority of strains produce only a single toxin type; however, occasional strains producing multiple toxins have been identified (70). Type A neurotoxin has a mouse LD_{50} by the intraperitoneal route of 0.00625 ng (67). Vegetative cells of *C. botulinum* contain on the order of 100-fold higher concentrations of botulinum toxin than do spores (71). The toxin does not escape from spores *in vivo*. These potent toxins are cytoplasmic proteins that are released when vegetative cells lyse (72).

Botulinum toxins exist in culture as macromolecular complexes, known as "progenitor toxins," which consist of a neurotoxic component and one or more nontoxic components, which for toxin types A, B, C, D, and G may include a hemagglutinin (67,73); sedimentation values for these progenitor toxins are 16S–19S (73). Sedimentation values for toxin types E and F, which lack the hemagglutinin, range from 10.3S to 11.6S (73). Dissociation of these progenitor toxins yields a deviative neurotoxin with a sedimentation value of 7S (5.9S for type F toxin) which corresponds to a molecular size of approximately 150 kD (67,73). The progenitor toxin appears to be critical to the pathogenesis of foodborne botulism, since the deviative neurotoxin is inactivated in the stomach (67,74).

The deviative neurotoxins are similar to each other and to tetanus toxin in molecular structure (67). The neurotoxin, which consists of a heavy chain of about 100 kD and a light chain of about 50 kD joined by a disulfide bond (Fig. 1), is synthesized as a single chain which has relatively low activity until it is cleaved or "nicked" by a

TABLE 2. *Selected characteristics of groups of* C. botulinum

Group	Toxin(s) produced	Proteolytic status	Lipase[a]	Heat resistance of spores	Disease occurrence
Group I	A, B, F	Proteolytic	+	High	Humans, severe disease
Group II	B, E, F	Nonproteolytic	+	Low	Humans, less severe disease
Group III	C, D	Nonproteolytic	+	Intermediate	Birds, nonhuman mammals, one infant
Group IV	G	Proteolytic	−	?	?

[a] Symbols: +, lipase-positive; −, lipase-negative.

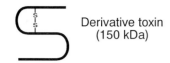

FIG. 1. Schematic representation of botulinum derivative toxin.

proteolytic enzyme (67) (Fig. 2). The carboxy-terminal end of the heavy chain appears to contain the binding site for the receptor on the nerve terminals, which may be a different ganglioside for each toxin type (73,75). The amino-terminal end of the heavy chain is believed to create channels in the membrane of the nerve terminal through which the light chain enters the cell (67,76,77). For Group I proteolytic strains, endogenous enzymes activate the toxins by cleaving the single chain; in contrast, for group II nonproteolytic strains, exogenous enzymes such as trypsin are required (67).

Amino acid compositions of types A, B, E, and F neurotoxins have been determined (78–81), and partial amino acid sequences have been identified (82–85, 85a,85b). For types A, B, and E toxin, amino acid sequences identified were similar (83,86). In addition, identified segments for botulinum and tetanus toxins were strikingly homologous (67,86,87).

Toxin types A, B, and E cause the vast majority of cases of human botulism of known toxin type; type F toxin is a rare cause of human disease. Types C and D cause disease in animals, especially birds, ducks, and chickens. Type C strains are subdivided to C-alpha and C-beta groups. C-alpha strains produce C_1 and C_2 toxins, whereas C-beta strains produce only C_2 toxin (67). C_1 toxin is a neurotoxin, whereas C_2 toxin has vascular permeability and lethal activities but is not neurotoxic (67,88,89). Type G organisms have been isolated from soil and from tissues obtained at autopsy from five individuals who died suddenly in Switzerland (90) and from nine cases of SIDS (91).

Although bacteriophages have been found in group I, II, and III strains, toxigenicity is associated with phages only for group III strains (67). Although plasmids have been found in strains in all four groups, a correlation between neurotoxin production and presence of plasmids has been observed only for group IV strains (67).

Spores of *C. botulinum* are heat-resistant. Strict anaerobic conditions are not required for spore germination and toxin production, but low-acid conditions (pH > 4.6) and low salt and sugar concentrations are necessary (12). Although toxin production is more efficient at ambient temperatures, toxin can be produced by nonproteolytic strains at refrigerator temperatures (12,92). Spores of group I organisms are most resistant to heat, followed by group III and then group II strains (93); spores of many strains of group I organisms survive boiling for 2 hr, whereas most spores of group II organisms fail to survive 80°C for 10 min (94). The toxins are heat-labile (i.e., they are inactivated by boiling) and are inactivated by alkali but are relatively resistant to acid (70).

Strains of *C. botulinum* causing foodborne and infant botulism have similar characteristics (95).

PATHOGENESIS AND PATHOPHYSIOLOGY

Foodborne botulism is caused by the ingestion of food contaminated with preformed botulinum toxin. The toxin is absorbed primarily in the upper small intestine. The toxin travels through the lymphatic system to the bloodstream (67) and binds rapidly and irreversibly to (a) receptors on cholinergic nerve fibers at a neuromuscular junction, (b) postganglionic parasympathetic nerve endings, and (c) autonomic ganglia (77,96) (Fig. 3). Following binding, the toxin enters the nerve endings by translocation through the membrane and irreversibly interferes with the release of acetylcholine (97,98), possibly by impairing calcium-induced exocytosis. However, the precise mechanism of this inhibition has not been defined (99), and a different mode of intercellular action may exist for type A and type B toxins (67). Recovery occurs with formation of new presynaptic end-plates and neuromuscular junctions (67). No host factors have been identified that predispose individuals to foodborne botulism.

Wound botulism results from spore germination and toxin production in contaminated wounds. Some cases have occurred in patients with clean wounds (37) and in spite of careful débridement resulting in removal of all apparent nonviable tissue and exogenous contaminants.

Infant botulism results from ingestion of spores that germinate and produce toxin in the infant's gastrointesti-

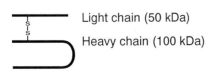

Light chain (50 kDa)

Heavy chain (100 kDa)

FIG. 2. Schematic representation of activation of botulinum toxin.

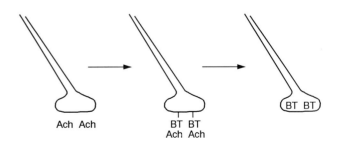

Ach Ach   BT BT   BT BT
                 Ach Ach

FIG. 3. Schematic representation of steps in action of botulinum toxin (Ach = acetylcholine; BT = botulinum toxin).

nal tract (8,100,101). Quantitative microbiologic studies of infants have identified 10^3–10^8 *C. botulinum* organisms per gram of feces, representing 0.01–3.3% of the fecal flora (102). Adult germ-free mice have been infected when fed 10 *C. botulinum* type A spores (103); these animals became resistant to colonization with 100,000 *C. botulinum* spores after spending 3 days in a room with normal mice (103), indicating that susceptibility is dramatically reduced in the presence of normal fecal flora. Conventional adult mice became susceptible to botulism following ingestion of spores when the animals were pretreated with metronidazole by the oral route (104). Results of an autopsy of an infant who died from infant botulism revealed that the colon was the site of colonization and toxin production (105). By 12 months of age, susceptibility of the human gastrointestinal tract to colonization by *C. botulinum* appears to have passed (67).

Adult infectious botulism results from germination of spores in the intestinal tract, with subsequent toxin release and absorption. Most cases have occurred in patients with underlying gastrointestinal disease (106,107).

PATHOLOGY

There are no specific gross pathologic findings in any of the botulism syndromes (108). Examination of neuromuscular junctions of mice following local injection of sublethal quantities of botulinum toxin revealed (a) evidence of sprouting from nerve terminals (109,110) in the absence of Nissl substance dispersion, (b) increase in cell body size, and (c) alterations in microfilaments as seen after axotomy (110). Muscle biopsies from three patients with type A foodborne botulism in Japan revealed group atrophy of skeletal muscle fibers. Electron-microscopic studies revealed end-plates denuded of their nerve terminals, a decrease in total nerve terminal area, and an increase in the ratio of postsynaptic to presynaptic membrane length (Fig. 4) (111).

CLINICAL MANIFESTATIONS

Foodborne Botulism

Symptoms and signs of foodborne botulism vary by toxin type (Table 3). The occurrence of acute gastrointestinal symptoms simultaneously with or just before the onset of descending weakness or paralysis strongly suggests the diagnosis of foodborne botulism. The first symptoms may appear from 6 hr to 8 days after ingestion of the toxin; however, the majority of patients become ill in 18–36 hr following exposure. The severity of illness is inversely proportional to the length of the incubation period (112). The initial symptoms may be gastrointestinal (nausea, vomiting, abdominal cramps, or diarrhea) or neurologic. Constipation is common once the neurologic syndrome is well established, but nausea and vomiting occur in 50% of the patients and diarrhea occurs in 20–25% early in the course of illness (113–116).

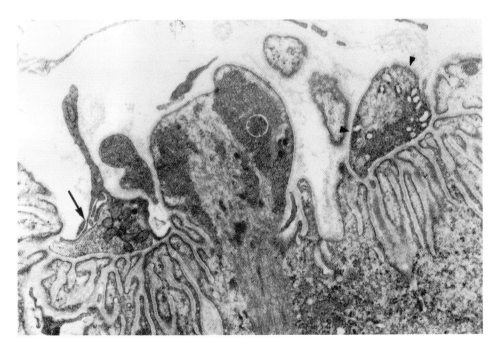

FIG. 4. Electron micrograph of motor end-plate in patient with botulism showing normal region (*arrow*) and abnormal region with postsynaptic region denuded of nerve terminal and replaced by part of a distorted muscle fiber (arrowheads). Bar = 1 μm. (From ref. 111, with permission.)

TABLE 3. *Range of reported frequency of clinical features of types A, B, and E foodborne botulism in outbreaks and patient series*[a]

	Type A disease (%) (115, 121, 122, 127)	Type B disease (%) (17, 34, 112, 114, 115, 124)	Type E disease (%) (17, 113)
Neurologic symptoms			
Dysphagia	25–96	77–100	63–90
Dry mouth	26–83	96–100	55–88
Diplopia	50–90	57–100	85
Dysarthria	25–100	69–100	50
Arm weakness	16–86	64–86	—
Leg weakness	16–76	64–86	—
Blurred vision	8–100	42–100	63
Dyspnea	35–91	34	88
Paresthesias	20	12–14	—
Gastrointestinal symptoms			
Constipation	73	17–100	25–38
Nausea	73	57–86	88–100
Vomiting	70	50–100	88–100
Abdominal cramps	33	46–86	—
Diarrhea	35	8–14	10
Miscellaneous symptoms			
Fatigue	8–92	69–100	—
Sore throat	75	29–50	38
Dizziness	8–86	30–100	63
Physical findings			
Ptosis	25–96	33–100	55
Extraocular muscle weakness	25–87	46–100	0
Facial nerve dysfunction	84	48–55	—
Hypoactive gag reflex	81	39–54	—
Tongue weakness	16–91	10–31	—
Pupils fixed or dilated	10–33	36–100	75
Extremity weakness	48–91	15–75	—
Nystagmus	8–44	4	—
Ataxia	24	13	—
Initial mental status			
Alert	88	93	—
Lethargic	4	4	—
Obtunded	8	4	—
Deep tendon reflexes			
Normal	33	71	—
Hypoactive or absent	54	29	—
Hyperactive	13	0	—

[a] Not all symptoms and signs documented in each report.

Initial neurologic symptoms are manifestations of cranial nerve dysfunction: blurred vision, diplopia, dysarthria, and dysphagia. Autonomic dysfunction may be more common with type B and type E than with type A disease (117–119). Muscle weakness progresses in a descending fashion, and, in severe cases, dyspnea occurs. Sore throat resulting from diminished salivation and dryness of mucous membranes frequently occurs early in the course of the illness. Some patients complain of fatigue and dizziness; an occasional patient may complain of paresthesias (115).

Cranial nerve dysfunction is typically manifested by ptosis, extraocular muscle palsies, facial muscle weakness, hypoactive gag reflex, and tongue weakness. How-ever, not all these findings are consistently present; a case characterized only by complete bilateral internal ophthalmoplegia has been reported (120). In severe cases, flaccid upper- and lower-extremity weakness and respiratory insufficiency are present. The weakness is typically symmetrical; however, mild degrees of asymmetry have been observed in some patients (112,115). Respiratory insufficiency may appear before significant arm and leg weakness. Manifestations of parasympathetic nervous system dysfunction include dryness of the mouth and paralytic ileus. Although pupils may be dilated or nonreactive, pupillary findings are frequently normal (121,122). Deep tendon reflexes are normal or hypoactive. Sensory signs are uncommon, but their presence does not exclude the diagnosis in an individual case (123). In the absence of complications, patients are usually alert and afebrile. However, some patients with type B botulism may be somnolent but are easily aroused (124). Muscle fasciculations are rarely observed (125).

The clinical spectrum of botulism varies from acute gastrointestinal symptoms without evidence of neurologic dysfunction to flaccid paralysis. Type A toxin produces severe disease more frequently than do types B and E. Patients with type A disease see a physician earlier in the course of illness, are more likely to require ventilatory support, and, on the average, are hospitalized longer than those with type B disease (115). Among adult patients with botulism reported to CDC between January 1979 and September 1982, 81% with type A disease, 47% with type B disease, and 39% with type E disease required mechanical ventilatory assistance (126). The case fatality rate for cases reported to CDC from 1976 to 1989 was approximately 7% and was higher for type A than for type B or E disease (Table 4).

In a large type A outbreak that occurred in New Mexico in 1978, respiratory failure occurred in 11 (32%) of 34 patients (127). Several important clinical lessons regarding recognition of patients at risk for respiratory failure were learned from this outbreak. Arterial blood gas measurements were of no value in predicting the subsequent occurrence of respiratory failure. Vital capacity was a more sensitive indicator of respiratory compromise; 25 (81%) of the 31 patients examined had decreased vital capacities at the time of initial evaluation. Respiratory failure developed insidiously; four of the patients who were not intubated at the time of initial examination subsequently had a respiratory arrest. The observation that all but one patient with vital capacities less than 30% of predicted values subsequently required mechanical ventilation supports recommendations that vital capacity be routinely measured and followed in patients with suspected botulism. The condition of all such patients should be closely monitored in an intensive care unit during the early stages of the illness (126).

In a large type B outbreak that occurred in Michigan in 1977, nine of 59 patients (15%) developed respiratory insufficiency (112). The triad of ptosis, medial rectus muscle palsy, and dilated, sluggishly reactive pupils was present in eight of nine patients who developed respiratory insufficiency. Respiratory insufficiency developed in eight of 11 patients (73%) with the triad and in only one of 34 patients (3%) with fewer than three of these findings (112). In a type B outbreak that occurred in England and Wales in 1989, the triad of impaired oropharyngeal functions, impaired ventilatory capacity, and paralytic illness was present in the most severe cases. Eight of 27 patients (30%) required ventilatory assistance; in each instance, ventilatory failure occurred within 12 hr of onset of third cranial nerve dysfunction (128).

Symptoms and signs of botulism are reversible. Respiratory failure may persist for months (129); one patient required mechanical ventilatory assistance for 6 months but eventually recovered (130). Symptoms of cranial nerve dysfunction and mild autonomic dysfunction may persist for more than a year (120,131). Follow-up over 2 years of patients involved in the 1978 New Mexico outbreak of type A disease revealed that many patients had persistent symptoms 2 years after the outbreak (132). Symptoms were more likely to persist in persons with severe disease. Diplopia, dysphagia, dysphonia, dry mouth, and generalized weakness were significantly more likely to persist after 2 years in patients with severe disease (132). Subsequent follow-up at nearly 5.5 years following the outbreak revealed that 11 of 19 patients had persistent symptoms, including dry mouth, dry eyes, dysphonia, dysphagia, blurred vision, and constipation (133).

Follow-up investigation of 13 patients who had type B foodborne botulism in Vancouver in 1985 (27) revealed that residual dyspnea and fatigue were common. Although lung function tests were normal, maximal oxygen consumption and maximal workload during exercise were reduced compared with those of controls, suggesting that reduced cardiovascular fitness, leg fatigue, or reduced motivation may have been responsible (134).

Wound Botulism

The disease is similar to foodborne botulism, except that nausea, vomiting, and diarrhea usually do not occur, fever due to wound infection may be present, and the incubation period is longer (median 7 days, range 4–18 days) (37). The clinical picture should cause little diagnostic confusion. Although tetanus frequently is considered, the differences in muscle tone observed in the two diseases permit differentiation. As for foodborne botulism, respiratory failure may be prolonged (135).

Infant Botulism

The earliest signs of infant botulism usually are constipation, which often appears 1–3 weeks before neurologic signs and poor feeding (136–139). Lethargy and listless-

TABLE 4. Case fatality rates for foodborne botulism cases reported to the Centers for Disease Control by toxin type, 1976–1989[a]

Toxin type	Cases	Deaths	Case fatality rate (%)
A	248	24	9.7
B	107	3	2.8
E	88	6	6.8
Totals	443	33	7.4

[a] Source: Centers for Disease Control, Atlanta, Georgia.

ness then appear, accompanied by a weak cry, a decreased gag reflex, decreased sucking, and drooling. The child may have difficulty holding its head erect and may develop ptosis and become floppy (136,137). This clinical picture is typical of infants hospitalized with infant botulism.

This type of disease, however, appears to have a much broader clinical spectrum, ranging from mild constipation to sudden death that is clinically indistinguishable from the SIDS. On occasion, an affected infant may appear to be comatose (43). The disease is reversible; complete recovery may begin before the concentrations of organisms and toxin in the gut decrease (140), and it typically occurs in several weeks to several months. Complications include otitis media, aspiration pneumonia, inappropriate secretion of antidiuretic hormone, and adult respiratory distress syndrome (141,142). Cases caused by type A and type B toxin have similar ages of onset and sex distributions (138). However, in one series of patients from states other than California, type B cases were more likely than type A cases to have dilated pupils, extraocular muscle paralysis, loss of facial expressions, and depressed patellar deep tendon reflexes (138). The mortality rate is 2–3% (141). For cases reported in California during 1988–1989, the average length of hospital stay was 4.9 weeks and the average hospital costs were over $62,000 (47).

Adult Botulism of Unknown Source

Clinical manifestations of botulism of unknown source are similar to those of foodborne botulism in adults. Such cases are sporadic. However, the presence of underlying gastrointestinal disease or a history of gastrointestinal surgery may provide a diagnostic clue.

APPROACH TO DIAGNOSIS

Foodborne Botulism

The diseases most frequently confused with botulism are food poisoning of other etiologies, myasthenia gravis, tick paralysis, and the Guillain–Barré syndrome, especially the Miller–Fisher variant (143,144). Patients with botulism typically have normal spinal fluid, although one patient with a total protein of 65 mg% has been reported (145); a normal spinal fluid may be useful in differentiating patients with botulism from those with Guillain–Barré syndrome, though the latter may also have normal spinal fluid early in the course of illness. An edrophonium chloride (Tensilon) test may be helpful in excluding the diagnosis of myasthenia gravis; however, patients with botulism may have transient responses that are usually less dramatic than those in patients with my-

asthenia gravis (115,122,146). Patients with botulism have normal motor conduction velocities and distal latencies. However, electromyography of involved muscle groups frequently reveals decreased amplitude of the muscle action potential and facilitation during rapid repetitive or post-tetanic stimulation (Fig. 5), similar to results in patients with the Eaton–Lambert syndrome (2,147–153).

Routine laboratory tests are not helpful in the diagnosis of botulism. A recently developed rapid enzyme-linked immunosorbent assay appears promising for detection of types A and B toxin in stools of patients with infant botulism (154–156) but requires further evaluation for use in adults. The most sensitive test for diagnosis of botulism is the mouse bioassay (93,157–160). Serum and stool and food extracts are inoculated intraperitoneally into mice; some mice are simultaneously given polyvalent and type-specific monovalent botulinum antitoxins (93). A positive test results in death within 24–48 hr of all mice except those protected by the polyvalent and type-specific antisera and those receiving inocula that have been heat-treated. Nonspecific patterns of mortality in mice may occur. One cause of such patterns is pyridostigmine, which can be removed from extract by dialysis prior to testing (161). The isolation of C. botulinum from the stool of an ill person also is considered confirmatory because the organism is rarely found in stools of normal individuals. Testing for botulinum toxin is performed in many state health department laboratories and at the CDC (see Appendix).

Wound Botulism

The approach to diagnosis involves testing serum for botulinum toxin and gram stain and culture of material

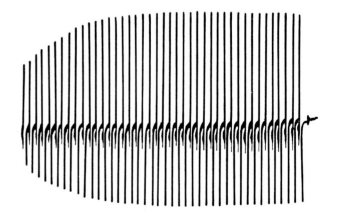

FIG. 5. Electromyogram from a patient with botulism showing increase in amplitude of muscle action potential during rapid repetitive stimulation at 50/second. (From ref. 121, with permission.)

from the wound. Electromyography of involved muscle groups may be helpful in confirming the diagnosis (162).

Infant Botulism

The differential diagnosis includes diseases producing hypotonia in infants (136,137). Sepsis, poliomyelitis, Epstein–Barr virus infections, and diphtheria must be considered. Tick paralysis, congenital myasthenia gravis, hypothyroidism, muscular dystrophy, and metabolic and toxic abnormalities may cause weakness and hypotonia. Guillain–Barré syndrome is rare in infants less than 6 months of age.

Diagnosis is by demonstration of *C. botulinum* or botulinum toxin in stool specimens (163–165). Organisms and toxin may persist in stool after recovery has begun. In contrast to adult botulism, in which serum specimens are frequently positive for botulinum toxin, infants are much more likely to have toxin detected in stool than in serum (165). The diagnosis may be supported by electromyography, in which a characteristic finding known as "brief, small abundant motor unit action potentials" (BSAP) is often observed (137,166); post-tetanic facilitation also may be present (167,168).

THERAPY

The mainstay of therapy for all forms of botulism is meticulous supportive care, with particular attention to monitoring vital capacity and prevention of nosocomial pulmonary and urinary tract infections. Because many patients will require ventilatory support for several days to several months, adequate nutritional support is essential. Death occurs early in persons in whom the diagnosis is unsuspected or in whom the potential gravity of the disease is unrecognized; late deaths usually result from respirator malfunction or nosocomial infection (115,126,127). Patients suspected of having botulism should be closely monitored in a critical care unit with serial measurements of vital capacity until the diagnosis is excluded.

Foodborne Botulism

If profound ileus is absent, an attempt should be made to remove unabsorbed toxin from the gastrointestinal tract by administering a cathartic or tap-water or saline enemas. Cathartics containing magnesium should probably be avoided because of the theoretical possibility that increased magnesium levels might enhance the action of botulinum toxin.

Although the efficacy of trivalent botulinum antitoxin has never been documented in a clinical trial, animal studies (169) and retrospective data suggest that antitoxin is effective in both types A and E disease (170) and

occasional dramatic responses have been reported (145). Data documenting efficacy in therapy of persons with type B botulism are not available, but antitoxin is generally administered (after diagnostic specimens are obtained) to patients with botulism caused by all three toxin types unless recovery has begun before diagnosis. Because the toxin binds irreversibly to nerve endings and only circulating toxin is neutralized, antitoxin should be given as early in the course of illness as possible. Trivalent botulinum antitoxin (A, B, and E) and clinical and laboratory consultation may be obtained from the CDC (see Appendix).

Because the antitoxin is of equine origin, patients must first be tested for hypersensitivity. If no evidence of hypersensitivity exists, adult patients may initially be given one vial of antitoxin intravenously and one intramuscularly. In severe cases or in those in which signs progress over the subsequent 4 hr, two additional vials may be given: one intravenously and one intramuscularly. Patients who appear to be sensitive to the equine serum should be desensitized prior to antitoxin administration. Serum levels of antitoxin obtained are substantially higher than those required to neutralize circulating toxin (171). Hypersensitivity reactions occur approximately in 10–20% of patients (13,172). A clinical trial of human botulism immune globulin in the treatment of infant botulism has been planned (47,173), but supplies are insufficient to conduct a trial in adults.

Guanidine hydrochloride has been reported to result in some clinical improvement in cranial nerve dysfunction or peripheral muscle strength (174–177) and electrophysiologic improvement in animals (178,179) and in humans (151). However, failures have also been reported (180,181), and one controlled trial failed to demonstrate efficacy (182). Use of this drug, as well as of guanoxan (a related drug for which a clinical response has recently been reported) (183) and of 3,4-diaminopyridine (which has recently been reported to be effective in the treatment of Eaton–Lambert syndrome) (184), should be considered experimental. There is no role for antimicrobial agents in the absence of infectious complications.

Wound Botulism

Therapy includes administration of botulinum antitoxin in the same manner as for patients with foodborne disease. Serum specimens should be obtained for botulinum toxin determination prior to antitoxin administration. After antitoxin is given, débridement of the wound should be performed to remove the focus of infection, even if the wound appears normal. During débridement, material should be collected for anaerobic culture for *C. botulinum*. High-dose penicillin therapy (10–20 million units per day, intravenously) is generally given, although its efficacy is not well documented.

Infant Botulism

Meticulous supportive care is the mainstay of therapy. Because serum specimens are rarely positive and there is a risk of hypersensitivity reactions, botulinum antitoxin has rarely been used. A clinical trial to evaluate the possible efficacy of human botulism immune globulin in infants has been planned in California (47). No role has been demonstrated for oral penicillin. In contrast to adults with respiratory insufficiency, who frequently require a tracheostomy, many infants have been managed successfully with endotracheal intubation. Although there is no evidence that the course of illness is influenced by the use of cathartics or enemas, this approach may be tried cautiously if profound ileus is absent. Aminoglycosides should be avoided if possible, because deterioration in clinical status has been temporally associated with their use (185–187).

PREVENTION

Foodborne Botulism

When the diagnosis of foodborne botulism is first considered, it is imperative to notify public health authorities because of the possibility that a commercial food product is responsible. Prompt reporting is necessary in order to facilitate (a) rapid investigation to prevent additional cases resulting from subsequent ingestion of contaminated food by others (27,188), (b) recognition of the rare outbreak caused by a commercial product in which single cases may occur over a large geographical area (189), and (c) identification of outbreaks caused by home-processed foods transported from one country to another, resulting in an international outbreak (190,191). Therefore, when a case is suspected, the state health department and the CDC should be promptly notified (see Appendix).

The disease may best be prevented by adherence to recommended home-canning and processing techniques. C. botulinum spores are not killed by boiling at 100°C; the higher temperature achieved under pressure as recommended for processing of low-acid fruits and vegetables is necessary. Because the toxin is heat-labile, it may be inactivated by thorough boiling of foods before consumption. Since the immunogenic dose is greater than the lethal dose (as with tetanus), second episodes of illness can occur (192). When unusual foods are implicated, further investigations may identify characteristics of the foods or of the procedures used to prepare or preserve the items that contributed to C. botulinum contamination and subsequent toxin production (25–32,193). In some cases, regulatory action (30) and major public education campaigns (191) have been based on the results of such studies.

Wound Botulism

The disease is best prevented by prompt and adequate débridement of contaminated wounds. Prophylactic use of antimicrobials cannot be relied on to prevent the disease.

Infant Botulism

Until the epidemiology and pathophysiology of infant botulism is better defined, few preventive recommendations are possible. However, infants 12 months of age or less should not be fed honey.

Infectious Botulism

Until the epidemiology and pathophysiology of this form of botulism are better understood, no specific preventive recommendations can be made.

Laboratory-Acquired Disease

A few cases of laboratory-acquired botulism have been reported from other countries. A phosphate-adsorbed pentavalent botulinum toxoid (ABCDE) manufactured by the Michigan Department of Public Health is available from the CDC (see Appendix) as an investigational new drug (IND) and should be administered to laboratory workers who routinely work with C. botulinum or its toxins in research laboratory settings.

The initial series involves deep subcutaneous injections of 0.5 ml at 0, 2, and 12 weeks, followed by a booster at 1 year. The toxoid is immunogenic (194,195), but titers decline over the year after the primary series (194). After the first booster, serum antitoxin titers persist to type A toxin, but titers decline in some persons to type B toxin (195). Subsequent boosters may be given at 2-year intervals if serum antitoxin levels against toxin type B or E are inadequate.

THERAPEUTIC USES OF BOTULINUM TOXIN

Local injection of small quantities of type A botulinum toxin has been found to be effective in the treatment of strabismus, blepharospasm, several other cranial–cervical dystonias, and constipation secondary to anismus by weakening or paralyzing involved muscles (196–200). The product (Oculinum) has been granted orphan drug status by the Food and Drug Administration (201) and has been approved for use in the treatment of strabismus and blepharospasm in patients over 12 years of age (197). Administration generally needs to be repeated periodically. No serious adverse effects have been reported (197).

APPENDIX

Cases of suspected foodborne botulism should be reported immediately to the state health department. Additional consultation may be obtained from the Centers for Disease Control (CDC) by calling 404-639-2206 (weekdays) or 404-639-2888 (evenings, weekends, and holidays). Consultation is available at the CDC on clinical and laboratory diagnosis and treatment for all types of botulism. Trivalent botulinum antitoxin is available through state health departments and through the CDC.

REFERENCES

1. Centers for Disease Control. Botulism in the United States, 1899–1977. *Handbook for epidemiologists, clinicians, and laboratory workers,* issued May 1979.
2. Cherington M. Botulism. *Semin Neurol* 1990;10:27–31.
3. Meyer KF. The rise and fall of botulism. *Calif Med* 1973;118:63–64.
4. van Ermengem E. A new anaerobic bacillus and its relation to botulism. *Rev Infect Dis* 1979;1:701–719. [Reprint of van Ermengem's original article, first published in 1897.]
5. Gunn RA. Botulism: from van Ermengem to the present. A comment. *Rev Infect Dis* 1979;1:720–721.
6. Meyer KF, Eddie B. *Sixty-five years of human botulism in the United States and Canada: epidemiology and tabulation of reported cases 1899–1964.* San Francisco: George Williams Hooper Foundation, University of California Medical Center, 1965.
7. Davis JB, Mattman LH, Wiley M. *Clostridium botulinum* in a fatal wound infection. *JAMA* 1951;146:646–648.
8. Midura TF, Arnon SS. Infant botulism: identification of *Clostridium botulinum* and its toxin in faeces. *Lancet* 1976;2:934–936.
9. Pickett J, Berg B, Chaplin E, et al. Syndrome of botulism in infancy: clinical and electrophysiologic study. *N Engl J Med* 1976;295:770–772.
10. Chia JK, Clark JB, Ryan CA, Pollack M. Botulism in an adult associated with food-borne intestinal infection with *Clostridium botulinum. N Engl J Med* 1986;315:239–241.
11. Lamanna C. The most poisonous poison: what do we know about the toxin of botulism? What are the problems to be solved? *Science* 1959;130:763–72.
12. Lund BM. Foodborne disease due to *Bacillus* and *Clostridium. Lancet* 1990;336:982–986.
13. Merson MH, Hughes JM, Dowell VR, et al. Current trends in botulism in the United States. *JAMA* 1974;229:1305–1308.
14. Blake PA, Horwitz MA, Hopkins L, et al. Type A botulism from commercially canned beef stew. *South Med J* 1977;70:5–7.
15. Centers for Disease Control. Botulism and commercial pot pie—California. *MMWR* 1983;32:39–40, 45.
16. Horwitz MA, Hughes JM, Merson MH, et al. Food-borne botulism in the United States, 1970–1975. *J Infect Dis* 1977;136:153–159.
17. Eisenberg MS, Bender TR. Botulism in Alaska, 1947 through 1974: early detection of cases and investigation of outbreaks as a means of reducing mortality. *JAMA* 1976;235:35–38.
18. Wainwright RB, Heyward WL, Middaugh JP, et al. Food-borne botulism in Alaska, 1947–1985: epidemiology and clinical findings. *J Infect Dis* 1988;157:1158–1162.
19. Meyer KF, Dubovsky BJ. The distribution of the spores of *C. botulinum* in the United States. *J Infect Dis* 1922;31:559–594.
20. Miller LG. Observations on the distribution and ecology of *Clostridium botulinum* type E in Alaska. *Can J Microbiol* 1975;21:920–926.
21. Smith LDS. The occurrence of *Clostridium botulinum* and *Clostridium tetani* in the soil of the United States. *Health Lab Sci* 1978;15:74–80.
22. MacDonald KL, Cohen ML, Blake PA. The changing epidemiol-

ogy of adult botulism in the United States. *Am J Epidemiol* 1986;124:794–799.
23. Midura TF, Nygaard GS, Wood RM, et al. *Clostridium botulinum* type F: isolation from venison jerky. *Applied Microbiol* 1972;24:165–167.
24. Green J, Spear H, Brinson RR. Human botulism (type F)—a rare type. *Am J Med* 1983;75:893–895.
25. Seals JE, Snyder JB, Edell TA, et al. Restaurant-associated type A botulism: transmission by potato salad. *Am J Epidemiol* 1981;113:436–444.
26. MacDonald KL, Spengler RF, Hatheway CL, et al. Type A botulism from sauteed onions: clinical and epidemiologic observations. *JAMA* 1985;253:1275–1278.
27. St Louis ME, Peck SHS, Bowering D, et al. Botulism from chopped garlic: delayed recognition of a major outbreak. *Ann Intern Med* 1988;108:363–368.
28. Sugiyama H, Woodburn M, Yang KH, et al. Production of botulinum toxin in inoculated pack studies of foil-wrapped baked potatoes. *J Food Protection* 1981;44:896–902.
29. Solomon HM, Kautter DA. Growth and toxin production by *Clostridium botulinum* in sauteed onions. *J Food Protection* 1986;49:618–620.
30. Morse DL, Pickard LK, Guzewich JJ. Garlic-in-oil associated botulism: episode leads to product modification. *Am J Public Health* 1990;80:1372–1373.
31. Centers for Disease Control. Botulism in New Mexico. *MMWR* 1978;27:138.
32. Centers for Disease Control. Botulism in New Mexico. *MMWR* 1978;27:145.
33. Mann JM, Martin S, Hoffman R, et al. Patient recovery from type A botulism: morbidity assessment following a large outbreak. *Am J Public Health* 1981;71:266–269.
34. Terranova W, Breman JG, Locey RP, et al. Botulism type B: epidemiologic aspects of an extensive outbreak. *Am J Epidemiol* 1978;108:150–156.
35. Dodds KL. Restaurant-associated botulism outbreaks in North America. *Food Control* 1990;1:139–141.
36. Centers for Disease Control. Foodborne disease outbreaks, 5-year summary, 1983–1987. In: CDC Surveillance Summaries, March 1990. *MMWR* 1990;39(SS-1):15–23.
37. Merson MH, Dowell VR Jr. Epidemiologic, clinical, and laboratory aspects of wound botulism. *N Engl J Med* 1973;289:1105–1110.
38. Cherington M, Ginsburg S. Wound botulism. *Arch Surg* 1975;110:436–438.
39. Swedberg J, Wendel TH, Deiss F. Wound botulism. *West J Med* 1987;147:335–338.
40. MacDonald KL, Rutherford GW, Friedman SM, et al. Botulism and botulism-like illness in chronic drug abusers. *Ann Intern Med* 1985;102:616–618.
41. Kudrow DB, Henry DA, Haake DA, et al. Botulism associated with *Clostridium botulinum* sinusitis after intranasal cocaine abuse. *Ann Intern Med* 1988;109:984–985.
42. Gunn RA. Epidemiologic characteristics of infant botulism in the United States, 1975–1978. *Rev Infect Dis* 1979;1:642–645.
43. Arnon SS. Infant botulism: anticipating the second decade. *J Infect Dis* 1986;154:201–206.
44. Midura TF, Snowden S, Wood RM, et al. Isolation of *Clostridium botulinum* from honey. *J Clin Microbiol* 1979;9:282–283.
45. Arnon SS. Infant botulism. *Annu Rev Med* 1980;31:541–560.
46. Spika JS, Shaffer N, Hargrett-Bean N, et al. Risk factors for infant botulism in the United States. *Am J Dis Child* 1989;143:828–832.
47. California Department of Health Services. Infant botulism in California, 1988–89. *Calif Morb* 1990;7/8.
48. Morris JG, Snyder JD, Wilson R, et al. Infant botulism in the United States: an epidemiologic study of cases occurring outside of California. *Am J Public Health* 1983;73:1385–1388.
49. Arnon SS, Damus K, Thompson B, et al. Protective role of human milk against sudden death from infant botulism. *J Pediatr* 1982;100:568–573.
50. Thompson JA, Glasgow LA, Warpinski JR, et al. Infant botulism: clinical spectrum and epidemiology. *Pediatrics* 1980;66:936–942.
51. Istre GR, Compton R, Novotny T. Infant botulism: three cases in a small town. *Am J Dis Child* 1986;140:1013–1014.

52. Hoffman RE, Pincomb BJ, Skeels MR, et al. Type F infant botulism. *Am J Dis Child* 1982;136:270–271.

53. Suen JC, Hatheway CL, Steigerwalt AG, et al. Genetic confirmation of identities of neurotoxigenic *Clostridium baratii* and *Clostridium butyricum* implicated as agents of infant botulism. *J Clin Microbiol* 1988;26:2191–2192.

54. Hall JD, McCroskey LM, Pincomb BJ, et al. Isolation of an organism resembling *Clostridium barati* which produces type F botulinal toxin from an infant with botulism. *J Clin Microbiol* 1985;21:654–655.

55. McCroskey LM, Hatheway CL, Fenicia L, et al. Characterization of an organism that produces type E botulinal toxin but which resembles *Clostridium butyricum* from the feces of an infant with type E botulism. *J Clin Microbiol* 1986;23:201–202.

56. Aureli P, Fenicia L, Pasolini B, et al. Two cases of type E infant botulism caused by neurotoxigenic *Clostridium butyricum* in Italy. *J Infect Dis* 1986;154:207–211.

57. Long SS. Epidemiologic study of infant botulism in Pennsylvania: report of the infant botulism study group. *Pediatrics* 1985;75:928–934.

58. Turner HD, Brett EM, Gilbert RJ, et al. Infant botulism in England. *Lancet* 1978;1:1277–1278.

59. Smith GE, Hinde F, Westmoreland D, et al. Infantile botulism. *Arch Dis Child* 1989;64:871–872.

60. Sinclair L, Haugh CA. Infant botulism. *Commun Dis Rep* 1990;90:4.

60a. Oguma K, Yokota K, Hayashisi et al. Infant botulism due to *Clostridium botulinum* type C toxin. *Lancet* 1990; 336:1449–1450.

61. Arnon SS, Damus K, Midura TF, et al. Intestinal infection and toxin production by *Clostridium botulinum* as one cause of sudden infant death syndrome. *Lancet* 1978;1:1273–1276.

62. Arnon SS. Breast feeding and toxigenic intestinal infections: missing links in crib death? *Rev Infect Dis* 1984;6:S193–S201.

63. Centers for Disease Control. Botulism—United States, 1978. *MMWR* 1979;28:73–75.

64. Bartlett JC. Infant botulism in adults. *N Engl J Med* 1986;315:254–255.

65. Sonnabend WF, Sonnabend OA, Grundler P. Intestinal toxicoinfection by *Clostridium botulinum* type F in an adult. *Lancet* 1987;1:357–361.

66. Isacsohn M, Cohen A, Steiner A, et al. Botulism intoxication after surgery in the gut. *Isr J Med Sci* 1985;21:150–153.

67. Hatheway CL. Toxigenic clostridia. *Clin Microbiol Rev* 1990;3:66–98.

68. Suen JC, Hatheway CL, Steigerwalt AG, et al. *Clostridium argentinense* sp. nov.: a genetically homogeneous group composed of all strains of *Clostridium botulinum* toxin type G and some nontoxigenic strains previously identified as *Clostridium subterminale* or *Clostridium hastiforme*. *Int J Syst Bacteriol* 1988;38:375–381.

69. Altwegg M, Hatheway CL. Multilocus enzyme electrophoresis of *Clostridium argentinense* (*Clostridium botulinum* toxin type G) and phenotypically similar asaccharolytic clostridia. *J Clin Microbiol* 1988;26:2447–2449.

70. Dowell VR. Botulism and tetanus: selected epidemiologic and microbiologic aspects. *Rev Infect Dis* 1984;6:S202–S207.

71. Smith LDS. *Botulism: the organism, its toxins, the diseases.* Springfield, IL: Charles C Thomas, 1977.

72. Suzuki JBR, Booth AB, Grecz N. Pathogenesis of *Clostridium botulinum* type A: study of *in vivo* toxin release by implantation of diffusion chambers containing spores, vegetative cells, and free toxin. *Infect Immun* 1971;3:659–663.

73. Sakaguchi G. *Clostridium botulinum* toxins. *Pharmacol Ther* 1983;19:165–194.

74. Ohishi I, Sugii S, Sakaguchi G. Oral toxicities of *Clostridium botulinum* toxins in response to molecular size. *Infect Immun* 1977;16:107–109.

75. Habermann E, Dreyer F. *Clostridium* neurotoxins: handling and action at the cellular and molecular level. *Curr Top Microbiol Immunol* 1986;129:93–179.

76. Hoch DH, Romero-Mira M, Ehrlich BE, et al. Channels formed by botulinum, tetanus, and diphtheria toxins in planar lipid bilayers: relevance to translocation of proteins across membranes. *Proc Natl Acad Sci USA* 1985;82:1692–1696.

77. Simpson LL. Molecular pharmacology of botulinum toxin and tetanus toxin. *Annu Rev Pharmacol Toxicol* 1986;26:427–473.

78. DasGupta BR, Moody MA. Amino acid composition of *Clostridium botulinum* type B neurotoxin. *Toxicon* 1984;22:312–315.

79. DasGupta BR, Rasmussen S. Purification and amino acid composition of type E botulinum neurotoxin. *Toxicon* 1983;21:535–545.

80. DasGupta BR, Rasmussen S. Amino acid composition of *Clostridium botulinum* type F neurotoxin. *Toxicon* 1983;21:566–569.

81. DasGupta BR, Sathyamoorthy V. Purification and amino acid composition of type A botulinum neurotoxin. *Toxicon* 1984;22:415–424.

82. Sathyamoorthy V, DasGupta BR. Partial amino acid sequences of the heavy and light chains of botulinum neurotoxin type E. *Biochem Biophys Res Commun* 1985;127:768–772.

83. Sathyamoorthy V, DasGupta BR. Separation, purification, partial characterization and comparison of the heavy and light chains of botulinum neurotoxin types A, B, and E. *J Biol Chem* 1985;260:10461–10466.

84. Schmidt JJ, Sathyamoorthy V, DasGupta BR. Partial amino acid sequence of the heavy and light chains of botulinum neurotoxin type A. *Biochem Biophys Res Commun* 1984;119:900–904.

85. Schmidt JJ, Sathyamoorthy V, DasGupta BR. Partial amino acid sequences of botulinum neurotoxins types B and E. *Arch Biochem Biophys* 1985;238:544–548.

85a. Binz T, Kurazono H, Wille M, et al. The complete sequence of botulinum neurotoxin type A and comparison with other clostridial neurotoxins. *J Biol Chem* 1990;265:9153–9158.

85b. Thompson DE, Brehm JK, Oultram JD, et al. The complete amino acid sequence of the *Clostridium* botulinum type A neurotoxin deduced by nucleotide sequence analysis of the encoding gene. *Eur J Biochem* 1990;189:73–81.

86. DasGupta BR, Datta A. Botulinum neurotoxin type B (strain 657): partial sequence and similarity with tetanus toxin. *Biochimie* 1988;70:811–817.

87. Eisel U, Jarausch W, Goretski K. Tetanus toxin: primary structure, expression in *E coli* and homology with botulinum toxins. *EMBO J* 1986;5:2495–2502.

88. Ohishi IL, Iwasaki M, Sakaguchi G. Vascular permeability activity of botulinum C_2 toxin components. *Infect Immun* 1980;31:890–895.

89. Simpson LL. A comparison of the pharmacological properties of *Clostridium botulinum* type C_1 and C_2 toxins. *J Pharmacol Exp Ther* 1982;223:695–701.

90. Sonnabend O, Sonnabend W, Heinzle R, et al. Isolation of *Clostridium botulinum* type G and identification of type G botulinal toxin in humans: report of five sudden unexpected deaths. *J Infect Dis* 1981;143:22–27.

91. Sonnabend OA, Sonnabend WF, Krech U, et al. Continuous microbiological study of 70 sudden and unexpected infant deaths: toxigenic intestinal *Clostridium botulinum* infection in 9 cases of sudden infant death syndrome. *Lancet* 1985;1:237–241.

92. Schmidt CF, Lechowich RV, Folinazzo JF. Growth and toxin production by type E *Clostridium botulinum* below 40°F. *J Food Sci* 1961;26:626–630.

93. Hatheway CL. Botulism. In: Balows A, Hausler WJ Jr, Ohashi M, Turano A, eds. *Laboratory diagnosis of infectious diseases: principles and practice.* New York: Springer-Verlag, 1988;111–133.

94. Hatheway CL. Bacterial sources of clostridial neurotoxins. In: Simpson L, ed. *Botulinum neurotoxin and tetanus toxin.* New York: Academic Press, 1989;3–23.

95. Dezfulian M, Dowell VR. Cultural and physiological characteristics and antimicrobial susceptibility of *Clostridium botulinum* isolates from foodborne and infant botulism cases. *J Clin Microbiol* 1980;11:604–609.

96. Sugiyama H. *Clostridium botulinum* neurotoxin. *Microbiol Rev* 1980;44:419–448.

97. Kao I, Drachman DB, Price DL. Botulinum toxin: mechanism of presynaptic blockage. *Science* 1976;193:1256–1258.

98. Simpson LL. The origin, structure, and pharmacological activity of botulinum toxin. *Pharmacol Rev* 1981;33:155–188.

99. Mallart A, Molgo J, Angaut-Petit D, et al. Is the internal calcium regulation altered in type A botulinum toxin-poisoned motor endings? *Brain Res* 1989;479:167–171.

100. Arnon SS, Midura TF, Clay SA, et al. Infant botulism: epidemiological, clinical, and laboratory aspects. *JAMA* 1977;237:1946.
101. Sugiyama H, Mills DC. Intraintestinal toxin in infant mice challenged intragastrically with *Clostridium botulinum* spores. *Infect Immun* 1978;21:59–63.
102. Wilcke BW, Midura TF. Quantitative evidence of intestinal colonization by *Clostridium botulinum* in four cases of infant botulism. *J Infect Dis* 1980;141:419–423.
103. Moberg LJ, Sugiyama H. Microbial ecological basis of infant botulism as studied with germfree mice. *Infect Immun* 1979;25:653–657.
104. Wang Y, Sugiyama H. Botulism in metronidazole-treated conventional adult mice challenged orogastrically with spores of *Clostridium botulinum* type A or B. *Infect Immun* 1984;46:715–719.
105. Mills DC, Arnon SS. The large intestine as the site of *Clostridium botulinum* colonization in human infant botulism. *J Infect Dis* 1987;156:997–998.
106. McCroskey LM, Hatheway CL. Laboratory findings in four cases of adult botulism suggest colonization of the intestinal tract. *J Clin Microbiol* 1988;26:1052–1054.
107. Freedman M, Armstrong RM, Killian JM, et al. Botulism in a patient with jejunoileal bypass. *Ann Neurol* 1986;20:641–643.
108. Petty CS. Botulism: the disease and the toxin. *Am J Med Sci* 1965;24:133–148.
109. Duchen LW. An electron microscopic study of the changes induced by botulinum toxin in the motor end-plates of slow and fast skeletal muscle fibres of the mouse. *J Neurol Sci* 1971;14:47–60.
110. Pamphlett R. Axonal sprouting after botulinum toxin does not elicit a histological axon reaction. *J Neurol Sci* 1988;87:175–185.
111. Tsujihata M, Kinoshita I, Mori M, et al. Ultrastructural study of the motor end-plate in botulism and Lambert–Eaton myasthenic syndrome. *J Neurol Sci* 1987;81:197–213.
112. Terranova W, Palumbo JN, Breman JG. Ocular findings in botulism type B. *JAMA* 1979;241:475–477.
113. Koenig MG, Spickard A, Cardella MA, et al. Clinical and laboratory observations of type E botulism in man. *Medicine* 1964;43:517–545.
114. Barker WH Jr, Weissman JB, Dowell VR Jr, et al. Type B botulism outbreak caused by a commercial food product. *JAMA* 1977;237:456–459.
115. Hughes JM, Blumenthal JR, Merson MH, et al. Clinical features of types A and B food-borne botulism. *Ann Intern Med* 1981;95:442–445.
116. Lecour H, Ramos MH, Almeida B, et al. Food-borne botulism: a review of 13 outbreaks. *Arch Intern Med* 1988;148:578–580.
117. Konig H, Gassman HB, Jenzer G. Ocular involvement in benign botulism B. *Am J Ophthalmol* 1975;80:430–432.
118. Jenzer G, Mumenthaler M, Ludin HP, et al. Autonomic dysfunction in botulism B: a clinical report. *Neurology* 1975;25:150–153.
119. Bradley WG, Ferrucci JT Jr, Shahani BT. Case records of the Massachusetts General Hospital: case 48-1980. *N Engl J Med* 1980;303:1347–1355.
120. Ehrenreich H, Garner CG, Witt TN. Complete bilateral internal ophthalmoplegia as sole clinical sign of botulism: confirmation of diagnosis by single fibre electromyography. *J Neurol* 1989;236:243–245.
121. Cherington M. Botulism: ten-year experience. *Arch Neurol* 1974;30:432–437.
122. Ryan DW, Cherington M. Human type A botulism. *JAMA* 1971;216:513–514.
123. Goode GB, Shearn DL. Botulism: a case with associated sensory abnormalities. *Arch Neurol* 1982;39:55.
124. Koenig MG, Drutz DJ, Mushlin AI, et al. Type B botulism in man. *Am J Med* 1967;42:208–219.
125. Badhey H, Cleri DJ, Amato RF. Two fatal cases of type E adult food-borne botulism with early symptoms and terminal neurologic signs. *J Clin Microbiol* 1986;23:616–618.
126. Hughes JM, Tacket CO. "Sausage poisoning" revisited. *Arch Intern Med* 1983;143:425–426.
127. Schmidt-Nowara WW, Samet JM, Rosario PA. Early and late pulmonary complications of botulism. *Arch Intern Med* 1983;143:451–456.
128. Critchley EMR, Hayes PJ, Isaacs PET. Outbreak of botulism in
North West England and Wales, June, 1989. *Lancet* 1989;2:849–853.
129. Paust JC. Respiratory care in acute botulism: a report of four cases. *Anesth Analg* 1971;50:1003–1009.
130. Colebatch JG, Wolff AH, Gilbert RJ, et al. Slow recovery from severe foodborne botulism. *Lancet* 1989;2:1216–1217.
131. Maroon JC. Late effects of botulinum intoxication. *JAMA* 1977;238:129.
132. Mann JM, Martin S, Hoffman R, et al. Patient recovery from type A botulism: morbidity assessment following a large outbreak. *Am J Public Health* 1981;71:266–269.
133. Mann J. Prolonged recovery from type A botulism. *N Engl J Med* 1983;309:1522–1523.
134. Wilcox P, Andolfatto G, Fairbarn MS, et al. Long-term follow-up of symptoms, pulmonary function, respiratory muscle strength, and exercise performance after botulism. *Am Rev Respir Dis* 1989;139:157–163.
135. Lewis SW, Pierson DJ, Cary JM. Prolonged respiratory paralysis in wound botulism. *Chest* 1979;75:59–61.
136. Polin RA, Brown LW. Infant botulism. *Pediatr Clin North Am* 1979;26:345–354.
137. Brown LW. Infant botulism. *Adv Pediatr* 1981;28:141–157.
138. Wilson R, Morris JG, Snyder JD, et al. Clinical characteristics of infant botulism in the United States: a study of the non-California cases. *Pediat Infect Dis* 1982;1:148–150.
139. Jagoda A, Renner G. Infant botulism: case report and clinical update. *Am J Emerg Med* 1990;8:318–320.
140. Paton JC, Lawrence AJ, Manson JI. Quantitation of *Clostridium botulinum* organisms and toxin in the feces of an infant with botulism. *J Clin Microbiol* 1982;15:1–4.
141. Long SS, Gajewski JL, Brown LW, et al. Clinical, laboratory, and environmental features of infant botulism in Southeastern Pennsylvania. *Pediatrics* 1985;75:935–941.
142. Kurland G, Seltzer J. Antidiuretic hormone excess in infant botulism. *Am J Dis Child* 1987;147:1227–1229.
143. Fisher M. An unusual variant of acute idiopathic polyneuritis (syndrome of ophthalmoplegia, ataxia and areflexia). *N Engl J Med* 1956;255:57–65.
144. Patel A, Pearce L, Hairston R. Miller Fisher syndrome (variant of Landry–Guillain–Barré–Strohl syndrome—ophthalmoplegia, ataxia, areflexia). *South Med J* 1966;59:171–175.
145. Whittaker RL, Gilbertson RB, Garrett AS. Botulism, type E: report of eight simultaneous cases. *Ann Intern Med* 1964;61:448–454.
146. Edell TA, Sullivan CP, Osborn KM, et al. Wound botulism associated with a positive Tensilon test. *West J Med* 1983;139:218–219.
147. Masland RL, Gammon GD. The effect of botulinus toxin on the electromyogram. *Pharmacol Exp Ther* 1949;97:499–506.
148. Gutmann L. Pathophysiologic aspects of human botulism. *Arch Neurol* 1976;33:175–179.
149. McQuillen MP, Johns RJ. The nature of the defect in the Eaton–Lambert syndrome. *Neurology* 1967;17:527–536.
150. Eaton LM, Lambert EH. Electromyography and electric stimulation of nerves in diseases of motor unit: observations on myasthenic syndrome associated with malignant tumors. *JAMA* 1957;163:1117–1124.
151. Cherington M. Botulism: electrophysiologic and therapeutic observations. In: Desmedt JE, ed. *New developments in EMG and clinical neurophysiology.* Basel: S Karger, 1973;375–379.
152. Martinez AC, Anciones B, Ferrer MT, et al. Electrophysiologic study in benign human botulism type B. *Muscle Nerve* 1985;8:580–585.
153. Pickett JB. AAEE case report #16: botulism. *Muscle Nerve* 1988;11:1201–1205.
154. Dezfulian M, Yolken R, Bartlett J. Rapid diagnosis of a case of infant botulism by enzyme immunoassay. *Pediatr Infect Dis* 1985;4:399–401.
155. Dezfulian M, Bartlett JG. Detection of *Clostridium botulinum* type A toxin by enzyme-linked immunosorbent assay with antibodies produced in immunologically tolerant animals. *J Clin Microbiol* 1984;19:645–648.
156. Dezfulian M, Bartlett JG. Selection isolation and rapid identification of *Clostridium botulinum* types A and B by toxin detection. *J Clin Microbiol* 1985;21:231–233.

157. Dowell VR Jr, McCroskey LM, Hatheway CL, et al. Coproexamination for botulinal toxin and *Clostridium botulinum. JAMA* 1977;238:1829.

158. Mann JM, Hatheway CL, Gardiner TM. Laboratory diagnosis in a large outbreak of type A botulism. *Am J Epidemiol* 1982;115:598.

159. Hatheway CL, McCroskey LM. Unusual neurotoxigenic clostridia recovered from human fecal specimens in the investigation of botulism. In: Hattori T, Ishida Y, Maruyama Y, et al., eds. *Recent advances in microbial ecology.* Proceedings of the 5th International Symposium on Microbial Ecology, Kyoto, Japan. Tokyo: Japan Scientific Societies Press, 1989;477–481.

160. Craig JM, Iida H, Inoue K. A recent case of botulism in Hokkaido, Japan. *Jpn J Med Sci Biol* 1970;23:193–198.

161. Horwitz MA, Hatheway CL, Dowell VR. Laboratory diagnosis of botulism complicated by pyridostigmine treatment of the patient. *Am J Clin Pathol* 1976;66:737–742.

162. de Jesus PV, Slater R. Neuromuscular physiology of wound botulism. *Arch Neurol* 1973;29:425–431.

163. Glasby C, Hatheway CL. Isolation and enumeration of *Clostridium botulinum* by direct inoculation of infant fecal specimens on egg yolk agar and *Clostridium botulinum* isolation media. *J Clin Microbiol* 1985;21:264–266.

164. Mills DC, Midura TF, Arnon SS. Improved selective medium for the isolation of lipase-positive *Clostridium botulinum* from feces of human infants. *J Clin Microbiol* 1985;21:947–950.

165. Hatheway CL, McCroskey LM. Examination of feces and serum from diagnosis of infant botulism in 336 patients. *J Clin Microbiol* 1987;25:2334–2338.

166. Cornblath DR, Sladky JT, Sumner AJ. Clinical electrophysiology of infantile botulism. *Muscle Nerve* 1983;6:448–452.

167. Enge WK. Brief, small, abundant motor-unit potentials: a further critique of electromyographic interpretation. *Neurology* 1975;25:173–176.

168. Clay SA, Ramseyer C, Fishman LS. Acute infantile motor unit disorder: infantile botulism? *Arch Neurol* 1977;34:236–243.

169. Karashimada TOT, Iida H. Studies on the serum therapy of type E botulism (part III). *Jpn J Med Sci Biol* 1970;23:177–191.

170. Tacket CO. Equine antitoxin use and other factors that predict outcome in type A foodborne botulism. *Am J Med* 1984;76:794–798.

171. Hatheway CH, Snyder JD, Seals JE, et al. Antitoxin levels in botulism patients treated with trivalent equine botulism antitoxin to toxin types A, B, and E. *J Infect Dis* 1984;150:407–412.

172. Black RE, Gunn RA. Hypersensitivity reactions associated with botulinal antitoxin. *Am J Med* 1980;69:567–570.

173. Lewis GE, Metzger JF. Botulism immune plasma (human). *Lancet* 1978;2:634–635.

174. Cherington M, Ryan DW. Botulism and guanidine. *N Engl J Med* 1968;278:931–933, 963.

175. Cherington M, Ryan DW. Treatment of botulism with guanidine. *N Engl J Med* 1970;282:195–197.

176. Oh SJ, Halsey JH, Briggs DD. Guanidine in type B botulism. *Arch Intern Med* 1975;135:726–728.

177. Puggiari M, Cherington M. Botulism and guanidine: ten years later. *JAMA* 1978;240:2276–2277.

178. Seaer RC, Tooker J, Cherington M. Effect of guanidine on the neuromuscular block of botulism. *Neurology* 1969;19:1107–1110.

179. Cherington M, Soyer A, Greenberg H. Effect of guanidine and germine on the neuromuscular block of botulism. *Curr Ther Res* 1972;14:91–94.

180. Faich GA, Graebner RW, Sato S. Failure of guanidine therapy in botulism A. *N Engl J Med* 1971;285:773–776.

181. Morris JG. Current trends in therapy of botulism in the United States. In: Lewis GE Jr, ed. *Biomedical aspects of botulism.* New York: Academic Press, 1981;317–326.

182. Kaplan JE, Davis LE, Narayan V, et al. Botulism, type A, and treatment with guanidine. *Ann Neurol* 1979;6:69–71.

183. Neal KR, Dunbar EM. Improvement in bulbar weakness with guanoxan in type B botulism. *Lancet* 1990;335:1286–1287.

184. McEvoy KM, Windebank AJ, Daube JR, et al. 3,4-Diaminopyridine in the treatment of Lambert–Eaton myasthenic syndrome. *N Engl J Med* 1989;321:1567–1571.

185. L'Hommedieu C, Stough R, Brown L, et al. Potentiation of neuromuscular weakness in infant botulism by aminoglycosides. *J Pediatr* 1979;95:1065–1070.

186. Schwartz RH, Eng G. Infant botulism: exacerbation by aminoglycosides. *Am J Dis Child* 1982;136:952.

187. Gay CT, Marks WA, Riley HD, et al. Infantile botulism. *South Med J* 1988;81:456–460.

188. Horwitz MA, Marr JS, Merson MH, et al. A continuing common-source outbreak of botulism in a family. *Lancet* 1975;2:861–863.

189. O'Mahony M, Mitchell E, Gilbert RJ, et al. An outbreak of foodborne botulism associated with contaminated hazelnut yoghurt. *Epidemiol Infect* 1990;104:389–395.

190. Slater PE, Addiss DG, Cohen A, et al. Foodborne botulism: an international outbreak. *Intern J Epidemiol* 1989;18:693–696.

191. Telzak EE, Bell EP, Kautter DA, et al. An international outbreak of type E botulism due to uneviscerated fish. *J Infect Dis* 1990;161:340–342.

192. Beller M, Middaugh JP. Repeated type E botulism in an Alaskan Eskimo. *N Engl J Med* 1990;322:855.

193. Rank E, Pflug IJ. Dry heat destruction of spores on metal surfaces and on potatoes during baking. *J Food Protection* 1977;40:608–613.

194. Siegel LS. Human immune response to botulinum pentavalent (ABCDE) toxoid determined by a neutralization test and by an enzyme-linked immunosorbent assay. *J Clin Microbiol* 1988;26:2351–2356.

195. Siegel LS. Evaluation of neutralizing antibodies to type A, B, E, and F botulinum toxins in sera from human recipients of botulinum pentavalent (ABCDE) toxoid. *J Clin Microbiol* 1989;27:1906–1908.

196. The Medical Letter. Botulinum toxin injection for ocular muscle disorders. *Med Lett Drugs Ther* 1987;29:101–102.

197. The Medical Letter. Botulinum toxin for ocular muscle disorders. *Med Lett Drugs Ther* 1990;32:100–102.

198. Kennedy RH, Bartley GB, Flanagan JC, et al. Treatment of blepharospasm with botulinum toxin. *Mayo Clin Proc* 1989;64:1085–1090.

199. Hallan RI, Melling J, Womack NR, et al. Treatment of anismus in intractable constipation with botulinum A toxin. *Lancet* 1988;2:714–716.

200. Jankovic J, Brin MF. Therapeutic uses of botulinum toxin. *N Engl J Med* 1991;324:1186–1194.

201. Nightingale SL. From the Food and Drug Administration: New therapy approved for strabismus and blepharospasm. *JAMA* 1990;263:793.

Infections of the Central Nervous System,
edited by W. M. Scheld, R. J. Whitley, and
D. T. Durack, Raven Press, Ltd., New York © 1991.

CHAPTER 25

Tetanus

Thomas P. Bleck

Tetanus is a serious but preventable affliction of humans and other vertebrates. Although the disease has become a curiosity in the industrial nations, it is still rampant in the third world. The dreadful clinical manifestations and high mortality make tetanus a subject of fear.

Yet, this disorder has been one of the most instructive in the history of medicine. The pathophysiology and pharmacology of tetanus intoxication have taught us an immense amount about normal motor control. The isolation of the responsible organism and of its toxin were cornerstones in the history of microbiology. Tetanus was one of the first bacterial conditions to be clearly prevented by immunization, representing a triumph in the application of research findings and public health measures.

HISTORICAL ASPECTS

Ancient physicians recognized the relationship between wounds and a disease producing spasticity, violent movements, and death. Case 7 in the Edwin Smith Surgical Papyrus discusses a patient with a penetrating skull wound who experiences trismus (Fig. 1) and nuchal rigidity (Fig. 2) (1). These findings were apparently well known to the Egyptian physician who used them to help formulate the prognosis. This is commonly accepted as the earliest recorded description of tetanus (2). Hippocrates described the disorder clearly; and his relative contemporary, Aretaeus, observed that these manifestations were "apt to supervene on the wound of a membrane, or of muscles, or of punctured nerves, when, for the most part, the patients die; for, 'spasm from a wound is fatal' "

(3). Galen noted that cutting a nerve in tetanus stopped the movement but paralyzed the innervated part.

The ensuing millennia saw some refinements in clinical observation. John of Arderne (1307–1380), often thought to be the first English surgeon–author, described a case of tetanus in which trismus ("taken with the cramp on his cheeks") began 11 days after a gardening injury (4). In the 18th century, tetanus was thought to be a consequence of nerve injury (5). However, the spasms of generalized tetanus were frequently confused with the convulsions of epilepsy. Sir Charles Bell, a noted illustrator as well as a surgeon, included a tetanus patient in his 1824 text (Fig. 3) (6).

Neonatal tetanus was called the "seven-day disease" in the Americas (7) and was known as the "nine-day fits" in Dublin (8). In 1846, Sims (9) proposed the "congestive" theory of neonatal tetanus. He thought that this condition resulted from placing infants on their backs, which compressed the occiput and occluded the veins of the medulla. Beumer (10) determined that the umbilicus was the portal of entry for tetanus in 1887.

The clinical advances of the 19th century culminated in this description by Sir William Gowers (11):

> Tetanus is a disease of the nervous system characterized by persistent tonic spasm, with violent brief exacerbations. The spasm almost always commences in the muscles of the neck and jaw, causing closure of the jaws (*trismus, lockjaw*), and involves the muscles of the trunk more than those of the limbs. It is always acute in onset, and a very large proportion of those who are attacked die.

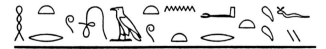

FIG. 1. Hieroglyphic of "the cord of his mandible is contracted," the first known description of trismus. (From ref. 1, with permission.)

T. P. Bleck: Departments of Neurological Sciences and Internal Medicine, Sections of Critical Care and Infectious Diseases, Rush Medical College, Chicago, Illinois 60612. *Present address:* Department of Neurology, University of Virginia School of Medicine, Charlottesville, Virginia 22908.

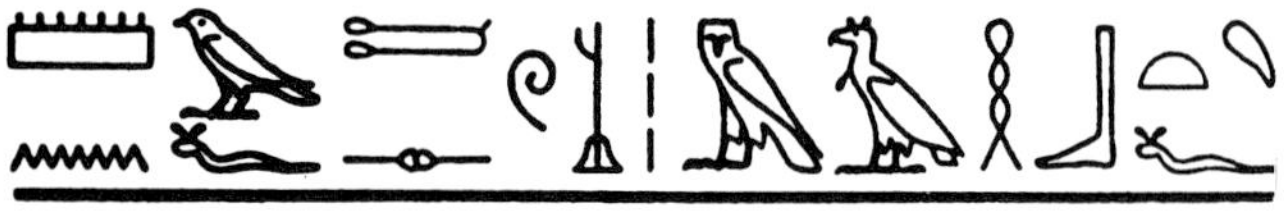

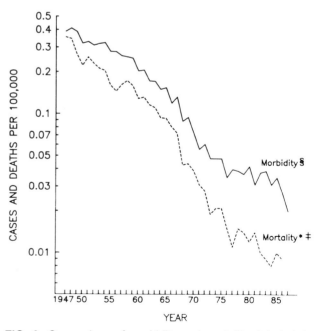

FIG. 2. Hieroglyphic of "while he suffers with stiffness in his neck," the first known description of nuchal rigidity in tetanus. (From ref. 1, with permission.)

Gowers, and many of his contemporaries, felt that nontraumatic tetanus accounted for up to 20% of cases; he blamed these on a sudden chill or a frightening episode. Although he recognized the similarity between tetanus and strychnine poisoning, he disparaged the notion of pathophysiologic similarity. In one of his few failures of insight, Gowers dismissed Nicolaier's first report of a strychnine-like toxin isolated from anaerobic soil bacteria (12). Six years later, Behring and Kitasato (13) proved that immunization with an inactivated derivative of this bacterial extract prevented tetanus.

Effective therapeutic suggestions for established tetanus also date from the 19th century. In 1829, Ceroli (14) described the use of morphine as a treatment for tetanus. Based on the observations of Claude Bernard, curare was employed with some rare successes (and some dramatic failures) in France (15), Germany (16), the United States (17), and England. Hutchinson and Jackson (18) of the National Hospital at Queen Square reported on the use of ether in tetanus in 1861. The lessons in long-term mechanical ventilation learned during the poliomyelitis epidemics of the 1950s finally made treatment with neuromuscular blockade feasible. Similarly, Gowers (11) gave a description of autonomic dysfunction in tetanus in 1888: "The pulse is increased in frequency, especially during the paroxysms, and is often very small. There is some reason to believe that the small size of the pulse is due to generalized vasomotor spasm." However, widespread recognition of the hypersympathetic state did not occur until the prolongation of survival of tetanus patients made possible by ventilatory management. Meltzer and Auer (19) employed magnesium salts to treat tetanus patients at the dawn of the 20th century.

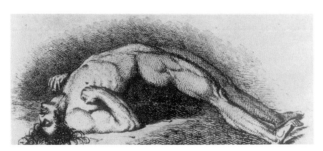

FIG. 3. Sir Charles Bell's sketch of a soldier with tetanus, demonstrating opisthotonus. (From ref. 6.)

EPIDEMIOLOGY

About one million cases of tetanus are thought to occur annually in the world (20), suggesting a global incidence of about 18 per 100,000 population per year. However, such estimates have large degrees of uncertainty. Published mortality figures underestimate the number of deaths but probably represent the most reliable data for much of the world. Cvjetanovic (21) cites annual mortality rates of 28 per 100,000 population in Africa, 15 per 100,000 in Asia, 0.5 per 100,000 in Europe, and less than 0.1 per 100,000 in North America. In the United States, reported cases per 100,000 population fell in a relatively linear fashion—from 0.28 in 1955 to 0.04 in 1975, with little change thereafter (22,23). About 70 cases have been reported to the Centers for Disease Control (CDC) each year for the past 5 years; this probably represents underreporting by about 50% for recognized cases. After an extensive analysis of reports to the CDC and the National Center for Health Statistics (NCHS), Sutter et al. (24) recently concluded that only 40% of cases are reported to the CDC, 60% are reported to the NCHS, and almost 25% are reported to neither one (Fig. 4). The majority of reported cases occur in patients over 60 years of age, confirming that waning immunity is a serious problem in this population (*vide infra*). Table 1 summarizes the etiologies of reported U.S. cases (25).

FIG. 4. Comparison of morbidity and mortality data in tetanus. The annual incidence reported to the CDC is represented by the solid line, whereas the mortality reported to the NCHS is represented by the dashed line. Asterisk (∗): Mortality data were not available for 1987. Double dagger (‡): NHCS underlying cause-of-death data. Section symbol (§): CDC incidence data. (From ref. 24, with permission.)

TABLE 1. *Etiology of U.S. tetanus cases, 1982–1984 (23, 25)*

Etiologic factor	Number of patients		Percentage
Neonatal tetanus	3		1.3
Acute injuries	166		69.5
Type of wound			
Punctures		85	51.2
Lacerations		81	48.8
Type of activity resulting in wound			
Indoor activity		68	41.0
Gardening or gardening-related		65	39.2
Animal-related		7	4.2
Major trauma		7	4.2
Other		19	11.4
Other identified conditions	53		22.2
Chronic wound		48	90.6
Parenteral drug abuse		5	9.4
No apparent source	17		7.1

Neonatal tetanus accounts for about half of all cases worldwide, and it has a 90% mortality rate (26,27). There is great variability in incidence of, and mortality from, the neonatal form of the disease, with an inverse relationship between the extent of maternal immunization and incidence (28).

ETIOLOGY

Clostridium tetani (Fig. 5) is a slender, obligatively anaerobic bacillus measuring 0.5–1.7 μm by 2.1–18.1 μm (29). Although it is usually classified as gram-positive, it may stain variably, especially in tissues or in older cultures (30). Most strains are sluggishly motile (31), and they have abundant peritrichous flagellae during growth (Fig. 6). The mature organism loses its flagellae (Fig. 7) and forms a spherical terminal spore (32), producing a profile like that of a squash racket (Fig. 8). The spores resist extremes of temperature and moisture, and they are stable at ambient oxygen tension; in addition, they survive indefinitely. [At least 10 other clostridial species form terminal spores, and many others form subterminal spores. Their differentiation has been reviewed (33).] They are viable after exposure to ethanol, phenol, and formalin, but they are killed by iodine, glutaraldehyde, or hydrogen peroxide. Strains vary in resistance; exposure to 100°C for 4 hr, or autoclaving at 121°C and 103 kPa (15 psi) for 15 min, is necessary to ensure sterility.

Spores can be isolated from the feces of many animals, and in small numbers are ubiquitous in soil and on carpets. Hence, any breach in skin defenses—for example, wounds, burns, animal or human bites, or even insect bites (34)—may result in the inoculation of spores. Certain types of injury are more prone to produce tetanus;

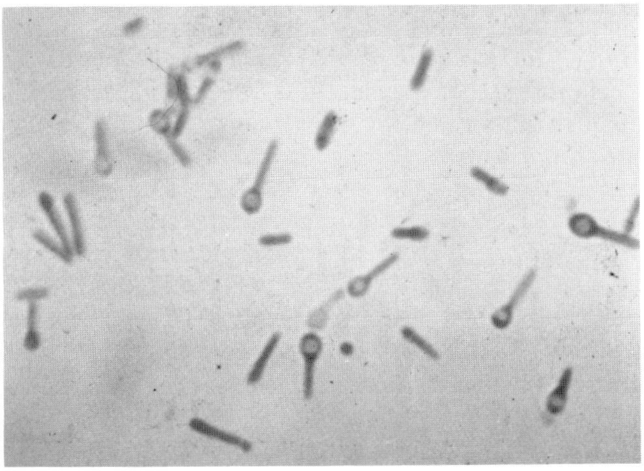

FIG. 5. Gram's stain of a culture of *C. tetani*. Original magnification: ×1000. (Courtesy of Paul C. Schrechenberger, Ph.D., and Alex Kuritza, Ph.D.)

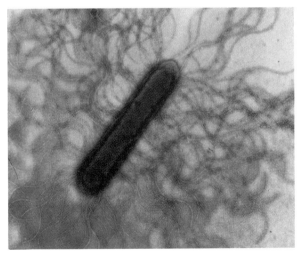

FIG. 6. Electron micrograph of a tetanus bacillus in growth phase [negatively stained with sodium phosphotungstate and bovine serum albumin (NaPTA–BSA)]. Original magnification: ×9000. (From ref. 32, with permission.)

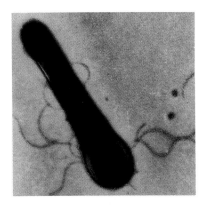

FIG. 7. Electron micrograph demonstrating early spore formation and loss of flagellae (negatively stained with NaPTA–BSA). Original magnification: ×9000. (From ref. 32, with permission.)

these are discussed below. Between 7% and 21% of tetanus cases are cryptogenic in most series (35).

In culture, growth occurs best at 37°C. *C. tetani* will grow on a variety of media if oxygen is excluded. When cultured on a solid medium such as blood agar, the organisms usually form a thin film over the entire surface ("swarming growth"). Routine anaerobic isolation techniques are sufficient if the tissue sample is rapidly placed in an anaerobic transport system. Clinical decisions should not be made on culture results in this disorder, because (a) cultures are commonly negative in patients with tetanus, (b) isolation of the organism is of no consequence in an immune host, and (c) routine bacteriologic studies will not indicate whether a strain of *C. tetani* carries the plasmid required for toxin production.

The spores germinate when introduced into a wound, and they will proliferate if the redox potential of the tissue is low. During growth, *C. tetani* produces two exotoxins: tetanospasmin and tetanolysin. The potential role of tetanolysin in human tetanus is unclear; at worst, it may damage otherwise viable tissue in the vicinity of an infected wound, lowering the redox potential and promoting the growth of anaerobic organisms (36). Tetanolysin can disrupt cell membranes, apparently by more than one mechanism. Rottem et al. (37) showed that it can form membrane channels, but it may also more directly damage membrane lipids (38). Although systemic administration of tetanolysin in animals produces electrocardiographic abnormalities and disseminated intravascular coagulation (39), the relevance of these findings to clinical tetanus is uncertain.

Tetanospasmin, the substance commonly called "tetanus toxin," is synthesized as a single 151-kD, 1315-amino-acid polypeptide chain (Fig. 9) (40–42). The genetic information for this molecule resides on a single large plasmid (Fig. 10) (43). Strains of *C. tetani* lacking this plasmid are not toxigenic. The native molecule has little or no toxic activity, but it becomes potent when nicked at serine-458 by a bacterial protease (44). This produces one heavy (100 kD) chain and one light (50 kD) chain, connected by a disulfide bridge. This bridge, as well as another one on the heavy chain, is required for the activity of the toxin (45). These chains or their various fragments are generally thought to affect different phases of toxin binding, cell entry, and toxicity. T-cell epitopes producing an immune response against two particular amino acid sequences from the amphipathic alpha-helical portion of the molecule are particularly common (46). The three-dimensional structure of tetanospasmin has recently been determined (Fig. 11) (47).

Investigators have proposed a wide range of nomenclatures for the various enzymatic digestion products (Fig. 12), but the clinical relevance of these products is uncertain. Now that the toxin molecule has been sequenced, reference to the specific amino acids of a fragment is preferred (48). The more commonly accepted fragments are those derived from papain treatment, which cleaves the heavy chain at lysine-865, about 50 kD from the carboxy-terminal end (49). This is termed the "C fragment," whereas the light chain and the amino-terminal end, still linked by the disulfide bridge, are variously called the "B fragment" or the "A–B fragment." Attachment and internalization of tetanospasmin is generally considered to be mediated by the heavy chain (50) or its C fragment (51), whereas the light chain is held responsible for inhibiting transmitter release (50,52). Fragment C may also be responsible for the

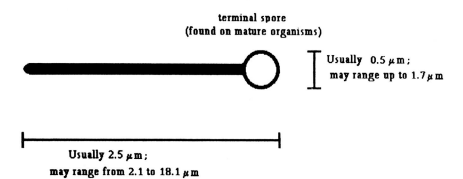

terminal spore
(found on mature organisms)

Usually 0.5 μm;
may range up to 1.7 μm

Usually 2.5 μm;
may range from 2.1 to 18.1 μm

FIG. 8. Schematic diagram of a mature *C. tetani* bacillus, illustrating the squash-racket morphology.

FIG. 9

```
     r-A    10          20           30          40           50          60
N- MPITINNFRY SDPVNNDTII MMEPPYCKGL DIYYKAFKIT DRIWIVPERY EFGTKPEDFH

         70          80           90         100          110         120
   PPSSLIEGAS EYYDPNYLRT DSDKDRFLQT MVKLFNRIKN NVAGEALLDK IINAIPYLGH

        130         140          150         160          170         180
   SYSLLDKFDT NSNSVSFNLL EQDPSGATTK SASMLTNLIIF GPGPVLNKNE VRGIVLRVDN

        190         200          210         220          230         240
   KNYFPCRDGF GSIMQMAFCP EYVPTFDNVI ENITSLTIGK SKYFQDPALL LMHELIHVLH

        250         260          270         280          290         300
   GLYGMQVSSH EIIPSKQEIY MQHTYPISAE ELFTFGGQDA NLISIDIKND LYEKTLNDYK

        310         320          330         340          350         360
   AIANKLSQVT SCNDPNIDID SYKQIYQQKY QFDKDSNGQY IVNEDKFQIL YNSIMYGFTE

        370         380          390         400          410         420
   IELGKKFNIK TRLSYFSMNH DPVKIPNLLD DTIYNDTEGF NIESKDLKSE YKGQNMRVNT

        430         440          450       r-460   B    470         480
   NAFRNVDGSG LVSKLIGLCK KIIPPTNIRE NLYNRTASLT DLGGELCIKI KNEDLTFIAE
                              L_ _ _ _ _ S-S _ _ _ _ _ _ ┘
        490         500          510         520         530         540
   KNSFSEEPFQ DEIVSYNTKN KPLNFNYSLD KIIVDYNLQS KITLPNDRTT PVTKGIPYAP

        550         560          570         580         590         600
   EYKSNAASTI EIHNIDDNTI YQYLYAQKSP TTLQRITMTN SVDDALINST KIYSYFPSVI

        610         620          630         640         650         660
   SKVNQGAQGI LFLQWVRDII DDFTNESSQK TTIDKISDVS TIVPYIGPAL NIVKQGYEGN

        670         680          690         700         710         720
   FIGALETTGV VLLLEYIPEI TLPVIAALSI AESSTQKEKI IKTIDNFLEK RYEKWIEVYK

        730         740          750         760         770         780
   LVKAKWLGTV NTQFQKRSYQ MYRSLEYQVD AIKKIIDYEY KIYSGPDKEQ IADEINNLKN

        790         800          810         820         830         840
   KLEEKANKAM ININIFMRES SRSFLVNQMI NEAKKQLLEF DTQSKNILMQ YIKANSKFIG
                              r-_ _ _ _ _ _→ C
        850         860          870         880         890         900
   ITELKKLESK INKVFSTPIP FSYSKNLDCW VDNEEDIDVI LKKSTILNLD INNDIISDIS

        910         920          930         940         950         960
   GFNSSVITYP DAQLVPGING KAIHLVNNES SEVIVHKAMD IEYNDMFNNF TVSFWLRVPK

        970         980          990        1000         1010        1020
   VSASHLEQYG TNEYSIISSM KKHSLSIGSG WSVSLKGNNL IWTLKDSAGE VRQITFRDLP

       1030        1040         1050        1060         1070        1080
   DKFNAYLANK WVFITITNDR LSSANLYING VLMGSAEITG LGAIREDNNI TLKLDRCNNN

       1090        1100         1110        1120         1130        1140
   NQYVSIDKFR IFCKALNPKE IEKLYTSYLS ITFLRDFWGN PLRYDTEYYL IPVASSSKDV

       1150        1160         1170        1180         1190        1200
   QLKNITDYMY LTNAPSYTNG KLNIYYRRLY NGLKFIIKRY TPNNEIDSFV KSGDFIKLYV

       1210        1220         1230        1240         1250        1260
   SYNNNEHIVG YPKDGNAFNN LDRILRVGYN APGIPLYKKM EAVKLRDLKT YSVQLKLYDD

       1270        1280         1290        1300         1310
   KNASLGLVGT HNGQIGNDPN RDILIASNWY FNHLKDKILG CDWYFVPTDE GWTND -C
```

FIG. 9. Amino acid sequence of tetanospasmin. **A:** Origin of the light chain. **B:** Origin of the amino portion of the heavy chain (H_1). **C:** Origin of the carboxy portion of the heavy chain (H_2). The N-terminal methionine is removed during processing of the toxin, and the amino acids are numbered starting with the adjacent proline. The disulfide bond connecting the light and heavy chains is illustrated (from cysteine-438 to cysteine-466). A second disulfide bond, connecting cysteine-1076 and cysteine-1092, is not shown. (From ref. 42, with permission; additional information can be obtained from ref. 44.)

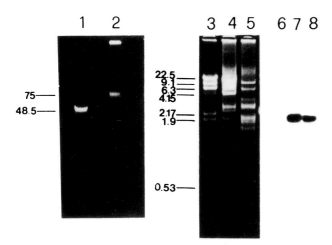

FIG. 10. Characterization of plasmid DNA from a toxigenic, nonsporulating Massachusetts strain of *C. tetani* on 0.8% agarose gel. **Lane 1:** Lambda DNA as a length marker. **Lane 2:** *C. tetani* plasmid E88 DNA digested with *Bam*HI. **Lanes 3–5:** Restriction fragments obtained by simultaneous digestion with *Sac*I/*Eco*RI (**lane 4**) or *Hind*III/*Eco*RI (**lane 5**) were separated together with *Hind*III-digested lambda markers (**lane 3**). **Lanes 6–8:** These lanes correspond to lanes 3–5, hybridized by the southern blot technique with radioactive oligonucleotides. (From ref. 43, with permission.)

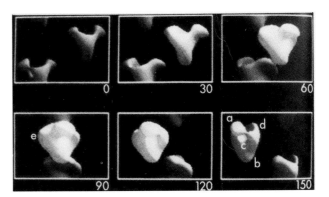

FIG. 11. A gallery of three-dimensional surface representations of tetanospasmin obtained by electron crystallography. The structure resembles a mitten: The "thumb" (*a*) rotates toward the viewer in successive views, and the "wrist" (*b*) points down in all views. Another prominent feature is the groove (*c*) which separates the thumb from the fingers (*d*). (From ref. 47, with permission.)

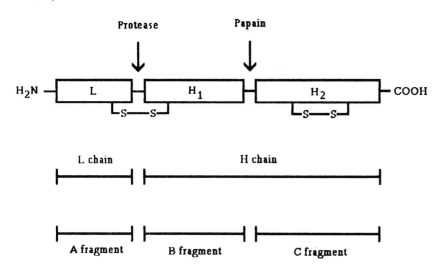

FIG. 12. Various nomenclatures of tetanospasmin fragments. (After ref. 42, with permission.)

transsynaptic transport of the toxin (53). However, some disagreement remains about these distinctions (54). This is a major area of interest in molecular neuroscience, because tetanospasmin and other toxins are extensively employed to probe the mechanisms underlying synaptic transmission.

All of the known clinical manifestations of tetanus result from the propensity of tetanospasmin to inhibit neurotransmitter release by a presynaptic terminal (55). This is a three-step process (Fig. 13): binding to the presynaptic membrane, translation of the toxin to the active site, and induction of paralysis (56). Because tetanospasmin avidly binds to gangliosides, these molecules were proposed as being the "receptors." Various lines of evidence reviewed by Middlebrook (57) now suggest that this binding is nonspecific. Experimental evidence does indicate that a nonganglioside receptor exists (58), but it has not been characterized. Similarly, the process by which the toxin breaches the cell membrane is less well understood than that for a variety of other bacterial toxins (59). The studies performed by Schwab and Thoenen (60) and Montesano et al. (61) suggest that tetanospasmin enters the cell via noncoated vesicles. This contrasts with botulinum toxin, which enters via clathrin-coated pits (62).

Once inside the presynaptic terminal, tetanospasmin can exert a local effect to inhibit transmitter release for several weeks. Although the synaptosomal content of gamma-aminobutyric acid (GABA) is not altered in epileptogenic cortical foci induced by tetanospasmin, the GABA release evoked by depolarization remains decreased for at least 3 weeks (63). Although this block probably occurs at a step after voltage-dependent calcium entry has taken place (64), even this point is debated. Gambale and Montal (65) recently demonstrated that native tetanospasmin or the isolated B fragment spontaneously forms channels in artificial membranes. After entering the cell, the toxin could produce a passive cation channel which would keep the cell depolarized

and therefore unable to release transmitter. Conversely, Aguilera and Yavin (66) reported that tetanospasmin translocates protein kinase C from its inactive cytoplasmic reservoir to its active location on the cell membrane, and then down-regulates it. Because protein kinase C is a crucial mediator of synaptic transmission, these changes may provide another mechanism for the action of tetanospasmin. A third alternative is the inhibition of cyclic guanosine monophosphate (cGMP) accumulation, a necessary step in neurosecretion (67). As Dreyer (68) wrote, "this section should begin with the confession that there is no indication whatever as to the molecular mechanism of action of tetanus toxin."

From the medical standpoint, one of the most important properties of intraneuronal tetanospasmin is its propensity to travel via the retrograde transport system back to the cell body, which allows access to a variety of other neurons (Fig. 14). This process is now known not only to extend from the periphery into the spinal cord, but also to occur across several orders of synaptically connected neurons in the brain (69). The particular clinical manifestations of tetanus depend on the classes and locations of the affected cells, as discussed in the section entitled "Pathogenesis and Pathophysiology," below.

MANIFESTATIONS

Tetanus is traditionally classified into four clinical types: *generalized, localized, cephalic,* and *neonatal.* These distinctions are useful diagnostically but do not reflect toxicologic differences. They do reflect variations in the site of toxin action, which predominate at the neuromuscular junction (NMJ) in some but in central inhibitory systems in others.

Although a portal of entry can be determined in most cases, and should be sought, the lack of a defined wound does not exclude the diagnosis of tetanus. Similarly, bacterial stains and cultures of wounds are of no conse-

1. Attachment to external surface of cell membrane (mediated by C fragment, probably by binding to a receptor molecule)

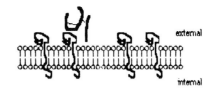

2. Internalization of toxin molecule

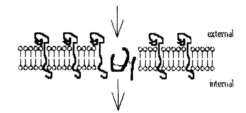

3. Uncoupling of calcium entry from transmitter release

    a. nerve terminal depolarizes normally

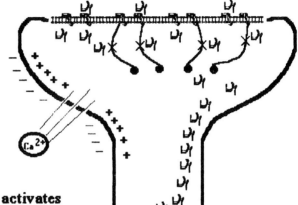

    b. calcium entry activates transmitter release system normally

    c. in the presence of tetanospasmin, transmitter vesicles (●) fail to fuse with the presynaptic membrane; transmitter is not released

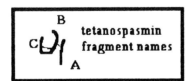

    B
  C   tetanospasmin fragment names
     A

FIG. 13. Steps in tetanospasmin binding, internalization, and activity.

quence in the diagnosis or management of tetanus. A "protective" titer of antitetanus antibody may help to exclude the diagnosis, but only in retrospect.

The temporal development of symptoms in each form of tetanus is of great prognostic significance. The *incubation period* extends from the time of spore inoculation to the first symptom, and the *period of onset* marks the time from that first symptom to the first reflex spasm. Regard-

less of the clinical type of tetanus, shorter periods indicate a poorer prognosis. The portal of entry is another important factor, with burns, umbilical stumps, surgical procedures, compound fractures, septic abortions, and intramuscular injections all associated with lesser chances for recovery. Narcotic addicts appear to develop particularly severe tetanus (70). Fever and tachycardia, if reflecting autonomic dysfunction rather than wound in-

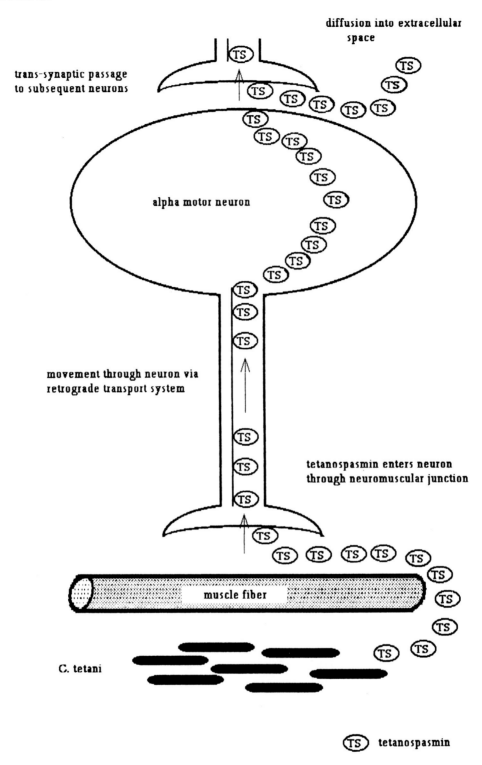

diffusion into extracellular space

trans-synaptic passage to subsequent neurons

alpha motor neuron

movement through neuron via retrograde transport system

tetanospasmin enters neuron through neuromuscular junction

muscle fiber

C. tetani

TS tetanospasmin

FIG. 14. Tetanospasmin diffuses from the site of introduction to the alpha motor neuromuscular junction. It moves via the retrograde transport system to the cell body, from which it diffuses out into the synapses and extracellular space within the spinal cord or brainstem.

TABLE 2. *Rating scale for tetanus*

Score one point for each:
A. Incubation period <7 days
B. Period of onset <48 hr
C. High-risk portal of entry (see text)
D. Generalized tetanus
E. Core temperature above 40°C (104°F)
F. Tachycardia (heart rate >120 in adults, >150 in neonates)

Severity and prognosis

Score	Severity	Mortality
0–1	Mild	<10%
2–3	Moderate	10–20%
4	Severe	20–40%
5–6	Very severe	>50%

Exceptions
A. Cephalic tetanus is always scored as severe or very severe.
B. Neonatal tetanus is always scored as very severe.

fection, are similarly dismal signs. Several authors have developed rating systems for severity and prognosis (71–73), which are summarized in Table 2.

Generalized Tetanus

This is the most commonly recognized form of the disease. It often complicates unrecognized local tetanus, because the focal symptoms are only retrospectively apparent. *Trismus* is caused by rigidity of the masseter muscles, producing inability to open the mouth (Fig. 15); its course can be followed by measuring the distance between the upper and lower teeth with the mouth maximally open. Trismus, or *lockjaw,* is the most common

presenting sign, although back or shoulder stiffness may have been present for hours. *Risus sardonicus,* "a sneering grin . . . thought of old to resemble the effect of a Sardinian ranunculus, which on being chewed contorted the face of the eater" (74), is often a subtle finding which may best be diagnosed by the family or friends of the patient. Physicians can diagnose risus sardonicus by comparison with photographs or in retrospect. Some degree of abdominal rigidity is usual on presentation. The typical generalized spasm resembles decorticate posturing, consisting of "a sudden burst of tonic contraction of muscle groups causing opisthotonos, flexion and adduction of the arms, clenching of the fists on the thorax, and extension of the lower extremities" (75). Although the spasms may be confused with posturing or epileptic seizures, they do not produce loss of consciousness and are extremely painful. Tetanospasmin is epileptogenic in experimental models, but true convulsive seizures in tetanus are probably confined to tetanus patients who have suffered severe hypoxia. Nonepileptiform electroencephalographic abnormalities have been noted, but they were attributed to hypoxia (76).

Respiratory compromise is the most serious early problem in generalized tetanus. Upper airway obstruction is common during spasms. The diaphragm and abdominal musculature are often involved, and they can produce apnea in inadequately treated patients in spite of mechanical ventilation. The NMJ effects of the toxin may produce diaphragmatic paralysis (72) or bilateral abductor vocal cord paralysis (77). With the advent of intensive respiratory care, autonomic dysfunction, usually a hypersympathetic state, is now frequently noted after several days of illness in patients with severe tetanus (78).

The severity of involvement may continue to increase for 10–14 days after diagnosis, reflecting the transport

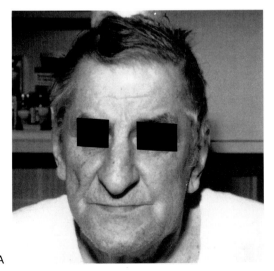
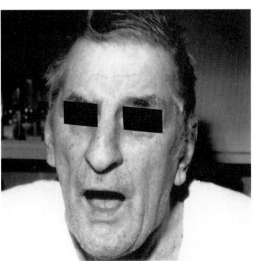

FIG. 15. A: Risus sardonicus. Note the straightened upper lip at rest. **B:** Trismus. The patient is instructed to open his mouth as fully as possible.

time of intraneuronal toxin into the central nervous system (CNS). Recovery then begins, usually requiring about 4 weeks. This period probably reflects the synthesis and transport of presynaptic constituents. In the absence of antitoxin, the disease persists as long as tetanospasmin is produced. The total amount of toxin produced is so small that it is inadequate to prompt an immune response; therefore, patients with newly diagnosed tetanus must be actively immunized. Recurrent tetanus is well documented if this is not done (79,80).

Localized Tetanus

Fixed rigidity of the muscles associated with a site of injury (which may include agonists, antagonists, and fixators) is the hallmark of localized tetanus. This may be mild, may persist for months without progression, and usually resolves spontaneously. The muscles involved may be painful, and deep tendon reflexes are enhanced. Neuromuscular transmission may be affected locally, producing weakness in addition to rigidity. Partial immunity to tetanospasmin may contribute to the development of local tetanus by decreasing the hematogenous spread of toxin (81). More commonly, however, local tetanus is the harbinger of the generalized form, unless treated.

Cephalic Tetanus

Cephalic tetanus is a form of localized tetanus which most commonly affects the lower-cranial-nerve musculature. Facial paresis is usually present (82), and it may be the presenting manifestation (83). Dysphagia has also been reported (84), and videofluoroscopy may be useful in its diagnosis and management (85). Although most series suggest a poor prognosis, a large report from India described many mild cases associated with chronic otitis media (86). This may represent colonization of the infected tissue with *C. tetani,* and subsequently the production of toxin. Cephalic tetanus has been described in a fully immunized patient (87). Rarely, extraocular movements are also affected, causing "ophthalmoplegic tetanus" (88) or supranuclear oculomotor palsies (89).

Neonatal Tetanus

Neonatal tetanus usually follows infection of the umbilical stump, often as a consequence of improper care. Because passively transferred maternal antibody is protective, the condition occurs only when the mother lacks immunity. Although ritual practices such as placing soil or cow dung on the stump may contribute (90), most cases probably arise from lack of aseptic technique in dividing the umbilical cord and dressing the stump. Four

factors are involved: (i) the length of the stump (longer appears to be safer), (ii) the care with which the cord is ligated, (iii) the cleanliness of the instruments and dressings, and (iv) the cleanliness of the environment and of the patient's and mother's clothing (91). Although these concerns are important on their own merits, active maternal immunization—or, if this should fail, passive immunization of the mother before delivery and of the child at birth—would eliminate the disease.

The most common presentation is weakness and inability to suck, usually presenting during the second week of life. Tetanic spasms and rigidity occur later, producing the typical opisthotonic posture. The hypersympathetic state occurs commonly in these infants, and it is often the cause of their death. Developmental retardation is common in survivors (92).

PATHOGENESIS AND PATHOPHYSIOLOGY

The actions of tetanospasmin predominantly involve three components of the nervous system: central motor control, autonomic function, and the NMJ. The central effects have been studied most intensively, and they provide paradigms for understanding the toxin's effects on other nervous system components.

Central Motor Control Effects

To express its toxic potential, tetanospasmin must gain access to its target neurons. The toxin appears to enter the nervous system predominantly through the NMJ of alpha motor neurons (93,94). Some toxin enters sensory and autonomic neurons, but the amount appears small and its contribution to symptoms is uncertain (95). It then moves, via the retrograde transport system, to the cell body (96). This system, consisting of microtubules and transport proteins, is normally used to bring signal molecules and exhausted presynaptic components back to the cell body for processing. It is also the mode of entry of some viruses, such as rabies and herpes simplex (97), into the CNS. The heavy chain or the C fragment of the toxin is necessary for retrograde transport (98). Tetanospasmin also spreads hematogenously from its site of production, but it still must enter via neurons (99). Toxin already in transit within the neuron is inaccessible to antitoxin, which partly explains the progression of the disease for several days after treatment. The intrathecal administration of human tetanus immunoglobulin (HTIG) represents an attempt to circumvent this problem (see section entitled "Immunotherapy," below).

Once transported to the spinal cord or the brainstem, the toxin then migrates transsynaptically into presynaptic inhibitory cells (100) which use either glycine or GABA as transmitters (Fig. 16) (101,102). The glyciner-

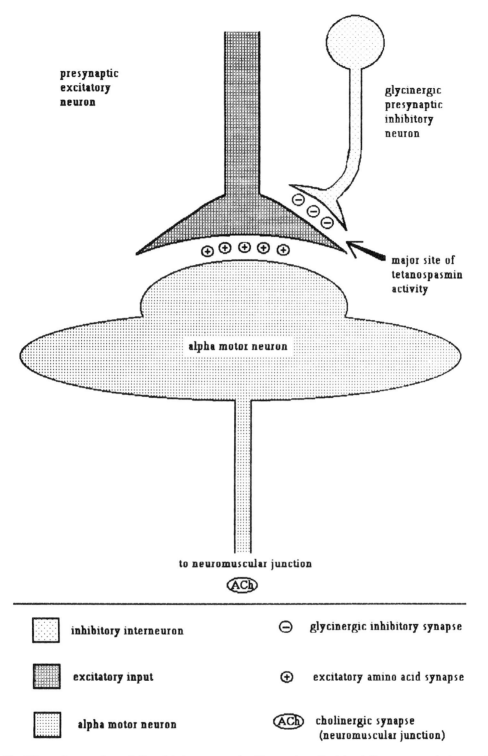

FIG. 16. Sites of synaptic activity of tetanospasmin. The major effect is at the synapse between the glycinergic presynaptic inhibitory neuron and the presynaptic excitatory neuron. The toxin can also inhibit the release of other transmitters, including those of excitatory amino acid synapses and of the neuromuscular junction.

gic cells are most important in the spinal cord, whereas the GABAergic cells are responsible for decreasing inhibition from the brainstem (103). Strychnine, which produces a similar clinical disorder, affects only the glycinergic cells. By preventing glycine or GABA release, tetanospasmin denies the alpha motor neuron its most essential inhibitory transmitters. This raises its resting firing rate, causing muscle rigidity. More seriously, the normal inhibition of other motor neurons during movements of a particular motor group depends on these inhibitory transmitters, as does the termination of reflexive contractions. Bereft of this inhibition, the motor system responds to an afferent stimulus with the intense, sustained contraction of a wide range of muscles that characterizes the tetanic spasm.

Histologic abnormalities have been reported in the brainstem nuclei in fatal cases (104), but the significance of these changes is unknown. They most likely reflect terminal hypoxia and autonomic dysfunction, rather than a direct effect of tetanospasmin. *Reversible* chromatolysis of motor neurons occurs in experimental tetanus when markedly suprathreshold doses of toxin are employed (105). Whether this is simply a manifestation of hypermetabolism or reflects another pathophysiologic process is unresolved.

Once transported into the CNS, the toxin can continue its rostral movement by further retrograde transport (106). This implies that structures above the brainstem could be affected by tetanospasmin; however, there is no evidence that this occurs in the natural history of tetanus. It is likely that generalized tetanus does involve some vertical movement of toxin within the neuraxis, but the widespread manifestations in this form are mostly due to the hematogenous dissemination of toxin to NMJs throughout the body. Tetanospasmin does inhibit the evoked release of norepinephrine (107), acetylcholine (108), and enkephalin (109) from brain tissue *in vitro*. Tetanospasmin is epileptogenic, producing (a) depolarizing shifts when added to CNS tissue in culture (110) and (b) partial seizures when injected intracerebrally (111). These seizures are associated with diminished extracellular GABA levels (112). Although these findings are intriguing, their clinical correlates are uncertain.

In addition to loss of inhibitory systems, excitatory transmission is also disrupted (113). This may partially explain the weakness associated with local tetanus.

Autonomic Nervous System Effects

Prior to modern intensive care, most patients with severe tetanus died quickly from ventilatory failure (114). Although autonomic involvement was mentioned in 1954 (115), the first major report of this aspect of tetanus appeared in 1968 (116). The latter group described "a

characteristic syndrome whose features include sustained but labile hypertension and tachycardia, irregularities of cardiac rhythm, peripheral vascular constriction, profuse sweating, pyrexia, increased carbon dioxide output, increased urinary catecholamine excretion, and, in some cases, the development of hypotension." Although these signs are usually present toward the end of the first week, they may develop during the second (117). Most are associated with elevated catecholamine levels. Domenighetti et al. (118) reported a patient with a plasma norepinephrine concentration of 14.1 nmol/liter (normal range: 1.2–2.9) and a plasma epinephrine concentration of 2.3 nmol/liter (normal range: 0.11–0.44). Kerr et al. (116) reported 24-hr urine catecholamine excretions ranging from 70 to 1000 μg/day, with a mean of 490 μg/day (normal range: up to 450 μg/day). Using a different assay, Kanerek et al. (119) described a patient whose 24-hr urinary catecholamine excretion was 225 μg/day (normal range: up to 25 μg/day). These manifestations resemble the effects of a pheochromocytoma; a similar cardiomyopathy is seen in both conditions (120).

Tetanospasmin disinhibits sympathetic reflexes at the spinal level, implying that the hyperadrenergic findings are not dependent on hypothalamic or brainstem dysfunction (121). The same group later showed that cutaneous stimulation of animals with local tetanus increased firing rates in renal sympathetic nerves (122). Conversely, the development of inappropriate antidiuretic hormone secretion may support hypothalamic involvement (123).

Clinical evidence suggests some disruption of parasympathetic function as well. Bradycardia is occasionally noted (124), as is hypotension without previous evidence of increased sympathetic tone. Although both of these findings can be reproduced by injection of tetanospasmin into a rat's third ventricle (125), a more peripheral mechanism appears likely in human tetanus. Gastric emptying is occasionally disrupted (71).

Neuromuscular Junction Effects

Because the central effects of tetanospasmin are so dramatic, the peripheral disorder it produces received scant clinical attention until 1977 (82). These investigators showed denervation changes in the muscle closest to the site of injury, which reflected failure of neuromuscular transmission. In fact, experimental studies by Harvey (126) had established the presence of neuromuscular blockade 40 years earlier. More recently, single-fiber electromyography has confirmed a presynaptic defect of acetylcholine release qualitatively similar to that of botulism (127). The NMJ may be permanently disabled by tetanospasmin; return of function requires sprouting of the terminal end to produce new synapses (128).

Tetanospasmin as a Research Tool

In addition to the usefulness of tetanospasmin in experimental studies of tetanus, a wealth of laboratory uses for this agent have been developed. These applications are of interest to the clinician not only because they cast light on disease mechanisms, but also because laboratory workers are exposed to the toxin. Because tetanospasmin binds avidly to the gangliosides of neurons, but not at all to non-neural cells of the nervous system, it is an important immunohistochemical marker (129) [tetanospasmin will label between 35% and 95% of neuroendocrine small-cell lung cancer cells (130), and most neuroblastomas and pheochromocytomas (131)]. Injection of tetanospasmin into the brain produces a robust model of epilepsy in both the limbic system (132) and the cerebral cortex (133). It can aid in the study of behavioral disorders (134), act as a probe of synaptic functions (135), and assist in determining the role of gangliosides in neurotransmission (136).

APPROACH TO DIAGNOSIS

Tetanus can only be diagnosed clinically; laboratory assistance is confined to the exclusion of other diagnoses, and to the determination of immunity. Electromyographic (EMG) studies may also be useful by showing evidence of denervation, reinnervation, and increased excitability of the motor neuron pool (137). Single-fiber EMG studies are mentioned above. Generalized and cephalic tetanus are easily recognized if one thinks of the disease. Localized tetanus is more difficult to detect early. The neonatal form is less easily recognized on initial presentation, but it rapidly becomes obvious.

Gowers (11), again, provided an unequaled clinical description in 1888:

The first symptom is usually a sense of stiffness in the neck or jaw, sometimes difficulty in swallowing, or stiffness of the tongue. . . . In the course of a few hours, or at most a day or two, the difficulty in separating the jaws becomes greater, and is clearly due to increasing rigidity of the masseters. With this there is also more stiffness in the neck, and the head is slightly bent backward from the preponderance of spasm in the extensor muscles. As the rigidity in the neck increases, it passes down the spinal muscles. . . . The legs may also become extended and rigid, but the arms are little affected.

A few patients have atypical features on presentation. The lack of an easily identified portal of entry, discussed above, does not exclude the diagnosis but makes prognostication more difficult because the incubation period cannot be determined. These patients should be carefully examined for signs of parenteral drug abuse, otitis, or rectal or vaginal instrumentation. Recent injections or minor surgical procedures may be uncovered by questioning. Lesions of the gastrointestinal tract are occasionally implicated, especially among inhabitants of rural areas among whom the carriage rate of *C. tetani* may be 20-fold higher than that of urban dwellers (138).

Differential Diagnosis

Although many disorders have small areas of overlap with tetanus, strychnine intoxication (139) is the only true mimic. This drug is a direct antagonist at the glycine receptor (140). Lack of abdominal rigidity between spasms may be more common with strychnine than with tetanus, and trismus may be absent in the former (74); otherwise, the clinical presentations are similar. For this reason, biochemical analyses of serum and urine for strychnine should be performed in suspected tetanus cases, and tetanus should be considered even when strychnine poisoning is likely. The initial symptomatic management of both conditions relies on benzodiazepines, but their subsequent treatments and complications differ substantially. Many other glycine and GABA antagonists have been exploited as experimental convulsant agents; although human poisoning has not been reported, conditions resembling tetanus may be expected.

Dystonic reactions to dopamine blockade usually involve torticollis, and oculogyric crises are common. Neither of these phenomena are part of tetanus, and reflex spasms are not seen. A rapid response to anticholinergic agents (benztropine, 1–2 mg; or diphenhydramine, 50 mg) and subsequent toxicologic studies confirm this diagnosis. A trial of anticholinergic agents is reasonable in suspected tetanus if the diagnosis is in doubt.

The nuchal rigidity of meningitis may resemble the neck stiffness of tetanus, but the other manifestations of each disorder should resolve any confusion. The cerebrospinal fluid is normal in tetanus. The other infection which may raise a question of tetanus is an alveolar ridge abscess producing trismus. Oral pain and tenderness is not characteristic of tetanus; the patient with a dental disorder will not display spasms or rigidity. Verma et al. (141) described a single case of unilateral trismus resulting from a tuberculoma of the brainstem.

Patients experiencing generalized convulsive status epilepticus may at first appear to have tetanic spasms, but the loss of consciousness and evolutionary movements of the former should quickly resolve any question.

Tetany precipitated by hypocalcemia or alkalosis will be accompanied by Chvostek's and Trousseau's signs. In contrast to tetanus, tetany involves the extremities more than the axial musculature.

Progressive fluctuating muscular rigidity (the "stiff-man" syndrome) has been likened to a chronic form of tetanus (142). This idiopathic syndrome has an insidious onset, usually has minimal cranial-nerve involvement, lacks trismus, and is relieved during sleep. Recent evidence links this disorder to autoantibodies against GABAergic neurons (143).

Although "pseudotetanus" has been used to describe a broad variety of disorders (144), analogy with "pseudoseizure" suggests that pseudotetanus be reserved for a psychogenic disorder in which the patient's movements resemble tetanus. The patient's posture may be complex or inconsistent; rigidity is lacking or obviously feigned, the patient is distractable, and some secondary gain is desired. We have cared for a tetanus patient who manifested pseudotetanus whenever removal of her tracheostomy was discussed. Preexisting psychologic problems may also complicate the diagnosis and management of tetanus (145).

Determination of Immunity

When properly administered and maintained, immunization with alum-adsorbed tetanus toxoid is highly effective, with an estimated failure rate of less than four per 100 million persons in immunocompetent populations (146). Therefore, a confirmed history of active immunization almost eliminates tetanus as a diagnosis. This includes both an acceptable initial series and a booster within 10 years.

The serum concentration of antitetanus antibodies can be measured by immunoassay or hemagglutination (147), but the results are seldom available in time to influence initial diagnosis and management. The results are quantitated in international units (IU) of antitoxin by reference to an arbitrary international standard. A recent report of a rapid test holds promise not only for the exclusion of tetanus but also for decisions regarding antitoxin administration (148); see section entitled "Therapy," below. In most epidemiologic studies, a level of 0.01 IU/ml is accepted as protective, based upon studies on guinea pigs reported in 1937 (149). Although this level has generally been held to be protective in humans, cases of tetanus have been reported with titers as high as 0.16 IU/ml (150). In one study of 64 tetanus patients, 24 had detectable antitoxin levels, and 10 had levels ≥ 0.01 IU/ml (151). The severity of tetanus tended to be less in the patients with higher levels, but six of the 10 required tracheostomy and mechanical ventilation. Some of the disparity among studies may reflect the insensitivity of the test systems to antibodies which are actually protective. In a bioassay, a mixture of several different monoclonal antibodies was necessary for protection; the most active single clone (that against the amino-terminal end of the heavy chain) was 100-fold less active than a polyclonal antiserum (152).

THERAPY

A patient with generalized tetanus requires the best possible intensive care. In this disease, the patient may become completely dependent on mechanical ventilation and the most extreme pharmacotherapy, yet stand a good chance of walking out of the hospital without deficits. Thus, patients with tetanus must be managed in facilities which can provide the high level of services required. Table 3 presents a time-based protocol which we have found effective in generalized tetanus. Some of the more important or controversial aspects are discussed below. In local tetanus, a similar approach is useful if adjusted for the patient's symptoms. Autonomic management in neonatal tetanus has not been studied, but it would likely be similar to that in older children and adults.

As the population at risk for tetanus becomes older, it becomes more important to recognize that elderly patients without serious chronic disease can survive generalized tetanus and its intensive therapy, and return to their premorbid state (153).

Portal of Entry

In most cases, the wound responsible for tetanus is still visible on presentation. If there is a surgical indication, débridement should be performed after spasms are controlled by benzodiazepines (and under local anesthesia). There is no apparent benefit of débridement for tetanus itself.

If no portal of entry is apparent, the patient should be carefully examined for ear infection, uterine disease, and foreign bodies.

Immunotherapy

Neutralization of tetanospasmin which has not yet entered the nervous system will shorten the course of the disease and may reduce its severity. HTIG should be administered as soon as spasms can be controlled. The retrospective studies of Blake et al. (154) have demonstrated the effectiveness of antitoxin. They also showed that a dose of 500 IU is as effective as the commonly recommended 3000- to 5000-IU dose. The smaller amount can be given as a single intramuscular injection. Because each injection is a potent stimulus for tetanic spasms, this is not a trivial point. In those rare areas where HTIG is not available, equine antitetanus serum is used after testing and desensitization.

Once the toxin has entered the motor neuron, it is no longer available for neutralization by the antibody. Intrathecal administration makes specific immunoglobulin available where the toxin diffuses out of the motor neuron into other CNS structures. Gupta et al. (155) showed 250 units of intrathecal HTIG to be superior to 1000 units administered intramuscularly. The HTIG preparations currently available in the United States are not licensed for intrathecal use, and they contain potentially neurotoxic preservatives.

TABLE 3. *Management protocol for generalized tetanus*

I. Diagnosis and stabilization: first hour after presentation
   A. Assess airway and ventilation. If necessary, prepare for endotracheal intubation under benzodiazepine sedation and neuromuscular blockade (e.g., vecuronium 0.1 mg/kg).
   B. Obtain samples for antitoxin level, strychnine and dopamine antagonist assays, electrolytes, blood urea nitrogen, creatinine, creatine kinase, and urinary myoglobin determination.
   C. Determine the portal of entry, incubation period, period of onset, and immunization history.
   D. Administer benztropine (1–2 mg, intravenously) or diphenhydramine (50 mg, intravenously) to rule out a dystonic reaction.
   E. Administer a benzodiazepine intravenously (diazepam in 5-mg increments, or lorazepam in 2-mg increments) to control spasm and decrease rigidity. Initially, employ a dose adequate to produce sedation and minimize reflex spasms. If this dose compromises the airway or ventilation, intubate using a short-acting neuromuscular blocking agent prior to transferring the patient to a quiet, darkened area of the intensive care unit.

II. Early management phase: first 24 hours
   A. Administer human tetanus immunoglobulin (HTIG), 500 units, intramuscularly.
   B. At a different site, administer adsorbed tetanus toxoid such as tetanus–diphtheria vaccine (0.5 ml) or diphtheria–pertussis–tetanus vaccine (0.5 ml), as appropriate for age, intramuscularly. Adsorbed tetanus toxoid without diphtheria toxoid is available for patients with a history of reaction to diphtheria toxoid; otherwise, the correct combination for the patient's age should be employed.
   C. Consider intrathecal administration of HTIG.
   D. Begin metronidazole—500 mg, intravenously, every 6 hr, for 7–10 days.
   E. Perform a tracheostomy after placement of an endotracheal tube and under neuromuscular blockade if spasms produce any degree of airway compromise.
   F. Débride wound if indicated for its own management.
   G. Place a soft, small-bore nasal feeding tube or a central venous hyperalimentation catheter.
   H. Administer benzodiazepines as needed to control spasms and produce sedation. If adequate control is not achieved, institute long-term neuromuscular blockade (e.g., vecuronium 6–8 mg/hr); continue benzodiazepines for sedation with intermittent electroencephalographic monitoring to ensure somnolence.

III. Intermediate management phase: next 2–3 weeks
   A. Treat sympathetic hyperactivity with labetalol (0.25–1.0 mg/min) or morphine (0.5–1.0 mg/kg/hr). Consider epidural blockade with local anesthetics. Do not use diuretics for blood pressure control, because volume depletion will worsen autonomic instability.
   B. If hypotension is present, place a pulmonary artery catheter and an arterial line, and administer fluids, dopamine, or norepinephrine.
   C. Sustained bradycardia usually requires a pacemaker. Atropine or isoproterenol may be useful during pacemaker placement.
   D. Begin prophylactic heparin.
   E. Use a flotation bed if possible, to prevent skin breakdown and peroneal nerve palsies. Otherwise, ensure frequent turning and employ antirotation boots.
   F. Maintain benzodiazepines until neuromuscular blockade, if employed, has been terminated and the severity of spasms has diminished substantially. Taper the dose over 14–21 days.
   G. Begin rehabilitation planning.

IV. Convalescent stage: 2–6 weeks
   A. When spasms are no longer present, begin physical therapy. Many patients require supportive psychotherapy.
   B. Before discharge, administer another dose of tetanus–diphtheria vaccine or diphtheria–pertussis–tetanus vaccine.
   C. Schedule a third dose of toxoid to be given 4 weeks after the second.

Active immunization is also required to prevent recurrent tetanus.

Corticosteroids

In 1954, Lewis et al. (156) attempted to show that steroids would diminish tetanus mortality. A group of 10 patients treated with oral cortisone (in a dose "that appeared to be just sufficient to counteract or prevent a rise in the temperature") experienced 60% survival; the 20 historical controls had only 15% survival. However, a group of five patients receiving intramuscular hydrocortisone all died. The question was later addressed by Paydas et al. (157); they found a trend toward a significant improvement in survival in 32 patients randomized to 40 mg of daily prednisolone when compared with 31

patients receiving placebo. The mechanism by which steroid treatment might improve survival in tetanus is obscure, and at present the use of such treatment should be considered experimental.

Airway Control and Ventilation

Because the upper airway is frequently occluded during tetanic spasms, it must be protected rapidly and effectively. An endotracheal tube may be passed under sedation and neuromuscular blockade. A soft, small-bore feeding tube should be placed concurrently. Because the endotracheal tube itself is a strong stimulus for spasms, some authors recommend that a tracheostomy be performed immediately (158). Although this procedure is often necessary, we believe that it can be decided individually. The patient may not require mechanical ventilation once the airway is secure and treatment has begun. Because pneumonia and pneumothorax occur commonly and produce fatalities, scrupulous pulmonary hygiene and ventilatory management are required (159). Tetanospasmin can inhibit macrophage function, but the relevance of this deficit to infectious complications is unknown (160).

Antibiotic Management

In vitro, C. tetani is sensitive to metronidazole, penicillins, cephalosporins, imipenen, macrolides, and tetracycline. However, the utility of antibiotic therapy for what is essentially an intoxication has often been questioned. Most authors recommending antibiotics have suggested large doses of penicillin. As a centrally acting GABA antagonist (161), penicillin may act synergistically with tetanospasmin to worsen spasms, and it could diminish benzodiazepine efficacy. High doses of penicillin might also lead to colonization of patients with resistant organisms, increasing morbidity from nosocomial infection. One study compared metronidazole (500 mg every 6 hr, orally) to penicillin (1.5 million units every 8 hr, intramuscularly); the metronidazole group demonstrated significantly less progression of disease, shorter hospitalization, and better survival (162). Although this may mean that metronidazole is superior to penicillin, it also suggests the possibility that penicillin is worse than no treatment at all. No placebo-controlled studies are available. At present, metronidazole should be used.

Antispasticity Agents

The benzodiazepines are the best agents currently available for the relief of spasms and rigidity. They are GABA$_A$ agonists, thereby indirectly antagonizing the effects of the toxin on inhibitory systems (163). Diazepam has received the greatest use, but lorazepam may be preferable because of its longer duration of action. The pharmacokinetics of these agents have not been studied at the exceptional doses and durations employed in treating tetanus. Doses in excess of 500 mg of diazepam (or 200 mg of lorazepam) may be required daily (164). Because such large doses, given intravenously, contain enough propylene glycol to induce metabolic acidosis (165), administration of benzodiazepines through a feeding tube should begin as soon as possible. Because midazolam does not require propylene glycol for solubility, it may become the agent of choice. It must be given by continuous infusion at a rate of 5–15 mg/hr because of its short half-life. Discontinuation of these agents may produce withdrawal symptoms, and they should therefore be tapered over 2 weeks.

Continuous intrathecal administration of baclofen (a GABA$_B$ agonist) may diminish the need for sedation and

ventilatory support and may therefore shorten hospitalization (166). This approach holds promise in regions where tetanus is relatively common, but it should probably not be considered a standard treatment in the more developed countries. Dantrolene, a direct muscle relaxant, may also be valuable in selected cases (167). It does not appear to have advantages over other therapeutic modalities, however.

Although barbiturates and neuroleptics have been employed for sedation of tetanus patients, they are inferior agents for this indication and are best avoided. Propofol, a new nonbarbiturate sedative, may prove to be a useful adjunct because of its short duration of action (168,169). However, since it lacks GABA agonist activity in the motor system, it should not be used as a single agent.

Neuromuscular Junction Blockade

When GABAergic agents are unable to control tetanus, neuromuscular blockade becomes necessary. Vecuronium (6–8 mg/hr) is the current agent of choice because it induces minimal autonomic instability (170). Atracurium has also been recommended (171). During the period of NMJ blockade, the patient must be adequately sedated to prevent the conscious perception and memory of this frightening situation (172). Because autonomic signs cannot be relied upon to signal inadequate sedation in this setting, electroencephalographic monitoring is indicated.

Therapy for Autonomic Dysfunction

Combined alpha- and beta-adrenergic blockade with labetalol is presently the treatment of choice for the hypersympathetic state in tetanus (118). Isolated beta-adrenergic blockade leaves the alpha-adrenergic vasoconstrictor response unopposed, and it should not be used. Buchanan et al. (173) described a child with tetanus who died after propranolol administration, probably from myocardial failure in the setting of a catecholamine-induced myocarditis. Clonidine may be a useful alternative (174). Morphine has also been shown to be effective, although the mechanism is uncertain (175). Tetanospasmin inhibits the release of enkephalins, which may play a modulatory role in the autonomic system. Epidural anesthesia is also effective, perhaps by decreasing adrenal stimulation (176).

Excessive parasympathetic function occurs rarely. If bradycardia or asystole occur, a pacemaker should be considered (177).

Nutrition

The nutritional requirements of tetanus patients are extraordinary, owing both to their muscular activity and to their excessive autonomic activity. The protein and calories required to maintain a positive nitrogen balance may exceed the maximal tolerable daily volume of enteral formulas (178). Gastric emptying may also be impaired. Thus, central venous nutrition may be necessary. However, we have successfully managed some patients with enteral feedings after controlling their neuromuscular and autonomic states.

COMPLICATIONS OF TETANUS

In the past, respiratory dysfunction was the most feared result of tetanus and was the major cause of death. The neuropathologic consequences of hypoxia (in concert with hyperthermia) probably accounted for earlier reports of brainstem neuronal destruction in this disease (104). However, the CNS and systemic consequences of hypoxia continue to occur, due to either delayed or inadequate treatment of respiratory problems (179). Cardiovascular consequences of autonomic instability, including cardiomyopathy, are still seen and may be less amenable to secondary prevention.

Phrenic and laryngeal neuropathies as a consequence of tetanus are discussed above (72,73). Other mononeuropathies probably occur. As in any sedated or paralyzed patient, care must be taken to prevent common peroneal nerve compression at the fibular head, which produces foot drop.

Rhabdomyolysis, which may lead to acute renal failure, is very common in generalized tetanus. If the serum creatine kinase level exceeds 5000 U/liter, or myoglobin is detected in the urine, hydration with normal saline and urinary alkalinization with sodium bicarbonate should be considered. Myositis ossificans circumscripta is a long-term complication of severe muscular hyperactivity, coupled with hematoma formation and anoxia (180). Vertebral compression fractures are common, especially in older patients. About 40% of patients have psychologic aftereffects, and 25% feel that their health has permanently worsened in some manner after recovery from tetanus (145).

PREVENTION

In the immunocompetent host, tetanus is an "inexcusable disease" (181). Active immunization with tetanus toxoid is one of the most effective preventive measures in medicine, and passive immunization may be performed at the time of any tetanus-prone wound.

Prophylactic Active Immunization

A series of three intramuscular injections of alum-adsorbed tetanus toxoid (10 lyophilized units; 0.5 ml) provides almost complete immunity to tetanus for at least 5 years. Other forms of toxoid are less immuno-

genic and should be avoided (182). If the immunization program began in infancy, a fourth dose should be administered 1 year after the third, with a fifth dose being administered upon elementary school matriculation. Some recent data suggest that the fourth dose may not be necessary (183); until this work is confirmed, it should still be given. The vaccine to be used varies with age: Children under the age of 7 years should receive combined diphtheria–tetanus–pertussis vaccine; if pertussis vaccine is considered to be contraindicated, diphtheria–tetanus adsorbed vaccine for pediatric use should be employed (184). In those over 7 years of age, tetanus–diphtheria vaccine is recommended. The complete series must be given; 30% of a group of elderly patients had inadequate antibody levels 4 years after a series of two injections (all who received three injections were protected) (185). Routine boosters should be given every 10 years; giving them more frequently may increase the risk of an adverse reaction (186). If *fluid* toxoid was used for previous immunizations, a dose of adsorbed toxoid should be given.

By introducing a plasmid encoding tetanospasmin fragment C into a *Salmonella typhimurium* aroA mutant carrier, Fairweather et al. (187) induced antitetanus immunity in mice by either oral or intravenous administration of the bacteria. This work suggests that a one- or two-dose oral vaccine may be available in the future.

In a small number of patients with humoral immunodeficiencies, the prescribed toxoid regimen does not produce immunity (188). Although antitetanus antibody is usually of the IgG1 subclass, three of six children with isolated IgG2 deficiency demonstrated poor responses to tetanus toxoid (189). This is also true of some patients infected with human immunodeficiency virus (HIV) (190). Whenever a question of immunity to tetanospasmin exists (whether it is due to failure of immunization or due to an underlying disorder of immunity), passive immunization is indicated after tetanus-prone injuries. Although limited *in vitro* evidence suggests that tetanus toxoid immunization may provoke HIV activation (191), there is no clinical evidence to suggest that patients with HIV infection should not receive tetanus toxoid when indicated. However, loss of response to soluble antigens like tetanus toxoid is one of the first immunologic consequences of HIV infection (192), suggesting that HIV-infected patients may not become immune after toxoid administration. Both HIV-1 and HIV-2 interfere with the proliferation of tetanus-specific T lymphocytes *in vitro* (193), raising the further concern that such patients may become unprotected even if they were previously adequately immunized. The gp120 envelope protein may be responsible for this effect (194). Administration of a monoclonal antibody which recognizes the leukocyte common antigen CD45 augments the response of peripheral blood mononuclear cells to tetanus toxoid *in vitro* (195), raising the possibility that a similar manipulation may be beneficial *in vivo*.

Immunization Following Injury

All patients who last received tetanus toxoid more than 10 years before an injury, or who do not recall their last immunization, should receive active immunization with tetanus–diphtheria vaccine for any injury that brings them to medical attention. If their wounds are considered tetanus-prone, they should be immunized after a 5-year interval. Tetanus-prone wounds include: those contaminated with dirt, feces, or saliva; punctures (including the use of unsterile needles, or injections through unprepared skin); missile wounds; burns; frostbite; avulsions; and crush injuries. Patients in whom the prior immunization history is incomplete or unknown should receive a full series of three monthly injections. Those with humoral immunodeficiencies should receive passive immunization after all such injuries unless immunity to tetanospasmin has been serologically demonstrated recently.

Clean, minor wounds are generally believed to carry such a low risk of tetanus that passive immunization is not recommended (146). A tetanus-prone wound in a patient with an incomplete or uncertain initial immunization history should prompt passive immunization with HTIG (250 units, intramuscularly). HTIG should also be considered for those whose immune status is in question.

Adverse Reactions to Tetanus Toxoid

A mild degree of local tenderness and edema is common after tetanus toxoid booster injections; fever is occasionally noted. Rare anaphylactoid responses, and delayed hypersensitivity to the preservative thiomersal, were documented in a large survey (196). Peripheral neuropathic complications (197), which may resemble the Guillain–Barré syndrome (198) or be relapsing (199), have been the subject of case reports.

ACKNOWLEDGMENTS

The author gratefully acknowledges the assistance of the following individuals: Paul C. Schrechenberger, Ph.D., University of Illinois, and Alex Kuritza, Ph.D., Rush Medical College, who provided Fig. 5; and Melvyn Wichter, M.D., Rush Medical College, who provided Fig. 15.

REFERENCES

1. Breasted JH. *The Edwin Smith surgical papyrus.* Chicago: University of Chicago Press, 1930.
2. Ghaliounggui P. *Magic and medical science in ancient Egypt.* London: Hodder & Stoughton, 1963.
3. Adams F. *The extant works of Aretaeus, the Cappadocian.* London: Publications of the Sydenham Society, 1856.
4. John of Arderne. De arte phisicali et de chirurgia of Master John Arderne, Surgeon of Newark, dated 1412. Cited in: Clendening L. *Source book of medical history.* New York: Paul B Hober, 1942.
5. Cullen W. First lines of the practice of physic. Dublin, 1791. Cited in: Mettler CA, Mettler FA. *History of medicine.* Philadelphia: Blakiston, 1947;157–175.
6. Bell C. *Essays on the anatomy and physiology of expression,* 2nd ed. London: J Murray, 1824.
7. de Ulloa A. Noticias Americanas: entretenimientos physicohistorios. Madrid, 1772. Cited in: Mettler CA, Mettler FA. *History of medicine.* Philadelphia: Blakiston, 1947;745–746.
8. Clarke J. An account of a disease which until lately proven fatal to a great number of infants in the Lying-In Hospital of Dublin. *Med Facts Observ* 1792;3:78–104. Cited in: Mettler CA, Mettler FA. *History of medicine.* Philadelphia: Blakiston, 1947. p. 746.
9. Sims JM. Trismus nascentium: its pathology and treatment. *Am J Med Sci* 1846;11:363–379.
10. Beumer O. Zur aitologischen Bedeutung der Tetanus-bacillen. *Berl Klin Wochenschr* 1887;00:541–543, 575–577. Cited in: Mettler CA, Mettler FA. *History of medicine.* Philadelphia: Blakiston, 1947.
11. Gowers WR. *A manual of diseases of the nervous system.* Philadelphia: Blakiston, 1888.
12. Nicolaier A. Ueber infectiösen tetanus. *Dtsch Med Wochenschr* 1884;10:842–844.
13. Behring E, Kitasato S. Ueber das zustandekommen der diphtherie-immunität und der tetanus-immunität bei thieren. *Dtsch Med Wochenschr* 1890;16:1113–1114.
14. Ceroli G. Storia di tetano sanato coll'acetato di morphina praticato guista il metodo endermico: guintair altea storia di neuralgia curata dello stesso modo. *Ann Univ Med Milano* 1829;50:239–247. Cited in: Mettler CA, Mettler FA. *History of medicine.* Philadelphia: Blakiston, 1947. p. 579.
15. Mollaret P. Prélude, choral et fugue au XIXe siècle de la curarisation dans le tétanos. *Presse Med* 1965;73:2313–2317.
16. Hoffman FA. Ein fall von tetanus traumaticus mit curare behandelt. *Berl Klin Wochenschr* 1879;16:637–638.
17. Meigs JF, Pepper W. *A practical treatise on the diseases of children,* 6th ed. Philadelphia: 1877. Cited in: Mettler CA, Mettler FA. *History of medicine.* Philadelphia: Blakiston, 1947. p. 776.
18. Hutchinson J, Jackson JH. On cases of recovery from traumatic tetanus. *Med Times Gazette* 1861;1:360–363.
19. Meltzer SJ, Auer J. The effects of intraspinal injection of magnesium salts upon tetanus. *J Exp Med* 1906;8:692–706.
20. Edsall G. Introduction. In: Edsall G, ed. *Proceedings of the fourth international conference on tetanus, Dakar.* Lyon: Fondation Merieux, 1975;19–20.
21. Cvjetanovic B. Public health aspects of tetanus control. In: Veronesi R, ed. *Tetanus: important new concepts.* Amsterdam: Excerpta Medica, 1981;1–7.
22. Centers for Disease Control. Summary of notifiable disease, 1988. *MMWR* 1989;38:39.
23. Centers for Disease Control. Tetanus—United States, 1982–1984. *MMWR* 1985;34:601–611.
24. Sutter RW, Cochi SL, Brink EW, Sirotkin BI. Assessment of vital statistics and surveillance data for monitoring tetanus mortality, United States, 1979–1984. *Am J Epidemiol* 1990;131:132–142.
25. Bleck TP. Tetanus: dealing with the continuing clinical challenge. *J Crit Illness* 1987;2:41–52.
26. Schofield F. Selective primary health care: strategies for control of disease in the developing world. XXII. Tetanus: a preventable problem. *Rev Infect Dis* 1986;8:144–156.
27. Cvjetanovic B, Grab B, Uemura K, Bytchenko B. Epidemiological model of tetanus and its use in the planning of immunization programmes. *Int J Epidemiol* 1972;1:125–137.
28. World Health Organization. *Expanded program on immunization* (September 1988 update). Geneva: WHO, 1988.
29. Cato EP, George WL, Finegold SM. Genus Clostridium prazemozski 1880, 23^AL. In: Smeath PHA, Mair NS, Sharpe ME, Holt JG, eds. *Bergey's manual of systematic bacteriology,* vol 2. Baltimore: Williams & Wilkins, 1986;1141–1200.
30. Hatheway CL. Bacterial sources of clostridial neurotoxins. In: Simpson LL, ed. *Botulinum neurotoxin and tetanus toxin.* San Diego: Academic Press, 1989;4–24.
31. Willis AT. Clostridium: the spore-bearing anaerobes. In: Parker

MT, ed. *Topley and Wilson's Principles of bacteriology, virology and immunity,* vol 2. Baltimore: Williams & Wilkins, 1983;442–475.

32. Hoeniger JFM, Tauschel HD. Sequence of structural changes in cultures of *Clostridium tetani* grown on a solid medium. *J Med Microbiol* 1974;7:425–432.

33. Smith LDS. The clostridia. In: Laskin AI, Lechevalier HA, eds. *CRC handbook of clinical microbiology,* vol 1, 2nd ed. Cleveland: CRC Press, 1977;337–345.

34. Tonge BL. Tetanus from chigger flea sores. *J Trop Pediatr* 1989;35:94.

35. Adams EB. The prognosis and prevention of tetanus. *S Afr Med J* 1968;42:739–743.

36. Smith JWG. Tetanus and its prevention. *Prog Drug Res* 1975;19:391–401.

37. Rottem S, Groover K, Habig WH, et al. Transmembrane diffusion channels in Mycoplasma gallisepticum induced by tetanolysin. *Infect Immun* 1990;58:598–602.

38. Blumenthal R, Habig WH. Mechanisms of tetanolysin-induced membrane damage: studies with black lipid membranes. *J Bacteriol* 1984;157:321–323.

39. Hardegree MC, Palmer AE, Duffin N. Tetanolysin: *in vivo* effects in animals. *J Infect Dis* 1971;123:51–60.

40. Craven CJ, Dawson DJ. The chain composition of tetanus toxin. *Biochim Biophys Acta* 1973;317:277–285.

41. Matsuda M, Yoneda M. Dissociation of tetanus neurotoxin into two polypeptide fragments. *Biochem Biophys Res Commun* 1976;57:1257–1262.

42. Matsuda M. The structure of tetanus toxin. In: Simpson LL, ed. *Botulinum neurotoxin and tetanus toxin.* San Diego: Academic Press, 1989;78.

43. Eisel U, Jarausch W, Goretzki K, Henschen A, Engels J, Weller U, Hude M, Habermann E, Niemann H. Tetanus toxin: primary structure, expression in *E. coli,* and homology with botulinum toxins. *EMBO J* 1986;5:2495–2502.

44. Bergey GK, Habig WH, Bennett JI, Lin CS. Proteolytic cleavage of tetanus toxin increases activity. *J Neurochem* 1989;53:155–161.

45. Krieglstein K, Henschen A, Weller U, Habermann E. Arrangement of disulfide bridges and positions of sulfhydryl groups in tetanus toxin. *Eur J Biochem* 1990;188:39–45.

46. Ho PC, Mutch DA, Winkel KD, et al. Identification of two promiscuous T cell epitopes from tetanus toxin. *Eur J Immunol* 1990;20:477–483.

47. Robinson JP, Schmid M, Morgan DG, Chiu W. Three-dimensional structural analysis of tetanus toxin by electron crystallography. *J Mol Biol* 1988;200:367–375.

48. Fairweather NF, Lyness VA. The complete nucleotide sequence of tetanus toxin. *Nucleic Acids Res* 1986;14:7809–7812.

49. Helting TB, Zwisler O. Structure of tetanus toxin. I. Breakdown of the toxin molecule and discrimination between polypeptide fragments. *J Biol Chem* 1977;12:1147–1153.

50. Mochida S, Poulain B, Weller U, Habermann E, Tauc L. Light chain of tetanus toxin intracellularly inhibits acetylcholine release at neuro-neuronal synapses, and its internalization is mediated by the heavy chain. *FEBS Lett* 1989;253:47–51.

51. Simpson LL. Fragment C of tetanus toxin antagonizes the neuromuscular blocking properties of native tetanus toxin. *J Pharmacol Exp Ther* 1984;228:600–604.

52. Bittner MA, Habig WH, Holz RW. Isolated light chain of tetanus toxin inhibits exocytosis: studies in digitonin-permeabilized cells. *J Neurochem* 1989;53:966–968.

53. Fishman P, Savitt JM. Transsynaptic transfer of retrogradely transported tetanus protein–peroxidase conjugates. *Exp Neurol* 1989;106:197–203.

54. Weller U, Dauzenroth ME, Meyer-zu-Heringdorf D, Habermann E. Chains and fragments of tetanus toxin. Separation, reassociation and pharmacological properties. *Eur J Biochem* 1989;182:649–956.

55. Bleck TP. Pharmacology of tetanus. *Clin Neuropharmacol* 1986;9:103–120.

56. Schmitt A, Dreyer F, John C. At least three sequential steps are involved in the tetanus toxin-induced block of neuromuscular transmission. *Naunyn Schmiedebergs Arch Pharmacol* 1981;317:326–330.

57. Middlebrook JL. Cell surface receptors for protein toxins. In: Simpson LL, ed. *Botulinum neurotoxin and tetanus toxin.* San Diego: Academic Press, 1989;95–119.

58. Yavin E, Nathan A. Tetanus toxin receptors on nerve cells contain a trypsin-sensitive component. *Eur J Biochem* 1986;154:403–407.

59. Morris RE, Saelinger CB. Entry of bacterial toxins into mammalian cells. In: Simpson LL, ed. *Botulinum neurotoxin and tetanus toxin.* San Diego: Academic Press, 1989;121–152.

60. Schwab ME, Thoenen H. Selective binding, uptake, and retrograde transport of tetanus toxin by nerve terminals in the rat iris. *J Cell Biol* 1978;77:1–13.

61. Montesano R, Roth J, Robert A, Orci L. Non-coated membrane invaginations are involved in binding and internalization of cholera and tetanus toxins. *Nature* 1982;296:651–653.

62. Black JD, Dolly JO. Interaction of ^{125}I-labeled botulinum neurotoxins with nerve terminals. II. Autoradiographic evidence for its uptake into motor nerves by acceptor-mediated endocytosis. *J Cell Biol* 1986;103:535–544.

63. Forchetti CM, Leheta B, Garant DS. *In vivo* and *in vitro* assessment of neurotransmitter amino acid function in tetanus toxin induced chronic seizure foci in rat hippocampus. *Soc Neurosci Abstr* 1990;16:948.

64. Mellanby J, Whittaker VP. The fixation of tetanus toxin by synaptic membranes. *J Neurochem* 1968;15:205–208.

65. Gambale F, Montal M. Characterization of the channel properties of tetanus toxin in planar lipid bilayers. *Biophys J* 1988;53:771–783.

66. Aguilera J, Yavin E. *In vivo* translocation and down-regulation of protein kinase C following intraventricular administration of tetanus toxin. *J Neurochem* 1990;54:339–342.

67. Sandberg K, Berry CJ, Eugster E, Rogers TB. A role of cGMP during tetanus toxin blockade of acetylcholine release in the rat pheochromocytoma (PC12) cell line. *J Neurosci* 1989;9:3946–3954.

68. Dreyer F. Peripheral actions of tetanus toxin. In: Simpson LL, ed. *Botulinum neurotoxin and tetanus toxin.* San Diego: Academic Press, 1989;179–202.

69. Manning KA, Erichsen JT, Evinger C. Retrograde transneuronal transport properties of fragment C of tetanus toxin. *Neuroscience* 1990;34:251–263.

70. Cherubin CE. Clinical severity of tetanus in narcotic addicts in New York City. *Arch Intern Med* 1968;121:156–158.

71. Habermann E. Tetanus. In: Vinken PJ, Bruyn GW, eds. *Handbook of clinical neurology,* vol 33. Amsterdam: North-Holland, 1978;491–547.

72. Veronesi R, Focaccia R. The clinical picture. In: Veronesi R, ed. *Tetanus: important new concepts.* Amsterdam: Excerpta Medica, 1981;183–206.

73. Bleck TP. Clinical aspects of tetanus. In: Simpson LL, ed. *Botulinum neurotoxin and tetanus toxin.* San Diego: Academic Press, 1989;379–398.

74. Wilson SAK. *Neurology.* London: Edward Arnold, 1940;625–638.

75. Weinstein L. Tetanus. *N Engl J Med* 1973;289:1293–1296.

76. Luisto M, Seppalainen AM. Electroencephalography in tetanus. *Acta Neurol Scand* 1989;80:157–161.

77. Bleck TP, Calderelli DD. Vocal cord paralysis complicating tetanus. *Neurology* 1983;33(Suppl 2):140.

78. Wright DK, Lalloo UG, Nayiager S, Govender P. Autonomic nervous system dysfunction in severe tetanus: current perspectives. *Crit Care Med* 1989;17:370–375.

79. Spenney JG, Lamb RN, Cobbs CG. Recurrent tetanus. *South Med J* 1971;64:859.

80. Brust JCM, Richter RW. Tetanus in the inner city. *NY State Med J* 1974;74:1735–1742.

81. Risk WS, Bosch EP, Kimura J, Cancilla PA, Fischbeck KH, Layzer RB. Chronic tetanus: clinical report and histochemistry of muscle. *Muscle Nerve* 1981;4:363–366.

82. Dastur FD, Shahani MT, Dastoor DH, Kohiyar FN, Bharucha EP, Mondkar VP, Kashyap GH, Nair KG. Cephalic tetanus: demonstration of a dual lesion. *J Neurol Neurosurg Psychiatry* 1977;40:782–786.

83. Mayo J, Berciano J. Cephalic tetanus presenting with Bell's palsy. *J Neurol Neurosurg Psychiatry* 1985;48:290.

84. Scholz DG, Olson JM, Thurber DL, Larson DE. Tetanus: an uncommon cause of dysphagia. *Mayo Clin Proc* 1989;64:335–338.

85. Lathrop DL, Griebel M, Horner J. Dysphagia in tetanus: evaluation and outcome. *Dysphagia* 1989;4:173–175.

86. Patel JC, Kale PA, Mehta BC. Otogenic tetanus: study of 922 cases. In: Patel JC, ed. *Proceedings of an international conference on tetanus, Bombay.* 1965;640–644.

87. Vieira BI, Dunne JW, Summers Q. Cephalic tetanus in an immunized patient. Clinical and electromyographic findings. *Med J Aust* 1986;145:156–157.

88. Saltissi S, Hakin RN, Pearce J. Ophthalmoplegic tetanus. *Br Med J* 1976;1:437.

89. Biglan AW, Ellis FD, Wade TA. Supranuclear oculomotor palsy and exotropia after tetanus. *Am J Ophthalmol* 1978;86:666–668.

90. Traverso HP, Bennett JV, Kahn AJ, Agha SB, Rahim H, Kamil S, Lang MH. Ghee application to the umbilical cord: a risk factor for neonatal tetanus. *Lancet* 1989;1(8636):486–488.

91. Schofield FD, Tucker VM, Westbrook GR. Neonatal tetanus in New Guinea: effect of active immunization in pregnancy. *Br Med J* 1961;2:785–789.

92. Anlar B, Yalaz K, Dizmen R. Long-term prognosis after neonatal tetanus. *Dev Med Child Neurol* 1989;31:76–80.

93. Price DL, Griffin JW, Peck K. Tetanus toxin: evidence for binding at presynaptic nerve sites. *Brain Res* 1977;121:379–384.

94. Green J, Erdmann G, Wellhoner HH. Is there retrograde axonal transport of tetanus toxin in both alpha and gamma fibers? *Nature* 1977;265:370.

95. Bizzini B. Axoplasmic transport and transynaptic movement of tetanus toxin. In: Simpson LL, ed. *Botulinum neurotoxin and tetanus toxin.* San Diego: Academic Press, 1989;203–229.

96. Price DL, Griffin J, Young A, Peck K, Stocks A. Tetanus toxin: direct evidence for retrograde axonal transport. *Science* 1975;188:945–946.

97. Cook ML, Stevens JG. Pathogenesis of herpetic neuritis and ganglionitis in mice: evidence for intraaxonal transport of infection. *Infect Immun* 1973;7:272–288.

98. Evinger C, Erichsen JT. Transsynaptic retrograde transport of fragment C of tetanus toxin demonstrated by immunohistochemical localization. *Brain Res* 1986;380:383–388.

99. Price DL, Griffin JW. Tetanus toxin: retrograde axonal transport of systemically administered toxin. *Neurosci Lett* 1977;4:61–65.

100. Schwab ME, Thoenen H. Electron microscopic evidence for a transsynaptic migration of tetanus toxin in spinal cord motoneurons: an autoradiographic and morphometric study. *Brain Res* 1976;105:213–227.

101. Curtis DR, Felix D, Game CJA, McCulloch RM. Tetanus toxin and the synaptic release of GABA. *Brain Res* 1973;51:358–362.

102. Price DL, Griffin JW. Immunocytochemical localization of tetanus toxin to synapses of spinal cord. *Neurosci Lett* 1981;23:149–155.

103. Davidoff RA, Hackman JC. Spinal inhibition. In: Davidoff RA, ed. *Handbook of the spinal cord,* vols 2 and 3. New York: Marcel Dekker, 1984;385–459.

104. Baker AB. The central nervous system in tetanus. *J Neuropathol Exp Neurol* 1942;1:394–405.

105. Tarlov IM, Ling H, Yamada H. Neuronal pathology in experimental tetanus. *Neurology* 1973;23:580–591.

106. Dumas M, Schwab ME, Thoenen H. Retrograde axonal transport of specific macromolecules as a tool for characterizing nerve terminal membranes. *J Neurobiol* 1979;10:179–197.

107. Bigalke H, Heller I, Habermann E. Effects of tetanus and botulinum A toxin on uptake and release of centrally acting neurotransmitters. *Naunyn Schmiedebergs Arch Pharmacol* 1980;313:R26.

108. Bigalke H, Ahnert-Hilber G, Habermann E. Tetanus toxin and botulinum A toxin inhibit acetylcholine release from but not calcium uptake into brain tissue. *Naunyn Schmiedebergs Arch Pharmacol* 1981;316:143–148.

109. Janicki PJ, Habermann E. Tetanus and botulinum toxins inhibit, and black widow spider venom stimulates the release of methionine-enkephalin-like material *in vitro. J Neurochem* 1983;41:395–402.

110. Bergey GK, MacDonald RL, Habig WH, Hardegree MC, Nelson PG. Tetanus toxin: convulsant action on mouse spinal cord neurons in culture. *J Neurosci* 1983;3:2310–2323.

111. Mellanby J, George G, Robinson A, Thompson PA. Epileptiform syndrome in rats produced by injecting tetanus toxin into the hippocampus. *J Neurol Neurosurg Psychiatry* 1977;40:404–414.

112. Garant DS, Chen Y-M, Bleck TP, Fariello RG. Long-term electrophysiologic and biochemical monitoring in the rat intra-amygdaloid tetanus toxin chronic model of epilepsy. *Soc Neurosci Abstr* 1989;15:1032.

113. Takano K, Kirchner T, Tiebert B, Terhaar P. Presynaptic inhibition of the monosynaptic reflex during local tetanus in the cat. *Toxicon* 1989;27:431–438.

114. Lassen HCA, Bjornboe M, Ibsen B, Neukirch F. Treatment of tetanus with curarization, general anesthesia, and intratracheal positive pressure ventilation. *Lancet* 1954;2:1040–1044.

115. Bjorneboe M, Ibsen B, Johnson S. Tetanus. A case treated with artificial respiration during 17 days. *Dan Med Bull* 1954;1:129–131.

116. Kerr JH, Corbett JL, Prys-Roberts C, Crampton Smith A, Spaulding JMK. Involvement of the sympathetic nervous system in tetanus. *Lancet* 1968;2:236–241.

117. Corbett JL, Harris PJ. Studies on the sympathetic nervous system in tetanus. *Naunyn Schmiedebergs Arch Pharmacol* 1973;276:447–460.

118. Domenighetti GM, Savary S, Striker H. Hyperadrenergic syndrome in severe tetanus responsive to labetalol. *Br Med J* 1984;288:1483–1484.

119. Kanerek DJ, Kaufman B, Zwi S. Severe sympathetic hyperactivity associated with tetanus. *Arch Intern Med* 1973;276:447–460.

120. Tsueda K, Oliver PB, Richter RW. Cardiovascular manifestations of tetanus. *Anesthesiology* 1974;40:588–592.

121. Parr GH, Wellhoner HH. The action of tetanus toxin in preganglionic sympathetic reflex discharges. *Naunyn Schmiedebergs Arch Pharmacol* 1973;276:437–445.

122. Parr GH, Wieland HJ, Wellhoner HH. The influence of tetanus toxin on sympathetic reflex discharges into the renal nerves. *Naunyn Schmiedebergs Arch Pharmacol* 1978;281:383–390.

123. Potgieter PD. Inappropriate ADH secretion in tetanus. *Crit Care Med* 1983;11:417–418.

124. Ambache N, Lippold OCH. Bradycardia of central origin produced by injections of tetanus toxin into the vagus nerve. *J Physiol (Lond)* 1949;108:186–196.

125. Nistico G, Gratteri S, Donato Di Paola E, Rossi F, Lampa E, Marmo E. Cardiovascular effects of tetanus toxin after systemic and intraventricular administration in rats. *Neuropharmacology* 1985;24:341–343.

126. Harvey AM. The peripheral action of tetanus toxin. *J Physiol (Lond)* 1939;96:348–365.

127. Fernandez JM, Ferrandiz M, Larrea L, Ramio R, Boada M. Cephalic tetanus studied with single fibre EMG. *J Neurol Neurosurg Psychiatry* 1983;46:862–866.

128. Duchen LW, Tonge DA. The effects of tetanus toxin on neuromuscular transmission and on the morphology of motor end-plates in slow and fast skeletal muscle of the mouse. *J Physiol (Lond)* 1973;228:157–172.

129. Mirsky R, Wendon LMB, Black P, Stolkin C, Bray D. Tetanus toxin: a cell surface marker for neurones in culture. *Brain Res* 1978;148:251–259.

130. Heymanns J, Neumann K, Havemann K. Tetanus toxin as a marker for small-cell lung cancer cell lines. *J Cancer Res Clin Oncol* 1989;115:537–542.

131. Berliner P, Unsicker K. Tetanus toxin labeling as a novel rapid and highly specific tool in human neuroblastoma differential diagnosis. *Cancer* 1985;56:419–423.

132. Jefferys JG. Chronic epileptic foci *in vitro* in hippocampal slices from rats with the tetanus toxin epileptic syndrome. *J Neurophysiol* 1989;62:458–468.

133. Garant D, Leheta B, Vern B, Bleck T. In vivo on-line analysis of cytochrome a, a₃ redox state with EEG and microdialysis in an unanesthetized cat cortical focal epilepsy model. *Soc Neurosci Abstr* 1990;16:1337.

134. Kryzhanovsky GN, Aliev MN. The stereotyped behavior syndrome: a new model and proposed therapy. *Pharmacol Biochem Behav* 1981;14:273–281.

135. Calabresi P, Benedetti M, Mercuri NB, Bernardi G. Selective depression of synaptic transmission by tetanus toxin: a comparative

study on hippocampal and neostriatal slices. *Neuroscience* 1989;30:663–670.

136. Wieraszko A, Seifert W. Evidence for the functional role of monosialoganglioside GM1 in synaptic transmission in the rat hippocampus. *Brain Res* 1986;371:305–313.

137. Woo E, Yu YL, Huang CY. Local tetanus revisited. Electrodiagnostic studies in 2 patients. *Electromyogr Clin Neurophysiol* 1988;28:117–122.

138. Heare BR, Shabot JM. Tetanus associated with carcinoma of the rectum. *Am J Gastroenterol* 1990;85:105–106.

139. Boyd RE, Brennan PT, Deng J-F, Rochester DF, Spykes DA. Strychnine poisoning. *Am J Med* 1983;74:507–512.

140. Johnson GAR. Neuropharmacology of amino acid neurotransmitters. *Annu Rev Pharmacol* 1978;18:269–289.

141. Verma A, Tandon PN, Maheshwari MC. Trismus caused by paradoxical activity of jaw-closing muscles in brainstem tuberculoma. *Oral Surg Oral Med Oral Pathol* 1988;65:675–678.

142. Morsch FP, Woltman HW. Progressive fluctuating muscular rigidity ("stiff-man syndrome"): report of a case and some observations in 13 other cases. *Mayo Clin Proc* 1956;421–427.

143. Solimena M, Folli F, Aparisi R et al. Autoantibodies to GABA-ergic neurons and pancreatic beta cells in stiff-man syndrome. *N Engl J Med* 1990;322:1555–1560.

144. Stoddart JC. Pseudotetanus. *Anaesthesia* 1979;34:877–881.

145. Edwards RA, James B. Tetanus and psychiatry: unexpected bedfellows. *Med J Aust* 1979;1:483–484.

146. Band JD, Bennett JV. Tetanus. In: Hoeprich PD, ed. *Infectious diseases.* Philadelphia: Harper & Row, 1983;1107–1114.

147. Kenrick KG, Wallace RC, Ismay SL. An improved assay for human tetanus anti-toxin and its use in the accession of human plasma for the production of high-titre tetanus immunoglobulin. *Vox Sang* 1990;58:35–39.

148. Mastroeni P, Leonardi MS, Gazzara D, Bizzini B. Rapid assessment of the antitetanus immune status of a subject using Dot-ELISA. *Eur J Epidemiol* 1989;5:97–100.

149. Sweath PAT, Kerslake EG, Scruby F. Tetanus immunity: resistance of guinea pigs to lethal spore doses induced by active and passive immunization. *Am J Hyg* 1937;25:464–476.

150. Passen EL, Andersen BR. Clinical tetanus despite a protective level of toxin-neutralizing antibody. *JAMA* 1986;255:1171–1173.

151. Goulon M, Girard O, Grosbius S, et al. Les anticorps antitétaniques. *Nouv Presse Med* 1972;1:3049–3050.

152. Trabaud MA, Lery L, Desgranges C. Human monoclonal antibodies with a protective activity against tetanus toxin. *APMIS* 1989;97:671–676.

153. Jolliet P, Magnenat J-L, Kobel T, Chevrolet J-C. Aggressive intensive care treatment of very elderly patients with tetanus is justified. *Chest* 1990;97:702–705.

154. Blake PA, Feldman RA, Buchanan TM, et al. Serologic therapy of tetanus in the United States. *JAMA* 1976;236:42–44.

155. Gupta PS, Kapoor R, Goyal S, Batra VK, Jain BK. Intrathecal human tetanus immune globulin in early tetanus. *Lancet* 1980;2:439–440.

156. Lewis RA, Satoskar RS, Joag GG, et al. Cortisone and hydrocortisone given parenterally and orally in severe tetanus. *JAMA* 1954;156:479–484.

157. Paydas S, Akoglu TF, Akkiz H, et al. Mortality-lowering effect of systemic corticosteroid therapy in severe tetanus. *Clin Ther* 1988;10:276–280.

158. Mukherjee DK. Tetanus and tracheostomy. *Ann Otol* 1977;86:67–72.

159. Edmondson RS, Flowers MWW. Intensive care in tetanus: management, complications, and mortality in 100 patients. *Br Med J* 1979;1401–1404.

160. Ho JL, Klempner MS. Tetanus toxin inhibits secretion of lysosomal contents from human macrophages. *J Infect Dis* 1985;152:922–929.

161. Clarke G, Hill RG. Effects of a focal penicillin lesion on responses of rabbit cortical neurones to putative neurotransmitters. *Br J Pharmacol* 1972;44:435–441.

162. Ahmadsyah I, Salim A. Treatment of tetanus: an open study to compare the efficacy of procaine penicillin and metronidazole. *Br Med J* 1985;291:648–650.

163. Tallman JF, Gallagher DW. The GABAergic system: a locus of benzodiazepine action. *Annu Rev Neurosci* 1985;8:21–44.

164. Vassa T, Yajnik VH, Joshi KR, Doshi HV, Shah SS, Patel SH. Comparative clinical trial of diazepam with other conventional drugs in tetanus. *Postgrad Med J* 1974;50:755–758.

165. Kapoor W, Carey P, Karpf M. Induction of lactic acidosis with intravenous diazepam in a patient with tetanus. *Arch Intern Med* 1981;141:944–945.

166. Müller H, Börner U, Zierski J, Hempelmann G. Intrathecal baclofen for treatment of tetanus-induced spasticity. *Anesthesiology* 1987;66:76–79.

167. Farquhar I, Hutchinson A, Curran J. Dantrolene in severe tetanus. *Intensive Care Med* 1988;14:249–250.

168. Langley MS, Heel RC. Propofol. A review of its pharmacodynamic and pharmacokinetic properties and use as an anaesthetic agent. *Drugs* 1988;35:334–372.

169. Orko R, Rosenberg PH, Himberg JJ. Intravenous infusion of midazolam, propofol and vecuronium in a patient with severe tetanus. *Acta Anaesthesiol Scand* 1988;32:590–592.

170. Powles AB, Ganta R. Use of vecuronium in the management of tetanus. *Anaesthesia* 1985;40:879–881.

171. Peat SJ, Potter DR, Hunter JM. The prolonged use of atracurium in a patient with tetanus. *Anaesthesia* 1988;43:962–963.

172. Roizen MF, Feeley TW. Pancuronium bromide. *Ann Intern Med* 1978;88:64–68.

173. Buchanan N, Smit L, Cane RD, De Andrade M. Sympathetic overactivity in tetanus: fatality associated with propranolol. *Br Med J* 1978;2:254–255.

174. Sutton DN, Tremlett MR, Woodcock TE, Nielsen MS. Management of autonomic dysfunction in severe tetanus: the use of magnesium sulphate and clonidine. *Intensive Care Med* 1990;16:75–80.

175. Rie M, Wilson RS. Morphine therapy controls autonomic hyperactivity in tetanus. *Ann Intern Med* 1978;88:653–654.

176. Southorn PA, Blaise GA. Treatment of tetanus-induced autonomic nervous system dysfunction with continuous epidural blockade. *Crit Care Med* 1986;14:251–252.

177. Brand GR, Breheny FX. Atrial pacing in tetanus. *Anaesth Intensive Care* 1984;12:63–65.

178. O'Keefe SJD, Wesley A, Jiala I, Epstein S. The metabolic response and problems with nutritional support in acute tetanus. *Metabolism* 1984;33:482–487.

179. Flowers MW, Edmondson RS. Long-term recovery from tetanus: a study of 50 survivors. *Br Med J* 1980;280:303–305.

180. Asa DK, Bertorini TE, Pinals RS. Myositis ossificans circumscripta: a complication of tetanus. *Am J Med Sci* 1986;292:40–43.

181. Edsall G. The inexcusable disease. *JAMA* 1976;235:62–63.

182. Levine L, McComb JA, Dwyer RC, Lathan WC. Active-passive tetanus immunization. *N Engl J Med* 1966;274:186–190.

183. Jones AE, Johns A, Magrath DI, Melville O, Smith M, Sheffield F. Durability of immunity to diphtheria, tetanus and poliomyelitis after a three dose immunization schedule completed in the first eight months of life. *Vaccine* 1989;7:300–302.

184. ACIP. Diphtheria, tetanus, and pertussis: guidelines for vaccine prophylaxis and other preventive measures. *MMWR* 1985;34:405–426.

185. Ruben FL, Fireman P. Follow-up study: protective immunization in the elderly. *Am J Public Health* 1983;73:1330.

186. Martin RR. Clostidium tetani. In: Mandell GL, Douglas RG, Bennett JE, eds. *Principles and practice of infectious diseases,* 2nd ed. New York: John Wiley & Sons, 1985;1355–1359.

187. Fairweather NF, Chatfield SN, Makoff AJ, et al. Oral vaccination of mice against tetanus by use of a live attenuated *Salmonella* carrier. *Infect Immun* 1990;58:1323–1326.

188. Webster ADB, Latif AAA, Brenner MK, Bird D. Evaluation of test immunization in the assessment of antibody deficiency syndromes. *Br Med J* 1984;288:1864–1866.

189. Shackelford PG, Granoff DM, Polmar SH, et al. Subnormal serum concentrations of IgG2 in children with frequent infections associated with varied patterns of immunologic dysfunction. *J Pediatr* 1990;116:529–538.

190. Furste W. The potential development of tetanus in wounded patients with AIDS: Tetanus toxoid and tetanus immune globulin. *Arch Surg* 1986;121:367.

191. Margolick JB, Volkman DJ, Folks TM, Fauci AS. Amplification of HTLV-III/LAV infection by antigen-induced activation of T cells and direct suppression of virus by lymphocyte blastogenic responses. *J Immunol* 1987;138:1719–1723.

192. Fuchs D, Shearer GM, Boswell RN, et al. Increased serum neopterin patients with HIV-1 infection is correlated with reduced *in vitro* interleukin-2 production. *Clin Exp Immunol* 1990;80:44–48.

193. Chirmule N, Saxinger C, Pahwa S. Influences of related retroviruses on lymphocyte function. *FEMS Microbiol Immunol* 1989;1:271–278.

194. Chirmule N, Kalyanaraman VS, Oyaizu N, Slade HB, Pahwa S. Inhibition of functional properties of tetanus antigen-specific T-cell clones by envelope glycoprotein GP120 of human immunodeficiency virus. *Blood* 1990;75:152–159.

195. Harris PE, Strba-Cechova K, Rubernstein P, et al. Amplification of T cell blastogenic responses in healthy individuals and patients with acquired immunodeficiency syndrome. *J Clin Invest* 1990;85:746–756.

196. Jacobs RL, Lowe RS, Lanier BQ. Adverse reactions to tetanus toxoid. *JAMA* 1982;247:40–42.

197. Baust W, Mayer D, Wachsmuth W. Peripheral neuropathy after administration of tetanus toxoid. *J Neurol* 1979;222:131–133.

198. Halliday PL, Bauer RB. Polyradiculoneuritis secondary due immunization with tetanus and diphtheria toxoids. *Arch Neurol* 1983;40:56–57.

199. Pollard JD, Selby G. Relapsing neuropathy due to tetanus toxoid. *J Neurol Sci* 1978;37:113–125.

Infections of the Central Nervous System,
edited by W. M. Scheld, R. J. Whitley, and
D. T. Durack, Raven Press, Ltd., New York © 1991.

CHAPTER 26

Bordetella pertussis and the Central Nervous System

Erik L. Hewlett

Pertussis (whooping cough) continues to be an infectious disease of major consequence worldwide. In developing nations where immunization is limited by factors such as vaccine cost, delivery, storage, and administration, pertussis is a serious contributor to childhood morbidity and mortality (1). In the developed world, pertussis is a problem for two reasons. Firstly, although pertussis vaccine has been generally effective in controlling the disease (2), concerns about efficacy and about the possibility of serious neurologic reactions have reduced vaccine acceptance, resulting in increases in the number of pertussis cases (3–8). Secondly, pertussis persists even in countries such as the United States where vaccine coverage has been maintained through mandatory childhood immunization. The inability to eliminate the disease is due to (a) infection of adults, in whom vaccine immunity has waned, and (b) transmission to infants who have yet to be adequately immunized (9–12). For these reasons, pertussis and pertussis vaccine are currently the focus of extensive research and development efforts worldwide (3,13,14).

In this chapter, clinical pertussis and the products of the organism will be discussed in order to consider the neurologic sequelae of the clinical infection. In addition, pertussis vaccine development and general reactogenicity will be presented as background for consideration of the data for and against the existence of pertussis-vaccine-induced encephalopathy. Several comprehensive sources on pertussis clinical disease, pathophysiology, and vaccine may be reviewed for additional information (3,15–20).

E. L. Hewlett: Division of Clinical Pharmacology, University of Virginia School of Medicine, Charlottesville, Virginia 22908.

INFECTION WITH *BORDETELLA PERTUSSIS*

Clinical Pertussis

Bordetella pertussis causes a localized infection of the respiratory tract. The organism is spread by exposure of a susceptible host to an actively infected individual; transmission is most likely via aerosol droplet, although fomites may be involved in some cases. There is an incubation period of 5–21 days (20). The clinical manifestations of infection begin with the catarrhal phase, during which the host experiences sneezing, lacrimation, coryza, a dry cough, and low grade fever. After 2–10 days the disease evolves into the paroxysmal stage, the stage which is most characteristic of pertussis. Individuals with typical disease (most frequently children with no prior immunity) exhibit paroxysmal cough followed by whooping, gagging, vomiting, and sometimes apnea and cyanosis. There is prolific saliva and mucus production. In severely affected patients, the number of paroxysms may exceed 20 per day, frequently followed by exhaustion and sleep. Depending on the state of immunity, the paroxysmal stage may be brief (few days) or prolonged (more than 6 weeks) and is followed by a convalescent period during which the frequency and severity of cough paroxysms decreases. The patient may be otherwise asymptomatic, but for up to 6 months he or she may experience recurrence of the paroxysmal cough either upon exposure to cold or in conjunction with development of a viral upper respiratory infection. It is generally during the paroxysmal phase that the complications of the disease, including those involving the central nervous system (CNS), occur. Several novel components of *B. pertussis* have been shown to be important virulence factors in animal systems, but the pathophysiology of pertussis in humans is poorly understood (14–16). The well-studied factors which are hypothesized to be important in clinical disease are listed in Table 1 and are discussed in the context of (a) their involvement in attachment of the bacterium to host cells, (b) evasion of host defenses, (c) development of local damage, and (d) production of systemic manifestations of disease.

Filamentous hemagglutinin (FHA) (21–23) and pertactin P.69 (24,25), and perhaps agglutinogens (26) and pertussis toxin (21), function as adhesins in the interaction of *B. pertussis* with host cells such as the ciliated cells of the respiratory mucosa and phagocytic immune effector cells. Tracheal cytotoxin is a disaccharide-tetrapeptide derived from peptidoglycan which causes ciliostasis and death of ciliated epithelial cells (27,28).

Adenylate cyclase (AC) toxin is a protein toxin which enters immune effector cells and others to catalyze the production of supraphysiologic levels of cyclic AMP (29,30). The AC toxin gene has been cloned and sequenced by Glaser et al. (31) and found to have sequence homology with *Escherichia coli* hemolysin. Both tracheal cytotoxin and AC toxin are felt to be major contributors to the evasion and disruption of host defenses necessary for virulence (14,15). Heat-labile (dermonecrotic) toxin, which elicits vascular smooth muscle contraction by an unknown mechanism, may also be involved in local damage to the respiratory tract (32,33). There is, however, no evidence for systemic dissemination of any of these molecules.

TABLE 1. *Virulence factors of* Bordetella pertussis, *their molecular actions, and their proposed roles in clinical disease*

Virulence factor	Composition	Size	Biological activity	Postulated role in pertussis[a]	References
Adenylate cyclase toxin (hemolysin)	Cell-associated protein	177 kD	Enters target cells and catalyzes cAMP production from host ATP; causes lysis of animal erythrocytes.	E, possibly L	29–31
Agglutinogens	Cell-surface proteins	Different proteins with a range of sizes	May be involved in attachment to target cells; serve as serologic markers.	Possibly A	3,21,26
Filamentous hemagglutinin	Cell-surface protein	220 kD	Involved in the attachment to ciliated respiratory cells and other cell types.	A	21–23
Heat-labile toxin (dermonecrotic, mouse lethal toxin)	Cell-associated (possibly intracellular) protein	102 kD	Causes contraction of vascular smooth muscle cells by unknown mechanism, dermonecrosis, and death of suckling mice.	Possibly L	32,33
Pertactin (P.69)	Cell-surface protein	69 kD (93 kD precursor)	Contributes to the attachment of *B. pertussis* to some target cells.	A	24,25
Pertussis toxin (lymphocytosis-promoting factor, islet-activating protein, pertussigen)	Protein, released from bacterium	105 kD	ADP-ribosylates several guanine-nucleotide-binding (G) proteins and blocks the cell function mediated by those G proteins; elicits lymphocytosis, sensitizes to histamine, enhances insulin secretion; is mitogenic for T lymphocytes and activates platelets by an ADP-ribosylation-independent process.	E, S, possibly A, possibly L	38–50
Tracheal cytotoxin	Disaccharide-tetrapeptide derived from peptidoglycan, released from bacterium	921 D	Damages tracheal epithelial cells, resulting in ciliostasis and cell death by unknown mechanism.	E	27,28

[a] A, attachment; E, evasion of host defenses; L, local damage; S, systemic disease; see ref. 14 for details.

Although it is believed by some that pertussis toxin (PT) is responsible for the clinical manifestations of this disease (34,35), *B. parapertussis,* a related organism which is unable to produce PT, causes a pertussis-like illness (36). Therefore, the exact role for PT in clinical pertussis remains unclear. PT is a member of the family of A/B protein toxins which affect target cell function by virtue of their ADP-ribosyltransferase activity. The gene for PT has been cloned and sequenced, confirming its heterodimeric structure (37,38). The action of PT—namely, transfer of ADP-ribose from NAD to a specific amino acid on target guanine-nucleotide-binding (G) proteins—results in an inactivation of those proteins and interruption of their signal transduction activities (39,40). The effects of PT in experimental animals include promotion of lymphocytosis, development of histamine sensitization, and enhancement of insulin secretion (39–42). At the level of isolated cells, PT-mediated ADP-ribosylation can block inhibition of adenylate cyclase, inhibit the activation of phospholipase, and reduce or prevent the opening of calcium or potassium channels by a variety of hormones and neurotransmitters (40,43–46). The intoxication of neuronal tissue *in vitro* by PT has led to the description of this molecule as a neurotoxin (47). The whole-animal and clinical data, however, do not support this nomenclature or concept.

Because a pertussis-like illness can occur in the absence of PT, it appears that a major role for the toxin is to increase the duration and severity of the illness, not to serve as the primary mediator of disease as is the case for toxins in tetanus or botulism. It may be that the host response to the localized infection is altered by PT such that the characteristic paroxysmal cough occurs. Slow turnover of the toxin-modified guanine-nucleotide-binding proteins could account for the persistence of symptoms beyond the time that organisms can be isolated from the host. PT has also been demonstrated to be mitogenic for T lymphocytes, able to activate platelets by binding to a cell-surface receptor, and independent of ADP-ribosylation (48–50). These activities are associated with a mobilization of calcium, but the mechanisms involved and the consequences to an infected host remain unknown.

The common complications of clinical pertussis are physical sequelae of the paroxysmal coughing (20). Subconjunctival hemorrhages, ulceration of the lingual frenulum, and, infrequently, pneumothorax and rectal prolapse occur. Infection is also a common problem; with the impaired pulmonary clearance mechanisms, secondary bacterial pneumonia is a major cause of morbidity. For example, of 4728 cases of pertussis reported to the Centers for Disease Control (CDC) in 1984–1985, 41% were hospitalized and 12% had pneumonia. For the patients less than 6 months of age, the figures were 74% and 20%, respectively (51). Frequent coughing and vomiting can result in dehydration and nutritional compromise, especially in infants and small children. The most serious complications of clinical pertussis affect the CNS, and they are discussed below.

The diagnosis of pertussis is suspected when one hears the characteristic paroxysmal cough—with or without whoop, vomiting, and cyanosis. The clinical impression is confirmed by culture, direct fluorescent antibody test, serology (antibody to PT or FHA), or, more recently, detection of products of *B. pertussis* by enzyme-linked immunosorbent assay (ELISA) or DNA probe (3). Treatment of *B. pertussis* infection using antibiotics is most effective when initiated early in the clinical course. Often, however, this is not possible because the diagnosis has not been made. The antibiotic of choice is erythromycin (40–50 mg/kg/day in four divided doses for 14 days), but limited data suggest that sulfatrimethoprim may also be effective in clearing the infection (52,53). Treatment for less than 2 weeks is associated with relapse rates of greater than 10%. Recently, it has been reported that antibiotic therapy initiated within 14 days of the onset of illness may reduce the duration and severity of symptoms (52). Adjunctive therapy with the β_2-adrenergic agonist, salbutamol, and/or with corticosteroids have been reported to reduce symptoms, but their use is not uniformly accepted (3,54).

Neurologic Abnormalities Associated with Acute Infection

A variety of acute neurologic abnormalities have been observed in pertussis patients, including seizures, paralysis, aphasia, deafness, and blindness (55–58). These complications are generally noted during the paroxysmal phase, and their onset may be either rapid or insidious. Patients with these signs and symptoms are often described as having pertussis encephalopathy. The frequency of CNS complications in the past has been quite high, with reported rates in excess of 5% of hospitalized patients (55). Even as recently as 1984–1985, data from the CDC (51) indicated that 1.7% of all reported pertussis patients had seizures (2.3% in children less than 1 year of age) and that 0.5% had encephalopathy (0.6% in children less than 6 months of age). There was no encephalopathy reported in patients who were ≥10 years of age (51,57).

Several pathophysiologic mechanisms have been proposed to account for CNS abnormalities that accompany acute pertussis (Table 2). Some of these are based upon pathologic or experimental data, whereas others represent speculation from knowledge of the actions of bacterial virulence factors. Focal hemorrhage in the CNS may occur as a result of increased intracranial pressure during severe cough paroxysms, and such lesions have been con-

TABLE 2. *Proposed mechanisms for neurologic abnormalities associated with infection by Bordetella pertussis*

1. CNS hemorrhage secondary to increased intracranial pressure during cough paroxysms.
2. Hypoxia occurring during cough paroxysms.
3. Hypoglycemia or metabolic imbalance as a result of pertussis-toxin-mediated increases in insulin secretion (accompanied by vomiting) in conjunction with cough paroxysms.
4. Vascular occlusion due to leukocytosis and/or platelet activation.
5. Secondary viral or bacterial infection of the CNS.
6. Direct effect of pertussis toxin in the CNS.
7. Inflammation of the CNS enhanced by the adjuvant effect of pertussis toxin (analogous to its role in experimental allergic encephalomyelitis).
8. Unrecognized, previously existing neurologic lesion.

sidered to be responsible for some focal deficits observed in pertussis patients (55–59). Massive intracerebral hemorrhage occurs rarely. Air emboli and nonhemorrhagic circulatory compromise have also been suggested (56). In addition, some pertussis patients clearly become hypoxic with coughing, and degenerative neuropathologic changes consistent with that etiology are sometimes seen (59). Although adults with pertussis may experience cough syncope, CNS complications are virtually unheard of in that age group.

PT is a potent enhancer of secretagogue-stimulated insulin secretion in animals injected with PT or in those infected with *B. pertussis* (34,41), and hypoglycemia is reported in children with pertussis (20). It is possible that hypoglycemia could occur as a result of increased insulin secretion and post-tussive vomiting. However, Furman et al. (60) measured plasma glucoses and insulins in 24 pertussis patients and 27 controls to address this issue. They found a slight hyperinsulinemia in the pertussis patients but no hypoglycemia in either group. Convulsions associated with hyponatremia have been reported in a 3-month-old child with pertussis (61). PT is also believed to be responsible for lymphocytosis which occurs during the disease and may result in a total white blood count exceeding 100,000 per cubic millimeter (42). Lymphocytic plugging of capillaries has been suggested as a possible mechanism of CNS damage and has been demonstrated pathologically in some cases (59).

PT is well recognized and is extensively used for its adjuvant effects (42). Its role in facilitating the development of experimental allergic encephalomyelitis (EAE) in mice injected with homogenized spinal cord has been demonstrated (62), although EAE can occur without the aid of pertussis vaccine or toxin (63). Nevertheless, EAE has been suggested as a model of pertussis neurotoxicity. This hypothesis is not supported by pathologic findings because encephalomyelitis is not common in patients with pertussis encephalopathy (59).

PT modifies the function of neuronal tissue *in vitro,* inhibiting glutamate release and establishing a condition in which stimulation of neurones may be unchecked (46,47). Such studies, however, have been conducted with high concentrations of PT (0.1–1.0 μg/ml), and there is no evidence that PT even enters the CNS during clinical disease. A case report by Davis et al. (64) of a 7-year-old boy with serologically diagnosed pertussis, however, has been used to support the hypothesis of toxin-induced encephalopathy. The child had delirium, semicoma, cortical blindness, and a normal brain biopsy, but he had little or no cough prior to development of neurologic abnormalities from which he eventually recovered completely. Finally, although it is rarely mentioned, some cases of encephalopathy occurring in infants and young children may reflect preexisting, unrecognized CNS lesions.

Because the mechanisms that underlie the CNS abnormalities associated with clinical pertussis are poorly understood and may well be multifactorial, it appears that the primary approach to avoiding neurologic sequelae is to prevent the disease with the use of pertussis vaccine. In the CDC data from the period 1979–1981, seizures during clinical pertussis occurred principally in unimmunized children less than 1 year of age and in only one child who had received ≥3 doses of vaccine (65). Therefore, the effect of immunization to reduce severity of disease appears to include prophylaxis against CNS manifestations. Intensive care of acutely ill infants, including prevention of hypoxia, should also reduce CNS complications.

IMMUNIZATION AGAINST PERTUSSIS

Vaccine Development

Although whooping cough was recognized as a clinical entity beginning in the 16th century, it was not until the early 20th century that the causative organism was identified and cultured by Bordet and Gengou (66). Soon thereafter, attempts were made to use killed, whole *B. pertussis* organisms to protect against the disease (20,67). These efforts were surprisingly successful and yielded the whole-cell pertussis vaccine which was used in the United States in the late 1940s and early 1950s (2,3). During the evaluation of pertussis vaccine before its general use, however, it was noted that some children experienced neurologic abnormalities following immunization. Madsen (67), for example, reported the death of two children who had received pertussis vaccine twice within the first few days of life. Subsequently, additional case reports were published, leading to the perception that pertussis vaccine caused encephalopathy (68–71). Nevertheless, clinical pertussis was such a common illness of young children that the benefit–risk relationship would clearly have been on the side of immunization, even if the vaccine had caused encephalopathy. In response to concerns about vaccine safety, efforts were made to extract the "protective antigen" from *B. pertussis* in order to produce a toxoid equivalent to tetanus and diphtheria toxoids (72). With the reduction in the incidence of pertussis achieved with whole-cell vaccine (2), there was increasing concern about vaccine reactogenicity, especially the possibility of vaccine-induced brain damage and death (73). Several major studies were conducted to address these issues, and efforts to develop a non-whole-cell (component or acellular) pertussis vaccine were continued. Progress was impeded, however, by (a) inability to identify a single protective antigen, (b) lack of understanding of the mechanisms by which whole-cell vaccine elicits immunity, and (c) absence of definitive information about serious systemic/neurologic problems occurring in association with vaccine administration.

In the winter of 1974–1975, pertussis immunization was suspended in Japan after two children died following vaccine administration (8,74). Although the vaccine was later absolved in these deaths, a decision was made to develop an acellular product for general use. In the meantime, the Japanese authorities raised the age of immunization to begin at 24 months. There were two types of acellular vaccines developed and used in Japan, both based upon the research of Sato and co-workers (8,75). The principal components were FHA and chemically inactivated PT (iPT), derived from supernatant culture medium following bacterial growth. This so-called T-type vaccine included more FHA than iPT and also contained other products from the culture medium, including pertactin and possibly agglutinogens. The B-type vaccine was composed of individually purified FHA and iPT, recombined in equal amounts. Since 1981, primarily T-type vaccine has been used in Japan for routine immunization of children beginning at 24 months of age. These vaccines appeared to be efficacious (76), but children less than 24 months of age were left unprotected. By 1984 the incidence of pertussis in the unimmunized children less than 24 months of age ($\sim$20 per 100,000 population) exceeded the values for the period 1970–1974 (74).

In order to evaluate acellular vaccine under conditions more applicable to those in the United States and other western nations, a cooperative efficacy study was carried out in Sweden in 1986 and 1987 with the support of the Swedish and U.S. governments and the Japanese manufacturers (77,78). Because pertussis vaccine was not being used routinely in Sweden as a result of efficacy concerns (4), it was possible to carry out a placebo-controlled study involving administration of B-type vaccines [JNIH-6 (approximately equal amounts of iPT and FHA) or JNIH-7 (iPT alone)] or placebo to children 5–11 months of age. The study revealed the efficacy of

two doses of JNIH-6 given 2 months apart to be 69% [95% confidence interval (CI), 47–82%], and it reported that of JNIH-7 to be 54% (95% CI, 26–72%) (3,77,78). These values were lower than would have been expected for whole-cell vaccine based upon historical controls, but a direct comparison was not done. Both of these iPT-containing vaccines were effective (79–80%) in protecting against severe disease as defined by cough of greater than 30 days' duration. These data support the proposal that PT is a contributor to the severity of clinical disease rather than being its sole cause (14). The acellular preparations contained 1–10% the amount of endotoxin present in whole-cell vaccine (as well as containing a smaller amount of active PT) and were associated with markedly lower rates of local reactions and fever than had been reported for whole-cell vaccine (77–79). There were, however, temporally associated neurologic events (79). Importantly, there was no correlation between the antibody response to PT or FHA and protection against infection with *B. pertussis* (77,78). Following this study, the Swedish Board of Health and Welfare decided not to license either of these vaccines for general use (80). At present, acellular pertussis vaccines are licensed and routinely used only in Japan.

In light of the unexpectedly low efficacy of the B-type acellular vaccine, consideration is being given to other antigens which might be more effective in preventing infection rather than just preventing severe disease (3,14). Pertactin (P.69 antigen) has been shown to be able to protect mice against aerosol challenge, as has AC toxin (81,82). Recombinant DNA methods for genetically toxoiding PT have been developed and incorporated into production of experimental acellular pertussis vaccine (83). A series of second-generation acellular vaccines containing one, two, three, or four components will be evaluated in several phase III efficacy trials in Europe beginning in 1991. It is clear from the information already at hand, however, that the evolution of acellular pertussis vaccine will not end soon, primarily because pertussis is simply not a single-toxin disease like tetanus and diphtheria.

Vaccine Reactogenicity

The reactogenicity of whole-cell pertussis vaccine was noted when this vaccine first came into use more than 50 years ago (3,67). A mouse toxicity test, measuring weight changes in mice 3 and 7 days after receiving one-half a single human dose of pertussis vaccine, was developed by Pittman and Cox (84) to monitor vaccine toxicity. This test does not measure any single component of *B. pertussis,* but results are influenced by PT and endotoxin content. There is a correlation between mouse toxicity and reactogenicity in children (85,86).

Most reports of whole-cell-vaccine reactogenicity in

the literature consisted of anecdotal collections of severe reactions associated with vaccine administration, rather than containing controlled studies to determine reaction rates attributable to pertussis by comparison of diphtheria–tetanus–pertussis (DTP) with diphtheria–tetanus (DT) alone (67–71,73). The only non-whole-cell vaccine licensed and marketed in the United States was a product named Tri-Solgen, made by extraction of *B. pertussis* organisms (3). This vaccine was introduced in 1962 and remained commercially available until 1977, when it was withdrawn from the market because the manufacturer decided to terminate its production of biologicals. Because of reports that it was less reactogenic, several studies were done to evaluate Tri-Solgen relative to whole-cell pertussis vaccine (87,88): 40–50% of whole-cell-vaccine recipients had local, systemic, or febrile reactions, as compared with approximately 30% for the extracted preparation.

In 1978–1979, Cody et al. (89) studied the nature and rates of adverse reactions occurring within 48 hr following 15,752 doses of DTP and 784 doses of DT. Their results for whole-cell vaccine, summarized in Table 3, were similar to those observed by Conner and Speers (87). Cody et al. (89) found that 37.4–50.9% of children experienced some form of local reaction. Systemic signs such as drowsiness, fretfulness, and fever (≥38°C) occurred at similar rates, in each case significantly more frequently than in DT recipients. Nine children had convulsions (seven of nine of these episodes were associated with fever), and nine had hypotonic/hyporesponsive episodes (HHEs) (seven of eight of those on whom data were available had fever). Although neither of these events were observed in the DT group, only 0–1 would be expected to occur, since the control (DT) group consisted of only 784 subjects. Other studies, of smaller size, have demonstrated similar rates of local and systemic reactions (90). Pollock et al. (91) reviewed reports of un-

toward events following DTP (124,700 doses) or DT (133,500 doses) vaccines. Of 33 severe episodes of anaphylaxis/collapse, four occurred following DT and six occurred following DTP.

In the Cody et al. (89) study, there was one non-sudden infant death syndrome (non-SIDS) death which occurred outside the 48-hr observation period, but there were no cases of encephalopathy. In order to address the issue of permanent neurologic damage, the authors were able to reevaluate 16 children 6–7 years after their episodes of convulsions or HHEs (92). No child had a significant neurologic deficit, although four had minor abnormalities on neurologic examination. In consideration of the mechanisms for the reactions associated with DTP vaccine, Baraff et al. (93) compared reaction rates with potency, toxicity (by mouse weight gain test), and endotoxin content of different vaccine lots using data from the original study. Endotoxin content was positively correlated with percentage of recipients experiencing fever, but negatively correlated with drowsiness. Local reactions and persistent screaming, however, were correlated positively with lower toxicity in the mouse weight gain test. These data indicate that with the exception of the expected relationship between endotoxin and fever, there is no clear etiology of the DTP reactions as a function of vaccine composition.

The first large study of encephalopathy following pertussis vaccine administration was carried out by Pollock and Morris (94) in the Northwest Thames region of England beginning in 1975. Of 1172 reports of reactions associated with DTP immunization, only 12 involved neurologic abnormalities, compared with two following DT immunization. Only four of the 12 occurred within 4 days of vaccination, and all four had an infection as the probable cause of the neurologic problem. The authors concluded that "no convincing evidence that DTP caused major neurological damage emerged from this large and lengthy study" (94).

The National Childhood Encephalopathy Study (NCES) was a case–control investigation of the association between acute neurologic events, as determined by hospital admissions, and receipt of pertussis vaccine (95). From July 1976 to June 1979, children in England, Scotland, and Wales between 2 and 35 months of age with the following acute neurologic problems were enrolled: encephalitis/encephalopathy, prolonged (>30 min) convulsions, infantile spasms, and Reye's syndrome. Two matched controls were selected for each case. The proximity of DTP or DT vaccine administration (≤72 hr, <7 days, <14 days, <28 days) to the onset of neurologic symptoms was assessed. In the first report, the authors described a relative risk of 2.4 for neurologic events occurring within 7 days of DTP immunization; for DT, the relative risk (1.5) was not statistically significant. Subsequently, Bellman et al. (96) determined that DTP immunization was not associated with an in-

TABLE 3. *Reactions following DTP and DT immunization[a]*

Reaction	Percentage of vaccine recipients experiencing reaction	
	DTP[b]	DT[c]
Redness	37.4	7.6
Swelling	40.7	7.6
Pain	50.9	9.9
Fever (≥38°C)	46.5	9.3
Drowsiness	31.5	14.9
Fretfulness	53.4	22.6
Persistent crying	3.1	0.7
Convulsion	0.06	0
Hypotonic, hyporesponsive episode	0.06	0

[a] Data taken from ref. 89. DTP, diphtheria–tetanus–pertussis; DT, diphtheria–tetanus.
[b] 15,752 DTP immunizations.
[c] 784 DT immunizations.

creased risk for infantile spasms, and therefore those cases were excluded from subsequent analyses of NCES data. In reanalyzing the data, the authors concluded that "children with encephalopathy were significantly more likely to have received DTP vaccine within seven days before onset and to have a history of whooping cough during the month of onset" (97). From these data, the attributable risks for an acute neurologic event were determined to be 1:140,000 (95% CI, 1:460,000 to 1:60,000) with DTP vaccine and 1:11,000 (95% CI, 1:40,000 to 1:4,000) with whooping cough. The risk of death or neurologic damage 12 months later was calculated to be 1:330,000 (95% CI, 1:18,000,000 to 1:50,000). Subsequent analysis of the data by others, however, revealed that after the apparent increase in risk of neurologic problems during the first 7 days following immunization, there is a decreased risk between 7 and 28 days, suggesting that either the vaccine is protective during the latter interval or, more likely, the apparent risk is merely a moving forward in time of an event which was due to occur subsequently (3).

The NCES results have been extensively cited and included in DTP vaccine package inserts and vaccination consent forms. Recently, there has been considerable debate and discussion of the data, with concern expressed about the number of patients upon which the attributable risk estimates were based (3,98–100). Several of the patients who had permanent damage at 12 months had other illnesses (such as viral infection and Reye's syndrome) which could have accounted for their neurologic problems. For these reasons, the CDC's Advisory Committee on Immunization Practices (ACIP) has recently recommended that the attributable risk figures be removed from general use in warnings and immunization consent forms.

The relationship between DTP immunization and specific neurologic abnormalities has been addressed in other studies. Several reports in addition to the NCES indicate that infantile spasms are not statistically associated with DTP vaccine administration (101,102). In an analysis of health records from Denmark, Shields et al. (103) determined that there is no relationship between pertussis immunization and the onset of epilepsy. A shift in the age of vaccine administration did not result in a change in the mean age of development of epilepsy in the population, indicating that DTP and DTP-associated convulsions are not etiologies of chronic seizure disorders. Griffin et al. (104) examined the risk of seizures and other neurologic disorders following more than 100,000 DTP immunizations. They found an increased risk of febrile seizures within 72 hr of immunization, but no onset of seizure disorder in a previously normal child and no occurrence of encephalopathy within 14 days.

Deaths have been reported following pertussis immunization, starting with the children who died during Madsen's field trial in the Faroe Islands (67). Several

etiologies have been proposed, and a link with SIDS has been suggested (105). The majority of epidemiological studies to address the relationship between DTP immunization and SIDS, however, have found no causal relationship (106–110).

The Case For and Against Pertussis Vaccine Encephalopathy

In the past, it was taken for granted that pertussis vaccine caused encephalopathy, based primarily on uncontrolled clinical reports plus knowledge of the toxins of B. pertussis and their actions in experimental animals and cultured cells. The change in the benefit–risk ratio for pertussis vaccination that accompanied the reduction in the level of disease in developed nations has, however, led to a reappraisal of the data concerning vaccine-associated CNS reactions. Although no one study provides information sufficient to make a decision about the existence of pertussis-vaccine-induced encephalopathy, the problem is one which has been extensively discussed in recent years (3,98–100,111–113).

Consideration of biological causation is a complex matter, involving a variety of perspectives. Sir Austin Bradford Hill (114) provided a set of useful criteria that can be applied to the case of pertussis vaccine encephalopathy. His nine criteria are: (i) strength of association, (ii) consistency, (iii) specificity, (iv) temporality, (v) biological gradient, (vi) plausibility, (vii) coherence, (viii) experimental data, and (ix) analogy with other examples.

Strength of association refers to the rate of occurrence of an event as a function of number of exposures. The example used by Bradford Hill (114) for comparison is the incidence of scrotal cancer in chimney sweeps in 19th-century England, which was 200 times that of the general population. The relative risk for pertussis-vaccine-associated encephalopathy within 7 days among previously apparently normal subjects was 2.9 in the NCES (97). This figure, upon which all reviewers of the NCES do not even agree, is very low relative to that of a strong relationship such as scrotal cancer in chimney sweeps. Therefore, although the NCES data do not exclude the possibility of vaccine-related encephalopathy, neither do they indicate a strong association.

The criterion of consistency requires that when several studies using different methodologies are used to address a question, the same result be observed (114). The exclusion of infantile spasms and SIDS from causal association with DTP immunization certainly represents an example of consistency among studies (101,102,106–110). Even after removal of the infantile spasms data from the NCES, however, the authors concluded that causation of serious acute neurologic illnesses and permanent brain damage by pertussis vaccine cannot be excluded. Others who reviewed the same material felt that the conclusion of a causal association was not warranted (98–100,112,113). Nevertheless, even if these events do occur "very rarely," their risk is far smaller than the risk of neurologic damage from disease. Additional studies to address this question have been considered, but their size and cost would exceed the benefits of the expected result. Therefore, the available studies are not sufficient to allow evaluation of consistency in consideration of a definitive decision for or against vaccine encephalopathy.

The likelihood of a causal relationship between two events is enhanced if there is a specific, unique pattern to the result—that is, the only condition under which the particular phenomenon occurs is following the alleged causal condition. This is not the case for pertussis vaccine and encephalopathy. In fact, a major flaw in the hypothesis has been the absence of a specific abnormality, laboratory test, or definable clinical syndrome upon which to base a diagnosis (3). Similarly, in the analysis of the neuropathology from pertussis-vaccine-associated deaths, no ". . . recurring pattern of inflammatory or other damage which could be accepted as a specific reaction to immunization against whooping cough" was observed (115). Therefore, this entity falls short on the issue of specificity.

Temporality is a critical aspect of causation because it is impossible to attribute an outcome to an event that does not precede it. In the case of neurologic events and pertussis vaccination, their temporal relationship is often the only association. The unresolved issue is length of time following immunization during which an acute event or insidiously progressing illness can be considered to be vaccine-associated. Many studies use 48–72 hr (89). This approach may be deceiving, however, because the NCES data revealed a reverse correlation (i.e., apparent vaccine protection) between 7 and 28 days following immunization (3). Since some components of pertussis vaccine (i.e., PT) have biological effects which last for months, the selection of short intervals may be too restrictive. The issue of temporal association is generally consistent with, but not strongly supportive of, pertussis-vaccine-induced encephalopathy.

A postulated causal interaction is strengthened by a demonstrable biological gradient or dose–response relationship. Whereas the activity of pertussis vaccine is well-documented to be dose-dependent in the mouse toxicity (mouse weight gain) test and in a study of local reactions in children (84,86), there is no basis for extrapolation from such reactions to severe neurologic problems (116). Furthermore, in studies of the reactogenicity of different lots of DTP vaccine, the only correlates found were between endotoxin content and fever and between local reactions and mouse toxicity, with the human reaction being associated with lower mouse toxicity (93). There were no correlates with HHEs or convulsions due to inadequate sample size. The only suggestion of a biological gradient for neurologic events comes from the studies of Hannik and Cohen (117). The authors reported the rate of pertussis-vaccine-associated encephalopathy for children in the Netherlands to be 1/400,000 over a 12-year period. When the concentration of organisms in the whole-cell vaccine was reduced in the subsequent 5-year period, there were no encephalopathies reported. The authors concluded, however, that the number of cases was too small to be reliable. Thus, there is no support for a biological gradient in vaccine-associated neurologic events.

Biological plausibility and coherence can be considered together as criteria in the establishment of causation. A proposed causal association should be plausible in the context of known biological mechanisms and should be consistent with known facts about the disease process itself. On the surface, it is not unreasonable to expect neurologic reactions in response to whole-cell pertussis vaccine, which is known to contain PT, endotoxin, heat-labile toxin, AC toxin, and other potentially active products (3,14–16). PT has, in fact, been termed "neurotoxin" by Pittman (47). When one considers, however, the limited quantities of these bacterial components, their form as part of the whole organism, and the route of administration of the vaccine relative to experimental studies of these isolated toxins in animals, the presumption of CNS interaction and/or damage is not supported by the data (118,119). For example, a dose of whole-cell vaccine contains ~5 μg of endotoxin and 0–400 ng of bioactive PT (120). When administered in the form of whole-cell vaccine, these materials elicited fever in less than 50% of vaccine recipients and caused lymphocytosis in none (89). This means that the bioavailability of these components is low. Even when very large doses of PT (0.5 or 1 μg/kg; that is, 100 times those given to vaccine recipients) were given intravenously to adult volunteers, there were no serious adverse effects and certainly no encephalopathy or neurologic abnormalities (121). These data indicate that it is unlikely that pertussis vaccine components can elicit encephalopathy in the concentrations present in the vaccine.

Epidemiological studies can be supported by experimental evidence from animal models. Several models have been proposed for study of pertussis vaccine encephalopathy. Injection of mice with neural tissue can elicit the development of EAE characterized by paralysis and death (62,63). Pertussis vaccine can enhance and accelerate the development of EAE by its adjuvant effect (62). It has been proposed that vaccine-associated events may reflect such an autoimmune process. In those studies, however, the injection of a CNS antigen was required, and pertussis vaccine or PT alone had no effect (62). Furthermore, the histopathology of CNS tissue from children who died following DTP immunization was not consistent with encephalitis (115).

While studying autoimmune reactions in the CNS, Steinman et al. (122) noted that mice given bovine serum albumin (BSA) and pertussis vaccine in sequential doses responded to the last dose of BSA with an acute reaction consisting of tachypnea, seizures, and death. This response appeared to be limited to injection with BSA and only occurred in genetically restricted mouse strains (122). PT could be substituted for whole-cell pertussis vaccine (123). This was proposed as a model for vaccine-associated encephalopathy and as an assay to monitor future vaccines for their encephalitogenic potential. Although these basic observations have been confirmed, other investigators concluded that the immunizing procedure was sensitizing for an acute anaphylactic reaction to BSA (124–126). It was known previously that PT was an adjuvant and could sensitize to histamine and other mediators of anaphylaxis (42). Thus this animal model appears to be not one of encephalopathy, but one of allergic reaction and death. It is, therefore, not relevant to most cases of vaccine-associated neurologic problems in humans.

The final factor for consideration in causation is analogy with other systems. Here again, a superficial similarity with neurologic sequelae of other vaccines (i.e., measles encephalitis) does not contribute, since pertussis vaccine has no live organisms to proliferate in the CNS and the histopathology does not support the diagnosis of encephalitis (115). Encephalopathy has been reported following DT administration, but the causal relationship in that case is even more tenuous and thus does not contribute to the understanding of this situation (127).

In considering the question of pertussis vaccine encephalopathy, there is no consistent pattern of neuropathologic findings, no biologically plausible model for its causation, and no biochemical marker of its having occurred (3,112,113,119). Although it is not always possible to explain the cause of a neurologic event in a child that occurs within 48–72 hr of pertussis vaccination, the available data are not adequate to conclude in any single case that the neurologic event can be attributed to the vaccine. This conclusion was supported by a judicial decision in the Loveday case in Great Britain (120). One must remember, however, that a negative result does not prove anything; it is essential to remain open-minded in anticipation of future data. As stated by Sir Austin Bradford Hill (114), "All scientific work is incomplete—whether it be observational or experimental. All scientific work is liable to be upset or modified by advancing knowledge."

SUMMARY

Pertussis is a serious illness for children and an annoyance for adults. The encephalopathy associated with clinical disease may be caused by several possible mechanisms. Whole-cell pertussis vaccine is temporal associated with acute neurologic events on rare occasions.

The data are inadequate, however, to conclude causation by the vaccine, and the extremely low rate of vaccine-associated encephalopathy may preclude definitive resolution of this question in the future.

REFERENCES

1. Six killers of children. *World Health* 1987;7.
2. Mortimer EA Jr, Jones PK. An evaluation of pertussis vaccine. *Rev Infect Dis* 1979;1:927–934.
3. Cherry JD, Brunell PA, Golden GS, Karzon DT. *Pediatrics report of the task force on pertussis and pertussis immunization,* vol 81. Illinois: American Academy of Pediatrics, 1988;939–984.
4. Romanus V, Jonsell R, Berquest SO. Pertussis in Sweden after the cessation of general immunization in 1979. *Pediatr Infect Dis J* 1987;6:364–371.
5. Fine PEM. Epidemiological consideration for whooping cough eradication. In: Wardlaw AC, Parton R, eds. *Pathogenesis and immunity in pertussis.* New York: John Wiley & Sons, 1988;451–467.
6. Cherry JD. The epidemiology of pertussis and pertussis immunization in the United Kingdom and the United States: a comparative study. *Curr Probl Pediatr* 1984;14:1–78.
7. Pollard R. Relation between vaccination and notification rates for whooping cough in England and Wales. *Lancet* 1981;1:1180.
8. Sato Y, Kimura M, Fukumi H. Development of a pertussis component vaccine in Japan. *Lancet* 1984;1:122–126.
9. Lambert HS. Epidemiology of a small pertussis outbreak in Kent County, Michigan. *Public Health Rep* 1965;80:365–369.
10. Linnemann CC Jr, Nasenbeny J. Pertussis in the adult. *Annu Rev Med* 1977;28:179–185.
11. Steketee RW, Wassilak SGF, Adkins WN Jr, et al. Evidence for a high attack rate and efficacy of erythromycin prophylaxis in a pertussis outbreak in a facility for the developmentally disabled. *J Infect Dis* 1988;157:434–440.
12. Hewlett EL. Pertussis in adults: possible use of booster doses for control. *Tokai Exp Clin Med* 1989;13:125–128.
13. Whooping cough vaccine research revs up. *Science* 1985;22:1184–1186.
14. Hewlett EL, Cherry JD. New and improved vaccines against pertussis. In: Woodlaw GC, Levine MM, eds. *New generation vaccines.* New York: Marcel Dekker, 1990;231–250.
15. Weiss AA, Hewlett EL. Virulence factors of *Bordetella pertussis. Annu Rev Microbiol* 1986;40:661–686.
16. Wardlaw AC, Parton R. *Pathogenesis and immunity in pertussis.* New York: John Wiley & Sons, 1988.
17. Kimura M, Manclark CR, eds. *Proceedings of the 5th international symposium on pertussis. Tokai J Exp Clin Med* 1988;13(Suppl).
18. Mebel S, Stompe H, Drescher M, Rushtenbach S, eds. *FEMS symposium on pertussis.* Berlin: Society of Microbiology and Epidemiology of the GDR, 1988.
19. Manclark CR, ed. *Proceedings of the sixth international symposium on pertussis.* Department of Health and Human Services United States Public Health Service, Bethesda, Maryland. 1990.
20. Lapin JH. *Whooping cough.* Springfield, IL: Charles C Thomas, 1943.
21. Tuomanen E. *Bordetella pertussis* adhesins. In: Wardlaw AC, Parton R, eds. *Pathogenesis and immunity in pertussis.* New York: John Wiley & Sons, 1988;75–94.
22. Kimura A, Mountzouros KT, Relman DA, Falkow S, Cowell JL. *Bordetella pertussis* filamentous hemagglutinin: evaluation as a protective antigen and colonization factor in a mouse respiratory infection model. *Infect Immun* 1990;58:7–16.
23. Relman D, Tuomanen E, Falkow S, Golenbock DT, Saukkonen K, Wright SD. Recognition of a bacterial adhesion by an integrin: macrophage CR3 (CD11b/CD18) binds filamentous hemagglutinin of *Bordetella pertussis. Cell* 1990;61:1375–1382.
24. Brennan MJ, Li ZM, Cowell JL, Bisher ME, Steven AC, Novotny P, Manclark CR. Identification of a 69-kilodalton nonfimbrial protein as an agglutinogen of *Bordetella pertussis. Infect Immun* 1988;56:3189–3195.
25. Charles IG, Dougan G, Pickard D, et al. Molecular cloning and

characterization of protective outer membrane protein P.69 from *Bordetella pertussis. Proc Natl Acad Sci* 1989;86:3554–3558.

26. Preston NW. Pertussis today. In: Wardlaw AC, Parton R, eds. *Pathogenesis and immunity in pertussis.* New York: John Wiley & Sons, 1988;1–18.

27. Goldman WE. Tracheal cytotoxin of *Bordetella pertussis.* In: Wardlaw AC, Parton R, eds. *Pathogenesis and immunity in pertussis.* New York: John Wiley & Sons, 1988;231–246.

28. Cookson BT, Cho HL, Herwaldt LA, Goldman WE. Biological activities and chemical composition of purified tracheal cytotoxin of *Bordetella pertussis. Infect Immun* 1989;57:2223–2229.

29. Confer DL, Eaton JW. Phagocyte impotence caused by an invasive bacterial adenylate cyclase. *Science* 1982;217:948–950.

30. Hewlett EL, Gordon VM. Adenylate cyclase toxin of *Bordetella pertussis.* In: Wardlaw AC, Parton R, eds. *Pathogenesis and immunity in pertussis.* New York: John Wiley & Sons, 1988;193–210.

31. Glaser P, Ladant D, Sezer O, Pichot F, Ullmann A, Danchin A. The calmodulin-sensitive adenylate cyclase of *Bordetella pertussis:* cloning and expression in *Escherichia coli. Mol Microbiol* 1988;2:19–30.

32. Endoh M, Nagai M, Nakase Y. Effect of *Bordetella* heat-liable toxin on perfused lung preparations of guinea pigs. *Microbiol Immunol* 1986;30:1239–1246.

33. Nakase Y, Endoh M. Heat-labile toxin of *Bordetella pertussis.* In: Wardlaw AC, Parton R, eds. *Pathogenesis and immunity in pertussis.* New York: John Wiley & Sons, 1988;211–229.

34. Pittman M, Furman BL, Wardlaw AC. *Bordetella pertussis* respiratory tract infection in the mouse: pathophysiological responses. *J Infect Dis* 1980;142:56–66.

35. Pittman M. The concept of pertussis as a toxin-mediated disease. *Pediatr Infect Dis* 1984;3:467–486.

36. Linneman CC Jr, Perry EB. *Bordetella pertussis. Am J Dis Child* 1977;131:560–563.

37. Locht C, Keith JM. Pertussis toxin gene: nucleotide sequence and genetic organisation. *Science* 1986;232:1258–1264.

38. Nicosia M, Perugini M, Franzine C, et al. Cloning and sequencing of the pertussis toxin genes: operon structure and gene duplication. *Proc Natl Acad Sci* 1986;83:4631–4635.

39. Katada T, Ui M. Direct modification of the membrane adenylate cyclase system by islet-activating protein due to ADP-ribosylation of a membrane protein. *Proc Natl Acad Sci USA* 1982;79:3129–3133.

40. Ui M. The multiple biological activities of pertussis toxin. In: Wardlaw AC, Parton R, eds. *Pathogenesis and immunity in pertussis.* New York: John Wiley & Sons, 1988;121–145.

41. Furman BL, Sidey FM, Smith M. Metabolic disturbances produced by pertussis toxin. In: Wardlaw AC, Parton R, eds. *Pathogenesis and immunity in pertussis.* New York: John Wiley & Sons, 1988;147–171.

42. Munoz JJ, Bergman RK. *Bordetella pertussis—immunological and other biological activities, vol 4. Immunology series.* New York: Marcel Dekker, 1977;1–234.

43. Gilman AG. G protein: transducers of receptor generated signals. *Annu Rev Biochem* 1987;56:615–649.

44. Fain JN, Wallace MA, Wojcikiewics RJH. Evidence for involvement of guanine nucleotide-binding regulatory proteins in the activation of phospholipases by hormones. *FASEB J* 1988;2:2569–2574.

45. Holz GG IV, Rane SG, Dunlop K. GTP-binding proteins mediate transmitter inhibition of voltage-dependent calcium channels. *Nature* 1986;319:670.

46. Dolphin AC, Prestwich SA. Pertussis toxin reverses adenosine inhibition of neuronal glutamate release. *Nature* 1985;316:148–150.

47. Pittman M. Neurotoxicity of *Bordetella pertussis. Neurotoxicity* 1986;2:53–68.

48. Tamura M, Nogimori K, Yajima M, K Ase, Ui M. A role of the B-oligomer moiety of islet-activating protein, pertussis toxin, in development of the biological effect on intact cell. *J Biol Chem* 1983;258:6756–6761.

49. Banga HS, Walker RK, Winberry LK, Rittenhouse SE. Pertussis toxin can activate human platelets: comparative effects of holo-toxin and its ADP-ribosylating S$_1$ subunit. *J Biol Chem* 1987;262:14871–14874.

50. Gray LS, Huber KS, Gray MC, Hewlett EL, Engelhard VH. Per-

tussis toxin effects on T lymphocytes are mediated through CD3 and not by pertussis toxin-catalyzed modification of a G protein. *J Immunol* 1989;142:1631–1638.

51. Centers for disease control. Pertussis surveillance, 1984–1985. *MMWR* 1987;36:168–171.

52. Bergquist SO, Bernander S, Dahnsjo H, Sundelof B. Erythromycin in the treatment of pertussis: a study of bacteriologic and clinical effects. *Pediatr Infect Dis* 1987;6:458–461.

53. Hoppe JE, Halm U, Hagedorn HJ, Kraminer-Hagedorn A. Comparison of erythromycin ethylsuccinate and co-trimoxazole for treatment of pertussis. *Infection* 1989;17:227–231.

54. Bass JW. Pertussis: current status of prevention and treatment. *Pediatr Infect Dis* 1985;4:614–619.

55. Litvak AM, Gibel H, Rosenthal SE, Rosenblatt P. Cerebral complication in pertussis. *J Pediatr* 1948;32:357–379.

56. Woolf AL, Caplin H. Whooping cough encephalitis. *Arch Dis Child* 1956;31:87–91.

57. Zellweger H. Pertussis encephalopathy. *Arch Pediatr* 1959;76:381–386.

58. Celemajer JM, Brown J. The neurological complication of pertussis. *Med J Aust* 1966;1066–1069.

59. Dolgopol VB. Changes in the brain in pertussis with convulsions. *Arch Neurol Psychiatry* 1941;46:477–503.

60. Furman BL, Walker E, Sidey FM, Wardlaw AC. Slight hyperinsulinaemia but no hypoglycemia in pertussis patients. *J Med Microbiol* 1988;25:183–186.

61. Harper JR, Maguire MJ. Hyponatraemia and convulsions in whooping-cough. *Lancet* 1975;1:1147.

62. Munoz JJ, Bernard CCA, Mackay IR. Elicitation of experimental allergic encephalomyelitis (EAE) in mice with the aid of pertussigen. *Cell Immunol* 1984;83:92–100.

63. Levine S, Saltzman A. The hyperacute form of allergic encephalomyelitis produced in rats without the aid of pertussis vaccine. *J Neuropathol Exp Neurol* 1989;48:255–262.

64. Davis LE, Burstyn DG, Manclark CR. Pertussis encephalopathy with a normal brain biopsy and elevated lymphocytosis-promoting factor antibodies. *Pediatr Infect Dis* 1984;3:448–451.

65. Centers for Disease Control. Pertussis surveillance, 1979–1981. *MMWR* 1982;31:333–336.

66. Bordet J, Gengou O. Le microbe del la coqueluche. *Ann Inst Pasteur* 1906;20:731–741.

67. Madsen T. Vaccination against whooping cough. *JAMA* 1933;101:187–188.

68. Byers RK, Moll FC. Encephalopathies following prophylactic pertussis vaccine. *Pediatrics* 1948;1:437–457.

69. Berg JM. Neurological complications of pertussis immunization. *Br Med J* 1958;2:24–27.

70. Kulenkampff M, Schwartzman JS, Wilson J. Neurological complications of pertussis inoculation. *Arch Dis Child* 1974;49:46–49.

71. Strom J. Is universal vaccination against pertussis always justified? *Br Med J* 1960;2:1184–1186.

72. Barta G. Soluble protective antigen from *Bordetella pertussis* prepared with sodium deoxycholate. *J Immunol* 1963;90:72–80.

73. Stewart GT. Vaccination against whooping-cough: efficacy versus risks. *Lancet* 1977;1:234–237.

74. Noble GR, Bernier RH, Esber EC, et al. Acellular and whole cell pertussis vaccines in Japan: report of a visit by US scientists. *JAMA* 1987;257:1351–1356.

75. Cowell JL, Sato Y, Sato H, Ander Lan B, Manclark CR. Separation, purification and properties of the filamentous hemagglutinin and the leukocytosis promoting factor-hemagglutinin from *Bordetella pertussis.* In: Robbins JB, Hill JC, Sadoff G, eds. *Seminars in infectious disease, vol 4: bacterial vaccines.* New York: Thieme-Stratton, 1982;371–379.

76. Aoyama T, Murase Y, Kato T, Iwata T. Efficacy of an acellular pertussis vaccine in Japan. *J Pediatr* 1985;107:180–183.

77. National Bacteriological Laboratory, Sweden. *A clinical trial of acellular pertussis vaccines in Sweden.* Technical Report, 1988.

78. Ad Hoc Group for the Study of Pertussis Vaccines. Placebo-controlled trial of two acellular pertussis vaccines in Sweden-protective efficacy and adverse effects. *Lancet* 1988;1:955–960.

79. Blennow M, Granstrom M. Adverse reactions and serologic response to a booster dose of acellular pertussis vaccine in children immunized with acellular or whole-cell vaccine as infants. *Pediatrics* 1989;84:62–67.

80. Olin P, Storsaeter J, Romanus V. The efficacy of acellular pertussis vaccine [Letter]. *JAMA* 1989;261:560.

81. Shahin RD, Brennan MJ, Li ZM, Meade BD, Manclark CR. Characterization of the protection capacity and immunogenicity of the 69-kD outer membrane protein of *Bordetella pertussis. J Exp Med* 1990;171:63–73.

82. Guiso N, Szatanik M, Rocancourt M. *Bordetella pertussis* adenylate cyclase: a protective antigen against colonization and lethality in immune respiratory and intra-cerebral models. In: *Proceedings of the sixth international symposium on pertussis,* 1990;208–211.

83. Pizza M, Covacci A, Bartoloni A, et al. Mutants of pertussis toxin suitable for vaccine development. *Science* 1989;246:497–500.

84. Pittman M, Cox CB. Pertussis vaccine testing for freedom-from-toxicity. *Appl Microbiol* 1963;13:447–456.

85. Hilton ML, Burland WL. Pertussis-containing vaccines: the relationship between laboratory toxicity tests and reactions in children. *Int Symp Pertussis* 1969;13:150–156.

86. Perkins FT, Sheffield F, Miller CL, Skegg JL. The comparison of toxicity of pertussis vaccines in children and mice. *Symp Ser Immunobiol* 1969;13:141–149.

87. Conner JS, Speers JF. A comparison between undesirable reactions to extracted pertussis antigen and to whole-cell antigen in DTP combinations. *J Iowa Med Soc* 1963;53:340–343.

88. Weihl C, Riley HD, Lapin JH. Extracted pertussis antigen: a clinical appraisal. *Am J Dis Child* 1963;106:210–215.

89. Cody CL, Baraff LJ, Cherry JD, et al. Nature and rates of adverse reactions associated with DTP and DT immunizations in infants and children. *Pediatrics* 1981;68:650–660.

90. Barkin RM, Pichichero ME. Diphtheria–pertussis–tetanus vaccine: reactogenicity of commercial products. *Pediatrics* 1979;63:256–260.

91. Pollock TM, Miller E, Mortimer JY, et al. Symptoms after primary immunization with DTP and with DT vaccine. *Lancet* 1984;2:146–149.

92. Baraff LJ, Shields WD, Beckwith L, Strome G, Marcy SM, Cherry JD, Manclark CR. Infants and children with convulsions and hypotonic–hyporesponsive episodes following diphtheria–tetanus–pertussis immunization: follow-up evaluation. *Pediatrics* 1988;81:789–794.

93. Baraff LJ, Manclark CR, Cherry JD, Christenson P, Marcy SM. Analyses of adverse reactions to diphtheria and tetanus toxoids and pertussis vaccine by vaccine lot, endotoxin content, pertussis vaccine potency and percentage of mouse weight gain. *Pediatr Infect Dis J* 1989;8:502–507.

94. Pollock TM, Morris J. A 7-year survey of disorders attributed to vaccination in Northwest Thames Region. *Lancet* 1983;1:753–757.

95. Miller DL, Ross EM, Alderslade R, et al. Pertussis immunization and serious acute neurological illness in children. *Br Med J* 1981;282:1595–1599.

96. Bellman MH, Ross EM, Miller DL. Infantile spasms and pertussis immunization. *Lancet* 1983;1:1031–1033.

97. Miller D, Wadsworth J, Diamond J, et al. Pertussis vaccine and whooping cough as risk factors in acute neurological illness and death in young children. *Dev Biol Stand* 1985;61:389–394.

98. McRea KD. Epidemiology, encephalopathy, and pertussis vaccine. In: Mebel S, Stompe H, Drescher M, Rustenbach S, eds. *FEMS symposium on pertussis.* Berlin: Society of Microbiology and Epidemiology of the GDR, 1988;302–311.

99. Stephenson, JBP. Pertussis vaccine on trial: science versus the law (high court of London). In: Mebel S, Stompe H, Drescher M, Rustenbach S, eds. *FEMS symposium on pertussis.* Berlin: Society of Microbiology and Epidemiology of the GDR, 1988;312–321.

100. Stephenson JBP. A neurologist looks at neurological disease temporally related to DTP immunization. *Tokai J Exp Clin Med,* 1988;13:125–128.

101. Melchior JC. Infantile spasms and early immunization against whooping cough: Danish survey from 1970 to 1975. *Arch Dis Child* 1977;52:134–137.

102. Fukuyama Y, Tomori N, Sugitate M. Critical evaluation of the role of immunization as an etiological factor of infantile spasms. *Neuropediatric* 1977;8:224–237.

103. Shields WD, Nielsen C, Buch D, et al. Relationship of pertussis immunization to the onset of neurologic disorders. *J Pediatr* 1988;113:801–805.

104. Griffin MR, Ray WA, Mortimer EA, Fenichel GM, Schaffner W. Risk of seizures and encephalopathy after immunization with the diphtheria–tetanus–pertussis vaccine. *JAMA* 1990;263:1641–1645.

105. Walker AM, Jick H, Perera DR, Knauss TA, Thompson RS. Neurologic events following diphtheria–tetanus–pertussis immunization. *Pediatrics* 1988;81:345–349.

106. Bernier RH, Frank JA Jr, Dondero TJ Jr, et al. Diphtheria–tetanus toxoids-pertussis vaccination and sudden infant deaths in Tennessee. *J Pediatr* 1982;101:419–421.

107. Baraff LJ, Ablon WJ, Weiss RC. Possible temporal association between diphtheria–tetanus toxoid–pertussis vaccination and sudden infant death syndrome. *Pediatr Infect Dis* 1983;2:7–11.

108. Mortimer EA Jr, Jones PK, Adelson L. DTP and SIDS. *Pediatr Infect Dis* 1983;2:492.

109. Walker AM, Jick H, Perera DR, et al. Diphtheria–tetanus–pertussis immunization and sudden infant death syndrome. *Am J Public Health* 1987;77:945–951.

110. Hoffman HJ, Hunter JC, Damus K, et al. Diphtheria–tetanus–pertussis immunization and sudden infant death: results of the national institute of child health and human development cooperative epidemiological study of sudden infant death syndrome risk factors. *Pediatrics* 1987;79:598–611.

111. Fenichel GM. The pertussis vaccine controversy: the danger of case reports. *Arch Neurol* 1983;40:193–194.

112. Cherry, JD. 'Pertussis vaccine encephalopathy': it is time to recognize it as the myth that it is [Editorial]. *JAMA* 1990;263:1679–1680.

113. Golden GS. Pertussis vaccine and injury to the brain. *J Pediatr* 1990;116:854–861.

114. Hill Sir AB. The environment and disease: association or causation. *Proc R Soc Med* 1965;00:295–300.

115. Corsellis JAN, Janota I, Marshall AK. Immunization against whooping cough: a neuropathological review. *Neuropathol Appl Neurobiol* 1983;8:261–270.

116. Blattner RJ, Feigin RD. Diphtheria, pertussis, and tetanus (DTP) immunization local reactions do not predict central nervous system reactions [Letter to the editor]. *Pediatrics* 1986;78:1168–1169.

117. Hannik CA, Cohen H. Pertussis vaccine experience in the Netherlands. In: Manclark CR, Hill JC, eds. *International symposium on pertussis.* US Department of Health, Education, and Welfare publication No. (NIH) 79-1830. Washington, DC: US Government Printing Office, 1979;279–282.

118. Amiel SA. The effects of *Bordetella pertussis* vaccine on cerebral vascular permeability. *Br J Exp Pathol* 1976;57:653–662.

119. Wardlaw, AC. Animal models for pertussis vaccine neurotoxicity. In: *The 5th international symposium on pertussis.* Copenhagen, 1988;13:171–175.

120. Robinson A, Irons LI, Ashworth LAE. Pertussis vaccine: present status and future prospects. *Vaccine* 1985;3:11–22.

121. Toyota T, Kai Y, Kakizaki M, et al. Effects of islet-activating protein (IAP) on blood glucose and plasma insulin in healthy volunteers (phase I studies). *Tohoku J Exp Med* 1980;130:105–116.

122. Steinman L, Sriram S, Adelman NE, et al. Murine model for pertussis vaccine encephalopathy: linkage to H-2. *Nature* 1982;299:738–740.

123. Steinman L, Weiss A, Adelman N, et al. Pertussis toxin is required for pertussis vaccine encephalopathy. *Proc Natl Acad Sci USA* 1985;82:8733–8736.

124. Hewlett EL, Cowell JL. Minireview. Evaluation of the mouse model for study of encephalopathy in pertussis vaccine recipients. *Infect Immun* 1989;57:661–663.

125. Wiedmeier SE, Chung HT, Cho BH, et al. Murine responses to immunization with pertussis toxin and bovine albumin challenge is due to an anaphylactic reaction. *Pediatr Res* 1987;22:262–267.

126. Munoz JJ, Peacock MG, Hadlow WJ. Anaphylaxis or so-called encephalopathy in mice sensitized to an antigen with the aid of pertussigen (pertussis toxin). *Infect Immun* 1987;55:1004–1008.

127. Greco D. Case–control study on encephalopathy associated with diphtheria–tetanus immunization in Campania, Italy. *Bull WHO* 1985;63:919–925.

128. Bowie C. Lessons from the pertussis vaccine court trial. *Lancet* 1990;335:397–399.

PART V

Spirochetal Infections of the CNS

Infections of the Central Nervous System,
edited by W. M. Scheld, R. J. Whitley, and
D. T. Durack, Raven Press, Ltd., New York © 1991.

CHAPTER 27

Central Nervous System Syphilis

Edward W. Hook III

Syphilis, as well as its propensity to attack the central nervous system (CNS), was well described in medical literature before the 16th century, long before the discovery of *Treponema pallidum* in 1905. Nonetheless, and despite years of study by prominent medical scientists, it remains a disease for which there are many gaps in understanding. Although for many modern clinicians the term "neurosyphilis" elicits an image of late, tertiary neurosyphilis manifest as either general paresis, tabes dorsalis, or gummatous involvement of the CNS, this very common assumption is incorrect. CNS involvement, as well as clinical signs and symptoms of CNS disease, occurs throughout all stages of syphilis. In the 1990s, as U.S. syphilis rates exceed those recorded over the past 40 years (1) and as the global pandemic of human immunodeficiency virus (HIV) infections (whose manifestations and epidemiology are intertwined with those of syphilis) progresses, the topic of CNS involvement and disease caused by syphilis has begun to be reappraised.

The term "neurosyphilis" has come to represent a spectrum of manifestations of CNS involvement in individuals with *T. pallidum* infection and, as such, tends to contribute to confusion in discussing the disease. In this chapter a distinction will be made between (a) CNS involvement as a manifestation of probable infection of the CNS by *T. pallidum* and (b) neurosyphilis, the clinically apparent disease processes which may result from involvement of the CNS by *T. pallidum*. Thus, as used in this chapter, asymptomatic patients in whom laboratory findings suggest CNS invasion by *T. pallidum* will be referred to as having CNS involvement rather than asymptomatic neurosyphilis. Patients with CNS involvement, if untreated, are at risk for development of clini-

cally apparent disease which will be referred to as "neurosyphilis."

PATHOGENESIS AND PATHOPHYSIOLOGY OF SYPHILITIC CNS INVOLVEMENT

For purposes of directing therapy, for helping to make decisions regarding partner notification, and for assessing the approximate duration of infection, it has been useful to divide syphilis into a series of stages defined largely on the basis of clinical signs whose presence roughly correlates with duration of infection (2,3). Primary syphilis occurs within days of acquisition of infection manifest by the presence of a syphilitic ulcer, the chancre, at the site of inoculation. Without therapy, over a period of 3–6 weeks the chancre will heal, after which the majority of patients progress to the secondary stage of disease in which systemic spirochetemia with *T. pallidum* becomes manifest by flu-like symptoms, accompanied by an array of clinical signs of which skin rash, generalized lymphadenopathy, and mucosal lesions are most common. Untreated, the findings of secondary syphilis also resolve following a period of weeks to months. Individuals with syphilis who do not develop secondary manifestations of infection, as well as patients with syphilis in whom the signs of secondary syphilis have resolved, then typically enter a latent stage in which there are no clinically apparent manifestations of infection. After a highly variable period ranging from months to years, about one-third of patients with untreated latent syphilis go on to develop tertiary manifestations of disease which may present as either cardiovascular syphilis, gummatous syphilis, or tertiary neurosyphilis (general paresis or tabes dorsalis). However, syphilitic invasion of the CNS occurs early in the disease, may be asymptomatically present throughout the entire course of infection, and may present as clinical neurosyphilis at

E. W. Hook III: Department of Medicine, Johns Hopkins University School of Medicine, Baltimore, Maryland 21205; and STD Clinical Services, Baltimore City Health Department, Baltimore, Maryland 21205.

any point in the natural history of infection beyond the primary stage (4–14).

Nearly all individuals who acquire syphilis do so as the result of direct inoculation of *T. pallidum* at cutaneous or mucous membrane sites. Following epithelial inoculation, during the earliest stages of infection the organism multiplies, disseminates hematogenously and to local lymphatic tissues, and elicits an initial polymorphonuclear leukocyte inflammatory response which is replaced shortly thereafter by lymphocytic infiltration at the site of the primary lesion (7,8). *T. pallidum* disseminates to the CNS during these earliest events, as evidenced by the ability to isolate the organism from the cerebrospinal fluid (CSF) of patients with primary syphilis and by the presence of CSF laboratory abnormalities in 5–9% of patients with seronegative primary syphilis (9,10). Systemic spirochetemia continues throughout the course of untreated early syphilis, and the increasing prevalence of CNS laboratory abnormalities observed in the successive stages of early syphilis is probably indicative of continued invasion of the CNS over the natural history of early stages of the disease.

T. pallidum is difficult to demonstrate microscopically in CSF, and culture for the organism is impractical for most purposes (see below). Thus current understanding of pathophysiologic events which occur due to CNS involvement in syphilis result from the relatively imprecise perspective generated from compilation of observations made by a number of investigators, many of whom worked early in the 20th century. In most instances, patients with primary or secondary syphilis and CNS invasion are asymptomatic or have only mild, relatively nonspecific symptoms (11). However, asymptomatic CNS involvement appears to predispose patients to subsequent development of clinically apparent neurosyphilis. Prospective studies conducted in the 1930s demonstrated the prognostic import of CSF abnormalities in patients with early syphilis (12–15). Moore and Hopkins (14) followed 123 syphilis patients with asymptomatic CNS involvement, subdividing them into three groups based on the intensity of their CSF abnormalities. Progression occurred in two (14%) of 14 patients with group I (the mildest) CSF changes and in five (7%) of 73 patients with group II changes, whereas 12 (33%) of the 36 patients with group III CSFs progressed to parenchymatous neurosyphilis (a substantial number of additional patients in each of the groups were considered to have "questionable" findings suggestive of, but not clearly diagnostic of, neurosyphilis). These data were generated with an average follow-up of only 7 years; this was particularly noteworthy because the mean time to development of parenchymatous neurosyphilis is felt to be 12–15 years. In contrast, these and other investigators also reported that patients without CSF abnormalities were unlikely to develop them and were at little or no risk for subsequent development of clinical neurosyphilis (12,13,15).

The pathologic bases for CSF laboratory abnormalities, as well as the gross and histologic CNS changes noted in patients with asymptomatic or symptomatic CNS involvement, reflect the fact that although the host response to infection often does not eradicate the infection, it does modify its clinical manifestations. As already mentioned, hematogenous dissemination of *T. pallidum* occurs during the earliest stages of disease; during the earliest stage of CNS invasion, pathologic changes are limited to perivascular and meningeal inflammation.

Because of the low mortality rate associated with early syphilis and also because there is no animal model of neurosyphilis, little is known about pathologic findings in the earliest stages of CNS involvement (4). In later stages of neurosyphilis, among the processes described are meningitis, ependymitis, and vasculitis involving vessels of all sizes as well as fibrotic changes and parenchymal neuron degeneration (4). It has been suggested that in some patients, vascular disease may be caused by immune complex vasculitis; it has also been suggested that in some instances, *T. pallidum* may directly damage neurons or other tissues (2,16,17). However, available data suggest the contribution of vascular damage to the origin of nearly all stages of CNS involvement in the disease (2). In patients with progressive vascular involvement, blood vessel inflammation goes on to result in endothelial damage which, in turn, leads to proliferation of subintimal fibroblasts which may ultimately progress to the point of luminal occlusion by thrombosis or the process itself. Progressive syphilitic vasculitis results in clinical signs and symptoms caused by (a) accompanying local inflammation, (b) transient vascular insufficiency related to spasm of involved vessels, (c) lasting tissue hypoxia related to irreversible vascular involvement, or (d) the fibrosis and scarring following hypoxic damage (2). The relationship of these general pathologic processes to each of the different clinical neurosyphilis syndromes will be further delineated in the portions of this chapter devoted specifically to those syndromes.

LABORATORY MANIFESTATIONS OF SYPHILITIC CNS INVOLVEMENT

T. pallidum, the causative agent of syphilis, is a spiral organism whose microbiologic characteristics have been a somewhat greater impediment to the study of this disease than have those of most other bacterial infections. The organism has an elongated spiral morphology, measuring 6–20 by 0.10–0.18 μm. The narrow width of *T. pallidum* precludes visualization of the organism by light microscopy with the stains used for visualization of other bacteria. The organism can be seen in clinical specimens using dark-field microscopy to identify its characteristic morphology and flexing "corkscrew" motility, or it may be identified in fixed tissues using silver stains or immunofluorescence microscopy. Although these techniques are useful for demonstration of *T. pallidum* in clinical specimens from cutaneous lesions, their utility is far less for diagnosis of CNS involvement in which the numbers of organisms present are thought to be relatively low and due to the susceptibility of such efforts to misidentification of artifacts as treponemes (11,18). In addition, *T. pallidum* cannot be cultivated readily in artificial media or in cell culture, further complicating efforts to study the spectrum, natural history, and extent of CNS infection. Although recently developed techniques using polymerase chain reaction technology to detect the presence of *T. pallidum* genetic material in clinical specimens hold great promise as tools for further study of this infection, at present the imperfect gold standard for demonstration of *T. pallidum* infection remains intratesticular inoculation of clinical specimens into rabbit testis. The sensitivity of rabbit inoculation is thought to be about 10 treponemes (11), making it sufficiently sensitive to be useful for proving the presence of infection. However, rabbit intratesticular inoculation is relatively expensive to perform and, more importantly, usually takes about 3 months to provide evidence of infection, limiting its clinical utility as a diagnostic test. Serologic testing, an approach which has a number of limitations, is the most widely used method of syphilis diagnosis. For diagnosis of CNS involvement in patients with syphilis, no single laboratory test is useful. Instead, the results of a battery of laboratory tests, interpreted in the context of the results of a carefully performed history and physical examination, are the most appropriate means of diagnosing CNS syphilis.

Laboratory testing of CSF from patients with syphilis may serve several distinct purposes which should be kept in mind as one interprets the results of such tests. In patients with neurologic signs or symptoms, laboratory testing for syphilis is useful for helping to attribute causation to syphilis. In the pre-penicillin era, lumbar puncture results were often used to determine the duration of therapy that patients would receive (2). This approach was based on observations that patients with CSF abnormalities were at risk for development of neurosyphilis whereas those with normal CSFs were not, and that treatment failures often presented with neurologic signs and symptoms (so-called neurorelapse). Since the mid-1940s, however, the great activity of penicillin against *T. pallidum* appears to have reduced the likelihood for development of neurosyphilis in early syphilis patients receiving this form of treatment; as a result, lumbar punctures, which were formerly used to evaluate patients with syphilis irrespective of clinical stage, are now being used primarily to help determine the need for neurosyphilis

therapy in patients with syphilis of more than 1 year's duration. Thus, CSF examination is now most often used either to (a) provide diagnostic information for patients with clinical findings which might be due to neurosyphilis or (b) diagnose asymptomatic CNS involvement in patients with untreated syphilis so that they might be treated to prevent progression to neurosyphilis. CSF examination for the former purpose is sometimes compromised by (a) the nonspecificity of some of the CSF abnormalities most commonly seen in syphilis patients with CNS involvement (elevations of CSF leukocyte or protein concentrations) and (b) the relatively low sensitivity of the more specific serologic test recommended for diagnostic purposes (the CSF VDRL; see below). For diagnosis of CNS involvement in asymptomatic patients, not all patients with CNS invasion by *T. pallidum* have abnormalities of commonly performed tests, an observation of uncertain significance. More recently, concerns about the diminished efficacy of benzathine penicillin for patients with early syphilis and concomitant HIV infection has made the issue of which patients might benefit from lumbar puncture more controversial than it was in the pre-HIV era.

Laboratory evidence of CNS involvement is far more common in syphilis patients than clinically apparent disease. Prior to the availability of effective therapy, as mentioned earlier, Moore and Hopkins (14) showed CSF laboratory abnormalities to be harbingers of clinical neurosyphilis. Since then, investigators have used a wide variety of tests ranging from simple measurement of CSF leukocytes or protein concentrations to any of a number of serologic tests or determinations of whether antibodies reacting in CSF syphilis serologic tests were produced in the CNS rather than being passively transferred across the meninges from serum to CSF. Unfortunately, much of this large body of work on serologic testing of CSF is difficult to interpret. In many of the studies the characteristics of the patient populations studied are relatively poorly defined and often include patients who have been previously treated. In addition, the relationship of test abnormalities to the presence or absence of *T. pallidum* in CSF or to the likelihood of progression to clinical neurosyphilis is unclear in nearly all recent studies of the problem.

Although a number of indirect parameters have been used to demonstrate CNS involvement in patients with all stages of syphilis, relatively few have been used in conjunction with measures to test for the presence of *T. pallidum*. Cultivation of *T. pallidum* from CSF is a relatively expensive, time-consuming process and has only been used occasionally in the study of CNS syphilis. Nonetheless, the data derived from the few studies which sought to cultivate treponemes from CSF of syphilis patients offer important insights into the frequency and pathogenesis of CNS invasion (11,19–22). Shortly following the first descriptions of *T. pallidum* as the causative agent of syphilis in 1905, investigators began to attempt to cultivate the organism. Other than the earliest report of successful isolation of *T. pallidum* by inoculation of CSF from a syphilis patient into the eyebrow of a chimpanzee, most investigators attempting to isolate spirochetes from patients have utilized rabbit intratesticular inoculation, probably because of convenience, lower cost, and the absence of data to suggest that other methods are more sensitive. In 1913, Nichols and Hough (19) reported the second successful isolation of *T. pallidum* from human CSF (and the first such report using rabbits) when they successfully cultivated the organism from CSF of a patient suffering neurologic relapse following treatment with salvarsan, the preferred treatment of the day. These authors also were among the first to suggest that the CNS may represent a site of treponemal infection less accessible to therapeutic agents than other parts of the body and that, as such, it might serve as a protected site from which relapse could originate following treatment. A second important contribution of their work was that the strain of *T. pallidum* isolated from their patient, now known as the "Nichols strain," has been serially passaged and disseminated among investigators since then, becoming the prototype strain of *T. pallidum* upon which most subsequent basic work on treponemal biology has been based. Likewise, the Nichols strain has served as the strain from which nearly all *T. pallidum*-based diagnostic tests have been derived.

Other investigators working in the second and third decades of the 20th century also used rabbit inoculation to describe events related to CNS syphilis, although the technique never became widely used for large studies of CNS involvement in syphilis patients (20,21). In 1924, Chesney and Kemp (21) performed lumbar punctures and rabbit inoculation of 34 patients with secondary syphilis and "normal" CSF (<9 WBCs/mm^3, normal CSF proteins, nonreactive CSF Wassermann reactions) and showed that five (15%) contained viable *T. pallidum*, thereby conclusively demonstrating that treponemes could invade the CNS of a substantial proportion of patients with early syphilis without being otherwise manifest. Unfortunately, no large studies have been done to clarify the relationship of viable *T. pallidum* in CSF, as determined by animal inoculation, to either the prevalence (or incidence) of subsequent laboratory abnormalities in syphilis patients or the likelihood of progression to clinically apparent disease. In 1988, Lukehart et al. (11) utilized rabbit inoculation studies to reevaluate the frequency of CNS invasion by *T. pallidum* in untreated syphilis patients and to study the relationship of other, more readily performed laboratory tests to treponemal isolation from CSF. These authors isolated treponemes from 12 (30%) of 40 patients with primary or secondary syphilis and none of 18 patients with latent syphilis. Of the 12 patients from whom treponemes were

cultivated, no commonly performed CSF laboratory tests (cell count, protein concentration, or CSF VDRL) were abnormal in four. Although CSF laboratory abnormalities were relatively common in patients with all stages of disease, no single laboratory test could be clearly related to successful isolation of *T. pallidum*. However, patients with any two CSF abnormalities (e.g., CSF leukocytosis, elevated CSF protein, or reactive CSF VDRL) were statistically more likely to have treponemes isolated than were patients with single or no abnormalities.

Given the difficulties associated with *T. pallidum* cultivation, it is not surprising that medical scientists have turned to more readily (and rapidly) available laboratory tests in efforts to diagnose CNS involvement in syphilis. Prior to the antibiotic era, determination of CSF pleocytosis, elevation of CSF protein (or globulins), and serologic tests on CSF [primarily the Wassermann test, a forerunner of currently utilized nontreponemal serologic tests such as the Venereal Disease Research Laboratory (VDRL) or rapid plasma reagin (RPR) tests] were used to validate clinical diagnoses of neurosyphilis and to identify patients at increased risk for progression to neurosyphilis. Several large series demonstrated CSF abnormalities (pleocytosis, increased globulins, or reactive CSF Wassermann reactions) in 5–9% of patients with seronegative primary syphilis, in 13–23% with seropositive primary syphilis, and in 20–32% of secondary syphilis patients (9,10,15), proving that CNS involvement occurred in substantial numbers of patients in the earliest stages of infection. In their more recent studies, Lukehart et al. (11) verified that despite questions as to whether the spectrum of neurologic involvement in syphilis patients had changed during the antimicrobial era (23–25), the frequency of CNS involvement in patients with early syphilis had not, reporting evidence of CNS involvement (CSF pleocytosis, elevated protein concentrations, or reactive CSF VDRL) in 43% of primary and 58% of secondary syphilis patients.

Although most of the patients included in studies of CNS involvement in early syphilis were asymptomatic or were noted to complain only of headache, in the preantibiotic era the CSF examination was a routine part of patient evaluation and the therapeutic choices were often influenced by the presence or absence of CSF abnormalities (2,26). At the time, it was also appreciated that serologic tests for syphilis (most often the Wassermann test, a reaginic complement fixation test) were nonreactive in a substantial proportion of patients with neurologic involvement (2,4). Thus in patients with syphilis, CNS involvement was often diagnosed based on CSF leukocytosis or elevated CSF protein concentrations. In the penicillin era, as a result of accumulating experience that penicillin therapy prevented the subsequent development of neurosyphilis in most patients (26), efforts to diagnose CNS involvement shifted from all patients to patients with syphilis of more than 1 year's duration.

In addition, subsequent to the availability of penicillin, a number of newly developed serologic tests for syphilis were evaluated as part of efforts to more accurately diagnose CNS involvement. The VDRL test came to replace the less sensitive and more time-consuming CSF Wassermann test; moreover, the newly developed treponemal tests such as the fluorescent treponemal antibody absorption (FTA-ABS) test replaced the more expensive and difficult *T. pallidum* immobilization (TPI) test as confirmatory tests. Unfortunately, the evaluations of these tests were often performed on relatively small numbers of patients and/or on study populations comprised of previously treated as well as untreated patients with a variety of clinical stages. Consequently, well-intended efforts to utilize newer, possibly improved tests for diagnosis of CNS involvement may have contributed to increasing confusion as to optimal measures for diagnosis of CNS involvement in syphilis patients.

The results of serologic testing of CSF in patients with syphilis are subject to confounding by several factors. CSF collected by lumbar puncture is contaminated by blood due to inadvertent puncture of nearby blood vessels in up to 10% of patients, providing an opportunity for contamination by seropositive blood to lead to false-positive CSF serologic test results (27,28). The likelihood of CSF serologic tests being altered by blood contamination is related to the relative amount of contamination, the antibody titers in blood, and the sensitivity of the test being considered. Several studies have addressed this issue, demonstrating that the CSF FTA test is more susceptible to artifactual change than the CSF VDRL, and that for patients with serum VDRL tests of 1:256 or less, sufficient contamination to be visible to the naked eye is required to cause spurious CSF VDRL test results (27,28). In general, however, in instances of traumatic lumbar punctures, repeated lumbar puncture is recommended for evaluation of patients whose CSF is contaminated by blood.

Although the specificity of the CSF VDRL for diagnosis of CNS involvement is generally accepted as high (6,29,30), a few patients with false-positive tests have been reported (31). However, the sensitivity of the CSF VDRL test for this purpose is thought to be low (6,29,30). Although no large series of confirmed neurosyphilis patients have been studied since the VDRL test became available, there are numerous studies performed in the first half of the 20th century which demonstrated that patients with neurosyphilis not uncommonly had nonreactive CSF Wassermann reactions (2,4). Since replacement of the Wassermann test by the more sensitive VDRL test for testing serum, it appears that the logical assumption was made that the VDRL test, while more sensitive, was nonetheless probably also occasionally nonreactive in patients with CNS involvement. This

supposition has been borne out by a number of studies performed in the past 30 years; however, precise definition of the true sensitivity of the CSF VDRL test is lacking. In recently published series of patients with neurosyphilis (23,25,32,33), more than one-third of patients have had nonreactive CSF VDRL tests, including a small proportion of patients with simultaneously nonreactive serum reaginic tests.

A number of authors have also explored the utility of the FTA or the FTA-ABS on CSF for diagnosis of neurosyphilis (30,33,40), applying the test to a variety of different patient populations. In general, these studies indicate the following: (a) the CSF FTA is more often reactive in syphilis patients than the CSF FTA-ABS, (b) both tests (the CSF FTA and CSF FTA-ABS) are more often reactive in syphilis patients than the CSF VDRL, (c) false-positive CSF FTA-ABS results are rare in patients who have not had syphilis (37), and (d) the CSF FTA-ABS is not infrequently the only abnormal CSF test in patients with (treated or untreated) syphilis. In one noteworthy study, Davis and Schmidt (33) reported on the use of the CSF FTA-ABS test as a screening test for neurosyphilis in 1,665 CSF specimens collected from patients undergoing lumbar puncture for any reason over a 10-year period. Forty-eight patients had reactive tests, and only 15 of these patients were felt to have active neurosyphilis. Most investigators agree with their conclusions that a nonreactive CSF FTA-ABS effectively rules out the likelihood of active neurosyphilis but that the specificity of a reactive test is far less than that of the CSF VDRL test. However, there are no compelling data which define the significance of a reactive CSF FTA-ABS as a useful parameter for making the diagnosis of neurosyphilis.

A number of investigators have attempted to evaluate the utility of alternative CSF tests, including (a) tests for anti-treponemal IgM in CSF or (b) tests designed to determine whether antibodies detected in CSF have been synthesized in the CNS or simply reflect diffusion of serum antibodies into CSF in patients with circulating anti-treponemal antibodies (30,41–44). The latter tests usually compare albumin and IgG concentrations in serum to those in CSF from the same patient, assuming that changes in their ratio relative to expected values reflect intrathecal synthesis of anti-treponemal antibodies. Some modifications of these tests refine this approach still further, measuring concentrations of specific treponemal antibodies. As is the case for most recent studies of serologic tests for CNS syphilis, the data on these tests have been derived from relatively small numbers of variably characterized patients, some of whom have previously received treatment for syphilis or who have other factors which complicate interpretation of the data.

At the present time, recently developed diagnostic tests for syphilis utilizing monoclonal antibody reagents for detection of treponemal antigens hold great but as yet unrealized promise for helping to diagnose CNS involvement with *T. pallidum* in syphilis patients, as do polymerase chain reaction tests for detection of treponemal DNA. Several studies exploring the utility of these new tests for diagnosis of CNS involvement in syphilis patients are being planned or are underway, but as yet there are no conclusive data on the utility of these promising diagnostic tools.

CLINICAL NEUROSYPHILIS SYNDROMES

Clinical neurosyphilis syndromes can be divided into several distinct clinical syndromes which tend to occur at somewhat different points in the natural history of untreated syphilis (4) (Table 1). Since the 1940s, when the increasing availability of penicillin and public health efforts to interrupt syphilis transmission began to dramatically reduce the numbers of new cases in North America and Europe, there may have been changes in the distribution of neurosyphilis syndromes (23,25).

TABLE 1. *Central nervous system involvement in syphilis patients—clinical classification*

Central nervous system involvement: Evidence of CNS invasion by *T. pallidum* may include (a) demonstration of *T. pallidum* in CSF or CNS tissue, (b) laboratory abnormalities due to CNS invasion, or (c) clinical syndromes resulting from CNS invasion. CNS involvement may be present at any time in the natural history of untreated infection and is frequently asymptomatic. CNS involvement may be further subdivided into five categories:

I. **Asymptomatic CNS involvement:** Occurs throughout the natural history of untreated syphilis. Patients with asymptomatic involvement are at risk for subsequent development of clinically apparent disease.
II. **Syphilitic meningitis:** Peak incidence 1–2 years following infection. Severe aseptic meningitis syndrome often associated with cranial nerve involvement. Usually resolves with effective therapy.
III. **Meningovascular syphilis:** Peak incidence 5–7 years following infection, presenting with focal neurologic deficits resulting from vasculitis involving small to medium-sized arterial blood vessels. Therapy halts progression, and often a degree of improvement follows.
IV. **Parenchymatous neurosyphilis (general paresis and tabes dorsalis):** Peak incidence 10–20 years following infection. Clinical deficits result from irreversible neuron damage either supratentorially (in paresis) or at the dorsal roots of the spinal column (in tabes). Therapy usually halts progression, but improvement of clinical signs is rare.
V. **Gummatous neurosyphilis:** Relatively rare occurrence of gummata, which may occur at nearly any time after infection and which may originate anywhere within the CNS. Signs and symptoms are due to the mass effect of the gummata. With therapy and resolution of gummata, clinical signs and symptoms may improve.

In addition, although the identification of patients having "asymptomatic neurosyphilis" on the basis of abnormal CSF laboratory tests was of prognostic import and was used to help guide decisions regarding therapy and follow-up in the preantibiotic era, its import today is less certain, at least for patients who do not have coexistent HIV infection (see section entitled "CNS Involvement in Syphilis Patients with HIV Infection," below). In the preantibiotic era, for patients in whom repeated lumbar punctures throughout the course of treatment could not be performed, it was emphasized that lumbar puncture at the time of follow-up was probably of greater prognostic import than that prior to treatment, since abnormal findings following treatment identified patients at increased risk for subsequent development of neurosyphilis (13). More recently, studies reporting post-therapy lumbar punctures in nearly 200 patients treated for early syphilis with 2.4 to 6 million units of penicillin (usually as daily injections of either penicillin aluminum monosterate or benzathine penicillin over a 1- to 2-week period) found almost no evidence of treatment failure (25), a finding which supported the impression of many clinicians that clinically apparent neurosyphilis following penicillin therapy was quite rare. Nonetheless, the substantial number of documented treatment failures in patients treated with recommended doses of benzathine penicillin (even prior to the advent of the HIV epidemic) indicate that some patients treated for early syphilis do fail therapy and that treatment failures not infrequently present as neurosyphilis (45–48). (This experience parallels experiences noted prior to the availability of penicillin, at which time CNS treatment failures sometimes occurred despite continued evidence of peripheral response to therapy as manifest by declining Wassermann reaction titers.)

It is useful to organize clinical neurosyphilis into four syndromes: syphilitic meningitis, meningovascular syphilis, parenchymatous neurosyphilis, and gummatous neurosyphilis, despite the fact that their clinical and laboratory findings often overlap (4–6). Although each syndrome may occur throughout the course of untreated syphilis, they vary as to time of peak incidence as well as with respect to the pathologic processes which lead to them (4,6). Syphilitic meningitis is thought to be the consequence of direct meningeal inflammation (Fig. 1), most likely due to a small-vessel arteritis and most often occurring within 2 years of acquisition of syphilis. These patients rarely have focal neurologic findings and may experience spontaneous resolution of disease. Meningovascular syphilis, which is most common 4–10 years following infection, is the consequence of vasculitis as well; however, meningovascular syphilis is due to proliferative endarteritis with transmural and perivascular infiltration of small to medium-sized vessels by lymphocytes and plasma cells and rarely resolves without therapy. If

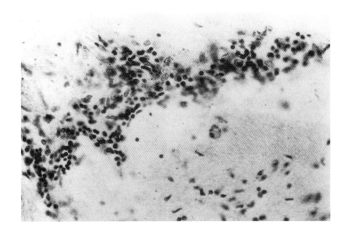

FIG. 1. Meningeal infiltration by lymphocytes and plasma cells from a patient with asymptomatic neurosyphilis. (From ref. 4, with permission.)

untreated, meningovascular syphilis may progress to fibrotic occlusion of blood vessels and permanent neurologic deficits. In patients with the third category of neurosyphilis, parenchymatous neurosyphilis (general paresis or tabes dorsalis), the pathologic processes most often become apparent 10–20 years following acquisition of infection and more directly involve neurons, leading to histologic findings of diminished neuron concentrations, demyelination, and astrocyte proliferation with accompanying gliosis. Finally, in the occasional patient with the fourth variant of neurosyphilis, gummatous neurosyphilis, the incidence peaks still later in the disease; moreover, neurologic deficits result from mass effect due to the presence of CNS gumma rather than from direct damage to neurons or their blood supply.

It is important to acknowledge several potential limitations to our current understanding of clinical neurosyphilis syndromes. The descriptions of the clinical syndromes that follow have mostly been compiled from studies published prior to the availability of penicillin, supplemented by more recently published case reports and small case series. Both prior to and subsequent to the availability of penicillin, descriptions of patients with neurosyphilis often included patients who had previously received some therapy or who were relapsing following earlier, apparently successful therapy. This limitation is difficult to avoid; furthermore, after careful study of the matter, I agree with my earlier and more experienced predecessors that there is little difference in clinical presentations between untreated patients and those who had received prior therapy, at least as far as the clinical descriptions of the syndromes goes. A second potential problem is that the classic descriptions of neurosyphilis as contained in the texts of Stokes (2) and Merrit et al. (4) were made at a time when the differential diagnosis of neurologic disease processes were far more limited than is currently the case. As a result, it is possible that in some instances, classic case series of patients with neurosyphilis syndromes also contain some patients with other diseases (6). Finally, there is debate as to whether the presentations of symptomatic neurosyphilis syndromes have been modified in the antibiotic era (possibly as the result of partially effective therapy or due to incidental therapy when patients with previously acquired syphilis are treated for other infections) or are simply less common than prior to the 1950s (23–33, 49–51).

Syphilitic Meningitis

Syphilitic meningitis is defined by the presence of signs and symptoms which are relatively common in patients with secondary syphilis but which are particularly intense in patients with the syndrome as classically described. The incidence of syphilitic meningitis is greatest in the first 2 years following infection (4,6,52). It is one of the least common neurosyphilis syndromes, having been estimated to occur in only 0.3–2.4% of syphilis cases (52). In 1935, Merritt and Moore (52) published their classic work on this syndrome, describing a total of 80 patients seen at four Boston Hospitals over a 15-year period. The most common symptoms in patients with syphilitic meningitis were severe headache, nausea, and vomiting. However, on the basis of additional signs and symptoms, these authors went on to further subdivide the syndrome into three variants, based on the area of the CNS predominantly affected. In acute syphilitic hydrocephalus the predominant findings were nonfocal and included headache, nausea, and vomiting, whereas in acute vertical syphilitic meningitis, additional abnormalities such as seizures, focal neurologic deficits (e.g., hemiplegia or aphasia which usually resolved with therapy), and delirium or confusion were usually present and were thought to result from inflammation which predominated on the vertex of the brain. The third variant, acute basilar syphilitic meningitis, was characterized primarily by the presence of cranial nerve involvement. Although these distinctions provide useful insight into the spectrum of manifestations which may occur in patients with syphilitic meningitis, they probably represent efforts to resolve this relatively rare syndrome to a degree which is not clinically useful. The predominant findings in patients with acute syphilitic meningitis are those of other aseptic meningitides. Headache, nausea, and vomiting were present in 73 (91%) of 80 patients, meningismus occurred in 59%, and fever occurred in less than 50%. In addition, a number of focal findings were also seen in these patients. Seizures occurred in 17% of patients with syphilitic meningitis; also occurring in these patients were less common focal abnormalities such as hemiplegia, aphasia, or mental status changes. Cranial nerve palsies occurred in 45% of patients with syphilitic meningitis.

Although syphilitic cranial nerve abnormalities are most common in patients with syphilitic meningitis (2,4,53–57), they are also well described in patients with meningovascular syphilis, patients with parenchymatous neurosyphilis, and patients who experience "neurorelapse" following insufficient treatment (2,4,58). In early syphilis and in patients with neurorelapse, the seventh and eighth cranial nerves are most commonly involved, followed in frequency by the optic and oculomotor nerves (Table 2). Although unilateral or bilateral involvement of individual cranial nerves is most common, 40–50% of patients have findings compatible with multiple nerve involvement (4). The onset of cranial nerve deficits may develop gradually or suddenly; following effective treatment, resolution usually occurs. The major exceptions to this statement are (a) optic atrophy, whose progression may be arrested by treatment but which is unlikely to improve, and (b) hearing deficits, which may improve following therapy but which not infrequently fail to return to normal.

CSF laboratory abnormalities are also common in patients with syphilitic meningitis. Perhaps partly because about one-third of patients in their series had previously received therapy of some sort, serologic (Wassermann) tests were more often reactive in CSF than in sera in the series reported by Merritt and Moore (52). In their series, 48 (60%) of 80 patients had reactive serum Wasserman reactions; however, the test was reactive in 69 (86%) CSF specimens from the same patients. Other CSF abnormalities seen in their series included mononuclear-cell-predominant CSF leukocytosis (79 of 80 patients had >10 CSF WBCs/mm^3), elevated CSF protein concentrations (78%), and mild decreases in CSF glucose (CSF glucose <50 mg% in 55% of patients). In contrast, descriptions of patients with isolated cranial nerve involvement from the pre-penicillin era indicate that normal

CSF findings are not unusual among this subset of patients (2,4,53).

The differential diagnosis of patients with syphilitic meningitis is that of aseptic meningitis and includes viral meningitis, tuberculous meningitis, and brain or epidural abscess, each of which may lead to signs and symptoms of increased intracranial pressure (headache, nausea, vomiting), as well as seizures or cranial nerve abnormalities. In general, the presence of a reactive serologic test for syphilis, as well as the relatively subacute onset of signs and symptoms, helps to differentiate this syndrome from other processes included in the differential diagnosis. Because the CSF may be normal in patients with isolated cranial nerve involvement, this circumstance in a patient with other evidence of syphilis may be one of the few situations in which the results of a therapeutic trial may be helpful for patients and diagnostically.

Patients with syphilitic meningitis tend to do well, and, unlike other neurosyphilis syndromes occurring later in the disease, syphilitic meningitis may resolve without therapy. In the pre-penicillin era, CSF abnormalities and clinical findings nearly uniformly resolved with treatment (2,4). The exception to this statement relates to the cranial nerve abnormalities seen in 45% of patients with syphilitic meningitis (4). Although most patients with cranial nerve abnormalities improved, residual abnormalities (particularly of the eighth cranial nerve) were not uncommon. Although a small proportion of patients with syphilitic meningitis went on to develop parenchymatous neurosyphilis (tabes dorsalis or general paresis) in the pre-penicillin era, and others have been reported subsequent to benzathine penicillin therapy, no instances of progression have been reported following modern, high-dose therapy.

Meningovascular Syphilis

Unlike other neurosyphilis syndromes, the proportion of neurosyphilis syndromes attributed to meningovascular neurosyphilis does not appear to have changed in the antibiotic era (25). Although estimates of the proportion of patients with CNS involvement who have meningovascular syphilis range from 3% to 15%, most recent authors find meningovascular syphilis to comprise 10–12% of individuals with CNS involvement at the present time (6,23,25). Meningovascular syphilis may occur as the presenting manifestation of syphilitic infection or may occur following ineffective therapy for early syphilis (4,59). Meningovascular syphilis is distinguished from meningeal syphilis temporally and on the basis of the focal neurologic findings which result from focal syphilitic arteritis, almost always occurring in combination with meningeal inflammation. Meningovascular syphi-

TABLE 2. *Cranial nerve involvement in acute syphilitic meningitis*[a]

Cranial nerve	Percent bilateral/unilateral involvement	Prevalence (%) in patients with cranial nerve
I	Unknown	2
II	100/0	27
III	0/100	24
IV	0/100	3
V	13/87	12
VI	22/78	22
VII	11/89	41
VIII	29/71	42
IX, X	20/80	6
XI, XII	0/100	4

[a] Data were taken from ref. 4.

lis occurs from months to years following syphilis acquisition, with peak incidence at about 7 years (4). In their series of meningovascular syphilis patients evaluated as part of their review of neurosyphilis patients seen at several Boston hospitals, Merritt et al. (4) found that 91% of meningovascular syphilis occurred in patients 30–60 years of age: 36% in patients 30–39 years old, 31% in those aged 40–49, and 24% in the 50- to 59-year age group.

Clinically, patients with meningovascular syphilis present with symptoms and signs of diffuse meningeal inflammation as well as with findings attributable to focal involvement of cerebral blood supply (2,4,59). Prior to development of neurologic deficits resulting from irreversible ischemia, most patients with meningovascular syphilis experience weeks to months of episodic prodromal signs and symptoms. These most commonly include headache or vertiginous episodes, personality changes (uncharacteristic apathy or inattention), behavioral changes (irritability or memory impairment), insomnia, or occasional seizures. Patients may also experience focal deficits reflecting episodes of ischemia to regions of the brain supplied by involved blood vessels. If untreated, progressive arterial insufficiency caused by meningovascular syphilis will lead to stroke syndromes with attendant irreversible neurologic deficits. Meningovascular syphilis may occur at virtually any location within the CNS, and, although cerebral angiography may demonstrate multifocal arterial narrowing (59), clinical deficits suggesting involvement of more than one vessel are relatively uncommon, occurring in only five of 42 patients (12%) reported by Merritt et al. (4). Similarly, although focal deficits may occur nearly anywhere within the cerebral blood supply, involvement of the middle cerebral artery is by far most common, occurring in 62% of the patients reported by Merritt et al. (4) [the next most common vessel involved in their series was the basilar artery, which was involved in five (12%) of 42 patients]. The lasting neurologic deficits in patients with meningovascular syphilis tend to be somewhat smaller than those occurring in patients with stroke syndromes arising from atherosclerotic disease, possibly because of the following: (a) Small and medium-sized vessels are most often involved in meningovascular syphilis, (b) individuals with meningovascular syphilis tend to be younger than patients with atherosclerotic cerebrovascular disease, and (c) the occlusive process which occurs in patients with meningovascular syphilis occurs over a period of time rather than suddenly, permitting establishment of collateral blood flow to ischemic areas. At the present time, the mortality associated with meningovascular syphilis is relatively low. In the preantibiotic era, however, patients debilitated by stroke syndromes caused by meningovascular syphilis occasionally died, less often as a result of their neurologic event than be-

cause their event left them predisposed to bedsores which often became infected, resulting in fatal sepsis.

Meningovascular syphilis may also, albeit rarely, involve the arterial supply to the spinal cord, affecting either the vertebral, anterior spinal, or posterior spinal arteries. Unlike in patients with cerebral meningovascular syphilis, in patients with the spinal variant the following facts apply: Prodromal signs and symptoms are uncommon, the onset of neurologic deficits is usually sudden, and these deficits are usually irreversible (4).

Clinically, patients with meningovascular syphilis have evidence of both meningeal and vascular involvement. Meningeal inflammation due to lymphocytic and plasma cell infiltration of small meningeal vessels is the likely source of CSF abnormalities (leukocytosis, elevated protein concentrations, reactive CSF VDRL tests) which are nearly uniformly present in meningovascular syphilis patients (4,6,59). In addition, however, arterial (syphilitic venous inflammation is very rare) inflammation affecting vessels of any size leads to the focal neurologic abnormalities which characterize meningovascular syphilis. Pathologically, in meningovascular syphilis the arteritis of medium and large arteries is referred to as "Heubner's arteritis" (Fig. 2), whereas arteriolar changes are referred to as "Nissl–Alzheimer arteritis" (4). In each the process is initially manifest by local infiltration of vessel walls with lymphocytes and plasma cells (including involvement of the vasa vasorum in larger arteries); however, the inflammatory process goes on to irreversibly damage arterial muscle fibers and elastic tissues in the medial layers of vessels. Without treatment, progres-

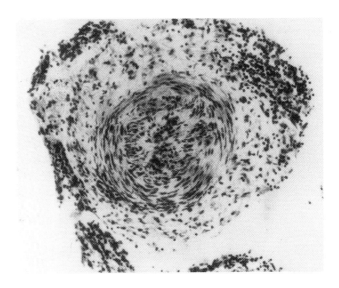

FIG. 2. Arterial inflammation from a patient with meningovascular syphilis. The arterial wall is infiltrated with lymphocytes and plasma cells, subintimal fibroblastic proliferation is present, and the vessel lumen is occluded by an organized thrombus. (From ref. 4, with permission.)

sive inflammation ultimately leads to proliferation of subendothelial fibrous material and irreversible occlusion of the vessel.

Although the differential diagnosis of progressive stroke syndromes in patients with known syphilis (usually manifest as a reactive serologic test for syphilis) is relatively narrow, the clinical syndromes associated with meningovascular syphilis may resemble those due to tuberculous meningitis, arteritis due to systemic vasculitis (e.g., systemic lupus erythematosus), or vasculitis due to CNS drug allergy (6,59).

Parenchymatous Neurosyphilis

In parenchymatous neurosyphilis, the latest of the true neurosyphilis syndromes to occur, general paresis and tabes dorsalis are distinguished from earlier forms of neurosyphilis in that they are manifestations of progressive neuron destruction rather than the direct result of ischemic changes caused by syphilitic involvement of CNS vasculature (4). The clinical manifestations of both syndromes are progressive and largely irreversible. Although both variants of parenchymatous neurosyphilis are relatively rare today (60) (even in comparison to other forms of neurosyphilis), both are still seen in most major hospitals and are among the most frequently misdiagnosed neurosyphilis syndromes. Tabes and general paresis differ substantially from each other in terms of time course, the sites of the nervous system predominantly affected, and their laboratory manifestations. In addition, patients may present with manifestations of both syndromes ("taboparesis"); moreover, it is likely that in the antibiotic era, modified presentations may occur as the result of inadvertent partial therapy at the time of treatment of other infectious illnesses (4).

General paresis (alternatively and equally descriptively referred to as "general paralysis of the insane" or "dementia paralytica") was described by Merritt et al. (4) as a chronic, progressive spirochetal meningoencephalitis which, while potentially occurring at any time beyond the first year of untreated infection, had its peak incidence at 10–20 years following infection. Prior to the widespread availability of penicillin, 5–15% of admissions to mental institutions were for patients with general paresis; since the advent of penicillin therapy, however, the disease has become far less common. Like other forms of neurosyphilis, general paresis is more common (four- to sevenfold) in males than in females. The clinical manifestations of general paresis are protean, often beginning insidiously with subtle deterioration of cognitive function presenting with difficulties in concentration, uncharacteristic irritability, or other subtle deficits in higher integrative function. During the earliest stages of general paresis, these subtle cognitive deficits may be the only manifestation of disease, and formal neurologic examination may otherwise be normal. Untreated, the cognitive abnormalities become progressively more marked and may lead to findings mimicking virtually any psychiatric disease. With further progression, patients may suffer loss of facial and extremity muscle tone, as well as fine motor control resulting in intention tremors or dysarthria. In the late stages of paresis, patients may suffer seizures and further loss of motor, bowel, and bladder control, leaving the patient paralyzed and incontinent in the period before the disease leads to the patient's death. Reflecting the generalized nature of the pathologic processes, it is noteworthy that focal neurologic deficits are distinctly unusual in paretic patients. While in some patients the onset can be quite abrupt and rapidly progressive, progression is more often subacute, occurring over a period of 3–4 years.

Examination of CSF in patients in whom paresis is suspected should contribute greatly to establishing the diagnosis, because CSF is said to be abnormal (leukocytosis, reactive serologic tests for syphilis, or elevation of protein concentrations) in 100% of untreated patients (4,6).

The pathologic changes seen in patients with general paresis reflect the progressive loss of neurons and accompanying gliosis which characterize the disease, manifest grossly as diffuse cortical atrophy (Fig. 3) and dilatation of the ventricles (4). Spirochetes may be demonstrated in the cortex of silver-stained preparations from 25–40% of patients with paresis. In addition, while the neurologic deficits in patients with general paresis are primarily due to pathologic processes occurring in the cerebral cortex, inflammatory thickening and chronic meningeal inflammatory changes are characteristic of this variant of neurosyphilis, as is the case for the others.

Tabes dorsalis or progressive locomotor ataxia, the other variant of parenchymatous neurosyphilis, like paresis, results from progressive degeneration of neurons; however, this disease differs from paresis in a number of ways (4,60). Tabes dorsalis is also more common in men than in women; however, it develops somewhat later than paresis, with the peak incidence occurring about 15–20 years following acquisition of infection. Unlike paresis, the onset of tabes dorsalis is often associated with characteristic symptomatology, and, rather than progressing rapidly to death, the progression of tabes is slower; death resulting from the primary disease process is rare.

In the early stages of the disease, patients with tabes dorsalis typically experience attacks of "lightning pains" in the distribution of single or multiple nerve roots (4). These lancinating pains are most common in the lower extremities, with attacks lasting minutes to hours. Lightning pains tend to occur episodically, and patients may experience periods of remission during which lightning pains do not occur. Merritt et al. (4) suggested that the unpredictability of recurrence of lightning pains,

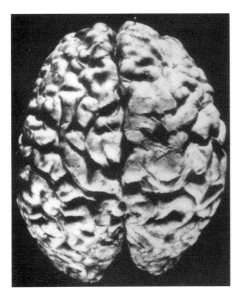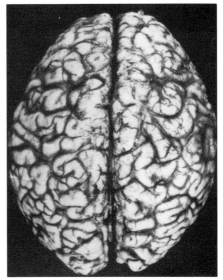

FIG. 3. Normal (**left**) and paretic (**right**) brains demonstrating diffuse cortical atrophy and meningeal clouding and thickening. (From ref. 4, with permission.)

rather than the intensity of the discomfort associated with them, was a major reason for their prominence as a feature of tabes. Ten to 20 percent of patients with tabes also experience "visceral crises" characterized by episodic attacks of abdominal pain. Early in the course of disease, 25% of patients with tabes experience paresthesias rather than lightning pains. Like lightning pains, the parethesias occurring in patients with tabes occurred episodically and with fluctuating intensity. With progression of the disease, patients experience progressive loss of sensation which may be manifest as patchy anesthesia and decreased proprioception. In addition, loss of vibration and loss of pain sensation occur, accompanied by diminution or loss of reflexes. Ultimately, the loss of proprioception and diminished sensation may lead to repeated inadvertent trauma, resulting in late manifestations of tabes such as Charcot joints. Other late findings occurring in tabetic patients include loss of urinary continence and ataxia due to loss of proprioception. Characteristically, patients compensate for proprioceptive loss by widening their gait, leading to the broad-based, shuffling gate characteristic of late tabes dorsalis. Although the lumbosacral spinal cord is the site most often involved in patients with tabes, cervical tabes has been described as well, and approximately 20% of patients have optic atrophy and/or involvement of oculomotor nerves as part of their disease. Ultimately, at least subtle pupillary changes can also be seen in the majority of patients with tabes. Although not limited in occurrence to tabes or even patients with syphilis, the Argyll Robertson pupillary changes in which one or both pupils constrict with accommodation but do not react to light was widely described in patients with tabes.

Unlike paresis, in which CSF abnormalities are nearly uniformly present, the CSF in patients with tabes dorsalis need not always be abnormal, nor is the magnitude of the abnormality as pronounced as in paresis (4,60). The potential absence of CSF changes may reflect the tendency of tabes to sometimes "burn out," leaving patients with residual deficits but disease which is no longer progressive. In their series of 100 patients, Merritt et al. (4) reported that the serum Wassermann reaction was positive in 88% of patients; in CSF, however, leukocytosis (>5 WBCs/mm^3) was present in only 50% of patients, protein concentrations were elevated in 53%, and the CSF Wassermann test was reactive in 72% of patients. These investigators also stated that the prevalence of CSF abnormalities tended to be lower in patients who had received prior therapy than in those who had not.

Pathologically, patients with tabes display (a) atrophic changes of the posterior columns of the spinal cord and the posterior nerve roots as they exit the spinal canal and (b) clouding of the meninges over involved regions of the spinal column (4). Microscopically, involved areas display diminished numbers of neurons and inflammatory infiltrates consisting largely of lymphocytes and plasma cells. Unlike paresis, in which spirochetes are histologically demonstrable in a substantial proportion of patients, efforts to demonstrate *T. pallidum* in tissue sections from patients with tabes are usually unsuccessful.

Gummatous Neurosyphilis

Gumma are late occurring manifestations of the tertiary stage of syphilis which may occur virtually anywhere, including the CNS (2,4,61). As such, gummatous neurosyphilis is a rare occurrence which does not reflect true CNS involvement by the disease process. Patients with gummatous neurosyphilis present with signs and symptoms of mass lesions at the sites where gumma or gummata occur.

THERAPY OF SYPHILIS PATIENTS WITH CNS INVOLVEMENT

Definition of Response to Neurosyphilis Therapy

The desired outcomes of therapy for syphilis patients with CNS involvement, as well as the measures of therapeutic effectiveness, vary with the clinical manifestations of disease being treated (62,63). In patients with CSF abnormalities but without clinically apparent disease syndromes, the goals are to prevent progression to symptomatic disease and to ameliorate the laboratory abnormalities thought to indicate disease activity. In contrast, for patients with clinical neurosyphilis syndromes, the goal may be either to reverse clinical signs and symptoms or to arrest disease progression (however, even "adequate" therapy may not prevent some degree of progression in patients with late stages of neurosyphilis; see below). Thus the outcomes of neurosyphilis therapy may be measured using a variety of different parameters. In addition, assessment of the adequacy of therapy is largely dependent on the need to conduct such assessments using indirect measures of outcome: Isolation of *T. pallidum,* which might potentially provide the most accurate assessment of therapeutic efficacy, is impractical because of (a) the lack of data regarding the relationship between *T. pallidum* isolation from CSF and the subsequent course of disease and (b) the other practical limitations already mentioned.

In the 1940s, the early descriptions of the utility of penicillin for syphilis therapy effectively ended decades of debate as to the relative merits of various therapeutic regimens for CNS syphilis utilizing arsenicals, bismuth, or fever therapy alone or in combination (64,65). Contrary to commonly held beliefs, however, the assessment of syphilologists whose careers spanned the period when heavy-metal therapy was replaced by penicillin was that the major benefit of penicillin was not increased efficacy (although penicillin therapy for neurosyphilis is probably more efficacious than earlier therapies). Rather, penicillin provided the convenience of dramatically shortened duration of therapy, marked reduction in the complications of therapy, and, related to these benefits, improved compliance with therapy, which, in turn, led to completion of planned courses of therapy by substantially more patients than had previously been the case

(64). These benefits were particularly apparent with respect to therapy of patients with CNS involvement, because these patients were often treated for nearly twice as long as those with other types of syphilis (e.g., therapy was planned for up to 2 years rather than the 60-week duration recommended for patients with uncomplicated syphilis). It is difficult to utilize data from the pre-penicillin era to describe the expected response of neurosyphilis to therapy, for several reasons: (a) These therapies had considerable toxicity associated with them; (b) the prolonged course of therapy administered contributed to difficulties in ascertaining to what degree the resolution of clinical or laboratory findings was due to the therapy administered as opposed to simply being a reflection of the natural history of the disease; and (c) the laboratory definition of adequate laboratory response to infection has changed from complete resolution of CSF abnormalities to "significant" improvement.

Therapeutic Agents for Neurosyphilis

As mentioned above, almost immediately following the first reports of its utility, penicillin became the preferred drug for neurosyphilis therapy and has remained so since that time. Although recent data have described variation in sensitivity to erythromycin among the few clinical isolates of *T. pallidum* tested (66), and other authors have described the presence of plasmid DNA in *T. pallidum* (68), a feature which suggests that the organism may have the capacity to develop antibiotic resistance, there are no data to currently suggest the presence of clinically significant penicillin resistance. Although based on testing of a limited number of strains, it is nonetheless widely accepted that penicillin in a concentration of 0.018 mg/liter is reliably treponemicidal (67). Consequently, given the time and difficulties in evaluation of response to therapy, a number of studies designed to evaluate therapy for CNS syphilis have focused on attainment or exceeding this penicillin level in CSF as endpoints, assuming that to do so will ensure effective therapy, provided that effective CSF levels of drug are sustained for sufficient duration.

Presently, considerable controversy remains as to the most appropriate dose of penicillin for neurosyphilis therapy (69,70). In the first 5–10 years following its introduction, penicillin formulations evolved rapidly, resulting in the use of penicillins with markedly different pharmacokinetics and bioavailability for many of the early penicillin treatment trials (65). Among the formulations utilized in the early trials were amorphous penicillin, penicillin G, penicillin in beeswax or peanut oil (for sustained release), procaine penicillin, procaine penicillin G in 2% aluminum monosterate, and benzathine penicillin G; each of these different formulations gave markedly different peak serum levels and yielded effective serum levels for periods varying from hours to days (65). In the late 1940s and early 1950s, the Cooperative Study Group formed by the Committee on Medical Research of the Office of Scientific Research and Development studied 26 different treatment schedules for syphilis therapy, exploring the import of variables such as duration of therapy, total dosage of penicillin over a 40-fold range, the interval between injections, the effect of combined therapy using penicillin in combination with other therapies (arsenicals, bismuth, fever), and the effect of formulations which delayed absorption (65). These data, in combination with the careful experimental observations of investigators such as Harry Eagle (71), began to define the principles which continue to guide syphilotherapy today with respect to duration of therapy (at least 8 days) and the belief that duration of therapy was a more important determinant of cure than were peak blood levels.

The studies conducted by the Cooperative Clinical Group remain among the largest and most important studies to evaluate the utility of penicillin for therapy of neurosyphilis (72,73). These studies evaluated over 700 patients with "asymptomatic neurosyphilis" using progression to clinically apparent neurosyphilis and resolution of laboratory abnormalities as outcome criteria. Participants in these studies were treated using a variety of penicillin formulations and administration schedules. Fifty-five percent of patients received between 2.4 and 9 million units of total therapy. Upon completion of their studies, the investigators concluded that patients treated with 2.4 to 5 million units of penicillin fared as well as patients receiving larger doses; in 1961 Richard Hahn, who authored a number of the reports of the Cooperative Study Group's trials (74), slightly modified his earlier conclusions, contending that 6–10 million units of penicillin administered in repository form was adequate therapy for most patients with neurosyphilis.

Although penicillin is widely accepted as the drug of choice for treatment of neurosyphilis, the total dose, most appropriate formulation, and duration of therapy remains a subject of debate. This debate focuses largely on the question of whether benzathine penicillin, which is convenient to use, is sufficient for therapy of CNS syphilis or whether other regimens which attain considerably higher serum and CSF drug levels are required. A number of investigators have clearly documented that 2.4 million units of benzathine penicillin does not reliably provide CSF penicillin levels in excess of 0.018 mg/liter, whereas alternative regimens using higher doses of intravenously administered penicillin G or oral amoxicillin more reliably accomplish this goal (75–80). Other pharmacologic studies evaluating the potential utility of procaine penicillin therapy for neurosyphilis have provided more variable results which suggest that adminis-

tration of procaine penicillin (a currently recommended alternate therapy) in doses of 600,000 to 2,400,000 units sometimes (but not always) achieves the desired CSF penicillin levels (80,81).

Advocates of benzathine penicillin regimens support their preference by pointing out that despite the frequent involvement of the CNS in the early stages of the disease, few patients treated with the currently recommended benzathine penicillin regimens fail therapy or go on to develop neurosyphilis. However, proponents of the use of regimens other than benzathine penicillin cite data from a study of 26 patients treated with 4.8 million units of benzathine penicillin for "active neurosyphilis" defined on the basis of CSF abnormalities which uniformly included CSF cell counts of more than $11/mm^3$ in whom two patients were defined as treatment failures, based on increasing CSF pleocytosis (45). Whereas the authors (45) felt that the observed failure rate compared favorably with results of studies conducted up to that time, many subsequent investigators feel it was too high. Further data leading to questions regarding the utility of benzathine penicillin are derived from case reports describing either neurosyphilitic presentations of treatment failures in patients treated for early syphilis with benzathine penicillin, the persistence of viable *T. pallidum* in the CSF of patients treated with benzathine penicillin, or persistent CSF abnormalities in patients treated for asymptomatic CNS involvement using benzathine penicillin (11,46–48). To summarize these data, it appears that a small but poorly defined proportion of patients treated for syphilis with benzathine penicillin go on to fail therapy, with treatment failures being manifest as either persistent CSF laboratory abnormalities or clinically apparent neurosyphilis. At the same time, the observations that many benzathine-penicillin-treated patients resolve their CSF abnormalities and do not progress have been made despite solid data which demonstrate that benzathine penicillin does not reliably attain CSF levels thought to be therapeutic for *T. pallidum*, suggesting that factors other than merely the amount of penicillin present also play an important role in the response to therapy. Final resolution of this debate awaits further study.

Although there is wide acceptance of penicillin and related drugs as effective therapy for neurosyphilis, there are no large studies evaluating alternative therapeutic agents. Recommendations for therapy in patients who cannot receive penicillin are based on case reports or small series, clinical experience, and extrapolation from observations made in studies of experimental animals. The tetracyclines, chloramphenicol, and ceftriaxone have all been described to be of potential utility for treatment in neurosyphilis in penicillin-allergic patients (63,82,83). Erythromycin had also been recommended; however, recent data describing increased treatment failures in erythromycin-treated patients has led to abandonment of the recommendation of erythromycin as alternate therapy for syphilis patients with or without CNS involvement.

The Effect of Penicillin on Manifestations of CNS Involvement in Syphilis Patients

Soon after the early descriptions of the efficacy of penicillin therapy, members of the Subcommittee on Venereal Disease from the Office of Scientific Research and Development targeted therapy of early infectious syphilis and neurosyphilis as research priorities (65). Although their work was compromised by poor standardization, imprecise definitions and criteria for defining therapeutic success, and other methodologic flaws, the data provided by the Cooperative Clinical Group remain among the largest and most important studies evaluating the utility of penicillin for therapy of CNS involvement in syphilis patients (65,72,73,84). These studies evaluated 765 patients with asymptomatic CNS involvement (defined by the presence of abnormal CSF serologic tests for syphilis, abnormal CSF colloidal gold tests, or elevations of CSF cell count or protein concentrations in patients with normal neurologic examinations and syphilis of more than 2 years' duration), using progression to clinically apparent neurosyphilis and resolution of laboratory abnormalities as outcome criteria (72,73). Participants in these studies were treated using a variety of penicillin formulations and administration schedules, with 55% receiving between 2.4 and 9 million units of total therapy. In these studies, in which 75% of participants were followed for more than 2 years and some for as long as 7 years following therapy, a maximum of 3.3% of patients were felt to progress to symptomatic neurosyphilis following therapy, with nine of 12 possible therapeutic failures occurring within 3 years of therapy. The authors qualified a number of the possible "progressions" as "dubious," questioning the significance of some neurologic changes classified as indicative of disease progression and stating that in at least some cases the disease progression was likely to have occurred despite that fact that the disease had been adequately treated.

For patients with clinically apparent neurosyphilis syndromes, the desired outcomes of therapy are variable and depend on the pathologic processes which underlie clinical findings. Thus for patients with syphilitic meningitis in whom signs and symptoms are reflections of meningeal irritation caused by acute inflammatory response, clinical findings other than cranial nerve abnormalities usually completely resolve. For patients with meningovascular syphilis (perhaps surprisingly because the focal neurologic deficits noted clinically often reflect

CNS hypoxic damage due to vascular insufficiency), the prognosis following therapy is relatively good as well. Although the precise reasons for the high degree of recovery among patients with meningovascular syphilis are unclear, a number of reasons have been suggested, including the following: (a) It predominantly results from focal arteritis involving small and medium vessels rather than large arteries, thereby permitting collateral flow to salvage proportionately larger areas of involvement than for diseases which affect larger vessels; (b) it is related to the fact that the deficits are in some cases the consequence of vascular spasm rather than irreversible occlusion; and (c) it is related to the ability of afflicted individuals to learn to compensate for the deficits caused by the relative small strokes which characterize this syndrome. Clearly, however, the larger the clinically apparent deficit which occurs prior to therapy, the more limited the recovery of the patient. Another goal of treatment for patients with meningovascular syphilis, however, is to prevent further ischemic events caused by neurosyphilis.

For patients with general paresis or tabes dorsalis, the probability of marked improvement is considerably lower than that for patients with other types of neurosyphilis, again reflecting the fact that in patients with these syndromes, most of the observed pathology is caused by irreversible neuron damage rather than being caused by CNS inflammation (4,62,84). Dattner et al. (62) reported that only 10% of patients with paresis showed "marked improvement" and that even for those in whom improvement occurred, resolution was a gradual process said to occur over a period of "weeks to months." In fact, despite therapy, it appears that a substantial proportion of patients with general paresis may experience progression of their disease. Wilner and Brody (85) reviewed the medical records of 100 patients with general paresis surviving for at least 10 years after treatment and reported that the rates of progression were similar irrespective of whether patients had been treated with regimens which included penicillin or not (64 of 100 had been treated with penicillin alone or in combination with malaria therapy, whereas the remaining 36 had been treated with malaria and heavy-metal therapy). These authors found that following therapy (which for those receiving penicillin therapy involved total doses of 3–30 million units), 39% of patients subsequently developed new neurologic signs. Progression, which occurred a mean of 12 years following therapy, was most often manifest as seizures but also included paraplegia, amyotrophy, tabes dorsalis, optic atopy, and oculomotor palsies. Disease progression in this series did not appear to be related to the type of therapy received or to the dose of penicillin administered. These authors felt that their data suggested that at least a portion of the damage caused by the paretic process would continue, perhaps due to scarring or other "healing" process despite eradication of viable *T. pallidum* from the afflicted individual.

The studies conducted by the Collaborative Clinical Group also provided important data regarding the response of CSF laboratory abnormalities to penicillin therapy (73). In their studies, the CSF cell count appeared to be the most sensitive index of response. Eighty-nine percent of the 454 patients who initially had 10 or more leukocytes per cubic milliliter of CSF had normalized their cell counts at the time of follow-up lumbar puncture 1 year following therapy, whereas among the 235 with abnormal pretreatment CSF protein concentrations, 69% had become normal at follow-up 1 year after therapy. They also observed that the intensity of the CSF abnormalities did not necessarily parallel the duration or the "severity" of the infection and that high pretest serologic test titers were not always present in patients with active CNS involvement (28% of patients in this study had titers of 1:2 or less). In addition, their studies confirmed the observations of previous investigators that the serologic response of patients to syphilotherapy may be disassociated from the response of CSF parameters, noting that neither the presence nor the rate of serologic response could be used to predict resolution of CSF abnormalities. Certain factors, however, were related to more rapid response to therapy. These included (a) the presence of abnormal CSF cell counts and (b) patients who were younger or with shorter duration of infection.

Thus although debate continues as to the optimal dose and duration of penicillin for therapy, its utility for arresting progression of disease, for promoting resolution of clinical findings associated with syphilitic meningitis, and for improving laboratory CSF abnormalities associated with CNS involvement in syphilis patients appears to have been reliably demonstrated. CSF laboratory abnormalities, which may respond somewhat slowly to therapy, appear to be a more reliable indicator of response to therapy than do changes in clinical findings. At the present time, the Centers for Disease Control recommend high-dose, parenteral penicillin as the drug of choice for therapy of syphilis patients with CNS involvement (86) (Table 3), erring on the side of caution with respect to the continuing debate regarding optimal therapy for this disease.

TABLE 3. *Recommended regimens for therapy of central nervous system syphilis*

Preferred regimen
Intravenous aqueous crystalline penicillin G, 12–24 million units daily in divided doses at 4-hr intervals for 10–14 days.

Alternate regimen
Procaine penicillin, 2.4 million units administered intramuscularly daily, plus probenecid, 500 mg orally, four times daily, both for 10–14 days.

CNS INVOLVEMENT IN SYPHILIS PATIENTS WITH HIV INFECTION

A number of recent studies have examined the potential interactions between syphilis and HIV infection, and several links between the two illnesses have been demonstrated (87–89). Both diseases are predominantly sexually transmitted, and patients with syphilis have been repeatedly demonstrated to be at increased risk for HIV infection. In addition, both diseases frequently invade the CNS, usually resulting in asymptomatic CSF abnormalities early in the course of the disease but also having the capacity to subsequently cause devastating progressive CNS disease as well. Culture diagnosis of the pathogens causing each disease is infrequently performed; as a result, CNS invasion by either *T. pallidum* or HIV is most often demonstrated by less specific indicators of infection, such as elevations of CSF leukocyte counts or protein concentrations. Consequently, in patients with both diseases, clinicians and investigators are often left in a quandary as to which disease has caused the abnormalities noted on CSF examination.

As discussed above, the clinical manifestations of syphilis as well as the response of the disease to therapy are markedly influenced by the interactions between the host's immunologic response to infection and *T. pallidum*. Thus it is not surprising that there are data to suggest that the clinical manifestations, course, and response to therapy of patients with neurosyphilis and concomitant HIV infection may differ from those described for patients without HIV infection (11,89–96). Although a number of case reports have suggested that CNS involvement is more common in HIV-infected syphilis patients than in those without concomitant HIV infection, the only systematically conducted, prospective study to examine this issue to date has been conducted by Lukehart et al. (11). In this study which set out to examine the frequency of CNS invasion in patients with syphilis, when patients with HIV infection were compared to those without it, the only significant difference noted in the frequency of CSF laboratory abnormalities was with regard to CSF leukocyte concentrations. In their study, 10 (67%) of 15 HIV-infected patients had >5 leukocytes per cubic millimeter of CSF, a finding present in only six (24%) of 25 HIV-seronegative patients. In addition, although isolation of *T. pallidum* was no more common in HIV-infected patients, of four patients with secondary syphilis from whom the organism was isolated prior to receipt of recommended single-dose therapy (2.4 million units of benzathine penicillin G) and evaluated with follow-up lumbar puncture, two HIV-infected patients had persistence of viable treponemes in CSF following therapy, and another who was in the process of converting to HIV seropositivity had a clinically significant increase in his serum VDRL and was thus considered a treatment failure despite the absence of persistent CSF treponemes. Of the four patients, the only one in whom unequivocable improvement of all serologic and CSF parameters occurred was HIV negative and remained so throughout the duration of the study.

A number of case reports and small case series have also described patients treated for early syphilis with benzathine penicillin in whom therapy was unsuccessful (11,90,91). In several of these reports, patients treated with benzathine penicillin experienced initial improvement of clinical signs and laboratory abnormalities, only to subsequently present with probable syphilitic meningitis or meningovascular syphilis. Other small series have suggested that the incidence of neurosyphilis in patients with syphilis and HIV infection may be higher and the course more rapid than is often thought to be the case for non-HIV-infected individuals. It is important to point out that, thus far, the presentations of HIV-infected patients with CNS involvement and syphilis are presentations which have been well described in the pre-HIV era. Although neurosyphilis may prove to be more common or to occur earlier in the course of disease, there are no data to suggest that presentations of CNS syphilis are substantially altered in HIV-infected persons who acquire syphilis.

Thus at the present time there is a sense on the part of many experts that patients with early syphilis and CNS invasion by *T. pallidum* may be more likely to fail therapy with single-dose benzathine penicillin than would non-HIV-infected patients. Proof of this belief, as well as quantification of the magnitude of the increased risk for treatment failure, is unclear and await the results of a recently initiated Centers for Disease Control-sponsored, multicenter trial designed to address these issues. Similarly, resolution of the question as to whether or not patients with HIV who acquire syphilis are at increased risk for development of neurosyphilis awaits carefully performed, prospective study.

REFERENCES

1. Centers for Disease Control. Syphilis and congenital syphilis—United States, 1985–88. *MMWR* 1988;37:486–489.
2. Stokes JH, Beerman H, Ingraham NR. *Modern clinical syphilology*, 3rd ed. Philadelphia: WB Saunders, 1944.
3. Hutchinson CM, Hook EW III. Syphilis in adults. *Med Clin North Am* 1990;74:1389–1416.
4. Merritt HH, Adams RD, Solomon HC. *Neurosyphilis.* New York: Oxford University Press, 1946.
5. Catterall RD. Neurosyphilis. *Br J Hosp Med* 1977;17:585–604.
6. Simon RP. Neurosyphilis. *Arch Neurol* 1985;42:606–613.
7. Lukehart SA, Baker-Zander SA, Lloyd RMC, Sell S. Characterization of lymphocyte responsiveness in early experimental syphilis. II. Nature of cellular infiltration and *Treponema pallidum* distribution in testicular lesions. *J Immunol* 1980;124:454–460.
8. Baker-Zander S, Sell S. A histopathologic and immunologic study of the course of syphilis in the experimentally infected rabbit: demonstration of long-lasting cellular immunity. *Am J Pathol* 1980;101:387–414.
9. Wile UJ, Hasley CK. Involvement of nervous system during primary stage of syphilis. *JAMA* 1921;8–9.
10. Mills C. Routine examination of the cerebrospinal fluid in syphilis. Its value in regard to more accurate knowledge, prognosis and treatment. *Br Med J* 1927;527–532.
11. Lukehart SA, Hook EW III, Baker-Zander SA. Invasion of the central nervous system by *Treponema pallidum:* implications for diagnosis and treatment. *Ann Intern Med* 1988;109:855–861.
12. Merritt HH. The early clinical and laboratory manifestations of syphilis of the central nervous system. *N Engl J Med* 1940;September:446–450.
13. Hahn RD, Clark EG. Asymptomatic neurosyphilis: a review of the literature. *Am J Syph Gonorrhea Vener Dis* 1946;30:305–316.
14. Moore JE, Hopkins HH. Asymptomatic neurosyphilis. VI. The prognosis of early and late asymptomatic neurosyphilis. *JAMA* 1936;95:1637–1641.
15. Moore JE, Faupel M. Asymptomatic neurosyphilis. V. A comparison of early and late asymptomatic neurosyphilis. *Arch Dermatol Syph* 1928;18:99–108.
16. Jorizzo JL, McNeely C, Baughn RE, et al. Role of circulating immune complexes in human secondary syphilis. *J Infect Dis* 1986;153:1014–1022.
17. Young EJ, Weingarten NM, Baughn RE, Duncan WC. Studies on the pathogenesis of the Jarisch–Herrheimer reaction: development of an animal model and evidence against a role for classical endotoxin. *J Infect Dis* 1982;146:606–615.
18. Montenegro ENR, Nicol WG, Smith JL. Treponemalike forms and artifacts. *Am J Ophthalmol* 1969;68:197–205.
19. Nichols HJ, Hough WH. Demonstration of *Spirochaeta pallida* in the cerebrospinal fluid. *JAMA* 1913;60:108–110.
20. Wile UJ. The spirochetal content of the spinal fluid of tabes, general paresis, and cerebrospinal syphilis. *Am J Syph* 1917;1:84–90.
21. Chesney AM, Kemp JE. Incidence of *Spirochaeta pallida* in cerebrospinal fluid during early stage of syphilis. *JAMA* 1924;83:1725–1728.
22. Collart P, Franceschini P, Piotevin M. et al. Modified method of filtering cerebrospinal fluid and aqueous humour for the detection of treponemes. Proof of the persistence of their vitality in rabbits. *Br J Vener Dis* 1974;50:251.
23. Hoshmand H, Escobar MR, Kopf SW. Neurosyphilis: a study of 241 patients. *JAMA* 1972;219(6):726–729.
24. Luxon L, Lees AJ, Greenwood RJ. Neurosyphilis today. *Lancet* 1979;1:90–95.
25. Hotson JR. Modern neurosyphilis: a partially treated chronic meningitis. *West J Med* 1981;135:191–200.
26. Fernando WL. Cerebrospinal fluid findings after treatment of early syphilis with penicillin. *Br J Vener Dis* 1965;41:168–169.
27. Izzat NN, Bartruff JK, Glicksman JM, et al. Validity of the VDRL test in cerebrospinal fluid contaminated by blood. *Br J Vener Dis* 1971;47:162–164.
28. Davis LE, Sperry S. The CSF-FTA test and the significance of blood contamination. *Ann Neurol.* 1979;6:68–69.
29. Rudolph AH. Examination of the cerebrospinal fluid in syphilis. 1976;17:749–752.
30. Jaffe HW, Kabins SA. Examination of cerebrospinal fluid in patients with syphilis. *Rev Infect Dis* 1982;4:S842–S847.
31. Madiedo G, Ho K, Walsh P. False-positive VDRL and FTA in cerebrospinal fluid. *JAMA* 1980;244(7):688–689.
32. Burke JM, Schaberg DR. Neurosyphilis in the antibiotic era. *Neurology* 1985;35:1368–1370.
33. Davis LE, Schmitt JW. Clinical significance of cerebrospinal fluid tests for neurosyphilis. *Ann Neurol* 1989;25:50–55.
34. Harris AD, Bossak HM, Deacon WE, Bunch WL. Comparison of the fluorescent treponemal antibody test with other tests for syphilis on cerebrospinal fluids. *Br J Vener Dis* 1960;36:178–180.
35. Harner RE, Smith JL, Israel CW. The FTA-ABS test in late syphilis. *JAMA* 1968;203(8):545–548.
36. Escobar MR, Dalton HP, Allison MJ. Fluorescent antibody tests for syphilis using cerebrospinal fluid: clinical correlation in 150 cases. *Am J Clin Pathol* 1970;53:886–890.

37. Jaffe HW, Larsen SA, Peters M, et al. Tests for treponemal antibody in CSF. *Arch Intern Med* 1978;138:252–255.
38. Traviesa DC, Prystowsky SD, Nelson BJ, et al. Cerebrospinal fluid findings in asymptomatic patients with reactive serum fluorescent treponemal antibody absorption tests. *Ann Neurol* 1978;4:524–530.
39. McGeeney T, Yount F, Hinthorn DR, Liu C. Utility of the FTA-Abs test of cerebrospinal fluid in the diagnosis of neurosyphilis. *Sex Transm Dis* 1979;6:195–198.
40. Duncan WP, Jenkins TW, Parham CE. Fluorescent treponemal antibody-cerebrospinal fluid (FTA-CSF) test. *Br J Vener Dis* 1972;48:97–101.
41. Lugar A, Schmidt BL, Steyrer K, Schonwald E. Diagnosis of neurosyphilis by examination of the cerebrospinal fluid. *Br J Vener Dis* 1981;57:232–237.
42. Vartdal F, Vandvik B, Michaelsen TE, et al. Neurosyphilis: intrathecal synthesis of oligoclonal antibodies to *Treponema pallidum.* *Ann Neurol* 1982;11:35–40.
43. Muller F, Moskophidis M. Estimation of the local production of antibodies to *Treponema pallidum* in the central nervous system of patients with neurosyphilis. *Br J Vener Dis* 1983;59:80–84.
44. Eijk RW, Wolters EC, Tutuarima JA, et al. Effect of early and late syphilis on central nervous system: cerebrospinal fluid changes and neurological deficit. *Genitourin Med* 1987;63:77–82.
45. Short DH, Knox JM, Glicksman J. Neurosyphilis, the search for adequate treatment. *Arch Dermatol* 1966;93:87–91.
46. Tramont EC. Persistence of *Treponema pallidum* following penicillin G therapy. Report of two cases. *JAMA* 1976;236:2206–2207.
47. Greene BM, Miller NR, Bynum TE. Failure of penicillin G benzathine in the treatment of neurosyphilis. *Arch Intern Med* 1980;140:1117–1118.
48. Moskovitz BL, Klimek JJ, Goldman RL, Fiumara NJ, Quintilliani R. Meningovascular syphilis after "appropriate" treatment of primary syphilis. *Arch Intern Med* 1982;142:139–140.
49. Wetherill JH, Webb HE, Catterall RD. Syphilis presenting as an acute neurological illness. *Br Med J* 1965;1:1157–1158.
50. Joffe R, Black MM, Floyd M. Changing clinical picture of neurosyphilis: report of seven unusual cases. *Br Med J* 1968;1:211–212.
51. Talbot MD, Morton RS. Neurosyphilis: the most common things are most common. *Genitourin Med* 1985;61:95–98.
52. Merritt HH, Moore M. Acute syphilitic meningitis. *Medicine* 1935;14:119–183.
53. Moore JE. Syphilitic iritis: a study of 249 patients. *Am J Ophthalmol* 1931;14:110–126.
54. de Souza EC, Jalkh AE, Trempe CL, Cunha S, Schepens CL. Unusual central chorioretinitis as the first manifestation of early secondary syphilis. *Am J Ophthalmol* 1988;105:271–276.
55. Willcox RR, Goodwin PG. Nerve deafness in early syphilis. *Br J Vener Dis* 1971;47:401–406.
56. Becker GD. Late syphilis: otologic symptoms and results of the FTA-ABS test. *Arch Otolaryngol* 1976;102:729–731.
57. Balkany TJ, Dans PE. Reversible sudden deafness in early acquired syphilis. *Arch Otolaryngol* 1978;104:6668.
58. Bayne LL, Schmidley JW, Goodin DS. Acute syphilitic meningitis. Its occurrence after clinical and serologic cure of secondary syphilis with penicillin G. *Arch Neurol* 1986;43:137–138.
59. Holmes MD, Zawadzki B, Simon RP. Clinical features of meningovascular syphilis. *Neurology* 1984;34:553–555.
60. Kampmeier RH. Whatever has happened to locomotor ataxy? [Editorial] *AVDA* 1976;3:51–53.
61. Kulla L, Russell JA, Thomas DO, et al. Neurosyphilis presenting as a focal mass lesion: a case report. *Neurosurgery* 1984;14,2:234–237.
62. Dattner B, Thomas EW, Mello LD. Criteria for the management of neurosyphilis. *Am J Med* 1951;463–467.
63. Rothenberg R. Treatment of neurosyphilis. *Sex Transm Dis* 1976;3:153–158.
64. Kampmeier RH. Syphilis therapy: an historical perspective. *Sex Transm Dis* 1976;3:99–107.
65. Kampmeier RH. The introduction of penicillin for the treatment of syphilis. *Sex Transm Dis* 1981;8:260–265.
66. Stapleton JT, Stamm LV, Bassford PJ Jr. Potential for development of antibiotic resistance in pathogenic treponemes. *Rev Infect Dis* 1985;7:S314–S317.
67. Idsoe O, Guthe T, Wilcox RR. Penicillin in the treatment of syphilis: the experience of three decades. *Bull WHO* 1972;47(Suppl);1–68.
68. Norgard MV, Miller JN. Plasmid DNA in *Treponema pallidum* (Nichols): potential for antibiotic resistance by syphilis bacteria. *Science* 1981;213:553–555.
69. Jordan KG. Modern neurosyphilis—a critical analysis. *West J Med* 1988;149:47–57.
70. Musher DM. How much penicillin cures early syphilis? *Ann Intern Med* 1988;109:849–851.
71. Eagle H. Speculations as to the therapeutic significance of the penicillin blood level. *Ann Intern Med* 1948;28:260–278.
72. Hahn RD, Cutler JC, Curtis AC, Gammon G, Heyman A, Johnwick E, et al. Penicillin treatment of asymptomatic central nervous system syphilis. I. Probability of progression to symptomatic neurosyphilis. *Arch Dermatol* 1956;74:355–366.
73. Hahn RD, Cutler JC, Curtis AC, Gammon G, Heyman A, Johnwick E, et al. Penicillin treatment of asymptomatic central nervous system syphilis. II. Results of therapy as measured by laboratory findings. *Arch Dermatol* 1956;74:367–377.
74. Hahn RD. Some remarks on the management of neurosyphilis. *J Chronic Dis* 1961;13:1–5.
75. Dunlop EM, Al-Egaily SS, Houang ET. Penicillin levels in blood and CSF achieved by treatment of syphilis. *JAMA* 1979;241:2538–2540.
76. Mohr JA, Griffiths W, Jackson R, Saadah H, Bird P, Riddle J. Neurosyphilis and penicillin levels in cerebrospinal fluid. *JAMA* 1976;236:2208–2209.
77. Schoth PEM, Wolters ECH. Penicillin concentrations in serum and CSF during high-dose intravenous treatment for neurosyphilis. *Neurology* 1987;37:1214–1216.
78. Morrison RE, Harrison SM, Tramont EC. Oral amoxycillin, an alternative treatment for neurosyphilis. *Genitourin Med* 1985;61:359–362.
79. Faber WR, Bos JD, Reitra PJ, Fass H, Van Erjk RV. Treponemacidal levels of amoxicillin in cerebrospinal fluid after oral administration. *Sex Transm Dis* 1983;10:148–150.
80. Goh BT, Smith GW, Samarasinghe L, Singh V, Lim KS. Penicillin concentrations in serum and cerebrospinal fluid after intramuscular injection of aqueous procaine penicillin 0.6 MU with and without probenecid. *Br J Vener Dis* 1984;60:371–373.
81. Van Der Valk PGM, Kraai EJ, Van Voorst Vader PC, Haaxma-Reiche H, Snijder JAM. Penicillin concentrations in cerebrospinal fluid (CSF) during repository treatment regimen for syphilis. *Genitourin Med* 1988;64:223–225.
82. Romanowski B, Starreveld E, Jarema AJ. Treatment of neurosyphilis with chloramphenicol: a case report. *Br J Vener Dis* 1983;59:225–227.
83. Hook EW III, Baker-Zander SA, Moskovitz BL, Lukehart SA, Handsfield HH. Centriaxone therapy for asymptomatic neurosyphilis. Case report and Western blot analysis of serum and cerebrospinal fluid IgG response to therapy. *Sex Transm Dis* 1986;13:185–188.
84. Hahn RD, Webster B, Weickhardt G, Thomas E, et al. The results of treatment in 1,086 general paralytics the majority of whom were followed for more than five years. *J Chronic Dis* 1958:209–227.
85. Wilner E, Brody JA. Prognosis of general paresis after treatment. *Lancet* 1968;1370–1371.
86. Centers for Disease Control. 1989 Sexually transmitted diseases treatment guidelines. *MMWR* 1989;38(Suppl 8):9.
87. Quinn TC, Cannon RO, Glasser D, et al. The association of syphilis with risk of human immunodeficiency virus infection in patients attending sexually transmitted diseases clinics. *Arch Intern Med* 1990;150:1297–1302.
88. Hook EW III. Syphilis and HIV infection. *J Infect Dis* 1989;160:530–534.
89. Musher DM, Hamill RJ, Baughn RE. Effect of human immunodeficiency virus (HIV) infection on the course of syphilis and on the response to treatment. *Ann Intern Med* 1990;113:872–881.
90. Johns DR, Tierney M, Felenstein D. Alteration in the natural his-

tory of neurosyphilis by concurrent infection with the human immunodeficiency virus. *N Engl J Med* 1987;316:1569–1572.

91. Berry CD, Hooton TM, Collier AC, et al. Neurologic relapse after benzathine penicillin therapy for secondary syphilis in a patient with HIV infection. *N Engl J Med* 1987;316:1587–1589.

92. Carter JB, Hamill RJ, Matoba AY. Bilateral syphilitic optic neuritis in a patient with a positive test for HIV. *Arch Ophthalmol* 1987;105:1485–1486.

93. Johns DR, Tierney M, Parker SW. Pure motor hemiplegia due to meningovascular neurosyphilis. *Arch Neurol* 1987;44:1062–1065.

94. Kase CS, Levitz SM, Wolinsky JS, Sulis CA. Pontine pure motor hemiparesis due to meningovascular syphilis in human immunodeficiency virus-positive patients. *Arch Neurol* 1988;45:832.

95. Terry PM, Page ML, Goldmeier D. Are serological tests of value in diagnosing and monitoring response to treatment of syphilis in patients infected with human immunodeficiency virus. *Genitourin Med* 1988;64:219–222.

96. Katz DA, Berger JR. Neurosyphilis in acquired immunodeficiency syndrome. *Arch Neurol* 1989;46:895–898.

Infections of the Central Nervous System,
edited by W. M. Scheld, R. J. Whitley, and
D. T. Durack, Raven Press, Ltd., New York © 1991.

CHAPTER 28

Lyme Disease

Louis Reik, Jr.

In 1975, the observations of two women from the small town of Lyme, Connecticut, triggered a series of investigations that led to the identification of a new clinical entity—Lyme disease.

In November of that year, the mother of a child diagnosed as having juvenile rheumatoid arthritis (JRA) reported to the Connecticut State Health Department that an unusual number of children in her neighborhood of Lyme had the same disease, and she questioned the diagnosis. The physician who took her call passed this information on to Dr. Allen Steere, who was then in the rheumatology group at Yale. Just a few days later, another woman from Lyme consulted the rheumatology clinic at Yale about two of her children, also diagnosed as having JRA. She, too, questioned the diagnosis, because she, her husband, and a number of neighborhood children all had a similar illness (1,2).

In response to these observations, physicians from the Health Department and Yale established a surveillance system in the three adjoining communities of Old Lyme, Lyme, and East Haddam, Connecticut, to identify all children with inflammatory joint disease. They found 39 children and 12 adults who had a characteristic remitting, relapsing, oligoarticular arthritis with onset between 1972 and 1976, usually in summer or early fall. The arthritis was epidemiologically distinct from JRA. Its prevalence among children was 12.2 per 1000, a frequency 100 times greater than that of JRA; and the cases were closely clustered geographically. All of those affected lived in sparsely settled, forested parts of the towns; and, in both Old Lyme and East Haddam, half of them lived on two adjacent country roads. Of the children living along these four roads, one in 10 had the illness. Moreover, six families had more than one affected member; and, within these families, the affected

members usually had the onset of symptoms in different years. These observations suggested an arthropod-transmitted disease (3).

In addition, 13 of these patients had noted an unusual skin lesion an average of 4 months before the arthritis started (3). The lesion began as an erythematous papule that expanded to form a red ring which resembled erythema chronicum migrans (ECM), a skin lesion described from Europe and known to follow the bite of the sheep tick, *Ixodes ricinus*. ECM was largely unknown at that time in North America: Only one case acquired in the United States (Wisconsin) had been reported before 1975 (4). But it was common in Europe, where it had been reported as early as 1909 and was thought to be infectious in origin (5). Its infectious nature had been demonstrated through transmission of ECM from patients to volunteers by inoculation of material from the edge of the lesion (6,7), but the infectious agent was not known. Viruses and rickettsiae had been suspected but not proved (8). Lennhoff (9), in 1948, had reported seeing spirochetes in mercury-stained sections of ECM (9); however, subsequent studies failed to confirm his findings (8). Yet Hollstrom (10,11) had successfully treated ECM patients with penicillin as early as 1948, and similar success with penicillin had led Hellerstrom (12) in 1951 to theorize that ECM was caused by a tick-transmitted spirochete.

In Europe, ECM was also known to be followed in many cases by a syndrome of chronic lymphocytic meningitis accompanied by cranial nerve palsies and painful radiculoneuritis (meningopolyneuritis, or Bannwarth's syndrome). The first case, described by Garin and Bujadoux (13) in 1922, was that of a man who developed meningoencephalitis, painful sensory radiculitis, paralysis of a deltoid muscle, and spreading erythema following a tick bite. Reports of chronic meningitis following ECM ensued (10,12,14). Then, in 1941 and 1944, Bannwarth (15,16) described 19 patients with intense radicular pain, lymphocytic meningitis (often without menin-

L. Reik, Jr.: Department of Neurology, University of Connecticut Health Center, Farmington, Connecticut 06032.

geal signs), and peripheral and cranial nerve palsies, especially facial palsy; some of these patients had preceding ECM. Subsequent reports by Schaltenbrand (17–19) and Bammer and Schenk (20) noted that the radicular pain often began, and was most intense, in the region of the tick bite; as a result, these investigators enlarged the spectrum of neurologic abnormalities to include myelitis and optic neuritis. Meanwhile, Hollstrom (10) and Hellerstrom (12) had reported that both the meningitis and the skin lesion responded to penicillin therapy. Finally, in 1973, Horstrup and Ackermann (21) published a detailed description of 47 patients with meningopolyneuritis. They confirmed the relationship between tick bite, ECM, and subsequent neurologic abnormalities; described the peak onset in summer months; and detailed the full spectrum of peripheral and cranial neuropathies.

But the Yale investigators were not yet aware of neurologic abnormalities in their patients, and ECM had not been associated with arthritis in Europe. When cultures and serologic tests performed on their Connecticut patients did not indicate infection with agents known to cause arthritis, the Yale investigators, believing they were describing a new disease, named it "Lyme arthritis" (3).

The following year, 1976, the Yale group prospectively followed patients who developed the skin lesion or Lyme arthritis (22). Twenty-four patients with the skin lesion were identified. Many later developed arthritis, but some also developed neurologic abnormalities (Bell's palsy, sensory radiculitis, lymphocytic meningitis) or cardiac conduction defects. In patients with both the skin lesion and arthritis, the skin lesion invariably occurred first; and its onset between May and August in all but one case strengthened the arthropod vector theory. Moreover, the usual location of the lesion on the thigh or buttock or in the axilla favored a crawling arthropod. Indeed, three patients recalled a tick bite at the site of the skin lesion up to 20 days before the lesion appeared. Thus the identity of the skin lesion which preceded Lyme arthritis was confirmed as ECM, and the similarity of its neurologic complications to those of Bannwarth's syndrome was noted.

Further prospective studies in 1977 confirmed the tick vector theory (23). The Yale group identified an additional 43 patients with the onset of ECM or Lyme arthritis or both. Nine of them had had an initial tick bite at the site of the skin lesion. One of them saved the tick: It was initially identified as *Ixodes scapularis* but was later reclassified as *Ixodes dammini*, a new species (24). Additional field studies, undertaken in the same year, showed that the geographical distribution of clinical cases paralleled that of the tick (25).

Subsequent clinical studies by Steere and his associates detailed the neurologic (26) and cardiac abnormalities (27) and confirmed the antibiotic responsiveness of ECM and its associated symptoms (28). In recognition of the multisystem nature of the illness, they renamed it "Lyme disease" (26). Meanwhile, the widespread distribution of Lyme disease became apparent as increasing numbers of cases were reported from outside Connecticut (29). But the identity of the infectious agent of Lyme disease remained unknown.

Then, in 1981, Willy Burgdorfer from the Rocky Mountain Laboratories in Hamilton, Montana, discovered the agent (30). Burgdorfer, in collaboration with Jorge Benach from the New York State Health Department, was trying to identify the tick vector for Rocky Mountain spotted fever on Shelter Island, New York, a known endemic area for Lyme disease. Attempts to demonstrate the spotted fever agent, *Rickettsia rickettsii,* in adult dog ticks, *Dermacentor variabilis,* had failed, and he began looking for *R. rickettsii* in *I. dammini.* He found no rickettsiae but did find microfilariae in the hemolymph of two female ticks. When he next examined Giemsa-stained midgut smears from the same two ticks to see if microfilariae were also present in the digestive tract, he found spirochetes. Burgdorfer then dissected an additional 124 ticks and found spirochetes in 60% of them. Remembering the earlier European literature, Burgdorfer realized he might have discovered the cause of Lyme disease (8).

Burgdorfer then enlisted the help of Alan Barbour, his colleague at the Rocky Mountain Laboratories. Barbour's success in culturing the *I. dammini* spirochete was the crucial next step. It allowed the investigators to demonstrate the antigen relatedness of the cultured spirochete to the agent of Lyme disease by both indirect immunofluorescence and western blot analysis of sera from patients with the illness (30,31). Animal inoculation showed that the spirochete caused a similar disease in, and could be recovered from, laboratory animals (30,32). Finally, the spirochetal etiology of the infection was proved when the *I. dammini* spirochete was cultured from the blood, skin lesions, and cerebrospinal fluid (CSF) of patients with Lyme disease (33,34) and demonstrated histologically in biopsies of ECM lesions (35).

In short order, identical spirochetes were isolated from *Ixodes pacificus* from the west coast of the United States (36), from *I. ricinus* from Europe (31,37), and from European patients with ECM (38) and with neurologic involvement (39,40). The spirochete was identified as a new species of *Borrelia* and was named *Borrelia burgdorferi* in honor of its discoverer (41).

Identification and culture of *B. burgdorferi* also led to the development of sensitive serologic tests which allowed the diagnosis of Lyme disease on laboratory as well as clinical grounds. Cases of neurologic involvement diagnosed serologically, without antecedent ECM or subsequent arthritis, were described (42); and two skin lesions of unknown cause, lymphocytoma cutis and acrodermatitis chronica atrophicans, were attributed to infection by *B. burgdorferi* on the same grounds (43). Finally, recognition of the spirochetal etiology of Lyme disease led to effective antibiotic treatments for the arthritis (44) and neurologic abnormalities (45).

EPIDEMIOLOGY

Lyme disease is a worldwide tick-transmitted spirochetosis now reported from five continents: North America, Europe, Asia, Africa, and Australia (46–51). The usual vectors are small, hard-bodied ticks of the genus *Ixodes* which have a three-host, 2-year life cycle. The seasonal patterns of tick activity, with active questing and feeding beginning in the spring, determines the seasonal pattern of illness onset, with symptoms usually beginning in late spring or summer. Because these ticks usually prefer the brushy understories of forests or their margins, the illness is more common in individuals with exposure to such areas. In some cases, pet ownership is also a factor, with the ticks presumably being transferred from pet to owner (23,52).

Lyme Disease in North America

The United States is the major focus of Lyme disease in North America, although cases acquired in Canada are now being recognized. From 1977 through May 1989, 25 cases of indigenous Lyme disease were reported to Canada's Laboratory Centre for Disease Control, with most of them coming from Ontario (17 cases) and Manitoba (five cases) (46a).

In the United States, Lyme disease is now the most commonly reported tick-transmitted illness, with 4,572 cases being reported to the Centers for Disease Control (CDC) in Atlanta in 1988 (46). The disease is endemic along the east coast from Maryland to Massachusetts, in the Midwest in Minnesota and Wisconsin, and on the Pacific coast in California and southern Oregon (46,47,53). In addition, there are increasing numbers of cases reported from southeastern and south-central

states; and Lyme disease has now been acquired in 43 states (53). However, 92% of the cases reported to the CDC in 1987–1988 were acquired in just eight states: Connecticut, Massachusetts, Minnesota, New Jersey, New York, Pennsylvania, Rhode Island, and Wisconsin (53). New York alone accounted for 2553 cases in 1988, more than half of the total; but the state with the highest incidence of Lyme disease was Rhode Island, with 9.9 cases per 100,000 population (53).

I. dammini, the deer tick (see color Fig. 1 on page 669), is the usual vector in the Northeast and Midwest. It ranges from southern Delaware northward to Massachusetts, mainly in coastal areas, and is common also in Wisconsin, Minnesota, and southern Ontario, Canada (Fig. 1) (54). In some areas, up to 80% of the ticks harbor spirochetes (55), explaining the very high attack rate in these locations. The tick develops in a 2-year cycle in three stages—larva, nymph, and adult, all of which bite humans (56). Immature ticks feed on a variety of small mammals and birds (especially the white-footed mouse, *Peromyscus leucopus*), whereas adult ticks feed mainly on deer (56–58). Domestic animals are parasitized too, and Lyme disease has been reported in dogs, cattle, and horses (59–61). But the presence of both deer and white-footed mice is key to maintaining disease transmission, and Lyme disease is most common in forested and suburban areas where both are common (62). Both deer and mice are readily infected after being bitten by infected ticks, but they do not appear to suffer pathology. Mice, in particular, remain highly infectious to larval ticks for most of their lifespan; and, in some areas, almost 90% of the mice are infected (58).

The ticks are infected by feeding on a spirochetemic host, usually a mouse. The spirochetes then proliferate in the midgut, only occasionally penetrating the gut wall to initiate a systemic infection. At the time of subsequent feeding, however, the borreliae multiply, enter the he-

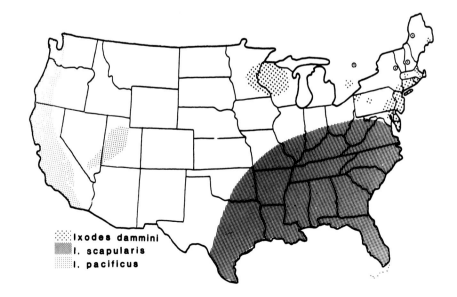

Ixodes dammini
I. scapularis
I. pacificus

FIG. 1. Geographic distribution of North American *Ixodes* vectors of Lyme disease. The circles with center dots indicate collection sites outside the main range of *I. dammini.* (Reproduced from ref. 54, with permission.)

mocele, and disseminate (63). Transmission to a new host then occurs via regurgitation of infected gut contents or saliva but generally takes some time: The rate of transmission is low, with less than 24 hr of attachment (64).

During dissemination, the ovaries can be invaded, but effective transovarial transmission of *B. burgdorferi* in *I. dammini* is probably rare. Infection has been reported in 3–25% of the unfed larval offspring of infected adult females, but the infection apparently is not maintained into the nymphal stage, suggesting a gradual die-off of the spirochetes (63). Transmission occurs horizontally instead, from infected nymphs to uninfected larvae through white-footed mice. Nymphs feed on and infect mice from May to July; larvae feed on the same mice in August and are infected in turn. Because the nymphs of *I. dammini* most often bite humans, Lyme disease begins most commonly in summer, in areas where *I. dammini* is the vector.

B. burgdorferi has also been isolated from the ticks *D. variabilis*, *Amblyoma americanum*, and *Hemaphysalis leporispalustris* and from horse flies, deer flies, and mosquitoes in the Northeast (57,65). These other ticks and biting insects may be secondary vectors in some areas.

I. pacificus, the western black-legged tick, is the usual vector of Lyme disease on the Pacific coast (36,52,54). It ranges along the seaboard from British Columbia to Mexico and is found also on the western slopes of the Sierra Nevada and Cascade Mountains and in Idaho, Nevada, and Utah (Fig. 2). Like *I. dammini*, *I. pacificus* is a three-host tick whose larvae and nymphs feed on a variety of small rodents, lizards, and birds while the adults feed on dogs, foxes, cattle, deer, and humans (54). But the nymphs of *I. pacificus* rarely attack humans, and fewer than 3% of ticks harbor spirochetes in most areas—hence the lower frequency of Lyme disease on the west coast (36,52).

The mechanics of spirochetal transmission are probably the same for *I. pacificus* as for *I. dammini*, except that disseminated infection of the ticks apparently is more common and transovarial transmission is more frequent (63). In one experiment, one of three naturally infected adult female *I. pacificus* produced 100% infected F_1 larvae which remained infected through all subsequent developmental stages and which, in the case of four of five F_1 females, eventually transmitted the infection transovarially to up to 97% of their own (F_2) progeny (63).

As in the eastern United States, secondary vectors may be important too: *B. burgdorferi* has been detected in *Dermacentor occidentalis*, the Pacific Coast tick, from California (52).

In the other areas of the United States where Lyme disease has been acquired, the vectors are less certain. Another ixodid tick, *I. scapularis*, the common black-legged tick, is widely distributed in southeastern and south-central states, with its range extending from the

Gulf of Mexico north to Kansas, Missouri, Iowa, Ohio, Indiana, and Maryland (Fig. 2) (54). It also is a three-stage tick which parasitizes a wide variety of animals, with members of all three stages attacking humans (54). *B. burgdorferi* has been isolated from *I. scapularis* from North Carolina (66), and larval *I. scapularis* have been shown to efficiently acquire and maintain *B. burgdorferi* infection (67,68). In Texas, however, *B. burgdorferi* was isolated from the ticks *A. americanum*, *Rhipicephalus sanguineus*, and *Dermacentor parumapertus* and from a flea, *Ctenocephalides felis*, collected off infected humans or from sites where human infection had occurred, but were not isolated from *I. scapularis* from the same sites (69).

Lyme Disease in Europe

B. burgdorferi infection is widespread and often very common in Europe (47,70). It is present in all four Scandinavian countries and is so common in Sweden that *B. burgdorferi* is the most frequent central nervous system (CNS) bacterial pathogen there (71). The infection is also prevalent in Austria, Switzerland, and the Federal Republic of Germany and occurs, but is less common, in Belgium, Czechoslovakia, France, Hungary, Italy, the Netherlands, Romania, Spain, the United Kingdom, the Soviet Union, and Yugoslavia (47,70).

I. ricinus, the sheep tick, is the usual vector in Europe (47,54,72), although cases acquired outside its range have been attributed to mosquito bites (73). *I. ricinus* is found from the British Isles and southern Scandinavia south through central Europe, France, Spain, Portugal, Italy, the Balkans, and European Soviet Union into northern Iran and North Africa (47,54). The tick favors (a) the brushy edges of forests and (b) clearings with high grass (72). Juveniles feed on a variety of small mammals (especially rodents), and the adults feed on larger wild and domestic animals. Peak feeding activity occurs in May and June and again in September and October, and cases of human infection peak in July and August (72). Infection rates for *I. ricinus* are intermediate between those of *I. dammini* and *I. pacificus*, ranging from 5% to 35% in areas where human infections are most common (47).

As with *I. pacificus*, *I. ricinus* may itself serve as a reservoir for *B. burgdorferi*, because transovarial transmission apparently does take place. One hundred percent of the F_1 larval progeny of three of 10 Austrian female *I. ricinus* were infected transovarially and maintained the infection into the nymphal stage (63,74).

Lyme Disease in Asia and Australia

Much less is known about the frequency and distribution of Lyme disease in Asia. A single case has been reported from Japan (48), whereas over 300 cases have been detected among Chinese forest workers in Heilongjiang Province (49), which is located in north central Manchuria and borders on the Soviet Union to the north. The vector in both areas is *Ixodes persulcatus,* another forest-dwelling ixodid tick. Because *I. persulcatus* ranges throughout the whole southern part of the forest zone of the Soviet Union from the Baltic to the Pacific (54,75), Lyme disease may prove to be widespread in at least the temperate parts of Asia. Indeed, in a recent report of Lyme disease from the Soviet Union, 16 of 90 cases were from Asiatic Russia, within the range of *I. persulcatus* (50).

In Australia, cases of Lyme disease have been acquired in several localities in New South Wales, including the Hunter Valley and the central and south coasts (47,76). Because ixodid ticks are not found in Australia, the vectors there are not known.

ETIOLOGY

B. burgdorferi is a slender, irregularly coiled spirochete 10–30 μm long and 0.2–0.3 μm wide (Fig. 2). Like other borreliae, it stains with Giemsa stain and can be demonstrated in tissues by silver impregnation techniques. It also shares with the other members of its genus a characteristic structure (Fig. 3). An outer slime layer surrounds the outer cell membrane which contains several species-specific but strain-variable proteins. Beneath this membrane are three to 14 periplasmic flagella antigenically similar to those of other borreliae. Interior to the flagella is the bacterial cell wall, composed of peptidoglycan, surrounding in turn the protoplasmic cylinder containing four to seven plasmids, both linear and supercoiled, in addition to the usual organelles (77,78).

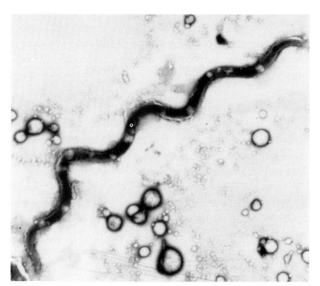

FIG. 2. Transmission electron micrograph of *Borrelia burgdorferi.* ×10,000. (Courtesy of Theodore G. Andreadis, Ph.D., Connecticut Agricultural Experiment Station, New Haven, Connecticut.)

B. burgdorferi also resembles other borreliae in its biochemistry and growth requirements. It is not an obligate intracellular parasite but prefers an extracellular existence and can be grown in culture in Barbour–Stoenner–Kelly (BSK) medium (79). Growth in BSK medium is most rapid between 30°C and 37°C: The doubling time is 12 hr at 35°C. The organism is catalase-negative and microaerophilic, and it ferments glucose to lactate via the Embden–Myerhof pathway.

B. burgdorferi also requires long-chain fatty acids for growth and incorporates these, unaltered, into its cellular lipids (77). Between 1.5% and 4% of the dry weight of the organism is composed of a lipopolysaccharide (LPS) similar to rough-form, gram-negative bacterial LPS (80). *B. burgdorferi* LPS partitions to the phenol phase after hot phenol–water extraction and consists of 35% carbohydrate, 44–51% lipid A, 3% 3-deoxy-D-mannooctulosonic acid, and 3–8% protein. On sodium dodecyl sulfate–polyacrylamide gel electrophoresis (SDS-PAGE) analysis, the extracted LPS shows a small number of diffuse bands with apparent molecular weights of 3200–4200 daltons. Like classic LPS, *B. burgdorferi* LPS is mitogenic for human and murine lymphocytes, is pyrogenic in rabbits, and produces cross-protective tolerance to an unrelated LPS (from *Escherichia coli* 0111:B4) after repeated injection. It also induces the production of large amounts of interleukin-1 (IL-1) and, typical of rough-form LPS, fails to initiate complement activation by either the classic or alternate pathways (80).

All *B. burgdorferi* isolates tested so far have been shown by DNA hybridization to belong to a single species of *Borrelia.* DNA hybridization of 10 isolates from the United States and Europe has shown a divergence of 0.0–0.1% and a relatedness of 58–98% (81). Although *B. burgdorferi* DNA is also 30–46% homologous with that of *Borrelia hermsii* (one of the North American tickborne relapsing fever borreliae), it is only 16% homologous with treponemal DNA and 1% homologous with leptospiral DNA (81).

A number of different strains of *B. burgdorferi* have been identified, however, on the basis of PAGE and western blot analysis of their protein components (82–86). All strains tested so far share two components of constant molecular weight: (i) a 60-kD protein which is common to treponemes and to other borreliae and (ii) a 41-kD flagellar antigen shared only with other borreliae. The strains vary in having one, two, or three other major proteins of lower molecular weight: (i) 31- to 32-kD outer surface protein A (osp A), (ii) 33- to 36-kD outer surface protein B (osp B), and (iii) 21- to 22-kD protein C (pC). Using monoclonal and polyclonal antibodies against these proteins, Wilske et al. (86) have characterized five serotypes of *B. burgdorferi* among North American and European patient isolates, plus two additional serotypes among tick isolates.

In general, European isolates differ antigenically from, and are more heterogeneous than, North American iso-

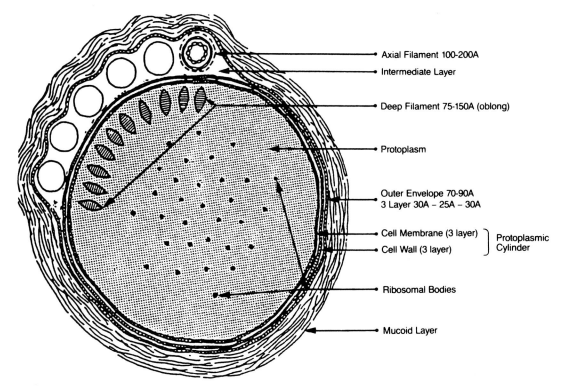

FIG. 3. Cross-sectional diagram of a spirochete containing six axial filaments (flagella). (From ref. 257, with permission.)

lates, supporting the theory that *B. burgdorferi* originated in Europe and spread later to North America (83) and suggesting one basis for reported clinical differences between European and North American patients with *B. burgdorferi* infection. In addition, European CSF isolates are more heterogeneous than European skin isolates. The occurrence of apparently seronegative CNS infections may be one consequence of this heterogeneity (86). Heterogeneity of surface proteins has also been observed among different generations of the same strain: osp B proteins can change during *in vitro* cultivation (82,87), but such a change has not yet been demonstrated within a host during the course of infection. Similar variability of surface proteins does occur during infection with relapsing fever borreliae and is thought to be the mechanism through which the spirochetes escape the host's immune response.

The genes coding for osp A and osp B are located on a single linear plasmid, and the variability of their expression is a reflection of the extreme variability of plasmid profiles among *B. burgdorferi* isolates. Although North American isolates are congruent for a 49-kb plasmid containing the genes for outer-membrane proteins, and European stains are congruent for a larger 53-kb plasmid coding for the same proteins, only two of 13 strains examined so far have had the same total plasmid profile (87). Moreover, strains passaged many times in culture have been shown to lose plasmids, indicating one way that outer-surface proteins could change during infection (87).

PATHOGENESIS AND PATHOPHYSIOLOGY

There is no single animal model which reproduces all of the clinical abnormalities of human Lyme disease. Some experimentally infected laboratory rats develop arthritis (88), as do naturally infected dogs (89), horses (60,61), and cattle (60). Experimentally infected rabbits (90) and naturally infected white-footed mice (91) develop skin lesions and spirochetemia. But there is no good model for human nervous system infection with *B. burgdorferi*. Although the organism has been isolated from the brain of a horse with encephalitis (92), no other nonhuman examples of nervous system disease have been described. In laboratory animals, nervous system infection without symptoms is more usual.

Among laboratory animals, the Syrian hamster is probably the best-studied experimental host for *B. burgdorferi*: The hamsters are easily infected but show no signs of disease (93,94). In hamsters infected by intradermal inoculation, *B. burgdorferi* proliferates locally, quickly enters the bloodstream and lymphatics, and disseminates to multiple organs, including the brain. Spirochetes can be isolated from the blood of cutaneously infected hamsters as early as the first day of infection and can be both isolated from and visualized in the gonads, lungs, kidneys, heart, eyes, and brain by the end of the first week. They remain mostly extracellular in the tissues and, once localized there, can persist for a long time: Hamsters remain infected for up to 14 months (94). Moreover, *B. burgdorferi* in the hamster retains the capacity for spirochetemia for a long time: The organisms have been visualized in heart blood after more than 6 months of infection (94).

In the human host, *B. burgdorferi* also first proliferates locally in the skin at the site of the tick bite, with the spirochete's presence and the host's reaction to it eventually producing the skin lesion, ECM (95). Within days or weeks, the organism spreads hematogenously throughout the body. A prominent immune response follows, characterized by proliferation of lymphocytes and plasma cells, production of increased serum levels of immunoglobulin M (IgM), the appearance of circulating immune complexes, and an often symptomatic hyperplasia of elements of the reticuloendothelial system, including the lymph nodes, spleen, and bone marrow. At this stage of the illness, spirochetes have been isolated from the blood and skin and have been demonstrated histologically in skin, bone marrow, spleen, lymph nodes, and liver; but it is not known whether they are in the nervous system. Nervous system abnormalities usually develop weeks to months later, after the acute reactive stage has largely resolved. Once neurologic abnormalities have developed, the organism can be demonstrated in, or isolated from, both brain parenchyma (95,96) and CSF (33,39,40,97).

During the stage of hematogenous dissemination, *B. burgdorferi* can also be transmitted transplacentally. Both congenital infection and fetal demise have now been reported; and spirochetes can be recovered from, or demonstrated histologically in, sparsely inflamed fetal tissues—including the liver, heart, adrenal, kidney, meninges, subarachnoid space, and brain (98,99).

Persistence is also a feature of human *B. burgdorferi* infection, just as it is in infection of laboratory animals. Arthritis develops months to years after the stage of early neurologic abnormalities and is characterized by the presence of organisms in synovium (100) and synovial fluid (101). Moreover, other progressive skin and nervous system abnormalities can begin years after the initial infection because of the persistence of live organisms. Spirochetes can be demonstrated in, or cultured from, late skin lesions (102–104); and they have been demonstrated by silver staining of CSF 15 months after the onset of neurologic symptoms (105). Although *B. burgdorferi* has not been cultured from the nervous system in late disease, the response of late neurologic disease to antibiotic therapy suggests that live organisms are present.

It is not entirely clear how *B. burgdorferi* is able to evade the host's immune defenses and persist for such long periods of time. Because the organisms remain extracellular (94,95), they should be vulnerable to immune attack. Possible escape mechanisms include: suppression of host immune defenses by the spirochete; antigenic mimicry or variation; and sequestration in immunologically privileged sites. There is evidence that each of these mechanisms may play a role.

Experimentally infected Syrian hamsters develop specific antibodies against *B. burgdorferi,* but the organism can persist in tissues despite the presence of these antibodies. Passive immunization with either rabbit or hamster anti-*B. burgdorferi* antibodies does protect the hamsters from challenge with the same strain of spirochetes against which the antibodies were raised, but only if the antibodies are administered prior to challenge (106). Hamsters immunized 17 hr after challenge are not protected, suggesting that the spirochete can be sequestered quickly in host tissues where it is either resistant to or inaccessible to the protective effect of antibody (106).

Experiments in passive immunization of hamsters also suggest that serum immunity to *B. burgdorferi* infection is strain-specific. Immunization of hamsters against a *B. burgdorferi* isolate from one geographic area does not protect against challenge with an isolate from another geographic area (106). Apparently, among strains of borreliae from different areas, the antigens that elicit formation of protective antibody are heterogeneous (106). The idea that humoral immunity to *B. burgdorferi* is strain-specific provides one explanation for human cases of reinfection (107). It also suggests that the antigenic shifts in outer-surface proteins observed among different generations of the same strain during *in vitro* cultivation (82,87) could protect the spirochetes from immune elimination if such shifts occur also *in vivo*.

In human hosts, both cellular and humoral immune responses occur during *B. burgdorferi* infection. The T-cell response occurs first (108,109). Lymphocytes from patients with Lyme disease proliferate *in vitro* in response to *B. burgdorferi* beginning early in the illness, often preceding measurable antibody production. Once established, the proliferative response is long-lasting and not related to disease activity. Moreover, patients with late Lyme disease who have had early but inadequate treatment with antibiotics are often seronegative while still showing a T-cell response: The early removal of the bulk of organisms apparently prevents the development of humoral, but not cellular, immunity (108,110,110a).

Most recent reports indicate a normal total number of lymphocytes and total number of T cells in Lyme disease (109), although conflicting data have been reported (111). But the numbers of cells in specific T-cell subsets is not normal. The natural killer (NK) cytotoxic ability of peripheral blood lymphocytes is below normal in patients with active disease but is normal in patients with early treated or seronegative disease (109,112). Because a similar inhibition of NK function is seen *in vitro* only in the presence of actively proliferating *B. burgdorferi,* it seems that inhibition of NK function is a result of interaction between proliferating organisms and the host immune system; however, the mechanism is not clear (112). Suppressor cell activity is affected also. Suppressor activity is increased early in the illness and then becomes depressed later on, explaining both an initial delay in the appearance of specific antibody and the eventual vigorous humoral response (109,113,114).

The human humoral response does develop more slowly. Specific antibody is usually not detectable when ECM appears (115). The IgM response becomes maximal 3–6 weeks later and then declines, although titers do sometimes remain high during late disease (115–118). The titer of specific IgM correlates well with total serum levels of IgM. At the same time, circulating immune complexes containing IgM, IgG, and components of complement often appear. Their presence is predictive of subsequent joint or nervous system disease, and their levels often parallel disease activity (22,26,119).

The appearance of specific IgG antibody is delayed, but measurable amounts are nearly always present during early neurologic or joint involvement (33,116). Once present, specific IgG antibody can persist in high titer for years, even during remission (33,116,117). Both the early IgM response and the initial IgG response are directed against the 41-kD flagellar antigen, but the IgG response expands as the disease progresses to include a broader range of antigens (117,120). This expansion of the immune response is not seen in patients with early disease successfully treated with antibiotics, and it ceases in patients with late disease once treatment is given. These observations suggest the prolonged persistence of live organisms allowing production of antibody to antigens not recognized in early disease (117). As in experimental animals, however, the development of humoral immunity does not eradicate *B. burgdorferi.* The demonstration of spirochetes in, and of their recovery from, patients with high titers of specific antibody, along with the expansion of the antibody response which ceases with antibiotic treatment of late disease, indicates the presence of live organisms despite high levels of specific antibody (121).

The exact mechanisms through which *B. burgdorferi* causes disease are not certain, but the direct inflammatory response to its presence is probably important. *B. burgdorferi* and both its osp A and flagellin components are chemotactic for neutrophil leukocytes (122), whereas its LPS component has endotoxin-like activity (81) and can stimulate the release of IL-1 from macrophages (123,124). The release of IL-1 may be responsible for many of the clinical abnormalities of Lyme disease. IL-1 mediates the acute-phase response characterized by fever, fatigue, anorexia, synthesis of acute-phase reactants, and leukocytosis. It also is chemotactic for neutro-

phils, stimulates antibody secretion, and stimulates lymphocytes to secrete IL-2. IL-2 may be responsible, in turn, for local increases in the number of lymphocytes and the release of lymphokines. Within joints, IL-1 causes the release of collagenase, proteases, prostaglandin E_2, and plasminogen activator from synovial cells and chondrocytes (124). Finally, the intradermal injection of IL-1 in the rabbit has produced ECM-like lesions (123).

Immunopathic tissue damage in response to the presence of living spirochetes also may be important. The demonstration of spirochetes in tissues, the ability to isolate them in culture (even in late disease), the expanding antibody response in late disease, and the antibiotic responsiveness of late disease all do point to the involvement of living organisms in the pathogenesis of Lyme disease. Yet the organisms are difficult to isolate from human material, and they appear few in number in tissue sections, suggesting that the number of spirochetes in the infected human is too small for *B. burgdorferi* to cause all of the clinical manifestations of Lyme disease directly. Therefore, the immune response to the presence of the organism could be another important element in pathogenesis. Possible mechanisms for immunopathic tissue damage in response to *B. burgdorferi* include: the cross-reaction of anti-*B. burgdorferi* antibodies with host antigens; the induction of cellular autoimmunity; the deposition of circulating immune complexes in tissues; and the uncontrolled local production of specific antibody because of loss of suppressor activity, leading to local formation of immune complexes and chronic inflammation. There is evidence that at least some of these mechanisms may cause nervous system disease.

Within the CNS, both the direct effects of the organism and the host's reaction to it are probably important. Meningitis most likely does result directly from invasion of the CSF by *B. burgdorferi:* The organism has been cultured from CSF (33,39,40), and antibiotics shorten the course (44). At least some CNS parenchymal abnormalities may result from direct invasion also. *B. burgdorferi* has been demonstrated histologically in, and has been isolated from, brain tissue (Fig. 4) (95,96).

Clinical evidence suggests, however, that some other CNS abnormalities are due to vasculopathy. This evidence includes: the diffuse and multifocal pattern of neurologic abnormalities in some patients (26); the occurrence of both apparent transient ischemic attacks and strokes in some patients with encephalopathy (125–127); the relatively high frequency of hemiparesis in some series (128); computerized tomographic (CT) abnormalities in some cases, suggesting cerebral infarction (127,129,130); and, in several cases, cerebral angiographic changes consistent with vasculitis (129,131,132). Although vasculitic changes have been demonstrated histologically in other tissues (95), such changes have not

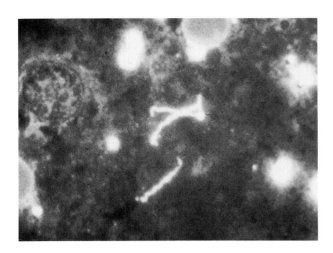

FIG. 4. *Borrelia burgdorferi* in a touch preparation of cerebral cortex taken at autopsy from a patient with dementia and stained with anti-*B. burgdorferi* monoclonal antibody. ×500. (Courtesy of Dr. Alan B. MacDonald, Department of Pathology, Southampton Hospital, Southampton, New York.)

yet been seen in the CNS, and the evidence for them is still indirect. Furthermore, the pathogenesis of this putative vasculopathy remains speculative. Possibilities include: (a) direct invasion of the vessel walls by *B. burgdorferi* and (b) the local deposition of immune complexes. However, *B. burgdorferi* has not been demonstrated in vessel walls, and immune complexes have not been localized to sites of vascular injury in the CNS or elsewhere. Immune complexes are present in the blood (22,26) and CSF (133) of some patients with Lyme disease and neurologic abnormalities, however.

Other, indirect immunopathic mechanisms may be operating within the CNS as well. Both CT and magnetic resonance imaging (MRI) scans from some patients with cerebral symptoms have shown changes consistent with demyelination (134–136), whereas the CSF of some patients with radiculomyelitis contains both (a) T-cell lines reactive to myelin basic protein, peripheral myelin, and galactocerebrosides and (b) *B. burgdorferi*-specific T-cell lines (137). Finally, serum of patients with neurologic abnormalities of Lyme disease contains IgM anti-*B. burgdorferi* antibodies that cross-react with neuronal antigens (138).

Similarly, *B. burgdorferi* may damage the peripheral nervous system (PNS) both directly and indirectly. Spinal radiculitis and cranial neuritis could result from direct extension of infection and inflammation from the meninges and subarachnoid space to the nerve roots (139). But clinical patterns (mononeuritis simplex and multiplex; asymmetrical radiculoplexitis) again suggest a vascular cause (26,140). Moreover, examination of biopsied nerves has shown vasculopathy (see below) (141–143); and, in many cases, electrophysiologic testing has shown multifocal axonal injury (42,139,141,144). Yet, in others, the electrophysiologic changes indicate de-

myelination (139,145,146); and severe weakness in Lyme disease can recover in weeks (26,42,139,147), a time course more consistent with repair of segmental demyelination than with regeneration after wallerian degeneration. Therefore, both segmental demyelination and axonal injury apparently do occur in the PNS in Lyme disease. Whether both are caused by the same vasculopathy is not clear. The identification of T-cell lines reactive to peripheral myelin in the CSF of patients with neurologic abnormalities of Lyme disease (137) suggests that demyelination may result from indirect immunopathological mechanisms, however.

PATHOLOGY

The histopathological picture in Lyme disease, particularly in its late stages, also suggests immunologic damage in response to persistence of the organism (95). The typical histologic reaction is a perivascular infiltration of lymphocytes and plasma cells accompanied by varying numbers of macrophages, dendritic immune cells, and tissue mast cells. There is seldom tissue necrosis, and giant cells and gummas are not present. In later stages, vascular thickening and (sometimes) occlusion is prominent and, in the dermis, is accompanied by scleroderma-like collagen expansion (95).

During the earliest stage of the illness, perivascular round cell infiltration is confined to the area of initial skin involvement. Following dissemination, perivascular infiltrates are found in the secondary skin lesions (as are the spirochetes), and there is an accompanying proliferation of plasma cells and their precursors in the organs of the reticuloendothelial system (95). Subsequent cardiac involvement, usually beginning after hyperplasia of the reticuloendothelial system has subsided, is characterized by infiltration of all three cardiac layers by lymphocytes, plasma cells, and macrophages accompanied by obliterative endarteritis (95,148,149). Spirochetes are present in the myocardium (149). Obliterative endarteritis also occurs in small vessels of the synovium in Lyme arthritis, along with the usual lymphoplasmacytic infiltrate plus synovial cell and villous hypertrophy (100). Spirochetes are present in synovium and synovial fluid but are few in number (100,101). Similar vessel changes and inflammatory cell infiltrates occur in the skin lesions of late Lyme disease and may be accompanied by thickening of the dermis by excess collagen (95). Living spirochetes are still present in these skin lesions years after onset and can both be demonstrated histologically and be isolated in culture (102–104).

Less detail is known about the pathology of the nervous system in Lyme disease, particularly the CNS. The few fatal cases with early neurologic involvement have shown (a) band-like infiltration of lymphocytes and plasma cells in the meninges, (b) mild spongiform

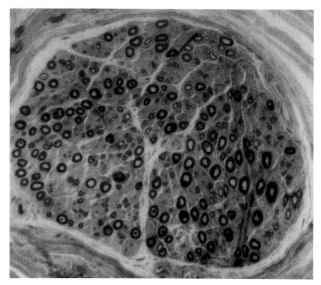

FIG. 5. Thick section of sural nerve biopsy specimen from a patient with Lyme disease and meningopolyneuritis, showing moderate loss of large and medium-sized myelinated fibers. Toluidine blue, ×100. (Courtesy of Dr. Margaret L. Grunnet, Department of Pathology, University of Connecticut Health Center, Farmington, Connecticut.)

changes in the cerebral cortex, and (c) increased numbers of oligodendrocytes, sometimes in cuffs around vessels (95). A brain biopsy specimen from one patient with encephalitis revealed microglial nodules and an increased number of round cells in the parenchyma; spirochetes were present in silver-stained specimens (95). To my knowledge, no pathologic material from cases of late neurologic involvement have been described.

Slightly more is known about the pathology of muscle

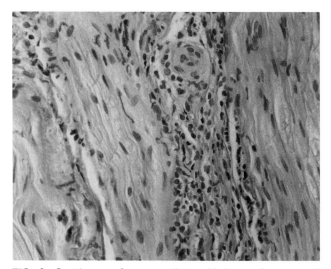

FIG. 6. Sural nerve from a patient with Lyme disease and meningopolyneuritis, showing cuffing and infiltration of perineural arteriole by lymphocytes and monocytes. Hematoxylin and eosin, ×400. (Courtesy of Dr. Margaret L. Grunnet, Department of Pathology, University of Connecticut Health Center, Farmington, Connecticut.)

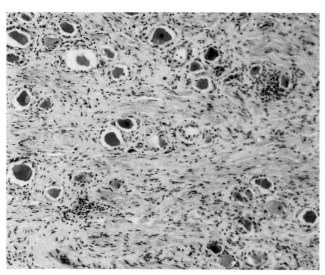

FIG. 7. Autonomic ganglion from a patient with stage II Lyme disease, showing patches of lymphocytes and plasma cells scattered throughout the ganglion. Hematoxylin and eosin. (Courtesy of Dr. Paul H. Duray, Department of Pathology, Fox Chase Cancer Center, Philadelphia, Pennsylvania.)

and peripheral nerve. Spirochetes have been demonstrated in muscle but not nerve, whereas the usual lymphoplasmacytic infiltrate is present in both (95). In muscle, these infiltrates are mainly perivascular, and the muscle cells themselves show minimal swelling but no other changes. In peripheral nerve, on the other hand, the nerve fibers themselves are clearly damaged. The histologic appearance is the same in biopsied nerves from patients with meningopolyneuritis, distal axonopathy of late Lyme disease, and the neuropathy which accompanies acrodermatitis chronica atrophicans (one of the skin lesions of late Lyme disease) (141–143). Typical changes include: axonal degeneration; loss of large myelinated fibers (Fig. 5); epineurial perivasculitis with occasional vessel wall infiltration (Fig. 6) and luminal thrombosis; and pericapillary plasma cell infiltrates in the perineurium (141–143,150,151). Aggregates and groups of lymphocytes can also infiltrate autonomic ganglia and their afferent and efferent rootlets (Fig. 7) (95).

CLINICAL MANIFESTATIONS

General Clinical Features

The skin, heart, nervous system, and joints are the organ systems most often involved, frequently in sequence; and the typical illness is said to have three stages: early skin lesions accompanied by systemic signs and symptoms (stage I), followed weeks to months later (in some patients) by neurologic or cardiac abnormalities (stage II), and weeks to years later by arthritis (stage III) (2). However, these organ systems are not always involved sequentially; clinical illness may begin in any one of them. Moreover, other skin lesions may develop in later stages, and late neurologic abnormalities may accompany arthritis. Nevertheless, the idea that Lyme disease develops in a series of stages in the typical case does provide a useful framework for understanding its clinical features (Table 1).

Stage I

The illness usually begins 3 days to 1 month after a tick bite, with a red macule or papule which starts at the site of the tick bite and which expands centrifugally to form an annular erythematous lesion with central clearing, known as "erythema chronicum migrans" (ECM) (see color Fig. 2 on page 669). ECM develops in about 80% of cases in the United States and is the best clinical marker for the disease (2,22).

The appearance of ECM can be variable, however (152,153): The initial papule occasionally ulcerates; target lesions and erythematous patches with varying intensities of red within the patch, but no definite clearing, can occur; and shades of blue are present in about 10% of the lesions. ECM is often entirely flat, but it can be raised slightly at the center, the edge, or both. The surface is normally smooth, is occasionally scaling, and is generally warmer than the surrounding skin. ECM is located most often on the thigh or in the groin or axilla (2,22,154). The lesion itself is frequently asymptomatic, but in up to one-third of cases it may itch or burn (152,153). Regional lymphadenopathy is common (40%), as are: mild systemic symptoms, usually fatigue, malaise, and lethargy (80%); fever and chills (60%); headache (65%); neck stiffness (50%); arthralgias (50%); and myalgias (45%) (2,22,152–154).

The disease usually remains localized to this single skin lesion in stage I, but in 25% of cases it disseminates to form multiple secondary annular lesions (see color Fig. 3 on page 669) (2,22,152,154) which ordinarily spare the palms, soles, and mucous membranes (152) but which do not always do so (155). Systemic signs and symptoms then intensify. Adenopathy becomes generalized; lethargy and fatigue are more severe; and there may be meningism, encephalopathy, migratory musculoskeletal pain, splenomegaly, sore throat, and cough (2,

TABLE 1. Clinical stages of Lyme disease

Stage	Clinical abnormality
I	Erythema chronicum migrans and systemic symptoms
II	Borrelial lymphocytoma Meningopolyneuritis Carditis
III	Lyme arthritis Acrodermatitis chronica atrophicans Tertiary neurologic abnormalities

22,154). Mild or severe, these early signs and symptoms generally last 3 or 4 weeks and then resolve, even without treatment.

Stage II

The nervous system is eventually involved in 10–15% of cases, either while ECM is still present or 1–6 months later (26,139). The typical neurologic abnormality at this stage is a lymphocytic meningitis accompanied by cranial and peripheral neuropathies and radiculopathies. Systemic symptoms may be present; but fever, ECM, and lymphadenopathy are usually absent by the time neurologic abnormalities develop (139). Neurologic involvement can occur without antecedent ECM and can be the first manifestation of the disease, however (42,139).

Another characteristic skin lesion sometimes develops in the second stage, especially in Europe (43,153). Called "lymphocytoma" or "lymphadenosis benigna cutis" (see color Fig. 4 on page 670), it is a solitary red or violaceous lesion ranging in size from a small nodule to a plaque several centimeters in diameter. Lymphocytoma is most commonly located on the ear lobe in children or on the nipple in adults and may appear at the site of, or remote from, the causative tick bite. The lesion consists of hyperplastic lymphoid follicles with germinal centers in the dermis. Spirochetes have been isolated (156) from, and demonstrated histologically within, the lesions (97). Lymphocytoma may occur together with, or be preceded by, ECM; but it also can develop 6–10 months after the bite and persist for months or years if untreated (153). Patients with lymphocytoma often have no systemic symptoms; but they sometimes do have regional lymphadenopathy, headaches, meningitis, choroiditis, cranial nerve palsies, or arthritis (153). When these other abnormalities accompany lymphocytoma, the skin lesion is a clue to their diagnosis.

Cardiac involvement also develops within several weeks of illness onset, affects about 8% of patients, and lasts from days to 6 weeks (27,148). The most common cardiac abnormality is a fluctuating atrioventricular block that may progress to asystole. Evidence for more diffuse cardiac involvement includes electrocardiographic changes suggesting myocarditis, decreased ejection fraction on radionuclide ventriculography, and increased myocardial gallium-67 uptake (27,148). Fibrinous pericarditis leading to constriction has also been described (95).

Stage III

Stage III is the chronic stage of Lyme disease. It begins months to years after the initial tick bite and is characterized by involvement of the joints, skin and subcutaneous tissue, and nervous system (2,95).

Lyme arthritis is a mono- or oligoarticular inflammatory arthritis which occurs in recurrent attacks and which begins between 1 month and 2 years after illness onset, often following (but occasionally preceding) stage II neurologic abnormalities (2,22). Arthritis eventually affects about 60% of patients in the United States with untreated ECM (2,22), but it is less common in Europe (43,107,157). One or two large joints—typically the wrist, shoulder, or, especially, the knee—are involved in attacks lasting weeks to months and sometimes recurring over years (2,22). During the attacks, the involved joints are swollen, hot, and painful but not usually red. Fatigue is common then, but other systemic symptoms are usually absent. The synovial fluid usually contains between 500 and 100,000 cells per cubic millimeter, as well as 3–8 g/dl of protein. In about 10% of those with arthritis, joint involvement may become chronic and cause erosion of cartilage and bone (2,22).

Stage III also has a characteristic skin lesion, more common in Europe, called "acrodermatitis chronica atrophicans" (ACA) (43,153). ACA is a chronic disorder with a gradual, insidious onset. It starts with inflammation, may proceed to atrophy, and mainly affects the elderly, particularly women. ACA usually begins asymmetrically on the distal parts of the extremities, in some cases (18%) on the same extremity where ECM was present 6 months to 10 years before. Occasionally, the trunk is extensively involved. The first change is a bluish-red discoloration and doughy swelling of the skin that can persist for years, or even decades (see color Fig. 5 on page 670). Unlike the earlier skin lesions of Lyme disease, ACA does not resolve spontaneously; and the inflammation is eventually replaced by atrophy of the skin and underlying structures. Polyneuropathy (40%), local joint deformity (30%), and fibrous nodules near joints can accompany the skin changes; and weight loss, fatigue, and personality change have been reported in conjunction with them (153). Hyperglobulinemia is common, the erythrocyte sedimentation rate (ESR) may be increased, and anti-*B. burgdorferi* antibodies are present. The clinical diagnosis is confirmed by skin biopsy: The typical histologic findings are telangiectases and perivascular lymphoplasmacytic infiltration of the dermis. Viable spirochetes are probably present regardless of the duration of ACA: They have been successfully cultured after up to 10 years of illness (102,103), and spirochetes are regularly present in silver-stained sections of both ACA and its accompanying fibrous nodules (104).

Other skin lesions also may develop in stage III. Sclerotic skin lesions, indistinguishable (on clinical and histopathological grounds) from localized scleroderma (morphea) and lichen sclerosus and atrophicus, are present in about 10% of patients with ACA (95,153). Moreover, elevated titers of anti-*B. burgdorferi* antibodies have been reported in patients with atrophoderma, eosinophilic fasciitis, and anetoderma (primary macular atrophy); and anetoderma-like areas of macular atrophy have developed in some patients with ACA (153). The majority of patients with these sclerotic skin lesions are not infected with *B. burgdorferi,* however; and their presence, unlike that of ECM or ACA, is not diagnostic for Lyme disease.

New neurologic abnormalities can appear during stage III. The abnormalities include: distal axonopathy in the PNS (142); an asymmetrical polyneuropathy in patients with ACA (143); chronic progressive encephalomyelitis (158); focal encephalitis (159); a mild organic brain syndrome (160); and, possibly, a multiple-sclerosis-like illness and psychiatric syndromes (136). These and the other neurologic abnormalities of Lyme disease are described in detail below and are summarized in Table 2.

Neurologic Abnormalities

Stage I

Patients with early Lyme disease frequently have headache, neck stiffness, lethargy, or mild encephalopathy along with their other systemic symptoms, particularly if

TABLE 2. *Neurologic abnormalities in Lyme disease by stage[a]*

Stage	Central nervous system	Peripheral nervous system
I	Headache Neck stiffness without pleocytosis	
II	Lymphocytic meningitis Encephalitis Myelitis	Cranial neuritis Radiculitis Plexitis Mononeuritis Guillain–Barré syndrome
III	Progressive encephalomyelitis Late mental changes with MRI abnormalities Latent CNS borreliosis ? Amyotrophic lateral sclerosis ? Others	Distal axonopathy Neuropathy of ACA

[a] MRI, magnetic resonance imaging; ACA, acrodermatitis chronica atrophicans; CNS, central nervous system.

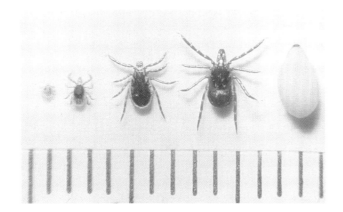

COLOR FIGURE 1. Larva, nymph, adult male, and adult female of *Ixodes dammini,* shown in comparison to a millimeter scale. The object on the right is a sesame seed. (Courtesy of M. Fergione, Pfizer Central Research, Groton, Connecticut.)

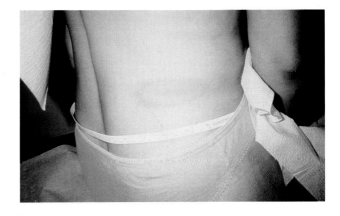

COLOR FIGURE 2. Single large erythema migrans lesion on the lateral trunk. (Courtesy of Dr. Steven W. Luger, Old Lyme Family Practice, Old Lyme, Connecticut.)

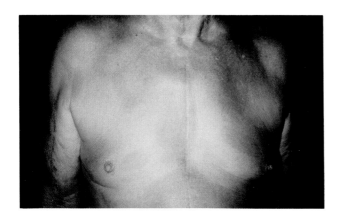

COLOR FIGURE 3. Multiple secondary lesions of erythema chronicum migrans. (Courtesy of Dr. Steven W. Luger, Old Lyme Family Practice, Old Lyme, Connecticut.)

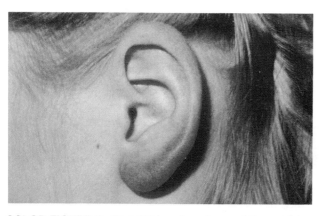

COLOR FIGURE 4. Borrelial lymphocytoma of the ear lobe. (From ref. 43, with permission.)

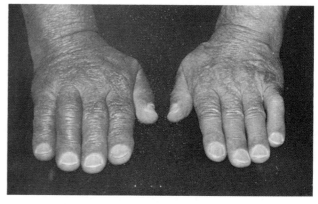

COLOR FIGURE 5. Acrodermatitis chronica atrophicans involving the right hand, which is erythematous and swollen. (From ref. 43, with permission.)

there are multiple secondary skin lesions (2,22,107, 154,157). But the CSF is usually normal at this stage of the illness. Occasionally, definite neurologic abnormalities do develop while ECM is still present; however, they develop most often in, and are one of the hallmarks of, the second stage.

Stage II

Meningitis

Meningitis is the most common neurologic abnormality of stage II and may be the first symptom of Lyme disease (42,139): It is preceded by ECM in only about 40% of cases overall (range: 10–90%), with preceding erythema being apparently more common in North America than in Europe. When meningitis does follow ECM, it usually does so by 2–10 weeks (26,42,71,128,139, 147,161–169).

At least 80% of patients with stage II neurologic abnormalities have CSF pleocytosis, although the number who are actually symptomatic is usually smaller. The percentage of cases reported with meningeal symptoms has been quite variable, ranging from 30% to over 90%, depending partly on the method of ascertainment and partly on their country of origin (26,42,71,128,139,147,161–169). In general, Swedish (71,128) and North American patients (26,139) seem to have more intense meningeal symptoms than do German (147) or Austrian (164) patients. Among German patients, children are more likely to be symptomatic than are adults (165,167).

Headache is the single most common symptom. It affects 30–90% of patients, is usually frontal or occipital, and ranges from mild to severe (or even disabling) in intensity. Neck stiffness is less common, affecting only 10–20% of those with CSF inflammation; but when it does occur, it is only present on extreme flexion. Kernig's and Brudzinski's signs are infrequent. Other meningeal symptoms—photophobia, nausea, and vomiting—are intermediate in frequency between headache and neck stiffness (20–30%) (26,42,71,128,139,147,161–169). Papilledema has been reported, but it is uncommon (26,42,147,167,170). Accompanying systemic symptoms, present in up to two-thirds of cases, include: malaise and fatigue (40%), myalgias (30%), fever (30%), arthralgias (20%), and involuntary weight loss (26,42,71,128,139,147,161–169). Fever is usually only low grade (37.5°C to 38.5°C) but is occasionally higher. The duration of symptoms in untreated cases ranges from 1 to 9 months; during this time the symptoms tend to fluctuate, particularly in North American cases (26,42,139). Typical patients experience recurrent attacks of severe meningeal symptoms lasting weeks, alternating with similar several-week periods of milder symptoms (26,42,139).

The CSF pressure may be increased. Typical changes in its contents include a pleocytosis of up to 3500 cells per cubic millimeter (usually <500); these cells are mostly lymphocytes (>90% lymphocytes in 75% of cases), although some plasma cells are often present also. The CSF protein is usually increased (up to 620 mg/dl), and it is even higher in cases of longer duration. Increases in CSF IgG, IgM, and IgA and the presence of oligoclonal bands are also common and similarly related to disease duration: It takes 4–5 weeks for these abnormalities to appear. The CSF glucose is most often normal; but it can be low (<50% of serum glucose), particularly in cases of longer duration (26,42,71,128,139, 147,161–173).

CNS Parenchymal Abnormalities

Mild cerebral symptoms are common in North American patients with stage II neurologic abnormalities (26,42,139). About 50% of those with meningitis have such symptoms: Somnolence, emotional lability, depression, impaired memory and concentration, and behavioral symptoms are most common. These tend to fluctuate in severity for weeks to months in untreated cases before resolving, sometimes in concert with the meningeal symptoms and sometimes independent of them. Cerebral symptoms of this type are less common in Europe: No more than 20% of European patients with stage II neurologic involvement have these mild mental changes (147,164,167). In both Europe and North America, however, most patients with such cerebral symptoms have abnormal electroencephalograms (EEGs): The nonspecific abnormalities reported include focal or generalized slowing and increases in sharp activity (26,42,139,147,165,167). Computerized tomography, on the other hand, is almost always normal.

More severe parenchymal abnormalities are less common in stage II; but they do occur, accompanied almost always by CSF pleocytosis and frequently by meningeal and systemic symptoms. Transverse myelitis, usually incomplete and either acute or subacute and progressive, is probably the single most common severe CNS abnormality at this stage. Spastic paraparesis, disturbance of micturition, and Babinski's signs are the most frequently reported findings; but spastic quadriparesis has also been reported. Sensory loss is apparently less frequent (26,42,71,162,164–169,174–178).

The brain is less often severely affected, but a variety of abnormalities do occur. These include: cerebellar ataxia, chorea, focal and secondary generalized seizures, hemiplegia (both sudden and gradual in onset), hallucinatory delirium, dementia, acute focal encephalitis, and cerebral demyelination (26,42,71,134,162,164,166–168,174,176,177,179–183). With prompt treatment, recovery may be complete; but irreversible dementia and demyelination, persistent seizures, and residual ataxia, hemiparesis, and paraparesis have all been reported (42,71,134,162,165,168,176,183,184). Computerized tomography in patients with severe cerebral involvement has shown both enhancing and nonenhancing low-density lesions, mass effect, and cerebral demyelination (Fig. 8) (42,134,166,183). Cerebral angiography in one patient with acute encephalitis showed only a shift of the anterior cerebral artery (134).

Cranial Neuropathies

Approximately 50% (up to 90% in some series) of patients with stage II neurologic involvement have cranial neuropathies, with the neuropathy usually beginning (along with headache and meningismus) several weeks after the onset of ECM (26,42,71,139,147,161–170,178,179). Because ECM itself can last for several weeks, the skin lesion and its associated systemic symptoms are sometimes still present when cranial nerve palsies debut.

Facial palsy is most common (26,42,71,139,147,161–170,178,179): It accounts for 80–90% of cranial nerve palsies overall, and it developed in 10% of all patients with Lyme disease in one large series (185). The facial weakness is rapid in onset (often evolving over 1 or 2 days) and is frequently accompanied by slight ipsilateral facial numbness or tingling or ipsilateral ear or jaw pain (139,163,185). Taste is commonly spared, suggesting that the point of involvement is distal to the chorda tympani (139,163,185). Facial palsy is bilateral in 30–70% of cases; the two sides are affected asynchronously in most cases, usually within a few days to 3 weeks of each other (166,186). Typically, other neurologic abnormalities are present and there is almost always an accompanying CSF pleocytosis. But facial palsy does occur alone, and it may be the presenting feature of Lyme disease and can therefore be confused with idiopathic Bell's palsy

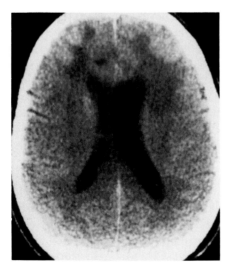

FIG. 8. Postcontrast cranial CT scan demonstrating extensive areas of low density in the white matter of the frontal lobes and centrum semiovale of a 38-year-old man with stage II Lyme disease and encephalitis.

(26,139,187–189). Indeed, Lyme disease so frequently results in facial weakness that it has been identified as the cause of 40% of Bell's palsy cases in Austria (188) and 20% of Swedish cases (189). During August and September the Swedish percentage reaches 45% (189); and it reaches 67% in Swedish children below age 15 (189), with the weakness often developing on the same side as an earlier facial ECM (190). Electrophysiologic testing of Lyme disease patients with facial palsy suggests demyelination (distal latencies four to seven times normal have been recorded), but denervation in facial muscles has also been detected (191). The rate of recovery also is consistent with demyelination: Facial weakness usually resolves completely (most often within 1 or 2 months), but recovery may take longer or may be incomplete (26,42,71,139,142,161–170,178,179).

Other cranial nerves are also involved in stage II, but less often than the seventh (26,42,71,139,147,161–170,178,179). Those most often affected are: II; III; the sensory portion of V; VI; and the acoustic portion of VIII. But abnormalities of all of the cranial nerves except the first have been reported. The nerves are often involved in multiples, frequently accompanied by other stage II neurologic abnormalities. As with facial weakness, recovery usually takes place within 2 months. Recovery may be incomplete, however: Permanent near-blindness (71), hearing loss, and Argyll Robertson pupils (134,180) have all been reported (192).

Peripheral Neuropathy

The peripheral nerves are involved in 30–50% of North American patients (26,42,139,163) and in up to 96% of adult European patients (71,147,161,162,164,166–169,178) with stage II neurologic abnormalities. Peripheral neuropathy is less common in European children with Lyme disease (165,167,190). There is frequently, but not always (164), an accompanying meningitis; and the nerves are usually involved asymmetrically.

The involvement begins with severe radicular pains, paresthesias, or hyperesthesias on the trunk or proximal limbs that typically start 5 or 6 weeks after ECM and persist for up to 2 months (26,139,141,147,162,166–168,170,186). During this time the pain may remain localized to the original area, may spread to involve additional areas, or may move completely to new areas. Associated back pain is common. In some European (but not North American) series (71,141,178,179), but not in others (147), the pain has begun and been most intense in the region of the initial tick bite or subsequent ECM. Symptoms begin acutely or subacutely, reaching a maximum in hours to a few days. The pain ranges from mild and migratory to severe and immobilizing and is described as drawing, stabbing, cutting, burning, or boring in quality. It is often worse at night (141,179,186).

Within days to weeks of the onset of pain (mean period of time: 3 weeks), motor weakness of the extremities appears in 10–75% of patients (26,139,141,147, 162,166–168,170,186). The weakness is focal or multifocal, typically asymmetrical, and often most marked in the vicinity of the initiating pain (147,178,179). It begins gradually and may progress over days to weeks. Separate extremities are usually affected asynchronously. Nerve roots, plexuses, and individual nerves may all be involved; and about half of those with motor weakness also have cranial nerve palsies, usually facial palsy. A variety of clinical patterns are common, including: motor radiculitis in the extremities, lumbar or brachial plexitis, and mononeuritis simplex and multiplex. Widespread depression of deep tendon reflexes may be present in patients whose clinical abnormalities are otherwise more localized (141,147,179), and at least one case resembling Guillain–Barré syndrome has been reported (145); both paralysis of the diaphragm (167,182) and paralysis of the abdominal muscles (167) have also been reported. Motor weakness without antecedent radicular pain can occur (10%), as can motor weakness without pleocytosis (10%) (164). Weakness may quickly progress to atrophy (139,174,193), but the outcome is favorable in most cases. Strength usually returns to normal within 2 months; occasionally, recovery takes longer or is incomplete.

Actual sensory loss, as opposed to sensory symptoms, is less common than motor weakness, occurring in 5–35% of patients with stage II neurologic abnormalities and then usually combined with weakness; sensory loss occurs alone in only about 5% of cases (26,139,141, 147,162,166–168,170,186). The most common pattern is of lower cervical or (particularly) thoracic sensory loss —usually between T8 and T12, often bilateral, and frequently asymmetrical. Initial intense pain in these areas is followed by dermatomal hypesthesia (or sometimes hyperesthesia) over one or two segments at about the same time that motor weakness develops. Less often, mild loss of superficial sensation occurs in paretic limbs. Wherever it occurs, sensory loss usually resolves completely within 1–2 months; residual hypesthesia is rare.

Electrophysiologic testing in patients with stage II peripheral neuropathy has shown evidence for both axonal injury and demyelination (42,139,141,144–146,163, 174,191,193). The most commonly reported abnormalities include: decreased sensory amplitude with mildly delayed sensory conduction velocity; slight prolongation of distal motor latency with normal or mildly slowed motor conduction velocity; and decreased amplitude of the compound action potential. Neurogenic interference patterns are also common, and denervation potentials in nerve and root patterns have been reported. Decreased amplitude of F waves, along with prolongation of these waves, has suggested root involvement. In other cases, marked slowing of conduction velocity in multiple nerves, combined with the absence of denervation potentials in weak muscles, has suggested demyelination.

Myositis

Myalgias are common in early Lyme disease (2,22,154), but no electrophysiologic testing of patients with myalgias, nor histologic examination of their muscle tissue, has been reported. A few cases of definite myositis in stage II have been described, however. Duray and Steere (95) refer to a syndrome of extreme pain in one or more proximal muscle groups, both at rest and during motion and accompanied by local swelling and tenderness, that is seen in European patients with late stage II disease independent of other nervous system involvement. The duration of this syndrome is not known, but one case of progressive, necrotizing inflammation of the quadriceps muscles beginning in stage II and lasting 8 years has been reported (129). In another case, muscle tenderness, increased serum creatine kinase, myopathic electromyographic changes, and myopathic changes plus lymphoplasmacytic perivascular infiltrates on biopsy occurred in a patient with otherwise typical meningopolyneuritis and resolved in weeks with antibiotic treatment (194).

Stage III

Accumulating evidence indicates that neurologic abnormalities, both central and peripheral, are not confined to stage II as was originally thought, but can also occur later on, sometimes associated with arthritis.

Progressive Borrelia *Encephalomyelitis*

The best-defined late CNS abnormality in Lyme disease is progressive *Borrelia* encephalomyelitis—a syndrome reported most often from Europe, where it has been described from a number of countries (125– 127,129–132,135,158,159,178). The largest and most detailed series was published by Ackermann et al. (158), who reported the findings in 44 German cases.

Men and women are equally affected, and the average age at onset is 45 years (range: 7–79) (158). There is often no history of a tick bite or ECM; but three reported cases have followed ECM by days to 1.5 years (126,130,131), one other began 3 months after a tick bite (132), and two additional cases began after a preceding illness characterized by fever, myalgias, and pharyngitis (127). In other instances, progressive *Borrelia* encephalomyelitis has begun following an earlier meningopolyneuritis; the interval between the two has been 9 months to 5 years (129,135,158).

Symptoms can begin acutely but are more commonly gradual in onset. Once started, they worsen progressively over months to years (up to 15 years), either gradually or in a stepwise fashion punctuated by sudden deteriorations with only partial improvement between attacks. In patients with mainly cerebral symptoms these attacks resemble transient ischemic attacks and strokes, and meningovascular syphilis is simulated (127,129,131, 132,135,158,178). When the spinal cord is mainly involved, multiple sclerosis (MS) is suggested (158). Unlike meningopolyneuritis, progressive *Borrelia* encephalomyelitis does not resolve spontaneously.

The most common neurologic symptoms are gait difficulties, ataxia, bladder dysfunction, visual changes, hearing loss, and poor memory and concentration (125–127,129–132,135,158,159,178). Headache, nausea, vomiting, and neck stiffness are less frequent but do occur. Systemic signs and symptoms are rare; but retarded growth and sexual development was seen in two teenagers whose disease began in childhood, one of whom also had kyphosis (158).

The neurologic abnormalities are diffuse and multifocal and reflect involvement of the brain, spinal cord, and cranial and peripheral nerves (125–127,129–132,135, 158,159,178). Myelitis is most common, affecting two-thirds of patients and usually developing gradually. Those affected have either paraparesis or quadriparesis, which is severe in about two-thirds. About one-third have bladder dysfunction, and an equal number have sensory change which is usually slight; but severe sensory loss has been reported. Half of the patients have cranial nerve palsies, most commonly facial palsy (usually unilateral) and hearing loss (usually bilateral); but abnormalities of nerves II, III, V, VI, IX, and XII have also been reported. Slightly fewer patients (40%) have cerebral abnormalities. Mild organic mental defects (behavioral change, poor memory and concentration) are usual. Less frequent abnormalities include: severe dementia, delirium, disorientation, somnolence, cerebellar ataxia, myoclonus, seizures, and bitemporal hemianopsia. The most common transient cerebral signs are hemiparesis and dysphasia, both of which can become permanent. The spinal nerve roots are affected least often (5%), but a progressive meningoradicular form does exist (105).

The CSF is almost always abnormal (125–127,129–132,135,158,159,178). Typical abnormalities include: a pleocytosis of up to 1125 cells per cubic millimeter (median: 145), mostly lymphocytes and plasma cells plus a few neutrophils; increased protein of up to 1114 mg/dl (median: 269); and a normal or low glucose concentration. Usually also present are: locally synthesized IgG and sometimes IgM and IgA; oligoclonal bands; and specific anti-*B. burgdorferi* antibody (158). Antibodies to myelin basic protein have been detected in the CSF of a few cases, as well (127).

The EEG in patients with cerebral symptoms has shown nonspecific generalized slowing or dysrhythmia, focal slowing, or no abnormality at all (126,135,158). CT scan is abnormal in a majority of those with cerebral symptoms. The abnormalities include: focal hypodensities located in the periventricular and subcortical white matter (130,135,158) that are occasionally contrast-enhancing but without mass effect; infarcts in the internal capsule, lentiform nucleus, and thalamus (127,129–131,135); communicating hydrocephalus (135); and cerebral atrophy with intracerebral calcifications (126). MRI scan has shown multifocal abnormalities in similar locations, suggesting demyelination as well as ventricular dilatation, caudate atrophy, periventricular and subinsular cavities, and atrophy of the pons and medulla (126,135). Myelography in one case demonstrated lumbar arachnoiditis (135). Cerebral angiography in several patients with progressive *Borrelia* encephalomyelitis has now shown changes consistent with vasculitis (Fig. 9): multiple segmental stenoses of intracerebral arteries with poststenotic dilatation (129); multiple occlusions of branches of the anterior and middle cerebral arteries (131); and occlusion of the basilar artery (132).

Because progressive *Borrelia* encephalomyelitis does not resolve spontaneously, the outcome depends on how early antibiotic treatment is initiated (127,129–132,135,158). Patients treated late when considerable neurologic damage has already accrued may recover little and be left disabled or may recover only partially. Patients treated early may recover completely.

Late Mental Changes and MRI Abnormalities

The grave neurologic abnormalities of progressive *Borrelia* encephalomyelitis may represent only the most

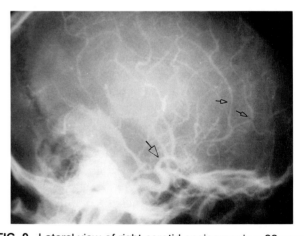

FIG. 9. Lateral view of right carotid angiogram in a 22-year-old woman with chronic lymphocytic meningitis and recurrent transient ischemic attacks due to Lyme disease. Note the marked narrowing of the supraclinoid carotid artery (*large arrow*), multiple areas of arterial narrowing and dilatation (*small arrows*), mural irregularities, and several abruptly terminated arterial branches. (Courtesy of Dr. Arnold S. Witte, Trenton, New Jersey.)

extreme cases of a more common but milder CNS inflammation in late Lyme disease: Many North American patients with late Lyme disease have far less dramatic CNS symptoms but are nonetheless disabled by them. Halperin et al. (160) have pointed out that most patients with chronic Lyme disease have incapacitating fatigue, often accompanied by defects in memory and concentration and usually without physical neurologic abnormalities on examination.

Neuropsychologic testing of 17 such nondepressed patients (average age, 39; average disease duration, 32 months), using a battery of sophisticated tests, documented a variety of abnormalities that correlated well with the patients' own perceptions of their disabilities (160). These deficits consisted of defects in the following: immediate and delayed auditory–verbal and visual memory, the ability to learn and retrieve new information, sustained attention and concentration, perceptual–motor performance, problem solving, and conceptual flexibility. None of these patients had physical evidence of CNS disease on examination; but four did have cranial or peripheral neuropathy or radiculopathy, two had EEG slowing, and two had CSF pleocytosis. The deficits had improved significantly when the patients were re-tested 5–28 weeks after antibiotic treatment.

MRI scan of 10 patients with these mental changes (average age, 39; average disease duration, 32 months) was abnormal in four of the five with the most severe subjective intellectual deficits and in three of four with moderate-to-severe deficits on neuropsychologic testing (160). Punctate hyperresonant areas, without mass effect, were detected in the cerebral white matter. These areas were dense on both T1- and T2-weighted images and resembled, but were smaller than, the similar lesions seen in patients with MS. Halperin et al. (160) have interpreted these MRI scans as indicating that a mild inflammatory encephalomyelitis may cause the cerebral dysfunction that they have observed in their patients with late Lyme disease, and they have suggested that other reported cases of more severe CNS disease may represent only the most extreme examples of the same process.

Other Late CNS Abnormalities

In two reports, Pachner (136,195) has also described a variety of CNS abnormalities in 26 patients with late Lyme disease. All of the reported patients had CNS abnormalities without other apparent cause, high titers of IgG anti-B. burgdorferi antibody in serum, and residence in an endemic area; most had either previous or simultaneous involvement of other organ systems typical of Lyme disease; and many improved with antibiotic therapy. In the earlier series (195), about half had an initial ECM and systemic symptoms, whereas the other half had typical stage II neurologic abnormalities. The stage

III neurologic involvement began a mean of 5 years after illness onset (range: 1.5–17 years). Three-quarters also had arthritis within a few to 10 years before neurologic abnormalities began.

The neurologic abnormalities reported ranged from mental changes without physical neurologic signs to severe, progressive multifocal CNS disease (136,195). Thirteen patients, nine of whom became ill in childhood, had diffuse chronic involvement (136). Difficulty with memory and concentration and changes in mood, personality, and behavior were most common. But also observed were: subacute encephalitis with severe confusion, disorientation, and agitation; simple dementia; and an anorexia-nervosa-like illness responsive to penicillin therapy. Overall, 10 of the 13 received intravenous penicillin, with clear improvement in five, possible improvement in three, and no response in two. Six patients had either progressive or remitting and relapsing focal CNS disease, both cerebral and spinal and resembling MS in some cases. One of them had a single pontine and multiple periventricular plaques on MRI scan, but the clinical findings were of progressive brainstem encephalitis. Although these patients resembled European patients with progressive Borrelia encephalomyelitis, not all of them responded to intravenous penicillin. Of the seven patients remaining, four had recurrent episodes of incapacitating fatigue without other abnormalities (except for a Babinski sign in one case), one had seizures alone, and two had progressive radiculoneuritis. CSF showed a pleocytosis in only four of 10 cases examined, the EEG was abnormal in only one of nine, CT scan was normal in eight of eight, and MRI was abnormal in only one of five (195).

One additional case of late focal encephalitis 6 years after stage II meningopolyneuritis has been reported; this patient appeared to respond to penicillin therapy (159).

The spectrum of severity in my own unpublished cases of stage III CNS disease is similar, ranging from mild mental changes alone to severe multifocal parenchymal abnormalities. The abnormalities include: mental changes with punctate cerebral white-matter abnormalities (Fig. 10), increased CSF IgG, and, in one case, an isolated Babinski sign; seizures, increased CSF IgG, and intrathecal anti-B. burgdorferi antibody synthesis; and both progressive focal and multifocal brainstem encephalitis with corresponding focal MRI abnormalities and multilevel remitting and relapsing cerebrospinal disease with CSF pleocytosis. The interval between earlier stage I disease and subsequent stage III neurologic abnormalities in these cases has been 8 months to 7 years, and all of the patients have either improved or stabilized with antibiotic (ceftriaxone) therapy.

In addition, one recent publication reported high titers of serum antibody to B. burgdorferi in four of 54 patients from Wisconsin and Illinois with motor neuron disease (196). We have not been able to confirm this relationship in our motor neuron disease patients from Connecti-

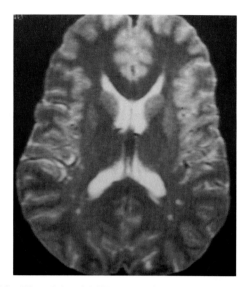

FIG. 10. T2-weighted MRI scan of the cerebrum of a 32-year-old man with fatigue, decreased memory, and poor concentration due to late Lyme disease, showing three punctate areas of increased signal intensity adjacent to the posterior horns of the lateral ventricles (TR = 2500, TE = 80).

cut, however, nor have investigators from Massachusetts (197).

Finally, Ackermann et al. (158) have found evidence for latent CNS infection in four patients, three of whom had had a spontaneously resolving stage II meningopolyneuritis 3, 6, and 12 years earlier. One patient had a slight residual facial palsy, one had a loss of Achilles tendon reflexes, and had one migrating pains without clinical signs. All four patients had intrathecally synthesized anti-*B. burgdorferi* antibody without other CSF abnormalities: CSF cell counts, protein, and IgG content were all normal.

Peripheral Neuropathy in Late Lyme Disease

Many patients with late Lyme disease also have a mild polyneuropathy that is distinct from stage II meningopolyneuritis (142,160). Up to 50% of patients with late disease complain of intermittent tingling paresthesias of their extremities, and up to one-fourth of those also have radicular pain. Physical signs of neuropathy are less frequent: About 25% of patients with paresthesias have a mild stocking/glove distal sensory loss, but motor weakness and reflex changes are rare. Nearly one-fourth also may have accompanying mild cerebral symptoms, usually without signs of CNS disease. In one series, three of seven patients tested had CSF pleocytosis and increased protein without increased IgG or oligoclonal bands (142). Nevertheless, symptomatic patients (and some others who are asymptomatic) almost always have electrophysiologic evidence for neuropathy even though physical signs are absent.

Halperin et al. (160) tested 82 patients with late Lyme disease (average age, 40; average disease duration, 30 months) electrophysiologically. Fifty-one had paresthesias, and 60 had electrophysiologic abnormalities, involving two or more nerves in 39 cases. Sensory nerve conduction velocity (CV) or amplitude, or both, were abnormal in 43 cases; distal motor latency or CV or amplitude, in 34; and F-wave latency, in 34. Twenty-one patients had electrophysiologic evidence for carpal tunnel syndrome. The authors have interpreted these changes as indicating multifocal axonal and (particularly) distal axonal disease (160). However, the F-wave abnormalities suggest that the nerve roots are also involved. Moreover, demyelination can occur too: One patient had severe slowing of conduction velocity and multiple areas of conduction block (142).

Patients improved symptomatically following antibiotic therapy (penicillin, chloramphenicol, or ceftriaxone), and the results of repeated electrophysiologic testing mirrored this improvement (142,160). There was statistically significant improvement in sensory nerve CV, sensory amplitude, and distal motor latency within 3–7 months after treatment, suggesting improved distal axonal function.

Peripheral neuropathy is equally common in European patients with ACA (143,153,198,199). Between 25% and 50% of ACA patients have neuropathic symptoms that are usually most marked in the vicinity of the skin lesions (143,198). The most frequent symptoms are paresthesias, mild-to-severe burning or sharp pains, hyperesthesia, weakness, and muscle cramps. Physical signs of neuropathy are nearly as prevalent (40%). Typical findings are: hypesthesia and hypalgesia in about 25% of cases, especially in areas of skin atrophy; impaired vibratory sense (20%); hyperpathia (5%); reflex changes (7–40%); muscle weakness (15%); and atrophy (5%) (198). As with the symptoms, the signs of peripheral neuropathy in patients with ACA are often asymmetrical and most marked near areas of skin involvement (143,198). Several clinical patterns of neuropathy have been described: cutaneous neuropathy with hypesthesia restricted to the distribution of a single cutaneous nerve; distal asymmetric polyneuropathy; and distal symmetric polyneuropathy (143). Profound fatigue and personality change may accompany ACA-associated neuropathy, but physical signs of CNS disease are absent (153). Yet CNS disease may occur: One-third of 26 ACA patients in one report had abnormal brainstem auditory evoked responses which returned to normal after antibiotic treatment (153). Systemic symptoms and signs are likewise sometimes present. Those most typical are: lymphadenopathy, subluxation of small joints in the hands or feet, and intermittent arthritis of the knee (153).

Electrophysiologic abnormalities have been recorded in most symptomatic patients and in up to 10% of those without symptoms (143,198). These include: mild slowing of motor and sensory nerve CV in most patients and prolongation of distal motor latency; decreased amplitude of compound action potential; and increased dispersion in many. As in the case of North American patients with late Lyme disease and polyneuropathy, these changes have been interpreted as indicating axonal damage (143). But demyelination probably occurs as well, inasmuch as at least two reported patients have had very slow motor nerve CVs (21 and 22 m/sec) (198).

The response of these electrophysiologic abnormalities to antibiotic treatment has not been reported, but signs and symptoms do improve. The frequency of clinical neuropathy is lower (28%) among patients first examined neurologically after treatment than among untreated patients (62%) (143). Even low-dose oral penicillin therapy (4 million units daily for 2 weeks) has improved symptoms in some patients, although others have progressed despite such therapy (198).

Differences Between European and North American *Borrelia burgdorferi* Infection

Early reports of Lyme disease emphasized a number of differences between North American and European patients with ECM and related disorders. North American patients were thought to develop neurologic abnormalities less often and to more often have ECM before neurologic involvement did develop, whereas European patients were thought not to have arthritis (22,26,139). But neurologic abnormalities do develop without antecedent ECM in the United States (42), and arthritis does occur in Europe (43,107,157,200,201); and it seems now that these reported differences were only an artifact of ascertainment bias and differences in treatment between the two continents (202). Because the earliest reports from the United States were of prospective studies of patients with either ECM or arthritis (2,22,23), they were biased toward overestimating the frequency of arthritis in Lyme disease and toward virtually guaranteeing that nearly every patient who developed neurologic abnormalities had already had ECM. Early European reports (15–21,147), on the other hand, focused primarily on the neurologic abnormalities, thus creating a bias toward overestimating their frequency while underestimating that of ECM. Moreover, European patients with ECM had been routinely treated with oral penicillin or tetracycline since the 1940s (10,11), whereas North American patients had not been until the 1980s (28). Because early treatment with oral antibiotics can prevent later arthritis but may be inadequate to eliminate all organisms from the nervous system, the frequency of arthritis in European Lyme disease may have been artificially lowered with respect to that of neurologic involvement (202).

Other reported differences between the patterns of neurologic abnormalities on the two continents have not yet been reconciled. The earliest description of neurologic abnormalities in North American Lyme disease emphasized mild cerebral symptoms which had not been appreciated in European patients (26). Although a subsequent report from the United States found these symptoms to be less frequent (139), it is now clear that they are common and quantifiable, at least later on in the illness (160). It remains unclear, therefore, whether North American Lyme disease patients really have cerebral involvement more often than their European counterparts or if European patients just haven't been tested thoroughly enough. Another unresolved issue is the relationship between radicular pain in stage II meningopolyneuritis and the initiating tick bite. Early European reports indicated that the radicular pain usually begins (and is most severe) in the same dermatomal segment as the bite and subsequent ECM (17–20,71,141,178,179), whereas reports from North America did not (26,139). However, more recent European reports (147) have not confirmed a relationship between the sites of the tick bite and the pain, and the relationship remains in question. In question also is the similarity of meningeal symptoms. In North American patients with meningitis due to Lyme disease, headache is intense, long-lasting, and nearly universal, and meningismus is frequent (26,42,139); but early European reports described the meningitis of Bannwarth's syndrome as often being asymptomatic (15,16). More recent reports indicate a higher frequency of meningeal symptoms, but a substantial discrepancy remains (71,128,147,161–169).

A final neurologic difference concerns progressive *Borrelia* encephalomyelitis which has been reported only from Europe. However, I believe that some of Pachner's published cases (136,195), as well as some of my own unpublished ones, fit the case definition, and I also believe that the syndrome occurs on both continents. Because Lyme disease apparently has been common in North America for a relatively short time, and because progressive *Borrelia* encephalomyelitis has a long incubation period, the syndrome is probably more common in Europe at present. With time and increased awareness, I expect more cases to be reported from North America.

Some other differences remain that could relate to strain variations between North American and European *B. burgdorferi*. In a careful prospective study, Asbrink and Olsson (203) have shown that multiple secondary skin lesions, severe systemic symptoms, and laboratory abnormalities were less common in Swedish patients with ECM than in their North American counterparts, whereas a prolonged course (>6 months) of ECM was more common. Moreover, lymphocytoma and ACA appear to be almost uniquely European (43,153), although a few cases of North American ACA have been described (204). It is worth noting, however, that the apparent greater frequency of ACA in Europe,

TABLE 3. *Neurologic conditions in which Lyme disease should be considered*

Acute aseptic meningitis	Cranial neuritis (Bell's palsy)
Chronic lymphocytic meningitis	Mononeuritis simplex or multiplex
Acute meningoencephalitis	Radiculoneuritis
Acute focal encephalitis	Plexitis
Brainstem encephalitis	Distal axonal neuropathy
Progressive encephalomyelitis	Demyelinating neuropathy
Cerebral demyelination	Carpal tunnel syndrome
Cerebral vasculitis	Focal myositis
Dementia	
Transverse myelitis	

like that of progressive *Borrelia* encephalomyelitis, may be due to both (a) the longer history of Lyme disease there and (b) a greater familiarity with the skin lesion among European dermatologists.

APPROACH TO DIAGNOSIS

Lyme disease should be suspected in any patient with chronic lymphocytic meningitis or mild meningoencephalitis with superimposed cranial neuritis or radiculitis. But patients with other neurologic abnormalities (Table 3) may have the same illness, especially those with Bell's palsy, unexplained distal axonal polyneuropathy, or progressive encephalomyelitis. When these other abnormalities follow ECM, accompany or follow Lyme arthritis, or accompany ACA, the diagnosis is straightforward (Table 4).

Nervous system involvement in Lyme disease can occur without either skin lesions or arthritis, however. Then a history of tick bite, onset in summer, or travel to or residence in an endemic area are clues to the diagno-

TABLE 4. *Minimal diagnostic criteria for Lyme neuroborreliosis*[a]

Definite neuroborreliosis
Compatible neurologic abnormality without other cause and with one of the following:
1. History of well-documented ECM
2. Presence of ACA
3. Serum *and* CSF immunoreactivity, or CSF reactivity alone, against *B. burgdorferi* by ELISA or western blot
4. Both other organ system involvement typical of Lyme disease (e.g., Lyme arthritis) and serum immunoreactivity to *B. burgdorferi*
5. Seroconversion or fourfold rise in titer of antibody to *B. burgdorferi* between acute and convalescent sera

Probable neuroborreliosis
Compatible neurologic abnormality without other cause and with serum immunoreactivity to *B. burgdorferi*

Possible neuroborreliosis
Compatible neurologic abnormality without other cause and with tick bite or travel or residence in an endemic area

[a] ECM, erythema chronicum migrans; ACA, acrodermatitis chronica atrophicans; CSF, cerebrospinal fluid; ELISA, enzyme-linked immunosorbent assay.

sis. Nonspecific laboratory clues in cases of stage II involvement include a high ESR, an increase in serum IgM, and the presence of serum cryoglobulins or circulating immune complexes, at least in North America (26). In cases of neuropathy, the presence of both axonal and demyelinating changes on electrophysiologic testing of the same patient is another clue, as is the presence of a pleocytosis or other typical CSF abnormalities in cases of cranial or peripheral neuropathy.

Once suspected on clinical, epidemiologic, or laboratory grounds, the diagnosis usually can be confirmed by detection of an immunologic response to *B. burgdorferi.*

Laboratory Diagnosis of Lyme Disease

The best laboratory test for diagnosing Lyme disease is the demonstration of specific antibody to *B. burgdorferi:* A positive test in a patient with compatible neurologic abnormality is strong evidence for the diagnosis.

Tests for antibody to *B. burgdorferi* are now widely available through a number of reference and commercial laboratories. In the United States at least, the tests also are routinely performed in local hospitals as well as state health department laboratories in endemic areas. Most laboratories now use the enzyme-linked immunosorbent assay (ELISA) technique with sonicated *B. burgdorferi* as antigen, but some still use the immunofluorescence (IF) technique. Both techniques give similar results (116,118,205), but the ELISA is probably the better test (116,206–208); it is more sensitive, more specific, and more easily standardized and automated; and its absorbance values can be statistically analyzed.

Even though these tests are widely used, they are not standardized (209), and there is apparently a great deal of interlaboratory variability (210). In one recent study (210a), results of serologic tests for Lyme disease performed on identical sera in four different laboratories, and at different times in the same large commercial laboratory, were compared. Levels of agreement were consistently low, both among the four laboratories (kappa statistic: 0.45 to 0.53) and within the commercial laboratory (kappa statistic: 0.50 to 0.54). Consequently, interpretation of serologic tests for Lyme disease in a clinical setting requires that the physician be certain of the reliability of the laboratory performing the test.

When the ELISA technique is used, levels of IgM and IgG antibodies are usually measured separately. Specific IgM antibody appears first: Serum levels typically peak 3–6 weeks after the onset of ECM and then decline slowly, although they may remain elevated for months to years (33,116–118,208). Measurable antibody is usually not present when the skin lesion first appears. The appearance of serum IgG antibody is even more delayed: Elevated levels are not detectable during the first 4–6 weeks of illness, the levels peak months to years later, and they can remain elevated for years after clinical remission (33,116–118,208). Therefore, by the time stage II or III Lyme disease develops, most patients have elevated serum levels of IgG anti-*B. burgdorferi* antibody, but the titer of IgM antibodies may or may not be elevated. Thus, elevated serum titers of specific IgM antibody generally indicate acute infection, whereas elevated titers of IgG antibody can indicate either active or past infection.

A positive test may indicate only exposure to *B. burgdorferi* rather than active infection with it, however. In hyperendemic areas, up to 8% of residents (211,212) and 15% of outdoor workers (213,214) with high risk for tick exposure have measurable antibody, and the ratio of symptomatic to asymptomatic infection in such areas is probably 1:1 (211,212).

Furthermore, false-positive reactions do occur. Positive tests have been obtained in sera from patients with rheumatoid arthritis (RA), Rocky Mountain spotted fever, infectious mononucleosis, tuberculous meningitis, leptospirosis, yaws, syphilis, and both louse-borne and tick-borne relapsing fever (33,116,206,208,215,216). With the exception of those in treponemal and other borrelial infections, all of the reported false-positive reactions have shown low titers of cross-reacting IgM antibodies alone. High titers of cross-reacting IgG antibodies have been detected only in patients with syphilis or relapsing fever (208); these illnesses usually can be excluded on clinical and laboratory grounds. Patients with syphilis and cross-reacting antibodies should have a positive reaginic test: A positive treponemal test is insufficient to diagnose syphilis in patients with high titers of anti-*B. burgdorferi* antibody, because nearly 10% of patients with Lyme disease have a positive fluorescent treponemal antibody-absorption (FTA-Abs) test (206,217,218). Relapsing fever can be excluded on epidemiologic grounds in most cases, or by the failure to see *Borrelia* on repeated peripheral blood smears in others (219).

The regular use of immunoblotting techniques could overcome some of the shortcomings of the ELISA. Immunoblots are more sensitive than the ELISA in cases of less than 2 weeks' duration, and they are less often falsely positive (117,215,220). Serum from occasional patients with systemic lupus, RA, Reiter's syndrome, syphilis, and relapsing fever does contain IgM reacting with the 41-kD flagellar antigen (117), but most patients with Lyme disease have antibodies reacting with several different antigens (220). Immunoblots are not generally available at present, however, and their use is unlikely to become routine. The greater difficulty of performing immunoblots is likely to limit their use to cases which are hard to diagnose and to sorting out false-positives.

The use of *B. burgdorferi* fractions (particularly the flagellin fraction) as antigen in the ELISA may also increase test sensitivity and specificity (221,222), as may the use of antibody-capture immunoassay (222a). Moreover, the detection of *B. burgdorferi* antigens in the urine of infected humans and mice by immunoassay with monoclonal antibodies has been reported (222b) and may eventually be applied to diagnosis. These tests are not yet in general use, however.

Specific antibody also appears in the CSF and may be detectable there in stage II disease before serum antibody tests are positive (217,223). Moreover, calculation of a specific antibody/IgG index for serum and CSF often indicates intrathecal synthesis of anti-*B. burgdorferi* antibody in both stage II meningopolyneuritis and stage III progressive encephalomyelitis (158,217,223–225). The most accurate method for determining this index appears to be that of Hofstad et al. (226), in which serum and CSF are first diluted to the same total IgG concentration before comparing the antibody activity of the two samples. The approximations and uncertainties of determining antibody titers are thus avoided because the ratio is arrived at directly. When the test is performed carefully in this way, it may prove useful in diagnosing other types of late nervous system disease, in identifying patients with latent CNS infection, and, perhaps, in separating patients with actual CNS infection from those with other neurologic illnesses who have been exposed to, but who are not actually infected with, the spirochete.

Seronegative Lyme Disease

Tests for serum antibody by ELISA or IF are not always positive when Lyme disease patients develop neurologic abnormalities. In Europe especially, but also in North America, diagnostic levels of serum antibody may not be present when stage II neurologic abnormalities first appear (71,128,217). Testing acute and convalescent sera may show a rise in titer (183), but testing paired sera has the disadvantage of leading to a delay in treatment if the diagnosis is in doubt clinically. Similarly, an immunoblot might be positive before serum antibody titers are diagnostic (117,215,220), but immunoblots are generally less available than ELISA or IF.

Testing the CSF for specific antibody can help. Initial antibody titers were elevated in both serum and CSF in

48% of cases of *Borrelia* meningitis in Sweden, whereas 16% were positive only in serum and 24% only in CSF. Positive antibody tests limited to the CSF were more common in cases of shorter duration (mean: 3 weeks). In cases of very short duration (1–3 weeks), both serum and CSF were often negative initially but could become positive later on (71,217). Thus, even if CSF antibody titers are routinely measured at the time of presentation in patients with stage II neurologic abnormalities, treatment in some cases will have to be prescribed without laboratory confirmation once a reasonable effort has been made to rule out other treatable causes for the illness.

Early treatment with oral antibiotics sometimes abrogates the antibody response to *B. burgdorferi* without eliminating the organism from the nervous system, and late Lyme disease may then develop in a seronegative patient (108,110). Although this situation is not common (<5% of Lyme disease patients seen in one large clinic population) (110), it can present a difficult diagnostic problem. Immunoblots are occasionally, but not usually, positive in patients with seronegative late disease (108).

However, the T-cell response to *B. burgdorferi* may be preserved even when the B-cell response is absent. Recent reports indicate that measurement of T-cell blastogenesis in response to *B. burgdorferi* can document exposure to the organism in some such patients and can therefore help to confirm the diagnosis (108,110). But a report from another laboratory has indicated an unusually high frequency of *B. burgdorferi* reactivity in normal, unexposed individuals from endemic areas, suggesting that the test may not be specific (110a). Because the test is not yet widely available, and because it is positive in only about 80% of apparently seronegative cases (110), treatment in some will have to be prescribed on clinical grounds alone, even if the test does prove reliable and becomes more generally available.

Diagnosing Late Lyme Disease

It seems likely that the full spectrum of late nervous system disease due to *B. burgdorferi* infection remains to be defined, and it is not yet clear how best to diagnose late nervous system borreliosis either. Because the presence of serum antibody really only indicates exposure, and because antibody can persist in high titer for years after apparently successful treatment, a positive serologic test may not be sufficient for diagnosis. Measurement of anti-*Borrelia* antibodies in the CSF may provide one clue. But it is not at all certain that CSF reactivity is the best measure of disease activity or the best predictor of response to antibiotic therapy as it is in CNS syphilis.

Until we have the answers to these questions, the neurologist's best weapons are a high index of suspicion and

the frequent use of serologic tests. Neurologic patients with a positive serum test should have a lumbar puncture and measurement of CSF antibody titer. Antibiotic treatment should be prescribed if pleocytosis, elevated protein, or locally synthesized anti-*Borrelia* antibodies are present. Patients with late polyneuropathy will often have normal CSF and should be treated regardless of its reactivity. It also seems prudent at present to prescribe the same treatment for patients with compatible CNS abnormalities, a positive serum antibody test, and a normal CSF but no explanation for their symptoms other than Lyme disease, especially if the deficits are progressive. Finally, in patients with neurologic abnormalities of unknown cause and a history of ECM but negative serology, the CSF should be tested for antibody; but antibiotics should probably be prescribed regardless of the result (140).

TREATMENT

The aims of treatment in Lyme disease are threefold: to stop ECM and its associated systemic symptoms; to prevent the development of late skin, joint, heart, or nervous system abnormalities; and to arrest and possibly reverse those late complications that do develop. The best antibiotic regimens for accomplishing these aims are not certain, however.

B. burgdorferi is sensitive to a number of antibiotics. *In vitro,* it is most sensitive to erythromycin, ceftriaxone, and cefotaxime; but it is also sensitive, though less so, to amoxicillin alone or with clavulanate, tetracycline, minocycline, doxycycline, lincomycin, imipenem, ciprofloxacin, and ofloxacin (227–230). In general, *in vivo* sensitivities in infected laboratory animals parallel those *in vitro*—except in the case of erythromycin, which is less active *in vivo* (229,230). *B. burgdorferi* is, at most, only moderately sensitive to penicillin, both *in vivo* and *in vitro* (229,230).

Treatment of Early Lyme Disease

Treatment with several of these antibiotics does shorten the course of ECM and its associated symptoms and reduces the incidence of subsequent arthritis, carditis, and neurologic abnormalities. In several reports based on nonrandomized patients, Steere et al. (2,28,231) found that ECM resolved more quickly (2–4 days) in patients treated with oral penicillin or tetracycline than in untreated patients (10 days), whereas erythromycin treatment had no such effect. They also found that none of 39 tetracycline-treated patients with ECM, only three of 40 treated with penicillin, and four of 29 treated with erythromycin developed late complications (231). Based on these observations, they recommended that adult patients with ECM receive tetracycline (250 mg, four times daily) for at least 10 days (up to 20 days if symptoms persisted or recurred) (2,231). They suggested that phenoxymethyl penicillin (500 mg, four times daily) could be substituted for tetracycline and recommended that children with ECM receive phenoxymethyl penicillin (50 mg/kg/day) for 10–20 days or, in cases of penicillin allergy, erythromycin (30 mg/kg/day) for 15–20 days (2,231).

Similarly, Neumann et al. (232) observed no late complications in 72 Austrian patients with ECM treated with phenoxymethyl penicillin (1.5 million units, three times daily) for 14 days, and Asbrink et al. (157) obtained the same results in over 200 Swedish patients treated with phenoxymethyl penicillin (2 g daily) for 10 days [or either tetracycline or erythromycin (1 g daily) for 10 days in penicillin-allergic patients].

Yet Weber, in Germany, found that 27% of his patients with ECM developed late extracutaneous manifestations after treatment with a variety of oral antibiotic regimens using penicillin, tetracycline, amoxicillin, or clavulanic acid (233). Moreover, Steere and his group in a later publication noted that despite oral antibiotic therapy, nearly 50% of their patients had minor late complications such as recurrent headaches, arthralgias, migratory musculoskeletal pains, and lethargy (234). The late complications generally appeared in those patients with more severe initial illness and sometimes recurred over several years. Berger (235) obtained similar results using either tetracycline or penicillin with or without probenecid to treat patients with ECM: He found that only two of 80 with minor illness required re-treatment, compared with 17 of 81 with more severe symptoms, four of whom did not respond at all.

It may be that tetracycline and penicillin are not the best oral antibiotics for treating early disease. The minimal inhibitory concentrations of both for some strains of *B. burgdorferi* are equivalent to or greater than the serum concentrations achieved by oral administration (236). Amoxicillin could be a better choice than penicillin: It is more active against *B. burgdorferi* than penicillin V, and it is more reliably absorbed than penicillin G (237). Moreover, oral amoxicillin given with probenecid can achieve treponemicidal levels in both serum and CSF in patients with syphilis (238) and therefore might be expected to better prevent late CNS abnormalities in patients with ECM and early disseminated disease. Similarly, doxycycline is probably a better choice than tetracycline HCl because it achieves higher tissue levels, has fewer gastrointestinal side effects, and can be given on a twice-daily schedule (237).

Clearly, there is some uncertainty about the best treatment for early Lyme disease, but the prompt administration of oral antibiotics is just as clearly the best defense against late complications. Based on the information available, adults with ECM should probably receive either doxycycline (100 mg) twice daily for 2–4 weeks,

depending on disease severity, or amoxicillin (500 mg) plus probenecid (500 mg) four times daily for a similar time period (Table 5). Children with ECM should receive amoxicillin and probenecid in age-appropriate doses. Penicillin-allergic children can be treated with erythromycin (30 mg/kg/day) in divided doses for 15–20 days, although there is no firm evidence to support its use.

Treatment of Late Lyme Disease

Once neurologic abnormalities develop, oral antibiotics are less active, and thus parenteral treatment is usually required. In patients with stage II meningitis or meningopolyneuritis, intravenous penicillin is usually effective. Steere et al. (45) first reported the use of high-dose intravenous aqueous penicillin G (20 million units daily for 10 days) in 12 patients with meningitis due to Lyme disease: All 12 improved clinically within 7–10 days, although five continued to have headaches for several weeks, and three continued to have frequent arthralgias, musculoskeletal pain, and fatigue. Several subse-

TABLE 5. *Antibiotic therapy of Lyme disease: early disease and neurologic abnormalities* [a]

Manifestation	Treatment
ECM and systemic symptoms	
Adults	Amoxicillin 500 mg p.o. q.i.d. for 2–4 weeks (plus probenecid 500 mg p.o. q.i.d.)[b]
	Doxycycline 100 mg p.o. b.i.d. for 2–4 weeks
Children (≤8 years)	Amoxicillin 20–40 mg/kg/day in four divided doses for 2–4 weeks
	Erythromycin 30 mg/kg/day in four divided doses for 2–4 weeks
Neurologic disease (stage II or III)	
Facial palsy alone	Oral antibiotics as for stage I
All others	
Adults	Ceftriaxone 2 g/day i.v. for 2–4 weeks
	Penicillin G 20–24 million units/day (i.v.) for 10–14 days
	Doxycycline 100 mg p.o. b.i.d. for 10–30 days or 200 mg (i.v.) for 2 days, then 100 mg/day (i.v.) for 8 days
Children	Ceftriaxone 50–80 mg/kg/day (i.v.) for 2–4 weeks
	Penicillin G 250,000 units/kg/day (i.v.) in divided doses

[a] ECM, erythema chronicum migrans; p.o., orally; q.i.d., four times per day; b.i.d., twice per day; i.v., intravenously.
[b] Optional.

quent European reports encompassing nearly 200 patients with stage II neurologic disease described similar success with intravenous penicillin G in doses of 15–20 million units daily for 10–14 days (162,239–241), although Kristoferitsch et al. (242) found the benefit to be restricted to those patients treated within 5 weeks of onset of neurologic symptoms.

When high-dose intravenous penicillin therapy is prescribed for stage II neurologic disease, pain and fever may worsen temporarily in the first 18 hours. This may be analogous to the Jarisch–Herxheimer reaction (45). Then meningeal and systemic symptoms generally begin to improve within days, whereas radicular pains decrease over weeks and motor deficits improve over many weeks (mean, 8; range, 1–24) (45,240). Stage II CNS abnormalities are arrested by treatment and may improve slowly, but some residual deficit is common (45,162,240). CSF cell counts are usually lower by the end of the course of treatment but may not return to normal for several months (45,240). The CSF protein concentration falls somewhat more slowly: It is usually lower by the end of therapy but may remain elevated for a year or more (45,240). CSF IgG titers are usually falling by 4 months (241).

Intravenous doxycycline (200 mg on day 1, then 100 mg daily for 10 days) has also been used to treat stage II meningitis, and some patients (but not all) have responded (241). A randomized trial of intravenous doxycycline (200 mg on the first 2 days, followed by 100 mg daily for 8 days) versus intravenous penicillin G (20 million units daily for 10 days) in 75 patients with both stage II and stage III neurologic abnormalities showed the two treatments to be equally effective, however (243). Moreover, in one additional small study, oral doxycycline (100 mg twice daily for 10–20 days) was effective in treating eight patients with stage II meningopolyneuritis (244).

Some others have failed to improve with intravenous penicillin therapy but have then responded to intravenous cefotaxime (2 g three times daily for 10 days) (245), ceftriaxone (2 g once or twice daily for 14 days) (246), or chloramphenicol (1 g four times daily for 2 weeks) (247). Finally, a small, randomized, prospective study of 21 patients with stage II meningopolyneuritis showed that intravenous penicillin G (20 million units daily for 10 days) and cefotaxime (2 g three times daily for 10 days) were equally effective (248).

Nonetheless, high-dose intravenous penicillin is very effective in stage II neurologic disease (especially when the meninges are inflamed), and most patients will respond. When the meninges are not inflamed, parenteral therapy may not always be necessary. Facial palsy in particular can occur without pleocytosis, and Steere et al. (45) have recommended oral tetracycline for patients with isolated facial weakness. Olsson et al. (189), how-

ever, have treated all patients with facial palsy with intravenous antibiotics, regardless of CSF abnormality. Still, it is probably sufficient to do a lumbar puncture on all Lyme disease patients with facial weakness and to treat with intravenous antibiotics (penicillin or ceftriaxone) if there is a pleocytosis or intrathecal antibody synthesis. If the CSF is normal, and there is no other extracutaneous disease, oral amoxicillin and probenecid or doxycycline can be prescribed as for stage I disease.

Like stage II meningopolyneuritis, progressive *Borrelia* encephalomyelitis responds to high-dose intravenous penicillin (127,129–132,135,158,241) and intravenous doxycycline (243). Most patients are stabilized by treatment, some improve partially, and a few become clinically normal. Pleocytosis resolves within about 3 months of treatment, and CSF protein content is usually falling by then also. Specific antibody may persist in the CSF for a year or more, however.

The other stage III neurologic abnormalities seem to respond less well to intravenous penicillin, perhaps because the infection is more parenchymal than meningovascular. Intravenous ceftriaxone appears to be much more effective. Dattwyler et al. (249) have shown a striking response to intravenous ceftriaxone (2 g once or twice daily for 14 days) in patients with arthritis, peripheral neuropathy, and/or encephalopathy due to late Lyme disease (disease duration: 27–39 months), both in a randomized comparison with high-dose intravenous penicillin and in a subsequent open trial. In the controlled trial, 50% of penicillin-treated patients failed to improve and continued to have arthritis, fatigue, and memory impairment. Eighty percent of the penicillin failures responded to ceftriaxone. Overall, only five of 44 ceftriaxone-treated patients failed to improve. Those who did fail were slightly older, had had the illness slightly longer, and were more likely to have had previous steroid therapy. Both cerebral and peripheral nerve symptoms improve in those who do respond, but the improvement is slow. Little change is apparent during the course of treatment itself; improvement develops over ensuing weeks. Objective changes in neuropsychologic and electrophysiologic tests can be measured within months and are usually complete within 6 months (140,162,249).

Less is known about the response to antibiotic treatment of the neuropathy associated with ACA. Kristoferitsch et al. (143) did find that neuropathy was less common among antibiotic-treated patients with ACA than among untreated patients (28% versus 62%), but no details of the prescribed treatment were given. Resolution of neurologic symptoms has been reported, however, in 30–50% of patients following treatment with phenoxymethyl penicillin, 4 million units daily for 2 weeks (198); and the edema and erythema, but not the skin atrophy of ACA itself, seem to respond to oral phenoxymethyl penicillin, 1 g three times daily for 3 weeks (250). However, analogy with the distal axonopathy seen in North American patients with late Lyme disease suggests that intravenous ceftriaxone may be a better treatment for the neuropathy.

In summary, patients with Lyme disease and neurologic abnormalities, with the possible exception of isolated facial palsy, should receive parenteral antibiotics (Table 5). High-dose intravenous penicillin is adequate in many, but not all, cases. Ceftriaxone (2 g daily for 2 weeks) is more reliably effective and appears to be the antibiotic of choice in late disease. Although the drug itself is more expensive than penicillin, ceftriaxone's long half-life allows once-daily dosing, facilitating cost savings through outpatient treatment. Many penicillin-allergic patients can still receive ceftriaxone. If not, doxycycline (100 mg twice daily) can be given for a month, or chloramphenicol (1 g four times daily) can be given for 2 weeks. If there is no response to ceftriaxone, or relapse occurs after an initial good response, re-treatment for a longer course (4 weeks) can be considered. It seems prudent at present to avoid corticosteroids because of their possible detrimental effect on outcome.

PREVENTION

A high level of awareness among the population at risk provides the best chance for the prevention of Lyme disease at present. Individuals likely to be exposed can avoid infection if they are knowledgeable about the patterns of disease transmission and about effective methods of personal protection. Preventive measures directed at control of the tick population (or of their vertebrate hosts) are secondary and likely to be useful only in special circumstances.

Some understanding of the epidemiology of Lyme disease is necessary for its prevention. In many areas, the disease is more common among those with outdoor occupational or recreational exposure (49,213,214,251), and such individuals need to be able to recognize the common tick vectors and be aware of the danger from their bites. They also need to beware of high-risk areas. In North America, *I. dammini* is most common in mixed hardwood forests with extensive shrub layers (62), particularly in areas inhabited extensively by deer (252,253). Avoidance of such areas should reduce the number of infective bites—especially during the warmer late spring and early summer months, when questing nymphs are most numerous and less protective clothing is likely to be worn. Visiting areas where deer are common is less likely to be a problem in the fall: More protective clothing is worn then; and adult ticks, the most active fall feeders, are larger, more easily noticed, and less numerous than the nymphs. The association between Lyme

disease and pet ownership (23,52) may also be important: Pets that spend time outdoors should be fitted with tick-repellent collars and inspected regularly for ticks.

A certain amount of exposure is still inevitable, however, even if high-risk areas are avoided. In North America, Lyme disease often occurs in suburbs near large tracts of undeveloped woodlands (62). Indeed, in Westchester County, New York, almost 70% of reported tick bites occur in the bitten individuals' own yards (89). If exposure is unavoidable, permethrin treatment of clothing is effective in repelling ticks that come in contact with it (253). If attachment occurs anyway, regular daily inspection for ticks after outdoor activities, and their removal by gentle traction, can still help to reduce disease transmission. Transmission is unlikely after fewer than 24 hr of attachment (64). Whether prophylactic penicillin or tetracycline treatment of those at risk would further reduce disease transmission has not been studied, nor is the value of presumptive antibiotic treatment of tick bites in endemic areas known. Because only about 4% of bites in such areas appear to lead to symptomatic infection (254,255), it is probably better to wait for symptoms to appear before initiating treatment.

Control of tick populations is also possible in some circumstances, but many of the methods tried so far are unlikely to be acceptable in many areas, and some are not environmentally safe. Burning, brush cutting, and residual application of acaricides (carbaryl, diazinon) have all been shown to temporarily reduce local populations of adult *I. dammini* for up to 1 year, but not thereafter (62,253). Biological controls are safer but have not been tested extensively. The one environmentally safe method of control (directed against juvenile *I. dammini*) that has been tested is the dispersal of plastic tubes containing permethrin-treated cotton batting (253,256). The cotton is harvested by white-footed mice for nesting material, and the permethrin kills the *I. dammini* larvae and nymphs in the nest, substantially reducing their numbers in the treated area for as long as a year. The tubes are now commercially available, but their expense and the need for repeated application will probably preclude their regular use.

Denial of tick access to animal hosts is another possible preventive strategy that may be of value in special circumstances. In one experiment, the near-total elimination of deer on Great Island, Massachusetts, was followed by a decrease in the numbers of larval and nymphal *I. dammini* in each of the next three summers, but the numbers of questing adults were increased (253). Similarly, in areas of Europe where *I. ricinus* adults depend entirely on sheep, pasture rotation led to a sharp decrease in the number of larval ticks (253).

Finally, even if these preventive measures fail, infection occurs, and Lyme disease does develop but is promptly recognized, nervous system infection can still be prevented by timely treatment with antibiotics as outlined above.

REFERENCES

1. Steere AC, Hardin JA, Malawista SE. Lyme arthritis: a new clinical entity. *Hosp Pract* 1978;13(4):143–158.
2. Steere AC, Malawista SE, Bartenhagen NH, et al. The clinical spectrum and treatment of Lyme disease. *Yale J Biol Med* 1984;57:453–461.
3. Steere AC, Malawista SE, Snydman DR. Lyme arthritis: an epidemic of oligoarticular arthritis in children and adults in three Connecticut communities. *Arthritis Rheum* 1977;20:7–17.
4. Scrimenti RJ. Erythema chronicum migrans. *Arch Derm* 1970;102:104–105.
5. Afzelius A. Erythema chronicum migrans. *Acta Derm Venereol (Stockh)* 1921;2:120–125.
6. Binder E, Doepfmer R, Hornstein O. Experimentelle Übertragung des Erythema chronicum migrans von Mensch zu Mensch. *Hautarzt* 1955;6:494–496.
7. Sonck CE. Erythema chronicum migrans with multiple lesions. *Acta Derm Venereol (Stockh)* 1965;45:34–36.
8. Burgdorfer W. Discovery of the Lyme disease spirochete and it relation to tick vectors. *Yale J Biol Med* 1984;57:515–520.
9. Lennhoff C. Spirochaetes in aetiologically obscure diseases. *Acta Derm Venereol (Stockh)* 1948;28:295–324.
10. Hollström E. Successful treatment of erythema chronicum migrans Afzelius. *Acta Derm Venereol (Stockh)* 1951;31:235–243.
11. Hollström E. Penicillin treatment of erythema chronicum migrans Afzelius. *Acta Derm Venereol (Stockh)* 1958;38:285–289.
12. Hellerström S. Erythema chronicum migrans Afzelius with meningitis. *Acta Derm Venereol (Stockh)* 1951;31:227–234.
13. Garin C, Bujadoux C. Paralysie par les Tiques. *J Med Lyon* 1922;71:765–767.
14. Lecinsky CG. Case of erythema chronicum migrans with meningitis. *Acta Derm Venereol (Stockh)* 1951;31:464–467.
15. Bannwarth A. Chronische lymphocytäre Meningitis, entzündliche Polyneuritis und "Rheumatismus". *Arch Psychiatr Nervenkr* 1941;113:284–376.
16. Bannwarth A. Zur Klinic und Pathogenese der "chronischen lymphocytären Meningitis". *Arch Psychiatr Nervenkr* 1944;117:161–185.
17. Schaltenbrand G. Radiculomyelomeningitis nach Zeckenbiss. *Münch Med Wochenschr* 1962;104:829–834.
18. Schaltenbrand G. Durch Arthropoden übertragene Infektionen der Haut und des Nervensystems. *Münch Med Wochenschr* 1966;108:1557–1562.
19. Schaltenbrand G. Durch Arthropoden übertragene Erkrankungen der Haut und des Nervensystems. *Verh Dtsch Ges Inn Med* 1966;72:975–1005.
20. Bammer H, Schenk K. Meningo-myelo-radiculitis nach Zeckenbiss mit Erythem. *Dtsch Z Nervenheilk* 1965;187:25–34.
21. Hörstrup P, Ackermann R. Durch Zecken übertragene Meningopolyneuritis (Garin–Bujadoux, Bannwarth). *Fortschr Neurol Psychiatr* 1973;41:583–606.
22. Steere AC, Malawista SE, Hardin JA, Ruddy S, Askenase PW, Andiman WA. Erythema chronicum migrans and Lyme arthritis: the enlarging clinical spectrum. *Ann Intern Med* 1977;86:685–698.
23. Steere AC, Broderick TF, Malawista SE. Erythema chronicum migrans and Lyme arthritis: epidemiologic evidence for a tick vector. *Am J Epidemiol* 1978;108:312–321.
24. Spielman A, Clifford CM, Piesman J, Corwin MD. Human babesiosis on Nantucket Island, USA: description of the vector, *Ixodes (Ixodes) dammini*, n. sp. (Acarina: Ixodidae). *J Med Entomol* 1979;15:218–234.
25. Wallis RC, Brown SE, Kloter KO, Main AJ. Erythema chronicum migrans and Lyme arthritis: field study of ticks. *Am J Epidemiol* 1978;108:322–327.
26. Reik L, Steere AC, Bartenhagen NH, Shope RE, Malawista SE. Neurologic abnormalities of Lyme disease. *Medicine (Baltimore)* 1979;58:281–294.
27. Steere AC, Batsford WP, Weinberg M, et al. Lyme carditis: cardiac abnormalities of Lyme disease. *Ann Intern Med* 1980;93:8–16.
28. Steere AC, Malawista SE, Newman JH, Spieler PN, Bartenhagen NH. Antibiotic therapy in Lyme disease. *Ann Intern Med* 1980;93:1–8.
29. Steere AC, Malawista SE. Cases of Lyme disease in the United States: locations correlated with distribution of *Ixodes dammini*. *Ann Intern Med* 1979;91:730–733.
30. Burgdorfer W, Barbour AG, Hayes SF, Benach JL, Grunwaldt E, Davis JP. Lyme disease—a tick-borne spirochetosis? *Science* 1982;216:1317–1319.
31. Burgdorfer W, Barbour AG, Hayes SF, Peter O, Aeschlimann A. Erythema chronicum migrans—a tickborne spirochetosis. *Acta Trop* 1983;40:79–83.
32. Kornblatt AN, Steere AC, Brownstein DG. Infection in rabbits with the Lyme disease spirochete. *Yale J Biol Med* 1984;57:613–614.
33. Steere AC, Grodzicki RL, Kornblatt AN, et al. The spirochetal etiology of Lyme disease. *N Engl J Med* 1983;308:733–740.
34. Benach JL, Bosler EM, Hanrahan JP, et al. Spirochetes isolated from the blood of two patients with Lyme disease. *N Engl J Med* 1983;308:740–742.
35. Berger BW, Clemmensen OJ, Ackerman AB. Lyme disease is a spirochetosis. *Am J Dermatopathol* 1983;5:111–124.
36. Burgdorfer W, Lane RS, Barbour AG, Gresbrink RA, Anderson JR. The western black-legged tick, *Ixodes pacificus:* a vector of *Borrelia burgdorferi. Am J Trop Med Hyg* 1985;34:925–930.
37. Barbour AG, Burgdorfer W, Hayes SF, Peter O, Aeschlimann A. Isolation of a cultivable spirochete from *Ixodes ricinus* ticks of Switzerland. *Curr Microbiol* 1983;8:123–126.
38. Asbrink E, Hederstedt B, Hovmark A. The spirochetal etiology of erythema chronicum migrans Afzelius. *Acta Derm Venereol (Stockh)* 1984;64:291–295.
39. Pfister H, Einhäupl K, Preac-Mursic V, Wilske B, Schierz G. The spirochetal etiology of lymphocytic meningoradiculitis of Bannwarth (Bannwarth's syndrome). *J Neurol* 1984;231:141–144.
40. Preac-Mursic V, Wilske B, Schierz G, Pfister HW, Einhäupl K. Repeated isolation of spirochetes from the cerebrospinal fluid of a patient with meningoradiculitis Bannwarth. *Eur J Clin Microbiol* 1984;3:564–565.
41. Johnson RC, Schmid GP, Hyde FW, Steigerwalt AG, Brenner DJ. *Borrelia burgdorferi* sp. nov.: etiologic agent of Lyme disease. *Int J Syst Bacteriol* 1984;34:496–497.
42. Reik L, Burgdorfer W, Donaldson JO. Neurologic abnormalities in Lyme disease without erythema chronicum migrans. *Am J Med* 1986;81:73–78.
43. Weber K, Schierz G, Wilske B, Preac-Mursic V. European erythema migrans disease and related disorders. New Haven: *Yale J Biol Med* 1984;57:463–471.
44. Steere AC, Green J, Schoen RT, et al. Successful parenteral penicillin therapy of established Lyme arthritis. *N Engl J Med* 1985;312:869–874.
45. Steere AC, Pachner AR, Malawista SE. Neurologic abnormalities of Lyme disease: successful treatment with high-dose intravenous penicillin. *Ann Intern Med* 1983;99:767–772.
46. Lyme disease—United States, 1987 and 1988. *MMWR* 1989;38:668–672.
46a. Lyme disease—Canada. *MMWR* 1989;38:677–678.
47. Schmid GP. The global distribution of Lyme disease. *Rev Infect Dis* 1985;7:41–50.
48. Kawabata M, Baba S, Iguchi K, Yamaguti N, Russell H. Lyme disease in Japan and its possible incriminated tick vector, *Ixodes persulcatus. J Infect Dis* 1987;156:854.
49. Chengxu A, Yuxin W, Yongguo Z, et al. Clinical manifestations and epidemiological characteristics of Lyme disease in Hailin County, Heilongjiang Province, China. *Ann NY Acad Sci* 1988;539:302–313.
50. Dekonenko EJ, Steere AC, Berardi VP, Kravchuk LN. Lyme borreliosis in the Soviet Union: a cooperative US–USSR report. *J Infect Dis* 1989;158:748–753.
51. Rousselle C, Floret D, Cochat P, Reignier F, Wright C.

Encéphalite aiguë à *Borrelia burgdorferi* (maladie de Lyme) chez un enfant algérien. *Pediatrie* 1989;44:265–269.

52. Lane RS, Lavoie PE. Lyme borreliosis in California: acarological, clinical, and epidemiological studies. *Ann NY Acad Sci* 1988;539:192–203.
53. Tsai TF, Bailey RE, Moore PS. National surveillance of Lyme disease, 1987–1988. *Conn Med* 1989;53:324–326.
54. Anderson JF. Epizootiology of *Borrelia* in *Ixodes* tick vectors and reservoir hosts. *Rev Infect Dis* 1989;11(Suppl 6):S1451–S1459.
55. Johnson SE, Klein GC, Schmid GP, Bowen GS, Feeley JC, Schulze T. Lyme disease: a selective medium for isolation of the suspected etiological agent, a spirochete. *J Clin Microbiol* 1984;19:81–82.
56. Spielman A, Levine JF, Wilson ML. Vectorial capacity of North America *Ixodes* ticks. *Yale J Biol Med* 1984;57:507–513.
57. Anderson JF, Magnarelli LA. Avian and mammalian hosts for spirochete-infected ticks and insects in a Lyme disease focus in Connecticut. *Yale J Biol Med* 1984;57:621–641.
58. Anderson JF. Mammalian and avian reservoirs for *B. burgdorferi*. *Ann NY Acad Sci* 1988;539:180–191.
59. Bosler EM, Cohen DP, Schulze TL, Olsen C, Bernard W, Lissman B. Host responses to *Borrelia burgdorferi* in dogs and horses. *Ann NY Acad Sci* 1988;539:221–234.
60. Burgess EC. *Borrelia burgdorferi* infection in Wisconsin horses and cows. *Ann NY Acad Sci* 1988;539:235–243.
61. Cohen D, Bosler EM, Bernard W, Meirs D, Eisner R, Schulze T. Epidemiologic studies of Lyme disease in horses and their public health significance. *Ann NY Acad Sci* 1988;539:244–257.
62. Schulze TL, Parkin WE, Bosler EM. Vector tick populations and Lyme disease: a summary of control strategies. *Ann NY Acad Sci* 1988;539:204–211.
63. Burgdorfer W, Hayes SF, Benach JL. Development of *Borrelia burgdorferi* in ixodid tick vectors. *Ann NY Acad Sci* 1988;539:172–179.
64. Piesman J, Mather TN, Sinsky RJ, Spielman A. Duration of tick attachment and *Borrelia burgdorferi* transmission. *J Clin Microbiol* 1987;25:557–558.
65. Magnarelli LA, Anderson JF, Barbour AG. The etiologic agent of Lyme disease in deer flies, horse flies and mosquitoes. *J Infect Dis* 1986;154:355–358.
66. Magnarelli LA, Anderson JF, Apperson CS, Fish D, Johnson RC, Chappell WA. Spirochetes in ticks and antibodies to *Borrelia burgdorferi* in white-tailed deer from Connecticut, New York State and North Carolina. *J Wildl Dis* 1986;22:178–188.
67. Burgdorfer W, Gage KL. Susceptibility of the black-legged tick, *Ixodes scapularis*, to the Lyme disease spirochete, *Borrelia burgdorferi*. *Zentralbl Bakteriol Mikrobiol Hyg [A]* 1986;263:15–20.
68. Piesman J. Vector competence of ticks in the southeastern United States for *Borrelia burgdorferi*. *Ann NY Acad Sci* 1988;539:417–418.
69. Rawlings JA. Lyme disease in Texas. *Zentralbl Bakteriol Mikrobiol Hyg [A]* 1986;263:483–487.
70. Stanek G, Pletschette M, Flamm H, et al. European Lyme borreliosis. *Ann NY Acad Sci* 1988;539:274–282.
71. Stiernstedt G, Gustafsson R, Karlsson M, Svenungsson B, Sköldenberg. Clinical manifestations and diagnosis of neuroborreliosis. *Ann NY Acad Sci* 1988;539:46–55.
72. Radda A, Burger I, Stanek G, Wewalka G. Austrian hard ticks as vectors of *Borrelia burgdorferi*. *Zentralbl Bakteriol Mikrobiol Hyg [A]* 1986;263:79–82.
73. Hard S. Erythema chronicum migrans (Afzelii) associated with mosquito bite. *Acta Derm Venereol (Stockh)* 1966;46:473–476.
74. Stanek G, Burger I, Hirschl A, Wewalka G, Radda A. *Borrelia* transfer by ticks during their life cycle: studies on laboratory animals. *Zentralbl Bakteriol Mikrobiol Hyg [A]* 1986;263:29–33.
75. Korenberg EI, Kryuchechnikov VN, Ananyina YV, Chernukha YG. Prerequisites of the existence of Lyme disease in the USSR. *Zentralbl Bakteriol Mikrobiol Hyg [A]* 1986;263:471–472.
76. Lawrence RH, Bradbury R, Cullen JS. Lyme disease on the NSW central coast. *Med J Aust* 1986;145:364.
77. Johnson RC, Hyde FW, Rumpel CM. Taxonomy of the Lyme disease spirochetes. *Yale J Biol Med* 1984;57:529–537.
78. Barbour AG, Hayes SF. Biology of *Borrelia* species. *Microbiol Rev* 1986;50:381–400.
79. Barbour AG. Isolation and cultivation of Lyme disease spirochetes. *Yale J Biol Med* 1984;57:521–525.
80. Habicht GS, Beck G, Benach JL, Coleman JL. *Borrelia burgdorferi* lipopolysaccharide and its role in the pathogenesis of Lyme disease. *Zentralbl Bakteriol Mikrobiol Hyg [A]* 1986;263:137–141.
81. Schmid GP, Steigerwalt AG, Johnson S, et al. DNA characterization of Lyme disease spirochetes. *Yale J Biol Med* 1984;57:539–542.
82. Barbour AG, Tessier SL, Hayes SF. Variation in a major surface protein of Lyme disease spirochetes. *Infect Immun* 1984;45:94–100.
83. Barbour AG, Heiland RA, Howe TR. Heterogeneity of major proteins in Lyme disease borreliae: a molecular analysis of North American and European isolates. *J Infect Dis* 1985;152:478–484.
84. Barbour AG, Schrumpf ME. Polymorphisms of major surface proteins of *Borrelia burgdorferi*. *Zentralbl Bakteriol Mikrobiol Hyg [A]* 1986;263:83–91.
85. Wilske B, Preac-Mursic V, Schierz G, Busch KV. Immunochemical and immunological analysis of European *Borrelia burgdorferi* strains. *Zentralbl Bakteriol Mikrobiol Hyg [A]* 1986;263:92–102.
86. Wilske B, Preac-Mursic V, Schierz G, Kühbeck R, Barbour AG, Kramer M. Antigenic variability of *Borrelia burgdorferi*. *Ann NY Acad Sci* 1988;539:126–143.
87. Barbour AG. Plasmid analysis of *Borrelia burgdorferi*, the Lyme disease agent. *J Clin Microbiol* 1988;26:475–478.
88. Barthold SW, Moody KD, Terwilliger GA, Duray PH, Jacoby RO, Steere AC. Experimental Lyme arthritis in rats infected with *B. burgdorferi*. *J Infect Dis* 1988;157:842–846.
89. Kornblatt AN, Urband PH, Steere AC. Arthritis caused by *Borrelia burgdorferi* in dogs. *J Am Med Vet Assoc* 1985;186:960–964.
90. Kornblatt AN, Steere AC, Brownstein DG. Experimental Lyme disease in rabbits: spirochetes found in erythema migrans and blood. *Infect Immun* 1984;46:220–223.
91. Magnarelli LA, Anderson JF, Chappell WA. Geographic distribution of humans, raccoons, and white-footed mice with antibodies to Lyme disease spirochetes in Connecticut. *Yale J Biol Med* 1984;57:619–626.
92. Burgess EC, Mattison M. Encephalitis associated with *Borrelia burgdorferi* infection in a horse. *J Am Vet Med Assoc* 1987;191:1457–1458.
93. Johnson RC, Marek N, Kodner C. Infection of Syrian hamsters with Lyme disease spirochetes. *J Clin Microbiol* 1984;20:1099–1101.
94. Duray PH, Johnson RC. The histopathology of experimentally infected hamsters with the Lyme disease spirochete, *Borrelia burgdorferi* (422251). *Proc Soc Exp Biol Med* 1986;181:263–269.
95. Duray PH, Steere AC. Clinical pathologic correlations of Lyme disease by stage. *Ann NY Acad Sci* 1988;539:65–79.
96. MacDonald AB, Miranda JM. Concurrent neocortical borreliosis and Alzheimer's disease. *Hum Pathol* 1987;18:759–761.
97. DeKoning J, Bosma RB, Hoogkamp-Korstanje JAA. Demonstration of spirochaetes in patients with Lyme disease with a modified silver stain. *J Med Microbiol* 1987;23:261–267.
98. MacDonald AB. Human fetal borreliosis, toxemia of pregnancy, and fetal death. *Zentralbl Bakteriol Mikrobiol Hyg [A]* 1986;263:189–200.
99. Schlesinger PA, Duray PH, Burke BA, Steere AC, Stillman MT. Maternal–fetal transmission of the Lyme disease spirochete, *Borrelia burgdorferi*. *Ann Intern Med* 1985;103:67–68.
100. Johnson YE, Duray PH, Steere AC, et al. Lyme arthritis: spirochetes found in synovial microangiopathic lesions. *Am J Pathol* 1985;118:26–34.
101. Snydman DR, Schenkein DP, Berardi VP, Lastavica CC, Pariser KM. *Borrelia burgdorferi* in joint fluid in chronic Lyme arthritis. *Ann Intern Med* 1986;104:798–800.
102. Asbrink E, Hovmark A. Successful cultivation of spirochetes from skin lesions of patients with erythema chronicum migrans Afzelius and acrodermatitis chronica atrophicans. *Acta Pathol Microbiol Immunol Scand [B]* 1985;93:161–163.
103. Asbrink E, Hovmark A, Hederstedt B. The spirochetal etiology of acrodermatitis chronica atrophicans Herxheimer. *Acta Derm Venereol (Stockh)* 1984;64:506–512.
104. Frithz A, Lagerholm B. Acrodermatitis chronica atrophicans, ery-

thema chronicum migrans and lymphadenosis benigna cutis—spirochetal diseases? *Acta Derm Venereol (Stockh)* 1983;63:432–436.

105. Wokke JHJ, de Koning J, Stanek G, Jennekens FGI. Chronic muscle weakness caused by *Borrelia burgdorferi* meningoradiculitis. *Ann Neurol* 1987;22:389–392.

106. Johnson RC, Kodner C, Russell M, Duray PH. Experimental infection of the hamster with *Borrelia burgdorferi*. *Ann NY Acad Sci* 1988;539:258–263.

107. Weber K, Neubert U. Clinical features of early erythema migrans disease and related disorders. *Zentralbl Bakteriol Mikrobiol Hyg [A]* 1986;263:209–228.

108. Dattwyler RJ, Volkman DJ, Halperin JJ, Luft BJ, Thomas J, Golightly MG. Specific immune responses in Lyme borreliosis: characterization of T cell and B cell responses to *Borrelia burgdorferi*. *Ann NY Acad Sci* 1988;539:93–102.

109. Dattwyler RJ, Thomas JA, Benach JL, Golightly MG. Cellular immune response in Lyme disease: the response to mitogens, live *Borrelia burgdorferi*, NK cell function and lymphocyte subsets. *Zentralbl Bakteriol Mikrobiol Hyg [A]* 1986;263:151–159.

110. Dattwyler RJ, Volkman DJ, Luft BJ, Halperin JJ, Thomas J, Golightly MG. Seronegative Lyme disease: dissociation of specific T- and B-lymphocyte responses to *Borrelia burgdorferi*. *N Engl J Med* 1988;319:1441–1446.

110a.Zoschke D, Kolstoe J, Skemp A. Positive lymphocyte proliferation to borrelia in Lyme disease—a cautionary note. *Arthritis Rheum* 1989;32:S46.

111. Moffat CM, Sigal LH, Steere AC, Freeman DH, Dwyer JM. Cellular immune findings in Lyme disease: correlation with serum IgM and disease activity. *Am J Med* 1984;77:625–632.

112. Golightly M, Thomas J, Volkman D, Dattwyler R. Modulation of natural killer cell activity by *Borrelia burgdorferi*. *Ann NY Acad Sci* 1988;539:103–111.

113. Thomas JA, Lipschitz R, Golightly MG, Dattwyler RJ. Immunoregulatory abnormalities in *Borrelia burgdorferi* infection. *Ann NY Acad Sci* 1988;539:431–433.

114. Sigal LH, Moffat CM, Steere AC, Dwyer JM. Cellular immune findings in Lyme disease. *Yale J Biol Med* 1984;57:595–598.

115. Shrestha M, Grodzicki RL, Steere AC. Diagnosing early Lyme disease. *Am J Med* 1985;78:235–239.

116. Craft JE, Grodzicki RL, Steere AC. The antibody response in Lyme disease: evaluation of diagnostic tests. *J Infect Dis* 1984;149:789–795.

117. Craft JE, Fischer DK, Shimamato GT, Steere AC. Antigens of *Borrelia burgdorferi* recognized during Lyme disease: appearance of a new immunoglobulin M response and expansion of the immunoglobulin G response late in the illness. *J Clin Invest* 1986;78:934–939.

118. Magnarelli LA, Anderson JF. Early detection and persistence of antibodies to *Borrelia burgdorferi* in persons with Lyme disease. *Zentralbl Bakteriol Mikrobiol Hyg [A]* 1986;263:392–399.

119. Steere AC, Hardin JA, Malawista SE. Erythema chronicum migrans and Lyme arthritis: cryoimmunoglobulins and clinical activity of skin and joints. *Science* 1977;196:1121.

120. Coleman JL, Benach JL. Isolation of antigenic components from the Lyme disease spirochete: their role in early diagnosis. *J Infect Dis* 1987;155:756–765.

121. Habicht GS. Lyme disease: antigens of *Borrelia burgdorferi* and immune responses to them. *Ann NY Acad Sci* 1988;539:112–114.

122. Benach JL, Coleman JL, Garcia-Monco JC, Deponte PC. Biological activity of *Borrelia burgdorferi* antigens. *Ann NY Acad Sci* 1988;539:115–125.

123. Beck G, Habicht GS, Benach JL, Coleman JL, Lysik RM, O'Brien RF. A role for interleukin-1 in the pathogenesis of Lyme disease. *Zentralbl Bakteriol Mikrobiol Hyg [A]* 1986;263:133–136.

124. Habicht GS, Beck G, Benach JL. The role of interleukin-1 in the pathogenesis of Lyme disease. *Ann NY Acad Sci* 1988;539:80–86.

125. Kohler J, Kasper J, Kern U, Thoden U, Rehse-Kupper B. *Borrelia* encephalomyelitis. *Lancet* 1986;2:35.

126. Bensch J, Olcen P, Hagberg L. Destructive chronic *Borrelia* meningoencephalitis in a child untreated for 15 years. *Scand J Infect Dis* 1987;19:697–700.

127. Weder B, Wiedersheim P, Matter L, Steck A, Otto F. Chronic progressive neurological involvement in *Borrelia burgdorferi* infection. *J Neurol* 1987;234:40–43.

128. Stiernstedt G. Tick-borne *Borrelia* infection in Sweden. *Scand J Infect Dis [Scand]* 1985;45:1–70.

129. Midgard R, Hofstad H. Unusual manifestations of nervous system *Borrelia burgdorferi* infection. *Arch Neurol* 1987;44:781–783.

130. Wokke JHJ, van Gijn J, Elderson A, Stanek G. Chronic forms of *Borrelia burgdorferi* infection of the nervous system. *Neurology* 1987;37:1031–1034.

131. Uldry P-A, Regli F, Bogousslavsky J. Cerebral angiopathy and recurrent strokes following *Borrelia burgdorferi* infection. *J Neurol Neurosurg Psychiatry* 1987;50:1703–1704.

132. Veenendaal-Hilbers JA, Perquin WVM, Hoogland PH, Doornbos L. Basal meningovasculitis and occlusion of the basilar artery in two cases of *Borrelia burgdorferi* infection. *Neurology* 1988;38:1317–1319.

133. Coyle PK, Schutzer SE. Cerebrospinal fluid immune complexes in Lyme disease. *Ann Neurol* 1988;24:142.

134. Reik L, Smith L, Khan A, Nelson W. Demyelinating encephalopathy in Lyme disease. *Neurology* 1985;32:1302–1305.

135. Kohler J, Kern U, Kasper J, Rhese-Küpper B, Thoden U. Chronic central nervous system involvement in Lyme borreliosis. *Neurology* 1988;38:863–867.

136. Pachner AR. *Borrelia burgdorferi* in the nervous system: the new "great imitator". *Ann NY Acad Sci* 1988;539:56–64.

137. Martin R, Ortlauf J, Sticht-Groh V, Bogdahn U, Goldmann SF, Mertens HG. *Borrelia burgdorferi*-specific and autoreactive T-cell lines from cerebrospinal fluid in Lyme radiculomyelitis. *Ann Neurol* 1988;24:509–516.

138. Sigal LH, Tatum AH. Lyme disease patients' serum contains IgM antibodies to *Borrelia burgdorferi* that cross-react with neuronal antigens. *Neurology* 1988;38:1439–1442.

139. Pachner AR, Steere AC. The triad of neurologic manifestations of Lyme disease: meningitis, cranial neuritis and radiculoneuritis. *Neurology* 1985;35:47–53.

140. Reik L. *Borrelia burgdorferi* infection: a neurologist's perspective. *Ann NY Acad Sci* 1988;539:1–3.

141. Vallat JM, Hugon M, Lubeau M, Leboutet MJ, Dumas M, Desproges-Gotteron R. Tick-bite meningoradiculoneuritis: clinical, electrophysiologic, and histologic findings in 10 cases. *Neurology* 1987;37:749–753.

142. Halperin JJ, Little BW, Coyle PK, Dattwyler RJ. Lyme disease: cause of a treatable peripheral neuropathy. *Neurology* 1987;37:1700–1706.

143. Kristoferitsch W, Sluga E, Graf M, et al. Neuropathy associated with acrodermatitis chronica atrophicans: clinical and morphological features. *Ann NY Acad Sci* 1988;539:35–45.

144. Lubeau M, Vallat JM, Hugon J, Dumas M, Desproges-Gotteron R. Tick bite meningoradiculitis: ten cases. *Zentralbl Bakteriol Mikrobiol Hyg [A]* 1986;263:321–323.

145. Sterman AB, Nelson S, Barclay P. Demyelinating neuropathy accompanying Lyme disease. *Neurology* 1982;32:1302–1305.

146. Graf M, Kristoferitsch W, Baumhackl U, Zeitlhofer J. Electrophysiologic findings in meningopolyneuritis of Garin–Bujadoux–Bannwarth. *Zentralbl Bakteriol Mikrobiol Hyg [A]* 1986;263:324–327.

147. Ackermann R, Horstrup P, Schmidt R. Tick-borne meningopolyneuritis (Garin–Bujadoux, Bannwarth). *Yale J Biol Med* 1984;57:485–490.

148. Reznick JW, Braunstein DB, Walsh RL. Lyme carditis: electrophysiologic and histopathologic study. *Am J Med* 1986;81:923–927.

149. Marcus LC, Steere AC, Duray PH, Anderson AE, Mahoney EB. Fatal pancarditis in a patient with co-existing Lyme disease and babesiosis. *Ann Intern Med* 1985;103:374–376.

150. Camponovo F, Meier C. Neuropathy of vasculitic origin in a case of Garin–Bujadoux–Bannwarth syndrome with positive *Borrelia* antibody response. *J Neurol* 1986;233:69–72.

151. Meier C, Grehl H. Vaskulitische Neuropathie bei Garin–Bujadoux–Bannwarth-Syndrom: ein Beitrag zum Verständnis der Pathologie und Pathogenese neurologischer Komplikationen bei Lyme-Borreliose. *Dtsch Med Wochenschr* 1988;113:135–138.

152. Berger BW. Erythema chronicum migrans of Lyme disease. *Arch Dermatol* 1984;120:1017–1021.
153. Asbrink E, Hovmark A. Early and late cutaneous manifestations in *Ixodes*-borne borreliosis (erythema migrans borreliosis, Lyme borreliosis). *Ann NY Acad Sci* 1988;539:4–15.
154. Steere AC, Bartenhagen NH, Craft JE, et al. The early clinical manifestations of Lyme disease. *Ann Intern Med* 1983;99:76–82.
155. Burke WA, Steinbaugh JR, O'Keefe EJ. Lyme disease mimicking secondary syphilis. *J Am Acad Dermatol* 1986;14:137–139.
156. Hovmark A, Asbrink E, Olsson I. The spirochetal etiology of lymphadenosis benigna cutis solitaria. *Acta Derm Venereol (Stockh)* 1986;66:479–484.
157. Asbrink E, Olsson I, Hovmark A. Erythema chronicum migrans Afzelius in Sweden: a study on 231 patients. *Zentralbl Bakteriol Mikrobiol Hyg [A]* 1986;263:229–236.
158. Ackermann R, Rehse-Küpper B, Gollmer E, Schmidt R. Chronic neurologic manifestations of erythema migrans borreliosis. *Ann NY Acad Sci* 1988;539:16–23.
159. Broderick JP, Sandok BA, Mertz LE. Focal encephalitis in a young woman 6 years after the onset of Lyme disease: tertiary Lyme disease? *Mayo Clin Proc* 1987;62:313–316.
160. Halperin JJ, Pass HL, Anand AK, Luft BJ, Volkman DJ, Dattwyler RJ. Nervous system abnormalities in Lyme disease. *Ann NY Acad Sci* 1988;539:24–34.
161. Ryberg B. Bannwarth's syndrome (lymphocytic meningoradiculitis) in Sweden. *Yale J Biol Med* 1984;57:499–503.
162. Stiernstedt GT, Sköldenberg BR, Vandvik B, et al. Chronic meningitis and Lyme disease in Sweden. *Yale J Biol Med* 1984;57:491–497.
163. Pachner AR, Steere AC. Neurologic findings of Lyme disease. *Yale J Biol Med* 1984;57:481–483.
164. Baumhackl U, Kristoferitsch W, Sluga E, Stanek G. Neurological manifestations of *Borrelia burgdorferi* infections. *Zentralbl Bakteriol Mikrobiol Hyg [A]* 1986;263:334–336.
165. Christen H-J, Hanefeld F. Neurologic complications of erythema-migrans-disease in childhood—clinical aspects. *Zentralbl Bakteriol Mikrobiol Hyg [A]* 1986;263:337–342.
166. Hansen K, Rechnitzer C, Pedersen NS, Arpi M, Jessen O. *Borrelia* meningitis in Denmark. *Zentralbl Bakteriol Mikrobiol Hyg [A]* 1986;263:348–350.
167. Pfister H-W, Einhäupl KM, Wilske B, Preac-Mursic V. Bannwarth's syndrome and the enlarged neurologic spectrum of arthropod borne borreliosis. *Zentralbl Bakteriol Mikrobiol Hyg [A]* 1986;263:343–347.
168. Stiernstedt GT, Sköldenberg BR, Garde A, et al. Clinical manifestations of *Borrelia* infections of the nervous system. *Zentralbl Bakteriol Mikrobiol Hyg [A]* 1986;263:289–296.
169. Wokke JHJ, Burgdorfer W. Bannwarth's syndrome in the Netherlands. *Zentralbl Bakteriol Mikrobiol Hyg [A]* 1986;263:351.
170. Hindfelt B, Jeppsson PG, Nilsson B, Olsson J-E, Ryberg B, Sörnäs R. Clinical and cerebrospinal fluid findings in lymphocytic meningo-radiculitis (Bannwarth's syndrome). *Acta Neurol Scand* 1982;66:444–453.
171. Krüger H, Englert D, Pflughaupt K-W. Demonstration of oligoclonal immunoglobulin G in Guillain–Barré syndrome and lymphocytic meningoradiculitis by isoelectric focusing. *J Neurol* 1981;226:15–24.
172. Felgenhauer K. Differentiation of the humoral immune response in inflammatory diseases of the central nervous system. *J Neurol* 1982;228:223–237.
173. Pohl PE, Schmutzhard E, Stanek G. Cerebrospinal fluid findings in neurological manifestations of Lyme disease. *Zentralbl Bakteriol Mikrobiol Hyg [A]* 1986;263:314–320.
174. Boudin G, Vernant J-C, Lanoé, Vojir Y. Les paralysies par morsure de tiques: arbovirose ou origine toxinique. *Ann Med Interne (Paris)* 1974;125:55–60.
175. Rousseau JJ, Lust C, Zangerle PF, Bigaignon G. Acute transverse myelitis as presenting neurological feature of Lyme disease. *Lancet* 1986;2:1222–1223.
176. Bendig JWA, Ogilvie D. Severe encephalopathy associated with Lyme disease. *Lancet* 1987;1:681–682.
177. Muhlemann MF, Wright DJM. Emerging pattern of Lyme disease in the United Kingdom and Irish Republic. *Lancet* 1987;1:260–262.
178. Sindic CJM, Depre A, Bigaignon G, Goubau PF, Hella P, Laterre C. Lymphocytic meningoradiculitis and encephalomyelitis due to *Borrelia burgdorferi*: a clinical and serological study of 18 cases. *J Neurol Neurosurg Psychiatry* 1987;50:1565–1571.
179. Morin B, Dordain G, Tournilhac M, Rey M. Méningo-radicultes après piqure de tique. *Presse Med* 1976;5:1965–1968.
180. Koudstaal PJ, Vermeulen M, Wokke JHJ. Argyll Robertson pupils in lymphocytic meningoradiculitis (Bannwarth's syndrome). *J Neurol Neurosurg Psychiatry* 1987;50:363–365.
181. Louis FJ, Schill H, LeBris H, et al. Deux formes neurologiques graves de maladie de Lyme. *Presse Med* 1987;16:32–33.
182. Melet M, Gerard A, Voiriot P, et al. Méningoradiculonévrite mortelle au cours d'une maladie de Lyme. *Presse Med* 1986;22:2075.
183. Feder HM, Zalneraitis EL, Reik L. Lyme disease: acute focal meningoencephalitis in a child. *Pediatrics* 1988;82:931–934.
184. Carlsson M, Malmvall B-E. *Borrelia* infection as a cause of presenile dementia. *Lancet* 1987;2:798.
185. Clark JR, Carlson RD, Sasaki CT, Pachner AR, Steere AC. Facial paralysis in Lyme disease. *Laryngoscope* 1985;95:1341–1345.
186. Meyer-Rienecker HJ, Hitzschke B. Lymphocytic meningoradiculitis. In: Vinken PJ, Bruyn GW, eds. *Handbook of clinical neurology,* vol 34. New York: Elsevier, 1978;571–586.
187. Asbrink A, Olsson I, Hovmark A, Carlsson B. Tick-borne spirochetes as a cause of facial palsy. *Clin Otolaryngol* 1985;10:279–284.
188. Schmutzhard E, Pohl P, Stanek G. Involvement of *Borrelia burgdorferi* in cranial nerve affection. *Zentralbl Bakteriol Mikrobiol Hyg [A]* 1986;263:328–333.
189. Olsson I, Engervall K, Asbrink E, Carlsson-Nordlander B, Hovmark A. Tick-borne borreliosis and facial palsy. *Acta Otolaryngol (Stockh)* 1988;105:100–107.
190. Jorbeck HJA, Gustafsson PM, Lind HCF, Stiernstedt GT. Tickborne *Borrelia* meningitis in children: an outbreak in the Kalmar area during the summer of 1984. *Acta Paediatr Scand* 1987;76:228–233.
191. Wulff CH, Hansen K, Strange P, Trojaborg W. Multiple mononeuritis and radiculitis with erythema, pain, elevated CSF protein and pleocytosis (Bannwarth's syndrome). *J Neurol Neurosurg Psychiatry* 1983;46:485–490.
192. Schmutzhard E, Stanek G, Pohl P. Polyneuritis cranialis associated with *Borrelia burgdorferi*. *J Neurol Neurosurg Psychiatry* 1985;48:1182–1184.
193. Uldry PA, Steck AJ, Regli F. Manifestations neurologiques des infections à *Borrelia burgdorferi*. *Schweiz Med Wochenschr* 1986;116:135–142.
194. Schmutzhard E, Willeit J, Gerstenbrand F. Menigopolyneuritis Bannwarth with focal nodular myositis: a new aspect of Lyme borreliosis. *Klin Wochenschr* 1986;64:1204–1208.
195. Pachner AR, Steere AC. CNS manifestations of third stage Lyme disease. *Zentralbl Bakteriol Mikrobiol Hyg [A]* 1986;263:301–306.
196. Waisbren BA, Cashman H, Schell RF, Johnson R. *Borrelia burgdorferi* antibodies and amyotrophic lateral sclerosis. *Lancet* 1987;2:332–333.
197. Mandrell H, Steere AC, Reinhart BN, et al. Anti-*Borrelia burgdorferi* (Lyme disease) antibodies are normal in amyotrophic lateral sclerosis. *Ann Neurol* 1988;24:178–179.
198. Hopf HC. Peripheral neuropathy in acrodermatitis chronica atrophicans (Herxheimer). *J Neurol Neurosurg Psychiatry* 1975;38:452–458.
199. Burgdorf WHC, Worret W-I, Schultka O. Acrodermatitis chronica atrophicans. *Int J Dermatol* 1979;18:596–601.
200. Huaux JP, Bigaignon G, Stadtsbaeder S, Zangerle PF, de Deuxchaisnes CN. Pattern of Lyme arthritis in Europe: report of 14 cases. *Ann Rheum Dis* 1988;47:164–165.
201. Schmidt R, Kabatzki J, Hartung S, Ackermann R. Erythema-migrans-Borreliose in der Bundesrepublik Deutschland. *Dtsch Med Wochenschr* 1985;10:1803–1807.
202. Dattwyler RJ, Volkman DJ, Luft BJ, Halperin JJ. Lyme disease in Europe and North America. *Lancet* 1987;1:681.
203. Asbrink E, Olsson I. Clinical manifestations of erythema chronicum migrans Afzelius in 161 patients: a comparison with Lyme disease. *Acta Derm Venereol (Stockh)* 1985;65:43–52.

204. Lavoie PE, Wilson AJ, Tuffanelli DL. Acrodermatitis chronica atrophicans with antecedent Lyme disease in a Californian. *Zentralbl Bakteriol Mikrobiol Hyg [A]* 1986;263:262–265.

205. Magnarelli LA, Meegan JM, Anderson JF, Chappell WA. Comparison of an indirect fluorescent-antibody test with an enzyme-linked immunosorbent assay for serological studies of Lyme disease. *J Clin Microbiol* 1984;20:181–184.

206. Russell H, Sampson JS, Schmid GP, Wilkinson HW, Plikaytis B. Enzyme-linked immunosorbent assay and indirect immunofluorescent assay for Lyme disease. *J Infect Dis* 1984;149:465–470.

207. Magnarelli LA. Serologic diagnosis of Lyme disease. *Ann NY Acad Sci* 1988;539:154–161.

208. Magnarelli LA, Anderson JF. Enzyme-linked immunosorbent assays for the detection of class-specific immunoglobulins to *Borrelia burgdorferi*. *Am J Epidemiol* 1988;127:818–825.

209. Wilkinson HW, Russell H, Sampson JS. Caveats on using non-standardized serologic tests for Lyme disease. *J Clin Microbiol* 1985;21:291.

210. Hedberg CW, Osterholm MT, MacDonald KL, White KE. An interlaboratory study of antibody to *Borrelia burgdorferi*. *J Infect Dis* 1987;155:1325–1327.

210a. Schwartz BS, Goldstein MD, Ribeiro JM, Schulze TL, Sahied SI. Antibody testing in Lyme disease: a comparison of results in four laboratories. *JAMA* 1989;262:3431–3434.

211. Hanrahan JP, Benach JL, Coleman JL, et al. Incidence and cumulative frequency of endemic Lyme disease in a community. *J Infect Dis* 1984;150:489–496.

212. Steere AC, Taylor E, Wilson ML, Levine JF, Spielman A. Longitudinal assessment of the clinical and epidemiological features of Lyme disease in a defined population. *J Infect Dis* 1986;154:295–300.

213. Wilske B, Schierz G, Preac-Mursic V, Weber K, Pfister H-W, Einhäupl K. Serological diagnosis of erythema migrans disease and related disorders. *Infection* 1984;12:331–337.

214. Münchhoff P, Wilske B, Preac-Mursic V, Schierz G. Antibodies against *Borrelia burgdorferi* in Bavarian forest workers. *Zentralbl Bakteriol Mikrobiol Hyg [A]* 1986;263:412–419.

215. Barbour AG, Burgdorfer W, Grunwaldt E, Steere AC. Antibodies of patients with Lyme disease to components of the *Ixodes dammini* spirochete. *J Clin Invest* 1983;72:504–515.

216. Magnarelli LA, Anderson JF, Johnson RC. Cross-reactivity in serological tests for Lyme disease and other spirochetal infections. *J Infect Dis* 1987;156:183–188.

217. Stiernstedt GT, Granström M, Hederstedt B, Sköldenberg B. Diagnosis of spirochetal meningitis by enzyme-linked immunosorbent assay and indirect immunofluorescent assay in serum and cerebrospinal fluid. *J Clin Microbiol* 1985;21:819–825.

218. Hunter EF, Russell H, Farshy CE, Sampson JS, Larsen SA. Evaluation of sera from patients with Lyme disease in the fluorescent treponemal antibody-absorption test for syphilis. *Sex Transm Dis* 1986;13:232–236.

219. Reik L. Spirochaetal infections of the nervous system. In: Kennedy PGE, Johnson RT, eds. *Infections of the nervous system*. London: Butterworths, 1987;43–75.

220. Grodzicki RL, Steere AC. Comparison of immunoblotting and indirect enzyme-linked immunosorbent assay using different antigen preparations for diagnosing early Lyme disease. *J Infect Dis* 1988;157:790–797.

221. Coleman JL, Benach JL. Isolation of antigenic components from the Lyme disease spirochete: their role in early diagnosis. *J Infect Dis* 1987;155:756–765.

222. Hansen K, Hindersson P, Pedersen NS. Measurement of antibodies to the *Borrelia burgdorferi* flagellum improves serodiagnosis in Lyme disease. *J Clin Microbiol* 1988;26:338–346.

222a. Bernardi VP, Weeks KE, Steere AC. Serodiagnosis of early Lyme disease: analysis of IgM and IgG antibody responses by using an antibody-capture enzyme immunoassay. *J Infect Dis* 1988;158:754–760.

222b. Hyde FW, Johnson RC, White TJ, Shelburne CE. Detection of antigens in the urine of mice and humans infected with *Borrelia burgdorferi*, etiologic agent of Lyme disease. *J Clin Microbiol* 1989;27:58–61.

223. Murray N, Kristoferitsch W, Stanek G, Steck AJ. Specificity of CSF antibodies against components of *Borrelia burgdorferi* in patients with menigopolyneuritis Garin–Bujadoux–Bannwarth. *J Neurol* 1986;233:224–227.

224. Rehse-Küpper B, Ackermann R. Demonstration of locally synthesized *Borrelia* antibodies in cerebrospinal fluid. *Zentralbl Bakteriol Mikrobiol Hyg [A]* 1986;263:407–411.

225. Wilske B, Schierz G, Preac-Mursic V, et al. Intrathecal production of specific antibodies against *Borrelia burgdorferi* in patients with lymphocytic meningoradiculitis (Bannwarth's syndrome). *J Infect Dis* 1986;153:304–314.

226. Hofstad H, Matre R, Nyland H, Ulvestad E. Bannwarth's syndrome: serum and CSF IgG antibodies against *Borrelia burgdorferi* examined by ELISA. *Acta Neurol Scand* 1987;75:37–45.

226a. Schutzer SE, Coyle PK, Belman AL, Golightly MG, Drulle J. Sequestration of antibody to *Borrelia burgdorferi* in immune complexes in seronegative Lyme disease. *Lancet* 1990;1:312–315.

227. Johnson SE, Klein GC, Schmid GP, Feeley JC. Susceptibility of the Lyme disease spirochete to seven antimicrobial agents. *Yale J Biol Med* 1984;57:549–553.

228. Berger BW, Kaplan MH, Rothenberg IR, Barbour AG. Isolation and characterization of the Lyme disease spirochete from the skin of patients with erythema chronicum migrans. *J Am Acad Dermatol* 1985;13:444–449.

229. Johnson RC, Kodner C, Russell M. *In vitro* and *in vivo* susceptibility of the Lyme disease spirochete, *Borrelia burgdorferi*, to four antimicrobial agents. *Antimicrob Agents Chemother* 1987;31:164–167.

230. Mursic VP, Wilske B, Schierz G, Holmburger M, Süss E. *In vitro* and *in vivo* susceptibility of *Borrelia burgdorferi*. *Eur J Clin Microbiol* 1987;6:424–426.

231. Steere AC, Hutchinson GJ, Rahn DW, et al. Treatment of the early manifestations of Lyme disease. *Ann Intern Med* 1983;99:22–26.

232. Neumann R, Aberer E, Stanek G. Treatment and course of erythema chronicum migrans. *Zentralbl Bakteriol Mikrobiol Hyg [A]* 1986;263:372–376.

233. Weber K, Preac-Mursic V, Neubert U, et al. Antibiotic therapy of early European Lyme borreliosis and acrodermatitis chronica atrophicans. *Ann NY Acad Sci* 1988;539:324–345.

234. Steere AC, Green J, Hutchinson GJ, et al. Treatment of Lyme disease. *Zentralbl Bakteriol Mikrobiol Hyg [A]* 1986;263:352–356.

235. Berger BW. Treatment of erythema chronicum migrans of Lyme disease. *Ann NY Acad Sci* 1988;539:346–351.

236. Luft BJ, Volkman DJ, Halperin JJ, Dattwyler RJ. New chemotherapeutic approaches in the treatment of Lyme borreliosis. *Ann NY Acad Sci* 1988;539:352–361.

237. Neu HC. A perspective on therapy of Lyme infection. *Ann NY Acad Sci* 1988;539:314–316.

238. Faber WR, Bos JD, Rietra TJ, Fass H, van Eljk VW. Treponemicidal levels of amoxicillin in cerebrospinal fluid after oral administration. *Sex Transm Dis* 1983;10:148–150.

239. Sköldenberg B, Stiernstedt G, Garde A, Kolmodin G, Carlström A, Nord CE. Chronic meningitis caused by a penicillin-sensitive microorganism? *Lancet* 1983;2:75–78.

240. Sköldenberg B, Stiernstedt G, Karlsson M, Wretlind B, Svenungsson B. Treatment of Lyme borreliosis with emphasis on neurological disease. *Ann NY Acad Sci* 1988;539:317–323.

241. Kohlhepp W, Mertens H-G, Oschmann P. Acute and chronic illness after tick-bite *Borrelia burgdorferi* infections: results of treatment. *Zentralbl Bakteriol Mikrobiol Hyg [A]* 1986;263:365–371.

242. Kristoferitsch W, Baumhackl V, Sluga E, Stanek G, Zeiler K. High-dose penicillin therapy in meningopolyneuritis Garin–Bujadoux–Bannwarth: clinical and cerebrospinal fluid data. *Zentralbl Bakteriol Mikrobiol Hyg [A]* 1986;263:357–364.

243. Kohlhepp W, Oschmann P, Mertens H-G. Treatment of Lyme borreliosis: randomized comparison of doxycycline and penicillin G. *J Neurol* 1989;236:464–469.

244. Dotevall L, Alestig, Hanner P, Norkrans G, Hagberg L. The use of doxycycline in nervous system *Borrelia burgdorferi* infection. *Scand J Infect Dis [Suppl]* 1988;53:74–79.

245. Pal GS, Baker JT, Wright DJM. Penicillin-resistant *Borrelia* encephalitis responding to cefotaxime. *Lancet* 1988;1:50–51.

246. Dattwyler RJ, Halperin JJ, Pass H, Luft BJ. Ceftriaxone as effective therapy in refractory Lyme disease. *J Infect Dis* 1987;155:1322–1325.

247. Diringer MN, Halperin JJ, Dattwyler RJ. Lyme meningoencephalitis—report of a severe, penicillin-resistant case. *Arthritis Rheum* 1987;30:705–708.

248. Pfister HW, Preac-Mursic V, Wilske B, Einhäupl M. Cefotaxime vs penicillin G for acute neurologic manifestations in Lyme borreliosis: a prospective randomized study. *Arch Neurol* 1989;46:1190–1194.

249. Dattwyler RJ, Halperin JJ, Volkman DJ, Luft BJ. Treatment of late Lyme borreliosis—randomised comparison of ceftriaxone and penicillin. *Lancet* 1988;1:1191–1194.

250. Asbrink E. Erythema chronicum migrans Afzelius and acrodermatitis chronica atrophicans: early and late manifestations of *Ixodes ricinus*-borne *Borrelia* spirochetes. *Acta Derm Venereol [Suppl] (Stockh)* 1985;118:1–63.

251. Smith PF, Benach JL, White DJ, Stroup DF, Morse DL. Occupational risk of Lyme disease in endemic areas of New York State. *Ann NY Acad Sci* 1988;539:289–301.

252. Wilson ML, Litwin TS, Gavin TA. Microgeographic distribution of deer and of *Ixodes dammini:* options for reducing the risk of Lyme disease. *Ann NY Acad Sci* 1988;539:437–439.

253. Spielman A. Prospects for suppressing transmission of Lyme disease. *Ann NY Acad Sci* 1988;539:212–220.

254. Falco RC, Fish D. A survey of tick bites acquired in a Lyme disease endemic area in southern New York State. *Ann NY Acad Sci* 1988;539:456–457.

255. Paul H, Gerth H-J, Ackermann R. Infectiousness for humans of *Ixodes ricinus* containing *Borrelia burgdorferi. Zentralbl Bakteriol Mikrobiol Hyg [A]* 1986;263:473–476.

256. Mather TM, Ribeiro JMC, Moore SI, Spielman A. Reducing transmission of Lyme disease spirochetes in a suburban setting. *Ann NY Acad Sci* 1988;539:402–403.

257. Wiegand SE, Stroebel PL, Glassman LH. Electron microscopic anatomy of pathogenic *Treponema pallidum. J Invest Dermatol* 1972;58:186–204.

PART VI

Fungal Infections of the CNS

Infections of the Central Nervous System,
edited by W. M. Scheld, R. J. Whitley, and
D. T. Durack, Raven Press, Ltd., New York © 1991.

CHAPTER 29

Pathogenesis and Pathophysiology of Fungal Infections of the Central Nervous System

John R. Perfect and David T. Durack

Fungi provide humankind with many benefits, both commercial and medicinal. They are essential for major domestic industries such as production of bread and beer. Current major roles in medical science include production of antibiotics and the study of eukaryotic genetics and molecular biology. However, fungi also can cause major problems for humans. Some plant fungi can inflict serious damage on crops; in addition, primary fungal pathogens such as *Cryptococcus, Histoplasma,* and *Blastomyces* can infect humans, causing local or disseminated disease including central nervous system (CNS) infections. Opportunistic fungal pathogens such as *Aspergillus* and *Candida* pose a serious threat to the enlarging pool of immunocompromised hosts, including: neonates, postsurgical patients, and those with malignancies, organ transplants, or the acquired immunodeficiency syndrome (AIDS). Many of these primary and secondary fungal pathogens can invade the CNS. This chapter will review the pathogenesis of CNS mycoses.

The brain and the subarachnoid space constitute an immunologically sequestered site. This site is located inside distinct anatomical and functional barriers which may exclude or modify certain immune responses. Some patients with a CNS fungal infection have no overt immune defect or underlying disease, but most have some flaw in their immune responses that allows invasion by fungi, most of which are relatively nonvirulent. Host defenses normally are highly effective in excluding fungi from the CNS, but certain conditions can lead to failure of this function. Some are obvious, such as direct inoculation of organisms into the brain following head injuries, whereas others are more subtle. Certain drug regimens

increase the frequency of CNS fungal infections; for example, neutropenia due to cancer chemotherapy can predispose to CNS candidiasis and aspergillosis, whereas corticosteroids predispose to cryptococcal meningitis. Infection with the human immunodeficiency virus (HIV) allows invasion of the CNS by fungi such as *Cryptococcus neoformans* and *Histoplasma capsulatum.* Finally, there are other underlying medical conditions such as diabetes, pregnancy, malignancies, and iron chelation therapy which suppress normal immune responses in various ways, favoring invasion by fungi. Table 1 provides a summary of the main conditions predisposing to fungal infections of the CNS.

In addition to their role in pathogenesis, the patients' immune responses and underlying diseases are the major factors determining outcome of CNS fungal infections.

A plethora of different fungal species can infect the CNS. For example, common environmental fungi occasionally cause meningitis in humans: *Alternaria* (1), *Rhodotorula* (2), *Acremonium* (3), *Dreschlera* (4), *Sependonium* (5), *Scedosporium* (6), *Schizophyllum* (7), *Paecilomyces* (8), and *Ustilago* (9). Such cases are interesting, but rare. Most cases of fungal CNS infections are caused by only a few important species, which can be classified into two groups (Table 2). First, all the primary fungal pathogens of humans can cause CNS infections. This group includes *C. neoformans* (10–12), *Coccidioides immitis* (13), *Blastomyces dermatitidis* (14,15), *Paracoccidiodes brasiliensis* (16), *Sporothrix schenckii* (17–19), *H. capsulatum* (20–24), *Pseudallescheria boydii* (25–28) and dematiaceous fungi (29,30). Second are the opportunists, which take advantage of immune defects. This group includes *Candida* species (31–35), *Aspergillus* species (36–40), the *Zygomycetes* (41,42) and *Trichosporon* species (43–45). This grouping

J. R. Perfect and D. T. Durack: Division of Infectious Diseases and International Health, Duke University Medical Center, Durham, North Carolina 27710.

TABLE 1. *Some factors predisposing to fungal infections of the CNS[a]*

Predisposing factors	Examples	Typical organisms
Prematurity		*Candida*
Inherited immune defects	CGD, SCID, etc.	*Candida, Cryptococcus, Aspergillus*
Acquired immune defects	Corticosteroids	*Cryptococcus, Candida*
	Cytotoxic agents	*Aspergillus, Candida*
	HIV infection	*Cryptococcus, Histoplasma*
	Alcoholism	*Sporothrix*
Iron chelator therapy	Desferoxamine	*Zygomycetes*
Intravenous drug abuse		*Zygomycetes, Candida*
Ketoacidosis		*Zygomycetes*
Trauma, surgery, foreign body, near-drowning		*Candida, Pseudallescheria,* dematiaceous fungi

[a] CNS, central nervous system; SCID, severe combined immune deficiency; HIV, human immunodeficiency virus; CGD (chronic granulomatous disease).

is not absolute; some overlap occurs (46–49). The rest of this chapter will discuss in more detail the pathogenesis of CNS infections caused by some of these fungi.

Cryptococcus neoformans

This encapsulated yeast is the most common cause of fungal meningitis. The first report of human cryptococcosis was published over 105 years ago; approximately 10 years later this yeast was identified as a CNS pathogen. A review of the incidence of systemic mycoses by selected hospitals in the United States showed an increase in the number of reported infections, including cryptococcosis, during the 1960s and 1970s (50). In the 1980s a further dramatic increase in numbers of cases of cryptococcosis in the United States and certain African countries occurred, directly related to the rising prevalence of HIV infections. In the United States, cryptococcal meningitis ranks as one of the five most common opportunistic infections in patients with AIDS. At Duke University Medical Center, approximately two new cases of invasive cryptococcosis are diagnosed each month.

This important pathogen is distributed worldwide. It is found in bird excreta, in soil, and in animals, and it can even colonize humans. The vast majority of initial infections occur through inhalation of small yeast forms from the environment. Once in the host, the cryptococci develop a large polysaccharide capsule which resists phagocytosis. Capsule production is stimulated by physiologic concentrations of carbon dioxide found in the lung (51), an exquisite adaptation favoring survival in a mammalian host. The inflammatory reaction to inhaled cryptococci produces a primary lung–lymph node complex (52), which usually limits spread of the organism. Most pulmonary infections are asymptomatic, but a clinically apparent pneumonia can occur on initial infection. This is of variable severity, often resolving slowly over weeks or months with or without treatment (53). Other patients develop focal or nodular pulmonary lesions. Cryptococci can remain dormant in the lung or lymph nodes until host defenses become weakened.

C. neoformans can spread from the lung and intrathoracic lymph nodes to circulate in the blood, especially if the host is immunocompromised. This can occur during the primary infection, or during reactivation years

TABLE 2. *Spectrum of involvement for fungi that can infect the CNS[a]*

Species	Incidence	Predilection to involve the CNS[b]	Chief pathological manifestations		
			Meningitis	Abscess or inflammatory mass	Infarct
Cryptococcus	Common	++++	++++	+	+
Coccidioides	Common	+++	++++	+	+
Candida	Common	++	++	++	−
Aspergillus	Occasional	++	+	+++	++++
Zygomycetes	Occasional	++	+	+++	++++
Histoplasma	Occasional	+	+	+	+
Blastomyces	Occasional	+	+	+	−
Sporothrix	Occasional	+	+	−	−
Paracoccidioides	Rare	±	±	±	−
Dematiaceous fungi	Rare	+++	±	++++	−
Pseudallescheria	Rare	+	++	++	−

[a] Key: ++++, common; ±, very rare; −, does not occur.
[b] Versus other body sites.

later. If distant infection occurs, the site most likely to be involved is the CNS.

The remarkable predilection for this encapsulated yeast to infect the subarachnoid space remains unexplained. It has been suggested that an important virulence factor for *C. neoformans* is its ability to produce melanin via a pathway which utilizes a unique phenoloxidase enzyme (54). Melanin has been shown to protect certain microorganisms from lysis after exposure to host defense cells. Substrates for the phenoloxidase enzyme include certain diphenolic compounds, including norepinephrine and other catecholamines which are highly concentrated in the CNS. This might partially explain the tropism of *C. neoformans* for this site. Recent investigations have found that diphenolic compounds do not provide substrate for growth of *C. neoformans* (55), but instead provide substrate for production of melanin which can be used to protect the yeast from host-derived oxidative damage (56). It has been shown convincingly in animal studies that the phenoloxidase enzyme and presence of the capsule are crucial for virulence (54).

Yeasts from the subarachnoid space can be identified by withdrawing cerebrospinal fluid (CSF) and mixing it with India ink on a slide for a simple microscopic examination. The yeast cells measure 4–6 μm in diameter, with a capsule ranging from 1 to 30 μm wide. A careful India ink examination of CSF will be positive in approximately half of the cases of cryptococcal meningitis. In patients with AIDS the yield is even higher. Quantitative counts from patients with meningitis reveal from 10^3 colony-forming units (CFU) to 10^7 CFU of yeasts per milliliter of CSF (11).

C. neoformans is divided into two varieties. The first is *C. neoformans* var. *neoformans,* which includes strains of polysaccharide capsular serotypes A and D. These serotypes represent the most common isolates from patients worldwide, including all but a few isolates from AIDS patients. The second variety is *C. neoformans* var. *gatti,* which includes serotypes B and C. These serotypes are predominantly found in clinical infections from Australia, Southeast Asia, Central Africa and southern California. Serotypes B and C are more likely to cause disease in nonimmunosuppressed hosts, and they seem to be more likely to invade the brain parenchyma, causing mass lesions called "torulomas."

We will discuss the subject of CNS infection by *C. neoformans* in depth because it is, in many respects, the best understood of all fungal CNS pathogens. Even so, some major questions regarding pathogenesis remain unanswered.

Many factors contribute to the pathogenesis of CNS cryptococcosis. The yeast has several phenotypic characteristics which appear to be associated with invasion of the CNS: phenoloxidase production, presence of polysaccharide capsule, and ability to thrive at host body temperatures (54). All three phenotypes have been associated with CNS invasion and mortality using the powerful tools of genetics. As previously mentioned, the ability to produce melanin is necessary for cryptococcal CNS invasion. Mutants which do not possess this phenoloxidase enzyme system are avirulent in murine models, and they only rarely cause meningitis in humans. Recent information suggests that melanin may act as an antioxidant protecting the organism from host damage.

The second major characteristic is the ability to produce a capsule which protects the yeast from host defenses, especially phagocytosis. Genetic studies have shown that acapsular mutants are not virulent in mice. A well-known acapsular mutant (namely, mutant 602) will not produce a progressive cryptococcal meningitis in immunosuppressed rabbits when introduced intracisternally. It also appears that it is not simply the presence or absence of a capsule. Dynamic regulation of capsule production by the yeast is likely to be important. A clone was isolated from a virulent, wild-type strain of *C. neoformans* which did not respond normally to physiological carbon dioxide concentrations by increasing production of polysaccharide capsular material. This clone had simultaneously lost its ability to establish infection in the subarachnoid space of rabbits (51). Therefore, it is likely that both the presence of capsule and regulation of its production are important factors for establishing infection in the CNS.

Another characteristic which appears important for CNS invasion is the ability of the yeast to grow at 37°C. *C. neoformans* is one of the few species of cryptococci which has adapted to human body temperature; genetic studies have demonstrated the importance of this phenotype for invasion.

Future studies are needed to dissect out the mechanisms by which these phenotypic characteristics confer virulence. It is likely that molecular techniques will allow identification of cryptococcal genes and their products which are specifically and uniquely necessary for invasion and growth in the CNS, an environment which is not particularly favorable for this yeast. Such studies could identify targets for therapeutic intervention.

The primary immune defects that predispose to cryptococcosis lie in the cell-mediated responses (57,58). Thus, most cases of cryptococcal meningitis occur in patients with apparent or potential defects in cell-mediated immunity: reticuloendothelial malignancy, sarcoidosis, organ transplantation, collagen vascular diseases, corticosteroid therapy, and AIDS. Lymphocyte functions are abnormal in most patients with disseminated cryptococcosis, and certain cell-mediated immune defects can persist after infection apparently has been eliminated (59). Animal studies have shown the potential importance of natural killer cells in eliminating the initial infection (60). In animals, cytotoxic lymphocytes could transfer protection (61), and suppressor cells have been shown to proliferate in response to polysaccharide antigens (62). Activated macrophages become potently fungistatic for *C. neoformans;* this is probably an important factor in the host's response (63). In the subarachnoid space of rabbits, the development of activated CSF macrophages correlates with the killing of yeast at this site (64). The high susceptibility of AIDS patients vividly illustrates the essential role of CD4 lymphocytes in preventing the occurrence of disseminated cryptococcosis, and of recurrence after treatment. Genetic defects in the cell-mediated immune system of beige (65) and nude mice (66) enhance their susceptibility to *C. neoformans* infections.

Humoral immunity appears to play a secondary role in host defenses against cryptococcosis. Both IgG and C3b bind to (and within) the capsule, enhancing phagocytosis. Experiments suggest that the presence of an intact complement system may be important in preventing dissemination (67). The role of antibody in this infection has received considerable study, with mixed results (68,69). Antibody-dependent killing of *C. neoformans* by human peripheral blood mononuclear cells has been documented (70,71), and measurable titers of serum antibody to *C. neoformans* were associated with a more favorable outcome (72). However, passive immunization of mice conferred little protection against challenge with the yeast (69). In a rabbit model of cryptococcal meningitis, immunization with capsule to produce significant serum antibody titers did not protect against subarachnoid challenge with yeasts (73).

It should be noted that many of these studies examined the antibody responses in serum, not in the CSF. It seems appropriate to examine the local immune response in the subarachnoid space. When this was done, specific anticryptococcal immunoglobulin was detected in the CSF of patients with cryptococcal meningitis (74,75). Also, in rabbits with cryptococcal meningitis, there is rapid local production of immunoglobulin in the CSF following infection which correlates temporally with killing of yeast at this site (76). This specific antibody production is halted if the animals receive corticosteroids or cyclosporine during infection (76).

In summary, it seems certain that humoral factors play a part in host defenses against *C. neoformans*. However, the rarity of cryptococcal meningitis in patients with either congenital or acquired deficiencies in antibody (77) or complement production argues that humoral immunity is much less important than cellular immunity for this yeast.

Two specific factors have been instrumental in elevating *C. neoformans* to prominence as the most common fungal pathogen in the CNS. These are corticosteroids and HIV infection. Excess corticosteroids produce a variety of immune defects which greatly increase the host's risk for disseminated cryptococcosis. Either endogenous overproduction of corticosteroid or exogenous treatment can do this (11). Rabbits, which are normally resistant to experimental cryptococcosis, can be rendered highly susceptible by corticosteroid treatment (78). Figure 1 shows the histopathology of infection in the rabbit model. It is primarily an infection of the subarachnoid space, with occasional yeasts seen in the brain parenchyma as cystoid collections. The normal animal has a brisk inflammatory response, whereas the immunosuppressed animal has few cells along with masses of yeasts. These findings are similar to those seen in patients with AIDS or receiving high-dose corticosteroids. This model has allowed examination of many local CSF factors important to immune responses at this site. The single most striking finding is the CSF leukopenia caused by corticosteroids. The number of polymorphonuclear cells and mononuclear cells (including T and B lymphocytes and macrophages) that migrate into the CSF of corticosteroid-treated rabbits inoculated with cryptococci is far lower than that in untreated controls (78). Both the number of yeasts and the reduction of inflammatory cell numbers in CSF are closely related to the dose of corticosteroid administered (78). CSF leukopenia caused by corticosteroids is partially explained by the inhibition of chemotactic factors produced locally in the subarachnoid space (79). Experimental cryptococcal meningitis in these corticosteroid-treated rabbits shows many similarities to CNS cryptococcosis in AIDS patients: low CSF cell counts, large burden of organisms, high antigen titers, and high mortality. On the other hand, treatment with another powerful suppressor of cellular immunity, cyclosporine, also predisposes rabbits to cryptococcal meningitis without inducing the severe CSF leukopenia seen in corticosteroid-treated animals (80).

The second major factor is HIV infection (81–87). The profound, progressive loss of CD4-helper cells in HIV-infected patients correlates with appearance of cryptococcosis, which is often the AIDS-defining illness. Clinical studies suggest that 6–13% of AIDS patients will develop cryptococcal meningitis. Many of these patients will present with a large burden of organisms, high polysaccharide antigen titers, and unusually low CSF leukocyte counts. Over half of AIDS patients will present with less than 20 leukocytes per cubic millimeter in CSF. This lack of the normal inflammatory response at the site of infection indicates both defective immunity and poor prognosis. Although the successful immune response of the immunocompetent host is comprised of many components, both corticosteroid-treated rabbits and AIDS patients demonstrate that adequate numbers of host cells in the subarachnoid space are necessary for recovery.

Despite availability of antifungal agents to treat this infection, treatment often fails. Better outcomes will likely require further understanding of local CNS host factors allowing specific or nonspecific treatment interventions. We still have little knowledge of the role of biological

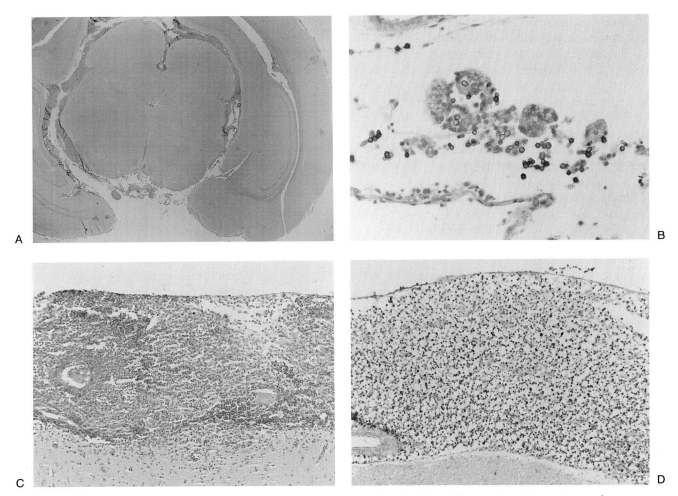

FIG. 1. Sections of brain and meninges from cortisone-treated rabbits with experimental cryptococcal meningitis, 1–2 weeks after inoculation of *C. neoformans*. **A:** A cross-section in the region of the pons, showing a widespread meningeal infiltration with large numbers of blue-staining yeasts. There are occasional collections of cryptococci within the brain parenchyma, but primarily this organism infects the subarachnoid space. Alcian blue, ×5. **B:** Host cells, particularly mononuclear phagocytes, ingesting yeasts in the subarachnoid space. Alcian blue, ×400. **C:** The subarachnoid space of an infected rabbit, not treated with cortisone, is packed with abundant mononuclear host cells (*pink*) and very few cryptococci (*blue*). Alcian blue, ×250. **D:** The subarachnoid space of an infected, cortisone-treated animal is packed with a multitude of yeasts (*blue*), but very few host inflammatory cells are present. Contrast this appearance with the normal cellular response in part C. Alcian blue, ×100. (From ref. 78, with permission.)

response modifiers at the site of CNS infection with this yeast. Manipulations of the immune system using modulators such as interleukins, granulocyte colony-stimulating factor (G-CSF), granulocyte–macrophage colony-stimulating factor (GM-CSF), tumor necrosis factor, or gamma interferon to improve cell function or recruitment of cells to the site of infection may be needed to improve results of treatment in immunocompromised hosts.

Coccidioides

Coccidioides immitis is a highly pathogenic dimorphous fungus which normally inhabits semi-acid soil. This limits its ecological distribution to certain areas in the southwestern United States and parts of Mexico, Central America, and South America. However, because of frequent travel into and out of these areas, the human infection—coccidioidomycosis—often is seen by clinicians outside the organism's natural geographic boundaries.

The infection begins with inhalation of arthroconidia, which can establish a primary pulmonary infection. The majority of such patients remain asymptomatic. In less than 0.2% of primary infections does the organism disseminate outside the respiratory tract. Up to one-third of this small proportion of extrapulmonary cases present as meningitis. The CNS frequently is the only site involved during dissemination, which usually occurs within the first several months after primary infection (13).

It is likely that an intact cell-mediated host response is important in the prevention of coccidioidal meningitis (88). The development of a positive skin test with the primary infection suggests that dissemination is unlikely to occur. However, the link between immune suppression and meningitis is not as conclusive as it is for *C. neoformans*. For example, the majority of patients are healthy before development of coccidioidal meningitis, and only 2% of patients had an underlying disease. Nevertheless, immunosuppressed patients may be at higher risk of dissemination after primary lung infection. For instance, corticosteroid treatment has been associated with dissemination of infection, and there have been a few cases of coccidioidal meningitis in AIDS patients (89).

Epidemiologic studies show that non-Caucasians are more likely to develop meningitis after a primary infection. Pregnancy is an adverse prognostic factor which increases the chance of dissemination to the CNS after a primary infection. The potential clinical significance of interactions between host hormones (such as estrogens) and fungi (which possess receptors for various hormones and pheromones) remains an area of active investigation which may yield important clues to understanding certain fungal virulence factors (90).

Histoplasma

Histoplasma capsulatum resides in the soils of the Ohio and Central Mississippi valleys and along the Appalachian mountains. Infection occurs after inhalation of spores. Skin testing in endemic areas shows that the majority of patients have minimal or no symptoms during primary infection in the lung. Rarely does the yeast disseminate. It has been estimated that when dissemination from the respiratory tract does occur, between one-tenth and one-quarter of these patients will develop CNS involvement.

Development of progressive disseminated histoplasmosis suggests that cell-mediated immune defenses are impaired. Approximately one-half of patients with disseminated histoplasmosis receive immunosuppressive therapy or have illnesses such as lymphoma, lymphocytic leukemia, hyposplenic disorders, or AIDS (20–24). Recent experience suggests that CNS involvement in disseminated histoplasmosis is more common in AIDS patients (91). Therefore, like *C. neoformans*, *H. capsulatum* infection reactivates and disseminates during immune suppression. When this occurs, the CNS is a prime location for invasion. In one patient with *Histoplasma* meningitis, immune suppression was demonstrated at the site of infection. An abundance of suppressor T cells in CSF was found during *Histoplasma* meningitis (92).

Blastomyces

Blastomyces dermatitidis is a dimorphic fungus which is endemic in parts of the United States: from the lower Mississippi valley up to the North Central states and into the mid-Atlantic states. Like the other fungi described above, primary infection is presumed to result from inhalation of spores from a soil source. However, it has been difficult to locate the fungus in the environment; only recently has it been found in nature and associated with an epidemic.

Disseminated blastomycosis is characterized by suppurative, granulomatous lesions of the lung, skin, or bone. This fungus invades the CNS in 6–33% of cases when dissemination occurs (14,15). Most patients with CNS blastomycosis have infection documented at other sites, but occasionally meningitis can present without evidence of extraneural disease. A few patients will develop a blastomycoma while showing no evidence of meningitis. Unlike cryptococcal meningitis and CNS infections with *Candida* and *Aspergillus* species, there are no known specific risk factors or immune defects for development of CNS blastomycosis. *B. dermatitidis* has only recently been identified as a potential fungal pathogen in AIDS patients (93). Invasion of the CNS appears to be a late complication of a systemic infection and thus should always be considered in patients with concomitant neurological symptoms and *Blastomyces* isolated from another body site (94).

Paracoccidioides

Paracoccidioides brasiliensis is a dimorphic fungus whose distribution is limited to subtropical areas of Central and South America. The lung is the primary site of infection. When the CNS is involved, the majority of patients have widely disseminated disease which is easily identified. Rarely, this infection has been reported to involve the CNS alone. CNS infection generally occurs in an apparently normal host (16). However, host responses against this organism remain poorly understood.

Sporotrichosis

Sporothrix schenckii is a fungus with worldwide distribution. The organism is found in soil or plant material (such as sphagnum moss) and enters the body via traumatic inoculation, such as a prick from a rose thorn. Sporotrichosis generally presents as an infection of skin and subcutaneous lymphatics after a primary skin inoculation; pulmonary disease following inhalation of spores is uncommon. Dissemination beyond the skin, lung, or joints is rare, but approximately a dozen cases of *Sporo-*

thrix meningitis have been reported. Particular risk factors for invasion into the CNS cannot be identified because these cases are so rare (17–19). However, certain patients may be more predisposed to disseminate from a local infection. Patients with myelodysplastic syndromes or ethanol abuse, or those receiving corticosteroid therapy, may be at increased risk for dissemination. Disseminated sporotrichosis has been described in a patient with AIDS (95).

Phaeohyphomycosis

This group of mycoses results from infection with one of a heterogeneous group of fungal species which form dematiaceous yeast-like cells, pseudohyphae, septated hyphae, or any combination of these forms. In most cases infections are limited to local disease, without dissemination. However, one organism, *Xylophypha bantiana* (synonyms: *Cladosporium bantianum, Cladosporium trichoides*) shows a remarkable predilection to infect the brain and meninges. Cerebral lesions may present as single, multilocular, or multiple abscesses. Histology of these CNS infections is similar to that seen in the subcutaneous form of infection, with a marked inflammatory reaction and necrosis. These dematiaceous fungi can cause CNS infections in both normal and immunocompromised hosts (29,30).

Hyalohyphomycoses

Pseudallescheria boydii is the most prominent species of this group with respect to CNS infections. It has a worldwide distribution in soil and contaminated water and is a common cause of mycetomas. It rarely causes meningitis (25,27). Although factors which predispose to invasion of the CNS with this fungus are not well-defined, cases presented in the literature suggest that corticosteroids may be a risk factor (26). Another potential risk factor for CNS infection is water immersion (28). Several cases of near-drowning have resulted in pneumonia caused by *Pseudallescheria boydii,* resulting from aspiration of contaminated material. Such pneumonia can serve as a nidus of infection which allows dissemination to the CNS. *Fusarium* species have also been found to cause disseminated infection in severely immunocompromised hosts, particularly in neutropenic patients. This species can invade the CNS (96).

The next four groups of microorganisms are considered opportunistic invaders of the CNS because most cases have occurred in immunocompromised hosts.

Candida

Candida species are part of the normal human microbial flora. They rarely cause CNS disease unless host defenses have been impaired. Many different factors can encourage spread of *Candida* into the blood, and potentially into the CNS. These include broad-spectrum antibiotic therapy, hyperalimentation, prematurity, malignancy, indwelling catheters, treatment with corticosteroids, neutropenia, abdominal surgery, diabetes, thermal injuries, and parenteral drug abuse (31–34). In the past, *Candida* infections were considered to be the most common cerebral fungal infection, based upon necropsy studies (35). This still is likely to be the case at institutions where large numbers of cancer patients are treated. However, with the increasing numbers of AIDS patients and the reduced duration of neutropenia associated with the use of biological growth factors, such as G-CSF and GM-CSF, *C. neoformans* may now have replaced *Candida* as the most common CNS mycosis.

Candida species have been found to be particularly susceptible to both oxidative and nonoxidative antimicrobial mechanisms of professional phagocytes. Therefore, neutropenia is a major risk factor for invasive *Candida* infections (35). The importance of the host response has been further emphasized by reports of *Candida* meningitis in both acquired and congenital immunodeficiency syndromes (97). Patients with chronic granulomatous disease of childhood may present with *Candida* meningitis (98,99). This specific underlying immune defect should be considered in any case of spontaneously occurring *Candida* meningitis (98,99). Cases of *Candida* meningitis or brain abscess have been reported in patients with severe combined immune deficiency (SCID) (100) and in AIDS patients. Finally, *Candida* can involve the brain and subarachnoid space by direct extension through trauma, ventriculostomy placements, or ventricular shunts, particularly if antibiotics have previously been used.

In prematures and neonates, meningitis is the most common form of CNS infection (101). In adults, *Candida* infection of the CNS often presents with brain abscesses rather than meningitis (see Chapter 32). Although *C. albicans* is the most common species of *Candida* involved, others such as *C. tropicalis* also occasionally produce CNS infection.

Aspergillus

Aspergillus fumigatus and *A. flavus* can cause CNS infections in humans. This can develop by direct extension from the paranasal sinuses; or following head trauma, surgery, or lumbar puncture; or through hematogenous spread in the immunocompromised host, particularly those with prolonged neutropenia (36–40). The risk of disseminated aspergillosis and subsequent brain involvement increases with the duration of neutropenia (102).

Invasion of the brain parenchyma with formation of abscesses and infarcts is a more common clinical presentation of these fungi than is meningitis. *Aspergillus* may also invade the CNS via local involvement of the vertebrae and direct extension into the subarachnoid space (98). This direct extension is seen most commonly in patients with chronic granulomatous disease of childhood. Although alveolar macrophages play a role in limiting initial infection of the lungs with this ubiquitous fungus, the polymorphonuclear leukocyte is likely the crucial host defense against CNS invasion. The virulence of some strains of *Aspergillus* may be caused, in part, by production of elastase (103), as well as by a phagocytosis or complement inhibitor (104,105) which may assist in CNS tissue invasion.

Zygomycosis

The ubiquitous molds of this group can cause CNS infection in immunocompromised hosts by direct extension or by hematogenous spread (41,42). The genus *Rhizopus* is responsible for most infections within this group. The angioinvasive nature of these fungi, similar to that of *Aspergillus* species, causes most CNS infections to present with symptoms of cerebral infarctions.

Certain patients are at risk for CNS invasion by *Zygomycetes*. Those with diabetes, those receiving immunosuppressive therapy, those using intravenous drugs, or those with an underlying malignancy are all at increased risk for this CNS mycosis. Patients who have become acidotic, especially from diabetic ketoacidosis, are at risk for *Zygomycetes* infection which could then extend from the nasal area and sinuses into the CNS. Some cases of disseminated zygomycosis, including brain involvement, have occurred in patients receiving desferoxamine therapy (106). It is suspected that these fungi, under conditions of low iron, can use this iron chelator as a siderophore. This could promote its growth and spread, possibly by blocking an important antimicrobial host factor, transferrin.

Trichosporonosis

Infections caused by *Trichosporon* species generally involve superficial skin or hair shafts. However, with the increasing number of immunocompromised hosts, a few disseminated infections with this organism have been reported. Infection of the CNS has been reported with *Trichosporon beigelii* (43–45).

REFERENCES

1. Ohashi Y. On a rare disease due to *Alternaria tenuis nees*. *Tohoku J Exp Med* 1960;72:78–82.

2. Pore RS, Chen J. Meningitis caused by *Rhodotorula*. *Sabouraudia* 1976;14:331–335.
3. Lavie CJ, Khandheria BK, Seward JB, Tajik AJ, Taylor CL, Ballard DJ. Factors associated with the recommendation for endocarditis prophylaxis in mitral valve prolapse. *JAMA* 1989;262:3308–3312.
4. Fuste FJ, Ajello L, Threlkeld R, Henry JE Jr. *Drechslera hawaiiensis:* causative agent of a fatal fungal meningo-encephalitis. *Sabouraudia* 1973;11:59–63.
5. Mukerji S, Patwardhan JR, Gadgil RK. Bacterial and mycotic infection of the brain. *Indian J Med Sci* 1971;25:791–794.
6. Watanabe S, Hironaga M. An atypical isolate of *Scedosporium apiospermum* from a purulent meningitis in man. *Sabouraudia* 1981;19:209–215.
7. Chaves-Batista A, Mala JA, Singer P. Basidioneuromycosis in man. Instituto de Micologia Publicacao No. 42. *Universidade de Recife Brasil* 1955:53–60.
8. Fagerburg R, Suh B, Buckley HR. Cerebrospinal fluid shunt colonization and obstruction by *Paecilomyces varoti*. *J Neursurg* 1981;54:257–260.
9. Moore M, Russell WO, Sachs E. Chronic leptomeningitis and ependymitis caused by Ustilago, probably *U. zeae* (corn smut); ustilagomycosis, second reported instance of human infection. *Am J Pathol* 1946;22:761–777.
10. Sabetta JR, Andriole VT. Cryptococcal infection of the central nervous system. *Med Clin North Am* 1985;69:333–344.
11. Perfect JR, Durack DT, Gallis HA. Cryptococcemia. *Medicine* 1983;62:98–109.
12. Perfect JR. Cryptococcosis. *Infect Dis Clin North Am* 1989;3:77–102.
13. Bouza E, Dreyer JS, Hewitt WL, Meyer RD. Coccidioidal meningitis: an analysis of thirty-one cases and review of the literature. *Medicine* 1981;60:139–172.
14. Gonyea EF. The spectrum of primary blastomycotic meningitis: a review of central nervous system blastomycosis. *Ann Neurol* 1978;3:26–39.
15. Buechner HA, Clawson C. Blastomycosis of the central nervous system, II. A report of nine cases from the Veterans Administration Cooperative Study. *Am Rev Respir Dis* 1967;95:820–826.
16. Pereira WC, Raphael A, Tenut RA. Localizacoa encefalico da blastomicose sul-americana: consideraooes a proposito de 9 casos. *Arg Neuropsiguiat* 1965;23:113–126.
17. Ewing GE, Bosl GJ, Peterson PK. *Sporothrix schenckii* meningitis in a farmer with Hodgkin's disease. *Am J Med* 1980;68:455–457.
18. Freeman JW, Ziegler DK. Chronic meningitis caused by *Sporothrix schenckii*. *Neurology* 1977;27:989–992.
19. Klein RC, Ivens MS, Seabury JH, Dascomb HE. Meningitis due to *Sporotrichum schenkii*. *Arch Intern Med* 1966;118:145–149.
20. Goodwin RA Jr, Shapiro JL, Thurman GH, Thurman SS, Des Prez KM. Disseminated histoplasmosis: clinical and pathologic correlations. *Medicine* 1980;59:1–33.
21. Karalakulasingam R, Arora KK, Adams G, Serratoni F, Martin DG. Meningoencephalitis caused by *Histoplasma capsulatum*. *Arch Intern Med* 1976;136:217–220.
22. Cooper RA Jr, Goldstein E. Histoplasmosis of the central nervous system. Report of two cases and review of the literature. *Am J Med* 1963;35:45–57.
23. Tynes BS, Crutcher JC, Utz JP. Histoplasma meningitis. *Ann Intern Med* 1963;59:619–621.
24. Wheat LJ, Batteiger BE, Sathapatayavongs B. *Histoplasma capsulatum* infections of the central nervous system. *Medicine* 1990;69:244–260.
25. Benham RW, Georg LK. *Alleschria boydii* causative agent in a case of meningitis. *J Invest Dermatol* 1948;10:99–110.
26. Yoo D, Lee WHS, Kwon-Chung KJ. Brain abscess due to *Pseudallescheria boydii* associated with primary non-Hodgkin's lymphoma of the central nervous system: a case report and literature review. *Rev Infect Dis* 1985;7:272–277.
27. Selby R. Pachymeningitis secondary to *Alleschria boydii*. *J Neursurg* 1972;36:225–227.
28. Dworzack DL, Clark RB, Padgett PJ. New causes of pneumonia, meningitis, and disseminated infections associated with immersion. *Infect Control Hosp Epidemiol* 1987;1:615–633.

29. Bennett JE, Bonner H, Jennings AE, Lopez RI. Chronic meningitis caused by *Cladosporium trichoides*. *Am J Clin Pathol* 1973;59:398–407.
30. Seaworth BJ, Kwon-Chung CJ, Hamilton JD, Perfect JR. Brain abscess caused by a variety of *Cladosporium trichoides*. *Am J Clin Pathol* 1983;79:747–752.
31. Bayer AS, Edwards JE Jr, Seidel JS, Guze LB. *Candida* meningitis. Report of seven cases and review of the English literature. *Medicine* 1976;55:477–485.
32. Chadwick DW, Hartley E, Mackinnon DM. Meningitis caused by *Candida tropicalis*. *Arch Neurol* 1980;37:175–176.
33. Chattopadhyay B. *Candida tropicalis* meningitis. A case report. *J Laryngol Otol* 1981;95:1149–1151.
34. Buchs S, Pfister P. *Candida* meningitis: course, prognosis and mortality before and after introduction of the new antimycotics. *Mykosen* 1983;26:73–81.
35. Parker JC Jr, McCloskey JJ, Lee RS. The emergence of candidosis. The dominant postmortem cerebral mycosis. *Am J Clin Pathol* 1978;70:31–36.
36. Iyer S, Dodge P, Adams RD. Two cases of *Aspergillus* infection of the central nervous system. *J Neurol Neurosurg Psychiatry* 1952;15:152–163.
37. Gordon MA, Holzman RS, Senter H, Lapa EW, Kupersmith MJ. *Aspergillus orzyme* meningitis. *JAMA* 1976;235:2122–2123.
38. Mukoyama M, Gimple K, Poser CM. Aspergillosis of the central nervous system. Report of a brain abscess due to *A. fumigatus* and review of the literature. *Neurology* 1969;19:967–974.
39. Goodman ML, Coffey RJ. Stereotaxic drainage of *Aspergillus* brain abscess with long-term survival: case report and review. *Neurosurgery* 1989;24:96–99.
40. Guisan von M. Sclerosing post-traumatic meningeal aspergillosis. *Schweiz Arch Neurol Psychiatr* 1962;90:235–254.
41. Jones PG, Gilman RM, Medeiros AA, Dyckman J. Focal intracranial mucomycosis presenting as chronic meningitis. *JAMA* 1981;246:2063–2064.
42. Meyers BR, Wormser G, Hirschman SZ, Blitzer A. Rhinocerebral mucormycosis premortem diagnosis and therapy. *Arch Intern Med* 1979;139:557–560.
43. Walsh TJ. Trichosporonosis. *Infect Dis Clin North Am* 1989;3:43–52.
44. Watson KC, Kallichurum S. Brain abscess due to *Trichosporon cutaneum*. *J Med Microbiol* 1970;3:191–193.
45. Surmont I, Vergauwen B, Marcelis L, Verbist L, Verhoef G, Boogaerts M. First report of chronic meningitis caused by *Trichosporon beigelii*. *Eur J Clin Microbiol* 1990;9:226–229.
46. Salaki JS, Louria DB, Chmel H. Fungal and yeast infections of the central nervous system. A clinical review. *Medicine* 1984;63:108–132.
47. Walsh TJ, Hier DB, Caplan LR. Fungal infections of the central nervous system: comparative analysis of risk factors and clinical signs in 57 patients. *Neurology* 1985;35:1654–1657.
48. Lyons RW, Andriole VT. Fungal infections of the CNS. *Neurol Clin* 1986;4:159–170.
49. Chernik NL, Armstrong D, Posner JB. Central nervous system infections in patients with cancer. *Medicine* 1973;52:563–581.
50. Fraser DW, Ward JI, Ajello L, Plikaytis BD. Aspergillosis and systemic mycosis. *JAMA* 1979;242:1631–1635.
51. Granger DL, Perfect JR, Durack DT. Virulence of *Cryptococcus neoformans*: regulation of capsule synthesis by carbon dioxide. *J Clin Invest* 1985;76:508–516.
52. Baker RD. The primary pulmonary lymph node complex of cryptococcosis. *Am J Clin Pathol* 1976;65:83–92.
53. Warr W, Bates JH, Stove A. The spectrum of pulmonary cryptococcosis. *Ann Intern Med* 1968;69:1109–1116.
54. Kwon-Chung KJ, Rhodes JC. Encapsulation and melanin formation as indicators of virulence in *Cryptococcus neoformans*. *Infect Immun* 1986;51:218–223.
55. Polachek I, Platt Y, Aronovitch J. Catecholamines and virulence of *Cryptococcus neoformans*. *Infect Immun* 1990;58:2919–2922.
56. Jacobson ES, Emery HS. Molecular basis of resistance to leukocytes [Abstract]. *International Conference on Cryptococcus and Cryptococcosis* 1989:S4.
57. Diamond RD, Bennett JE. Disseminated cryptococcosis in man:

58. Schimpff SC, Bennett JE. Abnormalities in cell-mediated immunity in patients with *Cryptococcus neoformans* infection. *J Allergy Clin Immunol* 1975;55:430–441.
59. Henderson DK, Bennett JE, Huber MA. Long-lasting specific immunologic unresponsiveness associated with cryptococcal meningitis. *J Clin Invest* 1982;69:1185–1190.
60. Hidore MR, Murphy JW. Correlation of natural killer cell activity and clearance of *Cryptococcus neoformans* from mice after adoptive transfer of splenic nylon wool-nonadherent cells. *Infect Immun* 1986;51:547–555.
61. Lim TS, Murphy JW. Transfer of immunity to cryptococcosis by T-enriched splenic lymphocytes from *Cryptococcus neoformans*-sensitized mice. *Infect Immun* 1980;30:5–11.
62. Murphy JW, Mosley RL, Moorhead JW. Regulation of cell-mediated immunity in cryptococcosis. II. characterization of first order T-suppressor cells (TS1) and induction of second order suppressor cells. *Infect Immun* 1983;130:2876–2881.
63. Granger DL, Perfect JR, Durack DT. Macrophage-mediated fungistasis *in vitro*: requirements for intracellular and extracellular cytotoxicity. *J Immunol* 1985;131:672–680.
64. Perfect JR, Hobbs MM, Granger DL, Durack DT. Cerebrospinal fluid macrophage cytotoxicity: *in vitro* and *in vivo* correlation. *Infect Immun* 1988;56:849–854.
65. Marquis G, Montplaisir S, Pelletier M. Genetic resistance to murine cryptococcosis: the beige mutation (Hediak–Higashi syndrome) in mice. *Infect Immun* 1985;47:288–293.
66. Cauley LK, Murphy JW. Response of congenital athymic (nude) and phenotypically normal mice to *Cryptococcus neoformans* infection. *Infect Immun* 1979;23:644–651.
67. Diamond RD, May JE, Kane MA. The role of the classical and alternative complement pathways in host defense against *Cryptococcus neoformans* infection. *J Immunol* 1974;112:2260–2270.
68. Graybill JR, Hague M, Drutz DL. Passive immunization in murine cryptococcosis. *Sabouraudia* 1981;19:237–244.
69. Louria DB, Kaminski T. Passively-acquired immunity in experimental cryptococcosis. *Sabouraudia* 1965;4:80–84.
70. Diamond RD, Allison AC. Nature of the effector cells responsible for antibody-dependent cell-mediated killing of *Cryptococcus neoformans*. *Infect Immun* 1976;14:716–720.
71. Miller GPG, Kohl S. Antibody-dependent leukocyte killing of *Cryptococcus neoformans*. *J Immunol* 1983;131:1455–1459.
72. Diamond RD, Bennett JE. Prognostic factors in cryptococcal meningitis. A study of 111 cases. *Ann Intern Med* 1974;80:176–181.
73. Perfect JR, Lang DR, Durack DT. Influence of agglutinating antibody in experimental cryptococcal meningitis. *Br J Exp Pathol* 1981;62:595–599.
74. Porter KG, Sinnamon DG, Gillies RR. *Cryptococcus neoformans*—special oligoclonal immunoglobulins in cerebrospinal fluid in cryptococcal meningitis. *Lancet* 1977;1:1262–1262.
75. Lamantia L, Salmaggi A, Tajoli L, et al. Cryptococcal meningoencephalitis: intrathecal immunological response. *J Neurol* 1986;233:362–366.
76. Hobbs MM, Perfect JR, Granger DL, Durack DT. Opsonic activity of cerebrospinal fluid in experimental cryptococcal meningitis. *Infect Immun* 1990;58:2115–2119.
77. Gupton S, Ellis M, Cesario T, Ruhling M, Vayuvegula B. Disseminated cryptococcal infection in a patient with hypogamma-globulinemia and normal T cell functions. *Am J Med* 1987;82:129–131.
78. Perfect JR, Lang SDR, Durack DT. Chronic cryptococcal meningitis: a new experimental model in rabbits. *Am J Pathol* 1980;101:177–194.
79. Perfect JR, Durack DT. Chemotactic activity of cerebrospinal fluid in experimental cryptococcal meningitis. *Sabouraudia* 1985;23:37–46.
80. Perfect JR, Durack DT. Effects of cyclosporine in experimental cryptococcal meningitis. *Infect Immun* 1985;50:22–26.
81. Kovacs JA, Kovacs AA, Polis M, et al. Cryptococcosis in the acquired immunodeficiency syndrome. *Ann Intern Med* 1985;103:533–538.
82. Zuger A, Louie E, Holzman RS. Cryptococcal disease in patients

with acquired immunodeficiency syndrome. *Ann Intern Med* 1986;104:234–240.

83. Eng RH, Bishburg E, Smith SM. Cryptococcal infections in patients with acquired immune deficiency syndrome. *Am J Med* 1986;81:19–23.

84. Chuck SL, Sande MA. Infections with *Cryptococcus neoformans* in the acquired immunodeficiency syndrome. *N Engl J Med* 1989;321:794–799.

85. Levy RM, Bredesen DB, Rosenblum MC. Neurological manifestations of the acquired immunodeficiency syndrome (AIDS): experience at UCSF and review of the literature. *J Neursurg* 1985;62:475–495.

86. Grant IH, Armstrong D. Fungal infections in AIDS. Cryptococcosis. *Infect Dis Clin North Am* 1988;2:457–464.

87. Weink T, Rogler G, Sixt C, et al. Cryptococcosis in AIDS patients: observations concerning CNS involvement. *J Neurol* 1989;236:38–42.

88. Catanzaro A, Spitler LE, Moser KM. Cellular immune response in coccidioidomycosis. *Cell Immunol* 1975;15:360–371.

89. Bronnimann DA, Adam RD, Galgiani JN, et al. Coccidioidomycosis in the acquired immunodeficiency syndrome. *Ann Intern Med* 1987;106:372–379.

90. Stevens DA. The interface of mycology and endocrinology. *J Med Vet Mycol* 1989;27:133–140.

91. Wheat LJ, Slama TG, Zeckel ML. Histoplasmosis in the acquired immune deficiency syndrome. *Am J Med* 1985;78:203–210.

92. Couch JR, Abdou NI, Sagava A. *Histoplasma* meningitis with hyperactive suppressor T cells in cerebrospinal fluid. *Neurology* 1976;28:119–123.

93. Pappas PG, Pottage JL, Topper ML, et al. Blastomycosis in AIDS patients. *Interscience Conf Antimicrob Agents Chemother* 1990;30:1166.

94. Roos KL, Bryan JP, Maggio WW. Intracranial blastomycoma. *Medicine* 1987;66:224–235.

95. Lipstein-Kresch E, Isenberg HD, Singer C, Cooke O, Greenwald RA. Disseminated *Sporothrix schenkii* infection with arthritis in a patient with acquired immunodeficiency syndrome. *J Rheumatol* 1985;12:805–808.

96. Steinberg GK, Britt RH, Enzmann DR. *Fusarium* brain abscess. Case report. *J Neursurg* 1983;58:598–601.

97. Oleske J, Minnefor A, Cooper R, et al. Immune deficiency syndrome in children. *JAMA* 1983;249:2345–2349.

98. Cohen MS, Isturiz RE, Malech HL, et al. Fungal infection in chronic granulomatous disease. *Am J Med* 1981;71:59–66.

99. Fleischmann J, Church JA, Lehrer RI. Case report: Primary *Candida* meningitis and chronic granulomatous disease. *Am J Med Sci* 1900;291:334–341.

100. Smego RA, Devoe PW, Sampson HA, Perfect JR, Wilfert CM, Buckley RH. *Candida* meningitis in two children with severe combined immunodeficiency. *J Pediatr* 1984;104:902–904.

101. Smego RA, Perfect JR, Durack DT. Combined therapy with amphotericin B and 5-fluorocytosine for *Candida* meningitis. *Rev Infect Dis* 1984;6:791–801.

102. Gerson SL, Talbot GH, Hurwitz S, Strom BL, Lusk EJ, Cassileth PA. Prolonged granulocytopenia: the major risk factor for invasive pulmonary *Aspergillus* in patients with acute leukemia. *Ann Intern Med* 1984;100:345–351.

103. Kathary MH, Chase T Jr, MacMillan JD. Correlation of elastase production by some strains of *Aspergillus fumigatus* with ability to cause pulmonary invasive *Aspergillus* in mice. *Infect Immun* 1984;43:320–325.

104. Mullbacher A, Eichner RD. Immunosuppression *in vitro* by a metabolite of a human pathogenic fungus. *Proc Natl Acad Sci* 1984;81:3835–3837.

105. Washburn RG, Hammer CH, Bennett JE. Inhibition of complement by culture supernatants of *Aspergillus fumigatus*. *J Infect Dis* 1986;154:944–951.

106. Windus DW, Stokes TJ, Julian BA, Fenves AZ. Fatal rhizopus infections in hemodialysis patients receiving deferoxamine. *Ann Intern Med* 1987;107:678–680.

Infections of the Central Nervous System,
edited by W. M. Scheld, R. J. Whitley, and
D. T. Durack, Raven Press, Ltd., New York © 1991.

CHAPTER 30

Chronic Meningitis

Tarvez Tucker and Jerrold J. Ellner

The relatively uniform clinical picture of chronic meningitis belies the diversity of its causes. Patients present with a distinctive syndrome: subacute onset of headache, fever, and stiff neck, often associated with signs of encephalitis such as confusion, disorientation, or lethargy. Cerebrospinal fluid (CSF) is abnormal, with pleocytosis (usually lymphocytic), elevated protein, and, on occasion, moderately low glucose. Some authors (1,2) define chronic meningitis as the persistence of these signs and symptoms with abnormal CSF for at least 4 weeks. In practice, however, the initial evaluation of the patient usually occurs before 4 weeks; important therapeutic decisions need to be made well before the patient reaches this empirical deadline.

The diagnosis of chronic meningitis warrants a thorough attempt to establish the underlying cause (Table 1) (1,3). The history is key: Chronic meningitis must be distinguished from recurrent meningitis in which acute exacerbations are separated by disease-free intervals. Recurrent meningitis usually does not represent an infectious disease; but it may indicate a congenital or acquired dural defect, or a parameningeal focus repeatedly discharging into the subarachnoid space (4). In the acquired immunodeficiency syndrome (AIDS) era, recognition that a patient is from a group at high risk of infection with human immunodeficiency virus (HIV) shifts the differential diagnosis of central nervous system (CNS) infection; therefore, chronic meningitis in HIV-infected patients must be considered separately.

Very little in the neurological presentation, history, or CSF formula clearly distinguishes the various causes of subacute or chronic meningitis. Rarely, a decisive historical clue or physical finding may be diagnostic. For example, a tick bite followed by erythema chronicum mi-

grans, then followed by meningitis, allows the clinical diagnosis of Lyme disease. Ophthalmological examination in a patient with subacute meningitis may reveal uveitis or granulomatous periphlebitis suggestive of sarcoidosis. These situations are exceptional. Most often, physicians are faced with a clinical picture typical of chronic meningitis without clear-cut clues from the medical history or physical examination as to the cause of the meningitis.

Whereas infection may be the first diagnostic consideration, particularly because of a natural focus on potentially treatable causes, noninfectious entities may present with a similar clinical and CSF picture. Two examples are systemic lupus erythematosus and subarachnoid hemorrhage. Therefore, algorithms for the diagnosis of chronic meningitis are difficult to formulate, and they need to rely on the absence of diagnostic clues as well as their presence. Certain diseases may be excluded by the lack of exposure to the infectious agent. For example, histoplasmosis is uncommon in the rural plains states. The absence of associated physical findings, such as a characteristic rash in Lyme disease or pulmonary infection in tuberculosis, can provide some diagnostic guidance. Demographics are only helpful on rare occasions. Granulomatous angiitis, for example, would be unlikely to occur in an individual older than 70 years or in a patient with a completely normal mental status. CSF parameters can also be used to exclude this diagnosis if the spinal fluid protein is normal or if there are large numbers of cells.

Some forms of chronic meningitis associated with systemic disease may occur in the absence of extraneural manifestations of these diseases. For example, tuberculous infection of the CNS may occur without chest x-ray abnormalities, tuberculin skin test reactivity, or positive AFB stains or cultures from blood, sputum, or other body fluids. Sarcoidosis can present with neurological manifestations (e.g., hypothalamic dysfunction) as its

T. Tucker and J. J. Ellner: Department of Neurology and Medicine, University Hospitals of Cleveland, Case Western Reserve University, Cleveland, Ohio 44106.

TABLE 1. *Relatively common causes of chronic meningitis*[a]

Infectious	Noninfectious
Mycobacterium tuberculosis	Carcinoma
Cryptococcus neoformans	Sarcoid
Treponema pallidum	Granulomatous angiitis
Coccidioides immitis	Systemic lupus erythmatosus
Histoplasma capsulatum	Behcet's disease
Borrelia burgdorferi	Vogt–Koyanagi–Harada syndrome

[a] In the non-AIDS patient, exposure history may greatly increase likelihood of parasitic infection (e.g., cysticercosis).

sole manifestation. Similarly, the symptoms of carcinomatous meningitis may precede the diagnosis of the primary cancer by weeks to months.

Some organization in the approach to a patient with chronic meningitis is helpful. First, do features of encephalitis accompany the signs and symptoms of meningitis? Certain infectious agents such as *Cysticercus* and *Toxoplasma* can present with a clinical picture of meningoencephalitis. On the other hand, alteration of consciousness in the absence of increased intracranial pressure is less common with specific fungal agents such as *Cryptococcus* or *Histoplasma* and is usually not found with spirochetal infections such as Lyme disease. Diseases which affect the basilar meninges, causing raised intracra-

nial pressure, hydrocephalus, and cranial neuropathy, include sarcoidosis and tuberculosis as well as some of the fungal meningitides. These conditions may present with alteration of mental status, ataxia, and nausea and vomiting in addition to headache and meningeal signs.

Involvement of specific cranial nerves can be helpful diagnostically. Oculomotor palsies or eighth-nerve dysfunction suggest granulomatous or inflammatory processes affecting the basilar meninges such as tuberculosis, sarcoidosis, fungal infections, or syphilis. In contrast, despite the basilar clustering of cysts in cysticercosis, this parasitic infection rarely presents as the racemose form with associated cranial nerve palsies. Some processes show a predilection for involvement of specific cranial nerves—for example, VII, VIII, and II in syphilis, VII in sarcoidosis. Unfortunately, however, even these physical findings can be misleading, because nonlocalizing sixth-nerve palsies may occur as a result of elevations of cerebral pressure due to causes other than direct infection, such as parameningeal foci of infection or hydrocephalus.

On rare occasions, the neurological clinical picture can be characteristic of one diagnosis. For example, leptomeningeal carcinomatosis frequently presents with a constellation of neurological signs and symptoms implicating multiple areas of involvement of the neuraxis: cranial nerves, nerve roots, and long tract signs. Few in-

TABLE 2. *CSF formula in chronic meningitis and related syndromes*[a]

Lymphocytic low-glucose:	<50–100 WBCs[b]:	Carcinoma
		Sarcoidosis
		Subarachnoid hemorrhage
	50–500 WBCs:	Tuberculosis
		Fungal
		Syphilis
		Parasitic (toxoplasmosis, cysticercosis)
		Viral (lymphocytic choriomeningitis, mumps meningoencephalitis)
Lymphocytic normal-glucose:	<50–100 WBCs[b]:	Sarcoidosis
		Chronic benign lymphocytic meningitis
		Vasculitis
		Intracranial mass lesions
		Multiple sclerosis
	50–500 WBCs:	Most fungal, viral, and parasitic infections
		Chemical meningitis
Pleocytosis with neutrophilic predominance:		Bacteria (*Nocardia, Actinomyces, Brucella*)
		Fungi (*Blastomyces, Coccidioides, Aspergillus, Zygomycetes, Cladosporium, Pseudoallescheria*)
		Systemic lupus erythematosus
		Chemical meningitis
		Discharge from epidermoid tumors or craniopharyngioma
		Intrathecal drugs, contrast agents
Pleocytosis with eosinophilic predominance:		Hodgkin's disease
		Parasites (*Angiostrongylus cantonensis, Cysticercus, Gnathostoma spinigerum*)
		Tuberculosis
		Coccidioides
		Chemical meningitis (e.g., ibuprofen, foreign bodies)

[a] Note that categorization is based on the typical cerebrospinal fluid (CSF) findings. Exceptions may occur.
[b] Usually <50; occasionally 50–100. WBCs, white blood cells.

fectious agents produce this characteristic clinical picture, and thus the correct diagnosis may be suggested even before confirmation by lumbar puncture.

It is helpful to organize CSF findings in chronic meningitis into three categories: lymphocytic low-glucose, lymphocytic normal-glucose (5), and pleocytosis with neutrophilic or eosinophilic predominance (5–8) (Table 2). Further subdivisions can be made according to the number of leukocytes. Patterns of CSF abnormalities are particularly helpful in approaching the patient with undiagnosed disease, as discussed below.

APPROACH TO THE PATIENT

The history, physical examination, and laboratory data may (a) focus the differential diagnosis around a few of the myriad of disease processes which can cause chronic meningitis, (b) indicate an extraneural site for biopsy which will have a high diagnostic yield, or (c) provide support for a therapeutic trial.

History

The travel and exposure history may suggest exposure to an infectious agent which is restricted in its geographic distribution. For example, *Histoplasma capsulatum* and *Blastomyces dermatiditis* are endemic in the Mississippi and Ohio River valleys. At least in the case of *Histoplasma*, latent foci of infection may reactivate years after the patient leaves the endemic area, particularly if immunosuppression supervenes. In the United States, *Coccidiodes immitis* is endemic in certain semi-arid areas of the Southwest. Similarly, areas of endemicity exist for fungi in other areas of the world. Point-source outbreaks of fungal infection also can occur if there is exposure to heavily contaminated environmental sources; a recent example is an epidemic of blastomycosis after exposure at a beaver pond in Wisconsin (9). The occurrence of Lyme disease is largely determined by the range of the tick vector. Although most Lyme disease occurs in the northeastern United States, sporadic cases have been reported in most geographic areas. Lyme disease is unique among causes of chronic meningitis in its seasonal occurrence; the peak prevalence in late summer and early fall reflects tick activity. Cysticercosis is endemic in Mexico and South America, and its occurrence in the United States is virtually restricted to immigrants from these areas.

Exposure history is important for other infectious agents, as well. Person-to-person spread occurs in tuberculosis. Most helpful is a history of a case of pulmonary tuberculosis in the household. Given the natural history of tuberculosis, the initial exposure may have occurred years previously. A history of previous tuberculo-

sis (particularly if not treated adequately) or of known positive tuberculin skin test reaction likewise provides a background for reactivation. *Brucella* infection follows ingestion of unpasteurized milk or dairy products. *Angiostrongylus cantonensis* is a common cause of eosinophilic meningitis (which may be chronic) in humans living in endemic areas in the Far East who ingest raw or undercooked mollusks or contaminated vegetables.

The history also may reveal antecedent systemic manifestations of the disease process currently involving the CNS; in fact, the systemic disease may have been diagnosed previously. Polyarthritis and pleuritis may represent systemic lupus erythematosus. Penile lesions, uveitis, and arthritis may anticipate CNS involvement with Behcet's syndrome. Previous genital lesions, usually long forgotten, may have represented the primary manifestation of syphilis. Skin rash may be a harbinger of CNS involvement in Lyme disease or syphilis. The prior diagnosis of lymphoma, adenocarcinoma, or malignant melanoma is a special case in point. The current disease may represent spread of the tumor, an opportunistic infection, or, where relevant, a chemical reaction to intrathecal drug administration. History of an opportunistic infection, Kaposi's sarcoma, or lymphoma also may indicate that a patient is infected with HIV, whether or not the individual admits to belonging to an at-risk group.

Physical Examination

Findings on physical examination generally are nonspecific. They may be more helpful in identifying a site for biopsy than in directly suggesting a diagnosis (Fig. 1). An exception is the rash of erythema chronicum migrans (ECM) in the patient with Lyme disease. Depigmentary choroidal tubercles are found in tuberculosis and sarcoidosis; uveitis also may be seen in Behcet's disease and Vogt–Koyanagi–Harada (VKH) syndrome, which are described below. Depigmentation of the skin and hair (vitiligo, poliosis) is the sine qua non of VKH syndrome. A skin rash consisting of macular-hyperpigmented lesions and also involving the palms and soles may be a manifestation of secondary syphilis. Sarcoidosis and disseminated mycoses may present with skin lesions. Most helpful diagnostically are subcutaneous nodules, abscesses, draining sinuses, or ulcerative lesions, as seen (for example) in blastomycosis. Palatal and other lesions involving the oral mucosa are sometimes found in histoplasmosis.

Lymphadenopathy, either generalized or regional, may provide a useful target for biopsy. The yield is greater if the involved nodes are large (>1.5–2.0 cm), abnormally firm or hard in consistency, noninguinal, and asymmetric. Adenopathy can be seen in most systemic diseases which cause chronic meningitis. The pres-

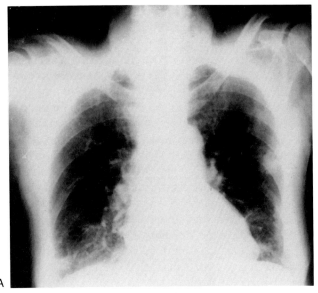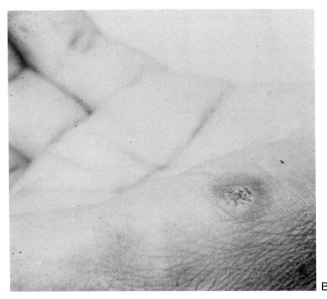

FIG. 1. Chest x-ray (**A**) and skin lesion (**B**) of a 73-year-old woman treated for chronic lymphocytic leukemia with corticosteroids and cytotoxic drugs. She presented with nodular pulmonary infiltrates and chronic meningitis. The diagnosis of cryptococcal meningitis was established by aspiration of the skin lesion, which revealed encapsulated yeast on India ink preparation. (From ref. 1, with permission.)

ence of hepatomegaly or hepatosplenomegaly also is a helpful finding; the yield of liver biopsy is likely to be higher if the liver is enlarged and the serum alkaline phosphatase is increased.

Laboratory Data

Certain laboratory tests and radiographic procedures should be performed routinely in patients with chronic meningitis. In addition to a complete blood count and serum chemistries, antinuclear antibody and antibody to HIV should be determined.

Cryptococcal polysaccharide antigen should be measured in serum and CSF of all patients. Serologic tests for *Brucella, Toxoplasma,* and HIV, as well as those for serum and CSF antibody titers against *Histoplasma* and *Coccidioides* must be obtained in the appropriate settings. All patients should have serologic tests for syphilis as well as determination of CSF-VDRL. *Coccidioides* and *Histoplasma* antibody determinations are particularly germane in individuals at risk of disease—that is, those who are, or who have been, living in geographic areas of high endemicity. *Brucella* requires the appropriate exposure, and *Toxoplasma* is more likely to occur in the immunocompromised host. Although the presence of IgM antibodies or high or increasing titers of IgG antibody to a specific agent supports the diagnosis, problems exist in terms of specificity and sensitivity. For example, CSF complement-fixing antibodies to *Histoplasma* are found in 25–50% of other fungal meningitides (10).

Some experimental tests which are neither widely available nor standardized for routine use can nonetheless have diagnostic value in individual cases. Most of these can be performed by special arrangement with an investigator working in the field. Most promising is the detection of *H. capsulatum* antigen in serum, urine, or CSF by radioimmunoassay (10). The yield is particularly high in immunocompromised patients (11). Tuberculostearic acid in CSF may be indicative of tuberculous meningitis (12). Many, if not most, infectious causes of chronic meningitis also are associated with selective compartmentalization of antigen-responsive lymphocytes and antibody-forming cells in the subarachnoid space. The CSF/blood (or CSF/serum) ratio with regard to lymphocyte reactivity to antigens and antibody levels, therefore, may be of diagnostic use.

Spinal fluid examination is the single most important test for diagnosis of chronic meningitis. Lumbar puncture should be repeated often enough to ensure adequate material for culture and cytologies and to follow the course of meningeal inflammation. India ink preparations of CSF are invaluable for the diagnosis of cryptococcal meningitis, particularly in immunosuppressed patients in whom yeast may outnumber white blood cells and/or when the presentation is acute to subacute. This test requires mixing India ink with the sediment of 3–5 ml of CSF; when the mixture is correct, newsprint can be read through the slide. The entire slide should be scanned under low-power, and suspicious areas should be viewed under high dry and oil-immersion lenses. Cryptococci appear as refractile yeasts, sometimes budding, with inclusions. The yeasts are surrounded by a large, round, regular capsule which is impermeable to ink particles (Fig. 2). At least three specimens of CSF for cytologic examination are necessary to assess the possibility of tumor. Staining of CSF lymphocytes with monoclonal antibodies also can be used to determine whether cells found in CSF are monoclonal, as in some lymphomas or leukemias.

Culture of CSF is the mainstay of diagnosis for infectious chronic meningitis. Cultures should be repeated at intervals until a diagnosis is achieved; the yield of microbes may improve with the passage of time. Samples should be cultured for bacteria, acid-fast bacilli, and fungi. Cultures of three samples of CSF should be adequate for the diagnosis of most bacteria and mycobacteria. Anaerobic culture conditions and increased CO_2 tension are necessary for *Actinomyces* and *Brucella*, respectively. Additional specimens should be cultured in their entirety for fungi. The yield from cultures containing few organisms can be improved by inoculating Sabouraud's agar layered on the bottom of Ehrlenmeyer flasks with large volumes of CSF. This allows culture for long periods while avoiding desiccation. It is appropriate to incubate fungal cultures for at least 4–6 weeks because growth of some organisms is exceedingly slow, particularly when the inoculum is low. The growth of even a single colony of an organism capable of causing chronic meningitis, such as *Sporothrix*, may be diagnostic (13).

Patients with chronic meningitis caused by tuberculosis, cryptococcosis, blastomycosis, or histoplasmosis frequently have occult disseminated disease. Therefore, even in the absence of signs of extraneural disease, it is useful to culture gastric washings, blood, sputum, and urine, and stool for mycobacteria and fungi. Biopsy speci-

mens should be obtained from skin lesions, and abnormal lymph nodes should they be detected on physical examination. In addition, biopsy of the bone marrow and liver are useful if tuberculosis, histoplasmosis, or other granulomatous disease is suspected. Biopsy specimens should be divided for culture and histology. Granulomas are an important finding in biopsies from several diseases associated with chronic meningitis. Demonstration of an acid-fast bacillus or yeast in a tissue may allow diagnosis, or at least support the initiation of specific therapy pending definitive cultures. The finding of granulomas with caseation is suggestive of tuberculosis, histoplasmosis, and coccidioidomycosis. Focal necrosis may be seen in brucellosis. Blastomycosis can produce a mixture of pyogenic and granulomatous inflammation.

If a craniotomy is to be performed for exploration of a mass lesion or to relieve symptomatic hydrocephalus, meningeal and brain biopsy specimens (and, if possible, a sample of ventricular fluid) should be obtained (see below).

Skin testing should include assessment of tuberculin reactivity and reactivity to an anergy panel. The presence of reactivity to intermediate-strength purified protein derivative (PPD) indicates that an individual is infected with *Mycobacterium tuberculosis,* thus increasing the likelihood that the chronic meningitis is tuberculous. A negative tuberculin skin test does not exclude tuberculous meningitis because up to 35% of patients with tuberculous meningitis will be nonreactive, often in the setting of generalized anergy. If the initial tuberculin skin test is nonreactive, the testing should be repeated after 2

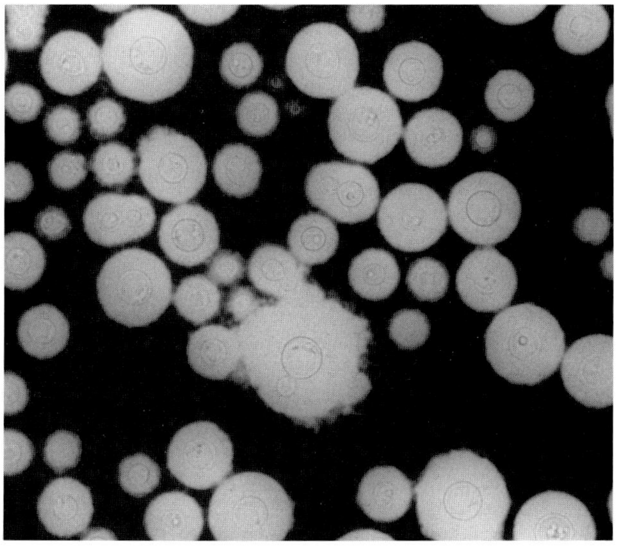

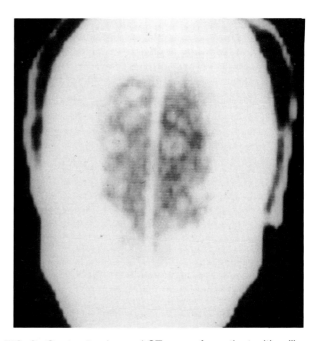

FIG. 2. India ink preparation of CSF showing many cryptococci. Encapsulated yeast cells far outnumber white blood cells, typical of an immunosuppressed patient with cryptococcal meningitis. Some yeast cells show budding.

FIG. 3. Contrast-enhanced CT scan of a patient with miliary tuberculosis, showing multiple contrast-enhancing areas indicative of granulomatous lesions.

weeks. Many anergic patients with tuberculosis will later develop positive skin tests, after antituberculous therapy has been instituted.

Computerized axial tomography (CT) scanning or magnetic resonance imaging (MRI) should be performed before lumbar puncture in all patients with chronic meningitis. Mass lesions, including brain abscesses, may present with a clinical picture identical to that of chronic meningitis. Nonspecific findings in chronic meningitis may be present, such as contrast enhancement over the convexities; the basilar cisterns may also be obscured by inflammatory cells. More helpful is the finding of contrast enhancement of granulomatous lesions (Fig. 3) or larger parenchymal lesions. CAT scanning also may show cerebral infarction due to vasculitis, or it may show hydrocephalus. Hydrocephalus is potentially reversible with treatment of the chronic meningitis, and thus its presence per se does not constitute a sufficient indication for surgery.

AN ALGORITHM FOR ENIGMATIC CASES

Not infrequently the clinician must choose between invasive diagnostic techniques (such as meningeal biopsy) and a therapeutic trial prior to obtaining a specific diagnosis. The need for such a choice may be prompted by clinical deterioration or serious functional impairment early in the course before the results of cultures and serologies are available or after the initial tests have proven negative.

Although it is difficult to generalize, certain principles may be useful in approaching the individual patient. Sometimes the history, physical examination, and laboratory data allow a presumptive clinical diagnosis. Treatment of the entity, if treatment exists, can be instituted pending confirmatory tests. The decision regarding whether to begin empirical therapy or perform invasive diagnostic tests in an attempt to establish a definitive diagnosis depends on the certainty of the clinical diagnosis, the severity of the illness, and the potential toxicity of the empirical therapy. If the presentation is suggestive of Lyme disease or brucellosis, for example, a therapeutic trial of ceftriaxone or daxycycline plus rifampin, respectively, is appropriate unless the patient is so ill that death seems likely should the diagnosis be wrong.

Algorithms for patient management can be constructed on the basis of the CSF formula (Table 2). If the pleocytosis is predominantly lymphocytic with 50–500 cells and the CSF glucose is depressed or normal, an infectious disease is extremely likely. Should a positive tuberculin skin test support the diagnosis of tuberculosis, empirical treatment is appropriate pending the outcome of cultures.

Should the tuberculin skin test be negative, it is appropriate to start antituberculous drugs and to measure cryptococcal polysaccharide antigen and various anti-

bodies in serum and CSF. Concurrently, however, arrangements should be made for additional diagnostic procedures to be performed. This should consist of cerebral angiography if vasculitis seems a reasonable possibility, followed by a meningeal biopsy (Fig. 4), possibly with aspiration of ventricular fluid for culture. Ventricular fluid may have a higher cultural yield than does lumbar CSF. Fungal meningitis is quite likely in this setting; and *Histoplasma, Blastomyces,* and *Sporothrix* typically cause chronic meningitis in which lumbar CSF is culture-negative (13,14). Untreated, fungal meningitis may progress to irreversible disease in a rapid and unpredictable fashion. Therefore, observing the patient for a response to antituberculous drugs is not an acceptable plan unless a biopsy procedure is contraindicated, perhaps because of bleeding diathesis, the patient's age, or underlying disease.

If the pleocytosis is predominantly lymphocytic but is lower grade (<50 cells), infectious disease is less likely. Furthermore, some such patients will have a benign course and improve spontaneously (15). In such a case, the impetus for meningeal biopsy is lessened by the dearth of treatable causes of chronic meningitis. Certainly, biopsy should be delayed until the results of cytologies, serologies, and cultures are available.

Empirical treatment with corticosteroids is not indicated because of its potential deleterious effects on unsuspected tuberculous or fungal meningitis. Empirical treatment with antifungal drugs is rarely indicated because of its toxicity and also because of uncertainty with regard to dose, duration, and route of administration in the absence of a defined infectious agent.

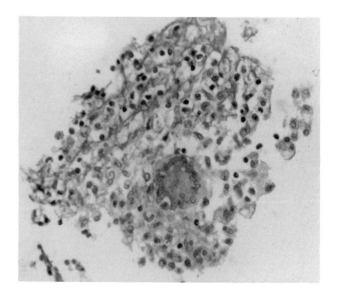

FIG. 4. Meningeal biopsy in a patient with cryptococcal meningitis. A multinucleated giant cell is present in a poorly defined granuloma. Periodic acid–Schiff stain demonstrated cryptococci in the biopsy specimen. Meningeal biopsy is still required for diagnosis in some patients with cryptococcal disease.

CHRONIC MENINGITIS IN THE IMMUNOCOMPROMISED PATIENT

CNS infection in immunosuppressed patients is increasing in importance (16). The number of immunocompromised patients is rising because of the AIDS epidemic and also because of increasingly sophisticated treatments which prolong survival in patients with cancer and autoimmune disease. The widespread use of immunosuppressive and radiation therapy for transplant recipients and cancer patients has created a large pool of patients at risk. Development of a CNS infection in a chronically immunosuppressed individual significantly worsens the prognosis, independent of the underlying diseases. In one recent series from the Massachusetts General Hospital, 30 of 49 patients died as a result of their CNS infection, in contrast to the otherwise good prognosis in 41 of these 49 immunocompromised patients (16).

Several factors make the recognition and management of chronic meningitis in the immunocompromised patient difficult:

1. Some patients, particularly transplant recipients and those with HIV infection, may develop simultaneous infections with more than one organism. Ring-enhancing lesions on cerebral CT scan in an HIV-positive individual may be due to simultaneous toxoplasmosis and cryptococcoma and/or *Candida* abscess, for example. In a large series at the University of California at San Francisco, 30% of patients with more than one abscess on cerebral CT scan were infected with organisms other than, or in addition to, toxoplasmosis (17). In addition, the same patient may have sequential infections with different infectious agents at different times.

2. The clinical manifestations of chronic infection of the nervous system differ in the immunosuppressed patient because the immune response is altered. The suspicion of infection must remain high despite the absence of clinical signs of meningitis such as meningeal irritation, fever, neck pain, or headache. Prompt diagnosis of meningeal infection in the immunocompromised patient can prolong useful survival. The CSF profile in cryptococcal meningitis in the immune competent patient is likely to be markedly abnormal with elevated protein, lymphocytic pleocytosis, and, at times, lowered glucose. In contrast, however, immunosuppressed patients, particularly those infected with HIV, are less likely to have abnormal CSF white blood cell counts or chemistries. Both groups of patients will, however, have abnormal specific tests such as cryptococcal antigen and culture. As another example, the *Toxoplasma* abscess in the immunocompromised patient may show less of a surrounding inflammatory reaction on histopathological examination, reflecting a diminished immune reaction to the organism.

3. The pathogenesis of chronic infection in this population may be altered by cofactors that may affect an individual's predisposition to a particular disease. For example, attention has focused on the role of other viruses in altering immune response and activation of HIV. Both cytomegalovirus and Epstein–Barr virus have been implicated in activating HIV from its latent state to a state in which transcription and protein synthesis may proceed, fostering replication of the virus. The replicative cycle of HIV is restricted at the DNA-integration stage into the host genome until the cell is activated by mitogenic, allogeneic, or antigenic stimulation (18). Semen, blood, or factor VIII transfusions may result in allogeneic stimulation. Antecedent exposure to other viruses, such as cytomegalovirus or herpes simplex virus, may provide antigenic stimulation, augmenting the expression of HIV replication.

4. Immunocompromised patients are susceptible to infection with organisms that normally do not cause disease in the immune competent host. Yet, susceptibility is selective: Within disparate groups of immunocompromised patients, the frequency of particular opportunistic infections varies. For example, *Listeria* and *Pseudomonas* are two important CNS bacterial pathogens for the CNS in patients with cancer or following organ transplantation. Yet, these agents rarely cause infection in AIDS. Instead, a disproportionate number of patients in the HIV-seropositive population are infected by *Toxoplasma* or *Pneumocystis carinii* or develop progressive multifocal leukoencephalopathy. Fungal infections also vary according to the host. Cryptococcus is seen in both AIDS and non AIDS groups of immunosuppressed patients. Yet, *Nocardia* and *Aspergillus* infections, prevalent in iatrogenically immunosuppressed patients, are uncommon in AIDS.

The basis for the selective susceptibility of patients with AIDS to certain infections is not yet known. Susceptibility to *Pneumocystis* infection may be explained in part by the predilection of HIV for the alveolar macrophage. The macrophage is relatively refractory to HIV-induced syncytia formation (18), a process which is lethal to infected lymphocytes. Therefore, macrophages may serve as a reservoir for viral persistence in the CNS. The specific vulnerability of tissues such as the lung and brain to opportunistic infections in AIDS may be explained by the characteristics of the macrophages which are specific to these tissues. For example, Kupffer cells are not targeted by HIV, perhaps because these liver macrophages do not transcribe viral RNA (19).

Chronic Meningitis in HIV Infection

Aseptic Meningitis

A self-limited syndrome of acute meningitis or meningoencephalitis may occur early after infection with HIV, at about the time of seroconversion. Acute HIV meningitis has been called "atypical" because it frequently is accompanied by long tract signs and cranial nerve deficits. On rare occasions, meningitis can persist or recur. Patients will periodically manifest headache and fever with mild CSF pleocytosis over a period of months after the onset of symptoms. Early invasion of the CNS by HIV is supported by recovery of this retrovirus from CSF in patients with atypical meningitis, as well as by the measurement of HIV-specific intrathecal antibody synthesis in neurologically asymptomatic HIV-seropositive patients (20–22).

Cryptococcal Meningitis

Cryptococcus neoformans is the third most common infectious agent that causes neurological disease in patients with AIDS, following HIV itself and *Toxoplasma gondii*. This yeast is the most frequent fungal infection of the CNS in AIDS.

Cryptococcal meningitis serves as an example of how an altered immune response may subdue the clinical presentation of infection. Cryptococcal meningitis may present in AIDS patients with nonspecific symptoms such as headache or lethargy alone. Although fever is common, meningeal signs occur only in a minority of patients. Stiff neck and photophobia are often absent. Similarly, the CSF is less likely to be abnormal in AIDS patients with cryptococcal meningitis than in the immunocompetent host. In the majority of patients in two recent series (23,24), the CSF white blood cell count was less than 5 per cubic millimeter. Modest protein elevations were seen; however, the glucose was greater than 40 mg/dl in most cases. In a small number of patients in both series, all CSF parameters were normal.

Fortunately, however, specific tests for *Cryptococcus*, such as culture and cryptococcal antigen, are positive in the CSF in AIDS patients. Cryptococcal antigen titer was greater than 1:8 in all 16 patients in the Kovacs et al. (23) series, and in 20 of 22 patients in the series by Zuger et al. (25). Serum cryptococcal antigen is often markedly elevated, with a median titer of 1:400 in all 21 patients in the Dismukes (24) study. In one study, the serum antigen test was slightly more sensitive than CSF titers in diagnosing cryptococcal meningitis (26).

Relapse rates and therapeutic failures following administration of amphotericin B, either alone or in combination with flucytosine, unfortunately are high. The initial response to amphotericin B is favorable in only about 58% of cases, and sustained clinical improvement occurs in only 20% (27). A recent study (26) has shown that two factors are predictors of shorter survival in cryptococcal meningitis: positive cultures of extrameningeal specimens for cryptococcus and serum hyponatremia. This same study showed no increased survival in patients treated with amphotericin plus flucytosine versus those patients treated with amphotericin alone. Long-term suppressive treatment with ketoconazole or amphotericin, although not always effective in preventing relapse, did improve overall survival. Long-term maintenance therapy with amphotericin B is usually necessary, and both amphotericin and flucytosine have dose-limiting side effects (26). In particular, leukopenia and thrombocytopenia limit flucytosine's usefulness. There is some evidence that cryptococcal antigen titers greater than 1:8 after therapy are associated with a higher relapse rate and worse prognosis (24), although other investigators have not confirmed this (26).

Early experience with fluconazole, a new oral triazole antifungal agent, shows favorable results as both initial treatment and suppressive therapy (28–30). Fluconazole CSF levels are 70–80% of simultaneous serum levels (31).

Toxoplasma Meningoencephalitis

Toxoplasma gondii, an intracellular protozoan, infects the brain of AIDS patients with striking frequency. It is the most commonly encountered neurological opportunistic infection, affecting up to 30% of AIDS patients who have antibodies to *T. gondii* (17,32). Because most adults in the United States have antibodies to this protozoan, indicating prior exposure, and because *Toxoplasma* encephalitis is rare in children with HIV infection, it is assumed that cerebral toxoplasmosis in the HIV-infected adult population represents reactivation of latent primary infection.

Cerebral toxoplasmosis generally presents focally with hemiparesis, aphasia, hemisensory loss, homonymous hemianopia, cranial nerve palsies, or seizures developing in a subacute course over days to weeks (32–34). Headache and mental status changes are frequent. Less commonly, *Toxoplasma* meningoencephalitis may present as a diffuse chronic meningitis with confusion, memory loss, lethargy, and cognitive decline indistinguishable from the AIDS dementia complex or other indolent causes of chronic meningitis in these immunocompromised patients.

CT scans show hypodense contrast-enhancing lesions with a predilection for the basal ganglia, the gray–white junction of the cerebral hemispheres, and the cerebellum. Ring enhancement of these lesions is characteristic, but not invariable. Magnetic resonance imaging (MRI) is more sensitive than CT in detecting the abscesses caused by toxoplasmosis, and multiple lesions may be seen on MRI scans when CT scans show only a solitary abscess (35). It is important, however, to recognize that multiple lesions may be due to multiple pathogens (33). Improvement in CT or MRI scans occurs with therapy, but may lag significantly behind clinical response. Steroids, given in addition to chemotherapy, may reduce edema surrounding cerebral *Toxoplasma* abscesses but are recommended with caution in this immunosuppressed population.

Information on CSF abnormalities in HIV-associated cerebral toxoplasmosis is limited because lumbar puncture is not performed routinely in the presence of a focal neurological examination or in the presence of mass lesions on CT or MRI scanning. Infrequently, *Toxoplasma* meningoencephalitis may present as a diffuse encephalopathy without localizing features, similar to the clinical picture of chronic meningitis due to other causes. CSF protein usually is mildly elevated, and there is a mononuclear pleocytosis of mild degree (36). There is some controversy over the value of serologic studies in serum and CSF in AIDS patients with toxoplasmosis. Although negative IgG titers make the diagnosis of toxoplasmosis less likely (32), in general neither positive nor negative blood CSF serologies are diagnostic of active infection. Although intrathecal production of antibodies to *T. gondii* occurs in patients with *Toxoplasma* encephalitis (37), specific IgG may be undetectable in the CSF and serum in patients with biopsy- or autopsy-proven CNS toxoplasmosis. However, certainly most patients with *Toxoplasma* encephalitis have positive IgG antibodies. Conversely, IgM *Toxoplasma* antibodies are likely to be high in patients with AIDS from geographic areas with a high prevalence of *Toxoplasma* antibodies.

Some authors advocate biopsy of single or even multiple cerebral mass lesions because in these immunocompromised hosts, simultaneous infection by multiple organisms is common. However, even the least invasive stereotactic biopsies of mass lesions guided by CT or real-time ultrasonography impart a risk to AIDS patients frequently ill with systemic or pulmonary disease, and often with thrombocytopenia. Therefore, most physicians caring for AIDS patients in whom toxoplasmosis is a diagnostic consideration will begin an empirical course of therapy with pyrimethamine and sulfadiazine. Pyrimethamine is a dihydrofolate reductase inhibitor, and sulfadiazine inhibits dihydrofolate synthetase. These drugs block folic acid metabolism synergistically in the proliferative form of *T. gondii* (32). The cyst form of the organism, however, is not affected by these medications. Therefore, withdrawal of initial therapy frequently results in recurrences of *Toxoplasma* encephalitis, commonly in the same area of the brain initially affected. Support for an empirical trial of therapy is based upon the high prevalence of this infection in AIDS patients with CNS symptoms and appropriate radiographic lesions (38). Initial response to two-drug therapy occurs in up to 90% of patients (27). Clindamycin often is substituted for sulfadiazine, however, because of the latter drug's toxicity, commonly a drug-induced rash or leukopenia. Lifelong maintenance therapy with pyrimethamine, in combination with sulfadiazine or clindamycin,

is recommended after 6–8 weeks of full-dose therapy (39). If the patient does not improve clinically or radiographically after 1–2 weeks of empirical therapy, consideration should then be given to brain biopsy for diagnosis.

The finding of *Toxoplasma* cysts or tachyzoites on biopsy is diagnostic. The inflammatory response varies from focal granulomatous lesions of lymphocytic infiltrates with central areas of necrosis to a more diffuse necrotizing encephalitis (32). Immunohistochemical staining with the peroxidase–antiperoxidase method can demonstrate the *Toxoplasma* antigen and the organism itself.

Other Infections

Chronic meningitis in AIDS patients also can be caused by *Candida albicans, M. tuberculosis, Aspergillus fumigatus, H. capsulatum,* and *C. immitis.* There are no clinical indicators for these fungal infections, and diagnosis is made by CSF culture or serologies as discussed below. These organisms may be suspected if a patient presents with the clinical and CSF profiles of a chronic meningitis such as that caused by *Cryptococcus,* with negative cryptococcal antigen determinations in blood and CSF. Fortunately, the empirical therapy for all the fungal infections is the same—that is, amphotericin B. *Mycobacterium avium intracellulare* (MAI) is commonly found in nervous tissue at autopsy, but it is not felt to be pathogenic. Tuberculous meningitis and meningomyelitis in AIDS usually respond to drug therapy (40,41).

Neurosyphilis

Treponema pallidum infection may take a clinically aggressive course in HIV-seropositive persons (42). Early neurosyphilis, presenting in the meningitic and meningovascular forms, is seen with increased frequency in the HIV-positive population, presumably because of the defects in cell-mediated immunity caused by this retrovirus. Most patients with syphilis and AIDS die before the classic parenchymal forms of the disease, general paresis or tabes dorsalis, have a chance to develop.

There have been several reports of patients who have received recommended therapy for early syphilis with benzathine penicillin but who later developed neurosyphilis (43,44). Benzathine penicillin may not reach treponemicidal levels in the CSF. Thus recommendations for treatment of early forms of syphilis in the HIV-infected population have been changed. Although there is not full agreement on this subject at present, most authorities recommend higher doses of antibiotics for longer periods, as is recommended for neurosyphilis. Repeat CSF examinations with serologies may be necessary to assess whether or not treatment has been adequate. Differentiating true relapse from reinfection in this sexually active population may be difficult. However, in one case of presumed inadequate treatment, the peripheral blood VDRL titer remained at 1:8, identical to its lowest level following benzathine penicillin therapy, thus making reinfection unlikely (45).

Lymphomatous Meningitis

Non-Hodgkin's lymphoma as seen in the HIV-infected population can spread to the leptomeninges, causing a lymphomatous meningitis (46–48). Patients present with symptoms and signs referrable to many locations of the neuraxis. Multiple cranial neuropathies, spinal root radicular syndromes, and pyramidal tract signs signal the diagnosis (47). This neurological picture is quite characteristic of leptomeningeal spread of malignancy, and may in fact presage the diagnosis of systemic lymphoma, warranting a thorough search for this disease.

The CSF may show a modest lymphocytic pleocytosis with slightly elevated protein. A lowered glucose level in an individual with the constellation of signs described above and with risk factors for this malignancy should raise the suspicion of lymphomatous meningitis. Initial CSF cytology may be negative; the yield is improved by sending larger quantities of fluid at the time of repeat lumbar punctures. In some cases, when the fluid and clinical picture is suggestive of this diagnosis yet cytology is negative, the yield may be improved by obtaining CSF from a cisternal C1–C2 spinal puncture, particularly if cranial nerve palsies are present, suggesting basilar meningeal disease.

SPECIFIC CAUSES OF CHRONIC MENINGITIS

Now that the general approaches to the different categories of patients have been discussed, the more common causes of chronic meningitis will be reviewed. Consideration of the characteristic presentation of specific diseases is useful in the patient with a presumptive diagnosis to assist in assigning a relative likelihood to the entity under consideration. In the patient with a confirmed diagnosis, it will provide some guidance for treatment as well as for prognosis. Some of the infectious causes of chronic meningitis are considered elsewhere in this text; therefore the noninfectious diseases will receive particular attention in this section.

Tuberculous Meningitis

Tuberculous meningitis develops when a parameningeal tuberculous focus ruptures or leaks into the subarachnoid space (49). The result is the equivalent of an *in situ* delayed-type hypersensitivity reaction with exuda-

tion of protein and cells into the CSF. The occurrence of tuberculous meningitis requires antecedent tuberculous infection; the actual breakdown of the so-called Rich focus is, however, a chance event.

The age-specific prevalence of tuberculous meningitis parallels infection with *M. tuberculosis* in the population. Where tuberculosis is common, meningeal involvement usually occurs in children 3 months to 5 years of age, as a consequence of hematogenous spread and miliary disease representing progressive primary tuberculosis (50). Associated pulmonary involvement is common, with hilar adenopathy occurring in 50–90% of cases. In countries such as the United States, the decreasing prevalence of tuberculous infection and the increasing age of patients with tuberculosis results in a greater proportion of cases in adults, usually representing delayed reactivation. In this setting, tuberculous meningitis may occur as an isolated finding with a normal chest x-ray, or in association with pulmonary or miliary infection.

In addition to a thick, exudative basilar meningitis, often spreading into the parenchyma as a meningoencephalitis, the hallmark of CNS tuberculosis is vasculitis. The vessels at the base of the brain are most involved. The changes tend to be diffuse, however, involving large, medium, and small arteries as well as veins, with most prominent vasculitis in the middle and anterior cerebral arteries. Approximately one-third of patients will have cerebral infarctions as a result of vasculitis. Hydrocephalus is a relatively constant finding in patients with tuberculous meningitis, although it may resolve with medical therapy and usually does not require surgical intervention.

The initial symptoms of tuberculous meningitis are nonspecific complaints which last 2 weeks or longer and usually consist of low-grade fever, lassitude, depression, confusion, and personality or behavioral changes (50–58). The next phase of the illness reflects meningeal involvement, with headache and stiff neck. Cranial nerve VI, III, IV, or I palsies are present in about one-third of patients. Focal signs may result from cerebral infarction.

The CSF formula usually is typical of chronic meningitis. Within the first few weeks of the onset of symptoms, the CSF may show a neutrophilic pleocytosis, which shifts spontaneously to a mononuclear pleocytosis of 100–500 cells per microliter (59,60). Hypoglycorrhachia is present in 50–95% of patients in the absence of antituberculous therapy, and serial lumbar punctures usually will show progressive depression of CSF glucose. Increased opening pressure, increased CSF protein, and hyponatremia may be present, with the latter being due to inappropriate secretion of antidiuretic hormone. CT scan may show the following: hydrocephalus; contrast enhancement of the basilar exudates, sometimes obliterating the cisterns; multiple contrast-enhancing granulomas; or ischemic infarction.

The tuberculin skin test can be useful when positive in areas of low prevalence of infection with *M. tuberculosis*.

About one-third of patients will have a negative tuberculin skin test at the time of initial presentation. The demonstration of acid-fast bacilli in a stained sediment of CSF is particularly useful in establishing the diagnosis. The yield has been extremely variable (10–87%) and is, in large part, technique-dependent. The yield may be as high as 85–91% if 10–20 ml of CSF are sedimented at 2,500 rpm for 30 min and a thick smear of the pellicle is examined for 30–90 min (61). The ultimate yield of culture of CSF is 47–87%. Cultures of sputum and gastric aspirates are positive in 21–50% of cases.

The detection of tuberculostearic acid (TBSA) in CSF shows great promise in the rapid diagnosis of tuberculous meningitis (62,63). TBSA is a constituent of mycobacteria and nocardia. Determinations of TBSA by frequency-pulsed electron-capture gas–liquid chromatography are currently available from the Centers for Disease Control; the test has a specificity of 91% and a sensitivity of 95% (63a). Moreover, TBSA has been present in CSF up to 8 months after starting antituberculous therapy, so that determinations also are of value in confirming the diagnosis in patients already begun on empirical therapy.

Empirical therapy often is necessary pending the results of cultures, which may be delayed for 4–6 weeks. Combination therapy with isoniazid and rifampin for 9 months should be effective unless drug resistance is suspected. In such a case, the addition of pyrazinamide and ethambutol would be appropriate. In view of the severity of the illness, it is common practice to use at least three drugs in most patients. Direct evidence is lacking for the efficacy of corticosteroids for treatment of adults with tuberculous meningitis. Possible indications include: severe illness with obtundation or coma; evidence of multiple cerebral infarctions; life-threatening increases in intracranial pressure; cranial neuropathy; and contrast-enhancing exudate in the basilar cisterns. If corticosteroids are to be used, moderate doses (1 mg/kg/day) for a limited period of time (approximately 4 weeks) are appropriate. As discussed above, if a patient presents with chronic meningitis and CSF abnormalities consistent with tuberculosis but the tuberculin skin test is negative, empirical antituberculous drugs should be started, and concurrently a thorough attempt must be initiated to establish a diagnosis definitively.

The prognosis of tuberculous meningitis depends largely on the extent of neurologic damage at the time of diagnosis. Mortality is 10–33%. Neurologic sequelae occur in 25–31% of adult cases and include hydrocephalus, learning disabilities, chronic cranial nerve damage, and focal signs such as hemiparesis (55).

Cryptococcal Meningitis

Even in the pre-AIDS era, cryptococcal meningitis was the most common CNS infection in chronically immunosuppressed patients (16), and approximately one-half of patients with this infection had an underlying disease associated with immunosuppression. *C. neoformans* is a common environmental saprophyte which grows luxuriantly in pigeon droppings because of their high creatine content. Exposure is widespread; however, cryptococcal disease is infrequent. The exposure history is not helpful because of the ubiquitous nature of the organism. Laboratory workers provide an example: They can have intense exposure to organisms and manifest delayed-type hypersensitivity on skin testing with cryptococcal antigenic preparations, presumably reflecting infection, but do not develop disease manifestations. Individuals at greatest risk of developing cryptococcal disease have an underlying disease associated with depression of the cell-mediated immune response. The classic associations are with Hodgkin's disease and lymphosarcoma and treatment with high doses of corticosteroids. These risk factors for cryptococcal meningitis have now been surpassed in frequency by AIDS (23,25). Even a relatively short course of corticosteroids as may be used for obstructive airways disease can suffice to predispose to cryptococcal meningitis, if the dose is high. Patients with renal allografts or transplantation of other organs also are at increased risk. Those individuals developing cryptococcal meningitis in the absence of the above predisposing conditions still may have an underlying process associated with some degree of immunocompromise: sarcoidosis, diabetes mellitus, chronic hepatic, or renal failure. Interestingly, even patients with no apparent underlying disease may fail to develop delayed-type hypersensitivity responses after treatment for cryptococcal meningitis, perhaps indicative of a selective defect in cellular immunity.

Almost invariably, the portal for entry of cryptococcosis is the lungs. The pulmonary focus may be active, in the form of nodular pulmonary lesions when the patient develops symptoms of CNS involvement. More often, the initial portal of entry of infection is not demonstrable, presumably because it has already regressed spontaneously. One perplexing presentation is that of pulmonary cryptococcosis which must be distinguished from cryptoccal colonization of the lower respiratory tract, a condition which may be associated with carcinoma of the lung. If the patient has invasive pulmonary cryptococosis and a significant underlying disease, occult dissemination to the CNS is likely. All patients with pulmonary cryptococcosus, therefore, require a lumbar puncture and determination of cryptococcal polysaccharide antigen in serum and CSF.

The most common presentation of cryptococcal meningitis is a subacute-to-chronic febrile syndrome with headache (64–68) (Table 3). Occasionally the onset of illness is even more indolent, in which case fever is unusual and the major finding is dementia or more subtle cognitive defects. Overall, confusion, irritability, and other personality changes reflecting meningoencephalitis are found in about one-half of patients. Other com-

TABLE 3. *Signs and symptoms caused by fungal organisms most frequently etiologic in chronic meningitis*[a]

Fungal organism	Fever (>101°F)	Headache	Stiff neck	Change in mentation	Focal signs	Visual disturbance
Blastomyces	+	+++	+++	+	++	+
Candida	+++	+++	++	+	+	+
Coccidioides	+	+++	+	++	++	++
Cryptococcus	+	+++	+++	+	+	+++
Histoplasma	++	+	++	+	+	+
Sporothrix	+	++	++	++	+	?

[a] Adapted from ref. 100. +, rare; ++, occasionally to moderately frequently; +++, usually.

plaints include generalized weakness and seizures. Ocular abnormalities present in 40% of patients include papilledema (with or without loss of visual acuity) and cranial nerve palsies. Cryptococcus is unusual among the causes of chronic meningitis in its propensity to invade the optic nerve directly. Focal granulomas or cryptococcal abscesses may present as a mass lesion, producing hemiparesis or other focal neurologic signs.

The CSF findings in patients with cryptococcal meningitis vary with the presence of an underlying disease and the nature of the CNS involvement. In the immunocompromised host, signs of inflammation may be minimal and the number of cryptococci often exceeds that of leukocytes. Overall, the white blood cell count usually ranges from 40 to 400 per microliter, with counts rarely above 800 per microliter. In over 50% of patients, the pleocytosis consists primarily of mononuclear leukocytes. The protein concentration is greater than 40 mg/dl and may be quite high. The glucose concentration is depressed in 55% of patients.

The India ink preparation of CSF is positive in one-third to one-half of patients with cryptococcal meningitis and is more likely to be positive in patients presenting acutely and in the setting of immunosuppression. Budding yeast forms may be seen in the latter cases, and the India ink preparation may show organisms even in the absence of a significant inflammatory response. The India ink test usually correlates with the magnitude of cryptococcal polysaccharide antigen which must be determined in serum as well as in CSF for all patients with chronic meningitis. The overlap yields the diagnosis in about 94% of patients. Unfortunately, this leaves some patients in whom serologies are negative, and the diagnosis may be delayed or missed entirely unless CSF cultures are positive or a meningeal biopsy is performed (Fig. 4). The initial culture of CSF is positive for *Cryptococcus* in three-quarters of patients. The cultural yield may, however, be delayed as long as 2–6 weeks. Additional cultures of CSF, as well as cultures of blood, sputum, urine, and stool, are appropriate in all patients with chronic meningitis. Cultures from extraneural sites may be positive even in the absence of clinical signs of dissemination or local end-organ involvement. Currently, cryptococcal meningitis is treated with amphotericin B (0.3

mg/kg/day, intravenously) and flucytosine (150 mg/kg/day) for 6 weeks, with careful monitoring of renal function and flucytosine levels. Patients with AIDS usually require lifelong suppressive treatment after primary therapy, to prevent relapse. Fluconazole is an oral drug which may prove effective in the initial therapy of cryptococcal meningitis, or as maintenance therapy. Cryptococcal meningitis can relapse despite apparently adequate therapy, especially in AIDS patients. Therefore, patients at risk for relapse, such as those with high levels of polysaccharide antigen at the completion of treatment, should have repeated lumbar punctures for examination and culture of CSF.

Coccidioidal Meningitis

Coccidioides immitis is a thermal, dimorphic fungus; this means that the organism exists in nature as a mycelial form but that it exists in the tissues of infected animals and humans, at body temperature, as spherules. Endemic areas are at low altitude, warm, and arid. In the United States, this includes large areas of California, New Mexico, and Texas.

Wind-borne arthrospores of *C. immitis* infect humans, through the respiratory route. Dissemination occurs in approximately one of 200 patients with symptomatic coccidioidomycosis, and one-half of such patients develop meningitis. Dissemination to the meninges occurs early in the course of disease, often within the first 3 months. Non-Caucasians, particularly Filipinos, are at greatly increased risk of dissemination (69).

The presentation of coccidioidal meningitis varies from acute to chronic (69–72). The most common symptoms are fever, headache, and weight loss. About one-half of patients develop disorientation, lethargy, confusion, or memory loss. One-third have a stiff neck. Papilledema, cranial nerve signs, and other focal findings also may be present. Extraneural lesions in the skin (one-third of patients) or lung (two-thirds of patients) may be helpful in reaching a specific diagnosis.

Variations in CSF findings reflect the stage of disease. Generally there is a lymphocytic pleocytosis with increased protein and hypoglycorrhachia (in 76%), and the mean cell count is 260 per microliter (range: 0–1,200).

Normal CSF does not exclude the possibility of coccidioidal meningitis. Culture of CSF is positive in up to 46% of patients; the yield may be increased by the technique of membrane filtration. Blood and urine cultures occasionally yield the organism. Nonetheless, serologies are critical to the diagnosis in most patients. A serum complement-fixation (CF) titer of greater than or equal to 1:16 is suggestive of disseminated coccidioidomycosis (73). Any CSF titer is suggestive of meningitis. Modified CF testing of CSF is positive in up to 95% of patients. Most patients will have a negative coccidioidin skin test, but this is of no clinical relevance.

Patients with coccidioidal meningitis must be treated with intravenous plus intrathecal amphotericin B (72,74). The local amphotericin is given three times weekly for 3 months, usually through a ventricular reservoir, followed by a tapering course. Therapy is discontinued after the CSF has been normal for at least 1 year on a once-every-6-weeks regimen. The CSF should, however, be followed at 6-week intervals for two additional years after treatment is stopped. Alternate modalities for therapy are badly needed in this disease.

Histoplasma Meningitis

Histoplasma capsulatum is a dimorphic fungus whose infectious mycelial phase is found in the soil of the Ohio and Mississippi River valleys. Disturbances of microfoci contaminated with the fungus (as occurs in construction sites) result in the airborne-spread of spores over wide areas. Not surprisingly, over one-half of adults in endemic areas have been infected with H. capsulatum—usually in an asymptomatic fashion, or manifest as a benign, self-limited illness. After inhalation, microconidia transform into yeast which disseminate hematogenously. The development of cell-mediated immunity leads to regression of infection, although delayed reactivation is possible. In the immunologically impaired host, or following massive exposure, infection often progresses.

Meningitis due to Histoplasma may represent an isolated site of infection or may be associated with progressive dissemination with fever, anorexia, weight loss, and involvement of multiple organs (hepatomegaly, splenomegaly, lymphadenopathy, mucosal or skin ulcers) (75). The presentation of chronic Histoplasma meningitis most commonly includes mental status abnormalities (reduced level of consciousness, confusion, personality changes, memory impairment) and headache (76–78). Cranial nerve palsies and focal signs are also common.

The CSF usually shows a lymphocytic pleocytosis (11–100 cells per microliter). It is unusual for the cell count to exceed 300 per microliter. CSF protein is increased and glucose is low in 79% of patients. Cultures of CSF are positive in up to 56% of patients. Large volumes of CSF, however, may be required to culture the organism.

In addition to CSF, fungal cultures of blood, bone marrow, sputum, and urine should be obtained, as well as biopsies of other tissues which are involved clinically. Although skin testing is contraindicated because it may falsely elevate serologies, the detection of antibody in serum and CSF and of Histoplasma antigen in urine, CSF, and serum is useful and may support the empirical use of amphotericin B pending the results of culture. The CF test using yeast and mycelial antigens is positive at dilutions of ≥1:8 of serum in 71% of reported cases. The test is not entirely specific, but it provides an early clue that chronic meningitis may be due to H. capsulatum. As in coccidioidal meningitis, antibodies are produced locally in infected meninges and can be detected in the CSF. Although a positive CF test or radioimmunoassay for antibodies to Histoplasma in CSF is found in at least two-thirds of patients, false positives occur in one-half of other chronic fungal meningitides, and serum antibodies may passively diffuse into the CSF (79).

In contrast to antibody detection, the radioimmunoassay for Histoplasma antigen is highly specific. A polysaccharide antigen is found in the urine of 90%, and in the blood of 50%, of patients with disseminated histoplasmosis (80). Antigen also has been found in the CSF of two of 10 patients with Histoplasma meningitis (10). In AIDS patients with disseminated histoplasmosis, high levels of antigen can be detected in the urine of 97%, and in the blood of 79%, of patients (11). Determination of Histoplasma antigen also may be useful in following the response to therapy in these patients.

These data suggest that detection of Histoplasma antigen in urine, CSF, or blood of a patient with chronic meningitis is a sufficient indication for treatment. Detection of high levels of anti-Histoplasma antibodies in serum or CSF also may warrant empirical therapy.

In patients with Histoplasma meningitis, amphotericin B should be administered intravenously over an 8- to 12-week period, for a total dose of 2.0 g. After the course of treatment is completed, the CSF must be examined regularly over a 2-year period for early diagnosis of relapse. Intraventricular amphotericin B is indicated in patients who fail to respond to intravenous drug (persistent CSF abnormalities) and in those who relapse more than once.

Blastomycotic Meningitis

Blastomyces dermatiditis is a dimorphic fungus which causes disease around the Mississippi river basin and Great Lakes, as well as in the Southeast. A recent microepidemic provided the first clear association between environmental source (soil from a beaver lodge and dam) and human disease, suggesting an ecologic niche (moist soil, high content organic material, acid pH, animal excreta) (14). Blastomycosis disseminates from a pulmonary focus, frequently involving the skin, bone, and prostate. CNS involvement usually occurs in the setting of dissemination, although it may be isolated.

Blastomycotic meningitis is usually associated with other manifestations of disseminated disease. Its clinical presentation may be acute and/or fulminant with headache, stiff neck, and focal signs predominating (1,14,81). The CSF usually shows a lymphocytic pleocytosis with cell counts which may exceed 1,200 per microliter. The CSF protein is increased and glucose may be depressed. Organisms may be seen on direct smear of the CSF. Cultures are positive in only about one-fourth of patients. Diagnosis, therefore, often requires culture from extraneural sites, particularly lung, skin, and biopsy material. Neither skin testing nor the generally available serologic assays are helpful because of low sensitivity and specificity. Recently, an enzyme-linked immunoassay to detect antibody to the A antigen of *B. dermatiditis* showed promise as a more sensitive test (77% positive), at least in acute disease (14). Intravenous amphotericin B is the drug of choice for treatment of blastomycotic meningitis. Experience is insufficient to know the optimal dose of drug, but at least 2 g seems necessary.

Sporothrix Meningitis

Sporothrix schenckii is a yeast-like fungus isolated from a number of environmental sources. Infections have usually followed implantation of the fungus from soil, plants, and timber, as well as from bites of animals, birds, and insects. Lymphocutaneous disease is most common, and it rarely disseminates. Pulmonary disease from inhalation of spores is also uncommon.

Only 15 patients have been reported with *Sporothrix* meningitis (13,82) (Fig. 5). The infection has been restricted to the CNS in most patients. The pathogenesis of spread to the meninges is unknown. Headache is a uniform feature of the presentation, and patients are usually afebrile. Gait disturbance and seizures have occurred. CSF pleocytosis is mainly lymphocytic (0–517 cells per microliter), protein concentrations are increased, and glucose levels are depressed. The delay between onset of symptoms and first lumbar puncture and diagnosis was 3–11 months in one series, resulting in a nearly 6.5-month delay in instituting treatment.

In the study by Scott et al. (13), enzyme immunoassay and latex agglutination showed CSF and serum antibodies to the causative agent. Recommended treatment of *Sporothrix* meningitis is amphotericin B intravenously,

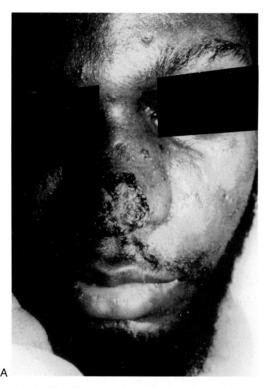
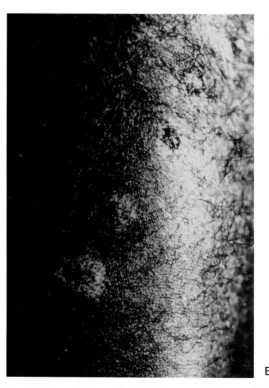

A   B

FIG. 5. Nasal lesion (**A**) and thigh lesions (**B**) in a patient with *Sporothrix* meningitis. He was a 26-year-old admitted with headache, lethargy, ataxia, and chronic lymphocytic meningitis with hypoglycorrhachia. Nine months after initial presentation, the diagnosis remained unknown, but a ventriculojugular (V–J) shunt was placed for hydrocephalus. Seven months later he was admitted with worsening headache, a fungating nose mass, multiple subcutaneous abscesses, a testicular mass, and reticulonodular densities in chest x-ray. Multiple cultures yielded *Sporothrix schenckii*. The initially localized CNS infection thus disseminated following placement of the V–J shunt.

for a total dose of at least 2.0 g. Some isolates are resistant to amphotericin B and the meningitis may be refractory to therapy, with persistent positive cultures.

Candida Meningitis

Candida meningitis is an infrequent complication of disseminated disease and usually is associated with intravenous drug abuse, indwelling venous catheters, abdominal surgery, and corticosteroid therapy (3,83,84). It also occurs in neonates, especially premature infants with other medical problems (81,82). Conspicuously absent in the list of predisposing conditions is hematologic malignancy; presumably in this situation the number of yeast cells in the blood is too low to infect the meninges. Overall, 71% of patients have active extraneural *Candida* infection; and an additional 14% have had antecedent procedures which may have introduced yeast into the subarachnoid space, such as ventricular shunting or lumbar puncture.

Onset of symptoms may be abrupt or insidious. Fever is an invariable part of the presentation. Major findings are headache and stiff neck; some patients have depressed mental status, confusion, and cranial neuropathies or other focal neurological signs. CSF findings are variable; pleocytosis may involve up to 2,000 white blood cells per microliter, with a mean in one series of 600 cells. Lymphocytes predominate in one-half of patients. Protein is elevated in most patients, and the glucose is depressed in 60%. Yeast are found on smears of CSF in 43% of the patients, and cultures of CSF should be positive. Extraneural culture may yield *Candida* as well. The treatment of *Candida* meningitis requires amphotericin B.

Brucella Meningitis

Brucellosis remains a common disease worldwide (85,86). For example, 8,698 cases were reported in Spain in 1984 (87). *Brucella* causes a zoonosis; the variety of livestock likely to be infected varies with the geographic distribution of strains. *Brucella melitensis,* which infects goats and sheep, is most common in Spain; some authors believe this species may have a particular meningotropism. Although most patients with CNS brucellosis report consumption of unpasteurized dairy products, contact with animals or animal products, or a previous episode of brucellosis, one-third do not have a clear exposure history.

If strict criteria are applied—namely, culture of *Brucella* from the CSF or demonstration of the presence of antibodies to *Brucella* (agglutinating or nonagglutinating) in the CSF along with other abnormalities—approximately 3.5% of patients with brucellosis have predominant involvement of the CNS.

Brucella meningitis may be associated with systemic symptoms (fever, arthralgias, myalgias, sweating, and malaise) or may be an entirely localized process. In one-third of patients, CNS involvement is the first manifestation of brucellosis. Meningitis usually is subacute to chronic and may be transient or recurrent, even in the absence of specific therapy. Associated cranial neuropathy may occur with involvement of nerves VI, VII, or VIII; eighth-nerve involvement, which may be cochlear or vestibular, is most common. Meningitis may be the main manifestation of CNS brucellosis, or there may be meningoencephalitis, myeloradiculitis, or neuritis. Most of the patients show motor abnormalities, although disordered mentation, sensory disturbances, spastic paraparesis, seizures, sciatica, or cervicobrachialgia may be present. Occasionally, vascular involvement attributed to vasculitis or spasm is associated with transient ischemic attacks or, rarely, subarachnoid hemorrhage. The CSF shows a mononuclear cell pleocytosis (20–500 white blood cells per microliter), with depressed glucose in two-thirds of cases and an increased protein. *Brucella* may be cultured from the CSF (particularly if the disease is localized), but it rarely is found concurrently in blood. The diagnosis hinges on demonstration of antibody to *Brucella* in CSF. In some series, agglutinating antibody, usually in titers below those found in serum, is present in CSF. Agglutinating antibodies, however, may not be present, particularly if disease is localized to the CNS. A more reliable finding is the presence of nonagglutinating antibody to *Brucella* in the CSF (and serum) as determined by a modified Coombs' test. Optimal treatment of CNS brucellosis probably should consist of doxycycline plus rifampin and must be continued for prolonged periods of time (>4 months), gauging duration by changes in the CSF. The response to antibiotics is variable, presumably reflecting the extent of irreversible neurological disease before institution of therapy.

Neurosyphilis

Although the antibiotic treatment of early forms of syphilis has reduced the prevalence of neurosyphilis considerably, this disease remains an important diagnostic consideration in patients with signs of meningeal inflammation and neurological deficits. The prevalence of primary and secondary forms of syphilis has increased worldwide in the past decade. Some of this increase is attributable to the increased occurrence of syphilitic infections in HIV-positive individuals. As described in the section on immunocompromised patients, syphilis in the HIV-infected patient may take a particularly aggressive clinical course. Even in immunocompetent hosts, the index of suspicion for syphilitic infection of the nervous system must remain high because atypical forms of the disease are prevalent; in most cases, the disease is treatable by high doses of antibiotics.

Most of the epidemiological analysis of the prevalence and characteristics of neurosyphilis have resulted from thorough studies in the 1930s and 1940s, particularly those by Merritt et al. (88) at Boston City Hospital. It is important to keep in mind that all of the classic manifestations of neurosyphilis occur because of active meningeal inflammation. Thus, abnormal CSF is the hallmark of this disease. The diagnosis of cerebrovascular syphilis or paretic neurosyphilis ("general paresis" or "dementia paralytica") cannot be made in the absence of abnormal CSF. An exception to this rule is tabes dorsalis which, in the late stages, can present with normal spinal fluid. This occurred, however, in only two of 100 cases of tabes reported by Merritt et al. (88).

Treponemal infection of the meninges causes a subacute leptomeningeal process which either presents with clinical evidence of meningitis or is asymptomatic. In the Merritt et al. (88) series, 31% of patients with evidence of meningeal inflammation (i.e., abnormal CSF examinations) were, in fact, neurologically asymptomatic within the first months or years of infection. When localized at the meninges at the base of the brain, infection causes either hydrocephalus or cranial nerve palsies as described below. Obliterative endarteritis affects cerebral blood vessels in meningovascular syphilis, causing narrowing and occlusion of these vessels and thereby causing cerebral infarction.

Infection of the nervous system occurs in about 10% of persons infected with *T. pallidum.* In clinical meningitis, infection may be asymptomatic, but it more commonly presents within 2 years of the initial primary stage. Fever may be absent. Headache, mental status changes, and signs of meningeal inflammation, however, are usually present. Cranial nerve palsies—particularly those involving nerves VII, VIII, and II—may occur when the meninges at the base of the brain are affected by the inflammatory process. Seizures may occur when the meninges over the cerebral convexities are involved. *Cerebrovascular syphilis,* occurring after a longer latency of several years following primary infection, usually presents with stroke syndromes. The clinical picture may be identical to stroke from nonsyphilitic cause such as hypertension or thromboembolism, but pre-ischemic prodomes also occur with headache, lethargy, or behavioral changes over weeks to months before the acute ischemic event. Angiography may show beading and concentric narrowing of both large and medium-sized cerebral vessels.

General paresis, the dementia that occurs after an even longer latency of 10–20 years, may be indistinguishable from dementia due to another cause such as Alzheimer's disease. The classical euphoric delusional psychosis originally described in this illness is less common than originally proposed. *Tabes dorsalis,* the fourth classical form of neurosyphilis, presents about 10 years after infection, with a triad of shooting or lightning pains, urinary dysfunction, and ataxia. On examination, Argyll Robertson pupils frequently are present, as is loss of posterior column function and areflexia. A transiently abnormal CSF cell count may occur in some patients after penicillin therapy (89).

The CSF in neurosyphilis is almost invariably abnormal, showing either (a) elevated opening pressure, (b) lymphocytic pleocytosis with values of 500 per microliter or greater, common in syphilitic meningitis, or (c) a less vigorous lymphocytic pleocytosis in the 50- to 200-per-microliter range in syphilitic vascular disease and general paresis. CSF pleocytosis is probably the most sensitive indicator of active disease. Protein commonly is elevated, though less than 200 mg/dl in most cases of neurosyphilis. It is most likely to be high in general paresis; additionally, gamma globulin also can be elevated in this form of CNS syphilis. As noted above, the spinal fluid in tabes dorsalis is usually abnormal, but it can be normal in rare cases.

The fluorescent treponemal antibody-absorbed (FTA) test of serum is a sensitive test for neurosyphilis, and it is reactive in more than 95% of patients with late syphilis (90). Unlike the nontreponemal flocculation test, the VDRL, the FTA remains reactive despite therapy. However, the VDRL test is more useful in the CSF as an indicator of active diseases. It is Simon's (90) opinion that patients with negative CSF serologies probably represent meningitis due to causes other than syphilis. If neurosyphilis is a diagnostic consideration, the CSF VDRL is an important parameter to obtain. However, a negative FTA antibody in the blood excludes the diagnosis of neurosyphilis and makes a lumbar puncture unnecessary (90).

The standard treatment regimens for neurosyphilis have recently been revised because of several reports of recurrence or persistence of the infection following what was thought to be adequate antibiotic therapy. Treatment recommended for late syphilis includes: aqueous penicillin G, 600,000 units (intramuscularly) per day for 15 days; penicillin G, 2–4 million units (intravenously) every 4 hr for 10–14 days; or penicillin G benzathene, 2.4 million units (intramuscularly) per week for 3 weeks. The latter protocol has been criticized by the World Health Organization (91). Treatment of the immunocompromised patient with neurosyphilis is discussed in an earlier section of this chapter.

Assessment of the adequacy of treatment regimens for neurosyphilis involves repeat lumbar punctures at 6, 12, and 24 months. The CSF pleocytosis should show resolution to normal within a period of 6 months. Both the serum and CSF VDRL return to nonreactive, although a low fixed titer in serum is seen on occasion. Relapse can occur, and thus any change in clinical status should prompt a repeat lumbar puncture, which, in most cases of relapse, shows an increasing CSF white blood cell count.

Lyme Disease

Lyme disease was originally described as an oligoarticular arthritis associated with a localized skin rash at the site of a tick bite. It is caused by a newly recognized spirochete, *Borrelia burgdorferi,* whose vector is a deer tick. Cases were originally described from Lyme, Connecticut, but other endemic areas in the United States include Long Island, Cape Cod, and central New Jersey, as well as southeastern Connecticut. The disease has a seasonal occurrence, prevalent in the late summer and early fall, especially August and September. A cluster has occurred around Wurzburg, West Germany, where the disease presents as a meningoradiculitis and is known as "Bannwarth's syndrome" (92). A tick bite is recalled by only a small proportion of patients. Specific immunoreactivity (i.e., serum antibody to *B. burgdorferi*) is prevalent in areas that are endemic for this disease. Therefore, the causal relationship between immunologic evidence of this spirochetal exposure and neurological disease has only recently been carefully explored.

The frequency of Lyme disease within a region is dependent upon the frequency of ticks infected with the organism. Deer appear to be a critical host, and the disease is common in areas where deer are common.

Although it is assumed that the organism traverses the blood–brain barrier early in the course of Lyme disease (perhaps at the time of initial signs and symptoms of meningeal inflammation), the exact mechanism of CNS invasion and infection are not known. Like the spirochete that causes syphilis, the Lyme disease organism has the capacity to lie latent within the CNS and become activated after a variable period of time. Factors that trigger activation in neurosyphilis and in Lyme disease are not fully understood.

The neurological manifestations of Lyme disease were originally described as those of a painful radiculopathy associated with a lymphocytic meningitis. Cranial neuritis, particularly unilateral or bilateral facial palsies, were also described. More recently, however, CNS and peripheral manifestations have been described (93,94).

Lyme disease may be divided into three stages in most patients. In the first stage, 60–80% of patients develop Erythema chronicum migrans ECM. Initially, a flu-like illness occurs shortly after infection, sometimes associated with the characteristic skin rash and meningoencephalitis. Cardiac or neurological involvement occurs in the second stage, generally weeks to months after the initial infection. The last stage, a mono- or oligoarthritis, has an even longer latency period: months to years after exposure. Neurological symptoms and signs may predominate in this final stage of the disease.

Patients may have symptoms of a meningoencephalitis during the first stage of the illness. Interestingly, signs of meningeal irritation—such as Kernig's and Brudzinski's signs, stiff neck, or neck pain—are frequently absent. Headache, however, is often present. CSF examination either is normal or reveals a mild lymphocytic pleocytosis. A more fulminant meningitis occurs several weeks after the initial infection in 10–15% of patients who have contracted Lyme disease. Once again, headache is the predominant symptom in this second stage of the illness, sometimes accompanied by a seventh-nerve palsy or radiculoneuritis; in addition, the CSF shows a lymphocytic pleocytosis with mildly elevated protein

and normal glucose. Many of these patients have anti-*B. burgdorferi* antibodies in the CSF, in a concentration exceeding that of serum, indicative of intrathecal synthesis (92).

The third (i.e., arthritic) stage of the infection, which occurs months to years after the original tick bite, can also cause prominent nervous system syndromes, including what has been described as a "multiple sclerosis-like syndrome" and encephalopathy. Abnormalities of memory and cognition were found in 22 of 85 patients recently studied in Long Island, New York. In 10 of the 13 patients in whom CSF was analyzed, intrathecal synthesis of anti-*B. burgdorferi* antibody was found (94). In addition, MRI scans showed hyperdense lesions in the white matter on T2-weighted images. Because the patients' symptoms and cognitive deficits improved following intravenous ceftriaxone (the recommended therapy for Lyme disease) and also because in some instances the MRI scans normalized, these clinical and radiographic findings were attributed to Lyme disease and were considered reversible with therapy. Other patients, with an episodic and chronic relapsing–remitting course suggestive of multiple sclerosis, did not have such a favorable response to therapy, and CSF in these patients showed elevations of IgG and oligoclonal bands but did not demonstrate intrathecal production of specific antibody to the Lyme agent.

The peripheral nervous system has also been involved asymmetrically in Lyme disease. The characteristic cranial nerve deficit is a facial palsy. When patients present with peripheral seventh-nerve deficits and a lymphocytic CSF pleocytosis, the Guillain–Barré syndrome is a diagnostic consideration. However, progressive motor weakness and areflexia do not develop in Lyme disease.

The CSF lymphocytic pleocytosis consists of a range of 6–700 white blood cells per microliter, with a median count of 166 (93). A plasma cell reaction has been described in the early stages of neurological involvement in Lyme disease. Total protein is usually mildly elevated; and immunoglobulin against *B. burgdorferi* is, as described above, most likely to be found in high titers in the later, more chronic neurological stages of the disease.

Because patients with syphilis may have falsely positive serologies to this species of *Borrelia,* serum fluorescent treponemal antibody-absorption (FTA-Abs) antibodies should be determined in patients suspected of having Lyme disease. The serologic diagnosis of Lyme disease has been confusing because of false negatives and false positives. During the first few weeks of illness, 30–40% of patients will have a positive indirect IgM enzyme-linked immunosorbent assay (ELISA) test. In convalescence, 60–80% have a positive-capture IgM ELISA. False positives, however, have been reported in normal individuals and patients with amyotrophic lateral sclerosis or multiple sclerosis, so that confirmatory western blotting is appropriate.

The initial stage of the illness is treated with oral tetracycline or penicillin. However, for neurological manifestations, intravenous penicillin G and (more recently) ceftriaxone are recommended (95). These antibiotics appear to be effective in shortening the duration of symptoms as well as in preventing the late complications of the disease, such as arthritis.

Cystercercosis

Worldwide, cysticercosis is the most common parasitic infection of the CNS. Most cases of cysticercosis are seen in the southwestern United States and are uncommon elsewhere in this country. Endemic areas include South and Central America, Mexico, Africa, India, eastern Europe, China, and Indonesia. The World Health Organization estimates that 2.5 million harbor the porcine tapeworm, *Taenia solium,* and that an even greater number are infected with the larval form, cysticercus.

Within the CNS, two distinct forms of cysticercosis occur. *Cysticercus cellulosae* occurs primarily in brain parenchyma; and *Cysticercus racemosus* occurs in grape-like clusters within the basilar cisterns, the ventricles, or subarachnoid space.

Clinical manifestations of neurocysticercosis may be diverse. The majority of patients present with either (a) seizures or (b) symptoms of increased intracranial pressure (96). Parenchymal cysticerci have a predilection for gray matter and subpial areas. Therefore, they may cause seizure disorders, both focal and generalized, and focal neurological signs, sometimes stroke-like in onset. If the number of cerebral cysts is extensive, more diffuse presentations such as those characteristic of encephalopathy or dementia may occur. In endemic areas, cysticercosis is one of the most frequent causes of epilepsy in young people. Parenchymal cysts which are clinically manifest solely as epilepsy are usually best treated with anticonvulsants alone. In time, even if untreated, seizures appear to resolve (97). Cognitive changes, movement disorders, cavernous sinus syndrome, and, rarely, myopathy may also occur.

When the cysts are located in the ventricle, hydrocephalus may ensue. Because intraventricular cysts may be mobile with position change, the striking clinical syndrome of episodic symptoms of raised intracranial pressure with position change can suggest the diagnosis.

Exceptionally, cysticercosis may occur in the spinal cord as both extramedullary and intramedullary cysts, usually with raised CSF protein.

The racemosus form of cysticercosis produces multiple cystic masses near the basal meninges, causing some of the most catastrophic symptoms of cerebral cysticercosis. The cysts may expand in the subarachnoid space, producing intracranial hypertension; may cause a meningitis and arachnoiditis with obstruction of the foramena of Luschka or Magendie; or may mimic tumors of the cerebellopontine angle, cisterna magna, or pituitary fossa. The chronic meningitis seen in this form of CNS cysticercosis may be subclinical, persisting over many years. Symptoms, therefore, may not appear in some pa-

tients from endemic areas for 10–15 years after immigration to the United States.

Interestingly, the meningitis associated with cysticerci usually presents without fever or cranial nerve palsies, distinguishing it from other inflammatory basilar meningeal processes such as tuberculosis or sarcoidosis. An indirect hemagglutination (IHA) test performed by the Centers for Disease Control is positive in the majority of patients with meningitis. However, patients with calcified, and therefore nonactive, lesions tend to have nondiagnostic titers. Although the CSF may be entirely normal, about one-half of patients will have a predominantly mononuclear pleocytosis. One-half of these patients also had hypoglycorrachia, and in one study (98) the presence of hypoglycorrachia presaged a poor prognosis. A recent study (99) found an ELISA of IgM antibodies against cysticercus antigens to be 87% sensitive in CSF samples. A helpful additional finding in the CSF is the presence of eosinophilia in 16–40% of patients. If the diagnosis of CNS cysticercosis is suspected, a Wright stain, therefore, should be performed on the CSF sample.

The diagnosis of CNS cysticercosis is more commonly made by CT scan than by CSF examination. Intracranial calcifications about 2–10 mm in diameter are the hallmark of the disease. The second most common lesions are cystic lesions, which with contrast may show ring enhancement. These lesions may progress to become isodense with brain parenchyma and later calcify, a process which may take many years.

The therapy of cerebral cysticercosis varies according to the clinical presentation. Seizures are usually responsive to anticonvulsants, which may, over a period of years, no longer be needed when the cysticercus calcifies. Calcified lesions are usually nonprogressive, and therefore they do not require surgical resection. Large cysts of the fourth ventricle, however, may require surgical extirpation for control of symptoms. Because resection of lateral and third-ventricular cysts may have a high complication rate, many patients are treated (with good outcome) with ventricular shunting alone. The clinical response to shunting procedures is often dependent upon the number, location, and activity of basilar and intracerebral cysts.

Treatment of CNS cysticercosis with larvicides such as praziquantel is controversial because many of the clinical symptoms are the result of an inflammatory response against already-lifeless cysts, and further killing of cysts may release antigenic substances which exacerbate the inflammatory reaction. Furthermore, in many cases, cerebral cysticercosis becomes clinically manifest only after the cysticercus has died. Giving a cysticercocidal agent at this point, therefore, may be unnecessary.

Other Infections of the CNS

All of the major fungi and yeasts are capable of producing focal parenchymal lesions, meningitis, or both

(75). *C. neoformans, C. immitis, H. capsulatum, B. dermatiditis,* and *C. albicans* most often present as meningitis or meningoencephalitis (Table 3).

A distinct group of organisms more commonly causes brain abscesses or focal granulomas. The clinical syndrome may, however, resemble chronic meningitis with prominent focal findings and focal lesions on neuroradiographic procedures; or, in rare instances, these organisms may cause an isolated meningitis (100,101). *Aspergillus* and *Zygomycetes* are ubiquitous environmental saprophytes and rarely cause disease unless the host is immunocompromised. Patients with sustained neutropenia and organ transplant recipients are at greatest risk for *Aspergillus* infection, whereas patients with diabetic ketoacidosis are at greatest risk for *Zygomycetes.* CNS involvement accompanies disseminated infection and is usually refractory to treatment. Exceptions occur in which these organisms cause disease in patients with lesser degrees of immunocompromise or even in the apparently healthy host, and CNS involvement may take the form of isolated meningitis. *Cladosporium trichoides* is a dematiacious fungus, the hyphae of which are darkly pigmented. When it causes CNS disease, the organisms are limited to the brain except for the occasional finding of lesions in the lung or ear (102). *Phialophora,* particularly *Phialophora pedrosoi* and *Phialophora dermatiditis,* cause chromoblastomycosis, a chronic cutaneous infection; when CNS disease occurs, it may be associated with skin lesions. *Paracoccidioides brasiliensis* is endemic to the subtropical regions of Central and South America. It causes South American blastomycosis, most often in young adult males who are laborers in rural areas and who presumably acquire the disease by contact with contaminated soil (103). CNS involvement usually produces increased intracranial pressure suggestive of a brain tumor. *Pseudoallescheria boydii* is found in soil, polluted water, and sewage worldwide. It usually causes a mycetoma. Dissemination may occur in the immunocompromised host.

In addition to these fungal organisms, *Nocardia, Actinomyces,* and *Arachnia* are bacteria which generally produce focal lesions but which may present with the clinical syndrome of chronic meningitis (104,105). *Nocardia* generally affects the immunocompromised host, particularly patients receiving treatment with high doses of corticosteroids or with conditions associated with depression of the cell-mediated immune response; curiously, *Nocardia* is not a frequent opportunistic agent in patients with AIDS in the United States, possibly because it is limited in the environment. It may prove to be more common in the setting of AIDS in other parts of the world. *Actinomyces* and *Arachnia* are anaerobic mouth flora which rarely cause CNS disease, and then usually as part of a mixed infection (106). *Nocardia* is weakly acid-fast, and *Actinomyces* form typical "sulfur granules" in tissue and are strictly anaerobic—properties which are useful in their isolation and identification.

Sarcoidosis

Sarcoidosis involves the nervous system in 5% of patients. In nearly one-half of these, the presenting manifestations of sarcoidosis are neurological (98). Cranial nerve palsies are common, due to the granulomatous inflammation of the meninges at the base of the brain. Peripheral seventh-nerve palsies are the most common cranial nerve lesions, and in some series they are the most frequent neurological manifestation of sarcoidosis overall (107,108). Eighth-nerve dysfunction takes the form of sensorineural hearing loss. The optic nerve also may be compressed by granulomas, or it may be affected by pressure caused by hydrocephalus. Hypothalamic dysfunction occurs, producing neuroendocrinological disease, most commonly affecting fluid balance. Elevated serum prolactin levels are found variably in CNS sarcoidosis.

A chronic aseptic meningitis also occurs, both at the time of neurological presentation in patients with sarcoidosis and as a recurrent syndrome. Headache and meningeal signs are present, and the CSF shows a lymphocytic pleocytosis in the range of 6–200 cells per microliter. In several large series of patients with neurosarcoidosis, approximately 70% of patients had pleocytosis, 70% had elevated protein (usually less than 200 mg/dl), and 20% had hypoglycorrhachia (108,109).

There is nothing pathognomonic in the CSF profile or clinical presentation. The diagnosis may be made by histological examination of enlarged lymph nodes, tissue obtained by transbronchial biopsy or mediastinoscopy, and, on some occasions, biopsy of salivary glands or conjunctiva. Elevated serum angiotensin-converting enzyme sometimes is helpful. A positive Kveim test would also be diagnostically useful. In many instances, however, extraneural sarcoid is not present. It is important to exclude other treatable disorders presenting with CSF parameters consistent with neurosarcoidosis. When mass lesions are present in the cerebrum, biopsy may yield a definitive diagnosis. Pursuit of histological confirmation is important, since the treatment for sarcoidosis, corticosteroid therapy, is contraindicated in other causes of chronic meningitis such as fungal or tuberculous infections which present with similar CSF and clinical pictures.

Vasculitis and Collagen Vascular Disease

Neurological manifestations of vasculitic and rheumatologic diseases are common, and they most often occur in the setting of systemic disease after the primary diagnosis has been established. CNS involvement in polyarteritis nodosa, for example, most often occurs late in the course of the systemic illness. However, CNS involvement may on occasion be the presenting feature of unrecognized systemic disease. Rarely, neurological syndromes may be the sole manifestation of the primary disease, as in granulomatous angiitis of the nervous system.

Localized Vasculitis of the Central Nervous System

Granulomatous Angiitis of the Nervous System

No specific clinical picture or laboratory parameter allows with certainty the diagnosis of cerebral angiitis. However, altered mental status, elevated protein, and cells in the CSF usually are present before the diagnosis is entertained. Having stated this, it should be noted that granulomatous angiitis has been reported in several patients in whom the entire CSF formula was normal (110) and in whom the diagnosis was confirmed by angiography or diagnostic biopsy. Granulomatous angiitis is characterized by granulomatous inflammation of the small arteries and arterioles of the parenchymal and leptomeningeal vessels. Giant cells of the Langhans and foreign-body type are associated with intimal proliferation. The histologic picture looks very much like giant cell arteritis, except that the vessel media may be spared.

Clinically, patients present with headache and encephalopathy, followed by progression to a stroke-like syndrome with hemiparesis or other focal signs such as cranial neuropathies (110,111,112). Although the mean age at diagnosis is 46 years (113), the prognosis is grim in most patients, with death within weeks to months of diagnosis. The use of corticosteroids and immunosuppressive agents in recent years seems to have improved the outcome (110).

The erythrocyte sedimentation rate is elevated variably. Similarly, other laboratory studies indicative of autoimmune disease cannot be counted on to confirm the diagnosis. If angiography shows no evidence of the characteristic symmetrical or segmental narrowing, irregularity of vessels, or "beading," a leptomeningeal biopsy may be necessary to make the diagnosis (110,114). CSF is frequently abnormal, characterized by elevated opening pressure, elevated total protein in approximately 80%, and a lymphocytic pleocytosis, usually less than 100 per microliter, in three-quarters of patients. Glucose is depressed rarely.

Vasculitis Associated with Herpes Zoster Ophthalmicus

Stroke, usually manifest as contralateral hemiplegia, may occur from 1 week to 2 years after ophthalmic zoster. At times, the facial nerve also is involved clinically. The CSF parameters are similar to those seen in granulomatous angiitis of the nervous system, with elevated numbers of lymphocytes and protein content. However, the prognosis is usually better than in patients with cerebral vasculitis. Significant resolution of neurological deficits is commonly observed.

Cogan's Syndrome

Cogan's syndrome, whose hallmark is vestibuloauditory dysfunction and interstitial keratitis presenting in young adults, may, on rare occasion, present with a meningoencephalitis. A mild CSF pleocytosis may occur in a small percentage of patients. The diagnosis usually is made by associated eighth-nerve involvement as well as visual loss due to keratitis. Although rare, this syndrome is important to diagnose because it responds, in some cases, to corticosteroids (115).

Systemic Vasculitides Affecting the Central Nervous System

Polyarteritis Nodosa

The CNS may be involved in polyarteritis nodosa (PAN), although less commonly than is the peripheral nervous system, where PAN is a classic cause of mononeuritis multiplex. Initial CNS symptoms include (a) headache, sometimes accompanied by fever and leukocytosis, and (b) cognitive changes which have been described as toxic delirium with confusion and disorientation. Abdominal pain, myalgias, or arthralgias may be present upon initial diagnosis. Less commonly, hemiparesis and seizures herald the onset of the disease. Neurasthenic symptoms such as weight loss, fatigue, anorexia, and generalized weakness are present in some patients at the time of diagnosis, as are upper respiratory symptoms such as sinusitis, mastoiditis, or otitis. The CSF may be normal or show a low-grade pleocytosis and elevated protein, usually less than 100 mg/dl. Interpretation of the CSF formula may be difficult because some patients present with seizure, stroke, or subarachnoid hemorrhage, syndromes which also may produce a mild pleocytosis in the CSF.

Systemic Lupus Erythematosus

Disturbed mental function is one of the most common neurological manifestations of systemic lupus erythematosus (SLE). Encephalopathy occurs in 10–30% of patients, usually manifest as acute confusional states, affective disorders, and perceptual disturbances. At times, it is difficult to attribute mental status changes to the primary disease process because other causes of encephalopathy associated with SLE are common. Metabolic dysfunction due to renal disease, ischemic events due to hypertension, corticosteroid-related psychotic changes, and CNS infection all occur in SLE and may produce cognitive changes. SLE may also present with seizures, migraine headache, stroke or transient ischemic attack (TIA) syndromes, transverse myelopathy, chorea, or peripheral neuropathies.

Recent evidence suggests that MRI may be more sensitive than CT in detecting evidence of active CNS disease (116). T2-weighted images show focal high-intensity areas, often in the white matter, possibly representing the vasculopathy and microinfarcts associated with SLE.

The CSF is abnormal in approximately one-fourth of patients with nervous system dysfunction, usually showing a mild elevation of protein and minimal pleocytosis. Glucose is uncommonly depressed; but interestingly, hypoglycorrhachia can be seen with the transverse myelopathy associated with SLE (113).

Histologically, microinfarcts and larger infarcts are seen in patients dying of nervous system disease in SLE. The infarcts are often hemorrhagic and frequently multiple. Because true vasculitis with perivascular infiltration of inflammatory cells is rare in SLE, other causative mechanisms of cerebral disease in SLE have been postulated. The circulating anticoagulant sometimes found in SLE, despite its name, is infrequently associated with hemorrhagic events but is associated with thrombotic tendencies (117). Lupus anticoagulants and anticardiolipin antibodies are antiphospholipin immunoglobulins which may interfere with neuronal function by binding to neurons or to neurotransmitters. In addition, autopsy studies show cardiac sources of emboli from Libman–Sacks endocarditis and mural thrombi. Arterial occlusions also occur during thrombocytopenic purpura, which may complicate the later stages of SLE.

Therapy for the primary disease process in SLE includes corticosteroids and other immunosuppressive agents. Antipsychotic drugs also are used for the acute delusional and delirious states associated with the encephalopathy once metabolic, toxic, or infectious causes have been excluded.

Sjogren's Syndrome

Like SLE, Sjogren's syndrome is a rheumatological disorder with frequent nervous system manifestations. Peripheral neuropathies occur in about 25% of patients. CNS dysfunction may be even more common, particularly if subtle cognitive change is assessed. Signs and symptoms of CNS disease include: stroke or transient ischemic events; seizures; movement disorders; encephalopathy; intermittent nervous system dysfunction similar to multiple sclerosis; and a recurrent aseptic meningitis.

Sjogren's syndrome is characterized by xerophthalmia (dry eyes), xerostomia (dry mouth), and drying of other mucous membranes as well as the skin. The sicca complex also may occur in association with other connective tissue disease such as rheumatoid arthritis, SLE, or progressive systemic sclerosis.

In the subset of patients whose disease mimics demyelinating disease, the CSF profile in Sjogren's syndrome may look quite similar to that of multiple sclerosis, char-

acterized by elevated IgG index, lymphocytic pleocytosis, and oligoclonal banding. However, preliminary data indicate the presence of anti-rho (SS-A) autoantibodies in the CSF of patients with Sjogren's syndrome and neurological symptoms (118). In addition, HLA studies in multiple sclerosis show the supertypic specificity HLA-DRw$_{53}$, whereas patients with Sjogren's syndrome have supertypic specificity HLD-DRw$_{52}$ (118). At autopsy, diffuse polymorphous meningitis is seen with microhemorrhages and mononuclear cell inflammation. As in SLE, vasculopathy with small-vessel thrombosis and necrosis is present, but it lacks prominent inflammatory response suggestive of vasculitis (119).

Oligoclonal bands are more frequently found in patients with Sjogren's syndrome and active CNS disease; they are infrequent in patients with Sjogren's syndrome without neurological symptoms or signs. MRI is sensitive in demonstrating focal neurological disease in Sjogren's syndrome. Even in patients with diffuse cognitive dysfunction, approximately 50% show abnormalities on MRI—most frequently small, hyperintense areas on T2-weighted images in subcortical white matter.

Behcet's Disease

Behcet's disease, a rheumatic disorder characterized by recurrent oral and genital ulceration with ocular lesions, also can be associated with neurological complications. Five to 10 percent of patients have neurological disease, usually late in the illness. In most cases, oral and genital ulcerations are present at the time of neurological symptoms. Like PAN, any part of the neuraxis may be involved. Seizures, encephalopathy, stroke-like syndromes, cranial nerve paresis, and a meningitis-like picture may occur. However, CSF is frequently abnormal, unlike that in PAN. Pleocytosis is present in a majority of specimens, although usually less than 60 cells per microliter (120). The pleocytosis may be of lymphocytic or polymorphonuclear predominance. Protein is usually mildly elevated. Glucose is normal.

Like those of Sjogren's syndrome, the neurological manifestations of Behcet's syndrome may follow an intermittent, exacerbating–remitting pattern similar to that of multiple sclerosis. Similarly, it may be difficult to distinguish the neurological syndromes of Behcet's disease from those of stroke due to atherosclerotic vascular disease or syphilis or other infiltrative meningeal process. The presence of ocular lesions and oral and genital ulcerations usually clarifies the diagnosis. In fact, without the triad of oral, genital, and ocular lesions, the neurological picture can simulate multiple sclerosis or stroke.

Rheumatoid Arthritis

CNS involvement in rheumatoid arthritis is uncommon, but features of toxic encephalopathy with lethargy, irritability, seizures, or meningeal signs have been described. Cerebral vasculitis in the setting of systemic rheumatoid disease is infrequent.

Vogt–Koyanagi–Harada Syndrome

Inflammation affecting the uvea, retina, meninges, and skin occurs in the Vogt–Koyanagi–Harada (VKH) syndrome (121,122). Meningeal signs and symptoms may be associated with this syndrome, and in one series they were noted in 61% of cases (123). Meningeal symptoms may either precede or follow the onset of ocular inflammation. Because of the occurrence of meningoencephalitis in this syndrome, it has also been called the "uveomeningoencephalitic syndrome" (124). The characteristic features of the syndrome are: (a) severe anterior and posterior uveitis, usually accompanied by detachment of the retina; (b) poliosis (whitening of eyebrows and eyelashes), alopecia, and vitiligo; and (c) dysacousis and tinnitus.

The meningeal phase of the illness begins acutely, usually within 10 days (before or after) of the uveitis. The patient develops low-grade fever, headaches, meningismus, and nausea and vomiting. Frequently there is papilledema, confusion, and fluctuating involvement of cranial nerves III–VII. The CSF shows a predominantly lymphocytic pleocytosis of variable intensity. The course usually is one of gradual remission of nervous system involvement.

As the uveitis resolves, the severe ocular complications may develop; these are glaucoma, cataracts, and phthisis bulbi. Three or more months into the disease the skin and auditory involvement becomes manifest.

VKH syndrome usually is considered an autoimmune disease directed against pigment-bearing tissue. Although controlled trials are lacking in this relatively rare syndrome, corticosteroids have been reported to preserve visual acuity and prevent multisystem involvement. The potential for severe CNS and ocular damage probably warrants such an aggressive approach to treatment, potentially even to include cytotoxic drugs.

Migraine with CSF Pleocytosis

Abnormal CSF is rare in uncomplicated migraine. However, in a subset of patients with migraine and transient neurological dysfunction with headache and focal symptoms, the CSF may be abnormal. A mononuclear pleocytosis occurs in a range from 40 to 233 cells, with an average of 121 (125). Protein levels are increased, usually reaching values of around 100 mg/dl, and glucose concentrations are normal. It is not clear whether the CSF abnormalities reflect an inflammatory process presenting as migraine, or are due to the migraine itself. Stroke of other cause, due to hypertensive vasculopathy

or atherosclerosis, may also cause a transient pleocytosis in the CSF, as may generalized seizures.

Chemical Meningitis

The intrathecal injection of several compounds may cause an inflammatory reaction in the leptomeninges, producing a chemical meningitis. Contrast agents for radiographic studies, as well as drugs such as chemotherapeutic agents, antibiotics, or local anesthetics, may produce a chemical meningitis. Among the contrast agents, the older, oil-based media such as Pantopaque were more likely to produce arachnoiditis than are the newer, water-soluble agents such as Metrizamide. The CSF may reflect a partial or complete spinal block with low opening pressure, elevated protein, and a lymphocytic pleocytosis. At times, fever and signs of meningeal irritation are prominent. The CSF abnormalities generally resolve in 1–2 weeks.

Multiple Sclerosis

The clinical picture of multiple sclerosis is usually distinct from that seen in subacute or chronic meningitis. Fever is generally not present; and the characteristic relapsing–remitting course, abnormalities on neurological examination, and historical evidence of hallmarks of the disease, such as optic neuritis or Lhermitte's sign, usually make the clinical distinction. However, the CSF profile in chronic meningitis and multiple sclerosis may be quite similar. A low level of mononuclear leukocytosis occurs in the CSF in about one-third of cases of multiple sclerosis. The white count is less than 16 per microliter in 95% of patients (126). The likelihood of finding a pleocytosis may be greater during clinical exacerbation. Although total protein is normal in most, mild elevations may be seen, although proteins in excess of 100 mg/dl warrant a search for another diagnosis. Because of increased intrathecal immunoglobulin synthesis, the CSF gamma-globulin content is increased over that in serum. Therefore, indices of gamma-globulin synthesis are increased, and electrophoresis shows the presence of oligoclonal bands in the vast majority of patients with clinically defined multiple sclerosis.

Chronic Meningitis Associated with Malignancies

Brain Tumors

Since the advent of cerebral CT and MRI scanning, it is rarely necessary to examine the CSF to aid in the diagnosis of primary or secondary malignancies of the brain. Lumbar puncture in the setting of a focal mass lesion may, of course, be hazardous, and it rarely assists in diagnosis. An exception to this is the importance of positive cytologies in patients with suspected leptomeningeal carcinomatosis, in whom morphological examination of the cellular CSF content may establish the diagnosis.

In the era preceding CT and MRI scans, brain tumors were not diagnosed as early and CSF examinations were sometimes diagnostic. The hallmarks of brain tumor were those of raised intracranial pressure and elevated CSF protein. Both features, however, may be absent early in the development of these tumors. Xanthrochromia can also occur from CSF protein concentrations greater than 150 mg/dl (127) or from bleeding, which can occur with particular cerebral metastases such as malignant melanoma, renal cell carcinoma, and choriocarcinoma. Of the primary brain tumors, oligodendrogliomas also may be responsible for subarachnoid bleeding.

Necrotic malignant gliomas, particularly those which invade ventricular walls, may be associated with very high CSF cell counts. Protein elevation, according to Fishman (127), is primarily a result of increased endothelial cell permeability associated with these tumors. Because neurofibromas are apparently more permeable to protein than are meningiomas, a CSF protein concentration greater than 200 mg/dl might favor the former diagnosis in patients with a cerebellopontine angle mass.

Leptomeningeal Metastases

Leptomeningeal spread of solid tumors can produce a CSF profile indistinguishable from that seen in chronic meningitis (128). In a series of 90 patients from Memorial Sloan–Kettering, the initial lumbar puncture was abnormal in all but three patients (129). The cell count, predominantly consisting of lymphocytes, was elevated in 51 patients; protein concentration was approximately 50 mg/dl in 73 patients. Hypoglycorrhachia was present in the initial examination in 28 patients. Definitive diagnosis was, of course, confirmed by the finding of malignant cells within the CSF. Positive cytologies were present on initial lumbar puncture in 49 of 90 patients (54%); but on subsequent spinal taps, cytology eventually became positive in 82%. Larger volumes of CSF, as opposed to small aliquots, are likely to yield the diagnosis with greater frequency. Because the recovery of malignant cells solidifies the diagnosis of leptomeningeal carcinomatosis, repeated lumbar punctures (sometimes six or more) have been performed in patients in whom the diagnosis is suspected.

Patients with breast and lung cancer and melanoma are most susceptible to carcinomatous meningitis. Among these, adenocarcinomas most commonly seed the leptomeninges. In the series of 90 patients from Memorial Sloan–Kettering, 73% suffered from adenocarcinoma.

The diagnosis is suggested clinically when neurologi-

cal deficits appear at multiple levels of the neuraxis—involving the cerebrum, cranial nerves, and spinal roots (128,129). Headache and encephalopathy, as well as seizures, may be present. The most common cranial nerve deficits are those involving: extraocular muscles causing diplopia; eighth-nerve dysfunction with hearing loss, dizziness, or vertigo; and seventh- and second-nerve involvement, causing facial numbness and diminished visual acuity. Radicular symptoms are also common: back pain radiating down one or both legs; leg weakness; and sphincter dysfunction. Paresthesias are also present. A cauda equina syndrome may be the presenting feature.

Supporting radiographic studies include myelography, CT, and MRI scans. Myelograms may show thickening and nodularity of the nerve roots, resulting from tumor seeding of the meninges in these areas. MRI is sensitive to these nodules also, and it may show tumor involvement of thickened nerve roots. CT scans of the head, even in the absence of metastatic focal lesions, may show hydrocephalus or enhancement of the basilar cisterns, possibly caused by occlusion of CSF absorptive pathways in the subarachnoid space.

Treatment for leptomeningeal metastases may actually cause a secondary meningoencephalitis or meningitis. After the administration of intraventricular methotrexate via an Ommaya reservoir, for example, an acute meningoencephalopathy may occur with headache, fever, cognitive changes, and meningeal signs. The CSF may show a pleocytosis greater than that at diagnosis with elevated protein, suggesting methotrexate toxicity. However, chemotherapy does result in improvement or stabilization of neurological symptoms in some patients.

Chronic Benign Lymphocytic Meningitis

Some patients with unexplained headache, depression, malaise, and lymphocytic pleocytosis have a self-limited illness (15). In the original description of this syndrome, patients with focal neurological findings specifically were excluded, although three of the seven patients had papilledema. Five of seven cases had a low-grade pleocytosis, with less than 100 mononuclear cells per microliter; protein levels were less than 120 mg/dl, and glucose concentrations were minimally depressed at some time in the course of three patients. The symptoms vacillated in these patients, with four undergoing complete clinical remission after 32–99 weeks; normalization of CSF was, however, documented in only one. There was no clear relationship between changes in the clinical course of a given patient and the CSF abnormalities.

The diagnosis of chronic benign lymphocytic meningitis certainly does not describe a uniform clinical syndrome attributed to a single cause. Consideration of the syndrome does seem to emphasize that some patients with unexplained chronic meningitis chosen to exclude those with fixed or progressive local signs will have a nonprogressive illness. This, of course, must be balanced by the fact that potentially life-threatening infectious disease may begin in a like manner. Nonetheless, following the algorithm for enigmatic cases presented above, most patients fulfilling the criteria for chronic benign lymphocytic meningitis would be observed rather than being required to undergo invasive diagnostic procedures because of the lack of serious functional impairment, the stable course, and low-grade pleocytosis.

REFERENCES

1. Wilhelm C, Ellner JJ. Chronic meningitis. *Neurol Clin* 1986; 4:115–141.
2. Ellner JJ, Bennett JE. Chronic meningitis. *Medicine* 1976; 55:341–369.
3. Swartz M. Chronic meningitis—many causes to consider. *N Engl J Med* 1987;317:957–959.
4. Hermans PE, Goldstein NO, Wellman WE. Mollaret's meningitis and differential diagnosis of recurrent meningitis. *Am J Med* 1972;52:128–140.
5. Hyslop NE Jr, Swartz MN. Bacterial meningitis. *Postgrad Med* 1975;58(3):120–128.
6. Koo J, Pieu F, Kliks MM. Angiostrongylus (Parastrongylus) eosinophilic meningitis. *Rev Infect Dis* 1988;10:1155–1162.
7. Kuberski T. Eosinophils in the cerebrospinal fluid. *Ann Intern Med* 1979;91:70–75.
8. Peacock JE Jr, McGinnis MR, Cohen MS. Persistent neutrophilic meningitis: report of four cases and review of the literature. *Medicine* 1984;63:379–395.
9. Klein BS, Vergeront JM, Weeks RJ, et al. Isolation of *Blastomyces dermatitidis* in soil associated with a large outbreak of blastomycosis in Wisconsin. *N Engl J Med* 1986;314:529–534.
10. Wheat LJ, Kohler RB, Tewari RP, Garten M, French MLV. Significance of Histoplasma antigen in the cerebrospinal fluid of patients with meningitis. *Arch Intern Med* 1989;149:302–304.
11. Wheat LJ, Connolly-Stringfield P, Kohler RB, Frame PT, Gupta MR. *Histoplasma capsulatum* polysaccharide antigen detection in the diagnosis and management of disseminated histoplasmosis in patients with acquired immunodeficiency syndrome. *Am J Med* 1989;87:396–400.
12. Daniel TM. New approaches to the rapid diagnosis of tuberculous meningitis. *J Infect Dis* 1987;155:599–602.
13. Scott EN, Kauman L, Brown AC, et al. Serologic studies in the diagnosis and management of meningitis due to *Sporothrix schenckii. N Engl J Med* 1987;317:935–945.
14. Kravitz GR, Davies SF, Eckman MR, Sarosi GA. Chronic blastomycotic meningitis. *Am J Med* 1981;71:501.
15. Hopkins AP, Harvey PKP. Chronic benign lymphocytic meningitis. *J Neurol Sci* 1973;18:443.
16. Hooper DC, Pruitt AA, Rubin RH. Central nervous system infection in the chronically immunosuppressed. *Medicine* 1982; 61:166–188.
17. Levy RM, Bredesen DE, Rosenblum ML. Neurological manifestations of the acquired immunodeficiency syndrome (AIDS): experience at UCSF and review of the literature. *J Neurosurg* 1985;62:475–495.
18. Ho DD, Pomerantz RJ, Kaplan JC. Pathogenesis of infection with human immunodeficiency virus. *N Engl J Med* 1987; 317:278–286.
19. Narayan O, Kennedy-Stoskopf S, Zink MC. Lentivirus–host interactions: lesions from visna and caprine arthritis–encephalitis viruses. *Ann Neurol* 1988;23(Suppl):S95–S100.
20. Ho DD, Rota TR, Schooley RT, Kaplan JC, et al. Isolation of HTLV-III from cerebrospinal fluid and neural tissues of patients with neurologic syndromes related to the acquired immunodeficiency syndrome. *N Engl J Med* 1985;313:1493–1497.
21. Scully RE, Mark EJ, McNeely BU. Case 43-1986. *Case Records of the Massachusetts General Hospital* 1986;315:1143–1154.
22. Goudsmit J, Wolters EC, Bakker M, Smit L, et al. Intrathecal synthesis of antibodies to HTLV-III in patients without AIDS or AIDS related complex. *Br Med J* 1986;292:1231–1234.
23. Kovacs JA, Kovacs AA, Polis M, et al. Cryptococcosis in the acquired immunodeficiency syndrome. *Ann Intern Med* 1985;103:533–538.
24. Dismukes WE. Cryptococcal meningitis in patients with AIDS. *J Infect Dis* 1988;157:624–628.
25. Zuger A, Louie E, Holzman RS, et al. Cryptococcal disease in patients with the acquired immunodeficiency syndrome. Diagnostic features and outcome of treatment. *Ann Intern Med* 1986;104:234–240.
26. Chuck SL, Sande MA. Infections with *Cryptococcus neoformans* in the acquired immunodeficiency syndrome. *N Engl J Med* 1989;321:794–799.
27. McArthur JC. Neurologic manifestations of AIDS. *Medicine* 1987;66:407–437.
28. Stern JJ, Hartman BH, Sharkey P, et al. Oral fluconazole therapy for patients with acquired immunodeficiency syndrome and cryptococcosis: experience with 22 patients. *Am J Med* 1988;85:477–480.
29. Sugar AM, Saunders C. Oral fluconazole as suppressive therapy of disseminated cryptococcosis in patients with acquired immunodeficiency syndrome. *Am J Med* 1988;85:481–489.
30. Byrne WR, Wajszczuk CP. Cryptococcal meningitis in the acquired immunodeficiency syndrome (AIDS): successful treatment with fluconazole after failure of amphotericin B. *Ann Intern Med* 1988;108:384–385.
31. Arndt CAS, Walsh TJ, et al. Fluconazole penetration into cerebrospinal fluid: implications for treating fungal infections of the central nervous system. *J Infect Dis* 1988;157:178–180.
32. Israelski DM, Remington JS. Toxoplasmic encephalitis in patients with AIDS. *Infect Dis Clin North Am* 1986;2:429–444.
33. Luft BJ, Remington JS. Toxoplasmic encephalitis. *J Infect Dis* 1987;157:1–6.
34. Carrazana EJ, Rossitch E Jr, Samuels MA. Cerebral toxoplasmosis in the acquired immune deficiency syndrome. *Clin Neurol Neurosurg* 1989;91:291–301.
35. De La Paz RL, Enzman D. Neuroradiology of acquired immunodeficiency syndrome. In: Rosenblum RL, Levy RM, Bredesen D, et al., eds. *AIDS and the nervous system.* New York: Raven Press, 1988;121–153.
36. Navia BA, Petito CK, Gold JWM, et al. Cerebral toxoplasmosis complicating the acquired immune deficiency syndrome: clinical neuropathological findings in 27 patients. *Ann Neurol* 1986; 19:224–238.
37. Potasman I, Resnick L, Luft BJ, Remington JS. Intrathecal production of antibodies against *Toxoplasma gondii* in patients with toxoplasmic encephalitis and the acquired immunodeficiency syndrome (AIDS). *Ann Intern Med* 1988;108:49–51.
38. Cohn JA, McMeeking A, Cohen W, et al. Evaluation of the policy of empiric treatment of suspected *Toxoplasma* encephalitis in patients with the acquired immunodeficiency syndrome. *Am J Med* 1989;86:521–527.
39. Leport C, Raffi F, Matheron S, et al. Treatment of central nervous system toxoplasmosis with pyrimethamine/sulfadiazine combination in 35 patients with the acquired immunodeficiency syndrome. *Am J Med* 1988;84:94–100.
40. Woolsey RM, Chambers TJ, Chung HD, McGarry JD. Mycobacterial meningomyelitis associated with human immunodeficiency virus infection. *Arch Neurol* 1988;45:691–693.
41. Bishburg E, Sunderam G, Reichman LB, Kapila R. Central nervous system tuberculosis with the acquired immunodeficiency syndrome and its related complex. *Ann Intern Med* 1986; 105:210–213.
42. Johns DR, Tierney M, Felsenstein D. Alteration in the natural history of neurosyphilis by concurrent infection with the human immunodeficiency virus. *N Engl J Med* 1987;316:1569–1602.
43. Emskitter TH, Jenzevski H, Pulz M, Spehn J. Neurosyphilis in HIV infection—persistence after high-dose penicillin therapy. *J Neuroimmunol* 1988;20:153–155.
44. Berry CD, Hooton TM, Collier AC, Lukehart SA. Neurologic relapse after benzathine penicillin therapy for secondary syphilis

in a patient with HIV infection. *N Engl J Med* 1987;316:1587–1589.
45. Bayne LL, Schmidley JW, Goodin DS. Acute syphilitic meningitis: its occurrence after clinical and serologic cure of secondary syphilis with penicillin G. *Arch Neurol* 1986;43:137–138.
46. Lowenthal DA, Straus DJ, et al. AIDS-related lymphoid neoplasia. *Cancer* 1988;61:2325–2337.
47. Rosenblum ML, Levy RM, Bredesen DE. *AIDS and the nervous system.* New York: Raven Press, 1988.
48. Ziegler JL, Beckstead JA, Volberding PA, et al. Non-Hodgkin's lymphoma in 90 homosexual men. *N Engl J Med* 1984;311:565–570.
49. Rich AR, McCordock HA. The pathogenesis of tuberculous meningitis. *Bull Johns Hopkins Hosp* 1933;52:5.
50. Molavi A, LeFrock JL. Tuberculous meningitis. *Med Clin North Am* 1985;69:315–331.
51. Lepper MH, Spies HW. The present status of the treatment of tuberculosis of the central nervous system. *Ann NY Acad Sci* 1963;106:106.
52. Weiss W, Flippin HF. The changing incidence and prognosis of tuberculous meningitis. *Am J Med Sci* 1965;50:46.
53. Barrett-Conner EB. Tuberculous meningitis in adults. *South Med J* 1967;60:1061.
54. Kennedy DH, Fallon FJ. Tuberculous meningitis. *JAMA* 1979;241:264–268.
55. Johnson J, Ellner JJ. Tuberculous meningitis. In: Evans RW, Baskin DS, Yatsu FM, eds. *Prognosis in neurological disease.* New York: Oxford University Press, 1990.
56. Weiss W, Flippin HF. The changing incidence and prognosis of tuberculous meningitis. *Am J Med Sci* 1965;250:80–93.
57. Ogawa SK, Smith MA, Brennessel DJ, Lowy FJ. Tuberculous meningitis in an urban medical center. *Medicine* 1987;66:317–326.
58. Klein NC, Damsker B, Hirschmann SZ. Mycobacterial meningitis: retrospective analyses from 1970–1983. *Am J Med* 1985;79:29–34.
59. Merritt HH, Fremont-Smith F. Cerebrospinal fluid in tuberculous meningitis. *Arch Neurol Psychol* 1935;33:516.
60. Jeren T, Beus I. Characteristics of cerebrospinal fluid in tuberculous meningitis. *Acta Cytol* 1982;26:678.
61. Stewart SM. The bacteriologic diagnosis of tuberculous meningitis. *J Clin Pathol* 1953;6:241–242.
62. Brooks JB, Daneshuar MI, Fast DM, Good RC. Selective procedures for detecting femtomole quantities of tuberculostearic acid in serum and CSF by frequency-pulsed electron capture gas–liquid chromatography. *J Clin Microbiol* 1987;25:1201–1206.
63. French GL, Chan CY, Cheung SW, et al. Diagnosis of tuberculous meningitis by detection of tuberculostearic acid in cerebrospinal fluid. *Lancet* 1987;2:117–119.
63a. Brooks JB, Daneshuar MI, Maherberger RL, Mikhail IA. Rapid diagnosis of tuberculous meningitis by frequency-pulsed electron-captured gas-liquid chromotography detection of cerbotylic acid in cerebeluspinal fluid *J Clin Med* 1990;28:989–997.
64. Stocksill MT, Kauffman CA. Comparison of cryptococcal and tuberculous meningitis. *Arch Neurol* 1983;40:81–85.
65. Spickard A, Butler WT, Andriole V, et al. The improved prognosis of cryptococcal meningitis with amphotericin B therapy. *Ann Intern Med* 1963;58:66.
66. Butler WT, Alling DW, Spickard A, et al. Diagnostic and prognostic value of clinical and laboratory findings in cryptococcal meningitis. A follow-up study of forty patients. *N Engl J Med* 1964;270:59.
67. Littman ML, Walter JE. Cryptococcosis: current status. *Am J Med* 1968;45:922.
68. Diamond RD, Bennett JE. Prognostic factors in cryptococcal meningitis. A study of 111 cases. *Ann Intern Med* 1974;80:176.
69. Bouza E, Dreyer JS, Hewitt WL, Meyer RD. Coccidioidal meningitis. An analysis of 31 cases and review of the literature. *Medicine* 1981;60:139–172.
70. Candill RG, Smith CE, Reinarz JA. Coccidioidal meningitis. A diagnostic challenge. *Am J Med* 1970;49:360.
71. Deresinski SC, Stevens DA. Coccidioidomycosis in compromised hosts. *Medicine* 1974;54:377.
72. Winn WA. The treatment of coccidioidal meningitis. The use of amphotericin B in a group of 25 patients. *Calif Med* 1964;101:75.
73. Smith CE, Saito MT, Simons SA. Pattern of 39,500 serologic tests in coccidioidomycosis. *JAMA* 1956;160:546.
74. Winn WA. Coccidioidal meningitis: a follow-up report. In: Ajello L, ed. *Coccidiomycosis.* Tucson: University of Arizona Press, 1967;55.
75. Smith JW, Utz JP. Progressive disseminated histoplasmosis. *Ann Intern Med* 1972;76:557.
76. Tynes BS, Crutcher JC, Utz JP. Progressive disseminated histoplasmosis. *Ann Intern Med* 1972;76:557.
77. Gilden DH, Miller EM, Johnson WG. Central nervous system histoplasmosis after rhinoplasty. *Neurology* 1974;24:874.
78. Gelfand JA, Bennett JE. Active *Histoplasma* meningitis of 22 years duration. *JAMA* 1975;233:1294.
79. Wheat J, French M, Batteiger B, et al. Cerebrospinal fluid *Histoplasma* antibodies in central nervous system histoplasmosis. *Arch Intern Med* 1985;145:1237.
80. Wheat LJ, Kohler RB, Tewari RP. Diagnosis of disseminated histoplasmosis by detection of *Histoplasma capsulatum* antigen in serum and urine specimens. *N Engl J Med* 1986;314:83.
81. Buechner HA, Clawson CM. Blastomycosis of central nervous system. II. A report of nine cases from the Veterans Administration Cooperative Study. *Am Rev Respir Dis* 1967;95:820.
82. Ewing GE, Bose GJ, Petersen PK. *Sporothrix schenckii* meningitis in a farmer with Hodgkin's disease. *Am J Med* 1980;68:455.
83. DeVita VT, Utz JP, Williams T, et al. *Candida* meningitis. *Arch Intern Med* 1966;117:527.
84. Bayer AS, Edwards JE Jr, Seidel JS, et al. *Candida* meningitis. *Medicine* 1976;55:477–486.
85. Fincham RW, Sahs AL, Joynt RJ. Protean manifestations of nervous system brucellosis. *JAMA* 1963;184:97.
86. Bouza E, Garcia de la Torre M, Parras F, et al. Brucellar meningitis. *Rev Infect Dis* 1987;9:810–822.
87. Pascual J, Combarios O, Polo JM, Verciano J. Localized CNS brucellosis: report of 7 cases. *Acta Neurol Scand* 1988;78:282–289.
88. Merritt HH, Adams RD, Solomon HC. *Neurosyphilis.* New York: Oxford University Press, New York, 1946.
89. Hooshmand H, Escobar MR, Kopf SW. Neurosyphilis: a study of 241 patients. *JAMA* 1972;219:726–729.
90. Simon RP. Neurosyphilis. *Arch Neurol* 1985;42:606–613.
91. Willcox RR. Treatment of syphilis. *Bull WHO* 1981;59:655–663.
92. Wilske B, Schierz G, Preac-Mursic V, et al. Intrathecal production of specific antibodies against *Borrelia burgdorferi* in patients with lymphocytic meningoradiculitis (Bannwarth's syndrome). *J Infect Dis* 1986;153:304–314.
93. Pachner AR, Steere AC. The triad of neurologic manifestations of Lyme disease: meningitis, cranial neuritis, and radiculoneuritis. *Neurology* 1985;35:47–53.
94. Halperin JJ, Luft BJ, Anand AK, et al. Lyme neuroborreliosis: central nervous system manifestations. *Neurology* 1989;39:753–759.
95. Abramowicz M, ed. Treatment of Lyme disease. *Med Lett Drugs Ther* 1989;31:31.
96. Loo L, Braude A. Cerebral cysticercosis in San Diego. *Medicine* 1982;61:341–359.
97. McCormick GF, Zee C-S, Heiden J. Cysticercosis cerebri. Review of 127 cases. *Arch Neurol* 1982;39:534–539.
98. Douglas AC, Maloney AFJ. Sarcoidosis of the central nervous system. *J Neurol Neurosurg Psychiatry* 1973;36:1024–1033.
99. Rosas N, Sotelo J, Nieto D. ELISA in the diagnosis of neurocysticercosis. *Arch Neurol* 1986;43:353–356.
100. Salaki JS, Louria DB, Chmel H. Fungal and yeast infections of the central nervous system: a clinical review. *Medicine* 1984;63:108–113.
101. Jones PG, Gilman RM, Medeiros AA, et al. Focal intracranial mucormycosis presenting as chronic meningitis. *JAMA* 1981;24:2063.
102. Bennett HE, Bonner H, Jennings AE, et al. Chronic meningitis caused by *Cladosporium trichoides.* *Am J Clin Pathol* 1973;59:398.
103. Pereira WC, Raphael A, Tehuto RA, et al. Localizacao encefalica da blastomicose sud-Americana: consideracoes a proposito de 9 casos. *Arq Neuropsiquiatr* 1965;23:113.
104. Richter RW, Silva M, Neu HC, et al. The neurological aspects of *Nocardia asteroides* infection. *Infect Nerv Syst* 1968;44:424.

105. King RB, Stoops WL, Fitzgibbon J, et al. *Nocardia asteroides* meningitis. A case successfully treated with large doses of sulfadiazine and urea. *J Neurosurg* 1966;24:749.

106. Smego RA Jr. Actinomycosis of the central nervous system. *Rev Infect Dis* 1987;9:855.

107. Stern BJ, Krumholz A, Johns C, et al. Sarcoidosis and its neurological manifestations. *Arch Neurol* 1985;42:909–917.

108. Delaney P. Neurologic manifestations in sarcoidosis. *Ann Intern Med* 1977;87:336–345.

109. Gaines JD, Eckman PM, Remington JS. Low CSF glucose level in sarcoidosis involving the central nervous system. *Arch Intern Med* 1970;125:333–336.

110. Cupps TR, Moore PM, Fauci AS. Isolated angiitis of the central nervous system. Prospective diagnostic and therapeutic experience. *Am J Med* 1983;74:97–105.

111. Reik L, Grunnet ML, Spencer RP, Donaldson JO. Granulomatous angiitis presenting as chronic meningitis and ventriculitis. *Neurology* 1983;33:1609–1612.

112. Nurik S, Blackwood W, Mair WGP. Giant cell granulomatous angiitis of the central nervous system. *Brain* 1972;95:133–142.

113. Sigal LH. The neurologic presentation of vasculitis and rheumatologic syndromes. A review. *Medicine* 1987;66:157–180.

114. Scully RE, Galdabini JJ, McNeelu BU. Case 43-1976. *N Engl J Med* 1976;295:944–950.

115. Vollertsen RS, McDonald TJ, Younge BR, et al. Cogan's syndrome: 18 cases and a review of the literature. *Mayo Clin Proc* 1986;61:344–361.

116. Jacobs L, Kinkel PR, Costello PB, et al. Central nervous system lupus erythematosus: the value of magnetic resonance imaging. *J Rheumatol* 1988;15:601–606.

117. Levine ST, Welch KMA. The spectrum of neurologic disease associated with antiphospholipid antibodies. *Arch Neurol* 1987;44:876–883.

118. Provost TT, Vasily D, Alexander E. Sjogren's syndrome. *Neurol Clin* 1987;5:405–426.

119. Alexander E, Provost TT. Sjogren's syndrome. Association of cutaneous vasculitis with central nervous system disease. *Arch Dermatol* 1987;123:801–810.

120. Schotland DL, Wolf SM, White HH, Dubin HV. Neurologic aspects of Behcet's disease. Case report and review of the literature. *Am J Med* 1963;34:544–553.

121. Cowper AR. Harada's disease and Vogt–Koyanagi syndrome. *Arch Ophthalmol* 1951;45:367.

122. Riehl J-L, Andrews JM. The uveomeningoencephalitis syndrome. *Neurology (Minn)* 1966;16:603.

123. Ohno S, Char DH, Kimura SJ, O'Connor GR. Vogt–Koyanagi–Harada syndrome. *Am J Ophthalmol* 1977;83:735–740.

124. Pattison EM. Uveomeningoencephalitic syndrome (Vogt–Koyanagi–Harada). *Arch Neurol* 1965;12:197.

125. Bartleson JD, Swanson JW, Whisnant JP. A migrainous syndrome with cerebrospinal fluid pleocytosis. *Neurology* 1981;31:1257–1262.

126. Tourtellotte WW. Cerebrospinal fluid in multiple sclerosis. In: Vinken PJ, Bruin GW, eds. *Handbook of clinical neurology*, vol 9. Amsterdam: Elsevier, 1979;324–382.

127. Fishman RA. *Cerebrospinal fluid in diseases of the nervous system.* Philadelphia: WB Saunders, 1980.

128. Gonzalez-Vitale JC, Garcia-Bunel R. Meningeal carcinomatosis. *Cancer* 1976;37:2906–2911.

129. Wasserstrom WR, Glass JP, Posner JB. Diagnosis and treatment of leptomeningeal metastases from solid tumors: experience with 90 patients. *Cancer* 1982;49:759–772.

Infections of the Central Nervous System,
edited by W. M. Scheld, R. J. Whitley, and
D. T. Durack, Raven Press, Ltd., New York © 1991.

CHAPTER 31

Diagnosis and Treatment of Fungal Meningitis

John R. Perfect

This chapter discusses an approach to diagnosis and treatment of fungal meningitis. These important central nervous system (CNS) infections comprise a diverse group of clinical situations, some well understood and others obscure. In some cases a diagnosis can be made in a few minutes with a simple India ink test, whereas in others even meningeal biopsy for histopathology and culture fails to yield the etiology. Information on treatment regimens ranges from extensive (in the case of cryptococcal meningitis, one of the most intensively studied CNS infections) to scanty or nonexistent (in the case of rare, opportunistic fungi). Treatment for fungal meningitis is more difficult than that for most forms of bacterial meningitis, and prognosis is worse. Fungal meningitis has become much more common in the past decade, due to the high frequency of cryptococcal meningitis in acquired immunodeficiency syndrome (AIDS) patients.

DIAGNOSIS

The clinical presentation of fungal meningitis is less stereotyped than that of bacterial meningitis. Patients most often present with the chronic meningitis syndrome, defined as meningitis which fails to improve or which progresses over at least 4 weeks of observation (1). Likely manifestations include some combination of fever, headache, lethargy, confusion, nausea, vomiting, stiff neck, or neurological deficits. Often, only one or two of the cardinal manifestations will be present at first. For example, patients may present with nothing more than a subacute dementia.

The time course of illness is a vitally important consideration in diagnosis of fungal meningitis. A few cases present as acute meningitis, many are subacute, and

some are chronic. Occasionally cryptococcal, coccidioidal, or histoplasmic meningitis cause symptoms persisting for years, even in the absence of treatment (2–5). Careful evaluation of the natural history and meticulous, repeated observation may be required before the diagnosis can be confirmed. In contrast, immunocompromised patients such as those receiving high doses of corticosteroids or those with human immunodeficiency virus (HIV) infection can develop severe symptoms and signs of cryptococcal meningitis within a few days.

Fungal meningitis always is a primary consideration in the differential diagnosis of a patient with the chronic meningitis syndrome (see Chapter 30). However, the differential diagnosis includes many other infectious and noninfectious conditions (Table 1). For instance, it may be particularly difficult to distinguish fungal meningitis from mycobacterial meningitis (6).

The cerebrospinal fluid (CSF) findings in fungal meningitis have been well studied (7). Most cases have a mononuclear pleocytosis, ranging from 20 to 500 cells per cubic millimeter. The proportion of polymorphonuclear leukocytes is variable, usually well below 50%. In a few cases, polymorphonuclear leukocytes predominate; this is most likely in CNS infections caused by species of *Aspergillus, Zygomycetes* or *Pseudallescheria.* In severely immunocompromised patients, especially those with AIDS or those on high-dose corticosteroids, very low or even normal leukocyte counts may be found during active cryptococcal meningitis. This syndrome is precisely mimicked by experimental cryptococcal meningitis in rabbits treated with cortisone (8). Although most cases present with a predominance of mononuclear cells, chronic neutrophilic meningitis can occur (9).

CSF protein levels generally are elevated. If very high protein concentrations (i.e., above 1 g/dl) are found, a subarachnoid block is likely to be present. CSF glucose levels in fungal meningitis often are reduced, but may be normal. Hypoglycorrhachia in a patient with meningitis

J. R. Perfect: Division of Infectious Diseases and International Health, Duke University Medical Center, Durham, North Carolina 27710.

729

TABLE 1. *Some important nonfungal conditions that can cause chronic meningitis*

Infectious	Noninfectious
Aseptic meningitis, due to viruses[a]	Aseptic meningitis, due to drugs or chemical inflammation (arachnoiditis)
Syphilis	Parameningeal infections
Lyme disease	Subarachnoid hemorrhage
Brucellosis	Systemic lupus erythematosus
Toxoplasmosis	Granulomatous arteritis
Nocardiosis	Carcinomatous meningitis
Actinomycosis	Sarcoidosis
Leptospirosis	Chronic benign lymphocytic meningitis
Helminthic meningitis	Behcet's disease
Mycobacterial infections	

[a] Most cases of viral meningitis are acute, producing self-limiting disease.

suggests an infectious cause, but noninfectious processes also can produce low CSF glucose levels. A list of various causes for hypoglycorrhachia is presented in Table 2. A fungal brain abscess may present with normal CSF parameters or with a mild pleocytosis and elevated protein, but glucose usually is normal (see Chapter 32).

Conclusive proof for a fungal CNS infection is provided by identification of the fungus in brain tissue or in CSF (Table 3). Unfortunately, CSF cultures are not always positive in fungal meningitis. Only one-quarter to one-half of patients with coccidioidal meningitis have positive CSF cultures. Blastomycotic meningitis rarely yields positive CSF cultures, and even at autopsy it is difficult to grow *Histoplasma* from the subarachnoid space. The best-studied cause of fungal meningitis, *Cryptococcus neoformans,* yields positive CSF cultures in approximately 75% of patients. Today, this figure is higher because the majority of new cases occur in AIDS pa-

TABLE 2. *Some conditions that can cause low CSF glucose concentrations*

Acute bacterial meningitis
Mycobacterial meningitis
Fungal meningitis
Subarachnoid hemorrhage
Carcinomatous meningitis
Meningeal cysticercosis/trichinosis
Drug-induced meningitis (nonsteroidal anti-inflammatories)
Acute syphilitic meningitis
Chemical meningitis (direct intrathecal injections)
Viral meningitis (occasionally; i.e., mumps)
Hypoglycemia
Rheumatoid meningitis
Lupus myelopathy
Amebic meningitis

tients, who have a higher proportion of positive CSF cultures—about 90%.

Clinicians should be aware that in certain cases of fungal meningitis it is extremely difficult to isolate fungi from the CSF despite multiple attempts. To improve the yield, large volumes of CSF (10–30 ml) should be withdrawn and sent for culture when fungal meningitis is considered likely but the routine CSF examination was negative. The microbiologist should be requested to centrifuge these specimens and to place the sediment onto appropriate culture media.

Candida species can be identified in the laboratory within a few days. *C. neoformans* will be identified in most cases from 2 to 10 days after the laboratory receives the specimen. Classic dimorphic fungi such as *Blastomyces, Histoplasma,* or *Coccidioides* will require several weeks for identification. Lysis–centrifugation culture methods for isolation of yeasts from blood have better detection capabilities than do routine or radiometric methods (10). Although this method is not likely to improve isolation of yeasts from CSF, it may be helpful in identifying yeasts in the blood in some patients who have systemic infection linked to the cause of the CNS infection. Unfortunately, except for *Candida, Cryptococcus,* and *Histoplasma* in AIDS patients, blood cultures usually are negative during fungal meningitis. Cultures of CSF from the lumbar space may be negative because the meninges are not involved at that site. Fungal meningitis commonly involves primarily the basilar meninges, and thus cisternal CSF may yield organisms when lumbar fluid is negative (11). Likewise, yeasts may be found growing in ventricular fluid during a ventricular shunt infection when the lumbar fluid is sterile. It is important to emphasize that in difficult cases of chronic meningitis, repeated lumbar fluid examinations or CSF from cisternal or ventricular fluid may be needed for diagnosis. Stereotaxic brain biopsies with culture and histological examination of the aspirate have been particularly successful in identifying fungal brain abscesses with organisms such as *Aspergillus* (12).

Although a positive culture is the gold standard for diagnosis of a fungal CNS infection, cultures may be negative or very slow to grow to the point where they can be identified in the laboratory. Therefore, adjunctive tests may be helpful. Serological tests are important in the diagnosis of some forms of fungal meningitis, especially cryptococcal infection. The latex agglutination test for cryptococcal polysaccharide antigen is both sensitive and specific (13–15). When samples are heated to eliminate rheumatoid factor (16) and proper controls for nonspecific agglutination and interfering substances (17) are performed, the antigen test is well over 90% sensitive and specific for *C. neoformans* infection. False-positive tests may occur if surface condensation from agar plates contaminates the assay slide (18). False-positive tests also can be associated with other infections. For

TABLE 3. *Some diagnostic and therapeutic characteristics of fungi that cause CNS infection*[a]

Microorganism	CSF cultures positive	CSF serologies	Primary antifungal therapy	References
Aspergillus species	Rare	Ab/An	AMB	99,108–110,126,127
Blastomyces dermatitidis	Rare	Ab	AMB	104,105,111
Candida species	50%	Ab/An	AMB/5FC	65,98,106,107,114,115
Coccidioides immitis	25–45%	Ab	IT AMB	21,45,87,88
Cryptococcus neoformans	75–80%	An	AMB/5FC	48,64,72,74,75,112,113
Dematiacious fungi	Rare	None	Surgery	101,102
Histoplasma capsulatum	50%	Ab	AMB	22,116–118,120
Paracoccidioides brasiliensis	Rare	Ab	KTZ	119
Pseudallescheria boydii	Rare	None	MCZ/KTZ	121,122
Sporothrix schenckii	Rare	Ab	AMB	123–125
Zygomycetes species	Rare	Ab	AMB	100,102

[a] Ab, antibody test; An, antigen test; AMB, amphotericin B; FC, flucytosine; MCZ, miconazole; KTZ, ketoconazole; IT, intrathecal.

example, false cryptococcal antigen titers can be found in disseminated *Trichosporon beigelii* infection (19), and they also have been reported in paravertebral bacterial infections (20).

Detection of this antigen in CSF demonstrates infection of the subarachnoid space, because the large polysaccharide molecules probably do not diffuse into CSF from serum. The polysaccharide antigen test may be positive early in the infection, even when the culture is negative. Titers of 1:8 or greater are usual, but any titer can be significant if proper controls are performed (15).

Antigen often can be found in serum as well as in CSF. In normal hosts with cryptococcal meningitis, serum titers usually are negative or are lower than in the CSF. In severely immunocompromised patients, especially AIDS patients with disseminated disease, serum titers may be extremely high; in such cases they often exceed the titer in CSF. Therefore, serum cryptococcal antigen detection has been effectively used in HIV-infected patients as a screen for possible CNS infection.

Although the latex test for cryptococcal antigen is one of the best diagnostic tests available for any fungal disease, it is not infallible. Rare false-positives occur. Therefore, if a patient whose clinical presentation does not seem compatible with cryptococcal meningitis proves to have a positive CSF cryptococcal antigen the test should be repeated before a diagnosis is made and treatment started, especially if the titer is very low. False-negative tests are uncommon; in most cases these are due to early infection with a low burden of organisms in the CSF, and they will eventually turn positive. Repeatedly negative titers over a period of a month or more virtually rule out the diagnosis of cryptococcal meningitis. Alternatively, a false-negative can represent a prozone phenomenon resulting from antigen excess.

The cryptococcal antigen test has been a major advance in diagnosis, but unfortunately its ability to assess response to treatment remains uncertain. Certainly it is reassuring if antigen titers drop during therapy, when compared with previous CSF specimens tested with the same commercial kit. However, guidelines for using titers to ensure success of treatment cannot be given.

Cryptococcal antibody titers are not presently useful in clinical practice.

For infection with *Coccidioides immitis,* elevated complement-fixing antibodies (CFAs) are the hallmark of disseminated disease. Serum CFA titers above 1:32–1:64 suggest disseminated disease. However, patients with coccidioidal meningitis may have low serum CFA titers when other body sites are not involved. In patients with meningitis, CFA titers are present in CSF from at least 70% of patients when infection is initially diagnosed, and from almost all patients as the infection progresses. If the patient does not have meningitis, CFA is usually negative in unconcentrated CSF even in the presence of high serum CFA titers associated with extraneural disease. Occasionally CFA is positive in CSF in the absence of meningitis when a parameningeal coccidioidal lesion abuts the dura mater.

In coccidioidal meningitis the CFA titers appear to parallel the course of meningeal disease. Therefore, they can be used as a basis for both diagnosis and treatment (21). Patients who relapse after initial response to therapy generally develop CSF pleocytosis or abnormal protein or glucose concentrations before detectable CSF antibody recurs.

Detection of specific antibodies in the CSF has been used for diagnosis of histoplasmic meningitis (22), *Sporothrix* meningitis (23), and *Zygomycetes* infections of the CNS (24). Because the CSF is culture-positive in less than 50% of cases of histoplasma meningitis, detection of antibodies to *Histoplasma* by both complement-fixation and radioimmune assays have been used for diagnosis. These tests have excellent sensitivity, but they are less specific. Cross-reactions with other fungal pathogens occur in approximately 50% of cases. Histoplasma antibodies can also be found in CSF when the blood–brain barrier is broken during meningitis caused by other pathogens if patients have preexisting antibody titers in their serum. A recent diagnostic approach has been the detection of histoplasma polysaccharide antigen (25), which was found in the CSF of 40% of patients with histoplasma meningitis in one series. Potentially it could be useful in the rapid diagnosis of infection in immunocompromised hosts, in whom antibody tests are less useful.

Sporothrix meningitis is extremely difficult to diagnose. Delays of up to 6–7 months from initial symptoms can occur when cultures are used as the basis for diagnosis. A latex agglutination test and enzyme immunoassay for *Sporothrix* antibodies has been successful in confirming diagnosis of this rare infection in the CSF (23). When a titer of 1:8 or greater was used, there was no cross-reaction with other pathogens. These serological tests for fungal antibodies and antigens should always be considered in the diagnostic work-up for difficult cases of chronic meningitis.

Several other potentially useful serological tests for fungi have not yet been formally studied in CSF. *Aspergillus* antibody testing has been used in identifying chronic lung infections; and *Aspergillus* antigen detection tests have been used in blood, sputum, and CSF of immunocompromised hosts (26). *Aspergillus* antigen detection has also been helpful in the detection of *Aspergillus* meningitis (9). Candida antibody and antigen tests are presently too insensitive to be consistently useful in predicting invasive candidiasis. No formal attempts have been used to study their value in CSF.

There are several other old and new techniques which could be useful for diagnosis of fungal meningitis. For cryptococcal meningitis, India ink examination of CSF remains a rapid, effective test. It is positive in approximately 50% of all cases; in patients with HIV infection, this increases to 80%. In some AIDS patients, the CSF contains more yeasts than leukocytes. One novel method to detect yeasts in the CNS is to test CSF samples for products of yeast metabolism, such as arabinitol and mannitol. Increased arabinitol and mannitol concentrations have been found in CSF of animals with experimental candida and cryptococcal meningitis, respectively (27,28). So far, this approach has not been studied in humans. Another unique method for determining the presence of certain fungi in the subarachnoid space is to examine the blastogenic response of lymphocytes separated from the CSF to specific fungal antigens (29). Several older tests may also be useful in the diagnosis of fungal meningitis. A cytological examination of cells spun down from CSF may occasionally reveal a fungus. When brain parenchyma is involved, a methenamine silver stain of an aspirate may be extremely helpful. For instance, *Zygomycetes* may be seen on histological or cytological preparations even though culture of the specimen is negative. Although not specific for fungal meningitis, CSF lactic acid concentrations are generally elevated (30).

TREATMENT

The treatment of fungal meningitis will be approached from three perspectives: (i) a review of some features, relevant to the CNS, of the main antifungal drugs, (ii) recommendations for treatment of specific fungal infections, and (iii) prognosis.

Amphotericin B

Amphotericin B has been used for over 30 years to treat many forms of fungal meningitis. The degree of success achieved has been remarkable in view of the fact that amphotericin B levels in the CSF during treatment are generally low or even unmeasurable (31–33). This observation suggests that the drug either (a) accumulates in affected CNS tissues (including the meninges) rather than in CSF or (b) stimulates or enhances the host's immune responses. Certainly, amphotericin B has some specific immunostimulatory effects. Because amphotericin B concentrations in the subarachnoid space following intravenous administration are so low, some clinicians have used intrathecal administration through subcutaneous reservoirs or directly into the cisternal or lumbar space to achieve higher drug levels (34,35). For example, intrathecal doses of 0.25–0.5 mg/day have been used to suppress coccidioidal meningitis or to treat severe cases of cryptococcal meningitis. However, administration of intrathecal amphotericin B carries certain risks. Side effects in the CNS include arachnoiditis, vasculitis, and secondary bacterial infections of subcutaneous reservoirs used to administer intrathecal amphotericin B (36).

Flucytosine

Flucytosine can be used to treat CNS fungal infections caused by *Candida, Cryptococcus,* and *Chromoblastomyces*. This drug penetrates well into CSF, achieving concentrations approaching 75% of simultaneous serum levels. Despite its excellent pharmacokinetics in the CNS, flucytosine should not be given alone for treatment of CNS fungal infections. Treatment failures with both meningitis and brain abscesses have occurred because fungi developed *in vitro* and *in vivo* resistance during single-drug therapy (37,38). Therefore, clinicians have generally used it in combination with amphotericin B for treatment of CNS infections.

Miconazole

This drug is a nonabsorbable imidazole which is usually used for topical therapy for treating candida or superficial dermatophyte infections. Experience with intravenous miconazole in treatment of CNS mycoses is limited. Both successes (39,40) and failures (41) in treatment of fungal meningitis have been reported. Because miconazole does not penetrate well into the subarachnoid space, intrathecal drug must be given for management of meningitis (42).

Ketoconazole

Ketoconazole is an oral imidazole which has proven effective in treatment of deep-seated infections of histoplasmosis, blastomycosis, paracoccidioidomycosis, and coccidioidomycosis (43). This drug has *in vitro* activity against many fungi which cause CNS infections, but poor penetration across the blood–CSF and blood–brain barrier limits its use in meningitis. Failures of ketoconazole treatment for fungal meningitis have occurred (44). Investigators have attempted to improve its efficacy in fungal meningitis by raising the dose to produce higher serum and CSF drug levels. Some improvement in patients with coccidioidal meningitis was reported using doses as high as 1,200 mg/day (45). This dose carries a high rate of side effects. Although no significant human experience with ketoconazole in combination with either amphotericin B or flucytosine has been reported, these regimens have succeeded in an animal model of meningitis (46).

Fluconazole

Fluconazole is a new, broad-spectrum triazole compound which has been used to treat cryptococcal and candidal infections (47). It possesses excellent properties for treatment of CNS infections. The drug passes easily across the blood–CSF barrier and has a long half-life in this CNS compartment, in both humans (48–50) and animals (51,52). It has been used successfully in the treatment of cryptococcal meningitis (52) in animals, as well as for suppressive therapy of this infection in AIDS patients (53–55).

Investigational Agents

Several investigational treatments may be useful for fungal meningitis. Liposomal amphotericin B appears to have reduced toxicity for the host and therefore can be administered in higher doses (56). If there is greater accumulation of drug in the CNS with higher doses, this preparation may represent an advance in treatment of fungal CNS infections. Itraconazole is a new triazole which has broad-spectrum *in vitro* inhibitory activity, which includes *Aspergillus* species (57,58). This agent shows very limited penetration into CSF (51), yet it has been successful in treatment of cryptococcal meningitis in animals (52) and in humans with AIDS (59,60). Its apparently

paradoxical effectiveness in treatment of CNS infections may be related to its potent antifungal activity and its lipophilic nature. This characteristic allows avid binding to host cells. Possibly, itraconazole could be transported directly to the site of infection by immune cells recruited to infiltrate infected tissue in the CNS. SCH 39304 is another investigational triazole which penetrates well into the CNS of animals and which has proven effective in treatment of fungal meningitis in animal models (61). Finally, cilofungin is a fungicidal lipopeptide derived from echinocandin B. This new agent has potent *in vitro* fungicidal activity against *C. albicans* and *C. tropicalis.* Its ability to treat candidal CNS infections has not been tested, but it shows limited penetration into the CNS unless given by constant infusion. It will likely remain a prototype for future derivatives because clinical investigations have been halted as a result of toxicity.

Combinations of Antifungal Drugs

Combination therapy for CNS fungal infections offers the potential of better results with less toxicity, by permitting use of lower doses of one or both components. Amphotericin B plus flucytosine has proven successful in the treatment of cryptococcal meningitis (62–64). A retrospective review suggests that this combination may also be effective for candida meningitis (65). Rifampin, which penetrates the blood–CSF barrier, has been added to amphotericin B *in vitro* to potentiate the activity of the polyene against yeasts (47). However, there are no definitive data to judge its effectiveness in fungal meningitis in humans.

The combination of amphotericin B with various azoles has given variable results. *In vitro* studies showed that amphotericin B and miconazole were antagonistic (66), whereas others have shown additive effects with amphotericin B and ketoconazole (67). *In vivo* results of treatment of cryptococcal meningitis in animals suggest that additive effects exist (46), but further studies of polyenes plus azole compounds for fungal meningitis are needed.

Another potentially active combination which should be studied is flucytosine plus an azole compound. The azole compound might prevent development of resistance to flucytosine. Some azoles—for example, fluconazole or SCH 39304—achieve high CSF drug levels, similar to flucytosine. Animal studies with the ketoconazole–flucytosine combination have been successful in cryptococcosis (68), and further animal and human studies of these new triazoles combined with flucytosine should be encouraged. A combination of two azoles (miconazole and ketoconazole) has been tried in *Pseudallescheria boydii* meningitis (69).

The following section describes specific antifungal treatment regimens for several of the more common fungi causing meningitis.

CRYPTOCOCCAL MENINGITIS

Although an occasional patient survived for many years (70), untreated cryptococcal meningitis was uniformly fatal. Introduction of amphotericin B produced cures in over 50% of patients with cryptococcal meningitis (71), at the expense of considerable drug-related toxicity during months of treatment. Because the combination of amphotericin B plus flucytosine had potent *in vitro* activity, trials were conducted to determine whether reduced doses of amphotericin B administered with flucytosine would be as effective as amphotericin B alone. A large collaborative trial comparing amphotericin B (0.4 mg/kg/day) alone for 10 weeks with amphotericin B (0.3 mg/kg/day) plus flucytosine (150 mg/kg/day) for 6 weeks found the overall outcomes to be similar (64). This drug combination routinely sterilized the CSF within 2 weeks and allowed treatment to be shortened to a total of 6 weeks. A follow-up study showed that approximately 85% of a selected group of patients were cured or improved with this regimen for cryptococcal meningitis (72). A 4-week combination regimen was found to be successful for those patients with no underlying diseases and good prognostic indicators at the beginning and end of therapy (72).

Amphotericin B nephrotoxicity is reduced at the lower doses used in this combined regimen, but flucytosine toxicity for the bone marrow, liver, and gastrointestinal tract is troublesome. Thus, the combination may be criticized on the grounds that it substitutes flucytosine toxicity for amphotericin B toxicity. In several large studies of cryptococcal meningitis, including patients with AIDS, between 30% and 50% of patients experienced some side effects attributable to flucytosine, with approximately half occurring in the first 2 weeks of therapy. It has been shown that bone marrow toxicity correlated with peak serum flucytosine levels above 100 μg/ml 2 hr after a dose (73). Therefore, it seems reasonable to conclude that most patients should have serum flucytosine concentrations measured when therapy continues for more than 1–2 weeks, and repeated if renal function worsens. Personal experience suggests that 100 mg/kg/day of flucytosine will result in acceptable therapeutic blood levels of 30–80 μg/ml in most patients. It is particularly important to reduce the dose of flucytosine in patients with renal dysfunction. Flucytosine toxicity is not necessarily greater in those patients with poor bone marrow reserves prior to treatment (73).

Fluconazole has been evaluated for primary treatment of cryptococcal meningitis (48,74,75). Experience suggests that it takes longer to sterilize the CSF with this triazole compared to treatments that use amphotericin B (76,77). This finding supported previous findings in the rabbit model (46,52). Clinical experience suggests that more failures may occur during the first few weeks of treatment with fluconazole than with amphotericin B plus flucytosine. However, the outcome after 1 year for cryptococcal meningitis in patients with AIDS is similar after either regimen. It should be emphasized that most of the studies with fluconazole were performed in HIV-infected patients who generally have a high burden of organisms, sometimes greater than 10^6 colony-forming units (CFU) per milliliter of CSF. The value of fluconazole or other triazoles for initial therapy of patients with a lower burden of organisms or different underlying diseases is unknown.

Other therapeutic interventions may be required in certain patients. Intraventricular amphotericin B has been used successfully in cases with a poor prognosis, but side effects must be considered. The development of hydrocephalus may require placement of a shunt (78). In some cases, it may be necessary to place a shunt for hydrocephalus while active infection is present. Although shunts can become infected with cryptococci (79), antifungal drug therapy sometimes controls infection so well that the shunt does not need to be removed (80).

Cryptococcomas in the brain parenchyma are much less common than meningeal disease. In cases where the lesions are small and multiple, antifungal chemotherapy alone is generally successful. Large lesions (greater than 3 cm in size) located in surgically accessible areas may be surgically removed (81). In AIDS patients, a ring-enhancing brain lesion in the presence of cryptococcal meningitis may represent a simultaneous infection with another organism such as *Toxoplasma gondii* (82) or *Nocardia* rather than a cryptococcoma.

Cryptococcal meningitis during pregnancy should be managed in a manner similar to that for other cases. Although no cases of congenital cryptococcosis have been described, both amphotericin B and flucytosine cross the blood–placenta barrier.

A major factor influencing the treatment of cryptococcal meningitis is the degree to which the host is immunosuppressed. The most troublesome iatrogenic factor in cryptococcal meningitis is concomitant corticosteroid administration. In management of patients with cryptococcal meningitis who must receive corticosteroids, the dose should be reduced rapidly, as far as the underlying disease will allow. A reasonable goal for most patients is to reduce the dose of steroid to the equivalent of 20 mg prednisone per day, or less. Patients receiving immunosuppressive regimens for an underlying disease require at least 6 weeks of treatment with amphotericin B and flucytosine.

Before the advent of AIDS, treatment of cryptococcal meningitis could be based upon well-established guidelines. With the emergence of the AIDS epidemic, management has changed (83–86). The profound and persistent immune suppression of HIV infection has caused a myriad of treatment failures and relapses. The largest studies of these patients disagree as to the outcome of initial therapy. One reported poor initial therapeutic results in greater than 50% (83), whereas another showed that 75% of patients successfully completed initial therapy (84). However, all experience confirms that the relapse rate is very high in this group of patients. Recent studies show a 15–25% relapse rate in non-AIDS patients with cryptococcal meningitis; in contrast, AIDS patients can be expected to relapse in over 50% of cases. Most relapses occur in the first 3–6 months after stopping therapy.

This experience favors the concept of lifelong suppressive or maintenance therapy after primary treatment of cryptococcal meningitis in AIDS patients (54,55). Fluconazole has become the drug of choice for this purpose, being more convenient and more effective than intermittent amphotericin B infusions (77). The length of suppressive treatment is not well-defined, but it seems advisable to administer suppression for as long as immunosuppression continues. For AIDS patients, the regimen should be continued indefinitely. The effect of new antiretroviral agents such as zidovudine or immune modulators on the host response may allow revision of these recommendations in the future. This approach probably should be extended to selected other immunosuppressed patients judged to be at high risk for relapse.

Unexpected deaths during the first week of treatment have been observed in some AIDS patients with cryptococcal meningitis. These patients deteriorated suddenly; some manifested dramatic increases in intracranial pressure. The pathophysiology of this catastrophic event remains unclear. It is unlikely to be a drug reaction, because it has been observed in patients treated with a variety of different drugs and regimens. It appears more likely to be due to some perturbation or reaction among the large burden of yeasts in the brain and CSF of these patients as treatment is started. One possibility is that a large amount of mannitol released by these yeasts could increase intracranial pressure via osmotic effects. Further studies are needed to understand and prevent this unfortunate complication. The benefit of a short course of corticosteroids to prevent cerebral edema may outweigh the risks, even in this immunosuppressed group.

COCCIDIOIDAL MENINGITIS

The primary mode of treatment for coccidioidal meningitis is intraventricular amphotericin B. Initially, doses of amphotericin B between 0.5 and 1.0 g are given intravenously, to treat occult disseminated foci of fungal infection. Primary control of CNS infection is subsequently achieved through the use of intrathecal amphotericin B. Therapy is begun with small doses of 0.01 mg/day; the dosage is then gradually increased as tolerated, up to 0.5 mg/day. Complications of therapy include radicular pain or paresthesias, myelopathy, headaches, and bacterial superinfection, particularly if a reservoir is used for intraventricular therapy.

Recommendations with regard to length of therapy are variable. Because of the poor prognosis for cure, many patients have been treated indefinitely. Treatment should probably continue for at least a year after obtaining a normal CSF. Clinicians have used the CSF leukocyte count to judge the need for continuing therapy, attempting to keep the cell count in CSF below 10 per cubic millimeter. A lowering of the CSF antibody titer also is considered a good prognostic sign. Vigilance for development of hydrocephalus or bacterial superinfection must be maintained throughout therapy.

Some positive results have been reported with systemic and local use of miconazole or with very high oral doses of ketoconazole (45). The most recent experience with newer triazoles which penetrate freely into the CSF, such as fluconazole, are encouraging (87,88). If these early successes are repeated, the use of an effective oral agent for long-term suppressive therapy may represent a major advance in management of this very recalcitrant infection. At present, the goal for most cases of coccidioidal meningitis remains not cure of, but suppression of infection.

CANDIDAL MENINGITIS

Unlike cryptococcal and coccidioidal meningitis, occasional spontaneous cures of candida meningitis may occur. Therefore, comparison of treatments is more difficult for this form of fungal meningitis. Nevertheless, clinical experience with amphotericin B and flucytosine suggests that the prognosis of candida meningitis has been much improved by treatment. As usual, amphotericin B is the primary therapeutic agent. The combination of amphotericin B with flucytosine is attractive for this infection because these two drugs have synergistic activity against *Candida in vitro,* and because flucytosine reaches high concentrations in CSF. Review of the literature suggests that this combination provides a good cure rate (65). Today, the mortality of candida meningitis has been reduced to approximately 10%.

HISTOPLASMOSIS OF THE CNS

The clinical presentations of CNS histoplasmosis range from intraparenchymal histoplasmomas to meningitis with or without evidence of dissemination to other sites. With the advent of AIDS, the frequency of disseminated histoplasmosis in association with meningitis has increased. Unlike cryptococcal meningitis, guidelines for treatment are based upon retrospective reports of small series of patients. A summary of current experience suggests that less than 50% of cases can be cured with antifungal treatment. However, outcome is somewhat better in patients who received at least 30–35 mg/kg of amphotericin B over the course of treatment (89).

To achieve these total doses, up to 0.7–1.0 mg/kg/day may be given, if tolerated. Intrathecal/intraventricular administration may be tried, but there is no proof that this is more efficacious.

Patients should be followed for at least 5 years to exclude relapse. Patients with a persistent immune deficiency such as AIDS will likely benefit from long-term suppressive treatment. The optimal regimen for suppression is unknown; intermittent amphotericin B or the newer triazoles, fluconazole and itraconazole, may be considered. Patients with histoplasmomas should be treated initially with systemic antifungal therapy, reserving surgical intervention for large masses or failure to respond.

OTHER FUNGI

Information on treatment regimens for *Blastomyces* and *Sporothrix* meningitis is limited because these CNS infections are uncommon. Some cases have been cured with amphotericin B, which remains the recommended primary therapy. Trials of oral agents would be desirable. *Aspergillus* infections of the CNS are very difficult to treat successfully. Occasionally, high doses of amphotericin B have been successful in arresting the infection, particularly if host responses improve. *Pseudallescheria boydii* CNS infections have been treated with miconazole and ketoconazole (69). Miconazole seems to be the drug of choice for this infection.

SURGICAL MEASURES

The management of fungal brain abscesses is not well standardized (90). Blastomycotic and histoplasma abscesses have been successfully removed surgically, with concomitant amphotericin B treatment. With regard to cryptococcomas, it has been suggested that size is a criterion for operative intervention. Small lesions may be treated medically, whereas lesions 2–3 cm or more across in accessible areas should be considered for surgical removal. In patients with *Zygomycetes* or *Aspergillus* infection invading the vessels of the brain with resulting infarction, direct surgical removal of infarcted tissue should be considered if lesions are surgically accessible. Some of these lesions have been successfully managed with stereotactic aspiration for diagnosis and systemic amphotericin B treatment (12). Dematiaceous fungi, for which little or no effective drug treatment is available, cause brain abscesses for which the only hope of cure is surgical removal (91). In AIDS patients with fungal meningitis and parenchymal lesions, more than one organism may be present. Biopsies may be necessary to establish the complete diagnosis.

Fungal infections of CSF shunts inserted for treatment of hydrocephalus and chronic meningitis are uncommon (92). If candida or cryptococcal meningitis develops in a patient with a shunt in place, eradication of infection is most likely to be achieved by removing the shunt and treating with antifungal agents (79,93). The shunt may be replaced after cure. Even if the clinical situation does not allow shunt removal or demands (re)placement of a shunt during active meningitis, medical treatment with amphotericin B and flucytosine may be successful (80).

Intracranial mycotic aneurysms are rare complications of CNS fungal infection. Aneurysms have been described in association with *Aspergillus, Zygomycetes, Coccidioides,* and *Candida* infections (94–96). Aneurysms associated with fungi tend to involve proximal intracranial vessels, particularly the large arteries at the base of the brain. Surgical treatment is warranted if discrete intracranial aneurysms bleed, cause significant mass effect, or enlarge despite optimal medical therapy.

PROGNOSIS

The prognosis for fungal meningitis depends primarily upon early diagnosis and treatment, plus control of significant underlying disease(s). The substantial clinical experience with cryptococcal, candidal, and coccidioidal meningitis allows identification of certain specific prognostic factors.

In cryptococcal meningitis, patients were more likely to fail amphotericin B therapy if they had the following features: (a) an initial positive CSF India ink test, (b) high CSF opening pressure, (c) low CSF leukocyte concentration (i.e., <20 per cubic millimeter), (d) cryptococci isolated from extraneural sites, (e) absent anticryptococcal antibody, (f) initial CSF or serum cryptococcal antigen titer greater than or equal to 1:32, (g) corticosteroid therapy, or (h) lymphoreticular malignancy. Patients were more likely to relapse after treatment if they had one or more of the following features: (a) a CSF glucose concentration which remained abnormal during 4 weeks or more of therapy, (b) low initial CSF leukocyte concentration (<20 per cubic millimeter), (c) cryptococci isolated from extraneural sites, (d) absent anticryptococcal antibody, (e) post-treatment CSF or serum cryptococcal antigen titers greater than or equal to 1:8, (f) no significant decrease in CSF and serum antigen titers during therapy, or (g) daily corticosteroid therapy equivalent to 20 mg of prednisone or more after completion of therapy (97).

A large collaborative study of treatment with combined amphotericin B and flucytosine identified several factors associated with a favorable response: (a) headache as a symptom, (b) normal mental status, and (c) CSF leukocyte count above 20 cells per cubic millimeter (72). These findings illustrate both the importance of early diagnosis and the adequacy of the host's immune responses.

The single most significant factor in determining the outcome of CNS mycoses is the patient's underlying disease. A study of cryptococcal meningitis illustrates this statement. Despite effective therapy for cryptococcal meningitis, patients with concomitant cancer (97) or HIV (83–86) infection rarely survive more than 2 years after onset of the fungal infection.

Prognostic factors for candida meningitis are less well studied, but several factors have been found to be associated with a poor prognosis. These are: (a) diagnostic interval after start of symptoms greater than 2 weeks, (b) CSF glucose levels below 35 mg/100 ml, and (c) development of intracranial hypertension and focal neurologic deficits (98).

Coccidioidal meningitis remains an extremely difficult infection to cure. At least 50% of patients will survive initial treatment. However, these survivors frequently require suppressive therapy, and many fail to recover sufficiently to return to their prior employment. Experienced clinicians will consider patients cured only after they have survived for more than 5–8 years without relapse. Factors portending an unfavorable outcome are: (a) hydrocephalus, (b) an underlying disease, and (c) non-Caucasian race. On the other hand, low or absent complement-fixation antibody titers in CSF at the end of therapy suggest a favorable outcome (21).

REFERENCES

1. Ellner JJ, Bennett JE. Chronic meningitis. *Medicine* 1976;55:341–369.
2. Campbel GD, Currier RD, Busey JF. Survival in untreated cryptococcal meningitis. *Neurology* 1981;31:1154–1157.
3. Rosen E, Belber JP. Coccidioidal meningitis of long duration: report of a case of four years and eight months' duration with necropsy findings. *Ann Intern Med* 1951;34:796–809.
4. Norman DD, Miller ZR. Coccidioidomycosis of the central nervous system. A case of ten years' duration. *Neurology* 1954;4:713–717.
5. Gelfand JA, Bennett JE. Active *Histoplasma* meningitis of 22 years' duration. *JAMA* 1975;233:1294–1295.
6. Stockstill MT, Kaufman CA. Comparison of cryptococcal and tuberculous meningitis. *Arch Neurol* 1983;40:81–85.
7. McGinnis MR. Detection of fungi in cerebrospinal fluid. *Am J Med* 1983;129–138.
8. Perfect JR, Lang SDR, Durack DT. Chronic cryptococcal meningitis: a new experimental model in rabbits. *Am J Pathol* 1980;101:177–194.
9. Peacock JE, McGinnis MR, Cohen MS. Persistent neutrophilic meningitis. *Medicine* 1984;63:379–395.
10. Brannon P, Kiehn TE. Large-scale clinical comparison of the lysis–centrifugation and radiometric systems for blood culture. *J Clin Microbiol* 1985;22:951–954.
11. Gonyea EF. Cisternal puncture and cryptococcal meningitis. *Arch Neurol* 1973;28:200–201.
12. Goodman ML, Coffey RJ. Stereotaxic drainage of *Aspergillus* brain abscess with long-term survival: case report and review. *Neurosurgery* 1989;24:96–99.
13. Goodman JS, Kaufman L, Loening MG. Diagnosis of cryptococcal meningitis: detection of cryptococcal antigen. *N Engl J Med* 1971;285:434–436.
14. Kaufman L, Blumer S. Latex–cryptococcal antigen test. *Am J Clin Pathol* 1973;60:285–286.
15. Snow RM, Dismukes WE. Cryptococcal meningitis: diagnostic value of cryptococcal antigen in cerebrospinal fluid. *Arch Intern Med* 1975;135:1155–1157.
16. Bennett JE, Bailey JW. Control for rheumatoid factor in latex test for cryptococcosis. *Am J Clin Pathol* 1971;56:360–365.
17. Stockman L, Roberts GD. Specificity of the latex test for cryptococcal antigen: a rapid, simple method for eliminating interference factors. *J Clin Microbiol* 1982;16:965–967.
18. Boom WH, Piper BJ, Ruoff KL, Ferraro MJ. New cause for false-positive results with the cryptococcal antigen test by latex agglutination. *J Clin Microbiol* 1985;22:856–857.
19. McManus EJ, Bozdeck MJ, Jones JM. Role of the latex agglutination test for cryptococcal antigen in diagnosing disseminated infections with *Trichosporon beigelii*. *J Infect Dis* 1985;151:1167–1169.
20. MacKinnon S, Kane JG, Parker RH. False positive cryptococcal antigen test and cervical prevertebral abscess. *JAMA* 1978;240:1982–1983.
21. Bouza E, Dreyer JS, Hewitt WL, Meyer RD. Coccidioidal meningitis: an analysis of thirty-one cases and review of the literature. *Medicine* 1981;60:139–172.
22. Wheat J, French M, Batteiger B, Kohler R. Cerebrospinal fluid *Histoplasma* antibodies in central nervous system histoplasmosis. *Arch Intern Med* 1985;145:1237–1240.
23. Scott EN, Kaufman L, Brown AC, Muchmore HG. Serologic studies in the diagnosis and management of meningitis due to *Sporothrix schenckii*. *N Engl J Med* 1987;317:935–940.
24. Pierce PF Jr, Solomon SL, Kaufman L, Garagusi VF, Parker RH, Ajello L. *Zygomycetes* brain abscess in narcotic addicts with serologic diagnosis. *JAMA* 1982;248:2881–2882.
25. Wheat LJ, Kohler RB, Tewari RP, Garten M, French ML. Significance of *Histoplasma* antigen in the cerebrospinal fluid of patients with meningitis. *Arch Intern Med* 1989;149:302–304.
26. Weiner MH, Talbot GH, Gerson SL, Filice G, Cassileth PA. Antigen detection in the diagnosis of invasive aspergillosis. *Ann Intern Med* 1983;99:777–782.
27. Scheld WM, Lee D, Bernard EM. CSF arabinitol in experimental *Candida albicans* meningitis [Abstract]. *Interscience Conf Antimicrob Agents Chemother* 1984;1168.
28. Wong B, Perfect JR, Beggs S, Wright KA. Production of the hexitol D-mannitol by *Cryptococcus neoformans in vitro* and in rabbits with experimental meningitis. *Infect Immun* 1990;58:1664–1670.
29. Plouffe JF, Silva J, Fekety R, Baird I. Cerebrospinal fluid lymphocyte transformations in meningitis. *Arch Intern Med* 1979;139:191–194.
30. Body BA, Oneson RH, Herold DA. Use of cerebrospinal fluid lactic acid concentration in the diagnosis of fungal meningitis. *Ann Clin Lab Sci* 1987;17:429–434.
31. Bindschadler DD, Bennett JE. A pharmacologic guide to the clinical use of amphotericin B. *J Infect Dis* 1969;120:427–436.
32. Dugoni B, Guglielmo BJ, Hollander H. Amphotericin B concentrations in cerebrospinal fluid of patients with AIDS and cryptococcal meningitis. *Clin Pharm* 1989;8:220–221.
33. Drutz DJ, Spickard A, Rogers DE, Koenig MG. Treatment of disseminated mycotic infections. *Am J Med* 1968;45:405–418.
34. Polsky B, Depman MR, Gold JW, Galicich JH, Armstrong D. Intraventricular therapy of cryptococcal meningitis via a subcutaneous reservoir. *Am J Med* 1986;81:24–28.
35. Labadie EL, Hamilton RH. Survival improvement by high-dose intrathecal amphotericin B. *Arch Intern Med* 1986;146:2013–2018.
36. Diamond RD, Bennett JE. A subcutaneous reservoir for intrathecal therapy of fungal meningitis. *N Engl J Med* 1973;288:186–188.
37. Bennett JE. Flucytosine. *Ann Intern Med* 1977;86:319–319.
38. Utz JP, Shadomy S, McGehee KF. 5-Flucytosine: experience in patients with pulmonary and other forms of cryptococcosis. *Am Rev Respir Dis* 1969;99:975–975.
39. Weinstein L, Irving J. Successful treatment of cerebral cryptococcoma and meningitis with miconazole. *Ann Intern Med* 1980;93:569–571.
40. Sung JP, Campbell GD, Grendahl JG. Miconazole therapy for fungal meningitis. *Arch Intern Med* 1978;35:443–447.

41. Fisher JF, Duma RJ, Markowitz SM, Shadomy S, Espinel-Ingroff A, Chew WH. Therapeutic failures with miconazole. *Antimicrob Agents Chemother* 1978;13:965–968.

42. Graybill JR, Levine HB. Successful treatment of cryptococcal meningitis with intraventricular miconazole. *Ann Intern Med* 1978;138:814–816.

43. Dismukes WE, Cloud G, Bowles C. Treatment of blastomycosis and histoplasmosis with ketoconazole: results of a prospective randomized clinical trial. *Ann Intern Med* 1985;103:861–861.

44. Perfect JR, Durack DT, Hamilton JD, Gallis HA. Failure of ketoconazole in cryptococcal meningitis. *JAMA* 1982;247:3349–3351.

45. Craven PC, Graybill JR, Jorgensen JH, Dismukes WE, Levine BE. High-dose ketoconazole for treatment of fungal infections of the central nervous system. *Ann Intern Med* 1983;98:160–167.

46. Perfect JR, Durack DT. Amphotericin B, 5-fluorocytosine and ketoconazole in experimental cryptococcal meningitis. *J Infect Dis* 1982;146:429–435.

47. Medoff G, Kobyashi GS, Kwan CN, Schlessinger D, Venkov P. Potentiation of rifampicin and 5-fluorocytosine as antifungal antibiotics by amphotericin B. *Proc Natl Acad Sci* 1972;69:196–199.

48. Foulds G, Brennan DR, Wajszczvk CP, et al. Fluconazole penetration into cerebrospinal fluid in humans. *J Clin Pharmacol* 1988;28:363–366.

49. Kinnier Wilson SA. *Neurology.* Baltimore: Williams & Wilkins, 1940.

50. Arndt CA, Walsh TJ, McCully CL, Balis FM, Pizzo PA, Poplack DE. Fluconazole penetration into cerebrospinal fluid: implications for treating fungal infections of the central nervous system. *J Infect Dis* 1988;157:178–180.

51. Perfect JR, Durack DT. Penetration of imidazoles and triazoles into cerebrospinal fluid of rabbits. *J Antimicrob Chemother* 1985;16:81–86.

52. Perfect JR, Savani DV, Durack DT. Comparison of itraconazole and fluconazole in treatment of cryptococcal meningitis and *Candida* pyelonephritis in rabbits. *Antimicrob Agents Chemother* 1986;29:579–583.

53. Dupont B, Drouhet E. Cryptococcal meningitis and fluconazole. *Ann Intern Med* 1987;106:778–778.

54. Sugar AM, Saunders C. Oral fluconazole as suppressive therapy of disseminated cryptococcosis in patients with acquired immunodeficiency syndrome. *Am J Med* 1988;85:481–489.

55. Stern JJ, Hartman BJ, Sharkey P, et al. Oral fluconazole therapy for patients with the acquired immunodeficiency syndrome and cryptococcosis: experience with 22 patients. *Am J Med* 1988;85:477–480.

56. Lopez-Berenstein G, Fainstein V, Hopfer R, et al. Liposomal amphotericin B for the treatment of systemic fungal infections in patients with cancer: a preliminary study. *J Infect Dis* 1985;151:704–710.

57. Viviani MA, Tortorano AM, Langer M, et al. Experience with itraconazole in cryptococcosis and aspergillosis. *J Infect* 1989;18:151–165.

58. Denning DW, Tucker RM, Hanson LH, Stevens DA. Treatment of invasive aspergillosis with itraconazole. *Am J Med* 1989;86:791–800.

59. Viviani MA, Tortorano AM, Giani PC, et al. Itraconazole for cryptococcal infection in the acquired immunodeficiency syndrome [Letter]. *Ann Intern Med* 1987;106:166–166.

60. Denning DW, Tucker RM, Hanson LH, Hamilton JR, Stevens DA. Itraconazole therapy for cryptococcal meningitis and cryptococcosis. *Arch Intern Med* 1989;149:2301–2308.

61. Perfect JR, Wright KA, Hobbs MM, Durack DT. Treatment of experimental cryptococcal meningitis and disseminated candidiasis with SCH 39304. *Antimicrob Agents Chemother* 1989;33:1735–1740.

62. Utz JP, Garrigues IL, Sande MA, et al. Therapy of cryptococcosis with a combination of flucytosine and amphotericin B. *J Infect Dis* 1975;132:368–373.

63. Jimbow T, Tejima Y, Ikemoto H. Comparison between 5-fluorocytosine, amphotericin B, and the combined administration of these agents in the therapeutic effectiveness for cryptococcal meningitis. *Chemotherapy* 1978;24:374–389.

64. Bennett JE, Dismukes W, Duma J. A comparison of amphotericin B alone and combined with flucytosine in the treatment of cryptococcal meningitis. *N Engl J Med* 1979;301:126–131.

65. Smego RA, Perfect JR, Durack DT. Combined therapy with amphotericin B and 5-fluorocytosine for *Candida* meningitis. *Rev Infect Dis* 1984;6:791–801.

66. Cosgrove RF, Beezer AE, Miles RJ. *In vitro* studies of amphotericin B in combination with the imidazole antifungal compounds clotrimazole and miconazole. *J Infect Dis* 1978;138:681–685.

67. Smith D, McFadden HW, Miller NG. Effect of ketoconazole and amphotericin B on encapsulated and non-encapsulated strains of *Cryptococcus neoformans. Antimicrob Agents Chemother* 1983; 24:851–855.

68. Craven PC, Graybill JR. Combination of oral flucytosine and ketoconazole as therapy for experimental cryptococcal meningitis. *J Infect Dis* 1984;149:584–590.

69. Schiess RJ, Coscia MF, McClellan GA. *Petriellidium boydii* pachymeningitis treated with miconazole and ketoconazole. *Neurosurgery* 1984;14:220–224.

70. Beeson PB. Cryptococcic meningitis of nearly sixteen years' duration. *Arch Intern Med* 1952;89:797–801.

71. Sarosi GA, Parker JD, Doto IL, Tosh FE. Amphotericin B in cryptococcal meningitis: long-term results of treatment. *Ann Intern Med* 1969;71:1079–1087.

72. Dismukes WE, Cloud G, Gallis HA, et al. Treatment of Cryptococcal meningitis with combination amphotericin B and flucytosine for four as compared with six weeks. *N Engl J Med* 1987;317:334–341.

73. Stamm AM, Diasio RB, Dismukes WE, et al. Toxicity of amphotericin B plus flucytosine in 194 patients with cryptococcal meningitis. *Am J Med* 1987;83:236–242.

74. Tozzi V, Bordi E, Galgani S, et al. Fluconazole treatment of cryptococcosis in patients with acquired immunodeficiency syndrome. *Am J Med* 1989;87:353.

75. Byrne WR, Wajszczvk CP. Cryptococcal meningitis in the acquired immunodeficiency syndrome (AIDS): successful treatment with fluconazole after failure of amphotericin B. *Ann Intern Med* 1988;108:384–385.

76. Larsen RA, Leal MAE, Chan LS. Fluconazole compared with amphotericin B plus flucytosine for cryptococcal meningitis in AIDS. *Ann Intern Med* 1990;113:183–187.

77. Galgiani JN. Fluconazole, a new antifungal agent. *Ann Intern Med* 1990;113:177–179.

78. Tang LM. Ventriculoperitoneal shunt in cryptococcal meningitis with hydrocephalus. *Surg Neurol* 1990;33:314–319.

79. Walsh TJ, Schlegel R, Moody MM, Costerton JW, Saloman M. Ventriculoatrial shunt infection due to *Cryptococcus neoformans:* an ultrastructural and quantitative microbiological study. *Neurosurgery* 1986;18:373–375.

80. Yadav YR, Perfect JR, Friedman A. Successful treatment of cryptococcal ventriculo-atrial shunt infection with systemic therapy alone. *Neurosurgery* 1988;23:317–322.

81. Fujita NK, Reynard M, Sapico FL, Guze LB, Edwards JE Jr. Cryptococcal intracerebral mass lesions. *Ann Intern Med* 1981;94:382–388.

82. Bahls F, Sumi SM. Cryptococcal meningitis and cerebral toxoplasmosis in a patient with acquired immune deficiency syndrome. *J Neurol Neurosurg Psychiatry* 1986;49:328–330.

83. Kovacs JA, Kovacs AA, Polis M, et al. Cryptococcosis in the acquired immunodeficiency syndrome. *Ann Intern Med* 1985;103:533–538.

84. Zuger A, Louie E, Holzman RS. Cryptococcal disease in patients with acquired immunodeficiency syndrome. *Ann Intern Med* 1986;104:234–240.

85. Eng RH, Bishburg E, Smith SM. Cryptococcal infections in patients with acquired immune deficiency syndrome. *Am J Med* 1986;81:19–23.

86. Chuck SL, Sande MA. Infections with *Cryptococcus neoformans* in the acquired immunodeficiency syndrome. *N Engl J Med* 1989;321:794–799.

87. Tucker RM, Denning DW, Dupont B, Stevens DA. Itraconazole therapy for chronic coccidioidal meningitis. *Ann Intern Med* 1990;112:108–112.

88. Tucker RM, Galgiani JN, Denning DW, et al. Treatment of coccidioidal meningitis with fluconazole. *Rev Infect Dis* 1990;12:s380–s389.

FUNGAL MENINGITIS / 739

89. Wheat LJ, Batteiger BE, Sathapatayavongs B. *Histoplasma capsulatum* infections of the central nervous system. *Medicine* 1990;69:244–260.
90. Young RF, Gade G, Grinell V. Surgical treatment for fungal infections in the central nervous system. *J Neursurg* 1985;63:371–381.
91. Seaworth BJ, Kwon-Chung CJ, Hamilton JD, Perfect JR. Brain abscess caused by a variety of *Cladosporium trichoides. Am J Clin Pathol* 1983;79:747–752.
92. Mangham D, Gerding DN, Peterson LR, Sarosi GA. Fungal meningitis manifesting in hydrocephalus. *Arch Intern Med* 1983;143:728–731.
93. Gower DJ, Crone K, Alexander E, Kelly DL. *Candida albicans* shunt infection: report of two cases. *Neurosurgery* 1986;19:111–113.
94. Kikuchi K, Watanabe K, Sugawara A. Multiple fungal aneurysms: report of a rare case implicating steroids as a predisposing factor. *Surg Neurol* 1985;24:253–259.
95. Hadley MN, Martin NA, Spetzler RF, Johnson PC. Multiple intracranial aneurysms due to *Coccidioides immitis* infection. *J Neursurg* 1987;66:453–456.
96. Shimosaka S, Waga S. Cerebral chromoblastomycosis complicated by meningitis and multiple fungal aneurysms after resection of a granuloma. Case Report. *J Neursurg* 1983;59:158–161.
97. Diamond RD, Bennett JE. Prognostic factors in cryptococcal meningitis. A study of 111 cases. *Ann Intern Med* 1974;80:176–181.
98. Bayer AS, Edwards JE Jr, Seidel JS, Guze LB. *Candida* meningitis. Report of seven cases and review of the English literature. *Medicine* 1976;55:477–485.
99. Guisan von M. Schlerosing post-traumatic meningeal aspergillosis. *Schweiz Arch Neurol Psychiatr* 1962;90:235–254.
100. Jones PG, Gilman RM, Medeiros AA, Dyckman J. Focal intracranial mucomycosis presenting as chronic meningitis. *JAMA* 1981;246:2063–2064.
101. Seaworth B, Kwon-Chung CJ, Hamilton JD, Perfect JR. Brain abscess caused by a variety of *Cladosporium trichoides. Am J Clin Pathol* 1983;79:747.
102. Salaki JS, Louria DB, Chmel H. Fungal and yeast infections of the central nervous system. A clinical review. *Medicine* 1984;63:108–132.
103. Lyons RW, Andriole VT. Fungal infections of the CNS. *Neurol Clin* 1986;4:159–170.
104. Gonyea EF. The spectrum of primary blastomycotic meningitis: a review of central nervous system blastomycosis. *Ann Neurol* 1978;3:26–39.
105. Buechner HA, Clawson C. Blastomycosis of the central nervous system, II. A report of nine cases from the Veterans Administration Cooperative Study. *Am Rev Respir Dis* 1967;95:820–826.
106. Buchs S, Pfister P. *Candida* meningitis: course, prognosis and mortality before and after introduction of the new antimycotics. *Mykosen* 1983;26:73–81.
107. Parker JC Jr, McCloskey JJ, Lee RS. The emergence of candidosis. The dominant postmortem cerebral mycosis. *Am J Clin Pathol* 1978;70:31–36.
108. Iyer S, Dodge P, Adams RD. Two cases of aspergillus infection of the central nervous system. *J Neurol Neurosurg Psychiatry* 1952;15:152–163.
109. Gordon MA, Holzman RS, Senter H, Lapa EW, Kupersmith MJ. *Aspergillus orzyme* meningitis. *JAMA* 1976;235:2122–2123.
110. Mukoyama M, Gimple K, Poser CM. Aspergillosis of the central nervous system. Report of a brain abscess due to *A. fumigatus* and review of the literature. *Neurology* 1969;19:967–974.
111. Kravitz GR, Davies SF, Eckman MR, Sarosi GA. Chronic blastomycotic meningitis. *Am J Med* 1981;71:501.
112. Sabetta JR, Andriole VT. Cryptococcal infection of the central nervous system. *Med Clin North Am* 1985;69:333–344.
113. Perfect JR, Durack DT, Gallis HA. Cryptococcemia. *Medicine* 1983;62:98–109.
114. Chadwick DW, Hartley E, Mackinnon DM. Meningitis caused by *Candida tropicalis. Arch Neurol* 1980;37:175–176.
115. Chattopadhyay B. *Candida tropicalis* meningitis. A case report. *J Laryngol Otol* 1981;95:1149–1151.
116. Goodwin RA Jr, Shapiro JL, Thurman GH, Thurman SS, Des Prez KM. Disseminated histoplasmosis: clinical and pathologic correlations. *Medicine* 1980;59:1–33.
117. Karalakulasingam R, Arora KK, Adams G, Serratoni F, Martin DG. Meningoencephalitis caused by *Histoplasma capsulatum. Arch Intern Med* 1976;136:217–220.
118. Cooper RA Jr, Goldstein E. Histoplasmosis of the central nervous system. Report of two cases and review of the literature. *Am J Med* 1963;35:45–57.
119. Pereira WC, Raphael A, Tenut RA. Localizacoa encefalico da blastomicose sul-americana: consideraooes a proposito de 9 casos. *Arq Neuropsiguiatr* 1965;23:113–126.
120. Tynes BS, Crutcher JC, Utz JP. *Histoplasma* meningitis. *Ann Intern Med* 1963;59:619–621.
121. Benham RW, Georg LK. *Allescheria boydii*, causative agent in a case of meningitis. *J Invest Dermatol* 1948;10:99.
122. Selby R. Pachymeningitis secondary to *Allescheria boydii. J Neursurg* 1972;36:225–227.
123. Ewing GE, Bosl GJ, Peterson PK. *Sporothrix schenckii* meningitis in a farmer with Hodgkin's disease. *Am J Med* 1980;68:455–457.
124. Freeman JW, Ziegler DK. Chronic meningitis caused by *Sporothrix schenckii. Neurology* 1977;27:989–992.
125. Klein RC, Ivens MS, Seabury JH, Dascomb HE. Meningitis due to *Sporotrichum schenkii. Arch Intern Med* 1966;118:145–149.
126. Chernik NL, Armstrong D, Posner JB. Central nervous system infections in patients with cancer. *Medicine* 1973;52:563–581.
127. Fraser DW, Ward JI, Ajello L, Plikaytis BD. Aspergillosis and systemic mycosis. *JAMA* 1979;242:1631–1635.

Infections of the Central Nervous System,
edited by W. M. Scheld, R. J. Whitley, and
D. T. Durack, Raven Press, Ltd., New York © 1991.

CHAPTER 32

Space-Occupying Fungal Lesions of the Central Nervous System

Kent Sepkowitz and Donald Armstrong

Fungal abscesses of the central nervous system (CNS) were once extremely rare. In the past 30 years, however, the increased administration of immunosuppressive drugs, broad-spectrum antibiotics, and corticosteroids has forced a change in the spectrum of infectious agents causing CNS disease. Now, fungal infection of the CNS often can be anticipated in specific clinical settings. Survival rates remain generally poor; however, with earlier diagnoses (1) and improvements in therapy (2), more successful treatment of fungal CNS abscess should become a reality.

The description of the first case of fungal brain abscess is credited to Pautlauf (3), who, in 1885, reported a case of cerebral mucormycosis. For many years thereafter, scattered case reports constituted the entire literature on this medical oddity. A review in 1933 reported 24 cases of mycotic CNS infection collected over 25 years (4). Nineteen were torulosis (cryptococcosis); there was one each of aspergillosis, oidiomycosis (blastomycosis), coccidiomycosis, endomycosis (candidiasis), and sporotrichosis. At least half of these were limited to the meninges, but several were true abscesses. In a review of more than 15,000 consecutive autopsies from 1919 to 1955, 88 cases of fungal disease were found (5). Less than 10 involved the CNS. A 1967 monograph summarized all reported cases of CNS mycoses, still a rare clinical entity (6). Meningitis was grouped with abscess; *Cryptococcus neoformans* was by far the most common organism.

Since then, there has been a steady increase in the diagnosis of intracranial fungal infection. Improvements in our ability to diagnose such infections account for

some of the increase. More important, though, is the increasing therapeutic use of immunosuppressive drugs and broad-spectrum antibiotics. A 1969 review based on data collected from two hospitals over a period of 7 years yielded 119 cases of deep-seated fungal infection, of which at least 14 were CNS infection (including meningitis and abscess) (7). A 1978 paper reviewed almost 9000 consecutive autopsies collected from 1964 to 1973 in a general hospital (8). Thirty-nine cases of fungal infection of the CNS were identified. *Candida* species were the predominant organisms, accounting for 49%, followed by *C. neoformans* (23%), mucormycoses (13%), *Aspergillus* species (5%), and *Histoplasma capsulatum* (5%). A review of CNS infections from Memorial Sloan–Kettering Cancer Center, covering the period 1955–1971, reported 11 (28%) cases of fungal abscess out of 39 total cases of abscess (9). *Aspergillus* species accounted for seven (64%), mucormycoses three (27%), and *Candida albicans* one (9%). Another review of CNS infections in immunocompromised hosts reported 55 cases of abscess; 15 were due to *C. neoformans,* seven were due to *Aspergillus* species, and one was due to mucormycosis (10).

A more recent review from two tertiary care medical centers reported 61 cases of CNS infection (meningitis plus abscess) collected over a 30-year period (11). There were 27 cases (44%) of *Candida* species, 17 cases (28%) of *Aspergillus* species, 14 cases (23%) of *C. neoformans,* two cases (3%) of mucormycoses, and one case (2%) of *H. capsulatum.*

These series underscore the emergence of *Candida* species, *Aspergillus* species, and other fungi as potential pathogens in the immunocompromised host. No similar change in spectrum has occurred in immunocompetent patients. Of 315 patients with brain abscess collected from seven series in general hospitals, only two patients

K. Sepkowitz and D. Armstrong: Infectious Disease Service, Memorial Sloan-Kettering Cancer Center, New York, New York 10021.

had a fungal pathogen (12). In a cancer hospital, *Aspergillus* species and *C. neoformans* can be expected to predominate, whereas in a community hospital, *Candida* species might be the most frequently isolated organism.

The type of clinical setting and presentation may allow the diagnosis of a specific fungus to be anticipated (13). However, diagnosis of fungal brain abscess is often unexpected, even in patients at risk; and many cases are discovered at autopsy. Frequently, the presenting signs and symptoms do not distinguish a patient with fungal abscess from one with bacterial abscess or tumor. Spinal fluid results are usually nonspecifically abnormal; and computerized tomographic (CT) and magnetic resonance imaging (MRI) scan, while quite sensitive, seldom show changes specific for fungal abscess (14,15). Diagnosis almost invariably requires biopsy of a lesion, with

prompt inspection of the specimen by Gram's stain, potassium hydroxide wet mount preparation, and appropriate cultures. Many patients at risk for invasive fungal infection, however, have an underlying coagulopathy that precludes a diagnostic biopsy.

Even with appropriate biopsy specimens, the diagnosis of fungal infection is often difficult. Many times, a fungus, such as a member of the Mucorales, is seen on examination of biopsied tissue yet fails to grow in culture; conversely, sometimes a fungal isolate, such as *C. albicans,* that was not seen on potassium hydroxide wet mount preparation or on histopathology will prove culture-positive in the microbiology laboratory. In these circumstances, serologic information may be helpful. Various tests for fungal antigen or antibody to a fungus are available. Of these, the test for cryptococcal antigen is

TABLE 1. *Comparison of pathogenic fungi as pathogens of the CNS[a]*

	Molds	*Candida* species	*Cryptococcus* species	Dimorphic fungi	Dematiacious fungi
Pathogens:	*Aspergillus* species Mucorales *P. boydii*	*C. albicans* *C. tropicalis* *C. parapsilosis*	*C. neoformans*	*B. dermatitidis* *P. brasiliensis* *H. capsulatum* *C. immitis*	*X. bantiana* *Bipolaris* species *Exserohilum* species *Curvularia* species
Less common pathogens:	*Fusarium* *S. griseus*	*T. glabrata* *C. krusei*		*S. schenckii*	*F. pedrosi* *R. obovoideum*
Immune status:	Compromised (neutrophil function) Normal acidosis IVDU	Compromised (neutrophil function)	Normal Compromised (T cells)	Normal Compromised (T cells)	Normal Compromised
Clinical setting:	Hematologic neoplasms Transplant Organ Marrow Diabetes Near-drowning	IVDU Intravenous catheters Prolonged therapy with broad-spectrum antibiotics Abdominal surgery	Community-acquired	Community-acquired	Community-acquired
Presentation:	Stroke syndrome Resembles bacterial abscess or infarct Rhinocerebral	Fever Altered mental status	Meningitis Resembles bacterial abscess	Meningitis	Resembles bacterial abscess
CSF:	RBCs Increased protein Increased WBCs (mono or poly) Stable or decreased glucose	No RBCs Increased protein Increased WBCs (mono or poly) Stable or decreased glucose	No RBCs Increased protein Increased WBCs (mono or poly) Stable or decreased glucose	No RBCs Increased protein Increased WBCs (mono or poly) Stable or decreased glucose	No RBCs Increased protein Increased WBCs (mono or poly) Stable or decreased glucose
Histopathology:	Vasculitis and infarct Cerebritis Granuloma (rare)	Meningitis Microabscess Vasculitis (rare)	Meningitis Granuloma	Miliary microabscess (resembles MTB)	Abscess/granuloma

[a] CNS, central nervous system; IVDU, intravenous drug use; CSF, cerebrospinal fluid; RBCs, red blood cells; WBCs, white blood cells; MTB, *Mycobacterium tuberculosis.*

the most sensitive and specific and has been used in routine clinical practice for decades. Either serum or cerebrospinal fluid (CSF) can be tested. Serologic tests for several other fungal infections, including histoplasmosis and coccidioidiomycoses, are also widely available, although their use in the diagnosis of CNS infection has not been established. Reliable serologic tests for aspergillosis, mucormycosis, and candidiasis, among others, are under development and may enter clinical practice in the near future. Their immediate applicability to the diagnosis of infections of the CNS, however, has not been well-investigated.

The role of susceptibility testing of clinical isolates remains to be determined in selecting antimicrobial agents. We would recommend using such tests as rough guidelines, especially in cases when a patient is not improving on a specific therapy. We employ a microtiter method using a 96-well plate. Increasing concentrations of antibiotic are placed in sequence across a row to which a standardized inoculum of fungus is added. The wells are examined at 24 and 48 hr for evidence of turbidity, which reflects fungal growth. Synergy studies may be done using a standard checkerboard technique, with increasing doses of each antifungal added to a fixed inoculum of fungus. Examination at 24 and 48 hr will allow interpretation of susceptibility.

There are four general categories of fungal infection: molds (hyphal yeasts), dimorphic yeasts, other yeasts (fungal yeasts), and dematiacious fungi. Fungal morphology, patients at risk, and clinical syndromes vary for each group (Table 1). In the brain, dimorphic and fungal yeasts are more likely to cause meningitis, whereas molds usually cause hyphal vasculitis and subsequent parenchymal infarction and abscess (16,17).

MOLDS

Molds are ubiquitous organisms found in soil, water, and decaying vegetation. The major pathogenic molds are *Aspergillus* species and the Mucorales. Morphologically, molds exist as hyphae both at room temperature and at 37°C. Patients at risk for infection include those on glucocorticoids and other immunosuppressive agents, those receiving long courses of broad-spectrum antibiotics, and those with prolonged episodes of neutropenia. Diabetic patients are at particular risk for mucormycosis. Cases have been described without obvious risk factor, but this remains exceptionally rare (18). Many infections of the CNS caused by molds occur by direct extension from an ongoing paranasal sinus infection, the so-called rhinocerebral syndrome. The predominant features of CNS infections caused by molds are summarized in Table 2.

Aspergillus Species

History

The first report of cerebral aspergillosis appeared in 1897 (19), describing a 37-year-old man who developed aspergillosis of the sphenoid sinus that extended posteriorly to involve the optic chiasm and internal carotid artery. Until the advent of immunosuppressive therapy, similar presentations—sinusitis extending to involve the frontal or temporal lobes of the brain—were the rule. However, in recent years, hematologic dissemination, usually from a primary lung infection, has become far more common. Several reviews have been published

TABLE 2. Pathogenic molds in the CNS

	Aspergillus species	Mucorales	*Pseudallescheria boydii*
Patients at risk:	Hematologic neoplasm Neutropenia on broad-spectrum antibiotics Corticosteroids Organ transplants Intravenous drug use Liver disease Post-craniotomy	Diabetes with ketoacidosis (>70%) Hematologic neoplasm Neutropenia on broad-spectrum antibiotics Renal transplant Intravenous drug use Desfuroxamine Acidosis	Near-drowning Intravenous drug use Neutropenia on broad-spectrum antibiotics Hematologic malignancy
Pathogenesis:	Hematogenous Direct extension, including rhinocerebral (rare)	Rhinocerebral Hematogenous	Hematogenous Direct extension Traumatic implantation
Microscopic appearance:	Septate hyphae Acute branching	Nonseptate hyphae Broad right-angle branching	Narrow septate hyphae with rare branching
Culture from CSF:	Rare	Never	Occasional
Treatment:	Surgery Amphotericin B ± Rifampin ? ± Fluconazole	Surgery Amphotericin B	Surgery Miconazole ? Amphotericin B

through the years (20–22). A recent review found 124 cases of intracranial aspergillosis in the world literature (23).

Etiologic Agent

Aspergillus was first described by Micheli, a priest, in 1729. Its name derives from its similarity, when viewed microscopically, to the aspergillum, a perforated globe used to sprinkle holy water in certain churches. Over 200 species of *Aspergillus* have been described; at least nine have caused CNS infection, including *A. fumigatus, A. flavus* (21), *A. amstelodami* (24), *A. candidus* (25), *A. oryzae* (26), *A. terreus* (meningitis only) (27), *A. glaucus* (28), *A. versicolor* (29), and *A. sydowii* (30). *A. fumigatus* accounts for most human infection (28).

Aspergillus species are ubiquitous molds found in soil, water, decaying vegetation, or any location with organic debris (31). Disease has been described in birds.

Aspergillus species have a characteristic microscopic appearance. The hyphae develop terminal buds, or vesicles, which crown the organism with multiple small conidiae. The organism remains a mold *in vivo* and *in vitro.*

Epidemiology

Cases of intracranial aspergillosis have been reported worldwide. India may be endemic for all forms of aspergillosis (32–35). There is no demonstrable predisposition by sex or race. Most reported cases occur in adults, although at least three cases have been reported in neonates (36).

Pathogenesis and Pathophysiology

The lungs are the usual site of primary infection because the airborne spore is continually inhaled. Intracranial seeding occurs during dissemination. Infection may also occur from direct innoculation by surgery (37) or trauma, or else by direct extension from the paranasal sinuses or eye (4,19,38–40). This latter route resembles the rhinocerebral form of mucormycosis and may present as an indolent disease with symptoms lasting for years (22,25,39).

Most cases of invasive aspergillosis have occurred in neutropenic patients who have an underlying hematologic neoplasm. Also, patients receiving organ transplants are at increased risk (41,42). Intracranial aspergillosis, however, may occur more commonly in patients without the usual risk factors for invasive disease; one review reported 53% of cases of *Aspergillus* brain abscess occurring in patients without common risk factors (11). Hepatic disease or Cushing's syndrome was present in many of these patients. Many patients with alcoholic

liver disease have been described (20,43–45). Some patients have no discernible risk factor (39,46).

Cases of intracranial aspergillosis have also been described in patients receiving chronic corticosteroid therapy for many reasons, including sarcoid (47), pulmonary tuberculosis (48), and bronchopulmonary aspergillosis (49). There is a report of a patient with diabetes mellitus developing intracranial infection via spread from a middle ear infection (50). One review reported several cases arising in postcraniotomy patients (10). Intravenous drug users with and without demonstrable endocarditis, as well as patients with prosthetic valve endocarditis, have been reported (51). Up to 56% of patients with *Aspergillus* species endocarditis may have discernible emboli (11,52).

Aspergillus is the second or third most common fungal cause of intracranial infection in most series. A survey of autopsies performed between 1956 and 1985 at two medical centers revealed 61 cases of CNS fungal infection, 17 (28%) of which were caused by *Aspergillus* (11). A report from Memorial Sloan–Kettering Cancer Center reviewed all patients with microbiologically proven CNS infection from 1955 to 1971 and reported 146 patients with CNS infection, 39 of whom had brain abscess. Of the abscesses, fungi caused 12 (31%), seven of which (18% of abscesses) were attributed to *Aspergillus* species (9). A follow-up study found 88 cases of CNS infection, including meningitis, of which *Aspergillus* accounted for 11 (9% of all cases) (53).

Three large reviews place the brain as the second or third most commonly involved organ in patients with aspergillosis (54–56). Concurrent intracranial involvement is seen in 13–16% of patients with pulmonary aspergillosis. Of patients with disseminated aspergillosis, brain involvement is found in 40–60% of cases (21,54,55,57).

Pathology

Two general patterns of infection are seen. In patients whose disease arises by direct extension from the paranasal sinuses, eye, or middle ear, a single or a few abscesses may form (50) (see Fig. 1). These lesions tend to occur in the frontal or temporal lobes, and symptoms may develop over years. In hematogenously spread infection, multiple small abscesses and microabscesses are seen, often at the junction of the gray and white matter. One report found abscesses to be common in the distribution of the posterior circulation (55). A regional focus of meningitis overlying the area of abscess is sometimes found. The progression of this type of infection is usually quite rapid.

Aspergillus species share in common with the other molds a propensity to invade blood vessels. Histopathological examination of involved brain tissue reveals hy-

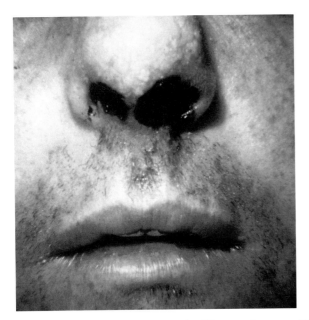

FIG. 1. Necrotic material in nares of a 30-year-old man with acute myelogenous leukemia who died of disseminated *Aspergillus*. At autopsy, multiple abscesses filled with septate hyphae were found in the brain.

phal angiitis with thrombosis in small and large vessels (see Figs. 2–4). Infarct and hemorrhage often result. The infection spreads centrifugally into fresh tissue while circumscribing an enlarging necrotic center. Meningeal blood vessels are occasionally involved. Meningitis without cerebritis is rare (10). The predilection to infect blood vessels also predisposes to formation of mycotic aneurysm (58,59).

Clinical Manifestations

The most common clinical sign in patients with *Aspergillus* brain abscess is a stroke syndrome referable to the involved area of brain (23). Headache and mild encephalopathy are also common. Seizures can occur.

Fever may or may not be present. Signs of meningeal irritation are rare (9,60). Patients with frontal lobe involvement may develop papilledema, visual field defects, and proptosis.

Evidence of *Aspergillus* involving other organs is common: 45 of 49 patients in combined series had evidence of pulmonary disease (7,10,11,54). A persistently neutropenic patient with pulmonary infiltrates who develops a stroke syndrome should have *Aspergillus* brain abscess included in the differential diagnosis. Isolated aspergilloma rarely has been described (44,58).

Diagnosis

Most cases of *Aspergillus* brain abscess are diagnosed at autopsy. Brain biopsy and, very rarely, CSF culture are currently the only ways to secure the diagnosis antemortem. CSF culture is only rarely positive (56). Serologic tests to detect *Aspergillus* antigen in the serum and/or CSF remain experimental (61,62).

CSF is usually nonspecifically abnormal. Elevated opening pressure, decreased glucose, and elevated protein may occur. Pleocytosis with no specific formula may be found. The presence of red blood cells in a patient with abscess is suggestive of possible intracranial aspergillosis (54). Normal CSF has also been described (6).

Radiologic imaging has proven a useful adjunct. CT scan appears quite sensitive (15,63) (see Figs. 5 and 6). A single false-negative has been reported; this occurred using a "first-generation" machine (14). Ring enhancement, if present, is slight in neutropenic patients. MRI scan appears more sensitive (64,65). Often several lesions are found, not all of which are clinically apparent. Imaging has been shown to allow earlier diagnosis and therefore earlier treatment, leading to improved survival (1). The finding of cerebral infarct in a patient with known risks for invasive aspergillosis should suggest the diagnosis.

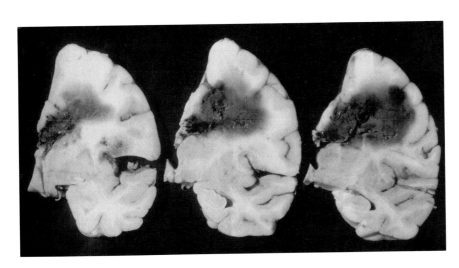

FIG. 2. Cerebral involvement with *Aspergillus* in a 28-year-old woman with neuroblastoma. (Courtesy of Dr. Marc Rosenblum.)

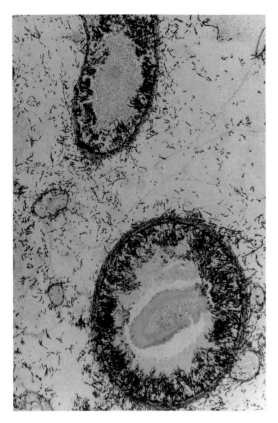

FIG. 3. Leptomeningeal vessel from patient in Fig. 2. Note hyphal forms filling the small vessels. (Courtesy of Dr. Marc Rosenblum.)

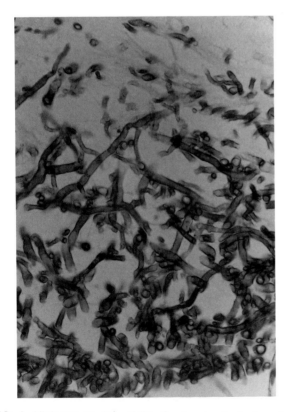

FIG. 4. High-power view of Fig. 3, showing typical septate hyphae. (Courtesy of Dr. Marc Rosenblum.)

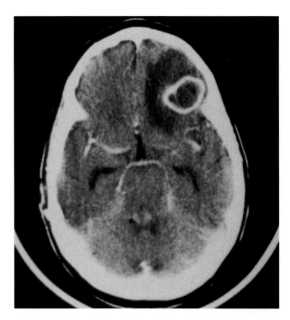

FIG. 5. CT scan of an aspergilloma in a 9-year-old boy with glioblastoma multiforme. The patient was receiving high-dose steroids and had a normal white blood cell count.

Treatment

The best therapy for *Aspergillus* brain abscess, as with other brain abscesses, is extirpation or drainage (66). However, given the patient population most likely to develop this infection, this may not be possible because of an underlying coagulopathy.

The mainstay of medical therapy remains intravenous amphotericin B, 0.6–1 mg/kg/day. In confirmed cases that appear unresponsive to this dose, up to 1.25 mg/kg/day may be effective. Duration of therapy is not known. In patients who have survived, over 3 g of amphotericin B has been given. Radiographic resolution may lag behind clinical improvement.

Concomitant therapy with rifampin (600 mg/day, orally) or 5-fluorocytosine [100–150 mg/kg/day (orally) in four divided doses, adjusted according to serum and CSF levels] has been tried, although no controlled studies have been done. We prefer the use of rifampin because of *in vitro* susceptibility studies which often show synergy. High-dose (1200 mg/day) ketoconazole was given successfully along with amphotericin B and 5-fluorocytosine in one patient (67). There are no reports of treatment of CNS infection with other imidazoles.

Mucormycosis (Phycomycosis)

History

Mucormycosis is perhaps the most acute, fulminant fungal infection known. CNS infection with the Muco-raceae was first described in 1885, in a man with multi-

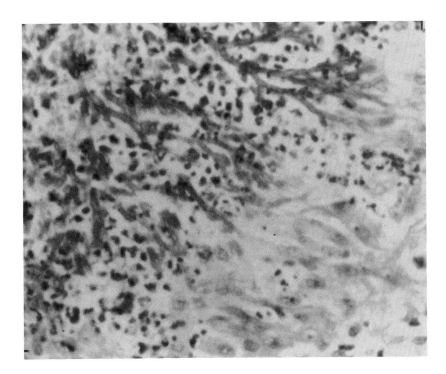

FIG. 6. Microscopic view of the aspergilloma shown in Fig. 5. Note the hyphae at the edge of the abscess, entering uninfected brain tissue.

ple brain abscesses who died with widely disseminated infection (3). In 1943, the description of three cases established the classic triad of mucormycosis: diabetes mellitus, orbital infection, and meningoencephalitis in patients in ketoacidotic coma (68).

Mucormycosis was initially a uniformly fatal disease. The first survivor, reported in 1955, was a 14-year-old girl with diabetes who was treated successfully by rigid control of her diabetes and, possibly, administration of systemic iodides (69). The efficacy of amphotericin B was demonstrated in 1958, and a new era of therapy began (70). Since then, survival rates for mucormycosis have steadily improved (71). Many excellent reviews have been published, all stressing the need for early diagnosis and prompt therapy (72–77).

Etiologic Agent

The Mucoraceae are ubiquitous fruit and bread molds that thrive in soil, in manure, and on decaying material. The hyphae are characteristically thick and ribbon-like and have irregular, nonseptate walls and acute right-angle branching.

The nomenclature used to describe this infection can be confusing (78). The class Phycomycetes (Zygomycetes) includes the families Mucoraceae, Cunninghamellaceae, Saksenaeaceae, and Entomophthoracae. The family Mucoraceae includes the pathogenic genera *Rhizopus, Mucor,* and *Absidia.* Brain abscess has also been caused by Cunninghamellaceae (79) and Saksenaeaceae (80). The term "mucormycosis" is used interchangeably with "phycomycosis" and "zygomycosis"; we prefer the term "mucormycosis." These terms describe any infection caused by a member of the family Mucoraceae.

Infections caused by Entomophthoracae are not considered mucormycoses; these rare infections usually occur in normal hosts residing in tropical climates and are characterized by eosinophilia and granuloma seen on histopathology of infected sinus tissue. Such infections seldom invade the CNS. Occasionally, confusion between Mucoraceae and Entomophthoraceae has led to the misdiagnosis of mucormycosis in a normal host (75).

Epidemiology

Cases of mucormycosis have been reported worldwide and in all ages. Both sexes are equally affected, and there appears to be no racial predilection to infection.

Pathogenesis and Pathophysiology

Many predispositions to mucormycosis have been described, and for each group of patients a single form of CNS disease predominates. Less than 5% of cases occur in normal hosts (71,77,81–85).

1. Patients with diabetes mellitus comprise at least 70% of all reported cases and consist uniformly of the rhinocerebral form of mucormycosis. Acidosis and not hyperglycemia appears to be the important predisposition to infection (86). However, rare cases of mucormycosis have been reported in diabetic patients with tight glycemic control (75). These patients may have a slowly progressing form of mucormycosis (87). Other cases of

slowly progressive mucormycosis, without apparent underlying diabetes mellitus, have been described (85,88).

2. Other patients who are acidemic from profound systemic illnesses—including sepsis, severe dehydration or diarrhea, or chronic renal failure—also may develop the rhinocerebral form (71,81,89,90).

3. Patients with hematologic neoplasms are more likely to develop pulmonary and/or disseminated mucormycosis and CNS involvement by hematogenous seeding (91). One review of autopsies reported no cases of mucormycosis among 4000 solid-tumor patients (91). All reported patients with disseminated mucormycosis have been in relapse. Most (three of four in one series) reported cases of rhinocerebral mucormycosis in patients with hematologic neoplasms occur in patients with concurrent diabetes mellitus (91). In disseminated disease, either multiple or solitary mass lesions may be found in the CNS. Isolated brain abscess in the absence of demonstrable disease elsewhere has been described (91,92).

4. Renal transplant patients are also at risk (93). These patients almost exclusively contract the rhinocerebral form of the disease. In one report, at least five of 14 patients had diabetes mellitus; and all were receiving immunosuppressive agents, including prednisone, azathioprine, and cyclosporine. The onset of mucormycosis occurred within a median time of 2 months after transplant, and nine of 14 died (93).

5. CNS mucormycosis may rarely occur after neurosurgery or direct trauma (94).

6. Mucormycosis is the most common cause of intracerebral fungal abscess in intravenous drug users (51,76,95–97). Abscess may occur with or without underlying endocarditis (98).

7. Use of deferoxamine may predispose patients to development of rhinocerebral mucormycosis (99). Many of these patients, however, may have other metabolic and hematologic predispositions for mucormycosis.

Pathology

The Mucorales, like many other pathogenic molds, invade arteries, causing thrombosis and infarction. Gross examination reveals clean lines of demarcation between vital areas and dry, gangrenous tissue. The mold may spread quickly along the lamina propria of small and medium-sized arteries and eventually extend beyond the sinuses and into the brain (98). The infection may involve all structures along its path, including the orbit, the eye, bone, and brain tissue. Rapidly expanding cerebritis rather than well-circumscribed granuloma formation is the rule.

Microscopically, hyphae can be seen invading into and through the arterial walls and spreading into uninfected tissue. The internal carotid artery is thrombosed

in one-third of autopsied patients (18,100). Cavernous sinus thrombosis may develop via direct extension from infected carotid arteries (101).

Clinical Manifestations

The appearance of a patient with severe rhinocerebral mucormycosis is not easily mistaken (see Fig. 7). The sight of enlarging areas of black mucosal or even facial necrosis is among the most dramatic in medicine. Before progressing to this stage, however, an infected patient may have many suggestive signs and symptoms. Any unusual complaint referable to the eyes or sinuses in a patient with diabetes mellitus should alert the treating physician to the possibility of rhinocerebral mucormycosis. The complaints may include headache, facial pain, diplopia, lacrimation, or nasal stuffiness or discharge (74,91,92,102,103). Less specific complaints may include fever and lethargy. Some patients present with newly diagnosed diabetes mellitus and concurrent mucormycosis (75). Any diabetic patient presenting in hyperglycemic ketoacidotic coma who does not awaken upon correction of metabolic imbalance should be suspected of having mucormycosis (75).

Initial signs more specific to rhinocerebral mucormycosis include development of a nasal ulcer, either hyperemic from early inflammation or else blackened from ischemic necrosis. Facial swelling and nasal discharge, followed by exophthalmosi, may ensue as the infection begins to spread posteriorly to involve the orbit. Cranial nerve abnormalities are common. Blindness may occur as a result of vascular compromise rather than as a result of direct invasion of the eye or optic nerve. Development of focal neurologic deficits—including hemiparesis, seizure, or monocular blindness—suggests more far-advanced disease and carries a worse prognosis (71).

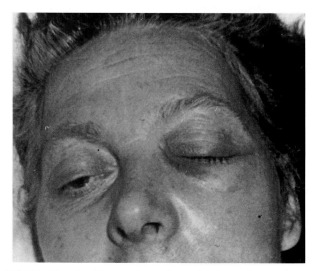

FIG. 7. Discoloration and swelling of left eyelid in woman who developed mucormycosis with brain involvement.

A recent review of 22 cases of nonrhinocerebral brain abscess caused by the Mucorales reported fever, headache, or focal neurologic signs to be present in over half of the patients (76). Fifty percent of the patients were intravenous drug users; of these, the basal ganglia were the most commonly infected site (83%). Seven patients survived. Patients with hematologic neoplasm who develop abscess during hematogenous seeding may have symptoms referable to the infected area of brain or may be without specific localizing signs (91).

Diagnosis

Diagnosis can be made by swabbing, scraping, or biopsying an involved area. A nasal or palatal ulcer specimen, "black pus" from a surgically drained sinus, or tissue from a brain biopsy should reveal, on potassium hydroxide wet mount preparation, the typical ribbon-like, broad, nonseptated hyphae. The organism grows on most culture media.

The CSF is usually nonspecifically abnormal, although patients with normal parameters have been reported (76,104). Elevated opening pressure, elevated protein, and pleocytosis with at least 50% polymorphonuclear cells are the most common abnormalities. Glucose is usually normal relative to the often-elevated serum glucose. One report of patients with hematologic neoplasms described red blood cells in the CSF of infected patients (91). Recovery of mucorales from CSF has not been reported.

There are several radiographic clues to diagnosis. Plain sinus radiographs seldom reveal an air–fluid level as can be seen in acute bacterial sinusitis (75). However, bony erosion may be found. Both CT scan and nuclear magnetic resonance imaging may show characteristic changes, including sinus opacification, erosion of bone, and obliteration of deep fascial planes (63,105–108). Frontal lobe involvement may show little or no ring enhancement.

A recently developed serum immunodiffusion test for antibody may prove helpful (95,109,110). The sensitivity and specificity of the test have not yet been established.

Therapy

Recovery from rhinocerebral mucormycosis was described before introduction of amphotericin B (69). This was achieved primarily by correcting the underlying metabolic abnormality. Several other successful treatments were subsequently described (90,111), but mortality remained at least 90% until the introduction of amphotericin B. This antibiotic given intravenously (0.6–1.0 mg/kg/day), along with aggressive surgical débridement and correction of underlying metabolic abnormalities, re-

mains the cornerstone of therapy. The amphotericin B therapy should be continued until there is clinical and radiologic evidence of resolution as well as correction of any metabolic or hematologic abnormalities that may have predisposed the patient to this infection.

Two reviews from the 1980s pointed out an increasing survival for all patients with mucormycosis (71,92). The underlying illness appears to be the most important predictor of outcome. In one review, 60% of patients with diabetes mellitus survived, compared to 20% of patients with other diseases (71). Amphotericin B use increased survival in both groups. One study (92) found survival before 1970 to be 6% and after 1970, 73%. Up to 70% of surviving patients are left with residual impairment (71). There is at least one case report of a patient with in vitro evidence of amphotericin B resistance. The patient, who progressed while given first 713 mg of amphotericin B and then 8 days of intravenous miconazole, finally improved on 600 mg/day of ketoconazole given for 5 months (112).

Patients with cerebritis, especially those with carotid artery and/or cavernous sinus involvement, have a much graver prognosis, although some survivors have been reported (113–117).

Hyperbaric oxygen therapy has been reported to be a useful adjunct, although no prospective, controlled studies have been performed (118).

Treatment with the new imidazoles has not been reported.

Infections Caused by *Pseudallescheria boydii*

History

Pseudallescheria boydii is best known as a common cause of "Madura foot," a chronic suppurative infection of the extremities. It was first reported to cause brain abscess in 1964 (119). Since then, approximately 25 additional cases have been reported (120,121).

Etiologic Agent

Pseudallescheria boydii (formerly *Petriellidium boydii* or *Allescheria boydii*; sexual form *Scedosporium apiospermium,* formerly *Monosporidium apiospermium*) is a common mold readily isolated from soil. It also may be cultured from polluted water, sewage sludge, and the manure of poultry and cattle. The association between near-drowning and subsequent illness from *P. boydii* may derive from the pathogen's presence in contaminated water and manure (121,122). It forms septate hyphae with rare branching and may be impossible to distinguish from *Aspergillus* species when examined in tissue.

Epidemiology

Although infection in the immunocompromised host is more common, brain abscess caused by *P. boydii* has been described in normal hosts as well (120,121,123). There is no evident age, race, or sex predilection to infection.

Pathogenesis and Pathophysiology

P. boydii may enter the CNS in at least four ways: (i) direct entry from trauma (124); (ii) hematogenous dissemination from a pulmonary route, including aspiration into lungs, especially implicated in near-drowning victims (121,125,126); (iii) via an intravenous catheter (127); and (iv) via direct extension from infected sinuses (128).

Pathology

Like other molds, *P. boydii* has a proclivity to invade blood vessels and, from the initial area of angiitis, to extend centrifugally and form abscess. An active granulomatous response with encapsulation is often seen, unlike the disorganized areas of cerebritis frequently found with mucormycosis.

In approximately one-half of reported cases, no sites of *P. boydii* infection other than the CNS were found (120,121).

Clinical Presentation

In the immunocompromised host, infection with *P. boydii* occurs in the same clinical settings one might anticipate for *Aspergillus* species infection: patients with hematologic neoplasms (129) and those receiving immunosuppressive agents, including cyclophosphamide, azathioprine, and corticosteroids (126,130). Signs and symptoms of a space-occupying lesion, including headache, fever, and focal neurological deficits, suggest the presence of brain abscess.

Patients who develop *P. boydii* infection after an episode of near-drowning tend to develop clinical signs and symptoms 15–30 days later (121). Often they will have endured an episode of bacteremia, diagnosed and treated beginning on admission. Metastatic skin lesions may herald the fungemia. *P. boydii* has been isolated from these papular lesions (121).

CSF findings are nonspecific. Mild-to-moderate elevations in protein and decreases in glucose may be seen along with a moderate-to-marked pleocytosis with a preponderance of polymorphonuclear leukocytes. A CT scan of the head may show the abscess(es) at any stage of development, beginning as nonspecific edema and progressing to well-circumscribed abscesses. Single or multiple lesions may be found.

Diagnosis

A certain diagnosis can only be made upon aspiration and culture of the abscess. *P. boydii* has been successfully cultured from blood of patients with endocarditis (121) but not from blood of those with brain abscess. A serologic test to measure antibody has aided in diagnosis in at least one case (128).

Therapy

Several patients have survived infection with *P. boydii,* although the mortality rate remains quite high. Survival may be better in patients with single rather than multiple lesions (121,126). Surgical drainage of the abscess remains the cornerstone of effective therapy, although antibiotic therapy may play an increasing role.

P. boydii shows *in vitro* resistance to amphotericin B; however, it is usually quite sensitive to miconazole (0.5–1.0 g intravenously, three times per day) (121,124,130,131). Several reports have shown clinical improvement (and, in some cases, cure) by giving intrathecal and/or intravenous miconazole. Therapy often must be given for many months, and relapses are common (121). In addition, dose increases often must be made during therapy; this is because miconazole blood levels begin to drop on stable doses of drug, long after a steady-state should have been achieved. This may be due to hepatic enzyme induction.

There has been a single report of partial response to fluconazole (600–800 mg/day, orally) (131a).

Other Hyphal Fungi (Molds)

Brain abscess from *Fusarium* species (132,133), *Paecilomyces* species (134,135), *Streptomyces griseus* (136), *Acremonium alabamensis* (137), and *Penicillium* species (138) have all been described. The diseases occurred in patients with expected predisposing illnesses. No clinical clue predicted the infection, and diagnosis was made in each case either at biopsy or autopsy.

The list of pathogenic molds certainly will continue to lengthen as more intensive chemotherapeutic regimens are given, indwelling catheters are used, higher doses of corticosteroids are administered, and the ability to diagnose CNS lesions with increasingly sensitive brain scans continues to improve. Hope for improved survival rates will continue to depend upon prompt diagnosis and institution of effective therapy, including surgical intervention and antifungal agents.

INFECTIONS CAUSED BY *CANDIDA*

History

Brain abscess caused by *Candida* species was first reported in 1895 (139), but it was not until 1943 that *Candida* was successfully cultured from a cerebral lesion (140). *Candida* remained a relatively infrequent CNS pathogen until the 1960s, when use of chemotherapeutic agents, glucocorticoids, and intravenous drugs rendered increasing numbers of patients susceptible to opportunistic infections. A 1978 review of 9,000 autopsies disclosed that *Candida* had surpassed *Cryptococcus* as the most common CNS fungal pathogen, accounting for half of the 39 cases described (8).

Etiologic Agent

Candida species are small, round yeasts that reproduce by budding. In tissue, *Candida* may exist as yeast, pseudohyphae, and (with *C. albicans* only) hyphae. Mucocutaneous candidiasis is a common ailment of (a) patients receiving antibiotics, (b) diabetics, (c) obese patients, (d) infants, and (e) patients with immunodeficiencies, including T-helper-cell dysfunction.

C. albicans accounts for 90% of the cases of candidal brain abscess. Intracranial infection has also been described with *C. tropicalis, C. guilliermondii, C. stellatoidea,* and *C. parapsilosis* (6,141,142).

Epidemiology

Invasive candidiasis occurs only in patients with an immunodeficiency. Some reports have found intracranial candidal infection to occur two times more frequently in men than in women (143,144). However, other reviews have reported an equal distribution (141,142). There is an increased incidence of both disseminated candidiasis and CNS involvement in the newborn (145,146). Pediatric cases accounted for 29% (12 of 42) of cases of CNS infection in one series (143). After infancy, there is no demonstrable increase in likelihood of infection with regard to age or race.

The CNS is frequently involved in patients with disseminated disease, although there is wide variation in reported incidence: from 18% (144) to 90% (147). Many reviews have reported CNS involvement in the setting of disseminated candidiasis to be approximately 50% (141,142). Most surveys ranking organ involvement in disseminated disease place the brain second only to the kidney (18).

Pathogenesis and Pathophysiology

Candida species are part of normal intestinal flora. Microabscesses provoked by chemotherapy and/or thrombocytopenia, as well as antibiotic-induced alteration in the balance of gut flora, allow seeding of *Candida* from the intestinal lumen into the bloodstream. In addition, an intravenous catheter placed into a central vein may serve as an entry site for *Candida* species. Also, patients (including intravenous drug users) with candidal endocarditis may develop subsequent CNS infection up to 80% of the time (141,142).

Pathology

Candida may involve the CNS in many ways. Most commonly, multiple microabscesses are seen, typically in the distribution of the middle cerebral artery (8). Noncaseating granuloma are also found, although less commonly. Macroabscesses occur in up to 14% of cases (141).

Vascular involvement with apparent fungal invasion of the vessel wall, as is seen in infection with molds such as *Aspergillus* species and mucormycosis, has also been described (143,148). Local areas of thrombosis and infarction may result, and *Candida* may be found in the necrotic tissue.

Mycotic aneurysm has been described with *C. albicans* and *C. parapsilosis* (59,141).

Multiple fungus balls of the temporal lobes have been described in one patient who also had disseminated cerebral aspergillosis (141). At autopsy, the fungus balls were packed with candidal hyphae forms.

Meningitis and ependymitis occur concomitantly with or separately from, parenchymal infection. One series of 42 patients with CNS candidal infections found 27 (64%) to have meningitis only and found the remaining 15 (36%) to have abscesses (143). Later series have placed the incidence of meningitis much lower, probably less than 15% (141,142).

Clinical Presentation

Any patient predisposed to develop disseminated candidiasis, including those with appropriate immunodeficiencies and those on immunosuppressive agents, may develop intracranial candidiasis. Nonspecific symptoms such as confusion, drowsiness, or stupor may be the only indication of CNS infection. However, fever is more often seen with CNS candidal infections than with other fungal infections of the CNS (18). In addition, classic meningeal signs such as nuchal rigidity, headache, and photophobia, which also are unusual in other intracranial mycoses, may be found (18). Focal neurologic deficits corresponding to involved areas of the brain may be seen in patients with large abscesses.

One autopsy review found that a major operation during the terminal admission had occurred in 12 of 19 patients with candidal infection of the CNS (8). Treatment for gram-negative bacteremia was given in 100% of patients who subsequently developed candidal brain abscess.

Diagnosis

Diagnosis is still most often made at autopsy. However, premorbid diagnosis has been made from biopsy; and, rarely, the organism has been recovered from CSF (141,149). In the absence of meningeal involvement, a positive CSF culture is rare unless parenchymal involvement develops subjacent to the subarachnoid space or ependyma. Nonspecific changes in CSF formula—including a mild decrease in glucose, a mild elevation in protein, and a pleocytosis—may be seen. Normal CSF is also described (6). Use of hypertonic media may enhance recovery of *Candida* from cultures (150).

Recovery of *Candida* from other sites—including urine, sputum, bone marrow, and pleural and peritoneal fluid—should suggest the possibility of dissemination and, therefore, the possible involvement of the CNS.

Radiologic diagnosis of candidal brain abscesses has been described, although there are no features typical of *Candida* that allow ready distinction from other causes of brain abscess (151,152).

Serologic tests for candidal precipitins in both CSF and serum have been used with variable results (153). Both immunodiffusion and counterimmunodiffusion electrophoresis (CIE) tests have been developed. The nonspecificity of current tests have made routine use of these tests unadvisable.

Therapy

A 1970 review of the world literature revealed 16 cases of candidal brain abscess; only one patient had survived (143). Since then, at least four additional adult survivors have been described (141,151,152). A report of 14 neonates with CNS candidal infection described survival of eight (146). Patients with well-circumscribed solitary lesions have responded well to surgical removal (151). Successful therapy with intravenous amphotericin B (0.6–1.0 mg/kg/daily) with and without oral flucytosine (100–150 mg/kg/day in four divided doses, adjusted for CSF and serum levels) has been reported (141,149,152). Many of the successfully treated neonates received both amphotericin B and flucytosine after worsening on therapy with amphotericin B alone (146). There is one report of successful treatment using amphotericin B, flucytosine, and itraconazole (154). No other cases using the imidazoles have been described.

INFECTIONS CAUSED BY TORULOPSIS GLABRATA

At least three cases of intracranial infection with *Torulopsis glabrata* have been described (155–157). *T. glabrata* is a member of the family Cryptococcaceae and is increasingly being recognized as a pathogen in the immunocompromised host. It is a part of normal intestinal flora, allowing apparent entry into the bloodstream. *T. glabrata* may also enter the bloodstream via an intravenous catheter.

Intracranial infection with *T. glabrata* has been described in both immunocompromised and noncompromised patients. All patients became progressively obtunded over weeks to months. Two of the patients had disseminated *T. glabrata,* and the third apparently had infection limited to the CNS. One patient had positive blood cultures for *T. glabrata*. In another patient, yeast was seen in, but not grown from, the CSF. A serologic test aided the diagnosis (156). Treatment with amphotericin B, flucytosine, ketoconazole, and itraconazole has been reported. The one surviving patient responded to flucytosine alone after failing therapy with intravenous amphotericin B (156). No surgery was attempted on any of the three reported patients.

INFECTIONS CAUSED BY CRYPTOCOCCUS

History

The first reports of intracerebral cryptococcoma appeared in the 1900s, although some dispute still exists concerning the exact taxonomy of the reported organisms (158,159). Since then, approximately 60 cases of space-occupying lesions due to *Cryptococcus neoformans* have been reported. Combined with cases of meningitis, *C. neoformans* was the most common fungal infection of the CNS (6) until the early 1970s, when autopsy studies established that *Candida* species had become a more prevalent CNS pathogen (8). With the human immunodeficiency virus (HIV) epidemic, cryptococcal CNS infections again lead all the rest. Most of the reviews of cryptococcoma were completed prior to the onset of the HIV epidemic, and therefore the following information refers (except where specifically stated) to a population not known to be infected with HIV.

Older names include *Torulopsis histolytica* and European blastomycosis.

Etiologic Agent

C. neoformans accounts for all reported cases of cryptococcal brain abscess. *C. neoformans* is a ubiquitous encapsulated yeast found in soil. It is present in high concentrations in the feces of pigeons and chickens, although it does not appear to cause disease in these animals. It has also been recovered from the skin and mucous membranes of noninfected humans (160). Disease in horses, cows, cats, and other mammals has been described.

In humans, the organism typically causes opportunistic infection. Prior to the HIV epidemic, over 50% of patients with meningitis (not cryptococcoma) had underlying illnesses associated with immune deficits, including hematologic neoplasms, diabetes mellitus, systemic lupus erythematosis, and organ transplantation. This association does not hold true for cryptococcoma, which occurs 95% of the time in normal hosts.

C. neoformans exists as a yeast both in culture and in tissue. It reproduces by budding and is taxonomically related to the *Candida* species.

Epidemiology

Unlike many other fungal diseases of the CNS, which occur equally in men and women, cryptococcal infection is far more frequent in men (approximately 80% of reported cases). This trend was established long before the HIV epidemic, and it holds true for both cryptococcal meningitis and cryptococcoma. The reasons are unknown, although occupational exposure to soil may be partially responsible.

There is no clear age or race predilection. Some authors have described an increased incidence among patients in their teens and twenties (161), whereas others have discerned an increase in the fourth and fifth decades (162). Most reported cases have come from the United States, Europe, and Australia (163). Cases are also regularly reported from China, India, and Southeast Asia (164).

Pathophysiology and Pathogenesis

Cryptococcus enters the body through the respiratory tract. No alternative routes (e.g., intravenous catheters or direct inoculation) have been postulated. Once established in the lungs, it may disseminate and seed the meninges, similar to *Mycobacterium tuberculosis*. Intraparenchymal lesions are felt to arise when a single miliary lesion begins to expand (165,166). It is not known why most patients develop meningitis while very few develop cryptococcoma.

Pathology

The brain, including the meninges, is by far the most common organ affected in cryptococcosis. At autopsy, 90% of all patients with cryptococcosis have CNS involvement (6). The lungs are involved at autopsy in 50% (162).

Grossly, a cryptococcoma may have a honey-combed or soap-suds appearance. One review has described four appearances of cryptococcoma (162): (i) a well-circumscribed pseudocystic lesion, similar to pyogenic abscess, containing inflammatory cells and cryptococci (9% of cases); (ii) a gelatinous mass composed mostly of cryptococci, with scant inflammatory response (24%);

(iii) a fibrogranulomatous lesion consisting mostly of fibrous reaction, with rare cryptococci (15%); and (iv) a mixed type (43%). Nine percent of lesions could not be classified. No neuroanatomic area appears more frequently involved. A few cases of intraventricular cryptococcoma, probably initiating in the choroid plexus, have been described (165,167–169).

Clinical Presentation

Cryptococcoma has a wide range of potential presentations. Reviews of cases of cryptococcal meningitis estimate the concurrent existence of cryptococcoma to be 4–8% (161,163,165). No estimate of meningitis with concurrent cryptococcoma has been made in acquired immunodeficiency syndrome (AIDS) patients, although one report described six undiagnosed lesions seen among 58 patients with cryptococcosis who received a CT scan (170). Conversely, cryptococcoma occurs with concurrent meningitis in approximately 63% of cases (162); the remaining 37% have cryptococcoma with no evidence of other CNS cryptococcosis.

Of particular note is that less than 5% of patients with cryptococcoma (with or without concurrent meningitis) have evidence of an underlying disorder which might have compromised their immune system—as opposed to greater than 50% of patients with cryptococcal meningitis who do have an underlying immune disorder (162).

Among presenting complaints, the most common is headache (73%). Multiple other symptoms—including fatigue, fever, seizures, confusion or other altered mental state, visual disturbances, or unsteady gait—occur variably; each symptom is reported in less than one-third of cases. As many as 18% of patients have no complaint referable to the CNS (162). Up to 5% of cases have been incidentally discovered at autopsy. Neurologic exam may demonstrate a focal deficit or may be normal.

Diagnosis

Cryptococcal disease can be diagnosed more readily than many other fungal illnesses because of its unique appearance on histopathology and the existence of a highly sensitive and specific latex agglutination test for cryptococcal capsular antigen.

CSF may be completely normal; but usually there is some abnormality, including elevated protein, decreased glucose, or a modest pleocytosis. A review of CSF cultures in 25 patients with cryptococcoma who had undergone neurosurgery reported the following results: 52% had positive initial India ink smears or cultures, 32% were culture- and smear-negative, and the cultures from the remaining 16% became positive after craniotomy (171).

There are no reports on the sensitivity and specificity of the cryptococcal capsular antigen test in the CSF of patients with cryptococcoma; however, absent cryptococcal antigen titers have been described in the presence of cryptococcoma.

CT scan of the head may reveal several different patterns according to the enhancement properties. The mass may enhance circumferentially, homogeneously, or not at all (172–175). Distinction from pyogenic abscess or tumor is seldom possible, but a patient with a granuloma seen on chest x-ray and one or several mass lesions on head CT should be suspected of having cryptococcoma.

Treatment

Surgical excision was the mainstay of therapy until the 1970s, when improvement in diagnostic capability and the introduction of effective antifungal agents made medical therapy possible. Now, therapy with both surgery and antifungal agents or with antifungal agents alone may be effective. Although survival may approach 50%, over half of the survivors may be left with a neurologic deficit (162). Patients who are at higher risk include those with concurrent meningitis and those in their forties or older (162). Surgery without subsequent antifungal therapy, even in the absence of meningitis, is probably not advisable (162).

Intravenous amphotericin B (0.3–1.0 mg/kg/daily, with the lower dose reserved for those patients receiving concomitant flucytosine) remains an effective treatment (176) with or without flucytosine (100–150 mg/kg/day in four divided doses, adjusted for serum and CSF flucytosine levels) (177). Duration of therapy is unknown but should extend well after there is clinical and radiologic evidence of resolution. Successful treatment with flucytosine alone has also been reported (161). One report described a patient who did not respond to combination amphotericin B and flucytosine but who was cured upon introduction of intravenous miconazole (178). Therapy with the newer imidazoles has not been fully evaluated in cryptococcal meningitis; thus far, there are no reports in cryptococcoma.

DIMORPHIC YEASTS

The intracranial presentation of the dimorphic yeasts is often similar to that of CNS infection with *Mycobacterium tuberculosis*. Dimorphic yeasts include *Blastomyces dermatitidis, Histoplasma capsulatum, Coccidioides immitis,* and *Paracoccidioides brasiliensis.* They are so grouped because of their growth characteristics: They have a mycelial form at room temperature and grow as yeast at 37°C. The dimorphic yeasts typically cause disease in the meninges of a normal host and seldom involve the CNS. Unlike the hyphal fungi, which cause vasculitis and infarction with resultant cerebritis

and/or brain abscess, the dimorphic yeasts usually cause a chronic meningitis (8,17). Occasionally, multiple microgranulomata may be seen, presumably from miliary seeding from a primary lung focus. Chronic meningitis may also give rise to asymptomatic local cerebritis in the subjacent parenchyma. True abscesses have rarely been described with dimorphic yeasts, either in normal or abnormal hosts.

Blastomyces dermatitidis

History

The first cases of *B. dermatitidis* infection of the brain were reported in the second decade of this century (179). Some authors (171,180) feel that earlier reports of intracranial blastomycosis (158,159) referred to *C. neoformans* rather than to *B. dermatitidis;* others count these as early cases of intracranial blastomycosis (6,181). A 1939 review found only 16 cases of blastomycosis with CNS involvement, many of which were limited to the meninges (182).

Etiologic Agent

Once known as "North American blastomycosis" or "Gilchrist's disease," *B. dermatitidis* infection is now known to occur worldwide. It is a typical dimorphic yeast with a mycelial or filamentous phase at room temperature and a yeast form in living tissue. Its environmental niche is probably the soil, but attempts to culture it have only rarely been successful (183,184). A canine form of blastomycosis resembles the human form, suggesting another possible source of exposure.

Epidemiology

The absence of a reliable skin test has thwarted attempts to delineate the extent of blastomycosis. Several small epidemics have been reported in Wisconsin, North Carolina, and other locations. Rare cases of intracranial infection have been reported worldwide (185,186). Blastomycosis is endemic to the south and south-central United States and to the Great Lakes area. Of sporadic cases, men outnumber women 9 to 1 (143). Most cases occur in middle-aged persons. There is no evident racial predilection.

Pathophysiology and Pathogenesis

Fungal spores enter the body via the respiratory tract and may cause subclinical infection or a pneumonitis. Certain patients may then develop disseminated disease, with potential seeding of the CNS. Immunocompromised patients do not appear to be at higher risk for dissemination.

Pathology

The lung is the most frequently involved organ, showing evidence of infection in at least 95% of autopsied cases (180). Skin lesions from presumed dissemination are found in 50%. Other frequently involved organs include bone and prostate.

The CNS is involved in approximately 5% (187) of cases and in up to 25% of cases with disseminated disease (6,188,189). The most common CNS finding is meningitis, which typically occurs late in the course of disseminated disease (180). A recent extensive review of intracranial blastomycoma found 31 cases reported in the world literature (181), although several of the early cases may actually have been cryptococcomas (180). The early reports excluded cases of involvement secondary to overlying osteomyelitis of the skull, a not infrequent presentation. Fifteen of 31 (48%) were solitary lesions, and the others were multiple. No anatomic area of the brain appeared more susceptible. All patients appeared to have disease in sites other than the CNS.

Microscopically, an abscess may have a fibrous capsule circumscribing necrotic tissue, inflammatory cells, and yeasts. Multinucleated giant cells are usually present; microabscesses with caseous necrosis may also be seen, mimicking tuberculosis (6). Occasionally, perivascular inflammation may occur (190).

Clinical Symptoms

Most patients with CNS blastomycosis exhibit evidence of pulmonary disease. The CNS abscess may cause increased intracranial pressure with or without localizing signs (6,181). Some patients are asymptomatic. The site of CNS involvement correlates with the specific neurologic deficit.

Diagnosis

Diagnosis of blastomycosis can only be made by isolating the organism by biopsy. To date, no reliable serologic test has been established, although several reports of newer tests appear promising (191,192).

CSF culture is rarely positive, even in cases of *B. dermatitidis* meningitis. In cases of abscess, opening pressure may be elevated and the CSF formula may be nonspecifically abnormal, including elevated protein, normal glucose, and slight pleocytosis without particular predominance of polymorphonuclear cells (180).

CT scan may show isodense or slightly hyperdense lesions with surrounding edema and uniform enhancement after contrast administration (181). Confusion with tumor is common (180).

Treatment

Intravenous amphotericin B (0.6–1.0 mg/kg/day) is the only established therapy for intracranial blastomycoma (180,181). Duration of therapy is not known but should extend until clinical and radiologic improvement. Intrathecal therapy is probably not required (181). High-dose (800 mg/day) ketoconazole has been given to one patient (186), with apparent improvement. The patient, however, declined to continue taking the medicine and died. There are no other reports of using the imidazoles to treat CNS blastomycosis.

Histoplasma capsulatum

History

Although histoplasmosis remains the most common deep-seated fungal infection in North America, development of a CNS abscess continues to be exceptionally rare. A recent review found only nine cases of cerebral histoplasmoma (193). Since then, at least three additional cases have been reported (194,195).

Etiologic Agents

H. capsulatum and *H. duboisii* are the causitive agents for, respectively, American and African histoplasmosis. No cases of brain abscess caused by *H. duboisii* have been described. *H. capsulatum* is a typical dimorphic yeast, existing in a mycelial form at room temperature and as a yeast at 37°C. It has been isolated from soil of endemic areas and is highly concentrated in bird and bat feces. Illness in other mammals, including dogs, has been described and may represent another route of exposure (195).

Epidemiology

H. capsulatum is endemic to river valleys, including the Ohio, the Mississippi, and the St. Lawrence; it is also endemic along the Appalachian Mountains and in North Carolina and Virginia (18). Serosurveys have revealed that most adults in endemic areas have been infected. There is a bimodal incidence of disseminated disease; about half of the cases occur in infants and young children, and the remainder occur in people over 40 years of age. In cases of dissemination after infancy and of intracranial histoplasmoma, men outnumber women approximately 5 to 1. The increased incidence in men is likely due to occupational exposures (193). No racial predisposition is apparent.

Pathogenesis and Pathophysiology

Infection is established upon inhalation of airborne spores. Once present in the lung, the infection may disseminate and establish a focus in the CNS. One case of probable postsurgical inoculation has been reported (196).

Of the reported cases of intracranial histoplasmoma, over one-third have occurred in immunocompromised patients; underlying diseases have included diabetes mellitus (197), Hodgkin's disease (198), cirrhosis (199), and systemic lupus erythematosis in a patient receiving prednisone (193). The contribution of the immune deficit to subsequent development of an intracranial histoplasmoma is uncertain.

Pathology

Most cases of histoplasmosis are limited to the lungs. In disseminated disease, involvement of the adrenals and bone marrow is common and oropharyngeal ulcers may be found.

CNS involvement in histoplasmosis, including meningitis, is seen in up to 7.6% of all cases and in 24% of patients with disseminated disease (200,201). Up to half, however, are cases of subclinical focal meningitis (201), and many of the others are limited to meningitis. Solitary abscess is more common than multiple lesions, but both may occur (193). Only one case of intracranial histoplasmoma without other organ involvement has been described (197). The patient, however, had extensive pulmonary tuberculosis which may have obscured a primary focus of H. capsulatum.

In addition to changes seen with meningitis, intracranial histoplasmosis may appear microscopically as miliary noncaseating granulomas along small veins or as larger granulomata (histoplasmoma) (201). In histoplasmoma, giant cells and other inflammatory cells surround an area of necrosis, often caseous. Histiocytes within the abscess contain H. capsulatum.

Clinical Presentation

All reported cases of CNS histoplasmoma have presented with neurologic findings, including seizure, hemiparesis, altered mental status, and ataxia (193). Constitutional signs of disseminated histoplasmosis, including fever, weight loss, and malaise, are often present which, combined with a lesion seen on CT scan, may mistakenly give the picture of metastatic carcinoma.

Diagnosis

The only certain way to make the diagnosis is with biopsy. However, culturing H. capsulatum from the bone marrow, a lymph node, or an oropharyngeal ulcer of an individual with evidence of a brain abscess should strongly suggest H. capsulatum as the etiologic agent of the intracranial lesion.

A reliable complement-fixing antibody test is available for H. capsulatum. Its utility, however, is limited by the extremely high prevalence of seropositive persons in endemic areas. A new radioimmunoassay (RIA) antigen test may be a more specific indicator of active disease (202). Complement-fixing antibody tests of the CSF may be negative in cases of intracranial histoplasmoma despite positive serum results (194). Culture of CSF has rarely yielded H. capsulatum (198).

CT scan findings are not specific. Intracranial lesions may show ring enhancement and surrounding edema indistinguishable from tumor.

Therapy

Of 12 reported patients with histoplasmoma, eight have survived, all treated with a combination of (a) surgical drainage or extirpation and (b) amphotericin B intravenously (0.6–1.0 mg/kg/day) (193–195). Duration of therapy is not known but should extend until there is evidence of clinical and radiologic improvement. No patient has survived with surgery alone. Amphotericin B therapy alone has not been attempted. A patient treated with ketoconazole (194) had progression of lesions and improved when amphotericin B therapy was instituted.

Coccidioides immitis

The first reports of C. immitis involving the brain appeared in the 1900s (159,203). Since then, the frequent occurrence of meningitis in patients with disseminated coccidiomycosis has been well-documented (204,205). Meningitis remains the predominant form of CNS coccidiomycosis.

C. immitis is a typical dimorphic yeast, endemic to parts of Arizona and the San Joaquin Valley. It is found in soil and enters the body through the respiratory tract, causing (in most patients) a self-limited respiratory illness. Rarely, it may disseminate and infect other organ systems, including the CNS. Pregnancy, diabetes mellitus, and other immunodeficient states may predispose to dissemination (204).

Meningitis may occur with or without underlying cerebritis. One review of CNS coccidiomycosis reported 13% (four of 32) with meningitis alone, 78% (25 of 32) with meningitis and concurrent cerebritis, and 9% (three of 32) with scattered miliary granulomas resembling tuberculomas (205). Another study reported scattered parenchymal granuloma in one of 31 autopsied patients (204). One of seven patients with AIDS and disseminated disease had intracranial granulomata (206), but

more than a year of treatment. One patient who survived longer than 2 years received ketoconazole in addition to amphotericin B and flucytosine (235). The use of other imidazoles has not been reported.

Other Dematiacious Fungi

Drechslera species (including *hawaiiensis, specifera,* and *halodes*) have recently been reclassified as either *Bipolaris* species or *Exserohilum* species. Several cases of cerebral abscess caused by these organisms have been described, with all but one occurring in immunocompetent hosts (220,236–239). Invasive pulmonary disease is usually seen in immunocompromised hosts (220).

Drechslera-Bipolaris-Exserohilum species resemble *Aspergillus* species in certain clinical respects, despite their lack of taxonomic relationship. They all may cause disseminated disease (in immunocompromised hosts) that is characterized by diffuse hyphal vasculitis; they may cause sinusitis in immunocompetent hosts; and all are associated with allergic bronchopulmonary disease (220).

A patient with brain abscess may present with signs and symptoms typical of a space-occupying lesion. CT scan may show abscess or, as seen in one case, temporal lobe changes suggestive of herpes simplex encephalitis (238).

Treatment with aggressive surgical débridement and intravenous amphotericin B (0.6–1.0 mg/kg/day) with or without flucytosine [100–150 mg/kg/day (orally) in four divided doses, adjusted according to serum and CSF flucytosine levels] has cured some patients. Maintenance ketoconazole therapy has been given to one survivor (237).

Several intracranial abscesses due to *Curvularia* species, including *lunata* and *pallescens,* have been reported, many in patients with concurrent pneumonitis (240–244). Most have occurred in normal hosts; one patient had an unexplained T-cell defect (241). The lone survivor received 12.2 g of amphotericin B (241). Neither ketoconazole nor flucytosine was beneficial in this patient.

Cases of brain abscess caused by *Fonsecaea pedrosoi* (*Phialophora pedrosoi*), *Wangiella dermatitidis, Dactylaria constricta,* and *Ramichloridium obovoideum* have been reported; one of these cases was accompanied by concurrent *X. bantiana* infection (245,246). All occurred in apparently normal hosts (although one patient had a short-bowel syndrome), and all died within weeks despite aggressive surgical and medical therapy. Primary infection may have been pulmonary. Differentiation of *F. pedrosoi* from the genera *Rhinocladiella* and *Ramichloridium* was made after careful testing, but confusion among these genera may exist.

MISCELLANEOUS

At least one case of brain abscess due to *Trichosporon cutaneum* has been reported (247). The patient was a 39-year-old woman with untreated adenocarcinoma of the lung metastatic to brain. Autopsy of the brain disclosed multiple lesions consisting of metastatic tumor with yeast-like organisms seen at the periphery. Cultures grew *T. cutaneum.* The infection appeared limited to the CNS. *T. cutaneum* typically causes white piedra of hair and occasional nail infections. It is found in soil and may be a normal colonizer of human skin. *T. beigelii* more commonly causes cutaneous disease. In a recent review that included this organism, no cases of CNS involvement with *T. beigelii* were noted (248).

A few cases of intracranial infection with *Trichophyton* species have been reported (249,250). In one case, a man with a possible T-cell immune defect developed invasive *T. mentagrophytes.* After over 5 years of chronic invasive disease, he finally died of widely disseminated fungal infection, including brain abscess (249).

One patient with disseminated *Microsporum audouinii* had intracranial involvement (251). Treatment with amphotericin B and plasma infusions cleared the infection.

Rhinosporidium seeberi, a fungus of uncertain classification, is endemic to India. At least one case of disseminated disease has been described (252).

Sepondium species were cultured from a fungating intraventricular mass of a 2-year-old boy who died of a fulminant neurologic infection (253). Hyphal organisms were seen on wet mount preparation. *Staphylococcus aureus* was also cultured from the lesion.

REFERENCES

1. Rosenblum ML, Hoff JT, Norman D, Weinstein PR, Pitts L. Decreased mortality from brain abscesses since the advent of computerized tomography. *J Neurosurg* 1978;49:658–668.
2. Saag MS, Dismukes WE. Azole antifungal agents: emphasis on new triazoles. *Antimicrob Agents Chemother* 1988;32:1–8.
3. Pautlauf A. Mucosis mucorina. *Virchows Arch [A]* 1885;102:543.
4. Freeman W. Fungus infections of the central nervous system. *Ann Intern Med* 1933;6:595–607.
5. Keye JD, Magee WE. Fungal diseases in a general hospital. *J Clin Pathol* 1956;9:1235–1253.
6. Fetter BF, Klintworth GK, Hendry MS. *Mycoses of the central nervous system.* Baltimore: Williams & Wilkins, 1967.
7. Hart PD, Russell E, Remington JS. The compromised host and infection. II. Deep fungal infection. *J Infect Dis* 1969;120:169–191.
8. Parker JC, McCloskey JJ, Lee RS. The emergence of candidiosis: the dominant post-mortem cerebral mycosis. *Am J Clin Pathol* 1978;70:31–36.
9. Chernik NL, Armstrong D, Posner JB. Central nervous system infections in patients with cancer. *Medicine* 1973;52:563–581.
10. Beal MF, O'Carroll P, Kleinman GM, Grossman RI. Aspergillosis of the nervous system. *Neurology* 1982;32:473–9.
11. Walsh TJ, Hier DB, Caplan LR. Aspergillosis of the central nervous system: clinicopathological analysis of 17 patients. *Ann Neurol* 1985;18:574–582.

12. Chun CH, Johnson JD, Hofstetter M, Raff MJ. Brain abscesses: a study of 45 consecutive cases. *Medicine* 1986;65:415–431.
13. Walsh TJ, Hier DB, Caplan LR. Fungal infections of the central nervous system: comparative analysis of risk factors and clinical signs in 57 patients. *Neurology* 1985;35:1654–1657.
14. Enzmann DR, Brant-Zawadzki M, Britt RH. CT of central nervous system infections in immunocompromised patients. *Am J Neuroradiol* 1980;1:239–243.
15. Whelan MA, Stern S, deNapoli RA. The CT spectrum of intracranial mycosis: correlation with histopathology. *Radiology* 1981;141:703–707.
16. Parker JC, McCloskey JJ, Solanki KV, Goodman NL. Candidiosis: the most common post-mortem cerebral mycosis in an endemic fungal area. *Surg Neurol* 1976;6:123–128.
17. Bell WE. Treatment of fungal infections of the central nervous system. *Ann Neurol* 1981;9:417–422.
18. Salaki JS, Louria DB, Chmel H. Fungal and yeast infections of the central nervous system. *Medicine* 1984;63:108–132.
19. Oppe W. Zur Keuntniss der Schimmelykosen beim Menschem. *Zentralbl Allg Pathol* 1897;8:301.
20. Mukoyama M, Gimple K, Poser CM. Aspergillosis of the central nervous system. *Neurology* 1969;19:967–974.
21. Khoo TK, Sugai K, Leong TK. Disseminated asperillosis. *Am J Clin Pathol* 1966;45:697–703.
22. Yanai Y, Wakao T, Fukamachi A, Kunimine H. Intracranial granuloma caused by *Aspergillus fumigatus. Surg Neurol* 1985;23:597–604.
23. Matsumura S, Sato S, Takamatsu HFH, et al. Cerebral aspergillosis as a cerebral vascular accident. *No To Shinkei* 1988;40:225–232.
24. David M, Charlin A, Morice J, Naudascher J. Infiltration mycosique à *Aspergillus amsteloidami* du lobe temporal simulant un abces encapsule. Ablation en masse. Guerison operatoire. *Rev Neurol (Paris)* 1951;85:121–124.
25. Linares G, McGarry PA, Baker RD. Solid solitary aspergillotic granuloma of the brain. *Neurology* 1971;21:177–184.
26. Ziskind J, Pizzolato P, Buff EE. Aspergillosis of the brain. *Am J Clin Pathol* 1958;29:554–559.
27. Stein SC, Corrado ML, Friedlander M, Farmer P. Chronic mycotic meningitis with spinal involvement (arachnoiditis): a report of five cases. *Ann Neurol* 1982;11:519–524.
28. Young RC, Jennings A, Bennett JE. Species identification of invasive *Aspergillus* in man. *Am J Clin Pathol* 1972;58:554–557.
29. Venugopal PV, Venugopal TV, Thiruneelakantan K, Subrabanian S, Shetty BMV. Cerebral aspergillosis: report of two cases. *Saburadia* 1977;15:225–230.
30. Zimmerman LE. Fatal fungus infections complicating other diseases. *Am J Clin Pathol* 1955;25:46–65.
31. Rinaldi MG. Invasive aspergillosis. *Rev Infect Dis* 1983;5:1061–1077.
32. Mohandas S, Ahuja GK, Sood VP, Virmani V. Aspergillus of the central nervous system. *J Neurol Sci* 1978;38:229–233.
33. Mukerji S, Patwardhan JR, Gadgil RK. Bacterial and mycotic infection of the brain. *Indian J Med Sci* 1971;25:791–796.
34. Makik R, Malhotra V, Gondal R, et al. Mycopathology of cerebral mycosis. *Acta Neurochir* 1985;78:161–163.
35. Banerjee AK, Singh MS, Kak VK, Talwar P, Rout D. Cerebral aspergillosis: report of 8 cases. *Indian J Pathol Microbiol* 1977;20:91–100.
36. Rhine WD, Arvin AM, Stevenson DK. Neonatal aspergillosis. *Clin Pediatr* 1986;25:400–403.
37. Ouammou A, El Ouarzazi A, Belghmaidi M, El Faidouzi M. Cerebral aspergillosis and encephalomeningocele. *Child's Nerv Syst* 1986;2:216–218.
38. DeMicco DD, Reichman RC, Violette EJ, Winn WC. Disseminated aspergillosis presenting with endophthalmitis. *Cancer* 1984;53:1995–2001.
39. Iyer SI, Dodge PR, Adams RD. Two cases of *Aspergillus* infection of the central nervous system. *J Neurol Neurosurg Psychiatry* 1952;15:152–163.
40. Lowe J, Bradley J. Cerebral and orbital *Aspergillus* infection due to invasive aspergillosis of the ethmoid sinus. *J Clin Pathol* 1986;39:774–778.
41. Britt RH, Enzmann DR, Remington JS. Intracranial infection in cardiac transplant recipients. *Ann Neurol* 1981;9:107–119.
42. Hooper DC, Pruitt AA, Rubin RH. Central nervous system infection in the chronically immunosuppressed. *Medicine* 1982;61:166–188.
43. Shapiro K, Tabaddor K. Cerebral aspergillosis. *Surg Neurol* 1975;4:465–471.
44. Klein HJ, Richter H-P, Schachenmayr W. Intracerebral *Aspergillus* abscess: case report. *Neurosurgery* 1983;13:306–309.
45. Bettoni BL, Gabrielli M, Lechi LA, Trabattoni G. Cerebral mycosis: clinicopathological report of four cases observed in fifteen months. *Ital J Neurol Sci* 1984;V:427–443.
46. Goldhammer Y, Smith JL, Yates BM. Mycotic intrasellar abscess. *Trans Am Ophthalmol Soc* 1974;72:65–78.
47. Polatty C, Cooper KR, and Kerkering TK. Spinal cord compression due to an aspergilloma. *South Med J* 1984;77:645–648.
48. Spens N, Tartersall WH. Fungal infection of the central nervous system supervening during routine chemotherapy for pulmonary tuberculosis. *Br Med J* 1965;2:862.
49. Starke ID, Keal EE. Cerebral aspergilloma in a patient with allergic bronchopulmonary aspergillosis. *Br J Dis Chest* 1980;74:301–305.
50. Perlmutter I, Perlmutter D, Hymans PJ. Fungal infection of the brain. *South Med J* 1980;73:499–501.
51. Kasantikul V, Shuangshoti S, Taecholarn C. Primary phycomycosis of the brain in heroin addicts. *Surg Neurol* 1987;28:468–472.
52. Kammer RB, Utz JP. *Aspergillus* species endocarditis. *Am J Med* 1974;56:506–521.
53. Chernik NL, Armstrong D, Posner JB. Central nervous system infections in patients with cancer: changing patterns. *Cancer* 1977;40:268–274.
54. Meyer RD, Young LS, Armstrong D, Yu B. Aspergillosis complicating neoplastic disease. *Am J Med* 1973;54:6–15.
55. Young RC, Bennett JE, Vogel CL, et al. Aspergillosis: the spectrum of the disease in 98 patients. *Medicine* 1970;49:147–173.
56. Jinkins JR, Sequeira E, Al-Kawi MZ. Cranial manifestations of aspergillosis. *Neuroradiology* 1987;29:181–185.
57. Carbone PP, Sabesin SM, Sidaransky H, Frei E. Secondary aspergillosis. *Ann Intern Med* 1964;45:697–703.
58. Visudhiphan P, Bunyaratavej S, Khantanaphar S. Cerebral aspergillosis. *J Neurosurg* 1973;38:472–476.
59. Mielke B, Weir B, Oldring D, von Westarp C. Fungal aneurysm: case report and review of the literature. *Neurosurgery* 1981;9:578–581.
60. Armstrong D, Wong B. Central nervous system infections in immunocompromised hosts. *Annu Rev Med* 1981;33:293–308.
61. Fisher BD, Armstrong D, Yu B, Gold JWM. Invasive aspergillosis: progress in early diagnosis and treatment. *Am J Med* 1981;71:571–577.
62. Murrow R, Wong B, Finkelstein WE, Sternberg SS, Armstrong D. Aspergillosis of the cerebral ventricles in a heroin abuser. *Arch Intern Med* 1983;143:161–164.
63. Centeno RS, Bentson JR, Mancuso AA. CT scanning in rhinocerebral mucormycosis and aspergillosis. *Radiology* 1981;140:383–389.
64. Mikhael MA, Rushovich AM, Ciric I. Magnetic resonance imaging of cerebral aspergillosis. *Comput Radiol* 1985;9:85–89.
65. Nov AA, Cromwell LD. Computed tomography of neuraxis aspergillosis. *J Comp Assist Tomogr* 1984;8:413–415.
66. Goodman ML, Coffey RJ. Stereotactic drainage of *Aspergillus* brain abscess with long-term survival: case report and review. *Neurosurgery* 1989;24:96–99.
67. Kwong YL, Yu YL, Chan FL, et al. High dose ketoconazole in the treatment of cerebral aspergilloma. *Clin Neurol Neurosurg* 1987;89:193–196.
68. Gregory JE, Golden A, Haymaker W. Mucormycosis of the central nervous system. *Johns Hopkins Med J* 1943;73:405–415.
69. Harris JS. Mucormycosis: report of a case. *Pediatrics* 1955;16:857–867.
70. Chick EW, Evans J, Baker RD. Treatment of experimental mucormycosis (*Rhizopus oryzae* infection) in rabbits with amphotericin B. *Antibiot Chemother* 1958;8:394–399.

71. Blitzer A, Lawson W, Meyers BR, Biller HF. Patient survival in paranasal sinus mucormycosis. *Laryngoscope* 1980;90:635–648.

72. Ferry AP. Cerebral mucormycosis (phycomycosis). *Surv Ophthalmol* 1961;6:1–24.

73. Meyers BR, Wormser G, Hirschman SZ, Blitzer A. Rhinocerebral mucormycosis. *Arch Intern Med* 1979;139:557–560.

74. Eisenberg L, Wood T, Boles R. Mucormycosis. *Laryngoscope* 1977;87:347–356.

75. Meyer RD, Armstrong D. Mucormycosis—changing status. *CRC Crit Rev Clin Lab Sci* 1973;4:421–451.

76. Stave GM, Heimberger T, Kerkering TM. Zygomycosis of the basal ganglia in intravenous drug users. *Am J Med* 1989;86:115–117.

77. Straatsma BR, Zimmerman LE, Gass JDM. Phycomycosis: a clinicopathologic study of fifty-one cases. *Lab Invest* 1962; 11:963–985.

78. Baker RD. The phycomycoses. *Ann NY Acad Sci* 1970;174:592–605.

79. Brennan RO, Crain BJ, Proctor AM, Durack D. *Cunninghamella*: a newly recognized cause of rhinocerebral mucormycosis. *Am J Clin Pathol* 1983;80:98–102.

80. Kaufman L, Padhye AA, Parker S. Rhinocerebral zygomycosis caused by *Saskenaea vasiformis*. *J Med Vet Mycol* 1988;26:237–241.

81. McNulty JS. Rhinocerebral mucormycosis: predisposing factors. *Laryngoscope* 1982;92:1140–1143.

82. Whalen MJ, Beyt BE. Cryptic cerebral phycomycosis. *Ann Intern Med* 1979;91:655.

83. Watson DF, Stern BJ, Levin ML, Dutta D. Isolated cerebral phycomycosis presenting as focal encephalitis. *Arch Neurol* 1985;42:922–923.

84. Tang L-M, Ryu S-J, Chen T-J, Cheng S-Y. Intracranial phycomycosis: case reports. *Neurosurgery* 1988;23:108–111.

85. Blodi FC, Hannah FT, Wadsworth JAC. Lethal orbito-cerebral phycomycosis in otherwise healthy children. *Am J Ophthalmol* 1969;67:698–705.

86. Abramson E, Wilson D, Arky RA. Rhinocerebral phycomycosis in association with diabetic ketoacidosis. *Ann Intern Med* 1966;66:735–742.

87. Finn DG, Farmer JC. Chronic mucormycosis. *Laryngoscope* 1982;92:761–763.

88. Tay AGC, Tan CT. Mucormycosis and chronic brain abscess. *Med J Aust* 1986;144:725–726.

89. Morris DJ, Altus P. Rhinocerebral mucormycosis in an anephric patient. *South Med J* 1988;81:400–403.

90. Kurrein F. Cerebral mucormycosis. *J Clin Pathol* 1954;7:141–144.

91. Meyer RD, Rosen P, Armstrong D. Phycomycosis complicating leukemia and lymphoma. *Ann Intern Med* 1972;77:871–879.

92. Parfrey NZ. Improved diagnosis and prognosis of mucormycosis. *Medicine* 1986;65:113–123.

93. Morduchowicz G, Shmueli D, Shapira Z, et al. Rhinocerebral mucormycosis in renal transplant recipients. *Rev Infect Dis* 1986;8:441–446.

94. Ignelzi RJ, Vander Ark GD. Cerebral mucormycosis following open head trauma. *J Neurosurg* 1975;42:593–596.

95. Pierce PF, Solomon SL, Kaufman L, et al. Zygomycetes brain abscesses in narcotic addicts with serological diagnosis. *JAMA* 1982;248:1881–1882.

96. Woods KF, Hanna BJ. Brain stem mucormycosis in a narcotic addict with eventual recovery. *Am J Med* 1986;80:126–128.

97. Hameroff SB, Eckholdt JW, Linderberg R. Cerebral phycomycosis in a heroin addict. *Neurology* 1970;20:261–265.

98. Chlmel H, Grieco MH. Cerebral mucormycosis and renal aspergillosis in heroin addicts without endocarditis. *Am J Med Sci* 1973;266:225–231.

99. Daly AL, Velasquez LA, Bradley SF, Kaufman CA. Mucormycosis: association with deferoxamine therapy. *Am J Med* 1989;87:468–471.

100. Anaissie EJ, Shikhani AH. Rhinocerebral mucormycosis with internal carotid occlusion: report of two cases and review of the literature. *Laryngoscope* 1985;95:1107–1113.

101. Johnson EV, Kline LB, Julian BA, Garcia JH. Bilateral cavernous sinus thrombosis due to mucormycosis. *Arch Ophthalmol* 1988;106:1089–1092.

102. Maniglia AJ, Mintz DH, Novak S. Cephalic phycomycosis: a report of eight cases. *Laryngoscope* 1982;92:755–760.

103. Pillsbury HC, Fischer ND. Rhinocerebral mucormycosis. *Arch Otolaryngol* 1977;107:600–604.

104. Lehrer RI, Howard DH, Sypherd PS, et al. Mucormycosis. *Ann Intern Med* 1980;93:93–108.

105. Lazo A, Wilner HI, Metes JJ. Craniofacial mucormycosis: computed tomographic and angiographic findings in two cases. *Radiol* 1981;139:623–626.

106. Anderson D, Matick H, Naheedy MH, Stein K. Rhinocerebral mucormycosis with CT scan findings: a case report. *Comput Radiol* 1984;8:113–117.

107. Narang AK, Dina TS. Cerebral mucormycosis: a case report. *Comput Med Imag Graphics* 1988;12:259–262.

108. Anderson D, Matick H, Naheedy MH, Stein K. Rhinocerebral mucormycosis with CT scan findings. *Comput Radiol* 1984;8:113–117.

109. Marchevsky AM, Bottone EJ, Geller SA, Giger DK. The changing spectrum of disease, etiology and diagnosis of mucormycosis. *Hum Pathol* 1980;11:457–464.

110. Jones KW, Kaufman L. Development and evaluation of an immunodiffusion test for diagnosis of systemic zygomycosis (mucormycosis): preliminary report. *J Clin Microbiol* 1978;7:97–103.

111. McBride RA, Carson JM, Dammin GJ. Mucormycosis. *Am J Med* 1960;28:832–846.

112. Barnert J, Behr W, Reich H. An amphotericin B resistant case of rhinocerebral mucormycosis. *Infection* 1985;13:134–136.

113. Ferry AP, Abedi S. Diagnosis and management of rhino-orbito-cerebral mucormycosis. *Ophthalmology* 1983;90:1096–1104.

114. Soloniuk DS, Moreland DB. Rhinocerebral mucormycosis with extension to the posterior fossa. *Neurosurgery* 1988;23:641–643.

115. Ochi JW, Harris JP, Feldman JI, Press GA. Rhinocerebral mucormycosis: results of aggressive surgical débridement and amphotericin B. *Laryngoscope* 1988;98:1339–1342.

116. Hamill R, Oney LA, Crane LR. Successful therapy for rhinocerebral mucormycosis with associated bilateral brain abscess. *Arch Intern Med* 1983;143:581–583.

117. Smith JL, Stevens DA. Survival in cerebro-rhino-orbital zygomycosis and cavernous sinus thrombosis with combined therapy. *South Med J* 1986;79:501–504.

118. Ferguson BJ, Mitchell TG, Moon R, Camporesi EM, Farmer J. Adjunctive hyperbaric oxygen for treatment of rhinocerebral mucormycosis. *Rev Infect Dis* 1988;10:551–559.

119. Rosen F, Deck JHN, Newcastle NB. *Allescheria boydii*—unique systemic dissemination to thyroid and brain. *Can Med Assoc J* 1965;93:1125–1127.

120. Berenguer J, Diaz-Mediavilla J, Urra D, Munoz P. Central nervous system infection caused by *Pseudallescheria boydii*. *Rev Infect Dis* 1989;11:890–896.

121. Dworzack DL, Clark RB, Borkowski WJ, et al. *Pseudallescheria boydii* brain abscess: association with near-drowning and efficacy of high-dose, prolonged miconazole therapy in patients with multiple abscesses. *Medicine* 1989;68:218–224.

122. Travis LB, Roberts GD, Wilson WR. Clinical significance of *Pseudallescheria boydii*: a review of ten years' experience. *Mayo Clin Proc* 1985;60:531–537.

123. Fry VG, Young CN. A rare fungal brain abscess in an uncompromised host. *Surg Neurol* 1981;15:446–448.

124. Anderson RL, Carroll TF, Harvey JT, Myers MG. *Petriellidium boydii* orbital and brain abscess treated with intravenous miconazole. *Am J Ophthalmol* 1984;97:771–775.

125. Fisher JF, Shadomy S, Teabeaut JR, et al. Near-drowning complicated by brain abscess due to *Petriellidium boydii*. *Arch Neurol* 1982;39:511–513.

126. Dubeau F, Roy LE, Allard J, et al. Brain abscess due to *Petriellidium boydii*. *Can J Neurol Sci* 1984;11:395–398.

127. Perez RE, Smith M, McClendon J, Kim J, Eugenio N. *Pseudallescheria boydii* brain abscess. *Am J Med* 1988;84:359–362.

128. Bryan CS, DiSalvo AF, Kaufman L, et al. *Petriellidium boydii*

infection of the sphenoid sinus. *Am J Clin Pathol* 1980;74:846–851.

129. Yoo D, Lee WHS, Kwon-Chung KJ. Brain abscesses due to *Pseudallescheria boydii* associated with primary non-Hodgkin's lymphoma of the central nervous system: a case report and review of the literature. *Rev Infect Dis* 1985;7:272–277.

130. Winston DJ, Jordan MC, Rhodes J. *Allescheria boydii* infections in the immunosuppressed host. *Am J Med* 1977;63:830–835.

131. Lutwick LI, Galgiani JN, Johnson RH, Stevens DA. Visceral fungal infections due to *Petriellidium boydii*. *Am J Med* 1976;61:632.

131a.Bailey T, Graham MB, Powderly W. Disseminated *Pseudallescheria boydii* infection treated with fluconazole. *Sixth International Symposium on Infections in the Immunocompromised Host, Peebles, Scotland, 1990.* Abstract 71.

132. Steinberg GK, Britt RH, Enzmann DR, Finlay JL, Arvin AM. *Fusarium* brain abscess. *J Neurosurg* 1983;56:598–601.

133. Richardson SE, Bannatyne RM, Summerbell RC, et al. Disseminated fusarial infection in the immunocompromised host. *Rev Infect Dis* 1988;10:1171–1181.

134. Ho KL, Allevato PA, King P, Chason JL. Cerebral *Paecilomyces javanicus* infection. *Acta Neuropathol* 1986;72:134–141.

135. Uys CJ, Don PA, Schrire V, Barnard CN. Endocarditis following cardiac surgery due to the fungus *Paecilomyces*. *South Afr Med J* 1963;37:1276–1280.

136. Clarke PRR, Warnock GBR, Blowers R, Wilkonson M. Brain abscess due to *Streptomyces griseus*. *J Neurol Neurosurg Psychiatry* 1964;27:553–555.

137. Wetli CV, Weiss SD, Cleary TJ, Gyori E. Fungal cerebritis from intravenous drug abuse. *J Forensic Sci* 1983;29:260–268.

138. Huang SN, Harris LS. Acute disseminated penicilliosis. *Am J Clin Pathol* 1963;39:167–174.

139. Heller A. Beitrag zur Lehre vom Soor. *Dtsch Arch Klin Med* 1895;55:123–140.

140. Miale JB. *Candida albicans* infection confused with tuberculosis. *Arch Pathol* 1943;35:427–37.

141. Lipton SA, Hickey WF, Morris JH, Loscalzo J. Candidal infection in the central nervous system. *Am J Med* 1984;76:101–108.

142. Parker JC, McCloskey JJ, Lee RS. Human cerebral candidosis—a post-mortem evaluation of 19 patients. *Hum Pathol* 1981;12:23–28.

143. Black JT. Cerebral candidiasis: case report of brain abscess secondary to *Candida albicans* and review of the literature. *J Neurol Neurosurg Psychiatry* 1970;33:864–870.

144. Myerowitz RL, Pazin GJ, Allen CM. Disseminated candidiasis: changes in incidence, underlying disease and pathology. *Am J Clin Pathol* 1977;68:29–38.

145. Haruda F, Bergman MA, Headings D. Unrecognized *Candida* brain abscess in infancy: two cases and a review of the literature. *Johns Hopkins Med J* 1980;147:182–185.

146. Faix RG. Systemic *Candida* infection in infants in intensive care nurseries: high incidence of CNS involvement. *J Pediatr* 1984;105:616.

147. Crislip MA, Edwards JE. Candidiasis. *Infect Dis Clin North Am* 1989;3(1):103–136.

148. Parker JC, McCloskey JJ, Knauer KA. Pathobiologic features of human candidiasis. *Am J Clin Pathol* 1976;65:991–1000.

149. Wietholter H, Thron A, Scholz E, Dichgans J. Systemic *Candida albicans* infection with cerebral abscess and granulomas. *Clin Neuropathol* 1984;3:37–41.

150. Igra-Siegman Y, Louria DB, Armstrong D. "Culture-negative" meningitis: isolation of organisms in hypertonic medium. *Isr J Med Sci* 1981;17:383–384.

151. Ilgren EB, Westmoreland D, Adams CBT, Mitchell RG. Cerebellar mass caused by *Candida* species. *J Neurosurg* 1984;60:428–430.

152. Thron A, Wietholter H. Cerebral candidiasis: CT studies in a case of brain abscess and granuloma due to *Candida albicans*. *Neuroradiology* 1982;23:223–225.

153. Filice G, Yu B, Armstrong D. Immunodiffusion and agglutination tests for *Candida* in patients with neoplastic disease: inconsistent correlation of results with invasive infections. *J Infect Dis* 1977;135:349–357.

154. Foreman NK, Mott MG, Parkyn TM, Moss G. Mycotic intracranial abscesses during induction treatment for acute lymphoblastic leukaemia. *Arch Dis Child* 1988;63:436–438.

155. Minkowitz S, Koffler D, Zak F. *Torulopsis glabrata* septicemia. *Am J Med* 1963;34:252–255.

156. Wurzel B, Goldberg P, Caroline L, Bozza AT, Kozinn PJ. *Torulopsis glabrata* meningoencephalitis treated with 5-fluorocytosine. *Ann Intern Med* 1973;77:815–816.

157. Van Cutsem E, Boogaerts MA, Tricot G, Verwilghen RL. Multiple brain abscesses caused by *Torulopsis glabrata* in an immunocompromised patient. *Mykosen* 1986;29:306–308.

158. LeCount ER and Myers J. Systemic blastomycosis (cryptococcosis). *J Infect Dis* 1907;4:187–200.

159. Evans N. Coccidioidal granuloma and blastomycosis (cryptococcosis) in the central nervous system. *J Infect Dis* 1909;6:523–536.

160. Carton CA, Mount LA. Neurosurgical aspects of cryptococcosis. *J Neurosurg* 1951;8:143–156.

161. Arumugasamy N. Intracerebral cryptococcomas. *Ann Acad Med* 1985;14:16–21.

162. Fujita NK, Reynard M, Sapico FL, Guze LB, Edwards JE. Cryptococcal intracerebral mass lesions. *Ann Intern Med* 1981;94:382–388.

163. Harper CG, Wright DM, Parry G, O'Connor MJ. Cryptococcal granuloma presenting as an intracranial mass. *Surg Neurol* 1979;11:425–429.

164. Reddy DR, Prabhakar V, Rao D, Laxmi CR. A case of cryptococcal abscess of the brain. *Indian J Med Sci* 1971;25:546–549.

165. Vijayan N, Bhatt GP, Dreyfus PM. Intraventricular cryptococcal granuloma. *Neurology* 1971;21:728–734.

166. Krainer L, Small JM, Hewlitt AB, Deness T. A case of systemic *Torula* infection with tumor formation in the meninges. *J Neurol Neurosurg Psychiatry* 1946;9:158–162.

167. Manganiello LOJ, Nichols P. Intraventricular toruloma granuloma. *J Neurosurg* 1955;12:306–310.

168. Maurice-Williams RS. Intraventricular cryptococcal granuloma. *J Neurol Neurosurg Psychiatry* 1975;38:305–308.

169. Penar PL, Kim J, Chyatte D, Sabshin JK. Intraventricular cryptococcal granuloma. *J Neurosurg* 1988;68:145–148.

170. Chuck SL, Sande MA. Infections with *Cryptococcus neoformans* in the acquired immunodeficiency syndrome. *N Engl J Med* 1989;321:794–799.

171. Selby RC, Lopes NM. Torulomas on the central nervous system. *J Neurosurg* 1973;38:40–46.

172. Tress B, Davis S. Computed tomography of intracerebral toruloma. *Neuroradiology* 1979;17:223–226.

173. Garcia CA, Weisberg LA, Lacorte WSJ. Cryptococcal intracerebral mass lesions: CT–pathologic considerations. *Neurology* 1985;35:731–734.

174. Bateson EM. Computed tomography of intracranial torulosis in the Australian aboriginal. *Australas Radiol* 1986;30:92–95.

175. Kanter SL, Friedman WA, Ongley JP. Pitfalls in the CT diagnosis of toruloma. *Surg Neurol* 1984;21:113–118.

176. Sapico FL. Disappearance of focal cryptococcal brain lesion on chemotherapy alone. *Lancet* 1979;1:560.

177. Bayardelle P, Giard N, Maltais R, Delorme J, Brazeau M. Success with amphotericin B and 5-fluorocytosine in treating cerebral cryptococcoma accompanying cryptococcal meningitis. *Can Med J* 1982;127:732–733.

178. Weinstein L, Jacoby I. Successful treatment of cerebral cryptococcoma and meningitis with miconazole. *Ann Intern Med* 1980;93:569–571.

179. Krost RA, Moes MJ, Stober AM. A case of systemic blastomycosis. *JAMA* 1908;50:184–188.

180. Gonyea EF. The spectrum of primary blastomycotic meningitis: a review of central nervous system blastomycosis. *Ann Neurol* 1978;3:24–39.

181. Roos KL, Bryan JP, Maggio WM, Jane JA, Scheld WM. Intracranial blastomycoma. *Medicine* 1987;66:224–235.

182. Martin DS, Smith DT. Blastomycosis—a review of the literature. *Am Rev Tuberc* 1939;39:275–304.

183. Sarosi GA, Davies SF. Blastomycosis. *Am Rev Respir Dis* 1979;120:911–938.

184. Klein BS, Vergeront JM, Weeks RJ, et al. Isolation of *Blasto-*

myces dermatitidis in soil associated with a large outbreak of blastomycosis in Wisconsin. *N Engl J Med* 1986;314:529–534.

185. Raftopoulos C, Flament-Durand J, Coremans-Pelseneer J, Noterman J. Intracerebellar blastomycosis abscess in an African man. *Clin Neurol Neurosurg* 1986;88(3):209–212.

186. Cooper K, Lalloo UG, Naran HK. Cerebral blastomycosis. *S Afr Med J* 1988;74:521–524.

187. Buechner HA, Clawson CM. Blastomycosis of the central nervous system. *Am Rev Respir Dis* 1967;95:820–827.

188. Schwartz J, Baum GL. Blastomycosis. *Am J Clin Pathol* 1951;21:999–1029.

189. Busey JF, Baker R, Birch L, et al. Blastomycosis: a review of 198 cases from the Veterans Administration hospitals. *Am Rev Respir Dis* 1964;89:659–672.

190. Morse HG, Nichol WP, Cook DM, Blank NK, Ward TT. Central nervous system and genitourinary blastomycosis. *West J Med* 1983;139:99–103.

191. Tang TT, Marsik FJ, Harb JM, et al. Cerebral blastomycosis: an immunodiagnostic study. *Am J Clin Pathol* 1984;82:243–246.

192. Klein BS, Vergeront JM, Kaufman L, et al. Serological tests for blastomycosis: assessments during a large point-source outbreak in Wisconsin. *J Infect Dis* 1987;155:262–268.

193. Vakili ST, Eble JN, Richmond BD, Yount RA. Cerebral histoplasmoma. *J Neurosurg* 1983;59:332–336.

194. Walpole HT, Gregory DW. Cerebral histoplasmosis. *South Med J* 1987;80:1575–1577.

195. Venger BH, Landon G, Rose JE. Solitary histoplasmoma of the thalamus: case report and literature review. *Neurosurgery* 1987;20:784–787.

196. Gilden DH, Miller EM, Johnson WG. Central nervous system histoplasmosis after rhinoplasty. *Neurology* 1974;24:874–877.

197. White HW, Friztlen TJ. Cerebral granuloma caused by *Histoplasma capsulatum. J Neurosurg* 1962;19:260–263.

198. Allo MD, Silva J, Kaufman CA, Dicks RE. Enlarging histoplasmomas following treatment of meningitis due to *Histoplasma capsulatum. J Neurosurg* 1979;51:242–244.

199. Bridges WR and Echols DH. Cerebellar histoplasmoma. Case report. *J Neurosurg* 1967;26:261–263.

200. Goodwin RA, Shapiro JL, Thurman GH, Thurman SS, Des Prez RM. Disseminated histoplasmosis: clinical and pathological correlations. *Medicine* 1980;59:1–33.

201. Cooper RA, Goldstein E. Histoplasmosis of the central nervous system. Report of two cases and review of the literature. *Am J Med* 1963;35:45–57.

202. Wheat LJ, Kohler RB, Tewari RP. Diagnosis of disseminated histoplasmosis by detection of *Histoplasma capsulatum* antigen in serum and urine specimens. *N Engl J Med* 1986;314:83–8.

203. Ophuls W. Further observations on a pathogenic mould formerly described as a protozoon (*Coccidioides immitis, Coccidioides pyogenes*). *J Exp Med* 1905;6:443–485.

204. Bouza E, Dreyer JS, Hewitt WL, Meyer RD. Coccidioidal meningitis. *Medicine* 1981;60:139–172.

205. Sobel RA, Ellis WG, Nielsen SL, Davis RL. Central nervous system coccidiomycosis. *Hum Pathol* 1984;15:980–985.

206. Bronnimann DA, Adam RD, Galgiani JN, et al. *Coccidioides* in the acquired immunodeficiency syndrome. *Ann Intern Med* 1987;106:372–379.

207. Levy RM, Bredesen DE, Rosenblum ML. Neurological manifestations of the acquired immunodeficiency syndrome (AIDS): experience at UCSF and review of the literature. *J Neurosurg* 1985;62:475–495.

208. de Carvalho CA, Allen JN, Zafranis A, Yates AJ. Coccidioidal meningitis complicated by cerebral infarction. *Hum Pathol* 1980;11:293–296.

209. Jarvik JG, Hesselink JR, Wiley C. Coccidioidomycotic brain abscess in an HIV-infected man. *West J Med* 1988;149:83–86.

210. Guerreiro CAM, Chuluc SSD, Branchini MLN. A new treatment for large cerebral paracoccidioidomycosis. *Arq Neuropsiquiatr* 1987;45:419–423.

211. Rippon JW. Paracoccidioides. In: Rippon JW, ed. *Medical mycology: the pathogenic fungi and pathogenic actinomycetes.* Philadelphia: WB Saunders, 1988;506–531.

212. Pereira WC, Raphael A, Sallum J. Lesoes neurologicas na blasto-

micose sul-americana: estudo anatomopatologico de 14 casos. *Arq Neuropsiquiatr* 1965;23:95–112.

213. Araujo JC, Werneck L, Cravo MA. South American blastomycosis presenting as a posterior fossa tumor. *J Neurosurg* 1978; 49:425–428.

214. Minguetti G, Madalozzo LE. Paracoccidioidal granulomatosis of the brain. *Arch Neurol* 1983;40:100–102.

215. Pereira WC, Raphael A, Tenuto RA, Sallum J. Localizacao encefalica da blastimicose sul-americana: consideracoes a proposito de 9 casos. *Arq Neuropsiquiatr* 1965;23:113–126.

216. Gullberg RM, Quintanilla A, Levin ML, Williams J, Phair JP. Sporotrichosis: recurrent cutaneous, articular, and central nervous system infection in a renal transplant patient. *Rev Infect Dis* 1987;9:369–375.

217. Satterwhite TK, Kageler WV, Conklin RH, Portnoy BL, DuPont HL. Disseminated sporotrichosis. *JAMA* 1978;240:771–772.

218. Dixon DM, Walsh TJ, Merz WG, McGinnis MR. Infections due to *Xylohypha bantiana* (*Cladosporium trichoides*). *Rev Infect Dis* 1989;11:515–525.

219. Seaworth BJ, Kwon-Chung KJ, Hamilton JD, Perfect JR. Brain abscess caused by a variety of *Cladosporium trichoides. Am J Clin Pathol* 1983;79:747–752.

220. Adam RD, Paquin ML, Petersen EA, et al. Phaeohyphomycosis caused by the fungal genera *Bipolaris* and *Exserohilum. Medicine* 1986;65:203–217.

221. Rippon JW. Chromoblastomycosis and phaeohyphomycosis. In: Rippon JW, ed. *Medical mycology: the pathogenic fungi and pathogenic actinomycetes.* Philadelphia: WB Saunders, 1988; 276–324.

222. McGinnis MR. Chromoblastomycosis and phaeohyphomycosis: new concepts, diagnosis, and mycology. *J Am Acad Dermatol* 1983;8:1–16.

223. Banti G. Sopra un caso di oidiomicosi cerebrale. *Atti Accad Medicofis Fiorentina* 1911, p. 49 (cited in ref. 6).

224. Saccardo PA. Torula fungine bantiana. *Ann Mycopathol* 1912;10:320–321 (cited in ref. 6).

225. Binford CH, Thompson RK, Gorham ME. Mycotic brain abscess due to *Cladosporium trichoides,* a new species. *Am J Clin Pathol* 1952;22:525–542.

226. Sandhyamani S, Bhatia R, Mohapatra LN, Roy S. Cerebral cladosporiosis. *Surg Neurol* 1981;15:431–434.

227. Chandramukhi A, Ramadevi MG, Shankar SK. Cerebral cladosporiosis—a neuropathological and microbiological study. *Clin Neurol Neurosurg* 1983;85:245–253.

228. Salem FA, Kannangara W, Nachum R. Cerebral chromomycosis. *Ann Neurol* 1983;40:173–174.

229. Middleton FG, Jurgenson PF, Utz JP, Shadomy S, Shadomy HJ. Brain abscess caused by *Cladosporium trichoides. Arch Intern Med* 1976;136:444–448.

230. Duque O. Meningoencephalitis and brain abscess caused by *Cladosporium* and *Fonescaea. Am J Clin Pathol* 1961;36:505–517.

231. Kim RC, Hodge CJ, Lamberson HV, Weiner LB. Traumatic intracerebral implantation of *Cladosporium trichoides. Neurology* 1981;31:1145–1148.

232. Kasantikul V, Shuangshoti S, Sampatanukul P. Primary chromoblastomycosis of the medulla oblongata: complication of heroin addiction. *Surg Neurol* 1988;29:319–321.

233. Bennett JE, Bonner H, Jennings AE, Lopez RI. Chronic meningitis caused by *Cladosporium trichoides. Am J Clin Pathol* 1972;59:398–407.

234. Shimosaka S, Waga S. Cerebral chromoblastomycosis complicated by meningitis and multiple fungal aneurysms after resection of a granuloma. *J Neurosurg* 1983;59:158–161.

235. Naim-Ur-Rahman, Mahgoub ES, Aisha HA, et al. Cerebral Phaeohyphpmycosis. *Bull Soc Pathol Exot* 1987;80:320–328.

236. Pratt MF, Burnett JR. Fulminent *Drechslera* sinusitis in an immunocompetent host. *Laryngoscope* 1988;97:1343–1347.

237. Ruben SJ, Scott TE, Seltzer HM. Intracranial and paranasal sinus infection due to *Drechslera. South Med J* 1987;80:1057–1058.

238. Fuste FJ, Ajello L, Threlkeld R, Henry JE. *Drechslera hawaiiensis:* causative agent of a fatal fungal meningoencephalitis. *Sabouraudia* 1973;11:59–63.

239. Yoshimori RN, Moore RA, Itabashi HH, Fulikawa DG. Phaeo-

hyphomycosis of brain: granulomatous encephalitis caused by *Drechslera spicifera. Am J Clin Pathol* 1982;77:363–370.

240. de la Monte SM, Hutchins GM. Disseminated *Curvularia* infection. *Arch Pathol Lab Med* 1985;109:872–874.

241. Pierce NF, Millan JC, Bender BS, Curtis JL. Disseminated *Curvularia* infection: additional therapeutic and clinical considerations with evidence of medical cure. *Arch Pathol Lab Med* 1986;110:959–961.

242. Lampert RP, Hutto JH, Donnelly WH, Shulman ST. Pulmonary and cerebral mycetoma caused by *Curvularia pallescens. J Pediatr* 1977;91:603–605.

243. Friedman AD, Campos JM, Rorke LB, Bruce DA, Arbeter AM. Fatal recurrent *Curvularia* brain abscess. *J Pediatr* 1981;99:413–415 (follow-up of ref. 242).

244. Rohwedder JJ, Simmons JL, Colfer H, Gatmaitan B. Disseminated *Curvularia lunata* infection in a football player. *Arch Intern Med* 1979;139:940–941.

245. Al-Hedaithy SSA, Jamjoom ZAB, Saeed ES. Cerebral phaeohyphomycosis caused by *Fonsecaea pedrosoi* in Saudi Arabia. *Acta Pathol Microbiol Immunol Scand* [*Suppl*] 1988;3:94–100.

246. Naim-Ur-Rahman Mahgoub ES, Chagla AH. Fatal brain abscesses caused by *Ramichloridium obovoideum:* report of three cases. *Acta Neurochir (Wien)* 1988;93:92–95.

247. Watson KC, Kallichurum S. Brain abscess due to *Trichosporon cutaneum. J Med Microb* 1970;3:191–193.

248. Anaissie E, Bodey G, Kantarjian H, et al. New spectrum of fungal infections in patients with cancer. *Rev Infect Dis* 1989;11:369–378.

249. Hironaga M, Okazaki N, Saito K, Watanabe S. *Trichophyton mentagrophytes* granulomas. *Arch Dermatol* 1983;119:482–490.

250. Araviysky AN, Araviysky RA, Eschkov GA. Deep generalized trichophytosis. *Mycopathologica* 1975;56:47–65.

251. Allen DE, Snyderman R, Meadows L, Pinnell SR. Generalized *Microsporidium audouinii* infection and depressed cellular immunity with a missing plasma factor required for lymphocyte blastogenesis. *Am J Med* 1977;63:991–1000.

252. Rajam RV, Viswanathan GS, Rao AR, Rangiah PN, Anguli VC. Rhinosporidiosis—a study with report of a fatal case of systemic dissemination. *Indian J Surg* 1955;17:269–298.

253. Mukerji S, Patwardhan JR, Gadgil RK. Bacterial and mycotic infection of the brain. *Indian J Med Sci* 1971;791–796.

PART VII

Protozoal and Helminthic Infections of the CNS

Infections of the Central Nervous System,
edited by W. M. Scheld, R. J. Whitley, and
D. T. Durack, Raven Press, Ltd., New York © 1991.

CHAPTER 33

Protozoal Infections of the Central Nervous System

J. Peter Cegielski and David T. Durack

Protozoa cause some of the most prevalent and debilitating infections that afflict mankind. Some of these protozoa can invade the central nervous system (CNS). Cerebral malaria and sleeping sickness are common in certain geographic areas, where they cause high morbidity and mortality. Cerebral amebiasis and primary amebic encephalitis (PAM), although rare, carry a mortality approaching 100%. This chapter will describe our present understanding of these important CNS diseases.

CEREBRAL MALARIA

Introduction

Malaria remains a leading cause of human suffering and death. Over 1 billion people live in malarious areas. Each year this results in over 100 million cases worldwide, with 1 million deaths in Africa alone (1). The frequency of CNS involvement varies from 1% to 10% in different reports, depending upon the population sampled and the definition used for cerebral malaria (2–4). Cerebral malaria has a mortality rate ranging from 20% to 50% (2,5–7), thus accounting for up to 80% of the total deaths attributable to malaria (8).

Cerebral malaria is an encephalopathy which occurs in some patients infected with *Plasmodium falciparum.* Definitions of cerebral malaria vary, a fact which confounds the interpretation of reports from different groups in different regions of the world. Most experienced clinicians in malarious areas would regard any central neurologic dysfunction in a patient with *P. falci-*

J. P. Cegielski and D. T. Durack: Division of Infectious Diseases and International Health, Duke University Medical Center, Durham, North Carolina 27710.

parum parasitemia as evidence of cerebral involvement, and they would treat accordingly. This is appropriate. However, patients presenting with delirium or convulsions may not be comparable to patients presenting in coma, because fever alone can cause some of these findings. Warrell et al. (6) suggested a uniform definition of cerebral malaria to be used for the purposes of research. This has been supported by the World Health Organization Malaria Action Program (3). The definition requires all three of the following: (a) unarousable coma, with the best motor response being nonlocalizing or absent, (b) infection with *P. falciparum,* and (c) no other identifiable cause of coma.

Even though it has been studied for more than a century (9), the pathogenesis of this disease has not yet been fully unraveled. Recent scientific advances have shed light on some aspects of the pathogenesis of cerebral malaria, but a host of new questions based on these findings have surfaced. Here we will review the epidemiology, pathology, pathogenesis, clinical features, diagnosis, management, and prevention of the CNS manifestations of malaria. We will concentrate on data gleaned from human studies, because an ideal animal model for human cerebral malaria has not been identified (9,10).

Epidemiology

Cerebral malaria is thought to be caused only by infection with *Plasmodium falciparum.* There have been isolated case reports of *P. vivax* causing cerebral malaria (11–14), but in most of these, coinfection by *P. falciparum* or other causes of coma were not ruled out (14,15). This leaves a few reports which suggest that *P. vivax* malaria cannot be dismissed entirely as a cause of cerebral malaria (11,16). For the purposes of this chapter, however, the diagnosis of cerebral malaria requires the presence of *P. falciparum* infection.

Accordingly, the geographic domain of *P. falciparum* defines the territory of endemic cerebral malaria. Within these tropical and subtropical zones, the pattern of distribution of cases varies according to local endemicity. In holoendemic areas (for example, much of sub-Saharan Africa), malaria transmission is stable throughout the annual cycle (17). Here, the disease occurs mostly in infants and young children, in whom the infection rate is extremely high. By 18 months of age, approximately 90% of randomly sampled children outside Lagos, Nigeria had malaria parasites in their blood (4,18). They comprise most of the susceptible population because they have not yet developed the protective immunity that follows repeated malaria infections. A numerically smaller group at risk for disease consists of nonimmune visitors or immigrants, or returning adults who have lost their immunity by living for some years in nonmalarious areas.

In these holoendemic areas, mortality in children in the first 3 years of life may be as high as 12% (19). Malaria usually spares the youngest children (up to the first 6 months of life) because of the persistence of transplacentally transmitted maternal antibody. By 5 years of age, most of the survivors are semi-immune, so that older children and adults rarely have clinically apparent attacks of malaria (4,17,18,20). Defining the true incidence and prevalence of cerebral malaria in holoendemic regions is extremely difficult. Data from the Garki Project in northern Nigeria show that the prevalence of *P. falciparum* infection was between 30% and 55% in different groups. The infant mortality rate was approximately one-tenth the rate of *P. falciparum* infection and varied in parallel with it (21). Bruce-Chwatt (4) and Hendricks and King (22) showed that cerebral malaria accounted for 50% of the malaria deaths (Table 1).

In contrast, in areas of unstable malaria transmission, all age groups can suffer the consequences of severe malaria infection. In a 2-year hospital-based study in the Philippines (7), 83% of malaria occurred in people between the ages of 10 and 50 years. Seven percent of *P.*

falciparum cases had cerebral involvement. The overall mortality rate in patients with *P. falciparum* malaria was 0.04%, whereas that in patients with cerebral malaria was 20%. Similarly, in Southeast Asia (23), Latin America, and parts of Africa, where malaria is seasonally epidemic, cerebral malaria occurs in both children and adults. In India, Gautam et al. (24) reported that CNS symptoms occurred in 5% of children with malaria, including convulsions in 2% and coma in 3%.

Paradoxically, children who are severely malnourished may be less likely to acquire cerebral malaria and are less likely to die from it (18,20,25–27; J. P. Cegielski, *personal observations*). This has been attributed to abnormalities in iron metabolism (25,28), riboflavin deficiency, (29,30), and thymic atrophy (27), all characteristics of severe protein-calorie malnutrition.

Some data are available on the occurrence of cerebral malaria among nonimmune soldiers exposed while overseas during wartime. In World War II (2), reported incidence of cerebral malaria ranged from 0.25% in British troops in Africa to 2.3% among U.S. and allied troops in the Pacific, expressed as a percentage of all cases of *P. falciparum* malaria. Spitz (8) reported on fatal cases of *P. falciparum* malaria studied by necropsy during World War II. Cerebral involvement occurred in approximately 10% of cases and accounted for 80% of malaria deaths. Daroff et al. (2) studied 1200 cases of *P. falciparum* malaria which occurred among U.S. soldiers in South Vietnam during a 10-month period. Nineteen of these (1.6%) had cerebral malaria, defined as signs of cerebral dysfunction without other explanation. Mortality in the World War II Pacific theater ranged from 8% to 41%, but no deaths occurred in the Vietnam study. Daroff et al.'s definition may have included less severe cases, because only eight of their patients were stuporous or comatose.

In the United States, 1760 cases of imported malaria, most of which were caused by *P. falciparum*, were reported in the 22 years ending 1987, with a case fatality rate of 3.8%. Neurologic symptoms were reported in 37% of patients. An upward trend in both the number of cases and mortality was evident over this period (31).

TABLE 1. *Cerebral and noncerebral malaria as a cause of death in children at necropsy in Lagos, Nigeria, 1933–1950[a]*

	Age (years)						Total
	<1	1–2	3–4	5–7	8–10	11–15	
Cerebral malaria:	43 (23%)	77 (41%)	44 (24%)	14 (7%)	4 (2%)	5 (3%)	187 (100%)
Percent of total necropsies:	4.9	8.7	6.8	3.0	1.4	1.3	5.3
Noncerebral malaria:	31 (19%)	48 (29%)	47 (29%)	27 (17%)	8 (5%)	2 (1%)	163 (100%)
Percent of total necropsies:	3.5	5.4	7.3	5.8	2.8	0.5	4.6
Total malaria:	74 (21%)	125 (36%)	91 (26%)	41 (12%)	12 (3%)	7 (2%)	350 (100%)
Percent of total necropsies:	8.4	14.2	14.2	8.8	4.3	1.8	9.9
Total:	877 (25%)	881 (25%)	643 (18%)	467 (13%)	282 (8%)	390 (11%)	3540 (100%)

[a] Adapted from ref. 4.

Pathology

Our present understanding of the pathology of cerebral malaria is built upon necropsy studies spanning at least a century. Several problems arise in assessing the pathologic findings. First, varying definitions of cerebral malaria have been used, as discussed previously. Second, because most patients with cerebral malaria recover without neurologic sequelae (3), pathologic changes in the CNS must be either reversible or trivial in most cases. Therefore, pathologic findings in fatal cases will represent the most extreme changes. Third, because no ideal animal model for cerebral malaria exists (9,32–34), conclusions drawn from pathologic studies on animals may be misleading.

Clark and Tomlinson (35) reported on findings from 487 fatal cases of *P. falciparum* malaria in Panama and Honduras. In their experience, the brain was generally edematous and heavy, with widening and flattening of the gyri and congestion of the cortical and meningeal vessels. The brain parenchyma often was discolored. In cases of extreme parasitemia and congestion, an intense pink hue was present in the cortex. This is the so-called "pink brain" of cerebral malaria. In other cases the cortex took on a slate-gray appearance, resulting from the accumulation of malarial pigment in capillaries of the highly vascular cortex. In severe cases, sufficient pigment would accumulate in the white matter and the brainstem, giving these a gray color also. In many cases, petechial hemorrhages were found in the subcortical white matter (Fig. 1). These authors emphasized the lack of correlation between gross pathologic changes in the brain and the clinical manifestations of cerebral involvement. Spitz (8) at the Army Institute of Pathology reported a series of 50 consecutive autopsies on soldiers dying of *P. falciparum* malaria. She described engorgement of the cerebral vessels in 46 of the cases. In 41 of these 46, the engorged vessels contained large numbers of parasitized erythrocytes. Other viscera such as heart, lung, and intestines showed a similar degree of parasitization of erythrocytes in engorged vessels. In 15 of the 50 cases, multiple petechial hemorrhages were present, located in the subcortical white matter and occasionally in the gray matter of the brainstem. Spitz (8) also described the presence of so-called malarial granulomas in 12 of these 15 cases, but she did not report their presence in any of the other 35 cases in this series.

Few authors have attempted to correlate the gross pathologic findings with the clinical manifestations of cerebral malaria. Thomas (36) reviewed all cases of pathologically proven cerebral malaria from Mulago Hospital in Kampala, Uganda over a 4-year period. Malarial pigment was present in all 30 cases, sometimes providing the only basis for the histologic diagnosis. White-matter edema was present in most cases. Petechial

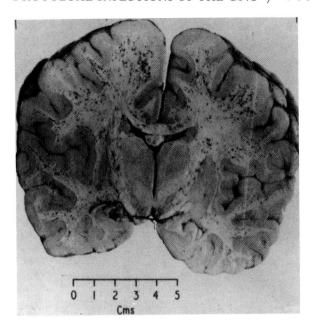

FIG. 1. Cerebral malaria. Coronal section of the brain, showing multiple petechial hemorrhages in white matter. (From ref. 36, with permission.)

hemorrhages were present in 17 of the cases (Fig. 1), and in most of these the brain was heavy and edematous when compared to age and sex-matched norms or when compared to the 13 cases without petechial hemorrhages. On reviewing the clinical records of these patients, Thomas (36) found that 14 of the 17 with cerebral malaria had syndromes compatible with this diagnosis and that most were diagnosed correctly antemortem. None of the 13 without petechial hemorrhages were diagnosed as having cerebral malaria before death. He concluded that presence of petechial hemorrhages correlated strongly with the clinical syndrome of cerebral malaria.

A well-known study by Oo et al. (37) from Burma using a strict definition for cerebral malaria reported similar pathologic findings in 19 patients. Generally the brains were gray-pink, with flattened gyri. Gross edema was present in seven (37%), and hemorrhages were found in nine (47%). Focal infarcts, spotty hemorrhages, and occasional massive intracerebral hemorrhages have been reported (15).

Microscopically, cerebral capillaries and venules are consistently packed with parasitized and uninfected red blood cells (38) (Fig. 2). A disproportionate number of erythrocytes in the cerebral capillaries are parasitized when compared with erythrocytes in the peripheral circulation (36). Parasitized red blood cells in the systemic circulation contain mainly ring forms and early trophozoite stages, with only occasional gametocytes and rare schizonts. In contrast, the parasitized erythrocytes filling

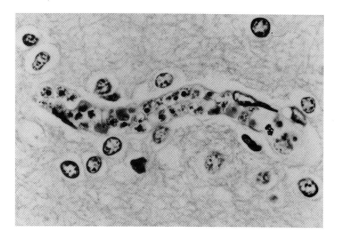

FIG. 2. Cerebral malaria. Capillary packed full of parasitized erythrocytes. (From ref. 37, with permission.)

the cerebral capillaries and venules contain primarily late trophozoites and schizonts. In the venules and larger vessels, these parasitized red blood cells are seen closely apposed to the endothelium (i.e., marginated), sometimes in clumps (Fig. 3). In many cases the capillaries appear to be distended or engorged, often with a clear halo suggesting edema. These observations led to the conclusion that the vessels are functionally occluded. This concept is supported by the occasional finding of dilated arterioles proximally in areas of cerebral edema.

The petechial hemorrhages consist of an annulus of extravasated red cells, usually with an identifiable central vessel (8,37) (Fig. 4). A zone of necrotic, demyelinized tissue surrounds the vessel inside the round or oval ring of blood cells. Interestingly, the red blood cells in

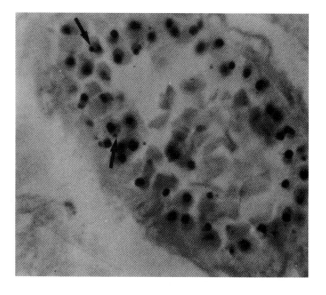

FIG. 3. Cerebral malaria. Small vessel with marginated, parasitized erythrocytes. (From ref. 211, with permission.)

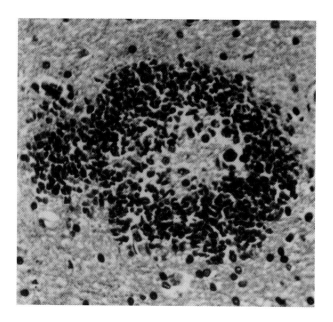

FIG. 4. Cerebral malaria. Ring hemorrhages in the brain. (From ref. 36, with permission.)

these "ring hemorrhages" are not parasitized (8). Ring hemorrhages are seen in patients who survive at least 10 days (38,39). In some cases, endothelial cell damage and necrosis of the vessel wall is evident (37), but in most it is conspicuously absent (8). The same can be said of frank thrombosis. Clear-cut thrombosis of small vessels does occur, but only in a minority of cases (8,35,36). Oo and Than (40) have proposed a pathogenetic mechanism to explain the phenomenon of ring hemorrhages. Extravasation of red cells may be caused by vascular endothelial damage, resulting in markedly increased permeability. Systolic arterial pressure forces the highly deformable unparasitized red cells to leak out of the vessel. After the central vessel becomes obstructed, only plasma can filter out, pushing out the previously extruded erythrocytes away from the central vessel to form a peripheral ring of red blood cells. The proteinaceous plasma thus forms the central pale acellular area inside the ring (40).

In patients who survive longer, a granulomatous inflammatory response is seen at the site of these hemorrhages. First described by Durck in 1923 (15), they are now known as "Durck nodules" or "malarial granulomas" (Fig. 5). These inflammatory lesions show an accumulation of glial cells and mononuclear phagocytes in the demyelinized zone inside the red cell ring (15,38,39). The presence of inflammatory cells and the fact that they occur later in the course of disease than do ring hemorrhages has given rise to the concept that they are part of the process of tissue repair (8,15).

Only one study systematically compared brain histology from patients with cerebral malaria to that of fatal cases of noncerebral malaria, in a small number of pa-

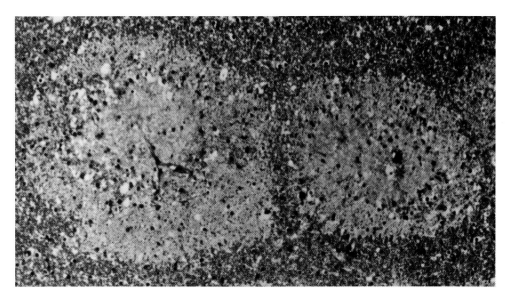

FIG. 5. Cerebral malaria. Malarial granulomas in cerebral tissue, showing multiple circumscribed foci of demyelinization and glial proliferation. (From ref. 212, with permission.)

tients (41). In cerebral malaria, three times as many vessels contained parasitized red blood cells, the proportion of red blood cells which were parasitized was higher, the red blood cells were packed much tighter in vessels, and the proportion of tightly packed vessels was much higher than in noncerebral malaria patients (Table 2). In a small number of patients in both groups, endothelial damage, fibrillar deposits, and endothelial pseudopodia were present. These authors noted interesting differences between the CNS and other tissues: In cerebral malaria patients, a much higher proportion of red blood cells were parasitized in the brain (45%) than in the heart (20%), liver (17%), kidney (5%), or lung (4%). The parasites in the pulmonary capillaries were nearly all ring forms and early trophozoites, and there were numerous polymorphonuclear and mononuclear leukocytes, whereas in the cerebral capillaries there were gametocytes, schizonts, and few leukocytes (41). Additionally, in cerebral malaria patients the proportion of parasitized red blood cells in peripheral venous blood, in capillary blood ob-

tained by finger prick, and in skin biopsy specimens was significantly lower than that in a group of patients with uncomplicated malaria.

Pathogenesis

Intense efforts have been directed toward understanding the pathogenesis of cerebral malaria based on these histopathologic features. The prevailing view at present is that during schizogony, parasitized erythrocytes adhere to the endothelium of cerebral capillaries, mechanically occluding them. Previously, it was thought that red blood cells containing late asexual stage *P. falciparum* occluded capillaries because the enlarging parasites made the red cell less pliable (3) and the rigid cells were unable to squeeze through the capillary network. This resulted in tissue anoxia and necrosis and perhaps initiated an inflammatory response that contributed to tissue damage and edema. This theory could not explain (a)

TABLE 2. *Comparison of cerebral vessels in patients with and without cerebral malaria[a]*

Patient group	Percentage of PRBCs[b]	Degree of packing[c]	Percentage of vessels with 3+ packing[d]	Percentage of vessels with PRBCs	Percentage of vessels with endothelial damage
Cerebral malaria	43%	2.24	59%	63%	58%
Noncerebral malaria	17%	0.71	8%	15%	29%
p value[e]	<0.05	<0.01	<0.01	<0.01	Not significant

[a] Adapted from ref. 41.
[b] PRBCs, parasitized red blood cells.
[c] Packing defined on a scale of 0–3.
[d] 3+ packing, vessel filled with PRBCs with obvious distortion of cell outlines.
[e] Calculated by Mann–Whitney U test.

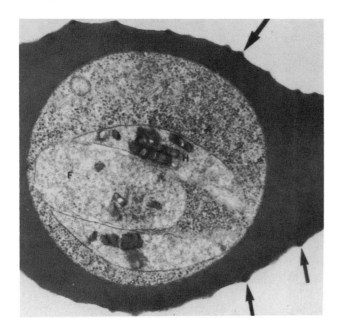

FIG. 6. Erythrocyte from *in vitro* culture, showing a late trophozoite of *Plasmodium falciparum* intracellularly and also exhibiting knobs on the surface (*arrows*). Electron micrograph, ×45,600. (From ref. 213, with permission.)

why parasitized red blood cells are concentrated in the venules as well as in the capillaries, instead of being trapped upstream from the proposed occlusion, (b) why there is preferential sequestration in cerebral capillaries as opposed to other organs, (c) why red blood cells infected by *Plasmodium vivax,* which are considerably larger, do not occlude cerebral capillaries and cause cerebral malaria, and (d) why there is a disproportionate number of parasitized erythrocytes in the red cell mass stacked up upstream from the obstruction. Thus a theory of pathogenesis based upon rheologic considerations seems inadequate. Rheologic factors may contribute, but they probably do not alone account for sequestration and the clinical severity of cerebral malaria.

Another theory, based on the occasional finding of a thrombosed vessel at the center of a ring hemorrhage, proposes that a form of disseminated intravascular coagulation causes the vascular occlusion and tissue damage. This theory is partly based upon findings in simian malaria caused by *P. knowlesi.* However, simian malaria does not appear to be a good model for acute *P. falciparum* malaria in humans (42). Histologic and laboratory evidence supports the occurrence of intravascular coagulation in some cases of severe malaria (42). These authors found (a) thrombocytopenia associated with hypofibrinogenemia, (b) a prolongation of the partial thromboplastin time, and (c) elevation of fibrin degradation products, in a small series of patients (42,43). However, trials with heparin in human cerebral malaria have caused hemorrhages which may have contributed to

death (42). In summary, while disseminated intravascular coagulation does occur in some cases of severe *P. falciparum* malaria, it appears to be a complication that occurs in only a minority of patients. Therefore, use of anticoagulants is not recommended (42).

Adherence of mature asexual stage parasitized red blood cells to endothelial and other cells must involve specific changes in the red cell membrane. Uninfected red blood cells and red cells containing ring forms do not adhere. At the ultrastructural level, the infected erythrocyte membrane develops cone-shaped protrusions, 40–80 nm in size (Figs. 6 and 7). These so-called knobs appear on the erythrocyte surface while the plasmodia are at the trophozoite stage, and they increase in number as the parasites mature during schizogony (37,44). Knobs appear to be a point of attachment between the red cell membranes and the endothelial cell membranes (37,41,44,45). Mediation of cytoadherence by these knobs may be responsible, at least in part, for the sequestration of *P. falciparum*-infected erythrocytes in the deep organ microvasculature during schizogony. Electron-microscopic studies have shown parasitized red blood cell membranes in intimate contact with endothelial cells at sites both with and without knobs. Electron-dense strands of material appear to run between the parasitized red blood cell and the endothelial cell, more frequently from the knobs themselves than from the membrane in between the knobs (41) (Fig. 8). The development of surface knobs, the adherence to host cells, and the sequestration of mature *P. falciparum* infected red blood cells during schizogony appear to be tightly correlated events. All wild-type isolates of *P. falciparum* induce knobs on the surface of red blood cells, which then demonstrate cytoadherence. Furthermore, the *P. falciparum*-like simian plasmodia, *P. fragile* and *P. coatneyi,*

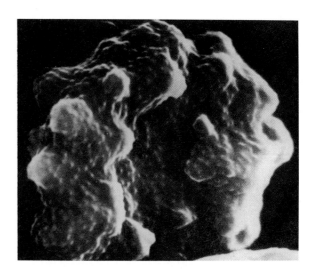

FIG. 7. Parasitized erythrocyte showing numerous knobs on the surface. Scanning electron micrograph, ×16,000. (From ref. 45, with permission.)

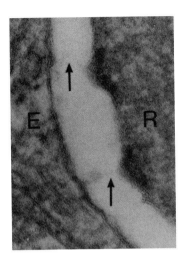

FIG. 8. Cerebral malaria. Sections from brain at postmortem, showing parasitized red blood cell (R) membrane with knobs, adjacent to the surface of an endothelial cell (E). Electron-dense material bridges the intervening space (*arrows*). (From ref. 41, with permission.)

which also induce knobs, cytoadhere whereas *P. vivax* and the simian *P. cynomolgi* do not induce knobs and do not cytoadhere. However, the correlation is not perfect, because knob-bearing red blood cells parasitized with two other plasmodia, *P. malariae* and *P. brasilianum,* do not adhere to host cells. Moreover, laboratory strains of *P. falciparum* and other xenotypic malarias have been described recently in which the association breaks down between the knob-expressing phenotype and cytoadherence (46). Some of these laboratory-derived strains may not reflect naturally occurring infection with wild-type *P. falciparum.* However, these findings do underscore the fact that surface knobs themselves probably do not provide the entire explanation of cytoadherence, sequestration, and microvascular occlusion.

Researchers are investigating the molecular basis for the apparent interactions between the knobs on parasitized red cells and the endothelial cell membrane. Species-specific host receptor molecules and parasite-induced surface molecules on *P. falciparum*-infected red blood cells that have been identified may be involved in cytoadherence. Although a detailed discussion of this subject is beyond the scope of this chapter, recent findings will be summarized. Three such putative host receptors have been identified: the extracellular matrix protein thrombospondin (32,47,48), the leukocyte differentiation antigen CD36 (3,47,49), and the intracellular adhesion molecule ICAM-1 (32,47). These three proteins share no evident sequence homology, and the structural basis for their binding by parasitized red blood cells is unknown. Considerable evidence exists supporting a role for each of these three receptors. Chulay and Ockenhause (47) hypothesize that there may be three

distinct receptors, because malaria parasites have developed redundant mechanisms to survive in the hostile environment of the immunologically competent host. Precedent for this exists in that *P. falciparum* merozoites have at least two alternative pathways by which to invade erythrocytes (47). The capacity to interact with more than one host receptor molecule may be an example of alternative mechanisms allowing for successful parasitism.

The surface molecules on the parasitized red blood cells which are involved in cytoadherence have been intensively studied (50). Three candidate membrane-associated proteins, along with a secreted protein, have been described. The knob-associated proteins are identified by the acronyms Pf-EMP1 (*P. falciparum*–erythrocyte membrane protein), Pf-EMP2, and Pf-HRP1 (*P. falciparum*–histidine-rich protein). The secreted protein is identified by the acronym Pf-HRP2. First identified by Leech et al. (51), Pf-EMP1 appears to be a strain-specific protein on the surface of parasitized erythrocytes that mediates cytoadherence *in vitro.* More extensive study by Howard et al. (52) substantiates this view. Recent progress on the identity of the attachment ligand has been summarized by Barnwell (48) and by Howard et al. (50). Pf-HRP1 appears to be a submembrane protein associated with an electron-dense structure located beneath the surface knobs. Pf-EMP1 appears to be strongly correlated with cytoadherence in wild-type isolates. Furthermore, Pf-EMP1 has multiple different forms distinguished by their molecular weight and adherence phenotype. This protein has been identified with molecular weights ranging from 240,000 to 350,000 daltons. The 240,000-dalton form of the molecule, while still associated with knobs, does not confer cytoadherence on the parasitized red blood cell. However, the higher-molecular-weight forms do confer the adherence phenotype. Thus the adherence phenotype appears to be associated with specific molecular forms of Pf-EMP1. This protein has also been shown to be antigenically diverse (53).

These studies illuminate important mechanisms by which *P. falciparum*-infected red blood cells adhere to endothelial cells, thereby sequestering in the brain and obstructing blood flow. However, the question remains as to how these molecular events cause cerebral dysfunction. Numerous theories have been proposed. One theory hypothesized that the fundamental pathophysiologic abnormality was increased capillary permeability (3) resulting in cerebral edema and increased intracranial pressure. However, numerous lines of evidence have been delineated which militate against this hypothesis. First one must keep in mind the bias inherent in necropsy material; one should not generalize from fatal cases to the pathophysiology of cerebral malaria. In addition to this selection bias, postmortem findings might partly represent agonal events or postmortem degenerative changes. However, more direct evidence has been obtained from clinical studies. When lumbar puncture is performed on patients with cerebral malaria, the CSF opening pressure is consistently less than 200 mm, within the normal range. In addition, papilledema is distinctly uncommon in cerebral malaria. Thirdly, a recent computerized tomographic imaging study (54) showed evidence of cerebral edema in only two of five fatal cases and in none of the survivors.

The prevailing theory at present is straightforward: Vascular obstruction leads directly to cerebral anoxia and coma. Evidence for this hypothesis comes from several studies. In 1985, White et al. (55) showed that cerebrospinal fluid (CSF) lactate levels were significantly elevated in 44 of 45 patients with cerebral malaria. Furthermore, lactate concentrations were higher in patients who died than in those who survived, and they were higher in comatose patients than in the same patients after they regained consciousness. Elevated CSF lactate levels were thought to result from cerebral hypoxia and resulting anaerobic metabolism. In the few patients where it was possible to measure arterial blood gases, they were normal. Thus the CSF findings were not caused by systemic hypoxemia and hypercapnia.

Warrell et al. (56) studied this question directly. They found significantly decreased cerebral oxygen consumption and significantly decreased arteriovenous oxygen content difference in comatose patients with cerebral malaria. Cerebral vascular resistance and jugular venous partial pressure of oxygen were increased. Although cerebral blood flow was within the normal range for healthy controls, it was subnormal relative to the metabolic demands imposed by fever, anemia, seizures, and reduced cerebral oxygen transport. These studies support the concept that cerebral circulation is mechanically obstructed by the parasitized erythrocytes.

Another theory of pathogenesis holds that the host immune response plays a major role in the pathogenesis of cerebral malaria. Vasoactive substances such as kinins and cytokines, other mediators such as tumor necrosis factor (TNF), and complement activation all have been studied in this regard. In rodent models of malaria, immunologically mediated damage plays a significant role in the pathogenesis of certain severe manifestations of the disease (57,58). However, murine malaria differs distinctly from human cerebral malaria in this regard, so these models may be misleading. On the other hand, activation of complement is a consistent feature in human cerebral malaria (3,43). Complement activation by the classic pathway appears to result from the formation of immune complexes following schizont rupture and the release of merozoites. The degree of hypocomplementemia correlates with the magnitude of parasitemia (59). Molyneux (60) summarizes data suggesting that TNF and other cytokines from activated macrophages are important in the pathogenesis of cerebral malaria.

TNF levels are high in children with profound coma caused by malaria. TNF has been shown to both up-regulate expression of one of the putative receptor molecules (ICAM-1; see above) for parasitized erythrocytes and to increase cytoadherence in vitro. This may be consistent with the role of TNF in modulating leukocyte-endothelial cell adherence. Histologic evidence for immune complex vasculitis is absent in fatal cases of P. falciparum malaria (3). The typical pathologic marker of an immune complex disease, proliferative glomerulonephritis, is not clinically significant in severe malaria. Rather, acute tubular necrosis is the usual lesion (3,61).

In addition to these considerations, it must be remembered that malarial involvement of the CNS does not occur in isolation. Many systemic or extracranial disturbances of other organ functions may contribute to cerebral dysfunction. Hypoglycemia, severe anemia, pulmonary edema, renal failure, bacterial superinfection, and metabolic acidosis commonly coexist in individuals with severe malaria. Hypoglycemia, potentially severe, occurs frequently in P. falciparum malaria. White et al. (62) identified two groups at risk for significant hypoglycemia associated with P. falciparum infection: (i) pregnant women and (ii) patients with life-threatening disease. In their experience, it occurred in 8% of patients with cerebral malaria. Glucose levels were often less than 5 mg/dl. In some cases, hypoglycemia may be caused by quinine therapy, because quinine is a potent insulin secretagogue. The study by White et al. (62) in Thai adults supported this mechanism. Kawo et al. (63) at Muhimbili Medical Centre in Dar es Salaam, Tanzania put forth a different view. In their study of hypoglycemia in children, the frequency of hypoglycemia did not differ significantly between patients with cerebral malaria and controls with other severe illnesses. Nor did it differ between comatose and conscious patients with malaria and controls. Insulin levels were appropriately low in hypoglycemic patients. The strongest correlate with hypoglycemia was the time since the last meal consumed by the patient. In addition, depressed level of consciousness and death were significantly correlated with length of time since the last food intake. This study indicated that hypoglycemia was not a specific complication of malaria, nor of antimalarial treatment, but was characteristic of severely ill, fasted children. Another recent study by Taylor et al. (64), working in Malawi, supported this conclusion. They studied glycemia before and after treatment of cerebral malaria with intravenous quinine. Twenty percent of patients were hypoglycemic before treatment. The hypoglycemic patients had low plasma insulin levels. Hypoglycemia recurred in over one-third of patients with pretreatment hypoglycemia, but it did not recur in any of the children who were initially normoglycemic. In addition, the children who were initially hypoglycemic had higher mortality and a higher frequency of neurologic sequelae. They concluded that hypoglycemia was a frequent complication of severe *P. falciparum* malaria, that it affected the severity of the disease, and that it indicated a poor prognosis. Hypoglycemia did not appear to be a complication of quinine treatment.

Endotoxemia may complicate severe malaria, contributing to the clinical manifestations. Tubbs (65) demonstrated endotoxemia in children with malaria. Endotoxin may originate from coinfection with gram-negative bacilli, which occurred in 11 of 16 patients in one series (66), or from absorption of bacterial products from the gut (67). Endotoxin or an endotoxin-like substance may originate from the malaria parasite itself (66,68).

Clinical Manifestations

The clinical features of cerebral malaria are diverse. Fever is nearly universal, but hypothermia has been reported. Often the picture is complicated by co-morbidity arising from malaria's effects on other organ systems, as well as from other causes. Because cerebral malaria occurs in only 1–2% of outpatients with *P. falciparum* or in approximately 10% of inpatients, other features may be pronounced. These might include: severe anemia; jaundice; oliguria caused by renal insufficiency; severe hyperpyrexia; pulmonary edema; hypoglycemia as discussed above; associated infections such as aspiration pneumonia or septicemia; bleeding from disseminated intravascular coagulation; vomiting and diarrhea leading to further hypovolemia; and shock. Splenomegaly or hepatomegaly are also commonly present in patients with malaria.

The severe stages of malaria develop most often in a patient who has been ill for several days with fever and other nonspecific symptoms. Cerebral malaria may follow this pattern, or it may occur suddenly with a generalized convulsion followed by persistent coma. As stated previously, most experienced clinicians working in tropical and subtropical regions of the world regard any new CNS signs developing in the presence of *P. falciparum* parasitemia as evidence of possible cerebral malaria, and they would treat accordingly. A cardinal feature is a decreased level of consciousness, ranging from lethargy to stupor to coma. An acute organic brain syndrome such as delirium, confusion, disorientation, agitation, hostile behavior, other personality changes, and frank psychoses may occur. Convulsions are common; they may be single or recurrent and are more prominent as a feature of cerebral malaria in children (69). In the pediatric population, it may be difficult to distinguish convulsions due to fever itself from convulsions due to cerebral malaria. Motor disorders such as ataxia, tremor, myoclonus, chorea, athetosis, and bruxism are frequently present. Focal neurologic deficits, though distinctly uncommon, have also been described. These include monoplegia, he-

miplegia, cerebellar ataxia, deafness, and blindness. The latter two may occur more frequently in children than in adults (70,71). Marsden and Bruce-Chwatt (70) described 921 African children with cerebral malaria, seven of whom lost their sight. Five of these children recovered their vision within 4 months. Agitation, confusion, delirium, and paranoid psychoses may all occur during the recovery stage as well.

Diagnosis

Demonstration of parasitemia and confirmation of species identity are best accomplished by an experienced microscopist examining thick and thin blood smears stained with Giemsa stain. In areas with limited resources, the simpler and more rapid Field's stain for thick films is used commonly. In most cases of cerebral malaria, there will be pronounced parasitemia; however, cerebral malaria may occur with a low peripheral parasite count. When the parasites sequester in the brain to undergo schizogony, they may be absent from the peripheral blood. In addition, partial treatment with antimalarials, which are widely available without prescription in many tropical countries, may decrease the peripheral parasitemia to the extent that they are difficult to find. The patients' relatives can be helpful in determining whether the patient has received any treatment. To rule out *P. falciparum* with certainty, blood smears should be repeated every 6–12 hr for 48 hr.

It is important to obtain CSF (provided there is no papilledema) in order to rule out other causes of encephalopathy. In malaria, the CSF is clear and the opening pressure is less than 200 mm in 80% of cases (16). Microscopy is normal and there are rarely more than 10 lymphocytes per microliter of CSF, though lymphocytosis of up to 150 cells has been reported (16). Neutrophils in the CSF should suggest another diagnosis because they are not a feature of cerebral malaria. The CSF-to-serum glucose ratio is normal. The protein concentration may be slightly elevated, sometimes reaching as high as 150 mg/dl.

Depending upon the resources available, blood glucose should be measured immediately to assess glycemia as a potential factor contributing to the neurologic picture. This can be done simply with glucose oxidase sticks if a chemistry laboratory is not available. Hematocrits also can be determined quickly and simply, even in some rural dispensaries and in most rural hospitals and clinics. If possible, a complete blood count, electrolytes, blood urea, and creatinine should be determined, and blood should be cultured to exclude bacteremia.

The differential diagnosis of febrile coma or febrile CNS disturbances in the tropics and subtropics includes the following: bacterial and viral meningitis; encephalitis; typhoid fever; hypoglycemia; diabetic hyperglycemia; uremia; trauma with closed head injury; eclampsia; epilepsy; stroke; poisonings and other forms of intoxication; and intracranial mass lesions such as neoplasms, abscesses, and tuberculomas. Alcoholic intoxication and malaria may coexist, so that the odor of alcohol on the breath of a stuporous patient may be misleading. It does not obviate the need for a blood smear and other diagnostic tests. In some areas of Africa, trypanosomiasis also must be considered. An appropriate and detailed history from relatives or friends accompanying the patient, along with physical examination and basic laboratory studies, can sort out these differential diagnostic considerations. In nonmalarious areas, an accurate travel history is crucial. In locations where advanced technology is available, computerized tomography can rule out intracranial mass lesions and help to assess whether there is elevation of intracranial pressure.

Treatment

Cerebral malaria is a medical emergency requiring rapid intervention. An initial abbreviated assessment can be accomplished quickly in order to confirm the diagnosis by blood smear and to establish the presence of other manifestations of severe malaria. Other diseases which require urgent treatment should be quickly ruled out, including acute bacterial meningitis, trypanosomiasis, diabetic coma, or eclampsia. If parasitologic confirmation is likely to be delayed, treatment should begin immediately. A more thorough assessment can follow.

Treatment for cerebral malaria can be divided into three categories: (i) specific antimalarial chemotherapy, (ii) supportive measures for coexistent complications of severe malaria, and (iii) treatment of associated conditions such as septicemia or aspiration pneumonia. Choice of antimalarial drug treatment depends on local patterns of susceptibility of P. falciparum. Chloroquine remains the drug of choice in the areas where the parasite is still susceptible. Unfortunately, this is a diminishing geographic circle and, as of this writing, includes only Mexico, Central America, Egypt, and parts of the Middle East (72). In much of Latin America, Africa, and Asia, P. falciparum is resistant to chloroquine. In these areas, quinine is the drug of first choice. Quinidine, the stereoisomer of quinine, is equally effective (73). Finally, quinine resistance is common in parts of Southeast Asia, and thus the addition of tetracycline or a folate antagonist is advocated. Three new antimalarials hold promise for treatment of resistant P. falciparum: mefloquine, halofantrine, and artemisinine (3,16).

Chloroquine is the most widely used, most widely available, and most effective agent against chloroquine-susceptible parasites (74). Chloroquine is generally safe, including use in pregnant women; moreover, it is well tolerated when given by the oral route. In some cases,

particularly in pediatric patients, vomiting will follow chloroquine administration, so that children must be observed to see if they have received the treatment effectively. In African patients, 50% will experience severe pruritus following chloroquine administration. Studies have shown that chloroquine is rapidly and completely absorbed from the gut in healthy adults and children and in comatose children given the drug by nasogastric tube (5). Recent work highlighted the potential cardiovascular toxicity of parenterally administered chloroquine, leading to a recommendation that it no longer be given by this route (3). However, White et al. (5) in The Gambia showed that chloroquine was both safe and effective with appropriate dosing regimens. In each of their seven trial regimens, the total cumulative dose was the standard 25 mg of chloroquine base per kilogram of body weight. Three parenteral regimens emerged as superior: continuous intravenous infusion of 0.83 mg of chloroquine base per kilogram of body weight over 30 hr and 3.5 mg of chloroquine base per kilogram given intramuscularly or subcutaneously every 6 hr. Chloroquine syrup administered by nasogastric tube resulted in similar rates of parasite clearance, reduction of fever, and adequate, timely blood levels when given by the following regimen: an initial dose of 10 mg base per kilogram, followed by doses of 5 mg base per kilogram 6, 24, and 48 hr later. This is critically important for rural health outposts where parenteral therapy may not be possible.

In areas of chloroquine resistance, quinine should be used. Our practice in Tanzania is to administer quinine dihydrochloride at a dose of 10 mg base per kilogram diluted in 10 ml per kilogram of isotonic fluid by intravenous infusion over 4 hr, every 8 hr. The dose and dilution volume is the same for children as for adults, on a per-kilogram basis. This regimen is supported by two authoritative reviews (3,75). A loading dose of 20 mg base per kilogram infused intravenously over 4 hr may be used initially in patients who have not received quinine before coming to medical attention (76). This schedule achieves therapeutic blood levels more safely and rapidly. Once the patient regains consciousness, he or she may be switched to oral quinine sulfate tablets at the same dose, or roughly 600 mg every 8 hr. Young children usually can swallow a suspension or syrup, or it can be given by nasogastric tube. Quinine is rapidly and completely absorbed from the gut. In most areas of the world, a 5- to 7-day course of therapy is sufficient. In Southeast Asia, 7–10 days is no longer effective; furthermore, oral tetracycline (250 mg four times daily in adults) or pyrimethamine-sulfadoxine (Fansidar) must be added. Tetracycline should be avoided in children and pregnant women. Recent work supports the substitution of quinidine for quinine (73). Quinidine may be more readily available in North America and western Europe, where it is commonly used in the treatment of cardiac arrhythmias.

Ancillary drugs that have been used in the past in the treatment of cerebral malaria include the following: dexamethasone; osmotic diuretics such as mannitol; heparin; and low-molecular-weight dextran. Dexamethasone has clearly been shown to be deleterious in the treatment of cerebral malaria (6); its use should be abandoned. The use of heparin, mannitol, dextrans, and corticosteroids are based on (a) outmoded concepts of the pathogenesis of cerebral malaria and (b) anecdotal reports of their successful use. More recently, some potential harmful effects of these treatments have been emphasized; they should no longer be used (3,6,16).

Supportive measures are vitally important to the successful treatment of cerebral malaria. These should first take into account other manifestations of severe malaria. Hypoglycemia is common, as discussed previously. It can occur despite use of 5% dextrose infusions. Early and frequent blood glucose monitoring is essential. Single injections of glucose may be insufficient (63). Multiple intravenous boluses or infusion of a higher concentration of glucose (10%) should be given. Acute pulmonary edema, a variant of adult respiratory distress syndrome, can occur as a direct effect of *P. falciparum* malaria. Careful fluid management is essential for prevention and treatment of this complication. Central venous pressure monitoring or pulmonary capillary wedge pressure monitoring should be instituted, if possible, when this complication occurs. Tracheal intubation and mechanical ventilation with positive airway pressure may be necessary if available.

Metabolic acidosis can result from obstruction of systemic and visceral capillaries. The blood pH may decrease out of proportion to the degree of hypoxia. Treatment is with sodium bicarbonate. Hyperparasitemia can be treated with exchange transfusions, provided that risks for transmission of acquired immunodeficiency syndrome (AIDS) and viral hepatitis are controlled. Oliguric renal failure requires careful monitoring of fluid balance and hemodynamic status. Urethral catheterization should be used to assess urine output. If severe anemia complicates the clinical picture, the patient should be transfused with whole blood or packed red blood cells. Convulsions, especially in children, are common and may be treated with diazepam. Prevention of seizures with phenobarbitone or diphenylhydantoin has been advocated. Hyperpyrexia can be treated with tepid sponging and acetaminophen. Septicemia occurs not uncommonly, generally arising from gut flora. Treatment with antibiotics effective against gram-negative bacilli and anaerobic intestinal flora should be instituted in these cases. Drugs commonly available in tropical and subtropical areas of the world include (a) gentamicin with chloramphenicol or (b) gentamicin with metronidazole. Aspiration pneumonia can be treated with parenteral penicillin. Because vomiting is common, patients should be nursed on their side to minimize the risk of aspiration.

Prevention

Prevention of cerebral malaria is synonymous with prevention of *P. falciparum* malaria. There are many facets to this endeavor, including individual chemoprophylaxis, individual behavioral preventive measures, vaccination, and large-scale malaria control. In-depth discussion of each of these measures is beyond the scope of this chapter. Considerable research is being directed toward the development of a malaria vaccine, without success to date.

Recommendations for malaria chemoprophylaxis depend upon the local pattern of *P. falciparum* susceptibility. In areas where the parasite remains sensitive, chloroquine should be taken in a weekly dose of 300 mg base. For travelers going to malarious areas, chloroquine chemoprophylaxis should begin 2 weeks prior to the traveler's departure and should continue for 6 weeks after return. In areas where the parasite is resistant to chloroquine, the new antimalarial mefloquine is advocated by the United States Centers for Disease Control, at a once-per-week oral dose of 250 mg beginning 2 weeks prior to departure and continuing for 4 weeks after return. Alternative regimens include chloroquine or amodiaquine (300 mg base once per week) in combination with proguanil (100–200 mg daily) or chlorproguanil (20 mg per week) in areas where chloroquine resistance is not widespread or is of a low degree. In areas where chloroquine resistance is widespread and of high degree, chloroquine or amodiaquine (300 mg base once per week) plus one of the following is recommended: sulfadoxine-pyrimethamine (Fansidar or Metakelfin), one tablet per week; pyrimethamine alone; proguanil, 200 mg daily; or chlorproguanil, 20 mg weekly. Tetracycline and quinine are not advocated as chemoprophylactic drugs. Behavioral measures for the prevention of malaria include the following: the use of mosquito repellant containing at least 30% *N,N*-diethyl-3-methylbenzamide (DEET); wearing clothing that covers most of the skin during periods when anopheline mosquitos are active; using bed nets; and excluding mosquitos from living quarters by screening doors and windows. Avoiding outdoor activities during periods of the day when anopheline mosquitos are active, especially dawn and dusk during wet seasons, also may be helpful.

TRYPANOSOMIASIS OF THE CNS

Introduction

The term "trypanosomiasis" encompasses two distinct entities: African and American trypanosomiasis. African trypanosomiasis (sleeping sickness) is caused by trypanosomes of the brucei group. CNS involvement is the major clinical concern in human African trypanosomiasis; it is common, and it is fatal if untreated. Trypanosomiasis in Africa also affects animals, especially domestic cattle. American trypanosomiasis, or Chagas' disease, is caused by *Trypanosoma cruzi.* CNS involvement is a relatively minor clinical consideration in this disease.

Historical Note

Sleeping sickness among Africans and their livestock has had a major impact on the history of human activities on that continent. The tsetse fly, transmitter of this disease, effectively excluded large areas from human settlement (77). It limited the incursions of Islamic traders from the North, as well as Portuguese and Boer settlers from the South (78). The susceptibility of domestic cattle excluded pastoralists from tsetse-infested areas. In addition, it prevented the use of ox-drawn vehicles and plows among agricultural tribes in many areas, perpetuating the use of head loads and primitive hand-held hoes (78).

Trypanosomiasis causes endemic disease, but also has the potential to break out into devastating epidemics. Major outbreaks of sleeping sickness were described by Arab writers as early as the 14th century (78). Around the turn of this century, major epidemics killed approximately half a million people in Zaire and about two-thirds of the population around Lake Victoria (79). The only control measure then available was evacuation. These epidemics attracted the interest of European researchers, who first described the pathologic features of this important systemic and CNS infection.

In this chapter we will review the epidemiology and parasitology, pathology, pathogenesis, clinical features, diagnosis, and treatment of human meningoencephalitic trypanosomiasis. Our knowledge is incomplete in many of these areas. Because trypanosomiasis is largely a rural disease, cases rarely occur near large academic medical centers, where laboratory and postmortem investigations can be systematically undertaken. Few cases come to necropsy today, due to the advent of effective chemotherapy. Animal models have been widely used, but they are inexact replicas of human disease. Fortunately, the application of modern molecular techniques in Kenya and in other laboratories far from the endemic areas promises to answer many of these problems.

Parasitology

Human African trypanosomiasis results from infection with hemoflagellate protozoans of the genus *Trypanosoma,* subgenus *Trypanozoon,* species *brucei,* and the two subspecies *gambiense* and *rhodesiense.* These two are morphologically identical to each other and to *T. (T.) b. brucei,* the third member of the *brucei* group (Fig. 9). The latter subspecies infects domestic and wild ungu-

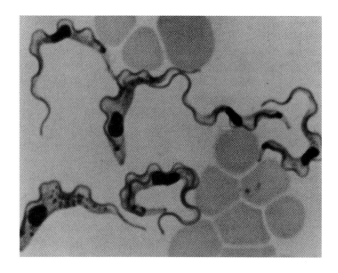

FIG. 9. African trypanosomiasis. Trypomastigote forms of *Trypanosoma rhodesiense* in a blood film. (From ref. 214, with permission.)

lates, causing a wasting disease similar to sleeping sickness, called "Nagana." It is distinguished by its inability to survive in humans and will not be described further here. The quadrinomial nomenclature is cumbersome, so for the purposes of this chapter the parasite names will be abbreviated according to common practice to *T. gambiense* and *T. rhodesiense.*

These parasites are transmitted by blood-sucking flies of the genus *Glossina*—the tsetse fly. *T. rhodesiense* is transmitted by the morsitans group of the *Glossina* genus. These flies are woodland and savannah dwellers (78). They feed primarily on large mammals, who are the major reservoir of this parasite in nature. In contrast, *T. gambiense* is transmitted by the palpalis group of *Glossina,* which occupy a riverine ecological niche. They feed primarily on humans, who provide up to 40% of their blood meals (79). Animals may harbor the parasite, but they probably are not an important reservoir. Transmission has also been reported as occurring through vertical (congenital), mechanical, and transfusion-related mechanisms (80).

The parasite has a complex life cycle which involves major morphological changes through the different stages of development, which occur in human and arthropod hosts. The details of this life cycle are well described in recent authoritative sources (78,81).

Epidemiology

The two main pathogenic subspecies are named for the geographic origin of the first reported respective cases. This reflects the geographic distribution of the parasites, and the names are commonly used to distinguish the two forms of the disease. *T. gambiense* occurs in

West and Central sub-Saharan Africa, from the Atlantic coast of Mauritania and Senegal eastward to Lake Victoria and southward to Angola. *T. rhodesiense* occurs in East and Southeast Africa from southern Ethiopia south to Mozambique and Zimbabwe and as far west as Eastern Zaire, Angola, and Nambia. Areas of overlap exist, especially around Lake Victoria. Within these broad regions, the disease is patchy in distribution, with approximately 200 known hyperendemic foci of sleeping sickness within tsetse-infested areas of sub-Saharan Africa (82). For example, in Tanzania, trypanosomiasis is reported from 11 of the 21 political regions, but in only five of these, geographically widely separated, does it occur annually. In only one of these, the Kigoma region, including the historically well-known Malagarasi River focus, are there more than 100 cases per year (Tanzania National Institute of Medical Research, *unpublished data*). The differing geographic distribution and ecologic niches help explain the distinct epidemiology of the two forms of trypanosomiasis. Humans are infected during certain activities such as: hunting; gathering food, honey, or firewood; herding livestock; collecting water; or bathing and washing in the habitat of tsetse flies, away from settled areas. Peridomestic transmission is uncommon. Incidence increases markedly in the dry months, especially in West Africa, when people concentrate around the diminishing number of available water sources (83).

At present, an estimated 25–50 million people and 35 million cattle live in areas of Africa where this disease is endemic (79,82). Detailed incidence and prevalence data are not widely available, partially because of the predominantly rural nature of this disease and the limited public health infrastructure of many African countries. The official incidence figure of 20,000 to 25,000 cases per year may be a substantial underestimate, considering that over 7000 patients were diagnosed in 1987 alone in the current Ugandan epidemic (84). A comprehensive study of trypanosomiasis in the Lambwe Valley of southwestern Kenya, on the northeast shore of Lake Victoria, was recently published by Wellde et al. (85). This study is unique in its depth and breadth. The population of this region increased from approximately 1300 in 1960 to 11,000 in 1982–1983. A total of 912 primary cases and 97 relapses had been recorded or reported during the 25 years from 1959 to 1984. This represents an average of 35 per year, with a range of 3–89 per year (83). Relapses may indicate occult or inadequately treated CNS disease. A point prevalence survey of 1340 volunteers in 1978 revealed only two cases (0.15%) of patent parasitemia (86). This contrasts with the rate of malaria parasitemia in the same area, which was 43% in children under 10 and 11% in adults over 20 (86). Twenty-one of those surveyed gave a history of sleeping sickness, and all of these were blood-smear negative. Thirteen (1%) of the surveyed individuals developed smear positive *T. rhode-*

siense infection over the next 6 years (86). An outbreak occurred in 1980–1984, resulting in 209 primary cases and 45 relapses. Cases were identified by passive surveillance at the hospital and active surveillance by field teams. The attack rate for this 5-year period was 5.4% overall, with considerable variability between areas of Lambwe Valley and between demographic groups (83). Of 96 patients admitted to the district hospital with primary sleeping sickness, 70% had abnormalities in the CSF, indicating CNS involvement. These included: increased leukocyte count (>5 per microliter); increased protein concentration (>45 mg/dl); or detection of parasites in CSF either by microscopy or by subinoculation into laboratory mice (87). This included 57% of patients with mild illness which did not significantly limit normal daily activities. Thirty-four relapses were identified, all of which had abnormal CSF (87). The high number of relapse cases, along with the finding of abnormal CSF in so many mild primary cases, indicates early invasion of the CNS in a substantial proportion of cases.

Similar data are available from Tanzania, though they are not as detailed. Outbreaks of sleeping sickness in the Kigoma region prompted active field surveillance of over 60,000 individuals in 1985–1986. Less than 1% had patent parasitemia (E. Komba, *personal communication*). In 1987, 216 primary cases were reported in Tanzania, with four relapses and 11 deaths (Tanzania National Institute of Medical Research, *unpublished data*). The majority (85%) of these cases were from the Kigoma region. One district of 9000 km² with 300,000 people contributed over 80% of these cases. Two hospitals and five free standing outpatient facilities served this district. For the 32 months ending in August 1988, one hospital reported 135 new cases and 22 relapses. Of the primary cases, 74 (55%) had CNS involvement (J. P. Cegielski, *unpublished data*). Veeken et al. (87a) reported from the same hospital during an outbreak in 1985 that 109 of 158 cases (69%) had meningoencephalitic disease. Patients in this area are thought to be infected with *T. rhodesiense.*

Comparably detailed studies on the Gambian form of the disease are not available. Some data have been published from Nigeria, which has a well-developed trypanosomiasis control program. Thomson (88) reported on the situation up until 1967 in northern Nigeria. In an area of 350,000 km² with 13 million people, fewer than 2000 cases were found annually. Active and passive surveillance in 1967 found 1355 cases, a prevalence nadir, among the three endemic and 12 epidemic foci in that region. Active surveys in 1967–1968 in outbreak areas found prevalence rates of sleeping sickness as high as 2.7–15.3% in four hamlet areas. Prevalence figures for CNS involvement were not given in this report. Weir et al. (89) described their experience at a rural mission hospital in southern Nigeria in an area where sleeping sickness had not been previously recognized. From 1983 to

1985, they saw 60 cases, 47 parasitologically confirmed, all from one area along the Ethiope River. Seventy-four percent of the confirmed cases had CNS involvement. Active surveillance undertaken in 1985 found up to 10% of inhabitants in some areas to be serologically positive for *T. gambiense*. A more recent, larger survey in that region found that 6.7–12.5% of individuals were seropositive using two different methods. Three percent of the total were parasitologically confirmed (90).

There are no data to indicate that subsets of the population are disproportionately susceptible or resistant to trypanosomiasis according to sex, age, race, tribe, or other genetic factors, except as related to their exposure to tsetse flies through their patterns of outdoor activity.

Pathology and Pathogenesis

The pathologic changes in the CNS resulting from infection with *T. rhodesiense* were described in a classic study by Calwell (91) from Tanganyika. In all 17 of his cases, trypanosomes were isolated from the CSF antemortem, and the patients died despite therapy. In general, the dura mater and the leptomeninges were adherent, especially at the vertex, with variable quantities of a sticky, milky exudate present. In only one case was the meningitis basilar in distribution. This contrasts with earlier studies of fatal Gambian sleeping sickness, in which the meningitis was typically basilar. The brain was edematous, and congestion of cerebral vessels was seen. The typical histologic lesion was infiltration of the leptomeninges and the perivascular spaces (particularly the Virchow–Robin spaces) with mononuclear inflammatory cells, namely, lymphocytes and plasma cells. The inflam-

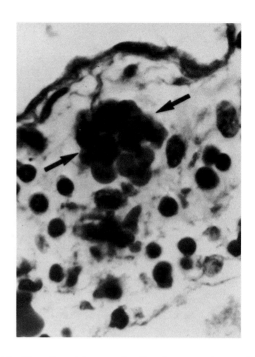

FIG. 11. Sleeping sickness. Section from meninges showing morular cell (*between arrows*) and numerous lymphocytes and plasma cells, characteristic of African trypanosomiasis. ×1140. (From ref. 215, with permission.)

matory infiltrate was marked in 14 of his 17 cases, and it was mild in three. The perivascular infiltrates are shown in Fig. 10. Glial cell proliferation was common; and morular cells, originally described by Mott in 1906, were present in the inflammatory foci in all cases. They were abundant in 11 of the cases. The morular cells (Fig. 11) have subsequently been shown to be modified plasma cells containing vacuoles full of immunoglobulin. In Calwell's series, the choroid plexus of sleeping sickness victims showed round-cell infiltrates, fibrosis, fibrinous exudates, and edema. Glial proliferation was seen in some brains. Perivascular demyelinization was seen in the subcortical white matter of 11 of 14 brains in which it was sought. There were no evident changes in the neuronal population of cells. No trypanosomes were seen in any of the specimens, but all patients had been treated.

Manuelidis et al. (92) and Poltera et al. (93), working in Uganda, supported and extended these findings. They emphasized the sparing of neuronal elements and the prominence of swollen astrocytes seen by special stains. The intense lymphocytic–plasmacytic perivascular and meningeal infiltrates seen by these workers are the histopathologic hallmarks of cerebral involvement by African trypanosomes (93,94). The meningocortical disease correlated clinically with earlier stages of CNS involvement, whereas cerebral white matter and basal ganglia lesions were involved in later stages. Neurons were similarly spared. In contrast to Calwell's study, however, these and other workers (94,95) found little or no cho-

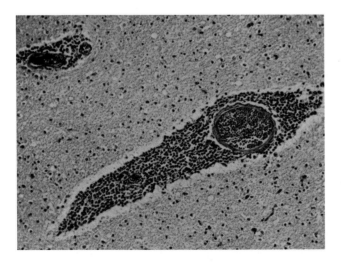

FIG. 10. Sleeping sickness. Perivascular infiltrates in the temporal cortex, with increased numbers of lymphocytes and astrocytes in the white matter. ×100. (From ref. 215, with permission.)

roid plexus involvement. Again, parasites were not seen. Nonetheless, studies using limiting dilution techniques and column chromatography on homogenates of brain tissue (96) and electron microscopy (97) in rodents and primates confirm that they are present in small numbers.

Another pattern of CNS pathology is a severe hemorrhagic leukoencephalopathy. Adams et al. (95), studying *T. gambiense* disease in the Ivory Coast, reported 13 of 16 cases with the typical picture described above. However, in three cases there was no cellular meningoencephalitis. Instead, there was fibrinoid necrosis of vessel walls in the brain but not in other organs, resulting in parenchymal hemorrhages (Fig. 12). These three cases occurred among 10 who had developed acute reactive arsenical encephalopathy. Manuelidis et al. (92) also reported a small series of cases in which hemorrhagic encephalopathy of the basal ganglia and brainstem was associated with melarsoprol (arsenic) toxicity.

In summary, the consistent pathologic features of CNS trypanosomiasis are lymphocytic–plasmacytic meningoencephalitis, especially in a perivascular distribution, glial proliferation, and sparing of neuronal elements. In some fatal cases, demyelinization and choroid plexus involvement occur. An acute hemorrhagic encephalopathy, possibly resulting from arsenic-induced vasculitis, is seen as well. Though the parasites invade the brain tissue they are rarely found in the CNS by light microscopy.

The pathogenesis of trypanosomiasis, particularly as it relates to the development of CNS disease, is poorly understood. Virtually all treatises on this subject start with a similar disclaimer. Numerous hypotheses have been advanced, but few firm data are available upon which to base a cohesive explanation of the mechanisms which result in trypanosomal CNS disease. In order to describe the processes which may operate in cerebral trypanoso-

miasis, a brief overview of the pathogenesis of this disease as a whole is necessary.

At the site where the biting fly inoculates parasites, an inflammatory nodule appears within several days. Active parasite replication and invasion of local tissues occurs, and a mononuclear cell infiltrate appears. The trypanosomes enter the lymphatics, causing lymphadenopathy, and the bloodstream, causing patent parasitemia (stage I). The most striking feature of this hemolymphatic stage of illness is the recurrent cycles of parasitemia (Fig. 13), associated with fever and constitutional symptoms. African trypanosomes are densely coated with a glycoprotein called the "variant surface glycoprotein" (VSG), which shields underlying structures from host antibodies. All of these glycoprotein molecules expressed on the surface of an individual parasite at a particular point in time are the same; that is, only a single VSG is expressed at one time. However, pathogenic trypanosomes have the striking ability to change this surface antigen coat (81). The host mounts an IgM response to this antigenic surface, so that the parasites disappear, or nearly disappear, from the blood. A new wave of parasitemia follows, resulting from the growth of a new population of parasites with an entirely new, antigenically different VSG. Each parasite has over 1000 different VSG genes (81). Thus a very large number of different antigenic types is possible. This cycle of parasite proliferation and humoral immune response is repeated again and again; it can continue for years in the more indolent West African disease. With each antigenically new population of trypanosomes, a corresponding wave of immunoglobulins is generated until massive hypergammaglobulinemia results. In a primate model reported by Fink et al. (98), serum IgM levels rose from the normal range of 850–3350 mg/liter to 15,000–35,000 mg/liter, corresponding to periods of high parasitemia.

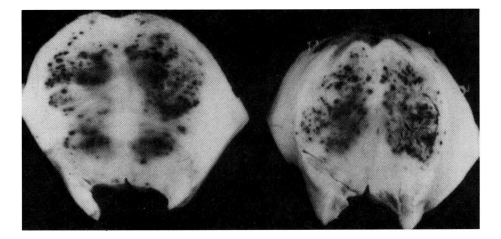

FIG. 12. Sleeping sickness. Section of the pons showing acute hemorrhagic leukoencephalopathy with numerous discrete and confluent hemorrhages in a patient who had been treated with melarsoprol. (From ref. 95, with permission.)

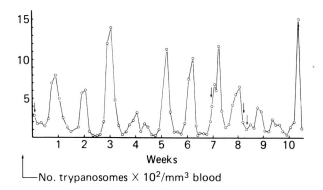

FIG. 13. African trypanosomiasis. Graph showing cycles of parasitemia with wide fluctuations in the number of parasites in the blood of a patient with sleeping sickness. (From ref. 215, with permission.)

IgG levels also rose 25–100%. However, these antibodies are not all VSG-specific. Marked polyclonal B-cell activation generates both specific and unrelated antibodies, including autoantibodies and immune complexes (80,81,99).

Eventually the trypanosomes invade the CNS to cause meningoencephalitis (stage II). Precisely how the parasites enter the brain parenchyma is not known. Alternative hypotheses have been proposed (94). They may enter the CSF via the choroid plexuses, circulating around the brain to reach the Virchow–Robin spaces and penetrate there. This is consistent with the pathologic findings. The parasites may also penetrate the brain substance by exiting from damaged, inflamed, or permeable meningeal or parenchymal vessels or via the ventricular ependymal cells. Following invasion of the CNS, immunoglobulin concentrations rise strikingly in the CSF (98). This can be used diagnostically (100). Some of these antibodies are directed against antigenic structures of the brain tissue itself (101). These antibodies are produced within the CNS of patients with stage II sleeping sickness; they do not reach the CSF by leaking across the blood–brain barrier from the systemic circulation (99).

The mechanism by which trypanosomes damage their mammalian hosts is still an unanswered question. Three general modes of pathogenesis have been proposed. First, toxin production by trypanosomes, leading to vascular permeability, has been observed in experimental models and may contribute to the thrombocytopenia and hemolytic anemia commonly seen in African trypanosomiasis (99). Second, metabolic derangements have been described by Seed et al. (102). They have presented data supporting the hypothesis that parasite-induced metabolic changes are important pathogenetic components of the disease. Their work demonstrates that African trypanosomes catabolize all three aromatic amino acids to compounds which are toxic *in vitro* and *in vivo*. These compounds are excreted in greatly ele-

vated concentrations in infected animals, presumably reflecting elevated blood and tissue levels. These metabolic pathways may generate toxic intermediates and deplete the precursor aromatic amino acids, as well as their biologically active metabolites, from the host's brain and other tissues (102). These include neurotransmitters, hormones, and protein precursors. Third, the most important disease-causing mechanism may be immunologic. Autoantibody production was previously mentioned; it is a consistent feature of African trypanosomiasis (81,99). Antibodies against human brain myelin proteins are found much more frequently in patients with CNS disease (71%) than in patients without CNS disease (23%) (101). Host antibodies form immune complexes with variant antigen types or autoantigens. Trypanosomes are found to invade the same organs in which immune complexes deposit (80,99). Complement is activated by both classic and alternative pathways. Immunofluorescent studies have shown deposition of complement and immunoglobulins in brain tissue (103). Finally, an immunoproliferative state, particularly of B lymphocytes, may be operative (81,99). The massive polyclonal B-cell activation, infiltration of tissues, and immunoglobulin secretion may result from a direct trypanosome B-cell mitogen or from interference with host T-cell control over B-cell function. A consistent feature of patients with trypanosomiasis is a poor immune response to recall antigens and to vaccination with, for example, tetanus toxoid or typhoid vaccine (81). A generalized state of humoral and cellular immunocompromise develops which is characteristic of African trypanosomiasis (104). This results in frequent, superimposed infectious complications. The kallikrein–kinin system is also activated (80,99,103) and may contribute significantly to vascular permeability, edema, hemostasis, and tissue hypoxia (105).

Clinical Manifestations

The clinical features of the East African and West African forms of sleeping sickness differ, albeit with considerable overlap. In general, *T. rhodesiense* causes an acute or subacute disease with chancre, fever, and early CNS involvement. Lymphadenopathy is minimal. Hemolymphatic and meningoencephalitic stages cannot be clearly distinguished. Death occurs within weeks to months in untreated cases. Gambian disease is an indolent process that is characterized by prominent lymphadenopathy, a gradual onset, chronic progressive course, and late CNS involvement. Enlargement of the posterior cervical lymph nodes is often conspicuous, being well known as "Winterbottom's sign." In contrast to the Rhodesian form, this disease may last months to years. Wellde's et al.'s classic study in Kenya (87) found that 54% of patients had mild illness at diagnosis (defined as no limitation in normal daily activities). Thirty-seven percent were moderately ill (ambulatory but in obvious distress, with limitation of normal daily activities), and 9% had severe disease (stupor, coma, and severe debility). Presenting clinical features are summarized in Table 3.

Following the tsetse bite, the chancre characteristically develops within 2 weeks. It is a painful inflammatory nodule, 2–5 cm in diameter, which resolves within 2–3 weeks. It may ulcerate spontaneously. It is more common in *T. rhodesiense* infection and much more common in non-Africans.

The hemolymphatic stage is highly variable. Bouts with fever, corresponding to waves of parasitemia, alternate with periods of well-being. African trypanosomiasis, along with malaria, are two of the very few causes of true intermittent fever. Nonspecific symptoms and signs, including headache, dizziness, arthralgia, malaise, weight loss, pruritus, and rash, occur during febrile episodes. Cardiac involvement is prominent in *T. rhodesiense* disease. It manifests as a myocarditis or pancarditis and can result in early mortality.

Major CNS symptoms include headache, alterations in mentation and behavior, abnormalities in the sleep–wake cycle for which the disease is named, motor disorders, and progressive deterioration of consciousness. The headache is often frontal or bilateral, is usually persistent, and progresses to become severe. Psychological and behavioral changes may be subtle or they may be flagrant. Changes in mood vary from apathy to excitation. Cognitive function may deteriorate; in addition, irritability, personality changes, and bizarre or inappropriate behavior occur. Lambo (106) describes the neuropsychiatric syndromes associated with trypanosomiasis

in Africa. These include personality disorders, psychoses, major affective disorders, and organic brain syndromes. Between 10% and 18% of patients diagnosed primarily with mental illnesses were found to have CNS trypanosomiasis. Conversely, 36–95% of patients with trypanosomiasis had mental syndromes in the psychiatric sense. The nature of the sleep disturbance is highly variable. However, generally, there is episodic daytime somnolence with nocturnal insomnia. Excessive sleeping increases as the disease progresses. At diagnosis, 61% of patients admitted to the hospital with East African trypanosomiasis sleep excessively whereas 9% are unable to sleep (87). Extrapyramidal symptoms and signs, cerebellar ataxia, parkinsonian rigidity, and convulsions are common as the disease progresses to later stages, as is papilledema (79). Cranial nerve palsies and long tract signs are uncommon. In the late stages, patients are wasted and increasingly obtunded (Fig. 14). Stupor and coma ultimately supervene in patients in whom treatment fails or in the absence of effective treatment. Mortality in the recent study from Tanzania was 12% overall (91). Mortality from both East and West African disease approaches 100% if untreated.

Diagnosis

Anemia and thrombocytopenia are common, whereas leukocytosis and eosinophilia are rare. The definitive diagnosis of human African trypanosomiasis depends on demonstration of the parasite in fluid aspirated from the chancre or lymph nodes or in blood, bone marrow, or CSF. In ascending order of complexity, cost, and sensitivity, wet blood films for motile parasites, Giemsa-stained

TABLE 3. Presenting clinical features of 96 Rhodesian sleeping sickness patients before treatment (58 males, 38 females)[a]

Symptom	Number (%)	Sign	Number (%)
Headache	92 (95.8)	Lymphadenopathy	83 (86.4)
Weakness	89 (92.7)	Fever (>98.6°F)	35 (36.4)
Joint pain	85 (88.5)	Enlarged spleen	31 (32.3)
Weight loss	78 (81.2)	Edema	28 (29.2)
Back pain	71 (74.9)	Presence of chancre	15 (15.6)
Abnormal sleep	68 (70.8)	Enlarged liver	12 (12.5)
Abnormal appetite	66 (68.7)	Abnormal coordination or reflexes	11 (11.4)
Abnormal vision	64 (66.7)	Clinical anemia	4 (4.2)
Abdominal pain	56 (58.3)	Dehydration	4 (4.2)
Pruritus	51 (53.1)	Tachycardia	3 (3.1)
Constipation	50 (52.1)	Tender abdomen	3 (3.1)
Abnormal coordination	49 (51.0)	Ascites	2 (2.1)
Abnormal speech	37 (38.5)	Coma	2 (2.1)
Amenorrhea[b]	18 (81.8)	Jaundice	0 (0.0)
Impotency[c]	32 (69.6)		

[a] Adapted from ref. 87.
[b] Sixteen of the 38 women were excluded from calculations, because of the following reasons: recent delivery (5), post-menopause (5), juvenile (4), pregnancy (2).
[c] Twelve of the 58 males were juveniles and were excluded from calculation.

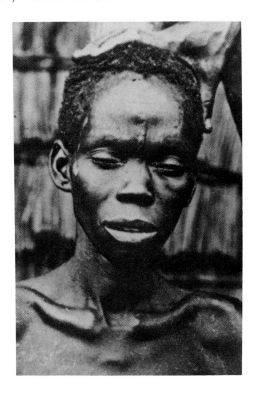

FIG. 14. Sleeping sickness. Characteristic appearance of a patient with advanced disease, showing somnolence and wasting. (From ref. 214, with permission.)

thick blood films, microhematocrit capillary tube centrifugation techniques, and anion-exchange chromatography columns are used for the diagnosis of trypanosomiasis. These tests are appropriate for field, clinical, and research conditions, respectively. Repeated examination may be necessary because of the cyclical nature of the parasitemia. Animal inoculation may be the most sensitive diagnostic test, especially for research applications

(107). Lumbar puncture should be performed in virtually all cases of trypanosomiasis except in the case of primary chancres found in isolation. Diagnosis of CNS disease by microscopic identification of the parasite can be accomplished by any one of the above methods. However, in the presence of demonstrated hemolymphatic disease, any elevation of CSF protein content or white cell content should be taken as evidence of CNS involvement. Analysis of CSF specimens is shown in Tables 4 and 5. Fifty-seven percent of patients with clinically mild disease, 73% of patients with clinically moderate disease, and 100% of patients with clinically severe disease had elevated CSF leukocyte counts and/or protein levels. Microscopically visible trypanosomes were present in 2.5%, 4.5% and 16.7% of patients in these same three categories, respectively. CSF immunoglobulin M levels were also progressively increased from 20% to 34% to 92% through these three clinical grades. A double-centrifugation technique for increased sensitivity of CSF diagnosis of trypanosomiasis has recently been described (108).

The antigenic variability of these parasites presents a major problem for application of immunologic diagnostic techniques. However, diagnosis of trypanosomiasis by serologic techniques such as card agglutination tests and indirect immunofluorescent antibody tests have been developed, with sensitivity rates of about 90%, mostly in *T. gambiense* disease (107,109). The use of procyclic forms as a source of antigens for the immunofluorescent test may improve sensitivity in *T. rhodesiense* disease (110). Newly developed enzyme-linked immunosorbent assays are a promising tool presently undergoing evaluation for the diagnosis of both *T. gambiense* and *T. rhodesiense* (109) (E. Komba, *personal communication*). These enzyme-linked immunosorbent assays and immunofluorescent antibody tests allow detection of antibodies in the CSF (100,109).

TABLE 4. *Analysis of cerebrospinal fluid samples from primary Rhodesian sleeping sickness patients[a]*

		Clinical grade: mild Number of cases: 40	moderate 44	severe 12	Total 96
Leukocytes	Protein				
N	N	17 (42.5)	12 (27.3)	0 (0.0)	29 (30.2)
E	N	16 (40.0)	16 (36.4)	5 (41.7)	37 (38.5)
N	E	0 (0.0)	1 (2.3)	1 (8.3)	2 (2.1)
E	E	7 (17.5)	15 (34.1)	6 (50.0)	28 (29.2)
Detectable immunoglobulins[d]					
IgM		8 (20.0)	15 (34.1)	11 (91.7)	34 (35.4)
IgA		4 (10.0)	10 (22.7)	6 (50.0)	20 (20.8)
IgG		36 (90.0)	43 (97.7)	12 (100.0)	91 (94.8)
Detectable trypanosomes					
Microscopy (sediment)		1 (2.5)	2 (4.5)	2 (16.7)	5 (5.2)
Subinoculation		2 (5.0)	2 (4.5)	2 (16.7)	6 (6.2)

[a] From ref. 87, with permission.
[b] N = normal (≤5 cells/μl); E = elevated (>5 cells/μl).
[c] N = normal (≤45 mg/dl); E = elevated (>45 mg/dl).
[d] Number of patients with detectable immunoglobulin (%).

TABLE 5. *Levels of leukocytes, total protein, and immunoglobulins in the cerebrospinal fluid of primary Rhodesian sleeping sickness patients[a]*

	Clinical condition: 2	3	4	Total
	Number of cases: 40	44	12	96
Leukocytes[b]				
Mean	46	64	147	67
Range	0–302	0–610	1–550	0–610
Distribution[c]				
0–5	17 (42.5)	13 (29.5)	1 (8.3)	31 (32.3)
6–30	13 (32.5)	18 (40.9)	2 (16.7)	33 (34.4)
31–100	8 (20.0)	4 (9.1)	5 (41.7)	17 (17.7)
>100	2 (5.0)	9 (20.4)	4 (33.3)	15 (15.6)
Total protein[d]				
Mean	32	47	76	44
Range	11–96	13–155	18–192	11–192
Distribution[c]				
10–45	33 (82.5)	28 (63.6)	5 (41.7)	66 (68.7)
46–70	6 (15.0)	6 (13.6)	4 (33.3)	16 (16.7)
71–100	1 (2.5)	8 (18.2)	1 (8.3)	10 (10.4)
>100	0 (0.0)	2 (8.3)	2 (16.7)	4 (4.1)
Immunoglobulins[e]				
IgM	1.8 (0–22)	5.1 (0–34)	17.3 (0–52)	5.1 (0–52)
IgA	0.2 (0–3)	0.9 (0–8)	3.4 (0–10)	0.9 (0–10)
IgG	15.3 (0–31)	18.4 (4–31)	33.5 (17–90)	19.0 (0–90)

[a] From ref. 87, with permission.
[b] Leukocytes/μl CSF, normal value, 0–5/μl.
[c] Distribution—number of patients (%) having CSF leukocytes counts or total protein at various levels.
[d] Total protein in mg/dl CSF, normal value, 10–45 mg/dl.
[e] Mean (range) for immunoglobulin levels in mg/dl.

Treatment

The specific drug treatment of cerebral trypanosomiasis is difficult. It must be viewed in the context of treatment of the hemolymphatic stage. Three key drugs are the mainstay of chemotherapy of African trypanosomiasis: suramin, pentamidine, and melarsoprol. Of these, only melarsoprol penetrates the CNS and is effective in CNS disease.

Intravenous suramin is the standard treatment of stage I human African trypanosomiasis. Suramin is also known as antrypol, germanin, and Bayer 205, as well as by other names. This drug clears the parasitemia; in the absence of CNS invasion, cure rates near 100% are achieved (79,111). A test dose of 100–200 mg is given initially because of the potential for severe idiosyncratic reactions. The dosage of 20 mg per kilogram of body weight in children and adults up to a maximum of 1 g is given promptly after reconstitution of the drug, by slow intravenous injection on days 1, 3, 7, 14, and 21. Suramin is toxic; one in 2000–4500 patients will have a sudden idiosyncratic reaction with vomiting, circulatory collapse, and shock, with or without seizures. Death results in a minority of these reactions (111)—hence the need for a test dose. Less severe reactions are common. Nephrotoxicity occurs, manifested as albuminuria. Suramin's mechanism of action is unknown, though inhibi-

tion of the parasite specific enzyme L-α-glycerophosphate oxidase is probably important (111).

Pentamidine isethionate or pentamidine dimethane sulfonate may be used in early cases of *T. gambiense* disease. Results are not as good as with suramin (79), and it is ineffective in *T. rhodesiense* disease. The dose is 3–4 mg of the base per kilogram of body weight, given intramuscularly daily for 7–10 days. Nephrotoxicity in the form of decreased glomerular filtration rate, and hypoglycemia may occur. Pentamidine in a dose of 4 mg of base per kilogram given intramuscularly every 3–6 months can be used prophylactically in West and Central Africa. Interference with nucleic acid synthesis has been identified as a potential mechanism of action (111), and selective uptake into parasite cells confers therapeutic specificity.

Melarsoprol, also called arsobal, melarsen oxide-BAL, and mel B, is the only treatment for CNS disease. Its use is complicated by the 10–18% incidence of a severe, reactive arsenical encephalopathy that often results in permanent neurologic damage or death (111,112). There are three characteristic syndromes of arsenical encephalopathy: status epilepticus with acute cerebral edema; rapidly progressive coma without seizures; and nonfatal cognitive abnormalities without neurologic signs (113). Corticosteroids are ineffective in preventing or treating these complications. Even though it is active in all stages of disease, melarsoprol's use should be restricted to patients with CNS involvement. It is given as a single daily intravenous injection of 3.6 mg/kg, up to a maximum of 180 mg daily, for 3 days. This schedule is repeated three times, with a rest period of 7 days between courses. Some authorities advise a graduated schedule. In the first course, 1.8 mg/kg is given on the first day, followed by 2.1 mg/kg on the second day and 2.4 mg/kg on the third day. For the second course, 2.7 mg/kg, 3.0 mg/kg, and 3.3 mg/kg are given on the 3 successive days. In the third course, the full dose of 3.6 mg/kg is given daily for the 3 days. Patients with severe disease should receive an abbreviated course of suramin prior to receiving melarsoprol. This consists of 250–500 mg of suramin daily (or every other day) for 4 days. Melarsoprol may be used if suramin or pentamidine treatment fails. It can also be repeated in the same patient on the same schedule for patients who relapse; in such cases, CNS involvement is highly likely.

Tryparsamide has been used in early *T. gambiense* disease, as have berenil in early disease of both forms and melarsonyl (mel W) in late-stage disease of both forms (111). The newest development in the treatment of meningoencephalitis is the use of difluoromethylornithine (DFMO, eflornithine). This compound irreversibly inhibits ornithine decarboxylase, the key enzyme in the synthesis the polyamines spermidine and putrescine from ornithine. These compounds are critical to the differentiation and proliferation of trypanosomes. Numerous reports indicate that this may be a promising new alternative to melarsoprol (114–118).

American Trypanosomiasis

American trypanosomiasis (Chagas' disease) is caused by infection with *Trypanosoma cruzi*, which is transmitted by reduviid bugs of the genus *Triatoma*. It occurs primarily in Latin America, extending as far north as southernmost Texas. Acute infection generally occurs in children. It is often asymptomatic or nonspecific, except that a characteristic unilateral orbital edema (Romaña's sign) occurs in some cases. Transmission to the fetus occurs in 2% of pregnancies if the mother is seropositive, resulting in congenital infection. The major pathologic features, seen mostly in adults, are cardiac and gastrointestinal, resulting in the two principal syndromes of the chronic form of the disease—congestive heart failure and megaesophagus or megacolon. Symptomatic CNS disease is very rare.

Even though CNS involvement was first recognized by Carlos Chagas himself, very little has been written on CNS disease. Acute CNS disease is most commonly a complication of congenital infection. Thus, the majority of cases involving the CNS are in children under 1 year old (119). Parasites can be found in the CSF following

acute infection at any age, but clinical or pathologic meningoencephalitis is rare (89). When it does occur, it is usually fatal. Histologically scattered granulomas are seen consisting of microglia and mononuclear inflammatory cells (119). The distribution and intensity of these lesions is highly variable. Amastigote forms of the parasite are seen inside glial cells (in the absence of inflammation) or in the center of granulomas.

The pathogenetic mechanisms underlying Chagasic encephalitis are unclear. Organotypic culture studies (120) have shown that trypomastigote forms invade the supporting glia, but not the neurons themselves. Nonetheless, this results in progressive abnormalities in neuron morphology and eventual neuron destruction *in vitro*. This effect is not transferred by culture supernatant alone, indicating that it is not related to secreted products of the parasites such as toxins. Immunologically mediated damage has also been proposed. Antitrypanosomal antibodies can be found in the CSF of patients with acute Chagas' disease (121). Some of the surface antigens of *T. cruzi* mimic antigens in mammalian brain and nerve tissue, and antibodies to these antigens are cross-reactive (122). These common antigens may include sulfated lipids present on both the *T. cruzi* surface and in mammalian brain (123).

Clinically, acute Chagasic encephalitis manifests itself as signs ranging from slight tremors to spasticity to generalized convulsions. Development is impaired. In these infants the diagnosis can be established by finding parasites in the blood, tissues, or CSF. Serologic testing can be helpful. The differential diagnosis includes toxoplasmosis, congenital syphilis, and cytomegalic inclusion disease. The trypanocides nifurtimox (Lampit) and benzonidazole (Rochagan) are used to treat this infection.

CNS involvement in the chronic forms of American trypanosomiasis was also described by Chagas, but it has been inadequately documented and investigated. Direct involvement of the CNS in chronic Chagas' disease must be differentiated from the indirect effects on the brain of severe Chagasic cardiomyopathy, including chronic hypoxia and thromboembolic phenomena. In addition, neuronal loss in the acute phase can result in cerebral and cerebellar atrophy (124). Chronic CNS infection can manifest as tumor-like lesions, described by De Quieroz (125) in 1973. These tumor-like lesions have also been seen in immunosuppressed patients (126,127). The other form of CNS involvement in chronic Chagas' disease is a granulomatous encephalitis (119). It was found at necropsy in three of 31 randomly chosen cases of fatal Chagasic carditis. In one of these cases the granulomas were perivascular, and amastigotes were seen. In the other two the lesions were less intense and appeared to be in a stage of repair. Clinically, epilepsy (128), spastic paralysis, cognitive impairment, and cerebellar syndromes (129) have all been described with chronic Chagas' disease, each in only a small number of cases. Thus the existence of chronic neurologic syndromes specifically caused by American trypanosomiasis remains controversial.

In summary, acute granulomatous encephalitis resulting from infection with *T. cruzi* is rare, occurring primarily as a result of congenital infection. It is usually fatal. Mass lesions of the brain in chronic Chagas' disease have been described, as have granulomas, but specific clinical CNS syndromes due to *T. cruzi* have not been proven.

AMEBIC INFECTIONS OF THE CENTRAL NERVOUS SYSTEM

Pathogenic amebae can invade the CNS, causing rare but highly fatal infections (Table 6). *Entamoeba histolytica* can spread from the intestine to cause amebic abscesses in liver, lung, and occasionally elsewhere, including the brain. Free-living amebae rarely cause disease in humans, but they can invade the CNS directly to cause a condition termed "primary amebic meningoencephalitis." These CNS infections have unique features which have drawn much attention from clinicians, pathologists, and researchers.

PRIMARY AMEBIC MENINGOENCEPHALITIS

Fowler and Carter (130) first reported human infection by free-living amebas in 1965. Four patients in South Australia developed an acute meningoencephali-

tis caused by amebae (later shown to be *Naegleria fowleri*), which proved rapidly fatal in all four cases (130). This devastating CNS disease has since become known as "primary amebic meningoencephalitis" (PAM). Additional cases have since been identified from many parts of the world, including infections caused by *Acanthamoeba* (131) and leptomyxid amebae (132). *N. fowleri* usually causes acute PAM, whereas *Acanthamoeba* usually causes subacute or chronic PAM, also termed "granulomatous amebic encephalitis" (GAE). The spectrum of disease caused by free-living amebae has expanded to include keratoconjunctivitis (133), skin ulcers (134), and disseminated infection (135,136). Fortunately, PAM remains rare. Less than 200 human cases have been reported, yet the unique features of CNS diseases caused by free-living amebae have stimulated a large number of clinical and experimental publications on the subject.

Etiology

Hundreds of species of free-living amebae are known, but only a few have been reported to infect humans. The most important of these are included in two genera: *Naegleria* and *Acanthamoeba* (Table 6). These protozoa are widely distributed, particularly in moist soils and warm fresh waters. Although they have been recovered from a variety of plant or animal sites, such as the fur of aquatic mammals or the guts of fish (137), true animal or plant reservoirs have not been identified (138). Recently, Visvesvara et al. (132) have implicated another group,

TABLE 6. *Pathogenic potential of various amebae*[a]

Nomenclature	Pathogen	Host	Disease	References
Order Amoebida				
Family Endamoebidae				
Entamoeba histolytica	Yes	Humans	Colitis, hepatic abscess, brain abscess	207, 209, 210
Endolimax nana	No	Humans	None	
Iodamoeba butschlii	No	Humans	None	
Family Acanthamoebidae				
Acanthamoeba culbertsoni, A. polyphaga, A. castellanii, A. astronyxis, A. palestinensis, A. rhysodes	Yes	Humans, mice	Subacute or chronic PAM, GAE, keratoconjunctivitis, skin ulcers, mandibular abscess	136, 172, 184, 185, 194
Order Schizopyrenida				
Family Vahlkampfiidae				
Naegleria fowleri	Yes	Humans and animals	Acute PAM	134
Naegleria australiensis	Yes	Mice	Experimental PAM	216
Naegleria gruberi	No	None known	None known	134, 217
Naegleria lovaniensis	No	None known	None known	134
Vahlkampfia	Unproven	? Humans	? Subacute PAM	186
Order Leptomyxida				
Leptomyxid amebae	Yes	Humans, primates, sheep	Subacute or chronic PAM	132

[a] Adapted from refs. 132, 134, and 185. PAM, primary amebic meningoencephalitis; GAE, granulomatous amebic encephalitis.

the leptomyxid amebae, as a cause of CNS infection in humans and animals.

Naegleria fowleri, the main pathogen causing acute PAM in humans, exists in three forms: trophozoites, flagellates, and cysts (Fig. 15). The trophozoite is a highly motile ameba, 7–20 μm in size. Electron micrographs reveal an ultrastructure which is typical for eukaryotic cells. Features include ribosomes, endoplasmic reticulum, a primitive Golgi apparatus, and membrane-bound organelles (138). The nucleus is single, with a large dark karyosome lying within a clear halo, with a fine nuclear rim; it is found in all three stages of *Naegleria.*

N. fowleri flourishes over a wide range of temperatures, from 15°C to 45°C, and tolerates a wide pH range, from 4.6 to 9.5 (138). *N. fowleri* grows best at 37°C to 44°C; however, it can be maintained at room temperature, which is appropriate for nonpathogenic strains such as *N. gruberi.* In the laboratory, *N. fowleri* can be propagated in defined or enriched liquid media, on agar, on tissue cultures, or by passage in susceptible animals (138–142). *Naegleria* species can be grown axenically in tubes or wells containing Chang's medium, which contains yeast and liver extract, casein, bovine serum, hemin, and L-methionine (142). The trophozoites reproduce vigorously, with generation times from 5 to 14 hr (143). An alternative culture method is to place amebae onto agar upon which a heavy inoculum of Enterobacteriaceae organisms has been spread (138,140). The growing amebae ingest the Enterobacteriaceae organisms for food, spreading centrifugally across the plate until all the bacteria have been consumed. *Naegleria*

species flourish in iron-containing waters; they require iron for growth, which can be inhibited by iron chelators (144). Trophozoites are quickly killed by drying or freezing, whereas cysts are more resistant.

These amebae actively ingest food and other particles from their environment. *N. fowleri* trophozoites grown on Vero cells show many food vacuoles containing ingested material, indicating great phagocytic activity (138,139). Electron micrographs show many pinocytotic vesicles (139) and specialized structures called "food cups" or "amebastomes" (Fig. 16) (138,145). Amebastomes function as a kind of mouth through which the amebae ingest bacteria, yeasts, and cellular debris and even parts of living mammalian cells (Fig. 17) (138). The food cup is apparently not a virulence factor, because the number of amebastomes observed on trophozoites decreases as virulence is increased by means of serial animal passage (145). The motility of *N. fowleri* trophozoites increases if they are exposed to potential foods such as mammalian cells or bacteria *in vitro* (146). These responses are complex, involving (a) chemokinesis and formation of amebastomes and (b) chemotaxis (146). The locomotive ability of *N. fowleri,* measured by rate of migration *in vitro,* correlates with virulence for mice (147).

When *Naegleria* trophozoites are placed in distilled water, some change into the flagellate form (Fig. 15). The flagellates contain a nucleus and a single contractile vacuole. They are highly motile, propelled by two to six flagellae located anteriorly. Thus, flagellates formed from trophozoites *in vitro* can be easily identified by their

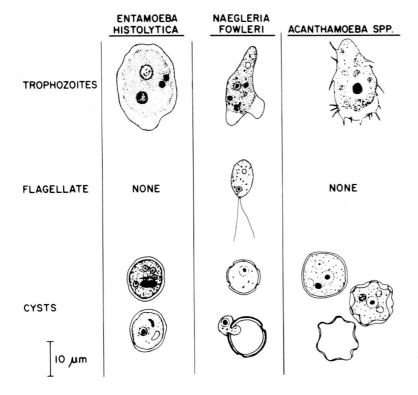

FIG. 15. Diagram showing the comparative morphology of three pathogenic amebae: the intestinal parasite, *Entamoebae histolytica;* and two free-living amebae, *N. fowleri* and *Acanthamoeba* species. (From ref. 134, with permission.)

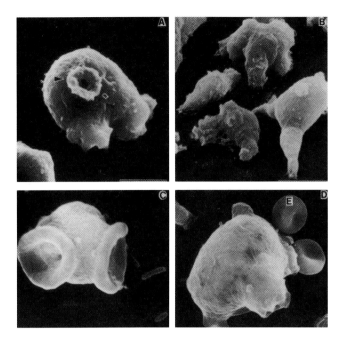

FIG. 16. Scanning electron micrographs of *N. fowleri.* **A:** A trophozoite in laboratory medium, showing a single food cup or amebastome (*arrowhead*). **B:** Virulent trophozoites after mouse passage; note absence of food cups. **C:** Trophozoite ingesting bacteria via food cups. **D:** Trophozoite attaching to and ingesting erythrocytes (E). (From ref. 138, with permission.)

rapid linear progress across a microscopic field. The regulation of differentiation by factors such as protozoal calmodulins is currently being studied at the molecular level (148,149).

Naegleria species form cysts (Fig. 15) in response to nutritionally deficient or otherwise stressful conditions such as desiccation, which rapidly kill trophozoites. The

cyst of *N. fowleri* is smaller than the other two stages of this species, being approximately 5 μm in diameter. It has a central karyosome and is surrounded by a thick, rounded, ridged, double-layered wall. Pores can be found in this wall, through which the protozoan excysts when it reverts to the trophozoite form (138). Cyst morphology varies considerably between species (150). The primary stimulus for excystment appears to be molecular carbon dioxide (151), which could be an effective signal indicating that the environment contains bacteria and other nutrients favorable for the growth of trophozoites.

Acanthamoeba species occur as trophozoites or cysts, but they do not form flagellates (Fig. 15). The trophozoite is somewhat larger than *Naegleria,* and it is distinguished by the formation of fine (filose) pseudopodia at the leading edge as it migrates (Fig. 18). The genus name, describing these thorn-like spikes, is derived from the Greek word for thorn, *akantha. Acanthamoeba* cysts are stellate rather than round, with opercula through which excystation occurs to form trophozoites. *Acanthamoeba* species can be grown axenically in Neff's medium. The optimal temperature for growth of *Acanthamoeba* species is about 33°C, but some are tolerant of higher temperatures. Considerable variation exists between strains for important characteristics such as animal virulence (152).

Recently, another free-living ameba from the order Leptomyxida (not yet taxonomically defined) has been isolated from the tissues of patients and animals with fatal CNS infections (132). The morphology of the pathogen(s) is distinctive (132). Application of an antileptomyxid antiserum to preserved tissue specimens resulted in reclassification of several cases which had previously been attributed to *Acanthamoeba* infection (135,153–

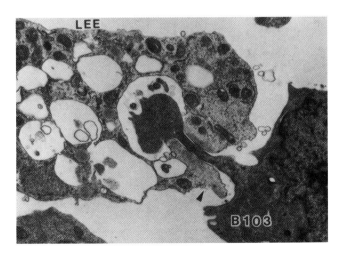

FIG. 17. Electron micrograph showing a trophozoite of *N. fowleri* (LEE strain) ingesting a portion of a target nerve cell (B103) in tissue culture. (From ref. 138, with permission.)

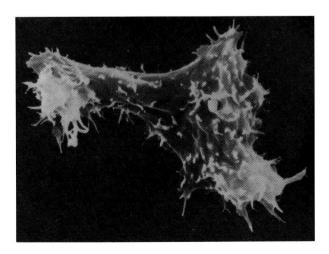

FIG. 18. Scanning electron micrographs of a trophozoite of *Acanthamoeba castellanii,* showing thorn-like pseudopodia. Bar represents 10 μm. (From ref. 134, with permission of Dr. David T. John.)

156). Further studies will be needed in order to define the relative frequency and importance of CNS and other infections caused by these amebae.

Epidemiology

Free-living amebae are widely distributed in soil throughout the world. They flourish in warm, moist conditions, and most cases of human infection have come from the warmer climates (134,143). Strains of *N. fowleri,* of varying virulence, have been recovered from lakes, puddles, pools, ponds, rivers, sewage sludge, tap water, air-conditioner drains, and soils (134,137,157, 158). Thermal pollution, in the form of warm-water effluents from factories, encourages growth of these temperature-tolerant protozoa (157,159).

Asymptomatic carriage by humans can occur. Wang and Feldman (160) recovered free-living amebae from the throats of otherwise-healthy subjects during the course of surveillance for viral respiratory infections, especially from children 2 years of age or less during the warmer months. Lawande et al. (161) recovered soil amebae, including two isolates of *N. fowleri,* from the nasal passages of 12 of 50 healthy children during the dusty harmattan period in Nigeria.

Sporadic cases of acute PAM occur when children swim or play in water containing the amebae (134). Outbreaks have occurred when swimming pools (134) or water supplies (140) have become contaminated, often through failure of chlorination. Males are affected more often than females, in a ratio of about 2:1 for *Naegleria* and 5:1 for *Acanthamoeba* (143). Acute PAM usually affects children and young adults, with the youngest reported patient being only 4 months old (156). GAE occurs at any age.

Pathogenesis

In 1961 Culbertson (162), on the basis of experimental studies, correctly predicted that free-living amebae might cause disease in humans, including CNS infections and granulomatous inflammation. In the same year, the first of Fowler and Carter's four cases of PAM occurred in South Australia, although the etiology was not reported until 1965 (130).

Pathogenic free-living amebae cause CNS infection similar to the human disease when inoculated intranasally or intracisternally into a variety of experimental animal species such as mice, guinea pigs, rabbits, baboons, and monkeys (132,138,140,163,164). Virulence varies widely for different species of amebae and for strains within species (Table 6) (134,138,140). Laboratory-adapted strains can lose virulence (134,138,164), which can be regenerated by animal passage (140).

The reason why these free-living amebae have a special predilection to infect the CNS is unknown. However, the route of infection has been described. *N. fowleri* enters the nasal cavity during swimming or diving in fresh water. When one considers that many children and adults repeatedly swim in contaminated fresh water in warm climates, invasion from the nasal cavity to the CNS must be a rare event. However, in some patients the amebae invade the roof of the nasal cavity, crossing the olfactory epithelium and ascending into the anterior cranial fossae through the cribrifom plate via the extensions of the olfactory nerve known as "fila olfactoria" (140). Martinez et al. (165) studied the details of invasion in mice infected by instillation of a drop of medium containing virulent *N. fowleri* into the nasal cavity. Their elegant ultrastructural studies showed amebae invading the mucosa (Fig. 19) and ascending to the brain via fila olfactoria (Fig. 20) and along blood vessels (Fig. 21) (165). In this way, amebae reach the meninges surrounding the frontal lobes, where they multiply, spread, and destroy CNS tissue. Virulent and avirulent strains of *Naegleria* are cytopathogenic for neural cells in tissue culture (166–168).

The motile amebae spread through the meninges, invade the parenchyma directly or along vascular pathways, and induce extensive, florid, necrotizing inflammation. *Acanthamoeba* species also may enter the CNS by this route, but more often they appear to invade the CNS by way of the bloodstream. *Acanthamoeba* species also can invade the CNS from a primary corneal infection of the eye (169).

These pathogenic amebae elaborate many enzymes which may be directly or indirectly involved in pathogen-

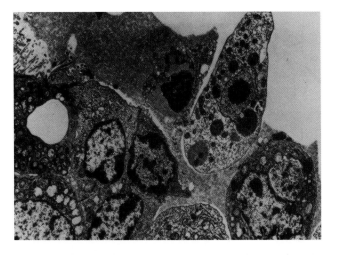

FIG. 19. Electron micrograph showing a trophozoite of *N. fowleri* (*upper right*) invading the olfactory mucosa of a mouse after instillation into the nasal cavity. (From ref. 165, with permission.)

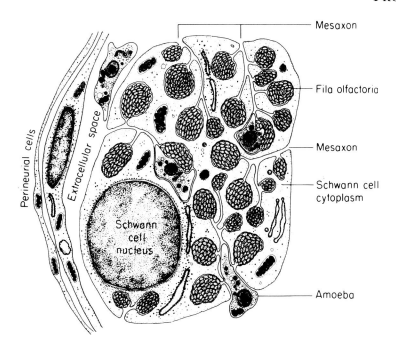

Mesaxon

Fila olfactoria

Mesaxon

Schwann cell cytoplasm

Amoeba

FIG. 20. Diagram of the olfactory submucosal nerve plexus showing fila olfactoria and invasion by several amebae located in the mesaxon and extracellular space. (From ref. 165, with permission.)

esis of tissue damage, including aminopeptidases, hydrolases (170), esterases, acid and alkaline phosphatases, and dehydrogenases (138,171). Analysis of these enzymes yields "zymograms" which correlate with species differences and with pathogenicity (172). Visvesvara and Balamuth (152) related the production of phospholipase by strains of *Acanthamoeba* to the severity of the cytopathic effect they produced on monkey kidney tissue culture cells (152). Lowrey and McLaughlin (173,174) demonstrated potent hemolytic/cytotoxic activity associated with the surface membrane of *N. fowleri*.

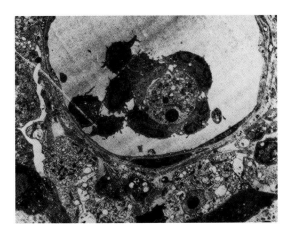

FIG. 21. Electron micrograph showing a trophozoite of *N. fowleri* in the lumen of a blood vessel in the olfactory mucosa of a mouse, surrounded by neutrophils. The blood vessel is surrounded by amebae, some containing erythrocytes. (From ref. 165, with permission.)

Because these amebae ingest bacteria as food and can carry viruses in their cytoplasm, the possibility that amebae could act as carriers or vectors for pathogenic microbes has been raised. Newsome and Wilhelm (144) showed that under certain experimental conditions, *Legionella pneumophila* can survive, and even multiply, inside *N. fowleri*. This potential mechanism of pathogenesis remains speculative.

The role of host immunity in these infections is an important and complex issue. Activated macrophages can damage *N. fowleri* by direct cytolysis and also by antibody-dependent cellular cytotoxicity (175). Macrophage amebicidal activity is mediated by soluble proteins derived from the activated macrophages (176). Ferrante and Mocatta (177) showed that human neutrophils could kill *N. fowleri in vitro*, but only if the neutrophils were first conditioned with medium from phytohemagglutinin-stimulated mononuclear cells.

Amebae activate the complement system, generating chemotactic factors (178). The trophozoites are susceptible to complement lysis (138). Agglutinating antibody enhances lysis, and virulent strains are relatively resistant to complement lysis (179).

Mice develop agglutinating antibodies after intravenous inoculation of *N. fowleri* (180). They can be partially protected against experimental PAM by immunization or transfer of immune serum (181). Lallinger et al. (182) passively protected rabbits by treatment with immunoglobulin G prepared from polyclonal immune serum, or with a monoclonal antibody to *N. fowleri*. Cursons et al. (183) found IgG and IgM antibodies to amebae in all normal subjects tested in New Zealand.

Whether this represents evidence of prior asymptomatic infection or nonspecific cross-reactivity is uncertain.

Acute PAM caused by *N. fowleri* usually occurs in previously healthy hosts (134). Martinez (136,184) has pointed out that subacute or chronic PAM (GAE) caused by *Acanthamoeba* is more likely to occur in patients with preexisting diseases or immunosuppression. This has been widely quoted by others (143,185); however, like many generalizations, it is only partly true. Subacute or chronic PAM can develop in normal hosts (153,156,186,187). Moreover, some of the underlying conditions, such as alcoholism (188,189), drug addiction (190), skin ulcers (184), antibiotic therapy, and pneumonia were nonspecific and not clearly immunosuppressive. Whether these conditions were truly the significant predisposing factor is uncertain. Other patients with GAE had definite immunosuppression, including renal transplantation (136) or AIDS (135).

Pathology

Inspection of the brain of a patient who has died of PAM presents a striking picture. The meninges are diffusely hyperemic, with focal or diffuse superficial hemorrhages (140,185). A diffuse purulent exudate of varying severity is present, especially at the base of the brain (Fig. 22). The involvement is often maximal around the olfactory bulbs, consistent with the site of entry of the amebae (see above). There may be frank necrosis, sometimes extensive, of the superficial cerebral parenchyma. The temporal and frontal lobes are most severely affected, but extensive damage can occur in the brainstem, cerebellum, and elsewhere.

Histologic sections show extensive inflammation with a heavy influx of polymorphonuclear leukocytes, hemorrhage, and necrosis. Many trophozoites are present in

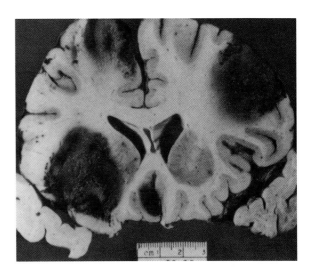

FIG. 23. Granulomatous amebic encephalitis. Coronal section showing multifocal areas of encephalomalacia in cerebral cortex, subcortical white matter, and basal ganglia. (From ref. 134, with permission.)

subarachnoid and perivascular spaces, although identification can be difficult because fixed trophozoites resemble host cells. Fluorescent antibodies can be used to positively identify amebae. Cysts and flagellate forms are not seen in sections of tissue infected by *N. fowleri* (186). Demyelination may be seen, even at a distance from amebae or inflammation, possibly because of the action of phospholipases or other enzymes elaborated by the protozoa (140).

Organs other than the CNS are usually unaffected in PAM, but myocarditis may occur (191,192). In one patient who died of meningoencephalitis and pulmonary edema, acute diffuse myocarditis was present (191). Although myocarditis appeared to be directly related to the patient's *Naegleria* infection, no amebas could be found in the inflamed areas of the heart (191). Markowitz et al. (192) found focal or diffuse myocarditis in seven of 16 (44%) cases of PAM (including the case above), whereas myocarditis was present in only two of 20 (10%) controls who died of bacterial meningitis or subarachnoid hemorrhage. The pathogenesis of myocarditis in PAM is uncertain, because no amebae were found in any of these cases despite a careful search (192).

Infection by *Acanthamoeba* can cause acute meningitis like *N. fowleri*, but more commonly *Acanthamoeba* causes focal GAE, or single or multiple brain abscesses. On inspection, a focal inflammatory mass or abscess(es) may be seen (Fig. 23). Histology shows granulomatous inflammation with mononuclear cells, histiocytes, and giant cells (134,186). Necrotizing vasculitis occurs, resulting from invasion of arterial walls by trophozoites (134,189). In one case, the inflammatory response to invasion of arterial walls by amebae led to the formation of mycotic aneurysms at the base of the brain (186).

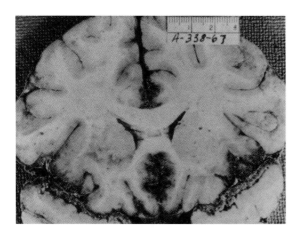

FIG. 22. Acute primary amebic meningoencephalitis caused by *N. fowleri*. Coronal section showing distribution of the most severe lesions, primarily in the basal meninges and adjacent cortex. (From ref. 134, with permission.)

Cysts are occasionally found in CNS tissue in GAE (186,188), but in most cases they are much less numerous than trophozoites (154). In one patient, a previously healthy 7-year-old girl with GAE, only cysts were found (193). In addition to the usual mononuclear and histiocytic granulomatous reaction with giant cells, the biopsy in this case showed a striking radial alignment of histiocytes around *Acanthamoeba* cysts (193).

Although the CNS and corneas are preferentially involved, disseminated infection has been reported (135,194); this seems most likely to occur in immunosuppressed patients. Amebae were recovered from brain, lung, lymph nodes, adrenals, and other tissues of a renal transplant recipient (194). Three cases have been reported in AIDS patients (135).

Clinical Manifestations

The acute form of PAM presents with sudden onset of high fever, photophobia, headache, and progression to stupor or coma, especially in a child who has been swimming in warm fresh waters. The initial presentation usually is indistinguishable from acute bacterial meningitis. Focal signs are more common than in bacterial meningitis, and seizures are common. Because the olfactory area is usually first involved, early symptoms of abnormal smell or taste sensation may be reported (140). Confusion, irritability, and restlessness progress to delirium, stupor, and, finally, coma. In most cases the patient is diagnosed as having bacterial meningitis with negative Gram stain, and he or she is treated with antibiotics. However, there is no response to treatment, and the patient deteriorates, often surviving only 2–4 days (143). Herniation of the brainstem is a common terminal event.

Subacute or chronic PAM (including GAE) presents more insidiously, with subacute or gradual onset of symptoms suggesting a brain tumor or abscess. Low-grade fever, headache, and focal signs are found. The patient usually deteriorates over a period of 2–4 weeks until death. Longer duration has been reported: One child was ill for 5 months (153) and another for 6 months (154) before death. Cleland et al. (195) reported a patient who survived for at least 18 months after diagnosis.

Acanthamoeba keratitis, first described in 1973, has been diagnosed with increased frequency since 1985 (196). Stehr-Green et al. (196), reviewing 208 cases reported to 1988, found that 85% of the patients wore contact lenses, mostly soft, extended-wear lenses which were kept in home-made saline solutions. This ocular infection is difficult to diagnose, often being confused with herpes keratitis (133). It is also difficult to treat, being likely to relapse after drug treatment or corneal grafting (133,197). Penetrating keratoplasty is needed for cure (133). Rarely, the amebae can spread intracranially from the eye to cause GAE (169).

Diagnosis

The key initial investigation in patients with acute PAM is usually a spinal tap for CSF examination. At first sight, the CSF appears to be consistent with the clinical syndrome of acute bacterial meningitis, showing leukocytosis with neutrophil predominance, low glucose, elevated protein concentration, and red blood cells. However, the Gram stain is always negative. If PAM is suspected before death, examination of fresh, warm specimens of CSF can reveal the ameboid movements of the motile trophozoites. After death, trophozoites can be demonstrated in the brain, by light or electron microscopy.

Patients with subacute or chronic PAM caused by *Acanthamoeba* or other species show a less florid inflammatory response in the CSF. Opening pressure is usually elevated, as is the protein concentration. The glucose concentration is often normal or only slightly reduced, whereas leukocytes are present in only low or moderate numbers. The majority of leukocytes present are mononuclear cells. No trophozoites are found in CSF in this form of PAM. Computerized tomographic scanning or magnetic resonance imaging shows focal lesions.

The main differential diagnosis for acute PAM is acute bacterial meningitis with negative Gram stain and culture, a condition which is much more common than PAM. Another diagnostic possibility is brain abscess with rupture into the CSF. Because the disease is rare and because amebae can be difficult to identify in fixed specimens, some cases of PAM undoubtedly must have been misclassified over the years as acute meningitis, or as meningoencephalitis, of undetermined etiology (198).

The differential diagnosis for subacute and chronic PAM is much wider, because it can present features of focal brain lesions as well as meningitis. It includes brain abscess, benign and malignant tumors, subacute and chronic meningitis, encephalitis, fungal infections, stroke, arteritis, and many other CNS conditions. For example, one case of GAE masqueraded as neurocysticercosis (153).

Because amebae are not found in CSF in GAE, specific diagnosis usually requires examination of a biopsy or necropsy specimen. Even then, the diagnosis is likely to be missed unless the pathologist is alerted in advance to consider this rare condition. This is illustrated by the fact that pathologic diagnoses of PAM often are made only in retrospect, sometimes years after the patient has died (132,155). In such cases, definitive speciation of the etiologic amebae is difficult or impossible (188).

Treatment

Free-living amebae are inhibited by a variety of antimicrobial agents and other drugs. Amphotericin B, tetracyclines, imidazoles (199), qinghaosu (200), and rifampin all are active *in vitro.* Amphotericin B is amebicidal for *N. fowleri* at low concentrations (201), but it is much less active against *Acanthamoeba.* Phenothiazines are amebicidal *in vitro* at concentrations of 100 μM, and it is amebastatic at lower doses; the mechanism of action is unknown (202). Trimethoprim is inhibitory for avirulent strains of *N. fowleri,* but it is inactive against virulent strains (203).

Only three or four patients have survived after treatment for acute PAM (204). All received amphotericin B, as well as various other antimicrobial agents. The best-documented survivor received amphotericin B and miconazole intravenously and intrathecally, rifampin, sulfizoxazole, and dexamethasone (204).

The optimal drug regimen for PAM is currently unknown; clearly, however, amphotericin B should be included. The authors' suggestion is to treat acute PAM with amphotericin B parenterally at maximum tolerated dosage, together with intracisternal injection of amphotericin B and concomitant administration of rifampin and tetracycline. Addition of experimental therapies such as phenothiazine (202) or qinghaosu (200) may be justified on the grounds that no effective regimen has been established.

Prognosis

Almost all patients with PAM die of the disease. Many are undiagnosed before death, whereas others die despite treatment. As noted above, the fact that there were four survivors indicates that aggressive treatment with amphotericin B and other drugs is warranted (204).

Because of its slower course, subacute or chronic PAM provides greater opportunity for antemortem diagnosis by brain biopsy, as well as for attempted treatment. There is no proven effective treatment other than surgical excision of focal granulomatous encephalitis or abscess. A previously healthy 7-year-old girl recovered from GAE after excision of a large inflammatory mass from the parietal lobe, followed by treatment with amphotericin B and ketoconazole (193). Callicott et al. (205) reported one patient with acute meningitis due to *Acanthamoeba* who recovered completely without receiving any therapy active against amebae.

Further research to discover effective antiamebic therapy and to define the optimal treatment regimens is needed.

Prevention

The primary means of prevention is to avoid swimming in contaminated fresh water containing free-living amebae. This is difficult to achieve, because children living in hot climates love to swim and dive in any available body of water. Education of children to reduce certain behaviors (such as jumping into water upright from a height) that might force large quantities of water into the nasal cavity under pressure has been attempted (134). Use of nose clips to reduce inhalation of water has been advocated. Public swimming pools and potable water supplies require monitoring for adequate chlorination. No method of prophylaxis with antimicrobials is known, nor is it needed because this disease is so rare. No effective vaccine has been produced.

CEREBRAL AMEBIASIS

Entamoeba histolytica is a common intestinal parasite of humans living in endemic areas. *E. histolytica* trophozoites colonize the large bowel, and they differentiate into cysts which pass in the feces. Commensal infections [called "luminal amebiasis" (206)] are common, being recognized by identification of trophozoites or cysts in stool of asymptomatic persons. Invasion of the colonic wall by trophozoites causes amebic dysentery (also called "invasive amebiasis"), associated with flask-shaped ulcers burrowing into the mucosa. The motile, histotoxic amebae actively destroy tissue and characteristically ingest red cells, a feature which assists in their identification by microscopy. The amebae can invade beyond the bowel wall, causing hepatic abscesses in a subgroup of patients. Less commonly, amebic abscesses develop in the lung or at other sites, including the CNS.

Orbison et al. (207) reviewed the chronology of medical recognition of cerebral amebiasis. The first observation of a brain abscess associated with a tropical liver abscess was made in 1838. The first demonstration of amebae in a brain abscess was reported in 1904. A study of 45 cases, with extensive clinical data, was published by Legrand in 1912 (207a). In 1951, Orbison et al. (207) reviewed a total of 88 cases from their personal experience and from the literature. They emphasized that only 27 (31%) of these cases were proven by direct demonstration of amebae in CNS tissue.

Epidemiology

Walsh (208) estimated that in any one year about 480 million people are infected with *E. histolytica.* The majority remain asymptomatic or have only mild symptoms of colitis, but about 36 million (8%) develop disabling colitis or extraintestinal abscesses. Although the death rate is only about 0.1% among these patients, amebiasis is so common that it causes about 40,000 deaths annually. If these estimates are correct, amebiasis is third in importance to malaria and schistomiasis as a cause of death worldwide (208).

Liver abscess is the most common extraintestinal lesion, occurring in up to 10% in necropsy series of patients with intestinal amebiasis, confirmed at necropsy.

The true incidence of hepatic abscess is, of course, much lower in the majority of patients with intestinal amebiasis, who do not come to necropsy. The lungs and pleura are next in frequency as sites of extraintestinal involvement. Amebic brain abscesses occur in less than 10% of patients with hepatic abscesses. The incidence has been reported to range from 0.7% to 8% in various studies (207,209). Thus, most patients with amebic liver abscess do not have a brain abscess; conversely, most patients with an amebic abscess of the CNS also have hepatic amebiasis. In 17 cases of amebic brain abscess reported by Lombardo et al. (209), all 17 had a liver abscess, and eight had a lung abscess. Orbison et al. (207) reviewed six cases of proven or probable amebic brain abscess that apparently occurred in isolation, in patients who did not have extraintestinal disease elsewhere.

Cerebral amebiasis occurs only in patients who have had intestinal infection. The patient must have previously ingested E. histolytica cysts while visiting or living in an endemic area. Intestinal amebiasis is endemic in the southern United States, but with low prevalence. Therefore, most patients presenting in this country with invasive amebiasis have a history of travel to an area such as Mexico, Latin America, Southeast Asia, Africa, or other areas where the intestinal infection is common. Sixty to 90 percent of patients have a history of previous amebic dysentery (207). The reported frequency of concurrent active colitis in patients with cerebral amebiasis is variable, from none of 17 cases in one series (209) to all of four in another (210).

Most patients with amebic brain abscess are young adults between 20 and 40 years of age (207,209). As in the case of liver abscess, males are affected much more frequently than females, in a ratio of 10–20 to 1. The reason for male predominance among patients with extraintestinal amebiasis is unknown.

Pathogenesis and Pathology

Amebic infection of the CNS originates from the colon, but the route by which trophozoites reach the CNS is not proven. The fact that cerebral amebic abscesses are frequently multiple, and located at the gray-matter-white-matter junction, strongly favors spread to the CNS via the bloodstream (207,210). Once in the CNS, the histotoxic and phagocytic properties of this invasive amebae produce destructive focal lesions. The cerebral hemispheres are most often involved, but cerebellar lesions are fairly common; the brainstem is hardly ever involved (207,209).

At necropsy, the brain is often swollen as a result of local or generalized cerebral edema, and terminal brain herniation may have occurred. Areas of focal meningitis can be seen overlying lesions which reach the surface (210), and generalized meningitis sometimes occurs

(209). On inspection, the cut surface of the brain shows focal, rounded lesions with irregular, poorly demarcated margins surrounding central necrotic tissue (Fig. 24). These lesions vary in size from 2 to 60 mm in diameter, and the number of lesions varies from one to 20. In one series, four of 17 (24%) brain abscesses were single (209). These lesions are frequently hemorrhagic, with varying degrees of peripheral edema (210).

Although these lesions are usually called "abscesses," they are quite distinct from a fully developed bacterial abscess, which has a rind of connective tissue surrounding a central cavity full of pus. In cerebral amebiasis, the center of the "abscess" is frequently not pus but rather gray, brown, or hemorrhagic necrotic tissue (210). In some cases, a true cavity containing liquid pus forms. Instead of a fibrous wall, the inner wall of the cavity is rough and ragged as a result of necrosis, lined with small shreds and scraps of dead tissue. In more chronic cases, a fibrous capsule begins to form. Rupture into the ventricular system can occur.

Histologically, the necrotic center shows an amorphous granular appearance. The wall of the lesion shows cellular infiltration of mononuclear cells, compound granular cells (Gitter cells), lymphocytes, plasma cells, and red blood cells. Amebae may be identified, but they may be easily missed if the pathologist is not alert to this diagnosis. In longer-lasting cases, granulation tissue with fibroblasts is found in the wall. Several authors have commented that the degree of inflammation seems relatively minor, compared with the extent of necrosis (209,210).

Clinical Manifestations

Patients with cerebral amebiasis may present with various combinations of findings. In addition to sys-

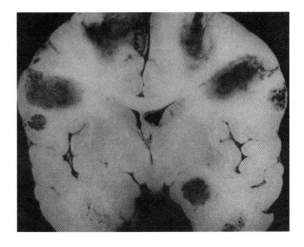

FIG. 24. Cerebral amebiasis. Coronal section of the brain showing multiple focal, hemorrhagic, necrotic lesions. Trophozoites of E. histolytica were seen on sections stained with periodic acid–Schiff stain. (From ref. 210, with permission.)

temic symptoms of infection and the manifestations of focal intracranial inflammatory lesions, there may be findings of invasive amebiasis elsewhere, especially in the liver and possibly in the lungs or colon. In the series of 17 cases reported by Lombardo et al. (209), fever occurred in 71%, loss of weight occurred in 65%, and anorexia occurred in 53%. Gastrointestinal symptoms were very common: Abdominal pain and hepatomegaly occurred in 65% of the patients, and diarrhea occurred in 53%. Respiratory symptoms were also common, with dyspnea and pleural effusion occurring in 65% of the patients, cough occurring in 53%, and hemoptysis occurring in 24%. Neurologic symptoms include headache, vomiting, meningeal signs, lethargy, seizures, and stupor progressing to coma.

Diagnosis

The presence of a focal CNS lesion in a febrile patient with hepatic or intestinal findings should suggest the possibility of cerebral amebiasis, especially if history of travel to an endemic area is obtained. In the absence of these clues, the patient will probably be diagnosed at first as having a bacterial brain abscess or possible brain tumor. The CSF may be normal, or it may show nonspecific changes (210). The serologic test for antiamebic antibodies is likely to be positive, because most of the patients have a concomitant liver abscess (206). It is not known whether patients with isolated cerebral amebiasis would have positive serology, because this condition is so rare. Imaging of brain, liver, and lungs will be important in establishing the diagnosis and in determining the extent of intracranial and extracranial disease.

Treatment and Prognosis

Up to the present, nearly all reported patients with cerebral amebiasis have died (207,209,210). It is likely that prompt treatment with metronidazole coupled with surgical aspiration and/or excision of accessible lesions will save some patients in the future. Metronidazole should be the drug of choice, because it is highly active against amebae and penetrates well into the CNS (206). However, as with other forms of brain abscess, aspiration or surgical excision is probably essential for optimal management. For prevention of cerebral amebiasis, the following measures should be taken: (a) eradication of intestinal amebiasis by drug therapy and (b) maintenance of a high level of sanitation to prevent ingestion of fecal cysts.

REFERENCES

1. Wyler DJ. Malaria-resurgence, resistance, and research. *N Engl J Med* 1983;308:875-878, 934-938.
2. Daroff RB, Deller JJ Jr, Kastl AJ Jr, Blocker WW Jr. Cerebral malaria. *JAMA* 1967;202:679-682.
3. Chongsuphajaisiddhi T, Gilles CHM, Krogstad DJ, et al. Severe and complicated malaria. *Trans R Soc Trop Med Hyg* 1986;80:3-51.
4. Bruce-Chwatt LJ. Malaria in African infants and children in southern Nigeria. *Ann Trop Med Parasitol* 1952;46:173-200.
5. White NJ, Miller KD, Churchill FC, et al. Chloroquine treatment of severe malaria in children. Pharmacokinetics, toxicity, and new dosage recommendations. *N Engl J Med* 1988;319:1493-1540.
6. Warrell DA, Looareesuwan S, Warrell MJ, et al. Dexamethasone proves deleterious in cerebral malaria. A double-blind trial in 100 comatose patients. *N Engl J Med* 1982;306:313-319.
7. Buck RL, Alcantara AK, Uylangco CV, Cross JH. Malaria at San Lazaro Hospital, Manila, Philippines, 1979-1981. *Am J Trop Med Hyg* 1983;32:212-216.
8. Spitz S. The pathology of acute *falciparum* malaria. *Milit Surg* 1946;99:555-572.
9. Yoeli M. Cerebral malaria—the quest for suitable experimental models in parasitic diseases of man. *Trans R Soc Trop Med Hyg* 1976;70:24-35.
10. Aikawa M. Human cerebral malaria. *Am J Trop Med Hyg* 1988;39:3-10.
11. Sachdev HS, Mohan M. *Vivax* cerebral malaria. *J Trop Pediatr* 1985;31:213-215.
12. Verma KC, Magotra ML. *Vivax* cerebral malaria in Jammu. *Indian Pediatr* 1976;112:229-231.
13. Dhayagude RG, Purandare NM. Autopsy study of cerebral malaria with special reference to malarial granuloma. *Arch Pathol* 1943;36:550-558.
14. Gilles HM. The differential diagnosis of malaria. In: Wernsdorfer WH, McGregor I, eds. *Malaria: principles and practice of malariology.* Edinburgh: Churchill Livingstone, 1988;769-780.
15. Boonpucknavig V, Boonpucknavig S. The histopathology of malaria. In: Wernsdorfer WH, McGregor I, eds. *Malaria: principles and practice of malariology.* Edinburgh: Churchill Livingstone, 1988;673-708.
16. White NJ, Warrell DA. The management of severe malaria. In: Wernsdorfer WH, McGregor I, eds. *Malaria: principles and practice of malariology.* Edinburgh: Churchill Livingstone, 1988;865-888.
17. Bruce-Chwatt LJ. *Essential malariology,* 2nd ed. New York: John Wiley & Sons, 1985.
18. Edington GM. Pathology of malaria in west Africa. *Br Med J* 1967;March 25:715-718.
19. Bruce-Chwatt LJ. Malaria. In: Jellife DB, Stanfield JP, eds. *Diseases of children in the subtropics and tropics,* 3rd ed. London: Edward Arnold, 1978;827-856.
20. Hendrickse RG, Hasan AH, Olumide LO, Akinkunmi A. Malaria in early childhood. *Ann Trop Med Parasitol* 1971;65:1-20.
21. Molineaux L, Gramiccia G. *The Garki Project: research on the epidemiology and control of malaria in the Sudan savanna of west Africa.* Geneva: World Health Organization, 1980.
22. Hendrickse RG, King MAR. Anaemia of uncertain origin in infancy. *Br Med J* 1958;2:662-669.
23. Harinasuta T, Bunnag D. The clinical features of malaria. In: Wernsdorfer WH, McGregor I, eds. *Malaria: principles and practice of malariology.* Edinburgh: Churchill Livingstone, 1988;709-734.
24. Gautam OP, Thawrani YP, Mathur PS. Pattern of malaria in children and its therapeutic evaluation. *Indian Pediatr* 1980;17:511-514.
25. Murray MJ, Murray NJ, Murray AB, Murray MB. Refeeding-malaria and hyperferraemia. *Lancet* 1975;1:653-654.
26. Murray MJ, Murray MB, Murray AB, Murray CJ. Somali food shelters in the Ogaden famine and their impact on health. *Lancet* 1976;1:1283-1285.
27. McGregor IA. Malaria and nutrition. In: Wernsdorfer WH, McGregor I, eds. *Malaria: principles and practice of malariology,* 1st ed. Edinburgh: Churchill Livingstone, 1988;753-767.
28. Murray MJ, Murray AB, Murray NJ, Murray MB. Cerebral malaria, hyperferremia and folate deficiency [Abstract]. *Am Soc Clin Nutr* Atlantic City, New Jersey. May 3, 1975; 475A.

29. Dutta P, Pinto J, Rivlin R. Antimalarial effects of riboflavin deficiency. *Lancet* 1985;2:1040–1043.
30. Anonymous. Riboflavin deficiency inhibits multiplication of malarial parasites. *Nutr Rev* 1984;42:195–196.
31. Greenberg AE, Lobel HO. Mortality from *Plasmodium falciparum* malaria in travelers from the United States, 1959 to 1987. *Ann Intern Med* 1990;113:326–327.
32. Aikawa M, Iseki M, Barnwell JW, Taylor D, Oo MM, Howard RJ. The pathology of human cerebral malaria. *Am J Trop Med Hyg* 1990;43:30–37.
33. Cox FEG. Major animal models in malaria research: rodent. In: Wernsdorfer WH, McGregor I, eds. *Malaria: principles and practice of malariology*, 1st ed. Edinburgh: Churchill Livingstone, 1988;1503–1543.
34. Collins WE. Major animal models in malaria research: simian. In: Wernsdorfer WH, McGregor I, eds. *Malaria: principles and practice of malariology*, 1st ed. Edinburgh: Churchill Livingstone, 1988;1473–1501.
35. Clark HC, Tomlinson WJ. The pathologic anatomy of malaria. In: Boyd MF, ed. *Malariology. A comprehensive survey of all aspects of this group of diseases from a global standpoint*. Philadelphia: WB Saunders, 1949;874–903.
36. Thomas JD. Clinical and histopathological correlation of cerebral malaria. *Trop Geogr Med* 1971;23:232–238.
37. Oo MM, Aikawa M, Than T, et al. Human cerebral malaria: a pathological study. *J Neuropathol Exp Neurol* 1987;46:223–231.
38. Winslow DJ, Connor DH, Sprinz H. Malaria. In: Marcial-Rojas RA, ed. *Pathology of protozoal and helminthic diseases with clinical correlation*, 2nd ed. Huntington, NY: Robert E Krieger, 1975;195–224.
39. Kreier JP. *Malaria, vol 2: Pathology, vector studies, and culture*. New York: Academic Press, 1980.
40. Oo MM, Than T. Pathogenesis of ring-haemorrhage in cerebral malaria. *Ann Trop Med Parasitol* 1989;83:555–557.
41. MacPherson GG, Warrell MJ, White NJ, Looareesuwan S, Warrell DA. Human cerebral malaria. A quantitative ultrastructural analysis of parasitized erythrocyte sequestration. *Am J Pathol* 1985;119:385–401.
42. Fletcher KA, Gilles HM. The chemical pathology of malaria. In: Wernsdorfer WH, McGregor I, eds. *Malaria: principles and practice of malariology*. Edinburgh: Churchill Livingstone, 1988;647–672.
43. Houba V. Specific immunity, immunopathology and immunosuppression. In: Wernsdorfer WH, McGregor I, eds. *Malaria: principles and practice of malariology*. Edinburgh: Churchill Livingstone, 1988;621–638.
44. Dayal-Drager R, Lambert P-H. Plasmodial antigens implicated in stage-specific immune protection. In: Wernsdorfer WH, McGregor I, eds. *Malaria: principles and practice of malariology*, 1st ed. Edinburgh: Churchill Livingstone, 1988;1675–1720.
45. Aikawa M. Fine structure of malaria parasites in the various stages of development. In: Wernsdorfer WH, McGregor I, eds. *Malaria: principles and practice of malariology*, 1st ed. Edinburgh: Churchill Livingstone, 1988;97–129.
46. Udomsangpetch R, Aikawa M, Berzins K, Wahlgren M, Perlmann P. Cytoadherence of knobless *Plasmodium falciparum*-infected erythrocytes and its inhibition by a human monoclonal antibody. *Nature* 1989;338:763–765.
47. Chulay JD, Ockenhouse CF. Host receptors for malaria-infected erythrocytes. *Am J Trop Med Hyg* 1990;43:6–14.
48. Barnwell JW. Minireview. Cytoadherence and sequestration in *falciparum* malaria. *Exp Parasitol* 1989;69:407–412.
49. Barnwell JW, Asch AS, Nachman RL, Yamaya M, Aikawa M, Ingravallo P. A human 88-kD membrane glycoprotein (CD36) functions *in vitro* as a receptor for a cytoadherence ligand on *Plasmodium falciparum*-infected erythrocytes. *J Clin Invest* 1989;84:765–772.
50. Howard RJ, Handunnetti SM, Hasler T, et al. Surface molecules on *Plasmodium falciparum*-infected erythrocytes involved in adherence. *Am J Trop Med Hyg* 1990;43:15–29.
51. Leech JH, Barnwell JW, Miller LH, Howard RJ. Identification of a strain-specific malarial antigen exposed on the surface of *Plasmodium falciparum*-infected erythrocytes. *J Exp Med* 1984;159:1567–1575.
52. Howard RJ, Barnwell JW, Rock EP, et al. Two approximately 300 kilodalton *Plasmodium falciparum* proteins at the surface membrane of infected erythrocytes. *Mol Biochem Parasitol* 1988;27:207–223.
53. Knowles DMII, Tolidjian B, Marboe C, D'Agati V, Grimes M, Chess L. Monoclonal anti-human monocyte antibodies OKM1 and OKM5 possess distinctive tissue distributions including differential reactivity with vascular endothelium. *J Immunol* 1984;132:2170.
54. Looareesuwan S, Warrell DA, White NJ, et al. Do patients with cerebral malaria have cerebral oedema? A computed tomography study. *Lancet* 1983;1:434–437.
55. White NJ, Looareesuwan S, Phillips RE, Warrell DA, Chanthavanich P, Pongpaew P. Pathophysiological and prognostic significance of cerebrospinal-fluid lactate in cerebral malaria. *Lancet* 1985;1:776–778.
56. Warrell DA, Veall N, Chanthavanich P, et al. Cerebral anaerobic glycolysis and reduced cerebral oxygen transport in human cerebral malaria. *Lancet* 1988;2:534–537.
57. Wright DH. The effect of neonatal thymectomy on the survival of golden hamsters infected with *Plasmodium berghei*. *Br J Exp Pathol* 1968;49:379.
58. Wright DH, Masembe RM, Bazira ER. The effect of antithymocyte serum on golden hamsters and rats infected with *Plasmodium berghei*. *Br J Exp Pathol* 1971;52:465.
59. McGregor IA, Wilson RJM. Specific immunity: acquired in man. In: Wernsdorfer WH, McGregor IA, eds. *Malaria: principles and practice of malariology*, 1st ed. Edinburgh: Churchill Livingstone, 1988;559–620.
60. Molyneux M. Cerebral malaria in children: clinical implications of cytoadherence. *Am J Trop Med Hyg* 1990;43:38–41.
61. Stone WJ, Hanchett JE, Knepshield JH. Acute renal insufficiency due to *falciparum* malaria. *Arch Intern Med* 1972;129:620.
62. White NJ, Warrell DA, Chanthavanich P, et al. Severe hypoglycemia and hyperinsulinemia in *falciparum* malaria. *N Engl J Med* 1983;61:66.
63. Kawo NG, Msengi AE, Swai AB, Chuwa LM, Alberti KG, McLarty DG. Specificity of hypoglycemia for cerebral malaria in children. *Lancet* 1990;336:454–457.
64. Taylor TE, Molyneux ME, Wirima JJ, Fletcher KA, Morris K. Blood glucose levels in Malawian children before and during the administration of intravenous quinine for severe *falciparum* malaria. *N Engl J Med* 1988;319:1040–1047.
65. Tubbs H. Endotoxin in human and murine malaria. *Trans R Soc Trop Med Hyg* 1980;74:121–123.
66. Kyaw-Zaw A, Maung-U K, Thwe M. Endotoxaemia in complicated *falciparum* malaria. *Trans R Soc Trop Med Hyg* 1988;82:513–514.
67. Clarke IA. Correlation between susceptibility to malaria and babesia parasites and endotoxicity. *Trans R Soc Trop Med Hyg* 1982;76:4.
68. Usawattanakul W, Tharavanij S, Warrell DA, et al. Factors contributing to the development of cerebral malaria. II. Endotoxin. *Clin Exp Immunol* 1985;61:562–568.
69. Chongsuphajaisiddhi T. Malaria in paediatric practice. In: Wernsdorfer WH, McGregor I, eds. *Malaria: principles and practice of malariology*. Edinburgh: Churchill Livingstone, 1988;889–902.
70. Marsden PD, Bruce-Chwatt LJ. Cerebral malaria. *Contemp Neurol Ser* 1975;12:29–44.
71. Olurin O. Cortical blindness following convulsions and fever in Nigerian children. *Pediatrics* 1970;46:102–107.
72. Centers for Disease Control. Recommendations for the prevention of malaria among travelers. *MMWR* 1990;39:1–10.
73. Miller KD, Greenberg AE, Campbell CC. Treatment of severe malaria in the United States with a continuous infusion of quinidine gluconate and exchange transfusion. *N Engl J Med* 1989;321:66–70.
74. Salako LA, Sowunmi A, Laoye OJ. Evaluation of the sensitivity *in vivo* and *in vitro* of *Plasmodium falciparum* malaria to quinine in an area of full sensitivity to chloroquine. *Trans R Soc Trop Med Hyg* 1988;82:366–368.
75. Zimmerman WJ, Steele JH, Kagan I. Trichinosis in the U.S. population, 1966–1970. *Public Health Rep* 1973;88:606–623.

76. White NJ, Looareesuwan S, Warrell DA, et al. Quinine loading dose in cerebral malaria. *Am J Trop Med Hyg* 1983;32:1–5.
77. Foulkes JR. Human trypanosomiasis in Africa. *Br Med J* 1981;283:1172–1174.
78. Beaver PC, Jung RC, Cupp EW. The blood and tissue flagellates. In: *Clinical Parasitology.* Philadelphia: Lea & Febiger, 1984;55–100.
79. Spencer HC. Trypanosomiasis. In: Strickland GT, ed. *Hunter's tropical medicine,* 6th ed. Philadelphia: WB Saunders, 1984;553–564.
80. Poltera AA. Pathology of human African trypanosomiasis with reference to experimental African trypanosomiasis and infections of the central nervous system. *Br Med Bull* 1985;41:169–174.
81. Hajduk SL, Englund PT, Smith DH. African trypanosomiasis. In: Warren KS, Mahmoud AAF, eds. *Tropical and Geographical Medicine,* 2nd ed. New York: McGraw-Hill, 1990;268–281.
82. Kuzoe FA. Current knowledge on epidemiology and control of sleeping sickness. *Ann Soc Belg Med Trop* 1989;69:217–220.
83. Wellde BT, Chumo DA, Reardon MJ, et al. Epidemiology of Rhodesian sleeping sickness in the Lambwe Valley, Kenya. *Ann Trop Med Parasitol* 1989;83:43–62.
84. Power J. Sleeping sickness research and control. In: Not Given, ed. *TDR News.* Not given: Not given, 1989;3.
85. Wellde BT, Reardon MJ, Chumo DA, et al. Demographic characteristics of the Lambwe Valley population. *Ann Trop Med Parasitol* 1989;83:29–42.
86. Wellde BT, Chumo DA, Hockmeyer WT, et al. Sleeping sickness in the Lambewe Valley in 1978. *Ann Trop Med Parasitol* 1989;83:21–27.
87. Wellde BT, Chumo DA, Reardon MJ, et al. Presenting features of Rhodesian sleeping sickness patients in the Lambwe Valley, Kenya. *Ann Trop Med Parasitol* 1989;83:73–89.
87a. Veeken HJG, Ebeling, MCA, Dolmans WMV. Tripanosomiasis in a rural hospital in Tanzania. *Trop Geogr Med* 1989;41:113–117.
88. Thomson KDB. The present sleeping sickness situation in the northern states of Nigeria. *J Trop Med Hyg* 1969;72:27–32.
89. Weir AB, Agbowu J, Ajayi N. Hyperendemic West African trypanosomiasis in a rural hospital setting. *J Trop Med Hyg* 1985;88:307–311.
90. Edeghere H, Olise PO, Olatunde DS. Human African trypanosomiasis (sleeping sickness): new endemic foci Bendel State, Nigeria. *Trop Med Parasitol* 1989;40:16–20.
91. Calwell HG. The pathology of the brain in Rhodesian trypanosomiasis. *Trans R Soc Trop Med Hyg* 1937;30:611–624.
92. Manuelidis EE, Robertson DHH, Amberson JM, Polak M, Haymaker W. *Trypanosoma rhodesiense* encephalitis. Clinicopathological study of five cases of encephalitis and one of mel B hemorrhagic encephalopathy. *Acta Neuropathol* 1965;5:176–204.
93. Poltera AA, Owor R, Cox JN. Pathological aspects of human African trypanosomiasis (HAT) in Uganda. A post-mortem survey of fourteen cases. *Virchows Arch* 1976;373:249–265.
94. de Raadt P, Atayi L, Adams H, et al. Informal meeting on the pathology of African trypanosomiasis. *TDR/WHO* Abidjan, Ivory Coast, Sep. 12–16, 1983.
95. Adams JH, Haller L, Boa FY, Doua F, Dago A, Konian K. Human African trypanosomiasis (*T. b. gambiense*): a study of 16 fatal cases of sleeping sickness with some observations on acute reactive arsenical encephalopathy. *Neuropathol Appl Neurobiol* 1986;12:81–94.
96. Mulumba PM, Wery M. Experimental infection with two stocks of *Trypanosoma brucei gambiense.* Study of the evolution by elution techniques of tissues. *Contrib Microbiol Immunol* 1983;7:120–129.
97. Rudin W, Poltera AA, Jenni L. An EM study on cerebral trypanosomiasis in rodents and primates. *Contrib Microbiol Immunol* 1983;7:165–172.
98. Fink E, Sayer P, Schmidt H. IgG and IgM—levels in serum and CSF of *T. rhodesiense*-infected vervet monkeys. *Contrib Microbiol Immunol* 1983;7:183–189.
99. Greenwood BM, Whittle HC. The pathogenesis of sleeping sickness. *Trans R Soc Trop Med Hyg* 1980;74:716–725.
100. Smith DH, Dailey JW, Wellde BT. Immunodiagnostic tests on cerebrospinal fluid in the diagnosis of meningoencephalitic *Try-*
101. Asonganyi T, Lando G, Ngu JL. Serum antibodies against human brain myelin proteins in Gambian trypanosomiasis. *Ann Soc Belg Med Trop* 1989;69:213–221.
102. Seed JR, Hall JE, Price CC. A physiological mechanism to explain pathogenesis in African trypanosomiasis. *Contrib Microbiol Immunol* 1983;7:83–94.
103. Poltera AA. Immunopathological and chemotherapeutic studies in experimental trypanosomiasis with special reference to the heart and brain. *Trans R Soc Trop Med Hyg* 1980;74:706–715.
104. Bancroft GJ, Askonas BA. Immunobiology of African trypanosomiasis in laboratory rodents. In: Tizard I, ed. *Immunology and pathogenesis of trypanosomiasis,* 1st ed. Boca Raton, FL: CRC Press, 1985;75–101.
105. Boreham PFL. Autocoids: their release and possible role in the pathogenesis of African trypanosomiasis. In: Tizard I, ed. *Immunology and pathogenesis of trypanosomiasis,* 1st ed. Boca Raton, FL: CRC Press, 1985;45–66.
106. Lambo TA. Neuro-psychiatric syndromes associated with human trypanosomiasis in tropical Africa. *Acta Psychiatrica Scandinavia,* 1966;42:474–484.
107. Wellde BT, Chumo DA, Reardon MJ, et al. Diagnosis of Rhodesian sleeping sickness in the lambwe Valley (1980–1984). *Ann Trop Med Parasitol* 1989;83:63–71.
108. Cattand P, Miezan BT, de Raadt P. Human African trypanosomiasis: use of double centrifugation of cerebrospinal fluid to detect trypanosomes. *Bull WHO* 1988;66:83–86.
109. Van Meirvenne N, Le Ray D. Diagnosis of African and American trypanosomiases. *Br Med Bull* 1985;41:156–161.
110. Katende JM, Nantulya VM, Musoke AJ. Comparison between bloodstream and procyclic form trypanosomes for serological diagnosis of African human trypanosomiasis. *Trans R Soc Trop Med Hyg* 1987;81:607–608.
111. Gutteridge WE. Existing chemotherapy and its limitations. *Br Med Bull* 1985;41:162–168.
112. Arroz JOL. Short Report. Melarsoprol and reactive encephalopathy in *Trypanosoma brucei rhodesiense. Trans R Soc Trop Med Hyg* 1987;81:192–192.
113. Haller L, Adams H, Merouze F, Dago A. Clinical and pathological aspects of human African trypanosomiasis *T. b. gambiense* with particular reference to reactive arsenical encephalopathy. *Am Soc Trop Med Hyg* 1986;35:94–99.
114. McCann PP, Bitonti AJ, Bacchi CJ, Clarkson AB. Use of difluoromethylornithine (DFMO, eflornithine) for late-stage African trypanosomiasis. *Trans R Soc Trop Med Hyg* 1987;81:701–701.
115. Petru AM, Azimi PH, Cummins SK, Sjoersma A. African sleeping sickness in the United States. Successful treatment with eflornithine. *Am J Dis Child* 1988;142:224–228.
116. Pepin J, Milord F, Guern C, Schechter PJ. Difluoromethylornithine for arseno-resistant *Trypanosoma brucei gambiense* sleeping sickness. *Lancet* 1987;2:1431–1433.
117. Doua F, Boa FY, Schechter PJ, et al. Treatment of human late stage *gambiense* trypanosomiasis with alpha-difluoromethylornithine (eflornithine): efficacy and tolerance in 14 cases in Cote d'Ivoire. *Am J Trop Med Hyg* 1987;37:525–533.
118. Taelman H, Schechter PJ, Marcelis L, et al. Difluoromethylornithine, an effective new treatment of Gambian trypanosomiasis. *Am J Med* 1987;82:607–614.
119. Pittella JEH. Brain involvement in the chronic cardiac form of Chagas' disease. *J Trop Med Hyg* 1985;88:313–317.
120. Tanowitz HB, Brosnan C, Guastamacchio D, et al. Infection of organotypic cultures of spinal cord and dorsal root ganglia with *Trypanosoma cruzi. Am J Trop Med Hyg* 1982;31:1090–1097.
121. Spina-Franica A, Livramento JA, Machado LR, Yasuda N. *Trypanosoma cruzi* antibodies in the cerebrospinal fluid: a search using complement fixation and immunofluorescence reactions. *Arq Neuropsiquiatr* 1988;46:374–378.
122. Van Voorhis WC, Eisen H. F1-160. A surface antigen of *Trypanosoma cruzi* that mimics mammalian nervous tissue. *J Exp Med* 1989;169:641–652.
123. Petry K, Nudelman E, Eisen H, Hakomori S. Sulfated lipids represent common antigens on the surface of *Trypanosoma cruzi* and mammalian tissues. *Mol Biochem Parasitol* 1988;30:113–121.

124. Alengar AA, Freitas MR. Neuropathology of Chagas' disease. *Neurol Neurochir Psiquiatr (Mexico)* 1977;18:375–390.

125. De Queiroz AC. Tumor-like lesion of the brain caused by *Trypanosoma cruzi. Am J Trop Med Hyg* 1973;22:473–476.

126. Del Castillo M, Mendoza G, Oviedo J, Perez Bianco RP, Anselm AE, Silva M. AIDS and Chagas' disease with central nervous system tumor-like lesion. *Am J Med* 1990;88:693–694.

127. Leiguarda R, Roncoroni A, Taratuto AL, et al. Acute CNS infection by *Trypanosoma cruzi* (Chagas' disease) in immunosuppressed patients. *Neurology* 1990;40:850–851.

128. Jardim E, Takayanagui OM. Epilepsy and chronic Chagas' disease. *Arq Neuropsiquiatr* 1981;39:32–41.

129. Manson-Bahr PEC, Bell DR. American trypanosomiasis (Chagas' disease). In: Manson-Bahr PEC, Bell DR, eds. *Manson's tropical diseases,* 19th ed. London: Ballière Tindall, 1987;74–86.

130. Fowler M, Carter RF. Acute pyogenic meningitis probably due to *Acanthamoeba* sp.: a preliminary report. *Br Med J* 1965;740–742.

131. Robert VB, Rorke LB. Primary amebic encephalitis, probably *Acanthamoeba. Ann Intern Med* 1973;79:174–179.

132. Visvesvara GS, Martinez AJ, Schuster FL, et al. Leptomyxid ameba, a new agent of amebic meningoencephalitis in humans and animals. *J Clin Microbiol* 1990;28:2750–2756.

133. Cohen EJ, Buchanan HW, Laughrea PA, et al. Diagnosis and management of *Acanthamoeba* keratitis. *Am J Ophthalmol* 1985;100:389–395.

134. Martinez AJ. *Free-living amebas: natural history, prevention, diagnosis, pathology, and treatment of disease,* 1st ed. Boca Raton, Florida, FL: CRC Press, 1985.

135. Anzil AP, Rao C, Wrzolek A, Sher JH, Kozlowski PB. Acanthamebic meningoencephalitis in an AIDS patients—an autopsy report. *J Neuropathol Exp Neurol* 1989;48:313.

136. Martinez AJ. Acanthamoebiasis and immunosuppression. *J Neuropathol Exp Neurol* 1982;41:548–557.

137. Franke ED, Mackiewicz JS. Isolation of *Acanthamoeba* and *Naegleria* from the intestinal contents of freshwater fishes and their potential pathogenicity. *J Parasitol* 1982;68:164–166.

138. Marciano-Cabral F. Biology of *Naegleria* spp. *Microbiol Rev* 1988;52:114–133.

139. Visvesvara GS, Callaway CS. Light and electron microscopic observations on the pathogenesis of *Naegleria fowleri* in mouse brain and tissue culture. *J Protozool* 1990;21:239–250.

140. John DT. Primary amebic meningoencephalitis and the biology of *Naegleria fowleri. Annu Rev Microbiol* 1982;36:101–123.

141. Carter RF. Primary amoebic meningo-encephalitis. An appraisal of present knowledge. *Trans R Soc Trop Med Hyg* 1972;66:193–208.

142. Chang SL. Etiological, pathological, epidemiological, and diagnostical considerations of primary amoebic meningoencephalitis. *Crit Rev Microbiol* 1974;3:135–159.

143. Duma RJ. Primary amebic meningoencephalitis. In: Warren KS, Mahmoud AAF, eds. *Tropical and geographical medicine,* 2nd ed. New York: McGraw-Hill, 1990;321–326.

144. Newsome AL, Wilhelm WE. Inhibition of *Naegleria fowleri* by microbial iron-chelating agents: ecological implications. *Appl Environ Microbiol* 1983;45:665–668.

145. John DT, Cole TB Jr, Bruner RA. Amebostomes of *Naegleria fowleri. J Protozool* 1985;32:12–19.

146. Marciano-Cabral F, Cline M. Chemotaxis by *Naegleria fowleri* for bacteria. *J Protozool* 1987;34:127–131.

147. Thong YH, Ferrante A. Migration patterns of pathogenic and nonpathogenic *Naegleria* spp. *Infect Immun* 1986;51:177–180.

148. Mar J, Lee JH, Shea D, Walsh CJ. New poly(A) + RNAs appear coordinately during the differentiation of *Naegleria gruberi* amebae into flagellates. *J Cell Biol* 1986;102:353–361.

149. Fulton C, Cheng KL, Lai EY. Two calmodulins of *Naegleria* flagellates: characterization, intracellular segregation, and programmed regulation of mRNA abundance during differentiation. *J Cell Biol* 1986;102:1671–1678.

150. Schuster FL. Ultrastructure of cysts of *Naegleria* spp: a comparative study. *J Protozool* 1975;22:352–359.

151. Averner M, Fulton C. Carbon dioxide: signal for excystment of *Naegleria gruberi. J Gen Microb* 1966;42:245–255.

152. Visvesvara GS, Balamuth W. Comparative studies on related free-living and pathogenic amebae with special reference to *Acanthamoeba. J Protozool* 1975;22:245–256.

153. Matson DO, Rouah E, Lee D, Armstrong RT, Parke JT, Baker CJ. *Acanthamoeba* meningoencephalitis masquerading as neurocysticercosis. *Pediatr Infect Dis J* 1988;7:121–124.

154. Wessel HB, Hubbard J, Martinez AJ, Willaert E. Granulomatous amebic encephalitis (GAE) with prolonged clinical course, C.T. scan findings, diagnosis by brain biopsy, and effect of treatment [Abstract]. *Neurology* 1980;30:442.

155. Carter RF, Cullity GJ, Ojeda VJ, Silberstein P, Willaert E. A fatal case of meningoencephalitis due to a free-living ameba of uncertain identity-probably *Acanthamoeba* sp. *Pathology* 1981;13:51–68.

156. Cox EC. Amoebic meningoencephalitis caused by *Acanthamoeba* species in a four month old child. *JSC Med Assoc* 1980;76:459–462.

157. De Jonckherre J, van De Voorde H. The distribution of *Naegleria fowleri* in man-made thermal waters. *Am J Trop Med Hyg* 1977;26:10–15.

158. Griffin JL. The pathogenic amoeboflagellate *Naegleria fowleri:* environmental isolations, competitors, ecologic interactions, and the flagellate-empty habitat hypothesis. *J Protozool* 1983;30:403–409.

159. De Jonckheere J, Van Dijck P, van De Voorde H. The effect of thermal pollution on the distribution of *Naegleria fowleri. J Hyg* 1975;75:7–13.

160. Wang SS, Feldman HA. Isolation of *Hartmannella* species from human throats. *N Engl J Med* 1967;277:1174–1179.

161. Lawande RV, Abraham SN, John I, Egler LJ. Recovery of soil amebas from the nasal passages of children during the dusty harmattan period in Zaria. *Am J Clin Pathol* 1978;71:201–203.

162. Culbertson CG. Pathogenic *Acanthamoeba (Hartmanella). Am J Clin Pathol* 1961;35:195–202.

163. Phillips BP. *Naegleria:* another pathogenic ameba studies in germfree guinea pigs. *Am J Trop Med Hyg* 1974;23:850–855.

164. Dempe S, Martinez AJ, Janitschke K. Subacute and chronic meningoencephalitis in mice after experimental infection with a strain of *Naegleria fowleri* originally isolated from a patient. *Infection* 1982;10:5–8.

165. Martinez AJ, Duma RJ, Nelson EC, Moretta FL. Experimental *Naegleria* meningoencephalitis in mice. Penetration of the olfactory mucosal epithelium by *Naegleria* and pathologic changes produced: a light and electron microscope study. *Lab Invest* 1973;29:121–133.

166. Marciano-Cabral F, John DT. Cytopathogenicity of *Naegleria fowleri* for rat neuroblastoma cell cultures: scanning electron microscopy study. *Infect Immun* 1983;40:1214–1217.

167. Marciano-Cabral FM, Bradley SG. Cytopathogenicity of *Naegleria gruberi* for rat neuroblastoma cell cultures. *Infect Immun* 1982;35:1139–1141.

168. Fulford DE, Bradley SG, Marciano-Cabral F. Cytopathogenicity of *Naegleria fowleri* for cultured rat neuroblastoma cells. *J Protozool* 1985;32:176–180.

169. Jones DB, Visvesvara GS, Robinson NM. *Acanthamoeba polyphaga* keratitis and *Acanthamoeba* uveitis associated with fatal meningoencephalitis. *Trans Ophthalmol Soc UK* 1975;95:221–232.

170. Lowrey DM, McLaughlin J. Subcellular distribution of hydrolases in *Naegleria fowleri. J Protozool* 1985;32:616–621.

171. Marciano-Cabral F, Stanitski S, Radhakrishna V, Bradley SG. Characterization of a neutral aminoacyl-peptide hydrolase from *Naegleria fowleri. J Protozool* 1987;34:146–149.

172. Pernin P, Cariou ML, Jacquier A. Biochemical identification and phylogenetic relationships in free-living amoebas of the genus *Naegleria. J Protozool* 1985;32:592–603.

173. Lowrey DM, McLaughlin J. A multicomponent hemolytic system in the pathogenic amoeba *Naegleria fowleri. Infect Immun* 1984;45:731–736.

174. Lowrey DM, McLaughlin J. Activation of a heat-stable cytolytic protein associated with the surface membrane of *Naegleria fowleri. Infect Immun* 1985;50:478–482.

175. Cleary SF, Marciano-Cabral F. Activated macrophages demonstrate direct cytotoxicity, antibody-dependent cellular cytotoxic-

ity, and enhanced binding of *Naegleria fowleri* amoebae. *Cell Immunol* 1986;98:125–136.

176. Cleary SF, Marciano-Cabral F. Soluble amoebicidal factors mediate cytolysis of *Naegleria fowleri* by activated macrophages. *Cell Immunol* 1986;101:62–71.

177. Ferrante A, Mocatta TJ. Human neutrophils require activation by mononuclear leucocyte conditioned medium to kill the pathogenic free-living amoeba, *Naegleria fowleri*. *Clin Exp Immunol* 1984;56:559–566.

178. Rowan-Kelly B, Ferrante A, Thong YH. Activation of complement by *Naegleria*. *Trans R Soc Trop Med Hyg* 1980;74:333–336.

179. Whiteman LY, Marciano-Cabral F. Susceptibility of pathogenic and nonpathogenic *Naegleria* spp. to complement-mediated lysis. *Infect Immun* 1987;55:2442–2447.

180. Haggerty RM, John DT. Serum agglutination and immunoglobulin levels of mice infected with *Naegleria fowleri*. *J Protozool* 1982;29:117–122.

181. Thong YH, Ferrante A, Shepherd C, Rowan-Kelly B. Resistance of mice to *Naegleria* meningoencephalitis transferred by immune serum. *Trans R Soc Trop Med Hyg* 1978;72:650–652.

182. Lallinger GJ, Reiner SL, Cooke DW, et al. Efficacy of immune therapy in early experimental *Naegleria fowleri* meningitis. *Infect Immun* 1987;55:1289–1293.

183. Cursons RTM, Brown TJ, Keys EA, Moriarty KM, Till D. Immunity to pathogenic free-living amoebae: role of humoral antibody. *Infect Immun* 1980;29:401–407.

184. Martinez AJ. Is *Acanthamoeba* encephalitis an opportunistic infection? *Neurology* 1980;30:567–574.

185. Gutierrez Y. The Free-Living Amebae: *Naegleria* and *Acanthamoeba*. In: Gutierrez Y, ed. *Diagnostic pathology of parasitic infections with clinical correlations*, 1st ed. Philadelphia: Lea & Febiger, 1990;80–93.

186. Martinez AJ, Sotelo-Aveila C, Alcala H, Willaert E. Granulomatous encephalitis, intracranial arteritis and mycotic aneurism due to a free-living ameba. *Acta Neuropathol* 1980;49:7–12.

187. Lawande RV, MacFarlane JT, Weir WRC, Awunor-Renner C. A case of primary amebic meningoencephalitis in a Nigerian farmer. *Am J Trop Med Hyg* 1980;29:21–25.

188. Hoffmann EO, Garcia C, Lunseth J, McGarry P, Coover J. A case of primary amebic meningoencephalitis. Light and electron microscope and immunohistologic studies. *Am J Trop Med Hyg* 1978;27:29–38.

189. Rutherfoord GS. Amoebic meningo-encephalitis due to a free-living amoeba. *S Afr Med J* 1986;69:52–55.

190. Patras D, Andujar JJ. Meningoencephalitis due to *Hartmannella* (*Acanthamoeba*). *Am J Clin Pathol* 1966;46:226–233.

191. Duma RJ, Ferrell HW, Nelson EC, Jones MM. Primary amebic meningoencephalitis. *N Engl J Med* 1969;281:1315–1323.

192. Markowitz SM, Martinez AJ, Duma RJ, Shiel FOM. Myocarditis associated with primary amebic (*Naegleria*) meningoencephalitis. *Am J Clin Pathol* 1974;62:619–628.

193. Kwame Ofori-Kwakye S, Sidebottom DG, Herbert J, Fischer EG, Visvesvara GS. Granulomatous brain tumor caused by *Acanthamoeba* [Abstract]. *J Neurosurg* 1986;64:505–509.

194. Visvesvara GS, Mirra SS, Brandt FH, Moss DM, Mathews HM, Martinez AJ. Isolation of two strains of *Acanthamoeba castellanii* from human tissue and their pathogenicity and isoenzyme profiles. *J Clin Microbiol* 1983;18:1405–1412.

195. Cleland PG, Lawande RV, Onyemelukwe G, Whittle HC. Chronic amebic meningoencephalitis. *Arch Neurol* 1982;39:56–57.

196. Stehr-Green JK, Bailey TM, Visvesvara GS. The epidemiology of *Acanthamoeba* keratitis in the United States [Abstract]. *Am J Ophthalmol* 1989;107:331–336.

197. Moore MB, McCulley JP, Luckenbach M, et al. *Acanthamoeba* keratitis associated with soft contact lenses. *Am J Ophthalmol* 1985;100:396–403.

198. Dos Santos NJG. Fatal primary amebic meningoencephalitis: a retrospective study in Richmond, Virginia. *Am J Clin Pathol* 1970;54:737–742.

199. Jamieson A. Effect of clotrimazole on *Naegleria fowleri*. *J Clin Pathol* 1975;28:446–449.

200. Cooke D, Lallinger G, Durack D. *In vitro* sensitivity of *Naegleria fowleri* to qinghaosu and dihydroqinghaosu. *J Parasitol* 1987;73:411–413.

201. Schuster FL, Rechthand E. *In vitro* effects of amphotericin B on growth and ultrastructure of the amoeboflagellates *Naegleria gruberi* and *Naegleria fowleri*. *Antimicrob Agents Chemother* 1975;8:591–605.

202. Schuster FL, Mandel N. Phenothiazine compounds inhibit *in vitro* growth of pathogenic free-living amoebae. *Antimicrob Agents Chemother* 1984;25:109–112.

203. Cerva L. *Naegleria fowleri*: trimethoprim sensitivity. *Science* 1980;209:1541–1541.

204. Seidel JS, Harmatz P, Visvesvara GS, Cohen A, Edwards J, Turner J. Successful treatment of primary amebic meningoencephalitis. *N Engl J Med* 1982;306:346–348.

205. Callicott JH Jr, Nelson C, Jones MM, et al. Meningoencephalitis due to pathogenic free-living amoebae. Report of two cases. *JAMA* 1968;206:579–582.

206. Martinez-Paloma A, Ruiz-Palacios G. Amebiasis. In: Warren KS, Mahmoud AAF, eds. *Tropical and geographic medicine*, 2nd ed. New York: McGraw-Hill, 1990;327–344.

207. Orbison JA, Reeves N, Leedham CL, Blumber JM. Amebic brain abscess. Review of the literature and report of five additional cases. *Medicine* 1951;30:247–282.

207a.Legrand H. Les abces dysenteriques du cerveau. *Arch Provinciales de Chir* 1912;21:1–35, 75–84, 212–239, 625–639.

208. Walsh JA. Problems in recognition and diagnosis of amebiasis: estimation of the global magnitude of morbidity and mortality. *Rev Infect Dis* 1986;8:228–238.

209. Lombardo L, Alonso P, Arroyo LS, Brandt H, Mateos JH. Cerebral amebiasis. Report of 17 cases. *J Neurosurg* 1964;21:704–709.

210. Banerjee AK, Bhatnagar RK, Bhusnurmath SR. Secondary cerebral amebiasis. *Trop Geogr Med* 1983;35:333–336.

211. von Lichtenberg F. Infectious Disease. In: Cotran RS, Kumar V, Robbins SL, eds. *Robbins pathologic basis of disease*, 4th ed. Philadelphia: WB Saunders, 1989;307–433.

212. Connor DH, Neafie RC, Hockmeyer WT. Malaria. In: Binford CH, Connor DH, eds. *Pathology of tropical and extraordinary disease: an atlas*, 1st ed. Washington, DC: Armed Forces Institute of Pathology, 1976;273–283.

213. Sun T. *Pathology and clinical features of parasitic diseases.* New York: Masson, 1982.

214. Hutt MRS, Wilks NE. African Trypanosomiasis (Sleeping Sickness). In: Marcial-Rojas RA, ed. *Pathology of Protozoal and Helminthic Diseases.* Huntington, NY: Robert E. Kreiger, 1975;57–68.

215. Vickerman K. Antigenic Variation in African Trypanosomes. In: Porter P, Knight J, eds. *Parasites in the Immunized Host: Mechanisms of Survival. Ciba Foundation Symposium 25 (new series).* Amsterdam: Associated Scientific Publishers, 1974;53–80.

216. De Jonckheere JF, Aerts M, Martinez AJ. *Naegleria australiensis*: experimental meningoencephalitis in mice. *Trans R Soc Trop Med Hyg* 1983;77:712–716.

217. Josephson SL, Weik RR, John DT. Concanavalin A-induced agglutination of *Naegleria*. *Am J Trop Med Hyg* 1977;26:856–858.

Infections of the Central Nervous System,
edited by W. M. Scheld, R. J. Whitley, and
D. T. Durack, Raven Press, Ltd., New York © 1991.

CHAPTER 34

Toxoplasmosis of the Central Nervous System

Carol S. Dukes, Benjamin J. Luft, and David T. Durack

Toxoplasma gondii is an important intracellular protozoan pathogen of humans and animals. Although most infections are mild or asymptomatic, this pathogen can cause significant morbidity and mortality in both humans and animals. The incidence of human infection, as measured by seropositivity, differs around the world, depending upon the following: dietary habits, especially the amount of meat consumed and whether eaten rare, raw, or well done; number of stray cats living in close proximity to humans; climatic conditions, in that moderate temperatures and high humidity favor survival of oocysts in soil; and the overall level of sanitation and hygiene. Among pregnant women, seropositivity rates have been found to vary: 84% in Paris, 32% in New York City (1), and 22% in London (2). Seroprevalence is 50–60% in the regions of Africa and Central and South America which have been studied, and it is low in China, Japan, and Australia (3).

Most human infections with *T. gondii* are asymptomatic. However, this protozoan can infect the central nervous system (CNS), where it causes four syndromes: (i) meningoencephalitis during primary infection in an immunocompetent host, (ii) encephalitis and retinochoroiditis as a result of transplacental infection of the fetus, (iii) retinochoroiditis associated with primary infection or reactivation of an earlier infection, and (iv) intracerebral mass lesions or encephalitis in immunocompromised hosts.

CNS infection with *T. gondii* was first described by the Czechoslovakian, Jankû (cited in ref. 3), in 1923, when he observed parasitic cysts in the retina of an 11-month-old child with congenital hydrocephalus and microphthalmos. Prior to this, the organism had been known as a pathogen only in animals. In 1937, Wolf and Cowen brought the disease to the attention of pediatricians; they described a fatal case of a protozoan encephalomyelitis in an infant (4) and established *T. gondii* as the etiologic agent (5–7). They and their colleagues later proved that the infection was acquired congenitally (8,9), and they provided details of the associated cerebral and retinal pathology (7). Sabin (10) and Pinkerton and Henderson (11) independently described the first cases of noncongenitally acquired toxoplasmic encephalitis in 1941; and Sabin (cited in ref. 12), in 1942, described the first series of children presenting beyond infancy with sequelae of congenital toxoplasmosis. Frenkel (13), in 1957, described the phenomenon of reactivation of latent toxoplasmosis in immunocompromised patients. Reactivation of latent infection was uncommon until the epidemic of acquired immunodeficiency syndrome (AIDS) began in 1981. A review published in 1968 found only 20 reported cases of reactivation toxoplasmosis, all associated with malignancies (13a). In patients with AIDS, toxoplasmosis is next only to *Cryptococcus neoformans* in frequency as a cause of opportunistic CNS infections (14), and it is currently the most common cause of focal CNS disease (15).

This chapter will focus on the epidemiology, pathogenesis, pathological findings, and clinical manifestations of CNS toxoplasmosis in each of the four main syndromes. A general discussion of diagnostic procedures, treatment options, and aspects of prevention will follow.

THE PARASITE

Toxoplasma gondii is a coccidian in the family Sarcocystidae. It was first identified in 1908 by Nicolle and Manceaux (cited in ref. 16) in North Africa, and independently by Splendore (cited in ref. 17) in Brazil. The parasite exists in several distinct forms: (i) the tachyzoite or endozoite (formerly called a trophozoite), which is the

C. S. Dukes and D. T. Durack: Division of Infectious Diseases and International Health, Duke University Medical Center, Durham, North Carolina 27710.

B. J. Luft: Division of Infectious Diseases, State University of New York—Stony Brook, Stony Brook, New York 11794.

TABLE 1. Toxoplasma gondii: *some characteristics of different stages of the life cycle*

Name(s)	Size	Characteristics	Hosts	Relevance to human disease
Tachyzoite (trophyzoite, endozoite)	2–4 by 4–8 μm	Cell-invasive Proliferative form Multiplies by endodyogeny Haploid Can become bradyzoite	All mammals Birds Possibly reptiles	Spreads infection from cell to cell, but not from animal to animal Elicits antibody production and inflammation; causes clinical disease states
Bradyzoite (cystozoite)	2–4 by 4–8 μm	Noninvasive Long-lived in tissue cysts Slowly multiplies by endodyogeny Haploid Can become tachyzoite	Same as tachyzoite	Forms tissue cyst (below)
Tissue cyst	10–200 μm	Collection of bradyzoites (up to 3000) in one cyst Formed within host cell vacuole, then free in tissue	Same as tachyzoite	Infectious upon ingestion Maintains chronic infection in humans Common in brain and in skeletal and heart muscle May break down and release tachyzoites
Oocyst	10–12 μm	Diploid; sexual stage; produced only in definitive host's (feline) gut by mating of gametocytes Sporulation occurs after passage in cat feces thus producing infectious organisms	Definitive host (felines)	Infectious for mammals after sporulation

cell-invasive, rapidly proliferating form; (ii) the tissue cyst, which contains intracystic bradyzoites or cystozoites; and (iii) the oocyst, which produces infectious sporozoites (Table 1). The size of these organisms varies: Tachyzoites measure 2–4 by 4–8 μm; oocysts are larger, 9–11 by 11–14 μm. Small tissue cysts may contain only a few bradyzoites, but these cysts may enlarge to 200 μm in size, enclosing up to 3000 organisms (3). Sabin and Olitsky described their obligate intracellular location in 1937, but it was not until 1970 that Frenkel and co-workers (18,19) reported experiments which delineated the life cycle of the organism.

The only definitive hosts for *T. gondii* are domestic cats, *Felis domestica,* and related species of Felidae. Cats become infected by eating animals (usually rodents) which contain cysts in their tissues, or by ingesting oocysts passed in the feces of other cats. The sexual phase, which occurs only in the feline gut, begins when a cat ingests either oocysts or tissue cysts (Fig. 1). The enteroepithelial cycle begins when the protozoa infect epithelial cells in the small intestine and develop into merozoites, which, in turn, infect other epithelial cells. Some merozoites develop into gametocytes which fuse and form diploid oocysts. Millions of oocysts are excreted in the feces, over a period of 2–3 weeks. Under favorable conditions such as a humid and warm climate, the oocysts may remain infectious in the environment for more than a year. Sporogony occurs 2–21 days after the oocysts have been discharged into the environment.

Only after the oocyst sporulates does it become infectious (20).

The asexual phase of the parasite's life cycle occurs in incidental hosts as well as in felines, and it is largely extraintestinal. After oocysts have been ingested, sporozoites are released into the small intestine, penetrate the gut wall, replicate, and are then spread hematogenously throughout the body. The organism is remarkable for its ability to nonselectively invade and multiply inside most mammalian cell types (Figs. 2 and 3), with the possible

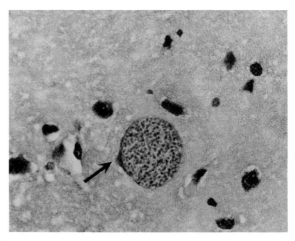

FIG. 1. A tissue cyst of *T. gondii* in brain (*arrow*), containing many bradyzoites. Note the absence of inflammatory response around the cyst. (From ref. 170, with permission.)

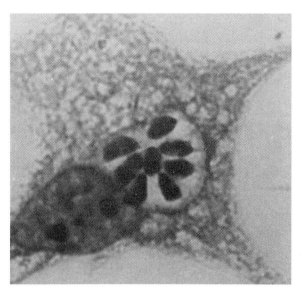

FIG. 2. A rosette of *T. gondii* tachyzoites, multiplying in a parasitophorous vacuole in a mammalian cell *in vitro*. (From ref. 169, with permission.)

exception of non-nucleated erythrocytes. Once inside a macrophage, or any other cell, the sporozoite transforms into a tachyzoite which multiplies by endodyogeny, a process in which two daughter cells develop within a mother cell. Binary fission continues; the tachyzoites proliferate intracellularly until many organisms accumulate, at which time the host cell ruptures. The tachyzoites released invade adjacent cells, and then the cycle is repeated until host immunity develops, limiting further multiplication.

Tachyzoites may form pseudocysts, structures consisting of aggregates of the organisms which accumulate in host cells for a time. Over time, these form true tissue cysts. Tissue cysts contain bradyzoites which divide slowly by endodyogeny. The complex outer membrane of the cyst has been investigated by several groups and appears to combine contributions from both host and parasite (17,21). The tissue cyst appears to be immunologically inert; in the chronically infected host, it is rare

to find any inflammatory response surrounding a cyst (13). Although a specific tissue tropism for *Toxoplasma* has never been demonstrated, tissue cysts are found most commonly in the nervous system and muscles of the host. It is believed that cysts may persist in tissue for the life of the host. The mechanisms that result in transformation of actively dividing tachyzoites into slowly dividing bradyzoites (and vice versa) are not known.

Control of toxoplasmic infection by humans depends primarily on cell-mediated immunity (22), which successfully limits replication of tachyzoites but fails to kill all the organisms. Some transform into bradyzoites and become dormant tissue cysts, which retain the potential to resume multiplication if cell-mediated immunity wanes.

This organism has evolved several complex mechanisms which circumvent immune responses and allow it to survive indefinitely in the host (22,23). These include: ability to actively invade most mammalian cells; ability to avoid triggering the oxidative burst of some professional phagocytes (24); ability to prevent phagosome–lysosome fusion (25) and acidification (26); production of catalase and superoxide dismutase, scavengers of toxic oxygen metabolites (27); and ability of the parasite itself to induce a down-regulation of the immune response (22). Thus, tachyzoites phagocytosed by human macrophages do not trigger the generation of reactive oxygen species and are thus able to survive and replicate within these cells. Human monocytes, on the other hand, do generate toxic oxygen metabolites after invasion by *Toxoplasma* and usually can eliminate intracellular infection (24).

Lymphokines such as gamma interferon activate macrophages and other cells to kill *Toxoplasma* (28), and exogenous gamma interferon confers resistance against *Toxoplasma* in the murine model (29). Interleukin-2 has also been found to have a protective effect against *T. gondii* infection in mice (22). Passive administration of anti-gamma interferon to animals acutely infected with *T. gondii* (22,30) has a detrimental effect on the host's ability to resist infection and may lead to recrudescence

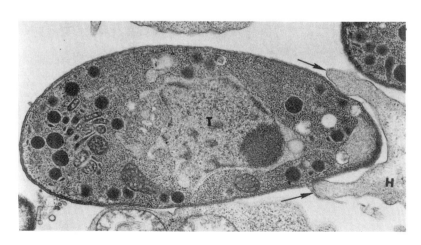

FIG. 3. A tachyzoite (T) of *T. gondii* invaginating the membrane of a host cell (H) prior to internalization. Pseudopods of the host cell (arrows) extend around the invading tachyzoite. Transmission electron micrograph ×25,000. (From ref. 48, with permission.)

of infection in chronically infected animals. Agents such as corticosteroids, cytotoxic drugs, and antilymphocytic agents which impair cell-dependent immunity depress the host's ability to control acute infection and can allow reactivation of latent infection with *T. gondii* (22). In addition, malignancies of the reticuloendothelial and hematological systems which cause defects in cell-mediated immunity are strongly associated with more severe disease due to *T. gondii* (31). AIDS patients who have advanced CD4 T-cell lymphopenia with resulting abnormalities in lymphocyte function have a particular propensity to develop toxoplasmic encephalitis.

TOXOPLASMOSIS IN NON-IMMUNOCOMPROMISED HOSTS

Epidemiology

Transmission of *T. gondii* to humans occurs commonly, most often by eating undercooked meats (32,33) or by inadvertent ingestion of oocysts from cat feces (34). Because infection can occur during the communal activity of eating, there have been numerous reports of common source outbreaks within families (33,35,36). Unpasteurized milk, particularly goat's milk (35), and contaminated water (37) can transmit the infection.

The prevalence of seropositivity in human populations, indicating previous infection, varies greatly from place to place. Factors favoring higher prevalence include: warm, humid climates; poor sanitation; exposure to cats; and partiality for raw or undercooked meats. The rate of seropositivity increases with age, but younger subjects have higher titers (38). Rates in males are similar to those in females (38). Serosurveys in U.S. military recruits (age 17–26 years) in 1962 revealed that 13% had evidence of previous infection (39). There were significant differences according to the geographic location of origin: rates of 16–20% were prevalent in the eastern states, and low rates (6%) were prevalent in the mountain zone. In the United States, representative rates of seropositivity are 20–40%, depending on location. In France, up to 80% of adults are seropositive (40).

Symptomatic CNS toxoplasmosis rarely develops during primary infection in normal hosts. In 1975, Townsend et al. (41) described six cases and reviewed 39 others from the literature. Fifteen (33%) of these patients had no evidence of immune dysfunction. Since this review, several other reports of acute toxoplasmic encephalitis in normal hosts have appeared (42–45). Luft and Remington (46) recently reviewed 48 cases from the world literature. Perkins (47) reviewed the literature on acquired lymphadenopathic toxoplasmosis to determine what proportion had ocular involvement. CNS involvement occurred in 4.3% of these cases. Retinochoroiditis occurred in only 1.2% of patients who presented with lymphadenopathy, but in 16% of those with CNS involvement (47). A more recent review of 107 cases of toxoplasmic lymphadenopathy in immunocompetent people found only one patient who appeared to have CNS involvement (43).

Pathogenesis

Systemic parasitemia occurs following invasion of the gut lining by *Toxoplasma*. The mechanisms by which this protozoan achieves chronic intracellular residence, and the host responses which limit its multiplication, have been studied in detail. These investigations have provided insights into macrophage function and intracellular parasitism.

There has been considerable debate about the mechanism by which *T. gondii* enters cells. Jones et al. (25) demonstrated that both professional phagocytes (macrophages) and nonprofessional phagocytes (HeLa cells and fibroblasts) engulf the organism, which then resides in a parasitophorous vacuole. Aikawa et al. (48) performed electron-microscopic studies focusing on the organism's anterior organelles; these include the rhoptries, which, according to the authors, are important in the process of active penetration of host cells (Fig. 2) (48). Nichols and O'Connor (49) studied this phenomenon after blocking macrophage phagocytosis, concluding that active invasion is the primary mechanism by which the parasite enters the cell.

Wilson et al. (24) investigated the finding that activated macrophages or freshly isolated human blood monocytes rapidly destroy *Toxoplasma*, whereas resting macrophages allow intracellular replication and survival. They found that cellular entry of the parasite failed to trigger the normal oxidative metabolic burst by macrophages. Sibley et al. (26) demonstrated that live tachyzoites modify the parasitophorous vacuole to prevent normal fusion with lysosomes and lowering of internal pH. The mechanisms whereby the parasite subverts these two microbicidal processes was recently studied by Joiner et al. (50), who showed that the dysfunction is induced by live parasites at the time of entry into cells rather than as a result of active secretion of fusion-inhibiting enzymes within the vacuole. This may occur as a result of membrane alteration of the parasitophorous vacuole at the time of entry.

Pathology

Because acute toxoplasmic encephalitis in normal hosts is uncommon and very rarely fatal, few reports of the pathological findings have been published, especially during recent years. Histological abnormalities in the brain in patients with multiple organ involvement ranged from relatively mild areas of perivascular inflammation and microglial nodules to extensive inflammation with foci of necrosis throughout white and gray matter (10,11,51,52). Sabin (10) described the brain lesion in a 6-year-old child who died from acquired toxoplasmic encephalitis as "a moth-eaten, necrotic and honeycombed area which was infiltrated with a varying number of cells which had irregular, pyknotic nuclei." Pinkerton and Henderson (11) noted that these lesions are reminiscent of the typhus nodules seen in rickettsial infections of the CNS (see Chapter 17). Gliosis and other nonspecific findings are common. Biopsy of a focal lesion in brain may reveal free tachyzoites, but this is quite unusual in immunocompetent patients. In one patient, a few toxoplasmas were seen in association with mononuclear perivascular infiltrates, along with tissue cysts and pseudocysts (51). This picture is markedly different from the florid necrotizing encephalitis that can occur in congenital toxoplasmosis. Nor were there any of the calcifications typical of congenital CNS infection. In some patients, the pathologic process caused by *T. gondii* is an indolent, localized necrotizing granulomatous reaction (53,54). This may be difficult to differentiate from a neoplastic process on frozen sections.

Clinical Manifestations

Primary infection with *T. gondii* in the immunocompetent normal host is usually asymptomatic. The most common manifestation is generalized lymphadenopathy, which can be found in only 10–20% of patients acutely infected with *T. gondii*. Some patients have low-grade fever. This diagnosis should be considered in a person with a seronegative mononucleosis-like illness (43). A maculopapular rash, described as being similar to the exanthem of Rocky Mountain spotted fever, may occur (11,54), but is rare. In fact, one of the early reports of acute toxoplasmosis in adults emphasized the need to differentiate toxoplasmosis and typhus–spotted fever (11).

Rarely, *Toxoplasma* can produce severe or even fatal infection in an apparently immunocompetent host (10,56). When the CNS is involved, drowsiness, confusion, irritability, and dysphasia progressing to coma and seizures have been reported (42,44). Patients may also present with signs of meningeal irritation, but this is uncommon. Physical exam often reveals hyperreflexia and signs of upper motor neuron involvement. Luft and Remington (46) reviewed 48 case reports on toxoplasmic encephalitis in normal hosts, finding two patterns of infection. The first is widely disseminated disease with encephalitis and multiple organ failure (56). A maculopapular rash is frequently seen in this form of infection. The severity of CNS involvement is variable, from mild and self-limiting to devastating. The second is confined to the brain, with no evidence of disease in other organs (46,57). The lesions may be diffuse or localized; the more focal form of disease may be difficult to distinguish from

a tumor. Acute toxoplasmic retinochoroiditis may precede or accompany the CNS process.

Results of cerebrospinal fluid (CSF) analysis reveals a mild pleocytosis, elevated protein, and normal glucose. Diagnosis has usually been made on the basis of increasing or markedly elevated serum and CSF antibody titers.

CONGENITAL TOXOPLASMOSIS

Epidemiology

The probability of becoming primarily infected with toxoplasmosis during pregnancy differs according to geographic and cultural circumstances. The incidence of congenital infection in any given population is dependent upon the yearly rate of acquisition of primary infection and the number of women of childbearing age who are seronegative, and therefore at risk for transmitting toxoplasmosis to the fetus (3). The seroprevalence rate in pregnant women in France was 87% in the years 1960–1970, decreasing to 70% by 1985. These data were generated using the Sabin–Feldman dye test (2). In contrast, prevalence rates in London and the United States are lower. When a pregnant woman experiences a primary infection with *T. gondii,* several outcomes are possible. She may be infected and seroconvert, but not pass the infection to her fetus. Alternatively, the fetus may be infected as evidenced by positive serologies after birth, but be asymptomatic; or the fetus may have the clinical picture of congenital toxoplasmosis. Desmonts and Couvreur (2) in France studied placentas from 202 women who either seroconverted during pregnancy or had high titers to toxoplasmosis before pregnancy; these authors demonstrated parasites in 26% of the placentas from the former group and in only 2% of those from the latter group. Of 11 women who seroconverted or had a significant rise in titer during pregnancy, two had offspring with clinical toxoplasmosis.

Pathogenesis

Risk for congenital toxoplasmosis begins when a nonimmune woman ingests the organisms encysted in animal meat or swallows oocysts emanating from infected cats. Maternal parasitemia is reflected in placental infection and transmission of tachyzoites via the umbilical vein to cause fetal parasitemia. The organisms become widely disseminated, forming many small lesions as first noted by Paige et al. (7) with multiple manifestations: pneumonia, myocarditis, myositis, hepatitis, and encephalitis. Despite widespread parasitemia, encephalitis may be the only manifestation. It may progress slowly so that it is not noted at birth, but causes in mental deterioration of a seemingly normal infant. Frenkel (58) related this to two observations regarding the differences in rapidity of clearing of infection from various organ systems: (i) in animals recovering from infection, organisms diminish in number first in blood, then in extraneural tissues, and last in the brain and eye; (ii) in neonates it has often been observed that a resolving toxoplasmic pneumonia and hepatitis exist concurrently with progressing CNS and retinal lesions.

The manifestations of congenital toxoplasmosis depend upon the rate of proliferation of the organism, the anatomical locations where this proliferation occurs, and the competency of the immune system. In fetuses, maternal antibody may be helpful in protecting against organisms which can cross the placental barrier. However, it has been clearly demonstrated that immunity to *T. gondii* is dependent primarily on cellular immunity, which in the neonate is immature and not transferrable between mother and fetus. When a pregnant woman becomes acutely infected, the frequency of congenital infection is directly related to the duration of gestation. The later in pregnancy the mother becomes infected, the more likely that the fetus will become infected (3). On the other hand, the severity of congenital infection is inversely related to the time during gestation in which the infection was acquired. Infections acquired early in gestation are more severe, often causing hydrocephalus and profound mental retardation. In contrast, infections acquired during the later part of gestation tend to be mild or subclinical at the time of birth (3).

Proliferating tachyzoites destroy parasitized cells. Loss of cells in those organs which have limited capacity for regeneration, such as the CNS, naturally leads to the most severe damage. Furthermore, the CNS appears to be preferentially infected, at least in neonates. The tachyzoites parasitize brain parenchymal cells and then enter the ventricular system, infecting ependymal cells and subependymal tissue. These destructive periventricular lesions have been described by Sabin (10). Inflammation consisting mainly of cellular components such as macrophages, monocytes, and lymphocytes ensues, producing ulcerations in the ependymal surface. With increased inflammation and edema, the ventricular system can become obstructed, trapping proliferating organisms and inflammatory cells in the lateral and third ventricles. Frenkel (58) referred to such an inflamed, damaged, and obstructed ventricle as an "abscess cavity". He proposed that at least some of the inflammation may occur as a result of the interaction of the antigenic load presented by the toxoplasmosis-laden ventricular fluid with maternal antibody circulating in fetal blood. The inflammatory response is often perivascular; direct parasite involvement of the vessel walls may cause a perivascular cellular infiltration or even a frank vasculitis. Increased vascular permeability and subsequent thrombosis may lead to anoxia, cell death, and tissue necrosis.

Another result of obstruction of the ventricular system is chronic hydrocephalus, which further diminishes neuronal function and contributes to mental retardation.

The periventricular lesions often calcify, and thus they can be seen on plain radiographs of the head (Fig. 4).

Retinochoroiditis frequently accompanies severe congenital toxoplasmosis but may also be seen in older children and adults who are otherwise asymptomatic (see section entitled "Ocular Toxoplasmosis," below). In autopsies of children dying with congenital toxoplasmosis, both healed and active retinal lesions can be seen. Microscopically, tachyzoites and cysts were found in and around the lesions (58).

Pathology

CNS lesions tend to be most intense in the cortex, basal ganglia and periventricular areas, and spinal cord. There may be a dense cellular reaction consisting predominantly of round cells in the leptomeninges. Calcification within the areas of necrosis occurs in the cortex, varying from broad bands to fine particles. Toxoplasmic tachyzoites (Figs. 2 and 3) and tissue cysts (Fig. 1) are usually seen in the periphery of the necrotic lesions, in proximity to glial nodules. Hydrocephalus may develop as a result of obstruction of the aqueduct of Sylvius or the foramen of Monroe by active ependymitis or by the deposition of large amounts of necrotic tissue within the ventricular spaces. Periventricular and periaqueductal vasculitis and necrolysis is almost pathognomonic for congenital toxoplasmosis and is frequently associated with calcification. The hypothalamus may also be involved.

The findings described above are the pathological features found in infants with severe congenital toxoplasmosis, many of whom succumb after birth. The lesions that cause their gross neurological defects are obvious. Many cases are less severe; the pathological changes in these instances have been less well studied because the babies survive. Infants born with subclinical infection

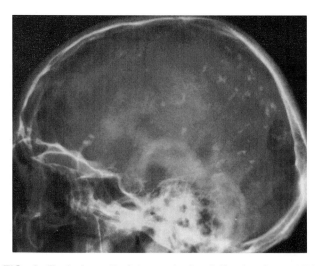

FIG. 4. Typical spotty intracerebral calcification in a child with congenital toxoplasmosis. (Radiograph provided by the Department of Radiology, Duke University Medical Center.)

may have abnormalities in their CSF. In some of these infants, clinical signs of subacute encephalitis may appear only months or even years after birth. The pathological features in such cases, which must be much milder than in severe cases of congenital toxoplasmosis, have not been delineated.

Clinical Manifestations

The spectrum of findings associated with documented intrauterine toxoplasmic infection ranges from asymptomatic or subclinical infection to severe, necrotizing encephalitis and systemic infection (Table 2). The classic triad of findings in an infant with congenital toxoplasmosis includes hydrocephalus, cerebral calcifications, and retinochoroiditis. These were present in the first case of congenital toxoplasmosis, which was described in 1937 (4,7); subsequent series, however, show this triad to be rather uncommon (1,59). *Toxoplasma* is not teratogenic and therefore is not associated with the development of fetal malformations; instead, clinical disease is due to encephalitis associated with destruction of brain tissue.

Presence of signs of infection at birth usually indicates severe infection which has already caused significant neurological damage. The disease may not be noted, however, until a few months after birth or until childhood, or occasionally not until reactivation of disease much later in life. The initial manifestations of toxoplasmosis in newborns with clinically apparent disease can be categorized either as predominantly neurological disease or as generalized disease. There is considerable overlap in these arbitrary classifications. The principal findings in both groups are retinochoroiditis, convulsions, abnor-

mal CSF, and anemia. The neurological group has a higher incidence of cerebral calcifications and hydrocephalus. In addition, because of the propensity for *Toxoplasma* to involve the periventricular area, there may be evidence of hypothalamic dysfunction resulting in wide fluctuations in body temperature. The generalized form is characterized by fever, jaundice, vomiting, diarrhea, rash, splenomegaly, lymphadenopathy, hepatomegaly, and pneumonitis. Though the initial presentation may differ, long-term follow-up reveals that mental retardation, seizures, and motor abnormalities occur with near-equivalent frequency in both groups of patients.

Based on serological studies, most intrauterine infections either appear to be asymptomatic or are associated with less specific outcomes such as premature birth or decreased birth weight. Alford et al. (59) prospectively screened 7,500 infants and found 10 with proven congenital toxoplasmosis, based on persistently positive serologies. Only one child had signs or symptoms suggestive of toxoplasmosis at birth. This newborn had obvious and severe disease with bilateral retinochoroiditis, intracranial calcifications, hepatomegaly, and jaundice. He died at 4 months of age as a result of severe hydrocephalus. Although there were no obvious signs of infection in any of the other infants at birth, careful ophthalmologic exams in the seropositive infants revealed unilateral retinochoroiditis in one other child. Furthermore, lumbar punctures were performed on eight of these asymptomatic children: All the CSF samples were found to be abnormal, with a pleocytosis and elevated protein levels. Striking abnormalities were found in two infants, one being the severely affected newborn mentioned above. The second infant was normal at birth, but by 2.5 months of age this infant had decreased head circumference, generalized intracranial calcifications by skull x-rays, and retinochoroiditis. By age 4 years, the child demonstrated marked developmental retardation. The other eight children were followed for 2.5 years and developed normally. In another study, it appeared that between 40% and 70% (depending on therapy) of congenitally infected children who appeared normal at the time of birth went on to develop significant neurological sequelae of toxoplasmosis later in life. These sequelae included such severe abnormalities as hydrocephalus, microcephalus, seizure disorders, and severe psychomotor retardation. As discussed in the section entitled "Ocular Toxoplasmosis" (below), another study found retinochoroiditis in 85% of seropositive but asymptomatic newborns, at a mean age of 3.7 years (60). Other neurologic sequelae developed in 54% of these children (60).

OCULAR TOXOPLASMOSIS

Epidemiology

Ocular toxoplasmosis is one of the most important causes of retinochoroiditis in humans. Ocular toxoplas-

TABLE 2. *Frequencies of various clinical manifestations of congenital toxoplasmosis*

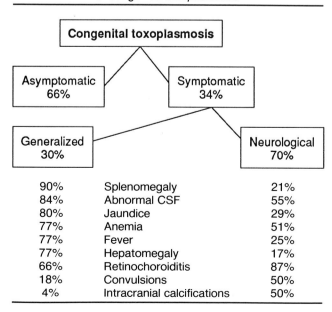

90%	Splenomegaly	21%	
84%	Abnormal CSF	55%	
80%	Jaundice	29%	
77%	Anemia	51%	
77%	Fever	25%	
77%	Hepatomegaly	17%	
66%	Retinochoroiditis	87%	
18%	Convulsions	50%	
4%	Intracranial calcifications	50%	

mosis can result from acquired lymphadenopathic toxoplasmosis, the most common form of symptomatic acquired toxoplasmosis; however, this complication is infrequent (61,62). Perkins (47) extensively reviewed reported cases of acquired lymphadenopathic toxoplasmosis and concluded that only 1.5% of these patients had associated retinochoroiditis. When ocular involvement occurs with acquired toxoplasmosis, it is most commonly associated with the less frequent clinical presentations, especially those of primary CNS disease. It has also been reported as occurring concurrently with toxoplasmic myocarditis and pulmonary disease.

Ocular toxoplasmosis is a very common finding in infants with symptomatic congenital toxoplasmosis. Retinochoroiditis has been reported in 87% of infants presenting with neurological disease and in 66% of infants with generalized toxoplasmosis (Table 2). A study of 24 infants with positive serology indicating congenital toxoplasmosis, but with no clinical signs of infection at birth, reported that 85% developed retinochoroiditis, at a mean of 3.7 years (60).

The third setting in which toxoplasmic retinochoroiditis occurs is in the immunocompetent older child or adult, but unassociated with acute toxoplasmosis. Here it is thought to represent reactivation of latent cysts left over from asymptomatic congenital infection (Fig. 1) (63). It is this ability of latent cysts to become active and cause clinical disease that makes studies of the epidemiology of ocular toxoplasmosis imprecise. Epidemiologic evidence that most adult cases of toxoplasmic retinochoroiditis occur as a result of reactivation of subclinical congenital infection rather than acquired infection is as follows: (a) serological surveys indicate that the incidence of acquired toxoplasmic infection continues to increase with age; (b) despite increasing serological prevalence of infection, retinochoroiditis consistent with toxoplasmic infection peaks in the second and third decades of life and is quite rare after age 50; (c) serological titers in patients with toxoplasmic uveitis are not higher than titers in asymptomatic persons—evidence against recent, acquired infection (47); and (d) prospective studies of infants born to women who seroconverted during pregnancy have found that many develop retinitis later in life (2,60).

Reactivation of toxoplasmic infection in immunocompromised patients more commonly presents as focal cerebral disease, but it also may rarely be seen in the eyes. In this setting, it may be difficult to differentiate from other causes of retinitis such as cytomegalovirus infection.

Pathogenesis

T. gondii infection in the nonimmune host causes widespread parasitemia and indiscriminate intracellular multiplication of tachyzoites, resulting in destruction of host cells and subsequent invasion into contiguous cells. When this occurs *in utero,* the ocular and CNS findings at birth can be attributed to damage during the acute infectious process. When the dormant, encysted organisms are not manifest until adulthood, however, the pathogenetic mechanisms are less clear.

The toxoplasmic cyst begins as a parasitized host cell, with organisms replicating within a parasitophorous vacuole. Eventually, the organisms fill up and distend the entire cell, which is no longer viable. The host cell wall fuses with the wall of the parasitophorous vacuole. This may account for the host's apparent immune tolerance for the cysts, which may remain dormant for years without provoking any inflammatory response (26).

Dormant cysts can be found in many tissues, including the retina, and appear to elicit very little inflammatory response in either human (13) or animal (64) tissues (Fig. 1). Rupture of the cyst, however, does induce inflammation, which may contribute to retinal damage. Though actual cyst rupture has not been directly observed in humans, there is circumstantial evidence to implicate this mechanism as the event which leads to reactivation retinochoroiditis (65). For instance, histological studies of infected retinal tissues in humans show free organisms and clusters of cysts, suggesting previous cyst rupture (65,66). In addition, toxoplasmic cysts can be found in the retina adjacent to scars typical of old toxoplasmic retinitis. Cyst rupture causes the release of proliferating trophozoites and is followed by invasion and destruction of surrounding retinal cells, with associated inflammation. This may occur as a "slow leak" of organisms causing chronic ocular involvement and long-term inflammation which may lead to painful glaucoma, even necessitating enucleation of the eye. Alternatively, there may be a transient acute episode (or episodes) following the sudden release of organisms after cyst rupture. Other pathogenetic mechanisms which have been proposed include possible elaboration of an antigenic toxin by *Toxoplasma.* Such toxins, however, have not been confirmed (64). Delayed hypersensitivity may play a role, especially in the pathogenesis of anterior chamber dysfunction, but this has not been proven (13).

The host–parasite relationship that permits the dormant cyst to survive silently for many years until a subtle shift in the balance allows reactivation resulting in retinal damage must be intricate. It still is not well understood.

Pathology

Congenital ocular lesions differ somewhat, depending on the gestational age at time of infection. Primary lesions usually begin in the retina, characteristically near the posterior pole of the eye, with vitreous and choroid pathology being secondary phenomena. The parasites are thought to gain access to the retina by lodging in the capillaries of the inner layers of the retina, where they invade the endothelium and adjacent tissues. Inflammation and edema ensues, resulting in disorganization and disruption of the retinal layers with undermining and sometimes complete destruction of retinal supporting and neural tissues (Fig. 5). Retinal cells may be displaced into the subretinal space, and cells from the inner nuclear layers may be displaced into adjacent vitreous. Eventually, proliferation of the organisms is halted and gliosis, fibrosis, and granulation take place. There may be proliferation of the pigment bordering the lesion over time (Fig. 6). Large lesions may show marked atrophy of the retina and choroid in the central part of the lesion. Retina and choroid become adherent after the inflammation subsides and scarring is completed. Parasites may be seen in the retina and sometimes in the choroid, either extracellularly or as intracellular pseudocysts (67).

The vitreous may be involved with serofibrinous exudate and inflammation secondary to extension through the inner limiting membrane of the retina. Granulation tissue and capillary proliferation may occur. The optic disk may show evidence of inflammation in adjacent retina causing papillitis. If hydrocephalus is present, there may be papilledema.

Ocular lesions in the adult are characterized by a focal necrotizing retinochoroiditis; they often occur in small clusters, though they occasionally occur as solitary lesions about the size of the optic disk (64). The classic lesion of severe toxoplasmic retinochoroiditis is that of a granuloma. There is usually marked inflammation with cuffs of inflammatory cells seen along the retinal arteries and veins (Fig. 5). This inflammation may be secondary to antigen–antibody reaction, which has been experimentally demonstrated in guinea pigs (13). Retinal edema, and especially macular and peripapillary edema, is nearly always present.

Anterior uveitis may occur secondary to intense inflammation. This may lead to increased intraocular pressure and to cataract formation. It is thought that this may be secondary to an antibody–antigen reaction or hypersensitivity, because *Toxoplasma* organisms have never been demonstrated in the anterior uvea of human subjects (68).

Ocular toxoplasmic infection in patients with AIDS has been reported as causing diffuse necrotizing retinochoroiditis with marked vitreitis, similar to the acute retinal necrosis syndrome (69).

Clinical Manifestations

In congenital toxoplasmosis, ocular abnormalities are very common. They are typically bilateral, though not necessarily symmetrical. If the infection occurred very early, microphthalmus may result. Nystagmus is a fre-

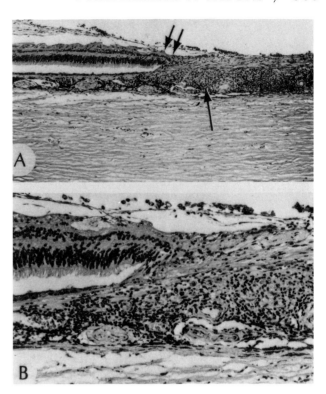

FIG. 5. A and B: Retinal toxoplasmosis. Abrupt transition from relatively normal retina on left to area of retinal necrosis on right, indicated by *double arrows*. A granulomatous inflammatory reaction (shown at higher magnification in part B) is present in the choroid under the necrotic infected retina, indicated by the *single arrow*. (From ref. 168, with permission.)

quent finding secondary to either the retinitis or the CNS involvement; similarly, strabismus may occur either from direct involvement of the extraocular muscles or from CNS disease. The iris and ciliary body may become dysfunctional because of inflammatory damage, leading to decreased pupillary accommodation. Cataract formation secondary to anterior and posterior uveitis occurs.

The timing of the clinical manifestations of congenital toxoplasmosis is of interest. One study followed asymptomatic congenital-toxoplasmosis-infected infants prospectively for a mean of 8.5 years (60). Group I consisted of 13 children who underwent serological studies for toxoplasmosis either because of routine screening procedures or because of other nonspecific reasons; of these, 85% developed sequelae of their disease, and retinochoroiditis was the initial manifestation in all of these at a mean age of 3.7 years (range: 1 month to 9.3 years). Group II consisted of 10 children who initially presented with eye or neurological abnormalities; in all of these patients, retinitis was present on examination. They presented at a mean of 4 months of age.

Funduscopic exam reveals lesions most commonly in the posterior portion of the eye; the macular region is frequently affected, though peripheral lesions also are common. Acute lesions are gray or gray-yellow and fairly well circumscribed (Fig. 6A). The retina is edema-

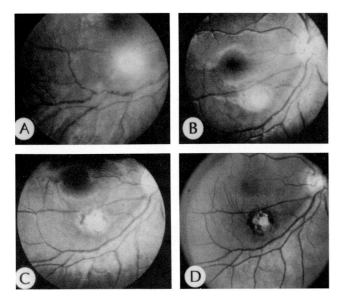

FIG. 6. Ocular toxoplasmosis. **A:** Acute lesion in the retina of a 12-year-old girl. The white spots on blood vessels represent cellular reaction on the surface of the retina. **B:** The same lesion 4 months later, with early pigmentation present. **C:** Three years later. **D:** Seventeen years after the initial attack —classic late lesions of ocular toxoplasmosis, with white center and dark peripheral pigmentation. (From ref. 168, with permission.)

tous; small hemorrhages and exudates may be seen, and fibrous stranding into the vitreous is not uncommon. As the acute inflammation subsides, the lesion becomes more distinct (Fig. 6B and 6C). A proliferation of the pigmented layer occurs at the margins. Completely

healed lesions are large, with an irregular border and marked central atrophy. They are often densely pigmented (Fig. 6D). Frequently, there are multiple lesions in various stages of inflammation and healing (67). Panuveitis may accompany retinochoroiditis. Papillitis may be seen in the setting of CNS disease. Acquired toxoplasmic ocular disease differs in that it is more often unilateral.

Visual acuity is affected if the macula or its fibers are involved. Congenital lesions outside this area will not be symptomatic unless reactivation occurs. Acute retinochoroiditis may present with blurred vision, pain, photophobia or scotoma. The symptoms resolve over time in the immunocompetent host, usually with some loss of visual acuity. Relapses are frequent. As mentioned earlier, chronic retinochoroiditis may result as painful glaucoma necessitating enucleation.

TOXOPLASMOSIS IN IMMUNOCOMPROMISED HOSTS

Epidemiology

In the past, reactivation toxoplasmosis of the CNS occurred most often in patients with lymphatic and hematological malignancies (70). Because most of these patients receive immunosuppressive or cytotoxic therapy, the relative contribution of malignancy-associated versus drug-associated immune dysfunction in predisposing to toxoplasmosis is difficult to define (71). There is at least one report of CNS toxoplasmosis occurring in a

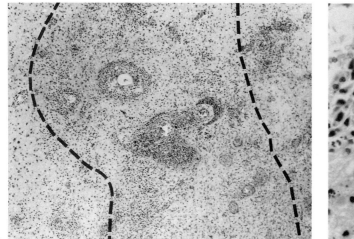
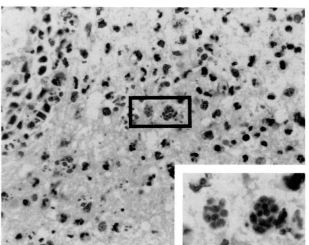

FIG. 7. Histopathology of a toxoplasma abscess in a patient with AIDS. **A:** Low-power view showing three zones of involvement. Left-hand zone: relatively normal brain, with some mild perivascular inflammation. Middle zone: severe perivascular inflammation. Right-hand zone: coagulative necrosis with thrombosed blood vessels. **B:** Higher power view showing a blood vessel with perivascular inflammation on the upper left, and two nearby cysts of *T. gondii* (small box). These are shown at higher power in the box at lower right. Sections provided by Dr. Douglas Anthony, Department of Pathology, Duke University.

patient with untreated Hodgkin's disease (72). CNS toxoplasmosis also can occur in those receiving immunosuppressive chemotherapy after organ transplantation (73–78) or for collagen vascular disorders such as systemic lupus erythematosus (79). In addition to the risk of reactivation of latent cysts, transplant recipients may also be primarily infected by cysts transferred to the patient in the allograft. Two groups evaluating cardiac transplant patients found that a seronegative recipient of a seropositive donor heart was at highest risk for seroconversion and development of severe toxoplasmosis (75,80). In one of these studies, seven of the seronegative patients were prophylactically treated with pyrimethamine, and none of them became ill with toxoplasmosis (75). Disseminated acute acquired toxoplasmosis has also been reported in renal and liver transplant patients (78,81,82).

Since 1981, the number of cases of CNS toxoplasmosis has increased dramatically (83,84). Toxoplasmosis has become one of the most common and most important opportunistic infections in patients with AIDS (Figs. 7–9). The prevalence of this complication of immunosuppression varies markedly from place to place, probably reflecting the underlying seroprevalence in a given population (85,86). A cancer hospital in New York City reported that 20% of their patients with AIDS had positive serologies to T. gondii by immunofluorescent antibody testing, and that 30% of these developed CNS toxoplasmosis (87). It was reported to occur in 40% of Haitians with AIDS (88), but in only 2.5% of all the AIDS patients reported to the Centers for Disease Control (CDC) as of 1987 (14). A very crude estimate from Western Congo indicated a rate of 20% in their AIDS patients (89). It has been estimated that by 1991 there could be as many as 20,000 to 40,000 cases of toxoplasmic encephalitis in patients with AIDS (40) in the United States.

There have been several reports of congenital toxoplasmosis occurring as a result of presumed recrudescent toxoplasmosis in human immunodeficiency virus (HIV)-infected mothers. In one report, all three mothers had positive immunoglobulin G (IgG) and negative immunoglobulin M (IgM) serologies. Only one mother had clinical evidence of active toxoplasmosis (90). In the pre-AIDS era, large studies showed that latent toxoplasmosis in an asymptomatic IgG-seropositive pregnant woman carried essentially no risk of transmission to the fetus. Evidently, this does not hold true for HIV-infected mothers (91).

Pathogenesis

The mechanisms by which mammalian hosts normally prevent reactivation of tissue cysts is not well understood. These mechanisms must depend primarily upon cellular immune function, because of the observed high frequency of recurrence in patients who develop abnormalities of cellular immunity, but not in humoral deficiency states. Certainly, the lymphocyte–monocyte–macrophage axis plays a dominant role in host defenses against Toxoplasma (22).

Our knowledge of the pathogenesis of toxoplasmic infection in the immunocompromised host is largely dependent on studies in animal models. After infection of animals the tachyzoites disseminate throughout the body, multiply, and eventually transform into tissue cysts. It has been proposed that toxoplasmic tachyzoites are less efficiently cleared from the brain of mice than from extraneural sites, making them more likely to persist in the CNS despite maturation of the normal cell-mediated and humoral immune response which limits or eliminates the protozoa elsewhere in the body. Exclusion of antibodies by the blood–brain barrier may favor proliferation of the organism in the CNS. After development of cell-mediated and humoral immunity, tachyzoites are destroyed and the tissue cyst becomes the only demonstrable form of the organism. There is also evidence to suggest that in chronically infected animals, active recurrent infection is responsible for the lifelong persistence of antibodies and cell-mediated immunity to Toxoplasma. Lainson (17) and Van der Waaij (21) studied the sequence of development of tissue cysts in the brains of mice and showed that daughter cysts develop in close proximity to larger cysts and that no inflammatory reaction accompanied this process. Therefore it seems that chronic infection in animal models is not a static state in which tissue cysts persist in a state of total inactivity through the lifespan of the host. Rather, there are intermittent cycles of cyst rupture with release of organisms and the formation of new cysts. This process may cause persistent antigenic stimulation, which could account for the persisting high titers of antibody characteristic of this infection.

The effect of immunosuppression on the pathogenesis of toxoplasmic encephalitis has been studied by numerous investigators. There is convincing experimental evidence that pharmacological suppression of cell-mediated immunity can trigger recrudescence of infection in animals chronically infected with T. gondii (22). Passive administration of antibody to gamma interferon to mice chronically infected with T. gondii caused recrudescence of encephalitis (30). The pathological features in these animals are similar to those seen in humans. Histologically, the encephalitis is a focal necrotizing process consistent with the rupture of tissue cysts in close proximity to one another. This causes the release of tachyzoites which infect surrounding neurons and astrocytes, inducing an inflammatory infiltrate. The centers of the inflammatory foci are necrotic, while toward the periphery there is inflammation with large numbers of tachyzoites.

In humans the pathogenesis of encephalitis in the immunocompromised host can be inferred from our knowledge of the natural history of the various forms of toxoplasmosis, as well as from the experimental findings described above. Although toxoplasmic encephalitis has been reported to occur in association with a variety of underlying conditions, malignancies of the reticuloendothelial system account for more than 50% of the non-AIDS cases (31). The combination of immunological abnormalities resulting from the malignancy plus cytotoxic chemotherapy favors recrudescence of latent infection leading to development of necrotizing toxoplasmic encephalitis. The most convincing evidence that recrudescence of latent infection is the mechanism which leads to development of toxoplasmic encephalitis has come from recent studies in AIDS patients and bone marrow transplant recipients. Virtually all AIDS patients and bone marrow transplant recipients who developed toxoplasmic encephalitis were seropositive for *T. gondii* prior to the onset of encephalitis. In contrast to these patient populations, there is strong epidemiological evidence that cardiac transplant recipients acquire toxoplasmosis rather than reactivate it (80,92). The donor heart is the principal source of infection. Cardiac transplant recipients who are seronegative for toxoplasmic antibodies prior to transplantation with a heart from a seropositive donor are likely to develop life-threatening toxoplasmosis. Clinically significant disease does not develop in those patients who are seropositive prior to transplantation. In addition, of four renal transplant recipients who developed toxoplasmic encephalitis, none had toxoplasmic antibody prior to transplantation. In these cases, as in transfusion-associated toxoplasmosis, the infection involved multiple organs.

The evidence for reactivation as the pathogenesis of CNS toxoplasmosis in the immunocompromised patient is severalfold. It is rare to find CNS involvement with toxoplasmosis during documented acute infections in immunocompetent hosts (93,94). Autopsy studies have demonstrated incidental findings of tissue cysts in various organs of immunocompetent patients (13), and animal and human studies have provided indirect evidence that disintegrating cyst-like structures are found in close proximity to CNS lesions (93,95). In patients with AIDS, the evidence for reactivation as the pathogenesis comes from the observation that CNS toxoplasmosis rarely develops in patients who are seronegative for IgG antibodies (83). Admittedly, the evidence for reactivation is mostly circumstantial. The manifestations of acute infection in an immunocompromised host might be different from that in a normal host; if so, the clinical distinction between reactivation and an atypical acute infection could be impossible.

Pathology

CNS infection with *Toxoplasma* causes vascular proliferation and endothelial hyperplasia associated with peri-

vascular inflammatory infiltrate which may progress to a frank vasculitis with associated necrosis (Fig. 7). There may be a profound microglial response with formation of nodules. These microglial nodules may not be associated with any other evidence of acute inflammation, but in the same brain there may be large areas of necrosis in areas remote from these nodules. By using routine histopathological stains, it is occasionally possible to demonstrate toxoplasmic tachyzoites adjacent to the microglial nodules. However, Conley et al. (97), using the highly sensitive peroxidase–antiperoxidase staining method, have shown that tachyzoites or toxoplasmic antigens are frequently associated with microglial nodules but are not found in surrounding parenchyma. Although focal areas of encephalitis separated by normal brain tissue (consistent with recrudescence of latent infection by excystment) is the usual finding, recent reports of diffuse necrotizing encephalitis in AIDS (98) may indicate that hematogenous spread of the organism also can occur.

The severity of the histopathological changes are variable and dependent on the severity of the underlying immunodeficiency. Changes can vary from a well-localized, indolent, granulomatous process (54,99) to a widely diffused necrotizing encephalitis (41,100). In patients who are severely immunocompromised, the ability to contain the infection and develop an encapsulated abscess may be diminished. The lesions can be unifocal or multifocal and may vary in size from microscopic to hemispheric. Both the white matter and the gray matter

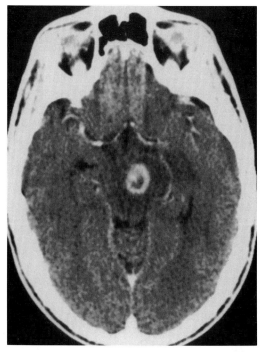

FIG. 8. Typical contrast-enhancing intracerebral lesion of *T. gondii* with associated edema in the region of the basal ganglia in a patient with AIDS. (Radiograph provided by the Department of Radiology, Duke University.)

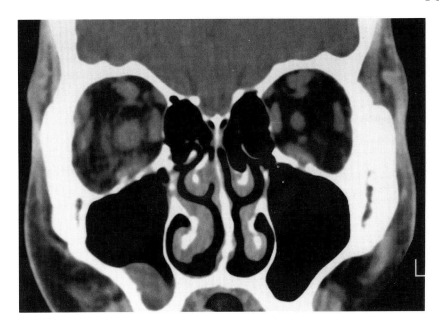

FIG. 9. CT scan showing unilateral edema and thickening of the rectus muscles and retro-orbital tissues in the right eye of an AIDS patient with isolated ocular toxoplasmosis. The eye was enucleated and showed severe retinochoroiditis with retinal necrosis. (Radiograph provided by the Department of Radiology, Duke University.)

as well as every part of the CNS may be involved. There is a propensity for lesions to localize in the basal ganglia (Fig. 8), the corticomedullary interface, the thalamus, and the white matter. The pituitary gland and the hypothalamus may be involved. In contrast to congenital toxoplasmosis, the meninges are usually not involved (71), except as part of a localized reaction to the underlying cortical process.

In 1967 The National Cancer Institute (NCI) reviewed the pathological findings in six patients with CNS toxoplasmosis (70). The main lesions were areas of focal necrotizing encephalitis in gray matter (Fig. 7). Perivascular inflammation was prominent towards the periphery of these lesions. Glial nodules composed of microglial cells and astrocytes were common. *Toxoplasma* organisms were also found within various types of cells throughout the gray matter. In general, inflammation was sparse, being more intense in earlier lesions where *T. gondii* organisms were present. There was usually a striking lack of meningitis (71) and little inflammatory cellular response (99).

The findings in patients with AIDS, now well-documented, are similar. The typical lesions of focal necrotizing encephalitis are often called "abscesses." Cysts and extracellular free tachyzoites are a hallmark of this disease process. Histopathologically, the most intense inflammation is associated with these cysts and tachyzoites (31,101–104). Three distinct zones have been identified (102) (Fig. 7). The central zone is an amorphous, avascular, necrotic area containing few identifiable organisms. When blood vessels are seen, they are necrotic and occluded by thrombi. Huang and Chou (105) examined the ring-enhancing lesions from four AIDS patients and

one other immunocompromised patient and found, by immunohistochemical staining, tachyzoites within the arterial walls associated with acute necrotizing arteritis in early lesions. In advanced lesions, more concentric fibrosis of the vessel wall was found, along with associated thrombosis and necrosis. These were associated with more tachyzoites. An intermediate zone contains engorged blood vessels, areas of patchy necrosis, numerous intracellular and extracellular tachyzoites, and variable numbers of cysts. There is prominent perivascular cuffing by round cells, with endothelial cell swelling and proliferation. In the outer zone, necrosis is rare and vascular lesions are minimal. In these areas, the organism most often appears in the form of tissue cysts, which are usually less numerous than in the middle zone. Examination of biopsies with standard histological stains may not reveal the organisms, but tachyzoites and *Toxoplasma*-specific antigens can be easily identified by immunohistologic methods (106). Multiple granulomas and diffuse (rather than focal) abscesses may be seen in some cases (98,103).

Clinical Manifestations

The clinical presentation is variable, ranging from an insidious process evolving over weeks to acute onset of a confusional state. The initial neurological symptoms and signs may be focal, nonfocal, or both. Focal abnormalities such as homonymous hemianopsia, diplopia, cranial nerve palsies, hemiparesis, hemiplegia, hemisensory loss, aphasia, focal seizures, personality changes, movement disorders, and cerebellar dysfunction correlate with the anatomical areas involved. Because *Toxoplasma* has a predilection to localize in the region of the basal ganglia and brainstem (Fig. 8), extrapyramidal symptoms resembling Parkinson's disease (as well as movement disorders such as hemichorea and hemiballismus) have been reported. In general, patients who present with nonfocal abnormalities usually develop signs of focal neurological disease as the infection progresses. However, a few patients develop a diffuse, rapidly fatal encephalitic process with no focal abnormalities seen on neuroradiographic studies (98). Nonfocal evidence of neurological dysfunction—including generalized weakness, headache, confusion, lethargy, alteration of mental status, personality changes, and coma—may predominate. Furthermore, focal neurological problems may at first be subtle and transient, evolving over time into persistent focal neurological deficits. It may be difficult to differentiate cerebral toxoplasmosis from herpes encephalitis. Panhypopituitarism (107) and hyponatremia resulting from inappropriate antidiuretic hormone secretion can occur. When patients present with global cognitive impairment associated with attention deficits, impaired recent memory, and slowness of motor responses, toxoplasmosis may be difficult to differentiate from other neurological processes, including the AIDS dementia syndrome itself. Because infection of the CNS by *Toxoplasma* is predominantly parenchymal, evidence of meningeal inflammation is rare. Toxoplasmic infection in the immunocompromised host is characterized by progressive CNS symptoms. Untreated, the course of the infection—from the initial manifestation of encephalitis until death—varies from days to months.

The pathogenesis of the infection may determine the clinical presentation. For example, toxoplasmic encephalitis in transplant recipients is often nonfocal. These patients often have diffuse, disseminated systemic disease (78); *T. gondii* may be found in the heart, lung, and bone marrow (80,81,108). Retinochoroiditis in a patient on long-term corticosteroid therapy has also been noted (66). CSF is remarkable for elevated protein concentrations in the range 100–230 mg/100 mg, few white blood cells (mainly mononuclear cells), and normal glucose levels (71). Early signs and symptoms include lethargy, confusion, decreased responsiveness, generalized seizures, and headache. Occasionally the initial clinical manifestations may include focal abnormalities; however, localizing neurological signs tend to occur late in the course of the infection in transplant recipients or not at all. Histopathologically, encephalitis tends to be diffuse and there is evidence of multiple organ involvement. As a result, in the early stages of encephalitis there may be no abnormalities on neuroimaging studies. In such cases, the etiology of the encephalitis may be indicated only by biopsy of another affected organ, or at necropsy. These findings may reflect the fact that in these patients, toxoplasmosis was acquired acutely during the peritransplant period. The course of the encephalitis in transplant patients is

variable, ranging from indolent progress over several months to fulminant disease that results in death within 2 weeks of the initial presentation. There is one report of apparent self-limited toxoplasmic parasitemia after liver transplantation, diagnosed by isolating the organisms from the patient's buffy-coat cells (109).

The presentation of toxoplasmic encephalitis in patients with underlying malignancies, such as Hodgkin's disease, is evenly distributed between focal and nonfocal manifestations of encephalitis. Twelve of 20 cases reviewed in the 1967 NCI study (70) had prominent CNS symptoms, with complaints of headache, disorientation, and drowsiness (70). Several patients demonstrated focal abnormalities (such as hemiparesis, cranial nerve palsies, long-track signs, and coma) which correlated with autopsy findings of focal toxoplasmic lesions within the brain. Also seen were convulsions, nausea and vomiting, papilledema, and nystagmus. CNS toxoplasmosis was associated with fever in eight of 20 of the cases. In a subsequent study of cases associated with underlying neoplasms, fever was a prominent (and sometimes the only) sign of toxoplasmosis (110).

Today, the number of cases of toxoplasmic encephalitis associated with cancer and transplants is minuscule compared with the number in AIDS patients. This can be the first manifestation of HIV infection, especially in areas where toxoplasmic seroprevalence is high (88,111). In the United States, CNS toxoplasmosis is the AIDS-defining illness in approximately half of those individuals who develop this complication of HIV infection.

Patients with AIDS often present with nonspecific signs such as neuropsychiatric complaints, headache, disorientation, confusion, and lethargy. Associated fever and weight loss are common but nonspecific in this population. The typical course is subacute, progressing over 2–8 weeks. Eventually the patients often develop evidence of a focal lesion and mass effect with ataxia, aphasia, hemiparesis, visual field loss, vomiting, or a more generalized encephalitis with increasing confusion, dementia, and stupor (112). Seizures are common and may be the presenting manifestation of the illness (113). In the majority of AIDS patients, the clinical manifestations of toxoplasmosis tend to be limited to the brain; however, cases of widely disseminated infection with multiple organ involvement have been reported. The CSF profile is characterized by a mild mononuclear cell pleocytosis and elevated protein levels. CSF glucose concentration is usually normal, but it may be reduced (114).

A report early in the AIDS epidemic identified toxoplasmic retinochoroiditis in a patient 6 months before cerebral toxoplasmosis became symptomatic (115). This sequence appears to be unusual. Rarely, isolated ocular toxoplasmosis occurs (Fig. 9). Other unusual presentations include unilateral akathisia (116) and panhypopituitarism (107).

The differential diagnosis of CNS disease in patients

with AIDS includes other infections such as cryptococcal meningitis, tuberculosis, nocardial, or bacterial abscess, progressive multifocal leukoencephalopathy (PML) (117), and malignancies, predominantly primary CNS lymphomas. It should be noted that CNS toxoplasmosis may occur as one of two or more concurrent, treatable CNS infections (113,118,119).

Early in the AIDS epidemic, focal CNS lesions were usually biopsied to determine appropriate treatment (120–122). Within a few years, the high incidence of toxoplasmosis versus other diagnoses in these patients led many physicians to begin empirical therapy without biopsy. Patients with no other evident diagnosis and neuroradiologic findings consistent with toxoplasmosis (see Chapter 37) were treated empirically for CNS toxoplasmosis and followed clinically and radiographically. A good response to therapy was often used as a positive diagnostic test. A retrospective evaluation of this practice of empirical therapy found that 68% (26 of 38) of patients responded to empirical therapy within 2–4 weeks of therapy. There were 12 nonresponders; further evaluation after 2–4 weeks of therapy led to the diagnosis of CNS tuberculosis in two patients and primary CNS lymphoma in another two. PML was diagnosed presumptively from radiographic appearance in another six. Patients who responded to therapy had a significantly longer median survival than did nonresponders: 311 days versus 79 days, $p = 0.05$ (123).

Empirical treatment for presumed toxoplasmosis could delay treatment of other rare but treatable CNS infections such as tuberculosis or nocardiosis. However, the other leading causes of focal CNS lesions, primary CNS lymphoma and PML, both have a dismal prognosis with or without treatment. The choice of empirical therapy versus brain biopsy remains controversial, requiring an individual decision on risks and benefits for each patient.

DIAGNOSIS

Serology

Serological testing is useful for population studies of prevalence of toxoplasmic infection (39). Its value for diagnosis of toxoplasmic encephalitis in a given patient is largely dependent upon the type of patient. In the nonimmunocompromised host, acute acquired toxoplasmosis is usually established by a fourfold rise in antibody titer. The Sabin–Feldman dye test is the standard test for IgG antibodies. In immunocompetent hosts, a single high titer is a sensitive indicator of acute infection (93%) if a titer of $\geq 1{:}1024$ is used as the criterion. The IgG–immunofluorescent antibody test (IgG-IFA) correlates well with the dye test. Neither of these tests is specific for acute infection, however, because 62% of patients will continue to have this high titer at 12 months (124). An

exception to this is the case of one nonimmunocompromised patient who eventually died of toxoplasmic encephalitis but who had no antitoxoplasmic antibody in the serum; however, toxoplasmic antibody was found in the CSF. The diagnosis in this patient was established by direct demonstration of organisms in the CSF (31).

Although the presence of a high antibody titer suggests acute infection, such titers may persist for years after acute infection. Therefore, the presence of IgM antibody directed against *T. gondii* may be useful for the diagnosis of acute acquired toxoplasmosis. The double-sandwich IgM enzyme-linked immunoabsorbent assay (DS-IgM-ELISA) is more sensitive and specific for acute infection than is the IgM-IFA assay (124). A positive result usually indicates infection within the prior 3–4 months. There are many exceptions, however; IgM antibody titers may remain elevated for as long as 9 months after acute infection (125). Conversely, subacute disease may not be investigated before the IgM has already decreased. One study reviewing patients with biopsy-proven toxoplasmic lymphadenopathy, who had serologies tested within 6 months of clinical symptoms, showed that 12% were negative by DS-IgM-ELISA. Recent data indicate that the presence of elevated antitoxoplasmic IgA antibody may be a more specific indicator of acute acquired infection. This latter test may be particularly useful in pregnant patients, in whom it is important to ascertain whether toxoplasmosis has been acquired during a relatively short period of gestation (126). Santoro et al. (127) have also reported an assay which uses monoclonal antibodies to purified p30 parasite protein in an IgM-capture ELISA which was relatively specific for acute toxoplasmosis.

The diagnosis of congenital toxoplasmic infection is complicated by (a) the high prevalence of IgG antibodies in the general population and (b) the frequency of asymptomatic congenital toxoplasmosis at birth. Nevertheless, it is often investigated and eventually diagnosed by serological methods. It is important to discern whether antibody present in the serum of the infant is present because of passive transfer of maternal antibody or because of an immunological reaction by the infant to active infection. The presence of antitoxoplasmic IgM antibody is useful in determining congenital infection. The highly sensitive DS-IgM-ELISA detects antibody in 75% of babies with congenital toxoplasmosis, whereas the IgM-IFA is positive in only 25% (124,128). At times, the development of an IgM response may be negative at birth, only to be detected after the first few weeks of life. It is important to be aware that IgM antibody may be present as a result of a placental leak; however, because of the short half-life of this class of antibody, the titer will decay rapidly over the first few weeks after birth. Determining whether the presence of IgG antibody is a result of passive transfer or a result of reaction by the infant to an ongoing infection is more difficult. This is complicated by several factors, including: the relatively longer half-life of IgG antibody, approximately 21 days; persistence of maternal antibody in the circulation of the infant for as long as 1 year; and the fact that antitoxoplasmic chemotherapy will delay antitoxoplasmic antibody synthesis in the infant. As a rule of thumb, if the infant is left untreated, significant rises in levels of antitoxoplasmic antibody should be seen by 3 months of age; if the infant is treated, these rises may not be obvious for 6–9 months. Antibody levels may fluctuate during the first year of life; therefore, antitoxoplasmic antibody titers should be assessed relative to the total IgG level.

The serological diagnosis of toxoplasmic encephalitis in the immunocompromised host requires an understanding of the pathogenesis of the infection in different groups at risk. For instance, in heart (and probably renal) transplant recipients, toxoplasmic encephalitis most often follows acute acquisition of the organism, usually as a result of receiving an organ from a donor who had been previously infected with *T. gondii* (78,80,129). The usefulness of antibody serology in predicting the development of significant disease due to *T. gondii* has been studied prospectively (80). Patients who were seronegative for *Toxoplasma* prior to transplantation and who received a heart from a seropositive donor seroconverted and developed severe symptomatic disease. In contrast, patients who were seropositive prior to transplantation often developed significant IgG and IgM antibody titers to *T. gondii* after transplantation but remained asymptomatic. In such instances, a rise in antibody titer did not indicate significant disease due to *T. gondii.* Obviously, knowledge of the serological status of the organ donor and recipient is necessary in order to identify high-risk patients, match donors and recipients, and interpret subsequent serologies. Significant rises in antibody titers have been demonstrated in a variety of immunocompromised patients without specific evidence of active infection (130). Therefore, clinicians should be careful in making a diagnosis of toxoplasmosis in patients with underlying immunocompromising conditions and nonspecific signs such as persistent fever and malaise. In these cases, confirmation of active toxoplasmosis should be sought by detection of parasitemia (131) or by histopathological demonstration of the organism.

Instead of rising or high titers, many immunocompromised patients may have low or absent antitoxoplasmic antibody titers. Sometimes this is because toxoplasmic encephalitis occurs as a result of a recrudescence of a latent infection in a patient who has been severely immunocompromised. This is evident in bone marrow transplant and AIDS patients (132). Because toxoplasmic encephalitis occurs most often as a result of a recrudescence of a latent infection in these patients, one can almost uniformly demonstrate the presence of antitoxoplasmic antibody prior to the development of the encephalitis. In addition, rises in antibody titer can be demonstrated in only a minority of cases, and titers may even decline as the encephalitis progresses. Antitoxoplasmic

IgM antibody is also rarely found in these patients, even when they have toxoplasmic encephalitis (88). In the non-AIDS immunocompromised host with a low frequency of toxoplasmic encephalitis, serology is of little or no value. A positive diagnosis usually requires immunohistochemical examination of biopsy material.

In the case of HIV-infected patients, in whom toxoplasmic encephalitis is a leading opportunistic infection of the brain, special attention should be paid to the interpretation of serology. More than 97% of patients with AIDS and toxoplasmic encephalitis have antibody titers against *T. gondii* which vary from 1:8 to >1:1024. The level of antitoxoplasmic antibody as measured by the Sabin–Feldman dye test or the indirect fluorescent assay is not discernibly different than that found in the AIDS patient without evidence of encephalitis. However, the predictive value of a positive serology in a patient with characteristic abnormalities on radiographic studies may be as high as 80% in the United States (123). Therefore, many physicians would initiate a therapeutic trial of antitoxoplasmic chemotherapy in an AIDS patients who is seropositive for *T. gondii* and who has a characteristic neuroradiographic abnormality. Bishburg et al. (133) questioned this approach on the grounds that the early statistics on *Toxoplasma* as a cause of CNS lesions in AIDS patients were drawn from populations with high prevalence of latent infection, such as Haitians. Their retrospective review of (largely) intravenous-drug-using AIDS patients showed more variation in the appearance of brain images and less predictive value for the pathogen ultimately found on biopsy. In populations in whom other CNS processes are more prevalent, the predictive value of a positive serology may be much lower (113). Also, in populations where the overall seroprevalence for *T. gondii* is very high, the ability of a positive serology to distinguish toxoplasmic encephalitis from other infectious and noninfectious etiologies which cause similar neuroradiologic abnormalities would be lowered. Efforts to introduce more sophisticated techniques (such as western blot analyses) to see if specific antibody fractions correlate with acute infection have not proven useful so far (134).

A useful adjunctive test may be the determination of antitoxoplasmic antibodies in the spinal fluid (135). For this technique, it is important to determine whether there is intrathecal production of antitoxoplasmic antibody. This can be determined by the following formula: [CSF dye test titer (reciprocal)/total CSF globulin] × [total serum globulin/serum dye test titer (reciprocal)]. Using this formula, a value of >1 is indicative of intrathecal production of antitoxoplasmic antibody in the immunocompromised host. The utility of this test decreases in patients with high serum levels of antitoxoplasmic antibody.

In summary, interpretation of serological tests for toxoplasmosis is dependent upon the clinical situation, the prior probability of disease, the clinician's understanding of the pathogenesis of the infection, and the patient's underlying conditions.

Imaging

Plain skull radiographs of infants with congenital toxoplasmosis may show characteristic spotty intracerebral calcification. Computerized axial tomography (CAT) and magnetic resonance imaging (MRI) are both extremely useful for diagnosis of CNS toxoplasmosis (102,136,137). Characteristically, CAT shows rounded isodense or hypodense lesions with ring enhancement after administration of contrast material (Fig. 8). The enhancement seems to correlate pathologically to vascular proliferation and surrounding inflammation. Although ring enhancement of toxoplasmic lesions is common, homogeneous enhancement or no enhancement also can be seen (112). In approximately 75% of cases (102), the lesions are multiple, often involving the corticomedullary junction and the basal ganglia, (Fig. 8) although any part of the CNS may be involved. The lesions are frequently associated with marked edema and mass effect. Some investigators believe that a double-dose delayed-contrast study may be a more sensitive method for delineating the true extent of disease. As a rule, however, CAT scans underestimate the number of lesions found at autopsy (112). In several cases, the immediate CAT scan was reported as negative whereas the delayed study demonstrated enhancing lesions. With increasing use of MRI, it has been shown that the CAT scan has limitations in defining the full extent of disease (136,137). MRI has detected lesions in patients with active toxoplasmic encephalitis whose CAT scans were normal. Therefore, it is recommended that an MRI be performed on patients with neurological symptoms and antibody to *Toxoplasma* whose CAT scans show no abnormality.

The features of the images seen in patients with toxoplasmic encephalitis are not pathognomonic; furthermore, they can be seen in a variety of infectious and noninfectious processes, including primary CNS lymphoma, Kaposi's sarcoma, and tuberculoma. In addition, toxoplasmosis may present with unusual CAT appearances, such as hydrocephalus without focal lesions (138). It has been suggested that multiple lesions suggest toxoplasmosis whereas single lesions are more consistent with lymphoma; however, this differentiation is weak.

MRI and CAT scans are useful for assessment of response to therapy, which is often used to confirm a clinical diagnosis of toxoplasmic encephalitis. This is especially true in AIDS patients. Although resolution of all or most abnormalities on CAT scan may take as long as 6 months, patients who respond to therapy will usually have radiographic evidence of improvement within 3 weeks of initiation of therapy (112). Oftentimes, radiographic response to therapy lags behind the clinical response. There is an impression that peripheral CNS lesions tend to resolve more quickly than deeper lesions. Because other processes, both infectious and malignant, can occur concomitantly with toxoplasmic encephalitis, a persistent or enlarging lesion, even in a patient in whom there has been an overall clinical and neuroradiographic response, should be considered for biopsy.

Identification and Isolation of the Organism

Toxoplasmic encephalitis is frequently diagnosed presumptively in patients with AIDS and in heart transplant patients. However, definitive diagnosis requires the demonstration of organisms in a clinical specimen. Occasionally, patients with toxoplasmic encephalitis may have a concomitant pneumonitis, with the pathogen being detected in bronchoalveolar lavage fluid (139). Also, in the rare patient in whom there is evidence of meningoencephalitis, the organism may be isolated from CSF (140). Recently, the organism has also been isolated in blood cultures of patients with and without evidence of an ongoing encephalitis (131). In the past, isolation of *T. gondii* from clinical specimens required inoculation of the specimen into laboratory animals, most commonly mice (139). However, this technique is labor-intensive and requires as long as 6 weeks to demonstrate the organism. Another diagnostic method, currently being explored by Boothroyd and co-workers (141), is selective amplification by polymerase chain reaction of DNA products specific to *T. gondii*. This latter technique may provide a sensitive and specific assay for the direct identification of *T. gondii* in clinical specimens. This may be particularly useful in the detection of *Toxoplasma* in the amniotic fluid of women with acutely acquired toxoplasmosis and congenital transmission of the infection to the fetus. The clinical utility of this extremely sensitive technique in identifying the pathogen in CSF (in an infection which is predominantly encephalitic rather than meningitic) remains to be demonstrated.

At present, the definitive diagnosis of toxoplasmic encephalitis during life usually requires a brain biopsy. Intraoperative sonography and needle biopsy with a stereotactic device have proven useful in identifying the site of infection and decreasing the morbidity from biopsy. However, the size of the biopsy is small, and this limits the extent to which immunohistochemical studies can be performed. Given that the histological changes associated with *Toxoplasma* may sometimes closely resemble those of viral encephalitis and that tachyzoites may be difficult to discern from nuclear debris, diagnosis of toxoplasmic encephalitis often requires specialized immunohistochemical techniques in order to detect the organism or its antigens. The immunofluorescence technique described by Sun et al. (142), using monoclonal antitoxoplasmic antibodies on brain touch preparations and CSF, were found to be more sensitive than hematoxylin–eosin or Giemsa stains for rapid diagnosis of CNS toxoplasmosis. In addition, the reactive round-cell infiltrate in toxoplasmic encephalitis may be difficult to differentiate from an intracerebral lymphoma. Therefore, it is recommended that if a needle biopsy does not definitively diagnose *T. gondii* infection or lymphoma, further tissue should be obtained for more extensive studies using pathogen and cell-specific antibodies (97,142). Pseudocysts and tachyzoites that are easily identifiable by histopathological stains may not be found in the center of the necrotic lesion and are best identified at the periphery of the lesion or within normal brain.

TREATMENT

Pyrimethamine and Sulfadiazine

The mainstay of therapy for toxoplasmic encephalitis is the combination of pyrimethamine, a dihydrofolate reductase inhibitor, and sulfadiazine, a dihydrofolate synthetase inhibitor (143,144). These two drugs sequentially block folic acid metabolism and thereby act synergistically against *T. gondii*. Therefore, in infections of the brain in which diffusion of the drug to the site of infection may be compromised, these drugs should be used in combination. Among the sulfonamides, sulfadiazine, sulfamethazine, and sulfamerazine are equally efficacious.

Pyrimethamine is well-absorbed after oral administration and has a half-life of approximately 4 days in the normal host. However, in recent studies in patients with AIDS and toxoplasmic encephalitis, pyrimethamine levels were found to be unpredictable (145,146). Recently, the pharmacokinetics of pyrimethamine in five patients with toxoplasmic encephalitis treated with 75 mg of pyrimethamine per day were studied (B. J. Luft, *unpublished data*). The half-life of pyrimethamine varied between 26 and 90 hr in these patients, and the serum levels varied between 500 and 2000 ng/ml. Therefore, it becomes apparent that our knowledge of the factors which determine serum pyrimethamine levels and the half-life of the drug is limited. Furthermore, there have been no studies performed which correlate the levels of antitoxoplasmic chemotherapeutic agents found in the serum to the response to therapy as well as to toxicity. Sulfadiazine is rapidly absorbed in the gastrointestinal tract, and serum levels peak within 3–6 hr after ingestion. Both pyrimethamine and sulfadiazine have been found to penetrate the blood–spinal fluid barrier.

Currently, pyrimethamine is administered as a 100- to 200-mg loading dose and 50–75 mg/day by mouth for the first 3–6 weeks of therapy. The latter dosage has been shown to maintain levels fairly consistently within the therapeutic range. Sulfadiazine is given at a dose of 4–6 g/day in four divided doses by mouth.

The combination of these drugs is highly effective

against tachyzoites, but they have no effect on the cyst form. Therefore, because both tachyzoites and cysts are present during active encephalitis (Figs. 1, 3, 7) patients who remain severely immunocompromised frequently relapse upon discontinuation of therapy. A multicenter retrospective review of toxoplasmic encephalitis in patients with AIDS found that 50% relapsed after discharge from the hospital (147). Therapy is therefore usually continued until adequate cell-mediated immunity has been reestablished, or, in the case of AIDS, for life (145). The maintenance phase of therapy usually requires much lower doses of pyrimethamine and sulfadiazine. A variety of regimens have been administered for maintenance therapy, including pyrimethamine (25–50 mg) plus sulfadiazine (2–4 g), given daily or two or three times weekly (145). Further studies are needed to determine the optimal doses and dosing intervals of these agents for both acute and long-term therapy.

The toxicity associated with pyrimethamine and sulfadiazine has been formidable. Up to 60% of patients with AIDS treated with these agents will develop a significant level of toxicity, often necessitating discontinuation of therapy (147). During the acute phase of treatment, skin rash is the most prominent dose-limiting toxicity and is expected to occur in up to 20% of patients with active encephalitis. The drug-induced hematologic toxicity associated with antitoxoplasmic therapy usually occurs in later stages of therapy and may be exacerbated by concomitant antiretroviral chemotherapy given to AIDS patients. With careful monitoring for evidence of hematologic toxicity, patients who are on long-term suppressive therapy for toxoplasmic encephalitis often can tolerate concomitant 3'-azido-3'-deoxythymidine (AZT) at a dose of 500 mg/day. In addition, recent *in vitro* and animal studies have shown that AZT antagonizes the effect of low concentrations of pyrimethamine on the parasite and reverses the usual synergism of pyrimethamine and sulfadiazine against *T. gondii*. This effect was also demonstrated in acutely infected mice (148). There have been no adequate studies in humans to evaluate the significance of this finding in the management of patients.

Folinic acid (e.g., leucovorin) supplements are often given in hopes of decreasing hematologic side effects seen, when pyrimethamine and sulfadiazine are used in combination. There is *in vitro* evidence that it reverses toxicity for bone marrow precursor cells (149). Leucovorin has been used to rescue patients given high-dose methotrexate for treatment of malignancies, but its value has not been proven in humans receiving antiprotozoal therapy. Bygbjerg et al. (150) compared folic acid and folinic acid supplements in patients receiving trimethoprim–sulfamethoxazole. These treatments did not abolish drug-related cytopenias, and folinic acid was of less benefit than folic acid. Although no control group was included, these authors recommended routine use of a 5-mg/day folic acid supplement (150). Sattler et al.

(151) found no difference between 80- and 160-mg leu-covorin daily supplements, given to reduce hematologic toxicity in patients treated with trimetrexate. In practice, many clinicians administer folate supplements to patients receiving treatment for toxoplasmosis, but evidence of efficacy is incomplete and optimal regimens have not been defined.

New Agents

The toxicity associated with standard antitoxoplasmic chemotherapy has stimulated a search for new chemotherapeutic agents. Clindamycin has long been recognized to be an effective drug for the treatment of murine toxoplasmosis (152). There have been several reports of patients with AIDS and toxoplasmic encephalitis who were effectively treated with pyrimethamine at doses of 25–75 mg/day plus oral or intravenous clindamycin at doses of 1200–4800 mg/day (153–155). Recently, a prospective study by the California University-wide Task Force on AIDS reported that clindamycin (1200 mg every 6 hr, intravenously) plus pyrimethamine (75 mg/day, orally) were equivalent in efficacy to pyrimethamine plus sulfadiazine for the treatment of toxoplasmic encephalitis (156). Furthermore, there appears to be a trend toward less toxicity with this regimen.

New and old chemotherapeutic agents have been recently shown to have efficacy in murine models of infection (157). These have included macrolides such as roxithromycin (158,159), and azithromycin (160). Roxithromycin has also been found to be synergistic with gamma interferon in the treatment of murine toxoplasmic encephalitis (161). A purine analogue, arprinocid, has also been studied. It is a competitive inhibitor of hypoxanthine transmembrane transport, an essential function in *Toxoplasma* organisms because they cannot synthesize purines *de novo* (162). It remains to be determined if these drugs will be efficacious in humans with toxoplasmic encephalitis. Other experimental agents that may prove to be useful for the treatment of toxoplasmic encephalitis are the highly lipid-soluble dihydrofolate reductase inhibitors such as trimetrexate or piritrexin (163,164). These drugs have a higher affinity for toxoplasmic dihydrofolate reductase than does pyrimethamine. However, it has been reported that toxoplasmic encephalitis recurs during the course of treatment with trimetrexate, when used alone (165). These agents in combination with sulfadiazine may be useful for the treatment of toxoplasmic encephalitis—especially in the subpopulation of patients who appear to respond poorly to initial therapy with pyrimethamine or sulfadiazine, or in those who have poor prognostic indicators such as severe lethargy and coma. Piritrexin, an alternative dihydrofolate reductase inhibitor to pyrimethamine, may cause fewer side effects such as skin rash and headache because it has less inhibitory activity on histamine *N*-methyltransferase, thus causing less accumulation of histamine in tissues (164).

The treatment of ocular toxoplasmosis has also relied upon pyrimethamine and sulfonamides. In addition, clindamycin, both intraocular and systemic, has been used with reasonable success as primary therapy, as well as in patients who had failed pyrimethamine and sulfonamides (166). In patients treated for a mean of 3 weeks, results were good (167).

PREVENTION

The ecology of *T. gondii* infection is such that, so long as humans eat meat and remain in close contact with cats, we will continue to serve as incidental hosts to the parasite. Although primary infection is usually asymptomatic, primary infection during pregnancy or immunocompromised state may have devastating consequences. Prevention of infection may be facilitated by eating only meat which has been well-cooked or which has been frozen at −20°C and thawed (18). Cleaner, less crowded living conditions with fewer stray cats has probably contributed to the decreasing incidence of congenital toxoplasmosis observed in industrialized countries in recent decades (2). Consistent handwashing after handling cats or their feces should decrease the ingestion of oocysts. Pregnant women and immunocompromised hosts especially should avoid close contact with cats, and they should also guard against eating poorly cooked or raw meat.

Prevention of congenital toxoplasmosis has been attempted in France, where seroprevalence rates are very high. Seronegative women at risk for primary infection were treated during pregnancy with spiramycin and had decreased incidence of congenital toxoplasmosis in their newborns (2,3). Prevention of primary infection in organ transplant patients is approached as follows: Pretransplant donor and recipient IgG serologies are established. If possible, seronegative recipients only receive seronegative organs. If this is not possible, treatment with pyrimethamine–sulfadiazine may be considered. No information is available regarding the optimal duration of such therapy.

REFERENCES

1. Kimball AC, Kean BH, Fuchs F. Congenital toxoplasmosis: a prospective study of 4,048 obstetric patients. *Am J Obstet Gynecol* 1971;111:211–218.
2. Desmonts G, Couvreur J. Toxoplasmosis in pregnancy and its transmission to the fetus. *Bull NY Acad Med* 1974;50:146–159.
3. Remington JS, Desmonts G. Toxoplasmosis. In: Remington JS, Klein JO eds. *Infectious diseases of the fetus and newborn infant.* Philadelphia: WB Saunders, 1990;89–195.
4. Wolf A, Cowen D. Granulomatous encephalomyelitis due to an encephalitozoon (*Encephalitozoon encephalitis*). A new protozoan disease of man. *Bull Clin Neurosci* 1937;6:306–371.
5. Wolf A, Cowen D, Paige BH. Toxoplasmic encephalitis. Experi-

mental transmission of the infection to animals from a human infant. *J Exp Med* 1940;71:187–214.

6. Wolf A, Cowen D, Paige B. Human toxoplasmosis: occurrence in infants as an encephalomyelitis verification by transmission to animals. *Science* 1939;89:226–227.

7. Paige BH, Cowen D, Wolf A. Toxoplasmic encephalomyelitis. *Am J Dis Child* 1942;63:474–514.

8. Wolf A, Cowen D, Paige BH. Fetal encephalomyelitis: prenatal inception of infantile toxoplasmosis. *Science* 1941;93:548–549.

9. Paige BH, Cowen D, Wolf A. Toxoplasmic encephalomyelitis. V. Further observations of infantile toxoplasmosis; intrauterine inception of the disease; visceral manifestations. *Am J Dis Child* 1942;63:474–514.

10. Sabin A. Toxoplasmic encephalitis in children. *JAMA* 1941;116:801–814.

11. Pinkerton H, Henderson RG. Adult toxoplasmosis. A previously unrecognized disease entity simulating the typhus–spotted fever group. *JAMA* 1941;116:807–814.

12. Cowen D, Wolf A, Paige BH. Toxoplasmic encephalomyelitis. VI. Clinical diagnosis of infantile or congenital toxoplasmosis; survival beyond infancy. *Arch Neurol Psychiatry* 1942;48:689–739.

13. Frenkel JK. Pathogenesis of toxoplasmosis and of infections with organisms resembling *Toxoplasma. Ann NY Acad Sci* 1956;64:215.

13a. Vietzke WM, Gelderman AH, Grimley PM, Valsamis MP. Toxoplasmosis complicating malignancy. *Cancer* 1968;21:816–827.

14. Selik RM, Starcher ET, Curran JW. Opportunistic diseases reported in AIDS patients: frequencies, associations, and trends. *Aids* 1987;1:175–182.

15. Price RW, Brew B. Management of the neurologic complications of HIV infection and AIDS. *Infect Dis Clin North Am* 1988;2:359–372.

16. Katz M, Despommier DD, Gwadz RW. *Parasitic diseases.* New York: Springer-Verlag, 1989.

17. Lainson R. Observations on the development and nature of pseudocysts and cysts of *Toxoplasma gondii. Trans R Soc Trop Med Hyg* 1958;52:396–407.

17a. Sabin AB, Olitzky PK. Toxoplasma and obligate intracellular parasitism. *Science* 1937;85:336–338.

18. Dubey JP, Miller NL, Frenkel JK. The *Toxoplasma gondii* oocyst from cat feces. *J Exp Med* 1970;133:636–662.

19. Frenkel JK, Dubey JP, Miller NL. *Toxoplasma gondii* in cats: fecal stages identified as coccidian oocysts. *Science* 1970;167:893–896.

20. Sheffield HG, Melton ML. *Toxoplasma gondii:* the oocyst, sporozoite, and infection of cultured cells. *Science* 1970;167:892–893.

21. Van der Waaij D. Formation, growth and multiplication of *Toxoplasma gondii* cysts in mouse brains. *Trop Geogr Med* 1959;11:345–360.

22. Luft BJ. *Toxoplasma gondii.* In: Walzer PD, ed. *Parasitic infections in the immunocompromised host. Immunologic mechanisms and clinical applications,* 1st ed. New York: Marcel Dekker, 1988;179–279.

23. Murray HW. How protozoa evade intracellular killing. *Ann Intern Med* 1983;98:1016–1018.

24. Wilson CB, Tsai V, Remington JS. Failure to trigger the oxidative metabolic burst by normal macrophages. Possible mechanism for survival of intracellular pathogens. *J Exp Med* 1980;151:328–346.

25. Jones TC, Yeh S, Hirsch JG. The interaction between *Toxoplasma gondii* and mammalian cells: mechanism of entry and intracellular fate of the parasite. *J Exp Med* 1972;136:1157–1172.

26. Sibley LD, Weidner E, Krahenbuhl JL. Phagosome acidification blocked by intracellular *Toxoplasma gondii. Nature* 1985;315:416–419.

27. Murray HW, Nathan CF, Cohn ZA. Macrophage oxygen-dependent antimicrobial activity. IV. Role of endogenous scavengers of oxygen intermediates. *J Exp Med* 1980;152:1610–1624.

28. Pfefferkorn ER, Guyre PM. Inhibition of growth of *Toxoplasma gondii* in cultured fibroblasts by human recombinant gamma interferon. *Infect Immun* 1984;44:211–216.

29. McCabe RE, Luft BJ. Effect of murine interferon gamma on murine toxoplasmosis. *J Infect Dis* 1984;150:961–962.

30. Suzuki Y, Orellana MA, Schreiber RD, Remington JS. Interferon-gamma: the major mediator of resistance against *Toxoplasma gondii. Science* 1988;240:516–518.

31. Luft BJ, Brooks RG, Conley FK, McCabe R, Remington JS. Toxoplasmic encephalitis in patients with acquired immune deficiency syndrome. *JAMA* 1984;252:913–917.

32. Weinman D, Chandler AH. Toxoplasmosis in man and swine—an investigation of the possible relationship. *JAMA* 1956;161:229–232.

33. Masur H, Jones TC, Lempert JA, Cherubini TD. Outbreak of toxoplasmosis in a family and documentation of acquired retinochoroiditis. *Am J Med* 1978;64:396–402.

34. Teutsch SM, Juranek DD, Sulzer A. Epidemic toxoplasmosis associated with infected cats. *N Engl J Med* 1979;300:695–699.

35. Sacks JJ, Roberto RR, Brooks NF. Toxoplasmosis infection associated with raw goat's milk. *JAMA* 1982;248:1728–1732.

36. Luft BJ, Remington JS. Acute *Toxoplasma* infection among family members of patients with acute lymphadenopathic toxoplasmosis. *Arch Intern Med* 1984;144:53–56.

37. Benenson MW, Takafuji ET, Lemon SM, Greenup RL, Sulzer AJ. Oocyst-transmitted toxoplasmosis associated with ingestion of contaminated water. *N Engl J Med* 1982;307:666–669.

38. Feldman HA, Miller LT. Serological study of toxoplasmosis prevalence. *Am J Hyg* 1956;64:320–335.

39. Feldman HA. A nationwide serum survey of United States military recruits, 1962. *Toxoplasma* antibodies. *Am J Epidemiol* 1965;81:385–391.

40. Luft BJ, Remington JS. AIDS commentary. Toxoplasmic encephalitis. *J Infect Dis* 1988;157:1–6.

41. Townsend JJ, Wolinsky JS, Baringer JR, Johnson PC. Acquired toxoplasmosis. A neglected cause of treatable nervous system disease. *Arch Neurol* 1975;32:335–343.

42. Bach MC, Armstrong RM. Acute toxoplasmic encephalitis in a normal adult. *Arch Neurol* 1983;40:596–597.

43. McCabe RE, Brooks RG, Dorfman RF, Remington JS. Clinical spectrum in 107 cases of toxoplasmic lymphadenopathy. *Rev Infect Dis* 1987;9:754–774.

44. Grant SC, Klein C. *Toxoplasma gondii* encephalitis in an immunocompetent adult. A case report. *S Afr Med J* 1987;71:585–587.

45. Cottrell AJ. Acquired toxoplasma encephalitis. *Arch Dis Child* 1986;61:84–85.

46. Luft BJ, Remington JS. Toxoplasmosis of the central nervous system. In: Remington JS, Swartz MN, eds. *Current topics in infectious diseases,* vol 6. New York: McGraw–Hill, 1985;315–358.

47. Perkins ES. Ocular toxoplasmosis. *Br J Ophthalmol* 1973;57:1–17.

48. Aikawa M, Komata Y, Asai T, Midorikawa O. Transmission and scanning electron microscopy of host cell entry by *Toxoplasma gondii. Am J Pathol* 1977;87:285–290.

49. Nichols BA, O'Connor GR. Penetration of mouse peritoneal macrophages by the protozoan *Toxoplasma gondii.* New evidence for active invasion and phagocytosis. *Lab Invest* 1981;44:324–335.

50. Joiner KA, Fuhrman SA, Miettinen HM, Kasper LH, Mellman I. *Toxoplasma gondii:* fusion competence of parasitophorous vacuoles in Fc receptor-transfected fibroblasts. *Science* 1990;249:641–646.

51. Callahan WP Jr, Russell WO, Smith MG. Human toxoplasmosis. A clinicopathologic study with presentation of five cases and review of the literature. *Medicine* 1946;25:343–397.

52. Kass EH, Andrus SB, Adams RD, Turner FC, Feldman HA. Toxoplasmosis in the human adult. *Arch Intern Med* 1952;89:759–782.

53. Bobowski SJ, Reed WG. Toxoplasmosis in an adult presenting as a space-occupying cerebral lesion. *Arch Pathol* 1958;65:460.

54. Koeze TH, Klingon GH. Acquired toxoplasmosis. *Arch Neurol* 1964;11:191–197.

55. Arriagada C, et al. Neurotoxoplasmosis adquirido en adultos. *Acta Neurol Latinoam* 1960;6:257.

56. Hooper AD. Acquired toxoplasmosis. *Arch Pathol* 1957;64:1–9.

57. Tognetti F, Galassi E, Gaist G. Neurological toxoplasmosis presenting as a brain tumor. *J Neurosurg* 1982;56:716–721.

58. Frenkel JK. Pathology and pathogenesis of congenital toxoplasmosis. *Bull NY Acad Med* 1974;50:182–191.

59. Alford CA Jr, Stagno S, Reynolds DW. Congenital toxoplasmosis: clinical, laboratory, and therapeutic considerations, with special reference to subclinical disease. *Bull NY Acad Med* 1974;50:160–181.

60. Wilson CB, Remington JS, Stagno S, Reynolds DW. Development of adverse sequelae in children born with subclinical congenital *Toxoplasma* infection. *Pediatrics* 1980;66:767–774.

61. Michelson JB, Shields JA, McDonald PR, Manko MA, Abraham AA. Retinitis secondary to acquired systemic toxoplasmosis with isolation of the parasite. *Am J Ophthalmol* 1978;86:548–552.

62. Gump DW, Holden RA. Acquired chorioretinitis due to toxoplasmosis. *Ann Intern Med* 1979;90:58–60.

63. Frenkel JK, Jacobs L. Ocular toxoplasmosis. *Arch Ophthalmol* 1958;59:260–279.

64. Dutton GN. The causes of tissue damage in toxoplasmic retinochoroiditis. *Trans Ophthalmol Soc UK* 1986;105:404–411.

65. Rao NA, Font RL. Toxoplasmic retinochoroiditis. *Arch Ophthalmol* 1977;95:273–277.

66. Nicholson DH, Wolchok EB. Ocular toxoplasmosis in an adult receiving long-term corticosteroid therapy. *Arch Ophthalmol* 1976;94:248–254.

67. Hogan MJ. *Ocular toxoplasmosis.* New York: Columbia University Press, 1951.

68. O'Connor GR. Manifestations and management of ocular toxoplasmosis. *Bull NY Acad Med* 1974;50:192–210.

69. Parke DW, Font RL. Diffuse toxoplasmic retinochoroiditis in a patient with AIDS. *Arch Ophthalmol* 1986;104:571–575.

70. Vietzke WM, Gelderman AH, Grimley PM, Valsamis MP. Toxoplasmosis complicating malignancy. *Cancer* 1968;21:816–827.

71. Carey RM, Kimball AC, Armstrong D, Lieberman PH. Toxoplasmosis—clinical experiences in a cancer hospital. *Am J Med* 1973;54:30–38.

72. Green JA, Spruance SL, Cheson BD. Favorable outcome of central nervous system toxoplasmosis occurring in a patient with untreated Hodgkin's disease. *Cancer* 1980;45:808–810.

73. Luft BJ, Conley F, Remington JS. Outbreak of central-nervous-system toxoplasmosis in Western Europe and North America. *Lancet* 1983;:781–783.

74. Ruskin J, Remington JS. Toxoplasmosis in the compromised host. *Ann Intern Med* 1976,84.193–199.

75. Hakim M, Esmore D, Wallwork J, English TAH. Toxoplasmosis in cardiac transplantation. *Br Med J* 1986;292:1108–1108.

76. Stinson EB, Bieber CP, Griepp RB, Clark DA, Shumway NE, Remington JS. Infectious complications after cardiac transplantation in man. *Ann Intern Med* 1971;74:22–36.

77. Frenkel JK. Immunosuppression and *Toxoplasma* encephalitis. Clinical and experimental aspects. *Hum Pathol* 1975;6:97–111.

78. Reynolds ES, Walls KW, Pfeiffer RI. Generalized toxoplasmosis following renal transplantation. *Arch Intern Med* 1966;118:401–405.

79. Deleze M, Mintz G, Carmen Majia MD. *Toxoplasma gondii* encephalitis in systemic lupus erythematosus, a neglected cause of treatable nervous system infection. *J Rheumatol* 1985;12:994–996.

80. Luft BJ, Naot Y, Araujo FG, Stinson EB, Remington JS. Primary and reactivated *Toxoplasma* infection in patients with cardiac transplants. *Am Coll Physicians* 1983;99:27–31.

81. Anthony CW. Disseminated toxoplasmosis in a liver transplant patient. *J Am Med Wom Assoc* 1972;27:601–603.

82. de Morais CF. Cerebral toxoplasmosis after renal transplantation. *Pathol Res Pract* 1986;181:339–341.

83. Wong B, Gold JWM, Brown AE, et al. Central-nervous-system toxoplasmosis in homosexual men and parenteral drug abusers. *Ann Intern Med* 1984;100:36–42.

84. Vilaseca J, Arnau JM, Bacardi R, Mieras C, Serrano A, Navarro C. Kaposi's sarcoma and *Toxoplasma gondii* brain abscess in a Spanish homosexual. *Lancet* 1982;1:572.

85. Feldman HA. Breaking the transmission chain of *Toxoplasma:* a program for the prevention of human toxoplasmosis. *Bull NY Acad Med* 1974;50:236–239.

86. Clumeck N, Sonnet J, Taelman H, et al. Acquired immunodeficiency syndrome in African patients. *N Engl J Med* 1984; 310:492–497.

87. Gold JWM, Armstrong D, Grant IH. Risk of CNS toxoplasmosis in patients with acquired immune deficiency syndrome. *Abstr ICAAC* 1986.

88. Pitchenik AE, Fischl MA, Dickinson GM, et al. Opportunistic infections and Kaposi's sarcoma among Haitians: evidence of a new acquired immunodeficiency state. *Ann Intern Med* 1983;98:277–284.

89. Carme P, M'Pele P, Mbitsi A, et al. Parasitoses et mycoses opportunistes AU COURS DU SIDA—Leurs frequences a Brazzavill (Congo). *Bull Soc Pathol Exot Filiales* 1988;81:311–316.

90. Mitchell CD, Erlich SS, Mastrucci MT, Hutto SC, Parks WP, Scott GB. Congenital toxoplasmosis occurring in infants perinatally infected with human immunodeficiency virus 1. *Pediatr Infect Dis J* 1990;9:512–518.

91. Medlock MD, Tilleli JT, Pearl GS. Congenital cardiac toxoplasmosis in a newborn with acquired immunodeficiency syndrome. *Pediatr Infect Dis J* 1990;9:129–132.

92. Nagington J, Martin AL. Toxoplasmosis and heart transplantation. *Lancet* 1983;679–679.

93. Remington JS. Toxoplasmosis in the adult. *Bull NY Acad Med* 1974;50:211–227.

94. Krick JA, Remington JS. Toxoplasmosis in the adult—an overview. *N Engl J Med* 1978;298:550–553.

95. Frenkel JK, Escajadillo A. Cyst rupture as a pathogenic mechanism of toxoplasmic encephalitis. *Am J Trop Med Hyg* 1987; 36:517–522.

96. Vollmer TL, Waldor MK, Steinman L, Conley FK. Depletion of T-4 lymphocytes with monoclonal antibody reactivates toxoplasmosis in the central nervous system: a model of superinfection in AIDS. *J Immunol* 1987;138:3737–3741.

97. Conley FK, Jenkins KA, Remington JS. *Toxoplasma gondii* infection of the central nervous system. *Hum Pathol* 1981;12:690–698.

98. Gray F, Gherardi R, Wingate E, et al. Diffuse "encephalitic" cerebral toxoplasmosis in AIDS. *J Neurol* 1989;236:273–277.

99. Ghatak NR, Sawyer DR. A morphologic study of opportunistic cerebral toxoplasmosis. *Acta Neuropathol* 1978;42:217–221.

100. Fisher MA, Levy J, Helfrich M, August CS, Starr SE, Luft BJ. Detection of *Toxoplasma gondii* in the spinal fluid of a bone marrow transplant recipient. *Pediatr Infect Dis J* 1987;6:81–83.

101. Israelski DM, Remington JS. Toxoplasmic encephalitis in patients with AIDS. *Infect Dis Clin North Am* 1988;2:429–445.

102. Post MJD, Chan JC, Hensley GT, Hoffman TA, Moskowitz LB, Lippmann S. *Toxoplasma* encephalitis in Haitian adults with acquired immunodeficiency syndrome: a clinical–pathologic–CT correlation. *AJR* 1983;140:861–868.

103. Millard PR. AIDS: histopathological aspects. *J Pathol* 1984; 143:223–239.

104. Farkash AE, Maccabee PJ, Sher JH, Landesman SH, Hotson G. CNS toxoplasmosis in acquired immune deficiency syndrome: a clinical–pathological–radiological review of 12 cases. *J Neurol* 1986;49:744–748.

105. Huang TE, Chou SM. Occlusive hypertrophic arteritis as the cause of discrete necrosis in CNS toxoplasmosis in the acquired immunodeficiency syndrome. *Hum Pathol* 1988;19:1210–1214.

106. Wanke C, Tuazon CU, Kovacs A, et al. Toxoplasma encephalitis in patients with acquired immune deficiency syndrome: diagnosis and response to therapy. *Am J Trop Med Hyg* 1987;36:509–516.

107. Milligan SA, Katz MS, Craven PC, Strandberg DA, Russell IJ, Becker RA. Toxoplasmosis presenting as panhypopituitarism in a patient with the acquired immune deficiency syndrome. *Am J Med* 1984;77:760–764.

108. Lowenberg B, Van Gijn J, Prins E, Polderman AM. Fatal cerebral toxoplasmosis in a bone marrow transplant recipient with leukemia. *Transplantation* 1983;35:30–34.

109. Kusne S, Dummer JS, Ho M, et al. Self-limited *Toxoplasma* parasitemia after liver transplantation. *Transplantation* 1986;44:457–458.

110. Hakes TB, Armstrong D. Toxoplasmosis—problems in diagnosis and treatment. *Am Cancer Soc* 1983;52:1535–1540.

111. Chan JC, Moskowitz LB, Olivella J, Hensley GT, Greenman RL,

Hoffman TA. *Toxoplasma* encephalitis in recent Haitian entrants. *South Med J* 1983;76:1211–1215.

112. Navia BA, Petito CK, Gold JWM, Cho E, Jordan BD, Price RW. Cerebral toxoplasmosis complicating the acquired immune deficiency syndrome: clinical and neuropathological findings in 27 patients. *Ann Neurol* 1986;19:224–238.

113. Levy RM, Bredesen DE, Rosenblum ML. Neurological manifestations of the acquired immunodeficiency syndrome (AIDS): experience of UCSF and review of the literature. *J Neurosurg* 1985;62:475–495.

114. Mills J. *Pneumocystis carinii* and *Toxoplasma gondii* infections in patients with AIDS. *Rev Infect Dis* 1986;8:1001–1011.

115. Alonso R, Heiman-Patterson T, Mancall EL. Cerebral toxoplasmosis in acquired immune deficiency syndrome. *Arch Neurol* 1984;41:321–323.

116. Carrazana E, Rossitch E Jr, Martinez J. Unilateral "akathisia" in a patient with AIDS and a toxoplasmosis subthalamic abscess. *Neurology* 1989;39:449–450.

117. Snider WD, Simpson DM, Nielsen S, Gold JWM, Metroka CE, Posner JB. Neurological complications of acquired immune deficiency syndrome: analysis of 50 patients. *Ann Neurol* 1983; 14:403–418.

118. Bahls F, Sumi SM. Cryptococcal meningitis and cerebral toxoplasmosis in a patient with acquired immune deficiency syndrome. *J Neurol Neurosurg Psychiatry* 1986;49:328–330.

119. Fischl MA, Pitchenik AE, Spira TJ. Tuberculous brain abscess and *Toxoplasma* encephalitis in a patient with the acquired immunodeficiency syndrome. *JAMA* 1985;253:3428–3430.

120. Handler M, Ho V, Whelan M, Budzilovich G. Intracerebral toxoplasmosis in patients with acquired immune deficiency syndrome. *J Neurosurg* 1983;59:994–1001.

121. Anderson KP, Atlas E, Ahern MJ, Weisbrot IM. Central nervous system toxoplasmosis in homosexual men. *Am J Med* 1983;75:877–881.

122. Horowitz SL, Bentson JR, Benson F, Davos I, Pressman B, Gottlieb MS. CNS toxoplasmosis in acquired immunodeficiency syndrome. *Arch Neurol* 1983;40:649–652.

123. Cohn JA, McMeeking A, Cohen W, Jacobs J, Holzman RS. Evaluation of the policy of empiric treatment of suspected *Toxoplasma* encephalitis in patients with the acquired immunodeficiency syndrome. *Am J Med* 1989;86:521–527.

124. Brooks RG, McCabe RE, Remington JS. Role of serology in the diagnosis of toxoplasmic lymphadenopathy. *Rev Infect Dis* 1987;9:775–782.

125. Naot Y, Guptill DR, Remington JS. Duration of IgM antibodies to *Toxoplasma gondii* after acute acquired toxoplasmosis. *J Infect Dis* 1982;145:770–770.

126. Stepick BP, Thulliez P, Araujo FG, Remington JS. IgA antibodies for diagnosis of acute congenital and acquired toxoplasmosis. *J Infect Dis* 1990;162:270–273.

127. Santoro F, Afchain D, Pierce R, Cesbron JY, Ovlaque G, Capron A. Serodiagnosis of *Toxoplasma* infection using a purified parasite protein (P30). *Clin Exp Immunol* 1985;62:262–269.

128. Naot Y, Desmonts G, Remington JS. IgM enzyme-linked immunosorbent assay test for the diagnosis of congenital *Toxoplasma* infection. *J Pediatr* 1981;98:32–36.

129. Rose AG, Uys CJ, Novitsky D, Cooper DKC, Barnard CN. Toxoplasmosis of donor and recipient hearts after heterotopic cardiac transplantation. *Arch Pathol Lab Med* 1990;107:368–373.

130. Peacock JE Jr, Folds J, Orringer E, Luft B, Cohen MS. *Toxoplasma gondii* and the compromised host. *Arch Intern Med* 1983;143:1235–1237.

131. Shepp DH, Hackman RC, Conley FK, Anderson JB, Meyers JD. *Toxoplasma gondii* reactivation identified by detection of parasitemia in tissue culture. *Ann Intern Med* 1985;103:218–221.

132. Jehn U, Fink M, Gundlach P, et al. Lethal cardiac and cerebral toxoplasmosis in a patient with acute myeloid leukemia after successful allogeneic bone marrow transplantation. *Transplantation* 1984;38:430–433.

133. Bishburg E, Eng RHK, Slim J, Perez G, Johnson E. Brain lesions in patients with acquired immunodeficiency syndrome. *Arch Intern Med* 1989;149:941–943.

134. Weiss LM, Udem SA, Tanowitz H, Wittner M. Western blot analysis of the antibody response of patients with AIDS and *Toxo-*

plasma encephalitis: antigenic diversity among *Toxoplasma* strains. *J Infect Dis* 1988;157:7–13.

135. Potasman I, Resnick L, Luft BJ, Remington JS. Intrathecal production of antibodies against *Toxoplasma gondii* in patients with toxoplasmic encephalitis and the acquired immunodeficiency syndrome (AIDS). *Ann Intern Med* 1988;108:49–51.

136. Jarvik JG, Hesselink JR, Kennedy C, et al. Acquired immunodeficiency syndrome. *Arch Neurol* 1988;45:731–736.

137. Gill PS, Graham RA, Boswell W, Meyer P, Krailo M, Levine AM. A comparison of imaging, clinical, and pathologic aspects of space-occupying lesions within the brain in patients with acquired immune deficiency syndrome. *Am J Physiol Imag* 1986;1:134–141.

138. Nolla-Salas J, Ricart C, Dolhaberriague L, Gali F, Lamarca J. Hydrocephalus: an unusual CT presentation of cerebral toxoplasmosis in a patient with acquired immunodeficiency syndrome. *Eur Neurol* 1987;27:130–132.

139. Derouin F, Sarfati C, Beauvais B, Iliou M, Dehen L, Lariviere M. Laboratory diagnosis of pulmonary toxoplasmosis in patients with acquired immunodeficiency syndrome. *J Clin Microbiol* 1989;27:1661–1663.

140. DeMent SH, Cox MC, Gupta PK. Diagnosis of central nervous system *Toxoplasma gondii* from the cerebrospinal fluid in a patient with acquired immunodeficiency syndrome. *Diagn Cytopathol* 1987;3:148–151.

141. Burg JL, Grover CM, Pouletty P, Boothroyd JC. Direct and sensitive detection of a pathogenic protozoan, *Toxoplasma gondii*, by polymerase chain reaction. *J Clin Microbiol* 1989;27:1787–1792.

142. Sun T, Greenspan J, Tenenbaum M, et al. Diagnosis of cerebral toxoplasmosis using fluorescein-labeled antitoxoplasma monoclonal antibodies. *Am J Surg Pathol* 1986;10:312–316.

143. Frenkel JK, Weber RW, Lunde MN. Acute toxoplasmosis. Effective treatment with pyrimethamine, sulfadiazine, leucovorin calcium, and yeast. *JAMA* 1960;173:1471–1476.

144. Kayhoe DE, Jacobs L, Beye HK, McCullough NB. Acquired toxoplasmosis. Observations on two parasitologically proved cases treated with pyrimethamine and triple sulfonamides. *N Engl J Med* 1957;257:1247–1254.

145. Leport C, Raffi F, Matheron S, et al. Treatment of central nervous system toxoplasmosis with pyrimethamine/sulfadiazine combination in 35 patients with the acquired immunodeficiency syndrome. Efficacy of long-term continuous therapy. *Am J Med* 1988;84:94–100.

146. Weiss LM, Harris C, Berger M, Tanowitz HB, Wittner M. Pyrimethamine concentrations in serum and cerebrospinal fluid during treatment of acute *Toxoplasma* encephalitis in patients with AIDS. *J Infect Dis* 1988;157:580–583.

147. Haverkos HW. Assessment of therapy for *Toxoplasma* encephalitis. The TE Study Group. *Am J Med* 1987;82:907–914.

148. Israelski DM, Tom C, Remington JS. Zidovudine antagonizes the action of pyrimethamine in experimental infection with *Toxoplasma gondii*. *Antimicrob Agents Chemother* 1989;33:30–34.

149. Golde DW, Bersch N, Quan SG. Trimethoprim and sulphamethoxazole inhibition of hematopoiesis *in vitro*. *Br J Haematol* 1978;40:363–367.

150. Bygbjerg C, Lund JT, Hording M. Effect of folic and folinic acid on cytopenia occurring during co-trimoxazole treatment of *Pneumocystis carinii* pneumonia. *Scand J Infect Dis* 1990;20:685–686.

151. Sattler FR, Allegra CJ, Verdegem TD, et al. Trimetrexate–leucovorin dosage evaluation study for treatment of *Pneumocystis carinii* pneumonia. *J Infect Dis* 1990;161:91–96.

152. Araujo FG, Remington JS. Effect of clindamycin on acute and chronic toxoplasmosis in mice. *Antimicrob Agents Chemother* 1974;5:647–651.

153. Westblom TU, Belshe RB. Clindamycin therapy of cerebral toxoplasmosis in an AIDS patient. *Scand J Infect Dis* 1988;20:561–563.

154. Rolston KV, Hoy J. Role of clindamycin in the treatment of central nervous system toxoplasmosis. *Am J Med* 1987;83:551–554.

155. Podzamczer D, Gudiol F. Clindamycin in cerebral toxoplasmosis. *Am J Med* 1988;84:800.

156. Dannemann BR, Israelski DM, Remington JS. Treatment of

toxoplasmic encephalitis with intravenous clindamycin. *Arch Intern Med* 1988;148:2477–2482.

157. Harris C, Salgo MP, Tanowitz HB, Wittner M. *In vitro* assessment of antimicrobial agents against *Toxoplasma gondii. J Infect Dis* 1988;157:14–22.

158. Chang HR, Pechere JF. Effect of roxithromycin on acute toxoplasmosis in mice. *Antimicrob Agents Chemother* 1987;31:1147–1149.

159. Chan J, Luft BJ. Activity of roxithromycin (RU 28965), a macrolide, against *Toxoplasma gondii* infection in mice. *Antimicrob Agents Chemother* 1986;30:323–324.

160. Araujo FG, Guptill DR, Remington JS. Azithromycin, a macrolide antibiotic with potent activity against *Toxoplasma gondii. Antimicrob Agents Chemother* 1988;32:755–757.

161. Hofflin JM, Remington JS. *In vivo* synergism of roxithromycin (RU 965) and interferon against *Toxoplasma gondii. Antimicrob Agents Chemother* 1987;31:346–348.

162. Luft BJ. Potent *in vivo* activity of aprinocid, a purine analogue, against murine toxoplasmosis. *J Infect Dis* 1986;154:692–694.

163. Kovacs JA, Chabner BA, Lunde M, et al. Potent effect of trimetrexate, a lipid-soluble antifolate, on *Toxoplasma gondii. J Infect Dis* 1987;155:1027–1032.

164. Araujo FG, Guptill DR, Remington JS. Concise communications. *In vivo* activity of piritrexin against *Toxoplasma gondii. J Infect Dis* 1987;156:828–830.

165. Polis MA, Masur H, Tuazon C, et al. Salvage trial of trimetrexate–leukovorin for treatment of cerebral toxoplasmosis in AIDS patients. *Clin Res* 1989;37:437A–437A.

166. Tate GW Jr, Martin RG. Clindamycin in the treatment of human ocular toxoplasmosis. *Can J Ophthalmol* 1977;12:188–185.

167. Lakhanpal V, Schocket SS, Nirankari VS. Clindamycin in the treatment of toxoplasmic retinochoroiditis. *Am J Ophthalmol* 1983;95:605–613.

168. Yanoff M, Fine BS. Granulomatous inflammation. In: Andresen W, ed. *Ocular pathology. A text and atlas,* 3rd ed. Philadelphia: JB Lippincott, 1989;67–101.

169. McCabe RE, Remington JS. Toxoplasma gondii. In: Mandell GL, Douglass RG, Bennett JE, eds. *Principles and practice of infectious diseases, 3rd ed.* New York: Churchill Livingstone, 1991;2090–2103.

170. Klintworth GK. Protozoal infections. In: Garner A, ed. *Pathobiology of occular disease. A dynamic approach.* New York: Marcel Dekker, 1982;345–358.

Infections of the Central Nervous System,
edited by W. M. Scheld, R. J. Whitley, and
D. T. Durack, Raven Press, Ltd., New York © 1991.

CHAPTER 35

Helminthic Infections of the Central Nervous System

Miriam L. Cameron and David T. Durack

Some 20 species of helminths can invade or involve the human central nervous system (CNS) (Table 1). The diseases that result are mostly restricted in geographic distribution, but immigration, refugee movements and modern travel cause cases to appear sporadically all over the world. Some of these diseases are common—for example, neurocysticercosis (1,2). Others are exotic or extremely rare—for example, lagochilascariasis (3). When helminths affect the CNS, they can cause significant morbidity (especially recurrent epilepsy) and some mortality.

This chapter is not intended to provide a full description of these helminths and all the diseases that they cause; instead, its purpose is to focus on CNS involvement. We review neurocysticercosis and echinococcosis in some detail, and we summarize the main features of other CNS diseases caused by helminths.

CNS DISEASES CAUSED BY CESTODES

Neurocysticercosis

History

Cysticercosis has been known since ancient times. The ancient Vedic texts describe helminthic intestinal infection and parasitic infestations of the head and eyes (4). The Greek physicians Hippocrates (460–377 B.C.) and Theophrastus (372–287 B.C.) were aware of human infection with tapeworms (5). During the same era, Aristophanes (448–386 B.C.) and Aristotle (384–322 B.C.) described cysticerci in pigs (4,5). It was not until about

1550 that Paranoli described a case of human CNS infection with cysticerci in a patient who had involvement of the corpus callosum (5). Laennec coined the term "cysticercosis," which comes from the Greek words "kystic" and "kercos," meaning bladder and tail, respectively (5). In 1686, Redi and Malpighi identified the cysticerci as parasites (5). The life cycle of *Taenia solium* and part of its relationship to human infection was determined by Küchenmeister in 1855, when he fed cysticerci from infected pigs to a criminal and then recovered adult tapeworms from the same person 4 months later (4,5). The pathology of the meningeal form of neurocysticercosis was described by Gessner and Rumler in 1558 with the presentation of a case of dura mater infection (5). Further contributions to the early understanding of neurocysticercosis were made by Virchow, Zenker, Griesinger, Volovatz, and other physicians in the late 19th century and early 20th century (5). In more modern times, larger series of neurocysticercosis have been described (6).

Etiology and Epidemiology

The cestode *Taenia solium* is a common intestinal tapeworm, widely distributed across the world. Cysticercosis is endemic in some parts of all continents except for Antarctica and Australia (7), where only imported cases have been reported (152). Neurocysticercosis occurs with some frequency in Mexico (10), Central and South America (8,9,11), Poland (12), China (13), Africa (14,15), India (16,17), and New Guinea (18,19). In addition, there are scattered case reports in natives of the United States (20–22), France (23), and Italy (24) who have not traveled to endemic areas. Most cases in developed countries occur in immigrants or travelers (25,26). The actual prevalence of neurocysticercosis is unknown,

M. L. Cameron and D. T. Durack: Division of Infectious Diseases, Duke University Medical Center, Durham, North Carolina 27710.

TABLE 1. *Helminths that can invade the central nervous system*

Etiologic species	Disease
Cestodes	
Taenia solium (larvae *Cysticercus cellulosae, C. racemose*)	Cysticerosis
Taenia (Multiceps) multiceps, T. serialis (larvae *Coenurus cerebralis*)	Coenurosis
Echinococcus granulosus	Cystic hydatid disease
Echinococcus multilocularis	Alveolar hydatid disease
Echinococcus vogeli	Polycystichydatid disease
Spirometra mansonoides, S. ranarum, S. mansoni, S. erinacei	Sparganosis
Nematodes	
Angiostrongylus cantonensis	Eosinophilic meningitis
Gnathostoma spinigerum	Gnathostomiasis
Trichinella spiralis	Trichinosis
Strongyloides stercoralis	Strongyloidiasis
Toxocara canis, Baylisascaris procyonis	Visceral larva migrans
Lagochilascaris minor	Lagochilascariasis
Trematodes	
Schistosoma haematobium, S. japonicum, S. mansoni	Schistosomiasis
Paragonimus westermani, P. mexicanus	Paragonimiasis

but autopsy series in Mexico reveal that up to 3.6% of the population may be affected (27). The incidence of known previous or concurrent presence of an intestinal tapeworm in patients with neurocysticercosis ranges from 2% to 16.9% (8,28,29). Immunocompromised hosts are not more susceptible to neurocysticercosis, though the disease has been found in a renal transplant recipient (30).

Pathogenesis

Man is both the definitive host and an intermediate host for the cestode *Taenia solium* (Fig. 1). Some species of monkeys and laboratory hamsters also can be definitive hosts. The disease "cysticercosis" is caused by *Cysticercus cellulosae* and *Cysticercus racemose,* the larval forms of *T. solium* (Table 2). "Taeniasis" is infestation of the small intestine by the adult tapeworm. Ingestion of pork infested with cysticerci, the tissue larval stage of *T. solium,* leads to taeniasis. Ingested cysticerci invaginate into the mucosa of the small intestine and then develop to adulthood. *T. solium* attaches to the mucosa of the small intestine by its scolex or head, which consists of four suckers and two rows of hooklets (Fig. 2). The adult worm consists of a scolex, a neck, and a strobila comprised of a string of 700–1000 proglottids. The worm elongates through the process of strobilization, a term for the formation of a string of proglottids. The proglottids mature and become gravid, moving progressively further away from the scolex as new, immature proglottids are added from the neck above. The entire worm may measure 2–7 m in length and may survive *in situ* for up to 25 years (27).

The terminal, gravid proglottids break off from the adult tapeworm and are then excreted in the feces. The gravid proglottids contain numerous eggs of *T. solium,* which are released into the environment (31–33). Pigs become the intermediate host for *T. solium* when they ingest food or water contaminated with human feces containing tapeworm eggs. The eggs hatch into true larvae, called "hexacanth embryos" or "oncospheres," in the porcine small intestine. The embryos migrate through the intestinal mucosa into blood vessels and then circulate to various tissues, including muscle. In the tissues, the oncospheres develop into cysticerci or infective bladder worms, also called "bladder larvae" (31–33). Humans then complete the cycle by ingesting the infected pork.

Humans, like pigs, can become intermediate hosts if fresh vegetables, uncooked food, or water contaminated with human feces are ingested (33). Theoretically, humans may also become intermediate hosts by autoinoculation, which occurs when gravid proglottids are regurgitated and swallowed or when eggs are spread by fecal–oral self-contamination (31,33). Autoinoculation of humans probably occurs only rarely with this parasite. In humans, as in pigs, the eggs hatch in the small intestine and the embryos migrate through the mucosa to the circulation, and from there they travel to various tissues (33). Cysticerci have a predilection to migrate to the CNS, to the eyes, and to striated muscle (34). The high glucose or glycogen content of these tissues may explain their tropism for cysticerci (35,36). Neurocysticercosis occurs when CNS or ocular involvement predominates.

Clinical Manifestations

Taeniasis (presence of the adult worm in the small bowel) is usually asymptomatic. Therefore, in most cases

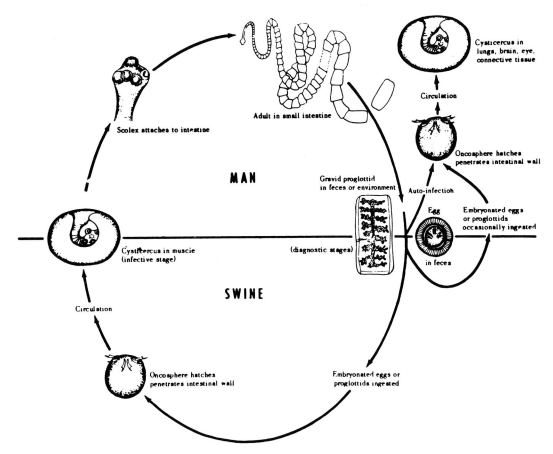

FIG. 1. Life cycle of *Taenia solium*. (From Ref. 283, with permission.)

a diagnosis is made only if proglottids or eggs are noticed in stools. Cysticercosis may or may not be symptomatic. Acute symptoms, including fever and headache during the phase of tissue invasion by larvae, have been described (6). However, in most cases, symptoms develop much later. Neurocysticercosis can become symptomatic 1–30 years after infection, with a median onset at 5–7 years (6).

Neurocysticercosis has a variety of clinical manifestations (Table 3). These are determined by the following

TABLE 2. *Terminology for cysticercosis and hydatid disease*

Disease:	Taeniasis	Echinococcosis
	Cysticercosis	Hydatid disease
	Neurocysticercosis	Hydatidosis
Etiology:	*Taenia solium*	*E. granulosus*
	Larval forms	*E. multilocularis*
	Cysticercus cellulosae	*E. vogeli*
	Cysticercus racemose	*E. oligarthrus*
Definitive host:	Humans	Dogs
	Some species of monkeys	Other canids
	Laboratory hamsters	
Intermediate host:	Humans	Sheep
	Pigs	Pigs
	Rodents	
	Other mammals	
Accidental host:		Humans
Developmental forms:	Oncosphere or true larva in tapeworm eggs	Oncosphere or true larva in tapeworm eggs
	Bladder larva/cysticercus in tissues of intermediate host, containing a protoscolex	Metacestode/hydatid cyst in tissues of intermediate or accidental host, containing protoscoleces
	Adult tapeworm in human intestine	Adult tapeworm in dog intestine

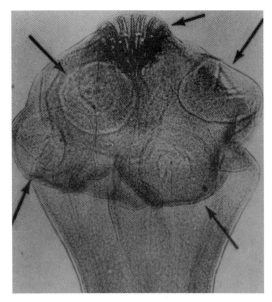

FIG. 2. Photomicrograph of *Taenia solium* scolex showing four suckers (*long arrows*) and a double row of hooklets (*short arrow*). (From ref. 33, with permission.)

factors: the burden of organisms; location of encystation; whether the organisms are alive, dying, or dead; the host response to infection; and, possibly, the sex of the patient (1,37–41). Neurocysticercosis may be active or inactive based on these factors. Six main clinical syndromes occur:

1. asymptomatic neurocysticercosis,
2. parenchymal neurocysticercosis,
3. subarachnoid neurocysticercosis,
4. intraventricular neurocysticercosis,
5. spinal neurocysticercosis, and
6. ocular neurocysticercosis.

In addition, many patients have mixed forms of neurocysticercosis, which are combinations of two or more of the above.

TABLE 3. *Initial symptoms and signs of neurocysticercosis*[a]

Symptoms and signs	Approximate frequency (%)
Headache	23–98
Seizures	37–92
Papilledema	48–84
Meningeal signs	29–33
Nausea/vomiting	74–80
Altered mental status	9–47
Dementia	1–6
Psychosis	1–17
Focal sensory or motor deficits	3–36
Cranial nerve palsies	1–36
Altered vision	5–34
Ataxia	5–24
Spinal cord compression	<1

[a] Adapted from refs. 6, 8, 12, 13, 26, 28, 29, and 47.

Asymptomatic Neurocysticercosis

The true incidence of asymptomatic infection is unknown. Autopsy studies from Mexico found neurocysticercosis in 1.9–3.6% of cases (27,42). A study of 500 patients from Brazil found only six (1%) asymptomatic patients (28), whereas 25% of 753 patients from Mexico had normal neurologic function (43). Asymptomatic neurocysticercosis has been diagnosed in Mexican children (44,45). Studies defining the ratio between the proportion of the population who actually have the disease and the total population at risk in areas of high endemicity are lacking. Cultural, economic, and religious factors strongly affect the endemicity of cysticercosis in any particular geographic area.

Parenchymal Neurocysticercosis

This form of CNS cysticercosis occurs when cysticerci develop within the brain, predominantly at the gray-matter–white-matter junction (46). The cysts may be alive (active) or dead (inactive). Living cysts are present in 13.2% of patients (43). Calcification, a marker of inactive or dead cysts, is found in 57.6% of cases (43). A variety of clinical syndromes have been described, including seizures, focal neurologic deficits, and alterations of mental status. Seizures affected 36–92% of subjects from large series of patients with neurocysticercosis (6,13,28,29,43,47). In Mexico, neurocysticercosis is the single most common cause of late-onset seizures (48). Focal seizures are most common; they are either simple motor or sensory in type, depending upon the location of the lesion (1,13). Generalized tonic–clonic seizures are also very common; they are preceded by focal symptoms in two-thirds of cases (13). Partial complex seizures and status epilepticus are less common (13). The likelihood of seizures may increase during therapy because the death of cysticerci releases larval antigens which can stimulate an inflammatory host response (49).

Focal neurologic deficits are determined by the location and size of cysticerci as well as by the host response. Small cysts and calcified cysts often are silent. Focal neurologic deficits are associated with larger intracerebral cysts or with surrounding edema or infarction (29). Parenchymal neurocysticercosis can cause a vast array of focal neurologic deficits, including hemiplegia, monoplegia, quadriplegia, aphasia, homonymous hemianopia, facial palsy, other cranial nerve deficits, vertigo, nystagmus, ataxia, Parinaud's syndrome, pyramidal tract signs, dysmetria, intention tremor, and hyper- or hypoesthesias (6,25,26,28,29,43,50–52). Pyramidal tract signs were the most common focal signs in several series, followed by brainstem dysfunction, cerebellar ataxia, involuntary movements, and sensory deficits (1,28).

Intellectual or mental status deterioration and coma

can occur in patients with parenchymal neurocysticercosis. Progressive dementia in some patients in mental institutions in Mexico has been found to be caused by neurocysticercosis (53–55). In a 15-year-old girl with previously normal intellect, severe dementia developed as a result of extensive miliary parenchymatous neurocysticercosis (56). Extensive involvement of brain parenchyma by cysticerci is one mechanism causing intellectual deterioration (29,56); however, other complications of neurocysticercosis, such as hydrocephalus (25) and severe meningitis or arachnoiditis (8,28), also may lead to dementia.

Encephalitis may complicate extensive or miliary parenchymal neurocysticercosis (37,38,57). Progressive dementia, focal deficits, and seizures may all occur in conjunction with the encephalitis, which can be fatal (38). Encephalitis occurs more commonly in females than in males (38). Sex-related differences in brain inflammation have been found (37) and may be due to differences in attachment of human leukocyte antigens on the surface of the parasites (59).

Subarachnoid Cysticercosis

Whereas parenchymal neurocysticercosis usually presents with seizures, subarachnoid neurocysticercosis usually presents with signs of meningitis and increased intracranial pressure. Headache is a frequent initial symptom (8,13,25,28,29,40,47). Papilledema, optic atrophy, vomiting, coma, dementia, and cranial nerve deficits also may occur (8,13,25,28,29,40,47). Papilledema was the most frequent sign in one series (28). Hydrocephalus is a common and severe complication of subarachnoid neurocysticercosis, occurring in up to 26% of cases (43). Brain herniation can complicate subarachnoid neurocysticercosis (29).

Cysticercosis of the basilar cisterns is a particularly severe and frequently fatal form of subarachnoid cysticercosis. This variant is caused by the racemose form of cysticercosis, which can cause obstruction of the fourth ventricle (29). Syringomyelia and syringobulbia have been described in a fatal case of subarachnoid and ventricular neurocysticercosis (60).

Subarachnoid cysticercosis can cause specific neurologic syndromes when large lesions are located in the cerebellopontine angle (61), at the sylvian fissure (62), or at the cerebral convexity (63). Cysticercosis rarely may mimic a pituitary tumor when it is located in the sella turcica (64–66).

Subarachnoid cysticercosis may have an associated vasculitis (43). Usually there is occlusion of small terminal arteries (43). Other vasculo-occlusive syndromes are rare; these have included internal carotid artery occlusion (29,67) and middle cerebral artery occlusion (68,69).

Intraventricular Cysticercosis

This form of neurocysticercosis is frequently found in conjunction with subarachnoid neurocysticercosis. Some series (8,47) categorize these two clinical syndromes together. Intraventricular neurocysticercosis may occur in up to 20% of patients or even more (13,25), but one large series from Mexico found only 0.7% with intraventricular neurocysticercosis (43). The fourth ventricle appears to be the most common site of involvement (13,25,43). Intraventricular neurocysticercosis most commonly presents as a syndrome of subacute hydrocephalus and increased intracranial pressure. Hydrocephalus and intracranial hypertension are due to obstruction of the ventricular foramen by cysticerci or by ependymitis (70,71,125). Hydrocephalus may occur subacutely without focal deficits, or it occasionally can present acutely with sudden death (71,73,125). Free-floating cysts in the ventricles cause Bruns' syndrome; this condition is characterized by intermittent foramen obstruction leading to episodic recurrent headaches, vertigo, occasional ataxia, and (rarely) drop attacks (13,25,73,74). An intermittently obstructing fourth ventricle cyst with arachnoiditis has mimicked pheochromocytoma (75). Intraventricular cysts may cause a granular ependymitis which may also be associated with hydrocephalus (76) and progressive midbrain dysfunction (77).

Spinal Neurocysticercosis

This is a rare but severe form of neurocysticercosis. It reportedly occurred in 1.5–2.7% of patients in older series (78–80), but in recent large series it accounted for less than 1% of the total (13,29,43). Intradural extramedullary cysticerci in the cervical region are most common (81). Extramedullary cysticercosis is thought to occur when cysticerci migrate through the subarachnoid space (81). Intramedullary spinal neurocysticercosis, which occurs even more rarely, has been documented in the literature in at least 32 patients (16,17). This form of spinal neurocysticercosis occurs most often in the thoracic region (17). Regional spinal blood flow and arachnoid membrane architecture are important factors in the pathogenesis of intramedullary spinal neurocysticercosis (80). Symptoms of spinal cysticercosis include Brown–Sequard syndrome, paresis, sensory deficits, dysesthesia, incontinence, radicular or nerve root pain, and cauda equina syndrome (6,13,16,17,286).

Ocular Cysticercosis

This syndrome is not well described in most series of patients with neurocysticercosis; however, it has been fully documented in the ophthalmologic literature, with reports dating back to 1866 (82). Extraocular intraorbital cysticercosis is rather rare because of circulation and space considerations (83). Conjunctival and palpebral cysticercosis can occur (83). Cysts in this location can cause proptosis, chronic conjunctivitis, ptosis, and intra-ocular muscle paresis (84). Intraocularly, cysticerci have been found in the anterior chamber, the lens, the vitre-ous body, and subretinally (83,85). The most common location of ocular neurocysticercosis is subretinal, in proximity to the macula (83). Symptoms may include (a) the perception of movement in the vitreous body, (b) visual deficits, or (c) sudden complete blindness (83). When the cysts are alive, complications of intraocular cysticercosis include foreign-body reactions, chronic or-bital edema, and cataract (83). Intraocular death of the cysticerci can lead to other complications such as eosino-philic infiltration, abscesses, panophthalmitis, fibrosis, necrosis, degeneration, and atrophy (83).

In addition to the six main clinical syndromes, there are case reports of neurocysticercosis which escape this classification. These unusual presentations of neurocys-ticercosis include skeletal muscle pseudohypertrophy (13) and subdural hematomas (86).

Though specific clinical syndromes can be described based on the six main anatomic locations where cysti-cerci develop in the CNS, it is important to remember that many patients have mixed forms of neurocysticer-cosis (43) and that the type and severity of disease mani-festations are related to the activity of the parasite and the host response (43). Patients with mixed forms of neurocysticercosis have various combinations of symp-toms and syndromes.

Pathology

Comprehensive pathologic descriptions can be found in several reviews (32–34,46,87). The location and activ-ity of cysts determine the pathologic picture. At nec-ropsy, the brain may weigh more than normal (33,87). The cut surface may exhibit a single cyst or may show as many as thousands of small cysts (33) (Fig. 3). The brain may show signs of hydrocephalus with or without her-niation (33). Areas of hemorrhage may be present. Some-times the brain appears normal to inspection.

Parenchymal cysts have been classified as developing through four stages: (i) vesicular, (ii) colloidal stage of the vesicular form, (iii) granular nodular form, and (iv) nodu-lar calcified form (34). Cysticerci in the brain paren-chyma are usually about 1 cm in size. They are fluid-filled lucent cysts with a "white spot" which is the scolex or cyst body itself (33). A giant cyst 60 cm in diameter has been described (88). The cysticerci may be surrounded by a fibrous membrane (33). Sometimes a smooth-walled fibrous capsule may be found, with either (a) no remaining evidence of the cysticercus itself or (b) only degenerated remnants (33,34). Parenchymal cysts may be uncalcified (active) or calcified (inactive) (43).

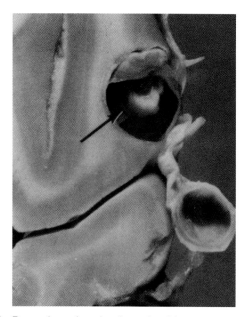

FIG. 3. Parenchymal and subarachnoid neurocysticercosis. Cut surface of brain exhibiting a cyst containing an intact sco-lex at the gray-matter–white-matter junction (*arrow*) and also exhibiting an empty cyst in the meninges. (From ref. 33, with permission.)

Subarachnoid and intraventricular cysts tend to be of the racemose form (33,34), though free-floating cysts oc-casionally are found in the ventricles (34). The racemose form of neurocysticercosis is a collection of transparent, translucent membranes which may form a cluster simi-lar to a bunch of grapes (34) (Fig. 4). The cyst body is missing; hence, this is thought to be a form fruste of *Cysticercus cellulosae* (33,34). Because of its location, the racemose form frequently causes an intense inflam-matory reaction leading to dense fibrous thickening of the racemose cysts and surrounding tissue, which causes communicating hydrocephalus. Occasionally, only the remnant of attachment of a degenerated racemose cyst may be found on the wall of the ventricle (87), or there may only be evidence of granular ependymitis (1,34,87). Supratentorial cysts are usually found in the sulci, but, though often located in the leptomeninges, they are rarely as large as the racemose cysts (87). These cysts, particularly as they degenerate, may be associated with fibrotic thickening.

Spinal cysts are most frequently intradural and extra-medullary in location, though intramedullary cysts can occur (81,89). These cysts are more likely to be large and racemose in nature when extramedullary (87). Evidence of spinal cord compression can result from cysts in either location (81,89,286).

Intraocular or periocular cysticerci can be seen during life if there is involvement of the sclera, conjunctiva, or vitreous body. Occasionally, a free-floating cyst may be seen in the vitreous body (34).

The microscopic pathology of neurocysticercosis is

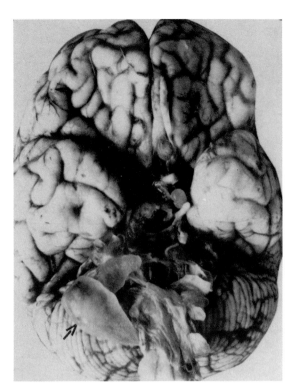

FIG. 4. *Cysticercus racemose.* Large grape-like clusters of cysts at the base of the brain (*arrow*). A smaller cyst is visible just medial to the left temporal lobe. (From ref. 34, with permission.)

determined by the location of the cysticerci, the degree of cyst activity, and the host response. The lifespan of cysticerci is thought to vary from 1 to 30 years (6), though some authors have reported a narrower lifespan ranging from 5 to 7 years (6,29,34). During this time, the cysticerci seem to elude host immunity by mechanisms that are not well understood. Other parasites have the ability to coat themselves with host antigens, thus escaping immune surveillance (72); cysticeri also use this mechanism (58). As cysticerci die and degenerate, their antigens are exposed to the host immune system, eliciting a response. For parenchymal and supratentorial cysts (*Cysticercus cellulosae*), this response ranges from an acute inflammatory reaction to a more chronic inflammation with perivascular cuffing, which is characterized by infiltration with lymphocytes, plasma cells, eosinophils, and some neutrophils surrounding the cysticerci (87). Microscopic evidence of edema may also be present (46). As the cysticerci continue to evolve, encapsulation with a dense fibrous capsule occurs, with subsequent calcification. There may be a narrow surrounding zone of granulation tissue with astrogliosis, plasma cells, lymphocytes, giant cells, macrophages, and capillary proliferation (87).

As the cysticerci evolve, their histologic appearance changes. Initially, the vesicular membrane may be intact, with three layers: the tegument, the muscle layer,

and the mesenchyme (33) (Fig. 5). The scolex with its two rows of hooklets can be clearly demonstrated, particularly in squash preparations (34,90). The tegument of the scolex stains strongly eosinophilic with hematoxylin and eosin (33). Calcareous corpuscles, found in the body of cysticerci, are important histologic markers that stain positively with stains for calcium such as von Kossa's stain (33). Later, when the cysticerci have died and degenerated, it may be difficult to make a histologic diagnosis unless residual hooklets or calcareous corpuscles are present (33).

Subarachnoid and intraventricular infection by *Cysticercus racemose* is easier to diagnose by gross inspection than by microscopy. The cyst may show the three vesicular membrane layers as found in *Cysticercus cellulosae,* and it has typical budding of the vesicular wall, but it frequently has degenerated as described above (33). Some authorities believe that *Cysticercus racemose* may actually be due to a variety of different cestodes, including *T. solium, T. multiceps, T. serialis,* or other yet undescribed species (91). The racemose form is usually sterile, lacking protoscoleces. Degenerated scoleces have been found in some racemose specimens, pointing to *T. solium* as an etiologic agent (34,88). The host response to the racemose form is remarkable for more intense granulomatous inflammation (87). Before cyst degeneration, there is loss of the ependymal lining along with subependymal gliosis, granulomatous ependymitis, and perivascular cuffing (87). Later, after cyst degeneration, granulomatous ependymitis and fibrosis may be the only residual histologic findings.

Ocular cysticerci cause microscopic changes similar to

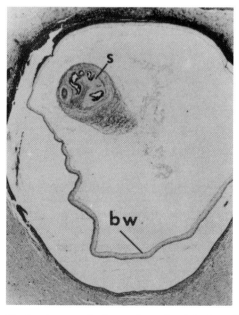

FIG. 5. Photomicrograph of a section of an intact cysticercus from brain. The scolex (s) and the three-layered bladder wall (bw) are shown. (From ref. 33, with permission.)

those seen in parenchymal and subarachnoid/intraventricular disease. Again, as the cyst dies it releases antigens, at which time the inflammatory reaction is most intense (33,83). On microscopic sectioning of the eye, the cysticercus often is located in the posterior pole of the eye (33,83) (Fig. 6). As for all other forms of neurocysticercosis, the pathology is intimately dependent on anatomic location, cyst activity, and host immune response.

Diagnosis

The diagnosis of neurocysticercosis during life is based upon clinical, radiographic, and serologic findings. According to the tests available, this diagnosis can be made with different levels of sensitivity and specificity. Accurate diagnosis is essential to allow appropriate choice of treatment.

Clinically, neurocysticercosis should be considered in the differential diagnosis of any patient who has subacute onset of headaches or seizures and who has a history of exposure in an endemic area (43,48). The history might include occupational exposure to infected pork (13,56), prior or present history of taeniasis, or a family history of taeniasis (6,8,13). Depending upon the series, the incidence of taeniasis in patients with neurocysticercosis ranges from 2% to 17% (8,28,29). Palpable or radiographically proven calcified subcutaneous intramuscular nodules are found in less than 5% in modern series of patients (13,92,93), though up to 54% of patients in an older series had nodules (6). Tongue nodules have also been described (94). Certainly, the absence of nodules does not rule out neurocysticercosis. Neurocysticercosis may mimic tumors, strokes, intracerebral hemorrhage,

other focal neurologic syndromes, mental illness, dementia, pseudotumor cerebri, and pheochromocytoma.

Most routine laboratory tests are normal in neurocysticercosis. Peripheral blood eosinophilia is inconstant, being reported in 0–37% of patients in various series (13,25,29). *T. solium* eggs can be found in stool samples from only a minority of patients (8,28,29). Cerebrospinal fluid (CSF) analysis may be normal in 19–60% of patients (13,28,43). Abnormal CSF findings include increased protein in 5–30% (13,25), pleocytosis of >10 white blood cells per cubic millimeter in 10–53% (13,25), and hypoglycorrhachia in 18–25% (25,43). Initially, the white blood cells may be predominantly polymorphonuclear (29), but later they are predominantly mononuclear (29). Eosinophils can be demonstrated in the CSF in some patients, but the frequency varies widely between studies, between less than 1% and 57% of patients (13,25,28,29,43). Hypoglycorrhachia may be moderate (<45 mg/dl) or occasionally extreme (<10 mg/dl). Very low CSF glucose concentrations were associated with higher morbidity and mortality in some series (25,29).

Serologic and CSF tests are important in the diagnosis of neurocysticercosis. Complement fixation was the first serologic test developed, as early as 1910–1912, but it did not achieve much success until 1927–1930 (53). An improved version of the complement fixation test was developed in 1956 (95). Immunoprecipitation also was tried in the mid-1930s (96). More recently, areas of active research into useful modalities for serologic diagnosis have included antibody and antigen detection systems and measurement of oligoclonal immunoglobulin or IgE (97,98). Various antibody detection systems include complement fixation (53,95,99), immunofluorescence (100), enzyme-linked immunosorbent assay (ELISA) (101–108), an erytholectin immunotest (99), indirect hemagglutination (100,109), and enzyme-linked immunoelectrotransfer blot (110,111). Cysticeral antigen detection systems include ELISA (112), latex agglutination (147) polyacrylamide gel electrophoresis, and electroimmunoblotting (106). Presently, antigen detection remains a research tool because it is not widely available.

Synthesis of IgG within the blood–brain barrier has been demonstrated in a small series of patients with neurocysticercosis (97). Oligoclonal IgG bands were present in CSF but were absent in serum (97). IgG levels in the spinal fluid are more frequently elevated when cysts are active and intact rather than calcified and inactive (103). IgE concentrations in CSF (113) and serum (98) have been measured in patients with neurocysticercosis. IgE levels were found to be elevated in the CSF of 63% of patients in a small series; however, Mexican control subjects without neurocysticercosis had increased CSF IgE in 26.6%, and non-Mexican control subjects with various diseases, including meningitis, multiple sclerosis, seizures, syringomyelia, and pseudotumor cerebri,

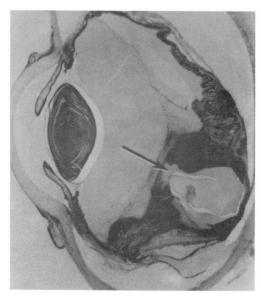

FIG. 6. Photomicrograph of a sagittal section of an eye showing a cysticercus in the posterior pole (*arrow*). (From ref. 33, with permission.)

also sometimes had increased IgE titers (113). A more recent study of serum IgE concentrations showed that 52% of 50 patients with neurocysticercosis had elevated serum IgE when compared to that of normal Mexican controls (98). Elevated serum IgE levels have been described in other helminthic infections, such as echinococcosis (114); furthermore, specific antiparasitic IgE has been found in other parasitic diseases, such as schistosomiasis (115). Unless an assay is developed for specific anticysticercal IgE in serum or CSF, measurement of IgE seems to be a nonspecific test of low sensitivity.

For both cysticercal antibody and antigen detection systems, sensitivity and specificity depend upon whether the specimen tested is CSF or serum, upon cyst activity (alive/active versus calcified/inactive), and upon the method of detection. There is a paucity of comparative studies of these assays (99,100,112,116). Table 4, a compilation of various CSF serologic studies and patient series, shows the ranges of specificities and sensitivities for the various antigen and antibody detection assays. Serologic studies may be unreliable (42,117–119) and may demonstrate false-positive results in uninfected persons living in areas of high endemicity (42,119). CSF serology is more sensitive and specific. CSF complement fixation is positive in 83% of patients with evidence of inflammation, but in only 22% of patients without evidence of inflammation (43). The specificity for CSF complement fixation is high, but false-positives can occur with neurosyphilis and meningeal tuberculosis (43,95). A fairly recently developed ELISA for anticysticercal IgM shows good specificity of 95% and sensitivity of 87% in the CSF of patients with active forms of neurocysticercosis (108). Serum results of this ELISA are as disappointing as previous serologic assays. The combination of CSF complement fixation and IgM ELISA probably increases the overall sensitivity and specificity of serologic assays (1). A more recent assay, the enzyme-linked immunoelectrotransfer blot (EITB), has a specificity of 100%, a sensitivity of >93% in serum, and a sensitivity of about 80% in CSF (111). At the present time, this assay is used by the Centers for Disease Control for serologic diagnosis or confirmation of neurocysticercosis (110,111).

Imaging techniques are of central importance in diagnosis of neurocysticercosis. Plain skull roentgenograms demonstrate intracerebral calcifications (29) and evidence of increased intracranial pressure such as suture diastasis and sella turcica changes (93). Plain soft-tissue roentgenograms may show typical cigar-shaped calcifications, particularly in the thighs (29). Pneumoencephalography, cerebral arteriography, radionucleotide scans, and myelography were also used in the past (29,120, 121). Except in special situations, these techniques have been replaced by computerized tomography (CT) and magnetic resonance imaging (MRI). Neither CT nor MRI are 100% sensitive or specific for neurocysticercosis. Radiographic diagnosis is very much dependent on cyst location, size, activity, and the host inflammatory response.

The CT appearances of neurocysticercosis can be grouped according to clinical syndrome. Asymptomatic neurocysticercosis may show parenchymal calcifications (43). Parenchymal neurocysticercosis has four different appearances on CT (1,122), which reflect disease and cyst activity. These radiographic patterns are as follows: (a) parenchymal calcifications/granulomas predominantly at the gray-matter–white-matter junction (Fig. 7); (b) low-density rounded lesions which are unenhanced by contrast; (c) hypodense or isodense rounded masses with surrounding edema which show ring or nodular enhancement with contrast (Fig. 8); and (d) diffuse brain edema with small lateral ventricles with multiple nodular enhancing lesions after contrast injection (38,93,122,123). Parenchymal calcifications represent inactive cysts. Low-density nonenhancing lesions repre-

TABLE 4. Comparison of CSF serologic assays for cysticercosis[a]

Assay	CSF Sensitivity (%)	Specificity (%)	References
Antibody detection			
EITB	80	100	111
CF	48–72	90.4	99, 100
ELISA IgG	80–97.6	98.9–100	100, 103–105,107
IgM	50	95	108
LA	77		281
HA	88.7	96.6	100,109
IF	87.2	98.9	100,116
Erythro-Lit	92	100	99
Antigen detection			
ELISA	68–77	100	112,282
Dot-ELISA	59	100	112

[a] CSF, cerebrospinal fluid; EITB, enzyme-linked immunoelectrotransfer blot; CF, complement fixation; ELISA, enzyme-linked immunosorbent assay; LA, latex agglutination; HA, hemagglutination; IF, immunofluorescence; Erythro-Lit, erythrolectin immunotest.

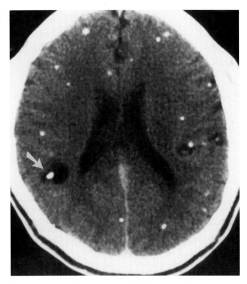

FIG. 7. Non-contrast-enhanced CT scan showing extensive parenchymal neurocysticercosis, with multiple calcified (inactive) lesions. An active cyst containing a scolex (*arrow*) is also demonstrated.

sent cysts which have not elicited an inflammatory reaction (1). The other two radiographic appearances of parenchymal cysticercosis are associated with encephalitic syndromes (1,124). Literally hundreds or thousands of intraparenchymal lesions may be demonstrated by CT in severe fatal encephalitis (38).

On CT, subarachnoid cysticercosis most frequently exhibits hydrocephalus (125). The hydrocephalus may be communicating or noncommunicating. Other radiographic abnormalities include: (a) contrast enhancement of the tentorium and basilar cisterns secondary to fibrotic reaction and arachnoiditis (126), (b) infarction secondary to occlusion or vasculitis, and (c) hypodense

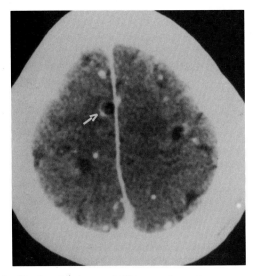

FIG. 8. Contrast-enhanced CT scan from the same patient as in Fig. 7, showing ring enhancement of an active cyst (*arrow*).

lesions in the sella turcica, sylvian fissure, and cerebello-pontine angle (61,63,65,67–69). *Cysticercus racemose* of the basilar cisterns appears radiographically as a large cyst or multiple cysts with a "bunch of grapes" appearance, which enhance after contrast (123). In general, serologic diagnosis is more important than radiography in confirming subarachnoid neurocysticercosis (1).

Intraventricular cysticerci are difficult to diagnose definitively by CT. Obstructive hydrocephalus is usually present and may occur in the presence of low-density intraventricular lesions. The actual cysticerci are difficult to demonstrate by CT without contrast (1,127), but they may enhance with positive CT contrast (128). Also, contrast enhancement of intraventricular cysticerci has been associated with granular ependymitis and adhesive arachnoiditis (127). Air-contrast pneumoencephalography (93) and CT metrizamide ventriculography are more sensitive (127) for demonstration of intraventricular cysts. Metrizamide enhances intraventricular cysts (127). Intraventricular cyst migration has occurred during pneumoencephalography (121) and CT ventriculography (127).

Spinal neurocysticercosis can be demonstrated by myelography, tomography (17,129), and CT myelography (129). Metrizamide myelography of extramedullary spinal neurocysticercosis demonstrates rounded filling defects (129) and irregularities consistent with arachnoiditis (129). Cranial CT may exhibit hydrocephalus (129). Metrizamide myelography with CT demonstrates findings similar to those obtained by regular myelography; in a series of four patients, CT did not improve the ability to make a diagnosis (129). Metrizamide can enter extramedullary spinal cysticerci, producing a radiographic appearance similar to that of spinal arachnoid cysts (129). Intramedullary spinal neurocysticercosis may show up on metrizamide myelography as total or partial block suggestive of extradural compression (17) or as cord enlargement suggestive of intramedullary tumor (17). Metrizamide does not enhance intramedullary cysts (17). Contrast spinal CT may also be useful to demonstrate an intramedullary cysticercus (130).

Ocular neurocysticercosis can be demonstrated by plain roentgenograms, ultrasound, and CT (83). Mixed forms of neurocysticercosis exhibit radiographic appearances appropriate for the anatomic locations involved, cyst activity, and host immune response.

MRI is currently proving to be useful in diagnosis of neurocysticercosis (131–137). As for the other diagnostic techniques, cyst location and activity, and host response determine the sensitivity and specificity of MRI. Viable parenchymal cysts have intensity similar to that of CSF on both T1- and T2-weighted images (131). Degenerated parenchymal cysts have increased signal intensity in T1-weighted images (131). Recently, MRI has been used to try to distinguish the four forms of parenchymal cysts: vesicular, colloidal, granular nodular, and nodular calcified (34,134). Cysts thought to be in the vesicular stage had signal intensity equivalent to CSF, no evidence of edema, and a discrete asymmetric nodule in the cyst wall which was thought to be the scolex (134). Colloidal cysts showed increased signal intensity, nonvisualization of a scolex, and evidence of surrounding edema (132,134). MRI characteristics of the granular nodular stage are not known. Calcified cysts are less well seen on MRI than on CT (131). During acute cysticercotic encephalitis, which can develop as the cysts degenerate, the MRI may show multiple lesions of the same signal intensity as CSF on T2-weighted images with associated periventricular hyperintensity, but it may show minimal lesions on T1-weighted imaging because as the cysts degenerate they become isodense with brain (136). Subarachnoid neurocysticercosis is better seen on MRI than on CT. MRI is also better than CT for detection of cisternal cysts (134). T1-weighted images are better for evaluating cisternal cyst walls, but T2-weighted images are better for showing inflammation and edema from arachnoiditis (134). Gadolinium-DTPA contrast may enhance the leptomeninges on T1-weighted images, suggesting inflammation (135). Racemose cysts have the same signal intensity as CSF (137). Intraventricular cysticerci may be difficult to image, as previously discussed, but their presence is suspected when hydrocephalus is present. Only small studies have been done, but MRI is probably superior to CT in the diagnosis of intraventricular cysts (133,134,137), though MRI occasionally does not show the cysts (134). On T1-weighted images, the cyst wall, a high-intensity mural nodule representing the scolex, and increased signal intensity cyst fluid may be visualized (134). Spinal cysticercosis has also been visualized by MRI (134). An asymptomatic lumbosacral cyst was found in the thecal sac in a patient with cisternal and intraventricular cysticerci (134). Hence, MRI may be superior to CT and ventriculography for imaging of certain parenchymal, subarachnoid, and intraventricular cysticerci.

A direct pathologic diagnosis of neurocysticercosis often is made at surgery for diagnosis or treatment of a mass lesion which was thought to be a tumor preoperatively, or sometimes during ventricular shunting for hydrocephalus. In asymptomatic patients, the diagnosis is made only as an incidental finding at necropsy.

Treatment

Appropriate therapy for neurocysticercosis depends on the clinical syndrome, neurologic impairment, location of cysticerci, activity of cysticerci, and host immune response. Asymptomatic neurocysticercosis found incidentally premortem requires no specific therapy. For therapeutic purposes, it is useful to classify the other forms of neurocysticercosis as "benign" or "malignant" (40,41). Benign neurocysticercosis is a chronic condition

in which there are either (a) no symptoms or (b) seizures only. Parenchymal cysticercosis is usually benign if small numbers of cysts are present, if cysts are predominantly calcified, or if isolated granulomas without edema are present (40). Hydrocephalus and arachnoiditis are absent or rare in benign neurocysticercosis. Surgery is rarely required for benign neurocysticercosis, but pharmacologic intervention may be indicated. Specific anticysticercal therapy is appropriate for viable cysticerci with minimal or no surrounding inflammation (1). Anticysticercal drugs include flubendazole (138), praziquantel (43,139–142), and albendazole (143). An inflammatory reaction resulting from death of cysticerci may lead to signs of increased intracranial pressure after drug treatment (49). Dexamethasone may be used to treat this syndrome, but prophylactic steroids are not recommended (1) because dexamethasone may decrease praziquantel bioavailability by about 50% (144). Calcified parenchymal cysticerci neither require nor respond to anticysticercal drug treatment, but symptomatic therapy with anticonvulsants may be necessary. Prior to the discovery of specific anticysticercal drug therapy, indium-113-labeled anticysticercal antibodies were used with some evidence of success (120).

The term "malignant neurocysticercosis" refers to more serious acute or subacute findings, to which hydrocephalus, arachnoiditis, multiple cysts, large cysts, intraventricular cysts, and signs of increased intracranial pressure may contribute (17,41). Severe diffuse parenchymal neurocysticercosis, arachnoid cysticercosis, intraventricular cysticercosis, and spinal neurocysticercosis all may present as the malignant form of the disease. Unlike benign neurocysticercosis, surgical therapy in addition to medical therapy is usually required for malignant neurocysticercosis. Surgical therapy includes ventricular shunting, cyst extirpation, and brain decompression. Ventricular shunting is indicated for hydrocephalus (71,125,145–147). Cyst extirpation or drainage is indicated for racemose cysticercosis (145,146,149) and for intraventricular neurocysticercosis (70,145,146). One case of intraventricular cysticercosis was successfully treated with albendazole alone (150). Solitary cysts that cause uncontrollable seizures should be surgically excised (145,146), after which the epileptogenic area may be ablated with electrocorticography (145). Solitary cysts that cause significant mass effects (146,147) or extramedullary spinal cysticerci are usually removed surgically (151). Intramedullary spinal cysticerci are usually removed surgically during the initial diagnostic procedure (1). Acute encephalitic cysticercosis that is unresponsive to medical therapy may require subtemporal decompressive craniotomy, and it occasionally requires temporal lobe resection (145,151). Optic chiasm arachnoiditis may require surgical débridement of adhesions and decompression (66). Occasionally, patients who initially respond to medical therapy with praziquantel may later require surgical therapy because of clinical deterioration (151). Patients with ocular neurocysticercosis require surgical removal of ocular cysts prior to drug therapy because the post-therapeutic inflammatory reaction may lead to loss of vision (83).

Specific anticysticercal medical therapy includes flubendazole (138), metrifonate (153), praziquantel (139–142), and albendazole (150,154,155). Flubendazole and metrifonate have only been tried in small series (138,153) and presently have no role in the routine therapy of patients with neurocysticercosis. Praziquantel is probably the drug of choice in the United States at present, although albendazole is rapidly taking over this role (143). More clinical experience is available with praziquantel, and this drug is more readily available in the United States; however, albendazole may have slightly better anticysticercal activity and has been used to treat patients with an incomplete response to praziquantel (143). Albendazole is the drug of choice in Mexico (143). Different regimens have been used (156). The usual dose for praziquantel is 50 mg/kg daily for 15 days, divided into three equal doses (140,157,158). A longer duration of therapy with praziquantel or repeated courses have been used for patients with very large cysts, numerous cysts, or lack of response to therapy (140,156). The dose for albendazole is 15 mg/kg daily for 1 month (150), though a recent report suggests that 8 days of therapy may be adequate (143). Symptomatic therapy, including steroids (159), osmotic diuretics, and anticonvulsants, are indicated when appropriate, again with the caveat that the steroids may decrease praziquantel bioavailability. Other factors such as cyst activity and CNS inflammation may also affect praziquantel bioavailability (160). No data have been published in reference to albendazole activity in the presence of corticosteroid therapy.

In general, the therapeutic approach to a patient with neurocysticercosis must be individualized. In its most acute and severe forms, in which increased intracranial pressure or spinal cord compression is present, medical and surgical therapy aimed at reducing edema, hydrocephalus, compression, and the risk of herniation take precedence over anticysticercal therapy. Various authors believe that exacerbation of symptoms reflecting cyst death and subsequent inflammation stimulated by antigen release is an early sign of response to therapy (49,159). Thus efficacy of drug therapy can be inferred if there is an early exacerbation of symptoms such as seizures, headaches, and vomiting. Efficacy is also assessed by follow-up imaging and CSF examinations. Repeat CT examinations have been used at different time intervals to assess response to therapy. The most appropriate time to repeat the CT scan and spinal tap for routine follow up is about 3 months after drug therapy, because prior to this time there may be residual inflammation (1,149,

158). Spinal neurocysticercosis should be followed up in the same way about 3 months after treatment (1).

Prognosis

The overall prognosis of neurocysticercosis has improved with the advent of modern imaging techniques and the availability of praziquantel and albendazole for use in combined medical–surgical treatment regimens. Nevertheless, the prognosis for certain forms of neurocysticercosis remains poor despite these innovations in diagnosis and therapy.

Parenchymal neurocysticercosis has a variable prognosis in different series (9,40,156–158,160). Benign parenchymal neurocysticercosis has a good prognosis. In one series of patients from Mexico, 2 weeks of praziquantel therapy led to disappearance of 90% of cysts (40). In another series, 91% of patients with parenchymal cysticercosis were improved by CT and CSF serologic analysis. Total cyst remission was achieved in 54%, and partial cyst remission was achieved in 37%. No change was found in 9% (157). An autopsy study of three patients treated with praziquantel showed complete resolution of cysts in patients who received 15 days of therapy (161). Complete cyst resolution has occurred in patients with solitary cysts (20).

Subarachnoid, intraventricular, spinal, and mixed forms of neurocysticercosis are more malignant and tend to have worse outcomes in terms of both morbidity and mortality (40,41,70,71,125,147,162). Morbidity after treatment includes failure to improve, shunt infections (160), peritonitis (160), and development or persistence of hydrocephalus and intracranial hypertension (125,158,160,163). Mortality may be as high as 50% in patients with arachnoiditis (125), though one series of patients with various forms of neurocysticercosis reported only 16% mortality (160,163). Mortality most frequently seems to be a result of intracranial hypertension complicated by ventricular obstruction or adhesive ependymitis (160). Shunt obstruction and bacterial meningitis are also frequent causes of mortality in this subgroup of patients (125).

In a series of 141 patients from Mexico, the long-term prognosis for all forms of neurocysticercosis 5 years after praziquantel therapy (with or without surgery, as appropriate) was reasonably good. Fifty-three percent of patients had complete cures with cyst/nodule disappearance or calcification. About 25% of patients exhibited clinical and radiographic improvement. The remaining 22% of patients were unchanged or became worse. During the follow-up period, 17 patients (12%) died of complications of neurocysticercosis or of complications related to its therapy (158).

Prevention

Neurocysticercosis is an eminently preventable disease. Adequate cooking of pork to 50°C (164) or freezing below −20°C (165) kills the cysticerci. *Taenia solium* infection of pork can be prevented by feeding pigs food uncontaminated with human feces. Vaccination can prevent infection in animal models (166).

Provision of sanitary water supplies uncontaminated by human feces is probably the most important preventative intervention. In addition, education about appropriate sanitary practices such as handwashing is important. Patients found to have *T. solium* intestinal infections should be treated to prevent spread of disease to family members or contacts. The low incidence of neurocysticercosis in natives of developed countries shows that neurocysticercosis can be virtually eliminated by a combination of these measures.

Coenurosis

Coenurosis is the disease caused by the larvae of several species of dog tapeworms: *Taenia* (also called *Multiceps*) *multiceps, T. serialis, T. brauni,* and *T. glomerata.* The pathogenesis of these diseases is conceptually similar to that of cysticercosis, except that the definitive host for the adult worm is a canid instead of a human. For *T. multiceps,* which is common in Europe, Africa, and Brazil (33), the intermediate hosts are sheep, goats, and occasionally other herbivora; thus, coenurosis is most likely to occur in sheep-raising areas. The predominant species in Canada and the United States is *T. serialis,* for which the intermediate hosts are rabbits, hares, and rodents. *T. brauni* and *T. glomerata,* two species found in Africa, usually do not cause CNS infection in humans and will not be discussed here.

In a typical cycle, the eggs of *T. multiceps* in dog feces are ingested by sheep. The oncospheres hatch and exit the sheep's intestine, migrating through vessels and tissues until they reach the CNS. There the larva develops, forming a fluid-filled, bladder-like cyst within which multiple scoleces develop. Such a structure is called a "coenurus"—hence the name of the disease. This species has a remarkable tropism for the CNS; in fact, it may be incapable of developing normally except in the brain, meninges, spinal cord, or eye (167). The mechanism(s) by which migrating larvae identify neural tissue and preferentially locate in CNS is unknown. In the CNS the coenurus enlarges slowly, causing a fatal disease in sheep called "blind staggers." The life cycle is completed if a dog eats sheep brains or other infected tissues, following which the scoleces can attach to the dog's intestinal wall and mature into adult tapeworms.

Occasionally, humans become accidental intermediate hosts for the larvae of these tapeworms by ingesting the eggs. Although only about 50 cases have been reported, the larvae apparently retain their tropism for neural tissue in humans because most of these cases involved the CNS (33). In order of frequency, coenuri were found in brain, subcutaneous or intermuscular tissues, eye, or spinal cord (168).

CNS coenurosis is usually diagnosed in adults 18–55 years of age, but a few cases have been described in young children (167). The usual onset is subacute or indolent, with symptoms related to a basal arachnoiditis caused by a coenurus cyst or cysts in the subarachnoid space. These symptoms include: occipital headache, vomiting, sixth-nerve palsies, and sometimes seizures, often related to obstructive hydrocephalus. Other focal signs, resulting from an intracranial mass, may occur. Cysts in the spinal canal can cause arachnoiditis. CSF examination shows a nonspecific profile indicating subacute nonbacterial inflammation. Moderate hypoglychorrhachia with glucose concentrations below 40 mg/dl occurs in about half the cases; occasionally the glucose levels fall to values as low as 10 mg/dl (167). Imaging reveals a cystic mass, often in the ventricles or in the subarachnoid space, suggesting the differential diagnosis of a parasitic infection (169). The only recognized treatment is surgical exploration and removal of cysts. At present, the diagnosis can be made only by pathologic examination of the excised coenurus by a specialist; even then, however, precise speciation of the parasite may be impossible.

Echinococcosis

Hydatid disease is an important zoonosis in many parts of the world, especially where humans live in close contact with dogs and sheep. The etiologic parasites are tapeworms of the genus *Echinococcus* which live in the gut of mammals, especially canines. The larval cysts (metacestodes) of these cestodes can cause hydatid disease when they develop in the tissues of intermediate hosts, especially herbivores. The word "hydatid" derives from the Latin word *hydatis,* meaning a drop of water; this refers to the fluid-filled cysts which contain the larvae and cause disease. These cysts most often develop in the liver, lungs, or other tissues, but occasionally they involve the CNS—one of the most serious complications of hydatid disease.

Etiology and Epidemiology

Echinococcosis is caused by tapeworms of the genus *Echinococcus,* common parasites of dogs, other canids, and felines. Four species can affect humans: *E. granulosus* causes cystic hydatid disease, *E. multilocularis* causes alveolar hydatid disease, and *E. vogeli* causes polycystic hydatid disease. *E. oligarthrus* is only rarely associated with human disease. *E. granulosus* is widely distributed in all climates—hence its importance in human and veterinary medicine. Countries around the Mediterranean Sea, such as Greece, Lebanon, and Turkey, have a high incidence in rural areas where sheep and dogs are found. Other highly endemic areas are East Africa, southern Africa, parts of the Soviet Union, and some countries in South America. Many interesting local variations in the predominant definitive (canid) and intermediate (mammalian) host species have been described (170). *E. multilocularis* is a tapeworm of foxes and cats, whose intermediate hosts are various rodents.

Pathogenesis and Pathology

The small adult worms, only 2–5 mm in length, live in the definitive host's small intestine and discharge large numbers of eggs into the feces. These eggs spread widely over the surroundings, beyond the actual range of the animal's movements. Each egg contains an oncosphere or true larva. When ingested by a suitable mammalian intermediate host, the oncosphere activates, penetrates the gut wall, and travels in veins or lymphatics draining the gut wall to other tissues, most often the liver or lungs (171). Once located in the final tissue site, the organism forms a slowly enlarging cyst, containing increasing numbers of protoscoleces. The anatomic details of development and growth vary for each species of *Echinococcus*. In the case of *E. granulosus*, the protoscoleces form within brood capsules which bud off the inner surface of the germinal membrane into the growing cyst (171). These protoscoleces form the characteristic "hydatid sand" which spills out when and if the cyst ruptures. Each protoscolex is an "embryonic" tapeworm which can remain dormant within the cyst for years or which can develop in either of two very different ways, according to the fate of the cyst. If the cyst or its contents are ingested by a suitable definitive host such as a dog, the protoscoleces can grow into adult tapeworms; if the cyst ruptures in tissue, they can develop into daughter (secondary) cysts (171).

Echinococcal cysts can develop almost anywhere in the body. Most form in the liver (50–70%) or lungs (20–30%), reflecting the lymphatic and venous drainage of the small bowel. Less than 10% are found elsewhere, such as in spleen, heart, and bones. Only a small minority develop in the CNS. Involvement of the CNS is diagnosed in about 2% of cases of echinococcosis (172). Both cystic (172,173) and alveolar (174) hydatids can develop in the brain.

The cyst of *E. granulosus* comprises two component layers (Fig. 9). Externally is the ectocyst, contributed by

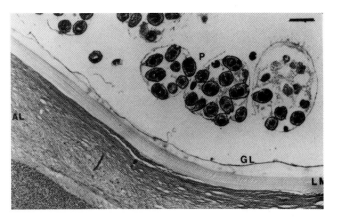

FIG. 9. Portion of a hydatid cyst showing protoscoleces (P) in brood capsules within an echinococcal cyst. Three layers of the cyst wall are labeled: germinative layer (GL), laminated membrane (LM), and adventitial layer (AL). Hematoxylin and eosin; bar represents 100 μm. (From ref. 171, with permission.)

the host's tissue reaction. It consists mainly of fibrous connective tissue with variable degrees of inflammation. Internally is the endocyst, contributed by the parasite. This is made up of an outer laminated membrane of mucopolysaccharide, lined inside by a germinal layer of cells. These cells reproduce and form brood capsules inside the cyst. Protoscoleces develop slowly by budding into the brood capsule. The cyst enlarges at a rate of 1–5 cm per year, and it may eventually contain many liters of fluid if not limited by anatomic factors, as in the case of CNS cysts.

E. multilocularis forms aggregates of alveoli, which are clusters of small grape-like cysts. These develop when this parasite's germinal membranes actively invade adjacent tissues, stimulating an inflammatory reaction which eventually forms laminated membranes around the cysts. These cysts contain many protoscoleces.

Clinical Manifestations

The symptoms of echinococcosis are primarily caused by the enlarging physical mass of the cyst or cysts. These mass effects are obviously of particular relevance when the cyst is located in the CNS. Additional, totally distinct symptoms may be caused by an acute allergic reaction to antigens released from the interior of the cyst.

In the CNS, cysts are usually located in the brain parenchyma and grow slowly to large size (Fig. 10). In the early stages, most cysts are asymptomatic. Eventually, symptoms develop, usually related to the focal lesion itself or to secondary raised intracranial pressure. Thus headache, papilledema, nausea and vomiting, focal or generalized seizures, hemipareses, dysarthrias, and cranial nerve palsies all are common.

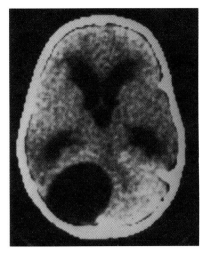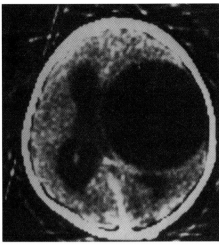

FIG. 10. CT scans from two patients showing hydatid cysts in brain. Note sharp spherical border with lack of rim enhancement or perifocal edema. The cyst contents have the same characteristics as CSF. (From ref. 176, with permission.)

Diagnosis

Although rare, hydatid disease of the brain enters the differential diagnosis of any patient who has a mass lesion in the CNS and who has lived in an endemic area. Specific preoperative diagnosis is highly desirable because special procedures are needed to prevent inadvertent spillage of fluid from the cyst during surgical removal, which might result in formation of secondary cysts. This mishap could convert a curable lesion into a progressive, incurable disease.

Skull roentgenograms are usually normal (174). In some cases, bony changes result from pressure exerted by large cysts (173). A small proportion of hydatid cysts implant and grow in bone, with local destruction evident on x-ray. Approximately half of all hydatid cysts found in bone are in the vertebrae, where they can cause vertebral collapse and spinal cord compression. When a collapsed vertebra is diagnosed in a relatively young patient from an endemic area, hydatid cyst is a likely cause (175). Alveolar hydatids can invade adjacent bone as the cysts extend into host tissues.

CT is the key imaging technique for diagnosis of CNS hydatids (Fig. 10). CT most often reveals a single large spherical cystic lesion, often with ventricular distortion and midline shift (176). There is no associated edema or ring enhancement. The cyst fluid has the same density as CSF. These features are almost diagnostic, distinguishing hydatids from more common lesions such as brain abscesses or tumors. Multiple primary cysts can occur (173). In rare instances, multiple cysts result from intracardiac rupture of a myocardial hydatid (172). Multiple cysts also could result from rupture of a primary cyst during earlier surgery, as noted above.

Adjunctive diagnostic findings include the presence of cysts elsewhere (especially in liver or lungs), which suggests this diagnosis. Peripheral blood eosinophilia occurs, but it is found in less than half the cases. The Ca-

soni skin test, much used in the past, is now considered obsolete because it lacked sensitivity. It has been replaced by various serologic tests. These are useful if positive (171); however, they are not sensitive enough to exclude echinococcosis, especially in patients with hyaline lung cysts. The best approach is to use a sensitive ELISA screening test, with confirmation of positive assays by a more specific test using a hydatid antigen known as the "arc-5" antigen. This can be performed by a double-diffusion technique in agar using a known positive control against arc-5 antigen prepared from sheep hydatid cyst fluid (177). An ELISA test for antibody to *E. multilocularis* is 95% sensitive, and antigens are available to distinguish false-positive results due to cross-reaction with *E. granulosus* (171). False-positives due to cross-reaction can occur in patients with cysticercosis.

Treatment

The primary therapy of CNS hydatids remains surgical excision. To cure a patient, the problems of brain tissue destruction during removal of large hydatids, possible spillage of cyst contents with daughter cyst formation, and other postoperative complications must be faced. However, excellent clinical results often can be achieved (176). Removal of an intact cyst is highly preferable to the alternatives of cyst aspiration or injection of killing solutions, because these procedures increase the risk of spilling brood capsules onto healthy tissues. Careful techniques, such as counterpressure, intraoperative adjustment of the patient's position, and injection of saline to separate the tissue planes between the cyst and the brain, facilitate separation and delivery of an intact cyst by the surgeon (Fig. 11) (172). For cysts that cannot be removed entirely, measures used include (a) injection of cysts with 20% saline, formalin, cetrimide, or silver nitrate to kill protoscoleces and (b) topical applications of

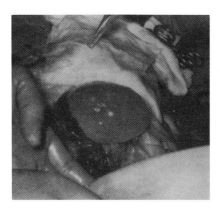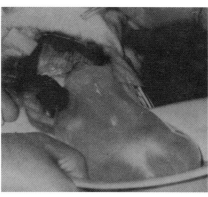

FIG. 11. Two sequential views showing surgical removal of a single large hydatid cyst from brain. (From ref. 172, with permission.)

20% saline or silver nitrate to tissues contaminated by spilled cyst contents. Aydin et al. (174) recently reported successful surgical removal of alveolar CNS hydatids as large as 7 cm in size from four patients who lived in rural areas of Turkey.

Hydatid disease does respond to currently available drug therapy, but the results are variable and imperfect. The benzimidazoles mebendazole and albendazole can penetrate into cysts in concentrations which can kill the protoscoleces, thus sterilizing the cyst. For example, treatment of naturally infected sheep with albendazole for 1 month killed most cysts (178). Microscopic studies of cysts resected from humans following treatment with albendazole showed damage to the germinal membrane (179). Follow-up of treated patients often showed regression in size or collapse of cysts. Furthermore, abendazole damaged the germinal membrane of small *E. granulosus* cysts maintained *in vitro,* and it reduced cyst growth and survival (180). Praziquantel was not effective in this assay system.

Initial studies in 12 Kenyans treated with albendazole for inoperable hydatid disease showed marked regression of cysts in most cases after 8 weeks of treatment (181). Later, more extensive studies on treatment of cystic hydatid disease with benzimidazoles showed that long-term therapy for 6 months or more was necessary, and they also showed that follow-up for at least 12 months was needed for realistic assessment of results. About one-third of patients treated with albendazole responded well, and about one-third improved (182). Cerebral echinococcosis is rare enough that drug treatment trials are difficult to perform. Davis et al. (182) reported successes in "a few patients with echinococcal cysts in the . . . brain," but no details were given. Thus, definitive data on drug therapy for hydatids in the CNS are not yet available. Surgery remains the treatment of choice.

Prognosis

Most information available regarding prognosis derives from patients with cysts located outside the CNS. Many cysts remain asymptomatic and undetected. Lung cysts sometimes resolve spontaneously, especially if the cyst ruptures and the germinal membrane is coughed up and expectorated. Up to one-third of known cysts may regress spontaneously without any treatment (183). Despite this, cystic hydatid disease has high morbidity and mortality; in the study cited above, one-fifth of 27 untreated patients died of the disease, with a median survival of about 3 years (183). Cysts in bone and brain are particularly difficult to cure.

Results of surgery are often excellent if complete excision without spillage of cyst contents is achieved. Long-term evaluation of the results of drug therapy are underway.

Prevention

Public health measures and animal husbandry could potentially reduce the prevalence of tapeworms and larvae in canids and intermediate hosts to a point where transmission would no longer occur. Treatment of dogs with praziquantel is highly effective in killing the adult worms in the gut, but unless mass treatments are used, reinfection will occur. Prevention of secondary cyst formation following cyst rupture during surgery is important.

Sparganosis

Sparganosis is a disease caused by larval tapeworms. Originally, the term "sparganum" was used to describe a larval tapeworm found in tissue, whose parent species was unknown. Later, it was discovered that these larvae originated from cestodes of the genus *Spirometra.*

Epidemiology

Sparganosis is a rare disease. Most cases occur in China, Korea, Japan, and Southeast Asia, but sporadic case reports have appeared from Europe, India, and other countries (33,184). Human sparganosis is caused by the genus *Spirometra,* which are tapeworms of dogs and cats. *Spirometrum mansonoides* is distributed in the Western Hemisphere, so that cases of sparganosis acquired in the United States are usually caused by this species (185). In the Far East, *S. ranarum* is the most common species, but infections by *S. mansoni* and *S. erinacei* also can occur (33).

The Parasite

The life cycle of these tapeworms is complex, because two intermediate hosts are involved (33). After eggs are shed in the feces of dogs or cats into fresh water, they are ingested by the first intermediate host, *Cyclops,* which are minute copepod crustaceans. In this host the procercoid larva develops. Certain vertebrates, including frogs, snakes, and mammals, can become the second intermediate host when they ingest *Cyclops.* In this stage, the motile plerocercoid larva (called a "sparganum") develops and migrates in the tissues. When a dog or cat eats spargana in infected tissues, the cycle is completed by the development of an adult tapeworm in the intestine.

Humans can serve as accidental second intermediate hosts. Humans also might be infected by eating uncooked meat of second intermediate host animals whose tissue contains spargana (33). After reaching the human intestine, the worm's scolex can attach to and penetrate the intestinal wall; at this point, the worm can migrate into the tissues, where it can grow back to full size. Occasionally, infection may follow direct application of infected animal flesh to humans as part of traditional medical treatments for sore eyes. A living sparganum can invade directly from such a poultice into the conjunctiva.

The spargana are quite wrinkled, flattened worms measuring 3–50 cm in length, broader at the anterior end (184). When extracted alive, they are motile, elongating, and contracting vigorously. This explains their ability to migrate through tissues. The organism can be distinguished from other tapeworm larvae by its rudimentary scolex without hooks, solid noncavitated body, and ridged tegument.

To identify the parent species of the parasite, a complicated procedure is required: The living larva must be extracted from tissue, fed to a suitable definitive host (usually a cat), and allowed to develop to maturity in the intestine. Some months later, the cat is killed and opened so that the adult tapeworm can be recovered for identification.

Pathogenesis and Pathology

The motile larvae can migrate to any tissue. Most reach the subcutaneous tissues, forming firm 1- to 2-cm nodules which may be migratory or fixed (33). Organisms have been found also in the abdominal cavity, perirenal fat, breast, scrotum, ureter, lymphatics, orbit, and CNS. In tissue, the tapeworm larvae cause nodules with variable inflammatory reactions. An excised nodule consists of fibroadipose tissue from which the living larva can be dissected out. When the parasite dies in tissue, a prominent inflammatory reaction results, producing an abscess-like lesion filled with necrotic material which contains the remains of the parasite. Thus, the parasite appears to stimulate a stronger inflammatory reaction when dead than when alive.

Clinical Manifestations and Surgical Treatment

Sparganosis only rarely involves the CNS (186). The first neurologic case from the United States was reported in 1984 (185), by which time a total of approximately 65 U.S. cases of sparganosis had been described. This patient had been born in Greece and exposed to dogs and cats. She presented with seizures, and CT revealed a nodule which did not respond to treatment for possible tuberculosis. At surgery, the nodule within a cyst was removed. Pathologic examination showed a coiled sparganum embedded in fibrous connective tissue surrounded by a mixed inflammatory exudate (185).

Holodniy et al. (184) recently reported another case of CNS sparganosis. Their patient was a 21-year-old man who lived in northern India until age 19 and who presented in the United States with episodes of confusion, generalized seizures, and homonymous hemianopia. CT revealed a cystic, multiloculated, thick-walled, ring-enhancing lesion in the occipital lobe. Biopsy yielded a mononuclear inflammatory infiltrate with occasional eosinophils, along with fragments of a helminth consistent with *Spirometra* larva. These authors also reviewed 17 cases from the literature (184). The diagnosis was made at surgery in each case; the mortality rate was about 25%, and survivors did well. In addition to these 18 intracerebral cases, there have been three cases of intradural and two of extradural spinal canal involvement (184).

A rare subgroup of this infection is termed "proliferative sparganosis" (187). Less than a dozen cases have been reported, mostly from Japan. This larva can multiply in tissues—hence the name. A case of proliferative sparganosis involving the spinal cord has been reported from Taiwan (187). A patient with back pain and lower-extremity paralysis showed multiple filling defects in the spinal canal at myelography. Surgical exploration revealed hundreds of small budding and branching cestode larvae, 2–3 mm in diameter. This larva has been named *Sparganum proliferum,* but taxonomy is doubtful because the parent tapeworm species for this rare form of sparganosis is unknown.

CNS DISEASES CAUSED BY NEMATODES

Angiostrongyliasis

Infection of humans by the larvae of a nematode, *Angiostrongylus*, can cause eosinophilic meningitis. This striking syndrome is characterized by headache and paresthesias, CSF leukocytosis with a high proportion of eosinophils, and low mortality.

Parasite and Life Cycle

Rats are the definitive hosts for *A. cantonensis*. This nematode normally lives in the main branches of the pulmonary arteries; hence it often is called the "rat lungworm." The adult worms, measuring 2–3 cm in length, deposit eggs into the pulmonary arterial blood. These eggs move into the lungs, embryonate, and hatch to release first-stage larvae into pulmonary alveoli. These larvae migrate up the rat's trachea, and then they travel down through the gastrointestinal tract to pass out in the feces. These larvae infect a variety of mollusks, often freshwater snails or slugs, which are the intermediate hosts. Within the mollusks, the larvae develop into second- and third-stage larvae by undergoing two moults. Up to several hundred larvae can be recovered from a single snail (188). The larvae re-enter the definitive host when a rat eats the infected mollusks, but a complicated migration within the rat's body is necessary before the parasites reach their final home in the pulmonary arteries. Third-stage larvae invade the gut wall and pass into the portal venous system, and then they pass through the right heart and pulmonary blood vessels to reach the arterial circulation. At this point, the remarkable proclivity of the larvae to reach the CNS of the host becomes apparent. The larvae invade the brain either (a) directly from the bloodstream or (b) after migrating through other organs before reaching the spinal cord and brain. In the CNS, the larvae move about and grow, undergoing a third moult to yield fourth-stage larvae. Remaining within the CNS, these larvae moult again to form adult worms which migrate through the brain tissues. After some time, they reach the venous system and travel back to the right side of the heart, completing the life cycle by colonizing the pulmonary arteries. The CNS phase of development can prove fatal for rats if a sufficient number of larvae are present. The reason why migration through the CNS should form an important part of this nematode's life cycle is unknown, but predilection for the brain is retained when humans ingest the larvae. Humans can become accidental hosts if they eat mollusks containing living third-stage larvae.

Epidemiology

The parasite is widespread; it was first recovered from rats in Canton in 1945 (189). Punyagupta et al. (190) showed that about 20% of *Pila* snails carry the larvae of *A. cantonensis* in parts of Thailand where eosinophilic meningitis is common. In these areas, *Pila* snails are eaten raw as an appetizer along with alcoholic drinks on social occasions. An outbreak occurred in American Samoa when a party of fishermen ate raw *Achatina fulica* snails (191).

Human infections are fairly common, having been reported from many parts of the world, especially areas with warmer climates. Many cases have been reported from Thailand (190,192,193); smaller numbers have been reported from India, Malaysia, Vietnam, Indonesia, Papua New Guinea, and the Pacific Islands, including Hawaii. Rosen et al. (194) reported 1,054 confirmed cases from French Polynesia between 1957 and 1965. Further cases have been reported from Madagascar, the Ivory Coast, Cuba, and Egypt. The fact that rats move freely from port to port in ships suggests that the parasite will spread to many other countries (188). For example, the parasite was recently described in rats in New Orleans (195). However, human cases acquired in the United States have not been described.

Pathogenesis and Pathology

The etiologic role of *A. cantonensis* in human eosinophilic meningitis was first indicated by recovery of worms from the brain or CSF of rare fatal cases (194).

As in rats, larvae ingested by humans migrate to the CNS; however, in humans the life cycle cannot continue beyond the CNS, and the worms presumably die there (188). Pathologic studies are few because few patients die of this disease. Rosen et al. (196) studied the brain of one patient who died of eosinophilic meningitis. They found leptomeningitis and recovered seven nematodes from the brain. Five of these were still alive. Inflammatory changes, including the presence of mononuclear cells and eosinophils, were found in relation to the parasites. Perivascular inflammatory cells, including lymphocytes and eosinophils, were found around vessels in the white matter. A small abscess, formed where a nematode had died, contained inflammatory cells including eosinophils, neutrophils, and foreign-body giant cells, and parasitic debris (196). In another case (193), five *A. cantonensis* worms were found in the brain, together with many worm tracks in the brain and spinal cord. These tracks were less than 0.1 mm in size. These tracks are much smaller and associated with less tissue destruction than the tracks caused by gnathostome worms (see below). This presumably explains why gnathostomiasis, which can also cause eosinophilic meningitis, causes more severe symptoms, higher mortality rates, and longer-term sequelae than does angiostrongyliasis (192). In another case (191), the brain showed edema with dilated meningeal vessels and diffuse subarachnoid hemorrhages. Numerous nematodes were found in the spinal cord but were not found in the brain. The pattern of cellular re-action suggested that viable worms cause less inflammatory reaction in CNS tissue than do decaying worms (191).

TABLE 5. *Cerebrospinal fluid findings in eosinophilic meningitis caused by* Angiostrongylus cantonensis[a]

Parameter	Mean (range)
Opening pressure (mm)	203 (155–250)
White blood cells (mm^{-3})	572 (300–1250)
Eosinophils (%)	49 (16–72)
Protein (mg/dl)	106 (52–205)
Glucose (mg/dl)	44 (31–56)

[a] Adapted from ref. 188.

Clinical Manifestations and Treatment

Symptoms begin 6–30 days after ingesting raw mollusks or other sources of the parasite (190). Patients with eosinophilic meningitis caused by *A. cantonensis* present with nonspecific findings of meningitis (197). These include severe headache (in 90%), stiff neck (56%), paresthesias (54%), and vomiting (56%). Fever is absent in about half the cases (190); when present, it is usually of moderate degree (197). The CSF shows characteristic changes: (a) moderate leukocytosis with 16–72% eosinophils and (b) increased protein concentration (Table 5). Prognosis is generally good; two of 34 patients in one series died of pneumonia, but most series report little or no mortality (190). Most patients recover within 1–2 weeks; sometimes resolution of symptoms takes longer (188).

Symptomatic treatment for symptoms such as headache, nausea, and vomiting is indicated. Corticosteroid therapy is of doubtful value (188). Benzimidazoles have been tried without definite benefit for humans, even though thiabendazole cleared *A. cantonensis* from rats (188).

Gnathostomiasis

Gnathostomiasis is the disease caused by *Gnathostoma spinigerum,* a nematode which parasitizes the stomachs of dogs and cats. The invasive, highly motile larva of this worm, ingested in raw or partially cooked animal flesh, can migrate through human tissues. Most of the clinical manifestations are caused by subcutaneous parasites, but invasion of the CNS is the most serious form of this disease.

Parasite and Life Cycle

The adult worm parasitizes the stomach of dogs or cats. Several adult worms, 2–3 cm in length, embed headfirst in the animal's gastric mucosa, which becomes hyperplastic and forms a pseudotumor with a central cavity into which the tails of the worms protrude and discharge eggs (198). These eggs pass out in the feces of the cat or dog, hatch in fresh water, and form small first-stage larva, 0.3 mm in size. These tiny larvae are eaten by *Cyclops,* a freshwater copepod crustacean in which they develop into second-stage larvae.

The next stage in the life cycle occurs when certain species of freshwater fish, frogs, snakes, and eels feed on *Cyclops* containing second-stage larvae. The larvae penetrate the stomach wall of these intermediate hosts and migrate into skeletal muscle, where they encyst. Birds (including domestic chickens) who eat infected intermediate hosts can also become infected, as can other animals. When a cat or dog eats muscles infected with cysts, the larvae penetrate their stomach wall and migrate in skeletal muscle and connective tissue during a period of development which lasts approximately 3 months. Then the mature larvae re-enter the stomach from the serosal surface and attach to the gastric mucosa, developing into adult worms.

Humans can become infected when they ingest raw fish, frogs, or snakes, the first intermediate hosts. However, the most common mode of infection is through eating the raw or undercooked flesh of ducks or chickens, which become second intermediate hosts if they eat the fish, frogs, or snakes mentioned above (198). The third-stage larvae cannot complete their cycle after ingestion by humans; however, they can migrate actively through tissues, causing irritation, inflammation, and mechanical damage.

Epidemiology

Gnathostoma spinigerum is widely distributed in the Far East. Most human cases have been reported from Thailand and Japan. The first case of CNS invasion was reported in 1967 from Thailand (199), where the disease has since become well known to neurologists and pathologists (192,200,201).

Pathogenesis and Pathology

Two forms of this nematode have been recovered directly from human tissue. The adult is a short tubular worm, 1–2 cm in length, with a small retractable head carrying four circumferential rows of spines. Regular rows of spines also cover the anterior half of the body of the worm. These spines are all directed tailward in a regular orientation, presumably to assist in directed forward movement of the worm through tissues. Both larval worms and sexually immature adults have been found in patients' tissues, but the worms do not develop to full maturity in humans. After ingestion of undercooked meat containing gnathostome cysts, digestion in the stomach "frees the larva for its subsequent, aimless migration" (198). Larvae migrate from the gastrointestinal tract to the liver (less commonly to the lungs), and from there they travel to skeletal muscle and subcutaneous tissues. During this migration, the motile worms cause local necrosis, acute inflammation, and hemorrhage. Within 1–2 days after ingestion, the patient may experience nonspecific nausea and vomiting, itching and urticaria, and upper abdominal discomfort or pain. The worms continue to migrate over a period of several weeks, usually reaching a subcutaneous site within 1–2 months. Areas most often affected are the head, trunk, upper limbs, and thighs. During this period, the patient may have peripheral blood eosinophilia. Presence of the worm in subcutaneous tissue causes intermittent development of red, warm, itchy swellings. These swellings change in position with the movement of the parasite, which can travel as fast as 1 cm/hr. In a few cases, the larvae cause subcutaneous creeping eruption. Occasionally, the worm will break out to the surface through the center of such a swelling, allowing removal and diagnosis. Episodes of local edema resolve over 1–2 weeks, but they recur at intervals of 2–6 weeks. Histologic examination shows the track made by the moving parasite, with associated edema and hemorrhage. After the worm has moved on, the tract becomes infiltrated with inflammatory cells, including eosinophils. When the worm remains stationary, a local connective tissue response with inflammatory reaction, giant cells, and necrosis surrounding the parasite develops.

CNS Involvement

Although localization of gnathostomes in the CNS is much less common than in subcutaneous sites, this is the most serious complication of the disease. The nematode can cause a variety of neurologic syndromes, most notably radiculomyelitis, encephalitis, and subarachnoid or intracerebral hemorrhage. The highly motile larvae or worms invade nerve roots, migrating to the spinal canal or into the spinal cord itself. From this site, they often move caudad into the brain, within which they continue to migrate. This explains the pattern of diverse clinical findings, which include radicular pain, radiculomyelitis or transverse myelitis, eosinophilic meningitis, encephalitis, and subarachnoid hemorrhage. Cranial nerve palsies also can occur. Among 24 patients with proven or probable gnathostomiasis, Boongird et al. (200) found 12 cases with radiculomyelitis, five with radiculomyelitis and encephalitis, two with encephalitis alone, and five with subarachnoid hemorrhages. Table 6 lists the syndromes observed in a further 39 patients (192).

Thus the lumbar, thoracic, cervical, and cranial nerve roots probably form the portal of entry for the worm to reach the CNS. After a period of 1–5 days, the radicular pain gradually resolves, often being replaced by headache if the nematode reaches the brain. Hemiplegia, paraplegia, or monoplegia is common because of the movement of worms in the spinal cord. Pathologic examination often shows hemorrhagic tracts in the spinal cord or brain. In a few cases, the worm itself has been found, either in the CNS or subcutaneously after recently exiting the CNS (200).

Clinical Findings and Diagnosis

In endemic areas such as Thailand or Japan, the history of painless migratory subcutaneous edema with recurrences is highly suggestive of the subcutaneous form

TABLE 6. *Findings in 39 patients with CNS gnathostomiasis*[a]

Clinical syndromes	Number of cases	Percentage
Meningitis	16	41
Cranial nerve palsy	16	41
Encephalitis	12	30
Subarachnoid hemorrhage	10	26
Transverse myelitis	8	20
Radiculitis	6	15
Optic nerve lesion	6	15
Radiculomyelitis	4	10
Intracranial hemorrhage	3	5
Transient obstructive hydrocephalus	1	3

CSF findings	Median	Range
Opening pressure	200 mm	90–350 mm
White blood cells	920/mm³	110–3000/mm³
Eosinophils	54%	15–90%
Protein (nonbloody CSF, $n = 29$)	0.80 g/liter	0.43–1.80 g/liter
Protein (bloody CSF, $n = 6$)	4.96 g/liter	3.45–9.00 g/liter
Glucose = CSF	0.51 g/liter	0.18–1.00 g/liter
= blood	1.04 g/liter	0.71–1.78 g/liter

[a] Adapted from ref. 192.

of gnathostomiasis. Patients are likely to come from rural areas and to give a history of consuming raw or poorly cooked food (200). CNS involvement is most often suggested by sudden onset of very severe radicular pain, followed by pareses, headache, cranial nerve palsies, or signs of subarachnoid or intracranial hemorrhage. Subarachnoid hemorrhage can be the presenting manifestation; at one hospital in Thailand, 6% of all subarachnoid hemorrhages were attributed to gnathostomiasis (192). The rapid migration of the parasite explains progression and multiplicity of symptoms.

Typical CSF findings include a moderate leukocytosis, with a high percentage of eosinophils (Table 6). Elevated protein, elevated blood cell counts, and xanthochromia may be present. Most of the tissue damage caused by gnathostomes is due to direct mechanical injury with tearing and destruction of neural tissue and vessels (200). However, release of hemolysin, hyaluronidase, and an acetylcholine-like substance may play a role.

Treatment and Outcome

No specific drug treatment has as yet been established. Patients usually receive symptomatic care, analgesia, and often systemic steroids to reduce inflammation and edema. In a few cases, the worms can be located and surgically removed. Subcutaneous involvement is not fatal, but the mortality of CNS invasion ranges from 8% to 25% (192,200,201). A median mortality rate of 10–15% is representative. Among survivors of CNS gnathostomiasis, about two-thirds recovered fully while the remainder had long-term sequelae, including pareses, nerve root lesions, and cranial nerve lesions (192).

Prevention

Effective prevention of gnathostomiasis could be achieved by proper cooking of food that might contain gnathostome cysts or larvae.

Trichinosis

Trichinosis is an important parasitic disease of humans and many other mammals caused by the nematode, *Trichinella spiralis.* Humans usually become infected by eating undercooked pork containing trichinella cysts. Trichinosis was extremely common in the United States during the first half of the 20th century, but the incidence has fallen dramatically since 1950 as a result of effective sanitary and public health measures.

Parasite and Life Cycle

The adult parasites are small nematodes which live in the mammalian small bowel. The adult female is 3–4

mm in length and 60–95 μm in diameter, whereas the male is only about half that size. These nematodes colonize the intestinal crypts and mucus layer lining the duodenum and jejunum, where the male copulates with and fertilizes the female with ameboid spermatozoa. Within the body cavity of the female, eggs mature into tiny worm-like larvae which are expelled through a vulval opening located towards the anterior end of the worm. Each female produces 1000–5000 such larvae over a life-span of 3–5 weeks, after which the adult worm dies and passes out of the gut (202).

The motile larvae, 100–160 μm in length and 6–7 μm in width, pass through the bowel wall into lymphatic vessels. After draining into the bloodstream, they pass through the right side of the heart and the lungs to the arterial circulation, which distributes them throughout the body. By this route the larvae can reach any organ, where they come to rest and provoke a brisk inflammatory reaction. The larvae can develop further only in skeletal muscle; they penetrate individual muscle fibers, where they provoke an eosinophilic inflammatory reaction and slowly mature into cysts. The diaphragm, masseter, and extraocular muscles are preferentially parasitized, but any skeletal muscle can be involved. Eventually, the inflammatory reaction subsides, leaving mature cysts in skeletal muscle, where they can remain dormant for many years (202,203).

No further development occurs unless the infected muscle is eaten by another mammal. If this occurs, the gastric juice liberates living larvae from the cysts; after this, the larvae colonize the upper small bowel, undergo two moults, and develop into adult worms. Natural infection with *Trichinella* has been demonstrated in many mammals, including pigs, wild boars, polar bears, dogs, walruses, cows, and whales. Many other mammalian herbivores, carnivores, and rodents can become infected.

Epidemiology

Trichinosis occurs worldwide, with the exception of Australia and a few other areas. For humans, the most important source of infection has been undercooked pork from pigs fed on untreated garbage containing infected rats and other rodents. This infection was previously so common in the United States that *Trichinella* cysts were found in the diaphragms of 16% of a series of patients autopsied between 1936 and 1941. By 1973, this figure had fallen to 1.8% of patients less than 45 years of age (204).

Pathogenesis and Pathology

In the process of migration, arrest in tissues, and invasion of muscle, the larvae provide a strong antigenic stimulus which provokes a variety of cellular and humoral immune responses. Among these, eosinophilia is prominent. Peripheral blood eosinophilia is usually present during the period of larviposition (which corresponds with the acute illness in symptomatic cases), providing an important diagnostic clue to tissue invasion by *Trichinella*.

Once inside skeletal muscle fibers, the larvae become surrounded by sarcolemma which forms a membrane, corresponding with the appearance of a basophilic halo, around the larvae. Meanwhile, a brisk inflammatory reaction develops around the larvae, initially consisting of mononuclear cells and polymorphonuclear leukocytes surrounding the encysting larvae (202). Over the next few weeks, the mixed cellular infiltrate evolves to form granulomas containing Langhan's giant cells and increasing numbers of eosinophils. Encystment is completed over about 3 months, during which the inflammatory reaction gradually subsides. Repeated intestinal infections can lead to muscle invasion by sequential waves of larvae. Light infections, often asymptomatic, result in 10 cysts or less per gram of muscle, whereas in heavy infections there can be 50–100 cysts per gram. After long periods, the cysts die and may calcify.

Although the larvae can only encyst in skeletal muscle, they can provoke an inflammatory response in any part of the body; thus, prominent inflammation can occur in the heart and/or the CNS. Involvement of these organs can result in death in severe cases. Examination of the CNS in fatal cases shows a picture of acute encephalitis. There is severe hyperemia and edema of the meninges, but usually there is no inflammatory cellular reaction in the CSF. During the early stages of larviposition, larvae may be identified in the brain or even in the CSF (205). Punctate hemorrhages may be visible in the brain parenchyma. Histology shows edema, dilatation of perivascular and Virchow–Robin spaces, and perivascular inflammation. Within the small vessels, endothelial proliferation, thrombosis, rupture, and resulting hemorrhages can be seen. Intraparenchymal granulomas can develop around larvae, which most often localize in subcortical white matter.

Clinical Manifestations

The presence and severity of symptoms is closely related to the number of parasites ingested. The majority of infestations are entirely asymptomatic; it has been estimated that only about 5% of cases have symptoms of clinical significance (205). With heavier parasite loads, a spectrum of clinical findings develop which range from mild symptoms to death. Gastrointestinal symptoms (including cramps, vomiting, or diarrhea) attributed to nematodes in the upper intestine occur 2–10 days after ingestion of infested pork or meat in about 25% of symptomatic cases. Diarrhea is not a usual manifestation; however, it was prominent in some cases from the Canadian Arctic, perhaps because of a local variation in pathogenicity (203). Once larviposition begins, a striking systemic syndrome develops. Fever of 38–40°C occurs in 92% of cases, with prominent myalgias. The combination of gastrointestinal symptoms and systemic illness with fever has often led to misdiagnosis as typhoid fever. The muscle pains of trichinosis are often severe, and the muscles are often firm and tender to touch as a result of edema and inflammation. This sign should suggest the diagnosis, especially if the masseter and extraocular muscles are involved. Periorbital edema, associated with inflammation in extraocular muscles, occurs in 84% of cases (203). Headaches are common (56%), and subconjunctival hemorrhages and petechiae occur in 42%.

CNS involvement occurs only in a small proportion of cases. These are patients with unusually heavy infestations, producing enough larvae to reach the CNS in numbers sufficient to produce symptoms. The mortality is much higher for patients with CNS involvement: 10 patients (18%) died in a series of 56 cases collected from the literature by Dalessio and Wolfe in 1960 (205). In this series, mortality was lower in the most recent cases, possibly due to better supportive measures or to corticosteroid therapy. Neurologic findings included (a) delirium in 70% and (b) stiff neck and headache suggesting meningitis in 12%. Other findings were polyneuritis, seizures, monoplegia, hemiplegia, paraplegia, cranial nerve palsies, and organic psychoses (205).

Treatment

Specific treatment for trichinosis is provided by oral thiabendazole, 25 mg/kg, twice daily for 7 days. This kills intestinal nematodes and thus prevents further production of tissue larvae. However, it is not active against larvae that have invaded muscle, nor is it active against cysts. Therefore, by the time a diagnosis has been made, it often will be too late for effective treatment with thiabendazole. Mebendazole may be active against tissue forms and cysts (206). Corticosteroids are usually given in severe cases, especially those with CNS involvement, to reduce inflammation and edema.

Prevention

Trichinosis could be prevented entirely if meat products, especially pork, were thoroughly cooked. Prolonged freezing, for 3 weeks or more at −15°C or lower, kills the larvae. Pigs should not be fed unprocessed garbage, which can contain infected rats or mice.

Strongyloidiasis

Strongyloides stercoralis is a small nematode which can live free in moist soil or which can parasitize the small bowel of humans. The main parasitic cycle is perpetuated by hermaphroditic adult females, which live buried in the intestinal crypts of the duodenum and jejunum. They produce up to 40 eggs daily (207). These eggs release rhabditiform larvae which undergo moults to yield the next stage, namely, filariform or infective larvae. Most often the infective larvae develop in moist soil, where they either (a) mature into free-living males and females which mate to produce more eggs and infective larvae or (b) penetrate the skin of mammals to establish intestinal parasitism.

The invading infective larvae are highly motile, first moving rapidly through the skin and then traveling into the lymphatic system to reach the venous system (207). The next step is migration from pulmonary blood vessels into alveoli, up the airways to the glottis, then down the esophagus to reach the small bowel. However, the migrating larvae can travel to other tissue sites, especially if the number of larvae is large.

In addition to the free-living and parasitic cycles, the larvae can also accomplish an endogenous cycle within the body of a single host. If some rhabditiform larvae develop into infective filariform larvae before leaving the bowel, these can re-invade the same host's tissues by passing through the bowel wall or the skin around the anus without reaching the environment (207). This process is called "autoinfection"; it explains why chronic parasitism can be maintained in some humans for many years after leaving an endemic area to live in an environment free of eggs and larvae (208,209). Strongyloidiasis has been detected in veterans exposed during military service in the Far East, long after they have returned to the United States (208). Normally, only small numbers of larvae achieve this "fast track" back to the small bowel, but if cellular immunity is compromised, the number of recycling larvae can increase enormously. This can produce the hyperinfection syndrome (207), in which larvae not only reach large numbers in lung and bowel, but disseminate to many other sites as well. The hyperinfection syndrome can involve the CNS.

The infective (filariform) larvae are adapted to invade skin and move through tissues at speeds of up to 10 cm/hr (210). The mechanisms by which the tiny, frail larvae cross the skin are not known in detail, but both mechanical and enzymatic factors are involved (211). Rege and Dresden (211) demonstrated that several species of *Strongyloides* produce enzymes with collagenolytic activity. McKerrow et al. (210) recently described a protease with elastase activity which is elaborated by infective larvae. The mobile larvae can carry bacteria from the bowel with them in their travels. This explains why bacteremias and meningitis caused by enteric bacteria occur during disseminated strongyloidiasis.

In the hyperinfection syndrome, the normal cycle of autoinfection is enormously escalated, presumably because of failure of an immunologic control mechanism. The number of infective larvae cycling from the intestine into the tissues and back to the intestine becomes so great that dissemination to other organs is inevitable. Larvae can be found in many tissues in addition to the upper intestine and lung, especially lymph nodes, liver, peritoneal cavity, adrenals, heart, and CNS (212–214). The diseases that predispose to hyperinfection with *Strongyloides* are diverse, including chronic infections, chronic renal disease, malnutrition, alcoholism, and other debilitating conditions. In most cases, immunosuppressive or cytotoxic chemotherapy, especially corticosteroids, have been used. An exception to this is patients with human immunodeficiency virus (HIV) infection, who can develop disseminated strongiloidiasis in the absence of steroids or other immunosuppressive therapy (215).

CNS Manifestations

Under normal conditions, *Strongyloides* infection does not involve the CNS. However, in the hyperinfection syndrome with disseminated strongyloidiasis, CNS involvement may be prominent. The leading CNS manifestation is bacterial meningitis caused by enteric bacteria. In the majority of cases, this is secondary to seeding of the meninges during persistent or recurrent bacteremias associated with the migration of infective larvae. It is postulated that the larvae carry organisms such as *Escherichia coli, Klebsiella, Serratia,* and enterococci in "piggyback" fashion on their surface as they exit the intestine. Alternatively, the larvae may carry the enteric organisms within their own gastrointestinal tracts. The fact that larvae are seldom found in the CNS, even when bacterial meningitis has occurred, suggests that the meningitis is secondary to seeding during bacteremias rather than being secondary to direct invasion. However, larvae occasionally have been found in the meninges. Owor and Wamukota (214) found larvae associated with gram-negative rods in the subarachnoid space of a 45-year-old Ugandan male who had a chronic wasting illness with lymphoid depletion, terminating in disseminated strongyloidiasis and acute bacterial meningitis. [Incidentally, this patient almost certainly was a very early case of acquired immunodeficiency syndrome (AIDS)]. Rarely, larvae are found within the parenchyma of the brain. Neefe et al. (216) described a patient receiving corticosteroids who developed hyperinfection syndrome with extensive involvement of the CNS. Larvae reaching the CNS by the hematogenous route impacted in small blood vessels, causing microinfarction. On inspection, the brain was edematous and a focal hemorrhage with necrosis was found in the cerebellum. Microinfarcts with slight inflammatory infiltrate were scattered through the parenchyma of the brain, surrounded by a zone of demyelination and microvacuolation (216). Serial sections occasionally showed degenerating larvae within microinfarcts, sometimes within capillaries. Apparently viable larvae without associated necrosis or inflammation were found throughout the brain, especially in the cerebellum. Larvae were also seen in the perivascular spaces, the dura, and the epidural, subdural, and subarachnoid spaces. This patient did not, however, develop bacterial meningitis (216). These authors felt that the observed distribution of larvae indicates that some of them reached the brain via migration by way of the spinal canal, moving upwards toward the brain.

The possibility of hyperinfection syndrome with *Strongyloides* should be kept in mind in any patient who has been in an endemic area and later becomes immunosuppressed, should he or she develop an unexplained febrile illness. Most patients reported so far have died, often with the diagnosis of disseminated strongyloidiasis being made only at necropsy (212,214,216). However, if the diagnosis is made before death and treatment given with thiabendazole 25 mg/kg twice daily, some patients can be saved from this serious opportunistic infection (207). Arroyo and Brown (217) showed that thiabendazole penetrated into the CSF of a patient with disseminated strongyloidiasis and *Serratia* meningitis.

Toxocariasis

Toxocariasis is caused by nematodes of the genus *Toxocara,* which are common parasites of dogs and cats. Adult worms live in the intestines of dogs and discharge millions of eggs daily into the animals' feces. These eggs become widely distributed; up to 30% of soil samples contain them (218). The larvae are efficiently transmitted to puppies by transplacental and transmammary routes, as well as by ingestion of eggs in soil. Thus, more than 90% of all puppies are infected within the first few weeks of life. *Toxocara cati* is a very similar species which parasitizes cats.

Humans become infected when they ingest soil containing ova, which hatch in the small intestine, producing larvae which pass through the intestinal wall and migrate to various tissues. The pathologic and immunologic response to migrating larvae produces the disease known as "visceral larva migrans" (VLM) (219,220). The organs most often affected are liver and lung, but the brain and other tissues also can be invaded. Migration of a larva into the eye produces an important, sight-threatening complication known as "ocular larva migrans" (OLM) (221).

Epidemiology

Because dog and cat ownership is so prevalent, and because these pets are nearly always infected with *Toxo-*

cara species early in life, it is not surprising that human infection with *Toxocara* is common (220,222). ELISA tests for antibody to these nematodes provide evidence regarding the prevalence of human infection. Seroprevalence varies widely according to the population tested, from 3.6% in Japan to 6.4% in the United States, 51% in Taiwan, and 83% in Saint Lucia (220). Seroprevalence is higher in young children than in older subjects (223).

The larvae elicit granulomatous inflammation associated with eosinophilia (219). When larvae are moving rapidly through tissues, they leave tortuous tracks which contain necrotic material with minimal associated inflammation (219). When the larvae come to rest, necrosis develops in the surrounding tissue, with infiltration by polymorphonuclear leukocytes, eosinophils, histiocytes, and lymphocytes. This focal infiltrate progresses to form granulomas, with multinucleated giant cells and epithelioid cells. The larvae can remain viable for years and may continue their migration; thus many granulomas do not contain larvae (220). In time, the granulomas resolve with complete healing; thus residual toxocaral lesions are not common as an incidental finding at necropsy in older adults.

Because toxocariasis is rarely fatal, only a few descriptions of CNS pathology have been published (219,224–227). However, there are several experimental animal models for toxocariasis which allow quantitative and descriptive studies. For example, Burren (228) infected mice by giving 1000 embryonated *Toxocara* eggs by stomach tube. They found *T. canis* larvae in 100% of the brains, 42% of spinal cords, and 5% of eyes of mice examined 1–20 weeks after infection with *T. canis*. Interestingly, larvae were found in the CNS in only 8% of mice infected with a similar number of *T. cati* eggs (228). It appears that granulomas are less readily formed in response to *Toxocara* larvae in the CNS than in liver or other sites (219). The usual microscopic finding is tracks made by larvae as they move through the CNS, with focal tissue necrosis and a minor infiltrate of inflammatory cells, including eosinophils. An exhaustive search using multiple sections may be required in order to find larvae, without which the diagnosis cannot be certain. Hill et al. (227) found nematode larvae in the pons, frontal lobe, and cerebellum of a 2-year-old child who died of trauma. The larvae were surrounded by an inflammatory infiltrate, in some cases forming granulomas with giant cells (227).

Clinical Manifestations of CNS Toxocariasis

The fact that seropositivity by ELISA is quite common in serosurveys (220,223) indicates that many cases remain asymptomatic. In young children with heavy infections, VLM manifests as a syndrome with diverse, often confusing symptoms such as abdominal pain, hepatomegaly, anorexia, nausea, vomiting, lethargy, sleep and behavior disturbances, pneumonia, cough, wheeze, sore throat, lymphadenopathy, and fever (219,223). Striking eosinophilia is a hallmark of VLM and should suggest the diagnosis, but eosinophilia is not present in every case (223).

The most common CNS symptom in VLM is headache, which is present in a majority of cases (223) but which may be unrelated to direct invasion of the CNS and is of little specific diagnostic value. Encephalopathy with seizures has been described (224); very rarely, death may result (225,226).

Children with idiopathic epilepsy have anti-toxocaral antibodies more often than do controls (229,230). This association raises the hypothesis that toxocariasis may be an etiologic factor in epilepsy. After much discussion, this question remains unresolved (230). On the one hand, toxocariasis could be the etiology of an important subgroup of patients with seizures (218). However, this infection could result from altered behavior in children who already have epilepsy (202). Further studies will be necessary in order to determine the etiologic role, if any, of toxocariasis in idiopathic epilepsy.

A variant of VLM can be caused by a related ascarid, *Baylisascaris procyonis,* a common intestinal round worm of raccoons. The life cycle and mode of infection for baylisascariasis are probably analogous to those of toxocariasis. The larvae of this nematode produces fulminant eosinophilic meningocephalitis in monkeys (231). Hugg et al. (231) described a 10-month-old boy who developed eosinophilic meningitis and encephalitis, which proved fatal. The child had been exposed to an environment contaminated with raccoon droppings. At necropsy, granulomas containing larvae of *B. procyonis* were found in various tissues, especially the brain. Numerous well-formed granulomas contained coiled larvae.

Lagochilascariasis

Human lagochilascariasis (232–234) is a rare disease reported in Brazil, Venezuela, Costa Rica, Columbia, Surinam, and Trinidad (235). Lagochilascariasis is usually characterized by neck, mastoid, and sinus abscesses, though pulmonary involvement has been described (235). A single case of CNS involvement by *Lagochilascaris minor* has been reported (3). There are several other species of the nematode, *Lagochilascaris,* but *Lagochilascaris minor* is the organism implicated in human disease. Little information is available or known about the life cycle of *Lagochilascaris* or its preferred hosts, though *Lagochilascaris* species have been found in opossums, raccoons, ocelots, dogs, and cats (236–240).

The single case of CNS involvement occurred in a 14-year-old boy from Brazil who had tetralogy of Fallot (3). He presented with headache and signs of meningismus.

His routine laboratory studies were unremarkable except for mild eosinophilia and a mildly increased erythrocyte sedimentation rate. His CSF initially showed a minimally increased protein but was otherwise normal. Two weeks after presentation, he developed papilledema, hemiparesis, and mental deterioration which progressed to coma and death. He had a brain CT scan which showed multiple areas of hemorrhage and infarction. His CSF showed progressive increases in white blood cells (which were predominantly mononuclear) and in red blood cells. Autopsy revealed multiple areas of hemorrhage and necrosis in the meninges and brain parenchyma. Numerous larvae and adult worms were found in the areas of hemorrhage. He also had extensive infestation of his lungs.

Diagnosis of lagochilascariasis is based on finding the adult worms in the tissues. Occasionally the eggs may be found in the feces (234). Therapy for CNS lagochilascariasis is unknown. Thiabendazole, mebendazole, and levamisole have been used with varying degrees of success to treat sinus, neck, and tonsillar lagochilascariasis (232,233). Levamisole may be more effective, though no comparative studies have been done (233,234).

The mortality for lagochilascariasis involving the CNS is probably high, but this cannot be confirmed from a single case report. Specific preventive measures cannot be recommended because the epidemiology and life cycle of the parasite are not well characterized. Certainly, provision of clean water and sanitation would be appropriate because the patients with *Lagochilascaris* lived under unsanitary, impoverished conditions (3).

CNS DISEASES CAUSED BY TREMATODES

Schistosomiasis

Schistosomiasis is one of the most important parasitic diseases, occurring in more than 200 million people worldwide. It has afflicted humans since ancient times: schistosome eggs have been found in Egyptian mummies dating from 1200 B.C. to 1090 B.C. Three different species of the trematode *Schistosoma* cause human disease: *Schistosoma japonicum* is found in Japan, China, Philippines, and Southeast Asia; *S. mansoni* is found in Africa, parts of Southwest Asia, the Caribbean, and South America; and *S. haematobium* is found in Africa and Southwest Asia. The disease occurs predominantly in countries between the latitudes of 36° north and 34° south (241).

Parasite and Life Cycle

Schistosoma are digenetic trematodes which have a complicated life cycle. They differ from other flukes in that (a) the adult worms live in blood vessels, (b) the eggs are nonoperculated, and (c) the worms lack an encysted metacercarial stage. Humans are the definitive hosts for the three main species of *Schistosoma*. Adult worms live in blood vessels in specific anatomic sites, according to the species: *S. mansoni* inhabits the inferior mesenteric veins, *S. haematobium* lives in the veins around the bladder, and *S. japonicum* inhabits the superior mesenteric veins. Adult worms mate in the blood vessels of the vertebrate host, after which the female worm migrates against normal blood flow into venules around the intestine or bladder. She lays hundreds to thousands of incompletely embryonated eggs, about half of which migrate upstream to small venules in the intestine (in the case of *S. mansoni* and *S. japonicum*) or in the bladder (in the case of *S. haematobium*). The rest of the eggs attach to venule endothelium and subsequently migrate through to the intestine or bladder. Some of the eggs incite an inflammatory reaction which leads to calcified granuloma formation. Other eggs pass into the urine or feces and are excreted into the environment. Eggs that reach fresh water under the appropriate conditions will hatch into miracidia. These ciliated miracidia will enter the appropriate intermediate host, namely, specific fresh water snails. In the snail, each miracidium develops into a mother sporocyst which produces motile daughter sporocysts. These sporocysts migrate to the snail's hepatic and gonadal tissues, where they develop into cercariae which migrate through vascular sinuses and exit through the snail's mantle. The tailed cercariae swim towards the surface in their search for their definitive hosts, namely, human beings. Cercariae attach to skin, penetrate, lose their tails and become schistosomula. Schistosomula subsequently migrate to the heart; then they travel to the lungs and finally to the liver, where they develop into adult worms which then migrate to their preferred sites, depending upon the species. There are no true reservoir hosts for *S. mansoni* or *S. haematobium*, though *S. mansoni* is found in rodents, baboons, and insectivores in Africa and in South America (241). *S. haematobium* is rarely found in other hosts. Domestic animals such as dogs, cats, cattle, water buffalo, pigs, goats, sheep, and horses are important reservoirs in the transmission of *S. japonicum*.

Pathogenesis and Pathology

The pathogenesis of chronic schistosomiasis is determined by tissue location of the eggs and the resulting local inflammatory response. CNS schistosomiasis usually follows egg migration into the spinal cord or brain vasculature, leading to infarction or granuloma formation (242). Because of their smaller size, *S. japonicum* eggs are more likely to reach the brain; they cause 60% of all intracranial lesions, whereas the larger eggs of

S. mansoni cause most spinal cord lesions. *S. haematobium* also causes mainly spinal cord disease, but it is more likely to be found in the brain than is *S. mansoni* (242). Deposition of *S. mansoni* eggs in the brain is probably impeded by their larger size, lateral spine, and production of a fibroblast-secreting factor which causes sclerosis (243). Even more rarely, adult worms may aberrantly localize in spinal cord vasculature or cerebral vessels (242). Schistosome eggs reach the spinal cord venules by means of retrograde flow from the iliac veins and inferior vena cava via the valveless venous plexus of Batson (242), with predominant localization of eggs in the lumbosacral venous plexus. Deposition of eggs in the brain appears to occur from embolization through the vertebral venous plexus, particularly in patients with cor pulmonale (242,244).

The tissue response to schistosome eggs may be either (a) totally absent, (b) moderate inflammation characterized by an infiltrate with lymphocytes, eosinophils, and macrophages with perivascular infiltration (245,246), or (c) a florid granulomatous reaction (244). Focal and diffuse vasculitis also can be found (244,247).

Schistosome eggs have localized to the following areas: leptomeninges; parietal (248), occipital, and temporal lobes; basal ganglia; hippocampus; brainstem; cerebellum; and choroid plexus (245,247,249). Apparently, significant granulomas rarely develop in the brain (242). Asymptomatic eggs are also found in the spinal cord, but granulomas (242), hypersensitivity reactions (247,250), and anterior spinal arterial occlusions occur (242).

Clinical Manifestations

Schistosomiasis may present acutely as Katayama fever; however, it is most prevalent in its chronic forms, including hepatosplenic, intestinal, urinary tract, and cardiopulmonary schistosomiasis. CNS involvement is well recognized but relatively rare (242). The site of CNS involvement by schistosomes depends upon the etiologic species, as do the clinical manifestations of the schistosomiasis.

Acute schistosomiasis occurs predominantly in children, adolescents, and young adults. Neurologic syndromes may occur in nonimmune individuals with Katayama fever, probably as a result of an immunologic reaction to the cercariae, schistosomula, and eggs (242). Mental confusion, seizures, coma, visual deficits, and papilledema may occur. More rarely, hemiplegia and opisthotonos occurs. Myelopathy may also occur, characterized by ataxia, muscle weakness, paresthesias, sensory deficits, and loss of sphincter control (242). The CSF is usually normal, though occasionally there may be an increase in pressure and mildly increased protein concentration with lymphocytosis and eosinophilia (249).

Neurologic symptoms are rare or absent in most patients with cerebral schistosomiasis (242). CNS involvement by schistosomiasis caused by *S. mansoni* and *S. haematobium* has been well described in necropsy series, but minimal clinical correlation is available (242). Symptoms attributed to CNS schistosomiasis include headache, vertigo, confusion, extremity pain, seizures, visual changes, tremors, and incoordination (242,251, 252). Clinical CNS syndromes described in case reports include seizures (244), cerebral hemorrhage (253), subarachnoid hemorrhage (254), encephalitis, meningitis, hemiplegia (251), hemianopia, visual-field deficit, optic neuritis (252), cerebellar and vestibular syndromes (255), tumor-like mass lesion syndromes (248,256), and cerebral edema syndromes (257).

Schistosomal myelopathy is more likely to be symptomatic than is cerebral schistosomiasis. The conus medullaris is the most common site of involvement by an intramedullary granuloma (242). Multiple nodules on the spinal cord, cord compression by a meningeal schistosome granuloma, and cord necrosis have occurred (247,258,259). Cauda equina and thoracic involvement are rare. Symptoms depend upon the site of involvement; they include flaccid paraplegia, sphincter dysfunction, areflexia, spasticity sensory deficit, radiculopathy, back pain (242), and transverse myelitis (260–262).

Diagnosis

Diagnosis is based on epidemiologic history of potential exposure and supporting laboratory data. Routine laboratory studies are not particularly helpful, though blood and CSF eosinophilia occur (242). CSF xanthochromia is found in some patients with myelopathy (258,259). Mild lymphocyte pleocytosis and occasional granulocytosis occurs, usually with myelopathy and sometimes with encephalopathy (242). CSF protein levels may be mildly to markedly elevated (242). CSF glucose is usually normal (242). Patients with cerebral schistosomiasis frequently have hepatosplenic involvement and cor pulmonale (242). Patients with schistosomal myelopathy rarely have overt clinical evidence of schistosomiasis, but directed diagnostic studies such as fecal examination, rectal snips, or urine examination reveal schistosome eggs in about 25% (242). Serologic tests such as complement fixation, hemagglutination, and ELISA demonstrate exposure to schistosomiasis but are not diagnostic. Imaging is useful. CT studies during Katayama fever have shown cerebral edema and multiple lucencies (263). Intracerebral schistosome eggs can be demonstrated by CT and by MRI (264,265). Findings may include edema and cerebral atrophy (266). Myelography or spinal CT demonstrate partial or complete spinal cord block with an intramedullary cord swelling (267), though occasionally the myelogram may be normal (260).

Therapy

Neurologic disease during Katayama fever responds to steroids (263) with or without concurrent anti-schistosomal therapy (249). Cerebral schistosomiasis may require surgery for tumor-like masses (255,269). Praziquantel has been used successfully to treat cerebral *S. japonicum* (257). Treatment of myelopathy usually requires a combination of laminectomy and drug therapy (242). Successful drug therapy includes oxamniquine or praziquantel for *S. mansoni* and praziquantel or metrifonate for *S. haematobium* (242,270,271). Whether corticosteroids should be used in patients with myelopathy is controversial (242).

Prognosis

The prognosis of cerebral and spinal schistosomiasis is hard to determine accurately from available series and case reports. Mortality in recent series of cases of spinal schistosomiasis is reported to be about 12% (242). Significant long-term morbidity including permanent neurologic impairment can occur.

Prevention

Prevention of schistosomiasis is a public health priority in endemic areas. Personal preventive measures depend upon avoidance of wading or bathing in water that could contain cerceriae. Major efforts have been expended on environmental measures intended to interrupt the life cycle of the parasite and improve the safety of bodies of fresh water.

Paragonimiasis

Paragonimiasis occasionally causes serious neurologic disease in inhabitants of Southeast Asia, particularly Korea (272), Japan (273–275), and China (276). The disease is also present in certain parts of Africa, India, and Central and South America. *Paragonimus westermani,* the oriental lung fluke, is the most common etiologic agent in Asia and throughout the world, though occasionally other species such as *Paragonimus mexicanus* (277) and *Paragonimus miyazakii* (278) may cause CNS infection.

Parasite and Life Cycle

Humans are accidental hosts for the infection, which is usually acquired from ingestion of infected raw or pickled freshwater crayfish or crabs. Ingestion of contaminated water or preparation of food contaminated with metacercariae are other possible routes of infection. Reservoirs for *Paragonimus* include tigers, other felines, dogs, foxes, opossums, humans, and other mammals who ingest crayfish and crabs. The adult worms reside in cysts in the host animal's lungs. Eggs are coughed up, swallowed, and then pass into the feces. On reaching fresh water, the eggs hatch into miracidia which penetrate into snails, where they develop into cerceriae. These cerceriae are subsequently released into the water, following which they invade the tissues of crayfish or crabs. Humans or other hosts complete the cycle by eating the infected crayfish or crabs (279). Ingested metacercariae excyst in the small intestine, penetrate the bowel wall, and migrate through the peritoneal cavity; then they travel through the diaphragm and into the lungs, where the metacercariae develop into adult worms. The brain is the most common ectopic site for *Paragonimus*. Migration occurs through the jugular foramen. Cysts tend to localize in the temporal and occipital lobes (279), though parietal and spinal involvement have occurred.

Clinical Manifestations

Cerebral paragonimiasis may present with six different clinical syndromes: (i) epilepsy, (ii) meningitis, (iii) tumor-like syndrome, (iv) subacute progressive encephalopathy, (v) infarction, and (vi) chronic brain syndrome. Common symptoms include headache, visual disturbances, focal motor defects, mental status changes, and nausea and vomiting. In one study from Korea, 58% of the patients also had pulmonary symptoms, including a cough that produced "rusty" sputum (272). The ophthalmologic exam is important; abnormalities found include optic atrophy, papilledema, decreased visual acuity, and homonymous hemianopia (272).

Diagnosis

The diagnosis of cerebral paragonimiasis is based upon epidemiologic history, clinical findings, laboratory data, and imaging. Routine laboratory tests are not helpful, except for the fact that eosinophilia occurs in 42% of patients (272). CSF eosinophilia is rarer (272). CSF findings are variable and mimic other diseases, including tuberculosis and syphilis (272). If pulmonary paragonimiasis is also present, eggs may be found in the sputum and feces. Biopsy of a CNS lesion may also show the eggs. An intradermal skin test has been used in the past with good results (272). A complement fixation test can be done on both serum and CSF (175). Imaging is useful, particularly skull roentgenograms which show characteristic "soap bubble" calcifications (272). CT may also show "soap bubble" calcifications and other findings, including ventricular dilatation (280).

Treatment and Prognosis

Both medical and surgical therapies are important in treatment of cerebral paragonimiasis. Bithionol was the available drug therapy in the past, but it has now been replaced with praziquantel. The optimal dose is unknown, but for pulmonary paragonimiasis the recommended dose is 25 mg/kg three times per day for 2 days. As for certain other CNS parasitic diseases, surgery is the major therapeutic modality. The prognosis for acute disease is reasonably good with therapy, but chronic disease responds poorly (272).

Prevention

Prevention should be aimed at dietary education, interruption of the parasite's life cycle by environmental measures, and early detection of infection (175).

REFERENCES

1. Del Brutto OH, Sotelo J. Neurocysticercosis: an update. *Rev Infect Dis* 1988;10:1075–1087.
2. Grisolia JS, Wiederholt WC. CNS cysticercosis. *Arch Neurol* 1982;39:540–544.
3. Rosemberg S, Lopez MBS, Masuda Z, Campos R, Viera Bressan MCR. Fatal encephalopathy due to *Lagochilascaris minor* infection. *Am J Trop Med Hyg* 1986;35:575–578.
4. Ramesh V. Cysticercosis. *Int J Dermatol* 1984;23:348–350.
5. Nieto D. Historical notes on cysticercosis. In: Flisser A, Williams K, Laclette JP, Larralde C, Redadura C, Beltran F, eds. *Cysticercosis. Present state of knowledge and perspectives.* New York: Academic Press, 1982;1–7.
6. Dixon HBF, Lipscomb FM. Cysticercosis: an analysis and follow-up of 450 cases. *Med Res Counc Spec Rep Ser* 1961;299:1–58.
7. Mahajan RC. Geographical distribution of human cysticercosis. In: Flisser A, Williams K, Laclette JP, Larralde C, Redadura C, Beltran F, eds. *Cysticercosis: present state of knowledge and perspectives.* New York: Academic Press, 1982;39–46.
8. Egas FA, Escalante L, Suarez J, et al. Neurocistercosis: revision de 65 pacientes. *Arch Neurobiol* 1988;51:252–268.
9. Mitchell WG, Snodgrass SR. Intraparenchymal cerebral cysticercosis in children: a benign prognosis. *Pediatr Neurol* 1985;1:151–156.
10. Lombardo L, Mateos JH. Cerebral cysticercosis in Mexico. *Neurology* 1961;11:824–828.
11. Acha PN, Aguilar FJ. Studies on cysticercosis in Central America and Panama. *Am J Trop Med Hyg* 1964;13:48–53.
12. Stephen L. Cerebral cysticercosis in Poland: clinical symptoms and operative results in 132 cases. *J Neurosurg* 1962;19:505–513.
13. Wei GZ, Cun-jiang L, Jia-mei M, Ming-chen D. Cysticercosis of the central nervous system. A clinical study of 1400 cases. *Chin Med J* 1988;101:493–500.
14. Powell SJ, Proctor EM, Wilmot AJ, MacLeod IN. Cysticercosis and epilepsy in Africans: a clinical and serological study. *Ann Trop Med Parasitol* 1966;:152–158.
15. Gelfand M, Jeffrey C. Cerebral cysticercosis in Rhodesia. *J Trop Med Hyg* 1973;76:87–89.
16. Sharma S, Banerjee AK, Kak VK. Intramedullary spinal cysticercosis. Case report and review of literature. *Clin Neurol Neurosurg* 1987;89:111–116.
17. Venkataramana NK, Jain VK, Das BS, Rao TV. Intramedullary cysticercosis. *Clin Neurol Neurosurg* 1989;91:337–341.
18. Gajdusek DC. Introduction of Taenia solium into West New Guinea with a note on an epidemic of burns from cysticercus

epilepsy in the Ekari people of the Wissel Lakes area. *Papua New Guinea Med J* 1978;21:320–342.

19. Muller R, Lillywhite J, Bending JJ, Catford JC. Human cysticercosis and intestinal parasitism among the Ekari people of Irian Jaya. *J Trop Med Hyg* 1987;90:291–296.

20. Rawlings D, Ferriero DM, Messing RO. Early CT reevaluation after empiric praziquantel therapy in neurocysticercosis. *Neurology* 1989;39:739–741.

21. Grossman EA. Cysticercosis acquired in the United States, without compatible travel history. *Neurology* 1986;36:305–305.

22. Earnest MP, Reller LB, Filley CM, Grek AJ. Neurocysticercosis in the United States: 35 cases and a review. *Rev Infect Dis* 1987;9:961–979.

23. Mahieux F, Roullet E, Marteau R. La cysticercose cerebrale: quatre cas. *Ann Med Interne (Paris)* 1987;138:298–300.

24. Bussone G, Mantia L, Frediani F, et al. Neurocysticercosis: clinical and therapeutic considerations. Review of italian literature. *Ital J Neurol Sci* 1986;7:525–529.

25. McCormick GF, Zee C, Heiden J. Cysticercosis cerebri. Review of 127 cases. *Arch Neurol* 1982;39:534–539.

26. Loo L, Braude A. Cerebral cysticercosis in San Diego: a report of 23 cases and a review of the literature. *Medicine* 1982;61:341–359.

27. Costero I. Enfermedades producidas por hongos y animales parasitos. In: Barcelona SA, ed. *Tratado de Antomia Pathologica.* Barcelona: Salvat Editores, 1946;1431–1514.

28. Takayanagui OM, Jardim E. Aspectos clincos da neurocisticercose. Analise de 500 casos. *Arq Neuropsiquiatr* 1983;41:51–63.

29. McCormick GF. Cysticercosis—review of 230 patients. *Bull Clin Neurosci* 1985;50:76–101.

30. Gordillo-Paniagua G, Munoz-Arizpe R, Ponsa-Molina R. Unusual complication in a patient with renal transplantation: cerebral cysticercosis. *Nephron* 1987;45:65–67.

31. Zavala, JT. Etiology of cysticercosis. In: Palacios E, Rodriquez-Garbajal J, Taveras JM, eds. *Cysticercosis of the central nervous system.* Springfield, IL: Charles C Thomas, 1983;18–26.

32. Gutierrez Y. Introduction to cestodes. In: *Diagnostic pathology of parasitic infections with clinical correlations.* Philadelphia: Lea & Febiger, 1990;423–431.

33. Gutierrez Y. Cysticercosis, coenurosis and sparganosis. In: *Diagnostic pathology of parasitic infections with clinical correlations.* Philadelphia: Lea & Febiger, 1990;432–459.

34. Escobar A. The pathology of neurocysticercosis. In: Palacios E, Rodriguez-Carbajal J, Taveras JM, eds. *Cysticercosis of the central nervous system.* Springfield, IL: Charles C Thomas, 1983;27–54.

35. Lopez-Albo W. Cisticercosis racemosa de la base del cerebro (periquisamatica y perihipofisiaria). Eosinofilia y glucorraquia. *Gac Med Esp (Madrid)* 1934;8:569–580.

36. Nieto D. Sobre la histopathologia de la cisticercosis cerebral. *Bol Estud Med Biol* 1942;2:73–82.

37. Del Brutto OH, Garcia E, Talamas O, Sotelo J. Sex-related severity of inflammation in parenchymal brain cysticercosis. *Arch Intern Med* 1988;148:544–546.

38. Rangel R, Torres B, Del Bruto OH, Sotelo J. Cysticercotic encephalitis: a severe form in young females. *J Trop Med Hyg* 1987;36:398–392.

39. Estanol B. Controversias en cisticercosis cerebral. *Gac Med Mex* 1983;119:461–466.

40. Estanol B, Corona T, Abad P. A prognostic classification of cerebral cysticercosis: therapeutic implications. *J Neurol* 1986;49:1131–1134.

41. Estanol B, Corona-Vazquez T, Abad-Herrera P. Clasificacion pronostica de la cisticercosis cerebral. Implicaciones terapeuticas. *Gac Med Mex* 1989;125:105–111.

42. Flisser A, Woodhouse E, Larralde C. The epidemiology of human cysticercosis in Mexico. In: Palacios E, Rodriguez-Carbajal J, Taveras JM, eds. *Cysticercosis of the central nervous system.* Springfield, IL: Charles C Thomas, 1983;7–17.

43. Sotelo J, Guerrero V, Rubio F. Neurocysticercosis: a new classification based on active and inactive forms. *Arch Intern Med* 1985;145:442–445.

44. Lopez Hernandez A, Garaizar C. Childhood cerebral cysticerco-

sis: clinical features and computed tomographic findings in 89 Mexican children. *Can J Neurol Sci* 1982;:401–407.

45. Lopez-Hernandez A, Garaizar C. Manifestations of infantile cerebral cysticercosis. In: Palacios E, Rodriguez-Carbajal J, Taveras JM, eds. *Cysticercosis of the central nervous system.* Springfield, IL: Charles C Thomas, 1983;69–83.

46. Thomas JA, Knoth R, Schwechheimer K, Volk B. Disseminated human neurocysticercosis. A morphologic analysis of two cases. *Acta Neuropathol* 1989;78:594–604.

47. Scharf D. Neurocysticercosis. Two hundred thirty-eight cases from a California hospital. *Neurology* 1988;45:777–780.

48. Medina MT, Rosas E, Rubio-Donnadieu F, Sotelo J. Neurocysticercosis as the main cause of late-onset epilepsy in Mexico. *Arch Intern Med* 1990;150:325–327.

49. Sotelo J, Escobedo F, Rodriquez-Carbajal J, Torres B, Rubio-Donnadieu F. Therapy of parenchymal brain cysticercosis with praziquantel. *N Engl J Med* 1984;310:1001–1007.

50. Cavalcanti CE. Cisticercos calcificados em ganglios da base E syndrome parkinsoniana. Registro de um caso. *Arq Neuropsiquiatr* 1984;42:183–186.

51. Barinagarrementeria F, Del Brutto OH. Lacunar syndrome due to neurocysticercosis. *Neurology* 1989;46:415–417.

52. Barinagarementia F, Del Brutto OH, Otero E. Ataxic hemiparesis from cysticercosis [Letter]. *Arch Neurol* 1988;45:246.

53. Nieto D. Cysticercosis of the nervous system: diagnosis by means of the spinal fluid complement fixation test. In: Palacios E, Rodriguez-Carbajal J, Taveras JM, eds. *Cysticercosis of the central nervous system.* Springfield, IL: Charles C Thomas, 1983;55–62.

54. Velasco-Suarez M. Cysticercosis: Personal impact and socioeconomic significance. In: Palacios E, Rodriguez-Carbajal J, Taveras JM, eds. *Cysticercosis of the central nervous system.* Springfield, IL: Charles C Thomas, 1983;3–6.

55. Schenone H, Villarroel F, Rojas A, Ramirez R. Epidemiology of human cysticercosis in Latin America. In: Flisser A, Williams K, Laclette JP, Larralde C, Redadura C, Beltran F, eds. *Cysticercosis: present state of knowledge and perspectives.* New York: Academic Press, 1982;25–38.

56. Rosselli A, Rosselli M, Ardila A, Penagos B. Clinical case report. Severe dementia associated with neurocysticercosis. *Int J Neurosci* 1988;41:87–95.

57. Stepien L, Chorobski J. Cysticercosis cerebri and its operative treatment. *Arch Neurol Psychiatry* 1949;61:499–521.

58. Correa D, Gorodesky C, Castro L, Raviela MT, Flisser A. Detection of MHC products on the surface of *Taenia solium* cysticerci from humans. *Rev Latinoam Microbiol* 1986;28:373–379.

59. Correa D, Gorodesky C, Castro L, Raviela MT, Flisser A. Detection of MHC products on the surface of *Taenia solium* cysticerci from humans. *Rev Latinoam Microbiol* 1986;28:373–379.

60. Escobar A, Vega J. Syringomyelia and syringobulbia secondary to arachnoiditis and fourth ventricle blockage due to cysticercosis. A case report. *Acta Neuropathol* 1981;VII:389–391.

61. Munoz C, Rodriquez-Carbajal J, Santoyo A, Zenteno MA. Lesiones del angulo ponto-cerebeloso y su demonstracion tomografica y comparacion con los estudios radiologicos. *Neurol Neurocir Psiquiatr (Mexico)* 1984;25:13–22.

62. Martinez-Lopez M, Ferrari FQY. Cysticercosis. *J Clin Neuro Ophthalmol* 1985;5:127–143.

63. Ramina R, Hunhevicz SC. Cerebral cysticercosis presenting as mass lesion. *Surg Neurol* 1986;25:89–93.

64. Prosser PR, Wilson CB, Forsham PH. Intrasellar cysticercosis presenting as a pituitary tumor: successful transsphenoidal cystectomy with preservation of pituitary function. *Am J Trop Med Hyg* 1978;27:976–978.

65. Rafael H, Gomez-Llata S. Intrasellar cysticercosis. Case report. *J Neurosurg* 1985;63:975–976.

66. Del Brutto OH, Guevara J, Sotelo J. Intrasellar cysticercosis. *J Neurosurg* 1988;69:58–60.

67. McCormick GF, Giannotta S, Zee CS, Fisher M. Carotid occlusion in cysticercosis. *Neurology* 1983;33:1078–1080.

68. Rodriquez-Carbajal J, Palacios E, Azar-Kla B, Churchill R. Radiology of cysticercosis of the central nervous system including computed tomography. *Comput Tomogr* 1977;125:127–131.

69. Rodriquez-Carbajal J, Palacios E, Zee C. Neuroradiology of cysticercosis of the central nervous system. In: Palacios E, Rodri-

quez-Carbajal J, Taveras JM, eds. *Cysticercosis of the central nervous system.* Springfield, IL: Charles C Thomas, 1983;101–143.

70. Apuzzo MLJ, Dobkin WR, Zee CS, Chan JC, Giannotta SL, Weiss MH. Surgical considerations in treatment of intraventricular cysticercosis. An analysis of 45 cases. *J Neurosurg* 1984;60:400–407.

71. Estanol B, Kleriga E, Lloyd M, et al. Mechanisms of hydrocephalus in cerebral cysticercosis: implications for therapy. *Neurosurgery* 1983;13:119–123.

72. Damien RT. Molecular mimicry antigen sharing by parasite and host and its consequences. *American Naturalist* 1964;98:129–150.

73. Bickerstaff ER. Cerebral cysticercosis—common but unfamiliar manifestations. *Br Med J* 1955;1:1055–1058.

74. Bickerstaff ER, Small JM, Woolf AL. Cysticercosis of the posterior fossa. *Brain* 1956;79:622–634.

75. Rajatanavin R, Dheandhanoo D, Siridej N, Somburanasin R. Cerebral cysticercosis simulating pheochromycytoma: a case report. *J Med Assoc Thai* 1981;64:351–355.

76. Simms NM, Maxwell RE, Christenson PC, French LA. Internal hydrocephalus secondary to cysticercosis cerebri: treatment with a ventriculoatrial shunt. Case report. *J Neurosurg* 1969;30:305–309.

77. Salzar A, Sotelo J, Martinez H, Escobedo F. Differential diagnosis between ventriculitis and fourth ventricle cyst in neurocysticercosis. *J Neurosurg* 1983;59:660–663.

78. Briceno CE, Biagi F, Martinez B. Cysticercosis. Observaciones sobre 97 casos de autopsia. *Prensa Med Mex* 1961;26:193–197.

79. Canelas HM, Cruz RD, Escalante OAD. Cysticercosis of the nervous system: Less frequent forms. III. Spinal cord forms. *Arq Neuropsiquiatr* 1963;21:77.

80. Queiroz LDS, Filho AP, Callegaro D, De Faria LP. Intramedullary cysticercosis. Case report, literature review and comments on pathogenesis. *J Neurol Sci* 1975;26:61–70.

81. Trelles JO, Caceres A, Palomino VL. La cysticercose medullaire. *Rev Neurol* 1970;123:187–202.

82. von Graefe A. Bemer kungen uber cysticercus. *Arch Ophthalmol* 1866;12:174.

83. Elizondo DL. Ophthalmic cysticercosis. In: Palacios E, Rodriguez-Carbajal J, Taveras JM, eds. *Cysticercosis of the central nervous system.* Springfield, IL: Charles C Thomas, 1983;84–100.

84. Malik SRK, Gupta AK. Ocular cysticercosis. *Am J Ophthalmol* 1968;66:1168–1171.

85. Junior L. Ocular cysticercosis. *Am J Ophthalmol* 1949;32:523–548.

86. Feinberg WM, Valdivia FR. Cysticercosis presenting as a subdural hematoma [Abstract]. *Neurology* 1984;34:1112–1113.

87. Itabashi HH. Pathology of CNS cysticercosis. *Bull Clin Neurosci* 1983;48:6–17.

88. Berman JD, Beaver PC, Cheever AW, Quindlen EA. Cysticercus of 60-milliliter volume in human brain. *Am J Trop Med Hyg* 1981;616–619.

89. Akiguchi I, Fujiwara T, Matsuyama H, Muranaka H, Kameyama M. Intramedullary spinal cysticercosis. *Neurology* 1979;29:1531–1534.

90. Escobar A. Cerebral cysticercosis [Letter]. *N Engl J Med* 1978;298:403–404.

91. Jung RC, Rodriquez A, Beaver PC, Schenthal JE, Levy RW. Racemose cysticercus in human brain. A case report. *Am J Trop Med Hyg* 1981;30:620–624.

92. Falanga V, Kapoor W. Cerebral cysticercosis: diagnostic value of subcutaneous nodules. *J Am Acad Dermatol* 1985;12:304–307.

93. Handler LC, Mervis B. Infections and Infestations. Cerebral cysticercosis with reference to the natural history of parenchymal lesions. *AJNR* 1983;4:709–712.

94. Webb J, Seidel JS, Correll RW. Multiple nodules on the tongue of a patient with seizures. *JADA* 1986;112:701–702.

95. Nieto D. Cysticercosis of the nervous system. Diagnosis by means of the spinal fluid complement fixation test. *Neurology* 1956;6:725–738.

96. Rothfeld J. Uber die pracipitationsreaktion bei Hirncysticerkose. *Dtsch Z Nervenheilk* 1935;137:93–102.

97. Miller BL, Staugaitis SM, Tourtellotte WW, et al. Intra-blood-brain barrier IgG synthesis in cerebral cysticercosis. *Arch Neurol* 1985;42:782–784.

98. Gorodezky C, Diaz ML, Escobar-Gutierrez A, Flisser A. Concentracion de IgE en el suero sanguineo de enfermos con neurocisticercosis. *Arch Invest Med* 1987;18:225–227.

99. Rossi CL, Prigenzi LS, Livramento JA. Erythro-lectin immuno test (ERYTHRO-LIT) in the immunodiagnosis of neurocysticercosis. *Braz J Med Biol Res* 1989;22:69–75.

100. Pialarissi CS de M, Vaz AJ, de Souza AMC, et al. Estudo comparativo de testes sorologicos no diagnostico immunologico da neurocisticercose. *Rev Inst Med Trop Sao Paulo* 1987;29:367–373.

101. Chang KH, Kim WS, Cho SY, Han MC, Kim C. Comparative evaluation of brain CT and ELISA in the diagnosis of neurocysticercosis. *AJNR* 1988;9:125–130.

102. Mohammad IN, Heiner DC, Miller BI, Goldberg MA, Kagan IG. Enzyme-linked immunosorbent assay for the diagnosis of cerebral cysticercosis. *J Clin Microbiol* 1984;20:775–779.

103. Espinoza B, Ruiz-Palacios G, Tovar A, Sandoval MA, Plancarte A, Flisser A. Characterization by enzyme-linked immunosorbent assay of the humoral immune response in patients with neurocysticercosis and its application in immunodiagnosis. *J Clin Microbiol* 1986;24:536–541.

104. Corona T, Pascoe D, Gonzalez-Barranco D, Abad P, Landa L, Estanol B. Anticysticercous antibodies in serum and cerebrospinal fluid in patients with cerebral cysticercosis. *J Neurol* 1986;49:1044–1049.

105. Diwan AR, Coker-Vann M, Brown P, et al. Enzyme-linked immunosorbent assay (ELISA) for the detection of antibody to cysticerci of *Taenia solium*. *Am J Trop Med Hyg* 1982;31:364–369.

106. Estrada JJ, Estrada JA, Kuhn RE. Identification of *Taenia solium* antigens in cerebrospinal fluid and larval antigens from patients with neurocysticercosis. *Am J Trop Med Hyg* 1989;41:50–55.

107. Ramirez G, Pradilla G. Use of enzyme-linked immunosorbent assay in the diagnosis of cysticercosis. *Arch Neurol* 1987;44:898–898.

108. Rosas N, Sotelo J, Nieto D. ELISA in the diagnosis of neurocysticercosis. *Arch Neurol* 1986;43:353–356.

109. Ueda M, Vaz AJ, Camargo ED, de Souza AMC, Benelli RMF, da Silva MV. Passive haemagglutination test for human neurocysticercosis immunodiagnosis. II. Comparison of two standardized procedures for the passive haemagglutination reagent in the detection of anti-*Cysticercus cellulosae* antibodies in cerebrospinal fluids. *Rev Inst Med Trop Sao Paulo* 1988;30:57–62.

110. Tsang VCW, Brand JA, Boyer AE. An enzyme-linked immunoelectrotransfer blot assay and glycoprotein antigens for diagnosing human cysticercosis (*Taenia solium*). *J Infect Dis* 1989;150:50–59.

111. Wilson M, Schantz P. Nonmorphologic diagnosis of parasitic infections. In: *Manual of clinical microbiology,* 5th ed. 1990;1–11.

112. Tellez-Giron E, Ramos MC, Dufour L, Alvarez P, Montante M. Detection of *Cysticercus cellulosae* antigens in cerebrospinal fluid by dot enzyme-linked immunosorbent assay (DOT-ELISA) and standard ELISA. *J Trop Med Hyg* 1987;37:169–173.

113. Goldberg AS, Heiner DC, Firemark HM, Goldberg MA. Cerebrospinal fluid IgE and the diagnosis of cerebral cysticercosis. *Bull Los Angeles Neurol Soc* 1981;46:21–25.

114. Kojima S, Vokogawa M, Tada T. Raised levels of serum IgE in human helminthiases. *Am J Trop Med Hyg* 1972;21:913–918.

115. Ottesen EA, Poindexter RW, Hussain R. Detection, quantitation, and specificity of antiparasite IgE antibodies in human *Schistosomiasis mansoni. Am J Trop Med Hyg* 1981;30:1228–1237.

116. Rydsewski AK, Chisholm AK, Kagan IG. Comparison of serologic tests for human cysticercosis by indirect hemagglutination, indirect immunofluorescent antibody and agar gel precipitin test. *J Parasitol* 1975;61:154–155.

117. Flisser A, Perez-Montfort R, Larralde C. The immunology of human and animal cysticercosis: a review. *Bull WHO* 1979;57:839–856.

118. Flisser A, Rivera L, Trueba J, et al. Immunology of human neurocysticercosis. In: Flisser A, Williams K, Laclette JP, Larralde C, Redadura C, Beltran F, eds. *Cysticercosis: present state and knowledge perspectives.* New York: Academic Press, 1982;549–563.

119. Coker-Vann MR, Subianto DB, Brown P, et al. ELISA antibodies to cysticerci of *Taenia solium* in human populations in New Guinea, Oceania, and Southeast Asia. *Southeast Asian J Trop Med Public Health* 1981;12:499–505.

120. Skromne-Kadlubik G, Celis C. Cysticercosis of the nervous system. Treatment by means of specific internal radiation. *Arch Neurol* 1981;38:288–298.

121. Zee CS, Ahmadi J, Mehringer CM, Becker TS, Segall HD. Neuroradiology of Intraventricular cysticercosis. *Bull Clin Neurosci* 1983;48:85–92.

122. Bouilliant-Linet E, Brugieres P, Coubes P, Gaston A, Laporte P, Marsault C. Cysticercose cerebrale. Interet diagnostique de la scanographie. A propos de 117 observations. *J Radiol (Paris)* 1988;69:405–412.

123. Rodacki MA, Detoni XA, Teixeira WR, Boer VH, Oliveira GG. CT features of *Cellulosae* and *Racemosus neurocysticercosis*. *J Comput Assist Tomogr* 1989;13:1013–1016.

124. Rodriquez-Carbajal J, Salgado P, Gutierrez-Alvarado R, Escobar-Izquierdo A, Aruffo C, Palacios E. The acute encephalitic phase of neurocysticercosis: computed tomographic manifestations. *AJNR* 1983;4:51–55.

125. Sotelo J, Marin C. Hydrocephalus secondary to cysticercotic arachnoiditis. A long-term follow-up review of 92 cases. *J Neurosurg* 1987;66:686–689.

126. Zee C, Segall HD, Miller C, et al. Unusual neuroradiological features of intracranial cysticercosis. *Neuroradiology* 1980;137:397–407.

127. Zee C, Segall HD, Apuzzo MLJ, Ahmadi J, Dobkin WR. Intraventricular cysticercal cysts: further neuroradiologic observations and neurosurgical implications. *AJNR* 1984;5:727–730.

128. Madrazo I, Renteria JAG, Paredes G, Olhagaray B. Diagnosis of intraventricular and cisternal cysticercosis by computerized tomography with positive intraventricular contrast medium. *J Neurosurg* 1981;55:947–951.

129. Zee CS, Segall HD, Ahmadi J, Tsai FY, Apuzzo M. CT myelography in spinal cysticercosis. *J Comput Assist Tomogr* 1986;10:195–198.

130. Holtzman RN, Hughes JE, Sachdev RK, Jarenwattananon A. Intramedullary cysticercosis. *Surg Neurol* 1986;26:187–191.

131. Teitelbaum GP, Otto RJ, Lin M, et al. MR imaging of neurocysticercosis. *AJR* 1989;153:857–866.

132. Spickler EM, Lufkin RB, Teresi L, Lanman T, Levesque M, Bentson JR. High-signal intraventricular cysticercosis on T1-weighted MR imaging (case report). *AJNR* 1989;10:S64.

133. Rhee RS, Kumasaki DY, Sarwar M, Rodriquez J, Naseem M. MR imaging of intraventricular cysticercosis. *J Comput Assist Tomogr* 1987;11:598–601.

134. Zee CS, Segall HD, Boswell W, Ahmadi J, Nelson M, Colletti P. MR imaging of neurocysticercosis. *J Comput Assist Tomogr* 1988;12:927–934.

135. Suh DC, Chang KH, Han MH, Lee SR, Han MC, Kim CW. Unusual MR manifestations of neurocysticercosis. *Neuroradiology* 1989;31:396–402.

136. Brutto OHD, Zenteno MA, Salgado P, Sotelo J. MR imaging in cysticercotic encephalitis. *AJNR* 1989;10:S18–S20.

137. Suss RA, Maravilla KR, Thompson J. MR imaging of intracranial cysticercosis: comparison with CT and anatomopathologic features. *AJNR* 1986;7:235–242.

138. Tellez-Giron E, Ramos MC, Dufour L, et al. Treatment of neurocysticercosis with flubendazole. *J Trop Med Hyg* 1984;33:627–631.

139. Lawner PM. Medical management of neurocysticercosis with praziquantel. *Bull Clin Neurosci* 1983;48:102–105.

140. Vasconcelos D, Cruz-Segura H, Mateos-Gomez H, Alanis GZ. Selective indications for the use of praziquantel in the treatment of brain cysticercosis. *J Neurol* 1987;50:383–388.

141. King CH, Mahmoud AAF. Diagnosis and treatment. Drugs five years later: praziquantel. *Ann Intern Med* 1989;110:290–296.

142. Groll E. Cisticercosis humana y praziquantel: una apreciacion panoramica de las primeras experiencias clinicas. *Bol Chil Parasitol* 1981;36:29–37.

143. Sotelo J, Penagos P, Escobedo F, Del Brutto OH. Short course of albendazole therapy for neurocysticercosis. *Arch Neurol* 1988;45:1130–1133.

144. Vazquez ML, Jung H, Sotelo J. Plasma levels of praziquantel decrease when dexamethasone is given simultaneously. *Neurology* 1987;37:1561–1562.

145. Rueda-Franco F. Surgical considerations of neurocysticercosis. *Childs Nerv Syst* 1987;3:212–212.

146. Locke GE, Byrd SE, Zant JD. Cerebral cysticercosis: surgical considerations. *Bull Clin Neurosci* 1983;48:93–101.

147. Velasco O, Bracho CG, Quiroz MG, Romero V, Pulido RM. Comparacion de una tecnica de deteccion de antigenos solubles de cisticercus cellulosae. *Salud Publica Mex* 1983;25:205–208.

148. Torrealba G, Del Villar S, Tagle P, Arriagada P, Kase CS. Cysticercosis of the central nervous system: clinical and therapeutic considerations. *J Neurol* 1984;47:784–790.

149. Leblanc R, Knowles KF, Melanson D, MacLean JD, Rouleau G, Farmer JP. Neurocysticercosis: surgical and medical management with praziquantel. *Neurosurgery* 1986;18:419–427.

150. Del Brutto OH, Sotelo J. Albendazole therapy for subarachnoid and ventricular cysticercosis. Case report. *J Neurosurg* 1990;72:816–817.

151. Tentori NV. La cirugia en casos de neurocysticercosis tratados con praziquantel. *Salud Publica Mex* 1982;24:661–677.

152. McDowell D, Harper CG. Neurocysticercosis—two Australian cases. *Med J Aust* 1990;152:217–218.

153. Trujillo-Valdes VM, Gonzalez-Barranco D, Villanueva-Diaz G, Sandoval-Islas ME, Orozco-Bohne R. Chemotherapy of human cysticercosis using metrifonate. In: Flisser A, Williams K, Laclette JP, Lavralde C, Redadura C, Beltran F, eds. *Cysticercosis: present state of knowledge and perspectives.* New York: Academic Press, 1982;219–226.

154. Escobedo F, Penagos P, Rodriguez J, Sotelo J. Albendazole therapy for neurocysticercosis. *Arch Intern Med* 1987;147:738–741.

155. Sotelo J, Escobedo F, Penagos P. Albendazole vs praziquantel for therapy for neurocysticercosis. A controlled trial. *Arch Neurol* 1988;45:532–534.

156. Spina-Franca A, Nobrega JPS, Machado LR, Livramento JA. Neurocisticercose e praziquantel. Evolucao a longo prazo de 100 pacientes. *Arq Neuropsiquiatr* 1989;47:444–448.

157. Sotelo J, Torres B, Rubio-Donnadieu F, Escobedo F, Rodriguez-Carbajal J. Praziquantel in the treatment of neurocysticercosis: long-term follow-up. *Neurology* 1985;35:752–755.

158. Robles C, Sedano M, Vargas-Tentori N, Galindo-Virgen S. Long-term results of praziquantel therapy in neurocysticercosis. *J Neurosurg* 1987;66:359–363.

159. de Ghetaldi LD, Norman RM, Douville AW Jr. Cerebral cysticercosis treated biphasically with dexamethasone and praziquantel. *Ann Intern Med* 1983;99:179–181.

160. Robles C. Mortalidad en 100 enfermos con neurocisticercosis tratatos con praziquantel. *Salud Publica Mex* 1982;24:629–632.

161. Mata AD. Resultado de las necropsias de tres pacientes con diagnostico de cisticercosis, tratados con praziquantel. *Salud Publica Mex* 1982;24:643–648.

162. Salpietro F, Caruso G, Cipri S, Gambardella G, Cannavo S. Failure of praziquantel treatment in cerebral cysticercosis. *J Neurosurg* 1987;31:187–190.

163. Robles C. Resultados tardios en el tratamiento de la cisticercosis cerebral por praziquantel. *Salud Publica Mex* 1982;24:625–627.

164. Cook G. Neurocysticercosis: parasitology, clinical presentation, diagnosis, and recent advances in management. *Q J Med* 1988;68:575–583.

165. Sotelo J, Rosas N, Palencia G. Freezing of infested pork muscle kills cysticerci. *JAMA* 1986;256:893–894.

166. Rickard MD, Williams JP. Hydatidosis/cysticercosis: immune mechanisms and immunization against infection. *Adv Parasitol* 1982;21:229–280.

167. Proctor NSF. Coenurosis. In: Marcial-Rojas RA, ed. *Pathology of protozoal and helminthic diseases with clinical correlation,* 1st ed. Huntington, NY: Robert E Krieger, 1971;627–634.

168. Kurtycz DFI, Alt B, Mack E. Incidental coenurosis: larval cestode presenting as an axillary mass. *Am J Clin Pathol* 1983;80:735–738.

169. Pau A, Turtas S, Brambilla M, Leoni A, Rosa M, Viale GL. Computed tomography and magnetic resonance imaging of cerebral coenurosis. *Surg Neurol* 1987;27:548–552.

170. Poole JB, Marcial-Rojas RA. Echinococcosis. In: Marcial-Rojas

RA, ed. *Pathology of protozoal and helminthic diseases with clinical correlation,* 1st ed. Huntington, NY: Robert E Krieger, 1971;635–657.

171. Schantz PM, Okelo GBA. Echinococcosis (hydatidosis). In: Warren KS, Mahmoud AAF, eds. *Tropical and geographic medicine,* 2nd ed. New York: McGraw-Hill, 1990;505–518.

172. Arana-Iniguez R, Lopez-Fernandez JR. Parasitosis of the nervous system, with special reference to echinococcosis. *Clin Neurosurg* 1966;14:123–144.

173. Sharma A, Abraham J. Multiple giant hydatid cysts of the brain. Case report. *J Neurosurg* 1982;57:413–415.

174. Aydin Y, Barlas O, Yolas C, et al. Alveolar hydatid disease of the brain. Report of four cases. *J Neurosurg* 1986;65:115–119.

175. Bia FJ, Barry M. Parasitic infections of the central nervous system. *Neurol Clin* 1986;4:171–206.

176. Abbassioun K, Rahmat H, Ameli NO, Tafazoli M. Computerized tomography in hydatid cyst of the brain. *J Neurosurg* 1978;49:408–411.

177. Coltorti EA, Varela-Diaz VM. Detection of antibodies against *Echinococcus granulosus* arc 5 antigens by double diffusion test. *Trans R Soc Trop Med Hyg* 1978;72:226–229.

178. Morris DL, Clarkson MS, Stallbaumer MF, et al. Albendazole treatment of pulmonary hydatid cysts in naturally infected sheep: a study with relevance to man. *Thorax* 1985;40:453–458.

179. Morris DK, Dykes PW, Marriner X, et al. Albendazole: objective evidence of response in human hydatid disease. *JAMA* 1985;253:2053–2057.

180. Taylor DH, Morris DL, Richards KS. *Echinococcus granulosus:* in vitro maintenance of whole cysts and the assessment of albendazole sulphoxide and praziquantel on the germinal layer. *Trans R Soc Trop Med Hyg* 1989;83:535–538.

181. Okelo GBA. Hydatid disease: research and control in Turkana, III. Albendazole in the treatment of inoperable hydatid disease in Kenya—a report on 12 cases. *Trans R Soc Trop Med Hyg* 1986;80:193–195.

182. Davis A, Dixon H, Pawlowski ZS. Multicenter clinical trials of benzimidazole-carbamates in human cystic echinococcosis (phase 2). *Bull WHO* 1989;67:503–508.

183. Zhongxi Q, Shuyuan G, Guoxue T, et al. Immediate and long-term results of surgical treatment of intrathoracic hydatid cysts. *Clin Med J* 1980;93:569–572.

184. Holodniy M, Almenoff J, Loutit J, Steinberg GK. Cerebral sparganosis: Case report and review. *Rev Infect Dis* 1991;13:155–159.

185. Anders K, Foley K, Stern WE, Brown WJ. Intracranial sparganosis: an uncommon infection. Case report. *J Neurosurg* 1984;60:1282–1286.

186. Chan S-T, Tse CH, Chan YS, Fong D. Sparganosis of the brain. Report of two cases. *J Neurosurg* 1987;67:931–934.

187. Lo Y-K, Chao D, Yan S-H, et al. Spinal cord proliferative sparganosis in Taiwan: a case report. *Neurosurgery* 1987;21:235–238.

188. Koo J, Pien F, Kliks MM. *Angiostrongylus (Parastrongylus)* eosinophilic meningitis. *Rev Infect Dis* 1988;10:1155–1162.

189. Beaver PC, Rosen L. Memorandum of the first report of *Angiostrongylus* in man, by Nomura and Lin, 1945. *Am J Trop Med Hyg* 1964;13:589–590.

190. Punyagupta S, Bunnag T, Juttijudata P, Rosen L. Eosinophilic meningitis in Thailand. Epidemiologic studies of 484 typical cases and the etiologic role of *Angiostrongylus cantonensis. Am J Trop Med Hyg* 1970;19:950–958.

191. Kliks MM, Kroenke K, Hardman JM. Eosinophilic radiculomyeloencephalitis: an angiostrongyliasis outbreak in American Samoa related to ingestion of *Achatina fulica* snails. *Am J Trop Med Hyg* 1982;31:1114–1122.

192. Schmutzhard E, Boongird P, Vejjajiva A. Eosinophilic meningitis and radiculomyelitis in Thailand, caused by CNS invasion of *Gnathostoma spinigerum* and *Angiostrongylus cantonensis. J Neurol Neurosurg Psychiatry* 1988;51:80–87.

193. Tangchai P, Nye SW, Beaver PC. Eosinophilic meningoencephalitis caused by angiostrongyliasis in Thailand. Autopsy report. *Am J Trop Med Hyg* 1967;16:454–461.

194. Rosen L, Loison G, Laigret J, Wallace GD. Studies on eosinophilic meningitis. 3. Epidemiologic and clinical observations on Pacific Islands and the possible etiologic role of *Angiostrongylus. Am J Epidemiol* 1967;85:17–44.

195. Campbell BG, Little MD. The finding of *Angiostrongylus cantonensis* in rats in New Orleans. *Am J Trop Med Hyg* 1988;38:568–573.

196. Rosen L, Chappell R, Laqueur GL, Wallace GD, Weinstein PP. Eosinophilic meningoencephalitis caused by a metastrongylid lung-worm of rats. *JAMA* 1962;179:126–130.

197. Kuberski T, Wallace GD. Clinical manifestations of eosinophilic meningitis due to *Angiostrongylus cantonensis. Neurology* 1979;29:1566–1570.

198. Swanson VL. Gnathostomiasis. In: Marcial-Rojas RA, ed. *Pathology of protozoal and helminthic diseases with clinical correlation,* 1st ed. Huntington, NY: Robert E Krieger, 1975;871–879.

199. Chitanondh H, Rosen L. Fatal eosinophilic encephalomyelitis caused by the nematode *Gnathostoma spinigerum. Am J Trop Med Hyg* 1967;16:638–645.

200. Boongird P, Phuapradit P, Siridej N, Chirachariyavej T, Chuahirun S, Vejjajiva A. Neurological manifestations of gnathostomiasis. *J Neurol Sci* 1977;31:279–291.

201. Bunnag T, Comer DS, Punyagupta S. Eosinophilic myeloencephalitis caused by *Gnathostoma spinigerum.* Neuropathology of nine cases. *J Neurol Sci* 1970;10:419–434.

202. Ribas-Mujal D. Trichinosis. In: Marcial-Rojas RA, ed. *Pathology of protozoal and helminthic diseases with clinical correlation,* 1st ed. Huntington, NY: Robert E Krieger, 1971;677–710.

203. Kazura JW. Trichinosis. *Trop Geogr Med* 1990;2:442–445.

204. Zimmerman WJ, Steele JH, Kagan I. Trichinosis in the U.S. population, 1966–1970. *Public Health Rep* 1973;88:606–623.

205. Dalessio DJ, Wolfe HG. *Trichinella spiralis* infection of the central nervous system: report of a case and review of the literature. *Arch Neurol* 1960;4:407–417.

206. Levin ML. Treatment of trichinosis with mebendazole. *Am J Trop Med Hyg* 1983;32:980–983.

207. Scowden EB, Schaffner W, Stone WJ. Overwhelming strongyloidiasis. An unappreciated opportunistic infection. *Medicine* 1978;57:527–544.

208. Pelletier LL, Gabre-Kidan T. Chronic strongyloidiasis in Vietnam veterans. *Am J Med* 1985;78:139–140.

209. Keefer CS. Subacute bacterial endocarditis: active cases without bacteremia. *Ann Intern Med* 1937;11:714–734.

210. McKerrow JH, Brindley P, Brown M, Gam AA, Staunton C, Neva FH. *Strongyloides stercoralis:* identification of a protease that facilitates penetration of skin by the infective larvae. *Exp Parasitol* 1990;70:134–143.

211. Rege AA, Dresden MH. *Strongyloides* spp: demonstration and partial characterization of acidic collagenolytic activity from infective larvae. *Exp Parasitol* 1987;64:275–280.

212. Brown HW, Perna VP. An overwhelming *Strongyloides* infection. *JAMA* 1958;168:1648–1651.

213. Wilson S, Thompson AE. A fatal case of strongyloidiasis. *J Pathol Bacteriol* 1964;87:169–176.

214. Owor R, Wamukota WM. A fatal case of strongyloidiasis with *Strongyloides* larvae in the meninges. *Trans R Soc Trop Med Hyg* 1976;70:497–499.

215. Schainberg L, Scheinberg MA. Recovery of *Strongyloides stercoralis* by bronchoalveolar lavage in a patient with acquired immunodeficiency syndrome. *Am J Med* 1989;87:486.

216. Neefe LI, Pinilla O, Garagusi VF, Bauer H. Disseminated strongyloidiasis with cerebral involvement. *Am J Med* 1973;55:832–838.

217. Arroyo JC, Brown A. Concentrations of thiabendazole and parasite-specific IgG antibodies in the cerebrospinal fluid of a patient with disseminated strongyloidiasis. *J Infect Dis* 1987;156:520–523.

218. Arpino C, Gattinara GC, Piergili D, Curatolo P. *Toxocara* infection and epilepsy in children: a case–control study. *Epilepsia* 1990;31:33–36.

219. Gutierrez Y. *Toxocara*—visceral larva migrans. In: Gutierrez Y, ed. *Diagnostic pathology of parasitic infections with clinical correlations,* 1st ed. Philadelphia: Lea & Febiger, 1990;262–272.

220. Schantz PM. *Toxocara* larva migrans now. *Am J Trop Med Hyg* 1989;41(Suppl):21–34.

221. Shields JA. Ocular toxocariasis, a review. *Surv Ophthalmol* 1984;28:361–381.

222. Glickman LT. Toxocariasis and related syndromes. *Trop Geograph Med* 1990;2:446–455.
223. Taylor MRH, Keane CT, O'Connor P, Mulvihill E, Holland C. The expanded spectrum of toxocaral disease. *Lancet* 1988;1:692–695.
224. Mikhael NZ, Montpetit VJA, Orizaga M, Rowsell HC, Richard MT. Toxocara canis infestation with encephalitis. *Can J Neurol Sci* 1974;1:114–120.
225. Beautyman W, Beaver PC, Buckley JJC, Woolf AL. Review of a case previously reported as showing an ascarid larva in the brain. *J Pathol Bacteriol* 1966;91:271–273.
226. Schochet SS. Human *Toxocara canis* encephalopathy in a case of visceral larva migrans. *Neurology* 1967;17:227–229.
227. Hill IR, Denham DA, Scholtz CL. *Toxocara canis* larvae in the brain of a British child. *Trans R Soc Trop Med Hyg* 1985;79:351–354.
228. Burren CH. The distribution of *Toxocara* larvae in the central nervous system of the mouse. *Trans R Soc Trop Med Hyg* 1971;65:450–453.
229. Woodruff A, Bisseru B, Bowe J. Infection with animal helminths as a factor causing poliomyelitis and epilepsy. *Br Med J* 1966;1:1576–1579.
230. Glickman L, Cypress R, Crumrine I, Gitlin D. Toxocara infection and epilepsy in children. *J Pediatr* 1979;94:75–78.
231. Hugg D, Neafie R, Binder M. The first fatal *Baylisascaris* infection in humans: an infant with eosinophilic meningitis. *Pediatr Pathol* 1984;2:345–352.
232. Oostburg BF, Varma AA. *Lagochilascaris minor* infection in Surinam. Report of a case. *Am J Trop Med Hyg* 1968;17:548–550.
233. Botero D, Little MD. Two cases of human *Lagochilascaris* infection in Colombia. *Am J Trop Med Hyg* 1984;33:381–386.
234. Volcan GS, Ochoa FR, Medrano CE, de Valera Y. *Lagochilascaris minor* infection in Venezuela. Report of a case. *Am J Trop Med Hyg* 1982;31:1111–1113.
235. Moraes MA, Arnaud MV, de Lima PE. New cases of human infection by *Lagochilascaris minor* Leiper, 1909, found in the state of Para, Brazil. *Rev Inst Med Trop Sao Paulo* 1983;25:139–146.
236. Bowman DD, Smith JL, Little MD. *Lagochilascaris sprenti* sp. n. (*Nematoda ascarididae*) from the opossum, *Didelphis virginiana* (*Marsupilalia didelphidae*). *J Parasitol* 1983;69:754–760.
237. Craig T, Robinson RM, McArthur NH, Ward RD. *Lagochilascaris major* in a raccoon. *J Wildl Dis* 1980;16:67–70.
238. Romero JR, Led JE. A new case of *Lagochilascaris major* (Leiper 1910) in the Argentine Republic parasitizing the cat (*Felis catus domesticus*). *Zentralbl Veterinarmed* 1985;32:575–582.
239. Craig TM, O'Quinn BO, Robinson RM, McArthur NH. Parasitic nematode (*Lagochilascaris major*) associated with a purulent draining tract in a dog. *J Am Vet Med Assoc* 1982;181:69–70.
240. Brenes-Madrigal RR, Ruiz A, Frenkel JK. Discovery of *Lagochilascaris* sp. in the larynx of a Costa Rican ocelot (*Felis paradalis mearnsi*). *J Parasitol* 1972;58:978.
241. Laughlin LW. Schistomiasis. In: Strickland GT, ed. *Hunter's tropical medicine*, 6th ed. Philadelphia: WB Saunders, 1984;708–740.
242. Scrimgeour EM, Gajdusek DC. Involvement of the central nervous system in *Schistosoma mansoni* and *S. Haematobium* infection. *Brain* 1985;108:1023–1038.
243. Wyler DJ, Wahl SM, Wahl LM. Hepatic fibrosis in schistosomiasis: egg granulomas secrete fibroblast stimulating factor *in vitro*. *Science* 1978;202:438–440.
244. Pittella JE, Lana-Peixoto MA. Brain involvement in hepatosplenic *Schistosomiasis mansoni*. *Brain* 1981;104:621–632.
245. Aleman G. Localization ectopica aparentemente asintomatica de huevos de *Schistosoma mansoni* en el encefalo. *Arch Hosp Vargas* 1966;8:71–84.
246. Luyendijk W, Lindeman J. *Schistosomiasis (bilharziasis) mansoni* of the spinal cord simulating an intramedullary tumor. *Surg Neurol* 1975;4:457–460.
247. Quieros AC. O envolvimento do sistema nervoso central na *Esquistossomose mansonica*. *Rev Patol Trop* 1974;3:255–261.
248. Andrade AN. Neuroschistosomiasis. *Arq Neuropsiquiatr* 1986; 44:275–279.
249. Gelfand M. Neurological complications of parasitic disease. In: Spillane JD, ed. *Tropical neurology*, 1st ed. London: Oxford University Press, 1973;247–258.
250. Lechtenberg R, Vaida GA. Schistosomiasis of the spinal cord. *Neurology* 1977;27:55–59.
251. Levy LF, Baldachin BJ, Clain D. Intracranial bilharzia. *Cent Afr J Med* 1975;21:76–84.
252. Piganiol G, Herve A, Pourpre X. Complications cerebrales de la bilharziose a *Schistosoma mansoni*. *Bull Soc Pathol Exot* 1956;49:450–455.
253. Raso P. Hemorragia cerebral macica devida ao *Schistosoma mansoni*. *Hosp Rio de Janiero* 1964;65:537–551.
254. Pompeu F, Sampaio de Lacerda PR. Subarachnoid hemorrhage due to *Schistosoma mansoni*: a rare etiology. *J Neurol* 1979;221:203–207.
255. Cabral G, Pittella JE. Tumoural form of cerebellar *Schistosomiasis mansoni*. Report of a surgically treated case. *Acta Neurochir* 1989;99:148–151.
256. Gjerde IO, Mork S, Larsen JL, Huldt G, Skeidsvoll H, Aarli JA. Cerebral schistosomiasis presenting as a brain tumor. *Eur Neurol* 1984;23:229–236.
257. Watts G, Adapon B, Long GW, Fernando MT, Ranoa CP, Cross JH. Praziquantel in treatment of cerebral schistosomiasis. *Lancet* 1986;2:529–532.
258. Hershkowitz A. Spinal cord involvement with *Schistosoma mansoni*: case report. *J Neurosurg* 1972;36:494–498.
259. Gama C. Compression granuloma of the spinal cord caused by *Schistosoma mansoni* ova: epiconus; conus medullaris; cauda equina: report of a case. *J Int Coll Surg* 1953;19:665–671.
260. Anonymous. Acute schistosomiasis with transverse myelitis in American students returning from Kenya. *MMWR* 1984; 33:445–447.
261. Suchet I, Klein C, Horwitz T, Lalla S, Doodha M. Spinal cord schistosomiasis: a case report and review of the literature. *Paraplegia* 1987;25:491–496.
262. Boyce TG. Acute transverse myelitis in a 6-year-old girl with schistosomiasis. *Pediatr Infect Dis J* 1990;9:279–284.
263. Kirchhoff LV, Nash TE. A case of *Schistosomiasis japonica*: resolution of CAT-scan detected cerebral abnormalities without specific therapy. *Am J Trop Med Hyg* 1984;33:1155–1158.
264. Mao SC, Ye XC, Liu JX, Zhang JW. CT brain scanning in the diagnosis and localisation of cerebral schistosomiasis. *Chung Hua Shen Ching Ching Shen Ko Tsa Chih (Chinese J Neurol Psychiatry)* 1989;7:115–118.
265. Masson C, Rey A, Ast G, Cambier J, Masson M. Schistosomiasis of the spinal cord. Contribution of magnetic resonance imaging. *Presse Med* 1990;19:1223–1224.
266. Khalil HH, Abdel WM, el Deeb A, et al. Cerebral atrophy: a schistosomiasis manifestation? *Am J Trop Med Hyg* 1986; 35:531–535.
267. El-Banhawy A. Schistosomiasis of the spinal cord, conus and cauda. *Neurol Med Chir (Tokyo)* 1971;11:17–33.
268. Houpis J, Oexman J, Martin J, Jacobi G, Reardon J, Waterman G. Acute schistosomiasis with transverse myelitis in American students returning from Kenya. *MMWR* 1984;33:445–447.
269. Bambirra EA, de Souza AJ, Cesarini I, Rodriques PA, Drummond CA. The tumoral form of schistosomiasis: report of a case with cerebellar involvement. *Am J Trop Med Hyg* 1984;33:76–79.
270. Peregrino AJ, de Oliveira SP, Porto CA, et al. Meningomyeloradiculitis caused by *Schistosoma mansoni*. Research protocol and report of 21 cases. *Arq Neuropsiquiatr* 1988;46:49–60.
271. Efthimiou J, Denning D. Spinal cord disease due to *Schistosoma mansoni* successfully treated with oxamniquine. *Br Med J* 1984;288:1343–1344.
272. Oh SJ. Cerebral paragonimiasis. *Trans Am Neurol Assoc* 1967;92:275–277.
273. Miyazaki I. Cerebral paragonimiasis. *Contemp Neurol Ser* 1975;12:109–132.
274. Suzuki Y, Itoh H, Yonemaru M, et al. A case of *Paragonimus westermani* infection with repeated spontaneous pneumothorax and cerebellar infarction—a review of the clinical feature in cases of paragonimiasis reported in Japan for the last 15 years. *Nippon*

Kyobu Shikkan Gakkai Zasshi (J Jpn Assoc Thorac Dis) 1987;25:119–124.

275. Kinoshita K, Koga T. Cerebral paragonimiasis with peculiar calcified foci: a case report. *No Shinkei Geka* [*Neurol Surg (Tokyo)*] 1986;14:669–672.

276. Yang QD. Clinical types and bitin treatment of paragonimiasis of the central nervous system—an analysis of 24 cases. *Chung Hua Shen Ching Ching Shen Ko Tsa Chih (Chin J Neurol Psychiatry)* 1983;16:1–4.

277. Brenes MR, Rodriquez-Ortiz B, Vargas SG, Ocamp OEM, Ruiz SPJ. Cerebral hemorrhagic lesions produced by *Paragonimus mexicanus.* Report of three cases in Costa Rica. *Am J Trop Med Hyg* 1982;31:522–526.

278. Soutsu M, Nishida S, Nakamura N, Katakura K, Kobayashi A, Araki K. Surgical treatment of cerebral paragonimiasis miyazakii. *No Shinkei Geka* [*Neurol Surg (Tokyo)*] 1984;12:865–870.

279. Markell EK, Goldsmith R. Trematode infections exclusive of schistosomiasis. In: Strickland GT, ed. *Hunter's tropical medicine,* 6th ed. Philadelphia: WB Saunders, 1984;740–758.

280. Yoshida M, Moritaker K, Kuga S, Anegawa S. CT findings of cerebral paragonimiasis in the chronic state. *J Comput Assist Tomogr* 1982;6:195–196.

281. Velasco O, Bracho CG, Quiroz MG, Romero V, Pulido RM. Comparacion de una tecnica de deteccion de antigenos solubles de *Cisticercus cellulosae. Salud Publica Mex* 1983;25:205–208.

282. Estrada JJ, Kuhn RE. Immunochemical detection of antigens of larval *Taenia solium* and anti-larval antibodies in the cerebrospinal fluid of patients with neurocysticercosis. *J Neurol Sci* 1985;71:39–48.

283. Melvin DM, Brooke MM, Sadun EH. *Common intestinal helminths of man.* Atlanta: DHEW publication no. [CDC] 72-8286, 1964.

284. Trelles JO, Trelles L. Cysticercosis of the nervous system. In: Vinken PJ, Bruyn GW, Klawans HL. eds. *Handbook of Clinical Neurology. Infections of the Nervous System—Part III.* New York: North-Holland Publishing Co, 1978;291–321.

PART VIII

Diagnostic Evaluation of CNS Infections

Infections of the Central Nervous System,
edited by W. M. Scheld, R. J. Whitley, and
D. T. Durack, Raven Press, Ltd., New York © 1991.

CHAPTER 36

Cerebrospinal Fluid in Central Nervous System Infections

John E. Greenlee

Infections within the central nervous system (CNS) frequently, although not invariably, produce changes in ventricular or lumbar cerebrospinal fluid (CSF). The changes produced may provide invaluable information as to the nature of the infectious process and, in many cases, may permit specific identification of the offending organism. Despite the great diagnostic value of CSF analysis, however, injudicious attempts to obtain CSF (as in the setting of brain abscess) may cause severe injury or death, and casual handling of the CSF obtained may render CSF analysis useless.

This chapter is divided into three parts. The first part reviews the anatomy of the CSF spaces, the physiology of CSF production and reabsorption, and the effect of infection on CSF physiology and composition. The second part discusses methods of CSF analysis in CNS infections. The third part summarizes the CSF analysis in specific CNS infections.

ANATOMY OF THE CSF COMPARTMENT

CSF is contained within two connecting compartments, the cerebral ventricles and the subarachnoid space (1,2). Both compartments may be affected by infectious organisms and may also reflect changes produced by infectious or parainfectious processes within meninges, brain, or spinal cord. In normal adults, total CSF volume is roughly 125 ml, of which approximately 22 ml (range: 7–56 ml) is contained within the ventricles (1–3).

J. E. Greenlee: Neurology Service, Veterans Affairs Medical Center, Salt Lake City, Utah 84148; and Department of Neurology, University of Utah School of Medicine, Salt Lake City, Utah 84132.

The Ventricular System

The cerebral ventricular system represents, in greatly elaborated form, the remnants of the embryological neural tube. The ventricles are lined by a single layer of neuroglially derived cells, the ventricular ependyma; these are backed by a dense network of astrocytic foot processes. The ventricular system is comprised of two lateral ventricles, the third ventricle, and the fourth ventricle (Fig. 1). The lateral ventricles are located within the cerebrum and consist of frontal, temporal, and occipital horns; these join at the ventricular trigone within the parietal lobe. The third ventricle is an elongated, slit-like cavity which lies within the midbrain and is bounded inferiorly by the hypothalamus. The fourth ventricle overlies the brainstem from the level of the mid-pons to the extreme rostral end of the spinal cord. The roof of the fourth ventricle is the cerebellum posteriorly and the superior and inferior medullary veli anteriorly. The fourth ventricle is roughly diamond-shaped and is widest at the lateral recesses which lie between the superior and middle cerebral peduncles.

The cerebral ventricles are connected to each other and with the subarachnoid space through a series of small openings. Each lateral ventricle drains into the third ventricle through the foramen of Monro, located in the inferomedial wall of the frontal horn. The third and fourth ventricles are connected by the aqueduct of Sylvius, which extends through the midbrain. The fourth ventricle drains into the subarachnoid space through three small openings, the foramina of Luschka and the foramen of Magendie. The foramina of Luschka are located in the lateral recesses of the fourth ventricle and are absent in up to 20% of the population (4). The foramen of Magendie is located in the midline and, in most persons, represents the major communication between the

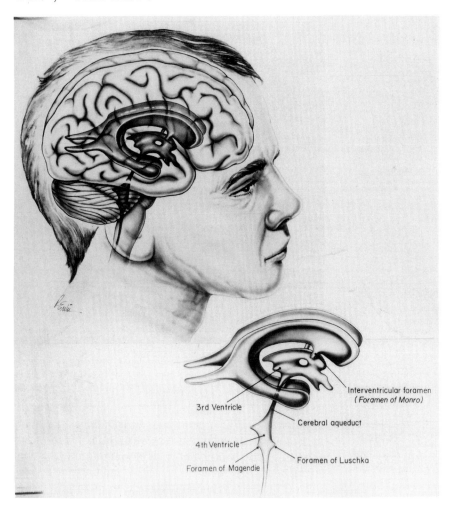

FIG. 1. The cerebral ventricles. The inset shows the structure of the fourth ventricle and the locations of the foramina of Luschka and Magendie. (From ref. 6, with permission.)

3rd Ventricle

4th Ventricle

Foramen of Magendie

Cerebral aqueduct

Interventricular foramen (Foramen of Monro)

Foramen of Luschka

fourth ventricle and the subarachnoid space (5). As will be discussed below, these narrow openings are important in CNS infections, since they represent the sites at which obstruction of CSF flow may most easily occur.

The Meninges and Subarachnoid Space

The brain and spinal cord are surrounded by three layers of meninges. The outermost layer of the meninges is a tough, fibrous membrane, the dura mater. Within the skull, the dura forms the inner layer of the cranial periosteum and is tightly adherent to bone. Below the foramen magnum, the dura and periosteum diverge and are separated by a fat-filled epidural space. The middle layer of meninges, the arachnoid, is held against the dura by the outward pressure of brain and CSF to form a potential subdural space. The arachnoid covers the brain and spinal cord loosely and extends outward along the course of cranial and spinal nerves. The third layer of meninges, the pia mater, is continuous with the surface of the brain and spinal cord. The pia mater also follows vessels into brain and spinal cord parenchyma and projects into the ventricles to form the choroid plexuses.

The pia mater and the ventricular ependyma merge at the foramina of Luschka and Magendie. CSF is contained in the subarachnoid space, enclosed between the arachnoid and the pia. The subarachnoid space surrounds the brain and extends within the spinal canal to the level of the second sacral vertebra. Within the skull, the subarachnoid space widens into cisterns where pia and arachnoid are more widely separated by irregularities in the contour of the brain. The largest of these, the cisterna magna, surrounds the brainstem and the cerebellum at the base of the skull and is occasionally used as a source of CSF for analysis and culture. The subarachnoid space is crossed by trabecular extensions of the arachnoid itself, by cranial nerves, by a network of small arteries, the rete mirabile, and by numerous bridging veins, which connect the meningeal veins with the deeper intracranial venous system (6).

The subarachnoid space is normally a closed system. Occasionally, however, congenital or post-traumatic communications may exist between the subarachnoid space and superficial tissues and may provide a route for single or recurrent episodes of meningitis. Congenital defects are due to incomplete closure of the neural tube. These defects may extend for variable distances into subcutaneous tissues or to the cutaneous surface and are most common in the upper cervical regions and over the sacrum. Their presence may be suggested by a cutaneous dimple or a patch of hair. Traumatic communications into the subarachnoid space are most frequently associated with basilar skull fractures. The most common sites of involvement are (a) the thin layers of bone which separate the cranial cavity from the paranasal sinuses and (b) the petrous bone which separates the auditory canals and mastoid from the cranial cavity. In rare instances, traumatic defects may occur over the cranial convexities or along the spinal column.

PHYSIOLOGY OF CSF PRODUCTION AND REABSORPTION

CSF is produced by the choroid plexuses of the lateral, third, and fourth ventricles and, to a lesser extent, by extrachoroidal sites (1,2,7). The choroid plexuses are specialized projections of vessels and pia mater into the ventricular cavities. Each choroid plexus branches into frond-like villi, each of which contains a capillary surrounded by loose connective tissue and a layer of specialized ependymal cells termed "choroidal epithelium." Choroidal epithelial cells, in contrast to ependymal cells elsewhere in the ventricular system, are columnar in shape and are covered on their ventricular surfaces by a brush border of microvilli. The villous structure of the choroid plexus and the presence of microvilli greatly increase the surface area available for secretion of CSF (8). In the normal adult, CSF production occurs at a high rate—approximately 20 ml/hr.

CSF formation involves both filtration and active transport (2,9–14). Filtration of CSF varies inversely with serum osmolality. In experimental animals, and possibly also in humans, CSF production changes 7% for each 1% change in serum osmolality (9–12). Active secretion of CSF involves Na,K-ATPase-mediated transport of sodium across choroidal epithelium into the ventricular lumen, with water, chloride, and bicarbonate ions following through facilitated transport. Ouabain, which binds to Na,K-ATPase, greatly reduces CSF formation in experimental animals, although the doses required for this effect are toxic in humans (14,15). The carbonic anhydrase inhibitor, acetazolamide, reduces CSF secretion by approximately 50%, as does furosemide (16–18). Simultaneous use of both agents reduces CSF formation by 75% (17,18).

Reabsorption of CSF occurs through arachnoid villi. The majority of these are located along the superior sagittal sinus. Smaller numbers of arachnoid villi are found along other intracranial venous sinuses and around spinal nerve roots (1,2). During health, the arachnoid villi along the superior sagittal sinus provide the major site of CSF uptake. The arachnoid villi along other sinuses and

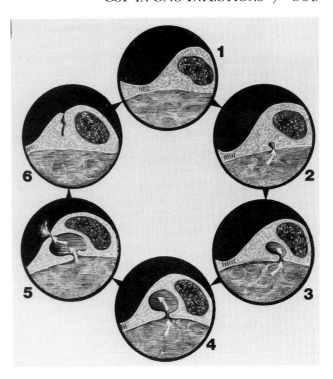

FIG. 2. Uptake of CSF by an arachnoid villus. (From ref. 2, with permission.)

surrounding spinal nerve roots are thought to provide alternative sites of CSF absorption following superior sagittal sinus thrombosis.

Each arachnoid villus represents an extension of the arachnoid membrane through the dura mater into the lumen of the venous sinus and functions as a one-way valve, permitting unidirectional flow from CSF into blood. Early work by Welch and co-workers (19–22) demonstrated that the arachnoid villi have a critical *in vitro* opening pressure of 2–5 cm H_2O; these studies also demonstrated that particles up to the size of erythrocytes readily pass from CSF into blood, whereas particles larger than 7.5 μm are excluded. Although these early data suggested that the arachnoid villi might provide a direct communication between CSF and blood, studies using electron microscopy have demonstrated that arachnoid villi and venous sinuses are separated by a layer of endothelial cells connected by tight junctions and that movement of CSF and particulate matter across the arachnoid villi occurs by transport within giant vesicles (23–26) (Fig. 2). These giant vesicles, although providing efficient transfer of CSF into blood under normal circumstances, can become obstructed by bacteria and inflammatory cells during meningitis or by red blood cells during subarachnoid hemorrhage (27,28).

BARRIER SYSTEMS

The brain and CSF are contained within a series of barrier systems. These prevent entry of fluids, electrolytes, and other substances from blood into CSF or brain by simple diffusion and also isolate the CNS from systemic immune responses. The blood–brain barrier is formed by tight junctions between endothelial cells of CNS capillaries and is further reinforced by a surrounding layer of astrocytes, whose processes terminate in overlapping fashion on the capillary walls. Unlike brain capillary endothelial cells, the endothelial cells of the choroid plexuses and arachnoid are separated by gap junctions which allow diffusion of substances across the vessel wall, so that the blood–CSF barrier is formed by tight junctions between cells of the arachnoid membrane and similar tight junctions between the epithelial cells of the choroid plexus. A CSF–brain barrier exists at the pia mater. The cells of the pia mater, like those of choroid plexus and arachnoid capillaries, are separated by gap junctions; entry of substances from CSF into brain is modulated by a basement membrane subjacent to the pia and by a continuous layer of astrocytes beneath the basement membrane.

The barrier systems which surround spinal cord and brain exclude from the CNS most of the immunological mechanisms which provide host defense elsewhere in the body. Normally, T cells and B cells are present in very small numbers in CSF and only rarely in brain; immunoglobulins and complement are largely excluded from both CSF and brain; and opsonic activity of CSF, even in the presence of meningitis, is far less than that of serum (29–32). CNS infections thus begin—and progress—in tissue which is poorly equipped to halt their spread.

Recent work has demonstrated that the barrier systems which isolate CSF, brain, and spinal cord from blood are not static systems but, instead, are highly dynamic in their ability to interact with and transport a wide variety of substances (13). In addition, it is increasingly recognized that the endothelial cells and astrocytes of the blood–brain and blood–CSF barriers are important sources of cytokines (including tumor necrosis factor and interleukins) and that astrocytes, in addition to their abilities to regulate solute entry into brain, have the ability to act as antigen-presenting cells. As is discussed in Chapters 14 and 16, release of cytokines by endothelial cells and astrocytes in response to bacterial endotoxins and other bacterial products is fundamental in the production of CNS inflammation and injury during infections (33–45).

MAINTENANCE OF CSF HOMEOSTASIS

The blood–brain and blood–CSF barriers maintain the cellular and chemical elements of the CSF within narrow ranges (13). Lipid-soluble substances within blood readily diffuse across choroidal epithelium or vascular endothelium into CSF or brain. Passage of fluid and ionically polar substances, however, requires mechanisms for transport and facilitated diffusion. Sodium enters CSF both by Na,K-ATPase-mediated transport during secretion of CSF and by passive diffusion. Potassium is secreted into CSF by active transport mechanisms and is also actively removed from CSF into brain by transport mechanisms which are believed to be located in astrocyte foot processes. Movement of calcium, magnesium, and phosphorus into CSF and brain also occur predominantly by active transport, and the concentrations of these substances is relatively independent of their concentrations in serum. Chloride and bicarbonate, like potassium, are actively secreted into, and actively removed from, CSF. Glucose, amino acids, amines, and thyroid hormone enter the brain by carrier-mediated transport mechanisms (13). Insulin and transferrin require receptor-mediated transport. Although lipids complexed to proteins were once thought to be excluded from the CNS, it is now known that complexed lipids undergo dissociation from their carrier proteins at the blood–brain interface and may enter the CNS without significant exodus of protein from brain capillaries.

Chloride represents the major anion in CSF. Normal CSF chloride concentration is 15–20 mEq/liter higher than serum. Early workers observed that CSF chloride concentrations were lowered in tuberculous meningitis; for many years, levels of CSF chloride were used to diagnose and follow the course of this infection (2). It is now recognized, however, that the lowered CSF chloride observed in tuberculous meningitis is nothing more than a reflection of lowered serum chloride values and has no diagnostic or prognostic utility (2,46).

The acid–base balance of the CSF, like its electrolyte concentration, tends to remain fairly constant despite fluctuations in systemic acid–base balance. In CSF as opposed to plasma, however, movement of CO_2 occurs readily by diffusion, whereas movement of bicarbonate occurs more slowly by carrier-mediated transport. The discrepancy in the rate of movement of these two cations may produce delayed (and, at times, paradoxical) responses in CSF pH as compared to systemic pH during rapid changes in bicarbonate concentration (2). CSF acid–base balance is also maintained by the choroid plexuses, which possess transport mechanisms capable of removing weak organic acids—including antibiotics such as the penicillins, cephalosporins, and aminoglycosides—from CSF (47–49). Choroid plexus transport of antibiotics and other weak organic acids can be blocked by probenecid.

ALTERATIONS OF CSF DYNAMICS AND PRESSURE IN CNS INFECTIONS: HYDROCEPHALUS, INTRACRANIAL HYPERTENSION, AND BRAIN HERNIATION

Acute or chronic CNS infections may produce profound alterations in intracranial pressure (ICP) by obstructing CSF flow or reabsorption, by behaving as space-occupying lesions, by altering CSF, or by producing hemorrhage or cerebral edema. These pathological consequences of infection, acting individually or together, may cause brain herniation and death.

Alteration of CSF Circulation in CNS Infections

Impairment of normal CSF circulation may result in ventricular enlargement and hydrocephalus. Interruption of CSF reabsorption produces communicating hydrocephalus, with normal circulation of CSF through the ventricular system and into the subarachnoid space. Communicating hydrocephalus is a common complication of bacterial meningitis and, in most cases, results from obstruction of the arachnoid villi by bacteria and white blood cells (27). Communicating hydrocephalus may also result from functional occlusion of arachnoid villi by fungi or by red blood cells in the course of subarachnoid hemorrhage from mycotic aneurysm (28). Thrombosis of the superior sagittal sinus may also block CSF reabsorption and thereby produce communicating hydrocephalus. Occlusion of a large portion of the superior sagittal sinus usually produces catastrophic, often hemorrhagic, cerebral infarction. Involvement of the anterior third of the sinus, however, may be clinically silent, except for the development of hydrocephalus (50).

Obstructive hydrocephalus results from interruption of CSF flow within the ventricular system or at its point of exit into the subarachnoid space. This may be the consequence of infection of the ventricular ependyma or basilar meninges or may result from extrinsic compression of the ventricular system by infection within brain parenchyma. Lesions producing obstructive hydrocephalus most commonly involve the ventricular system at its narrowest points: the foramina of Luschka and Magendie, the fourth ventricle, the aqueduct of Sylvius, and the foramina of Monro. Obstruction of the foramina of Luschka and Magendie is characteristic of exudative, basilar meningitides such as those caused by *Mycobacterium tuberculosis, Coccidioides immitis,* and *Cryptococcus neoformans* but may also be seen in bacterial meningitis. Hydrocephalus due to obliteration of the fourth ventricle is almost always extrinsic and is the result of ventricular compression by large cerebellar mass lesions, such as cerebellar abscess or hemorrhage. Occlusion of the aqueduct of Sylvius by granulomatous ependymitis may occur as a complication of tuberculosis, fungal infections, or sarcoidosis. Mumps virus, which replicates in ventricular ependymal cells, has been shown to produce congenital aqueductal stenosis in experimental animals (51). Rare cases of acquired aqueductal stenosis have also been reported following mumps meningoencephalitis in humans (52). Extrinsic compression of the aqueduct of Sylvius may be produced by abscesses or other localized infections within the pons or midbrain. Involvement of the foramen of

Monro is almost always unilateral and is the consequence of severe brain shifts caused by abscess, focal encephalitis, or hemorrhage. Hydrocephalus due to the occlusion of one foramen of Monro is particularly dangerous, because the CSF trapped within the involved lateral ventricle acts as a unilateral space-occupying lesion, greatly increasing the risk of transtentorial brain herniation.

Computerized tomography (CT) and magnetic resonance imaging (MRI) are invaluable in demonstrating the presence of hydrocephalus and in determining its cause. Ventricular dilatation—so-called hydrocephalus *ex vacuo*—is common in the elderly and is characterized by symmetrical ventricular dilatation accompanied by evidence of cerebral cortical atrophy. In contrast, hydrocephalus due to impaired CSF circulation is accompanied by loss of cortical markings visible on CT or MRI, as the brain is forced outward against the skull, and by periventricular areas of increased lucency, representing transependymal leakage of CSF. Communicating hydrocephalus and hydrocephalus due to obstruction of the foramina of Luschka and Magendie are characterized by symmetrical enlargement of all four ventricles. Hydrocephalus due to occlusion of the fourth ventricle or aqueduct of Sylvius results in loss of that structure on CT or MRI, with dilatation of the third and lateral ventricles. Hydrocephalus following compression of the foramen of Monro is almost invariably associated with an identifiable space-occupying lesion and a prominent midline shift. Thrombosis of the superior sagittal sinus may be difficult to detect as a cause of communicating hydrocephalus. CT in this setting, even with enhancement, is unreliable; also, the "empty delta" sign characteristic of superior sagittal sinus obstruction on CT is not always seen (50). In this setting, the diagnostic method of choice at present is MRI (53,54). The diagnostic value of MRI is based on the finding that protons carried within flowing blood pass rapidly out of the plane of radiographic section whereas protons within clotted blood do not. Thus, blood moving within vessels produces a signal void, whereas clotted blood produces an increased signal on both T1- and T2-weighted images. Magnetic resonance (MR) angiography, still in its early stages, will unquestionably increase the diagnostic yield of MRI in detection of venous sinus thrombosis.

Intracranial Hypertension and Brain Herniation

The normal mechanisms of CSF secretion and drainage maintain CSF pressure at a level of <150 mm of CSF in most patients (see below). Infection, however, greatly alters these homeostatic mechanisms; moreover, death during the acute stages of central CNS infections frequently results from extreme elevation in ICP, followed by brain herniation and respiratory arrest.

For a period of time, the intracranial contents are able

to compensate in response to space-occupying lesions before a rise in ICP occurs. This compensatory ability is termed "compliance" (dV/dP) and represents the ratio of changes in volume (dV) to changes in pressure (dP) (55–57). Compliance in response to space-occupying intracranial lesions is comprised of several factors. These include: increased rate of reabsorption of CSF (this may be prevented in meningitis by obstruction of the arachnoid villi by cells and exudate); displacement of CSF; reduction in the total volume of intracranial blood, predominantly by compression of veins and venous sinuses; and, finally, plasticity of the brain itself (58–62). Compliance is extremely limited when infection is accompanied by a rapid rise in ICP, such as during acute bacterial meningitis. In contrast, the ability of CNS compliance to compensate for increased ICP may be extensive where space-occupying lesions develop over time (6). Once compliance is exceeded, however, the rise in pressure in chronic lesions may occur with a rapidity similar to that seen in more acute processes. Compliance can be measured experimentally and clinically by determining the amount of artificial CSF which must be instilled into the subarachnoid or ventricular spaces before a rise in pressure occurs (56,59–63). In normal individuals, instillation of large volumes of artificial CSF has little effect on ICP. Once intracranial compliance is exhausted, administration of very small amounts of artificial CSF (1 ml or less) may cause a precipitous rise in ICP. Although measurement of compliance may provide a more accurate assessment of patient status than does measurement of ICP, the technique is not in routine use (63).

The elevation in CSF pressure seen in infections and other pathological conditions is not constant but, instead, fluctuates considerably. This fluctuation is usually not observed during the brief period of measurement provided by lumbar puncture but becomes an important parameter to observe during monitoring of ICP. Minor variation in pressure occurs during Cheyne–Stokes respiration and also during variations in blood pressure produced by Hering–Breuer reflexes. More major variations in ICP occur during plateau waves. These are abrupt elevations in ICP (usually lasting 5–20 min) in which ICP may reach 600–1300 ml of CSF (50–100 mmHg) (64). Although plateau waves may be without any detectable clinical effect, they may also be associated with signs of brainstem compression and impending herniation.

Increased pressure which exceeds intracranial compliance causes downward and backward shifting of the cerebrum and brainstem (65). Minimal degrees of shift are well-tolerated, but more extensive shift may cause herniation of the cingulate gyrus beneath the falx cerebri, herniation of the uncus of the temporal lobe over tentorium cerebelli, and, ultimately, herniation of the lower brainstem and cerebellar tonsils into the foramen magnum. Herniation of the cingulate gyrus is usually asymptomatic. Uncal herniation, however, initially produces compression of the third cranial nerve as it passes beneath the tentorium; it subsequently causes compression of the midbrain, with the onset of coma. The aqueduct of Sylvius is frequently occluded during uncal herniation, and the resultant hydrocephalus increases the mass effect already present. Herniation of the cerebellar tonsils through the foramen magnum, with compression of medullary respiratory centers and respiratory arrest, is frequently the terminal event in CNS infections. Occasionally, space-occupying lesions within the cerebellum cause upward herniation of posterior fossa contents through the foramen magnum (66). Extreme elevation of CSF pressure may elevate ICP above systemic arterial perfusion pressure, producing global cerebral and brainstem infarction.

Elevation in CSF pressure, as monitored by ICP monitoring devices, may provide an indication of prognosis in bacterial meningitis and possibly also in other CNS infections. Rebaud et al. (67) found that CSF pressures were significantly higher in patients who succumbed to meningitis or encephalitis than in patients who survived, and they also found that cerebral perfusion pressure was significantly lower in the former than in the latter. Goitein and Tamir (68) found that all patients with meningitis or encephalitis who had a cerebral perfusion pressure of >30 mmHg survived whereas those with lower pressures died.

CEREBROSPINAL FLUID ANALYSIS IN CNS INFECTIONS

Indications for Lumbar Puncture

Lumbar puncture is essential in the diagnosis of bacterial, viral, or fungal meningitis and may provide valuable information in encephalitis. Lumbar puncture is also used to detect subarachnoid blood in bacterial endocarditis with mycotic aneurysm or other potentially hemorrhagic infectious conditions. The procedure is of little specific diagnostic value in the diagnosis of brain abscess or parameningeal infections. There are no absolute contraindications to lumbar puncture. Nonetheless, inappropriate lumbar puncture can cause patient death or serious neurological injury, and the procedure should never be initiated without consideration of its potential danger to the patient.

Complications of Lumbar Puncture

Brain Herniation

Lumbar puncture normally results in a mild, transient lowering of lumbar CSF pressure which is rapidly communicated throughout the entire subarachnoid space.

Space-occupying lesions within the skull, however, produce a relative pressure gradient, with downward displacement of the cerebrum and brainstem (65,69). Lumbar puncture may increase this pressure gradient and precipitate brain herniation. Herniation rarely occurs at the time of the lumbar puncture itself; instead, it usually develops within a few hours of the procedure, as CSF continues to leak through the arachnoid at the site of puncture.

The likelihood of brain herniation following lumbar puncture in the setting of elevated ICP is greatly influenced by the nature of the underlying pathological process and its degree of severity. With rare exceptions, there is little risk of herniation following lumbar puncture in the setting of viral meningitis. Similarly, lumbar puncture can safely be performed in patients with subarachnoid hemorrhage, unless extensive parenchymal hemorrhage is present as well. Brain abscess, in contrast, represents a rapidly expanding space-occupying lesion in which focal brain displacement is present from the outset, and the risk of herniation following lumbar puncture is 10–20% (70,71). Subdural empyema, which represents an even more rapidly expanding lesion, presents a similar or greater risk. Herniation may also follow lumbar puncture in obstructive hydrocephalus (in which trapped intraventricular CSF behaves as a mass lesion), in patients with large intracranial hemorrhages, and in conditions associated with extensive cerebral edema, such as severe herpes simplex encephalitis or Reye's syndrome.

Lumbar puncture is a routine and necessary procedure in the diagnosis of acute meningitis and can usually be accomplished without difficulty or danger. Nonetheless, tonsillar herniation remains a major cause of death during the acute stages of illness, and bacterial meningitis is frequently accompanied by a number of conditions which render brain herniation likely to occur. These include: cortical encephalitis, with or without microabscesses; cerebral edema; hydrocephalus; and cortical venous or venous sinus thrombosis with hemorrhage (72–75). Horwitz et al. (75), in a review of 302 infants and children with bacterial meningitis, found that brain herniation occurred in 18 patients—that is, 6% of those studied. In all patients, herniation occurred within 8 hr following lumbar puncture. Lumbar puncture should thus be approached with caution in patients with bacterial meningitis and suspected severe intracranial hypertension. In such patients, a 22- or 25-gauge needle should be used, the patient should be watched closely for signs of impending herniation during the hours following the procedure, and the use of dexamethasone, hyperventilation, and mannitol to lower ICP should be strongly considered, along with placement of a device to monitor ICP. In extreme cases, it may be most prudent to treat the presumed meningitis with broad-spectrum antibiotics, achieve medical control of intracranial hy-

pertension, and defer lumbar puncture until the patient is more stable.

Patients with suspected meningitis who also have focal findings suggesting brain abscess present a significant clinical dilemma. Lumbar puncture in such patients is of obvious diagnostic use, but the need to rule out localized infection by CT or MRI may delay lumbar puncture and institution of antibiotic therapy for as long as several hours. *Where concern exists that both meningitis and brain abscess may be present, presumptive antibiotic therapy should be started immediately. CT or MRI should then be obtained emergently to exclude abscess, and the patient should undergo lumbar puncture after loculated infection or impending herniation from the meningitis itself has been excluded.*

Cortical Blindness

Downward displacement of the brainstem in states of increased intracranial pressure may compress the posterior cerebral arteries against the edge of the tentorium cerebelli, causing ischemic infarction of the occipital lobes and cortical blindness (65). Although this complication of intracranial hypertension is often accompanied by signs of uncal or tonsillar herniation, compression of the posterior cerebral arteries may also occur before other signs of herniation appear (75–77). Prognosis for return of vision is poor.

Cervical Spinal Cord Infarction

Rarely, lumbar puncture in the setting of bacterial meningitis may be followed within a few hours by respiratory arrest accompanied by flaccid tetraplegia (76–80). Similar instances of cervical spinal cord infarction have been observed following lumbar puncture in Reye's syndrome and, prior to lumbar puncture, in subdural empyema (81). A variety of mechanisms, including hypotension and vasculitis, have been postulated as the cause of cervical cord ischemia in these patients. In most patients, however, it is likely that displacement of the cerebellar tonsils through the foramen magnum as the result of greatly elevated intracranial pressure compresses the anterior spinal artery or its penetrating branches, with resultant ischemic infarction of the upper cord (80).

Spinal Hematoma with Cord Compression

Lumbar puncture in patients with severe disorders of blood coagulation or in patients anticoagulated with heparin or Coumadin may be complicated by continued bleeding at the site of puncture (82). Epidural or subdural collections of blood may compress the cauda equina, thereby producing permanent neurological injury (82,83). Where it is absolutely essential that lumbar puncture be performed in patients with abnormal coagulation, the procedure should be carried out by an experienced person using a 22- or, ideally, 25-gauge needle. Efforts should then be made to correct the defects in coagulation, and the patient should be monitored carefully for the appearance of neurological deficit. In general, lumbar puncture should be avoided in such patients until their clotting mechanisms can be transiently or permanently returned to an acceptable range.

Introduction of Infection into the Subarachnoid Space

Inadvertent lumbar puncture through an area of infection overlying the spinal canal may result in seeding of the subarachnoid space and meningitis. This is a particular risk in spinal epidural abscess or subdural empyema but may occasionally occur in the setting of superficial or deep paraspinal infections. The problem can be avoided by entering the subarachnoid space at a level well-removed from the site of presumed infection. Thus, in patients with known or suspected focal lumbar infection, spinal fluid should be obtained under fluoroscopic guidance by high cervical (C2) or cisternal puncture, whereas the lumbar route should be used in patients with suspected cervical or upper thoracic infections.

A long-standing concern in the evaluation of febrile patients with suspected CNS infection has been that lumbar puncture in the setting of bacteremia might result in meningitis (84–89). This concern is based, in part, on experimental work by Petersdorf et al. (90), who demonstrated that 81% of dogs undergoing cisternal puncture in the presence of severe bacteremia ($>10^3$ organisms per milliliter of blood) developed meningitis, whereas meningitis did not develop in similarly bacteremic control animals not undergoing cisternal puncture. Bacteremia at levels above 10^3 organisms per milliliter of blood, although unusual in adult infections, may occur in up to 30% of cases of neonatal sepsis, and it is of note that investigators have reported an association between meningitis and lumbar puncture in the setting of bacteremia in children less than 1 year of age but not in older children (91,92). Although these cases are of interest, normal CSF at the time of initial lumbar puncture does not exclude the possibility that meningitis was already present in its early stages. The diagnostic usefulness of lumbar puncture in the evaluation of febrile patients with suspected CNS infection far outweighs any small risk that the procedure itself might lead to meningitis.

Onset of Signs of Spinal Cord Compression Following Lumbar Puncture in the Setting of Spinal Block (Spinal Epidural Abscess or Subdural Empyema)

In occasional patients, it may be difficult to differentiate on the basis of neurological examination alone be-

tween meningitis and spinal epidural abscess or subdural empyema (93). In this setting, presumptive antibiotic therapy should be initiated, and MRI or CT myelography should be obtained on an emergent basis. Spinal fluid should be obtained at the time of myelography or after a compressive lesion has been ruled out by MRI. If MRI is not available, and if strong suspicion of epidural abscess or subdural empyema arises at the time of lumbar puncture, then the spinal needle should be left in place and the patient should be taken to myelography immediately.

Development of Intraspinal Epidermoid Tumor

This has been reported as an extremely rare complication of lumbar punctures in which the spinal needle was used without its stylet, allowing a small plug of skin to be inserted into the spinal canal (94).

Post-Lumbar-Puncture Headache

In approximately 10% of patients, lumbar puncture is followed by the development of severe, often pounding headache. The headache is characteristically absent when the patient is recumbent and rapidly appears when the patient stands upright or strains. Post-lumbar-puncture headache is believed to be due to low CSF pressure, caused by continued lumbar leakage of CSF. The headache usually resolves spontaneously within hours to days. In persistent cases, a blood patch may be used to seal the site of puncture (95).

Technique of Lumbar Puncture

Numerous reviews have been devoted to techniques of the lumbar puncture, and a detailed description of the procedure will not be given here (1,2,96). It should be kept in mind, however, that the purpose of the lumbar puncture is to obtain an accurate measurement of CSF pressure and collect quantities of CSF adequate for all studies required. These two objectives, although obvious, may be forgotten or approached in haphazard fashion in the urgency of initiating therapy in a critically ill patient. Thus, prior to carrying out the procedure, it is essential to decide on the studies which will be required, to make certain that adequate numbers of tubes are on hand to collect the samples needed, and to discuss with the appropriate laboratories any studies which may require advance preparation. The need for simultaneous evaluation of blood glucose should be kept in mind. Because CSF glucose equilibrates with blood glucose over time (see below), blood glucose should be drawn prior to, rather than after, the lumbar puncture. Fluid should be delivered promptly to the technicians performing the individual cultures and other tests. The lumbar puncture should be carefully noted in the patient's record, and the tests ordered should be listed. The results of these tests should be added to the procedure note as they become available. A flow sheet of spinal fluid results should be developed where multiple spinal fluid examinations are anticipated. Where one is dealing with chronic or unusual CNS infections, blood and CSF should be frozen and saved for future serological and other tests. Because many clinical laboratories routinely discard samples after 1–3 months, these samples should be placed in a location known to be secure, and their specific locations should be noted in order to prevent future loss.

Alternative Routes of Obtaining CSF

Cisternal, high cervical (C2), and ventricular approaches may be used to obtain CSF or to perform myelography if a lumbar approach is contraindicated by infection or is technically impossible (1,2). Cisternal puncture has been used in cases of chronic meningitis, and in a few cases it has yielded organisms when organisms could not be detected by the lumbar route (97–99). However, it is not clear whether cisternal puncture is more useful in the setting of chronic meningitis than is lumbar puncture with removal of large volumes (40–50 ml) of CSF, and cultures of large volumes of fluid obtained by the lumbar route have yielded organisms after cultures of cisternal fluid have been negative (100). Spinal puncture at the level of the second cervical vertebra has been suggested as a less hazardous approach than cisternal puncture, but its actual value remains unproven. Ventricular CSF may be of great diagnostic value where there is a predominantly intraventricular infection with obstructive hydrocephalus.

Routine Studies of CSF

Studies routinely obtained at the time of lumbar puncture include: measurement of CSF pressure; gross examination of the fluid for turbidity or changes in color; measurement of CSF protein and glucose concentrations; cell count; Gram's and/or acid-fast stains of CSF sediment; and submission of the fluid for Gram's stain and bacterial culture. Differentiation of bacterial meningitis from viral, mycobacterial, or fungal meningitis on the basis of CSF abnormalities is presumptive unless an organism is seen, and it rests not upon any single one of these tests but rather upon their sum. Amounts of CSF required by most laboratories for commonly obtained determinations are listed in Table 1. Because clinical laboratories differ somewhat in the amounts of CSF required for individual tests, it is important that the clinician determine the amounts of CSF required by his or her hospital laboratory for each intended test before performing the lumbar puncture.

TABLE 1. *Minimal volumes of CSF required for common diagnostic tests*[a]

Test	Volume of CSF required
Bacterial culture antigen detection, and limulus lysate assay	3–5 ml[b]
Acid-fast culture; fungal culture (includes acid-fast smear and India ink preparation)	See below[c]
Cell count and differential	0.5–5.0 ml[d]
Glucose and protein	0.5 ml[e]
VDRL	0.5 ml
Cryptococcal antigen	0.5 ml
Oligoclonal bands	2 ml + serum[f]

[a] Volumes required represent minimal quantities of CSF required by most hospital laboratories. The clinician should determine the amounts of CSF required by his or her hospital laboratory for each intended test before performing the lumbar puncture.

[b] As little as 0.5 ml may be submitted for culture if there is great difficulty obtaining fluid. However, additional CSF will be required for antigen detection, and the use of centrifuged sediment from larger volumes of CSF will improve yield on culture in acute bacterial meningitis. The use of large volumes of CSF are essential in more chronic infections.

[c] Yield on culture for acid-fast bacilli and fungi is, in general, extremely poor unless large volumes of CSF (20 ml or more in adults) are cultured.

[d] Approximately 0.5 ml will be needed for cell count. Amount of CSF required for differential will vary, depending on whether cytocentrifugation is used or material from centrifuged CSF sediment is studied.

[e] Blood drawn before initiating the lumbar puncture should also be submitted with spinal fluid for determination of simultaneous blood glucose.

[f] Serum (2–5 ml) drawn before or after the lumbar puncture should be submitted for electrophoresis along with CSF.

CSF Pressure

CSF pressure must be measured in the lateral decubitus position—with the patient lying horizontally, on his or her side. The head of the bed should be flat rather than elevated. Variations in posture and patient size make measurement of ICP unreliable with the patient sitting. Opening CSF pressure in normal adults, with the patient in the lateral decubitus position, ranges in between 50 and 195 mm CSF (3.8–15 mmHg) (2,101,102). Values below 150 mm CSF are clearly normal, those between 150 and 200 mm are suspicious, and those above 200 mm are abnormal. Normal lumbar CSF pressures in neonates and prematures are significantly lower, with mean values of 100 mm H_2O and 95 mm H_2O, respectively (102). CSF pressure can be spuriously elevated by Valsalva maneuver in an anxious or combative patient and may be falsely lowered by hyperventilation. Delay in obtaining the pressure reading over several minutes may reduce pressure by allowing fluid to escape around the needle at its point of entry into the subarachnoid space

(96). Extreme elevation of CSF pressure may herald impending brain herniation. If significantly elevated pressure is found on lumbar puncture, serious consideration should be given to both (a) use of measures to lower ICP and (b) continuous monitoring of intracranial and arterial pressures. Occasionally, CSF pressure may be normal or even low in the setting of ongoing tonsillar herniation. The falsely low readings obtained in this setting are believed to reflect occlusion of the CSF space at the foramen magnum by the herniated tonsils wedged against the lower brainstem. The possibility of complete spinal block should be kept in mind if CSF pressure falls to zero during the procedure (see above).

Gross Appearance of the Spinal Fluid

Normal CSF is colorless and clear. Under pathological conditions, CSF may become turbid, discolored, or both. CSF may become turbid as a result of entry of cells, bacteria, or fat. CSF can be made turbid by as few as 200 white blood cells or 400 red blood cells per cubic millimeter (2,103–105). CSF containing red blood cells will be grossly bloody if 6000 or more red blood cells are present per cubic millimeter, and it will be cloudy and xanthochromic or pinkish if 400–6000 cells are present (2). In occasional patients, turbidity may be due to bacteria or fungi in the absence of cells. Rarely, epidural fat aspirated at the time of lumbar puncture can give a turbid appearance to the CSF (106).

CSF may be discolored by the presence of breakdown products of red blood cells, or by protein, bilirubin, or other pigments. Discoloration of CSF by intact red blood cells usually results in a reddish discoloration as well as in turbidity. Although the average lifespan of a red blood cell is 120 days in the circulation, rapid lysis of red blood cells occurs in CSF. This results in a yellowish discoloration termed "xanthochromia" or "xanthochromasia." In most patients, xanthochromia begins to appear approximately 2–4 hr after red blood cells have entered the subarachnoid space. In 10% of patients, however, the appearance of xanthochromia may be delayed for 2–4 hr and is occasionally not seen for as long as 12 hr (107). Because CSF may remain colorless during the first 2–4 hr following the onset of subarachnoid hemorrhage, the absence of xanthochromia during this period of time cannot be used as evidence of a traumatic puncture (107). Xanthochromia may also develop within 1 hr *in vitro* after CSF has been removed, an important consideration when the CSF obtained at lumbar puncture has been contaminated by a traumatic tap.

Xanthochromia resulting from lysis of red blood cells is initially due to oxyhemoglobin. After 12 hr, the pigment represents predominantly bilirubin (1). Leakage of methemoglobin from a chronic parenchymal or subdural hemorrhage may also produce xanthochromia.

Xanthochromia may also represent the presence of increased amounts of protein, as described below, or may be a consequence of systemic hyperbilirubinemia above 10–15 mg/dl. In rare instances, xanthochromia may be caused by malignant melanoma metastatic to the meninges (2).

Viscosity of CSF is usually relatively little affected by the presence of meningeal infection or irritation. Qualitatively appreciable change in CSF viscosity, however, may be seen in severe cryptococcal infections and is believed to be due to capsular polysaccharides (2). Similar viscosity may be produced by widespread metastasis of adenocarcinoma; in such cases, mucicarmine stain of dried CSF residue may be positive (2).

Cell Count and Differential (Table 2)

Enumeration and characterization of cells within spinal fluid is of crucial value in the diagnosis of CNS infections and is of great value in following the course of illness and response to treatment. Improperly handled or counted CSF, however, can be a dangerous source of error. The cell count in CSF tends to fall over time and may be falsely low if measured after 30–60 min. This fall in cell count is due, in part, to the fact that leukocytes and red blood cells settle out over time if the tube of CSF is allowed to stand. In addition, however, lysis of red blood cells, polymorphonuclear leukocytes, and, to a lesser extent, lymphocytes begins *in vitro* within 1–2 hr of the lumbar puncture and may occasionally occur even more rapidly. White blood cells also adsorb to the glass or plastic walls of the tube and are not easily dislodged by agitation. Because of these factors, the reduction in cell count which occurs over time is only partially reversible if the tube is vigorously agitated prior to counting. CSF destined for cell counting should thus be handled carefully and expeditiously. The physician should determine the CSF cell count personally if there is any question of delay or uncertainty as to the skill of the laboratory personnel responsible for the cell count and differential. Similarly, where serial tubes must be counted to exclude a traumatic tap, the samples must be handled in the same manner and counted at the same time by the same person.

White Blood Cell Count

Quantification of numbers of cells in CSF should be carried out by manual methods, using a Neubauer counting chamber. Electronic cell counters are inaccurate below 1000 cells per cubic millimeter and should not be used to count CSF (1). The accuracy of the cell count is open to question unless the specimen is examined immediately after the lumbar puncture has been completed. CSF normally contains less than five cells per

TABLE 2. *Normal CSF values of importance in infectious diseases of the nervous system: values in adults, term infants, and premature infants[a]*

Parameter	Adults	Term infants	Premature infants
Cell count (per cubic millimeter)	<5	9[b]	9[b]
Percent polymorphonuclear leukocytes	0[c]	61[c]	57[c]
Protein (mg/dl) (lumbar)			
Mean	30	90	115
Range	9–58	20–170	65–150
Glucose (mg/dl)			
Mean[d]	62	52	50
Range[d]	45–80	34–119	24–63
CSF:blood glucose ratio			
Mean	0.60	0.81	0.74
Range	0.5–0.8[d]	0.44–2.48	0.55–1.55

[a] Adapted from ref. 2.

[b] Cell counts in term and premature infants represent mean values. The range of cell counts found in normal neonates is 0–32 cells per cubic millimeter and in premature infants is 0–29, with 2 standard deviations encompassing a range of 0–22.4 cells per cubic millimeter in term and 0–24.4 cells per cubic millimeter in premature infants. By 1 month of age, normal CSF contains <10 cells per cubic millimeter (2).

[c] Rare polymorphonuclear leukocytes may be seen in cytocentrifuged samples of CSF from normal adults. This is not necessarily abnormal if the CSF leukocyte count is 4 cells per cubic millimeter or less and if protein and glucose are normal.

[d] Assumes a blood glucose of 70–120 mg/dl. At high blood glucose levels (700 mg/dl), normal lower limit of CSF:blood glucose ratios may approach 0.4 (see text).

cubic millimeter. The majority of these cells are small lymphocytes (nuclear diameter ~6–7 μm) with scant cytoplasm. The presence of polymorphonuclear leukocytes should be regarded with concern. Occasionally, however, one to two polymorphonuclear cells per cubic millimeter will be detected in an otherwise normal spinal fluid (1,2,108). Larger numbers of polymorphonuclear leukocytes are abnormal in uncentrifuged CSF. *Cryptococcus neoformans* is similar in size to small CSF lymphocytes and may be mistaken for these cells in the counting chamber, although not in stained cytocentrifuged or otherwise concentrated samples. Neonatal CSF normally contains eight to nine white blood cells per cubic millimeter, and up to 32 white blood cells per cubic millimeter has been reported in the absence of disease (109).

Differential White Blood Cell Count. A differential count of CSF leukocytes may be obtained following concentration of CSF through a millipore filter, centrifugation of a volume (usually 5 ml) of CSF, concentration by sedimentation, or cytocentrifugation. The differential normally contains a predominance of lymphocytes and approximately 14.5% neutrophils (110). Differential cell counts of CSF from normal neonates may yield up to 60% neutrophils (109). The number of neutrophils is increased in a variety of conditions. In adults with bacterial meningitis, neutrophils comprise an average of 86.4% of cells counted, with neutrophils comprising an average of 34.2% of cells counted in aseptic meningitis (1,2,110). Large lymphocytes and other mononuclear cells are rarely seen in normal, unspun CSF but may be present in

samples of CSF examined by cytocentrifugation. Plasma cells and eosinophils should not be present in normal CSF. Increased numbers of plasma cells are seen in both infectious and noninfectious disorders and have little diagnostic significance other than as an indicator of inflammation. CSF eosinophilia is particularly associated with infections by *Taenia solium* (cysticercosis) and, in patients with a history of residence in Southeast Asia or Pacific Islands, by *Angiostrongylus cantonensis* and *Gnathostoma spinigerum* (Table 3) (2,111–118). Other helminthic infections may also result in significant CSF eosinophilia. In addition, however, CSF eosinophilia has been reported in a wide variety of other infectious and noninfectious conditions (Table 3), so that detection of eosinophils within the CSF should not be taken to be pathognomonic of parasitic infestation (2,117,118).

Red Blood Cells

The presence of red blood cells in CSF may result from a traumatic lumbar puncture or may indicate subarachnoid or parenchymal hemorrhage. Grossly bloody fluid which clears visibly as CSF is collected suggests a traumatic tap. Differentiation between a traumatic lumbar puncture and subarachnoid blood as the result of intracranial or intraspinal pathology becomes more difficult if only small numbers of red blood cells are present. In such cases, one should compare numbers of red blood cells present in CSF obtained at the beginning of the lumbar puncture with numbers present in CSF obtained

TABLE 3. *Conditions associated with CSF eosinophilia[a]*

Parasitic infestations
Taenia solium (cysticercosis)
Angiostrongylus cantonensis
Gnathostoma spinigerum
Trichinella spiralis
Ascaris lumbricoides
Toxoplasma gondii
Toxcara cati
Toxocara canis
Other infectious agents or conditions
Mycobacterium tuberculosis
Treponema pallidum
Mycoplasma pneumoniae
Rocky Mountain spotted fever
Subacute sclerosing panencephalitis
Lymphocytic choriomeningitis virus
Fungal meningitides
Central nervous system disorders of noninfectious or unknown origin
Idiopathic eosinophilic meningitis
Granulomatous meningitis
Malignant lymphoma
Hodgkin's disease
Leukemia
Multiple sclerosis
Subarachnoid hemorrhage
Obstructive hydrocephalus with shunt

[a] Adapted from refs. 2, 111, and 112.

at the end of the study (e.g., one should count cells from tubes 1 or 2 and then from tubes 4 or 5). The presence of xanthochromia in samples centrifuged immediately after obtaining CSF argues against a traumatic tap, although it must be kept in mind that lysis of red blood cells *in vitro* in CSF obtained during a traumatic tap will produce xanthochromia if the specimen is allowed to sit. Crenation of red blood cells may occur *in vitro* and has no diagnostic significance (116,119). Blood entering CSF during spontaneous subarachnoid hemorrhage or as the result of a traumatic tap contains white blood cells as well as red blood cells, and the CSF leukocyte count will thus rise. Numbers of white blood cells relative to those of red blood cells in CSF after a traumatic tap should be consistent with the leukocyte count of the peripheral blood, and the differential count of CSF will be the same. In contrast, actual subarachnoid hemorrhage frequently produces a lymphocytic pleocytosis, with elevation in the numbers of cells and alteration in the differential count. A traumatic tap in the setting of CNS infection will increase the numbers of white blood cells already present by an amount which can be calculated by comparing the ratio of red and white blood cells in CSF with that seen in peripheral blood.

CSF Glucose (Table 2)

Most glucose present in CSF moves across the choroid plexus and across ventricular and subarachnoid capillar-

ies by facilitated transport. A smaller amount of glucose enters the CSF by simple diffusion. Glucose is removed from CSF through utilization by cells lining the ventricles and subarachnoid space and by transport across capillaries and arachnoid villi. Entry of glucose occurs over time, and a period of 2–4 hr is required before serum and CSF glucose levels reach equilibrium (2). In the absence of infection or other pathological conditions, CSF glucose levels are a predictable reflection of blood glucose, and the ratio of CSF to blood glucose concentrations is approximately 0.6. CSF glucose, equilibrated with a normal blood glucose of 70–120 mg/dl, thus ranges between 45 and 80 mg/dl. Levels of glucose in ventricular fluid are 6–18 mg/dl higher than those in lumbar fluid (111,120,121).

CNS infections may alter glucose transport across the blood–CSF barrier, resulting in low CSF glucose, termed "hypoglychorrhachia" (2). Further reduction in CSF glucose levels may result from glucose consumption by white blood cells and organisms (122). Reduction of CSF glucose relative to blood glucose is characteristic of meningitis due to bacteria, mycobacteria, or fungi (123,124). CSF glucose is usually normal during viral infections. However, low CSF glucose levels are occasionally observed in meningoencephalitis due to mumps, enteroviruses, lymphocytic choriomeningitis, herpes simplex, and herpes zoster viruses (125–132). Low CSF glucose values have also been described in CNS complications of *Mycoplasma pneumoniae* infection, carcinomatous meningitis, CNS sarcoidosis, and subarachnoid hemorrhage (124,133–136). During recovery from meningitis, CSF glucose levels tend to return toward normal more rapidly than do cell counts and protein levels, making CSF glucose levels an important parameter to follow in assessing response to therapy (137,138).

Both reduction in CSF glucose values and altered ratios of CSF:blood glucose levels are used as indicators of infection. However, in part because of the prolonged interval over which CSF glucose equilibrates with serum glucose, the literature contains a variety of recommendations as to the point at which CSF glucose should be considered abnormally low (109,120–123,126,139–141). In general, a CSF:blood glucose ratio of less than 0.5 should be considered abnormal. In premature and term infants, however, the normal CSF:blood glucose ratio is 0.74–0.96, and a ratio of 0.6 is usually considered abnormal (109,139). In severe hyperglycemia, transport of glucose into CSF may lag, and at a blood sugar level of 700 mg/dl the CSF:blood glucose ratio may approach 0.4. For this reason, a ratio of 0.3 has been suggested as abnormal in diabetics (140). Silver and Todd (128) addressed the problem of diagnostically significant hypoglychorrhachia in a study of 181 pediatric patients with CSF glucose levels of less than 50 mg/dl or a CSF:blood glucose ratio of less than 50%. Patients ranged in age from less than 1 week to 14 years, with an average age of

1.5 years. Their series included patients with bacterial meningitis, aseptic meningitis, subarachnoid hemorrhage, and CNS carcinomatosis but did not include patients with tuberculous or fungal meningitis. Blood for glucose analysis was obtained 1–114 min prior to the lumbar puncture (average interval: 30 min). Of 35 patients with bacterial meningitis in this series, 27 (77%) had CSF glucose levels of 20 mg/dl or below, whereas CSF glucose levels of 20 mg/dl or below were found in only 10 of 146 patients (7%) with other conditions; and of 37 patients with glucose levels of less than 20 mg/dl, 27 (73%) had bacterial meningitis. CSF glucose levels of less than 20 mg/dl or a CSF:blood glucose ratio of less than 0.30 was highly correlated with bacterial meningitis, whereas an absolute CSF glucose value of between 20 and 50 mg/dl was nonspecific; also, a CSF:serum glucose ratio of greater than 0.3 was felt to exclude most (but not all) cases of bacterial meningitis. More recently, Spanos et al. (142) have analyzed the records of 422 patients with acute bacterial or viral meningitis. These workers found that a CSF glucose level of less than 18 mg/dl (1.9 mmol/liter) or a CSF:blood glucose level of less than 0.23 were individual predictors of bacterial as opposed to viral meningitis, with 99% or better certainty (142).

CSF Protein (Table 2)

Protein is largely excluded from CSF by the blood–CSF barrier and reaches CSF by pinocytotic transport across capillary endothelia (2). Total CSF protein concentration in normal adult lumbar CSF is less than 40 mg, and the CSF:serum ratio of albumin is 1:200 (2,30). Mean values of lumbar CSF protein in normal children and adults have ranged from 23 to 38 mg/dl, and the extreme upper and lower concentrations have been 58 and 9 mg, respectively (2). CSF protein in premature and term neonates may range between 20 and 170 mg/dl, with a mean of 90 mg (109). Protein concentrations in cisternal and lumbar CSF are lower, ranging from 13 to 30 mg/dl (1). Elevation of CSF protein to above 150 mg/dl may cause the CSF to be xanthochromic. Extreme elevation of protein (to above 1.5 g/dl) may cause formation of a web-like surface pellicle or an actual clot, as may high levels of fibrinogen (2). Levels of CSF protein may be falsely elevated by deteriorating red blood cells following subarachnoid hemorrhage or traumatic lumbar puncture. The amount of increase is roughly 1 mg/dl per 1000 red blood cells. Accurate assessment of the contribution to total CSF protein made by red blood cells requires that the cell count and protein determination be carried out on the same tube of CSF (141).

Changes in the concentration of protein in CSF are the most common and least specific of CSF alterations in disease and are seen in a wide variety of infectious and noninfectious neurological conditions. An elevated CSF protein level, taken alone, thus has little specific value in the diagnosis of CNS infections. Elevation of CSF protein to levels of above 100 mg/dl, particularly if obtained on serial lumbar punctures, argues against viral infection, however, and Spanos et al. (142) have recently demonstrated that elevation of protein to a level of 220 mg/dl (2.2 g/liter) suggests bacterial as opposed to viral meningitis, with 99% or greater certainty (also see ref. 143). CSF protein levels return to normal more slowly than do glucose levels and cell count during recovery from meningitis and may remain abnormal for months after parenchymal infections. Although elevation of CSF protein is common in CNS infections, normal protein values are occasionally seen in all types of CNS infections, including bacterial meningitis.

CSF Immunoglobulins

Immunoglobulins are almost totally excluded from normal CSF, and the blood:CSF ratio of immunoglobulin G (IgG) in normal CSF is normally in the range of 500:1. Immunoglobulin M (IgM) is essentially excluded from CSF (30). Studies with radioiodinated IgG have demonstrated that CSF IgG in normal individuals is derived entirely from serum, requiring 3–6 days to reach equilibrium (144,145). Immunoglobulins enter CSF less readily than does albumin; and, in health, immunoglobulin:albumin ratios in CSF are reduced relative to those in serum. Elevation in CSF immunoglobulins may follow disruption of the blood–brain barrier, allowing passage of immunoglobulins across capillary endothelium, or may result from local antibody synthesis within brain. Increased levels of CSF IgG per se have little diagnostic value in CNS infections. Detection of oligoclonal IgG bands unique to CSF and not seen in serum on gel electrophoresis provides strong evidence for an ongoing immune response within brain. Oligoclonal bands have been described in a variety of acute and chronic CNS infections of bacterial, mycobacterial, fungal, and viral origins, as well as in a number of noninfectious neurological disorders, so that detection of oligoclonal bands in CSF cannot be taken as reliable evidence of infection (30).

Microscopic Methods for Detecting Infectious Organisms

Gram's Stain

Gram's stain is of crucial value in providing rapid identification of the offending organism in bacterial meningitis and should be an invariable part of the CSF evaluation. Diagnostic accuracy of properly prepared Gram's stain is a function of the number of organisms present. Work by LaScolea and Dryja (146) has shown that 25%

of smears will be positive with 10^3 or fewer colony-forming units (CFU) of bacteria per milliliter, 60% with 10^3–10^5 CFU/ml, and 97% with $>10^5$ CFU/ml. In general, Gram's stain is positive in 60–80% of untreated patients (146–150). The yield is approximately 20% lower in patients who have received prior antibiotic therapy (146–150). Several pitfalls exist in obtaining an accurate study, all of which are largely correctable with patience and experience. Haste in carrying out an examination of the material may allow the examiner to miss organisms present in small numbers. This is less true for gram-positive organisms than for gram-negative bacteria and is particularly true in the case of *Neisseria meningitidis,* which tends to be intracellular. *Staphylococcus aureus* may be mistaken for streptococci if present as individual organisms. *Listeria monocytogenes* may be mistaken for diphtheroid contaminants or for *Streptococcus pneumoniae.* False-positive Gram stains may result from bacteria present in the collecting tubes, slides, or reagents or, rarely, from bacterial contamination from a skin fragment excised by a spinal needle used without its stylet (149,150). An important consideration in preparing CSF for the Gram-stain procedure is that adequate sedimentation of bacteria may require a force of 10,000*g* for 10 min. This force equates to a centrifugation time of approximately 60 min (an unacceptably long time for most clinicians) in the usual laboratory bench-top centrifuge, which delivers a force of approximately 1,000*g* (151).

The sensitivity of the Gram-stain procedure varies to some extent with the offending organism. Organisms will be detected by Gram's stain in almost 90% of cases of pneumococcal or staphylococcal meningitis, 86% of cases due to *Hemophilus influenzae,* and 75% of patients with *Neisseria meningitidis* meningitis (152). In contrast, organisms are present on Gram's stain in only 50% of cases of gram-negative meningitis and in less than 50% of cases of meningitis due to *Listeria monocytogenes* or anaerobic organisms. Accuracy of the Gram-stain procedure can be increased, and specific identification of the offending organism achieved, in pneumococcal meningitis by use of the Quellung test, in which CSF is mixed with a antisera against all known serotypes of the organism (Fig. 3). A polyvalent omniserum, reactive with 83 serotypes of *Streptococcus pneumoniae,* is available through the Staten Serum Institute, Copenhagen, Denmark. Polyvalent, pooled antisera recognizing smaller numbers of serotypes are available through the Serum Institute or the Communicable Diseases Center, Atlanta, Georgia. The Quellung test, although still a useful diagnostic test, has been largely supplanted by tests based on detection of bacterial antigens (see below).

Acid-Fast Stain

The sensitivity of the acid-fast stain depends greatly upon the skill and persistence of the examiner and the amount of fluid concentrated. In general, as large a volume of CSF as possible—at least 20 ml—should be taken for smear and culture unless contraindicated by the presence of elevated ICP or focal mass lesion (124). In most series, acid-fast bacilli (AFB) have been detected in the first sample in less than 37% of cases, although organisms may be detected in up to 87% of cases if material from four different lumbar punctures is evaluated by experienced personnel (153). The likelihood of detecting organisms on acid-fast stain will be far less, however, if only 1 or 2 ml of CSF are used to prepare the smear, if the examiner is unskilled, or if insufficient time is spent examining the specimen. Barrett-Connor (154), in a retrospective review of pediatric patients with tuberculous meningitis, found that the AFB stain was positive in only two of 21 patients. Idriss et al. (155) in a similar study of 43 children with tuberculous meningitis, found a positive AFB stain in only five (12%). In the series by Roberts (156), all 13 samples sent for AFB stain from patients who were eventually found to have tuberculous meningitis were negative. Sensitivity of the acid-fast stain can be considerably increased by immunofluorescence methods using auramine-rhodamine (157).

Microscopic Detection of Fungi and Protozoa in CSF

Fungi, including *Cryptococcus neoformans, Blastomyces dermatitidis, Coccidioides immitis,* and *Candida albicans,* may occasionally be detected on Gram or silver stains of concentrated CSF (158). In many cases of fungal meningitis, however, organisms are too few in number to be readily detectable, and negative Gram or silver stains of CSF sediment in no way excludes the possibility of fungal infection. India ink preparations, in which CSF

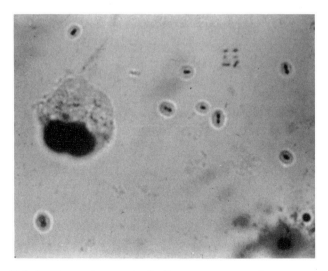

FIG. 3. Photomicrograph of a Quellung reaction. Capsules of *Streptococcus pneumoniae* are outlined by antibody.

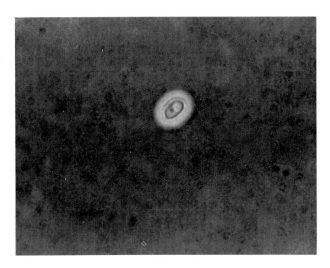

FIG. 4. India ink preparation of CSF, from a case of crypto-coccal meningitis. The capsule of a cryptococcal organism is clearly outlined by ink particles.

sediment from 3–5 ml of CSF is mixed with a drop of India ink, is a useful means of outlining the capsule of *Cryptococcus neoformans* in cases of cryptococcal meningitis (Fig. 4). Sensitivity of the India ink preparation is about 50%, although samples from several lumbar punctures may need to be examined before organisms are found (124,158–160).

Wet mount preparations have been successful in identifying motile trophozoites in the CSF of 14 of 16 patients with primary amebic meningoencephalitis (161). Search for motile organisms in wet mounts may be made more reliable by the use of phase-contrast microscopy (151).

CSF Culture for Bacteria and Fungi

Choice of culture media, methods of handling, and lengths of time over which cultures are to be maintained are thoroughly discussed in standard texts, such as the *Manual of Clinical Microbiology* by Lennette et al. (162) or the chapter by Krieg (141) in *Clinical Diagnosis and Management by Laboratory Methods*. The reader is referred to these sources for a detailed discussion of specific laboratory techniques. CSF should be submitted to the laboratory immediately after the procedure and should be placed in culture promptly to avoid loss of fastidious organisms such as *Hemophilus influenzae, Neisseria meningitidis,* or anaerobes. CSF cultured for bacteria should, at minimum, be plated on a blood-agar–chocolate-agar medium, or on a Fildes or Leventhal medium, and inoculated into broth. A minimum of 2 ml (ideally 5 ml or more) should be submitted for Gram's stain and bacterial culture.

If infection by *Mycobacterium tuberculosis* or fungi is

suspected, at least 20 ml of CSF should be submitted for culture if not contraindicated by intracranial mass lesions or hydrocephalus, and 40–50 ml should be cultured if at all possible. Frequently, a second lumbar puncture is performed to obtain these larger volumes. Cultures from most series of patients with tuberculous meningitis from Western countries are positive in 52–78% of cases (163,164). In contrast, mycobacterial cultures performed on patients in tropical countries are positive in less than 20% of cases (165). Sensitivity of cultures varies widely. *Cryptococcus neoformans* is cultured from the CSF in approximately 72% of cases on the first lumbar puncture and in over 90% on multiple attempts (124,165). Frequency of recovery of *Candida albicans* from CSF is also high (124,166,167). Isolation of other organisms such as *Histoplasma capsulatum* or *Brucella* species frequently proves difficult (124,168,169). In both mycobacterial and fungal infections, cultures of large volumes from multiple lumbar punctures may be required before an organism is identified (93,124).

In most bacterial and fungal infections, extraneural sites of possible infection should also be cultured. Depending on the organism being sought, these sites may include blood, urine, paranasal sinuses, ears, oropharynx, sputum, bone marrow, prostate, and/or abscess material.

Viral Culture

In general, overall yield of viral CSF culture is discouragingly low, and identification of viral agents in CSF by tissue culture or other methods is, at present, rarely (if ever) used to determine the need for antiviral therapy; in most cases, then, viral culture of CSF is used primarily for epidemiological purposes. This is in direct contrast to the role of brain biopsy in conditions such as herpes simplex virus encephalitis, where detection of the virus by tissue culture, immunohistological methods, or electron microscopy may be of great value in determining whether or not to continue antiviral therapy initiated acutely. Unlike bacterial and fungal cultures, where a standard battery of culture systems are routinely used, viral cultures must be carefully tailored to the individual clinical situation; furthermore, culture requirements should be carefully reviewed with the laboratory in advance of the lumbar puncture. Not all viral agents can be recovered from CSF (170,171). Enteroviruses, mumps virus, and lymphocytic choriomeningitis virus can frequently be grown from CSF samples, as can the agents of western, eastern, and Venezuelan equine encephalitides. Herpes simplex types 1 and 2 have been isolated from cases of meningitis but are only rarely recovered from CSF in cases of encephalitis. Herpes zoster, California, St. Louis, and Japanese B encephalitis viruses are rarely recovered (170).

ADJUNCTIVE STUDIES OF CSF IN THE DIAGNOSIS OF CNS INFECTION

The need for rapidly available, accurate diagnostic information in CNS infections, the poor sensitivity of microscopic examination of CSF sediment, and the delays inherent in obtaining results of CSF culture have led to the development of a wide variety of rapid diagnostic tests for CNS infections. Availability and accuracy of these tests varies from institution to institution, and the physician should learn which tests are readily available at his or her institution.

Bacterial Infections

Lactic Acid

Elevation of lactic acid levels in CSF occurs more frequently in bacterial than in viral meningitis, and a CSF lactate level of over 2.2 mmol/liter provides supportive evidence for a bacterial infection. However, viral infections may produce similar elevation of lactate levels, as may noninfectious conditions such as subarachnoid hemorrhage; in addition, the specificity of lactic acid determinations in bacterial meningitis is only 31% (172–174).

Limulus Lysate Test

The limulus lysate test is used to detect endotoxin produced by Neisseria meningitidis, Hemophilus influenzae, and other gram-negative bacteria. The assay is based on the finding that the lysate of amebocytes from the horseshoe crab (Limulus polyphemus) contains a cascade of clotting proteins which form a gel when exposed to minute quantities of endotoxin (175,176). The test is sensitive and simple to perform but does not detect gram-positive infections and does not provide specific identification of the gram-negative organism involved. The test may give false-positive results if material used for collection of CSF or the test reagents themselves are in any way contaminated with endotoxin.

Detection of Bacterial Antigens

A variety of immunological tests have been developed to provide rapid detection of bacterial surface antigens in spinal fluid (Table 4). These tests include countercurrent immunoelectrophoresis (CIE), coagglutination, latex agglutination, and enzyme-linked immunosorbent assay (ELISA) (177–180). CIE, the first of these tests made commercially available, is also the most technically demanding and has been replaced in many laboratories by one or more of the newer methods (177,178). Antigen detection tests have been most frequently employed to diagnose meningitis due to Hemophilus influenzae, Neisseria meningitidis, and Streptococcus pneumoniae but have also been used to identify Escherichia coli and Listeria monocytogenes. CIE has been found to provide positive results on initial examination of spinal fluid in 63–100% of cases of Hemophilus influenzae, 30–92% of cases of meningococcal meningitis, and 44–100% of cases of pneumococcal meningitis (177). The sensitivity of latex agglutination (which has largely superseded CIE) for these organisms is 78–100%, 71–88%, and 61–88%, and that of coagglutination methods is 57–100%, 33–49%, and 67–100%, respectively (177–179) (Table 4). Limited experience is available with the use of ELISA systems (which have a sensitivity 100–1000 times greater than latex agglutination methods) for detection of bacterial antigens in CSF (180). In general, antigen detection tests are less sensitive than bacterial culture, and their diagnostic reliability and usefulness may vary somewhat from institution to institution. Antigen detection tests frequently remain positive after cultures have become negative, and thus these tests are of particular value in distinguishing partially treated bacterial meningitis from viral meningitis.

Mycobacterial Infections

Measurement of Adenosine Deaminase Levels in CSF

Adenosine deaminase is an enzyme which is widely distributed in human tissues and is present in high con-

---

TABLE 4. *Sensitivity of CSF antigen detection tests against major organisms in meningitis*[a]

Organism	Countercurrent immunoelectrophoresis	Coagglutination	Latex agglutination
Group B streptococci	63–100	83	79–92
Hemophilus influenzae	63–100	57–100	78–100
Neisseria meningitidis	30–92	33–49	71–88
Streptococcus pneumoniae	44–100	67–100	61–88

[a] Adapted from ref. 177.
[b] Antisera used for clinical testing may also react with antigens of other bacteria. The cross-reactivity of the specific reagents used should be reviewed with the laboratory if clinical or other data are discordant with the organism identified.

centration in lymphocytes. Elevation of CSF adenosine deaminase levels may occur in a variety of neurological disorders, including bacterial meningitis and brain abscess. Elevated levels of lymphocyte adenosine deaminase are frequently present in the CSF of patients with tuberculous meningitis, and measurement of this enzyme has been used to provide presumptive evidence of *Mycobacterium tuberculosis* infection and to evaluate response to treatment (181–183). The test, although both sensitive and useful, is not specific, since it detects a component of host response and does not detect a structural component of the organism itself.

Detection of Mycobacterial Antigens and Antibodies

A variety of immunological tests have been developed to detect mycobacterial antigens and/or antibodies to mycobacterial products in the CSF of patients with tuberculous meningitis. The most promising of these have employed ELISA methods using as a substrate either (a) monoclonal antibodies to mycobacterial products or (b) antigens derived from bacillus Calmette–Guérin (BCG) or *Mycobacterium tuberculosis.* The sensitivity of these has ranged between 52% and 81.25%, with a diagnostic specificity of over 90% (184–187). These tests are of considerable potential value, because they are easy to perform; in addition, the reagents could readily be sold in kit form. At present, however, each of the above techniques remains experimental, and a standardized ELISA for mycobacterial infections of the nervous system is not yet in general use. The possible role of the polymerase chain reaction in detection of mycobacterial infection of the CNS is discussed below.

Lyme Disease

The overall sensitivity and specificity of tests for diagnosis of Lyme disease is still being determined, as is the accuracy of tests used to diagnose CNS involvement. Screening tests for Lyme disease usually employ serum in an ELISA system to detect IgM and IgG in serum. The antigen used in most commercially available ELISA kits for Lyme disease consists of sonicated, whole spirochetes. Preparations consisting of spirochetal subcomponents have been reported to provide greater accuracy but are not widely available (188). A western immunoblot test is used to confirm the diagnosis (188). Antibody to *Borrelia burgdorferi* may be absent early in the course of infection; and seronegative Lyme disease, diagnosed by T-cell proliferation to Lyme disease, has been reported (189). False-positive tests for Lyme disease may be seen in patients with infectious mononucleosis, positive serology for syphilis, and autoimmune conditions. Detection of antibody to *Borrelia burgdorferi* in CSF provides strong supporting evidence for CNS involve-

ment by the agent. However, not all patients develop CSF antibodies, and detection of CSF antibody is not essential for diagnosis (190–192). Accuracy and reliability of tests vary considerably from laboratory to laboratory; therefore, positive values reported by laboratories unfamiliar to the physician must be approached with caution and, if necessary, confirmed.

Fungal and Other Infections

Detection of cryptococcal antigen in spinal fluid is the single most useful diagnostic test for cryptococcal meningitis. The test has a high degree of specificity and sensitivity, being positive in 85–90% of cases (193,194). However, occasional patients may have false-negative values on one or more determinations, and occasional patients may have negative tests at low dilutions as a result of a prozone phenomenon. In such cases, repeat cryptococcal antigen determinations and cultures are essential (93,94,195). Complement-fixation antibodies are present in CSF in up to 95% of cases of meningitis due to *Coccidioides immitis* (196,197). ELISA for detection of antigens and antibodies have recently been developed for meningitis due to *Brucella* species and *Histoplasma capsulatum* (198–201). CSF antibody titers have been used to diagnose and follow CNS infections caused by *Toxoplasma gondii* in both acquired immunodeficiency syndrome (AIDS) and non-AIDS patients (202–205). Intrathecal synthesis of antibodies to *Toxoplasma gondii* may be detected in a subset of AIDS patients with toxoplasmic encephalitis, not all of whom will have a demonstrable elevation in serum antibody titers (204,205).

Viral Infections

Serological studies of CSF are seldom of diagnostic or therapeutic value during the initial stages of acute viral infections of the CNS. CSF antibody titers may, however, prove valuable in slow infections such as tropical spastic paraparesis, subacute sclerosing panencephalitis, or progressive rubella encephalitis (206–210). Comparison of serum versus CSF titers of antiherpesvirus antibodies has been proposed as a diagnostic test; but the test, which is dependent on intrathecal antibody synthesis, is only rarely of value at the time of presentation (211–213).

Other Adjunctive Tests in the Diagnosis of CNS Infections

Gas–Liquid Chromatography

Gas–liquid chromatography (GLC) has been used to provide rapid diagnosis of bacterial meningitis and to differentiate mycobacterial from fungal and viral meningitis and has been used with mass spectrometry to identify both the mycobacterial metabolite 3-(2-keto-hexyl)indoline and the mycobacterial component tuberculostearic acid (214–218). The study by French et al. (218) is of particular interest, because tuberculostearic acid was detected in the CSF of 21 out of 22 patients and was found in one patient after 237 days of therapy. The rather extensive technical requirements for accurate and reliable use of GLC, with or without mass spectrometry, limit these methods to a few specialized laboratories.

Animal Inoculation

Guinea-pig inoculation was formerly employed as a means of isolating *Mycobacterium tuberculosis* but is rarely used at present. Intraperitoneal inoculation of mice, with subsequent examination of ascitic fluid for organisms, may be used to propagate *Toxoplasma gondii* from CSF or other clinical samples (202). The risk of infection of laboratory personnel should be kept firmly in mind if animal inoculation is used to isolate *Toxoplasma gondii* or other organisms; infected animals should be properly isolated, and routines of sterile technique should be used meticulously.

Detection of Lymphokines in CSF

Tumor necrosis factor (TNF), interleukin-1 (IL-1), and other lymphokines have received increasing attention as mediators of the inflammatory response during bacterial meningitis (37,39,43,45). Leist et al. (37) have reported detection of TNF-α in the CSF of three of three patients with bacterial meningitis but in none of seven patients with viral meningitis. Mustafa et al. (42) have demonstrated that IL-1β can be detected in the CSF of 95% of infants and children with bacterial meningitis, and that levels of greater than 500 pg/ml were correlated with increased risk of neurological sequelae. These findings, although requiring both confirmation and amplification, suggest that analysis of TNF and other cytokines may prove of value in differentiating acute bacterial meningitis from viral meningitis and, possibly, in detecting patients at particular risk of adverse outcome.

Detection of Nucleic Acids in CSF

Radiolabeled or biotinylated probes have been used extensively to detect viral nucleic acids in biopsy specimens. Application of these techniques to the study of CSF has not received wide attention. In contrast, the polymerase chain reaction, which permits amplification of specified base sequences, appears to hold great promise as a diagnostic tool—particularly in chronic bacterial

or fungal infection, where numbers of organisms may be extremely small, and in infections caused by viral or other organisms which are difficult to culture *in vitro*. The polymerase chain reaction relies on the ability of the temperature-resistant enzyme, Taq polymerase, to facilitate repeated cycles of replication of oligonucleotides in response to a defined primer (219). In infections, the primer may be any defined, specific part of the agent's nucleic acid. The technique has been used experimentally to detect human immunodeficiency virus (HIV), human T-lymphotrophic virus 1 (HTLV-1), and *Toxoplasma gondii* nucleic acid sequences in CSF and has been reported to detect herpes simplex virus nucleic acid sequences in the CSF from four of four cases with herpes simplex virus encephalitis but to be negative in six patients with other CNS infections (219–221). The technique has also been used to identify *Mycobacterium tuberculosis* in lymph node cultures, at a level of sensitivity which would suggest that it might be successfully applied to CSF (222). The applications, strengths, and potential disadvantages of this technique are still being explored. A major disadvantage of the technique at present is that its extreme sensitivity may lead to false-positive results. In addition, the specificity of the technique—except in situations in which groups of organisms share common nucleic acid sequences—currently prevents its use as a broad diagnostic screen.

CHARACTERISTIC CSF FINDINGS IN MAJOR CNS INFECTIONS

CSF changes in CNS infections often provide provisional or suggestive diagnostic significance. It must be kept in mind, however, that CSF changes, in the absence of detectable organisms, are not pathognomonic of any group of conditions and that CSF findings must be interpreted in light of clinical, neurological, and neuroradiological findings. The need for caution is particularly important where there is a question of viral versus bacterial infections: Here an erroneous decision to withhold antimicrobial therapy based on CSF interpretation alone may result in death (142).

Bacterial Meningitis

Blood glucose (ideally drawn shortly prior to the lumbar puncture) and at least 5–7 ml of CSF should be obtained. At least 1 ml of CSF should be submitted for cell count and differential, and at least 0.5 ml (preferably 1–2 ml) of CSF should be used for glucose and protein determinations. A minimum of 3–5 ml should be submitted for bacterial culture, antigen detection, and, if gram-negative infection is suspected, limulus lysate assay. Bacterial meningitis characteristically produces a polymorphonuclear pleocytosis, a depressed level of glucose, and an elevated protein. Numbers of polymorphonuclear leukocytes may vary from a few to many thousand and usually range between 1000 and 10,000 cells. A predominantly (>50% of cells) lymphocytic pleocytosis has been reported in up to 14% of cases (223) and is more common in meningitis due to *Listeria monocytogenes* (224). A predominance of lymphocytes may also be seen in neonatal gram-negative meningitis (225). Leukocytes may be absent from CSF very early in the course of infection, in neonatal meningitis, or in severely immunocompromised patients (226–229). Glucose levels of less than 40 mg/dl or a CSF:blood glucose ratio of less than 0.4 should raise strong suspicion of bacterial meningitis, and less than 0.5 should be of concern. Glucose levels of less than 18 or a CSF:serum glucose ratio of 0.23 makes bacterial meningitis extremely likely (142). Normal glucose values will be obtained in approximately 9% of cases. Protein levels correspond with the intensity of meningeal inflammation but are between 100 and 500 mg/dl in most patients. Yield on Gram's stain varies from organism to organism (see above) but is positive in 60–80% of untreated patients.

Partially Treated Bacterial Meningitis

Requirements for CSF analysis are identical to those listed for acute bacterial meningitis without prior treatment. In general, antibiotics have little effect on CSF cell count, differential, protein, or glucose concentrations during the first 2–3 days of therapy (229–231). In a minority of patients, however, antibiotic therapy may result in a shift from a polymorphonuclear to a lymphocytic pleocytosis (232). Prior antibiotic therapy can be expected to reduce the diagnostic yield of Gram's stain by about 20% and of culture by about 30% (231,233). Immunological studies for bacterial antigens—and, in the case of gram-negative meningitis, limulus lysate assay—may permit identification of the infection as bacterial rather than viral.

Brain Abscess and Parameningeal Infection

Lumbar puncture in loculated parenchymal or parameningeal infections is usually unhelpful and is contraindicated by the risk of brain herniation. CSF findings are nonspecific and may include (a) a mixed, predominantly lymphocytic pleocytosis, (b) normal glucose, and (c) elevated protein. Organisms are not present unless there is accompanying meningitis, in which case CSF findings will be those of bacterial meningitis (71).

Tuberculous Meningitis

Volumes for routine bacterial culture, cell count, glucose, and protein are as described for bacterial meningi-

tis. Typical findings in tuberculous meningitis are (a) a pleocytosis with lymphocytic predominance, (b) lowered glucose, and (c) elevated protein (153,154,165,234). In approximately 70% of cases the cell count is between 100 and 400 cells (153). However, as many as 1000–1200 cells may be present, and in occasional patients the CSF is acellular despite the presence of organisms, elevation in protein, and hypoglycorrhachia. Although the majority of cells in the CSF are lymphocytes, relative numbers of lymphocytes and polymorphonuclear leukocytes may vary from lumbar puncture to lumbar puncture. Neutrophils predominate in approximately 27% of cases and are most likely to be present early in the course of infection or in severe infection (156). Small numbers of cells or acellular CSF may be found in patients with AIDS or other states of severe immune deficiency. Protein levels are 100–500 mg/dl in 65% of cases and may reach levels of 1000 mg or more if treatment is delayed (153,154). Elevation of CSF protein to levels greater than 1000 mg may result in xanthochromia. Extreme elevation of protein, accompanied by entry of fibrinogen into the CSF, may be accompanied by formation of a web-like clot or pellicle. In 25% of cases, protein levels are normal (153). Glucose levels are 30–45 mg/dl in 50% of cases and may occasionally be less than 10 mg/dl. In 17% of cases, CSF glucose levels are normal (153).

Mycobacterium tuberculosis may be extremely difficult to detect on smear or to recover by culture. Where tuberculous meningitis is strongly suspected, at least 20 ml of CSF should be submitted for acid-fast smear and culture unless contraindicated by increased ICP; larger volumes (40–50 ml) should be submitted if possible. Frequently, the need for a second lumbar puncture to obtain this large amount of CSF is first suggested by the abnormalities detected in the initial CSF sample. During appropriate therapy, CSF glucose returns toward normal before cell count or protein levels. CSF cell counts and protein levels may remain abnormal for protracted periods of time (153,154,163).

Fungal and Other Chronic Meningitides

Initial requirements for CSF analysis in suspected fungal infections are similar to those described above for tuberculous meningitis, and the same material may be sent for both mycobacterial and fungal culture. An additional 2 ml of CSF should be submitted for cryptococcal antigen and, if the patient has a history of residence in an endemic area, for complement-fixing antibodies to *Coccidioides immitis* or *Borrelia burgdorferi*. Additional samples of CSF, if obtainable, should be submitted for serological studies for *Histoplasma capsulatum, Brucella,* or other organisms as indicated by history and occupational exposure. Serum and CSF should be frozen and held for future serological studies. CSF findings in fungal infections are similar to those described in tuberculous meningitis, except that polymorphonuclear leukocytes may be found less frequently. The number of cells present may vary widely; and, as in tuberculous meningitis, CSF may be acellular in severely immunocompromised patients, including those with AIDS (235–237). An exception to this rule is seen in infections due to *Mucor,* where the extremely destructive nature of the infection may result in large numbers of neutrophils (238). As in tuberculous meningitis, CSF glucose may return towards normal before changes are seen in cell count and protein.

Neurosyphilis

Suspicion of neurosyphilis is predicated upon the presence of positive serum rapid plasma reagin (RPR) and fluorescent treponemal antibody-absorption (FTA-Abs) determinations. Amounts of CSF required are as described for bacterial meningitis. Additional CSF should be sent for VDRL determination (see Chapter 27). CSF may contain variable numbers of lymphocytes and an elevated protein during late primary and early secondary stages of the disease and during asymptomatic or symptomatic neurosyphilis (2). CSF findings are extremely variable, however; and normal CSF cell count, protein, and glucose values do not exclude active disease (236,237). Rarely, syphilis may present as an acute meningitis, with CSF findings similar to those of bacterial meningitis (2). False-negative CSF VDRL determinations which became positive with penicillin therapy have been described in neurosyphilis associated with AIDS (239).

Lyme Borreliosis

CSF requirements are as described for bacterial meningitis. CSF and serum should be sent for serological studies. CSF changes in Lyme neuroborreliosis are typically a mild lymphocytic pleocytosis, modest elevation of protein, and normal glucose. CSF may be normal, however, or, conversely, may occasionally exhibit changes identical to those seen in bacterial meningitis (188–194,240).

Viral and Other Acute Meningoencephalitides

Basic requirements for CSF analysis are identical to those for bacterial meningitis. The meningitis should be assumed to be bacterial until proven otherwise: Lumbar puncture should be performed immediately, and CSF should *always* be submitted for bacterial culture. Volumes and handling of CSF for viral culture should be reviewed with the laboratory, but the initial lumbar puncture should not be delayed if arrangements cannot be made immediately. Viral meningitis produces a lymphocytic pleocytosis, usually in the range of 10–1000 cells per cubic millimeter. Polymorphonuclear leuko-

cytes are frequently present in patients during the first 24–36 hr of the infection and may at times constitute over 50% of the cells (241–243). In some patients with Coxsackie virus infections of the CNS, polymorphonuclear leukocytes may constitute 90% of cells at the onset of infection, and the predominance of polymorphonuclear leukocytes may persist for longer than 24 hr. Protein is elevated in the range of 50–100 mg/dl but may sometimes be higher. Glucose is usually normal, but depression of glucose to levels approaching those of bacterial meningitis has been reported in infections due to herpes simplex virus 2, herpes zoster virus, mumps, and lymphocytic choriomeningitis virus (125–134). Spanos et al. (142) have recently developed a helpful nomogram for distinguishing between bacterial and viral meningitis. However, presumptive antibiotic therapy for bacterial meningitis should be initiated if the diagnosis of viral meningitis is in doubt (145). CSF and serum should be frozen for future serological testing.

Requirements for CSF analysis in cases of suspected viral encephalitis are similar to those for viral meningitis, and CSF findings are often similar. Polymorphonuclear leukocytes may be present in large numbers in severe encephalitides accompanied by extensive destruction of brain tissue. Herpes simplex virus classically produces a hemorrhagic encephalitis, and small amounts of blood may be seen in the spinal fluid. However, herpes simplex virus is not unique in its ability to produce hemorrhagic necrosis of brain, and red blood cells are frequently not detected; thus, the presence or absence of red blood cells cannot be used to differentiate herpes simplex virus encephalitis from other conditions. As in viral meningitis, serum and CSF should be held for future serological studies.

Acquired Immunodeficiency Syndrome

CSF abnormalities in HIV infection are protean and may reflect either (a) a response to CNS invasion by the agent itself, as in HIV-related meningitis, (b) meningitis or parenchymal infection by other agents, or (c) meningeal reaction to neoplastic or ischemic events within brain or spinal cord. The response to any of these conditions is frequently modified by the immunosuppressive effect of the virus (236). In HIV-infected individuals, normal findings on routine CSF studies do not exclude infectious disease of the nervous system. The neurological complications of HIV infection and the approach to the patient with suspected neurological involvement are discussed in detail in Chapter 10.

Slow Virus Infections

Two broad groups of slow infections occur in humans: (i) slow infections caused by conventional agents and (ii) transmissible spongiform encephalopathies, kuru, Creutzfeldt–Jakob disease, and Gerstmann–Straussler syndrome. CSF changes are minimal in slow infections caused by conventional agents. CSF is usually acellular, with normal or mildly elevated protein and normal glucose. In rare cases, progressive multifocal leukoencephalopathy may be accompanied by a modest lymphocytic pleocytosis. Oligoclonal bands and high titers of antiviral antibody are present in subacute sclerosing panencephalitis and progressive rubella panencephalitis and may also be present in HTLV-1-associated tropical spastic paraparesis (206–210). The transmissible spongiform encephalopathies do not elicit a cellular reaction in CSF, so that the presence of a CSF pleocytosis essentially excludes this group of diseases. Mild elevation of protein may occasionally be seen (244). CSF from cases of known or suspected Creutzfeldt–Jakob disease should be regarded as infectious and handled according to current guidelines (see Chapter 8) (245).

ACKNOWLEDGMENT

This work was supported, in part, by the U.S. Department of Veterans Affairs.

REFERENCES

1. Herndon RM, Brumback RA. *The cerebrospinal fluid.* Boston: Kluwer Academic Publishers, 1989.
2. Fishman RA. *Cerebrospinal fluid in diseases of the nervous system.* Philadelphia: WB Saunders, 1980.
3. Last RJ, Thompsett DH. Casts of the cerebral ventricles. *Br J Surg* 1953;40:525–543.
4. Alexander L. Die Anatomie der Seitentaschen der vierten Kirnkammer. *Z Gesamte Anat l. Z Anat EntwGesch* 1931;95:531–707.
5. Barr ML. Observations on the foramen of Magendie in a series of human brains. *Brain* 1948;71:281–289.
6. Greenlee JE. Anatomical considerations in central nervous system infections. In: Mandell GL, Douglas RG, Bennett JE, eds. *Principles and practice of infectious diseases,* 3rd ed. New York: Churchill Livingstone, 1990;732–741.
7. Bering EA Jr, Sato O. Hydrocephalus: changes in formation and absorption of cerebrospinal fluid within the cerebral ventricles. *J Neurosurg* 1963;20:1050–1063.
8. Voetmann E. On the structure and surface area of the human choroid plexuses. *Acta Anat* 1949;8(Suppl 10):1–116.
9. Dimattio J, Hochwald GM, Malhan C, Wald A. Effects of changes in serum osmolality on bulk flow of CSF into cerebral ventricles and on brain water content. *Pflugers Arch* 1975;359:253–264.
10. Hochwald GM, Wald A, Malhan C. The sink action of cerebrospinal fluid volume flow. Effect on brain water content. *Arch Neurol* 1972;33:339–344.
11. Cutler RWP, Page L, Galicich J, Watters GV. Formation and absorption of the cerebrospinal fluid in man. *Brain* 1968;91:707–720.
12. Heisey SR, Held D, Pappenheimer JR. Bulk flow and diffusion in the cerebrospinal fluid system of the goat. *Am J Physiol* 1968;203:775–781.
13. Partridge WM. Recent advances in blood–brain barrier transport. *Annu Rev Pharmacol Toxicol* 1988;28:25–39.
14. Cserr HF. Physiology of the choroid plexus. *Physiol Rev* 1971;51:273–311.
15. Vates TS Jr, Bonting SL, Oppelt WW. Na–K activated adenosine triphosphate formation of cerebrospinal fluid in the cat. *Am J Physiol* 1964;206:1165–1172.
16. Rubin RC, Henderson ES, Ommaya AK, Walker MD, Rall DP. The production of cerebrospinal fluid in man and its modification by acetazolamide. *J Neurosurg* 1966;25:430–436.
17. Buhrley LE, Reed DJ. The effect of furosemide on sodium-22 uptake into cerebrospinal fluid. *Exp Brain Res* 1972;14:503–510.
18. Reed DJ. The effects of furosemide on cerebrospinal fluid flow. *Arch Int Pharmacodyn* 1969;178:324–330.
19. Welch K. The principles of physiology of the cerebrospinal fluid in relation to hydrocephalus including normal pressure hydrocephalus. In: Friedlander WJ, ed. *Advances in neurology. Current reviews.* New York: Raven Press, 1975;345–375.
20. Welch K, Friedman V. The cerebrospinal fluid valves. *Brain* 1960;83:454–469.
21. Welch K, Pollay M. The spinal arachnoid villi of the monkeys *Ceropithecus aethiops sabaeus* and *Macaca irus. Anat Rec* 1963;145:43–48.
22. Welch K, Pollay M. Perfusion of particles through arachnoid villi of the monkey. *Am J Physiol* 1961;201:651–654.
23. Tripathi RC. Ultrastructure of the arachnoid mater in relation to the outflow of cerebrospinal fluid. A new concept. *Lancet* 1973;2:8–11.
24. Tripathi BS, Tripathi RC. Vacuolar transcellular channels as a drainage pathway for cerebrospinal fluid. *J Physiol* 1974;239:195–206.
25. Yamashima T. Functional ultrastructure of cerebrospinal fluid drainage channels in human arachnoid villi. *Neurosurgery.* 1988;22:633–641.
26. Krisch B. Ultrastructure of the meninges at the site of penetration of veins through the dura mater, with particular reference to Pacchionian granulations. Investigations in the rat and two species of New-World monkeys (*Cebus apella, Callitrix jacchus*). *Cell Tissue Res* 1988;251:621–631.
27. Scheld WM. Pathogenesis and pathophysiology of pneumococcal meningitis. In: Sande MA, Smith AL, Root RK, eds. *Contemporary issues in infectious diseases, 3. Bacterial meningitis.* New York: Churchill Livingstone, 1985;37–69.
28. Ellington E, Margolis G. Block of arachnoid villus by subarachnoid hemorrhage. *J Neurosurg* 1969;30:651–657.
29. Scheld WM. Bacterial meningitis in the patient at risk. Intrinsic risk factors and host defense mechanisms. *Am J Med* 1984;76(5A):193–207.
30. Leibowitz SL, Hughes RAC. *Immunology of the nervous system.* Croydon, Surrey: Edward Arnold, 1983.
31. Simerkoff MS, Moldover NH, Rahal JJ Jr. Absence of detectable bactericidal and opsonic activities in normal and infected human cerebrospinal fluids. A regional host defense deficiency. *J Lab Clin Med* 1980;95:362–372.
32. Zwahlen A, Nydegger UE, Vadaux P, et al. Complement-mediated opsonic activity in normal and infected human cerebrospinal fluid. *J Infect Dis* 1982;145:635–636.
33. Lieberman AP, Pitha PM, Shin HS, Shin ML. Production of tumor necrosis factor and other cytokines by astrocytes stimulated with lipopolysaccharide or a neurotropic virus. *Proc Natl Acad Sci USA* 1989;86:6348–6352.
34. Sawada M, Kondo N, Suzumura A, Marunouchi T. Production of tumor necrosis factor-alpha by microglia and astrocytes in culture. *Brain Res* 1989;491:394–397.
35. Frohman EM, Frohman TC, Dustin ML, Vayuvegula B, Choi B, Gupta A, van den Noort S, Gupta S. The induction of intercellular adhesion molecule 1 (ICAM-1) expression on human fetal astrocytes by interferon-gamma, tumor necrosis factor alpha, lymphotoxin, and interleukin-1: relevance to intracerebral antigen presentation. *J Neuroimmunol* 1989;23:117–124.
36. Lavi E, Suzumura A, Murasko DM, Murray EM, Silberberg DH, Weiss SR. Tumor necrosis factor induces expression of MHC class I antigens on mouse astrocytes. *Ann NY Acad Sci* 1988;540:488–490.
37. Leist TP, Frei K, Kam Hansen S, Zinkernagel RM, Fontana A. Tumor necrosis factor alpha in cerebrospinal fluid during bacterial, but not viral, meningitis. Evaluation in murine model infections and in patients. *J Exp Med* 1988;167:1743–1748.

38. Frei K, Leist TP, Meager A, Gallo P, Leppert D, Zinkernagel RM, Fontana A. Production of B cell stimulatory factor-2 and interferon gamma in the central nervous system during viral meningitis and encephalitis. Evaluation in a murine model infection and in patients. *J Exp Med* 1988;168:449–453.

39. Waage A, Halstensen A, Shalaby R, Brandtzaeg P, Kierulf P, Espevik T. Local production of tumor necrosis factor alpha, interleukin 1, and interleukin 6 in meningococcal meningitis. Relation to the inflammatory response. *J Exp Med* 1989;333–338.

40. Frei K, Malipiero UV, Leist TP, Zinkernagel RM, Schwab ME, Fontana A. On the cellular source and function of interleukin 6 produced in the central nervous system in viral diseases. *Eur J Immunol* 1989;19:689–694.

41. Mustafa MM, Mertsola J, Ramilo O, Saez-Llorens X, Risser RC, McCracken GH Jr. Increased endotoxin and interleukin-1 beta concentrations in cerebrospinal fluid of infants with coliform meningitis and ventriculitis associated with intraventricular gentamicin therapy. *J Infect Dis* 1989;160:891–895.

42. Mustafa MM, Lebel MH, Ramilo O, Olsen KD, Reisch JS, Beutler B, McCracken GH Jr. Correlation of interleukin-1 beta and cachectin concentrations in cerebrospinal fluid and outcome from bacterial meningitis. *J Pediatr* 1989;115:208–213.

43. McCracken GH Jr, Mustafa MM, Ramilo O, Olsen KD, Risser RC. Cerebrospinal fluid interleukin 1-beta and tumor necrosis factor concentrations and outcome from neonatal gram-negative enteric bacillary meningitis. *Pediatr Infect Dis J* 1989;8:155–159.

44. Helfgott DC, Tatter SB, Santhanam U, Clarick RH, Bhardwaj N, May LT, Sehgal PB. Multiple forms of IFN-beta 2/IL-6 in serum and body fluids during acute bacterial infection. *J Immunol* 1989;142:948–953.

45. Nadal D, Leppert D, Frei K, Gallo P, Lamche H, Fontana A. Tumour necrosis factor-alpha in infectious meningitis. *Arch Dis Child* 1989;64:1274–1279.

46. Schoen EJ. Spinal fluid chloride: a test 40 years past its prime. *JAMA* 1984;251:37–38.

47. Fishman RA. Blood–brain and CSF barriers to penicillin and related organic acids. *Arch Neurol* 1966;15:113–124.

48. Dixon RL, Owens ES, Rall DP. Evidence of active transport of benzyl-14C penicillin from cerebrospinal fluid to blood. *J Pharm Sci* 1969;58:1106–1109.

49. Spector R. The transport of gentamicin in the choroid plexus and cerebrospinal fluid. *J Pharmacol Exp Ther* 1975;194:82–88.

50. Greenlee JE. Suppurative intracranial phlebitis. In: Mandell GL, Douglas RG, Bennett JE, eds. *Principles and practice of infectious diseases,* 3rd ed. New York: Churchill Livingstone, 1990;793–795.

51. Johnson RT, Johnson KP. Hydrocephalus following viral infection: the pathology of aqueductal stenosis developing after experimental mumps virus infection. *J Neuropathol Exp Neurol* 1968;27:591–606.

52. Timmons GD, Johnson KP. Aqueductal stenosis and hydrocephalus after mumps encephalitis. *N Engl J Med* 1970;283:1505–1507.

53. Sze G, Simmons B, Krol G, Walker R, Zimmerman RD, Deck MD. Dural sinus thrombosis: verification with spin-echo techniques. *AJNR* 1987;9:679–686.

54. Bauer WM, Einhaupt K, Heywang SH, Vogl T, Seiderer M, Clados D. MR of venous sinus thrombosis: a case report. *AJNR* 1987;8:713–715.

55. Lofgren J, Swetnow NW. Cranial and spinal components of cerebrospinal fluid pressure. *Acta Neurol Scand* 1973;49:575–585.

56. Miller JD. Volume and pressure in the cerebrospinal axis. *Clin Neurosurg* 1975;22:76–105.

57. Marmarou A, Shulman K, Rosende RM. A nonlinear analysis of the cerebrospinal fluid system and intracranial pressure dynamics. *J Neurosurg* 1978;49:332–344.

58. Langfitt TW. Clinical methods for monitoring intracranial pressure and measuring cerebral blood flow. *Clin Neurosurg* 1975;22:302–320.

59. Mann JD, Butler AB, Rosenthal JE, et al. Regulation of intracranial pressure in rat, dog, and man. *Ann Neurol* 1978;3:156–165.

60. Leech P, Miller JD. Intracranial volume pressure relationships during experimental brain compression in primates. *J Neurol Neurosurg Psychiatry* 1974;37:1099–1104.

61. Miller JD, Garibi J, Pickard JD. Induced changes in cerebrospinal fluid volume. *Arch Neurol* 1973;28:265–269.

62. Shapiro HM. Intracranial hypertension: therapeutic and anesthetic considerations. *Anesthesiology* 1975;43:445–471.

63. Miller JD, Becker DP, Ward JD, et al. Significance of intracranial hypertension in severe head injury. *J Neurosurg* 1977;47:503–516.

64. Lundberg N, Cronquist S, Kjallquist A. Clinical investigations on inter-relationships between intracranial pressure and intracranial hemodynamics. *Prog Brain Res* 1968;30:69–81.

65. Plum F, Posner JB. *The diagnosis of stupor and coma,* 3rd ed. Philadelphia: FA Davis, 1980.

66. Cuneo RA, Caronna JJ, Pitts L, et al. Upward transtentorial herniation. Seven cases and a literature review. *Arch Neurol* 1979;36:618–623.

67. Rebaud P, Berthier JC, Hartemann E, Floret D. Intracranial pressure in childhood central nervous system infections. *Intensive Care Med* 1988;14:522–525.

68. Goitein KJ, Tamir I. Cerebral perfusion pressure in central nervous system infections of infancy and childhood. *J Pediatr* 1983;103:40–43.

69. Johnston IH, Rowan JO. Raised intracranial pressure and cerebral blood flow. Intracranial pressure gradients and regional cerebral blood flow. *J Neurol Neurosurg Psychiatry* 1975;37:585–574.

70. Duffy GP. Lumbar puncture in the presence of raised intracranial pressure. *Br Med J* 1969;1:407–409.

71. Wispelwey B, Scheld WM. Brain abscess. *Clin Neuropharmacol* 1987;10:483–510.

72. Rischbieth RH. Pneumococcal meningitis—a killing disease. *Med J Aust* 1960;1:578–581.

73. Williams CPS, Swanson AG, Chapman JT. Brain swelling with acute purulent meningitis. *Pediatrics* 1964;34:220–227.

74. Dodge PR, Schwartz MN. Bacterial meningitis—a review of selected aspects. II. Special neurologic problems, postmeningitis complications and clinicopathological correlations (concluded). *N Engl J Med* 1965;272:1003–1010.

75. Horwitz SJ, Boxerbaum B, O'Bell J. Cerebral herniation in bacterial meningitis in childhood. *Ann Neurol* 1980;7:524–528.

76. Harper JR, Lorber J, Smith H, Bowers DB. Timing of lumbar puncture in childhood meningitis. *Br Med J* 1985;291:651–653.

77. De Sousa AL, Kleinman MB, Mealey J Jr. Quadripegia and cortical blindness in *Hemophilus influenzae* meningitis. *J Pediatr* 1978;93:253–254.

78. Tal Y, Crichton JU, Dunn HG, Dolman CL. Spinal cord damage: a rare complication of purulent meningitis. *Aca Pediatr Scand* 1980;69:471–474.

79. Swart SS, Pye IF. Spinal cord ischemia complicating meningococcal meningitis. *Postgrad Med J* 1980;56:661–662.

80. Norman MG. Respiratory arrest and cervical spinal cord infarction following lumbar puncture in meningitis. *Can J Neurol Sci* 1982;9:443–447.

81. Herrick MK, Agamanolis DP. Displacement of cerebellar tissue into spinal canal: a component of respirator brain syndrome. *Arch Pathol* 1975;99:565–571.

82. Laglia AG, Eisenberg RL, Weinstein PR, Mani RL. Spinal epidural hematoma after lumbar puncture in liver disease. *Ann Intern Med* 1978;88:515–516.

83. Gutterman P. Acute spinal subdural hematoma following lumbar puncture. *Surg Neurol* 1977;7:355–356.

84. Wegefarth P, Latham JR. Lumbar puncture as a factor in the causation of meningitis. *Am J Med Sci* 1919;148:183–202.

85. Weed LH, Wegefarth P, Ayer JB, et al. The production of meningitis by release of cerebrospinal fluid during an experimental septicemia: preliminary note. *JAMA* 1919;72:190–193.

86. Weed LH, Wegefarth P, Ayer JB, et al. A study of experimental meningitis. IV. The influence of certain experimental procedures upon the production of meningitis by intravenous inoculation. *Monogr Rockefeller Inst Med Res* 1920;12:57–114.

87. Pray LG. Lumbar puncture as a factor in the pathogenesis of meningitis. *Am J Dis Child* 1941;62:295–308.

88. Torphy DE, Ray CG. Occult pneumococcal bacteremia. *Am J Dis Child* 1970;119:336–338.

89. Fischer GW, Brenz RW, Alden ER, Beckwith JB. Lumbar punctures and meningitis. *Am J Dis Child* 1975;192:590–592.

90. Petersdorf RG, Swarner DR, Garcia M. Studies on the pathogenesis of meningitis. II. Development of meningitis during pneumococcal bacteremia. *J Clin Invest* 1962;41:320–327.

91. Dietzman DE, Fischer GW, Schoenknecht FD. Neonatal *Escherichia coli* septicemia: bacterial counts in blood. *J Pediatr* 1974;85:128–130.

92. Telle DW, Dashefsky B, Rakusan T, et al. Meningitis after lumbar puncture in children with bacteremia. *N Engl J Med* 1981;305:1079–1081.

93. Greenlee JE. Epidural abscess. In: Mandell GL, Douglas RG, Bennett JE, eds. *Principles and practice of infectious diseases,* 3rd ed. New York: Churchill Livingstone, 1990;788–793.

94. Batnitsky S, Keucher TR, Mealey J, et al. Iatrogenic intraspinal epidermoid tumors. *JAMA* 1977;237:148–150.

95. Ostheimer GW, Palahniuk RJ, Schnider SM. Epidural blood patch for post-lumbar-puncture headache. *Anesthesiology* 1974;41:307–308.

96. Petito F, Plum F. The lumbar puncture. *N Engl J Med* 1974;290:225–226.

97. Gonyea EF. Cisternal puncture and cryptococcal meningitis. *Arch Neurol* 1973;28:200–201.

98. Berger MP, Paz J. Diagnosis of cryptococcal meningitis. *JAMA* 1976;236:2517–2518.

99. Craig WMcK, Carmichael FA Jr. Blastomycosis of the cerebellum. Report of a case. *Mayo Clin Proc* 1983;13:347–351.

100. Berlin L, Pincus JH. Cryptococcal meningitis. False negative antigen test results and cultures in immunosuppressed patients. *Arch Neurol* 1989;46:1312–1316.

101. Masserman JH. Cerebrospinal hydrodynamics. IV. Clinical experimental studies. *Arch Neurol Psychiatry* 1934;32:523–553.

102. Vidyasagar D, Raju TNK. A simple noninvasive technique of measuring intracranial pressure in the newborn. *Pediatrics* 1977;59:957–961.

103. Tourtellotte WW, Haerer AF, Heller GL, et al. *Post-lumbar puncture headaches.* Springfield, IL: Charles C Thomas, 1964.

104. Gooch WM III, Sotelo-Avila C. Meningitis in children: laboratory diagnosis. *J Tenn Med Assoc* 1976;69:563–564.

105. Patten BM. How much blood makes the cerebrospinal fluid bloody? [Letter] *JAMA* 1968;206:378.

106. Mealy J. Fat emulsion as a cause of cloudy cerebrospinal fluid. *JAMA* 1962;180:246–248.

107. Walton JN. *Subarachnoid hemorrhage.* Edinburgh: Livingstone, 1956.

108. Bonadio WA. Bacterial meningitis in children whose cerebrospinal fluid contains polymorphonuclear leukocytes without pleocytosis. *Clin Pediatr* 1988;27:198–200.

109. Sarff LD, Platt LH, McCracken GH Jr. Cerebrospinal fluid evaluation in neonates: Comparison of high-risk infants with and without meningitis. *J Pediatr* 1976;88:473–477.

110. Mengel M. The use of the cytocentrifuge in the diagnosis of meningitis. *Am J Clin Pathol* 1985;84:212–216.

111. Kuberski T. Eosinophils in the cerebrospinal fluid. *Ann Intern Med* 1979;91:70–75.

112. Scharf D. Eosinophilic meningitis in central nervous system cysticercosis [Letter]. *Arch Neurol* 1989;46:843.

113. Kolar OJ, Zeman W, Ciembroniewicz F, et al. Uber die Bedeutung der eosinophilen Leukocyten bei neurologische Krankheitungen. *Wien Z Nervenheilk* 1969;27:97–106.

114. Punyagupta S, Juttijudata P, Bunnag T. Eosinophilic meningitis in Thailand. Clinical studies of 484 cases probably caused by *Angiostrongylus cantonensis. Am J Trop Med Hyg* 1975;24:921–931.

115. Oehmichen M. *Cerebrospinal fluid cytology: an introduction and atlas.* Philadelphia: WB Saunders, 1976.

116. Bosch I, Oehmichen M. Eosinophilic granulocytes in the spinal fluid: analysis of 94 cerebrospinal fluid specimens and review of the literature. *J Neurol* 1978;219:93–105.

117. Crennan JM, Van Scoy RE. Eosinophilic meningitis caused by Rocky Mountain spotted fever. *Am J Med* 1986;80:288–289.

118. Weingarten JS, O'Sheal SF, Margolis WS. Eosinophilic meningitis and the hypereosinophilic syndrome. Case report and review of the literature. *Am J Med* 1985;78:674–676.

119. Matthews WF, Frommeyer WB Jr. The *in vitro* behaviour of erythrocytes in human cerebrospinal fluid. *J Lab Clin Med* 1955;45:508–515.

120. Fishman RA. Studies of the transport of sugars between blood and cerebrospinal fluid in normal states and in meningeal carcinomatosis. *Trans Am Neurol Assoc* 1963;88:114–118.

121. Meyers GC, Netsky MG. Relation of blood and cerebrospinal fluid glucose. *Arch Neurol* 1962;6:18–20.

122. Taylor LM, Smith HV, Vollum RL. Tuberculous meningitis of acute onset. *J Neurol Neurosurg Psychiatry* 1955;18:165–173.

123. Schwartz MN, Dodge PR. Bacterial meningitis—a review of selected aspects. I. General clinical features, special problems, and unusual meningeal reactions mimicking bacterial meningitis. *N Engl J Med* 1965;272:779–787.

124. Ellner JJ, Bennett JE. Chronic meningitis. *Medicine* 1976; 55:341–370.

125. Azimi PH, Shaban S, Hilty MD, Haynes RE. Mumps meningoencephalitis. Prolonged abnormality of cerebrospinal fluid. *JAMA* 1975;234:1161–1162.

126. Wilfert CM. Mumps meningoencephalitis with low cerebrospinal-fluid glucose, prolonged pleocytosis with elevation of protein. *N Engl J Med* 1969;280:855–858.

127. Adair CV, Gauld RL, Smadel JE. Aseptic meningitis, a disease of diverse etiology: clinical and etiologic studies on 854 cases. *Ann Intern Med* 1953;39:675–704.

128. Silver TS, Todd JK. Hypoglychorrhachia in pediatric patients. *Pediatrics* 1976;58:67–71.

129. Brenton DW. Hypoglychorrhachia in herpes simplex type 2 meningitis. *Arch Neurol* 1980;37:317.

130. Hevron JE. Herpes simplex type 2 meningitis. *Obstet Gynecol* 1976;49:622–624.

131. Wolf SM. Decreased cerebrospinal fluid glucose level in herpes zoster meningitis. *Arch Neurol* 1974;30:109.

132. Reimer LG, Reller B. CSF in herpes zoster meningoencephalitis. *Arch Neurol* 1981;38:688.

133. Klimek JJ, Russman BS, Quintiliani R. *Mycoplasma pneumoniae* meningoencephalitis and transverse myelitis in association with low cerebrospinal fluid glucose. *Pediatrics* 1976;58:133–135.

134. Gaines JD, Eckman PB, Remington JS. Low CSF glucose level in sarcoidosis involving the central nervous system. *Arch Intern Med* 1970;125:333–336.

135. Henson RA, Urich H. Carcinomatous meningitis. In: Henson RA, Urich H, eds. *Cancer and the nervous system. The neurological manifestations of systemic malignant disease.* Oxford: Blackwell, 1982;100–119.

136. Vincent FM. Hypoglychorrhachia after subarachnoid hemorrhage. *Neurosurgery* 1981;8:7–14.

137. Conley JM, Ronald AR. Cerebrospinal fluid as a diagnostic body fluid. *Am J Med* 1983;76:102–108.

138. Smellie J. The treatment of tuberculous meningitis without intrathecal therapy. *Lancet* 1954;2:1091.

139. Omene JAS, Okolo AA, Longe AC, Onyia DN. The specificity and sensitivity of cerebrospinal and blood glucose concentration in the diagnosis of neonatal meningitis. *Ann Trop Paediatr* 1985;5:37–39.

140. Powers WJ. Cerebrospinal fluid to serum glucose ratios in diabetes mellitus and bacterial meningitis. *Am J Med* 1981;71:217–220.

141. Krieg AF. Cerebrospinal fluid and other body fluids. In: Henry JB, ed. *Clinical diagnosis and management by laboratory methods,* 16th ed. Philadelphia: WB Saunders, 1979;635–657.

142. Spanos A, Harrell FE, Durack DT. Differential diagnosis of acute meningitis, an analysis of the predictive value of initial observations. *JAMA* 1989;2700–2707.

143. Lepow ML, Coyne N, Thompson LB. A clinical, epidemiologic, and laboratory investigation of aseptic meningitis during the 4-year period 1955–1958. *N Engl J Med* 1962;266:1118–1193.

144. Frick E, Scheid-Seydel L. Untersuchungen mit J131 markiertem Gamma-globulin zur Frage der Abstammung der Liquoreiweisskorper. *Klin Wochenschr* 1958;36:857–865.

145. Cutler RWP, Watters GV, Hammerstad J. The origin and turnover of cerebrospinal fluid albumin and gamma globulin in man. *J Neurol Sci* 1970;10:259–268.

146. LaScolea LJ Jr, Dryja D. Quantitation of bacteria in cerebrospinal fluid and blood of children with meningitis and its diagnostic significance. *J Clin Microbiol* 1984;19:187–190.

147. Dalton HP, Allison MJ. Modification of laboratory results by

partial treatment of bacterial meningitis. *Am J Clin Pathol* 1968;49:410–413.

148. Jarvis CW, Saxena KM. Does prior antibiotic treatment hamper the diagnosis of acute bacterial meningitis? An analysis of a series of 135 childhood cases. *Clin Pediatr* 1972;11:201–204.

149. Musher DM, Schell RF. False positive Gram stains of cerebrospinal fluid. *Ann Intern Med* 1973;79:603–604.

150. Joyer RW, Idriss ZH, Wilfert CM. Misinterpretation of cerebrospinal fluid Gram stain. *Pediatrics* 1974;4:360–362.

151. Washington JA, II. Bacteria, fungi and parasites. In: Mandell GL, Douglas RG Jr, Bennett JE, eds. *Principles and practice of infectious diseases,* 3rd ed. New York: Churchill Livingstone, 1990;160–193.

152. Graves M. Cerebrospinal fluid infections. In: Herndon RM, Brumback RA, eds. *The cerebrospinal fluid.* Boston: Kluwer Academic Publishers, 1989;143–165.

153. Kennedy DM, Fallon RJ. Tuberculous meningitis. *JAMA* 1979;241:264–268.

154. Barrett-Connor E. Tuberculous meningitis in adults. *South Med J* 1967;60:1061–1067.

155. Idriss ZH, Sinno AA, Kronfol NM. Tuberculous meningitis in childhood. Forty-three cases. *Am J Dis Child* 1976;130:364–367.

156. Roberts FJ. Problems in the diagnosis of tuberculous meningitis. *Arch Neurol* 1981;38:319–320.

157. Edberg SC, Samuels S. Conventional and molecular techniques for the laboratory diagnosis of infections of the central nervous system. *Neurol Clin* 1986;4:13–39.

158. McGinnis MR. Detection of fungi in cerebrospinal fluid. *Am J Med* 1983;75(1B):129–138.

159. Sabetta JR, Andriole VT. Cryptococcal infection of the central nervous system. *Med Clin N Am* 1985;69:333–344.

160. Butler WT, Alling DW, Spickard A, Utz P. Diagnostic and prognostic value of clinical and laboratory findings in cryptococcal meningitis: a follow-up study of 40 patients. *N Engl J Med* 1965;270:59–67.

161. Petri WA, Ravdin JI. Free-living amebae. In: Mandell GL, Douglas RG, Bennett JE, eds. *Principles and practice of infectious diseases,* 3rd ed. New York: Churchill Livingstone, 1990;2049–2056.

162. Lennette EH, Balows A, Hausler WJ Jr, Shadomy HJ. *Manual of clinical microbiology,* 4th ed. Washington, DC: American Society for Microbiology, 1985;687–693.

163. Lincoln EM, Sordillo SVR, Davies PA. Tuberculous meningitis in children: a review of 167 untreated and 74 treated patients with special reference to early diagnosis. *J Pediatr* 1960;57:807–823.

164. Sumaya CV, Simek J, Smith MHD, et al. Tuberculous meningitis in children during the isoniazid era. *J Pediatr* 1975;87:43–49.

165. Tandon PN. Tuberculous meningitis. In: Vincken PJ, Bruyn GW, Klawans HL, eds. *Handbook of clinical neurology,* vol 33. Amsterdam: North-Holland, 1978;195–262.

166. Bayer AS, Edwards JE, Seidel JS, Guze LB. *Candida* meningitis—review of 7 cases and review of the literature. *Medicine* 1976;55:477–486.

167. Tveten L. Candidiosis. In: Vincken PJ, Bruyn GW, eds. *Handbook of clinical neurology,* vol 35. Amsterdam: Elsevier/North-Holland, 1978;413–442.

168. Young EJ. Human brucellosis. *Rev Infect Dis* 1985;5:821–842.

169. Shakir RA, Al-Din ASN, Araj GF, et al. Clinical categories of neurobrucellosis. *Brain* 1987;110:213–223.

170. Lennette DA. Collection and preparation of specimens for virological examination. In: Lennette EH, Balows A, Hausler WJ Jr, Shadomy HJ, eds. *Manual of clinical microbiology,* 4th ed. Washington, DC: American Society for Microbiology, 1985;687–693.

171. Johnson RT. *Viral infections of the nervous system.* New York: Raven Press, 1982.

172. Rutledge J, Benjamin D, Hood L, Smith A. Is the CSF lactate measurement useful in the management of children with suspected bacterial meningitis? *J Pediatr* 1981;88:473–477.

173. Jordan GW, Statland B, Halsted C. CSF lactate in diseases of the CNS. *Arch Intern Med* 1983;143:85–87.

174. Yogev R. Advances in diagnosis and treatment of childhood meningitis. *Pediatr Infect Dis* 1985;4:321–325.

175. Jorgenson JH, Lee JC. Rapid diagnosis of gram-negative bacterial meningitis by the limulus lysate assay. *J Clin Microbiol* 1978;7:12–17.

176. Saubolle MA. Chromogenic limulus amoebocyte lysate assay as an aid in the diagnosis of meningitis. *Prog Clin Biol Res* 1985;189:369–385.

177. Fung JC, Tilton RC. Detection of bacterial antigens by counter-immunoelectrophoresis, coagglutination, and latex agglutination. In: Lennette EH, Balows A, Hausler WJ Jr, Shadomy HJ, eds. *Manual of clinical microbiology,* 4th ed. Washington, DC: American Society for Microbiology, 1985;883–904.

178. Wilson CB, Smith AL. Rapid tests for the diagnosis of bacterial meningitis. In: Remington JS, Swartz MN, eds. *Current topics in infectious diseases,* 7. New York: McGraw–Hill, 1986;134–156.

179. Sippel JE, Hider PA, Controni G, Eisenach KC, Hill HR, Rytel MW, Wasilauska BL. Use of the directigen latex agglutination test for detection of *Hemophilus influenzae, Streptococcus pneumoniae,* and *Neisseria meningitidis* antigens in cerebrospinal fluid. *J Clin Microbiol* 1984;20:884–886.

180. Sippel JE, Prato CM, Girgis NI, Edwards EA. Detection of *Neisseria meningitidis* group A, *Haemophilus influenzae* type B, and *Streptococcus pneumoniae* antigens in cerebrospinal fluid specimens by antigen capture enzyme-linked immunosorbent assays. *J Clin Microbiol* 1984;20:259–265.

181. Malan C, Donald PR, Golden M, Taljaard JJF. Adenosine deaminase levels in cerebrospinal fluid in the diagnosis of tuberculous meningitis. *J Trop Med Hyg* 1984;87:33–40.

182. Pyras MAS, Gakis C. Cerebrospinal fluid adenosine deaminase activity in tuberculous meningitis. *Enzyme* 1973;14:311–317.

183. Ribera E, Martinez-Vazquez JM, Ocana I, Segura RM, Pascual C. Activity of adenosine deaminase in cerebrospinal fluid for diagnosis and follow-up of tuberculous meningitis in adults. *J Infect Dis* 1987;155:603–607.

184. Sada E, Ruiz-Palacios GM, Lopez-Vidal Y, Ponce de Leon S. Detection of mycobacterial antigens in cerebrospinal fluid of patients with tuberculous meningitis by enzyme-linked immunosorbent assay. *Lancet* 1983;2:651–652.

185. Prabhakar S, Oommen A. ELISA using mycobacterial antigens as a diagnostic aid for tuberculous meningitis. *J Neurol Sci* 1987;78:203–211.

186. Watt G, Zaraspe G, Bautista S, Laughlin LW. Rapid diagnosis of tuberculous meningitis by using an enzyme-linked immunosorbent assay to detect mycobacterial antigen and antibody in cerebrospinal fluid. *J Infect Dis* 1988;158:681–686.

187. Chandramuki A, Allen PRJ, Keen M, Ivanyi J. Detection of mycobacterial antigen and antibodies in the cerebrospinal fluid of patients with tuberculous meningitis. *J Med Microbiol* 1985;20:239–247.

188. Steere A. Lyme disease. *N Engl J Med* 1989;321:586–595.

189. Datwyler RJ, Volkman DJ, Luft BJ, Halperin JJ, Thomas J, Golightly MG. Seronegative Lyme disease. Dissociation of specific T- and B-lymphocytic responses to *Borrelia burgdorferi. N Engl J Med* 1988;319:1441–1446.

190. Halperin JJ, Luft BJ, Anand AK, Roque CT, Alvarez O, Volkman DJ, Dattwyler RJ. Lyme neuroborreliosis: central nervous system manifestations. *Neurology* 1989;39:753–759.

191. Pachner AR, Duray P, Steere AC. Central nervous system manifestations of Lyme disease. *Arch Neurol* 1989;46:790–795.

192. Ackermann R, Rehese-Kupper B, Gollmer E, et al. Chronic neurologic manifestations of erythema migrans borreliosis. *Ann NY Acad Sci* 1989;539:16–23.

193. Goodman JS, Kaufman I, Koenig MG. Diagnosis of cryptococcal meningitis: value of immunologic detection of cryptococcal antigen. *N Engl J Med* 1971;285:434–436.

194. Snow RM, Dismukes WE. Cryptococcal meningitis: diagnostic value of cryptococcal antigen in cerebrospinal fluid. *Arch Intern Med* 1975;135:1155–1157.

195. Haldane DJM, Bauman DS, Chow AW, et al. False negative latex agglutination test in cryptococcal meningitis. *Ann Neurol* 1986;19:412–413.

196. Bouza E, Dreyer JS, Hewitt WL, Meyer RD. Coccidioidal meningitis. An analysis of thirty-one cases and review of the literature. *Medicine* 1981;60:139–172.

197. Kelly PC. Coccidioidal meningitis. In: Stevens DA, ed. *Coccidiomycosis, A text.* New York: Plenum Press, 1980;163–190.

198. Araj GF, Lulu AR, Saadah MA, et al. Rapid diagnosis of central nervous system brucellosis by ELISA. *Postgrad Med J* 1988;62:1077–1099.

199. Mousa ARM, Koshy TS, Araj GF, et al. *Brucella* meningitis: presentation, diagnosis and treatment. *Q J Med* 1986;223:873–875.

200. Bouza E, Garcia de la Torre M, Parras F, et al. Brucellar meningitis. *Rev Infect Dis* 1987;9:810–822.

201. Wheat LJ, Kohler RB, Tewari RP. Diagnosis of disseminated histoplasmosis by detection of *Histoplasma capsulatum* antigen in serum and urine. *N Engl J Med* 1986;314:83–88.

202. Luft BJ, Remington JS. Toxoplasmic encephalitis. *J Infect Dis* 1988;157:1–6.

203. Greenlee JE, Johnson WD, Campa JF, Adelman LS, Sande MA. Adult toxoplasmosis presenting as polymyositis and cerebellar ataxia. *Ann Intern Med* 1973;82:367–371.

204. Wong B, Gold JWM, Brown AE, Lange M, Fried R, Grieco M, Mildvan D, Giron J, Tapper ML, Lerner CW, Armstrong D. Central-nervous system toxoplasmosis in homosexual men and parenteral drug abusers. *Ann Intern Med* 1984;100:36–42.

205. Potasman I, Resnick L, Luft BJ, Remington JS. Intrathecal production of antibodies against *T. gondii* in patients with toxoplasmic encephalitis and AIDS. *Ann Intern Med* 1988;108:49–51.

206. Osame M, Matsumoto M, Usuku K, Izumo S, Ijichi N, Amitani H, Tara M, Igata A. Chronic progressive myelopathy associated with elevated antibodies to HTLV-I and adult T cell leukemialike cells. *Ann Neurol* 1987;21:117–122.

207. Ceroni M, Piccardo P, Rodgers-Johnson P, Mora C, Asher DM, Gajdusek DC, Gibbs CJ. Intrathecal synthesis of IgG antibodies to HTLV-I supports an etiological role for HTLV-I in tropical spastic paraparesis. *Ann Neurol* 1988;21(Suppl):S185–S187.

208. Vartdal F, Vandvik B, Norrby E. Intrathecal synthesis of virus-specific oligoclonal IgG, IgA, and IgM antibodies in a case of varicella-zoster meningoencephalitis. *J Neurol Sci* 1982;57:121–132.

209. Salmi AA, Norrby E, Panelius M. Identification of different measles virus-specific antibodies in the serum and cerebrospinal fluid from patients with subacute sclerosing panencephalitis and multiple sclerosis. *Infect Immun* 1972;6:248–254.

210. Townsend J, Baringer JR, Wolinsky JS, et al. Progressive rubella panencephalitis: late onset after congenital rubella. *N Engl J Med* 1975;292:990–993.

211. Levine DP, Lauter CB, Lerner AM. Simultaneous serum and CSF antibodies in herpes simplex encephalitis. *JAMA* 1978;240:356–360.

212. Nahmias AJ, Whitley RJ, Visintine AN, Takei Y, Alford CA, et al. Herpes simplex encephalitis: laboratory evaluations and their diagnostic significance. *J Infect Dis* 1982;145:829–836.

213. Koskiniemi M, Vaheri A, Taskinen E. Cerebrospinal fluid alterations in herpes simplex virus encephalitis. *Rev Infect Dis* 1984;6:608–618.

214. Brice JL, Tornabene TG, LaForce FM. Diagnosis of bacterial meningitis by gas–liquid chromatography. II. Analysis of spinal fluid. *J Infect Dis* 1979;140:453–464.

215. Craven RB, Brooks JB, Edman DC, Converse JD, Greenlee JE, Schlossberg D, Furlow T, Gwaltney JM, Miner WF. Rapid diagnosis of lymphocytic meningitis by frequency-pulsed electron capture gas–liquid chromatography: differentiation of tuberculous, cryptococcal and viral meningitis. *J Clin Microbiol* 1977;6:27–32.

216. Brooks JB, Choundhary G, Craven RB. Electron capture gas chromatography detection and mass spectrometry identification of 3-(2-ketohexyl)indoline in spinal fluid of patients with tuberculous meningitis. *J Clin Microbiol* 1977;5:625–628.

217. Mardh P-A, Larson L, Hoby N, Engbaek HC, Odham G. Tuberculostearic acid as a diagnostic marker in tuberculous meningitis. *Lancet* 1983;1:367.

218. French GL, Chang CY, Cheung SW, Teoh R, Humphries MJ, O'Mahoney GO. Diagnosis of tuberculous meningitis by detection of tuberculostearic acid in cerebrospinal fluid. *Lancet* 1987;2:117–119.

219. Eisenstein BI. The polymerase chain reaction: a new method of using molecular genetics for medical diagnosis. *N Engl J Med* 1990;322:178–183.

220. Burg GL, Grover CM, Pouletty P, Boothroyd JC. Direct and sensitive detection of a pathogenic protozoan, *Toxoplasma gondii*, by polymerase chain reaction. *J Clin Microbiol* 1989;27:1797–1792.

221. Rowley AH, Whitley RJ, Lakeman FD, Wolinsky SM. Rapid detection of herpes simplex-virus DNA in cerebrospinal fluid of patients with herpes simplex encephalitis. *Lancet* 1990;1:440–441.

222. Brisson-Noel A, Lecossier D, Nassif X, Gicquel B, Levy-Frebault, Hance AJ. Rapid diagnosis of tuberculosis by amplification of mycobacterial DNA in clinical samples. *Lancet* 1989;2:1069–1071.

223. Powers WJ. Cerebrospinal fluid lymphocytosis in acute bacterial meningitis. *Am J Med* 1985;79:216–220.

224. Lavetter A, Leedom JM, Mathies AW Jr, Ivler D, Wehrle PF. Meningitis due to Listeria monocytogenes, a review of 25 cases. *N Engl J Med* 1971;283:598–603.

225. Cherubin CE, Marr JS, Sierra MF, Becker S. Listeria and gram-negative bacillary meningitis in New York City, 1971–1979. *Am J Med* 1981;71:199–209.

226. Fishbein DB, Palmer DL, Porter KM, Reed WP. Bacterial meningitis in the absence of CSF pleocytosis. *Arch Intern Med* 1981;141:1369–1372.

227. Moore CM, Ross M. Acute bacterial meningitis with absent or minimal cerebrospinal fluid abnormalities. *Clin Pediatr* 1973;12:117–118.

228. Mangi RJ, Quintiliani R, Antriole VT. Gram-negative bacillary meningitis. *Am J Med* 1975;59:829–836.

229. Schwartz MN, Dodge PR. Bacterial meningitis—a review of selected aspects. I. General clinical features, special problems, and unusual meningeal reactions mimicking bacterial meningitis (continued). *N Engl J Med* 1965;272:779–787.

230. Jarvis CW, Saxena KM. Does prior antibiotic therapy hamper the diagnosis of acute bacterial meningitis? *Clin Pediatr* 1972;11:201–204.

231. Blazer S, Berant M, Alon U. Bacterial meningitis: effect of antibiotic treatment on cerebrospinal fluid. *Am J Clin Pathol* 1983;80:386–387.

232. Converse GM, Gwaltney JM, Strassburg DA, Hendley JO. Alteration of cerebrospinal fluid findings by partial treatment of bacterial meningitis. *J Pediatr* 1973;83:220–225.

233. Dalton HP, Allison MJ. Modification of laboratory results by partial treatment of bacterial meningitis. *Am J Clin Pathol* 1968,49.410–413.

234. Smith HV. Tuberculous meningitis. *Int J Neurol* 1964;4:134–157.

235. Kovacs JA, Kovacs AA, Polis M, Wright WC, Gill VJ, Tuazon CU, Gelman EP, Lane HC, Longfield R, et al. Cryptococcosis in the acquired immunodeficiency syndrome. *Ann Intern Med* 1985;103:533–538.

236. McArthur JC. Neurologic manifestations of AIDS. *Medicine* 1987;66:407–437.

237. Hooshmand H, Escobar RM, Kopf SW. Neurosyphilis. A study of 241 patients. *JAMA* 1972;219:726–729.

238. Johns DR, Tierney M, Felsenstein D. Alteration in the natural history of neurosyphilis by concurrent infection with the human immunodeficiency virus. *N Engl J Med* 1987;316:1569–1572.

239. Feraru ER, Aronow HA, Lipton RB. Neurosyphilis in AIDS patients: initial CSF VDRL may be negative. *Neurology* 1990;40:541–543.

240. Bourke SJ, Baird A, Bone FJ, Baird DR, Stevenson RD. Lyme disease with acute purulent meningitis. *Br Med J* 1988;297:460–461.

241. Feigin RD, Shackelford PG. Value of repeat lumbar puncture in the differential diagnosis of meningitis. *N Engl J Med* 1973;289:571–574.

242. Varki AP, Puthuran P. Value of second lumbar puncture in confirming a diagnosis of aseptic meningitis. *Arch Neurol* 1979;36:581–582.

243. Ratzan KE. Viral meningitis. *Med Clin North Am* 1985;69:399–413.

244. Roos R, Gajdusek DC, Gibbs CJ. The clinical characteristics of transmissible Creutzfeldt–Jakob disease. *Brain* 1973;96:1–20.

245. Committee on Health Care Issues, American Neurological Association. Precautions in handling tissues, fluids, and other contaminated materials from patients with documented or suspected Creutzfeldt–Jakob disease. *Ann Neurol* 1986;19:75–77.

Infections of the Central Nervous System,
edited by W. M. Scheld, R. J. Whitley, and
D. T. Durack, Raven Press, Ltd., New York © 1991.

CHAPTER 37

Imaging of Intracranial Infections

Robert A. Zimmerman

The introduction of new imaging techniques, first computerized tomography (CT) and then magnetic resonance imaging (MRI), has increased our ability to image the gross neuropathologic correlates of infectious processes that involve the brain and its enclosure (1). CT is rapid; scans can be performed in approximately 10–20 min, with each individual section requiring between 1 and 5 sec for data acquisition (2). Bone and blood (hematomas) are shown as areas of high density (white), whereas brain, cerebrospinal fluid (CSF), and air are shown as areas of lower density (gray to black). Routine plain CT is able to show the presence or absence of a mass, its location, and its effect on the CSF pathways. Abnormalities of the paranasal sinuses and cranial vault can be shown, such as (a) sinus opacification by infection and (b) bony defects due to fracture. CT, performed after the injection of an intravenous iodinated contrast media, shows abnormalities of the blood–brain barrier (BBB) by producing contrast enhancement (increased density, i.e., whiteness) at the site of such pathological processes (2). Thus, brain abscesses, infarcts, cerebral neoplasms, and a variety of other abnormalities can be demonstrated with a greater degree of sensitivity by postcontrast CT than by plain CT alone.

MRI is a modality which generates, in a direct fashion, images in all three planes (axial, coronal, sagittal). By manipulating the parameters involved in the setup of the MRI scan (Table 1), the images obtained can be optimized to provide information that addresses one or more of the following: (a) brain morphology; (b) brain pathology characterized by increased number of protons (free water); (c) blood products in the form of hematoma and/or its breakdown to hemosiderin; (d) blood flow within arteries and veins; and (e) disturbances of the BBB or enhancement at sites where the barrier does not

normally exist, such as in the pituitary gland, pineal gland, choroid plexus, and dura (3). Magnetic resonance (MR) images provide spatial resolution equal to that of CT, but they give contrast resolution that far exceeds that of CT. This is also true for the contrast enhancement that occurs with MR. MR has the following major disadvantages when compared to CT: (a) Data acquisition times for T1-weighted images (T1WIs) characterized by a short time to repetition (TR) and a short time to echo (TE) take several minutes, whereas T2-weighted images (T2WIs) characterized by a long TR and a long TE require many minutes. (b) Patient motion is a critical issue within the data acquisition time of the MR images: Motion will degrade studies to the point that they are not interpretable, thus requiring either patient cooperation, sedation, or general anesthesia. (c) Bone appears hypointense as does calcification, an intensity not easily separable from that of adjacent air and CSF; thus, abnormalities of the bone may be difficult to recognize. (d) Use of the magnetic fields and radiofrequency (RF) pulses to generate the images produces certain difficulties in the monitoring and support of ill patients or in the use of general anesthesia within the MR environment: Monitoring devices produce an RF output and degrade the MR scanner's image quality; ferromagnetic equipment introduced into the field of the magnet is pulled into the unit, acting as a projectile; and the magnetic field produces interference with the readout of devices, such as those using an electron gun, so that the display is not understandable (3). Despite these limitations, the high sensitivity of MR has, in many instances, made it the procedure of choice in the evaluation of patients with suspected intracranial infection (1).

CEREBRITIS

The earliest stage of purulent brain infection is cerebritis. This important CNS lesion is difficult to recognize

R. A. Zimmerman: Department of Radiology, Children's Hospital of Philadelphia, Philadelphia, Pennsylvania 19104.

TABLE 1. *Terminology used in magnetic resonance studies*

Term	Abbreviation	Meaning
Magnetic resonance imaging	MRI	An imaging modality in which high contrast is derived from inherent differences in the magnetic characteristics of tissues, most often protons of water.
T1-weighted image	T1WI	T1 is a time constant that describes the period of time required for 63% recovery (decay) of longitudinal magnetization from a higher energy state previously induced by a radiofrequency (RF) pulse. Contrast is created during recovery, because tissues that have a short T1 relaxation time recover more magnetization and produce a higher signal intensity than do those with longer T1 values.
T2-weighted image	T2WI	T2 is a time constant that describes the period of time required for the net transverse magnetization to decay to 37% of the value initially induced by the RF pulse. Contrast is created during the decay, because a tissue with a long T2 value retains its magnetization and is higher in signal intensity than are tissues with shorter T2.
Proton-density-weighted image	PDWI	Signal intensity is determined by magnetization within each tissue voxel proportional to its proton density. Imaging parameters are adjusted to produce a difference in image contrast between tissues of different proton densities.

with any degree of specificity on either CT (4,5) or MRI. On CT, the area of involvement needs to be relatively extensive so that the edema will create a low density or a mass effect that can be seen (Fig. 1). MRI is more sensitive to early edematous changes and petechial hemorrhages that occur in cerebritis. The edema is seen as a high signal intensity on the proton-density-weighted images (PDWIs) and T2WIs (Fig. 2). Mass effect is also

better appreciated on MRI because of better anatomic definition provided by multiplanar imaging, one that allows minimal compression of a gyrus or the ventricular structure to be identified. Large areas of petechial hemorrhages can be seen, with their appearance depending upon whether they are in the deoxyhemoglobin or methemoglobin state and upon the pulse sequence chosen (6). An area of deoxyhemoglobin is iso- to hypointense on

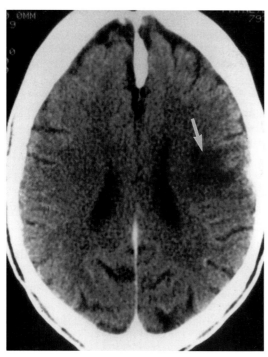

FIG. 1. Cerebritis. CT shows a vague area of hypodensity (*arrow*) in left frontoparietal region (axial non-contrast-enhanced CT).

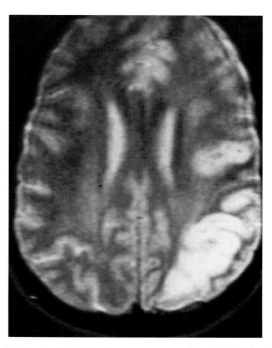

FIG. 2. Cerebritis. MR shows an area of cortical high signal intensity in left posterofrontal and parietal regions. The appearance suggests a cortical infarct (axial T2WI). In this case, this evolved into an area of cerebritis.

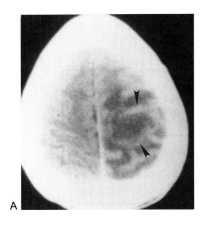
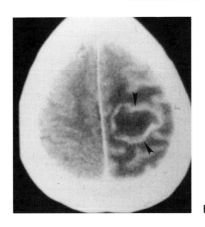

FIG. 3. Brain abscess. **A:** CT shows vasogenic edema in the left posterofrontal and parietal regions. There is a vague area of isodensity (*arrowheads*) that, in part B, becomes hyperdense following contrast administration (axial plain CT). **B:** CT shows enhancement of a thin-walled early abscess (*arrowheads*), surrounded by vasogenic edema (axial contrast-enhanced CT).

the T1WI and is markedly hypointense (black) on the T2WI. This marked hypointensity is a susceptibility effect resulting from the difference between the inherent magnetic fields within the deoxygenated red blood cell and those of the surrounding extracellular protons within the edema. The difference in the magnetic fields throws out of phase the spins of the protons that have been energized by the RF pulse. Thus no signal is returned, and the area appears black. If the petechial hemorrhages have already been oxidized from deoxyhemoglobin to methemoglobin, then the signal intensity will depend upon whether the methemoglobin is intra- or extracellular. Intracellular methemoglobin appears hyperintense (bright) on T1WI but is still hypointense on T2WI. This is because the intact red blood cell membrane creates two different areas of magnetic fields. If the red blood cell membrane has lysed as a result of the loss of nutrient supply, then the extracellular methemoglobin mixes with the surrounding edema, and the signal intensity is high on both T1WI and T2WI. The pulse sequence chosen can be optimized for identifying susceptibility effects from blood products. That is, when petechial hemorrhages cannot be seen on conventional MR images (spin echo), then gradient echo images (shorter flip angles) can be used to bring out the susceptibility effect of the petechial hemorrhages. The lack of a 180° refocusing pulse in the gradient echo image means that small areas of susceptibility effect will be emphasized as areas of marked hypointensity (6).

In an effort to better define the area of abnormality and to rule out an abscess within the zone of suspected cerebritis, it is appropriate with CT to take the examination to the next step, that of contrast enhancement (Fig. 3) (7). The same is true with MR. Gadolinium-DTPA (Magnevist, Berlex Laboratories, Cedar Knolls, New Jersey) can be injected intravenously and then imaged with multiplanar T1WI (8). Most often in the early stages, with CT or MR, there is little or no enhancement. In the later stages of cerebritis, enhancement is more marked, and the first findings suggestive of abscess formation are seen as an ovoid or round rim-like enhancement within the edematous zone (Fig. 3) (5). At this stage, the rim of enhancement is often quite thin, with the wall being ill-defined. It is important to emphasize that the radiographic findings on either CT or MR are not specific, and that the imaging findings must be interpreted in light of the clinical information. Given the situation where the imaging findings are consistent with the clinical findings and where cerebritis is suspected, either CT or MR play an important role during medical therapy in demonstrating either (a) a resolution of the process or (b) progression to brain abscess formation. When treatment has been successful, edema and any enhancement decrease and then disappear over the course of several months.

BRAIN ABSCESS

The radiographic appearance of a brain abscess is often highly suggestive, and in some instances it is rela-

TABLE 2. Brain abscess[a]

Finding	CT	MR	Sensitivity
Capsule	Isodense	T1WI: Iso- to hyperintense	Plain: MR > CT
	Enhances	T2WI: Hypo- to hyperintense	CE: MR > CT
Vasogenic edema	Hypodense	T1WI: Hypointense	Plain: MR > CT
		T2WI: Hyperintense	
Abscess contents	Hypodense	T1WI: Hypointense	Plain: MR = CT
		T2WI: Hyperintense	

[a] CT, computerized tomography; MR, magnetic resonance; T1WI, T1-weighted image; T2WI, T2-weighted image; CE, contrast-enhanced.

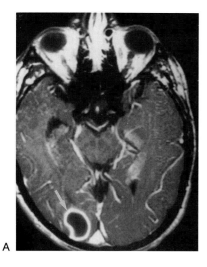

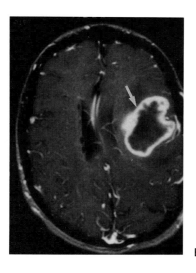

FIG. 4. Multiple brain abscesses. **A:** MR following gadolinium shows enhancement of an oblong, smooth-walled abscess (*arrow*) (axial T1WI). **B:** MR following gadolinium, at a higher level, shows a second abscess capsule (*arrow*). Note mass effect on the lateral ventricles (axial T1WI).

tively specific (Table 2). The most common finding with both CT and MR is that of a ring-enhancing mass surrounded by vasogenic edema (Figs. 3 and 4) (7,8). Most often, the mass lies at the corticomedullary juncture. Smaller, daughter rings may lie adjacent, often extending medially into the white matter. The overall amount of edema tends to be greater than the size of the abscess, and thus the mass effect is more prominent than expected for neoplasms other than glioblastoma multiforme and metastases. The thinnest portion of the contrast-enhancing ring is usually along the medial margin, in the direction of the white matter and ventricular system (9). This is thought to represent the point at which the middle collagen layer is less well developed during early abscess capsule formation (9). The abscess capsule on CT appears as a rim of tissue that is of greater density than surrounding edema or the central cavity. Thus, on the precontrast CT, the abscess wall can often be identified (Fig. 5A). This is different from the appearance of a malignant glioma, where the peripheral rim of tumor that enhances is lower in density on the preinjection study, so that it cannot be separated from the edema and necrosis. In the early stage of abscess formation the postcontrast study shows a thin rim of enhancement, whereas in the later stages the rim thickens. Chronic ab-

scess capsules can show calcification. Rarely, the abscess contains a gas-forming organism, and a gas fluid level or bubbles of gas within the abscess cavity may be seen. More often, a gas-containing abscess is one that is in continuity with a defect in a paranasal sinus or an operative site, with the air gaining access to the abscess in the same way as do the bacteria (Fig. 6).

MRI shows the edema that surrounds the abscess on PDWI and T2WI as a zone of marked high signal intensity (Fig. 7). Mass effect is graphically demonstrated. On T1WI the abscess capsule often appears as a discrete rim that is isointense to mildly hyperintense (Fig. 5B) (1). The central abscess cavity is of variable signal intensity, depending on the proteinaceousness of the fluid. On T1WI it is usually more intense than CSF, but less intense than normal brain. It is usually of increased intensity on T2WI. The abscess capsule may be either hypo- (Fig. 7) or hyperintense on T2WI. The etiology of the signal intensity changes in the abscess capsule are not precisely understood, but it may reflect signal intensities that originate from the presence of collagen and/or hemorrhage (1,9). Following the intravenous injection of gadolinium-DTPA, enhancement of the abscess capsule occurs on T1WI (Fig. 4) (10). This appears to be a very sensitive method for detecting small abscesses or multi-

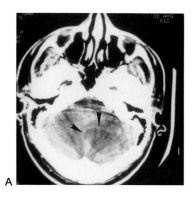

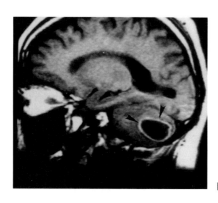

FIG. 5. Brain abscess in cerebellum. **A:** CT shows a faint rim of slightly increased density abscess capsule (*arrowheads*) in the left cerebellar hemisphere (axial noncontrast-enhanced CT). **B:** MR without contrast shows a thin-walled, hyperintense abscess capsule (*arrowheads*) (sagittal T1WI).

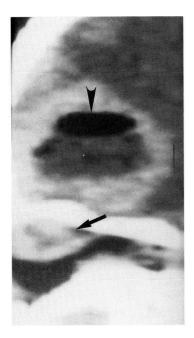

FIG. 6. Brain abscess. Sagittally reconstructed axial contrast-enhanced CT shows an air-containing brain abscess in the frontal region. Note that air (*arrowhead*) is more superior than the abscess capsule. A small collection of subperiosteal pus (*arrow*) is located in the roof of the orbit.

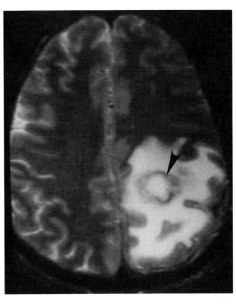

FIG. 7. Brain abscess. MR shows a high-signal-intensity mass effect in the left parietal lobe. The faint hypointense ring (*arrowhead*) is the abscess capsule (axial T2WI).

ple abscesses and for following their response to antibiotic therapy. It is important to remember that with both contrast-enhanced MRI and CT, steroids can decrease enhancement, giving a false sense of therapeutic accomplishment.

The first imaging choice for clinicians in evaluating a patient suspected of having a brain abscess is MRI. This

is because of its sensitivity. Both T2WI and pre- and post-gadolinium-enhanced T1WI should routinely be done. These should also be done at each follow-up visit. In a nonoperated early abscess of cerebritis or a surgically drained, more mature abscess, the MR studies should be repeated every 2 weeks as long as the patient is clinically improving or stable. It should also be repeated immediately if there is any sign of clinical worsening. Enhancement will continue for a prolonged period, usually several months, even when antibiotic therapy

TABLE 3. Acute meningitis[a]

Finding	CT	MR	Sensitivity
Sulcal dilatation	Hypodense CSF; enlargement of sulci	T1WI: Hypointense CSF in sulci T2WI: Hyperintense CSF in sulci	MR > CT
Leptomeningeal enhancement	CE: Increase in density of subarachnoid space	T1WI: CE: Marked increase in signal intensity	MR > CT
Ischemic cortical infarction secondary to vasculitis	Hypodense cortical mass effect CE: Subacute increase in density (enhancement)	T1WI: Hypointense cortex; mass effect T2WI: Hyperintense cortex; mass effect CE: Subacute enhancement; hyperintense on T1WI	MR > CT
Subdural collections	Hypodense peripheral CSF plus density collection CE: Hygroma—no Empyema—yes	T1WI: Hypointense peripheral collection CE: Hygroma—no Empyema—yes T2WI: Hyperintense peripheral collection	MR > CT

[a] CT, computerized tomography; MR, magnetic resonance; T1WI, T1-weighted image; CSF, cerebrospinal fluid; T2WI, T2-weighted image; CE, contrast-enhanced.

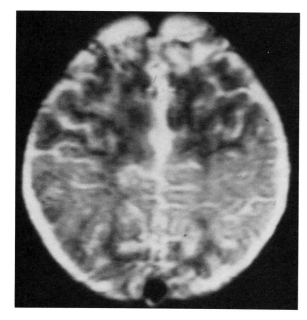

FIG. 8. Meningitis. MR shows distention of the subarachnoid space. Fluid is collected surrounding the brain. There is hypointensity in the subcortical white matter of both frontal lobes secondary to early hemorrhagic infarction from vasculitis (axial T2WI).

has been successful. Contrast-enhanced CT is a satisfactory alternative in the patient who is unable or unwilling to hold still for the MR study.

MENINGITIS

Acute Meningitis

Bacterial meningitis produces CT findings that vary from very subtle and nonspecific to overt (Table 3). Distention of the subarachnoid space on plain CT or MR is

the earliest finding (1). However, this can be difficult to read because in the adult, some degree of atrophy is common, and some normal prominence of the sulci is expected. In the first year and a half of life, sulci are also often generous. Nevertheless, enlarged sulci are usually the initial manifestation of bacterial meningitis (Fig. 8). Several days after the onset of infection, the pia covering the brain and the arachnoid lining the dura become vascularly congested so that following contrast injection, enhancement of these meninges may be seen (11). In showing this, contrast-enhanced CT is relatively less sensitive and contrast-enhanced MR is exceptionally sensitive (Fig. 9). Our own experience has been that small areas of leptomeningeal enhancement, as seen on CT, have not been harbingers of a bad outcome for the effectively treated patient. Less is known about the clinical significance of leptomeningeal enhancement seen on MR in meningitis (12). We have observed that the meninges may enhance dramatically on MR, even at a time when the infection appears to be under control. What is also not known is the time course of resolution of these MR findings following successful treatment of meningitis.

However, contrast enhancement of the cerebral cortex in the patient with bacterial meningitis is not a benign finding. It most often signifies that the walls of the blood vessels (arteries, veins, or both), bathed within the infected subarachnoid space, have become infected, so that occlusion has occurred, leading to infarction. When an artery is occluded, on plain CT this is seen as hypodense swollen areas of brain, often in a vascular distribution. On T2WI the infarcted brain shows an increase in signal involving cortex and adjacent white matter along with mass effect (Fig. 10) (13). On the contrast-enhanced CT, cortical enhancement due to infarction occurs. When the vascular involvement is that of a cortical vein,

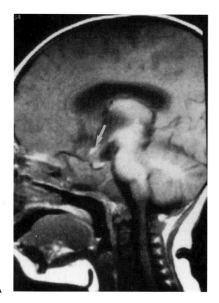

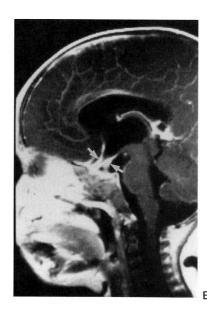

FIG. 9. Meningitis. **A:** MR without contrast shows obliteration of basilar cistern surrounding optic chiasm (*arrow*) (sagittal T1WI). **B:** MR following gadolinium shows enhancement of basilar meningitis in subarachnoid space (*arrows*) surrounding the optic chiasm. Note that hydrocephalus is present. Also note that there is enhancement of the subarachnoid space overlying the frontal lobes and on the surface of the corpus callosum (sagittal T1WI).

A

B

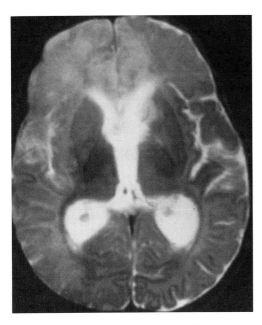

FIG. 10. Meningitis. MR shows high-signal-intensity changes in the cortex and subcortical white matter of both frontal lobes and in the right temporal lobe. There is also abnormal high signal intensity in the head of the left caudate nucleus. These findings are consistent with acute infarction due to vasculitis (axial T2WI).

the infarction is often hemorrhagic. On CT this appears as an area of high density, provided that the hemorrhagic component is significant relative to that of the edema and necrosis. MR is more sensitive than CT in demonstrating both the hemorrhagic (Fig. 11) and edematous changes (Fig. 10) of infarction due to meningitis (1). With the advent of MR angiography (14), it may be possible to demonstrate major vessel vasculitis associated with meningitis. Such findings have been shown prior to CT with carotid angiography. In patients who survive

the complications of meningitic vasculitis, the brain shows atrophic ventricular and sulcal dilatation as well as areas of cortical and subcortical infarction (Fig. 12).

In the newborn period, infants may develop neonatal meningitis due to gram-negative rods or gram-positive cocci. In this condition, ventriculitis with periventricular infarction and necrosis will occur, as will ventricular compartmentalization and hydrocephalus (15). MR is an ideal way of showing the changes of multicompartmental hydrocephalus.

Subdural collections, both infected (empyema) and sterile (hygroma), occur when the arachnoid necroses as a result of meningitis (11). The hygroma is characterized by an extracerebral peripheral CSF density (Fig. 13A) or intensity (Fig. 13B) collection that parallels the inner table of the skull, displacing the brain more centrally. Contrast enhancement is usually not seen on CT with the subdural hygroma. Our experience with contrast-enhanced MR is limited; but with the sensitivity of MR, it is possible that enhancement of the previously infected subarachnoid space would occur (Fig. 14). It would be expected that the noninfected subdural hygroma would not enhance (Fig. 13B). Pyogenic subdural collections appear to be higher in density than CSF, and they have dural and arachnoidal membranes that show enhancement (16,17). On T1WI, the signal intensity is higher than that of CSF; and on the long TR, short TE (PDWI), the signal intensity is higher than that of CSF (1). The pyogenic subdural empyema often has mass effect disproportionate to the size of the collection, and not infre-

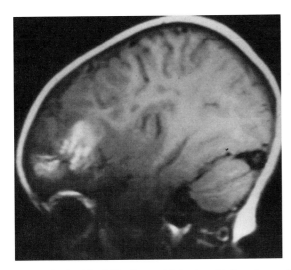

FIG. 11. Meningitis. MR shows high-signal-intensity methemoglobin in the frontal lobe at the site of cortical hemorrhagic infarction secondary to venous thrombosis from meningitis (sagittal T1WI).

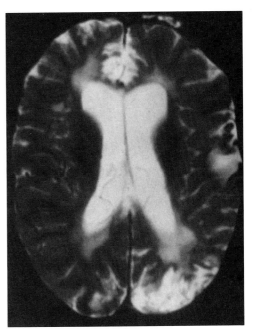

FIG. 12. Meningitis. MR shows multiple areas of old cortical and subcortical infarction, dilatation of the ventricles, and some sulci. The findings are secondary to prior meningitis with vasculitis (axial T2WI).

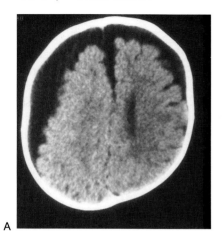
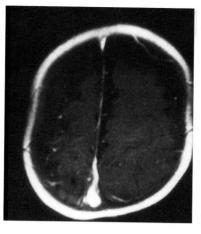

FIG. 13. Meningitis. **A:** CT shows bilateral extracerebral fluid collections compressing both frontal lobes (axial non-contrast-enhanced CT). **B:** MR following gadolinium shows no enhancement of the arachnoid, pia, or dura. Cortical veins are noted to be enhanced. The findings are consistent with a subdural hygroma (axial T1WI).

quently it is associated with underlying edema within the brain (17).

Chronic Meningitis

Blockage of the CSF pathways is a complication of meningitis and ventriculitis (Fig. 15). Blockage may occur anywhere, such as at the outlets of the fourth ventricle (foramina of Magendie and Luschka), at the tentorial incisura, around the sylvian fissures, or at the arachnoid granulations over the convexity of the brain (11). Such obstructions impede the reabsorption or the flow of CSF formed within the ventricles. Actual cystic loculations of CSF can occur within the subarachnoid space (18).

VENTRICULITIS

Ventriculitis most commonly occurs as a complication of ventriculoperitoneal shunting for hydrocephalus. Pyogenic infection of the ventricular cavity appears on CT as a loss of the distinctness of the ependymal margin (Fig. 16A) (1). Edema in the subependymal brain tissue is hypodense, so that it may not be easily distinguished from ventricular CSF. The margin of the ventricular wall also often becomes irregular. Pyogenic material within

the ventricle can be increased in density relative to non-infected CSF elsewhere. This increase in density is because of an increase in the protein content of the pyogenic ventricular fluid. Periventricular edema adds to the mass effect produced by the distention of the obstructed ventricular system. The lateral ventricles drain through the foramen of Monro into the third ventricle, which, in turn, drains through the aqueduct of Sylvius into the fourth ventricle. Both are sites of narrowing and potential obstruction. Fluid within the fourth ventricle drains through its outlets into the cisterna magna and cerebellopontine angles. These outlets, the foramina of Luschka and Magendie, are other sites of vulnerability for obstruction, which may result in acute or chronic hydrocephalus.

When the infected ependyma becomes hyperemic, enhancement occurs following intravenous contrast. Enhancement is better shown with MR (Fig. 17) but is often well shown with CT (Fig. 18). On MR, the tissue surrounding the ventricle is high in signal intensity on T2WI (Fig. 16B) (1). The margin of the ventricle appears irregular, and loculation of portions of the ventricle are common (Fig. 19). The content of the ventricles is higher in signal intensity than that of CSF on T1WI (Fig. 19A) and PDWI.

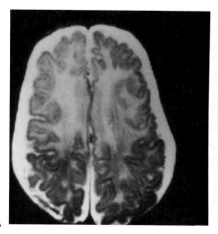
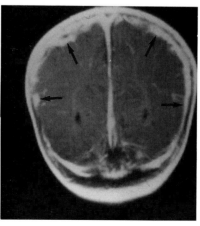

FIG. 14. Meningitis. **A:** MR shows marked distention of the subarachnoid and subdural spaces bilaterally (axial T2WI). **B:** MR following gadolinium shows marked enhancement of the subarachnoid and subdural spaces (*arrows*). The patient was clinically improving at this time and subsequently went on to a noneventful recovery (coronal T1WI).

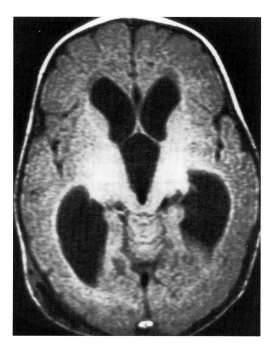

FIG. 15. Postmeningitic hydrocephalus. MR without contrast shows marked dilatation of the lateral and third ventricles down to the aqueduct. A shunt valve is present in the right occipital region. The patient has aqueductal stenosis secondary to meningitis (axial T1WI).

SUBDURAL AND EPIDURAL EMPYEMAS

Bacterial infections within the extracerebral spaces occur not only as complications of meningitis, but also as complications of sinusitis and other extracranial sources of infection. It is important to (a) recognize the intracranial infected collection, (b) recognize its need for treatment, and (c) identify its source. Abnormal density or signal intensity within the paranasal sinuses suggests, but does not guarantee, that the sinus is the origin of the

intracranial infection, because mucous retention cysts or allergic sinusitis can produce changes within the sinus but are not a source of infection. Occasionally, septic thrombophlebitis spreading from the paranasal sinus can actually be identified. Recognition of bony defects, such as those associated with fractures of the paranasal sinuses or calvarium, are best shown on CT (16). Both contrast-enhanced CT (Fig. 20) and MR (Fig. 21) are sensitive and reasonably specific, given the appropriate clinical circumstances. Signal intensity within these collections is high on PDWI, thereby causing them to stand out so that they can be recognized (Fig. 22) (1). A very small, yet significant, collection may be difficult to appreciate on CT. Multiplanar gadolinium-enhanced MR is probably the most sensitive test for identifying infected extracerebral collections. Underlying edema and swelling of the brain are other important signs to look for.

TUBERCULOMA

Tuberculoma appears on CT most often as a discrete, round lesion. It is usually found at the corticomedullary junction, and it contrast-enhances (Fig. 23) (19). The typical size is 5–15 mm in diameter. Occasionally, the lesion reaches such a size that it mimics a mass lesion such as a brain tumor. More often the lesion is multiple, less often solitary. Calcification, when present, is best seen by CT. On MR, the experience with tuberculomas has been relatively limited. Their appearance on MR has been that of a discrete corticomedullary juncture lesion which is hypointense on T1WI but which on T2WI tends to have a rim of surrounding hyperintensity (Fig. 24) (1,20). Enhancement with gadolinium-DTPA is often intense.

Tuberculous meningitis is seen on plain CT as an increase in density within the basilar subarachnoid space

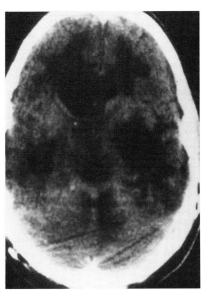

A

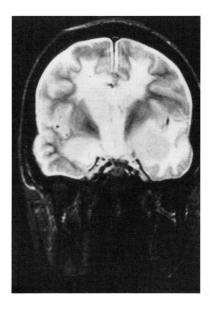

FIG. 16. Ventriculitis. **A:** CT shows indistinctness of the margins of the lateral ventricles due to subependymal, periventricular edema from ependymitis (axial CT). **B:** MR shows dilatation of the ventricular system with extensive surrounding vasogenic edema in the periventricular white matter
B (coronal T2WI).

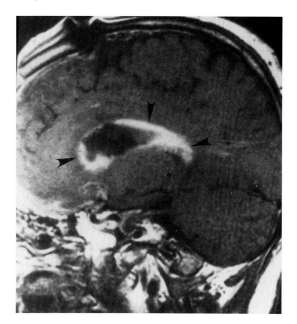

FIG. 17. Ventriculitis. MR following gadolinium injection shows marked enhancement of the ependymal surface (*arrowheads*) secondary to ventriculitis (sagittal T1WI).

(21,22). In conjunction, hydrocephalus, either obstructive or communicating, can be seen. A coexisting tuberculoma should be searched for (1). Following contrast injection, the basilar subarachnoid spaces enhance markedly, appearing thickened and distended (Fig. 23) (21,22). The tuberculoma that is associated with meningitis is often well shown following contrast (Fig. 23). With gadolinium-DTPA on T1WI the basilar meningitis enhances dramatically. In patients who have been successfully treated for tuberculous meningitis, CT may show (a) persistent hydrocephalus requiring shunting and (b) persistent obliteration of basilar subarachnoid space; it may even reveal calcification of these spaces.

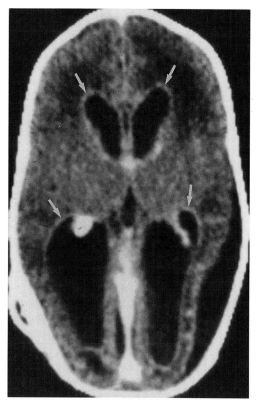

FIG. 18. Ventriculitis. Postcontrast CT shows marked enhancement (*arrows*) of the ependymal lining of both ventricles secondary to ventriculitis, as well as a left subdural hygroma and a right-sided posterior temporal shunt valve (axial CT).

CAVERNOUS SINUS THROMBOSIS

The cavernous sinuses are dural-covered structures lying on either side of the sella and pituitary gland. They contain large venous channels, the internal carotid arteries, and the cranial nerves 3, 4, the first and second

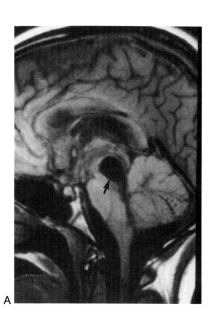

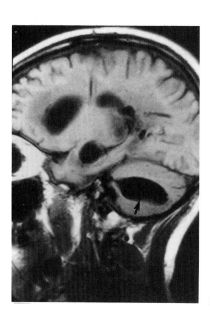

FIG. 19. Ventriculitis. **A:** MR without contrast through the region of the third ventricle shows filling of the third ventricular cavity by debris and loculation of CSF in the aqueductal region (*arrow*) (sagittal T1WI). **B:** MR further laterally shows marked irregularity and narrowing of the lateral ventricle and temporal horn and marked dilatation of the lateral recess of the fourth ventricle (*arrow*) (sagittal T1WI).

A

B

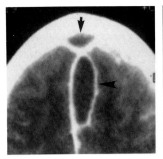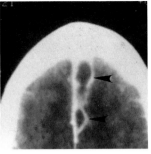

A

B

FIG. 20. Epidural and subdural empyemas secondary to sinusitis. **A** and **B:** Contiguous contrast-enhanced CT sections show an epidural collection (*arrow*) and left parafalcine subdural empyema (*arrowheads*).

divisions of 5, and 6. The bone of the body of the sphenoid containing the sphenoid sinus is positioned both medially and inferiorly. The cavernous sinuses transmit cranial nerves to the orbit and receive blood draining back from the orbit, paranasal sinuses, nasal cavity and nasopharynx, and face. The spread of bacterial or fungal infection either directly from the sphenoid sinus through osteomyelitis or along dehiscences in the bone, or retrograde extension of infection as a thrombophlebitis from the orbit or facial structures, can produce a septic cavernous sinus thrombosis. Radiographically, there are a number of ways to image both the structure of the cavernous sinus and the flow of blood within it. The patency of the venous channels within the cavernous sinus can be imaged by retrograde injection of dye from a scalp vein in the mid-forehead. By compressing scalp veins above the site of injection, and by compressing facial veins over the cheek, dye flows back through the angular veins into the orbit and through the superior ophthalmic veins to the cavernous sinuses. This method requires skill in cannulating the scalp vein in the forehead and in obtaining the proper compression of collateral venous routes. With this method, cavernous sinus patency or obstruction can

be demonstrated (23). A more invasive way of demonstrating the venous flow within the cavernous sinus is by retrograde catheterization of the inferior petrosal sinus. A catheter is placed either via the common femoral vein in the groin or via the jugular vein in the neck, retrograde into the inferior petrosal sinuses. By retrograde injection into the cavernous sinus, opacification is obtained. This method carries with it some element of risk, because rupture of intracranial veins has been known to occur. Carotid arteriography, via the femoral artery, can be performed for both carotids, demonstrating whether or not the intracavernous portion of the internal carotid artery is patent or narrowed. In patients with septic cavernous sinus thrombosis, frequently the intracavernous internal carotid artery is compressed or occluded. Today, magnetic resonance angiography (MRA) allows visualization of the intracavernous internal carotid artery flow, sufficient to rule out the need for conventional arteriography (14). By injecting intravenous gadolinium and then performing MRA, patency of the venous component of the cavernous sinus can be demonstrated.

For anatomic demonstration of the cavernous sinus structure unrelated to flow, the choice is between MR and CT (24). CT has the advantage of showing detail of the bony structures. With thin sections, cranial nerves 3 and 5 can be visualized as relative round hypodensities on an enhanced study. Enlargement of the cavernous sinus by clot can be shown. MR is more sensitive in the demonstration of clotted blood products within the cavernous sinus. In the coronal plane, anatomic demonstration of the cavernous sinus is often better with MR than with CT. With conventional MR, rapidly flowing blood within the internal carotid artery stands out (as a flow void) from the more slowly moving blood within the venous network. With septic thrombosis, cavernous sinuses appear distended and the signal intensity is dependent on the chemical composition of the clotted blood (Fig. 25).

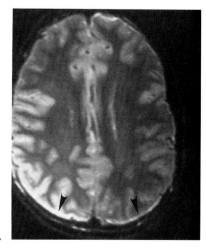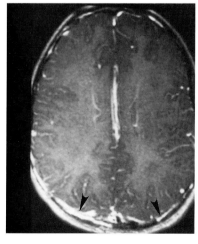

A

B

FIG. 21. Subdural empyema. **A:** MR shows a high-signal-intensity posterior peripheral extraaxial fluid collection (*arrowheads*) (axial PDWI). **B:** MR following gadolinium shows enhancement of the collections (*arrowheads*) (axial T1WI).

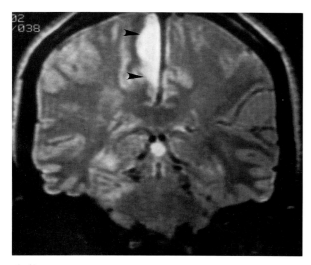

FIG. 22. Subdural empyema. MR shows a high-signal-intensity (*arrowheads*) right parafalcine subdural empyema (coronal PDWI).

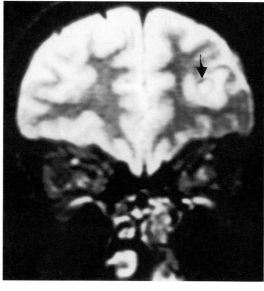

FIG. 24. Tuberculoma. MR shows a high-signal-intensity zone of edema surrounding a hypointense rim (*arrow*) containing a central high-intensity tuberculoma (coronal PDWI).

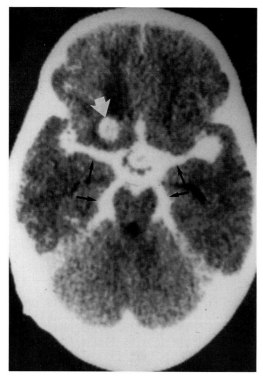

FIG. 23. Tuberculoma with tuberculous meningitis. CT shows a contrast-enhanced tuberculoma (*white arrow*) and marked enhancement of tuberculous meningitic granulomatous disease within the basilar cisterns (*black arrow*) (axial contrast-enhanced CT).

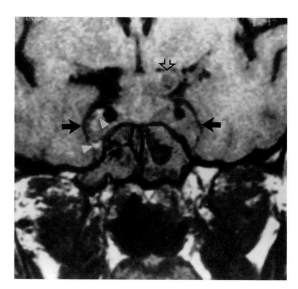

FIG. 25. Cavernous sinus thrombosis, suprasellar abscess, and sphenoid sinusitis. MR without gadolinium shows opacification of both air cells of the sphenoid sinus, bilateral distention of the cavernous sinus's dura (*arrows*), an area of high signal clot in the right cavernous sinus (*arrowheads*), and a left suprasellar mass (*open arrow*) adjacent to the optic chiasm (coronal T1WI).

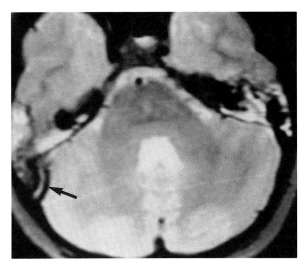

FIG. 26. Mastoiditis with right sigmoid sinus venous thrombosis. MR shows high-signal-intensity changes in both mastoid air cells. The right sigmoid sinus (*arrow*) shows variable curvilinear low and high signal intensities consistent with clot (axial T2WI).

EAR INFECTIONS

Acute mastoiditis is less common today, but the process can still be fulminant. Opacification of the mastoid air cells and development of soft tissue inflammation surrounding the mastoid are signs that can be demonstrated with CT or MR. Bony detail is seen only with CT; for this reason, it is the procedure of choice. Opacification of mastoid air cells is seen with both techniques, but it stands out more so on MR because of its sensitivity to water within the inflamed mucosa of the mastoid air cells (Fig. 26). The complications of mastoiditis include the development of brain abscesses within adjacent structures, such as (a) the temporal lobe above the petrous ridge or (b) the cerebellum behind it. An additional complication is thrombosis involving the sigmoid dural venous sinus. This occurs when infection perforates the sinus plate (a wall of the mastoid air cells), and involves the venous sinus. Also, the mastoid drains venous blood into the sigmoid sinus, and thus the extension of septic venous thrombosis from mastoid to venous sinus is an-

other possibility. Dural sinus thrombosis may lead to intracranial venous hypertension, hydrocephalus, and papilledema. Sigmoid dural venous sinus occlusion was previously demonstrated by arteriography or digital venous subtraction angiography, techniques which continue to be useful but which are now being supplanted by MR and/or MRA (14). Flowing blood in the sigmoid sinus is seen as an area of hypointensity on conventional MR. Isointensity or hyperintensity indicates absence of flow (Fig. 26). These findings, when put together with changes of inflammatory disease in the adjacent mastoid, indicate infection and its complication.

Malignant external otitis, an infection of the external auditory canal usually due to *Pseudomonas aeruginosa,* occurs in elderly patients who are often diabetic. With extension of the infection (via cartilage) into the hypotympanum, bacterial infection gains access to the cranial base and may produce jugular vein occlusion; as a result of osteomyelitis, this infection can extend intracranially into the posterior fossa in and around the basilar artery. CT is useful in showing bony destructive changes, opacification of air cells, and soft tissue swelling consistent with this invasive disease process (25). MR is useful in showing the changes of infection within the air-containing structures of the ear; it is also useful in demonstrating loculation of the abscess in the hypotympanum (with gadolinium enhancement), as well as in showing involvement of the jugular vein.

VIRAL INFECTIONS

Herpes Simplex

In the patient suspected of having herpes simplex infection due to reactivation of the virus, the methods of evaluation are either CT or MR, with or without enhancement (Table 4). CT changes are usually not seen before the fifth day after onset of symptoms (26,27). What is shown on CT, however, is hypodensity involving the anterior and medial aspects of the temporal lobe(s) and the inferior aspects of the frontal lobe(s) (Fig. 27) (26). These may be bilateral or unilateral. Smaller or larger areas of hemorrhage are also suggestive of herpes.

TABLE 4. *Findings on CT and MR imaging of patients with encephalitis*[a]

Finding	CT	MR	Sensitivity
Brain swelling	Hypodense mass effect	Mass effect T1WI: Hypointense T2WI: Hyperintense	MR > CT
Pial–parenchymal enhancement	CE: Increase in density	CE T1WI: Increase in signal	MR > CT
Hemorrhage	Hyperdensities	T1WI and T2WI: Hypo- to hyperintense foci	MR > CT

[a] CT, computerized tomography; MR, magnetic resonance; T1WI, T1-weighted image; T2WI, T2-weighted image; CE, contrast-enhanced.

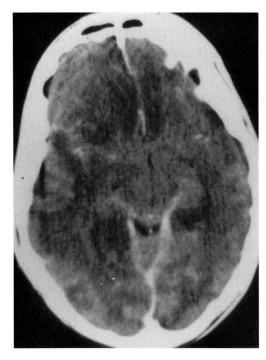

FIG. 27. Herpes simplex infection. CT shows hypodensity and mass effect involving the right temporal lobe and right frontal lobe (axial contrast-enhanced CT).

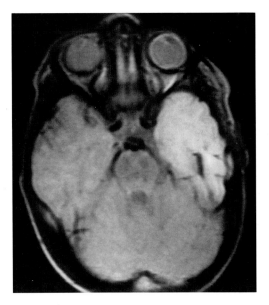

FIG. 28. Herpes simplex infection. MR shows marked high signal intensity in the left temporal lobe (axial PDWI).

However, such gross evidence of hemorrhage is unusual on CT (1). Involvement by low density of the island of Reil at the depths of the sylvian fissure, especially when it is bilateral, may be close to pathognomonic of herpes infection. Contrast enhancement of the pia and cortex can be seen once disruption of the BBB has occurred. With CT, this is usually not before the second week after onset of symptoms (28). In order for CT to be useful in subtle cases of herpes infection, the CT examination has to be optimized in order to prevent artifacts that often obscure the detail of the temporal lobe. The plane of slice should be angled parallel to the temporal lobe. The sec-

tion should be thin enough that partial voluming of temporal lobe with adjacent bone does not obscure a portion of the temporal lobe. Reconstructed coronal images or direct coronal images may be important in identifying subtle swelling and small hemorrhages.

MR gives unparalleled sensitivity to the increased water content that occurs with herpes infection. Thus the areas of involvement stand out as areas of increased signal intensity on PDWI and T2WI (Fig. 28). MR shows the temporal lobes and inferior frontal lobes to be swollen, and it also shows them to be of low signal intensity on T1WI and of high signal on PDWI and T2WI (Fig. 28) (1). Hemorrhages are shown with greater sensitivity by MR than by CT. MR has greater sensitivity than CT in showing involvement of the depths of the sylvian cortex as an area of high signal on PDWI (Fig. 29A) (10). T1WI with gadolinium enhancement shows cortical pial

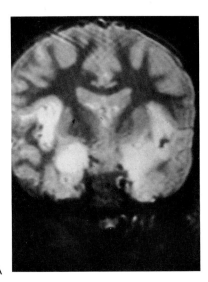

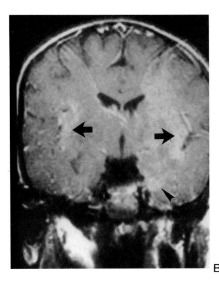

FIG. 29. Herpes simplex infection. A: MR shows bilateral involvement of the medial temporal lobes and insular cortex by high-signal-intensity changes (coronal PDWI). B: MR following gadolinium injection shows contrast enhancement of the sylvian cortex (arrows) bilaterally, and of the medial aspect of the left temporal lobe (arrowhead) (coronal T1WI).

A

B

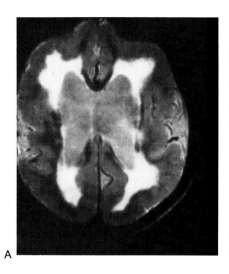

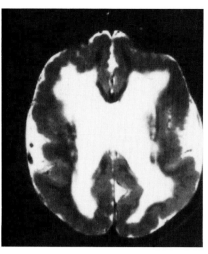

A

B

FIG. 30. Cytomegalic virus, congenitally transmitted. **A** and **B**: MR shows the following: a rather flat surface of the brain, consistent with a migrational abnormality; ventricular dilatation, consistent with atrophy; and high-signal-intensity changes in the periventricular white matter, consistent with gliosis (axial PDWI and T2WI).

and subpial abnormalities of the BBB (Fig. 29B). Follow-up studies have shown loss of substance, necrosis of brain, dilatation of the ventricles, and enlargement of sulci.

Cytomegalovirus

Congenital transmission of cytomegalovirus (CMV) before the third trimester of gestation can produce findings seen on both CT and MR in the newborn infant's brain. CT findings are those of subependymal and/or deeper white-matter calcification (29). Hypodensity within the white matter reflects gliosis and necrosis (29). Depending upon whether or not migration of neurons was interfered with by the transplacental CMV infection, there may be evidence of broad, flat gyri indicating a pachygyric-like change (probably micropolygyria) (30). MR is excellent at showing the destruction of the white matter and its involvement with gliosis as high signal intensity on T2WI (Fig. 30) (30). The calcification that is seen on CT is not seen on MR, except as a rare focal area of hypointensity. What is seen even better with MR than with CT is the appearance of a somewhat thickened and irregular cortex, a pachygyric-like change (Fig. 30B) (30).

Acute Disseminated Encephalomyelitis

This is a rare complication of a systemic viral infection, such as chickenpox. An immune reaction occurs, leading to white-matter demyelination in the CNS. Typically, symptoms develop 1–3 weeks after the viral infection. Areas of high signal intensity may be seen in the white matter, basal ganglia, brainstem, and cerebellum (Fig. 31). The most common pattern is one of an asymmetric distribution of lesions. These are best demonstrated on PDWI and T2WI (Fig. 31) (31,32). They are poorly (or not at all) seen on CT. Steroid therapy tends to

ameliorate the symptoms and to decrease the size and extent of the MR findings.

Human Immunodeficiency Virus (HIV) Infection and Acquired Immunodeficiency Syndrome (AIDS)

Subacute encephalopathy due to HIV infection has a range of manifestations on CT and MR that range from normal to atrophy, with a distinctly abnormal picture within the white matter (Fig. 32) (9). Shortly after the onset of symptoms of subacute encephalopathy, the CT and MR studies are often normal (Fig. 32A). Later, atrophy in the form of sulcal and ventricular enlargement is present. Eventually, one can see (a) hypodensity on CT within the white matter and (b) increased signal intensity

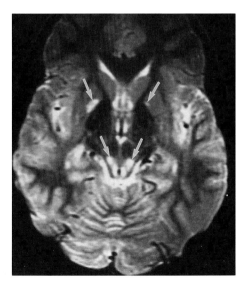

FIG. 31. Acute disseminated encephalomyelitis. MR shows high-signal-intensity foci (*arrows*) in both putamen and upper brainstem, consistent with acute demyelinating disease (axial T2WI).

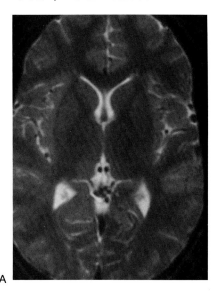

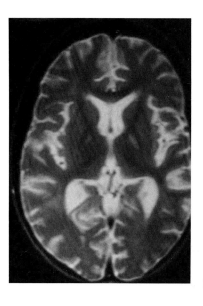

FIG. 32. AIDS. **A:** MR appears normal (axial T2WI). **B:** MR 6 months later shows dilatation of sulci and ventricles consistent with atrophy, along with focal areas of high signal intensity in the posterior limbs of the internal capsules bilaterally (axial T2WI).

on PDWI and T2WI (Fig. 32B). Contrast enhancement with CT and MR has not been a finding. Other causes of low density and high signal intensity within the white matter are seen in patients with HIV infection (33). These include progressive multifocal leukoencephalopathy (PML) due to JC papovavirus—a complication seen not only in AIDS patients, but also in patients with chronic lymphocytic leukemia and other immunocompromising conditions. The CT appearance of PML is that of multifocal areas of decreased density within the white matter, with peripheral contrast enhancement at some point. On PDWI and T2WI, the appearance of PML is one of increased signal intensity. Following gadolinium injection, at some point in the course of the disease, marginal contrast enhancement may be seen. Mass effect is most often not characteristic, but extension of the disease process along white-matter tracks and pathways is characteristic. In the congenital AIDS infection in the infant, calcification within the basal ganglia can be a finding. This is different from the calcification seen throughout the brain in the TORCH syndromes such as CMV and toxoplasmosis.

Imaging is essential for demonstration of opportunistic CNS infections due to viruses, fungi, parasites or bacteria in HIv-infected patients (9). Also there are the complications related to neoplasms that induce immunodeficiency, such as lymphomas. CMV produces meningitis, ependymitis, and areas of parenchymal infection. On CT and MR, CMV encephalitis produces edema and mass effect (33). Ependymitis suggests changes found in ventriculitis, but they are often less marked. Meningitis is usually not radiographically visible. However, with gadolinium-enhanced T1-weighted images, the pia and adjacent subarachnoid space may be seen to enhance in some patients.

The most common etiology of a focal parenchymal brain lesion in the patient with AIDS is *Toxoplasma gondii*. Ring or nodular contrast-enhancing multiple le-

sions, most often involving the basal ganglia, are the most frequent manifestation on CT (Fig. 33) (34). Prior to contrast injection they appear as low-density areas, with the toxoplasmic lesions often being indistinguishable from surrounding edema. Contrast enhancement separates the lesion from the surrounding edema. MR is much more sensitive than CT, showing vasogenic edema as hypointensity on T1WI and hyperintensity on T2WI. On T2WI the toxoplasmic lesion is often a ring of lesser intensity within the center of the edematous zone (Fig.

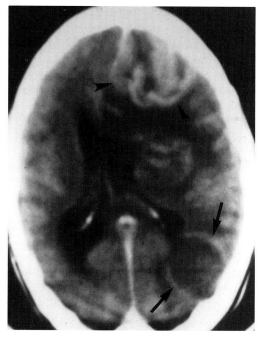

FIG. 33. *Toxoplasma* complicating AIDS. CT shows an irregular, ring-like, contrast-enhancing mass (*arrowheads*) in the left frontal lobe, surrounded by vasogenic edema. A ring-like lesion is also present (*arrows*) in the left parietal lobe. There is marked mass effect with displacement of the ventricles across the midline (axial contrast-enhanced CT).

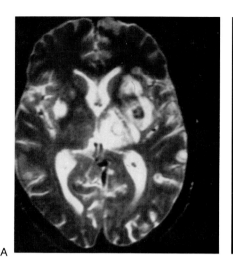
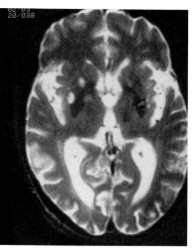

FIG. 34. *Toxoplasmosis* complicating AIDS, before and after treatment. **A:** MR shows multiple high-signal-intensity zones of edema with a central hypointensity (axial T2WI). **B:** One year later, following treatment for *Toxoplasma,* MR shows some atrophy with dilatation of the sylvian fissures but shows significantly reduced size of the toxoplasmic lesions (axial T2WI).

34A) (33). Gadolinium shows contrast enhancement of the toxoplasmic lesion. MR gives a sensitive method for following the response of the toxoplasmic lesion to treatment. Reduction in size of the lesion and in its enhancement can be graphically demonstrated (Figs. 34B and 35B). Differentiation of the toxoplasmic lesion from lymphoma is not possible on the basis of the imaging appearance. Lymphoma is more often a solid lesion, which on CT is slightly increased in density and enhances homogeneously, whereas the toxoplasmic lesion is more often low in density and enhances in a ring-like fashion. However, some lymphomas may show ring-like enhancement. The same is true for MR, since both lymphoma and *Toxoplasma* can appear on T2WI as an area of high signal intensity containing an area of focal lower signal intensity within it. Both lesions show gadolinium enhancement on T1WI. The differentiation of the two disease processes is based on either (a) biopsy or (b) the response of the toxoplasmic lesion to treatment.

A wide variety of other pathogens have been found in the brains of patients with AIDS. These include *Candida* and *Mycobacterium tuberculosis,* among others. Pyo-

genic bacterial infections are the only type of infection that are not common, because the immune deficit lies in cell-mediated, rather than humoral, immunity.

Cryptococcosis

Cryptococcal meningitis has only subtle signs on CT and MR (9). Studies may appear normal despite the presence of cryptococcal meningitis. Subtle dilatation of the subarachnoid space and the presence of hydrocephalus should suggest the possibility of cryptococcal meningitis.

Aspergillus Infection

Aspergillus, a ubiquitous mold in the environment, presents in the nonimmunocompromised patient most often as an inflammation of the sinus mucosa. This can be a chronic condition, in which the mucosa becomes polypoid and in which the bony wall becomes reactively sclerotic. Hemorrhagic changes in the infected sinus mu-

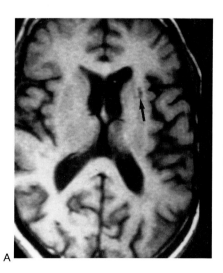
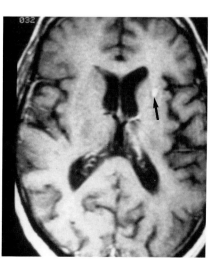

FIG. 35. *Toxoplasmosis* complicating AIDS. **A:** MR without gadolinium shows a small focal lucency (*arrow*) in the left basal ganglia (axial T1WI). **B:** MR following gadolinium injection shows focal enhancement of the small toxoplasmic lesion (*arrow*) (axial T1WI).

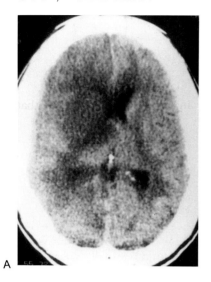
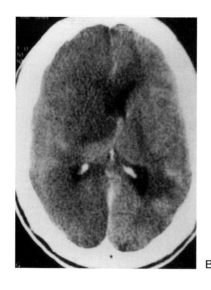

FIG. 36. Mucormycosis with infarction of brain. **A:** CT without contrast enhancement shows hypodensity and mass effect involving the right frontal and temporal lobes (axial CT). **B:** CT following contrast injection shows no evidence of enhancement (axial CT).

cosa are not uncommon. If the patient is then immunocompromised, the spread of *Aspergillus* beyond the confines of the paranasal sinus into structures such as the cavernous sinus and subarachnoid space may occur. Invasion of blood vessels with secondary thrombosis and

infarction are well-recognized complications (35). As a result, fungal brain abscesses may be seen. Because of the vasculitic component, hemorrhagic infarction is common; and because of extension of *Aspergillus* to the subarachnoid space, meningitis and meningoencephalitis

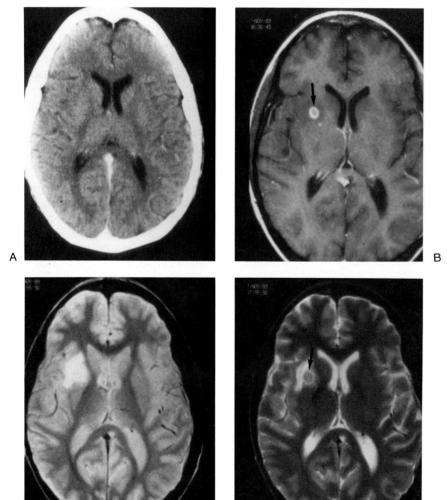

FIG. 37. Candidal abscess. **A:** Contrast-enhanced CT shows no abnormality 2 weeks prior to performing the MR scan shown in part B (axial CT). **B:** MR following gadolinium injection shows a focal, round, contrast-enhancing (*arrow*) lesion within the right putamen (axial T1WI). **C** and **D:** MR shows edema in the lateral basal ganglia, with the abscess appearing relatively hypointense (*arrow*) (PDWI and T2WI).

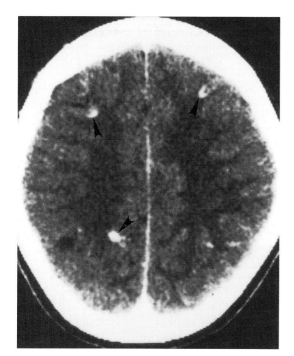

FIG. 38. Cysticercosis. Post-contrast-enhanced CT shows multiple gray-matter calcifications (*arrowheads*) (axial CT).

can occur. In the immunocompromised patient, the inflammatory response to the spread of infection is reduced, and the CT and MR studies reflect this compromise. The *Aspergillus* abscess grows rapidly; the ring enhancement seen in patients with normal defense mechanisms are often absent or minimal. Both CT and MR show hemorrhagic as well as nonhemorrhagic infarction.

Mucormycosis behaves in a fashion similar to that of

aspergillosis (35). It is a dreaded complication in the elderly diabetic. Sinus inflammation due to *Mucor* leads to invasion of the cavernous sinus and carotid arteries, with vascular dissemination and infarction (Fig. 36). *Candida* may produce meningitis or brain abscess (Fig. 37). *Cryptococcus, Histoplasma,* and *Coccidioides* are fungi that usually produce chronic meningitis.

PARASITIC DISEASES

Cysticercosis

In cysticercosis infection of humans, the brain is the second most common organ to be involved, after skeletal muscle. Clinical manifestations usually occur after the parasite dies; as a result, symptoms may not occur until many years after the onset of infection. Cysticerci are found within the subarachnoid space adherent to the meninges, within the ventricular system, and within the cerebral gray matter. An inflammatory response to the parenchymal cysticerci involves the following: fibroconnective tissue; granulation tissue; and chronic inflammatory cells, consisting of monocytes, plasma cells, lymphocytes, and eosinophils. Following death of the organism, a more marked inflammatory response occurs, leading to calcification of the organism (1). Calcifications can be seen on CT as focal hyperdensities at the appropriate location (Fig. 38) (36). On MR, calcification is poorly shown, and MR may only indicate the presence of the dead cysticerci as a zone of high signal intensity on T2WI in the brain surrounding the dead organism (1). The acute intraparenchymal phase of the cysticercosis is shown on CT as an area of low density that, following

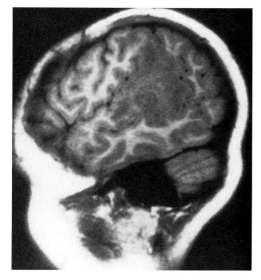 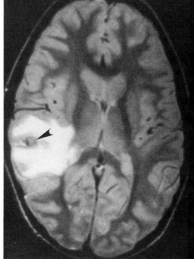 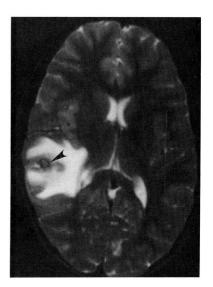

A B C

FIG. 39. Cysticercosis. **A:** MR shows a hypointense mass within the frontoparietal temporal juncture zone (sagittal T1WI). **B** and **C:** MR shows vasogenic edema and a more hypointense cysticercus cyst (*arrowheads*) (axial PDWI and T2WI).

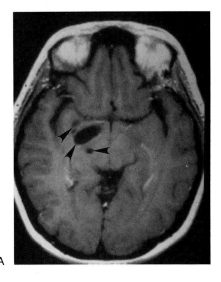

A

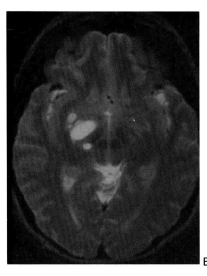

B

FIG. 40. Cysticercosis. A: MR following gadolinium injection shows multiple CSF intensity cysts (*arrowheads*) projecting from the basilar subarachnoid space into the brain parenchyma (axial T1WI). B: MR shows the same cysts to be the same signal intensity as CSF (axial T2WI).

contrast injection, enhances either homogeneously or in a ring-like pattern (37). This phase is shown on MR as high signal intensity edema of a vasogenic nature, surrounding the lesion on T2WI (Fig. 39). The cysticerci are seen as areas of lower signal intensity, often ring-like lesions on the T2WI (Fig. 39C). On T1WI the lesion is hypointense, as is the edema; following gadolinium injection, the cyst enhances, whereas the edema does not. The subarachnoid cysticerci are found as smaller or larger cysts either within the subarachnoid space (Fig. 40) or within the ventricular system. As a result of the obstruction of the CSF pathways, an obstructive or communicating hydrocephalus may be present, both of which can be shown by dilatation of the ventricles or subarachnoid pathways on CT (38) or MR. Recognizing the cyst within the ventricle on CT may be difficult. The contents have the same density as CSF; furthermore, the membranes are thin, and they usually do not enhance. Cysticercosis cysts within the basilar subarachnoid space can be outlined on CT performed after the instillation of water-soluble, iodinated contrast media as used for myelography. MR is able to show cysts within the basilar subarachnoid space with a higher degree of accuracy than does regular CT. Suss et al. (39) have reported the MR findings in cysticercosis. Cysts with live cysticerci within the brain have a reasonably characteristic configuration on T1WI MR. This is a low-intensity cystic lesion, with the fluid's signal intensity paralleling CSF, whereas the scolex within it is a much smaller mural high-signal-intensity nodule.

SUMMARY

The decision as to which imaging procedure to choose in the diagnostic evaluation of the patient with suspected intracranial infection depends on what pathology is expected and how it manifests itself, as well as on the status of the patient relative to the ability to tolerate the examination. CT remains the easiest examination, giving information regarding mass effect and the status of the ventricular system. Bony detail and calcifications are the province of CT. MR, while needing more time for data acquisition and being more complex in requirements for patient motion and support, offers a greater degree of sensitivity in demonstrating abnormalities of brain parenchyma and in showing changes that affect the meninges.

REFERENCES

1. Zimmerman RA, Bilaniuk LT, Sze G. Intracranial Infection. In: Brant-Zawadski M, Norman D, eds. *Magnetic resonance imaging of the central nervous system.* New York: Raven Press, 1987;235–257.
2. Gibby WA, Zimmerman RA. *X-ray computed tomography.* Contemporary Anatomy Series. FA Davis, 1991 in press.
3. Zimmerman RA, Bilaniuk LT, Hackney DB. Applications of magnetic resonance imaging in diseases of the pediatric central nervous system. *Magn Reson Imaging* 1986;4:11–24.
4. Zimmerman RA, Bilaniuk LT, Shipkin PM, et al. Evolution of cerebral abscess: correlation of clinical features with computed tomography—a case report. *Neurology* 1977;27:14–19.
5. Enzmann DR, Britt RH, Placone R. Staging of human brain abscess by computed tomography. *Radiology* 1983;146:703–708.
6. Barkovich AJ, Atlas SW. Magnetic resonance imaging of intracranial hemorrhage. *Radiol Clin North Am* 1988;26(4):801–820.
7. Whelan MA, Hilal SK. Computed tomography as a guide in the diagnosis and followup of brain abscess. *Radiology* 1980;135:663–671.
8. Haimes AB, Zimmerman RD, Morgello S, et al. MR imaging of brain abscesses. *AJNR* 1989;10:279.
9. Sze G, Zimmerman RA. The magnetic resonance imaging of infections and inflammatory diseases. *Radiol Clin North Am* 1988;26(4):839.
10. Zimmerman RA. Magnetic resonance imaging of intracranial infections. In: Wilkins RH, Rengachary SS, eds. *Neurosurgery update I: diagnosis, operative technique, and neuro-oncology.* McGraw-Hill, 1990;88–103.
11. Bilaniuk LT, Zimmerman RA, Brown L, Yoo HJ, Goldberg HI. Computed tomography in meningitis. *Neuroradiology* 1978;16:13–14.

12. Mathews VP, Kuharik MA, Edwards MK, et al. Gd-DTPA-enhanced MR imaging of experimental bacterial meningitis: evaluation and comparison with CT. *AJNR* 1988;9:1045.
13. Heier LA, Zimmerman RD, Deck MDF. Major vascular occlusion —an MR diagnosis [Abstract]. *AJNR* 1987;8:948.
14. Masaryk TJ, Modic MT, Ruggieri PM, Ross JS, Laub GA, Lenz GW, Tkach JA, Haacke EM, Selman WR, Harik SI. Three-dimensional (volume) gradient-echo imaging of the carotid bifurcation: preliminary clinical experience. *Radiology* 1989;171:801.
15. Naidich TP, McLone DG, Yamanouchi Y. Periventricular white matter cysts in a murine mode of gram-negative ventriculitis. *AJNR* 1983;4:461–465.
16. Carter BL, Bankoff MS, Fisk JD. Computed tomographic detection of sinusitis responsible for intracranial & extracranial infections. *Radiology* 1983;147:739–742.
17. Zimmerman RA, Bilaniuk LT. CT of orbital infection and its cerebral complications. *AJR* 1980;134:45–50.
18. Zimmerman RA, Patel S, Bilaniuk LT. Demonstration of purulent bacterial intracranial infections by computed tomography. *AJR* 1976;127:155–165.
19. Draouat S, Abdenabi B, Ghanem M, et al. Computed tomography of cerebral tuberculoma. *J Comput Assist Tomogr* 1987;11:594.
20. Gupta RK, Jena A, Sharma A, et al. MR imaging of intracranial tuberculomas. *J Comput Assist Tomogr* 1988;12:280.
21. Scott Casselman E, Hasso AN, Ashwal S, Schneider S. Computed tomography of tuberculous meningitis in infants and children. *J Comput Assist Tomogr* 1980;4:211–216.
22. Rovira M, Romeno F, Torrent O, et al. Study of tuberculosis meningitis by CT. *Neuroradiology* 1980;19:137–141.
23. Vignaud J, Clay C, Bilaniuk LT. Venography of the orbit—an analytical report of 413 cases. *Radiology* 1974;110:373–382.
24. Braffman BH, Zimmerman RA, Rabischong P. Cranial nerves III, IV, VI: a clinical/radiologic/anatomic approach to the evaluation of their dysfunction. *Semin Ultrasound* 1987;8(3):185–213.
25. Curtin HD, Wolfe P, May M. Malignant external otitis: CT evaluation. *Radiology* 1982;145:383.
26. Davis JM, Davis KR, Kleinman GM, et al. Computed tomography of herpes simplex encephalitis with clinicopathological correlation. *Radiology* 1978;129:419–427.
27. Enzmann DR, Ranson B, Norman D, et al. Computed tomography of herpes simplex encephalitis. *Radiology* 1978;129:419–425.
28. Zimmerman RD, Russel EJ, Leeds NE, Kaufman D. CT in the early diagnosis of herpes simplex encephalitis. *AJR* 1980;134:61–66.
29. Hayward J, Titelbaum DS, Clancy RR, Zimmerman RA. Lissencephaly–pachygyria associated with congenital cytomegalovirus infection. Presented at the Child Neurology Society Meeting in Halifax, Nova Scotia, September 1988.
30. Titelbaum DS, Hayward JC, Zimmerman RA. Pachygyriclike changes: topographic appearance at MR imaging and CT and correlation with neurologic status. *Radiology* 1989;173:663–667.
31. Dunn V, Bale JF, Zimmerman RA, Perdue Z, Bell WE. MRI in children with postinfectious disseminated encephalomyelitis. *Magn Reson Imaging* 1986;4:25–32.
32. Atlas SW, Grossman RI, Goldberg HI, Hackney DB, Bilaniuk LT, Zimmerman RA. MR diagnosis of acute disseminated encephalomyelitis. *J Comput Assist Tomogr* 1986;10(5):798–801.
33. Sze G, Brandt-Zawadzki M, Norman D, et al. The neuroradiology of AIDS. *Semin Roentgenol* 1987;22:42–53.
34. Kelly WM, Brandt-Zawadzki M. Acquired immunodeficiency syndrome: neuroradiologic findings. *Radiology* 1983;149:485–491.
35. Lyons RW, Andriole VT. Fungal infections of the CNS. *Neurol Clin* 1986;4:159–170.
36. Bradsford JF. *Cysticercus cellulosae*—its radiographic detection in the musculature and the central nervous system. *Br J Radiol* 1941;14:79–93.
37. Rodriguez-Carvajal J, Salgado P, Gutierrez-Alvarado R, Escobar-Izquierdo A, Aruffo C, Palacios E. The acute encephalitis phase of neurocysticcosis: computed tomographic manifestations. *AJNR* 1983;4:51–55.
38. Zee CS, Segall HD, Apuzzo MLJ, et al. Intraventricular cysticercal cysts: further neuroradiologic observations and neurosurgical implications. *AJNR* 1984;5:727–730.
39. Suss RA, Maravilla KR, Thompson J. MR imaging of intracranial cysticercosis: comparison with CT and anatomopathologic features. *AJNR* 1986;7:235–242.

Subject Index

A

A/New Jersey/76 vaccine, 262
Abdominal infections, 500
Abdominal pain, tabes, 649
Abductor vocal cord paralysis, 611
Abortion, *see* Spontaneous abortion
Abscess, *see* Brain abscess
Acanthamoeba keratitis, 793
Acanthamoeba species
  comparative morphology, 788
  immunosuppression role, 792
  pathogenic potential, 787
  pathologic effects, 792–793
Acellular pertussis vaccine, 629
Acetaminophen, and zidovudine, 222
Acetylcholine
  botulism, 592–593
  rabies virus, 12, 130
  tetanospasmin, 614
N-acetylglucosamine, 316
Achatina fulica snails, 842
Acid base balance, CSF, 864
Acid-fast stain, 874
Acquired aqueductal stenosis, 865
Acquired immunodeficiency syndrome,
  see AIDS
Acquired toxoplasmosis, 808, 810
Acremonium alabamensis, 693, 752
Acridine orange stain, CSF, 380
"Acrodermatitis chronica atrophicans"
  antibiotic response, 682–683
  appearance, 668
  Europe versus North America,
    677–678
  and peripheral neuropathy, 676
Actinobacillus actinomycetemcomitans,
  495, 501
Actinomyces israelii
  epidural abscess, 501
  subdural empyema, 495
Actinomyces species, meningitis, 350,
  721
Active transport, 11
Acute aseptic meningoencephalitis,
  209–210
Acute bacterial meningitis, *see* Bacterial
  meningitis
"Acute brain syndrome," *see* "Toxic"
  encephalopathy
Acute disseminated encephalopathy,
  901
Acute febrile cerebrovasculitis, 420–421
  computerized tomography, 421
  rickettsial disease similarity, 420–421
Acute inflammatory demyelinating
  polyneuropathy, *see* Guillain-
  Barre' syndrome
Acute meningitis, *see also* Bacterial
  meningitis

imaging, 891–894
syndrome recognition, 2–3
Acute necrotizing arteritis, 540
"Acute phase reactants," 323–324
Acute polyradiculopathy syndrome, 217
Acute suppurative meningitis, 550
Acyclovir
  chickenpox, 63–65
  combination therapy, 56
  herpes B virus treatment, 74
  herpes simplex encephalitis, 53–56,
    177–178
  herpes zoster, 64–65, 217
  neonatal herpes, 177–178
  oral versus intravenous, 65
  perinatal varicella-zoster, 187
  and relapse, 55
  toxicity, 55
Acyloxyacyl hydrolase, 356, 360
Adenocarcinoma, 725
Adenosine deaminase test
  evaluation, 876–877
  tuberculous meningitis, 435–436
S-adenosylmethionine, 209
Adenylate cyclase toxin
  acellular vaccine use, 629
  molecular actions, 626
Adhesion
  bacitracin use, 580
  bacteria pathogenesis, 298–299, 352,
    569
  CSF shunts, bacteria, 306–307, 569,
    580
Adjunctive therapy
  bacterial meningitis, 392–394
  tuberculous meningitis, 447
Adrenal insufficiency, AIDS, 206–207
Adrenocorticotropic hormone, 272
Adult botulism of unknown source,
  589–602
Aedes mosquitoes
  Eastern equine encephalitis, 89
  La Crosse encephalitis, 100–101
  Tahyna virus, 102
  Venezuelan encephalitis, 92
Aerosol infection, rabies, 131–133
African meningitis belt, 339–340, 344
African trypanosomiasis
  clinical manifestations, 782–783
  diagnosis, 783–785
  epidemiology, 778–780
  history, 778
  mortality, 783
  parasitology, 778
  pathology and pathogenesis, 780–782
Agammaglobulinemia, 25
Age factors
  bacterial meningitis, 336, 342–343
  brain abscess, 458

Guillain-Barre' syndrome, 274
herpes encephalitis outcome, 53–54
infective endocarditis, 516, 526
shunt infection, 569
subdural empyema, 490
Agglutinogens, 626
AIDS; *see also* HIV infection
  brain abscess, 458, 462–463, 481
  children, 212–213
    vaccines, 223
  chronic meningitis, 709–712
  clinical staging, 206–207
  Cryptococcus infection, 710, 734–735
  cytomegalovirus, 68
  fungal infections, 711
  herpesvirus infections, 217
  imaging, encephalopathy, 901–903
  median survival, 206
  meningeal diseases, 217–218,
    709–711
  neurological manifestations, 201–232
  ocular toxoplasmosis, 809–810
  parenchymal disease, 213–217
  primary amebic meningoencephalitis,
    792
  reactivated toxoplasmosis, 811–812
  serologic tests, toxoplasmosis, 816
  toxoplasmosis, 809–817, 902–903
    empirical therapy, 814–815
    imaging, 902–903
  treatment, 221–223
  tuberculosis, 427, 449–450
    treatment, 450
Aids dementia complex
  CSF p24 antigen, 209
  diagnosis, 210
  neuropathology, 210–211
  pathophysiology, 211–212
  zidovudine treatment, 222
Alaska, pneumococcal meningitis,
  342–343
Albendazole, 835–836
  hydatid cysts, 840
  neurocysticercosis, 835–836
Albumin
  blood-brain-barrier, 358–359
  Guillain-Barre' syndrome, 273
Alcoholics
  aspergillosis, 746
  meningococcal disease, 342
  pneumococcal meningitis, 343
Algorithms, 708
Allodermanyssus sanguineus, 417
Allogeneic stimulation, 709
Alper's disease, 162
Alpha-1 acid glycoprotein, 324
Alpha-interferon, 237
Alpha motor neurons, 612–614
Alphaviruses, 88–93

909

Alphaviruses (*contd.*)
    encephalitis, 88–93
    infectious agents, 88–89
    pathology and pathogenesis, 89
Alternaria, 693
Alum-absorbed tetanus toxoid,
        616–617, 619–620
Alzheimer's disease, 158–159
Amblyomma americanum, 414, 660
Amblyomma cajennense, 414
"Amebastomes," 788
    function, 788–789
    ultrastructure, 788
Amebic dysentery, 794–795
Amebic infections, 787–794
American Samoa outbreak, 842
American trypanosomiasis, 786–787
    CNS manifestations, 786–787
    pathogenesis, 786
    treatment, 786
Amikacin
    CSF penetration, 574
    intraventricular administration, 327,
        579
    neonatal meningitis, 325–326
    recommended doses, 388
    shunt infection, 574–575, 579
Aminoglycosides
    CSF penetration, 574
    epidural abscess, 505
    infective endocarditis, 523
    intraventricular dosage, 575
    neonatal meningitis, 324–326
    shunt infection, 574–575
Amnesia, infective endocarditis, 529
Amniotic fluid
    bacteria acquisition, 315, 317
    group B streptococci, 317
    toxoplasmosis diagnosis, 817
Amodiaquine, 777
Amoxicillin
    infective endocarditis prevention, 525
    Lyme disease, 681–682
    neurosyphilis therapy, 651
Amphotericin B
    Aspergillus brain abscess, 748
    candidal infection, 754
    coccidioidal meningitis, 715, 735
    cryptococcal infections, 710, 714,
        734, 756
    drug combinations, 733–734
    fungal meningitis, 732–736
    Histoplasma meningitis, 715,
        735–736
    intrathecal administration, 732
    liposomal form, 733
    mucormycosis, 751
    primary amebic meningoencephalitis,
        794
    resistance, 751
    shunt infections, 579
    spongiform encephalopathies, 162
    toxicity, 734
Ampicillin
    dexamethasone combination, CSF,
        360
    group B streptococci prophylaxis,
        328–329
    Hemophilus influenzae, 387–388
    infective endocarditis, 523
    intracranial pressure effect, 361
    Listeria monocytogenes, 390
    neonatal meningitis, 324–326
    recommended doses, meningitis, 388

"Amyloid enhancing factor," 158
Amyloid plaques, 155–156
Anaerobic bacteria
    brain abscess, 458
    meningitis, 350
    treatment, 390–391
Aneurysms, *see* Intracranial mycotic
        aneurysm
Angiitis
    and AIDS, 217
    intracranial aspergillosis, 747
"Angiographic triad, 437
Angiography
    intracranial mycotic aneurysm,
        544–545
    Lyme disease, 672, 674
    tuberculoma, 439
    tuberculous meningitis, 437
Angiostrongyliasis, 842–843, 871
Angiostrongylus cantonensis, 842–843,
        871
Animal inoculation 878
Anorexia, Lyme disease, 675
Anterior epidural abscess
    outcome, 506,
    pathogenesis, 499–500
    surgery, 506
Anterior uveitis, 809
Anterograde transport, 13
Antibiotic resistance; *see also under
        specific antibiotics*
    neonatal meningitis, 327
Antibiotics; *see also specific antibiotics*
    bacterial meningitis, 386–397
    and blood-brain-barrier, 386–387
    CSF effect, meningitis, 381
    prophylactic use, 580–581
    susceptibility testing, 745
Antibody tests, HIV, 207–208, 213
Anticoagulant therapy
    and cerebral hemorrhage, 527, 533,
        538–540
    intracranial mycotic aneurysm, 543,
        546
    lumbar puncture danger, 867–868
    prosthetic valve surgery, 538–539
    and valvular surgery, 537
Anticonvulsant drugs, 396
Antigen detection tests, 876
    herpes simplex encephalitis, 52
    HIV, 207–209
    sensitivity, 876
    tuberculous meningitis, 436–437
Antigenic stimulation, 709
Anti-HIV antibody tests, 207–209
Antitetanus antibodies, 616
Anti-treponemal antibodies, 643
Antrypol, *see* Suramin
Aortic valve infection
    cerebral emboli, 526, 533
    echocardiography, 538
Aortic valve replacement, 527
Aqueduct of Sylvius, 865
Aqueductal stenosis
    magnetic resonance imaging, 895
    mumps virus, 116
Arabinitol, 732
Arachnia, 721
Arachnoid layer, anatomy, 862
Arachnoid villus, 863
Arachnoiditis, 319–320
Arboviruses, 21, 29–30
"Arc-5" antigen, 839
Areflexia, 268–269

Argyll Robertson pupillary changes,
        649, 672
Arprinocid, 819
Arsenic, *see* Melarsoprol
Artemisinine, 776
Arteriography, 471
Arterioles, cerebral malaria, 770
Arteritis, 647–648
Arthritis
    Lyme disease, 668, 682
    rubella, 189, 192
Arthropod-borne viruses, 87–104
    encephalitis, 87–104
    epidemic CNS infections, 8
Artificial CSF, 866
Ascending herpes simplex infection,
        169–170
Aseptic meningitis, 19–34
    arboviruses, 29–30
    and chronic meningitis, 709–710
    clinical manifestations, 24–25
    CSF findings, 379
    enteroviruses, 19–28
    epidemiology, 22–23
    etiology, 19–20
    lymphocytic choriomeningitis virus,
        31–32
    mumps, 30–31
    Mycoplasma pneumoniae, 289
    noninfectious causes, 34
    nonviral pathogens, 33–34
    and sarcoidosis, 721
    seasonal occurrence, 21, 23
    varicella virus, 60
Aspergilloma, 747–748
Aspergillus fumigatus, 746
Aspergillus species
    antifungal agents, 731, 733, 748
    antigen detection, 732
    autopsy study, 743, 746–747
    brain abscess, 461–463, 721, 743–748
    brain biopsy, 730, 746–747
    cerebral embolism, endocarditis, 533,
        746
    and chronic meningitis, 721, 732
    clinical manifestations, 747
    diagnosis, 747–748
    epidemiology, 746
    epidural abscess, 501
    extirpation, 748
    imaging, 903–905
    infectious agent, 746
    infective endocarditis, 528, 533
    pathogenesis, 699–700, 745–746
    pathology, 746–747
    spectrum of CNS involvement,
        693–694
Aspiration
    brain abscess, 479–481
    CT-guided, 479–481
    versus excision, 479
    fungal infections, 736
Asplenic states
    meningococcal disease, 342, 376
    pneumococcal meningitis, 343, 376
Astrocytes
    bacterial meningitis pathology,
        364–366
    CSF barrier system, 864
    cytokine release, 864
    scrapie, 155
    sleeping sickness, 780–781
Asymmetrical radiculoplexitis, 665
Asymptomatic herpes simplex, 170–171

Asymptomatic neurocysticercosis, 828
Asymptomatic syphilis
    classification, 644
    CNS involvement, 644–645
    penicillin therapy, 651–652
Ataxia, 370, 373
Athletes, aseptic meningitis, 23
Atracurium, 618
Attention, Lyme disease effect, 675
Attenuated vaccines, polio, 247–248
Atypical mycobacteria
    and AIDS, 450
    meningitis, 449
Auditory evoked potentials, 671
Australia
    Guillain-Barre' syndrome, 260–261
    Lyme disease, 660–661
Autoantibodies, 782
Autoimmunity, *Mycoplasma pneumon-
    iae*, 287
Autoinfection, strongyloidiasis, 847
Autonomic dysfunction
    botulism, 594–595
    tetanospasmin effects, 614
    therapy, tetanus, 618
Autonomic neuropathy
    and AIDS, 221
    Lyme disease, 666
"Axis cylinder" transmission, 13
Axonal injury
    HIV infection, children, 213
    Lyme disease, 665–666, 673, 676
Axons, CNS viral transport, 13
Azetazolamide, 863
Azithromycin, 819
AZT, *see* Zidovudine
Aztreonam, 477

B
B lymphocytes, 782
B-type pertussis vaccine, 629
B virus, 69–74
    assays, 73–74
    characteristics, 70
    CNS disease, 72–73
    diagnosis, 73–74
    epidemiology, 71–72
    history, 69–70
    latency, 71
    pathology and pathogenesis, 70–71
    person-to-person transmission, 72
    prevention and treatment, 74
    recurrence, 73
    replication, 70
    survival, 73
Bacillus cereus, 461
Bacitracin A
    bacterial adherence disruption, 580
    topical application, 580–581
"Back mutation," 22
Back pain, Lyme disease, 672
Baclofen, 618
Bacteremia
    brain abscess, 465
    and CSF invasion, 353
    infective endocarditis, 518–519, 521
    lumbar puncture danger, 868
    pathology, meningitis, 368
    and shunt infection, 568
Bacterial adhesion, *see* Adhesion
Bacterial cell walls
    inflammation mediation, 356–357
    and treatment, 393

Bacterial endocarditis, *see* Infective en-
    docarditis
Bacterial infections, 297–312; *see also
    specific infections*
Bacterial meningitis, 335–409; *see also*
    Neonatal bacterial meningitis
    brain abscess, 304
    cerebrospinal fluid, 378–382,
        878–879
    clinical manifestations, 368–376, 549
        adults, 373–374
        children, 368–373
        elderly, 374
    contrast enhancement, 892–893
    differential diagnosis, 376–378
    epidemiology, 336–343
    etiology, 343–351
    imagery, 891–894
    infant rat model, 297
    infective endocarditis cause, 529–530,
        546–550
    laboratory diagnosis, 378–386,
        878–879
    neonates, 313–333
    pathogenesis and pathophysiology,
        297–302, , 351–362, 548–549
    pathology, 362–368
    prevention, 397–402
    versus primary amebic meningoence-
        phalitis, 793
    simultaneous viral infection, 351
    and strongyloidiasis, 847–848
    subarachnoid space inflammation,
        302
    treatment, 386–397
    versus viral meningitis, 377
Bacterial polysaccharide immune glob-
    ulin, 399
Bacteroides fragilis
    brain abscess, 303–305, 467–468
    host defenses, brain, 304–305
    meningitis, 350
    synergistic infectivity, 303
Bacteroides species, brain abscess,
    459–461
Baltimore, Maryland, *H. influenzae*, 337
Bannwarth's syndrome, 657–658, 677,
    719
Barbiturates, drug interactions, 389
Basal ganglia
    abscess, 467, 751
    congenital AIDS, imaging, 902
    mucormycosis, 751
    toxoplasmosis, 812
Basilar cisterns
    contrast enhancement, 892
    cysticercosis, 834–835
Bat populations, rabies, 132
Bayer 205, *see*, Suramin
Baylisascariasis, 849
BCG vaccine
    and HIV infection, 223, 450
    meningitis cause, 448–449
    tuberculosis prevention, 451
Behcet's disease, 723
Bell's palsy, 672
Benign neurocysticercosis, 835
Benzalkonium chloride, 138
Benzathine penicillin
    and HIV infection, 653–654, 711–712
    recommended regimen, 718
    treatment failures, syphilis, 644, 651,
        711–712

Benzodiazepines, tetanus management,
    617–618
Beta-adrenergic blockage, tetanus, 618
Beta-adrenergic receptor, reovirus, 12
Beta-hemolysin, 318
Beta-interferon, 209
Beta-lactams
    and blood-brain-barrier, 386
    group B streptococci, 325
    intraventricular administration, 328
Beta2-microglobulin
    AIDS-dementia, 210
    HIV infection, 209
    primary CNS lymphoma, 216
Bethel, Alaska, *H. influenzae*, 337
Bicarbonate concentration, CSF, 864
Bicuspid aortic valve, 516
Binding domains, viral attachment, 12
Bioprosthetic valves
    and intracranial mycotic aneurysm,
        546
    neurologic complications, 527
Biopsy, *see* Brain biopsy
Bipolaris species, 761
Birth weight, and botulism, 590
Bithionol, 852
"Black pus," 751
Blacks
    H. influenzae meningitis, 337
    meningococcal disease, 342
    tuberculosis, 427, 446
Blastogenic response, cytomegalovirus,
    180
Blastomyces dermatitidis
    amphotericin B., 731, 736
    brain abscess, 756–757
    classification, 693–694
    CSF culture, 757
    enzyme-linked immunoassay, 716
    pathogenesis, 698, 715–716, 756–757
Blastomycoma, 757
Blastomycosis, 756–757
Blastomycotic meningitis
    CSF culture, 730
    pathogenesis, 698, 715–716
Blebs, 347
"Blind staggers," 837
Blindness, cerebral malaria, 775
    Blood-brain-barrier
    antibiotics, 386–387
    bacterial infection effects, 358–360,
        386–387
    brain abscess therapy, 476–477
    cerebrospinal fluid, 476, 863–864
    HIV passage, 209
    host defenses, bacteria, 300
    imaging, 900–901
    permeability changes, bacteria, 302
    viral infection dynamics, 10–11
Blood culture
    infective endocarditis, 522–523
    neonatal bacterial meningitis, 321
    shunt infection, 572
Blood donors, cytomegalovirus, 183
Blood transfusion
    group B streptococci, 325–326
    toxoplasmosis, 812
Bone development, congenital varicella,
    186
Bone marrow transplantation
    serology, toxoplasmosis, 816
    toxoplasmosis reactivation, 811
"Border-zone encephalitis," 429
Bordetella parapertussis, 627

Bordetella pertussis, 625–635
  infection with, 625–627
  virulence factors, 626
Borrelia burgdorferi; *see also* Lyme disease
  aseptic meningitis, 33
  brain tissue isolation, 664–665
  cerebrospinal fluid, 664–665, 719
  characteristics, 661–662
  discovery, 658
  Europe versus North America, 677–678
  false-positive results, 679, 719
  flagellin fraction, 679
  immunization, 663
  laboratory diagnosis, 678–679, 719
  persistence, 663
  strain-specific immunity, 663
  strains of, 661
  Syrian hamster host, 662–663
  transmission, 660
Botulinum antitoxin, 597
Botulinum toxin
  derivative, 591–592
  therapeutic uses, 598
Botulism, 589–602
  clinical manifestations, 593–596
  diagnosis, 596–597
  electromyography, 596–597
  epidemiology, 589–591
  etiology, 591
  fatality rates, 595
  pathogenesis and pathophysiology, 592–593
  prevention, 598
  progenitor toxin, 591
  syndrome of, 4
  tetanus toxin similarity, 591–592
  therapy, 577–598
Botulism immune globulin, 597–598
Boutonneuse fever
  characteristics, 412
  CNS manifestations, 416
  pathology, 413, 416
  rash, 416
  treatment, 416–417
Bovine spongiform encephalopathy, 153–162
  transmission, 154
Bracing, 506
Bradycardia, 614
Bradyzoites, 802–803
Brain abscess, 457–487
  amebiasis, 462, 794–796
  animal models, 303
  antimicrobial therapy, 476–478, 480–481
    duration of, 481
  bacterial infection, 302–306, 376, 458–463
  and bacterial meningitis, 304, 384
  clinical manifestations, 469–470, 549
  computerized tomography, 384, 470–476, 480, 547–548, 889–892
    sensitivity, 472–474
    specificity, 474–475
  diagnosis, 376, 470–476
  encapsulation, 467–469, 889–890
  epidemiology, 457–458, 547–548
  etiology, 458–463
  fungal etiology, 743–761
  host defenses, 304–306
  infective endocarditis, 547–550

initiation and natural history, 303–304
  injection method, animals, 303–304
  lumbar puncture contraindication, 470, 867
  magnetic resonance imaging, 548, 889–892
  management, 480–481
  mycotic aneurysm sequelae, 543
  neurologic sequelae, 481, 496
  nonoperative management, 480–481
  pathogenesis and pathophysiology, 463–467, 548–549
  pathologic stages, 304–305, 467–468
  pathology, 467–469
  prognosis, 481–482, 550
  staging by CT scan, 480
  subdural empyema sequelae, 496
  surgery, 478–481
Brain biopsy
  Creutzfeldt-Jakob disease, 158–159
  herpes simplex encephalitis, 50–51
  neonatal herpes, 175
  primary CNS lymphoma, 216
  subacute sclerosing panencephalitis, 148
  toxoplasmosis, 817–818
Brain edema, *see* Cerebral edema
Brain herniation
  CSF effect, 864–866
  lumbar puncture complication, 866–867
Brain parenchyma
  cryptococcomas, 734
  fungal infection diagnosis, 732
  Lyme disease, 671–672
  neurocysticercosis, 828–830, 833–835
  neurosyphilis, 640, 644, 648–649
  subdural empyema, CT scan, 492–493
  viral infection dynamics, 10
Brain tumor, versus abscess, CT scan, 475–476
Brain water content, 360–361, 366–367
Brainstem
  infective endocarditis, 529
  rabies virus, 130
Brainstem abscess
  clinical manifestation, 470
  CT-guided surgery, 479–480
  otogenic cause, 464
  pathology, 467
Brainstem auditory evoked potentials, 676
Brazil
  bacterial meningitis, 344
  N. mengitidis, 339–341
Brazilian Indians, herpes simplex, 48
Breast-feeding
  botulism, 590
  H. influenzae protection, 339
  herpes simplex transmission, 169
Breast milk, cytomegalovirus, 182–183
Brill-Zinsser disease, 418–419
Bromide partition test, 435–436
Bronchiectasis, 465
Brown dog tick, 414
Brucella meningitis, 717
Brucella species
  brain abscess, 461
  chronic meningitis, agent, 717
  infective endocarditis, 521
  meningoencephalitis, 33
Brucellosis, 262
Brudzinski's signs, 368, 373

Bruns' syndrome, 829
Bulbar palsy, 269–270
Bulboparetic syndrome, 97
Bunyaviruses, 99–103
  aseptic meningitis, 29
  background, 99–100
  pathology and pathogenesis, 100
  structural features, 100
Burkitt's lymphoma, 66
"Burning feet," 221
Burr hole drainage
  intracranial epidural abscess, 511
  subdural empyema, 495

C

C-reactive protein
  bacterial meningitis test, 379, 382
  brain abscess, 470
  neonatal meningitis, 322–323
C3 breakdown products, 354
C3 receptors, 11
C5a
  chemotactic factor, 354–355
  pneumococcal meningitis, CSF, 300, 354–355
Caddenhill vaccine, 192
Calcifications, *see* Intracranial calcifications
Calcified cysts, MRI, 834–835
Calcified mitral annulus, 517
California serogroup viruses
  clinical disease, 101–102
  diagnosis, 102
  epidemiology, 101
  history, 100–101
  prevention and treatment, 102
Campylobacter fetus, 495
Campylobacter infections, 261
Canada, Lyme disease, 659
Canadian Arctic, trichinosis, 846
Candida albicans, 753–754
Candida parapsilosis, 753
Candida species
  autopsy study, 743, 754
  biopsy difficulties, 744
  brain abscess, 461–463, 743–744, 753–754
    imaging, 904–905
  clinical manifestations, 753–754
  CSF culture, 730–731, 754
  CSF serology, 730–731, 754
  diagnosis, 730–731, 754
  epidemiology, 753
  etiologic agent, 753
  and meningitis, 717, 735, 737
  pathogenesis, 699, 753
  pathology, 753
  spectrum of CNS infections, 693–694, 699
  therapy, 731, 735, 754
Canine model, brain abscess, 303–304
Capillaries, *see* Cerebral capillaries
Capsular polysarrcharide
  antibodies, 328
  antigen test, 730–731
  E. coli pathogenesis, 318–319
  genetic basis, 318
  meningococcal virulence, 347
  pneumococcal virulence, 348, 352
Capsule formation, *see* Encapsulation
Carageenan, 162
Carbamazepine, 34
Cardiac defects, rubella, 191

Cardiac dysfunction
    Lyme disease, 665–667
    sleeping sickness, 783
Cardiac surgery, 535–537
Cardiac transplant
    acquired toxoplasmosis, 811–812
    serology, toxoplasmosis, 816
Cardiac valves, see also Valvular surgery
    endocarditis pathogenesis, 517–519
Cardiopulmonary bypass
    cerebral embolism risk, 536–537
    and intracranial mycotic aneurysm,
        546
Carpal tunnel syndrome, 676
"Case infection rate," 564–565
Cataracts, neonatal herpes, 174
Catecholamines, tetanospasmin effects,
    614
Cats, Toxoplasma gondii host, 802, 804,
    819
Cavernous sinus aneurysms, 545
Cavernous sinus thrombosis
    brain abscess, 464, 750
    imaging, 896–898
C4b deficiency, 342
CD4, 12, 202
    and AIDS progression, 208
    cerebrospinal fluid, 209
    cryptococcosis, 696
    dideoxyinosine effects, 222
    HIV infection, 204, 208
    treatment strategies, 204
CD4:CD8 ratio, 208–209
CD36, 773
CDC AIDS diagnosis, 206–207
Cefotaxime
    brain water content effect, 361
    children, 391
    versus ceftriaxone, 326
    CSF penetration, 574
    H. influenzae, 388 389
    Lyme disease, 682
    neonatal meningitis, 325–326
    recommended doses, meningitis, 388
    shunt infection, 574
Ceftazidime
    H. influenzae, 388–389
    neonatal meningitis, 325
    neurosurgery use, 392
    P. aeruginosa, 390
    recommended doses, meningitis, 388
    shunt infection, 574
Ceftriazone
    brain water content, 361
    versus cefotaxime, 326
    CSF lipopolysaccharides, 357
    CSF penetration, 574
    H. influenzae, 388–389
    infective endocarditis, 523
    Lyme disease, 681–683
    N. meningitidis prophylaxis, 400
    recommended doses, 388–389
    shunt infection, 574
Cefuroxine, 388–389
Cell count, CSF, 870–871
Cell-mediated immunity
    amebae, 791
    B. burgdorferi, 663
    bacterial meningitis, 375–376
    ongenital cytomegalovirus, 180
    crytococcosis, 695–696
    Guillain-Barre' syndrome, 267–268
    mumps, 117

rabies, 131
toxoplasmosis, 803–804, 811
Cell-wall challenge, see Bacterial cell
    walls
Center for Disease Control, AIDS diag-
    nosis, 206–207
Central retinal artery, 550
Centrum semiovale, 210–211
Cephalic tetanus, 608
Cephalosporins
    in children, 391
    CNS penetration, 574
    E. coli, neonates, CSF, 326
    epidural abscess, 505
    gram-negative bacilli, 390
    H. influenzae, 388–389
    intraventricular dosages, 575
    shunt infection, 574–575
Cephalothin, 575
Cercariae, 850, 852
Cerebellar abscess
    diagnosis, 376
    otogenesis, 464
    symptoms, 469
Cerebellar ataxia
    enteroviruses, 28
    Mycoplasma pneumoniae, 289
    subacute sclerosing panencephalitis,
        146
    varicella infection, 59
Cerebellar tonsils, herniation, 367, 866
Cerebral abscess, see Brain abscess
Cerebral amebiasis, 794–796
    clinical manifestations, 796
    diagnosis, 796
    epidemiology, 794–795
    pathogenesis and pathology, 795–796
    treatment and prognosis, 796
Cerebral angiography, see Angiography
Cerebral blood flow
    autoregulation disturbance, 367
    bacterial meningitis, 362, 367
    and intracranial pressure, 362
    malaria, 774
Cerebral capillaries
    malaria pathology, 796–772
    mycoplasmas, thrombosis, 287–288
Cerebral cortex, Lyme disease, 666
Cerebral edema
    bacteria reaction, 302, 360–362,
        366–367
    brain abscess, 467, 795
    computerized tomography, 384
    pathology, 366–367
Cerebral embolism
    AIDS, 217
    anticoagulants, 538–539
    and brain abscess, 548
    cerebrospinal fluid, 532, 535
    clinical presentation, 533–534
    diagnosis, 534–535
    echocardiography, 537–538
    incidence, 532–533
    infective endocarditis, 526–530,
        532–539
    intracranial hemorrhage cause, 540
    management, 535–539
    outcome, 539
    pathogenesis, endocarditis, 527–528,
        533
Cerebral hemorrhage, see Intracranial
    hemorrhage
Cerebral infarction, 528
Cerebral malaria, 767–777

clinical manifestations, 775
diagnosis, 775–776
epidemiology, 767–768
hypoglycemia, 774–775
mortality rates, 768
pathogenesis, 771–775
pathology, 769–771
prevention, 777
treatment, 776–777
uniform definition, 767
Cerebral perfusion pressure
    bacterial meningitis, 367
    and prognosis, 866
Cerebral sulci
    imaging, meningitis, 892–893
    purulence, 363
Cerebral toxoplasmosis, see Toxoplas-
    mosis
Cerebral vasculitis, 362
Cerebral ventricles, see Ventricular sys-
    tem
Cerebritis; see also Meningoencephalitis
    aspergillosis, 747
    and brain abscess, 304–305, 467–468
    computerized tomography, 384, 480,
        547–548, 887–892
    incidence, endocarditis, 547–548
    magnetic resonance imaging, 887–889
    management, 549
    mucormycosis prognosis, 751
Cerebrospinal fluid, 861–885
    anatomy, 861–864
    antibiotic effects, 381, 386–387, 879
    antitoxoplasmic antibodies, 816
    aseptic versus bacterial meningitis,
        378–379
    B. burgdorferi, 664
    bacterial meningitis, 300–302,
        321–322, 353–362, 366, 378–382
        diagnosis, 378–382
    barrier system, 863–864
    brain abscess, 470
    cerebral embolism, 535
    cerebral malaria, 775
    chronic meningitis, 704, 706–708
    congenital rubella, 192
    culture techniques, 875
    enteroviruses, 27–28
    fungal meningitis, 729–731
    gross appearance, 870
    Guillain-Barre syndrome, 270
    HIV infection, 209
        children, 212–213
    host defenses, 354–355
    hydrocephalus effect, 864–866
    inflammation induction, 355–358
    Lyme disease, 664, 671, 674, 682
        antibiotic effects, 682
    mumps virus, 119–120
    Mycoplasma pneumoniae, 286, 290
    neonatal herpes encephalitis, 173
    neurocysticercosis, 832–833
    in normal newborns, 322, 871
    outflow resistance, 360–361
    penetration of, 573–575
    physiology and production, 863–864
    purulent exudate blockage, 366
    red blood cells, 871–872
    shunt infection, 306–307
        treatment, 392
    sleeping sickness, 784–785
    subacute sclerosing panencephalitis,
        148
    syphilis diagnosis, 641–643, 646

Cerebrospinal fluid (*contd.*)
  trauma, recurrent meningitis, 374–375
  Treponema pallidum penetration, 640
  tuberculous meningitis, 433–434, 879
  viral cultures, 875
  viral infection dynamics, 10
  white blood cells, 870–871
Cerebrospinal fluid block
  bacterial meningitis, 360–361
  tuberculous meningitis, 429, 433
Cerebrospinal fluid pressure
  measurement, 869–870
  and prognosis, 866
Cerebrospinal fluid reabsorption, 865
Cerebrospinal fluid reservoirs, 565–566
Cerebrospinal fluid rhinorrhea, 374–375
Cerebrospinal fluid shunt infections, 561–585
  antibiotics, 392
  bacteria, 306–307, 375
  bimodal distribution, 566
  case rate, 564–565
  clinical manifestations, 569–571
  diagnosis, 571–573, 577
  device infection at surgery, 568–569
  duration of treatment, 578
  epidemiology, 564–566
  etiology, 566–567
  operative rate, 564–565
  and operative technique, 565
  pathogenesis, 567–569
  prevention/prophylaxis, 579–581
  proximal and distal, 570
  review articles, 564
  and revisions, 564–565
  treatment, 573–579
Cerebrospinal fluid shunts, 561–585
  adhesion, 306
  antibiotic incorporation in, 579–580
  bacterial adherence, 569
  history, 561–564
  infection, *see* Cerebrospinal fluid shunt infections
  loss of, treatment, 579
  replacement of, 575–576
  types of, 562–564
Cerebrovascular syphilis, 718; *see also* General paresis
Cervical spine
  epidural abscess, 500, 506
  infarction, 867
  tuberculous epidural abscess, 507
Cervical tabes, 649
Cervical traction halo immobilization, 465
Cervical tuberculomas, 442
Cesarean section, 175–176
Cestodes, 826–841
Chagas disease, *see* American trypanosomiasis
Chancre, sleeping sickness, 783
Charleston County, South Carolina, 337
Chemical meningitis, 724
Chicken meat, gnathostomiasis, 843
Chickenpox; *see also* Varicella-zoster virus
  CNS manifestations, 59–60
  congenital abnormalities, 186
  diagnosis, 62–63
  epidemiology, 58, 185–186
  perinatal infections, 185–187
  and pregnancy, 185–186
  treatment, 63–65, 187

Childbirth, *see* Delivery
Child-care personnel, cytomegalovirus, 182–183
Children; *see also under specific infections*
  antibiotics, meningitis, 391
  bacterial meningitis, 368–373, 391
  brain abscess sequelae, 481
  Guillain-Barre syndrome, 273–275
  malaria, 768
  shunt infection, 569
  tuberculous meningitis, 430–431
China, Lyme disease, 660–661
Chinese cucumber root extract, 223
Chloramphenicol
  anaerobes, 390–391
  blood-brain-barrier, 386
  brain abscess, 477–478
  Citrobacter meningitis, 326
  CSF penetration, 574
  drug interactions, 388–389
  E. coli meningitis, neonates, 326
  H. influenzae, 387–388
  intraventricular dosages, 575
  Lyme disease, 682–683
  recommended doses, meningitis, 388
  resistance, 387, 574
  Rocky Mountain spotted fever, 415
  shunt infection, 574–575
  subdural empyema, 495
Chloride levels
  cerebrospinal fluid, 864
  tuberculous meningitis, 433, 864
Chlorine bleach, 162
Chloroerythromycin, 819
Chloroquine
  cardiovascular toxicity, 776
  cerebral malaria, 776
  chemoprophylaxis, 777
  and rabies vaccination, 251
Chlorproguanil, 777
Cholesteatoma, 463
Cholinergic nerves, botulism, 592
Chorioretinitis
  congenital cytomegalovirus, 183–184
  cytomegalovirus, AIDS, 68
  neonatal herpes, 172, 174
Choroid plexus
  anatomy, 862
  bacteria invasion, 353
  CSF production, 863
  E. coli localization, 319
  entervirus spread, 22
  sleeping sickness, 780–781
  viral infection dynamics, 10
"Chromoblastomycosis," 759
Chromosomal abnormalities, 186
Chronic benign lymphocytic meningitis, 725–726
Chronic encephalitis syndrome, 2–3
Chronic fatigue syndrome, 65–66
Chronic granulomatous disease, 699
Chronic inflammatory demyelinating peripheral neuropathy, 220
Chronic meningitis
  causes, 712–726
  diagnostic complexities, 703–705, 729–732
  HIV infection, 709–712
  imaging, 894–895
  laboratory data, 706–708
  patient history, 705
  physical examination, 705–706
  syndrome recognition, 2–3

Chronic mononucleosis syndrome, 66
Chronic wasting disease, 153–162
Cicatricial skin scarring, 186
Cilofungin, 733
Ciprofloxacin
  Mycoplasma hominis, 291
  N. meningitidis prophylaxis, 400
  rickettsial infections, 415
  side effects, 400
Circle of Willis, 542
Cisterna magna
  anatomy, 862
  bacterial invasion, 353
  purulent exudate, 363–364
Cisternal cerebrospinal fluid
  fungal meningitis, 730
  infection indications, 869
  lumbar puncture, 868
Citrobacter diversus, 465
Citrobacter species
  brain abscess, 304, 461
  neonatal meningitis, 314–315
  treatment, 326
Cladosporium trichoides, 721, 759–761
Clavulanic acid, 681
Clindamycin
  brain abscess, 477
  CSF penetration, 574
  Mycoplasma hominis, 291
  shunt infection, 575
  toxoplasmosis, 711, 819
Clonidine, tetanus management, 618
Clostridium argentinense, 591
Clostridium baratii, 590
Clostridium botulinum, 589–598
  infectious agent, 591
  neurotoxins, 591–592
Clostridium butyricum, 590
Clostridium species, 350
Clostridium tetani
  characteristics, 605–606
  growth in culture, 606
Coagglutination test
  meningitis, diagnosis, CSF, 381–382
  sensitivity, 876
Cobalamin deficiency
  and neuropathies, 220
  vacuolar myelopathy, 219
Cocaine inhalation
  botulism, 590
  brain abscess, 464
  infective endocarditis, 517
Coccidioidal meningitis
  amphotericin B, 735
  complement fixation antibodies, 731
  CSF findings, 714–715, 630–731
  presentation, 714
  prognosis, 737
  treatment, 715, 731, 735
Coccidioides immitis
  amphotericin B, 731
  brain abscess, 463, 758–759
  classification, 693–694
  complement fixation, 731, 877
  epidemiology, 714
  pathogenesis, 697–698
Coccidiomycosis, 758–759
Coenurosis, 837
Cogan's syndrome, 722
Cognitive impairment; *see also* Mental status
  toxoplasmosis, 814
Cold hemagglutinins, 287

Collagen
    brain abscess encapsulation, 468–469
    computerized tomography, 890
    and neurologic syndromes, 721–722
Colloidal cysts, MRI, 834–835
Colorado tick fever
    and aseptic meningitis, 29
    clinical findings, 104
    diagnosis, 104
    epidemiology, 104
    history, 103
    pathology and pathogenesis, 103–104
    prevention and treatment, 104
    virus characteristics, 103
Coma
    bacterial meningitis, elderly, 374
    herpes encephalitis outcome, 53–55
    rabies, 135–136
Combination chemotherapy, 56
Communicating hydrocephalus
    bacterial meningitis, 366, 384
    computerized tomography, 384
    CSF effects, 865
    tuberculous meningitis, 429
Complement-fixation assay
    Coccidioides immitis, 731
    mumps, 121
    Mycoplasma pneumoniae, 290
    neurocysticercosis, 832–833
Complement system
    amebae, 791
    B. burgdorferi, 664
    bacteria reaction, 299–201, 354
    cerebral malaria, 774
    cryptococcosis, 696
    Guillain-Barre' syndrome, 267–268
    meningococcal disease, 342, 352–353
    sleeping sickness, 782
    subarachnoid space, 354
"Compliance," 866
Compound muscle action potential,
    271, 274
Computerized tomography, 887–907
    AIDS-dementia, 210
    AIDS encephalopathy, 212
        toxoplasmosis, 215, 710, 902–903
    aspergillosis, 747–748
    bacterial meningitis, 382, 891–894
    brain abscess, 384, 463, 470–476,
        479–480, 889–892
        sensitivity, 472–474
        specificity, 474–475
    cavernous venous thrombosis,
        896–897
    chronic meningitis, 707–708, 894
    congenital cytomegalovirus, 183–184
    Creutzfeldt-Jakob disease, 158
    epidural abscess, 503–504, 509–510
    epidural empyemas, 895
    herpes simplex encephalitis, 51–52
    hydatid diagnosis, 839
    infective endocarditis, 532
    intracranial mycotic aneurysm, 544
    Lyme disease, 665, 671–672, 674
    versus magnetic resonance imaging,
        492–493, 504, 548, 887–907
    neurocysticercosis, 833–834, 905–906
    primary CNS lymphoma, 215, 903
    Rocky Mountain spotted fever, 415
    subacute sclerosing panencephalitis,
        148
    subdural effusion, 382–383
    subdural empyema, 491–493,
        893–898

surgery guidance, 479–481, 506
toxoplasmosis, 810, 817, 902–903
tuberculoma, 439–440
ventriculitis, 894–896
    neonates, 327
Conduction velocity, 676–677
Confusion, 549
Congenital aneurysms, 542
Congenital coronary heart disease, 466
Congenital cytomegalovirus
    clinical presentation, 183–184
    diagnosis, 185, 901
    epidemiology, 180–183
    history, 178–179
    immunology, 180
    magnetic resonance imaging, 901
    mortality, 183–184
    pathogenesis, 179–180
    treatment, 185
Congenital heart diseases, 466, 516
Congenital infection; see also under
        specific infections
    B. burgdorferi, 663
    Chagas disease, 786
    cytomegalovirus, 178–185
    Epstein-Barr virus, 187
    herpes simplex, 168–170
Congenital malformations
    mumps, 118
    subarachnoid space, 862–863
    varicella-zoster, 186
Congenital rubella, 191–192
    clinical findings, 191–192
    diagnosis, 192
    encephalitis, 192
    epidemiology, 191
    history, 188
    maternal-fetal transmission, 190–191
    prevention, 192
    serology, 190
Congenital toxoplasmosis, 805–807
    clinical manifestations, 807
    epidemiology, 805
    pathogenesis, 805–806
    pathology, 806–807
    polymerase chain reaction diagnosis,
        817
    prevention, 819
    retinochoroiditis, 807–808
    serology, 815
Congestive heart failure, 521
Conjunctival cysticercosis, 830
Connective tissue disease, 34
Consciousness, see Level of conscious-
        ness
Contact lenses, 793
Continuous-flow plasma exchange, 274
Contralateral hemiplegia, 61
Contrast agents, chemical meningitis,
        724
Contrast enhancement, see Gadolinium
        enhancement
Convulsions; see also Seizures
    cerebral malaria, 775
    childhood meningitis, 370
    congenital toxoplasmosis, 807
Cooperative Study Group Trials,
        651–653
Corn syrup ingestion, botulism, 590
Corneal cells, rabies virus, 130–131
Corneal infection, Acanthamoeba, 790,
        793
Corneal transplantation, rabies, 11, 130,
        133

Cortical blindness
    infective endocarditis, 550
    intracranial hypertension, 867
Cortical infarction, 384–385
Corticosteroids; see also Dexametha-
        sone
    and AIDS, CNS tuberculosis, 450
    brain abscess, 481
    cerebral malaria, 777
    computerized tomography effect, 475
    cryptococcosis cause, 696, 734
    CSF leukopenia, 696
    herpes zoster treatment, 63
    inflammatory cytokine suppression,
        393–394
    neurocysticercosis, 835–836
    praziquantal availability, 835–836
    tetanus management, 617
    in toxoplasmosis, 215
    tuberculous meningitis, 447–448,
        450, 713
Coumarin, 539
Countercurrent immunoelectrophoresis
    group B streptococci, 322
    sensitivity, 876
Counterimmunoelectrophoresis, 377,
        381–382
"Cowdry type A" inclusions
    herpes simplex infection, 45
    subacute sclerosing panencephalitis,
        147–148, 237
Coxiella burnetii, 412–414, 419
Coxsackie virus B5, 23
Coxsackieviruses
    CSF measurement, 880
    polymerase chain reaction, 26
    receptor family, 22
    serotypes, 22
Cranial nerve palsy
    childhood bacterial meningitis, 370
    Lyme disease, 672, 674
    Mycoplasma pneumoniae, 289
    progressive Borrelia encephalomyeli-
        tis, 674
    tuberculous meningitis, 431, 446–447
Cranial neuropathy
    botulism, 594–595
    Guillain-Barre' syndrome, 268–270
    HIV infection, 219–220
    infective endocarditis, 529, 531, 550
    Lyme disease, 672
    neurosyphilis, 646
Cranial trauma, see Head trauma
Craniotomy
    intracranial epidural abscess, 511
    meningitis association, 375
    subdural empyema, 495–496
Creatine kinase test, 221
Creutzfeldt-Jakob disease, 153–162
    versus Alzheimer's disease, 158–159
    clinical manifestations, 155
    diagnosis, 158–159
    electroencephalography, 157–158
    epidemiology, 153–154
    etiology, 159–161
    genetics, 161–162
    iatrogenic transmission, 154
    laboratory diagnosis, 157–158
    pathogenesis, 156–157
    pathology, 154–156
    prevention, 162
    prion hypothesis, 159–161
    therapy, 162
    transmission, 153–154

Crowded conditions, 342
Cry quality, 369
Cryptococcal meningitis
   amphotericin B, 734
   CD4 lymphocyte role, 696
   clinical presentation, 217, 713–714
   corticosteroid role, 696, 713, 734
   CSF test, 877
   diagnosis, 217–218, 729–732
   fluconazole maintenance, AIDS, 735
   and HIV infection, 214, 696, 734–735
      prognosis, 737
      treatment, 734–735
   imaging, 903
   immune response, 695–696
   India ink test, 706–707, 732
   pathogenesis, 695–696
   prognosis, 736–737
   relapse rate, 735
   serum antigen test, 731
   treatment, 710, 714, 731, 734–735
Crytococcal polysaccharide antigen, 730–731
Cryptococcomas
   appearance, 755
   clinical presentation, 755
   and cryptococcal meningitis, 755
   diagnosis, 755–756
   epidemiology, 755
   history, 754
   pathology, 755
   treatment, 734, 736, 756
Cryptococcosis, 694–697
Cryptococcus neoformans, 694–697, 754–756
   autopsy study, 743
   brain abscess, 462–463, 743–744, 754–755
   chronic meningitis, 710, 713–714
   classification, 693–694
   CSF cultures, 730–731, 755–756
   immune system response, 695–696
   India ink test, 706–707, 732, 755
   laboratory data, 706–707, 714, 730–731
   latex agglutination test, 730–731
   and other pathogens, CSF, 449
   serum antaigen test, 731
   virulence factors, 695
Cryptococcus neoformans var. *gatti,* 695
Cryptococcus neoformans var. *neoformans,* 695
"CSF-oma," 571–572
Ctenocephalidis felis, 660
Culex mosquitoes
   Japanese encephalitis, 94, 97, 246
   Murray Valley encephalitis, 94, 97–98
   Rift Valley fever, 103
   St. Louis encephalitis, 94–95
   Venezuelan equine encephalitis, 92
   Western equine encephalitis, 89, 91
Culiseta annulata, 102
Culiseta melanura mosquitoes, 90–91
Cunninghamellaceae, 749
Curvularia species, 761
"Cushing's relex," 370
Cutaneous lesions, *see* Skin lesions
Cuteus aplasia, 186
"Cutter incident," 247
Cyclic GMP, tetanospasmin, 608
Cyclops, 841, 843
Cystic fibrosis, brain abscess, 465
Cysticercosis, *see* Neurocysticercosis

Cysticercus cellulosae, 826–827, 830–831
   in brain parenchyma, 720
   histological appearance, 831
   host immune response, 831
Cysticercus racemose, 826–827, 830–831
   microscopic appearance, 831
   radiography, 834
Cysts; *see also* Tissue cysts
   amebae form, 788–789
   echinococcosis, 838
   magnetic resonance imaging, 834–835
   meningoencephalitis pathology, 792–793
   neurocysticerosis, 828, 830
   trichinosis, 845–846
Cytomegalovirus; *see also* Congenital cytomegalovirus
   activation of, HIV, 709
   CNS complications, 68–69
   diagnosis, 69
   epidemiology, 68, 180–183
   and Guillain-Barre' syndrome, 261–262
   history, 67
   and HIV infection, 213, 217, 709
   imaging, 901
   pathology and pathogenesis, 67–68
   perinatal infection, 178–185
   and Rasmussen's encephalitis, 153
   seropositivity rates, women, 180–181
   structure and replication, 67
   treatament, 69
Cytosine arabinoside, 34
Cytotoxic T lymphocytes, mumps, 117

D

Dactylaria constricta, 761
Dakar, Senegal, meningitis, 344
Dantrolene, tetanus management, 618
Day-care setting
   cytomegalovirus, 182–183
   H. influenzae meningitis, 338, 397–398
Deafness, mumps complication, 119, 242
Decubitus ulcers, 500, 567
Deer tick, *see Ixodes dammini*
DEET, 777
Deferoxamine, 750
Degenerative heart disease, 517
Degenerative joint disease, 500
Delayed hypersensitivity, tuberculosis, 432–433
Delivery
   cytomegalovirus, 182
   herpes simplex infection, 171
Dementia
   Lyme disease, 671, 675
   neurocysticercosis, 828–829
Demyelination
   Guillain-Barre' syndrome, 263–265, 267–268
   Lyme disease, 665, 672–673, 677
   primary amebic meningoencephalitis, 792
Dendritic trees, HIV infection, 213
Dengue fever, 245
Denmark, rabies identification, 133
Dental defects, cytomegalovirus, 183–184

Dental infections, brain abscess, 463–464
Deoxyhemoglobin, 888–899
Dermecentor andersoni, 103–104, 414
Dermacentor occidentalis, 660
Dermacentor parumapertus, 660
Dermacentor variabilis, 414, 660
Dermatiacious fungi
   brain abscess, 759–761
   spectrum of CNS involvement, 693–694
   surgery, 736
Dermatomes, herpes zoster, 58
Dermonecrotic toxin, 626
Dexamethasone
   ampicillin combination, CSF, 360
   brain abscess, 305, 481
   brain water, 361
   cerebral malaria, 777
   and CSF lipopolysaccharides, 357
   inflammatory cytokine suppression, 393–394
   intracranial pressure, 361, 395
   neurocysticercosis, 835–836
   praziquantel availability, 835–836
Dextrans
   cerebral malaria, 777
   spongiform encephalopathies, 162
Dextrostix, 375
DFMO, 786
Diabetes
   CSF:blood glucose ratio, 872
   epidural abscess, 500
   intracranial aspergillosis, 746
   rhinocerebral mucormycosis, 749–751
   tuberculous meningitis, 447
   Zygomycetes, 721
Diagnostic approach, syndromes, 2–4
3,4-Diaminopyridine, botulism, 597
Diaphragmatic paralysis, 611
Diazepam
   seizure treatment, 396
   tetanus management, 617–618
Diclofenac sodium, 356
Dideoxycytidine, 222
Dideoxyinosine, 222
N,N-Diethyl-3-methylbenzamide, 77
Difluoromethylornithine, 786
Dihydrofolate reductase inhibitors, 819
Dimorphic yeasts, 756–759
Diphenolic compounds, 695
Diphtheria-tetanus-pertussis vaccine
   encephalopathy controversy, 631–633
   reactogenicity, 629–631
Diphtheria-tetanus vaccine, 630
Diphtheroid infections
   clinical manifestations, 571
   incidence, shunts, 566–567
Diplopia, 550
Dipyridamole, 223
Direct instillation of antibiotics, 478, 575
Disinfection
   HIV virus, 205
   spongiform encephalopathy, viruses, 162
Disoxaril, 28
Disseminated herpes simplex
   neonates, 172–173, 176
   pregnant women, 170
   treatment, neonates, 176–177
Disseminated tuberculosis, HIV, 218

"Distal" shunt infection
  clinical manifestations, 570
  diagnosis, 572–573
  treatment, 577
Distal, symmetric, sensory polyneuropathy, 220–221
Disulfiram, 223
DNA viruses
  replication, 13
  slow infection, 146
Dogs
  rabies bites, 131
  Toxocara canis, 848
Dorsal root ganglia, rabies, 130
Dot-blot hybridization, enteroviruses, 27–28
Double-dose delayed-contrast CAT, 817
Double-sandwich IgM-ELISA, 815
Doughnut lesion, 414, 471
Doxycycline
  Lyme diseae, 681–683
  Rocky Mountain spotted fever, 415
  toxoplasmosis, 819
Dreschlera species, 693, 761
Drug abusers, *see* Intraverous drug abusers
Drug resistance; *see also under specific drugs*
  Mycobacterium tuberculosis, 445
DS-IgM-ELISA, toxoplasmosis, 815
Duck, gnathostomiasis, 843
Duck embryo vaccine, 139
"Dumb" rabies, 135
Dura mater
  anatomy, 862
  and trauma, fistula, 374–375
"Durck nodules," 770
Dysphagia, tetanus, 612
Dysphasia, herpes simplex, 14

E

E-protein, flaviviruses, 94
E1 glycoprotein, rubella, 189
"E1a," 204
Early antigen diffuse antibody response, 67
Early antigen restricted antibody response, 67
East African sleeping sickness, 782–783
Eastern equine encephalitis, 89–91
  diagnosis, 90–91
  epidemiology, 89–90
  history, 89
  overwintering phenomenon, 90
  pathology and pathogenesis, 89
  prevention and treatment, 91
Eaton-Lambert syndrome, 596
Echinococcosis, 837–840
  clinical manifestations, 838
  diagnosis, 839
  etiology and epidemiology, 837–838
  pathogenesis, 838
  prognosis, 840
  treatment, 839–840
Echinococcus granulosus
  abendazole effect, 840
  anatomy, 838
  geographical distribution, 837–838
Echinococcus multilocularis
  anatomy, 838
  geographical distribution, 838–838
Echocardiography

embolism prediction, 537–538
  infective endocarditis, 522, 537–538
Echovirus 9 meningitis, 25
Echovirus 71 meningitis, 25
Edema, *see* Cerebral edema
Edmonston vaccine, 238
Egg allergies, measles vaccine, 238
Ehrlichia canis, 412, 414, 420
Ehrlichia sennetsu, 420
Ehrlichiosis, 412, 420
EITB assay, 833
Eighth-nerve function, streptomycin, 447
Eikenella corrodens, 461
Elderly
  antibiotics, 392
  bacterial meningitis, 374
  tuberculosis, 427
"Electric shock" root pain, 502
Electroencephalogram
  brain abscess, 470–471
  Creutzfeldt-Jakob disease, 157
  Lyme disease, 671, 674
  mumps, 121
  progressive rubella panencephalitis, 152
  subacute sclerosing panencephalitis, 148, 237
Electrolytes, tuberculous meningitis, 432
ELISA
  HIV infection, 207
  Lyme disease, 678–679
  mumps, 121
  neurocysticercosis, 832–833
  toxoplasmosis, 815
  tuberculous meningitis, 436
Embolic phenomena; *see also* Cerebral embolism
  infectious endocarditis, 521
"Empty delta" sign, 865
Encapsulation
  bacteria, 299, 305
  brain abscess, 305, 467–469
  C. neoformans, 695
  versus cerebritis, CT scan, 480
  computerized tomography, 480, 890–891
Encephalitis cysticercosis, 835
Encephalitis; *see also* Herpes simplex encephalitis; Toxoplasmic encephalitis
  enteroviruses, 28
  Lyme disease, 672
  measles, 8, 15, 234, 236
  mumps, 31, 113–125
  Mycoplasma pneumoniae, 289
  occurrence, 8
  Rocky Mountain spotted fever, 415
  rubella, 189–190
  syndrome recognition, 2–3
  varicella-zoster viruses, 60–61
Encephalomalacia, 168
Encephalomyelitis, 3
Endemic typhus, 412, 419
Endocarditis, *see* Infective endocarditis
Endocytosis, viral entry, 12
Endolimax nana, 787
Endophthalmitis, 551
Endothelial cells
  AIDS-dementia pathophysiology, 211
  in barrier systems, 864
  cerebral malaria pathogenesis, 771–773

cytokine release, 864
  red blood cell adherence, 771–773
  viral transport, 11
Endotoxins
  cerebral malaria, 775
  rickettsial disease, 413
Endotracheal tube, tetanus, 617
Enkephalin, 614
Entamoeba histolytica
  brain abscess, 462, 794–796
  comparataive morphology, 788
  infection rate, 794–795
  pathologic potential, 787
Enteral feeding, tetanus, 619
Enterobacter species
  epidural abscess, 501
  neonatal meningitis, 314–315, 326
  treatment, neonates, 326
Enterococcus faecalis, 519–520
Enterovirus meningitis, 19–28
  clinical manifestations, 24–25
  diagnosis, 25–28
  epidemiology, 22–23
  laboratory findings, 25–28
  long-term effects, 25
  polymerase chain reaction, 26, 28
  predisposing factors, 23
  prevention, 28
  seasonal variation, 21, 23
  simultaneous bacterial infection, 351
  treatment, 25, 28
Enteroviruses
  laboratory findings, 25–27
  pathogenesis, 20–22
  subgroups, 20
  virology, 20–21
Entomophthoraceae, 749
env gene, HIV, 201
Enzyme-linked immunoelectrotransfer blot, 833
Enzyme-linked immunosorbent assay, *see* ELISA
Eosinophilia
  in CSF, 871
  toxocariasis, 849
Eosinophilic meningitis
  Angiostrongylus infection, 842–843
  baylisascariasis, 849
  gnathostomiasis, 844
Ependymal cells, mumps, 116–117
Epidemic typhus, 412, 417–418
Epidermal growth factor receptor, 12
Epidural abscess, 499–514; *see also* Intracranial epidural abscess; Spinal epidural abscess
Epidural anesthesia, 262
Epidural empyema
  computerized tomography, 895, 897
  magnetic resonance imaging, 493, 895
Epidural ICP monitoring devices, 562
Epidural space, anatomy, 862
Epidural tuberculous granulomas, 42
Epiglottitis, *H. influenzae*, 337
Epilepsy
  and pertussis vaccine, 631
  tetanospasmin model, 615
  toxocariasis association, 84j9
"Episome," 202
Epstein-Barr virus, 65–67
  CNS complications, 66
  diagnosis, 67
  epidemiology, 66, 187

Epstein-Barr virus (contd.)
  and Guillain-Barre' syndrome, 261–262
  history, 65
  HIV activation, 709
  meningitis, 32
  pathology and pathogenesis, 65–66
  perinatal infection, 187–188
  and primary CNS lymphoma, 216
  and Rasmussen's encephalitis, 153
  structure and transcription, 65
  treatment, 67
Epstein-Barr virus nuclear antigens, 66
  Equine rabies antiserum 251
Erythema chronicum migrans
  antibiotic treatment, 680–681
  appearance, 667
  B. burgdorferi cause, 663
  versus bacterial meningitis rash, 377–378
  and cranial neuropathy, 672
  Europe versus North America, 677
  Lyme disease lesion, 657–658, 667
  and meningitis, 671
  and radicular pain, 677
Erythrocyte sedimentation rate
  brain abscess, 470
  infective endocarditis, 522
  neonatal meningitis, 324
Erythrocytes, *see* Red blood cells
Erythromycin
  Lyme diseae, 680–681
  Mycoplasma pneumoniae, 291
  neurosyphilis treatment, 651–652
  pertussis, 627
"Escape" inflammation, 304
Escherichia coli
  brain abscess, 303–304, 468
  cerebral edema, 302, 361
  clonality, 318
  CSF pressure, 361
  fimbriae, binding, 300
  K1, pathogenesis, 318–319
  laboratory tests, neonates, 321–322
  meningitis, adhesion, 298
  neonatal meningitis, 314–324
  pathogenesis, neonates, 318–320
  shunt infections, 566
  treatment, neonates, CSF, 326
Ethambutol
  CSF penetration, 443
  treatment regimen, 445
  tuberculous meningitis, 444–445, 713
Ethionamide, 444
Europe, *Borrelia burgdorferi*, 677, 678
Evoked potentials, 676
Excision
  versus aspiration, 479
  brain abscess, 479–480
"Exit pump," 387
Experimental allergic neuritis
  pathophysiology, 266–267
  pertussis toxin, 628
Exserohilum species, 761
Externalized shunts/ventriculostomy
  antibiotic prophylaxis, 580
  clinical manifestations, infection, 571
  complications, 576
  CSF shunt types, 562–564
  effectiveness, 576–579
  in neonates, 565
  retrograde type, 567
  risk, 576
Extracranial-intracranial bypass, 545

Extramedullary cysticercosis, 829, 835
Extraocular intraorbital cysticercosis, 829–830
Extraocular muscle, *Trichinella*, 845–846
Extrapyramidal symptoms, toxoplasmosis, 813–814
Eye infection, neonatal herpes, 174
Eye movements, AIDS-dementia, 210

F
F-wave
  Guillain-Barre' syndrome, 271
  Lyme disease, 676
Facial bites, rabies, 133–134
Facial nerve palsy
  antibiotic treatment, 682
  Guillain-Barre' syndrome, 268–269
  Lyme disease, 672, 682
  mumps, 119
Facial paresis, tetanus, 612
Falx cerebri, anatomy, 488
Familial Alzheimer's disease, 162
Fansidar, 776–777
Faroe Islands, *N. meningitidis*, 339
Father-to-child, herpes simplex, 169
Fatigue, Lyme disease, 671, 675–676
Fc receptors
  endothelial cells, 11
  group B streptococci, neonates, 317–318
  HIV binding, 204
Felis domestica, 802
Fermi vaccine, 133
Fetal monitors
  bacteria acquisition, 315
  herpes transmission, 170
Fetal rhesus kidney cells, 251
Fetus; *see also* Intrauterine infection
  Borrelia burgdorferi effect, 663
  Epstein-Barr infection, 187
  herpes simplex transmission, 169–170
  toxoplasmosis risk, 805–807
  varicella-zoster infection, 186
Fever
  bacterial meningitis, 320–321, 368–369
  brain abscess, 469
  cryptococcal meningitis, 713–714
  Lyme disease, 671
  mumps, CNS infection, 118–119
  shunt infection, 570–571
  sleeping sickness, 783
  subdural empyema, 490–491
  tuberculous meningitis, 431
Fibrinogen, 323
Fibrinous pericarditis, 667
Fibroblast growth factor receptor, 12
Fibronectin, 315
Filamentous hemagglutinin, 626, 629
"Filia olfactoria," 790–791
Filipinos, *Coccidioides immitis*, 714
Fimbriae
  bacterial adhesion, 298–300, 352
  binding mechanism, 353
  E. coli, choroid plexus, 319
Finland
  Hemophilus influenzae meningitis, 337–339
  Neisseria meningitidis, 340–341
  polio outbreak, 248
Fish products, botulism, 589

Flagellate
  amebae form, 788–789
  meningoencephalitis pathology, 792
Flagellin fraction, 679
Flaviviruses, 93–99
  aseptic meningitis, 29
  background, 93
  encephalitis, 93–99
  infectious agents, 93–94
  pathology and pathogenesis, 94
Flubendazole, 835–836
Fluconazole
  AIDS patients, 735
  coccidioidal meningitis, 735
  cryptococcal meningitis, 710, 714, 733–735
  Pseudallestheria boydii infection, 752
Flucytosine
  and amphotericin B, 734
  candidal infections, 754
  cryptococcal brain abscess, 756
  cryptococcal meningitis, 710, 714, 732, 734
  fungal meningitis, 732–734
  toxicity, 734
  treatment failures, 732
  X. bantiana brain abscess, 760
Fluid management, hyponatremia, 396
Fluorescent treponemal antibody absorption test
  Lyme disease, 719
  neurosyphilis, 643, 718
5-Fluorocytosine
  Asperigillus brain abscess, 748
  shunt infections, 579
Flying squirrel, 417
Folic acid supplement, 818–819
Folinic acid, toxoplasmosis, 215, 818
Fonsecaea pedrosoi, 761
"Food cups," 788–789
  Foodborne botulism, 589–602
  clinical mnanifestations, 593–595
  diagnosis, 596
  epidemiology, 589–590
  fatality rates, 595
  prevention, 598
  therapy, 597
Foramen of Luschka
  anatomy, 861–862
  obstructive hydrocephalus, 865
Foramen of Magendie
  anatomy, 861–862
  obstructive hydrocephalus, 865
Foramen of Monro
  anatomy, 861–862
  obstructive hydrocephalus, 865
Formic acid, 162
Formula-fed infants, botulism, 590–591
Foscarnet, 222
Fourth ventricle
  anatomy, 861–862
  magnetic resonance imaging, 896
  obstructive hydrocephalus, 865
Foxes
  immunization, 139
  rabies virus, 129–130, 132
Fresh-frozen plasma, 273
  Fresno County, California, meningitis, 337
Frontal lobe abscesses
  clinical manifestations, 469
  computerized tomography, 472–476
  etiology, 458–459

otogenesis, 464
and sinusitis, 464
Frontal sinusitis
computerized tomography, 492
intracranial epidural abscess, 508
subdural empyema, 488
FTA-ABS test, 643
Fulminant meningococcal septicemia, 370
differential diagnosis, 377
treatment, 393
Fungal infections, 693–702, 743–761
brain, 743–761
CSF culture, 875, 879–880
CSF shunts, 567, 571, 579
endocarditis, 517
epidural abscess, 501
microscopic dtection, 874–875
space-occupying lesions, 743–761
Fungal meningitis
chronic syndrome, 703–726
clinical presentation, 729
CSF cultures, 729–731, 879–880
diagnosis, 729–732
laboratory tests, 706–708
prognosis, 736–737
surgery, 736
time course, 729
treatment, 731–737
Fungemia, 551
Fungus balls, 753
"Furious" rabies, 135
Furosemide, 863
Fusarium species, 752
Fusidic acid, 478
Fusion glycoprotein
HIV, 202
measles, 234
mumps virus, 114
Fusobacterium species, 350

G
GABA, tetanospasmin effect, 608, 612–614
Gadolinium enhancement, 889
AIDS encephalopathy, 902–903
bacterial meningitis evaluation, 385–386, 893–894
blood-brain-barrier, 900–901
brain abscess, 476, 890–891
cerebritis, 889
epidural abscess, 504
extra-axial inflammatory disease, 493
herpes simplex, 900–901
HIV infection, 902
neurocysticercosis, 835
technique, 889
tuberculous meningitis, 438, 896
ventriculitis, 896
Galactosemia, 316
Gallium-67 citrate, 522
Gambian sleeping sickness, 780, 782
Gamma interferon, 803
Gammaglobulin, enterovrus meningitis, 25, 28
Ganciclovir
B virus, 74
cytomegalovirus treatment, 69, 185, 217
mental confusion, 223
Gangliosides, and tetanospasmin, 615
Garki Project, 768

Gas-containing abscess, imaging, 890–891
Gas-liquid chromatography, 877–878
Gastroenteritis, 262
Gastrointestinal symptoms, botulism, 594–595
"Gemistocytic" astrocytes, 366
General paresis, 648
CSF diagnosis, 718
pathological changes, 648
penicillin effect, 652
syndrome, 648
Generalized tetanus, 608, 611–612
Genetic engineering, vaccines, 176
Genital herpes simplex
epidemiology, 48
perinatal transmission, 169–171
viral shedding, pregnancy, 171
Genital lesions, HIV transmission, 205
Genital tract, cytomegalovirus, 183
Gentamicin
CSF penetration, 574
intraventricular administration, 327–328, 575, 579
neonatal meningitis, 324–325, 327–328
neurotoxicity, 328
recommended doses, 388, 575
shunt infection, 574–575, 579
Germanin, *see* Suramin
Gerstmann-Sträussler syndrome, 152–162
clinical manifestations, 155
diagnosis, 158–159
epidemiology, 153–154
genetics, 161
pathology, 155–156
Gestation, congenital toxoplasmosis, 806
Giant vesicles, CSF transport, 863
"Gilchrist's disease," 756
Gitter cells, 796
Glasgow coma score, 54–55
Glaucomys volans, 417
Glial cells
bacterial meningitis pathology, 364–365
herpes simplex infection, 45
herpes simplex transmission, 13–14
sleeping sickness, 780–781, 786
toxoplasmosis, 812–813
Gliomas
cerebrospinal fluid, 725
imaging, 890
Glossina, 778
Glucocorticoids
myopathies, 221
in toxoplasmosis, 215
Glucose levels, CSF, 871–873; *see also* Hypoglycorrhachia
bacterial meningitis, 379, 381, 873
blood glucose ratio, 872
cerebral malaria, 774–775, 777
chronic meningitis, 704, 708
mumps, 120
neonatal meningitis, 321–322
tuberculous meningitis, 433–434, 879
values of, 871–873
Glucose-6-phosphate dehydrogenase, 416
Glycinergic cells, tetanospasmin, 612–614
Glycocalyx, *see* "Slime"
Glycoprotein D, 43

Glycoproteins
herpes simplex virus, 43
rabies virus, 129
Gnathostoma spinigerum, 843, 871
Gnathostomiasis, 843–845
clinical findings, and idagnosis, 844–845
CNS involvement, 844
CSF findings, 844–845
epidemiology, 843
pathogenesis and pathology, 843–844
treatment and outcome, 845
Goat's milk, 804
Göteborg, Sweden area, meningitis, 342–343
gp41, 201–202
gp120
AIDS-dementia pathophysiology, 211
CD4 binding, 204
cytopathic effects, 205
HIV virion, 201–202
"Gradenigo's syndrome," 509
Gradual echo images, 889
Gram-negative bacteria
antibiotics, 390, 578
brain abscess, 459–462
children and adults, 348
epidural abscess, 501
inflammation, CSF, 301
morphology, 297–298
neonatal meningitis, 314–316
and neurosurgical procedures, 375
shunt infections, 566, 572, 578
staining method, 874
subdural empyema, 494
Gram-positive bacteria
inflammation inducer, 301
morphology, 297–298
neonatal meningitis, 313–314, 316–320
pathogenesis, neonates, 316–320
staining method, 874
Gram's stain
bacterial meningitis, CSF, 380
method, 873–874
sensitivity, 874
Granular ependymitis, 116–117
Granular nodular cysts, MRI, 834–835
Granuloma; *see also* Malarial granuloma
Chagas disease, 786–787
meningitis diagnosis, 707–708
retinal toxoplasmosis, 809
and sarcoidosis, 721
toxocariasis, 848–849
Granulomatous amebic encephalitis
Acanthamoeba, 787
clinical manifestations, 793
diagnosis, 793
pathogenesis, 792
pathology, 792–793
treatment and prognosis, 794
Granulomatous angiitis, 722
AIDS, 217
clinical manifestations, 722
herpes zoster encephalitis, 61
laboratory studies, 722
Group B streptococci
capsular polysaccharides, 316–317
cerebral embolism, endocarditis, 533
chemoprophylaxis, 328–329
children and adults, 348–349, 390
extracellular products, 317–318
immunization, 328

920 / SUBJECT INDEX

Group B streptococci (*contd.*)
  immunoprophylaxis, 329
  laboratory tests, neonates, 321–322
  neonatal meningitis, 313–318
  pathogenesis, neonates, 315–318
  and penicillin resistance, 390
  prognosis, 326
  serotypes, 316, 348–349
  treatment, 325–326, 390
Growth hormone, 154
Guanidine hydrochloride, 599
Guanoxan, botulism, 597
Guillain-Barre' syndrome, 259–279
  antecedent conditions, 261–263
  versus botulism, 596
  cerebrospinal fluid, 270
  clinical manifestations, 268–271
  diagnosis, 268, 270
  electron microscopy, 264–265
  electrophysiology, 271–272
  epidemiology, 259–261
  HIV infection, 220
  and Lyme disease, 673
  Myoplasma pneumoniae, 289
  pathogenesis and pathophysiology,
    265–268
  pathology, 263–265
  plasma exchange, 272–274
  plateau phase, 274–275
  prognosis, 274–275
  and rabies, 135, 251, 262
  treatment, 272–274
Guinea pig inoculation, 878
Guinea pig model, CSF shunt infection,
  306
Gummatous neurosyphilis, 644,
  649–650

H
H-reflex, 271
H9 cell culture, 204
"HACEK" group, 519–520
Hadera district, Israel, 248
Haitian immigrants
  CNS tuberculosis, AIDS, 449–450
  toxoplasmosis, AIDS, 811
Halofantrine, 776
Hamster model, mumps, 116–117
Hand-foot-mouth syndrome, 25
Haptoglobin, 323–324
Hboc vaccine, 399
Head trauma *see also* Post-traumatic
    infection
  brain abscess, 465
  epidural abscess, 509
  meningitis association, 374–375, 392
  subarachnoid space, 863
  subdural empyema cause, 489
Headache
  brain abscess, 469
  cryptococcal meningitis, 713–714
  infective endocarditis, 529–530
  intracranial mycotic aneurysm, 543,
    545
  lumbar puncture complication, 868
  neurocysticercosis, 828–829
  sleeping sickness, 783
  subdural empyema, 490
  tubercular meningitis, 430–431
Hearing loss
  ataxia association, 373
  congenital cytomegalovirus, 183–184
  congenital rubella, 191–192

dexamethasone protection, 393–394
enterovirus meningitis, 25
Lyme diseae, 672
mumps, 119
Heart murmur, 521
Heart transplant, *see* Cardiac transplant
Heat disinfection
  HIV virus, 205
  spongiform encephalopathy viruses,
    162
Heat-labile toxin, 626
Heel stick cultures, 321
Helminthic infections, 825–858
Helper T cells, 207
Hemagglutination inhibition
  alphaviruses, 88
  mumps, 121
Hemagglutinin-neuraminidase glyco-
    protein, 114
Hematogenous brain abscesses
  capsule formation, 468
  pathogenesis, 465–467
Hematogenous spread
  Aspergillus species, 746
  Borrelia burgdorferi, 663
  and brain abscess, 465–467
  overview, 8–11
  shunt infection, 567–568
  subdural empyema, 489
  tetanospasmin, 612–614
  viral pathogens, 8
Hemianopsias
  brain abscess, 469
  interhemispheric subdural empyema,
    491
Hemiparesis
  childhood bacterial meningitis, 370
  progressive *Borrelia* encephalomyeli-
    tis, 674
  subdural empyema, 490
  tuberculous meningitis, 431
Hemiplegia
  brain abscess, 469
  herpes simplex encephalitis, 14–15
  Mycoplasma pneumoniae, 289
  ophthalmicus zoster, 61
Hemodialysis, infective endocarditis,
  517
Hemolysin
  group B streptococci, 318
  and pertussis, 626
Hemophilus influenzae; see also *Hemo-
    philus influenzae* type b
  electrophetic types, 345
  epidemiology, 336–339
  etiological factors, 343–345
  neonatal meningitis, 314–315
Hemophilus influenzae Rd, 358–359
Hemophilus influenzae type b
  adhesion, 299
  adults, symptoms, 373–374
  age stratification, meningitis, 336
  bacterial meningitis model, 32, 297
  blood-brain-barrier effects, 320,
    358–360
  brain abscess, neonates, 465
  brain water, dexamethasone, 361
  carriage rates, 337–338
  ceftriaxone, CSF, 357
  cerebral blood flow, 362
  chemoprophylaxis, 397–398
  children, symptoms, 369, 370, 373
  complement cascade, 300, 352
  CSF inflammation, 301–302, 356

CSF invasion, 353
epidemiology, meningitis, 336–339
and Guillain-Barre' syndrome,
  262–263
immunoprophylaxis, 398, 400
intracisternal inoculation, 356–357,
  360
lipopolysaccharide, CSF, 356–357,
  360
meningeal invasion, 353
monoclonal antibodies, 354
nasopharyngeal colonization,
  351–352
passive prophylaxis, 399–400
pathology, meningitis, 367
postinfectious encephalomyelitis, 16
secondary infection risk, 397
shunt infection, 567–568
subdural empyema, 495
Hemophilus species
  brain abscess, 461
  infective endocarditis, 528
Hemorrhagic leukoencephalopathy, 781
Hemorrhagic stroke, AIDS, 216–217
Hemorrhagic ventriculitis, 367–368
Heparin
  cerebral malaria, 777
  Guillain-Barre' syndrome, 272
  infective endocarditis, 539–9546
Hepatic abscess, 795
Herd immunity
  rubella, 192
  polio, 247
Hereditary hemorrhagic telangiectasia,
  466–467
Hermaphroditic nematode, 847
Herpes B virus, *see* B virus
Herpes labialis, recurrences, 46
"Herpes" simiae, *see* B virus
Herpes simplex encephalitis, 41–75
  animal model, latency, 7
  antigen detection, 52
  versus bacterial meningitis, 377
  brain biopsy, 50–51
  costs, 50
  CSF measurement, 880
  diagnosis, 50–52
  hemiplegia, 14–15
  imaging, 899–901
  mortality, 53–55
  newborns, 1720173, 177
  occurrence, 8, 50
  pathogenesis, 47
  prognosis, 53
  relapse, 55
  seizures, 14
  serology, 51–52
  therapy, 52
  treatment of newborns, 177–178
Herpes simplex virus *see also* B virus;
    Herpes simplex encephalitis;
    Neonatal herpes simplex
  and AIDS, 217
  CNS transport, 13–14
  epidemiology, 47–50
  general characteristics, 41–44
  history, 42–43
  latency, 46
  neural transmission, 11
  pathogenesis, 45–47
  pathology, 44–45
  replication, 32
  structure, 41–43
  vaccines, 176

Herpes simplex virus type 1
  cell-to-cell transmission, 13–14
  CNS transport, 13
  epidemiology, recurrence, 49–50
  general charactristics, 42
  genital infections, 32, 48, 169
  pathogenesis, 45
  perinatal transmission, 169
Herpes simplex virus type 2
  epidemiology, 48–50
  general characteristics, 42
  genital infection, 32, 217
  pathogenesis, 45
  seroprevalence, 50
Herpes zoster (shingles); see also Vari-
    cella-zoster virus
  and AIDS, 217
  course of disease, 58–59
  diagnosis, 62–63
  encephalitis, 61
  epidemiology, 58–59
  meningitis, 32
  neurologic complications, 32, 60–62
  perinatal infection, 185–187
  and pregnancy, 186
  treatment, 63–65, 187
Herpes zoster ophthalmicus
  general characteristics, 61
  and vasculitis, 722
"Heubner's arteritis," 647
"Highlands J" virus, 91
Hip prosthesis infection, 568
Histoplasma capsulatum
  autopsy study, 743
  brain abscess, 743–744, 757–758
  chronic meningitis agent, 715
  classification, 693–694
  CSF culture, 730–731
  CSF serology, 730–731, 877
  epidemiology, 757
  laboratory data, 706, 715, 730–732,
    758
  pathogenesis, 698, 758
  radioimmunoassay, 715, 731–732,
    758
  treatment, 731, 735–736, 758
Histoplasma meningitis, 715
  antibody detection, 715, 731–732
  CSF culture, 715, 730–731
  treatment, 715, 735–736
Histoplasmic polysaccharide antigen,
    732
Histoplasmoma, 758
Histoplasmosis, 757–758
HIV-infected mothers, toxoplasmosis,
    811
HIV infection, 201–232; see also AIDS
  brain abscess, 462–463, 481
  cell biology, 204–205
  cerebral toxoplasmosis, 710–712
  children, 212–213
    vaccines, 223
  chronic meningitis, 709–712
  clinical manifestations, 205–207
  crytococcus, 734–735
  diagnosis, CNS, 213–214
  epidemiology, 205
  epidural abscess, 502
  and Guillain-Barre' syndrome, 262
  imagery, subacute encephalopathy,
    901–902
  laboratory tests, 207–208
    infants, 213
  and lymphomatous meningitis, 712

and measles vaccination, 238–239
meningitis, 32–33, 711–712
mumps vaccine, 121
neurological manifestations, 209–223
and neurosyphilis, 218, 653–654,
    711–712
overview of pathogenesis, 9–10
provirus expression, 202–204
staging, 205–207
and tetanus immunization, 619
toxoplasmosis serology, 816
transmission, 205
treatment, 221–223
and tuberculosis, 218, 427, 449–450
  treatment, 450
vaccines, 223
virion, 201–202
virus life cycle, 202–204
HIV-2 infection, 207
HIV protease, 201
Hodgkin's disease
  and crytococcal meningitis, 713
  toxoplasmosis, 810, 814
Homeless, tuberculosis, 427
Homonymous hemianopsia, 543
Homosexuals, cytomegalovirus excre-
    tion, 68
Honey infestion, botulism, 590
Horse serum, 138
Hospital personnel, bacteria transmis-
    sion, 315
HPA23, 162
HPV vaccine strains, 192
HSV-1, see Herpes simplex virus type 1
HSV-2, see Herpes simplex virus type 2
HTLV-1
  and HIV, myeloradiculopathy, 219
  meningitis, 33
  myopathy, 221
  as slow virus, 153
"HTLV-1-associated myelopathy," 153,
    219, 221
Human diploid cell vaccine
  adverse effects, 139
  cost, 139
  rabies prophylaxis, 137–139, 250–253
Human growth hormone, 154
Human herpesviruses 6 and 7, 74–75
Human rabies immune globulin, 251
Human T-cell leukemia virus 1, see
    HTLV-1
Human tetanus immunoglobulin,
    616–617, 620
Humoral immune system
  AIDS, 207
  bacterial infection, 299–300, 376
  Borrelia burgdorferi, 663–664
  congenital cytomegalovirus, 180
  cryptococcosis, 696
  Guillain-Barre' syndrome, 267–268
Hyalohyphomycoses, 699
Hyaluronidase, 447
Hybridization-based assays, 27–28
Hydatid disease, 837–841
"Hydatid sand," 838
Hydranencephaly, 172
Hydrocephalus
  computerized tomography, 384, 865
  congenital toxoplasmosis, 806–807
  CSF obstruction, 366, 864–866
  CSF shunts, 561–585, 734
  E. coli, neonates, 320
  magnetic resonance imaging, 865, 893
  mumps, 116

neurocysticercosis, treatment, 835
subarachnoid cysticercosis, 829
surgery, 448
tuberculous meningitis, 429, 431, 448
Hydrophobia, rabies, 135, 250
Hyperbaric oxygen treatment
  epidural abscess, 506
  mucormycosis, 751
Hyperesthesias, Lyme disease, 672, 676
Hypergammaglobulinemia
  HIV infection, children, 213
  sleeping sickness, 781–782
Hyperglycemia, CSF glucose, 872
Hyperimmune globulin, 399–400
Hyperinfection syndrome, 847
Hyperventilation
  intracranial pressure effect, 395
  primary CNS lymphoma, 215
Hypoglycemia
  cerebral malaria pathophysiology,
    774–775
  pertussis, 628
Hypoglycorrachia, 872
  brain abscess, 470
  causes of, 730, 872
  cystercercosis, 720
  fungal meningitis, 729–730
  neonatal meningitis, 321
  tuberculous meningitis, 433
Hyponatremia
  fluid management, 396
  H. influenzae meningitis, 373
Hypoplastic extremities, 186
Hypothermia, tuberculous meningitis,
    447
Hypotonic/hyporesponsive episodes,
    630

I
Ibc protein, 317–318
ICAM-1 adhesion molecule, 773–774
Identical contralateral reflex sign, 368
Idiopathic hypertrophic subaortic ste-
    nosis, 517
Idoxuridine, 52–53
Ilheus virus, 98
Imaging, 887–907; see also specific
    imaging methods
Imipenem-cilastatin, 477
Immune complexes
  cerebral malaria, 774
  in choroid plexus, 528
  congenital cytomegalovirus, 180
  Guillain-Barre' syndrome, 268
  infective endocarditis, 519, 521
  intracranial mycotic aneurysm cause,
    542
  Lyme disease pathogenesis, 665
  sleeping sickness, 782
Immune response; see also Cell-me-
    diated immunity; Humoral im-
    mune system
  congenital cytomegalovirus, 180
  mumps, 117–118
  sleeping sickness pathogenesis, 782
  spongiform encephalopathies, 157
Immune serum globulin
  aseptic meningitis cause, 34
  neonatal meningitis therapy, 325–326
Immunization, see Vaccines
Immunoassay techniques, enterovi-
    ruses, 27

Immunoblotting techniques, Lyme disease, 679
Immunocompromised host
  amebae infection, 792
  antibiotics, 392
  bacterial meningitis, 375–376, 392
  brain abscess, 305, 462–463, 743–744
  chronic meningitis, 709–712, 721
  crytococcal meningitis, 734–735
  cytomegalovirus, 68–69
  fungal brain infestation, 743–746
  herpes simplex, 47
  measles, 236
  mumps, 117
  reactivation toxoplasmosis, 812
  toxoplasmosis, 810–815
  varicella-zoster infection, treatment, 63–65
Immunofluorescence, Lyme disease, 678–679
Immunoglobulin, 187
  Immunoglobulin A
    Guillain Barre' syndrome, 268
    and mycoplasmas, adhesion, 299
    proteases, bacterial virulence, 347
    sleeping sickness, 784–785
  Immunoglobulin G
    bacterial meningitis, 354
    blood-to-CSF ratio, 354
    Borrelia burgdorferi, 664, 679
    congenital cytomegalovirus, 180
    congenital toxoplasmosis, 815–816
    CSF levels, 354, 873
    group B streptococci protection, 317, 325–326, 328–329
    Guillain-Barre' syndrome, 268
    HIV infection, infants, 213
    monoclonal antibody, 325–326
    mumps, 117
    neonates, 315, 317
    neurocysticercosis, 832–833
    sleeping sickness, CSF, 784–785
    subacute sclerosing panencephalitis, 147–148
  Immunoglobulin M
    bacterial meningitis, 324, 354
    Borrelia burgdorferi, 664, 679
    congenital cytomegalovirus, 180
    congenital rubella, 192
    CSF levels, 354
    Guillain-Barre' syndrome, 268
    HIV infection, 205
    Japanese encephalitis virus, 245
    mumps, 117
    neonatal meningitis, 324
    neurocysticercosis, 832–833
    sleeping sickness, 784–785
    subactue sclerosing panencephalitis, 147–148
    toxoplasmosis diagnosis, 815
Immunosuppression, *see* Immunocompromised host
Implanted CSF reservoirs, *see* Internal CSF reservoirs
in utero infection, *see* Intrauterine infection
Inactivated polio vaccine, 247–249
Inappropriate antidiuretic hormone, 25
Incubation period
  meningococcal disease, 342
  rabies virus, 131, 134–135
  tetanus, 609
India
  aspergillosis, 746

malaria, 768
rabies cases, 133
India ink test
  cryptococci, 706–707, 732
  method, 874–875
Indium-111-labeled platelets, 522
Indomethacin
  brain water, pneumococci, 361
  and CSF inflammation, cell walls, 356
Infant botulism, 589–602
  clinical manifestation, 595–596
  diagnosis, 597
  epidemiology, 590–591
  hospital costs, 596
  and SIDS, 591, 596
  therapy, 598
Infant-to-mother transmission, cytomegalovirus, 181
Infectious aneurysms, *see* Intracranial mycotic aneurysm
Infectious botulism, 589–602
Infectious mononucleosis, 66
Infective endocarditis, 515–559
  blood culture, 522
  and brain abscess, 465–466
  cardiac surgery, 535–537
  clinical manifestations, 521–522, 529–531, 533–534
  CNS complications, 525–551
  CSF examinations, 531–532
  diagnosis, 522–523, 531–532
  epidemiology, 515–516, 525–526
  epidural abscess source, 500
  etiologic agents, 519–521, 528
  history, 515
  intracranial mycotic aneurysm, 540–546
  metastatic infections, 546–550
  negative blood cultures, 520–521
  neurologic syndromes, 529
  outcome, 532
  pathogenesis, 517–519, 527–528, 533–534
  predisposing factors, 516–517
  surgery, 523–524
  treatment, 523
Inflammation
  and antibiotic kinetics, 387
  bacterial induction, CSF, 355–358
  bacterial meningitis pathology, 363–365
  Borrelia burgdorferi pathogenesis, 664
  brain abscess containment, 305
  congenital toxoplasmosis, 806
  tuberculous meningitis, 429
Influenza B, *see* *Hemophilus influenzae* type b
Influenza vaccine, 262
Infratentorial subdural empyemas
  anatomy, 488
  clinical features, 491
  pathogenesis, 488–489
"Inhibitory quotient," 575
Inoculum effect, 387
Inosiplex, 149, 237
Instillation of antibiotics, 478, 575
Insulin secretion, pertussis, 628
Interferons
  in chickenpox, 63–64
  in herpes zoster, 64
  HIV infection, CSF, 209
  levels in mumps infection 117
Interhemispheric subdural empyema

clinical features, 491
computerized tomography, 492
Interleukin-1
  bacterial cell wall induction, 356–357
  blood-brain-barrier, 360
  Borrelia burgdorferi pathogenesis, 664
  CSF inflammation, bacteria, 301–302, 356–358
  detection in CSF, 878
  after dexamethasone, CSF, 357–358
  suppression of, treatment, 393
Interleukin-2
  Guillain-Barre' syndrome, 267
  Toxoplasma effect, 803
Interleukin-6, 357–358
Interleukins, HIV infection, 209
Intermittent-flow plasma exchange, 274
Internal carotid artery
  cysticercosis, 829
  murcormycosis, 750
Internal CSF reservoirs
  diagnosis of infection 572
  infection rate, 565
Interstitial edema, 360, 367
Interstitial pneumonia, 182
Intestinal amebiasis, 795
Intestinal tract, spongiform encephalopathies, 156
Intracerebral hemorrhage, *see* Intracranial hemorrhage
Intracranial calcifications
  AIDS encephalopathy, children, 212–213
  congenital cytomegalovirus, 183
  congenital toxoplasmosis, 807
  congenital varicella infection, 186
  neurocysticercosis, 828
Intracranial compliance, 866
Intracranial epidural abscess, 508–511
  clinical manifestations, 376–377, 508–509
  diagnosis, 509–510
  epidemiology, 508
  microbiology, 508
  pathogenesis and pathology, 508
  prognosis, 511
  and subdural empyema, 508
  treatment, 509, 511
Intracranial hemorrhage, 539–540
  and acute necrotizing arteritis, 540
  and anticoagulants, 538–539
  cerebrospinal fluid, 531
  computerized tomography, 534–535
  infective endocarditis, 526–527, 529, 534, 539–540
  malaria, 769–770
  mycotic aneurysm sequelae, 543
  pathogenesis, 539–540
  prognosis, 540
Intracranial hypertension, 864–866
Intracranial mycotic aneurysm, 540–546
  amebae, 793
  antibiotic therapy alone, 545–546
  aspergillosis, 747
  brain abscess, 547–549
  Candida species, 753
  and cardiac valve surgery, 546
  clinical presentation, 543
  computerized tomography, 532–535
  diagnosis, 543–544
  incidence, 529–530, 540–541
  intracranial hemorrhage cause, 539–540

management, 541, 544–546, 736
meningitis, 546–547
microbiology, 542
outcome, 546
pathogenesis, 528, 541–542
pathology, 542–543
surgery, 736
Intracranial pressure
bacterial meningitis, 360–362, 367, 369–370
cerebral blood flow correlation, 362
and cerebral edema, 367
in children, 369–370
and cortical blindness, 867
CSF effect, 864–866
dexamethasone effect, 361, 395
increases in, symptoms, 369–370, 378, 394
and lumbar puncture, 378
mannitol infusion, 362, 395
measurement, 869–870
monitoring devices, 562–565
infection risk, 565
neurocysticercosis, treatment, 835–836
plateau waves, 395
treatment of increases in, 394–396
Intramedullary spinal neurocysticercosis, 829, 834–835
Intranuclear inclusions
herpes simplex infection, 45–46
subacute sclerosing panencephalitis, 147–148
varicella-zoster virus, 57
Intraocular cysticercosis, 829–830
Intraparenchymal ICP monitoring, 562
Intrapartum infection
cytomegalovirus, 182
herpes simplex, 168–171
transmission factors, herpes, 169–171
Intrasellar abscess
clinical manifestations, 470
pathology, 467
Intraspinal epidermoid tumor, 868
Intrathecal administration
amphotericin B, 732
gentamicin, infants, 328
monoclonal antibodies, 354
shunt infections, 575–576, 579
Intrathecal PPD, 447
Intrathecal tetanus antitoxin, 616
Intrauterine infection
cytomegalovirus, 179, 181–182
herpes simplex, 168–172
rubella vaccine, 192
varicella-zoster virus, 185–187
Intravascular coagulation, 772
Intravenous antibiotics
CSF effect, meningitis, 381
Lyme disease, 681–683
shunt infections, 575–576
Intravenous drug abusers
botulism, 590
brain abscess, endocarditis, 547
CNS tuberculosis, AIDS, 450
epidural abscess, 500
infective endocarditis, 517, 521, 527, 542
intracranial mycotic aneurysm, 542
mucormycosis, 750–751
tetanus severity, 609
Intravenous gamma globulin, 274
Intraventricular catheters, 375
Intraventricular drug administration

amphotericin B, 734
neonatal meningitis, 327–328
recommended dosages, 575
shunt infection, 574–575, 579
Intraventricular foramen, see Foramen of Monro
Intraventricular ICP monitoring, 562
Intraventricular neurocysticercosis, 829
computerized tomography, 834
magnetic resonance imaging, 835
pathology, 830–831
prognosis, 836
symptoms, 829
treatment, 835
Intubation, bacteria acquisition, 315
Iodamoeba butschlii, 787
Iridocyclitis, 531
Iron, and bacterial infection, neonates, 316
Iron metabolism, and malaria, 768
"Irreversible adhesion," 569
Irrigation-suction techniques, 506
Island of Reil, 900
Isoniazid
CSF penetration, 443
drug resistance, 445
side effects, 443
treatment regimens, 445
tuberculous meningitis, 218, 443, 713
tuberculous spinal epidural abscess, 508
Israel
Guillain-Barre' syndrome, 260–261
polio outbreak, 248–249
Itraconazole, 733, 754
Ixodes dammini, 658
Borrelia burgdorferi transmission, 660
geographical distribution, 659
prevention strategies, 683
Ixodes pacificus, 658
Borrelia burgdorferi transmission, 660
geographical distribution, 659
Ixodes persulcatus, 661
Ixodes ricinus, 657–658
and erythema chronicum migrans, 657
geographical distribution, 660
Lyme disease spirochetes, 658, 660
prevention strategies, 683
Ixodes scapularia, 659–660
Ixodes tics
encephalitis, 94, 98–99
Powassan encephalitis, 99

J
Jackal, rabies virus, 132
Jamestown Canyon virus
aseptic meningitis, 29
encephalitis, 102
epidemiology, 102
Janeway lesions, 521
Japanese encephalitis
clinical findings, 97, 244–245
dengue fever protection, 245
diagnosis, 97, 245
history, 96
occurrence, 8, 96–97, 243–244
in pregnancy, 244
prevention and treatment, 97, 245
prognosis, 97, 245
vaccination, 245
virology, 243
Jarisch-Herxheimer reaction, 682

JC virus, 216
JNIH-6/JNIH-7 vaccines, 629

K
K1 antigen, 318–319, 326
antibodis, therapy, 326
immune system activation, 352
virulence factor, 318–319
Kanamycin, 325
Katayama fever, 850–851
Kawasaki disease, 34
Kenya
Guillain-Barre' syndrome, 260–261
sleeping sickness, 779
Keratitis, 793
Keratoconjunctivitis, 174
Kernig's virus, 368, 373
Ketoconazole
Aspergillus brain abscess, 748
fungal meningitis, 733, 735
granulomatous amebic encephalitis, 794
mucormycosis, 751
3-(2'-Ketohexyl)indoline, 436
Kigoma region, Tanzania, 779
King County, Washington, meningitis, 337–338
Klebsiella species
children and adult infection, 348
shunt infection, 566
treatment, neonates, 326
Kuru, 153–162
clinical manifestations, 154–155
eidemiology, 153–154
intestinal tract, 156
pathogenesis, 156–157
pathology, 155–156

L
Labctalol, tctanus managcmcnt, 618
Laboratory workers
botulism prevention, 598
Eastern equine encephalitis, 91
herpes B virus, 72–74
rabies prophylaxis, 137
Rift Valley fever, 103
spongiform encephalopathies, 162
tic-borne encephalitis, 99
Labyrinthitis, 373
La Crosse virus
aseptic meningits, 29
clinical disease, 101–102
diagnosis, 102
epidemiology, 101
history, 100–101
prevention and treatment, 102
Lactate CSF level
bacterial meningitis diagnosis, 379–381
cerebral malaria, 774
diagnostic test, 876
fungal infections, 732
mannitol effect, 362
pneumococci, 361
Lagochilascariasis, 849
Lagochilascaris minor, 849
Lake Victoria, Africa, 779
Lambwe Valley, Kenya, 779
Laminectomy, epidural abscess, 505
Lampit, 786
Larimer County, Colorado, 260–261
Laryngeal neuropathy, tetanus, 619

LAT region, herpes simplex, 46
Latency
    animal models, herpes simplex, 7
    B virus, 71
    herpes simplex, 7, 46–47
"Latency-associated transcript," 46
Latent membrane protein, 66
Lateral ventricles, anatomy, 861–862
Latex agglutination test
    bacterial antigens, CSF, 379, 381–382
    cryptococcal polysaccharide antigen, 730
    sensitivity, 876
    tuberculous meningitis, 436
Learning disabilities, 25
Left-sided endocarditis
    brain abscess, 548–549
    host defenses, 519
    intravenous drug abusers, 527
    neurologic complications, 526–527, 548–549
Legionella pneumophila, 791
Lentiviruses, and HIV, 201
Leptomeningeal metastases, 725
Leptomeningitis
    occurrence, 8
    subdural meningitis, 494–495
Leptomyxid amebae, 787, 789–790
Leptospirosis, 33
Lethargy, meningitis sign, 368–369
Leu¹⁰² mutation, 161
Leucovorin supplements, 818–819
Leukemia patients, measles vaccine, 239
Leukocyte interferon, see Interferons
Leukocyte scintigraphy, 476
Leukocytes
    C5a role, 354–355
    cell count, CSF, 871
    epidural abscess, 502
    meningitis, 322–323, 354, 355, 363
        survival, 355, 363
    mumps diagnosis, 119–121
    sleeping sickness, CSF, 784–785
    in subarahnoid space, 355, 363
Leukopenia
    corticosteroid cause, 696
    and meningitis survival, 355
Levamisole, 849
Levels of consciousness
    bacterial meningitis, 369, 373–374
    cerebral malaria, 775
    herpes encephalitis outcome, 53–55
    infective endocarditis, 529–530
    subdural empyema predictor, 495
Lidocaine, 395
"Lightning pains," 648–649
Limbic system, rabies, 130
Limulus lysate test
    bacterial meningitis, 379, 382
    technique, 876
Lipid A, 301, 356
Lipopolysaccharides
    antibodies, 328
    binding sites, 356
    blood-brain-barrier, 360
    Borrelia burdorferi, 661
    E. coli pathogenesis, 318
    genetics, E. coli, 318
    Hemophilus influenzae, 345
    IgM monoclonal antibody, 326
    inducer of inflammation, CSF, 301–302, 356–357
    lipid A region, 356
    N. meningitidis, 346–347, 353

Liposomal amphotericin B, 733
Listeria monocytogenes
    brain abscess, 461–463
    children and adult infection, 349, 390
    epidural abscess, 501
    immunocompromised host, 376
    neonatal meningitis, 314
    transmission, 349
    treatment, 390
Listeriosis, 262
Liver abscess, 795
Liver transplant, toxoplasmosis, 810, 814
Local instillation of antibiotics, 478
"Localized agranulocytosis," 519
Localized tetanus, 608, 612
Lockjaw, see Trismus
Lone Star tick, 414
Long terminal repeat, HIV, 202–204
Lorazepam
    seizure treatment, 396
    tetanus management, 617–618
Louping ill, 99
Louse-borne typhus, 412, 417–418
Lumbar drain, 562–563
Lumbar intrathecal antibiotics, 327–328
Lumbar puncture, 866–875
    brain abscess contraindication, 470, 867
    and brain herniation, 866–867
    cerebral embolism, 535
    and coagulation defects, 867–868
    complications, 866–867
    controversy, children, meningitis, 370, 376, 378, 867
    epidural abscess cause, 500
    fungal meningitis, 730
    headache as complication, 868
    indications for, 866
    infective endocarditis, 531
    and intracranial pressure, 378, 867
    Lyme disease, 682
    neonatal bacterial meningitis, 321, 326–327
    recommendations, meningitis, 867
    subdural empyema, 493–494, 867
    syphilis evaluation, 641, 643
Lumbar spinal epidural abscess, 500, 503, 507
Lumboperitoneal shunt infection
    CSF shunt types, 562–563
    diagnosis, 572
    incidence, 565
    meningeal signs, 570
    microbiology, 566
Lumbosacral cysts, MRI, 835
Lung abscess, 465
Lyme disease, 657–689
    versus bacterial meningitis, symptoms, 377–378
    cerebrospinal fluid, 664–665, 671, 719
    clinical manifestations, 666–678, 719
    diagnosis, 678–680, 877
    electrophysiology, 676–677
    Europe versus North America, 677–678
    epidemiology, 659–661, 683, 718–719
    etiology, 661–662
    and Guillain-Barre' syndrome, 673
    history, 657–658
    laboratory tests, 678–679, 719
    late mental changes, 674–675
    magnetic resonance imagery, 665, 674–675

    and meningitis, 33, 719–720
    neurologic abnormalities, 668–678, 719
    pathogenesis and pathophysiology, 662–665
    pathology, 665–666
    peripheral neuropathy, 665, 669, 672–673, 676–677, 719
    prevention, 683–684
    seronegative tests, 679–680, 719, 877
    stages, 667–677, 719
    transmission, 660
    treatment, 680–683
Lyme neuroborreliosis, 880
Lymphadenopathy
    physical examination, 705
    sleeping sickness, 782–783
    toxoplasmosis, 805
"Lymphadenosis benigna cutis," 667
Lymphocytes
    bacterial meningitis, 363
    blastogenic response, 732
    Borrelia burgdorferi, 663
    cryptococcosis, 695–696
    enumeration of, HIV infection, 208
    Guillain-Barre' syndrome, 263–267
    HIV culture, 208
    meningitis diagnosis, CSF, 380
    mumps response, 117, 120
    sleeping sickness, 780–782
    toxoplasmosis, 812
Lymphocytic choriomeningitis virus, 21, 31–32
"Lymphocytoma," 667, 677
Lymphocytosis, 90
Lymphokines, 878
Lymphoma; see also Primary CNS lymphoma
    versus toxoplasmosis, imaging, 903
Lymphomatous meningitis
    and AIDS, 218, 712
    CSF findings, 712
Lymphosarcoma, 713
Lys²⁰⁰ mutation, 161
Lysosomes, 267
Lyssavirus genus, 128–129

M

M protein, see Matrix protein
Macaca monkeys, 70, 73
Macrophages
    AIDS-dementia, 211
    amebicidal activity, 791
    cryptococcosis, 696
    Guillain-Barre' syndrome, 263–268
    HIV-1 infection, 9–10, 209, 709
    rickettsial disease, 413–414
    Toxoplasma effect, 804
"Madura foot," 751
Magnetic resonance imaging; see also Gadolinium enhancement
    AIDS-dementia, 210
    AIDS encephalopathy, 902–903
    aspergillosis, 747
    bacterial meningitis, 385–386, 891–894
    brain abscess, 476, 889–892
    cavernous sinus thrombosis, 896–897
    cerebritis, 887–889
    versus computerized tomography, 492–493, 504, 509, 548, 887–907
    congenital cytomegalovirus, 183
    epidural abscess, 503–505

epidural empyemas, 895
herpes simplex, 899–900
infective endocarditis, 532
intracranial epidural abscess, 509–510
intracranial mycotic aneurysm, 544
Lyme disease, 665, 675
neonatal herpes encephalitis, 173
neurocysticercosis, 834–835, 905–906
subacute sclerosing panencephalitis, 148
subdural effusions, 386
subdural empyema, 491–493, 893–898
terminology, 888
toxoplasmosis, 710, 817, 902–903
tuberculoma, 439, 895–896, 898
tuberculous meningitis, 438
ventriculitis, 894–896
Major histocompatibility complex, 267–268
Malagarasi River, Tanzania, 779
Malaria, see Cerebral malaria
Malarial granuloma, pathology, 770–771
Malignant glioma, imaging, 890
Malignant neurocysticercosis, 835–836
Malnutrition, malaria protection, 768
Manitoba, Canada, Lyme disease, 659
Mannitol
cerebral malaria, 777
cryptococcal meningitis, death, 735
CSF concentrations, 732
intracranial pressure effect, 362, 395
Marseilles fever, see Boutonneuse fever
Mass immunity, rubella, 192
Mass spectrometry, 878
Masseter muscle, Trichinella, 845–846
Mast cells, 266
Mastitis, mumps, 118, 242
Mastoiditis
and brain abscess, 463–464
imaging, 899
intracranial epidural abscess, 508
subdural empyema, 489
Maternal cytomegalovirus
epidemiology, 180–182
and immunity, 182
seropositivity, 180
Maternal herpes simplex, 170–171
Maternal varicella-zoster, 185–186
Matrix protein
measles, 234
rabies virus, 129
Measles
atypical form, 235
epidemiology, 234–235
CNS syndrome, 9
complications, 9, 236–238
elimination of, 239–240
encephalitis, 8, 15, 234, 236
epidemiology, 234–235
history, 233
meningitis, 32
vaccination, 238–240
virus mutations, 237
"Measles inclusion body encephalitis," 236
Meat, and toxoplasmosis, 819
Mebendazole
hydatid cysts, 840
trichinosis, 846
Mechanical prosthetic valves
anticoagulants, 539
versus bioprosthetic valves, 527
neurologic complications, 526–527

Mediterranean spotted fever, see Boutonneuse fever
Mefloquine, 776–777
Melanin, C. neoformans, 695
Melarsoprol
hemorrhagic meningoencephalitis, 781
sleeping sickness treatment, 785–786
toxicity, 781, 785–786
Memory
Lyme disease, 675, 719
toxoplasmosis, 814
Meningeal biopsy, algorithm, 708
Meninges
anatomy, 862–863
and antibiotic kinetics, 387
HIV infection, 209, 217–218
Meningiomas, 725
Meningismus
infective endocarditis cause, 529–530
tuberculous meningitis, 431
Meningitis; see also Aseptic meningits; Bacterial meningitis; Chronic meningitis; Mumps meningitis; Neonatal bacterial meningitis; Pneumococcal meningitis; Tuberculous meningitis
and AIDS, 217–218
infective endocarditis cause, 546–550
Lyme disease, 671–677
mumps, 30–31, 113–125, 242
mycoplasmas, 285–286, 289
syndrome recognition, 2–3
"Meningitis belt," 339–340
Meningococcal meningitis; see also Neisseria meningitidis
adults, symptoms, 373
antibiotics, 389
capsular antibody levels, 341
chemoprophylaxis, 400–401
diagnosis, 376–386
differential diagnosis, rash, 377
epidemiology, 339–342
etiology, 343–347
immunizing process, 341–342
immunoprophylaxis, 401–402
pathology, 367
and viral infection, predisposition, 342
virulence factors, 347
Meningoencephalitis; see also Cerebritis
HIV infection, 209–210
mumps, 242
Mycoplasms pneumoniae, 289
rubella, 189–190
sleeping sickness, 780–782
Toxoplasma, 711
Meningopolyneuritis
antibiotics, 681–682
Lyme disease, 666–667, 676
Meningovascular syphilis
classification, 64
diagnosis, 645–658
penicillin effect, 652
and progressive Borrelia encephalomyelitis, 674
syndrome of, 646–648
Mental retardation
congenital rubella, 191
congenital toxoplasmosis, 806–807
Mental status; see also Psychiatric abnormalities
Histoplasma meningitis, 715
infective endocarditis, 529–531

Lyme disease, 674–675
neurocysticercosis, 828–829
sleeping sickness, 783
Metabolic acidosis, 777
Methemoglobin, 544, 888–889
Methenamine silver stain, 732
Methicillin, 505
Methionine, HIV infection, 209
Methylprednisolone
and CSF inflammation, cell walls, 356
CSF outflow resistance, 360
5-Methyltetrahydrofolate, 209
Metrifonate, 836, 851
Metrizamide, 724, 734
Metronidazole
brain abscess, 477–478, 796
cerebral amebiasis, 796
tetanus management, 618
MHC class II antigen, 267
Miconazole
fungal meningitis, 732–733, 735
P. boydii treatment, 752
Microabscesses
Candida species, 753
clinical presentation, 549
and endocarditis, 534, 547–548
incidence, 547–548
magnetic resonance imaging, 548
management, 549
Microangiopathy, 287–288
Microcephaly
AIDS encephalopathy, children, 212
congenital cytomegalovirus, 183–184
Microglia
AIDS-dementia, 211
bacterial meningitis, 364–365
HIV infection, 209
Lyme disease, 666
toxoplasmosis, 812–813
Microsporum audouinii, 761
Midazolam, tetanus management, 618
Middle cerebral artery
meningovascular syphilis, 647
mycotic aneurysms, 542
Migraine, CSF pleocytosis, 724
Miliary disease, 432
Minimum inhibitory concentration, 569
Minocycline, 400
Mitral valve infection
cerebral emboli, 526, 533, 537
echocardiography, 537
Mitral valve prolapse, 517
Mitral valve replacement, 527
Mixed infections, meningitis, 351
"Mobile" vegetations, 537
Molds, 745–752; see also specific molds
Mollaret's recurrent meningitis, 34
clinical presentation, 34
herpes viruses, 32, 34
Mondini's dysplasia, 374
Mongoose, rabies virus, 132
Monkey gamma globulin, 74
Monoclonal antibodies
immunoglobulin G, 325–326
intrathecal injection, 354
Mononeuritis multiplex, 550
Lyme diseae, 665, 673
Mononeuritis simplex, 673
Mononeuropathy multiplex, 220
Mononuclear leukocytes, 270
Mononucleosis syndrome
cytomegalovirus, 68, 183
Epstein-Barr virus, 65–66
HIV infection, 205

Moraten vaccine, 238
Morphine, tetanus management, 618
"Morula," 414
Motor nerve conduction, 271–272, 274
Motor neurons
    Lyme disease, 675–676
    tetanospasmin effects, 612–614
Motor unit action ptoential, 271–272
Motor weakness, Lyme disease, 673, 682
Mouse bioassay, botulism, 596
Mouse-brain vaccine, rabaies, 139
Mouse toxicity test, pertussis, 629
Mouth infection, neonatal herpes, 174
Movement disorder, toxoplasmosis,
    813–814
Moxalactam
    brain abscess, 477
    E. coli, neonates, CSF, 326
Mucoraceae family, 749
Mucormycosis
    clinical manifestations, 750–751
    diagnosis, 751, 904–905
    etiologic agent, 749
    history, 748–749
    imagery, 904–905
    intracranial epidural abscess, 508
    pathogenesis and pathophysiology,
        749–750
Multilocus enzyme electrophoresis
    group B streptococci, 349
    H. influenzae, 345
    N. meningitidis, 346
Multinucleated giant cells, 211
Multiple aneurysms, 541, 544, 546
Multiple brain absesses
    ambeiasis, 795
    clinical presentation, 549
    computerized tomography, 473
    incidence, endocarditis, 547–548
    pathology, 467
Multiple cerebral microemboli
    clinical manifestations, 534
    computerized tomography, 535
Multiple mycotic aneurysms, 541, 544,
    546
Multiple sclerosis, 724
    diagnosis, 724
    Lyme disease similarity, 674
    and Sjogren's syndrome, 723
Mumps, 113–125; *see also* Mumps
        meningitis
    and aseptic meningitis, 21, 30–31,
        113–125
    autopsy reports, 116
    cerebrospinal fluid, 120–121
    clinical presentation, 30–31,
        118–119, 241–242
    diagnosis and laboratory findings,
        119–121
    encephalitis, 113–125
    epidemiology, 30–31, 114–115,
        241–242
    history, 113, 240
    immune response, 117–118
    immunization, 121–122, 241–243
    infectious agent, 114
    natural history, 118–119
    neurological complications, 119,
        242–243
    pathogenesis, 115–117
    sex differences, 115
    therapy, 31, 121
    in unimmunized populations, 114

    vaccine, 121–122, 241–243
    virology, 30, 240–241
Mumps meningitis
    clinical presentation, 30–31,
        118–119, 242
    diagnosis, 119–121
    epidemiology, 30–31, 114–115
    parotitis severity, 118
    pathogenesis, 30, 115
    versus poliomyelitis, 119–120
    treatment and prevention, 31,
        121–122
Mumps-specific immunoglobulins, 117
Mural vegetations, 537
Murine typhus, 412, 419
Murray Valley encephalitis
    clinical disease, 98
    diagnosis, 98
    epidemiology, 98
    history, 97–98
    prevention and treatment, 98
Muscle pain, trichinosis, 846
Muscle pathology, Lyme disease, 666
Muscle weakness, botulism, 594–595
Myalgias, Lyme diseae, 673
Myasthesia gravis, 596
Mycobacterial antigen/antibody
        detection, 877
    tuberculous meningitis test, 435–436
Mycobacterium avium-intracellulare
    and AIDS, 450, 711
    brain abscess, 462–463
    meningitis, 449
    small bowel infection, 206
Mycobacterium bovis
    and HIV infection, BCG, 450
    meningitis, 448
Mycobacterium flavescens, 449
Mycobacterium gordonae, 449
Mycobacterium kansasii, 449
Mycobacterium scrofulaceum, 449
Mycobacterium tuberculosis, 427
    brain abscess, 440, 461–463
    characteristics, 428
    CSF detection, 879
    drug resistance, 445
    epidural abscess, 501, 506
    and immune compromise, 427
    measurement, 876–877
Mycoplasma gallisepticum, 283–284
    cerebrovascular effects, 287
Mycoplasma hominis
Mycoplasma hyorhynis, 286
Mycoplasma neurolyticum, 283, 286
Mycoplasma pneumoniae
    aseptic meningitis, 34
    autoimmunity, 287
    cerebrospinal fluid, 286, 289
    cerebrovascular effects, 286–288
    characterization, 284–285
    clinical manifestations, pneumonia,
        288–289
    diagnosis, 289–290
    and Guillain-Barre' syndrome, 262
    neurological complications, 284–290
    pathogenesis, 283–284, 286–288
    pathology, 287–288
    radiography, 288–289
    treatment and prevention, 291–292
Mycoplasma salivarium, 283
Mycoplasmas, 283–293
    characterization, 283–285
    clinical manifestations, pneumonia,
        288–289

    diagnosis, 289–291
    epidemiology, 284–286
    etiology, 283–284
    pathogenesis and pathology, 286–288
    treatment, 291
Mycotic aneurysm, *see* Intracranial my-
        cotic aneurysm
Myelin, Guillain-Barre' syndrome,
        264–265
Myelin basic protein
    experimental allergic neuritis, 266
    parenchymal disease, AIDS, 214
    peripheral neuropathy, AIDS, 220
Myelinization, HIV infection, 213
Myelitis
    herpes zoster association, 61
    mumps as cause, 31, 119
Myelodysplastic children, 571
Myelography
    epidural abscess, 503–504
    spinal tuberculosis, 441–442
Myelopathy
    HIV infection, children, 213
    schistosomiasis, 850–851
Myeloradiculopathy, 219
Myocarditis, *Naegleria* infection, 792
Myopathies, AIDS, 221
Myositis, Lyme disease, 673
Myositis ossificans circumscripta, 619

N

Naegleria fouteri
    comparative morphology, 788
    epidemiology, 790
    growth conditions, 788
    immune system role, 791–792
    meningoencephalitis, 787
    pathogenesis, 790–792
    pathology, 792
    as vector, 791
Naegleria species
    pathogenic potential, 787
    ultrastructure, 788
Nafcillin
    brain abscess, 478
    CSF penetration, 573–574
    intraventricular dosages, 575
    neonatal meningits, 325
    recommended doses, 388
    shunt infection, 573–575
    Staphylococcus aureus, 390
"Nagana," 788
Nape-of-the-neck sign, 368
Narcotic addicts, *see also* Intravenous
        drug abusers
    tetanus severity, 609
Nasal cavity, *N. fowleri*, 790–791
Nasal stuffiness, mucormycosis, 750
Nasopharyngeal carcinoma, 66
Nasopharyngeal invasion, 351–352
National Bacterial Meningitis Surveil-
        lance Study, 343–344
National Childhood Encephalopathy
        Study, 630–631
Native valve endocarditis
    cerebral emboli, 533, 536, 540
    etiologic agents, 519–521
    mortality, 532
    treatment, 523
Natural killer cells
    Borrelia burgdorferi, 663–664
    cryptococcosis defense, 695–696
Near-drowning, 751–752

Neck biopsy, rabies, 136
Neck infection, rabies, 130
Neck stiffness, Lyme disease, 671
Necrotizing myelitis, 289
Needle sticks, 205
Nef protein, HIV, 20
Negative-stranded RNA viruses, 13
Negishi virus, 99
Negri bodies, rabies virus, 131, 136, 250
Neisseria lactamica, 341
Neisseria meningitidis
　adhesion, 299, 352
　antibiotics, 389, 391–392
　capsular antibody levels, 341
　carriage rate, 340–341
　chemoprophylaxis, 400–401
　clonal analysis, 346–347
　complement deficiency, 300, 352–353
　epidemiology, 339–342
　etiological aspects, 343–347
　immunizing process, 341–342
　immunoprophylaxis, 401–402
　meningeal invasion, 353–354
　neonatal meningitis, 315
　pathology, 367
　serogroup B immunoprophylaxis,
　　401–402
　serogroups, disease causation, 346
　subdural empyema, 495
　ultrastructure, 346
　virulence factors, 347
Nemadine myopathy, 221
Nematodes, 842–849
Neonatal bacterial meningitis, 313–333
　brain abscess, 304, 464–466
　diagnosis, 290–291, 320–324
　early- versus late-onset, 320–321
　epidemiology, 313–315
　etiology, 314
　gram-negative organisms, 314–315
　gram-positive organisms, 313–315
　monitoring therapy, 326–327
　mycoplasmas, 285–286, 289–291
　pathogenesis, 315–320
　prevention, 292
　subdural empyema cause, 489
　treatment, 323–328
　treatment failure, 327–328
Neonatal brain abscess
　Candida species, therapy, 754
　and meningitis, 466
　pathogenesis, 464–466
　sequelae, 481
Neonatal herpes simplex
　Caesarean section, 175–176
　classification, 171
　clinical presentation, 171–174
　diagnosis, 175
　encephalitis, 173
　epidemiology, 170–174
　history, 167
　intrapartum infection, 168–169
　intrauterine infection, 168–169
　maternal infection role, 170–171
　pathology and pathogenesis, 167–170
　postnatal infection, 169–170
　prevention, 175–176
　prognosis, encephalitis, 173
　serologic diagnosis value, 175
　treatment, 176–178
　vaccination, 176
Neonatal shunt infection, 569
Neonatal tetanus, 608
　history, 603

incidence, 605
　manifestations, 612
Neonatal toxoplasmosis, 805–807
Neonatal varicella-zoster infection,
　186–187
Nephritis, 570–571
Nephrotoxicity, 734
Neuritis
　herpes simplex virus, 52
　mumps, 119
Neuroblastomas, 615
Neurocysticercosis, 720, 825–841
　brain abscess, 462
　chronic meningitis, 720
　clinical manifestations, 720, 826–830
　diagnosis, 832–835, 905–906
　eosinophilia, 871
　etiology and epidemiology, 825–826
　and granulomatous amebic encepha-
　　litis, 793
　history, 825
　imaging techniques, 833–835,
　　905–906
　pathogenesis, 826
　pathology, 830–832
　prognosis, 836
　serology, 832–833
　taeniasis prevalence, 832
　treatment, 720, 835–836
Neuroleptic malignant syndrome, 378
Neuromuscular junction
　blockade of, tetanus, 618
　tetanospasmin, 614
Neuronal transmission, 8–9, 11–12
Neurons
　herpes simplex transmission, 13–14
　HIV infection, 209, 211
Neuropsychological tests
　HIV infection, 209–210
　Lyme disease, 675, 682
Neurosarcoidosis, 721
Neurosurgery
　brain abscess, 478–480
　epidural abscess, 505–506
　hydatid disease, 839–840
　intracranial epidural abscess, 511
　neurocysticercosis, 835–836
　prophylaxis with antibiotics, 580
　subdural empyema, 495–496
　tuberculosis meningitis, 448
Neurosyphilis, 639–656
　cerebrospinal fluid, 880
　and chronic meningitis, 717–718
　clinical syndromes, 644–645, 718
　definition, 639
　and HIV infection, 218, 653–654
　laboratory measures, 640–644, 718,
　　880
　pathogenesis and pathophysiology,
　　639–640
　penicillin evaluation, 651, 718
　therapy, 650–653, 718
Neurotoxins, AIDS-dementia, 211
Neurotransmitter receptors, 12
Neutropenia
　bacterial meningitis, 376
　brain abscess, 462
Neutrophils
　amebicidal activity, 791
　bacterial meningitis pathology, 363
　cell count, CSF, 871
　neonatal meningitis, 322–323
　subarachnoid space, 354–355, 363
"Nichols strain," 642

Nifurtimox, 786
Nigeria, sleeping sickness, 779–780
"Nissl-Alzheimer arteritis," 647
Nocardia species
　brain abscess, 461–463
　chronic meningitis, 721
Nodular calcified cysts, MRI, 834–835
Nonbacterial thrombotic endocarditis,
　517–518
Non-Hodgkin's lymphoma, 712
Nonsteroidal anti-inflammatory drugs,
　34
Nontuberculous mycobacteria, 449–450
Nordihydroguaiaretic acid, 356
Norepinephrine, 614
North Asian tick typhus, 412, 416
Norway, Guillain-Barre' syndrome, 260
Nosocomial endocarditis, 517
Nosocomial transmission, herpes sim-
　plex, 169
Nuchal rigidity
　bacterial meningitis, 368–369,
　　373⅜74
　in elderly, 374
　subdural empyema, 490
　versus tetanus, 615
Nucleic acids, detection in CSF, 878
Nucleocapsid protein, mumps virus, 114
Nursery personnel, 169
Nystagmus, 550, 809

O
Obliterative endarteritis
　Lyme disease pathology, 665
　neurosyphilis, 718
Observational data, bacterial meningi-
　tis, 369
Obstructive hydrocephalus
　bacterial meningitis, 366, 384
　computerized tomography, 384
　CSF effects, 865
　lumbar puncture contraindication,
　　867
Ocular complications
　congenital cytomegalovirus, 183–184
　congenital rubella, 191
　congenital varicella-zoster, 186
　infective endocarditis, 550–551
　mumps, 119
Ocular cysticercosis, 829–830
　clinical menifestations, 829–930
　computerized tomography, 834
　pathology, 831–832
　treatment, 836
"Ocular larva migrans," 849
Ocular nerve palsy, mumps, 119
Ocular toxoplasmosis, 807–810
　clinical manifestations, 809–810
　computerized tomography, 810
　epidemiology, 807–808
　pathogenesis, 808
　pathology, 808–809
　reactivation, 808
　timing of clinical manifestations, 809
　treatment, 819
Odontogenic brain abscess, pathology,
　464
Oklahoma City, Oklahoma, meningitis,
　342–343
OKT3, 34
Olfactory mucosa, *N. fowleri* invasion,
　790–791

Olfactory system
  herpes simplex pathogenesis, 47
  HSV-1 transport, 14
  viral transmission dynamics, 11–12
Oligodendrocytes, 666
Olmstead County data, 259–260
One-way shunt valves, 567
Ontario, Canada, Lyme disease, 659
Oocysts, 802–803
Oophoritis, mumps, 118
Open heart surgery, 536–537
Opening pressure, CSF, 378–379
  bacterial meningitis, 378–379
  brain abscess, 470
  cerebral malaria, 774
  tuberculous meningitis, 434
  values, 869
"Opertive case rate," 564–565
Ophthalmic zoster, see Herpes zoster
      ophthalmicus
"Ophthalmoplegic tetanus," 612
Optic atrophy
  congenital cytomegalovirus, 183–184
  syphilitic meningitis, 646
  tuberculous meningitis, 447
Optic disk, toxoplasmosis, 809
Optochin, 347
Oral acyclovir, herpes zoster, 65
Oral polio vaccine, 247–249, 262
Orbital cellulitis, 508
Orbiviruses, 103–104
  aseptic meningitis, 29
  background, 103
  infectious agent, 103
  pathology and pathogenesis, 103–104
Orchitis, and mumps, 118
Organ transplant patients, see Immuno-
      compromised host
Organic brain syndrome; see also
      AIDS-dementia complex
  cerebral malaria, 775
  tuberculous meningitis, 447
Oropharyngeal cavity, 174
Osler nodes, 521
Osteomyelitis, see Vertebral osteomye-
      litis
Otitis media
  and brain abscess, 458, 463–464, 466,
      899
  Fusobacterium meningitis, 350
  H. influenzae meningitis risk,
      338–339
  imaging, 899
  measles complication, 236
  and pneumococcal meningitis, 343,
      373–374
  subdural empyema, 489
Otogenic infections
  brain abscess, 463–464, 466
  subdural empyema, 489, 492, 494
Outer-membrane proteins
  Hemophilus influenzae, 345, 353
  Neissera meningitidis, 346–347
  vaccine, 399
Outer-membrane vesicles, 360
Overwintering phenomenon, 90
Oxacillin
  neonatal meningitis, 325
  infective endcarditis, 523
  recommended doses, 388
  S. aureus, 390
  topical use, prophylaxis, 580
Oxaminiquine, 851

Oxindanac, 356
Oxygen levels, cerebral malaria, 774

P
PO glycoprotein, 266–267
P2 protein, 266–268
p24 antigen
  cerebrospinal fluid, 209
    infants, 212–213
  HIV infection, prognosis, 208
  tests for, 207–208
Pacemakers, and infective endocarditis,
      517
Paecilomcyes species, 693, 752
Pain
  Guillain-Barre' syndrome, 270
  Lyme disease, 672
Palpebral cysticercosis, 830
Pancreatitis, and mumps, 118, 242
Panhypopituitarism, toxoplasmosis, 814
Panophthalmitis, 531
Pantopaque, 724
Papilledema
  brain abscess, 469
  Guillain-Barre' syndrome, 269–270
  infective endocarditis, 550
  intracranial pressure, 370
  Lyme disease, 671
  neurocysticercosis, 829
  subdural empyema, 490
  tuberculous meningitis, 431
Para-aminosalicylic acid, 444
Paracoccidioides brasiliensis
  brain abscess, 759
  chronic meningitis, 721
  classification, 693–694
  pathogenesis, 698, 759
  symptoms, 759
  treatment, 759
Parafalcine subdural empyema, 491
Paragonimiasis, 851–852
Paragonimus, 851–852
Paralytic myelitis, 28
"Paralytic" rabies, symptoms, 135
Parameningeal abscess, 549
Paranasal sinusitis
  aspergillosis, 746
  and brain abscess, 458–459, 464, 746
  computerized tomography, 492–493
  imaging, 895
  intracranial epidural abscess, 508
  subdural empyema, 488–489,
      492–493, 895
Paraplegia, infective endocarditis,
      529–531
Parasaggital subdural empyema, 491
Parasitic infections, 501
Parenchymal abnormalities, see Brain
      parenchyma
Parenchymal neurocysticercosis,
      828–829
  clinical manifestations, 828–829
  computerized tomography, 833–834
  magnetic resonance imaging, 834–835
  pathology, 830
  prognosis, 836
Parenchymatous neurosyphilis
  classification, 644
  pathophysiology, 640
  syndrome, 648–649
Parenteral antibiotics, shunt infection,
      580

Parenteral drug abusers, see Intravenous
      drug abusers
Paresis, see General paresis
Paresthesias, Lyme disease, 672, 676
Parotitis
  mumps clinical course, 118
  and mumps CNS infection, 30,
      118–119
Particle agglutination, streptococci, 322
Passive immunization, B. burgdorferi,
      663
Passive transport, blood-brain-barrier,
      11
Pasteur vaccine, 139
Pasteurella multocida, 495
Patient examination, overview, 1–4
Pefloxacin, 390
"Pellicle," 433
Penicillin; see also Penicillin G
  botulism, 597–598
  epidural abscess, 505
  group B streptococci, 325, 328–329
  infective endocarditis, 523
  Lyme disease, 680–683
  neurosyphilis treatment, 218,
      650–651
    dosage, 650–651
  tetanus management, 618
  treatment failures, syphilis, 644
Penicillin G
  in adults, meningitis, 391–392
  anaerobes, 390–391
  brain abscess, 477–478
  direct instillation, 478, 575
  Lyme disease, 681–682
  meningococcal meningitis, 389
  neurosyphilis treatment, 651–653
    recommended regimens, 653, 718
  pneumococcal meningitis, 389–390
  recommended doses, meningitis, 388
  shunt infection, 575
  subdural empyema, 495
Penicillin V, Lyme disease, 681
Penicillium species, 752
Pentamidine
  sleeping sickness treatment, 785
  toxicity, 223, 785
Pentobarbital
  intracranial pressure, 395–396
  seizure treatment, 396
Peptidoglycan, 355
Perinatal infections, 167–200
  cytomegalovirus, 178–185
  Epstein-barr virus, 187–188
  herpes simplex, 167–178
  rubella, 188–192
  varicella-zoster, 185–187
Perinephric abscess, 500
Periodic lateralized epileptiform dis-
      charges, 51
Peripheral neuropathy
  antibiotic treatment, 682
  dideoxyinosine side effect, 222
  Guillain-Barre' syndrome, 263–265,
      267–268
  infective endocarditis, 531, 550
  Lyme disease, 665, 667, 672–673,
      676–677, 682
  rubella vaccination, 192
Peritoneal shunt infection; see Ventric-
      uloperitoneal shunt
Peritonitis, peritoneal shunts, 571
Perivascular cuffing, herpes simplex, 45,
      168

"Perivascular space," 364–365
Periventricular area, toxoplasmosis, 806–807
Periventricular edema, imaging, 894–896
Permethrin treatment, 683
Peromyscus leucopus, 659–660
Persistent generalized lympadenopathy, 205–206
Personality changes, *see* Mental status
Pertactin P.69, 626, 629
Pertussis, 625–635
    clinical manifestations, 625
    complications, 627
    diagnosis, 627
    immunization, 628–633
    neurologic abnormalities, 627–628
    treatment, 627
Pertussis toxin
    acellular vaccine use, 629
    illness role, 627
    molecular actions, 626
    neuronal effects, 628
    reactogenicity, 631–632
    virulence factor, 626–627
Pertussis vaccine, 628–633
    development of, 628–629
    encephalopathy controversy, 630–633
    reactogenicity, 629–631
    risk data, 631
Pet ownership, Lyme disease, 683
Petechial hemorrhages
    magnetic resonance imaging, 889
    pathology, malaria, 769–771
Petechial rash
    childhood bacterial meningitis, 370
    differential diagnosis, 377
pH, antibiotic penetration, CSF, 386
Phagocytosis
    bacteria in brain, 304–305
    CSF shunt effects, 307
Phase-contrast microscopy, 875
Phenobarbital
    chloramphenicol interactions, 389
    intracranial pressure, 395
    seizure treatment, 396
Phenoloxidase, 695
Phenothiazines, 794
Phenoxymethyl penicillin, 681–683
Phenytoin
    chloramphenicol interactions, 389
    seizure treatment, 396
Pheochromocytomas, 615
Phialophora dermatiditis, 721
Phialophora pedrosoi, 721, 761
Philippines, malaria, 768
Phlebitis
    E. coli, neonates, 320
    meningitis pathophysiology, 362
Phlebovirus, encephalitis, 102–103
Phospholipase, 791
Phosphonoformate, 222
Photophobia, Lyme disease, 671
Phycomycosis, *see* Mucormycosis
Physical examination, 2
Physical exercise, aseptic meningitis, 23
"Phytotic" mycotic aneurysm, 542
Pia mater
    anatomy, 862
    barrier system, 864
Picornaviruses, 9
Pila snails, 842
Pili, meningococcal virulence, 347
"Pink brain," 769

Pinocytotic vesicles, 358–359
Piritrexin, 819
Pituitary abscess, pathology, 467
Placenta, *see* Transplacental infection
Plain radiography
    epidural abscess, 503
    mucormycosis, 751
    neurocysticercosis, 833
Plasma, HIV culture, 208
Plasma exchange
    continuous flow machines, 274
    fulminant meningococcemia, 393
    Guillain-Barre' syndrome, 272–274
        children, 273
        and prognosis, 274
Plasma-to-CSF pH gradient, 386
Plasmapheresis, *see* Plasma exchange
Plasmodium brasilianum, 759, 773
Plasmodium coatneyi, 772–773
Plasmodium falciparum
    cerebral malaria, 767
    chloroquine resistance, 776
    cytoadherence, 771–773
    geographic domain, 768
    knob expression phenotype, 772–773
Plasmodium fragile, 772–773
Plasmodium knowlesi, 722
Plasmodium malariae, 773
Plasmodium vivax, 767, 772–773
"Plateau waves," 395
    and intracranial pressure, 866
Platelet count; *see also* Thrombocyto-penia
    neonatal meningitis, 323
Platelet-fibrin, 519
Pleocytosis
    brain abscess, 470
    chronic meningitis, 704, 708
    fungal meningitis, 729
    Guillain-Barre' syndrome, 270
    HIV infectin, 209
    Lyme disease, 671
    mumps, 115, 120
    subdural empyema, 494
    syphilis, 642
    tuberculous meningitis, 433–434
Pneumococcal meningitis
    adults, 373–374
    carriage rates, 343
    cerebral blood flow, 362
    CSF pressure, 361
    diagnosis, 376–386
    elderly, 374
    epidemiology, 342–343
    etiology, 343–344, 347–348
    immunoprophylaxis, 402
    inflammation induction, CSF, 355–357
    leukopenia, and survival, 355
    mortality, 373
    pathology, 367
    predisposition, 343
    virulence, 348
Pneumocystis infection, 709
Pneumoencephalography, 834
Pneumonia; *see also* Pneumococcal meningitis
    clinical manifestations, 288–289
    measles complication, 236
    neurological complications, 284–285
    pathology and pathogenesis, 286–288
    treatment, 291
Pneumonitis, varicella, pregnancy, 185–186

Polio vaccine, 247–249
    complications, 247–248
    and Guillain-Barre' syndrome, 262
    inactivated and oral form, 247–249
    indications and contraindications, 248
Poliomyelitis
    incidence, 8
    versus mumps, 119–120
    vaccine, 247–249
Poliovirus type 1, 26
Poliovirus type 2, 28
Polioviruses
    aseptic meningitis, 21
    laboratory findings, meningitis, 25–28
    pathogenesis, 22
    receptors, 22
Polyarteritis nodosa, 722
Polyclonal hypergammaglobulinemia, 205
Polymerase chain reaction
    cytomegalovirus, 69
    enterovirus meningitis, 26, 28
    HIV infection, 208, 213
    Mycoplasma pneumoniae, 290
    subacute sclerosing panencephalitis, 148, 152
    technique, 878
    Toxoplasma gondii, 817
Polymicrobial bacterial meningitis, 351
Polymorphonuclear leukocytes
    Guillain-Barre' syndrome, 264
    meningitis diagnosis, CSF, 379–380
    quantification, CSF, 871
Polymyositis myopathy, HIV infection, 221
Polymyxin
    inflammation block, 356
    intraventricular administration, 327
    lipopolysaccaride effect, 360
Polyneuropathy, infective endocarditis, 550
Polyomavirus, 9
Polyradiculopathy
    cytomegalovirus, 217
    HIV infection, 221
    Mycoplasma pneumoniae, 289
Polysaccharide, *see* Capsular polysac-charide
Pork
    cestode infection, 826
    trichinosis, 845–846
Positive-stranded RNA viruses, 13
Posterior epidural abscess
    outcome, 506
    pathogenesis, 499–500
    surgery, 506
Posterior fossa subdural empyema, 489
Posterior fossa tumor, 378
Postexposure rabies vaccination, 137–139, 250–251
Postherpetic neuralgia, 64–65
Postinfectious encephalomyelitis
    measles as cause, 8, 15
    Mycoplasma pneumonia, 289
    Reye's syndrome, 15–16
Postinfectious syndromes, 3–4
Postnatal infection; *see also* Neonatal *entries*
    cytomegalovirus, 183
    herpes simplex, 169–170
Post-operative infection
    antibiotics, 392
    brain abscess, 465

Post-operative infection (*contd.*)
  candidiasis, 753
  epidural abscess, 500, 508–509
  meningitis, 375, 392
  subdural empyema, 489
Post-traumatic infection; *see also* Head trauma
  etiology, 459–461
  intracranial epidural abscess, 508–509
  meningitis, 374–375
  pathogenesis, 465
  spine, 500
  treatment, 392
Post-traumatic meningitis, 374–375, 392
"Pott's paraplegia," 507
Powassan encephalitis, 99
Praziquantel
  neurocysticercosis, 835–836
  paragonimiasis, 852
  schistosomiasis, 851
Prednisolone
  Guillain-Barre' syndrome, 272
  tetanus management, 617
Preexposure rabies vaccination, 250–251
Pregnancy; *see also* Congenital *entries*; Neonatal *entries*
  cerebral malaria, glucose levels, 774
  cryptococcal meningitis, treatment, 734
  cytomegalovirus, 181–182
  Epstein-Barr infection, 187–188
  Guillain-Barre' syndrome, 263
  herpes simplex epidemiology, 170–171
  rubella infection, 188–192
  toxoplasmosis, 805, 811
  tuberculous meningitis prognosis, 446
  varicella-zoster infection, 185–187
Premature infants
  bacterial meningitis, CSF, 322
  externalized shunt infection, 565
  group B streptococci risk, 317
  varicella-zoster, 186
Primary amebic meningoencephalitis
  versus bacterial meningitis, 793
  clinical manifestations, 793
  diagnosis, 793
  epidemiology, 790
  etiology, 787–790
  immune system role, 791–792
  and myocarditis, 792
  pathogenesis, 790–792
  pathology, 792–793
  treatment and prognosis, 794
Primary CNS lymphoma
  and AIDS, children, 212–213
  diagnosis, AIDS, 213, 215–216
  non-AIDS versus AIDS, 216
  prognosis, 216
  versus toxoplasmosis, imaging, 903
Primary cytomegalovirus infection, 179
  in utero transmission risk, 181–182
  versus recurrent infection, fetus, 182
Primary herpes simplex
  pathogenesis, 45–46
  perinatal transmission, 169–170
  seroprevalence, 49
Prions
  and genetics, 161
  spongiform encephalopathy origin, 159–161
"PRIP" gene, 161

Probenecid, Lyme disease, 681–682
Procaine penicillin, 651, 653
Prodrome, rabies virus, 135
"Progenitor toxins," 591
Proglottids, 826–827
Progressive *Borrelia* encephalomyelitis, 673–674
  antibiotic treatment, 682
  epidemiology, 673
  Europe versus North America, 677
  symptoms and prognosis, 674
Progressive encephalopathy
  and AIDS, children, 212–213
  zidovudine treatment, 222
Progressive locomotor ataxia, 648–649
Progressive multifocal leukoencephalopathy
  and AIDS, children, 212–213
  diagnosis, AIDS, 213–214, 216, 902
  imaging, 902
  pathogenesis, 9
  as slow virus, 153
  survival, 216
Progressive polyradiculopathy, 221
Progressive rubella panencephalitis, 149, 152
  clinical manifestations, 149
  diagnosis, 149, 152
  histopathology, 152
  pathogenesis, 9, 149
Progressive syphilitic vasculitis, 640
ProHIBIT vaccine, 263
"Proliferative sparganosis," 841
Properdin deficiency, 342
Propionibacterium acnes
  brain abscess, 461
  meningitis, 350
Propofol, tetanus management, 618
Proguanil, 777
Prostaglandin E₂
  and brain water, indomethacin, 361
  complement effects, CSF, 300
  and CSF inflammation, 356
Prosthetic devices, 306–307, 568
Prosthetic valve endocarditis
  anticoagulant use, 538–539
  cerebral emboli, 533, 536
  epidemiology, 516–517
  etiologic agents, 521
  intracranial hemorrhage, 540
  intracranial mycotic aneurysm, 541
  mortality, 532
  neurologic complications, 527–528
  pathogenesis, 517–519
  prevention, 524
  treatment, 523
Prostitutes, herpes simplex, 49
Protease, strongyloidiasis infection, 847
Protein CSF levels
  assessment, 873
  bacterial meningitis, 379, 381, 873
  epidural abscess, 502
  sleeping sickness, 784–785
  subdural empyema, 494
  toxoplasmic encephalitis, 814
  tuberculous, 433–434
  values of, 873
Protein kinase C, 608
Proteus mirabilis, 465
Prothrombin times, 538
Proton-density-weighted image
  acute disseminated encephalomyelitis, 901
  brain abscess, 890–891

herpes simplex, 900
HIV infection, 902
meaning, 888
subdural empyema, 493, 895, 898
ventriculitis, 894
Protoscoleces, 838
Protozoal infections, 767–800, 874–875
"Proximal" shunt infections
  clinical manifestations, 570
  treatment, 577
Prozone phenomenon, 731
PRP-D vaccine, 263, 398–399
PRP-OMP vaccine, 399
PRP-T vaccine, 399
PRP vaccine, 398–399
"PrP33–35," 160–262
Pseudallescheria boydii
  brain abscess, 461, 751–752
  classification, 693–694
  clinical presentation, 752
  drug combinations, 733, 736
  epidemiology, 752
  etiologic agent, 751
  pathogenesis, 699, 752
  therapy, 752
Pseudobulbar palsy, 550
Pseudomonas aeruginosa
  brain abscess, 461–462
  ceftazidime treatment, 390
  children and adults, 348
  epidural abscess, 501
  mycotic aneurysm, 542, 547
  neonatal meningitis, 314–315
  and neutropenia, 376
Pseudomonas paucimobilis, 461
Pseudopodia, 789
"Pseudotetanus," 616
Psoas abscess, 500, 507
Psychiatric abnormalities
  infective endocarditis, 529–531, 549
  Lyme disease, 671–672
  multiple microemboli, 549
  sleeping sickness, 783
Psychological effects
  Lyme disease, 674–675
  sleeping sickness, 783
Psychomotor retardation, 183–184
Psychosis
  AIDS-dementia, 210
  cerebral malaria, 775
  Japanese encephalitis, 97
  Mycoplasma pneumoniae, 289
Pulmonary crytococcosis, 713
Pulmonary paragonimiasis, 852
Pupillary changes, tabes dorsalis, 649
Purified protein derivative, 218, 447
Purpuric rash, 370
Purulent exudate
  bacterial meningitis pathology, 363–366
  CSF obstruction, 366
  primary amebic meningoencephalitis, 792
Pyrazinamide
  CSF penetration, 443
  treatment regimen, 445
  tuberculous meningitis, 443–444, 713
Pyrimethamine
  pharmacokinetics, 818
  toxoplasmosis, 215, 711, 818
Pyrimethamine-sulfadoxine
  and AZT, 818
  cerebral malaria, 776–777
  maintenance treatment, 818

toxicity, 818
toxoplasmosis, 818

Q

Q fever, 419–420
  characteristics, 412
  CNS manifestations, 416, 420
  cytopathic effects, 413
  laboratory findings, 420
  pathology, 413–414
  treatment, 420
Qinghaosu, 794
Quadriparesis, 274
Queensland tick typhus, 412, 416–417
Quellung test, 874
Quinidine, 776
Quinine therapy
  cerebral malaria, 776
  and hypoglycemia, 774
Quiniolinic acid
  AIDS-dementia pathophysiology, 211
  HIV infection, 209
Quinolones, 390

R

RA-27 vaccine, 192
Rabbit intratesticular inoculation test,
    641–642
Rabbit model, infective endocarditis,
    517–518
Rabies-free countries, 132–133
Rabies immunoglobulin, 138, 251
Rabies vaccine, 250–253
  administration, 138–139
  complications, 251–252
  efficacy, 251
  and Guillain-Barre' syndrome, 135,
    251, 262
Rabies virus, 124–144
  acute neurologic findings, 135
  asymptomatic infection, 133
  clinical spects, 133–136, 250
  CNS infection, 15
  coma, 135
  corneal transplantation, transmission,
    11
  diagnosis, 136
  epidemiology, 131–133, 249–250
  history, 127–128, 249
  immune globulin, 251
  incubation period, 131, 134–135
  infectious agent, 128–129, 249
  mortality, 135–136
  neural transmission, 11, 15, 130–131
  nonbite transmission, 130–131
  organ system complication, 135–136
  pathogenesis, 129–131, 250
  pathology, 131
  prevention, 137–139
  receptor-mediated transmission, 130
  replication in vitro, 129
  risk algorithm, 137–138
  site and severity of bite, 133–134
  survival, histopathology, 131
  treatment, 136–137
  vaccine, 138–139, 249–253
Raccoons, rabies varus, 132
Racemose cysts
  extirpation, 835
  magnetic resonance imaging, 835
  pathology, 830–831

Radicular pain
  antibiotics, 682
  Lyme disease, 676–677
Radiculomyelitis, Lyme disease, 665
Ragged red fibers, 221
Ramichloridium obovoideum, 462, 761
Rapid plasma reagin test, 642
Rash
  bacterial meningitis, children, 370
  differential diagnosis, meningitis,
    377–378
  Mediterranean spotted fever, 416
  neonatal herpes, 174
Rasmussen's encephalitis, 152–153
"Rat lungworm," 842
Reactivated toxoplasmosis
  epidemiology, 808
  evidence for, 812
  immunocompromised hosts, 810–815
  pathogenesis, retina, 808
Reactivation retinochoroiditis, 808
Receptors, viral attachment, 12
Receptosome, viral entry, 12
Reciprocal contralateral reflex sign, 368
Recombinant DNA techniques
  herpes simplex vaccine, 176
  rabies vaccine, 252
Recurrent cytomegalovirus infection
    and fetus, 179
  intrauterine period, 179, 181–182
  versus primary infection, fetus, 182
Recurrent embolization, 536–537
Recurrent herpes simplex
  epidemiology, 49–50
  pathogenesis, 45–46
  transplacental infection, 169, 171
Recurrent meningitis
  versus chronic meningitis, 703
  and trauma, 374–375
Recurrent toxoplasmosis, see Reacti-
    vated toxoplasmosis
Red blood cells
  cerebral malaria, 769–773
  endothelial cell adherence, malaria,
    771–773
  quantification, CSF, 871–872
  ultrastructure, 772–773
"Red" neurons, 365
Redbook Committee, 239
Reiter's syndrome, 206
Remyelination, 264–265
Renal dysfunction
  amphotericin B, 734
  shunt infection complication,
    570–571
Renal immune complex disease, 68
Renal transplants
  amebae infection, 792–793
  neurocysticercosis, 826
  rhinocerebral mucormycosis, 750
  toxoplasmosis, 810
Respiratory failure
  botulism, 594–595
  Guillain-Barre' syndrome, 272, 274
  tetanus, 611, 617–618
Respiratory syncytial virus, 352
Respiratory tract infection, 500
Retinal hemorrhage, 550
Retinitis
  cytomegalovirus, 217
  ocular toxoplasmosis, 809–810
Retinochoroiditis
  congenital toxoplasmosis, 807–808
  ocular toxoplasmosis, 808–810

pathogenesis, 808
pathology, 809
reactivation, 808
"Retrograde" shunt infection, 567
Retrograde transport
  CNS viruses, 13
  herpes simplex, 45
  tetanospasmin, 608, 610, 612–614
Retropharyngeal abscess, 500, 503
Retroviruses, replication, 13
Rev protein, HIV, 204
Revisions, CSF shunt, 564–565
Reye's syndrome, 15–16
Rhabdomyolysis, 619
Rhesus monkeys, B virus, 71
Rheumatic diseases
  CNS manifestations, 723–724
  infective endocarditis, 516
  Mycoplasma pneumoniae, 287
Rhinocerebral mucormycosis
  clinical manifestations, 750–751
  epidural abscess, 508
  pathogenesis, 749–750
  treatment, 751
Rhinogenic brain abscess, 464
Rhinorrhea, cerebrospinal fluid,
    374–375
Rhinosporidium seeberi, 761
Rhipicephalus sanguineus, 414, 660
Rhode Island, Lyme disease, 659
Rhodesian sleeping sickness, 782–783
  clinical manifestations, 782–783
  diagnosis, CSF, 784–785
Rhodotorula, 693
Riboflavin deficiency, malaria, 768
Rickettsia australis, 412, 416–417
Riskettsia conorii, 412–417
Rickettsia japonica, 412, 417
Rickettsia montana, 417
Rickettsia mooseri, 412, 419
Rickettsia prowazekii, 411–414, 417
Rickettsia rickettsii, 411–412, 414
Ricketesia sibirica, 412, 416–417
Rickettsia tsutsugamushi, 412–413
Rickettsia typhi, 412–413, 419
Rickettsial infections, 411–424
  differential diagnosis, meningitis, 377
  immune system response, 413
  major diseases, summary, 412
  neurological manifestations, 416
  pathogenesis and pathophysiology,
    411–414
Rickettsialpox, 417
Rifampin
  amphotericin B combination, 733
  Aspergillus brain abscess, 748
  CSF penetration, 443, 574
  H. influenzae prophylaxis, 397–398
  N. meningitidis prophylaxis, 400
  primary amebic meningoencephalitis,
    794
  recommended doses, 388
  shunt infection, 574
  side effects, 443
  treatment regimen, tuberculosis, 445
  tuberculous meningitis, 43, 445, 713
  tuberculous spinal epidural abscess,
    508
Rift Valley fever, 102–103
Right-sided endocarditis
  host defenses, 519
  meningitis, 548–549
  neurologic complications, 526–527
  treatment, 523

"Ring enhancing," 215, 890–892
Ring hemorrhages, 770–771
Risus sardonicus, 611
RNA viruses
  replication, 13
  slow infections, 146
Rochagan, 786
Rocky Mountain spotted fever, 414
  CNS manifestations, 414–416
  diagnosis, 415
  differential diagnosis, meningitis, 377
  drug treatment, 415–416
  encephalitis, 415
  pathogenesis, 411–412
  pathology, 413
  prognosis, 416
Rod body myopathy, 221
Romaña sign, 786
Roth spots, 522, 551
Roxithromycin, 819
Rubella, 188–192; see also Congenital
      rubella
  CNS syndrome, 9
  encephalitis, 189, 192
  epidemiology, 191
  history, 188
  infectious agent, 189
  maternal-infant transmission,
      190–191
  natural history, 189–190
  pathogenesis, 189–190
"Russian spring-summer encephalitis,"
      152
"Rusty" sputum 852

S

S fimbriae, 353
Sabin-Feldman dye test, 214, 815
Saccades, AIDS-dementia, 210
Sacral ganglia, latent herpes, 46
Sacral spinal epidural absesses, 500
Saksenaeaceae, 749
Saliva
  cytomegalovirus transmission, 181
  rabies, 133–134
Salmonella species
  brain abscess, 461–462, 465
  epidural abscess, 501
  neonatal brain abscess, 465
  subdural empyema, 495
Salvador, Brazil, bacterial meningitis,
      344
Sao Paulo, Brazil, N. meningitidis,
      339–341
Sarcoidosis, 721
Sardinia, Guillain-Barre' syndrome,
      260–261
Scedosporium, 693
SCH 39304, 733
Schistosoma haematobium, 849–851
Schistosoma japonicum, 849–851
  brain abscess, 462
Schistosoma mansoni, 849–851
Schistosomiasis, 849–851
  clinical manifestations, 850–851
  diagnosis and therapy, 851
  pathogenesis and pathology, 950
  prognosis, 851
Schizophyllum, 693
Schwann cells, 264–265
Schwarz vaccine, 238

Scrapie, 150–162
  diagnosis, 158–159
  epidemiology, 154
  etiology, 159–161
  genetics, 161–162
  pathogenesis, 156–157
  pathology, 154–156
  prevention, 162
  prion hypothesis, 159–161
  transmission, 154
"Scrapie-amyloid precursor protein,"
      161
Scrapie-associated fibrils, 158–160
  protein component, 160–161
Scrub typhus, 412, 416, 419
Seddenhill vaccine, 192
Seizures; see also Convulsions
  bacterial meningitisk, 321
  brain abscess, 469, 481
  herpes simplex encephalitis, 14
  infective endocarditis, 529–550
  Lyme disease, 671
  neonatal meningitis, 321
  neurocysticercosis, 828
      treatment, 835–836
  pertussis vaccine, 630–631
  rabies, 135
  subdural empyema, 490
  toxocariasis, association, 849
  toxoplasmic encephalitis, AIDS, 814
  treatment of, 396
  tuberculous meningitis, 430–431,
      446–447
Semple vaccine, 139
Sensorineural hearing loss
  congenital cytomegalovirus, 183–184
  dexamethasone protection, 393–394
  mumps, 119, 242
Sensory loss, Lyme disease, 673
Sependonium, 693
Sepondium species, 761
Sepsis, neonatal meningitis, 321
"Sepsis screen," 3232
Septic emboli, 540
Seroconversion, HIV infection, 205
Seronegative Lyme disease, 679–680
Serous tuberculous meningitis, 434–435
Serratia marsescens, 495
Serum C-reactive protein, see C-reactive
      protein
Severe combined immune deficiency,
      699
Sex differences
  brain abscess, 458
  H. influenzae meningitis, 337
  infective endocarditis, 516, 526
  mumps CNS disease, 115
  subdural empyema, 488, 490
Sheep, coenurosis, 837
Sheep tick, see Ixodes vicinus
Shell vial technique, cytomegalovirus,
      69
Shunt infection, see Cerebrospinal
      shunt infection
Shunt nephritis, 570–571
Shunt replacement, 575–576
Shunt reservoir, see Internal CSF reser-
      voirs
"Shunt tap," 572
Sialic acid, 300, 316–317
Sicca complex, 723
Sickle cell disease, 343
Sigmoid sinus, imagery, 899
Simian malaria, 772

Sinusitis
  and brain abscess, 458–459, 463–464
  imaging, 895
  and pneumococcal meningitis, 343
  subdural empyema, 488–489, 895
Sjogren's syndrome, 723
Skeletal muscle, Trichinella, 845–846
Skin lesions
  Lyme disease, 667–668
  neonatal herpes, 174
  spinal epidural infection, 500
Skin preparation, shunts, 565, 567, 580
Skin vesicles, neonatal herpes, 172,
      174–175
Skunk, rabies virus, 130, 132
Sleeping sickness, see African trypano-
      somias
"Slime"
  composition, 569
  immune system inhibition, 307
  and shunt adhesion, bacteria,
      306–307, 569
Slow virus diseases, 145–166
  conventional forms, 145–153
  CSF assessment, 880–881
  prion hypothesis, 159–161
  syndrome, 3–4
  unconventional forms, 153–162
Smallpox vaccine, and HIV, 223
Smell abnormalities, 793
Snowshoe hare virus, encephalitis, 102
Soap, rabies transmission, 138
"Soap bubble" calcifications, 852
Socioeconomic status
  cytomegalovirus, 68
  Epstein-Barr virus epidemiology, 66
  and herpes infection, 48–49
  meningococcal disease, 342
Sodium hydroxide disinfection, 162
Sodium hypochlorite disinfection, 162
Soft tissue infection, 500
Somatosensory evoked potentials,
      271–272
South American blastomycosis, 721, 759
South Vietnam, malaria, 768
Space-occupying lesions, 2–4
Sparganosis, 840841
"Sparganum," 840–841
Sphenoid sinus, imaging, 897–898
Sphenoid sinusitis, 464
Spinal anesthesia, 262
Spinal block
  and lumbar puncture, 868
  spinal tuberculosis, 440–441
  steroid use, prevention, 448
  tuberculous meningitis, 429
Spinal canal
  space-occupying lesions, 4
  tuberculosis lesions, 442
Spinal cord
  and HIV infection, 219
  infective endocarditis, 529, 531, 550
  tuberculosis, 440–442
Spinal cord compression, 218–219
Spinal cord parenchyma, 441
Spinal epidural abscess, 499–514
  damage to spinal cord, 499–500
  diagnosis, 502–505
  differential diagnosis, 502–503
  epidemiology, 499
  laboratory tests, 502
  microbiology, 501
  pathogenesis and pathophysiology,
      499–500

prognosis, 506
sequelae, 506
treatment, 505–506
tuberculous form, 506–508
Spinal ganglia, rabies, 130
Spinal hematoma, 867–868
Spinal neurocysticercosis, 829–830
computerized tomography, 834
prognosis, 836
symptoms, 829
treatment, 835–836
Spinal radiculomyelopathy, 441
Spinal subdural empyema, 496–497
Spinal tuberculosis, 440–442
clinical manifestations, 441
diagnosis, 441
pathology, 441
treatment, 441–442
Spirometra genus, 840–841
Spiroplasma mirum, 283
Splenectomy, 376
Spongiform encephalopathies, *see* Subacute spongiform encephalopathies
Spontaneous abortion
herpes simplex infection, 170
Japanese encephalitis virus, 244
Sporothrix meningitis, 716–717
diagnosis, 716, 731–732
pathogenesis, 716
treatment, 731, 736
Sporothrix schenckii
brain abscess, 759
classification, 693–694
labortory tests, 732
pathogenesis, 698–699, 716
Spotted fever group, 412, 414–418
St. Louis encephalitis virus
aseptic meningitis, 29
clinical findings, 95–96
diagnosis, 96
epidemiology, 94–95
history, 94
pathogenesis, 94
prevention and treatment, 96
recent outbreak, 8
Staging, HIV infection, 205–207
Staphylococci
brain abscess, 458–460
infective endocarditis, 520
subdural empyema, 494
Staphylococcus aureus
adherence, 569
brain abscess, 303–305, 460–461,
464, 468
and cavernous sinus thrombosis, 464
cerebral emboli endocarditis, 533
children and adults, 350, 390
epidural abscess, 501–502, 505
infective endocarditis, 517,
519–521, 528
CNS complications, 528, 531, 533,
547–549
intracranial mycotic aneurysm, 542
neonatal meningitis, 314
polymer surface adhesion, 306–307
shunt infections, 566, 578
spinal subdural empyema, 497
treatment, 390
virulence, 304
Staphylococcus epidermidis
epidural abscess, 501
neonatal meningitis, 315
shunt infection, 306, 566

slime production, 307
synergistic infectivity, brain, 303
Static encephalopathy, 212
Status epilepticus, treatment, 396
Stereotactic biopsy, 479
Stereotaxic aspiration, *see* Aspiration
Sterile tuberculous meningitis, 434–435
Steroid-withdrawal phenomenon, 448
Steroids; *see also* Corticosteroids
epidural abscess prognosis, 500
Guillain-Barre' syndrome, 272
herpes zoster treatment, 63
spinal tuberculosis, 441–442, 448
subdural empyema, 495
tetanus management, 617
tuberculous meningitis, 447–448
"Stiffman" syndrome, 615
Strabismus
infective endocarditis, 550
ocular toxoplasmosis, 809
Streptobacillus moniliformis, 461
Streptococci; *see also* Group B streptococci
brain abscess, 459–461
epidural abscess, 501
infective endocarditis, 519–521, 524,
528
CNS complications, 528
subdural empyema, 494–495
Streptococcus bovis, 519–520
Streptococcus intermedius
brain abscess, 303
synergistic infectivity, 303
Streptococcus milleri group
brain abscess, 458–460
infective endocarditis, 519
virulence, 459–460
Streptococcus mitis, 350
Streptococcus pneumoniae
adhesion, 352
adults, meningitis, 373–374
age stratification, meningitis, 336, 342
antibiotics, 389–392
brain abscess, 461–465
carriage rates, 343
cell wall, inflammation, 356–357
cerebral edema, 302
epidemiology, 342–343
etiological aspects, 343–344, 347–348
immunoprophylaxis, 402
infective endocarditis, 528
inflammation induction, CSF,
355–356
neonatal meningitis, 314–315
pathology, meningitis, 367
serotypes, 347–348
subarachnoid space inflammation,
301
subdural empyema, 495
systemic invasion, 299
Streptomyces griseus, 752
Streptomycin
CSF penetration, 442
drug resistance, 445
ototoxicity, 444
treatment regimens, 445
tuberculous meningitis, 444
Stress, rabies incubation period, 135
Stroke
and AIDS, 216–217
clinical presentation, endocarditis,
533
infective endocarditis, 529, 532–539
intracranial aspergillosis, 747

and meningovascular syphilis, 647,
718
Strongyloides stercoralis, 847–848
and AIDS, 218, 847
Strongyloidiasis, 847–848
and AIDS, 218, 247
bacterial meningitis role, 847–848
hyperinfection syndrome, 847
pathogenesis, 847
Strychnine
differential diagnosis, tetanus, 615
and tetanospasmin, 614
Subacute meningitis, 2–3
Subacute sclerosing panencephalitis,
145–149
clinical manifestations, 146, 237
differential diagnosis, 149
epidemiology, 145–146, 234, 237
etiology, 149
laboratory diagnosis, 147–148, 152,
237
and measles, 234, 236–238
pathogenesis, 9, 147, 237
pathology, 146–147
prevention, 149, 237–238
staging, 237
therapy, 149, 237–238
Subacute spongiform encephalopathies,
153–162
clinical manifestations, 154–155
epidemiology, 153–154
etiology, 159–161
genetics, 161–162
iatrogenic transmission, 154
pathogenesis, 156–157
pathology, 155–156
prevention, 162
prion hypothesis, 159–161
therapy, 162
transmission, 154
virus decontamination, 162
Subarachnoid cysticercosis, 829
computerized tomography, 834
pathology, 830–831
prognosis, 836
treatment, 835
Subarachnoid hemorrhage
CSF effects, 872
differential diagnosis, meningitis, 378
gnathostomiasis, 845
infective endocarditis, 529
magnetic resonance imaging, 544
mycotic aneurysm sequelae, 543–544
Subarachnoid space
anatomy, 862–863
bacterial invasion, 353
C. neoformans, 695–697
congenital defects, 862–863
host defenses, bacteria, 300–301,
354–355
infection introduction, lumbar puncture, 868
inflammation consequences,
301–302, 355–358
magnetic resonance imaging, 892
purulent exudate, 363–366
Subcortical dementia, HIV, 210
Subdural effusions
childhood bacterial meningitis, 370,
382–383
computerized tomography, 382–383
magnetic resonance imaging, 386
treatment, 396–397
Subdural empyema, 487–498

Subdural empyema (contd.)
  anatomy, 488–489
  bacteriology, 494–495
  clinical features, 489–491, 501–502
  computerized tomography, 382,
      895–898
  diagnostic studies, 491–494
  differential diagnosis, 491
  and epidural abscess, 509
  history, 487
  lumbar puncture contraindication,
      493–494, 867–868
  magnetic resonance imaging, 386,
      895–898
  neurologic sequelae, 496
  outcome, 495–496
  pathogenesis, 488–489
  in spine, 496–497
  symptoms, 376
  treatment, 495–496
Subdural hematomas
  mycotic aneurysm sequelae, 543
  neurocysticercosis, 830
Subdural hygroma, 893–894, 896
Subdural ICP monitoring, 562
Subdural space, anatomy, 488
Sub-Saharan Africa, meningitis,
      339–340
Suckling hamsters, mumps, 116
Suckling mouse brain vaccine, 139
Sudden infant death syndrome
  and botulism, 591, 596
  purtussis vaccine, 630–631
Sulcal dilatation, imaging, 891–893
Sulfadiazine
  N. meningitidis prophylaxis, 400
  resistance, 400
  toxicity, 818
  toxoplasmosis, 215, 711, 818
Sulfatrimethoprim, 627
Superior sagittal sinus, 865
Suppression-burst EEG
  Creutzfeldt-Jakob disease, 158
  subacute sclerosing panencephalitis,
      148
Suramin
  sleeping sickness treatment, 785–786
  toxicity, 785
Surgeon's experience, shunts, 565
Surgery; see also Neurosurgery
  and bacterial colonization, 568
  infective endocarditis, 523–524, 532
  intracranial mycotic aneurysms,
      545–546
Susceptibility testing, antibiotics, 745
Suture infection, 568
Swan-Ganz catheters, 517
Sweden
  pneumococcal meningitis, 342–343
  Lyme disease, 660, 671–672, 677
Swimming pools, amebae, 790, 794
Swine influenza vaccine, 262
Synaptic transmission, 13–14
Synaptosome, HSV-1, 13
Syndrome of inappropriate secretion of
      antidiuretic hormone
  childhood bacterial meningitis, 373
  Rocky Mountain spotted fever, 415
  tetanospasmin, 614
  tuberculous meningitis, 432
Syndrome recognition, 2–4
Synergism, antibiotics, 387
Synergistic infectivity, 303
Synovium, B. burgdorferi, 663, 668

Syphilis, 639–656
  and HIV infection, 218, 653–654
  laboratory diagnosis, 641–644
  versus Lyme disease, diagnosis, 679
  pathogenesis, stages, 639–640
  therapy, 650–653
Syphilitic meningitis
  classification, 644
  clinical syndrome, 645
  diagnosis, 646
  incidence and symptoms, 645–646
  penicillin effect, 652
Syrian hamster, 662–663
Systemic lupus erythematosus, 722–723
  aseptic meningitis cause, 34
  neurologic manifestations, 722–723
  toxoplasmosis, 810

T
T lymphocytes
  in AIDS, 207
  Borrelia burgdorferi, 663, 680
  depletion effect, toxoplasmosis, 812
  Guillain-Barre' syndrome, 266–268
  mumps, 117
T-type pertussis vaccine, 629
T weighted images, 492–493, 504
  acute disseminated encephalomyeli-
      tis, 901
  bacterial meningitis, 892–894
  brain abscess, 890–891
  data acquisition times, 887
  herpes simplex, 900
  HIV infection, 902
  meaning of, 888
  neurocysticercosis, 834–835, 905–906
  toxoplasmosis, AIDS, 902–903
  ventriculitis, 894
T7 position, shunts, 565
Tabes dorsalis
  clinical manifestations, 648–649, 718
  pathology, 649
  penicillin effect, 652
"Tache noire," 416
Tachycardia, in tetanus, 609, 611
Tachyzoites
  AIDS pathology, 813
  characteristics, 801–803
  congenital toxoplasmosis, 806
  drug treatment, 818
  macrophage effect, 804
Taenia multiceps, 837
Taenia serialis, 837
Taenia solium, 720, 825
  eosinophilia, 871
  geographic distribution, 825–826
  hosts, 826
  life cycle, 826–827
  photomicrograph, 828
  prevention of infection, 837
  stool samples, 832
"Taeniasis," 826, 832
Tahyna virus, 102
Taiwan, polio outbreak, 248
Tanganyika, sleeping sickness, 780
Tanzania, sleeping sickness, 779
Tapeworm infections, 828–858
Taste abnormalities, 793
Tat protein, HIV, 204
TC83 vaccine, 93
Technetium-99 scan, 471, 548
Teichoic acid, 355

Temporal lobe abscess
  clinical manifestations, 469
  diagnosis, 376
  etiology, 459
  otogenesis, 464
  pathology, 466
Temporal lobe sclerosis, 7
Tensilon test, 596
Tetanolysin, 606
Tetanospasmin
  amino acid sequence, 606–607
  autonomic effects, 614
  characteristics, 606–608
  enzyme digestion fragments, 606–608
  immunotherapy, 616
  mechanism of action, 608–609
  motor control effects, 612–614
  neuromuscular junction, 614
  as research tool, 615
  retrograde transport, 608, 610,
      612–614
  structure, 606–607
Tetanus, 603–624
  botulism toxin similarity, 591–592
  complications, 619
  diagnosis, 615–616
  epidemiology, 604–605
  etiology, 605–608
  history, 603–604
  and HIV infection, 619
  immunization, 619–620
  infectious agent, 605–606
  manifestations, 608–611
  mortality rates, 604
  nutrition, 618–619
  prevention, 619–620
  rating systems, 611
  therapy, 616–619
Tetanus-diphtheria vaccine, 619–620
Tetanus toxoid, 616–617, 619–620
  adverse reactions, 620
Tetracycline
  cerebral malaria, 776
  facial palsy, 682
  Lyme disease, 680–682
  mycoplasmas, 291
  primary amebic meningoencephalitis,
      794
  Rocky Mountain spotted fever, 415
Tetralogy of Fallot, 466
Thailand
  Angiostrongylus infections, 842
  Gnathostroma spinigerum, 843
Thalamus
  abscess pathology, 467
  HIV infection, 209
Thalidomide, 223
Thiabendazole, 843
  angiostrongyliasis, 842
  strongyloidiasis, 848
  trichinosis, 846
Thoracic spine
  epidural abscess, 500, 504
  tuberculous spinal epidural abscess,
      507
Thrombocytopenia
  HIV infection, 205–206
  neonatal meningitis, 323
  rickettsial disease, 413
Thrombophlebitis of the cavernous
      sinus, 542
Thrombosis
  bacterial meningitis pathology,
      364–365

E. coli, neonates, 320
Mycoplasma pneumoniae, 287–288
Rocky Mountain spotted fever, 415
subdural empyema sequelae, 496
Thrombospondin, 773
Thrombotic stroke, AIDS, 216–217
Thrombotic thrombocytopenic purpura, 217
Thyphoid fever, 262
Thyroiditis, 118
Tic-borne encephalitis
  chronic form, 152
  clinical findings, 99, 152
  diagnosis, 99, 152
  epidemiology, 98–99, 152
  history, 98
  laboratory workers, 99
Ticarcillin, 325
Tick-borne relapsing fever, 679
Ticks; *see also* Tic-borne encephalitis
  Lyme disease epidemiology, 659–661
  rickettsial diseases, 412, 414
Tight junctions
  bacteria effect, 358–359
  barrier system anatomy, 10, 864
Tissue-cage model, 306–307
Tissue culture, HIV, 208, 213
"Tissue-culture-infective dose," 208
Tissue cyst
  AIDS pathology, 813
  characteristics, 802–803
  pyrimethamine-sulfadiazine effect, 818
  reactivation retinochoroiditis, 808
  sequence of development, brain, 811
Tobramycin
  CSF penetration, 574
  neonatal meningitis, 325
  recommended dosage, 388, 575
  shunt infection, 574–575
Togaviruses
  background, 87
  encephalitis, 87–99
  glycoproteins, rubella, 189
Tongue infection, 174
Tonsillar herniation, 367, 866
Topical antibiotics, 580
"Torulomas," 695
Torulopsis glabrata, 754
"Toxic" encephalopathy
  infective endocarditis, 529–530, 534
  magnetic resonance imaging, 548
  microemboli, 534
  outcome, 550
Toxic syndromes, 3–4
Toxocara canis, 848–849
Toxocara cati, 848
Toxocariasis, 848–849
  clinical manifestations, 848–849
  epidemiology, 848
Toxoplasma gondii
  AIDS patients, 710–711
  brain abscess, 462
  characteristics, 801–804
  immune system circumvention, 803
  pathogenesis, 802–804
  polymerase chain reaction, 817
  reactivation pathogenesis, 811
  serological testing, 815–817, 877
  seroprevalence, 801, 804
Toxoplasmic encephalitis
  brain biopsy, 817
  clinical manifestations, 813–814
  imaging, 817

immunosuppression effect, 811
nonimmunocompromised hosts, 805
pathology, 812–813
serology, 815–816
transplant recipients, symptoms, 814
treatment, 818–819
Toxoplasmosis, 801–823; *see also* Congenital toxoplasmosis
  AIDS patients, 710–711, 810–819, 902–903
  brain abscess, 462–463, 481, 813
  in children, 213
  computerized tomography, 215, 481, 902–903
  diagnosis, AIDS, 213–215, 815–818
  empirical therapy, AIDS, 815
  history, 801
  immunocompromised host, 709, 810–819, 902–903
  infectious agent, 801–804
  versus lymphoma, imaging, 903
  magnetic resonance imaging, 902–903
  nonimmunocompromised host, 804–805
  ocular form, 807–810
  prevention, 819
  reactivation, 808, 810–815
  serology, 815–817
  treatment, 215, 481, 818–819
Tracheal cytotoxin, 626
Tracheal suctioning, 315
Tracheostomy, tetanus, 617
Transesophageal echocardiography, 522, 537
Transient ischemic attacks
  clinical manifestations, 534
  intracranial hemorrhage, 540
  mycotic aneurysm sign, 543
Transmissible mink encephalopathy, 153–162
  transmission, 154
Transphenoidal pituitary surgery, 465
Transplacental infection
  antibody protection, herpes, 170
  herpes simplex, 168–170
  rubella, 191
  varicella-zoster, 186
Transplant recipients; *see also* Immunocompromised host; *specific types of transplant*
  toxoplasmosis, 812–814
Transport, *see* Viral transport
Transposition of the great vessels, 466
Transsynaptic transmission, 13–14
Transverse myelitis
  Lyme disease, 671
  Mycoplasma pneumoniae, 289
  tuberculosis, 441
  varicella infection, 60
Trauma, *see* Head trauma; Posttraumatic infection
Trematodes, 849–852
Treponema pallidum
  characteristics, 640–641
  chronic meningitis, HIV, 711–712, 718
  CSF cultivation, 641–642
  CSF invasion, early stages, 640
  and HIV infection, 653–654, 711–712
  penicillin sensitivity, 650–651, 718
Treponema pallidum immobilization test, 643
Trichinella spiralis, 845
Trichinosis, 845–846

clinical manifestations, 846
epidemiology, 845
pathogenesis and pathology, 845–846
treatment, 846
Trichosporon beigelii, 700, 731
  cerebral abscess, 761
Trichosporon cutaneum, 761
Trichosporon mentagrophytes, 761
Trichosporon species, 693–694, 700
Tricuspid valve endocarditis
  drug addicts, 521, 527
  neurologic complications, 526
Tricyclic antidepressants, AIDS, 223
Trigeminal ganglia, 45–47
  herpes simplex latency, 46–47
  HSV-1, 45
Trigeminal nerve, herpes simplex, 47
Trimetrexate, 819
Trimethoprim-sulfamethoxazole
  brain abscess, 477
  Citrobacter meningitis, 326
  Listeria monocytogenes, meningitis, 390
  Mycoplasma hominis, 291
  Naegleria fowleri, 794
  Plasmodium brasiliensis, 759
  recommended dosage, 388
  Staphylococcus aureus, 390
Trismus
  early descriptions, 603
  manifestations, 611
  anus diagnosis, 615
Tri-Solgen, 630
Trivalent botulinum antitoxin, 597
"Trojan horse" mechanism, 209
Trophozoites
  amebae form, 788
  meningoencephalitis pathology, 792–793
  nasal cavity invasion, 790–791
  phagocytic activity, 788–789
"Tropical spastic paraparesis," 153
Trypanosoma cruzi, 778, 786–787
Trypanosoma gambiense, 778
  antigenic variability, diagnosis, 784
  epidemiology, 778–780
  pentamidine, 785
  tryparsamide, 786
Trypanosoma rhodesiense, 778
  antigenic variability, diagnosis, 784
  clinical manifestations, 782–783
  epidemiology, 779
Trypanosomiasis, 777–787; *see also* African trypanosomias American trypanosomias
Tryparsamide, 786
Tsetse fly, 778
Tsutsugamushi disease, 419
Tubercles
  clinical sign, meningitis, 431
  in spinal canal, 442
  tuberculosis pathogenesis, 428
Tuberculin test
  chronic meningitis, 707–708, 713
  interpretation, 432–433, 712–713
Tuberculoma, 438–440
  and AIDS, IV drug users, 450
  and brain abscess, 440
  course of treated disease, 446
  epidemiology, 439
  imaging, 895–896, 898
  laboratory evaluation, 439–440
  pathogenesis, 438–439
  spinal canal, 442

Tuberculoma (*contd.*)
  symptoms, 439
  treatment, 440
  versus tuberculous meningitis, 439
Tuberculosis, 425–456
  CNS involvement, 425–456
  history, 425–426
  and HIV infection, 218, 427, 449–450
  and measles, 236
Tuberculostearic acid
  gas-liquid chromatography, 878
  tuberculous meningitis test, 435–436, 706
Tuberculous brain abscess
  diagnosis and treatment, 440
  IV drug users, AIDS, 450
Tuberculous encephalopathy, 429
Tuberculous meningitis, 425–456
  adjuvant chemotherapy, 447–448
  age-specific incidence, 712
  and AIDS, 218, 427, 449–450
  cerebrospinal fluid, 879
  chest X-ray, 432
  children, 430–431
  clinical presentation, 430–432
  course of treated disease, 446
  culture results, 434–435, 713, 879
  diagnostic tests, 432–437, 879
  duration of symptoms, 430
  epidemiology, 426–428
  etiology, 428
  extraneural cultures, 433
  exudate, 428–429
  mortality and prognosis, 445–446, 713
  pathogenesis, 428
  pathology and pathophysiology, 428–430
    chemotherapy effects, 429–430
  prevention, 450–451
  radiology, 432, 437–438
  sequelae, 446, 713
  smear diagnosis, 434
  surgery, 448
  symptoms, 712
  treatment, 442–448, 713
  tuberculoma difference, 439
Tuberculous spinal epidural abscess, 506–508
  clinical manifestations, 507–508
  pathogenesis and pathophysiology, 506–507
  treatment, 508
Tubulovesicular particles, 155–156
Tularemia, 262
Tumor necrosis factor
  bacterial cell wall induction, 356–357, 393
  blood-brain-barrier, 360
  cerebral malaria, 774
  CSF inflammation, bacteria, 301–302, 356–357
  CSF levels, meningitis, 27
  detection in CSF, 878
  HIV infection, CSF, 209
    children, 212–213
  and treatment, 393
Twins, *H. influenzae* meningitis, 338, 397
Two-dose measles vaccine, 239
Tympanic membrane, 463
Type A botulism, 589–595, 597
Type B botulism, 589–592, 594–595, 597

Type E botulism, 589, 591–592, 594, 597
Type F botulism, 589–592
Type G botulism, 591–592
Typhus
  CNS manifestations, 416–418
  nodules, 417–418
  pathogenesis, 411–412
  transmission, 417
  treatment, 418
Typhus nodules, 417–418

U

Uganda, sleeping sickness, 779
Uncal herniation, 866
United Kingdom, bacterial meningitis, 344
University of California at San Francisco staging system, 206
Ureaplasma urealyticus, 284
  CNS infections, 285–286, 290–291
  diagnosis, neonates, 290–291
  epidemiology, 285–286
  treatment, 291
Ureteral shunt infection, 567
Urinary tract infection, 500
Ustilago, 693
Uveitis, 809
Uveocyclitis, 215
"Uveomeningoencephalitic syndrome," 724

V

Vaccines, 233–257; *see also under specific disorders*
  CNS protection, 233
  congenital rubella, 192
  and Guillain-Barre' syndrome, 262
  H. influenzae, 398–399
  herpes simplex, 176
  HIV infection, 223
  Japanese encephalitis virus, 245
  measles, 238–240
  mumps, 241–243
  mycoplasmas, 291
  N. meningitides, 401–402
  pertussis, 628–633
  polio, 247–249
  rabies, 138–139, 249–253
  subacute sclerosing panencephalitis, 237–238
  tetanus, 619–620
Vacuolar myelopathy
  and AIDS, 211, 219
  diagnosis, 219
Vacuoles, 154–155
Val[117] mutation, 161
Valkampfia, 787
Valvular surgery
  cerebral embolism prevention, 535–537
  infective endocarditis management, 535–537
  intracranial mycotic aneurysm, 546
Vampire bat, rabies, 132
Vancomycin
  brain abscess, 477–478
  CSF penetration, 574
  epidural abscess, 505
  infective endocarditis, 523, 525
  intraventricular administration, 327, 575

neonatal meningitis, 325, 327–328
  pneumococcal meningitis, 390
  recommended doses, 388
  shunt infection, 573–575
Varicella pneumonitis, pregnancy, 185–186
Varicella-zoster virus; *see also* Chicken-pox; Herpes zoster
  CNS infections, 56–65
  cytopathic effect, 57
  laboratory diagnosis, 62–63
  pathology and pathogenesis, 57–58, 185
  perinatal infections, 185–187
  structural characteristics, 57
"Variant surface glycoprotein," 781
Vascular shunt infection
  clinical manifestations, 570–571
  pathogenesis, 567, 569
Vasculitides, 722–724
Vasculitis
  bacterial meningitis, 362, 893
  and CNS disease, 721–724
  E. coli, neonates, 320
  Lyme disease pathophysiology, 664–665, 674
  magnetic resonance imaging, 893
  perinatal cytomegalovirus, 180
  Rocky Mountain spotted fever, 415
  spinal lmeningitis, 441
  syphilis pathophysiology, 640
  tuberculous meningitis, 437, 712
Vasculopathy, Lyme disease, 665
Vasogenic edema, imaging, 889–891
VDRL test, 642–643, 718
Vecuronium, 618
Veneral Disease Research Laboratory test, 641–643, 718, 880
Venezuelan equine encephalitis
  clinical findings, 93
  diagnosis, 93
  history, 92–93
  pathology and pathogenesis, 89
  prevention and treatment, 93
Venous shunt infection, *see* Vascular shunt infection
Venous thrombosis
  bacterial meningitis, 364–365
  E. coli histopathology, neonates, 320
  intracranial epidural abscess, 509
  and lumbar puncture, 867
  magnetic resonance imaging, 893
  subdural empyema sequelae, 496
Ventricular dilatation, 865
Ventricular drainage, 448
Ventricular fluid
  diagnostic technique, 869
  fungal infections, 730
Ventricular septal defect
  and brain abscess, 466
  infective endocarditis, 516
Ventricular system
  congenital toxoplasmosis, 806
  intraventricular antibiotics, 327–328
  neonatal meningitis, 327–328
Ventriculitis
  bacterial meningitis pathology, 367–368
  computerized tomography, 327, 894–895
  magnetic resonance imaging, 893–896
  treatment, neonates, 327–328
Ventriculoatrial shunt infection
  CSF shunt types, 562–563

hydrocephalus, 448
  incidence, 565
  meningitis, 375
Ventriculocisternostomy, 561
Ventriculoperitoneal shunt infection
  clinical manifestations, 570–571
  CSF shunt types, 562–563
  diagnosis, 572–573
  gram-negative organisms, 566
  imaging, 894–896
  incidence, 565
  meningitis, 375, 570
  microbiology, 566
Ventriculopleural shunt infection
  clinical manifestations, 571
  CSF shunt types, 562–563
Ventriculostomy
  and CSF shunt types, 562–563
  antibiotic instillation, 573
Vero cell, rabies vaccine, 253
Vertebral osteomyelitis
  and antibiotics, 505
  epidural abscess, 500, 504–505, 549
  magnetic resonance imaging, 504
  surgery, 506
Vesicular cysts, MRI, 834–835
Vesicular rash, neonatal herpes, 172, 174
Vidarabine
  chickenpox, 63–65
  combination therapy, 56
  herpes simplex encephalitis, 53–56,
    177–178
  herpes zoster, 64–65
  neonatal herpes, 177–178
  oral versus intravenous, 65
  and relapse, 55
  toxicity, 55
Vietnam
  malaria study, 768
  N. meningitidis, 341
Viral attachment, 12–13
Viral entry, 12–13
Viral meningitis, 19–34; see also under
    specific viruses
  versus bacterial meningitis, 377
  CSF findings, 880
Viral replication
  in CNS, 12–14
  tropisms, 12
Viral shedding, 171
Viral transport
  blood-brain barrier, 11
  mechanisms, 13–14
"Virchow-Robin space"
  bacterial meningitis, 364–365
  sleeping sickness, 780–782

Viridans streptococci
  cerebral emboli, endocarditis, 533
  infective endocarditis, 520–521, 528,
    533, 547
  meningitis, endocarditis, 547
"Virinos," 160
"Viscera larva migrans," 848–849
"Visceral crises," 649
Visual disturbances, 531
Vitreous body, cysticercosis, 830
Vitreous fluid, toxoplasmosis, 809
Vogt-Koyanagi-Harada syndrome, 705,
    724
Vomiting
  bacterial meningitis sign, 368–369
  brain abscess, 469
  Lyme disease, 671
  mumps infection, 118–119

W
W135 meningococcal serogroup, 346
Wallerian degeneration, 264–265
Walter Reed HIV staging system, 206
Wangiella dermatitidis, 761
Wasserman test, 642
"Wasting disease," 154
Water supplies
  amebae, 790, 794
  Toxoplasma, 804
Waterhouse-Friderichsen syndrome,
    370
Wayson stain, 380
Weil's disease, 33
West African sleeping sickness, 782–783
Western Australia, 260–261
Western blot, HIV infection, 207
Western equine encephalitis, 89–92
  clinical findings, 91–92
  diagnosis, 92
  epidemiology, 91–92
  history, 91
  pathology and pathogenesis, 89
  prevention and treatment, 92
Western Norway, 260
Wet mounts, 875
White blood cells
  bacterial meningitis, 378–381
  epidural abscess, 501
  mumps, 120–121
  quantification, CSF, 870–871
  shunt infection, 572
  subdural empyema, 494
  toxoplasmic encephalitis, 814
  tuberculous meningitis, 433, 434
White-footed mouse, 659–660

White matter
  AIDS encephalopathy, children,
    212–213
  malaria pathology, 769–770
"White spot," 830
Whole-cell pertussis vaccine, 629–633
Whooping cough, 625–635; see also
    Pertussis
"WIN" drugs, 28
"Winterbottom's sign," 782
Wolf, rabies transmission, 129–130, 132
Wood tick, 414
World War II, malaria, 768
Wound botulism, 589–602
  clinical manifestations, 595
  diagnosis, 596–597
  epidemiology, 590
  therapy, 597–598
Wound infections, and shunts, 569, 571
Wurzburg, West Germany, 719

X
X-linked lymphoproliferative syn-
    drome, 66
"Xanthochromia," 379, 725, 870
Xylophypha bantiana, 699
  brain abscess, 759–761
  mortality, 760

Y
Yemen, botulism, 591
Yukon-Kusko-Kurin delta, 342–343

Z
Zaria, Nigeria, 340–341
Zidovudine
  dosage, 222
  in progressive encephalopathy, 222
  pyrimethamine antagonism, 818
  side effects, 222
Zidovudine-induced myopathy,
    221–222
Zoster ophthalmicus, see Herpes zoster
    ophthalmicus
Zygomycetes species
  antibody test, 731
  chronic meningitis, 721
  pathogenesis, 700
  spectrum of CNS involvement,
    693–694
  treatment, 731
Zygomycosis; see also Mucormycosis
  brain abscess, 461, 749
"Zymograms," 791